CARDIAC, VASCULAR, AND THORACIC ANESTHESIA

CARDIAC, VASCULAR, AND THORACIC ANESTHESIA

Editor
John A. Youngberg, M.D.
Professor of Anesthesiology
Director of Cardiac Anesthesiology
Tulane University Medical Center
New Orleans, Louisiana

Associate Editors

Carol L. Lake, M.D., M.B.A.
Professor of Anesthesiology
Assistant Dean
Indiana Unversity;
Chief of Staff
Roudebush VA Medical Center
Indianapolis, Indiana

Michael F. Roizen, M.D.
Professor and Chairman
Department of Anesthesia and Critical Care
Professor, Department of Medicine
The University of Chicago
Division of the Biological Sciences
Pritzker School of Medicine
Chicago, Illinois

Roger S. Wilson, M.D.
Professor of Anesthesiology
Weill Medical College of Cornell University;
Chairman
Department of Anesthesia and Critical Care Medicine
Memorial Sloan-Kettering Cancer Center
New York, New York

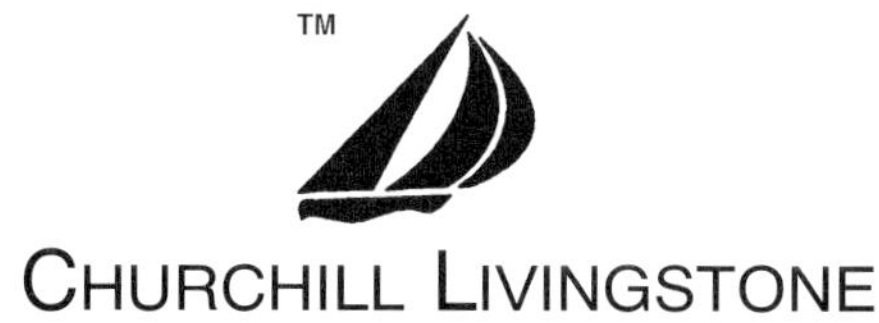

CHURCHILL LIVINGSTONE
A Division of Harcourt Brace & Company
New York • Edinburgh • London • Philadelphia • San Francisco

CHURCHILL LIVINGSTONE
A Division of Harcourt Brace & Company

The Curtis Center
Independence Square West
Philadelphia, Pennsylvania 19106

Library of Congress Cataloging-in-Publication Data

Cardiac, vascular, and thoracic anesthesia / edited by John A.
Youngberg . . . [et al.]. — 1st ed.
p. cm.
ISBN 0-0443-08920–5
1. Anesthesia. 2. Anesthesia in cardiology. 3. Chest—Surgery.
4. Blood-vessels—Surgery. 5. Cardiovascular system—Surgery.
I. Youngberg, John A.
[DNLM: 1. Anesthesia—methods. 2. Cardiac Surgical Procedures.
3 Vascular Surgical Procedures. 4. Thoracic Surgical Procedures.
WG 169 C2674 2000]
RD87.3.C37C367 2000
817.9′6—DC21
DNLM/DLC 98-20111
for Library of Congress

CARDIAC, VASCULAR, AND THORACIC ANESTHESIA ISBN 0-443-08920–5

Printed in the United States of America.

Last digit is the print number: 9 8 7 6 5 4 3 2 1

This textbook is dedicated to cardiac anesthesiologists and their patients worldwide.

Carol L. Lake, M.D., M.B.A.

My efforts on this volume are dedicated to cardiac, thoracic, and vascular patients and surgeons everywhere who benefit from the care and devotion of their anesthesiologists; to my parents and Bill Hamilton, who taught me to do what is right and to say what is fact and what is bias; and to Nancy, Jeffrey, and Jennifer and the members of the Department of Anesthesia and Critical Care at the University of Chicago, who allowed the time and sacrificed their own interests for the production of this work.

Michael F. Roizen, M.D.

To my mentors, Drs. Emanuel M. Papper and Richard J. Kitz, who have served as an inspiration for my academic development through the many years, and to my family, my wife Donna and children, Mark and Susan.

Roger S. Wilson, M.D.

This textbook represents the culmination of the influence that a number of individuals have had on my career: My father, Dameron A. Youngberg, who instilled a sense of desire to achieve goals and to make a contribution in my field of work; Max K. Mendenhall, M.D., who recruited me into the specialty of anesthesiology; and Joel A. Kaplan, M.D., and Robert R. Kirby, M.D., who served as both mentors and role models in my career development. I owe these individuals a debt of gratitude. I wish to thank my daughters Kristine and Michelle for their understanding and support.

John A. Youngberg, M.D.

Contributors

Donald Lea Akers, Jr., MD
Professor, Department of Surgery, Tulane School of Medicine; Director, Tulane Vascular Laboratory, Tulane University Medical Center; Director, McLand Vascular Laboratory, Medical Center of Louisiana at New Orleans; Vascular Staff, University Hospital, New Orleans, Louisiana
Endovascular Surgery

Paul Barash, MD
Professor, Department of Anesthesiology, Yale University School of Medicine; Attending Anesthesiologist, Yale New Haven Hospital, New Haven, Connecticut
Valvular Heart Disease

Steven J. Barker, MD, PhD
Professor and Head, Department of Anesthesiology, The University of Arizona; Director, Perioperative Services, University Medical Center, Tucson, Arizona
Monitoring Oxygenation and Ventilation

Elizabeth C. Behringer, MD
Associate Clinical Professor of Anesthesiology and Surgery, Department of Anesthesiology, University of California, Irvine; Director, Fellowship in Critical Care, University of California, Irvine, Orange, California
Tracheal Surgery

Steven D. Bell, MD
Assistant Professor of Anesthesiology, Jefferson Medical College, Thomas Jefferson University; Director of Critical Care, Managing Medical Director of Patient Testing Center, Thomas Jefferson University Hospital, Philadelphia, Pennsylvania
Postoperative Pain Management

David L. Brown, MD
Professor of Anesthesia, Department of Anesthesiology, University of Iowa, Iowa City, Iowa
Continuous Quality Improvement in Cardiac and Thoracic Anesthesia

Lawrence P. Cahalin, MA, PT
Clinical Associate Professor, Sargent College of Health and Rehabilitation Sciences, Boston University; Research Physical Therapist, Heart Failure and Cardiac Transplantation Service, Massachusetts General Hospital, Boston, Massachusetts
Preoperative Conditioning for the Thoracic Surgery Patient

Michael K. Cahalan, MD
Professor of Anesthesia, School of Medicine, Department of Anesthesia, University of California, San Francisco; Director, Anesthesia for Cardiac Surgery, School of Medicine, Department of Anesthesia, University of California, San Francisco, San Francisco, California
Transesophageal Echocardiography for the Anesthesiologist

Christopher L. Campese, MD
Assistant Professor of Anesthesiology, Albany Medical College; Attending Anesthesiologist, Albany Medical Center Hospital, Albany, New York
Respiratory, Renal, and Gastrointestinal Complications

Richard F. Davis, MD
Professor of Anesthesiology, Oregon Health Sciences University; Chief of Anesthesiology, Portland UAMC, Portland, Oregon
Cardiopulmonary Bypass: Technology, Pathophysiology, and Pharmacology

Steven R. Dryden, MD
Cardiac Anesthesiologist, Indiana Heart Institute, St. Vincent Hospital System, Indianapolis, Indiana
Minimally Invasive Coronary Artery Bypass Grafting

Jane Duggan, MD
Assistant Professor of Anesthesiology, School of Medicine, Emory University, Atlanta, Georgia
Peripheral Vascular Surgery

James B. Eisenkraft, MD
Professor of Anesthesiology, Mount Sinai School of Medicine of the City University of New York; Attending Anesthesiologist, The Mount Sinai Hospital, New York, New York
Monitoring Oxygenation and Ventilation

John E. Ellis, MD
Associate Professor, Director, Vascular-Thoracic Anesthesia, Department of Anesthesia and Critical Care, Division of the Biological Sciences, Pritzker School of Medicine, The University of Chicago Medical Center, Chicago, Illinois
Cost-Effectiveness and Benefit of Preoperative Work-up and Preparation for Vascular Surgery; Monitoring Cardiac Electrical Activity; Anesthesia for Abdominal Aortic Revascularization

Norig Ellison, MD
Professor of Anesthesia, Vice Chair, Department of Anesthesia, School of Medicine, University of Pennsylvania, Philadelphia, Pennsylvania
Coagulation and Coagulopathies

Lee A. Fleisher, MD
Associate Professor of Anesthesiology, Joint Appointment in Medicine (Cardiology) and Health Policy and Management, Johns Hopkins University School of Medicine; Attending Anesthesiologist, The Johns Hopkins Hospital, Baltimore, Maryland
Preoperative Assessment; Cost-Effectiveness and Benefit of Preoperative Work-up and Preparation for Vascular Surgery

Joseph F. Foss, MD
Clinical Assistant Professor, Department of Anesthesia and Critical Care, Division of the Biological Sciences, Pritzker School of Medicine, University of Chicago, Chicago, Illinois
Cost-Effectiveness and Benefit of Preoperative Work-up and Preparation for Vascular Surgery

Elyse Foster, MD
Associate Professor of Clinical Medicine and Anesthesia, School of Medicine, University of California, San Francisco; Director, UCSF Echocardiography, School of Medicine, University of California, San Francisco, San Francisco, California
Transesophageal Echocardiography for the Anesthesiologist

Thomas J. Gal, MD
Professor of Anesthesiology, University of Virginia; Attending Anesthesiologist, University of Virginia Health Sciences Center, Charlottesville, Virginia
Pulmonary Anatomy and Physiology

Melvin C. Gitlin, MD, FACPM
Professor of Clinical Anesthesiology, Tulane University School of Medicine; Director, Pain Management Center, Tulane University Hospital and Clinic, New Orleans, Louisiana
Postoperative Pain Management

Nikolaus Gravenstein, MD
Professor of Anesthesiology and Neurosurgery, Chairman, Department of Anesthesiology, University of Florida College of Medicine, Gainesville, Florida
Cardiac Complications

Raymond Hasel, MD
Department of Anaesthesiology, Lakeshore General Hospital, Pointe Claire, Quebec
Monitoring Ventricular Function

Paul M. Heerdt, MD
Associate Professor, Chief of Thoracic Anesthesia, Department of Anesthesiology, Weill Medical College of Cornell University; Associate Professor, Department of Anesthesiology, Memorial Sloan-Kettering Cancer Center, New York, New York
Lung Transplantation

Brad Hindman, MD
Associate Professor of Anesthesia, College of Medicine, University of Iowa, Iowa City, Iowa
Central Nervous System Complications

Roberta L. Hines, MD
Professor and Chairman, Department of Anesthesiology, Yale University School of Medicine; Chairman, Anesthesiology, Yale New Haven Hospital, New Haven, Connecticut
Monitoring Ventricular Function

Allen J. Hinkle, MD
Associate Professor of Anesthesiology and Pediatrics, Dartmouth Medical School, Hanover, New Hampshire; Corporate Medical Director and Senior Vice President, Blue Cross Blue Shield of New Hampshire, Manchester, New Hampshire
Continuous Quality Improvement in Cardiac and Thoracic Anesthesia

Jan C. Horrow, MD
Clinical Professor, Anesthesiology, Allegheny University of the Health Sciences, Philadelphia, Pennsylvania; Vice President, Clinical Development, IBEX Technologies Corporation, Malvern, Pennsylvania
Coagulation and Coagulopathies

Ira J. Isaacson, MD
Professor of Anesthesiology, School of Medicine, Emory University, Atlanta, Georgia
Peripheral Vascular Surgery

Eric Jacobsohn, MBChB, FRCPC
Assistant Professor, Departments of Anaesthesia, Surgery and Critical Care, Health Services Center, University of Manitoba, Winnipeg, Manitoba
Monitoring Cardiac Electrical Activity

Douglas C. Johnson, MD
Assistant Professor of Medicine, Harvard Medical School; Associate Physician, Massachusetts General Hospital, Boston, Massachusetts
Pulmonary Function Testing

Robert M. Kacmarek, PhD, RRT
Associate Professor, Department of Anesthesia, Harvard Medical School; Director, Respiratory Care, Massachusetts General Hospital, Boston, Massachusetts
Postoperative Ventilatory Support

David D. Kaemmer, AS, BS, CCP
Staff Perfusionist, Duke Heart Center, Duke University Medical Center, Durham, North Carolina
Low Cardiac Output States: Drugs, Intra-Aortic Balloon, and Ventricular Assist Devices

Colleen M. Kigin, MS, MPA, PT
Assistant Professor, MGH Institute of Health Professions; Director, Program Development, Center for Innovative Minimally Invasive Therapy, Massachusetts General Hospital, Boston, Massachusetts
Preoperative Conditioning for the Thoracic Surgery Patient

Anne C. Kolker, MD
Associate Professor of Clinical Anesthesiology, Weill Medical College of Cornell University; Associate Attending Anesthesiologist, Memorial Sloan-Kettering Cancer Center, New York, New York
Esophageal Surgery

David Kramer, MD
Department of Anesthesiology, Duke University Medical Center, Durham, North Carolina
Organ System Effects of Anesthetics

Jan Kramer, MD
Attending Anesthesiologist, Albert Einstein Medical Center, Philadelphia, Pennsylvania
Coronary Artery Disease

Carol L. Lake, MD, MBA
Professor of Anesthesia and Assistant Dean, Indiana University; Chief of Staff, Roudebush VA Medical Center, Indianapolis, Indiana
Cardiovascular Anatomy and Physiology; Heart and Lung Transplantation

C. Philip Larson, Jr., MDCM, MS
Professor of Clinical Anesthesiology, UCLA School of Medicine, Los Angeles, California; Professor-Emeritus of Anesthesia and Neurosurgery, Stanford University, Stanford, California
Cerebral Vascular Surgery

Noel W. Lawson, MD
Professor of Anesthesiology, Chairman, Department of Anesthesiology, The University of Missouri, Columbia, Missouri
Dysrhythmias

Philip D. Lumb, MB, BS, FCCM
Professor of Anesthesiology and Surgery, Chairman, Department of Anesthesiology, Albany Medical College; Anesthesiologist-in-Chief, Albany Medical Center Hospital, Albany, New York
Respiratory, Renal, and Gastrointestinal Complications

Carl Lynch III, MD, PhD
Professor of Anesthesiology, University of Virginia Health Sciences Center, Charlottesville, Virginia
Cardiovascular Anatomy and Physiology

Srinivas Mantha, MD
Additional Professor, Department of Anaesthesiology and Intensive Care, Nizam's Institute of Medical Sciences, Hyderabad, India; Visiting Scientist, Department of Anesthesia and Critical Care, The University of Chicago, Chicago, Illinois
Cost-Effectiveness and Benefit of Preoperative Work-up and Preparation for Vascular Surgery

Katherine Marschall, MD
Clinical Associate Professor of Anesthesiology, New York University School of Medicine; Director, Cardiac Anesthesia, NYU Medical Center, New York, New York
Intrathoracic Aortic Surgery

Robert G. Matheny, MD
Cardiothoracic Surgeon, Indiana Heart Institute, St. Vincent Hospital System, Indianapolis, Indiana
Minimally Invasive Coronary Artery Bypass Grafting

Joseph P. Mathew, MD
Associate Professor of Anesthesiology, Department of Anesthesiology, Duke University Medical Center, Durham, North Carolina
Valvular Heart Disease

Robert W. McPherson, MD*
Associate Professor, Department of Anesthesiology, Johns Hopkins University, Baltimore, Maryland
Monitoring Central and Peripheral Nervous System Function

---

*Deceased.

Mark F. Newman, MD
Associate Professor of Anesthesiology, Assistant Professor of Medicine, Duke University; Chief, Division of Cardiothoracic Anesthesia, Director, Neurologic Outcome Research Group, Duke Heart Center, Duke University Medical Center, Durham, North Carolina
Organ System Effects of Anesthetics

G. Alexander Patterson, MD
Joseph C. Bancroft Professor of Surgery, Washington University School of Medicine; Attending Physician, Barnes-Jewish Hospital of St. Louis, St. Louis, Missouri
Lung Transplantation

Joseph A. Proli, MD
Private Practice, Laurel, Mississippi
Invasive Cardiology: Diagnosis and Therapeutics

Michael F. Roizen, MD
Professor and Chairman, Department of Anesthesia and Critical Care, Professor, Department of Medicine, Division of the Biological Sciences, Pritzker School of Medicine, The University of Chicago, Chicago, Illinois
Cost-Effectiveness and Benefit of Preoperative Work-up and Preparation for Vascular Surgery; Anesthesia for Abdominal Aortic Revascularization

Joseph L. Seltzer, MD
Professor and Chairman, Department of Anesthesiology, Jefferson Medical College, Thomas Jefferson University; Chairman, Department of Anesthesiology, Thomas Jefferson University Hospital, Philadelphia, Pennsylvania
Postoperative Pain Management

Hiroshi Chris Shibutani, MD
Instructor, Weill Medical College of Cornell University; Clinical Assistant Anesthesiologist, Memorial Sloan-Kettering Cancer Center, New York, New York
Pulmonary Resection

Avner Sidi, MD
Associate Professor of Anesthesiology, Department of Anesthesiology, University of Florida College of Medicine, Gainesville, Florida
Cardiac Complications

Robert N. Sladen, MB, MRCP (UK), FRCPC
Professor of Anesthesiology, Vice Chairman, Department of Anesthesiology, Director of CT/SAICU, Columbia University College of Physicians and Surgeons; Director of CT/SAICU, Attending Intensivist and Anesthesiologist, Columbia Presbyterian Medical Center, New York, New York
Low Cardiac Output States: Drugs, Intra-Aortic Balloon, and Ventricular Assist Devices

Peter D. Slinger, MD, FRCPC
Associate Professor, Department of Anaesthesia, University of Toronto; Anaesthesia Staff, The Toronto Hospital, Toronto, Ontario
Lung Isolation

Mark Stafford Smith, MD, CM, FRCPC
Assistant Professor of Anesthesiology, Director of Cardiothoracic Anesthesia Fellowship Program, Duke Heart Center, Duke University; Attending Cardiothoracic Anesthesiologist, Duke Heart Center, Duke University Medical Center, Durham, North Carolina
Low Cardiac Output States: Drugs, Intra-Aortic Balloon, and Ventricular Assist Devices

John K. Stene, MD, PhD
Associate Professor of Anesthesia, Department of Anesthesia, College of Medicine, Penn State University; Co-director of Surgical Intensive Care Unit, Milton S. Hershey Medical Center, Penn State Geisinger Health System, Hershey, Pennsylvania
Thoracic Trauma

Paul E. Stensrud, MD
Instructor in Anesthesiology, Mayo Medical School, Rochester, Minnesota
Continuous Quality Improvement in Cardiac and Thoracic Anesthesia

Maria K. Sturaitis, MD
Assistant Professor, Department of Anesthesiology, Yale University School of Medicine, New Haven, Connecticut
Monitoring Central and Peripheral Nervous System Function

Alan N. Tenaglia, MD
Associate Professor of Medicine, Tulane University; Director, Cardiac Catheterization Laboratory, and Interventional Cardiology Program, Chief, Clinical Cardiology, Tulane University Medical Center, New Orleans, Louisiana
Invasive Cardiology: Diagnosis and Therapeutics

Stephen J. Thomas, MD
Professor and Vice Chair, Cornell University Medical College; New York Presbyterian Hospital, Cornell Campus, New York, New York
Coronary Artery Disease

B. Taylor Thompson, MD
Associate Professor of Medicine, Harvard Medical School; Director, Medical Intensive Care Unit, Massachusetts General Hospital, Boston, Massachusetts
Pulmonary Function Testing

John Thompson, MD
Staff Anesthesiologist, Southwest Washington Medical Center, Vancouver, Washington
Cardiopulmonary Bypass: Technology, Pathophysiology, and Pharmacology

Joseph D. Tobias, MD
Professor of Anesthesiology and Pediatrics, Director, Pediatric Anesthesiology/Pediatric Critical Care, The University of Missouri, Columbia, Missouri
Dysrhythmias

Anastasios N. Triantafillou, MD
Associate Professor of Anesthesiology, Washington University School of Medicine; Attending Physician, Anesthesiology, Barnes-Jewish Hospital of St. Louis, St. Louis, Missouri
Lung Transplantation

Hans J. Wilke, II, MD
Attending Anesthesiologist, Department of Anesthesiology, University Hospitals, Johann Wolfgang Goethe University, Frankfurt am Main, Germany
Monitoring Cardiac Electrical Activity

Roger S. Wilson, MD
Professor of Anesthesiology, Weill Medical College of Cornell University; Chairman, Department of Anesthesiology and Critical Care Medicine, Memorial Sloan-Kettering Cancer Center, New York, New York
Anesthesia for Bronchoscopy and Mediastinoscopy

Jacques YaDeau, MD, PhD
Assistant Professor of Anesthesiology, Cornell University Medical College; Assistant Attending Anesthesiologist, Hospital for Special Surgery, New York, New York
Coronary Artery Disease

Steven R. Young, MD
Assistant Clinical Professor, Department of Anesthesia, Indiana University School of Medicine; Chairman, Department of Anesthesia, Indiana Heart Institute, St. Vincent Hospital System, Indianapolis, Indiana
Minimally Invasive Coronary Artery Bypass Grafting

John A. Youngberg, MD
Professor of Anesthesiology, Director of Cardiac Anesthesia, Department of Anesthesiology, Tulane University Medical Center, New Orleans, Louisiana
Anesthesia for Abdominal Aortic Revascularization; Cerebral Vascular Surgery

James R. Zaidan, MD
Professor of Anesthesiology, Deputy Chairman for Education, Department of Anesthesiology, Emory University School of Medicine, Atlanta, Georgia
Pacemakers

William Zimmerman, MD
Fellow in Cardiac Anesthesiology, Yale University School of Medicine, New Haven, Connecticut
Valvular Heart Disease

Foreword

The world is allegedly divided into "lumpers" and "splitters." This has traditionally been true of medicine, leading to controversy about the roles of general physicians and specialists. The same types of arguments have occurred regarding the unity of anesthesiology. On the one hand, some believe that all anesthesiologists should be able to provide optimal anesthetic care for any patient undergoing any type of surgery, and should concentrate their efforts in the operating room. On the other hand, others suggest that specializing and concentrating on the specific problems posed by particular categories of patients or particular types of surgery will lead to development of greater knowledge and skills, ultimately improving patient care and outcomes.

A corollary to the latter contention is that the lessons learned in the management of a specific segment may then be applied to a wider population. For instance, philosophies of anesthetic management developed to provide safe conduct of patients through cardiac surgery for myocardial revascularization may be directly applicable to patients with coronary artery disease undergoing vascular surgery. (Or, for that matter, β-adrenergic blockade, which has been demonstrated to reduce death rates associated with myocardial infarction, might also reduce mortality of patients with coronary artery disease when they undergo stresses of surgery. Ironically, it took two decades to recognize and establish this principle, demonstrating a downside to splitting knowledge between cardiology and anesthesiology.)

The subspecialty of cardiac anesthesia was developed together with the surgical specialty of cardiac surgery. Originally, both were exotic, high-tech ventures of stubborn, dedicated physicians able to tolerate frequently being in dangerous situations no one had previously confronted, and the occurrence of high rates of failure and high death rates. The initial target population was largely limited to the relatively small number of patients with valvular or congenital heart disease—which most would not have considered a major public health problem. This changed dramatically with the advent of surgical procedures to address coronary artery disease, then the largest killer in the developed world and now projected soon to become the largest killer throughout the world. In similar fashion, vascular and thoracic anesthesia became recognized as distinct subspecialties linked, respectively, to the surgical specialties of general (or noncardiac) thoracic surgery and vascular surgery. Surely this marked the triumph of the splitters.

The organizers and editors of this textbook, each of whom concentrate in one of these anesthetic subspecialties, have taken a step toward the lumpers and away from the splitters. They have recognized the commonality of the areas of interest shared by these three anesthetic subspecialties. This represents a philosophical departure from the "splendid isolation" envisioned by many who pioneered the subspecialties. It also represents the confidence and maturity gained by hard work and success.

Will we now see a coalescing of the research-investigative-educational arms of these anesthetic subspecialties and merging of their clinical activities? Will the three transform into one, as perhaps predicted by the evolution of the journal now entitled *Journal of Cardiovascular and Thoracic Anesthesia*? Only time will tell. However, some lessons seem clear:

1. Focusing upon a concentrated area stimulates research and facilitates in-depth knowledge and superior care in that area.

2. Applying that knowledge to related problems in other areas may enhance care in these areas also.
3. Enhanced care will lead to medical, and in turn, scientific attacks on ever more challenging conditions within these areas.
4. These new challenges will stimulate concentration, focusing (or specializing) upon the issues posed by these new challenges.

Recognizing, studying, confronting, and solving health problems posed by progressively sicker patients represents one of the greatest joys and privileges of practicing medicine. In a single volume, the editors have gathered a great deal of information relative to the anesthetic management of patients with diseases of the circulatory and respiratory systems. This has the potential of not only educating the reader but also of stimulating some to further identify and approach new challenges, and further advance the science and practice of cardiovascular and thoracic anesthesia.

Edward Lowenstein, M.D.
Henry Isaiah Dorr Professor of Research and Teaching in Anaesthesia
Professor of Medical Ethics
Harvard Medical School

Provost
Department of Anesthesia and Critical Care
Massachusetts General Hospital
Boston, Massachusetts

Preface

The majority of anesthesiologists provide care for patients undergoing cardiac, vascular, or thoracic surgery. While a number of general anesthesiology textbooks are available—as are textbooks specializing in cardiac, vascular, or thoracic anesthesia—there was no textbook devoted to providing care in the three closely aligned areas of cardiac, thoracic, and vascular anesthesia. This textbook was written to fill that void and to be a reference source for practitioners involved in these challenging and often high-risk areas of patient care.

The text is comprised of 40 chapters written by over 65 contributing authors well recognized in their areas of interest and expertise. The text is divided into seven sections. Section I has seven chapters devoted to general areas of interest including anatomy, physiology, pharmacology, and preoperative conditioning. Also included are two closely related chapters on preoperative assessment and the cost-benefit effectiveness of preoperative preparation. Section II is devoted to monitoring and includes a full-color section. Section III deals with adult patients undergoing invasive or minimally invasive coronary artery revascularization procedures and valvular procedures and includes chapters on both cardiac and lung transplantation. Special areas of myocardial preservation and management of low cardiac output syndrome are addressed. Section IV is devoted to the area of vascular surgery and includes chapters addressing the specific considerations of patients undergoing endovascular, thoracic aortic, abdominal aortic, carotid artery, or peripheral artery procedures. Emphasis is placed on the risks and benefits of regional versus general anesthesia for these various procedures. Section V has six chapters that address a variety of thoracic procedures ranging from bronchoscopy and mediastinoscopy to esophageal surgery and one-lung ventilation. Special considerations in one-lung ventilation for lung transplantation, pulmonary resection, and lung isolation are emphasized.

The final two sections are also general interest sections with information of crossover interest to the three subspecialty areas of cardiac, vascular, and thoracic anesthesia. Section VI covers the general considerations of dysrhythmias, coagulation, and thoracic trauma. The chapter devoted to pacemakers addresses the various types and models of pacemakers and automatic internal defibrillators and the anesthesia considerations associated with each type. The final section addresses issues such as cardiac, central nervous system, respiratory, and renal complications. Additionally, chapters discussing pain management options and methods to predict outcome and design a quality improvement program are included.

The separation of the general purpose sections lessens the redundancy of material in the subspecialty sections and allows easier access to specific areas of interest for the reader.

This text would not have come to fruition if it had not been for the expertise and dedication of my colleagues and their endeavors: Carol L. Lake, M.D., M.B.A., Michael F. Roizen, M.D., and Roger S. Wilson, M.D. We are indeed indebted to each other and hope our efforts benefit you and your patients.

John A. Youngberg, M.D.
Professor of Anesthesiology
Director of Cardiac Anesthesia
Tulane Department of Anesthesiology

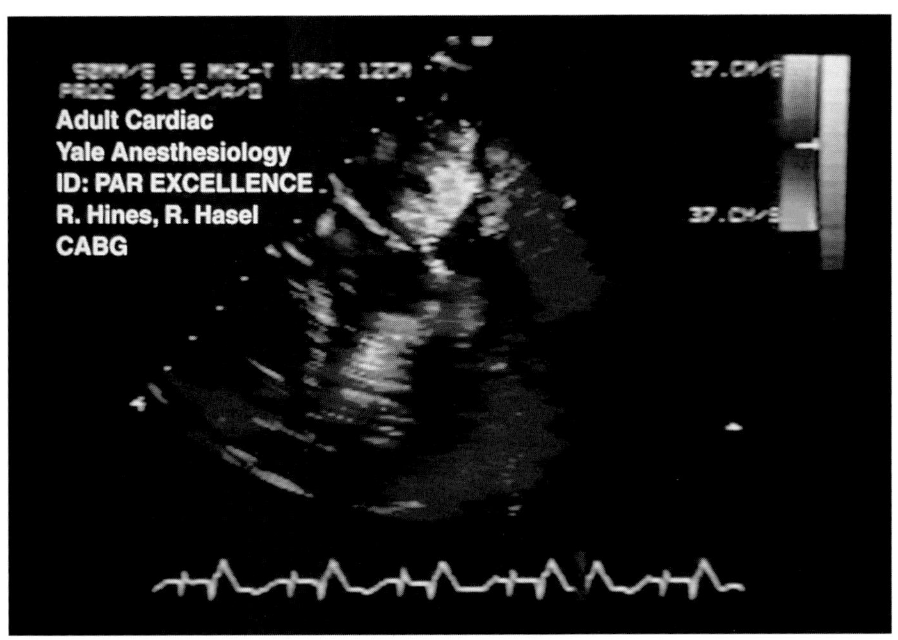

Figure 9–13. See page 260.

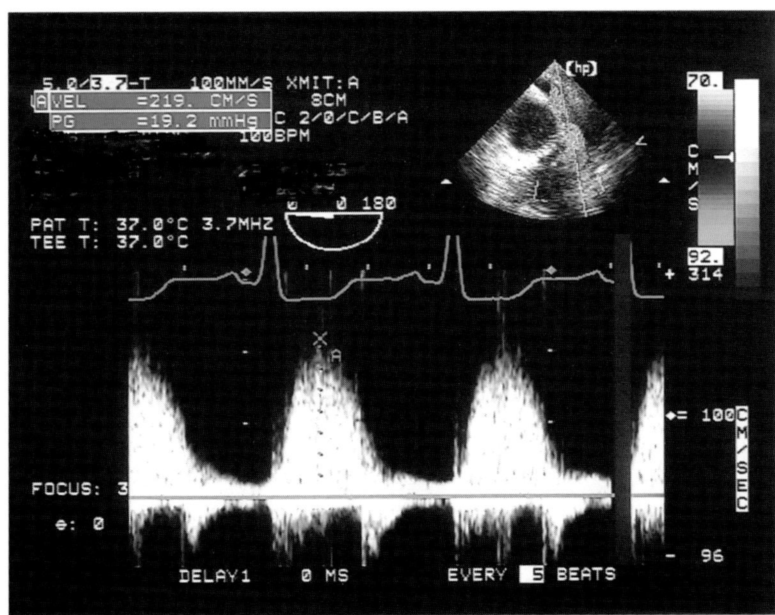

Figure 10–3. See page 276.

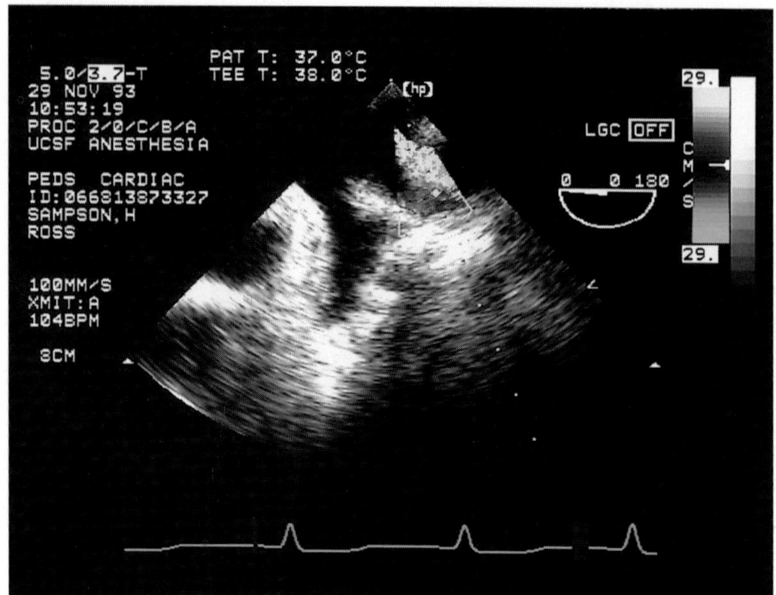

Figure 10–15. See page 289.

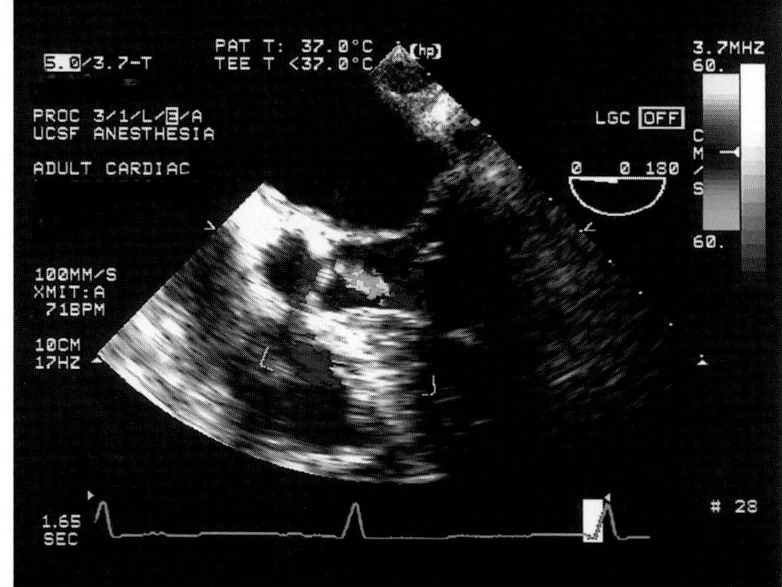

Figure 10–21. See page 299.

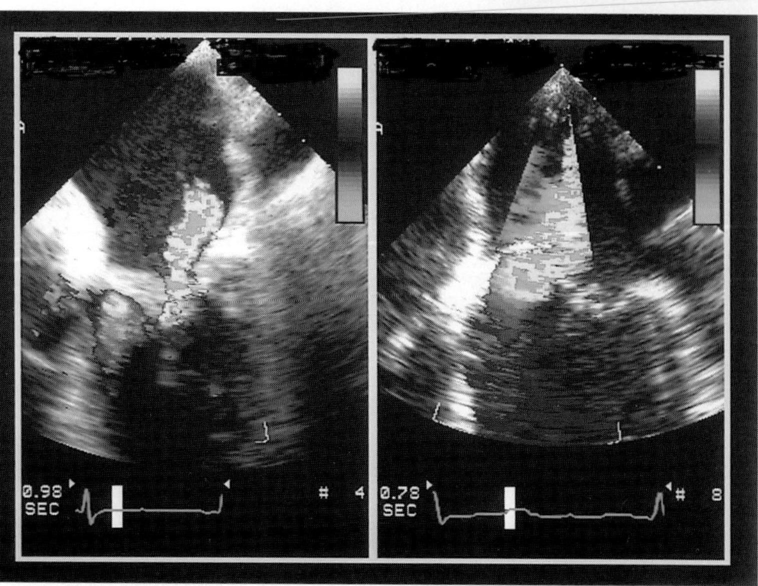

Figure 10–22. See page 300.

Contents

SECTION III

SECTION IV

SECTION V

SECTION I

INTRODUCTION

CHAPTER 1

Preoperative Assessment

Lee A. Fleisher, M.D.

Part and parcel of anesthesiologists' function in perioperative care is to reduce the patient's perioperative risk. In order to fulfill this function, the anesthesiologist establishes a database that includes the probability of disease based upon history, physical examination, and testing. The anesthesiologist often uses this information to modify perioperative care. In addition, the anesthesiologist can provide an assessment of risk to the patient and surgeon so that they may make an educated (informed) decision regarding the planned surgical procedure.

The preoperative database contains information obtained from the clinical history, physical examination, and laboratory testing. For example, the electrocardiogram (ECG) is routinely obtained in patients undergoing cardiac and thoracic surgery. Such testing is inexpensive and can provide important information.

The preoperative database should be complete and contain confirmatory evidence of the pertinent disease processes. Based upon the surgical procedure, specific organ systems may be targeted for a more extensive history. For example, the patient undergoing a carotid endarterectomy may have a more comprehensive neurologic evaluation than a patient undergoing femoral popliteal bypass grafting. A history of bleeding easily or for a prolonged time may require more extensive evaluation in the patient in whom an epidural anesthetic is planned than if general anesthesia is planned. The anesthesiologist frequently applies clinical judgment in the decision to further assess the probability of disease. Considering current constraints on medical economics, preoperative testing should only be performed when there is significant utility of the information. The potential benefit of the information must then be balanced against the risks and costs of obtaining the information. In this chapter, the clinical risk factors that raise the probability of disease and the use of tests to confirm the diagnosis will be outlined. In addition, issues of cost and benefit of a more detailed database will be discussed in this chapter and in the subsequent chapter.

Importance of Surgical Procedure

The surgical procedure has a significant impact on the amount of preoperative information required to perform anesthesia safely. Patients undergoing coronary artery bypass grafting (CABG) have definitive information regarding the coronary anatomy and ventricular function. Such information can be assimilated into an assessment of cardiovascular status.

For patients undergoing noncardiac surgery, the issues are often more complex. The cardiovascular and pulmonary status are usually less well defined prior to surgery. The decision to obtain noninvasive testing must take into account the potential benefits of a test against the known costs (monetary and potential complications). For surgical procedures that are not associated with significant organ system stress resulting in a high incidence of perioperative myocardial ischemia or morbidity, the risks (and costs) of the evaluation might be greater than any perceived benefits from the new information. For example, cataract surgery is associated with minimal organ system stress and exceedingly low morbidity and mortality rates even after the patient has suffered a recent myocardial infarction.[1] Similarly, transurethral resection of the prostate, a procedure frequently performed in patients with coronary artery disease (CAD), has a very low reported incidence of cardiac complications.[2] In the above examples, perioperative management is rarely changed by evaluation of the patient's cardiovascular status unless the patient demonstrates unstable angina or overt congestive heart failure. In contrast, patients undergoing procedures associated with significant organ system stress and increased morbidity can frequently benefit from a more extensive preoperative evaluation. For example, myocardial ischemia potential and incidence of perioperative cardiac morbidity increases with the ascending level of aortic cross-clamp in patients undergoing aortic revascularization.[3] In patients undergoing aortic surgery involving a suprarenal cross-clamp, the benefit of further evaluation and coronary artery revascularization may outweigh the associated costs or risks. Thus, the surgical procedure has important implications for the preoperative evaluation.

Historical Perspective

Preoperative evaluation of the patient undergoing cardiovascular and thoracic surgery has traditionally been approached from two perspectives: multifactorial risk indices and evaluation by new preoperative testing modalities. The first area was popularized by the pioneering work of the American Society of Anesthesiologists (ASA) (Physical Status Index) and then Dr. Lee Goldman and colleagues.[4] The second area has received extensive attention during the previous two decades with the advent of new noninvasive testing modalities.

In interpreting studies that develop a multifactorial index of risk, three basic assumptions are made. The first is that data on all of the potentially important variables are available. If angina was not included in the database, it could not be included in the final index. Second, eliminating variables from the model must be based upon biologic significance and not just statistical significance. In the original Goldman Cardiac Risk Index (CRI), New York Heart Association (NYHA) Class IV angina was not found to be a risk factor; however, the number of patients who fit this criterion was too small to achieve statistical significance.[4] Therefore, it was eliminated (? erroneously) from the model. Finally, if a factor is identified as placing the patient at significant risk, and the anesthesiologist can use the information to modify and reduce that risk, then the factor may no longer appear to be significant. For example, if perioperative hemodynamic management decisions did not include the hypertensive status of a patient, then lack of hypertensive management in subsequent patients may lead to increased morbidity.

Noncardiac Risk Indices

In 1977, Goldman and colleagues published their landmark article studying 1,001 patients undergoing noncardiac surgical procedures, excluding transurethral resection of the prostate (TURP).[4] The authors excluded TURP because of the authors' perception of a low morbidity rate when this procedure was performed under spinal anesthesia. The authors identified nine risk factors and gave each factor a certain number of points (CRI) (Table 1–1). Myocardial infarction by history and presence of an S_3 gallop were identified as the most significant risk factors. By adding up the total number of points, patients were placed in one of four classes. The patient's class could then be compared to the rates of morbidity and mortality from the original cohort (Table 1–2).

The CRI was subsequently validated in another cohort of patients; however, it has not been found to be predictive in patients undergoing major vascular surgery. Multiple studies have demonstrated that major vascular surgery is associated with a higher rate of morbidity and mortality compared to nonvascular surgery.[4–7] In order to rectify this problem, Detsky and colleagues proposed a modification of the CRI for vascular patients.[8]

Although both of these indices were useful when initially proposed, perioperative care has changed significantly in the intervening years. Goldman Class III and IV continue to represent a high-risk cohort; however, further stratification of the low-risk group is required. Several approaches to this risk stratification will be discussed throughout this chapter.

TABLE 1–1
Computation of the Cardiac Risk Index*

Criteria	Multivariate Discriminant Function Coefficient	"Points"
I. History:		
a. Age >70 yr	0.191	5
b. MI in previous 6 mo	0.384	10
II. Physical examination:		
a. S_3 gallop or JVD	0.451	11
b. Important VAS	0.119	3
III. Electrocardiogram:		
a. Rhythm other than sinus or PACs on last preoperative ECG	0.283	7
b. >5 PVCs/min documented at any time before operation	0.278	7
IV. General status: P_{O_2} < 60 or P_{CO_2} > 50 mmHg, K < 3.0 or HCO_3^- < 20 mEq/L, BUN > 50 or Cr > 3.0 mg/dl, abnormal SGOT, signs of chronic liver disease or patient bedridden from noncardiac causes	0.132	3
V. Operation:		
a. Intraperitoneal, intrathoracic, or aortic operation	0.123	3
b. Emergency operation	0.167	4
Total possible		53 points

*From Goldman L, Caldera DL, Nussbaum SR, et al: Multifactorial index of cardiac risk in noncardiac surgical procedures. N Engl J Med 297:845, 1977. Copyright 1977, Massachusetts Medical Society, with permission.

MI, myocardial infarction; JVD, jugular vein distention; VAS, valvular aortic stenosis; PACs, premature atrial contractions; ECG, electrocardiogram; PVCs, premature ventricular contractions; P_{O_2}, partial pressure of oxygen; P_{CO_2}, partial pressure of carbon dioxide; K, potassium; HCO_3, bicarbonate; BUN, blood urea nitrogen; Cr, creatinine; SGOT, serum glutamic oxalacetic transaminase.

Cardiac Surgery Risk Indices

Multiple studies have also examined risk stratification for cardiac surgery. Three large cooperative studies were begun in the 1970s to determine if CABG was superior to medical treatment: (1) the Coronary Artery Surgery Study (CASS), (2) the Veterans Administration Cooperative Study (VACS), and (3) the European Cooperative

TABLE 1–2
Cardiac Risk Index*

Class	Point Total	No or Only Minor Complication (*n* = 943)	Life-Threatening Complications† (*n* = 39)	Cardiac Deaths (*n* = 19)
I (*n* = 537)	0–5	532 (99)‡	4 (0.7)	1 (0.2)
II (*n* = 316)	6–12	295 (93)	16 (5)	5 (2)
III (*n* = 130)	13–25	112 (86)	15 (11)	3 (2)
IV (*n* = 18)	>26	4 (22)	4 (22)	10 (5.0)

*From Goldman L, Caldera DL, Nussbaum SR, et al: Multifactorial index of cardiac risk in noncardiac surgical procedures. N Engl J Med 297:845, 1977. Copyright 1977, Massachusetts Medical Society, with permission.
†Documented intraoperative or postoperative myocardial infarction, pulmonary edema, or ventricular tachycardia without progression to cardiac death.
‡Figures in parentheses denote %.

Study (ECS). Although not the primary goal of the studies, information regarding risk was obtained. Investigators involved in the CASS study performed multivariate analysis of clinical and angiographic factors that predicted perioperative mortality. Advanced age, female gender, symptoms of congestive heart failure, left main coronary artery stenosis, impaired left ventricular function, and nonelective surgery were all associated with increased perioperative mortality.[9] A similar multivariate logistic regression analysis was performed on the surgical patients in the Veterans Administration study, with priority of operation, age, peripheral vascular disease, great vessel repair, mitral valve replacement, and cardiomegaly being independent predictors of risk of poorer outcome.[10] With regard to gender, a later referral for catheterization and surgery for women has been suggested as a cause of the increased morbidity.[11]

Several models to predict perioperative morbidity and mortality have been reported.[12–14] Recently, O'Connor and colleagues studied data from 3,055 patients undergoing CABG at five clinical centers during the years 1987 to 1989.[14] The authors performed a logistic regression analysis to predict the risk of in-hospital mortality using data from the first 50% of the patients, and subsequently validated their model with data from the second group (50%) of patients. Similarly, Parsonnet and colleagues developed a risk stratification scheme at the Beth Israel Hospital in Newark.[15] The risk stratification schema was subsequently validated in a British hospital; however, the actual mortality rates were lower than predicted.[16] Investigators at the Cleveland Clinic developed a point system to predict morbidity and mortality (Table 1–3).[13] Risk stratification systems are useful in identifying patients at increased operative morbidity and mortality; however, the exact rate of complications may vary between institutions.

Assessment of Coronary Artery Disease in Patients Undergoing Noncardiac Surgery

For patients undergoing coronary artery bypass surgery, the probability of coronary artery disease is known. For patients undergoing noncardiac surgery, precise coronary anatomy and ventricular function are often less well defined. Several investigators have proposed a more functional approach to the preoperative evaluation.[17] The American Heart Association/American College of Cardiology (AHA/ACC) Task Force for Guidelines on the Perioperative Cardiovascular Evaluation for Noncardiac Surgery has proposed an algorithm that incorporates clinical history, exercise tolerance, and the surgical procedure in the decision to perform further evaluation.[18]

Known Coronary Artery Disease

Patients with known coronary artery disease (i.e., a probability of CAD of 100%) are patients with a prior myocardial infarction (MI) or classic angina with a positive stress test. Patients with a prior MI have coronary artery disease, although a small group of patients may sustain an MI from a nonatherosclerotic mechanism. Traditionally, risk assessment for noncardiac surgery was based upon the time interval between the MI and surgery. Multiple studies have demonstrated an increased incidence of reinfarction if the MI occurred within 6 months of the proposed surgical procedure (Table 1–4).[19–21] Improve-

TABLE 1–3
Clinical Severity Scoring System*

Preoperative Factors	Score
Emergency	6
Serum creatinine,	
≥141 and ≤167 μmol/L	
(≥1.6 and ≤1.8 mg/dl	1
≥168 μmol/L (≥1.9 mg/L)	4
Severe left ventricular dysfunction	3
Reoperation	3
Operative mitral valve insufficiency	3
Age ≥65 and ≤74 yr	1
Age ≥75 yr	2
Prior vascular surgery	2
Chronic obstructive pulmonary disease	2
Anemia (hematocrit ≤0.34)	2
Operative aortic valve stenosis	1
Weight ≤65 kg	1
Diabetes, on oral or insulin therapy	1
Cerebrovascular disease	1

*From Higgins T, Estafanous F, Loop F, et al: Stratification of morbidity and mortality outcome by preoperative risk factors in coronary artery bypass patients. JAMA 267:2344, 1992. Copyright 1992, American Medical Association, with permission.

TABLE 1–4
Reinfarction Rates in Different Studies and Number of Patients Studied

Time Elapsed Between Prior Myocardial Infarction and Operation (Months)	Reference		
	Tarhan et al. (1972)	Rao et al. (1983)	Shah et al. (1990)
0–3	37%, n = 18	5.8%, n = 52	4.3%, n = 23
4–6	16%, n = 19	2.3%, n = 86	0%, n = 18
>6	5.6%, n = 322	1.5%, n = 595	5.7%, n = 174
Time unknown	—	—	3.3%, n = 60

ments in perioperative care have decreased the risk of perioperative MI and shortened the safe time interval between an MI and elective surgery.

The importance of the intervening time interval may no longer be valid in the current era of thrombolytics, angioplasty, and risk stratification after an acute MI. Although many patients with an MI may continue to have myocardium at risk for subsequent ischemia and infarction, other patients may have their critical coronary stenosis either totally occluded or widely patent. The AHA/ACC Task Force has proposed the adoption of 30 days as the definition of an acute MI, while patients who have sustained a longer interval between the MI and surgery should have further evaluation and management based upon clinical symptoms.[18] For example, the patient with ongoing angina and a poor exercise tolerance might benefit from further evaluation and medical or surgical interventions. In contrast, a patient who sustained an MI 3 months previously and has a good exercise tolerance without the return of anginal symptoms may undergo all but the most extensive surgery without further evaluation or delay. In addition, the acute treatment of the MI and subsequent risk stratification should be included in the evaluation. For the nonsurgical patient, the use of percutaneous transluminal coronary angioplasty (PTCA) at the time of the MI has been associated with a lower in-hospital and 6-month morbidity and mortality compared to patients receiving thrombolytics. With proper risk stratification and stepped (stratified) appropriate management, vascular surgery has been performed with low morbidity and mortality.[22]

Patients with classic anginal symptoms have a near 100% probability of CAD. In such patients, it is important to determine the extent of myocardium at risk for ischemia and necrosis. Preoperative ischemia, both silent and symptomatic, has been associated with perioperative cardiac morbidity in noncardiac surgery patients.[5,23,24]

Patients with the diagnosis of chronic stable angina represent a continuum from those with a critical stenosis in a distal coronary artery to those patients who have left main disease. Although invasive and noninvasive testing can further define the extent of disease, clinical history can also provide important clues. Patients who develop shortness of breath or syncope with chest pain demonstrate evidence of left ventricular dysfunction. If patients experience such symptoms at minimal exercise, then the likelihood of *extensive* CAD is high. If the patient only develops angina with extremes of exercise and without concomitant symptoms (NYHA Class I), then the likelihood of *extensive* CAD is very low. In patients with either poor exercise tolerance without other symptoms, or excellent exercise tolerance with symptoms, the probability of extensive CAD is less well defined. Patients with unstable angina require urgent medical attention, since this syndrome frequently results in an MI unless treated. Shah and colleagues reported that patients with unstable angina experienced a 28% incidence of perioperative MI following noncardiac surgery.[25] Testing to define the extent of CAD will be discussed later in the chapter.

Patients with a Prior Revascularization

Patients who have previously undergone CABG are presumed to be at a lower risk. Although there have been no randomized trials, Foster and colleagues, and more recently Eagle and colleagues, examined the CASS database and reported that patients with a prior CABG had a significantly lower incidence of cardiac morbidity compared to a similar cohort of patients randomized to a group that received medical treatment alone.[26,26a] In addition, several investigators have reported low rates of cardiac morbidity and mortality when selective testing and revascularization are employed.[27,28] With regard to the optimal length of time between CABG and noncardiac surgery, Cruchley and colleagues reported that the rate of morbidity decreased significantly after 3 months.[29]

PTCA has recently been advocated as a means of reducing risk prior to noncardiac surgery. Similar to the case with CABG, no randomized trials have been conducted with PTCA; however, three case series have been reported. All three series demonstrated a very low incidence of perioperative morbidity and mortality in patients who had a PTCA at some time prior to noncardiac surgery (<2%).[30–32] Whether these cardiac complication rates would have been higher if PTCA was not performed will require further research. In the ambulatory population, most myocardial infarctions occur in areas distal to a noncritical stenosis.[33] If a similar pathophysiology underlies perioperative MI, then PTCA may be of limited benefit. Based upon these concerns, the AHA/ACC Guidelines advocate reserving the use of PTCA to those indications established for the nonoperative setting.

A secondary concern with regard to performing a PTCA before noncardiac surgery is the potential to develop thrombosis and acute closure. The perioperative period is associated with a hypercoagulable state, which increases this concern. There is anecdotal evidence and theoretical concerns that recent placement of a coronary stent may increase this risk.

Patients at Risk for CAD

For those patients without overt symptoms or history, the probability of CAD varies with the type and number of atherosclerotic risk factors present. Peripheral arterial disease has been shown to be associated with CAD in multiple studies. Hertzer and colleagues studied 1,000 consecutive patients scheduled for major vascular surgery and found that approximately 60% of patients had at least one coronary artery with a critical stenosis.[34] The presence of peripheral arterial disease, as assessed by the brachial–ankle blood pressure index (difference between pressure in brachial and ankle arteries) has been used as a marker for CAD. Therefore, the presence of peripheral atherosclerotic disease is a clue to uncover a high probability of CAD in a patient. Vascular surgery patients are frequently tested prior to noncardiac surgery to further define the diagnosis and potential extent of disease.[35–37]

Peripheral vascular disease also confers a high risk for patients undergoing CABG. This most likely reflects the higher incidence of diffuse arteriopathy. However, a subset of the patients undergoing aortic reconstructive surgery may represent a different pathophysiologic process from atherosclerosis, and may not be at the same risk. Tilson has demonstrated that the pathophysiologic process behind some aortic aneurysm formations may be a collagen vascular disease.[38] In the absence of other risk factors for CAD, these patients may represent a lower risk group.

Diabetic patients have a higher probability of CAD than nondiabetic patients.[39] The duration of the disease process and other associated end-organ dysfunction should be taken into account. Autonomic neuropathy has recently been found to be the best predictor of silent coronary artery disease and perioperative hemodynamic instability in patients with diabetes.[40] Diabetic patients are at very high risk for silent angina and for an MI. An electrocardiogram should be obtained to examine for the presence of Q waves and/or ischemia in the diabetic patient. Diabetes has been demonstrated to increase risk for both major vascular and cardiac surgery, and in multivariate models diabetes has been shown to be an independent predictor of subsequent morbidity.[5,41,42] The presence of diabetes is an important determinant that increases the utility of a test result by conferring a higher pretest probability.

Hypertension has also been associated with an increased incidence of silent myocardial ischemia and infarction.[39] Prys-Roberts and colleagues demonstrated that hypertensive patients had increased intraoperative hemodynamic derangements, particularly when preoperative medication was discontinued prior to surgery.[43] In the original study by Goldman and Caldera, hypertensive patients with a diastolic blood pressure greater than 110 mm Hg were suggested to be at increased risk; however, this was based upon a very small sample without poor outcomes.[44] Bedford and colleagues demonstrated that admission blood pressure was the best predictor of cardiovascular morbidity.[45] More recently, patients with left ventricular hypertrophy undergoing noncardiac surgery have been reported to be at a higher perioperative risk than nonhypertensive patients.[46] Investigators have suggested that the presence of a strain pattern on the ECG suggests a chronic ischemic state and that these patients might also be considered to have an increased probability of CAD.[47]

Several other risk factors have been used to suggest an increased probability of CAD. These include the atherosclerotic processes associated with tobacco use and hypercholesterolemia. When attempting to determine the overall probability of disease, the number and severity of the risk factors are important. In attempting to assess the risk of morbidity, exercise tolerance has long been advocated as providing important prognostic information. The wise old clinician of the 1960s and 1970s judged operability by walking their nonarteriopathic patients up two flights of stairs. In patients with an excellent exercise tolerance, all but the most strenuous procedures (i.e., high aortic temporary occlusion) are associated with low morbidity or mortality. McPhail and colleagues demonstrated that patients undergoing major vascular surgery who could exercise to 85% of their peak maximal heart rate were at a lower risk for cardiac morbidity when compared to those who were unable to reach the target heart rate, even in the presence of a positive stress test.[48] However, those patients who had a poor exercise tolerance had a high incidence of cardiac morbidity, and may require further definition of their risk.

As an alternative to formal exercise testing to determine maximal exercise tolerance, several activity-of-daily-living scales have been proposed. One such scale has been advocated by the AHA/ACC Guidelines (Table 1–5). By determining the maximal activity performed by a given patient, they can be stratified into two groups.

Risk Assessment for Patients Undergoing Cardiac Surgery

Several risk stratification indices have been proposed in patients undergoing coronary artery bypass grafting. Multiple factors are associated with increased risk including age, gender, presence of peripheral vascular disease, diabetes, and reoperation. One of the most consistent predictors of perioperative morbidity and mortality is impaired left ventricular function. Traditionally, an impaired ejection fraction was defined as less than 36%; however, more recent studies have lowered these limits. Christakis et al. studied 12,471 patients undergoing CABG and divided the patients into groups based upon their preoperative ejection fraction; greater than 40%, 20 to 40%, and less than 20%.[49] The perioperative mortality rates in these groups were 2.3, 4.8, and 9.8%, respectively.

Recently, attention has focused on identifying patients with impaired ejection fraction and the presence of "hibernating myocardium." Hibernating myocardium represents areas of tissue that are viable but have minimal or no contribution to ventricular function secondary to a

TABLE 1–5
Estimated Energy Requirement for Various Activities*

1 MET	Can you take care of yourself?	4 METs	Climb a flight of stairs or walk up a hill?
	Eat, dress, or use the toilet?		Walk on level ground at 4 mph or 6.4 km/hr?
	Walk indoors around the house?		Run a short distance
	Walk a block or two on level ground at 2–3 mph or 3.2–4.8 km/hr?		Do heavy work around the house like scrubbing floors or lifting or moving heavy furniture?
	Do light work around the house like dusting or washing dishes?		Participate in moderate recreational activities like golf, bowling, dancing, doubles tennis, or throwing a baseball or football?
4 METs		>10 METs	Participate in strenuous sports like swimming, singles tennis, football, basketball, or skiing?

*Adapted from the Duke Activity Status Index and AHA Exercise Standards. From Eagle K, Brundage B, Chaitman B, et al: Guidelines for perioperative cardiovascular evaluation of the noncardiac surgery. A report of the American Heart Association/American College of Cardiology Task Force on Assessment of Diagnostic and Therapeutic Cardiovascular Procedures. Circulation 93:1278, 1996, with permission.
MET, metabolic equivalent.

chronic ischemic state.[50] Areas of hibernating myocardium frequently improve in function after CABG. Testing employing both thallium imaging and positron emission tomography have been advocated to identify patients who would have a significant improvement in ejection fraction after revascularization.

The importance of preoperative angina and subsequent risk of CABG depends upon the pattern. While unstable angina is associated with a marked increase in risk, the importance of preoperative silent or symptomatic ischemia is debated. In the original work by Slogoff and Keats, the presence of prebypass ischemia was associated with a significantly higher rate of cardiac morbidity.[51,52] In contrast, the Study of Perioperative Ischemia (SPI) Research Group did not find an association between preoperative ischemia and perioperative morbidity.[53]

Emergent operations are also associated with a marked increase in risk. Unstable angina has been found to be associated with a 3.9% increased risk in the Coronary Artery Surgery Study.[9] In addition, CABG is now indicated in patients immediately after an acute MI. Patients who have suffered an acute MI may have any of the complications of an acute MI, such as papillary muscle rupture, mitral valve dysfunction, and septal infarction. With the increases in the use of PTCA, thrombolytics, and stents, patients who have acute closure or dissection of a coronary artery can present to the operating room, partially heparinized and demonstrating acute ischemia.

Testing to Confirm the Diagnosis and Determine the Extent of CAD

The decision to perform a test to confirm a diagnosis of CAD must be based on (1) the ability of the test to provide additional information, (2) the utility of the information to modify care, and (3) the risks and costs associated with the test and any perioperative interventions.[54] The ability of a test to provide additional information can be assessed by an application of Bayes' theorem. Bayes' theorem states that the posttest probability of disease is a function of the pretest probability of disease and the true-positive (sensitivity) and false-positive (specificity) rates of the test.[55] For example, in patients with a very low pretest probability of disease, a positive exercise electrocardiogram is frequently a false-positive test. Similarly, in patients with a very high pretest probability of disease, a negative exercise electrocardiogram is frequently a false-negative test.

The mathematical definition for sensitivity and specificity are:

$$\text{Sensitivity} = \frac{\text{TP}}{\text{TP} + \text{FN}}; \quad \text{Specificity} = \frac{\text{TN}}{\text{FP} + \text{TN}}$$

where TP = true-positive, TN = true-negative, FP = false-positive, and FN = false-negative. This lack of information of the test arises from the imperfect sensitivity and specificity of the test. Only a highly sensitive and specific test like coronary angiography would significantly change the likelihood of the diagnosis in patients with high and low pretest probabilities of disease. Using noninvasive testing to further define the probability of disease is only useful in the patient at moderate risk. L'Italien et al. has developed a two-step model in which the posttest probability of morbidity can be determined based upon the clinical risk profile and any subsequent testing.[56] By assessing clinical risk first, the value of subsequent noninvasive testing can be determined.

Although noninvasive testing is not useful for excluding disease in a high-risk population, a test still might provide important additional information by determining the extent of disease. Radionuclide imaging techniques can frequently quantify the area of risk. Since multiple studies have now demonstrated a relationship between quantity of myocardium at risk and perioperative morbidity in noncardiac surgery, this information might be useful depending on how one used the information to modify care, and how such modification affected outcome.[57–59]

If perioperative management decisions such as the requirement for invasive monitoring can be made on the basis of clinical history, further testing may not result in any change in care. There are circumstances, however, in which care would be modified if there was a change or confirmation of a diagnosis of cardiovascular disease. For example, using a central venous pressure monitor as opposed to a pulmonary artery catheter in a patient who has a negative stress test reduces the patient's risk and cost of the invasive monitor.[60] Additionally, the need for a postoperative intensive care unit bed may be modified by a more definitive diagnosis of cardiovascular disease.

Care may also be modified by the patient or surgeon based upon the results of a test. The patient or surgeon may require a precise assessment of cardiovascular risk in order to determine if the patient should undergo the planned surgical procedure. Axillobifemoral bypass has been advocated as an alternative to aortobifemoral bypass.[61] A patient may elect to forgo surgery because the risk of morbidity after elective surgery may be greater than the risk of not undergoing surgery. An 80-year-old patient with a 6-cm abdominal aortic aneurysm may elect to accept the future risk of aneurysm rupture as opposed to the immediate risk of perioperative morbidity.

The final issue is risk versus benefit. For noncardiac surgery, noninvasive testing is associated with a small though calculable risk. Testing frequently results in more invasive procedures. There are no randomized clinical trials to address the value of coronary revascularization before noncardiac surgery. An alternative approach to determining the optimal strategy for medical care in the absence of clinical trials is construction of a decision analysis. Two decision analyses have been published on this issue[62,63] (Fig. 1–1). Both assumed that patients with significant coronary artery disease would undergo coronary artery bypass grafting prior to noncardiac surgery. Both models found that the optimal decision was sensitive to local morbidity and mortality rates within the clinically observed range. These models suggest that preoperative testing for the purpose of coronary revascularization is not the optimal strategy if perioperative morbidity and mortality are low.

Importantly, the primary cost (in both dollars and morbidity) of preoperative testing and revascularization is the revascularization procedure itself. Therefore, the indications for revascularization and thus the frequency of its use has a significant impact on the model. Second, potential long-term benefits of coronary revascularization in this population were not included in the analysis, potentially biasing against the revascularization arm. Rihal et al. utilized the CASS database and found that coronary artery bypass grafting significantly improved survival in those patients with both peripheral vascular disease and triple-vessel coronary disease, especially the group with depressed ventricular function.[64] Therefore, identification of appropriate patients with diffuse disease or a significant left main stenosis amenable to surgery and acceptable risk should undergo CABG before noncardiac surgery. In this instance, the procedure is justified based on long-term benefit, and performing it before noncardiac surgery reduces the threat of perioperative myocardial infarction.

Selection of Patients Who Would Benefit from Further Testing

While almost all patients undergoing CABG surgery undergo preoperative coronary angiography, many patients undergoing noncardiac surgery do not have defined coronary circulation. Several algorithms have been proposed to determine which noncardiac surgery patients require further testing. Hertzer and colleagues suggested that all patients undergoing major vascular surgery in whom there is a suspicion of CAD should undergo coronary angiography, although they currently advocate noninvasive testing in selected patients.[34] Multiple authors have suggested noninvasive testing prior to vascular surgery; however, other authors have suggested that routine use of a noninvasive test loses its predictive value.[5,23,27,28,37,41,48,57,61,65–80] Testing is most useful in patients with a moderate probability of disease. Eagle and colleagues identified five clinical risk factors in patients undergoing vascular surgery: age greater than 70 years, Q waves on the electrocardiogram, history of diabetes, ventricular ectopic activity, and angina.[41] Dipyridamole thallium imaging had the greatest predictive value in patients with one or two risk factors. Patients without any of these five risk factors had such a low risk of perioperative morbidity that the test provided no additional information. Similarly, patients with three or more risk factors had such a high perioperative risk that a negative test was frequently falsely negative.

The algorithm proposed in the AHA/ACC Guidelines is shown in Figure 1–2.[18] An algorithm has been proposed that incorporates six steps. First, the clinician must evaluate the urgency of the surgery and the appropriateness of a formal preoperative assessment. Next, the clinician must determine if the patient has undergone a previous revascularization procedure or coronary evaluation. Those patients with unstable coronary syndromes should be identified, and appropriate treatment instituted. Finally, the decision to undergo further testing depends upon the interaction of the clinical risk factors, surgery-specific risk, and functional capacity (Table 1–6).

Tests to Better Confirm and Define Cardiovascular Disease (Table 1–7)

Exercise Electrocardiography

The exercise electrocardiogram has been the traditional method of evaluating individuals for the presence of coronary artery disease. The exercise ECG represents the least invasive and most cost-effective method of detecting ischemia, with a reasonable sensitivity (68 to 81%) and specificity (66 to 77%) for identifying coronary ar-

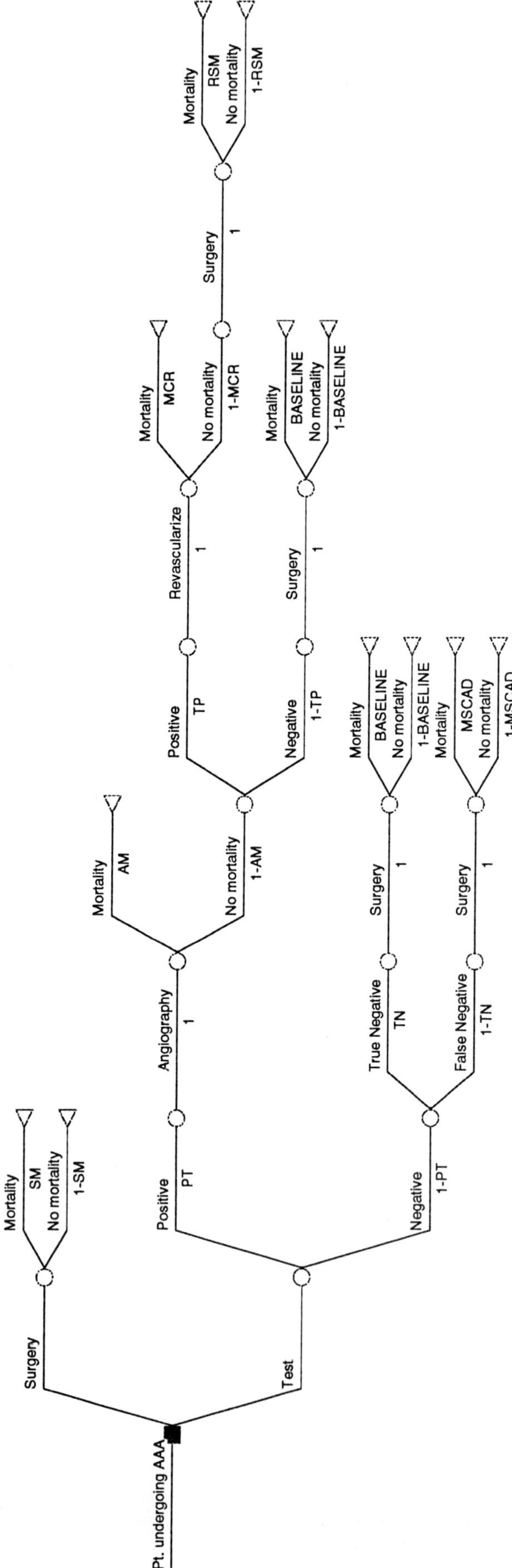

FIGURE **1–1.** Decision analysis evaluating the optimal strategy between abdominal aortic surgery (AAA) alone or cardiovascular testing and coronary revascularization prior to AAA surgery. The potential lower mortality for AAA surgery after coronary revascularization must be balanced against the mortality from the revascularization procedure itself. (From Fleisher LA, Skolnick ED, Holroyd KJ, Lehmann HP: Coronary artery revascularization before abdominal aortic aneurysm surgery: A decision analytic approach. Anesth Analg 79:661, 1994, with permission.)

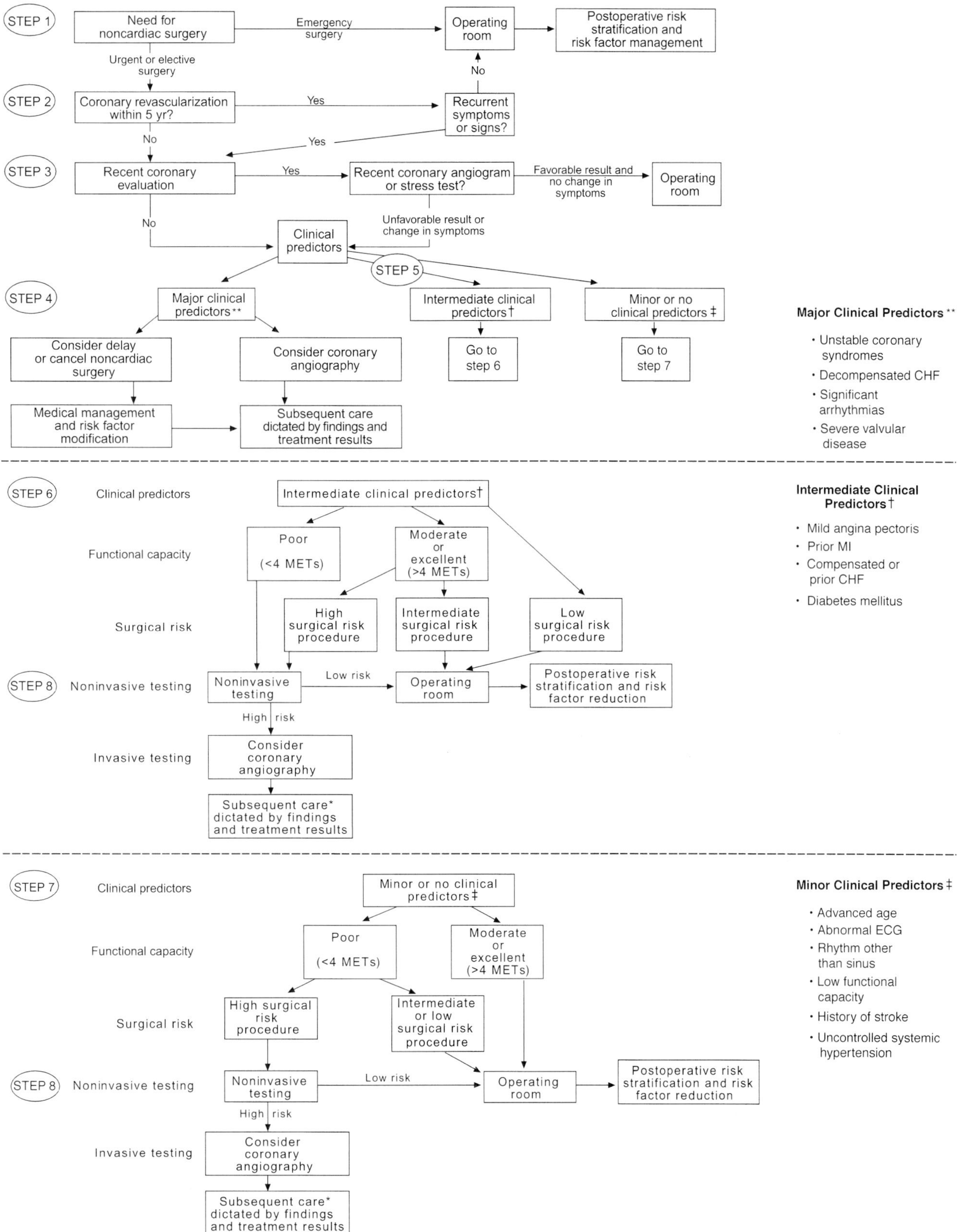

FIGURE **1–2.** The one algorithm proposed by the American Heart Association/American College of Cardiology Task Force on Perioperative Cardiovascular Evaluation for Noncardiac Surgery. The decision to perform further cardiovascular testing depends upon the clinical presentation of disease, surgery-specific risk, and exercise tolerance. (From Eagle K, Brundage B, Chaitman B, et al: Guidelines for perioperative cardiovascular evaluation of the noncardiac surgery. A report of the American Heart Association/American College of Cardiology Task Force on Assessment of Diagnostic and Therapeutic Cardiovascular Procedures. Circulation 93:1278, 1996, with permission.)

TABLE 1–6
Cardiac Risk Stratification for Noncardiac Surgical Procedures*†

High	(Reported cardiac risk often >5%) Emergent major operations, particularly in the elderly Aortic and other major vascular Peripheral vascular Anticipated prolonged surgical procedures associated with large fluid shifts and/or blood loss
Intermediate	(Reported cardiac risk generally <5%) Carotid endarterectomy Head and neck Intraperitoneal and intrathoracic Orthopedic Prostate
Low‡	(Reported cardiac risk generally <1%) Endoscopic procedures Superficial procedure Cataract Breast

*From Eagle K, Brundage B, Chaitman B, et al: Guidelines for perioperative cardiovascular evaluation of the noncardiac surgery. A report of the American Heart Association/American College of Cardiology Task Force on Assessment of Diagnostic and Therapeutic Cardiovascular Procedures. Circulation 93:1278, 1996, with permission.
†Cardiac risk is defined as combined incidence of cardiac death and nonfatal myocardial infarction.
‡Do not generally require further preoperative cardiac testing.

tery disease.[81] The goal of the test is to provoke ischemia by exercise. Electrocardiographic signs of myocardial ischemia and clinical signs of left ventricular dysfunction are considered positive. A decrease in blood pressure in response to exercise has been associated with global ventricular dysfunction in humans. Syncope during the test can also signify decreased cardiac output. Either sign signifies poor dynamic function, and is much more ominous than ST-segment depression alone.

Exercise electrocardiography can provide information concerning hemodynamic thresholds for ischemia. The heart rate and blood pressure at which ischemic changes developed might be noted by the anesthesiologist; however, ischemia *may not occur* at the same blood pressure and heart rate on the stress test as it would in daily life or under anesthesia. Most ischemia occurring intraoperatively may not be associated with any hemodynamic changes.[82,83] However, a positive exercise electrocardiographic stress test can alert the anesthesiologist that the patient is at risk for ischemia at a wide range of heart rates, with the greatest risk in those who develop ischemia at low workloads during the test.

TABLE 1–7
Sensitivity and Specificity of Various Diagnostic Tests for Detecting Coronary Artery Disease

Test	Sensitivity	Specificity
Exercise electrocardiography	81%	66%
Exercise thallium imaging		
Qualitative planar	84%	87%
Quantitative planar	89%	89%
SPECT	94%	82%
Dipyridamole thallium imaging	85%	90%
Stress echocardiography	80–90%	80–90%
Stress radionuclide angiography	70–80%	70–80%

SPECT, single photon emission computed tomography.

Exercise Thallium Imaging

The addition of nuclear imaging techniques to exercise increases the sensitivity and specificity of the noninvasive stress test. Currently, the most commonly used agent is thallium-201 (^{201}T1). ^{201}T1 is a radioactive perfusion agent that mimics potassium and is taken up by viable myocardial cells. There are currently two primary types of imaging, the traditionally planar imaging and the newer single photon emission computed tomography (SPECT) technology, which enables improved detection, localization, and determination of extent of the area of ischemia.[84] SPECT imaging offers higher contrast resolution and better separation of overlying myocardial segments. Because of the long period during which the patient needs to remain stationary, motion artifact may be more prevalent in SPECT imaging.

The uptake of ^{201}T1 in the myocardium is proportional to the coronary blood flow and myocardial extraction of ^{201}T1.[85] Initially, the patient is exercised to stress the myocardium. In patients who do not develop myocardial ischemia, the initial uptake of ^{201}T1 is therefore relatively homogeneous. Areas of scar (i.e., necrosed tissue) do not take up ^{201}T1, and demonstrate a defect on imaging. Areas distal to a significant coronary artery stenosis that attentuates flow during exercise, and therefore presumably at risk for myocardial ischemia during other stress (such as perioperative events), have a decreased coronary blood flow compared to the surrounding tissue, and have decreased initial ^{201}T1 uptake. These areas would also be represented with a defect on the initial (exercise) image. On subsequent imaging, the defect would fill-in from redistribution of the ^{201}T1 tracer after the blood flow returns to normal conditions (Fig. 1–3). Heterogeneity in flow, resulting in ^{201}T1 defects, may be induced earlier than the cellular alterations that result in ST-segment changes. This earlier appearance of flow redistribution may account for the higher incidence and greater prognostic implication of redistribution defects than electrocardiographic changes.

The sensitivity of exercise ^{201}T1 imaging depends upon the imaging technique. Qualitative visual ^{201}T1 imaging has an average sensitivity of 84% and specificity of 87% for detecting coronary artery disease.[86] The addition of quantitative analysis to planar ^{201}T1 increases the sensitivity and specificity to 89%.[84,87] Exercise ^{201}T1 SPECT imaging had an average 94% sensitivity, but only an 82% specificity in a multicenter study. Among centers, there is some individual variability in both the interpretation of the scans and the computer systems used for analysis.

Recent studies have focused on the previous inability to distinguish scar from severely ischemic tissue. Some areas of myocardium may be distal to a severe stenosis such that redistribution does not occur within the con-

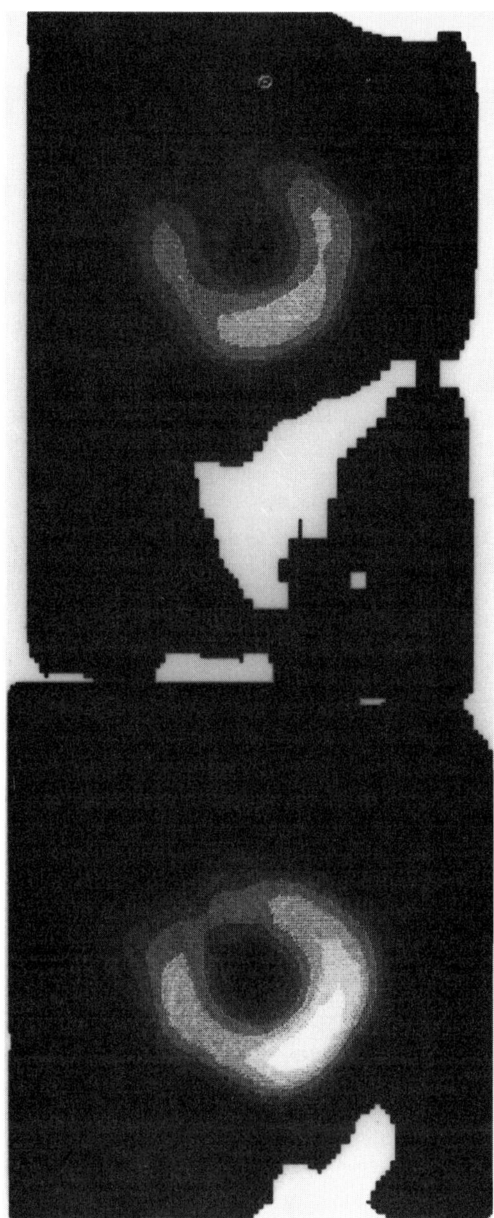

FIGURE 1–3. Thallium image demonstrating a defect on the top image associated with exercise or dipyridamole infusion. With time, viable myocardium takes up the thallium. Such a reversible defect represents an area at risk for myocardial ischemia.

ventional 4-hour period between first and second scans, and the second imaging demonstrates a persistent defect.[88] Investigators have suggested two techniques to determine if the fixed defect represents viable myocardium: (1) a 24-hour delayed image, (2) or a second dose of ^{201}Tl prior to the delayed imaging.[88,89] If the area was still viable, the defects were found to reperfuse. It is therefore important that one of these techniques is employed in patients with an initial apparently fixed defect.

Other measures to determine during stress ^{201}Tl imaging are size of defect, lung uptake, and left ventricular cavity size. An abnormally increased lung uptake of ^{201}Tl has been associated with myocardial ischemia that produces left ventricular dysfunction with a sudden rise in left ventricular end-diastolic pressure resulting in interstitial pulmonary edema during peak exercise.[90] The vast majority of patients who demonstrate abnormal lung uptake of ^{201}Tl have multivessel coronary artery disease or single-vessel disease involving either a dominant circumflex coronary artery or a high-grade proximal left anterior descending artery.[91] Another marker of severe coronary artery disease is transient left ventricular dilation, which is noted when the size of the left ventricular cavity is larger on the immediate poststress image than the delayed image, presumably as a result of myocardial ischemia.[92] Either marker is a harbinger of more severe disease and should alert the anesthesiologist to the possibility of perioperative ischemic left ventricular dysfunction.

Pharmacologic Stress Thallium Imaging

Exercise tolerance is an independent prognostic indicator in patients at risk for coronary artery disease, and therefore exercise stress testing is the optimal choice in those individuals who are able to exercise. However, a significant number of high-risk (arteriopathic) patients are unable to exercise, or exercise is contraindicated. In surgical patients, these limitations are most evident in those patients who experience claudication or have an abdominal aortic aneurysm. Although many patients with abdominal aortic aneurysms are able to exercise, many clinicians believe such exercise to be contraindicated due to the theoretical concern that the aneurysm may rupture during or following the high-cardiac-workload periods of the test. Pharmacologic stress testing has become popular, particularly as a preoperative test in vascular surgery patients.

Pharmacologic stress for the detection of coronary artery disease can be divided into two categories: (1) those that result in coronary artery vasodilatation, and (2) those that increase myocardial oxygen demand.[93] In the first category, dipyridamole and, more recently, adenosine are the agents employed. Of the agents that increase myocardial oxygen demand, dobutamine is the most common agent, although investigators have used isoproterenol and cardiac pacing to increase heart rate.

Coronary artery vasodilators are useful for defining myocardium at risk by producing differential flows in normal coronary arteries compared to those arteries with a stenosis. In a nonstressed situation, normal coronary arteries are vasoconstricted to deliver coronary flow to match myocardial oxygen demand. In areas of critical stenoses, the coronary artery vasodilates to increase flow distal to the stenosis. Therefore, the coronary artery with a critical stenosis has a diminished vasodilatory reserve.

Adenosine is a direct coronary artery vasodilator. Dipyridamole works by blocking adenosine reuptake, resulting in an increase in adenosine in the local coronary circulation. Prior to the availability of adenosine, dipyridamole was used in either intravenous or oral preparations (prior to U.S. Food and Drug Administration [FDA] approval of the intravenous preparation). The intravenous preparation is now approved for use with radionuclide testing. As experience with the newer adenosine reagent increases, it may replace the traditional dipyridamole test.[94,95] In the normal coronary artery, either agent will cause vasodilatation and a dramatic reduction in downstream resistance.[96] In the artery with the critical stenosis, vasodilatation will be limited and downstream resistance will be fixed at a level greater than the normal artery. Based upon the principles of flow and resistance starting at a single point, greater flow will go to the area distal to the normal coronary artery resulting in a redistribution of coronary flow. In addition, systemic vasodilatation may result from dipyridamole infusion, with a resultant fall in systemic blood pressure and a reflex increase in heart rate. Either agent can cause a transmural "coronary steal" by redistributing flow away from the endocardial layers to the epicardial region in the distribution of the critical coronary artery stenosis.

After infusion of the vasodilator, thallium, or more recently technetium, can be injected at peak dipyridamole or adenosine effect. If the difference in resistance between the two arteries is great, then flow to the myocardium distal to the critical stenosis may diminish below normal while flow to the area distal to the normal coronary artery will increase resulting in the area beyond a coronary stenosis appearing as a defect on thallium imaging. If the resultant flow is greater than oxygen demand but below that of a normal coronary artery, then there will be differential ^{201}T1 uptake, although myocardial ischemia will not develop. In either situation, there is diminished uptake and delayed clearance of the radioisotope in the stenotic zone, compared with increased uptake and more rapid clearance in normally perfused myocardium.

After the effects of the vasodilating agent dissipate, there will be faster washout of the areas of normal myocardium perfusion compared with areas supplied by stenosed vessels. This will result in "reperfusion" or filling-in of the defect on delayed imaging. Similar to the exercise stress test, nonviable myocardium will not take up radioisotope, resulting in an imaging defect that remains fixed on subsequent scans. Thus dipyridamole or adenosine radionuclide imaging is a means of assessing flow heterogeneity rather than provoking myocardial ischemia.

Several authors have reported that the presence of a redistribution defect is predictive of postoperative cardiac events in patients undergoing peripheral vascular surgery.[27,57,58,61,65,67,68,73,74,97] This work has recently been extended to include patients undergoing nonvascular surgery.[73]

There are several limitations to these imaging techniques. Defects that persist on delayed imaging (fixed defects) were thought in the past to represent an area of old infarction. Fixed defects on standard delayed imaging may, however, also occur in the presence of viable myocardium supplied by a critical stenosis. Additional imaging after a second resting injection of thallium imaging or delayed for 24 hours has been recently proposed to better define residual myocardial variability in the presence of a critical stenosis. However, significant morbidity has also been reported in patients with normal scans or fixed defects.[97–101] In rare circumstances, the test may appear normal in patients with severe three-vessel disease, since there is no normal myocardium to produce a maldistribution of flow.[101] Mangano and colleagues have questioned the sensitivity of the test to predict perioperative ischemia and cardiac events in vascular surgery patients when the clinicians were blinded to the results of the test; however, the authors were criticized for their patient selection and study design.[98] Baron and colleagues studied the largest (457) consecutive population of patients undergoing abdominal aortic surgery, and were also unable to demonstrate an association between thallium redistribution and perioperative cardiac morbidity.[102] Therefore, the value of the test in consecutive patients has been questioned.

In order to increase the predictive value of the test, several strategies have been suggested. As described above, the test demonstrates its best predictive value in the subgroup of patients at moderate clinical risk. L'Italien et al. constructed a Bayesian model using clinical risk factors and the results of dipyridamole thallium imaging.[56] The pretest (baseline) probability of an event can be calculated in a manner similar to cardiac risk indices, whereby clinical risk factors each are associated with a certain numeric weight that can be added to determine overall risk. The results of dipyridamole thallium imaging can then be used to modify the risk and determine the posttest probability of an event. In this manner, clinical risk factors can be used to determine if the test will raise the probability of morbidity above some threshold for action.

Lung uptake, left ventricular cavity dilation, and redistribution defect size have also been shown to increase the predictive ability of the diagnostic test. Fleisher et al. demonstrated that the delineation of "low-risk" and "high-risk" thallium scans markedly improved the test's predictive value.[103] They demonstrated that only patients with high-risk thallium scans demonstrated increased perioperative morbidity and long-term mortality.

An alternative method of increasing myocardial oxygen demand without exercise is to increase heart rate and blood pressure. Dobutamine can be used to achieve these parameters. Dobutamine thallium imaging has been shown to predict subsequent perioperative cardiac morbidity.[104] Atrial pacing with thallium imaging has also been used to stratify risk.[78]

Ambulatory Electrocardiography

The ambulatory ECG (AECG or Holter) provides a means of continuously monitoring the electrocardiogram for significant ST-segment changes during the preoperative period. Raby and colleagues monitored patients for 24 to 48 hours at some time prior to surgery, most frequently several days prior to surgery.[23] By contrast, we (Fleisher and colleagues) studied vascular surgery patients the evening prior to surgery and found a lower negative predictive value than the report by Raby.[5] Fleisher and colleagues suggest that their findings may be the result of the reduced ambulating the evening prior to surgery, particularly in vascular surgery patients who have had angiography. McPhail and colleagues compared dipyridamole thallium imaging and AECG monitoring in a cohort of vascular surgery patients and reported similar positive and negative predictive findings for the two testing modalities.[105] Fleisher and colleagues demonstrated a similar predictive value between Holter monitoring and dipyridamole thallium imaging for perioperative events; however, only high risk (large defects or increased lung uptake) on dipyridamole thallium imaging predicted those patients at risk for subsequent cardiac death within the next 2 years.[103] In comparing the two tests, it is important to realize that up to 33% of the patients undergoing major vascular surgery may have electrocardiographic abnormalities that prohibit the electrographic diagnosis of ischemia.[7] Therefore, further studies are required to determine the optimal use of ambulatory electrocardiography.

Assessment of Ventricular and Valvular Function

There are multiple methods to assess ejection fraction and valvular function. The least invasive method is echocardiography. Echocardiography can be employed to assess static function or can be combined with exercise or pharmacologic stress to assess dynamic function. Radionuclide angiography has been used as both a static and a dynamic measure of ejection fraction.

A preoperative resting echocardiographic evaluation can determine the presence of ventricular dysfunction, regional wall motion abnormalities, ventricular wall thickness, and valvular function. Pulsed wave Doppler can be used to obtain the velocity time integral. Ejection fraction can then be calculated by determining the cross-sectional area of the ventricle. Several investigators have examined the predictive value of ejection fraction using either echocardiographic or radionuclide measurements. Kazmers and colleagues found that a poor ejection fraction (<35%) was the best predictor of perioperative outcome after vascular surgery.[71] In contrast, Franco and colleagues found no difference in perioperative morbidity based upon ejection fraction.[106] Similarly, McEnroe and colleagues were unable to demonstrate a difference in perioperative morbidity based on ejection fraction.[97] There seems to be no consensus regarding the value of ejection fraction. This lack of agreement most likely reflects the static nature of the test.

More recently, stress echocardiography has received attention as a preoperative test. The appearance of new or worsened regional wall motion abnormalities is considered a positive test and represents areas of at-risk myocardium. The advantage of this test is that it is a dynamic assessment of ventricular function. Dipyridamole echocardiography has been used prior to vascular surgery and was found to have an 87% positive predictive value and a 99% negative predictive value.[79] Dobutamine echocardiography has also been studied and found to have among the best positive and negative predictive values.[107,108] In two recent meta-analyses, dobutamine stress echocardiography demonstrated the best predictive value for perioperative morbidity, although there was significant overlap in confidence intervals with the other diagnostic tests.[109,110]

Echocardiography can provide important information regarding valvular function, which may have important implication for both cardiac and noncardiac surgery, and is discussed more fully later in the book. In particular, aortic stenosis has been associated with a worse prognosis in noncardiac surgical procedures, and knowledge of valve lesions can lead to management choices and treatment of hemodynamic dysfunction.

Coronary Angiography

Coronary angiography represents the "gold standard" for defining coronary anatomy. Information regarding ventricular and valvular function can also be assessed. Finally, hemodynamic indices can be determined. For example, ventricular pressure and gradients across valves can be calculated.

In patients undergoing coronary artery bypass grafting, the information is routinely available. Certain lesions (i.e., left main disease) may be associated with greater perioperative risk. Certain disease types may also increase risk. Diffuse atherosclerosis in small vessels, as seen in patients with diabetes, may lead to incomplete revascularization and a risk for developing postbypass ischemia.

In patients undergoing noncardiac surgery, the decision to perform coronary angiography may be the result of a positive preoperative test or may be the first test in a patient with a very high probability of significant disease. Coronary angiography is then used by the cardiologist to determine if coronary artery revascularization is an option.

Unlike the exercise or pharmacologic stress tests described above, coronary angiography provides the clinician with anatomic, and not functional, information. Although a critical stenosis delineates an area at risk for developing myocardial ischemia, the functional response to that ischemia cannot be determined by angiography alone. Although coronary artery disease is undoubtedly the substrate for a perioperative MI, the critical stenosis may not be the underlying pathophysiology. In the ambulatory population, many infarctions are the result of acute thrombosis of a noncritical stenosis.[33] Therefore, the value of routine angiography prior to noncardiac surgery will depend upon the ability to correct the lesions that cause morbidity.

Assessment of Myocardial Viability

Increasing attention has been focused on the concept of stunned and hibernating myocardium.[50] After an episode of myocardial ischemia, the myocardium may not return to full function for several days. When function does return, the area continues to be at risk for developing ischemia. An example of this phenomenon is the development of new regional wall motion abnormalities that persist for several hours, but eventually return to full function. In patients who sustain an MI with postinfarct congestive heart failure, an assessment of ventricular dysfunction may demonstrate a very low ejection fraction. If such patients are reassessed at a later date after the failure resolves, the ejection fraction may be much higher. Therefore, these patients may have good ventricular function at rest, but poor function with stress.

For myocardium in a chronic ischemic state, one response is down-regulation of function (i.e., hibernating myocardium). Coronary artery bypass grafting to areas of hibernating myocardium will result in return of function.[111] This group of patients represents those who might benefit most from revascularization. Several new techniques are advocated for the assessment of myocardial viability in areas that appear nonfunctional. Dobutamine stress echocardiography has been advocated as a means of assessing viable myocardium.[112] The most common research tool is positron emission tomography (PET) scanning, in which glucose metabolism is evaluated.[113] Routine testing for the presence of hibernating myocardium may remain undeveloped for many years.

Assessment of Pulmonary Risk

As with the assessment of coronary artery disease, the assessment of pulmonary disease and risk traditionally has been dependent on the surgical procedure (see also Chapter 3). Patients undergoing thoracic surgery have usually undergone the most extensive assessment of risk, while patients undergoing peripheral arterial reconstruction frequently have undergone the least. These degrees of assessment may not be appropriate, as pulmonary complications may be the most common after peripheral vascular surgery, while many thoracic operations may depend on pulmonary vascular resistance and cardiovascular adaptation to it.

Tobacco use has the most profound impact on pulmonary function. Active tobacco use can decrease ciliary motion and mucus clearance, and leads to high levels of carbon monoxide. Tobacco use has been associated with an increased number of postoperative pulmonary complications.[114] These complications can range from atelectasis to severe pneumonia and increase the need for postoperative ventilation. Warner and colleagues studied the effects of smoking prior to CABG and found that the period from previous tobacco use is the critical factor.[115] Cessation of smoking for 24 hours reduces carbon monoxide and reduces complications. Cessation for greater than 24 hours but less than 6 weeks increases risk by decreasing mucociliary clearance. The authors suggest that the ideal situation is cessation for a minimum of 6 weeks prior to surgery.

Assessment of Neurologic Function

Although a neurologic examination is a routine part of the preoperative evaluation, the extensiveness can vary from a cursory examination to neuropsychometric testing. The need for this information varies greatly depending on the surgical procedure. Patients undergoing pulmonary resections or infrainguinal bypass procedures rarely develop neurologic morbidity postoperatively but motor and sensory assessment is mandatory if a regional block is planned. In contrast, carotid endarterectomy and CABG are associated with significant neurologic morbidity. Supraceliac cross-clamping is also associated with neurologic complications, although the complications are predominantly associated with spinal cord function.[116,117]

In patients scheduled for carotid endarterectomy, preoperative neurologic factors (crescendo transient ischemic attacks [TIAs]), TIAs while anticoagulated, multiple completed strokes, and ischemic symptoms <24 hours prior to surgery) or angiographic markers are indicators of high risk.[118] Therefore, a careful neurologic examination is important prior to this surgery. All of these patients have carotid Doppler and/or angiography. The results of such testing may influence perioperative management. For example, information regarding collateral blood flow to the area distal to the planned endarterectomy will help determine the probability of cerebral ischemia.

Similarly, coronary artery bypass grafting is associated with both transient and permanent neurologic dysfunction including psychomotor changes (see also Chapter 37). These changes may be related to both the low flow state and occurrence of emboli during or following cardiopulmonary bypass. Coronary artery disease is frequently associated with carotid artery disease, and patients with a critical carotid artery stenosis are therefore at greater theoretical risk of morbidity.[119] Preoperative evaluation should include questioning for any episodes of TIAs and examination for carotid bruits. Patients with symptoms or asymptomatic bruits will frequently be further evaluated with ultrasound studies.[120,121] The decision for obtaining such studies depends upon how the information will be used. The optimal decision regarding the appropriate scheduling of a patient with both coronary artery and carotid disease is more fully discussed in Chapter 37.[122–124]

As discussed above, the patient undergoing supraceliac cross-clamping is at risk for developing postoperative paraplegia. A thorough examination of both sensory and motor function preoperatively can assist in determining the etiology of any postoperative deficits.

Other Organ Systems

The need to assess the other major organ systems depends upon the preoperative history and planned surgery. A careful clinical history can be used to assess the probability of disease. If the probability of disease is unknown, or an abnormal state would result in changes in perioperative care, then further testing may be required. For example, patients on chronic aspirin therapy with a tendency for nose bleeds may not be suitable candidates for regional anesthesia. Further decision, such as the risk-benefit ratio of discontinuing aspirin and further studies, such as a bleeding time after 24 hours off aspirin, may be appropriate to obtain for such a patient. An assessment of the costs, benefits, and risks of testing is further discussed in Chapter 2.

Summary

In summary, the preoperative assessment of the patient undergoing cardiovascular and thoracic surgery depends upon how the information will be used to modify perioperative care. The anesthesiologist can serve as consultant by influencing the primary care physician, surgeon, and patient regarding how data from any area tested could impact perioperative care.

References

1. Backer CL, Tinker JH, Robertson DM, Vlietstra RE: Myocardial reinfarction following local anesthesia for ophthalmic surgery. Anesth Analg 59:257, 1980.
2. Ashton CM, Lahart CJ, Wray NP: The incidence of perioperative myocardial infarction with transurethral resection of the prostate. J Am Geriatr Soc 37:614, 1989.
3. Roizen MF, Beaupre PN, Alpert RA, et al: Monitoring with 2D transesophageal echocardiography: Comparison of myocardial function in patients undergoing supraceliac, suprarenal-infraceliac, or infrarenal aortic occlusion. J Vasc Surg 1:300, 1984.
4. Goldman L, Caldera DL, Nussbaum SR, et al: Multifactorial index of cardiac risk in noncardiac surgical procedures. N Engl J Med 297:845, 1977.
5. Fleisher L, Rosenbaum S, Nelson A, Barash P: The predictive value of preoperative silent ischemia for postoperative ischemic cardiac events in vascular and nonvascular surgical patients. Am Heart J 122:980, 1991.
6. Calvin JE, Kieser TM, Walley VM, et al: Cardiac mortality and morbidity after vascular surgery. Can J Surg 29:93, 1986.
7. Mangano DT, Browner WS, Hollenberg M, et al: Association of perioperative myocardial ischemia with cardiac morbidity and mortality in men undergoing noncardiac surgery. N Engl J Med 323:1781, 1990.
8. Detsky A, Abrams H, McLaughlin J, et al: Predicting cardiac complications in patients undergoing non-cardiac surgery. J Gen Intern Med 1:211, 1986.
9. Kennedy JW, Kaiser GC, Fisher LD, et al: Clinical and angiographic predictors of operative mortality from the Collaborative Study in Coronary Artery Surgery (CASS). Circulation 63:793, 1981.
10. Grover FL, Hammermeister KE, Burchfiel C, Surgeons AC: Initial report of the Veterans Administration Preoperative Risk Assessment Study for cardiac surgery. Ann Thorac Surg 50:12, 1990.
11. Khan S, Nessim S, Gray R, et al: Increased mortality of women in coronary artery bypass surgery: Evidence for referral bias. Ann Thorac Surg 38:563, 1990.
12. Hammermeister K, Burchfiel C, Johnson R, Grover F: Identification of patients at greatest risk for developing major complications of cardiac surgery. Circulation 82:IV-380, 1990.
13. Higgins T, Estafanous F, Loop F, et al: Stratification of morbidity and mortality outcome by preoperative risk factors in coronary artery bypass patients. JAMA 267:2344, 1992.
14. O'Connor G, Plume S, Olmstead E, et al: Multivariate prediction of in-hospital mortality associated with coronary artery by-pass graft surgery. Circulation 85:2110, 1992.
15. Parsonnet V, Dean D, Bernstein A: A method of uniform stratification of risk for evaluating the results of surgery in acquired adult heart disease. Circulation 79:I-3, 1989.
16. Nashef S, Carey F, Silcock M, et al: Risk stratification of open heart surgery: Trial of the Parsonnet system in a British hospital. Br Med J 305:1066, 1992.
17. Fleisher LA, Barash PG: Preoperative cardiac evaluation for noncardiac surgery: A functional approach. Anesth Analg 74: 586, 1992.
18. Eagle K, Brundage B, Chaitman B, et al: Guidelines for perioperative cardiovascular evaluation of the noncardiac surgery. A report of the American Heart Association/American College of Cardiology Task Force on Assessment of Diagnostic and Therapeutic Cardiovascular Procedures. Circulation 93:1278, 1996.
19. Tarhan S, Moffitt EA, Taylor WF, Giuliani ER: Myocardial infarction after general anesthesia. JAMA 220:1451, 1972.
20. Shah KB, Kleinman BS, Sami H, et al: Reevaluation of perioperative myocardial infarction in patients with prior myocardial infarction undergoing noncardiac operations. Anesth Analg 71: 231, 1990.
21. Rao TLK, Jacobs KH, El-Etr AA: Reinfarction following anesthesia in patients with myocardial infarction. Anesthesiology 59: 499, 1983.
22. Rivers SP, Scher LA, Gupta SK, Weith FJ: Safety of peripheral vascular surgery after recent acute myocardial infarction. J Vasc Surg 11:70, 1990.
23. Raby KE, Goldman L, Creager MA, et al: Correlation between perioperative ischemia and major cardiac events after peripheral vascular surgery. N Engl J Med 321:1296, 1989.
24. McFalls EO, Doliszny KM, Grund F, et al: Angina and persistent thallium defects: Independent risk factors in elective vascular surgery. J Am Coll Cardiol 21:1347, 1993.
25. Shah KB, Kleinman BS, Rao T, et al: Angina and other risk factors in patients with cardiac diseases undergoing noncardiac operations. Anesth Analg 70:240, 1990.
26. Foster ED, Davis KB, Carpenter JA, et al: Risk of noncardiac operations in patients with defined coronary disease: The Coronary Artery Surgery Study (CASS) Registry experience. Ann Thorac Surg 41:42, 1986.
26a. Eagle KA, Rihal CS, Mickel MC, et al: Cardiac risk of noncardiac surgery: Influence of coronary disease and type of surgery in 3368 operations. Circulation 96:1882, 1997.
27. Cambria RP, Brewster DC, Abbott WM, et al: The impact of selective use of dipyridamole-thallium scans and surgical factors on the current morbidity of aortic surgery. J Vasc Surg 15:43, 1992.
28. Blunt T: The role of a defined protocol for cardiac risk assessment in decreasing perioperative myocardial infarction in vascular surgery. J Vasc Surg 15:626, 1992.
29. Cruchley P, Kaplan J, Hug C, et al: Non-cardiac surgery in patients with prior myocardial revascularization. Can Anesth J 30: 629, 1983.
30. Allen J, Helling T, Hartzler G: Operative procedures not involving the heart after percutaneous transluminal coronary angioplasty. Surg Gynecol Obstet 173:285, 1991.
31. Eagle KA, Coley CM, Newell JB, et al: Combining clinical and thallium data optimizes preoperative assessment of cardiac risk before major vascular surgery. Ann Intern Med 110:859, 1989.
32. Huber KC, Evans MA, Bresnahan JF, et al: Outcome of noncardiac operations in patients with severe coronary artery disease successfully treated preoperatively with coronary angioplasty. Mayo Clin Proc 67:15, 1992.
33. Ambrose JA, Tannenbaum MA, Alexopoulos D, et al: Angiographic progression of coronary artery disease and the development of myocardial infarction. J Am Coll Cardiol 12:56, 1988.
34. Hertzer NR, Bevan EG, Young JR, et al: Coronary artery disease in peripheral vascular patients: A classification of 1000 coronary angiograms and results of surgical management. Ann Surg 199: 223, 1984.
35. Abraham SA, Coles NA, Coley CM, et al: Coronary risk of noncardiac surgery. Prog Cardiovasc Dis 34:205, 1991.
36. Gersh BJ, Rihal CS, Rooke TW, Ballard DJ: Evaluation and management of patients with both peripheral vascular and coronary artery disease. J Am Coll Cardiol 18:203, 1991.
37. Wong T, Detsky AS: Preoperative cardiac risk assessment for patients having peripheral vascular surgery. Ann Intern Med 116: 743, 1992.
38. Reilly JM, Tilson MD: Incidence and etiology of abdominal aortic aneurysms. Surg Clin North Am 69:705, 1989.
39. Kannel WB: New perspectives on cardiovascular risk factors. Am Heart J 114:213, 1987.
40. Burgos L, Ebert T, Asiddao C, Turner L: Increased intraoperative cardiovascular morbidity in diabetics with autonomic neuropathy. Anesthesiology 70:591, 1989.
41. Gottlieb A: The incidence of perioperative myocardial infarction in patients with prior percutaneous transluminal coronary angioplasty (PTCA). Anesthesiology 75:A52, 1991.
42. Charlson ME, MacKenzie CR, Gold JP, et al: Preoperative characteristics predicting intraoperative hypotension and hyperten-

sion among hypertensives and diabetics undergoing noncardiac surgery. Ann Surg 212:66, 1990.
43. Prys-Roberts C, Meloche R, Foex P: Studies of anaesthesia in relation to hypertension: I. Cardiovascular responses to treated and untreated patients. Br J Anesth 43:122, 1971.
44. Goldman L, Caldera DL: Risks of general anesthesia and elective operation in the hypertensive patient. Anesthesiology 50: 285, 1979.
45. Bedford R, Feinstein B: Hospital admission blood pressure, a predictor for hypertension following endotracheal intubation. Anesth Analg 59:367, 1980.
46. Hollenberg M, Mangano DT, Browner WS, et al: Predictors of postoperative myocardial ischemia in patients undergoing noncardiac surgery. The Study of Perioperative Ischemia Research Group. JAMA 268:205, 1992.
47. Pringle SD, MacFarlane PW, McKillop JH, et al: Pathophysiologic assessment of left ventricular hypertrophy and strain in asymptomatic patients with essential hypertension. J Am Coll Cardiol 13:1377, 1989.
48. McPhail N, Calvin JE, Shariatmadar A, et al: The use of preoperative exercise testing to predict cardiac complications after arterial reconstruction. J Vasc Surg 7:60, 1988.
49. Christakis GT, Weisel RD, Fremes SE, et al: Coronary artery bypass grafting in patients with poor ventricular function. J Thorac Cardiovasc Surg 103:1083, 1992.
50. Braunwald E, Rutherford JD: Reversible ischemic left ventricular dysfunction. Evidence for the hibernating myocardium. J Am Coll Cardiol 8:1467, 1986.
51. Slogoff S, Keats AS: Does perioperative myocardial ischemia lead to postoperative myocardial infarction? Anesthesiology 62: 107, 1985.
52. Slogoff S, Keats AS: Further observations on perioperative myocardial ischemia. Anesthesiology 65:539, 1986.
53. Leung JM, O'Kelly B, Browner WS, et al: Prognostic importance of postbypass regional wall-motion abnormalities in patients undergoing coronary artery bypass graft surgery. SPI Research Group. Anesthesiology 71:16, 1989.
54. Fleisher LA, Eagle KA: Screening for cardiac disease in patients having noncardiac surgery. Ann Intern Med 124:767, 1996.
55. Shuman P: Bayes' theorem: A review. Cardiol Clin 2:319, 1984.
56. L'Italien GJ, Paul SD, Hendel RC, et al: Development and validation of a bayesian model for perioperative cardiac risk assessment in a cohort of 1,081 vascular surgical candidates. J Am Coll Cardiol 27:779, 1996.
57. Lane SE, Lewis SM, Pippin JJ, et al: Predictive value of quantitative dipyridamole-thallium scintigraphy in assessing cardiovascular risk after vascular surgery in diabetes mellitus. Am J Cardiol 64:1275, 1989.
58. Lette J, Waters D, Lapointe J, et al: Usefulness of the severity and extent of reversible perfusion defects during thallium-dipyridamole imaging for cardiac risk assessment before noncardiac surgery. Am J. Cardiol 64:276, 1989.
59. Brown KA, Rowen M: Extent of jeopardized viable myocardium determined by myocardial perfusion imaging best predicts perioperative cardiac events in patients undergoing noncardiac surgery. J Am Coll Cardiol 21:325, 1993.
60. Isaacson IJ, Lowdon JD, Berry AJ, et al: The value of pulmonary artery and central venous monitoring in patients undergoing abdominal aortic reconstructive surgery: A comparative study of two selected, randomized groups. J Vasc Surg 12:754, 1990.
61. Boucher CA, Brewster DC, Darling RC, et al: Determination of cardiac risk by dipyridamole-thallium imaging before peripheral vascular surgery. N Engl J Med 312:389, 1985.
62. Fleisher LA, Skolnick ED, Holroyd KJ, Lehmann HP: Coronary artery revascularization before abdominal aortic aneurysm surgery: A decision analytic approach. Anesth Analg 79:661, 1994.
63. Mason JJ. Owens DK, Harris RA, et al: The role of coronary angiography and coronary revascularization before noncardiac surgery. JAMA 273:1919, 1995.
64. Rihal CS, Eagle KA, Mickel MC, et al: Surgical therapy for coronary artery disease among patients with combined coronary artery and peripheral vascular disease. Circulation 91:46, 1995.
65. Abraham SA, Coles NA, Coley CM, et al: Comparison of dipyridamole-thallium scintigraphy and ambulatory ECG monitoring in the preoperative assessment of cardiac risk for vascular surgery. J Am Coll Cardiol 17:204A, 1991.
66. Cutler BS: Prevention of cardiac complications in peripheral vascular surgery. Surg Clin North Am 66:281, 1986.
67. Cutler BS, Leppo JA: Dipyridamole thallium 201 scintigraphy to detect coronary artery disease before abdominal aortic surgery. J Vasc Surg 5:91, 1987.
68. Eagle KA, Singer DE, Brewster DC, et al: Dipyridamole-thallium scanning in patients undergoing vascular surgery. Optimizing preoperative evaluation of cardiac risk. JAMA 257: 2185, 1987.
69. Elliott BM, Robison JG, Zellner JL, Hendrix GH: Dobutamine-201T1 imaging. Assessing cardiac risks associated with vascular surgery. Circulation 84:III-54, 1991.
70. Fraedrich G, Wollschlager H, Schonbach B, Schlosser V: Reduction of the risk of surgery for abdominal aortic aneurysms by extended coronary diagnostics and therapy. Thorac Cardiovasc Surg 3:255, 1991.
71. Kazmers A, Moneta GL, Cerqueira MD, et al: The role of preoperative radionuclide ventriculography in defining outcome after revascularization of the extremity. Surg Gynecol Obstet 171: 481, 1990.
72. Leppo J, Plaja J, Gionet M, et al: Noninvasive evaluation of cardiac risk before elective vascular surgery. J Am Coll Cardiol 9:269, 1987.
73. Lette J, Waters D, Cerino M, et al: Preoperative coronary artery disease risk stratification based on dipyridamole imaging and a simple three-step, three-segment model for patients undergoing noncardiac vascular surgery or major general surgery. Am J Cardiol 69:1553, 1992.
74. McPhail NV, Ruddy TD, Calvin JE, et al: A comparison of dipyridamole-thallium imaging and exercise testing in the prediction of postoperative cardiac complications in patients requiring arterial reconstruction. J Vasc Surg 10:51, 1989.
75. Morise AP, McDowell DE, Savrin RA, et al: The prediction of cardiac risk in patients undergoing vascular surgery. Am J Med Sci 293:150, 1987.
76. Pasternack PF, Grossi EA, Baumann FG, et al: The value of silent myocardial ischemia monitoring in the prediction of perioperative myocardial infarction in patients undergoing peripheral vascular surgery. J Vasc Surg 10:617, 1989.
77. Reifsnyder T, Bandyk DF, Lanza D, et al: Use of stress thallium imaging to stratify cardiac risk in patients undergoing vascular surgery. J Surg Res 52:147, 1992.
78. Stratmann HG, Mark AL, Walter KE, Williams GA: Preoperative evaluation of cardiac risk by means of atrial pacing and thallium 201 scintigraphy. J Vasc Surg 10:385, 1989.
79. Tischler MD, Lee TH, Hirsch AT, et al: Prediction of major cardiac events after peripheral vascular surgery using dipyridamole echocardiography. Am J Cardiol 68:593, 1991.
80. Younis LT, Aguirre F, Byers S, et al: Perioperative and long-term prognostic value of intravenous dipyridamole thallium scintigraphy in patients with peripheral vascular disease. Am Heart J 119:1287, 1990.
81. Detrano R, Gianrossi R, Mulvihill D, et al: Exercise-induced ST segment depression in the diagnosis of multivessel coronary disease: A meta-analysis. J Am Coll Cardiol 14:1501, 1989.
82. Gordon MA, Urban MK, O'Connor T, Barash PG: Is the pressure rate quotient a predictor or indicator of myocardial ischemia as measured by ST-segment changes in patients undergoing coronary artery bypass surgery. Anesthesiology 74:848, 1991.
83. Leung JM, O'Kelly BF, Mangano DT, and SPI group: Relationship of regional wall motion abnormalities to hemodynamic indices of myocardial oxygen supply and demand in patients undergoing CABG surgery. Anesthesiology 73:802, 1990.
84. Maddahi J, Van Train K, Prigent F, et al: Quantitative single photon emission computed thallium-201 tomography for detection and localization of coronary artery disease: Optimization and prospective validation of a new technique. J Am Coll Cardiol 14:1689, 1989.
85. Bailey IK, Griffith LSC, Rouleau J: Thallium-201 myocardial perfusion imaging at rest and during exercise: Comparative sensitivity to electrocardiography in coronary artery disease. Circulation 55:79, 1977.
86. Gould KL: How accurate is thallium exercise testing for the diagnosis of coronary artery disease? J Am Coll Cardiol 14: 1487, 1989.

87. Berger BC, Watson DD, Taylor GJ, et al: Quantitative thallium-201 exercise scintigraphy for detection of coronary artery disease. J Nucl Med 22:585, 1981.
88. Rocco TP, Dilsizian V, McKusick KA, et al: Comparison of thallium reinjection with rest "reinjection" imaging for the detection of viable myocardium. Am J Cardiol 66:158, 1990.
89. Dilsizian V, Rocco TP, Freedman NMT, et al: Enhanced detection of ischemic but viable myocardium by the reinjection of thallium after stress-redistribution imaging. N Engl J Med 323: 141, 1990.
90. Homma S, Kaul S, Boucher CA: Correlates of lung/heart ratio of thallium-201 in coronary artery disease. J Nucl Med 28:1531, 1987.
91. Gibson RS, Watson DD, Carabello BA, et al: Clinical implications of increased lung uptake of thallium-201 during exercise scintigraphy 2 weeks after myocardial infarction. Am J Cardiol 49:1586, 1982.
92. Weiss AT, Berman DS, Lew AS, et al: Transient ischemic dilation of the left ventricle on stress thallium-201 scintigraphy: A marker of severe and extensive coronary artery disease. J Am Coll Cardiol 9:752, 1987.
93. Beller GA: Current status of nuclear cardiology techniques. Curr Probl Cardiol 16:447, 1991.
94. Coyne EP, Belvedere DA, Vande SP, et al: Thallium-201 scintigraphy after intravenous infusion of adenosine compared with exercise thallium testing in the diagnosis of coronary artery disease. J Am Coll Cardiol 17:1289, 1991.
95. Verani MS, Mahmarian JJ, Hixson JB: Diagnosis of coronary artery disease by controlled coronary vasodilation with adenosine and thallium-201 scintigraphy in patients unable to exercise. Circulation 82:80, 1990.
96. Beller GA, Holzgrefe HH, Watson DD: Effects of dipyridamole-induced vasodilation on myocardial uptake and clearance kinetics of thallium-201. Circulation 68:1328, 1983.
97. McEnroe CS, O'Donnell TF, Yeager A, et al: Comparison of ejection fraction and Goldman risk factor analysis to dipyridamole-thallium imaging 201 studies in the evaluation of cardiac morbidity after aortic aneurysm surgery. J Vasc Surg 11:497, 1990.
98. Mangano DT, London MJ, Tubau JF, et al: Dipyridamole thallium-201 scintigraphy as a preoperative screening test. A reexamination of its predictive potential. Study of Perioperative Ischemia Research Group. Circulation 84:493, 1991.
99. Fleisher L, Nelson A, Rosenbaum S: Failure of negative dipyridamole thallium scans to predict perioperative myocardial ischemia and infarction. Can J Anaesth 39:179, 1992.
100. Bertrand M, Coriat P, Baron JF, et al: Dipyridamole thallium scan is not accurate in detecting coronary stenosis in patients undergoing abdominal aortic surgery. Anesthesiology 73:A86, 1990.
101. Marwick TH, Underwood DA: Dipyridamole thallium imaging may not be a reliable screening test for coronary artery disease in patients undergoing vascular surgery. Clin Cardiol 13:14, 1990.
102. Baron JF, Mundler O, Bertrand M, et al: Dipyridamole-thallium scintigraphy and gated radionuclide angiography to assess cardiac risk before abdominal aortic surgery. N Engl J Med 330: 663, 1994.
103. Fleisher LA, Rosenbaum SH, Nelson AH, et al: Preoperative dipyridamole thallium imaging and ambulatory electrocardiographic monitoring as a predictor of perioperative cardiac events and long-term outcome. Anesthesiology 83:906, 1995.
104. Elliott BM, Robison JG, Zellner JL, Hendrix GH: Dobutamine-201T1 imaging. Assessing cardiac risks associated with vascular surgery. Circulation 84:III-54, 1991.
105. McPhail NV, Ruddy TD, Barber GG, et al: Cardiac risk stratification using dipyridamole myocardial perfusion imaging and ambulatory ECG monitoring prior to vascular surgery. Eur J Vasc Surg 7:151, 1993.
106. Franco CD, Goldsmith J, Veith FJ, et al: Resting gated pool ejection fration: A poor predictor of perioperative myocardial infarction in patients undergoing vascular surgery for infrainguinal bypass grafting. J Vasc Surg 10:656, 1989.
107. Lane RT, Sawada SG, Segar DS, et al: Dobutamine stress echocardiography for assessment of cardiac risk before noncardiac surgery. Am J Cardiol 68:976, 1991.
108. Eichelberger JP, Schwarz KQ, Black ER, et al: Predictive value of dobutamine echocardiography just before noncardiac vascular surgery. Am J Cardiol 72:602, 1993.
109. Mantha S, Roizen MF, Barnard J, et al: Relative effectiveness of four preoperative tests for predicting adverse cardiac outcomes after vascular surgery: A meta-analysis. Anesth Analg 79: 422, 1994.
110. Shaw LJ, Eagle KA, Gersh BJ, Miller DD: Meta-analysis of intravenous dipyridamole-thallium-201 imaging (1985 to 1994) and dobutamine echocardiography (1991 to 1994) for risk stratification before vascular surgery. J Am Coll Cardiol 27:787, 1996.
111. Brundage BH, Massie BM, Botvinick EH: Improved regional ventricular function after successful surgical revascularization. J Am Coll Cardiol 3:902, 1984.
112. Cigarroa CG, deFilippi CR, Brickner ME, et al: Dobutamine stress echocardiography identifies hibernating myocardium and predicts recovery of left ventricular function after coronary revascularization. Circulation 88:430, 1993.
113. Schelbert HR: Positron emission tomography for the assessment of myocardial viability. Circulation 84:I, 1992.
114. Holtz B, Bake B, Sixt R: Prediction of postoperative hypoxemia in smokers and nonsmokers. Acta Anaesth Scand 23:411, 1979.
115. Warner MA, Offord KP, Warner ME, et al: Role of preoperative cessation of smoking and other factors in postoperative pulmonary complications: A blinded prospective study of coronary artery bypass patients. Mayo Clin Proc 64:609, 1989.
116. McCullough JL, Hollier LH, Nugent M: Paraplegia after thoracic aortic occlusion: Influence of cerebrospinal fluid drainage. Experimental and early clinical results. J Vasc Surg 7:153, 1988.
117. Crawford ES, Svensson LG, Hess KR, et al: A prospective randomized study of cerebrospinal fluid drainage to prevent paraplegia after high-risk surgery on the thoracoabdominal aorta. J Vasc Surg 13:36, 1991.
118. Sieber FE, Toung TJ, Diringer MN, et al: Preoperative risks predict neurological outcome of carotid endarterectomy related stroke. Neurosurgery 30:847, 1992.
119. Craven TE, Ryu JE, Espeland MA, et al: Evaluation of the associations between carotid artery atherosclerosis and coronary artery stenosis. A case-control study. Circulation 82:1230, 1990.
120. Marshall WGJ, Kouchoukos NT, Murphy SF, Pelate C: Carotid endarterectomy based on duplex scanning without preoperative arteriography. Circulation 78:I-1, 1988.
121. Niederkorn K: Asymptomatic carotid artery disease detected by duplex scanning incidence and correlation with risk factors, cerebral blood flow and CT findings. Eur Neurol 30:61, 1990.
122. Schwartz RL, Garrett JR, Karp RB, Kouchoukos NT: Simultaneous myocardial revascularization and carotid endarterectomy. Circulation 66:I-97, 1982.
123. Jones E, Craver J, Michalik R, et al: Combined carotid and coronary operations: When are they necessary? J Thorac Cardiovasc 87:7, 1984.
124. Hertzer N, Loop F, Taylor P, Beven EG: Combined myocardial revascularization and carotid endarterectomy. J Thorac Cardiovasc Surg 85:577, 1983.

CHAPTER 2

Cost-Effectiveness and Benefit of Preoperative Work-up and Preparation for Vascular Surgery

Srinivas Mantha, M.D.
Lee A. Fleisher, M.D.
Michael F. Roizen, M.D.
John E. Ellis, M.D.
Joseph F. Foss, M.D.

Morbidity and mortality are higher after vascular surgery than after other types of noncardiac surgery. Outcome after vascular surgery depends primarily on patient factors (such as the aging of physiologic systems, including the arterial tree), surgical factors, and institution-specific factors (Table 2–1). Temperature fluctuations and stress responses also affect outcome. Of the postoperative complications reported for large series of patients, those related to the cardiovascular system have been the most common; 50 to 100% of deaths after vascular surgery have involved the cardiovascular or arterial system (Table 2–2). However, complications related to other systems also occur. A 1994 study reported a renal insufficiency rate of 17% and a respiratory failure rate of 8% after abdominal aortic surgery.[1] Serious morbidity or mortality due to central nervous system (CNS) causes has occurred in 0.2 to 33% of patients after carotid endarterectomy.[2]

The following adverse events are common after vascular surgery: cardiovascular events (cardiac-related death, myocardial infarction, dysrhythmias, and cardiogenic pulmonary edema; 2 to 8%), respiratory failure (0.5 to 10%), and renal failure (0.2 to 18%).[1,3–8] In one large study in California, the mortality rates at 30 days and 6 months after aortic or iliac surgery related directly to patient age: mortality increased by one natural logarithm per decade increase in age.[9] Although age itself is probably not responsible for the functional changes that occur with age, the arteriopathy of vascular surgery patients obviously varies with physiologic age. Mortality after vascular surgery varies directly, and increases logarithmically, with patient age.[9]

For any surgical procedure, the obvious goal of anesthesia is to minimize patient morbidity and to maximize the benefit of surgery. Achieving this goal for patients undergoing vascular surgery may not be easy because of the interplay of the many patient, surgical, and institution-specific factors influencing outcome. Nevertheless, the anesthesiologist can greatly influence morbidity after vascular surgery. Perhaps in no other area has mortality decreased so quickly—from a 6-day mortality rate of more than 25% at the best centers for major aortic reconstruction in the mid-1960s, to 8% in the 1970s, to 4% in the late 1980s, and to 1 to 2% today.[3,10] To reduce mortality further, some investigators have advocated preoperative evaluation that aims to decrease morbidity by recognizing, optimizing, and treating comorbid conditions.

Because asymptomatic coronary artery disease (CAD) is very prevalent among patients undergoing vascular surgery,[10] the goal is identification of this subgroup. To this end, more than 60% of the 570,000 patients in the United States each year who have vascular surgery[11] also undergo an expensive test to evaluate the risk of adverse perioperative cardiovascular events. The rationale is that preoperative identification of patients at increased risk would allow for important changes in perioperative care. However, given the costs and risks involved, subjecting all vascular surgery candidates to coronary angiography before vascular surgery may not be the most effective strategy. Moreover, conventional exercise electrocardiography may not be helpful if claudication of the lower extremities precludes the exercise load necessary for meaningful results. Therefore, other noninvasive tests are used to stratify cardiac risk before surgery[12–17]: dipyridamole-thallium scintigraphy (DTS),[18–35] estimation of ejection fraction by radionuclide ventriculography (RNV),[36–40] ambulatory electrocardiography (AECG),[24,41–45] and dobutamine stress echocardiography (DSE).[46–50]

This chapter discusses some of the concepts used in the technology assessment of various risk stratification methods that have been proposed. It also reviews the literature on cost-effectiveness and benefit of such strategies for patients undergoing noncardiac vascular surgery (repair of abdominal aortic aneurysms, procedures

TABLE 2–1
Factors Influencing Outcome after Vascular Surgery*

Category	Factor†
Patient factors[1,3–8]	Age ≥60 yr (68%) History of ciagarette smoking (88%) Coexisting diseases: Hypertension (40–68%) Coronary artery disease (40–60%) Dysrhythmias (36%) Diabetes mellitus (8–44%) Congestive heart failure (5–29%) Chronic obstructive airway disease (25–50%) Renal insufficiency (5–15%) Postoperative hypercoagulable state[121–123]
Surgical factors	Expertise of the surgeon Emergency/semiemergency state Major fluid shifts Clamping and unclamping of major vessels[124] Intraoperative hypotension Intraoperative hypertension
Institution-specific factors	University/community center Facilities for major preoperative work-ups Expertise in the interpretation of preoperative testing modalities, especially for coronary artery disease

*Adapted from Ellis JE, Roizen MF, Mantha S, Wilke H: Anesthesia for vascular surgery. In Barash PG, et al (eds): Clinical Anesthesia, 3rd ed. Philadelphia, Lippincott-Raven Publishers, 1997, p 871, with permission.
†Reported percentage of vascular surgery patients with factor.

TABLE 2–2
Perioperative Mortality Associated with Cardiac Events*

Aortic Reconstruction References (Yr)	Deaths/Total No. of Pts.	Mortality Caused by Cardiac Dysfunction
Szilagyi et al.[125] (1966)	59/401 (14.7%)	48%
Whittemore et al.[126] (1980)	1/110 (0.9%)	100%
Crawford et al.[127] (1981)	41/860 (4.8%)	54%
Benefiel et al.[128] (1986)	3/96 (3.1%)	67%
Johnston[129] (1989)	32/666 (4.8%)	69%
Golden et al.[26] (1990)	8/500 (1.6%)	75%
Krupski et al.[130] (1993)	1/53 (1.9%)	100%
Lachapelle et al.[131] (1992)	7/146 (4.8%)	71%
Suggs et al.[30] (1993)	3/247 (1.2%)	66%
Baron et al.[32] (1994)	20/457 (4.4%)	50%
L'Italien et al.[132] (1995)	16/321 (5.0%)	62%

*Adapted from Ellis JE, Roizen MF, Mantha S, Wilke H: Anesthesia for vascular surgery. In Barash PG, et al (eds): Clinical Anesthesia, 3rd ed. Philadelphia, Lippincott-Raven Publishers, 1997, p 871, with permission.

for aortic occlusive disease, lower extremity revascularization, and carotid endarterectomy). Finally, the chapter proposes a cardiac risk stratification sequence to maximize the benefit (i.e., improved outcome with decreased costs) for patients undergoing noncardiac vascular surgery.

Cardiac Morbidity and Mortality After Vascular Surgery

Two studies have shown a high prevalence of CAD in patients undergoing vascular surgery. Pooling data from 50 series representing more than 10,000 patients, Hertzer[51] found clinical evidence of CAD for approximately 50% (range, 22 to 70%) of patients scheduled for surgical repair of abdominal aortic aneurysm (AAA), carotid artery disease, or lower limb ischemia. Although the indications for coronary angiography and the definition of significant CAD varied among the series, significant CAD was found in approximately 60% of patients who underwent preoperative coronary angiography.[51]

In another study, Hertzer et al.[4] performed coronary angiography in 1,000 consecutive patients presenting for vascular surgery. Severe *correctable* CAD was identified in 25% of the entire series—specifically, in 31% of patients scheduled for AAA surgery, in 26% of patients with cerebrovascular disease, and in 21% of those with lower extremity ischemia. For the entire series, the incidence of significant CAD (stenosis >70%) was 37% for patients without clinical indications of CAD and 78% for those with CAD suspected clinically.

For both of these studies, the high prevalence of CAD in patients presenting for vascular surgery is consistent with the high risk of such patients for both short-term (30-day postoperative) and long-term mortality and morbidity that are related to cardiac sources.

Short-Term Morbidity and Mortality

The usual manifestations of cardiac-related morbidity and mortality after vascular surgery include cardiac-related death, myocardial infarction (MI), cardiogenic pulmonary edema, unstable angina, and dysrhythmias. The risk of these cardiac complications ranges from 5 to 40%.[13]

Three studies show that short-term morbidity and mortality occur commonly in all vascular surgery and are related to pre-existing CAD. Re-examining data from 20 studies, a 1994 meta-analysis reported the rates of cardiac morbidity and mortality for 1,891 patients who had not undergone myocardial revascularization before various vascular surgery procedures.[14] By procedure, the rates for cardiac morbidity and mortality were as follows: for aortic surgery, 51.3%; for lower extremity vascular surgery, 39.6%; and for carotid endarterectomy, 9.1%. Cardiac-related death occurred in 0 to 8% of patients; MI, in 0 to 15.3%; unstable angina, in 0 to 10.4%; and pulmonary edema, in 0 to 8.3%. Acceptance of the data for unstable angina and pulmonary edema must be guarded because of inconsistent reporting of these complications by some of the studies.

A 1992 report by Krupski et al.[6] compared the rate of cardiac complications for vascular surgery patients undergoing one of two types of procedure—aortic surgery (n = 53) or lower extremity vascular surgery (n = 87). Complications were defined as cardiac death, MI, unstable angina, congestive heart failure, or ventricular tachycardia. The rate of cardiac complications was 24% for aortic surgery and 28% for infrainguinal surgery; the rates of cardiac death were 2 and 3.5%, respectively. The percentage of patients who had a history of angina, congestive heart failure, diabetes, dysrhythmias, or digitalis therapy was significantly higher for those needing infrainguinal procedures than for those needing aortic surgery. The investigators attributed the high morbidity of infrainguinal procedures to a higher likelihood of preoperative cardiac risk factors for patients scheduled for those procedures than for patients scheduled for aortic surgery.

In a series consisting of 177 patients who underwent carotid endarterectomy, Rihal et al.[52] classified patients into three groups: those who had no clinically recognized CAD at the time of surgery (group 1; n = 93); those who had overt CAD at the time of surgery (group 2; n = 64); and those undergoing myocardial revascularization before surgery (group 3; n = 20). The rates of cardiac-related death, MI, pulmonary edema, and ventricular tachycardia were, respectively, as follows: for group 1—0, 2, 1, and 3%; for group 2—0, 3, 5, and 2%; and for group 3—0, 0, 10, and 0%. Three deaths occurred in group 1: one from stroke, one from pulmonary embolism, and one from aspiration pneumonia.

Long-Term Morbidity and Mortality

Although patients with and without CAD were not matched for physiologic functioning, data from four studies indicate that the presence of CAD decreases 5-year survival after vascular surgery by one half to one third. The first report studied 23 series representing 7,805 vascular surgery patients.[51] The 5-year mortality rate was 20% for those with "no overt CAD," 41% for those with suspected CAD, and 21% for those who had undergone prior coronary artery bypass graft (CABG) surgery. The second report was a population-based study having a 17-year follow-up on 131 patients who had repair of AAA.[53] Uncorrected CAD was associated with a twofold increase in the risk of death (hazard ratio, 1.79; 95% confidence interval, 1.06 to 3.00) and a fourfold increase in the risk of adverse cardiac events (hazard ratio, 3.71; 95% confidence interval, 1.79 to 7.69). For another geographically defined patient group (n = 173) having a follow-up period of up to 17 years after peripheral vascular surgery (aortoiliac, aortofemoral, femoropopliteal, or infrainguinal revascularization), the 5- and 10-year Kaplan-Meier survival rate was, respectively, 77 and 51% for those without overt CAD and 54 and 24% for those with overt CAD ($p < .001$).[54] The fourth report was also a population-based study.[52] The Kaplan-Meier estimate of 8-year relative survival after carotid endarterectomy was 89% for those without overt CAD and 75% for those with overt CAD. The authors noted that coronary rather than cerebrovascular disease was the most frequent cause of morbidity and mortality.

Two studies have discussed long-term survival after vascular surgery. A 1994 study compared a total of 1,561 patients who did (i.e., survivors) and did not have MI

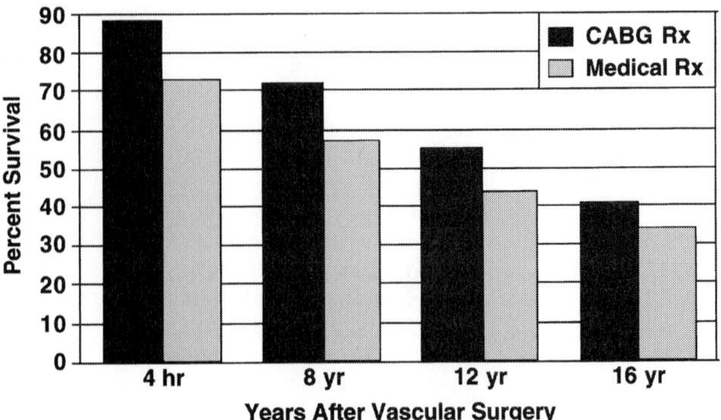

FIGURE 2–1. In the Coronary Artery Surgery Study (CASS), a survival advantage was evident for patients randomly allocated to surgical management (coronary artery bypass graft surgery, CABG Rx) versus medical management (medical Rx). (From Rihal CS, Eagle KA, Mickel MC, et al: Surgical therapy for coronary artery disease among patients with combined coronary artery and peripheral vascular disease. Circulation 91:46, 1995, with permission.)

after peripheral vascular surgery.[55] Although both groups had similar survival rates at 1 and 4 years, those who had MI had a higher incidence of subsequent adverse cardiac events and coronary artery revascularization than those who had surgery without MI. The second investigation was a 1995 study of a retrospective cohort analysis of 1,834 patients from the Coronary Artery Surgery Registry who had both peripheral vascular disease and CAD.[56] These patients underwent either CABG (n = 986) or medical therapy (n = 848) on a nonrandom basis. The estimated probability of survival at 4, 8, 12, and 16 years after surgery was significantly ($p < .001$) higher for the surgical group (88, 72, 55, and 41%, respectively) than for the medical therapy group (73, 57, 44, and 34%, respectively) (Fig. 2–1). That is, CABG revascularization gave the patient undergoing vascular surgery a survival advantage of approximately 3.8 years (in our current vernacular, such patients would be 3.8 years "younger" than vascular surgery patients who were treated medically). Multivariate analysis revealed that the type of therapy was independently associated with survival ($p < .0001$). Subgroup analysis suggested that benefits of surgical treatment on survival were limited to patients with three-vessel CAD and were inversely related to ejection fraction. The rate of survival free of MI was also significantly better for the surgical group. The authors concluded that surgical treatment provides long-term benefit for certain subgroups of patients who have both CAD and peripheral vascular disease (i.e., patients with triple-vessel CAD and poor ejection fractions). Thus, identification of, and therapy for, CAD prior to vascular surgery appears beneficial.

Cardiac Risk Stratification

Given the data for short- and long-term cardiac morbidity and mortality in patients undergoing vascular surgery, the desirability of detecting underlying CAD becomes evident. But what studies and methods of identification

TABLE 2–3
Risk Factors Predicting Adverse Cardiac Outcomes after Vascular Surgery

Component of Cardiac Risk Stratification	Risk Factor
History	Age >70 yr Previous myocardial infarction Diabetes mellitus Angina
Physical examination	Congestive heart failure, as evidenced by jugular venous distention or the presence of a third heart sound
Laboratory testing	On ECG: Dysrhythmias (frequent premature ventricular contractions or rhythms other than normal sinus) and Q waves on ECG On chest radiograph: Cardiomegaly On AECG: ST-segment depression of ≥1 mm or ST-segment elevation of ≥2 mm after J point (measured at 60 ms) lasting at least 1 min On RNV: Ejection fraction of ≤35% On DTS: Redistribution defects in at least one segment. Fixed defects may get converted to redistribution defects on delayed imaging at 18–24 hr On DSE: Development of new RWMAs or worsening of existing wall motion abnormalities in at least one segment during infusion of dobutamine

ECG, electrocardiogram; AECG, ambulatory electrocardiography; RNV, radionuclide ventriculography; DTS, dipyridamole-thallium scintigraphy; DSE, dobutamine stress echocardiography; RWMAs, regional wall motion abnormalities.

are appropriate? Historically, cardiac risk stratification has relied on patient history, physical examination, and laboratory testing. Table 2–3 shows the known predictors of adverse cardiac outcomes that can be revealed by each of these three components of cardiac risk stratification.[13,14,57–62] Thus, age over 70 years (i.e., calendar age, as physiologic age is not known), diabetes requiring treatment, dysrhythmias or congestive heart failure, and prior Q-wave infarction appear to indicate a high likelihood of CAD. In addition, Class IV angina (using the criteria of the Canadian Cardiovascular Society) or unstable angina indicates severe underlying CAD.[57]

Stratification of cardiac risk before vascular surgery has three main goals[13]:

1. For patients judged to be at high risk, the performance of a more conservative surgical procedure (e.g., peripheral or noninvasive reconstruction of a local area vs. major reconstruction of the aorta).
2. The performance of myocardial revascularization (CABG, percutaneous transluminal coronary angioplasty [PTCA], or an equivalent interventional therapy for CAD). Vascular surgery is usually performed a week after interventional therapy for CAD and 6 to 8 weeks after CABG. Alternatively, CABG could be combined with vascular surgery.[26,63,64] A retrospective 1994 study indicated that elective repair of AAA should be performed simultaneously or within 2 weeks of CABG because of the increased risk of AAA rupture after this period.[65] One study noted that the mortality rate for CABG was 2.4-fold higher for patients who had peripheral vascular disease, especially lower extremity arterial occlusive disease (7.7%; n = 796), than for those who did not have peripheral vascular disease (3.2%; n = 2,207).[66]
3. The identification of those patients who would benefit from the use of risk-reducing interventions such as intensive perioperative monitoring or modification of anesthetic techniques (Table 2–4). These morbidity-reducing strategies vary widely in costs and are used alone or in combination with other strategies. The choice of strategies generally depends on the surgical procedure, the discretion of the anesthesiologist and surgeons, and institutional protocols. However, there are no properly designed studies that would allow one to draw definitive conclusions about the superiority of one strategy over another.

TABLE 2–4
Perioperative Cardiac Risk-Reducing Strategies for Vascular Surgery Patients*

Cardiac Risk-Reducing Strategy	References
Perioperative clonidine	Ellis et al.[133]
β-Blocker therapy	Pasternack et al.[134] and Mangano et al.[153]
Regional or combined regional and general anesthesia technique	Tuman et al.[121] and Liu et al.[135]
Intraoperative monitoring with transesophageal echocardiography	Edwards and Reilly[136]
Perioperative use of a pulmonary artery catheter	Berlauk et al.[109]
Extended stay in an intensive care unit	Rao et al.[110]
Perioperative monitoring for myocardial ischemia	Mangano et al.[43] Raby et al.[137] Landesberg et al.[138]

*Perioperative cardiac risk-reducing strategies are not limited to those given in this table. These strategies are used alone or in combination with others. Choice of their usage depends on judgment of the anesthesiology and surgical teams at a particular institution.

The process of determining what stratification would be beneficial, and from what point of view, can be understood by using one of the many processes making up the general activity known as "technology assessment."

Technology Assessment and Economic Analyses

In the current era of cost containment, the primary goal of any strategy is to minimize cost while preserving or improving the quality of care. Regarding preparation for surgery, the primary goal is to minimize the cost of obtaining the best possible outcome produced by such preparation. To explain how one analyzes the process, one must use the terminology of technology assessment and economic analysis.[67–80] This chapter defines its terms in the following manner.

Efficacy

"Efficacy" refers to the probability of benefit to an individual from the use of a particular technology that is applied to a given medical problem under *ideal conditions* of use, such as research conditions. Efficacy studies are generally performed in tertiary care centers and have well-defined inclusion and exclusion criteria.

Effectiveness

"Effectiveness" refers to the benefit of a particular technology that is applied under conditions of *actual* use. Because effectiveness studies are used to determine the applicability of a technology in day-to-day clinical practice, conclusions reached by *efficacy* and *effectiveness* studies may differ.

Costs

In medical economic analysis, three dimensions need to be considered: the type of economic analysis being used, the characteristics of the cost-determination process, and the perspective from which the analysis is being made.

Types of Economic Analysis

Four types of economic analysis need definition.

Cost-Identification or Cost-Minimization Analysis. Cost-identification analysis determines the cost of an intervention (cost per service provided), assuming that the outcomes of the strategies being compared are equivalent. Because the goal is to identify the least expensive way of achieving the outcome, cost-identification analysis is also called cost-minimization analysis. This technique is not used if outcomes have not been shown to be similar, as concentrating only on costs poses the danger of ignoring differences in outcome and can produce misleading results.

Cost-Effectiveness Analysis (CEA). CEA measures and compares the costs and results of alternative interventions. CEA is used when the outcomes of different strategies (i.e., measures of effectiveness) vary but can be expressed in common natural units and, ideally, can be expressed in a single dimension, such as years of life saved or infection averted. With a common unit of outcome or effectiveness, different strategies can be expressed in terms of cost-per-unit outcome. The difference between an *incremental cost-effectiveness analysis*, a *marginal cost-effectiveness analysis*, and the *average cost-effectiveness ratio* must be noted.

Incremental Cost-Effectiveness Analysis. This type of analysis produces an "incremental cost-effectiveness ratio" (ICER), which is an estimate of the economic input per unit effectiveness of switching from one intervention to another mutually exclusive intervention; for example, from selective noninvasive cardiac testing (selection of tests based on clinical criteria) to a test-all strategy (testing of all patients irrespective of clinical criteria) before vascular surgery. In this case, the issue is whether the additional improvement in effectiveness is worth the additional economic burden. The numerator of the ratio represents the difference in economic burden of an intervention and its alternative, whereas the denominator represents the difference in effectiveness of the intervention and its alternative.

Marginal Cost-Effectiveness Analysis. This type of analysis is useful when the scale of intervention increases (e.g., more visits per patient or an expansion of ambulatory anesthesia services to accommodate a greater number of patients). When marginal returns are likely to decrease (i.e., when the net benefit per patient decreases), a marginal cost-effectiveness analysis would be needed. In other words, this term specifically refers to the change in economic input and outcome that comes from adding one unit of service.

Average Cost-Effectiveness Ratio. This ratio is estimated by dividing the cost of an intervention by a measure of effectiveness without regard to its competing alternatives (e.g., the cost per infection detected by means of a particular screening strategy). The average cost-effectiveness ratio has limited value because it cannot be used to set priorities between competing medical technology strategies.

Cost-Utility Analysis (CUA). This is a specific type of cost-effectiveness analysis in which the effects of the interventions are evaluated multidimensionally regarding both the quantity and quality of life, thereby allowing health outcomes to be measured in terms of quality-adjusted life years (QALYs). QALYs combine a particular utility-based measure of quality of life with a quantitative measure of life years to obtain a single measure of lifetime utility. One QALY is equal to 1 year at full health for that one individual.

Cost-Benefit Analysis (CBA). In this type of analysis, monetary value is placed on benefits or health outcomes. In other words, both the costs of providing care and effectiveness are measured in the same monetary unit, such as dollars. Results of a cost-benefit analysis could be expressed as the difference between economic input and benefit (expressed in monetary value, subtracting cost from benefit) or as the ratio of the two (the ratio of benefit to cost). In general, calculation of the net benefit is preferable to calculation of the benefit-to-cost ratio.

Cost Determination

Definition of Terms. The type of "cost" that must be used in the economic analysis depends on the perspective from which the analysis is being made (see section below). Therefore, three important terms related to "cost" need definition.

Charges. Charge is the amount the hospital, the clinic, the physician, or the pharmacy attempts to recover (or bills) for providing a service.

Payment. Payment is the amount actually paid by the individual or the third-party payer for the service.

Costs. The cost of a particular service is a function of all the resources consumed for that service. The types of relevant costs include direct, indirect, and intangible.

1. *Direct costs* consist of organizing and operational expenditures made in the delivery of medical care. These costs can be medical or nonmedical. *Direct medical costs* include those incurred by hospitalizations, drugs, physicians, and other relevant personnel. *Direct nonmedical costs* include family and patient expenses that result from illness, such as those for food, transportation, family lodging, and home help. These direct nonmedical costs, which can be substantial, are not usually covered to any significant degree by insurance companies and are therefore usually borne by the patient. Although such costs are not usually included in analyses, they should be included when pertinent to the perspective being used for analysis (e.g., the patient perspective, discussed below).
2. *Indirect costs* consist of the cost of loss of income (lost productivity) due to illness or death. These include those due to absence from work, lost wages, decreased earnings, and the need to change jobs. The indirect costs or productivity losses caused by an intervention should be contrasted with the indirect costs of illness. The indirect costs of an illness are usually measured by an extension of the human capital approach. Reduction in the indirect costs of illness is often estimated as a monetary benefit, especially for cost-benefit studies.
3. *Intangible costs* represent nonmonetary costs of illness such as pain, suffering, and grief, expressed in monetary terms. These costs are a part of the denominator in a cost-benefit analysis that uses the willingness-to-pay method. In cost-utility analysis, such items are not given a dollar value but are included in the determination of health outcomes (i.e., in the calculation of QALYs). Therefore, even in the cost-utility analysis, intangible costs become a part of the denominator.

Cost-Finding. An important aspect of cost determination is *cost-finding*, a term used to describe the highly complex procedure for delineation of costs. This procedure involves classification of costs as fixed or variable. *Fixed costs* are the ongoing costs of providing service and are unrelated to the volume of service provided. Examples would be the salaries of operating room managers and the cost of operating room and recovery room monitors. *Variable costs* are a function of the volume of service provided. Examples of variable costs in the operating room and recovery room would be those for supplies, drugs, and supplemental nursing services.

Perspective for Analysis

The "perspective for analysis" identifies from whose perspective the economic analysis of the strategy of interest is being evaluated. For example, a "societal perspective" implies economic analysis of a strategy regardless of who pays. Other typical perspectives are those of the hospital, the health maintenance organization (HMO), the third-party payer, or the individual patient. The type of costs that should be included in the economic analysis depends on the perspective being used. For example, an economic analysis from a societal perspective may include the cost of providing the service and of lost productivity due to illness, as well as any benefits that arise from future gains in productivity and the aversion of costs in the future. Thus, the cost to society would be the social opportunity cost (i.e., the result of having given up the opportunity to use the resources for some other purpose). Third-party payments (i.e., charges that are allowed by that payer) would be included in any economic analysis from the insurance company perspective. Hospital costs (i.e., the true costs of providing the service), regardless of the charge, would be included in a hospital perspective analysis. Cost to the patient is the amount he or she pays for the service (the portion not covered by insurance).

Discounting

"Discounting" is the adjustment for expected inflation and the time cost of money. This adjustment takes into account the fact that a future year is not worth as much monetarily as it is today or this year. Therefore, discounting incorporates the timing of events: a benefit occurring in the future is worth less than a benefit occurring now, and a harm delayed is not as bad as a harm occurring now. Also, money spent in the future is not as costly as money spent now. Discounting is an effort by which one obtains the present value of a number. Inflation is taken into account in a CEA by making all calculations in "today's" dollars or other currency.

In this chapter, a medical practice is said to be cost-effective if its benefits justify the costs, and if equal or greater benefits cannot be gained through less costly means. Alternatively, cost-effectiveness can be defined using the criterion of the relative value of the health outcome versus monetary cost. According to this view, one strategy is more cost-effective than another if it is less costly and at least as effective; it is more effective and more costly if its additional benefit is worth its extra cost; and it is less costly and less effective if the added benefit of the rival strategy is not worth its extra cost. A cost-effectiveness analysis is a process designed to help us make choices between alternatives (e.g., CABG prior to AAA vs. increased monitoring during AAA) when resources are limited and our goal is to use those results to maximize the overall health benefit while minimizing cost to the community.

Decision Analysis

"Decision analysis" is an explicit analytic tool designed to facilitate complex clinical therapeutic or diagnostic decisions in which many variables must be considered simultaneously. It is important to note the distinction between clinical decision analysis and policy applications of decision analysis. The former refers to application of clinical decisions to individual patients and can be performed at bedside. The latter refers to application of decisions to society, populations, or groups of patients. Decision analysis consists of six essential steps.

Constructing a Decision Tree

The first step in decision analysis is to construct a diagrammatic map of all relevant courses of action and their outcomes. The purpose of the resulting decision tree is to make explicit all possible outcomes and the cost of outcomes arising from each decision point. The tree is constructed from left to right and consists of branches, nodes, and outcomes. Branches are lines (conventionally drawn at right angles to nodes) that connect nodes with either other nodes or with outcomes. There are two kinds of nodes—decision nodes and chance nodes. A *decision node* (conventionally depicted as a square) is a point on a branch that represents a diagnostic or therapeutic decision. A *chance node* (conventionally depicted as a circle) is a point on a branch that represents a chance outcome not directly controlled by the physician. *Outcomes* are depicted as rectangles.

Assigning Probabilities

The second step is to assign values for probability for the events depicted at chance nodes of the decision tree. The probabilities of all events at a node must equal 1 (i.e., chance nodes define events that are mutually exclusive and jointly exhaustive).

Assigning Utilities to Each Potential Outcome

In this procedure, one assigns a numeric estimate of worth for each potential outcome on the decision tree. The "worth" represented by these values—"utility measures"—can be of various types, such as QALYs, costs, or 30-day postoperative survival. For the last type, for example, a utility value of 1 would be assigned for survival, and 0 would be assigned for death.

Determining the Expected Utility

The expected utility of each potential course of action on the decision tree is a function of both the probability of the outcome and the utility of the outcome. Multiplying the utilities by the probability of the outcome determines the expected utility of taking a particular action for each branch of the decision tree. The sum of expected utilities of all the branches gives the overall expected utility of a specific decision option. This process is called *averaging.* (In this type of analysis, for example, living with a stroke would have less value in life years than living in a healthy state. Therefore, a treatment that produced survival but with a stroke would be less valuable than a treatment that produced survival in a healthy state.)

Determining the Optimal Decision

Choosing the optimal decision on a decision tree depends on the type of utility. The optimal decision is the one having the highest overall expected utility with regard to survival or QALYs, and the lowest value with regard to cost.

Performing Sensitivity Analysis and Threshold Analysis

The final step in decision analysis consists of two other types of analyses.

Sensitivity analysis is a process that examines the stability of assumptions made in structuring the decision tree. It does this by assessing the impact of variations in probabilities and utilities on the final decision. The process consists of varying the assigned probabilities of one variable (one-way sensitivity analysis), of two variables (two-way sensitivity analysis), or of three variables (three-way sensitivity analysis) at a time.

Threshold analysis is a process that uses one-way sensitivity analysis to determine the threshold value at which a decision should be reconsidered with respect to two variables of interest. The threshold value is the point of intersecting values at which one would switch from selecting, for example, PTCA as therapy to selecting CABG.

Standards

A "standard" is a therapy or practice that should be performed on all patients having the condition in question. Standards are approved only after an assessment of the probabilities and utilities of the therapy indicates that the decision to choose the treatment or strategy would be virtually unanimous. In addition, designating a therapy or strategy a "standard" implies that it is considered cost-effective. Standards are meant to be applied rigidly.

Guidelines

A "guideline" is a therapy or practice that should be followed in most cases but that is applied more flexibly than a standard. Depending on the patient, setting, and other factors, guidelines can and should be tailored to individual needs. Finally, guidelines must also be cost-effective.

Options

An "option" is a therapy or practice that is recommended in a neutral fashion. Options merely note that different interventions are available, and that different people make different choices.

Interpretation of a Diagnostic Test

Our decisions about preoperative evaluation and work-up usually depend on the results of diagnostic tests. Therefore, understanding the principles for evaluating such tests is essential if preoperative assessment is to be cost-effective. Also, because this chapter considers clinical evaluation (i.e., history and physical examination) a form of testing, all the principles that apply to the interpretation of a diagnostic laboratory test also apply to clinical evaluation. Moreover, the *symptoms and signs obtained by clinical evaluation usually generate far more powerful tests of diagnostic hypothesis than can ever be derived from clinical laboratory tests.*[81]

Application of Bayes' Theorem to Diagnostic Testing

Definition of Terms

Definition of terms is necessary for an understanding of the application of Bayes' theorem to diagnostic testing.[14,81,82]

Prior Probability. This term refers to the likelihood that a patient already has a particular disease before performance of any test that might indicate the presence of that disease. "Prior probability" represents the proportion of patients in a given population who have the disease and is synonymous with the terms "pretest probability" and "prevalence."

Odds. "Odds" is another term used to express probability. If the probability of a particular event A is P, then the odds in favor of A (i.e., against *not-A*) can be defined as $P/(1 - P)$. The odds can be converted to probability using the following formula: Probability = odds/(1 + odds).

Posterior Probability or Posttest Probability. This value represents the revised likelihood that a patient has the disease, once test results have been taken into account. Specifically, application of Bayes' theorem allows one to revise the pretest probabilities when test results are known.[83] The general formula for Bayes' theorem is as follows:

$$\text{Posterior (or posttest) odds} = \text{prior (or pretest) odds} \times \text{likelihood ratio.}$$

Application of Bayes' Theorem

When Bayes' theorem is applied to diagnostic testing, the resulting likelihood ratio that is obtained for each test result can indicate either a positive test or a negative test, depending on the outcome of the test. Generation of a likelihood ratio greater than 1 produces a posttest probability that is higher than the pretest probability. Generation of a likelihood ratio that is less than 1 produces a posttest probability that is less than the pretest probability. Generation of a likelihood ratio of 1 means that pretest and posttest probabilities are the same. Test results having a high likelihood ratio virtually ensure the presence of the disease under study. Conversely, a test result that has a very low likelihood ratio (i.e., a ratio as close to 0 as possible) virtually rules out any chance that the patient has the disease in question. A positive test should be associated with a likelihood ratio that is as much greater than 1 as possible, and a negative test should be associated with a likelihood ratio that is, ideally, 0 or as close to 0 as possible.[13]

Let us demonstrate the application of Bayes' theorem to the outcome of DSE testing in a patient undergoing AAA surgery. The assumed values for variables are as follows: for the prior probability of CAD, 0.36; and for the sensitivity and specificity of DSE in detecting CAD, 0.81 and 0.83, respectively.

If the test is positive, the posttest probability of the patient having CAD may be calculated as follows:

$$\text{Prior probability} = 0.36$$

$$\text{Prior odds} = 0.36/(1 - 0.36) = 0.56$$

$$\text{Likelihood ratio (for a positive test)} = 0.81/(1 - 0.83) = 4.76$$

$$\text{Posterior odds} = 0.56 \times 4.76 = 2.67$$

$$\text{Posterior (posttest) probability} = 2.67/(1 + 2.67) = 0.73$$

If the test is negative, the posttest probability of the patient having CAD may be calculated as follows:

$$\text{Likelihood ratio (for a negative test)} = (1 - 0.81)/(0.83) = 0.23$$

$$\text{Posterior odds} = 0.56 \times 0.23 = 0.13$$

$$\text{Posterior (posttest) probability} = 0.13/(1 + 0.13) = 0.12$$

It is evident from the above formulas that the same test results can have different implications for patients who have different prior probabilities for the disease. Figure 2–2 presents this concept graphically. As prior probability increases, the predictive value of a positive test (the probability of disease in a patient with a positive test) increases, and the predictive value of a negative test (the probability that a patient with a negative test is normal) decreases. This decrease in the predictive value of a negative test implies that as prior probability increases, a negative test result need not necessarily indicate the absence of disease. In other words, as prior probability increases, the false-negative rate also increases.

Based on the principles of *Bayesian theory* discussed so far, one might infer that additional yield gained from testing progressively decreases as prior probability increases. When prior probability is high, the *quality* of information from a positive test may be excellent because of high predictive value of a positive test, but the *quantity* of information returned may be minimal because diagnostic certainty is already achieved before performance of the test. In addition, when prior probability is high, a negative test result may not necessarily indicate the absence of disease because of a high false-negative rate. Understanding these two concepts is extremely important if one is to save costs by avoiding unnecessary testing.

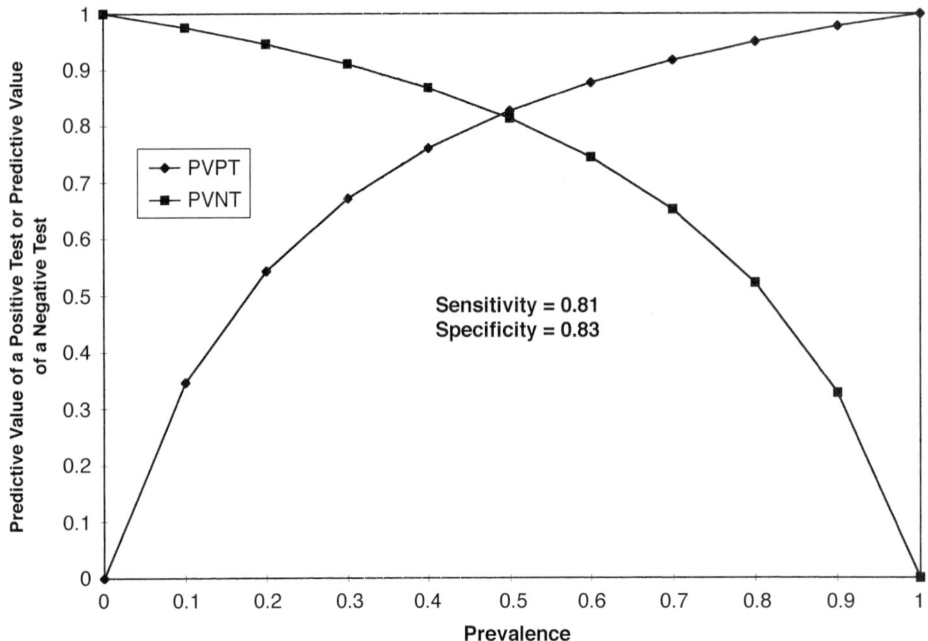

FIGURE **2–2.** The application of Bayesian principles to diagnostic testing. As prior probability ("prevalence") increases, the predictive value of a positive test (PVPT; i.e., the probability of disease in a patient with a positive test) increases and the predictive value of a negative test (PVNT; i.e., the probability that a patient with a negative test is normal) decreases. This decrease in the predictive value of a negative test means that as prior probability increases, the occurrence of a negative test result need not necessarily indicate the absence of disease. That is, as prior probability increases, the rate of false-negatives also increases.

Examples of Effectiveness, Cost-Effectiveness, and Benefit of Preoperative Tests for Cardiac Risk Stratification

In 1994 Mantha et al.[14] performed a meta-analysis of DTS, RNV, AECG, and DSE to evaluate their relative effectiveness in predicting cardiac death or MI occurring within 30 days of vascular surgery (Fig. 2–3 and Table 2–5). The evidence from different studies was combined using the concept of relative risk. Relative risk is an estimate of the predictive value of a particular test. It is the ratio of two probabilities: the probability of adverse cardiac events when the test is positive, and the probability of adverse cardiac events when the test is negative. For benefit to accrue from a test, the relative risk with the respective confidence intervals must be more than 1 (its effectiveness). That is, 1 is the value of an equal event occurring with either a negative or positive test result. Relative risk indicates the relative rate the patient is more likely to have an adverse event with a positive test than with a negative test; relative risk must be significantly greater than 1 for the test to have value.

According to this definition, all four tests were found to be effective (i.e., they had a relative risk greater than 1 with a confidence interval that did not include 1). However, it is difficult to determine which test is optimal because of an overlap of confidence intervals for the combined estimates. Based on the combined point estimate of relative risk for the four tests, the relative effectiveness (highest to lowest) of the tests is as follows: DSE, DTS, RNV, and AECG.

Likelihood ratios can also be used to evaluate the diagnostic abilities of particular tests: the largest likelihood ratio for a positive test and the smallest likelihood ratio for a negative test are beneficial.[13] Table 2–5 shows the likelihood ratios for different tests. With the exception of DSE, the bias for a better predictive ability (better relative risk or better likelihood ratio for a positive test) for studies done earlier in a test's "gestational life" can be noted in Table 2–5 and Figure 2–3. This finding is not surprising because of the possibility of *pretest referral bias*[84] in early studies in which patients were not recruited consecutively. Improvement in perioperative care over time may also explain the phenomenon of decreasing predictive value over time.

Bry et al.[31] attempted to define the cost-effectiveness of DTS screening prior to aortic and infrainguinal surgical procedures. To do so, these authors used the cost of cardiac death or MI that was averted within 30 days after surgery. Cost-effectiveness was represented by the ratio of two values. The numerator consisted of the difference between the total cost of DTS screening (including the cost of interventions following screening) and the total cost for unscreened patients. The denominator consisted of the difference between the number of deaths or MIs among unscreened patients and the number of deaths or MIs among screened patients. This calculation yielded a cost-effectiveness ratio of $392,253 per life saved and $181,039 per MI averted. Congestive heart failure and multiple reversible DTS defects were found to have predictive ability for adverse cardiac events.[31] Furthermore, clinical risk factors were minimally useful in the prediction of perioperative MI, cardiac-related death, or the need for myocardial revascularization. Although the model used to calculate the cost-effectiveness ratio is rather crude, and the alternative strategy (no screening) presents the projected incidence of MI and cardiac-related death without screening, the study was based on data over a 6-year period.

Fleisher et al.[85] used a decision analysis model to examine the benefit-effectiveness of preoperative screening with DTS for patients undergoing AAA surgery. They used 30-day cardiac-related mortality and survival, to

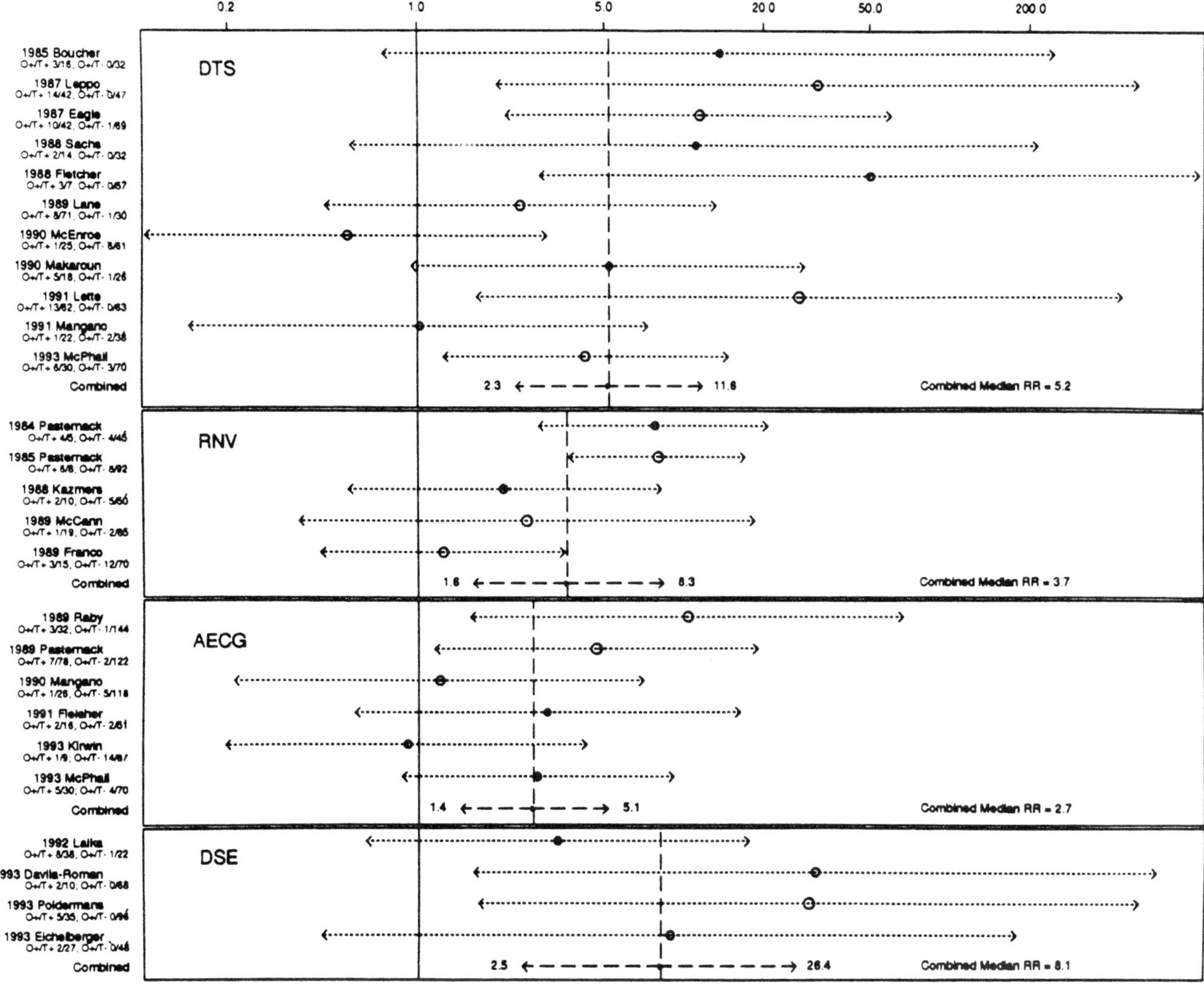

FIGURE **2–3.** Meta-analysis of studies in the literature that used one of four preoperative tests to predict the relative risk (RR; 95% confidence intervals) of adverse cardiac outcome after vascular surgery. In these studies, no myocardial revascularization procedures were performed before vascular surgery. The four preoperative tests were dipyridamole-thallium scintigraphy (DTS), estimation of ejection fractions by radionuclide ventriculography (RNV), ambulatory electrocardiography (AECG), and dobutamine stress echocardiography (DSE). In each panel, the center of the circle represents the point estimate of RR. The area of the circle is proportional to the study sample size for the respective test group. The *solid vertical line* represents an RR of 1 (i.e., when outcome is similar whether the test result is positive or negative). The *broken vertical line* represents the combined median RR for the studies. Because the higher the value for RR, the more predictive the test, the order of effectiveness was: DSE, DTS, RNV, and AECG. O+, a positive outcome; O−, a negative outcome; T+, a positive test result; T−, a negative test result. "Outcome" refers to cardiac death or myocardial infarction. References for the DTS studies are Boucher et al.,[154] Leppo et al.,[155] Eagle et al.,[19] Sachs et al.,[20] Fletcher et al.,[156] Lane et al.,[21] McEnroe et al.,[157] Makgroun MS et al.,[158] Lette et al.,[22] Mangano et al.,[23] and McPhail et al.[24] References for the RNV studies are Pasternack et al.,[36] Pasternack et al.,[37] Kazmers et al.,[38] McCann and Wolfe,[39] and Franco et al.[40] References for the AECG studies are Raby et al.,[41] Pasternack et al.,[42] Mangano et al.,[43] Fleisher et al.,[44] Kirwin et al.,[45] and McPhail et al.[24] References for the DSE studies are Lalka et al.,[46] Poldermans et al.,[47] and Eichelberger et al.[48] (Adapted from Mantha S, Roizen MF, Barnard J, et al: Relative effectiveness of four preoperative tests for predicting adverse cardiac outcomes after vascular surgery: A meta-analysis. Anesth Analg 79:422, 1994, with permission.)

TABLE 2–5
Relative Effectiveness of Four Noninvasive Tests in Predicting MI or Cardiac Death after Vascular Surgery

Test/Reference	Consecutive Pt. Selection	Blinding of MDs to Test Results	No. of Pts. in Study	MI or Cardiac Death (%)	Surgical Procedures (%)			Relative Risk (95% CI)*[,14]	Likelihood Ratio[†,13]	
					Aortic	LEVS	CEA		Neg.	Pos.
DTS studies										
Eagle et al.[19]	No	No	111	9.9	80.2	10.8	9	11.4 (2.1–60.4)	2.84	0.13
Sachs et al.[20]	?	Yes	46	4.3	37	34.7	28.3	11.0 (0.5–215.36)	3.66	0
Lane et al.[21]	No	No	101	8.9	8.9	91.1	0	2.4 (0.4–13.1)	1.30	0.35
Lette et al.[22]	Yes	No	125	10.4	71.2	22.4	6.4	27.4 (1.6–451.6)	2.28	0
Mangano et al.[23]	Yes	Yes	60	5.0	55.3	40	4.7	1.0 (0.1–7.2)	0.90	1.05
McPhail et al.[24]	No	Yes	100	9.0	91	9	0	4.2 (1.2–14.5)	2.53	0.45
								4.6 (2.1–10.4)[‡]		
RNV studies										
Pasternack et al.[36]	Yes	No	50	16.0	100	0	0	7.7 (2.8–20.7)	21.00	0.5
Pasternack et al.[37]	Yes	No	100	14.0	0	100	0	7.9 (3.7–16.9)	18.43	0.58
Kazmers et al.[38]	No	No	60	11.7	100	0	0	2.1 (0.5–8.1)	1.90	0.84
McCann and Wolfe[39]	No	No	104	2.9	100	0	0	2.6 (0.4–18.4)	1.87	0.81
Franco et al.[40]	Yes	No	85	17.6	0	100	0	1.2 (0.4–3.6)	1.17	0.96
								3.7 (1.6–8.3)[§]		
AECG studies										
Raby et al.[41]	Yes	Yes	176	2.2	32	52	16	10.2 (1.6–66.8)	4.44	0.30
Pasternack et al.[42]	Yes	No	200	4.5	33.5	26.5	40	4.6 (1.1–19.0)	2.09	0.35
Mangano et al.[43]	No	Yes	144	4.2	?	?	?	1.2 (0.2–6.9)	0.92	1.02
Fleisher et al.[44]	No	No	67	6.0	?	?	0	3.1 (0.6–16.1)	2.25	0.64
Kirwin et al.[45]	No	No	96	15.6	23.9	76.1	0	0.9 (0.2–4.3)	0.68	1.03
McPhail et al.[24]	No	Yes	100	9.0	91	9	0	2.8 (0.9–9.0)	2.02	0.61
								2.7 (1.4–5.1)[‖]		
DSE studies										
Lalka et al.[46]	No	No	60	15.0	100	0	0	3.3 (0.6–17.5)	1.51	0.27
Poldermans et al.[47]	Yes	Yes	131	3.8	71.3	28.7	0	29.6 (1.7–522.6)	4.2	0
Eichelberger et al.[48]	Yes	Yes	75	2.7	26.7	61.3	12	8.7 (0.4–175.8)	2.92	0
								8.1 (2.5–26.5)[¶]		

*Relative risk (RR) gives an estimate of the predictive value of a particular test. RR is the ratio of the probability of cardiac death or MI when the test is positive and the probability of these events when the test is negative. Ideally, RR and the respective CIs must be more than 1. An RR of 1 means that outcomes are similar when the test is positive or negative. For other computational details, see Mantha et al.[14]

†The likelihood ratio for a positive test = sensitivity/(1 − specificity); the likelihood ratio for a negative test = (1 − sensitivity)/(specificity). The likelihood ratio for a positive test must be as much greater than 1 as possible; for a negative test, the value would be, ideally, 0 or as close to 0 as possible. For more details, see text and Wong and Detsky.[13]

‡Combined median value for DTS.

§Combined median value for RNV.

‖Combined median value for AECG.

¶Combined median value for DSE.

MI, myocardial infarction; Aortic, aortic aneurysm surgery or aortofemoral graft surgery; LEVS, lower extremity vascular surgery; CEA, carotid endarterectomy; CI, confidence interval; DTS, dipyridamole-thallium scintigraphy; RNV, radionuclide ventriculography; AECG, ambulatory electrocardiograhy; DSE, dobutamine stress echocardiography; Neg., negative; Pos., positive.

which they assigned utilities of 0 and 1, respectively. The optimal decision regarding the performance of preoperative testing and myocardial revascularization prior to AAA surgery was a function of both the mortality rate for myocardial revascularization and the mortality rate for surgery performed without preoperative interventions. A two-way sensitivity analysis was performed by varying the probability of mortality for myocardial revascularization and the probability of mortality for AAA surgery performed in patients with CAD. The optimal decision regarding preoperative testing versus surgery alone depended on the interaction of these variables (Fig. 2–4).[85] The authors found that for patients with low prior probability of CAD, the preferred option was the performance of only vascular surgery with no prior screening with DTS. This analysis clearly demonstrates the importance of local institutional factors on the optimal preoperative strategy.

Strategies for Cardiac Risk Stratification in the Literature

Based on coronary angiographic data for 1,000 consecutive patients presenting for vascular surgery, Hertzer et al.[4] proposed that all patients symptomatic for CAD should have coronary angiography, and that asymptomatic patients should be screened by noninvasive testing for the detection of underlying CAD. After the first report of the usefulness of DTS noninvasive testing for cardiac risk stratification in vascular surgery patients,[18] this test gained wide popularity. Extensive experience with DTS resulted in authors from various institutions proposing strategies for cardiac risk stratification, the goal being to optimize preoperative screening for CAD (Table 2–6).

In addition, clinicians have proposed various algorithms that use the criteria of Eagle et al.[25] for optimizing

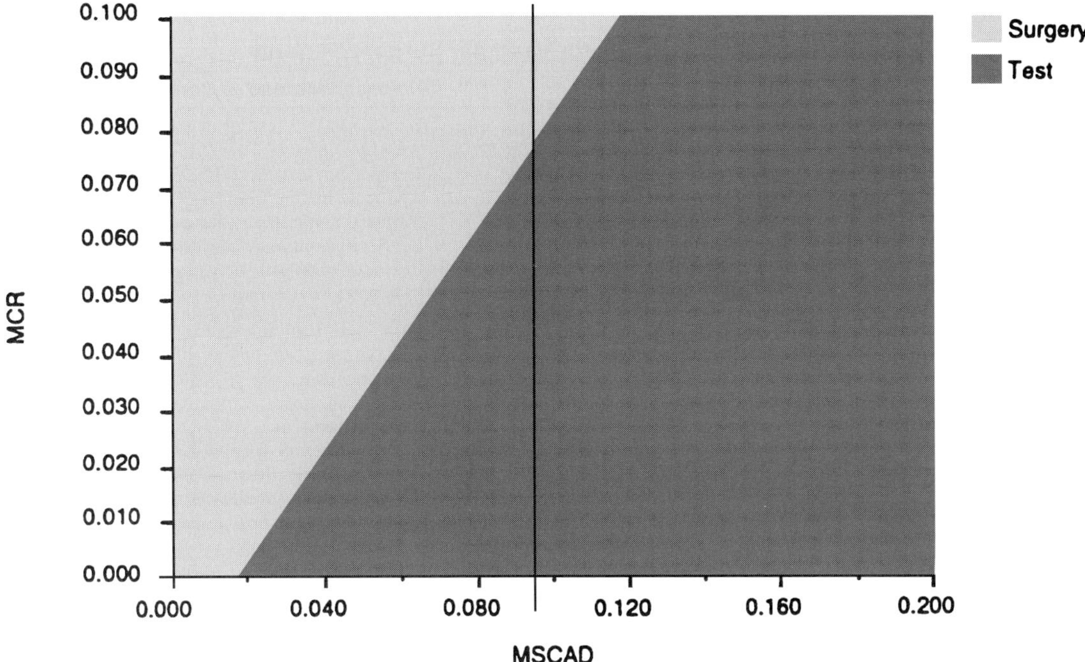

FIGURE **2–4.** The effect of local institutional factors on the optimal decision regarding preoperative testing with dipyridamole-thallium scintigraphy followed by myocardial revascularization ("test") versus vascular surgery alone without screening ("surgery"). The figure shows the results of a two-way sensitivity analysis performed by varying the probability of mortality for myocardial revascularization (MCR) and the probability of mortality for abdominal aortic aneurysm surgery performed in patients with coronary artery disease (MSCAD). It is evident from this figure that the optimal decision depends on the interaction of these variables. The *vertical line* indicates the probability (9.5%) of mortality from AAA surgery, for patients with CAD. (Adapted from Fleisher LA, Skolnick ED, Holroyd KJ: Coronary artery revascularization before abdominal aortic aneurysm surgery: A decision analytic approach. Anesth Analg 79:661, 1994, with permission.)

preoperative screening.[13,61] However, a few drawbacks of the study by Eagle and colleagues should be noted. This retrospective study evaluated 254 patients who underwent nuclear cardiology laboratory testing. For 44 of these patients, vascular surgery was canceled after screening with DTS; therefore, selection bias did exist. Moreover, because of the retrospective nature of the study, the authors were unable to confirm that ten patients had vascular surgery. When Lette et al.[22] evaluated 18 clinical variables and seven clinical scoring systems, they could not reproduce the findings of Eagle and colleagues, nor could they identify any other clinical variables for predicting adverse cardiac outcomes.

Furthermore, a 1993 study by Kresowik et al.[29] indicated that standard clinical markers of CAD, used alone, were not sensitive in detecting severe CAD in patients undergoing vascular surgery. In this study, 190 consecutive patients had DTS and RNV. Patients with unstable angina and recent (<12 months) myocardial revascularization were excluded. The authors compared the results of DTS, RNV, and coronary angiography in patients with and without clinical or electrocardiographic evidence of CAD. Redistribution defects were similar: 44.9% (35 of 78) for those with clinically evident CAD versus 46.4% (52 of 112) for those without clinically evident CAD. These results indicate that the clinical predictors used by these clinicians were inadequate. Also, redistribution defects were similar regardless of operative procedure—aortic, infrainguinal, or carotid. Coronary angiography identified triple-vessel or left-main CAD in 10.2% (8 of 78) of those with clinically evident CAD and in 14.3% (16 of 112) of those without clinically evident CAD. All 12 patients (6%) in the entire series whose ejection fractions were less than 35% on RNV had DTS defects (redistribution or fixed). Only two patients (8%) of 24 patients with left-main or triple-vessel CAD identified by RNV had ejection fractions of less than 35%. Sixteen (67%) of these 24 patients had ejection fractions of at least 50%. The authors also noted that if they had followed the recommendations of Eagle and co-workers, 6 (25%) of their 24 patients with left-main or triple-vessel CAD would have been overlooked.

Wong and Detsky[13] used the data of Lette et al.[22] to compute likelihood ratios for clinical scoring systems that try to predict cardiac death or MI after vascular surgery, such as the Goldman index[86] and the Detsky index.[87,88] A Goldman index of 5 or less (Class 1) and a Detsky index of 15 or less (Class 1) were associated with likelihood ratios of 0.73 and 0.99, respectively. The likelihood ratios for such low classes of risk should be, ideally, 0 or as close to 0 as possible. The occurrence of high likelihood ratios for patients in these two low classes of risk implies that adverse outcomes could still occur in the clinical low-risk category of patients. These

TABLE 2–6
Proposed Cardiac Risk Stratification Strategies for Vascular Surgery Patients

Reference	Study Design and Comments	Proposed Method of Cardiac Risk Stratification
Golden et al.[26]	500 consecutive patients presenting for AAA surgery Perioperative invasive hemodynamic monitoring (direct radial artery and PA pressure) to assist fluid or drug therapy starting a day before surgery	No noninvasive testing of patients having no evidence of CAD Noninvasive testing (DTS, AECG, RNV, or 2D echo) of patients having clinical or ECG evidence of CAD Coronary angiography for patients identified as very high risk after noninvasive testing and myocardial revascularization (before or coincident with AAA surgery)
Eagle et al.[25]	Retrospective observation of 200 patients presenting for all types of vascular surgery Possibility of selection bias, as 40 of initial 54 patients had cancellation of surgery after DTS testing	Initial stratification based on clinical risk factors (Q waves on ECG, history of ventricular ectopic activity, diabetes, age >70 yr, history of angina) DTS for intermediate-risk category (one or two clinical risk factors) DTS unnecessary for low-risk (no clinical risk factors) and high-risk (three or more risk factors) patients because adverse outcomes could be predicted by clinical information alone
Strawn and Guernsey[27]	Prospective evaluation of 68 consecutive patients presenting for AAA surgery Exclusion criteria: Patients at very high risk (e.g., MI within 6 mo, unstable or disabling angina, CHF, valvular heart disease)	Screening with DTS for patients at intermediate risk (history of MI >6 mo before surgery, stable angina, abnormal ECG findings) Screening not recommended for patients having no clinical or ECG evidence of CAD
Taylor et al.[89]	Prospective evaluation of 491 patients presenting for all types of vascular surgery Perioperative use of a PA catheter only for patients with CHF or poor LV function Intraoperative TEE monitoring not used Use of serial postoperative ECGs and cardiac enzymes for all the patients, to screen for postoperative MI	Screening with a noninvasive test (DTS, RNV, 2D echo) only for patients with severe symptoms (unstable angina, uncontrolled arrhythmias, CHF) Coronary angiography based on the findings of noninvasive tests followed by myocardial revascularization in appropriate cases No noninvasive tests in the absence of severe symptoms
Lette et al.[22]	Prospective evaluation of 125 consecutive patients presenting for all types of vascular surgery Evaluation of 18 clinical parameters and seven clinical scoring systems	Clinical parameters must not be used for risk stratification Quantitative interpretation of DTS based on the extent of redistribution defects to stratify intermediate-risk and high-risk subgroups Coronary angiography recommended for high-risk subgroup
Bunt[139]	Prospective evaluation of 630 consecutive patients presenting for all types of vascular surgery Routine daily assessment of postoperative ECGs and cardiac enzymes for 3 days	Routine use of RNV for all the patients Surgery for patients with negative cardiac history, normal ECG, and EF >50% DTS for patients with positive cardiac history, positive ECG findings, and EF <50% Coronary angiography for patients with positive DTS tests Above-stated strategy is of high utility in aortic procedures, of moderate utility in femorodistal bypass procedures, and of little utility in CEA procedures
Suggs et al.[30]	Retrospective evaluation of 263 patients presenting for AAA repair	Coronary angiography for patients with angina DTS for patients with other indicators of CAD No screening of patients without indicators of CAD

AAA, abdominal aortic aneurysm; AECG, ambulatory electrocardiography; CAD, coronary artery disease; CEA, carotid endarterectomy; CHF, congestive heart failure; 2D echo, two-dimensional echocardiography; DTS, dipyridamole-thallium scintigraphy; ECG, electrocardiogram, electrocardiographic; EF, ejection fraction; LV, left ventricular; MI, myocardial infarction; PA, pulmonary artery; RNV, radionuclide ventriculography; TEE, transesophageal echocardiography.

data indicate that, at least in these clinicians' hands, a clinical scoring system would be inadequate. The cynic could argue that perhaps in better clinical hands (e.g., Eagle and colleagues) such a system would be useful.

Authors who advocate testing with noninvasive tests only if patients are severely symptomatic argue that the current state of surgical, anesthetic, and perioperative care has made the cardiac morbidity rate after vascular surgery too low to warrant routine or selective screening.[89] A 1994 paper found that the presence of definite clinical evidence of CAD and old age were the most important predictors of an adverse cardiac outcome.[31] Proponents of aggressive risk stratification followed by myocardial revascularization in appropriate cases argue that CAD represents a lifetime risk, that CABG for such patients affords a 3.8-year survival advantage,[56] that referral for vascular surgery gives an opportunity for documentation and management of a potentially fatal condition,[56,59] and that management can result in a better long-term survival.

Methods and Problems Related to Technology Assessment of Research on Cardiac Risk Stratification

Despite an enormous amount of literature related to cardiac risk stratification before vascular surgery,[13,14] no clear conclusion results. The difference in conclusions may be attributable to differences in the following factors: pretest selection criteria; pretest probability of CAD because of inclusion of different vascular surgical procedures; experience in the interpretation of noninvasive screening tests; criteria chosen for selecting patients for coronary angiography after screening with noninvasive screening tests; perioperative care resulting in different cardiac outcomes; and different morbidity and mortality rates for myocardial revascularization at different institutions (Tables 2–5 and 2–6).

An ideal study of the predictive ability of a particular test to identify perioperative events would have the following design characteristics: a prospective study design, patient selection on a consecutive basis, and blinding of test results to physicians caring for the patients. A study by Mangano et al.[23] had such ideal characteristics but was limited by a sample size (n = 60) that was too small to gather adequate information. Bry et al.[31] discussed a prospective, randomized, multicenter study that was planned for the evaluation of cardiac risk stratification by means of DTS. The study would have had a sample size of 1,500, the minimum number required for evaluation of morbidity and mortality in this particular group of vascular surgery patients. Unfortunately, the attempt was unsuccessful because of unwillingness of some participants to blind clinicians to potentially high-risk scans.

A 1994 decision analysis by Fleisher et al.[85] demonstrated that the optimal preoperative strategy depended on local (hospital-specific) factors for planning preoperative testing and myocardial revascularization before AAA surgery. Therefore, a cost-effective strategy at one institution may prove ineffective at another, a fact that may be masked in a multi-institutional trial. Also, studies analyzing cardiac risk stratification prior to surgery are time consuming. By the time a study is completed, a new technology having better predictive and diagnostic abilities may have emerged.

Technology assessment studies may also suffer from *learning contamination bias.*[90] This is a bias against the use of a technology and results when the learning that occurs from inclusion of a technology in the care of some patients (e.g., monitoring, carotid endarterectomy) also improves the care of subsequent patients who are not even exposed to the technology. If this beneficial transfer of knowledge goes unrecognized and outcome for both the exposed and unexposed groups improves, the technology itself may be seen as unnecessary and its usefulness therefore underestimated.

Finally, unintentional crossover in prospective studies evaluating the long-term effects of different strategies can introduce obvious problems.[91] Unintentional crossover is very problematic in a number of studies. Major trials such as the Veterans Affairs Study, the European Coronary Surgery Study, and the Coronary Artery Surgery Study (CASS) examining the efficacy of CABG faced the problem of unintentional crossover. For example, in CASS, crossover rates after 5 years were 24% for medical allocations and 8% for surgical allocations.[92]

Problems associated with prospective studies and retrospective studies may force us to resort to meta-analysis, decision analysis, or other theoretical models.[13,14,70,71,93–98] Limitations of meta-analytic models can be attributed to inherent factors such as study design heterogeneity, duplicate or multiple publications bias, publication bias, pretest referral bias, and varying definitions of positive and negative test results and outcome measures.[99–101] Statistical methods such as use of *random effects models,*[14,102] *confidence profile models* (Bayesian or nonBayesian),[103] and other proposed guidelines for evaluating diagnostic tests[71,81,93,104–106] can control, to a certain extent, the limitations of meta-analysis.

Finally, even a well-designed technology assessment study supported by rigorous analysis cannot address some of the broader issues recently raised by a few experts. In an editorial commenting on a theoretical model that found cost per QALY to be excessive for routine use of pulmonary artery catheters in CABG patients, Thys[107] raised a very difficult question. Less usage of pulmonary artery catheters because of excessive costs can lead to reduced knowledge and experience with such catheters and can, in turn, adversely influence patient care when it is really needed—if you will, a form of the "learning contamination bias" problem. Thys questions whether a society can accept some of the sacrifices resulting from cost containment.

Areas for Future Research

A 1993 survey by Fleisher and Beattie[12] revealed that the mean incidence of preoperative testing to assess cardiac risk for each of the surgical categories was as high as 73% for aortic surgery, 59% for carotid endarterectomy, and 54% for lower extremity revascularization. DTS was the test most commonly used, and AECG was the least commonly used. There was no statistically significant difference in the percentage of patients undergoing testing in university versus private hospital settings. Given the extent of preoperative testing for cardiac risk stratification (>50% in the survey by Fleisher and Beattie[12]), and given the fact that approximately 570,000 patients in the United States undergo vascular procedures annually, the obvious question is, *Are the benefits worth the cost?*[108–110]

The central issue in cardiac risk stratification is not whether there is an appropriate role for coronary angiography among vascular surgery patients, but, rather, which patients should be selected for angiography in order to obtain maximum information on a realistic, cost-effective basis. A preponderance of data suggests that surgical treatment of CAD not only provides long-term benefit but also helps prevent subsequent adverse cardiac events in a subgroup of patients who have peripheral vascular disease.[51,56] Surgical treatment is most beneficial for patients who have triple-vessel CAD or ejection fractions of less than 35%. It is reasonable to believe that referral of patients with peripheral vascular disease for vascular surgery may be the best opportunity for us to identify the subgroup of patients who may gain a long-term benefit.

Our goal could be to create a cardiac risk stratification strategy ideally located in the lower right quadrant of a graph of cost versus QALY (Fig. 2–5).[77] Strategies located in the upper right and lower left quadrants must be compared with alternative strategies in order to obtain the incremental cost-effectiveness or incremental cost-utility ratio. Neither the profession of medicine nor society is accustomed to placing a dollar value on a life or on a year of life. However, assuming a societal willingness to pay, many analyses use $35,000 to $45,000 (in 1999 dollars) per QALY as the threshold value for judging a strategy to be cost-effective.[111] One 1994 study used a threshold value of $250,000 per life saved to judge the cost-effectiveness of administering streptokinase for acute MI.[112]

Although controversy still exists regarding the role of clinical risk factors in predicting cardiac events or optimizing noninvasive screening for CAD in vascular surgery patients, Pryor et al.[113] found basic clinical evaluation (clinical history, physical examination, electrocardiography, and chest radiography) quite valuable in predicting both the coronary anatomy at catheterization and 3-year survival in the general population with suspected CAD. However, because these investigators examined the general population with suspected CAD, their data cannot readily be extrapolated to vascular surgery patients.

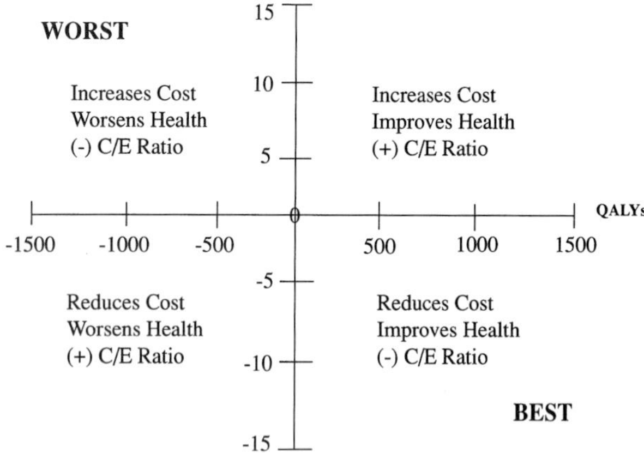

FIGURE **2–5.** Graph of cost versus quality-adjusted life years (QALYs). The best location for a cardiac risk stratification strategy on this graph would be the lower right quadrant. Strategies that fall into the upper right and lower left quadrants must be compared with alternative strategies in order to obtain the incremental cost-effectiveness (C-E) ratio or the incremental cost-utility ratio. A strategy falls into the worst location, the left upper quadrant, when the cost, morbidity, and mortality of the interventions of that strategy are high. (Adapted from Riegelman RK: The Measures of Medicine. Benefits, Harms, and Costs. Cambridge, MA, Blackwell Science, 1995, with permission.)

Of particular interest regarding patient history is the patient's ability to walk two blocks. Patients who cannot walk two blocks can be considered to be those at intermediate risk who might benefit from further noninvasive testing. If patients who can walk two blocks with no angina or dyspnea and have no other indicators of CAD, we can be quite certain they do not have left-main CAD, triple-vessel CAD, or severe left ventricular dysfunction (ejection fractions <35%). Such patients can proceed to vascular surgery without noninvasive testing because they are unlikely to be at risk of adverse perioperative outcomes. This assumption is our hypothesis and needs to be tested in future prospective studies with angiographic data.

It should be noted that MI and cardiac-related mortality are not always attributable to narrowed coronary arteries. Recent evidence suggests that the rupture of lipid-laden, macrophage-rich plaques can initiate unstable angina, acute MI, and sudden death. Plaque rupture occurs when the circumferential tension on a plaque exceeds its tensile strength, an event that cannot be predicted by coronary angiography.[114]

Pending information from well-designed prospective studies, the most powerful yet most flexible of the theoretical models (i.e., decision analysis models) may be employed to obtain further information regarding the effectiveness, benefit-effectiveness, and cost-effectiveness of cardiac risk stratification methods designed for vascular surgery patients. Decision analysis models can also help us to plan future studies. Decision analysts may consider some relevant data given in Table 2–7. Decision analysts attempting to look at the long-term effects may obtain relevant data from Farkouh et al.,[54] Roger et al.,[53] Gersh et al.,[59] and Rihal et al.[56] Markov models[115,116] can also be incorporated into analyses looking at long-term events.

Proposals for Optimizing Cardiac Risk Stratification for Vascular Surgery Patients

Because the literature does not provide sufficient information to guide the process of cardiac risk stratification, this chapter makes its own proposal regarding the reduction of costs without a compromise in quality. This proposal is based on our best possible estimate of outcomes informed by the published literature.

Many issues may need to be considered before choosing a particular test for cardiac risk stratification[117]:

1. *Technical issues*: Availability and quality of equipment, familiarity and level of comfort, and quality assurance.
2. *Interpretative issues*: Expertise in the interpretation of tests, ability to deal with artifacts, and sensitivity and specificity.

TABLE 2–7
Relevant Data for Interventions of Cardiac Risk Stratification Suited for Decision Analysis*

Variable	Baseline Estimate	Ranges that Could Be Tested in Sensitivity Analysis
Estimated mortality (%)		
For CABG[66]	7.7	5–10
For PTCA[140]	1	0–2
For coronary angiography[85]	0.1	0–0.3
For PA catheterization[141]	0.05	0.02–1.5
Estimated morbidity (%)		
For MI after CABG[56]	7.4	5–15
For MI after coronary angioplasty[142]	2.3	0–5
For stroke after CABG[56]	1.6	2–7.5
Characteristics of evaluative test[†]		
DSE		
Sensitivity[143]	0.81	0.7–1
Specificity[143]	0.83	0.7–1
DTS		
Sensitivity[143]	0.87	0.7–1
Specificity[143]	0.75	0.7–1
Costs (1991 U.S. dollars)[‡]		
Coronary angiography[94]	2,600	2,000–3,000
CABG[94]	22,400	20,000–25,000
Coronary angioplasty[94]	6,000	4,000–8,000
Cardiac death[144]	10,000	5,000–15,000
MI treatment[94]	9,000	5,000–15,000
Hospital cost of stroke treatment[145]	47,819	45,000–50,000
DSE[§]	407	350–800
DTS[§]	472	350–800

*Also refer to Fleisher et al.[85]
[†]Sensitivity and specificity refer to the diagnosis of significant coronary artery disease.
[‡]All costs were adjusted to 1991 U.S. dollars based on the medical care component of the consumer price index.
[§]Costs were calculated based on the cost-charge ratio of 1 : 2 used at the University of Chicago and were adjusted to 1991 U.S. dollars by use of the medical care component of the consumer price index. The 1994 charges, including charges for interpretation of DTS and DSE test results by physicians at the University of Chicago, were $1,450 and $1,250, respectively.
CABG, coronary artery bypass graft surgery; PTCA, percutaneous transluminal coronary angioplasty; PA, pulmonary artery; MI, myocardial infarction; DSE, dobutamine stress echocardiography; DTS, dypyridamole-thallium scintigraphy.

3. *Outcome issues*: Pretest probability of CAD, incremental value of the test, and other factors (see earlier section on interpretation of diagnostic tests).

The goal of the cardiac risk stratification strategy we now propose is to improve long-term outcome by identifying and performing CABG in the high-risk CAD subgroups (patients with three-vessel CAD, left-main CAD, or ejection fractions of <35%).

Of the four commonly used tests—RNV, AECG, DTS, and DSE—we recommend the last two for cardiac risk stratification because of their ability to diagnose or rule out significant CAD and to predict adverse cardiac outcomes. The choice of DTS versus DSE should depend on the availability of, and experience with, the test at a particular institution. When making a choice, physicians must also consider the advantages and disadvantages of these two tests (Table 2–8). Both DTS and DSE are amenable to semiquantitative interpretation (Table 2–9),[34,118] and such interpretation may help the clinician optimize coronary angiography in patients with positive test results.[119] Strongly positive results may effectively identify patients with severe CAD who might receive long-term benefit from surgical correction. We suggest that only patients with strongly positive results be recommended for coronary angiography. We believe such an approach can identify high-risk patients who may accrue long-term benefit from surgical correction of CAD. Patients with weakly positive test results may be subjected to surgery using perioperative risk-reducing strategies.

Our specific proposals, based on our review of the literature, are as follows. We propose that patients who can walk two blocks with no angina or dyspnea, and who have no other indicators of CAD (no prior MI; no current angina; no ECG evidence of MI; no history of congestive heart failure, arrhythmia requiring treatment, or diabetes), can proceed to surgery without noninvasive testing because they are unlikely to be at risk of adverse perioperative outcomes. Also, such patients are unlikely to have coronary lesions (triple-vessel CAD, left-main CAD, severe ventricular dysfunction) that would be benefited by surgical correction in the long run. Patients who cannot walk two blocks can be considered to be those at intermediate risk who might benefit from further noninvasive testing. In addition, we believe that basic evaluation (patient history, electrocardiography) helps segregate patients for cardiac risk stratification. Table 2–10 shows our proposals, based on the stated goal. The rationale for sending patients with very high likelihood of high-risk CAD (triple-vessel CAD, left-main CAD, or poor left ventricular function) directly to coronary angiography is based on Bayesian principles.[120] Such patients would not benefit from further noninvasive testing. In such high-risk patients, a positive noninvasive test does not provide additional information, and a negative test is also not helpful. We emphasize that our proposals are based on literature review and assumptions that need to be validated by prospective studies or explicit analysis.

Summary and Conclusions

Because of the interplay of many patient, surgical, and institution-specific factors that influence outcome, achieving the goal of the best long-term outcome is not easy regarding patients undergoing vascular surgery. Morbidity and mortality after vascular surgery is cardiac related because of the high prevalence of symptomatic and asymptomatic CAD. Severe CAD exists in more than 25% of patients presenting for vascular surgery, regardless of the type of surgical procedure being undertaken.[4] Risk stratification thus aims to identify patients with correctable CAD who would accrue long-term benefit (and a 3.8-year survival advantage) from changes in perioperative care. However, given the costs and risks involved, it is not practical to subject all vascular surgery patients to preoperative coronary angiography. There

TABLE 2–8
Important Features of DTS and DSE

Feature	DTS	DSE
Technique of evaluation	Evaluation of myocardium viable at risk, by pharmacologic induction of coronary vasodilation	Observation of regional wall motion abnormalities after pharmacologic stress induced by dobutamine infusion
Sensitivity*[,143]	0.87	0.81
Specificity*[,143]	0.75	0.83
Advantages	Ideal for vascular surgery patients who cannot exercise because of claudication No published report of death following DTS Amenable to semiquantitative interpretation[21,33–35] Safety of DTS regarding neurologic complications has been shown for 400 patients with cerebrovascular disease from seven centers[146]	Ideal for vascular surgery patients who cannot exercise because of claudication No published report of death following DSE Amenable to semiquantitative interpretation[118] DSE detects ischemia due to dynamic factors (stress) that can occur perioperatively The test takes <1 hr and can be done in an outpatient setting Sensitivity may be enhanced by addition of atropine[147]
Disadvantages	Requires overnight fasting Contraindicated for patients with unstable angina, recent myocardial infarction, bronchial asthma, or chronic obstructive pulmonary disease Requires delayed imaging at 3–4 hr and perhaps even at 18–24 hr[148] Reported failure to detect severe CAD and therefore to predict the cardiac events following vascular surgery[149,150] Possibility of cerebrovascular accident[151]	Possibility of life-threatening complications
Complications	Report of minor complications (chest pain, headache, nausea, dizziness) in 57 of 702 (8.1%) patients during DTS testing[14]	Per a prospective 1994 study on 2,949 tests from 24 laboratories: 0.5% of tests (1 in 210) had life-threatening events that required specific treatment, lasted >3 hr, or required new hospital admission[152]

*Sensitivity and specificity refer to the diagnosis or ruling out of significant CAD.
CAD, coronary artery disease; DTS, dipyridamole-thallium scintigraphy; DSE, dobutamine stress echocardiography.

fore, interest in other noninvasive preoperative tests for cardiac risk stratification has increased.[13,14] Commonly used preoperative noninvasive tests are RNV, AECG, DTS, and DSE.

Recommendations for cardiac risk stratification vary widely. Proponents of a highly selective noninvasive testing strategy argue that the current state of surgical, anesthetic, and perioperative care has reduced cardiac morbidity after vascular surgery to a point that is too low to warrant the use of routine or selective screening. Proponents of aggressive risk stratification followed by myocardial revascularization in appropriate cases argue that CAD represents a lifetime risk, and that referral for vascular surgery gives an opportunity for documentation and management of a potentially fatal condition.

In the current era of cost-consciousness, we need to address not only the issue of effectiveness but also cost-effectiveness. Unfortunately, well-designed prospective studies that address the issue of the cost-effectiveness of cardiac risk stratification for vascular surgery patients are still not available. Recent data suggest that surgical correction of CAD in patients with peripheral vascular disease provides long-term benefit, especially in patients with triple-vessel coronary disease or poor left ventricular function.[56] We believe that basic clinical information can segregate patients for angiography, DTS or DSE, and subsequent angiography and myocardial revascularization on a cost-effective basis. This basic clinical infor-

TABLE 2–9
Semiquantitative Interpretation of Test Results with DSE or DTS*

Test and Results	Manifestation
DSE	
Strongly positive	Occurrence of RWMAs at low infusion rate of dobutamine (<10 μg/kg/min), or low heart rate (<120 bpm); or Extensive ischemia and/or LV dysfunction in ≥3 LV segments during dobutamine infusion; or Multiple resting RWMAs involving more than one coronary artery territory (≥3 segments) worsening during dobutamine infusion
Negative	No echocardiographic changes during dobutamine infusion
Weakly positive	Intermediate between negative and strongly positive results
DTS	
Strongly positive	Redistribution defects in ≥4 myocardial segments in a 15-segment model or redistribution defects in ≥2 coronary territories
Negative	Absence of redistribution defects or the presence of a fixed defect
Weakly positive	Intermediate between negative and strongly positive results

*Data from Levinson et al.[34] and the ACC/AHA Task Force.[118]
DSE, dobutamine stress echocardiography; DTS, dipyridamole-thallium scintigraphy; LV, left ventricular; RWMAs, regional wall motion abnormalities.

TABLE 2–10
Proposed Interventions for the Stratification of Cardiac Risk in Patients Undergoing Vascular Surgery*

Criteria	Proposed Intervention[†]	Category of Proposal
Unstable angina or current CHF	***CATH***	Standard
Four or more risk factors on basic evaluation	***CATH***	Guideline
Inability to walk two blocks because of claudication or cardiac symptoms	***DTS*** or ***DSE***	
Two or three risk factors on basic evaluation	***DTS*** or ***DSE***	Option
Strongly positive DTS or DSE results	***CATH***	Guideline
Weakly positive DTS or DSE results	***Surgery with perioperative risk-reducing strategies; follow-up after surgery for progression of CAD***	Option
	or	
	CATH	Option
High-risk anatomic subgroups on CATH	***CABG***	Guideline
Two-vessel or single-vessel disease on CATH	PTCA or CABG, as appropriate	Option
	or	
	Surgery under perioperative risk-reducing strategies	Option

*The authors base their proposals on the following assumptions. The goal is to identify high-risk patients who would benefit from surgical correction of CAD even in the long run. High-risk patients are those with triple-vessel CAD, an ejection fraction >35%,[56] or left-main CAD. Basic evaluation of vascular surgery candidates would search for the following risk factors: myocardial infarction (by history or electrocardiography), age >70 yr, diabetes mellitus requiring treatment, stable angina, a history of CHF, or cardiomegaly on chest radiograph.

[†]Interventions shown in bold-face italic lettering are believed to be cost-effective or benefit-effective ways of achieving the stated goal.
CHF, congestive heart failure; CATH, coronary angiography; DTS, dipyridamole-thallium scintigraphy; DSE, dobutamine stress echocardiography; CAD, coronary artery disease; CABG, coronary artery bypass graft surgery; PTCA, percutaneous transluminal coronary angioplasty.

mation consists of the patient history, age greater than 70 years, diabetes, congestive heart failure, or arrhythmias requiring treatment, unstable angina, and Q wave MI on electrocardiograph. Furthermore, the value of such information in identifying those with high-risk CAD and in predicting long-term survival in the general population with suspected CAD has been documented.[113] Future studies to test the value of this proposal to improve long-term outcome are needed.

References

1. Martin LF, Atnip RG, Holmes PA, et al: Prediction of postoperative complications after elective aortic surgery using stepwise logistic regression analysis. Am Surg 60:163, 1994.
2. Ellis JE, Roizen MF, Mantha S, Wilke H: Anesthesia for vascular surgery. In Barash PG, et al (eds): Clinical Anesthesia, 3rd ed. Philadelphia, Lippincott-Raven Publishers, 1997, p 871.
3. Roizen MF, Ellis JE: Anesthesia for vascular surgery. In Barash PG, Cullen BF, Stoelting RK (eds): Clinical Anesthesia, 2nd ed. Philadelphia, JB Lippincott Co, 1992, p 1059.
4. Hertzer NR, Beven EG, Young JR, et al: Coronary artery disease in peripheral vascular patients. A classification of 1000 coronary angiograms and results of surgical management. Ann Surg 199: 223, 1984.
5. Cunningham AJ: Anaesthesia for abdominal aortic surgery—a review (part I). Can J Anaesth 36:426, 1989.
6. Krupski WC, Layug EL, Reilly LM, et al: Comparison of cardiac morbidity between aortic and infrainguinal operations. J Vasc Surg 15:354, 1992.
7. Clark NJ, Stanley TH: Anesthesia for vascular surgery. In Miller RD (ed): Anesthesia, 4th ed. New York, Churchill Livingstone, 1994, p 1851.
8. Cunningham AJ: Anaesthesia for abdominal and major vascular surgery. In Nimmo WS, Rowbotham DJ, Smith G (eds): Anaesthesia. London, Blackwell Scientific Publications, 1994, p 1042.
9. Glaser RB: Morbidity and mortality from major vascular surgery. In Roizen MF (ed): Anesthesia for Vascular Surgery. New York, Churchill Livingstone, 1990, p 1.
10. Roizen MF: Can the anesthesiologist reduce myocardial morbidity after vascular surgery? (Editorial). J Cardiothorac Vasc Anesth 5:424, 1991.
11. Szilagyi DE: Vascular surgery: A brief account of its past and present. In Veith FJ, Hobson RW II, Williams RA, Wilson SE (eds): Vascular Surgery. Principles and Practice, 2nd ed. New York, McGraw-Hill, 1994, p 3.
12. Fleisher LA, Beattie C: Current practice in the preoperative evaluation of patients undergoing major vascular surgery: A survey of cardiovascular anesthesiologists. J Cardiothorac Vasc Anesth 7:650, 1993.
13. Wong T, Detsky AS: Preoperative cardiac risk assessment for patients having peripheral vascular surgery. Ann Intern Med 116: 743, 1992.
14. Mantha S, Roizen MF, Barnard J, et al: Relative effectiveness of four preoperative tests for predicting adverse cardiac outcomes after vascular surgery: A meta-analysis. Anesth Analg 79: 422, 1994.
15. Fleisher LA, Hulyalkar A: Cardiovascular testing for the 1990s. Adv Anesth 11:27, 1994.
16. Leppo JA: Preoperative cardiac risk assessment for noncardiac surgery. Am J Cardiol 75:42D, 1995.
17. Blaustein AS: Preoperative and perioperative management of cardiac patients undergoing noncardiac surgery. Cardiol Clin 13: 149, 1995.
18. Boucher CA, Brewster DC, Darling RC, et al: Determination of cardiac risk by dipyridamole-thallium imaging before peripheral vascular surgery. N Engl J Med 312:389, 1985.
19. Eagle KA, Singer DE, Brewster DC, et al: Dipyridamole-thallium scanning in patients undergoing vascular surgery. Op-

timizing preoperative evaluation of cardiac risk. JAMA 257: 2185, 1987.
20. Sachs RN, Tellier P, Larmignat P, et al: Assessment by dipyridamole-thallium-201 myocardial scintigraphy of coronary risk before peripheral vascular surgery. Surgery 103:584, 1988.
21. Lane SE, Lewis SM, Pippin JJ, et al: Predictive value of quantitative dipyridamole-thallium scintigraphy in assessing cardiovascular risk after vascular surgery in diabetes mellitus. Am J Cardiol 64:1275, 1989.
22. Lette J, Waters D, Lassonde J, et al: Multivariate clinical models and quantitative dipyridamole-thallium imaging to predict cardiac morbidity and death after vascular reconstruction. J Vasc Surg 14:160, 1991.
23. Mangano DT, London MJ, Tubau JF, et al: Dipyridamole thallium-201 scintigraphy as a preoperative screening test. A reexamination of its predictive potential. Circulation 84:493, 1991.
24. McPhail NV, Ruddy TD, Barber GG, et al: Cardiac risk stratification using dipyridamole myocardial perfusion imaging and ambulatory ECG monitoring prior to vascular surgery. Eur J Vasc Surg 7:151, 1993.
25. Eagle KA, Coley CM, Newell JB, et al: Combining clinical and thallium data optimizes preoperative assessment of cardiac risk before major vascular surgery. Ann Intern Med 110:859, 1989.
26. Golden MA, Whittemore AD, Donaldson MC, Mannick JA: Selective evaluation and management of coronary artery disease in patients undergoing repair of abdominal aortic aneurysms. A 16-year experience. Ann Surg 212:415, 1990.
27. Strawn DJ, Guernsey JM: Dipyridamole thallium scanning in the evaluation of coronary artery disease in elective abdominal aortic surgery. Arch Surg 126:880, 1991.
28. Cambria RP, Brewster DC, Abbott WM, et al: The impact of selective use of dipyridamole-thallium scans and surgical factors on the current morbidity of aortic surgery. J Vasc Surg 15:43, 1992.
29. Kresowik TF, Bower TR, Garner SA, et al: Dipyridamole thallium imaging in patients being considered for vascular procedures. Arch Surg 128:299, 1993.
30. Suggs WD, Smith RB III, Weintraub WS, et al: Selective screening for coronary artery disease in patients undergoing elective repair of abdominal aortic aneurysms. J Vasc Surg 18:349, 1993.
31. Bry JDL, Belkin M, O'Donnell TF Jr, et al: An assessment of the positive predictive value and cost-effectiveness of dipyridamole myocardial scintigraphy in patients undergoing vascular surgery. J Vasc Surg 19:112, 1994.
32. Baron J-F, Mundler O, Bertrand M, et al: Dipyridamole-thallium scintigraphy and gated radionuclide angiography to assess cardiac risk before abdominal aortic surgery. N Engl J Med 330: 663, 1994.
33. Lette J, Waters D, Lapointe J, et al: Usefulness of the severity and extent of reversible perfusion defects during thallium-dipyridamole imaging for cardiac risk assessment before noncardiac surgery. Am J Cardiol 64:276, 1989.
34. Levinson JR, Boucher CA, Coley CM, et al: Usefulness of semiquantitative analysis of dipyridamole-thallium-201 redistribution for improving risk stratification before vascular surgery. Am J Cardiol 66:406, 1990.
35. Lette J, Waters D, Cerino M, et al: Preoperative coronary artery disease risk stratification based on dipyridamole imaging and a simple three-step, three-segment model for patients undergoing noncardiac vascular surgery or major general surgery. Am J Cardiol 69:1553, 1992.
36. Pasternack PF, Imparato AM, Bear G, et al: The value of radionuclide angiography as a predictor of perioperative myocardial infarction in patients undergoing abdominal aortic aneurysm resection. J Vasc Surg 1:320, 1984.
37. Pasternack PF, Imparato AM, Riles TS, et al: The value of the radionuclide angiogram in the prediction of perioperative myocardial infarction in patients undergoing lower extremity revascularization procedures. Circulation 72:II-13, 1985.
38. Kazmers A, Cerqueira MD, Zierler RE: The role of preoperative radionuclide ejection fraction in direct abdominal aortic aneurysm repair. J Vasc Surg 8:128, 1988.
39. McCann RL, Wolfe WG: Resection of abdominal aortic aneurysm in patients with low ejection fractions. J Vasc Surg 10:240, 1989.
40. Franco CD, Goldsmith J, Veith FJ, et al: Resting gated pool ejection fraction: A poor predictor of perioperative myocardial infarction in patients undergoing vascular surgery for infrainguinal bypass grafting. J Vasc Surg 10:656, 1989.
41. Raby KE, Goldman L, Creager MA, et al: Correlation between preoperative ischemia and major cardiac events after peripheral vascular surgery. N Engl J Med 321:1296, 1989.
42. Pasternack PF, Grossi EA, Baumann FG, et al: The value of silent myocardial ischemia monitoring in the prediction of perioperative myocardial infarction in patients undergoing peripheral vascular surgery. J Vasc Surg 10:617, 1989.
43. Mangano DT, Browner WS, Hollenberg M, et al: Association of perioperative myocardial ischemia with cardiac morbidity and mortality in men undergoing noncardiac surgery. N Engl J Med 323:1781, 1990.
44. Fleisher LA, Rosenbaum SH, Nelson AH, Barash PG: The predictive value of preoperative silent ischemia for postoperative ischemic cardiac events in vascular and nonvascular surgery patients. Am Heart J 122:980, 1991.
45. Kirwin JD, Ascer E, Gennaro M, et al: Silent myocardial ischemia is not predictive of myocardial infarction in peripheral vascular surgery patients. Ann Vasc Surg 7:27, 1993.
46. Lalka SG, Sawada SG, Dalsing MC, et al: Dobutamine stress echocardiography as a predictor of cardiac events associated with aortic surgery. J Vasc Surg 15:831, 1992.
47. Poldermans D, Fioretti PM, Forster T, et al: Dobutamine stress echocardiography for assessment of perioperative cardiac risk in patients undergoing major vascular surgery. Circulation 87:1506, 1993.
48. Eichelberger JP, Schwarz KQ, Black ER, et al: Predictive value of dobutamine echocardiography just before noncardiac vascular surgery. Am J Cardiol 72:602, 1993.
49. Dávila-Román VG, Waggoner AD, Sicard GA, et al: Dobutamine stress echocardiography predicts surgical outcome in patients with an aortic aneurysm and peripheral vascular disease. J Am Coll Cardiol 21:957, 1993.
50. Langan EM III, Youkey JR, Franklin DP, et al: Dobutamine stress echocardiography for cardiac risk assessment before aortic surgery. J Vasc Surg 18:905, 1993.
51. Hertzer NR: Basic data concerning associated coronary disease in peripheral vascular patients. Ann Vasc Surg 1:616, 1987.
52. Rihal CS, Gersh BJ, Whisnant JP, et al: Influence of coronary artery disease on morbidity and mortality after carotid endarterectomy: A population-based study in Olmsted County, Minnesota (1970–1988). J Am Coll Cardiol 19:1254, 1992.
53. Roger VL, Ballard DJ, Hallett JW Jr, et al: Influence of coronary artery disease on morbidity and mortality after abdominal aortic aneurysmectomy: A population-based study, 1971–1987. J Am Coll Cardiol 14:1245, 1989.
54. Farkouh ME, Rihal CS, Gersh BJ, et al: Influence of coronary heart disease on morbidity and mortality after lower extremity revascularization surgery: A population-based study in Olmsted County, Minnesota (1970–1987). J Am Coll Cardiol 24:1290, 1994.
55. Yeager RA, Moneta GL, Edwards JM, et al: Late survival after perioperative myocardial infarction complicating vascular surgery. J Vasc Surg 20:598, 1994.
56. Rihal CS, Eagle KA, Mickel MC, et al: Surgical therapy for coronary artery disease among patients with combined coronary artery and peripheral vascular disease. Circulation 91:46, 1995.
57. Roizen MF: Anesthetic implications of concurrent diseases. In Miller RD (ed): Anesthesia, 4th ed. New York, Churchill Livingstone, 1994, p 903.
58. Mangano DT: Perioperative cardiac morbidity. Anesthesiology 72:153, 1990.
59. Gersh BJ, Rihal CS, Rooke TW, Ballard DJ: Evaluation and management of patients with both peripheral vascular and coronary artery disease. J Am Coll Cardiol 18:203, 1991.
60. Fleisher LA, Barash PG: Preoperative cardiac evaluation for noncardiac surgery: A functional approach. Anesth Analg 74: 586, 1992.
61. Weitz HH: Cardiac risk stratification prior to vascular surgery. Med Clin North Am 77:377, 1993.
62. Maziak DE, Ralph-Edwards AC, Deitel M, Wooster DL: Preoperative cardiac evaluation of the patient with vascular disease. Can J Surg 37:95, 1994.

63. Reul GJ Jr, Cooley DA, Duncan JM, et al: The effect of coronary bypass on the outcome of peripheral vascular operations in 1093 patients. J Vasc Surg 3:788, 1986.
64. O'Connor MS, Licina MG, Kraenzler EJ, et al: Perioperative management and outcome of patients having cardiac surgery combined with abdominal aortic aneurysm resection. J Cardiothorac Vasc Anesth 8:519, 1994.
65. Blackbourne LH, Tribble CG, Langenburg SE, et al: Optimal timing of abdominal aortic aneurysm repair after coronary artery revascularization. Ann Surg 219:693, 1994.
66. Birkmeyer JD, O'Connor GT, Quinton HB, et al: The effect of peripheral vascular disease on in-hospital mortality rates with coronary artery bypass surgery. J Vasc Surg 21:445, 1995.
67. Finkler SA: The distinction between cost and charges. Ann Intern Med 96:102, 1982.
68. Udvarhelyi IS, Colditz GA, Rai A, Epstein AM: Cost-effectiveness and cost-benefit analyses in the medical literature. Are the methods being used correctly? Ann Intern Med 116:238, 1992.
69. Weinstein MC, Fineberg HV: Clinical Decision Analysis. Philadelphia, WB Saunders Co, 1980.
70. Pauker SG, Kassirer JP: Decision analysis. N Engl J Med 316: 250, 1987.
71. Petitti DB: Meta-Analysis, Decision Analysis, and Cost-Effectiveness Analysis. Methods for Quantitative Synthesis in Medicine. New York, Oxford University Press, 1994.
72. Franklin C: Basic concepts and fundamental issues in technology assessment. Intensive Care Med 19:117, 1993.
73. Weinstein MC, Stason WB: Foundations of cost-effectiveness analysis for health and medical practices. N Engl J Med 296: 716, 1977.
74. Doubilet P, Weinstein MC, McNeil BJ: Use and misuse of the term "cost effective" in medicine. N Engl J Med 314:253, 1986.
75. Detsky AS, Naglie IG: A clinician's guide to cost-effectiveness analysis. Ann Intern Med 113:147, 1990.
76. Fuchs VR, Garber AM: The new technology assessment. N Engl J Med 323:673, 1990.
77. Riegelman RK: The Measures of Medicine. Benefits, Harms, and Costs. Cambridge, MA, Blackwell Science, 1995.
78. Robinson R: What does it mean? BMJ 307:670, 1993.
79. Eddy DM: Designing a practice policy. Standards, guidelines, and options. JAMA 263:3077, 1990.
80. Shomaker TS: Practice policies in anesthesia: A foretaste of practice in the 21st century. Anesth Analg 80:388, 1995.
81. Sackett DL, Haynes RB, Guyatt GH, Tugwell P: Clinical Epidemiology: A Basic Science for Clinical Medicine, 2nd ed. Boston, Little, Brown & Co, 1991.
82. Ingelfinger JA, Mosteller F, Thibodeau LA, Ware JH: Biostatistics in Clinical Medicine, 3rd ed. New York, McGraw-Hill, 1994.
83. Goldman L: Cardiac risk in noncardiac surgery: An update. Anesth Analg 80:810, 1995.
84. Rozanski A, Diamond GA, Berman D, et al: The declining specificity of exercise radionuclide ventriculography. N Engl J Med 309:518, 1983.
85. Fleisher LA, Skolnick ED, Holroyd KJ: Coronary artery revascularization before abdominal aortic aneurysm surgery: A decision analytic approach. Anesth Analg 79:661, 1994.
86. Goldman L, Caldera DL, Nussbaum SR, et al: Multifactorial index of cardiac risk in noncardiac surgical procedures. N Engl J Med 297:845, 1977.
87. Detsky AS, Abrams HB, McLaughlin JR, et al: Predicting cardiac complications in patients undergoing non-cardiac surgery. J Gen Intern Med 1:211, 1986.
88. Detsky AS, Abrams HB, Forbath N, et al: Cardiac assessment for patients undergoing noncardiac surgery. A multifactorial clinical risk index. Arch Intern Med 146:2131, 1986.
89. Taylor LM Jr, Yeager RA, Moneta GL, et al: The incidence of perioperative myocardial infarction in general vascular surgery. J Vasc Surg 15:52, 1991.
90. Roizen MF, Toledano A: Technology assessment and the "learning contamination" bias (Editorial). Anesth Analg 79:410, 1994.
91. Diamond GA, Denton TA: Alternative perspectives on the biased foundations of medical technology assessment. Ann Intern Med 118:455, 1993.
92. CASS Principal Investigators and Their Associates: Coronary Artery Surgery Study (CASS): A randomized trial of coronary artery bypass surgery. Survival data. Circulation 68:939, 1983.
93. Simes J: Meta-analysis: Its importance in cost-effectiveness studies. Med J Aust 153(Suppl):S13, 1993.
94. Cohen DJ, Breall JA, Ho KKL, et al: Evaluating the potential cost-effectiveness of stenting as a treatment for symptomatic single-vessel coronary disease. Use of a decision-analytic model. Circulation 89:1859, 1994.
95. Spackman TN: A theoretical evaluation of cost-effectiveness of pulmonary artery catheters in patients undergoing coronary artery surgery. J Cardiothorac Vasc Anesth 8:570, 1994.
96. Patterson RE, Eisner RL, Horowitz SF: Comparison of cost-effectiveness and utility of exercise ECG, single photon emission computed tomography, positron emission tomography, and coronary angiography for diagnosis of coronary artery disease. Circulation 91:54, 1995.
97. Richardson WS, Detsky AS, for the Evidence-Based Medicine Working Group: Users' guides to the medical literature. VII. How to use a clinical decision analysis. A. Are the results of the study valid? JAMA 273:1292, 1995.
98. Richardson WS, Detsky AS, for the Evidence-Based Medicine Working Group: Users' guides to the medical literature. VII. How to use a clinical decision analysis. B. What are the results and will they help me in caring for my patients? JAMA 273: 1610, 1995.
99. Felson DT: Bias in meta-analytic research. J Clin Epidemiol 45: 885, 1992.
100. Boden WE: Meta-analysis in clinical trials reporting: Has a tool become a weapon (Editorial)? Am J Cardiol 69:681, 1992.
101. Mantha S: Duplicate publications (Letter). J Cardiothorac Vasc Anesth 9:349, 1995.
102. DerSimonian R, Laird N: Meta-analysis in clinical trials. Control Clin Trials 7:177, 1986.
103. Eddy DM, Hasselbald V, Shachter R: Meta-analysis by the Confidence Profile Method. The Statistical Synthesis of Evidence. Boston, Academic Press, 1992.
104. Irwig L, Tosteson ANA, Gatsonis C, et al: Guidelines for meta-analyses evaluating diagnostic tests. Ann Intern Med 120:667, 1994.
105. Goel V and the Health Services Research Group: Decision analysis: Applications and limitations. Can Med Assoc J 147:413, 1992.
106. Feinstein AR: Clinical judgment revisited: The distraction of quantitative models. Ann Intern Med 120:799, 1994.
107. Thys DM: Can our patients afford the cost of cost containment (Editorial)? J Cardiothorac Vasc Anesth 8:487, 1994.
108. Roizen MF: Preoperative evaluation of vascular patients: Are the benefits worth the cost? (Letter). J Cardiothorac Vasc Anesth 7: 645, 1993.
109. Berlauk JF, Abrams JH, Gilmour IJ, et al: Preoperative optimization of cardiovascular hemodynamics improves outcome in peripheral vascular surgery. A prospective, randomized clinical trial. Ann Surg 214:289, 1991.
110. Rao TLK, Jacobs KH, El-Etr AA: Reinfarction following anesthesia in patients with myocardial infarction. Anesthesiology 59: 499, 1983.
111. Goldman L: Cost awareness in medicine. In Isselbacher KJ, Braunwald E, Wilson JD, et al (eds): Harrison's Principles of Internal Medicine, 13th ed. New York, McGraw-Hill, 1994, p 38.
112. Midgette AS, Wong JB, Beshansky JR, et al: Cost-effectiveness of streptokinase for acute myocardial infarction: A combined meta-analysis and decision analysis of the effects of infarct location and of likelihood of infarction. Med Decis Making 14: 108, 1994.
113. Pryor DB, Shaw L, McCants CB, et al: Value of the history and physical in identifying patients at increased risk for coronary artery disease. Ann Intern Med 118:81, 1993.
114. MacIsaac AI, Thomas JD, Topol EJ: Toward the quiescent coronary plaque. J Am Coll Cardiol 22:1228, 1993.
115. Beck JR, Pauker SG: The Markov process in medical prognosis. Med Decis Making 3:419, 1983.
116. Sonnenberg FA, Beck JR: Markov models in medical decision making: A practical guide. Med Decis Making 13:322, 1993.

117. Kaul S: Technical, economic, interpretative, and outcomes issues regarding utilization of cardiac imaging techniques in patients with known or suspected coronary artery disease. Am J Cardiol 75:18D, 1995.
118. American College of Cardiology/American Heart Association Task Force on Practice Guidelines (Committee on Perioperative Cardiovascular Evaluation for Noncardiac Surgery): Guidelines for perioperative cardiovascular evaluation for noncardiac surgery. Circulation 93:1278, 1996.
119. Iskandrian AS, Heo J: Optimizing patient selection for coronary angiography. Am J Cardiol 75:14D, 1995.
120. Schulman P: Bayes' theorem—a review. Cardiol Clin 2:319, 1984.
121. Tuman KJ, McCarthy RJ, March RJ, et al: Effects of epidural anesthesia and analgesia on coagulation and outcome after major vascular surgery. Anesth Analg 73:696, 1991.
122. Rosenfeld BA, Beattie C, Christopherson R, et al: The effects of different anesthetic regimens on fibrinolysis and the development of postoperative arterial thrombosis. Anesthesiology 79: 435, 1993.
123. Gibbs NM, Crawford GPM, Michalopoulos N: Thrombelastographic patterns following abdominal aortic surgery. Anaesth Intensive Care 22:534, 1994.
124. Gelman S: The pathophysiology of aortic cross-clamping and unclamping. Anesthesiology 82:1026, 1995.
125. Szilagyi DE, Smith RF, DeRusso FJ, et al: Contribution of abdominal aortic aneurysmectomy to prolongation of life. Ann Surg 164:678, 1966.
126. Whittemore AD, Clowes AW, Hechtman HB, Mannick JA: Aortic aneurysm repair. Reduced operative mortality associated with maintenance of optimal cardiac performance. Ann Surg 192:414, 1980.
127. Crawford ES, Saleh SA, Babb JW III, et al: Infrarenal abdominal aortic aneurysm. Factors influencing survival after operation performed over a 25-year period. Ann Surg 193:699, 1981.
128. Benefiel DJ, Roizen MF, Lampe GH, et al: Morbidity after aortic surgery with sufentanil vs isoflurane anesthesia (Abstract). Anesthesiology 65:A516, 1986.
129. Johnston KW: Multicenter prospective study of nonruptured abdominal aortic aneurysm. Part II. Variables predicting morbidity and mortality. J Vasc Surg 9:437, 1989.
130. Krupski WC, Layug EL, Reilly LM, et al: Comparison of cardiac morbidity rates between aortic and infrainguinal operations: Two-year follow-up. Study of Perioperative Ischemia Research Group. J Vasc Surg 18:609, 1993.
131. Lachapelle K, Graham AM, Symes JF: Does the clinical evaluation of the cardiac status predict outcome in patients with abdominal aortic aneurysms? J Vasc Surg 15:964, 1992.
132. L'Italien GJ, Cambria RP, Cutler BS, et al: Comparative early and late cardiac morbidity among patients requiring different vascular surgery procedures. J Vasc Surg 21:935, 1995.
133. Ellis JE, Drijvers G, Pedlow S, et al: Premedication with oral and transdermal clonidine provides safe and efficacious postoperative sympatholysis. Anesth Analg 79:1133, 1994.
134. Pasternack PF, Grossi EA, Baumann FG, et al: Beta blockade to decrease silent myocardial ischemia during peripheral vascular surgery. Am J Surg 158:113, 1989.
135. Liu S, Carpenter RL, Neal JM: Epidural anesthesia and analgesia. Their role in postoperative outcome. Anesthesiology 82: 1474, 1995.
136. Edwards ND, Reilly CS: Detection of perioperative myocardial ischaemia. Br J Anaesth 72:104, 1994.
137. Raby KE, Barry J, Creager MA, et al: Detection and significance of intraoperative and postoperative myocardial ischemia in peripheral vascular surgery. JAMA 268:222, 1992.
138. Landesberg G, Luria MH, Cotev S, et al: Importance of long-duration postoperative ST-segment depression in cardiac morbidity after vascular surgery. Lancet 341:715, 1993.
139. Bunt TJ: The role of a defined protocol for cardiac risk assessment in decreasing perioperative myocardial infarction in vascular surgery. J Vasc Surg 15:626, 1992.
140. Landau C, Lange RA, Hillis LD: Percutaneous transluminal coronary angioplasty. N Engl J Med 330:981, 1994.
141. Practice guidelines for pulmonary artery catheterization. A report by the American Society of Anesthesiologists Task Force on Pulmonary Artery Catheterization. Anesthesiology 78:380, 1993.
142. Hamm CW, Reimers J, Ischinger T, et al: A randomized study of coronary angioplasty compared with bypass surgery in patients with symptomatic multivessel coronary disease. N Engl J Med 331:1037, 1994.
143. O'Keefe JH Jr, Barnhart CS, Bateman TM: Comparison of stress echocardiography and stress myocardial perfusion scintigraphy for diagnosing coronary artery disease and assessing its severity. Am J Cardiol 75:25D, 1995.
144. Krumholz HM, Pasternak RC, Weinstein MC, et al: Cost effectiveness of thrombolytic therapy with streptokinase in elderly patients with suspected acute myocardial infarction. N Engl J Med 327:7, 1992.
145. Oster G, Huse DM, Lacey MJ, Epstein AM: Cost-effectiveness of ticlopidine in preventing stroke in high-risk patients. Stroke 25:1149, 1994.
146. Lette J, Carini G, Tatum JL, et al: Safety of dipyridamole testing in patients with cerebrovascular disease. Am J Cardiol 75:535, 1995.
147. McNeill AJ, Fioretti PM, El-Said EM, et al: Enhanced sensitivity for detection of coronary artery disease by addition of atropine to dobutamine stress echocardiography. Am J Cardiol 70:41, 1992.
148. Kiat H, Berman DS, Maddahi J, et al: Late reversibility of tomographic myocardial thallium-201 defects: An accurate marker of myocardial viability. J Am Coll Cardiol 12:1456, 1988.
149. Chin W, Go R, Lenehan S, Underwood DA: Failure of dipyridamole-thallium myocardial imaging to detect severe coronary disease. Cleve Clin J Med 56:587, 1989.
150. Fleisher LA, Nelson AH, Rosenbaum SH: Failure of negative dipyridamole thallium scans to predict perioperative myocardial ischaemia and infarction. Can J Anaesth 39:179, 1992.
151. Whiting JH Jr, Datz FL, Gabor FV, et al: Cerebrovascular accident associated with dipyridamole thallium-201 myocardial imaging: Case report. J Nucl Med 34:128, 1993.
152. Picano E, Mathias W Jr, Pingitore A, Previtali M, on behalf of the Echo Dobutamine International Cooperative: Safety and tolerability of dobutamine-atropine stress echocardiography: A prospective, multicenter study. Lancet 344:1190, 1994.
153. Mangano DT, Layug EL, Wallace A, Tateo I: Effect of Atenolol on mortality and cardiovascular morbidity after noncardiac surgery. N Engl J Med 335:1713, 1996.
154. Boucher CA, Brewster DC, Darling RC, et al: Determination of cardiac risk by dipyridamole-thallium imaging before peripheral vascular surgery. N Engl J Med 312:389, 1985.
155. Leppo J, Plaja J, Gionet M, et al: Noninvasive evaluation of cardiac risk before elective vascular surgery. J Am Coll Cardiol 9:269, 1987.
156. Fletcher JP, Antico VF, Gruenewald S, Kershaw LZ: Dipyridamole-thallium scan for screening of coronary artery disease prior to vascular surgery. J Cardiovasc Surg 29:666, 1988.
157. McEnroe CS, O'Donnell TF, Yeager A, et al: Comparison of ejection fraction and Goldman risk factor analysis to dipyridamole-thallium 201 studies in the evaluation of cardiac morbidity after aortic aneurysm surgery. J Vasc Surg 11:497, 1990.
158. Makaroun MS, Shuman-Jackson N, Rippey A, et al: Cardiac risk in vascular surgery: the oral dipyridamole-thallium stress test. Arch Surg 125:1610, 1990.

CHAPTER 3

Pulmonary Function Testing

Douglas C. Johnson, M.D.
B. Taylor Thompson, M.D.

Pulmonary function testing (PFT) is very helpful in assessing patients with symptoms of dyspnea, cough, or wheezing; in guiding therapy and in following the course of patients with lung disease; and in evaluating preoperative patients. PFTs include spirometry, after bronchodilator spirometry, lung volume measurement (by helium dilution or plethysmography), single-breath diffusing capacity, and respiratory muscle forces. Measures of gas exchange include arterial blood gases and oximetry, which can be performed both at rest and with activity. Tests used less commonly include methacholine challenge testing, exercise testing, pulmonary compliance measurements, and determination of dead space and shunt.

Several pulmonary symptoms, and types of disease that can cause these symptoms, are listed in Table 3–1. Pulmonary function testing can differentiate among many of these diseases. There are characteristic PFT findings with emphysema, asthma, upper airway obstruction, cystic fibrosis, interstitial lung disease, restrictive lung disease without interstitial lung disease, and respiratory muscle weakness.

Spirometry

Spirometry is the basic screening pulmonary function test. Spirometry measures the volume and flow of air during inspiration and expiration. Measurements are typically made either with a spirometer, which moves as it fills with expired air, or with a device that measures gas flow as it comes out from the mouth. Recommended criteria for the equipment have been published.[1] Depending upon the device, flow is calculated from the rate of change of volume, or volume is calculated from the integrated flow. Volume and flow values must be corrected to body temperature pressure saturated (BTPS) units to reflect changes in the lung.

Spirometry is typically performed using a maximal expiratory effort after the subject has inspired completely. Several parameters are obtained from spirometry. The total volume of air expired is the forced vital capacity (FVC). The amount of air expired in the first second after extrapolated time zero[2] is the forced expired volume in 1 second (FEV_1). The FEV_1/FVC ratio and several flow rates are generally reported. These include the peak expiratory flow rate (PEFR), the average flow during the middle 50% of expired volume (the maximal mid expiratory flow [MMEF], and flows at 50 and 75% of expiration (FEF_{50} and FEF_{75}). The peak inspiratory flow rate (PIFR) is usually the only parameter reported for the maximal inspiratory effort.

There are standard guidelines for performing spirometry[1] which include performing multiple maneuvers, with FEV_1 and VC results ideally reproducible to within 5%. The best values for FEV_1, VC, PEFR, and PIFR are reported, with other flows determined from the best effort (usually the effort with the best sum of FEV_1 and FVC).

Normal values and their ranges have been established from studies with large groups of healthy subjects with multiple demographic characteristics. Predicted values are determined separately for males and females from regression equations using height and age. There are differences among racial groups, with predicted values for blacks generally 10 to 15% below those for whites of the same age, sex, and height.[3] The confidence intervals about the predicted values vary depending upon which test is being evaluated, and by age.

The flow-volume loop allows visual evaluation of flow in relation to volume throughout an expiratory and inspiratory maneuver (Fig. 3–1). Since many disease conditions limit volume and/or flow, interpretation of spirometry can suggest these diseases, and evaluate the degree of limitation. Flow-volume loop patterns are characteristic of certain types of lung disease.

Interstitial lung diseases (Fig. 3–2) have a characteristic appearance of the flow-volume loop due to the increased lung elastic recoil and lung restriction. There typically is a reduced vital capacity, but elevated flow rates relative to the expiratory volume, resulting in increased PEFR/VC and FEV_1/VC ratios. With early interstitial lung disease the PEFR may be above normal, while with progressive interstitial disease as the VC falls

TABLE 3–1
Pulmonary Symptoms and Associated Diseases

Shortness of breath
- Obstructive lung disease
- Restrictive lung disease
- Interstitial lung disease
- Respiratory muscle weakness
- Pulmonary vascular disease
- Cardiovascular disease

Cough
- Obstructive lung disease
- Interstitial lung disease
- Lung cancer
- Infection

Wheezing
- Obstructive lung disease (asthma, COPD, cystic fibrosis, upper airway obstruction)
- Vocal cord dysfunction

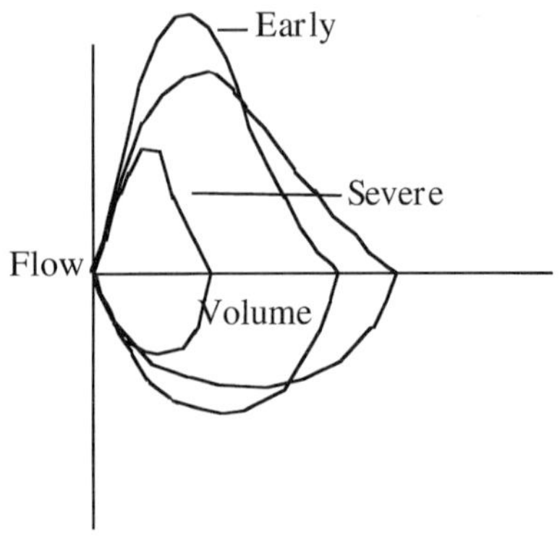

FIGURE **3–2.** Interstitial lung disease (ILD) flow-volume loops with early and with severe ILD. Other PFT findings with ILD include spirometry, $\downarrow$ VC, preserved or elevated flows, $\uparrow$ FEV$_1$/VC; lung volumes, reduced; DLco, reduced; ABG, hypoxia with exercise or if severe ILD, P_{CO_2} usually $\downarrow$ or normal unless severe disease.

there are reductions in the PEFR and FEV$_1$. Restrictive lung diseases due to pleural or chest wall abnormality (Fig. 3–3) have reduced VC, but flow rates are not increased, since lung elastic recoil is normal.

Upper airway obstruction (Fig. 3–4) yields a distinctive appearance of the flow-volume loop with a plateau in the inspiratory and/or expiratory flow. Since the extrathoracic upper airway tends to open during expiration and close during inspiration, extrathoracic upper airway obstruction limits inspiratory flows more than expiratory flows. The relative reduction is reversed with intrathoracic upper airway obstruction; during expiration the pressure is less in the airway than outside the airway, narrowing the airway and reducing flows. Obstruction in a mainstem bronchus yields the appearance of a normal appearing loop for the first half of the vital capacity, then a plateau followed by the expected reduction of flows related to small airway resistance and reduced lung elastic recoil at lower lung volumes.

Other obstructive lung diseases include asthma and chronic obstructive pulmonary disease (COPD). Flow rates, particularly expiratory flow rates, are reduced in both asthma (Fig. 3–5) and COPD (Fig. 3–6) leading to reductions in FEV$_1$ and FEV$_1$/FVC. With more significant obstruction, FVC falls as well. Response to bronchodilator and the single-breath diffusing capacity of carbon monoxide (DLco) results can help differentiate between asthma (reversible and relatively normal DLco) and COPD/emphysema (not as reversible and low DLco).

Bronchodilator spirometry assesses whether there is an acute improvement in flows following administration of a bronchodilator, usually of an inhaled β-agonist. Significant improvement in FEV$_1$, FVC, and flow rates indicate that bronchodilator therapy should help the patient. Improvement to bronchodilator, often to normal values, is characteristic of asthma. Improvement to bronchodilator, but to below normal values, is common with COPD (many patients who benefit from long-term bronchodilator therapy may not show a significant response to acute inhalation of a β-agonist).

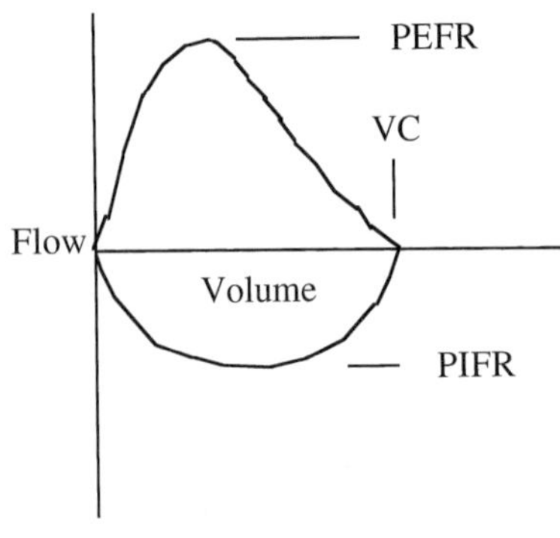

FIGURE **3–1.** Normal flow-volume loop, showing a maximal expiratory effort from total lung capacity followed by a maximal inspiratory effort. PEFR, peak expiratory flow rate; PIFR, peak inspiratory flow rate; VC, vital capacity.

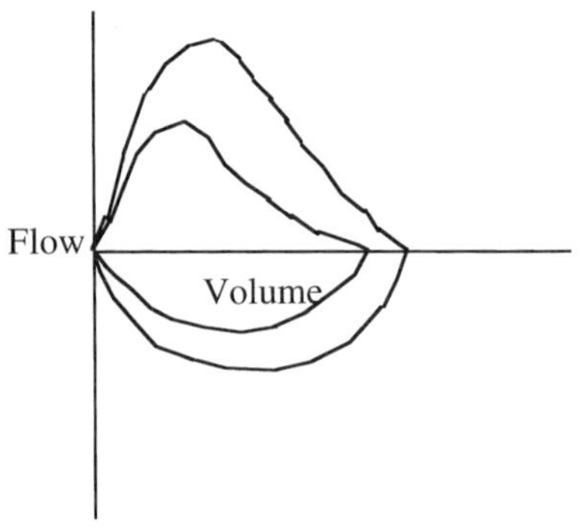

FIGURE **3–3.** Restrictive lung disease due to pleural or chest wall abnormality flow-volume loop. Other PFT findings include spirometry, $\downarrow$ VC and therefore $\downarrow$ FEV$_1$, flows preserved but not elevated; lung volumes, reduced; DLco, mildly reduced, with elevated DLco/lung volume; ABG, normal unless severe disease.

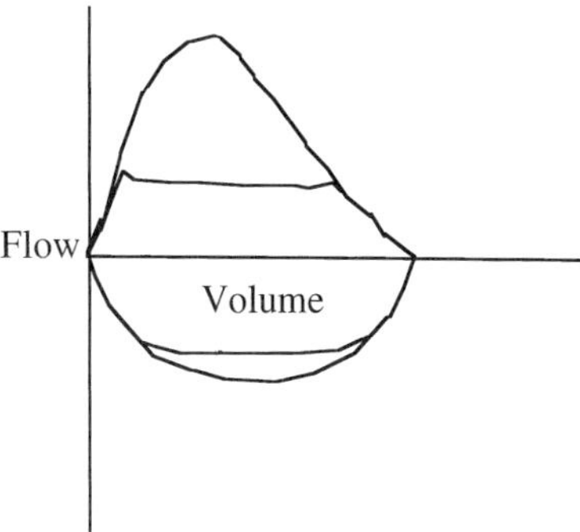

FIGURE **3–4.** Upper airway obstruction flow-volume loop. Other PFT findings include spirometry, ↓ peak flows, expiratory plateau with intrathoracic obstruction, inspiratory plateau with extrathoracic obstruction, ↑ FEV_1/PEFR; lung volumes, normal; DLco, normal.

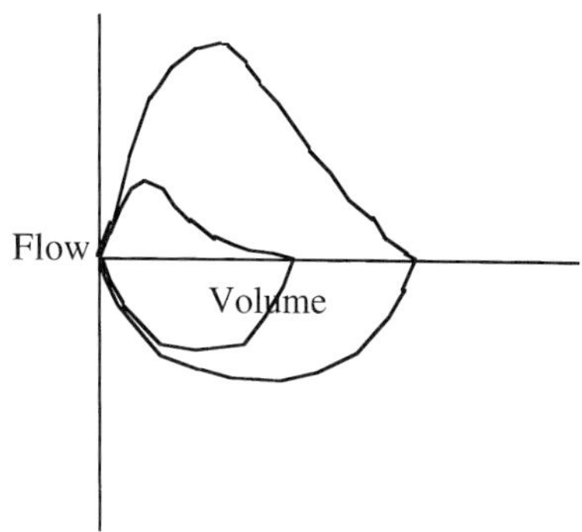

FIGURE **3–6.** COPD flow-volume loop. Other PFT findings with COPD include spirometry, ↓ flows, ↓ FEV_1, ↓ FEV_1/VC, lower expiratory than inspiratory flows; lung volumes, ↑ TLC; DLco, reduced; ABG, often hypoxia, ↑ P_{CO_2} in some with severe COPD.

Lung Volumes

The lung volume is determined by a balance of the lung, the chest wall, the diaphragm, and the respiratory muscles. While most interstitial lung diseases reduce lung volumes, most obstructive lung diseases increase lung volumes. Upper airway obstruction should not affect lung volumes.

The total lung capacity (TLC) is the lung volume after a maximal inhalation, the functional lung capacity (FRC) is the volume at the end of a normal exhalation, and the residual volume (RV) is the volume after a maximal exhalation (Fig. 3–7). The expiratory reserve volume (ERV) is the difference between the FRC and RV. The two standard techniques of measuring FRC are helium dilution and plethysmography.

Helium dilution can determine lung volume, since helium is not absorbed by the lung. The lung volume can be determined from the initial volume (V_1) and the concentrations of helium before (C_1) and after (C_2) equilibration with the lung:

$$V_1 \times C_1 = (V_1 + V_{lung}) \times C_2$$

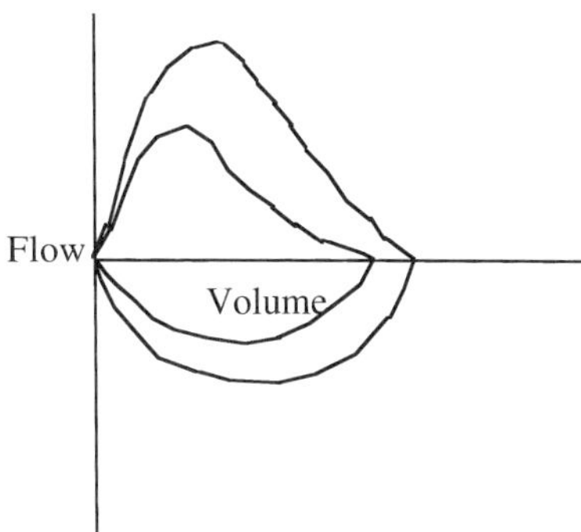

FIGURE **3–5.** Asthma flow-volume loop. Other PFT findings with asthma include spirometry, ↓ flows, ↓ FEV_1, ↓ FEV_1/VC, improvement with bronchodilator; lung volumes, ↑ TLC; DLco, normal; ABG, hypoxia if severe, ↑ P_{CO_2} only if very severe; methacholine challenge test, positive (even if mild asthma).

It is important to absorb carbon dioxide (CO_2), add oxygen (O_2) to keep the volume constant, mix the gas during testing, and wait sufficient time for equilibration. Insufficient equilibration time, which is more common in severely obstructed patients, will lead to underestimation of the lung volume.

Plethysmography depends upon the concept of Boyle's law—that $P_1 \times V_1 = P_2 \times V_2$. With the subject in an enclosed box breathing into a mouthpiece, a shutter is closed when the lung volume is at FRC. During panting against the closed mouthpiece, with inspiration the pressure in the lung becomes lower (ΔP) and the lung expands. With lung expansion, the pressure in the box increases. Since the volume of air in the box is known, the amount of lung expansion (ΔV) can be calculated from the box pressure change. Other types of plethysmography use other techniques to determine the change in lung volume. The initial pressure (P_1) is atmospheric. The pressure at the mouth is measured and assumed to reflect the pressure throughout the lung. Therefore the equation $P_1 \times V_1 = (P_1 + \Delta P) \times (V_1 + \Delta V)$ can be solved for V_1, the lung volume at which the mouth shutter was closed. With significant airway obstruction, pressure changes at the mouth may underestimate the pressure changes in the lung. This will lead to overestimation of lung volume. This problem can be reduced by having

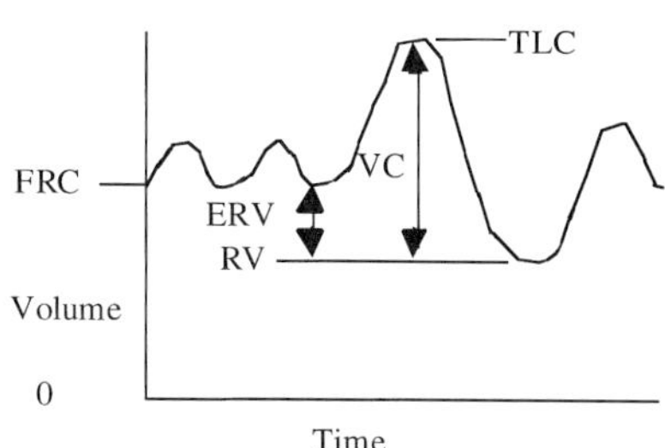

FIGURE **3–7.** Lung volumes, showing tidal breathing, then inspiration to TLC, then expiration to RV, then tidal breathing. ERV, expiratory reserve volume; FRC, functional residual capacity; RV, residual volume; TLC, total lung capacity; VC, vital capacity.

the subject pant more slowly (e.g., once per second), with the lower flow rates within the lung reducing any pressure differences between the lung and the mouth.

Once the FRC is determined by either helium dilution or plethysmography, the RV is calculated by subtracting the ERV from the FRC, and TLC is calculated by adding the VC to the RV.

Diffusing Capacity

The transfer of gas across the blood-gas barrier occurs by diffusion. The rate of this transfer is called the diffusing capacity. The diffusing capacity is lowered in conditions that damage or destroy alveoli such as emphysema, block off the pulmonary circulation such as pulmonary embolism, or cause scarring in the lung parenchyma such as interstitial lung diseases. Both anemia[4] and reduced lung volumes[5] lower DLco, but their effects can be accounted for by determining the predicted DLco for the patient's hemoglobin and lung volume. Pulmonary hemorrhage can elevate DLco.[6] Patients with asthma who have airway obstruction but normal alveoli and pulmonary capillaries have a normal or elevated DLco. The diffusing capacity is especially useful to assess lung function in interstitial lung diseases, and in differentiating asthma from emphysema.

The DLco provides a measure of the ability of the lung to take up O_2, since the diffusing capacity of O_2 is about 1.23 times that for CO. The diffusing capacity of any gas is the rate of uptake divided by the pressure gradient of the gas. For most gases, it is very difficult or impossible to know the pressure gradient from alveolus to blood, because the pressure in blood changes rapidly as the blood moves through the pulmonary capillary. CO, however, is very tightly bound by hemoglobin, resulting in a very low back-pressure of CO. Ignoring the back-pressure, the DLco equals the rate of CO uptake divided by the alveolar CO pressure.

For the single-breath technique, the subject expires to RV, breathes in to TLC a mixture of helium and CO, holds his breath for about 10 seconds, and then expires.[7] A sample of gas is collected during exhalation after an initial volume is discarded. The concentrations of CO and helium are measured in the inspired and expired samples. From these values and the inspired volume, one can calculate the lung volume (VA) in which the helium was distributed, the initial alveolar CO pressure, and the DLco. The DLco/VA or KCO is often reported as well. KCO changes even more than DLco with reductions in lung volume,[5] so it is important to use predicted values that account for lung volume.

Respiratory Muscle Forces

Respiratory muscle (diaphragm and chest wall) strength can be assessed by measuring the maximal pressures a subject can generate at different lung volumes. The pressures are typically evaluated at TLC, RV, and FRC. As the lung volume increases, the maximal inspiratory pressure (MIP) decreases, and maximal expiratory pressure (MEP) decreases. The pressures decrease with age, and are lower in females than in males.[8,9]

Arterial Blood Gases and Oximetry

Assessment of oxygenation is an important component in the evaluation of the patient with dyspnea. It is well documented that providing supplemental oxygen to hypoxemic patients with COPD leads to improved clinical status and survival,[10] so it is important to recognize and treat hypoxemia.

Oximetry measures the level of arterial hemoglobin saturation from fluctuations in transmission of different wavelengths of light through tissue. This process is an effective screening test for hypoxemia, with an O_2 saturation below 90% corresponding to a PO_2 below 60 mm Hg in patients with normal acid-base status. Oximetry is often used to determine whether desaturation occurs with activity or during sleeping.

There are five physiologic causes of hypoxemia. These include low inspired oxygen (e.g., high altitude), low alveolar O_2 due to elevated alveolar CO_2 (e.g., hypoventilation due to drug overdose), areas of the lung with low alveolar O_2 due to low ventilation-perfusion ($\dot{V}/\dot{Q}$) ratios, shunting of venous blood bypassing the pulmonary capillaries (e.g., pulmonary arteriovenous [AV] malformation), and severe reductions in diffusing capacity (e.g., severe interstitial lung disease). A low mixed venous PO_2, such as occurs with exercise, will worsen the arterial PO_2 if shunt or low DLco are present.

The alveolar PO_2 can be estimated from the inspired O_2, the alveolar PCO_2 (generally assumed equal to the arterial PCO_2), and the respiratory quotient (the ratio of CO_2 production to O_2 consumption). Increased gradients between alveolar and arterial PO_2 are expected with hypoxemia due to low $\dot{V}/\dot{Q}$, shunting, or low diffusing capacity; while normal gradients are expected with low inspired oxygen or elevated alveolar PCO_2. Breathing 100% O_2 will raise the alveolar PO_2 to high values throughout the lung, including those areas with low $\dot{V}/\dot{Q}$. Therefore, checking the PO_2 with the patient breathing 100% O_2 can differentiate between hypoxemia due to low $\dot{V}/\dot{Q}$ (fully corrected PO_2) or due to shunt (only partially corrected PO_2).

Arterial blood gas measures PO_2, PCO_2, and pH, thus providing information on oxygenation, ventilation, and acid-base status. The arterial PCO_2 is determined by a balance between CO_2 production and alveolar ventilation. Measurement of PCO_2 and pH enables interpretation of acid-base status. The normal PCO_2 is 40 mm Hg, and normal pH is 7.40. With acute changes in PCO_2, a fall of 0.08 pH units is expected for a 10-mm Hg rise in PCO_2. For chronic changes, the expected fall is 0.03 pH units for a 10-mm Hg rise in PCO_2. With primary metabolic changes, there is an expected rise in PCO_2 of 7 mm Hg for a 10-mEq/L rise in bicarbonate.

Methacholine Challenge Testing

Methacholine challenge testing is most commonly used to evaluate patients suspected of having asthma, but without significant airways obstruction on spirometry testing. Individuals with asthma typically experience a drop in their FEV_1 by more than 20% at inhaled nebulized methacholine concentrations of below 8 mg/ml, while only 3% of normals react below this dose.[11,12] Those with mild reactive airways may respond at below 16 mg/ml, while only 8% of normals respond below this dose. Most patients with moderate to severe COPD will have reactive airways as assessed by methacholine challenge testing.

Preoperative Pulmonary Testing

Postoperative pulmonary complications, including atelectasis, retained secretions, bronchitis, pneumonia, or progressive respiratory failure are important causes of morbidity and mortality following major surgery. These complications have been reported to occur in 3 to 20% of patients with normal preoperative vital capacities and 70% of those with a significantly reduced vital capacity. Ninety-five per cent of all postoperative pulmonary complications occur in patients with abnormal preoperative spirometry.[13,14]

Following upper abdominal and certain thoracic surgery, vital capacity is reduced 50%, functional residual capacity 20%, and expiratory reserve volume approximately 30%. Functional residual capacity falls below closing volume, leading to small airways collapse and atelectasis. Ventilatory patterns are also abnormal after upper abdominal and thoracic surgery, manifest by a 20% reduction in tidal volume and an increase in respiratory rate, with diminished sighs. In addition, reflex activation of expiratory musculature occurs, resulting in active expiration. The rapid, shallow ventilatory pattern with active expiration further reduces functional residual capacity and predisposes to atelectasis. Postoperative maneuvers to increase functional residual capacity, such as incentive spirometry or deep breathing exercises, have been shown in prospective studies to reduce postoperative pulmonary complications.[13–15]

The role of pulmonary function testing in screening patients for postoperative pulmonary complications is controversial. As noted above, spirometry is very sensitive in detecting a group of patients likely to suffer complications. However, spirometry is nonspecific, and many patients with abnormal preoperative spirometry undergo surgery without complications. Because of this lack of specificity, routine spirometry cannot be recommended for all patients undergoing high-risk surgical procedures. However, in patients with a history of cigarette smoking, chronic lung disease, or unexplained preoperative pulmonary symptoms (Table 3–1), pulmonary function testing is indicated to either define previously undiagnosed lung disease or to guide preoperative treatment of reversible forms of lung disease such as reactive airways disease.

Spirometry is indicated for all patients undergoing thoracic resection. When combined with regional studies of lung function (ventilation or perfusion lung scanning), spirometry allows for calculation of postoperative pulmonary function. Postoperative FEV_1 can be calculated by multiplying the preoperative FEV_1 times the percent of ventilation or perfusion in the uninvolved lung. Correlation coefficients of approximately .9 are obtained when the predicted postoperative FEV_1 is compared to the actual postoperative FEV_1. If preoperative pulmonary function testing and lung scanning predict a postoperative FEV_1 of less than 800 ml, thoracic resection is relatively contraindicated.[16] The predicted postoperative product of D_{LCO} and FEV_1 has recently been shown to be an even better predictor of mortality with thoracic resection.[17]

Recent studies have evaluated the relationship between an impaired cardiovascular response to stress and postoperative pulmonary complications. The surgical procedure per se along with postoperative physical therapy provide a cardiovascular stress requiring an increase in oxygen delivery. If the increase in O_2 consumption cannot be met, then an oxygen debt may occur, lactic acidosis may ensue, wound healing may be impaired, and multiple organ failure may develop should the added stress of postoperative infection develop. When $\dot{V}O_2max$ is below 12 ml/kg, postoperative complications and mortality are increased after major cardiac or thoracic surgery. Preoperative $\dot{V}O_2max$ can be measured directly by exercise testing with analysis of inhaled and exhaled gases or inferred by cycle ergometry at predetermined workloads. A simple exercise evaluation, such as asking the patient to climb two flights of stairs, has been shown in some studies to be very predictive of successful results of cardiothoracic surgery. Patients able to climb two flights of stairs (equivalent to an O_2 consumption of 16 ml/kg/min for a 70-kg man walking 20 steps/min) usually do well with cardiothoracic surgery.[18,19]

Summary

Spirometry, arterial blood gas analysis, regional measures of lung function including ventilation and perfusion lung scanning, and some measurement of exercise capacity are helpful to better characterize previously unidentified cardiopulmonary diseases preoperatively, to guide preoperative surgical preparation, and to identify at-risk patients for postoperative complications. Other than thoracic resection, routine screening of pulmonary function in asymptomatic nonsmokers is not indicated. However, in symptomatic patients or in patients with a prior smoking history, preoperative characterization of the patient's lung disease and cardiovascular limitation is indicated.

References

1. American Thoracic Society: Standardization of spirometry—1987 update. Am Rev Respir Dis 136:1285, 1987.

2. Gardner RM, Baker CD, Broennle AM, et al: ATS Statement—Snowbird workshop on standardization of spirometry. Am Rev Respir Physiol 33:367, 1979.
3. Ghio AJ, Crapo RO, Elliott CG: Reference equations used to predict pulmonary function. Chest 97:400, 1990.
4. Clark EH, Woods RL, Hughes JMB: Effect of blood transfusion on the carbon monoxide transfer factor of the lung in man. Clin Sci Mol Med 54:727, 1978.
5. Stam H, Hrachovina V, Stijnen T, Versprille A: Diffusing capacity dependent on lung volume and age in normal subjects. J Appl Physiol 76:2356, 1994.
6. Ewan PW, Jones HA, Rhodes CG, Hughes JMB: Detection of intrapulmonary hemorrhage with carbon monoxide uptake. N Engl J Med 295:1391, 1976.
7. American Thoracic Society: Single-breath carbon monoxide diffusing capacity (transfer factor): Recommendations for a standard technique—1995 update. Am J Respir Crit Care Med 152:2185, 1995.
8. Leech JA, Ghezzo H, Stevens D, Becklake MR: Respiratory pressures and function in young adults. Am Rev Respir Dis 128:17, 1983.
9. Enright PL, Kronmal RA, Manolio TA, et al: Respiratory muscle strength in the elderly: Correlates and reference values. Am J Respir Crit Care Med 149:430, 1994.
10. Nocturnal Oxygen Therapy Trial Group: Continuous or nocturnal oxygen therapy in hypoxemic chronic obstructive lung disease: A clinical trial. Ann Intern Med 93:391, 1980.
11. Juniper FE, Frith PA, Hargreave FE: Airway responsiveness to histamine and methacholine: Relationship to minimum treatment to control symptoms of asthma. Thorax 36:575, 1981.
12. Malo JC, Pineau L, Cartier A, Martin RR: Reference values of the provocative concentrations of methacholine that cause 6% and 20% changes in forced expiratory volume in one second in a normal population. Am Rev Respir Dis 128:8, 1983.
13. Tisi G: Preoperative evaluation of pulmonary function: Validity, indications and benefits. Am Rev Respir Dis 119:293, 1979.
14. Celli BR: What is the value of preoperative pulmonary function testing? Med Clin North Am 77:309, 1993.
15. Celli BR, Rodriguez KS, Snider GL: A controlled trial of intermittent positive pressure breathing, incentive spirometry and deep breathing exercises in preventing pulmonary complications after abdominal surgery. Am Rev Respir Dis 130:12, 1984.
16. Bria WF, Kanarek DJ, Kazemi H: Prediction of postoperative pulmonary function following thoracic operations. J Thorac Cardiovasc Surg 82:186, 1983.
17. Pierce RJ, Copland JM, Sharpe K, Barter CE: Preoperative risk evaluation for lung cancer resection: Predicted postoperative product as a predictor of surgical mortality. Am J Respir Crit Care Med 150:947, 1994.
18. Gilbrith EM, Weisman IM: Role of exercise stress testing in preoperative evaluation of patients for lung resection. Clin Chest Med 15:389, 1994.
19. Bollinger CT, Jordon P, Soler M, et al: Exercise capacity as a predictor of postoperative complications in lung resection candidates. Am J Respir Crit Care Med 151:1472, 1995.

CHAPTER 4

Preoperative Conditioning for the Thoracic Surgery Patient

Colleen M. Kigin M.S., M.P.A., P.T.
Lawrence P. Cahalin, M.A., P.T.

Substantial evidence in the last decade indicates that increased preoperative functional capacity and exercise tolerance can greatly reduce morbidity and mortality and improve functional outcome of thoracic surgery patients.[1–13] These benefits have been documented in individuals undergoing lung resection and pneumonectomy[1–13] and awaiting cardiac transplantation.[14]

Across the United States, many centers now provide interdisciplinary, integrated programs including preoperative evaluation and targeted preoperative conditioning for such patients. Preoperative evaluation often includes functional and conditioning evaluations done economically, yet offering a great deal of information regarding the patient's physical status and general ability to undergo the operative procedure.

This chapter will review the spectrum of preoperative evaluation and treatment programs that through prediction allow prevention of postoperative complications. The chapter will include some reference to immediate postoperative care and the need for postoperative conditioning to maximize functional outcomes.

Clearly, if conditioning is important to perioperative outcome, then measures of preoperative condition should correlate with outcome, and interventions that improve condition should improve outcome. While no direct evidence proves such, this chapter reviews the data that indicate such a hypothesis is likely to be found valid.

Preoperative Assessment

Evaluation of General Health

The Medical Outcomes Study Short-Form Health Survey (SF-36)

Obtaining data regarding the patient's functional status and general health prior to the initial clinic visit can be helpful in identifying patients at greater risk for peri- or postoperative complications. One such easily administered tool is the SF-36 questionnaire.[15]

The SF-36 is a 36-item questionnaire that evaluates eight related health profiles including physical functioning, social functioning, role limitations due to physical problems, role limitations due to emotional problems, mental health, energy/fatigue, bodily pain, and general health perception (Fig. 4–1).[15] Two summary scores of physical and mental health and the eight related health profile scores are calculated on a scale of 0 to 100 and reported as a percentage of the total possible score for the profile or summary score. The higher the score, the better the health in all of the categories except for bodily pain.[15–17]

The SF-36 was adapted from the Medical Outcomes Study Long-Form Health Status Scale[18] and the Medical Outcomes Study Short-Form (SF-20) Scale[15] and demonstrated a high degree of precision for measures that the Long-Form evaluated.[16] The SF-20 was found to be reliable in evaluating six health measures in 2,008 healthy subjects (range, 0.76 to 0.88) and in 11,186 patients (range, 0.81 to 0.88) with a variety of chronic medical conditions (hypertension, diabetes, congestive heart failure [CHF], recent myocardial infarction, and depression).[15] Subsequent studies of the precision and reliability of the SF-36 in healthy subjects and patients with chronic medical or psychiatric conditions have shown good levels of performance that were comparable to other measurement tools.[16,17] A recent study found all of the eight scales of the SF-36 to be valid measures that were highly correlated to psychometric testing of 22,462 patients with hypertension, diabetes, CHF, and recent myocardial infarction (MI).[18]

Although the SF-36 was not specifically developed for the thoracic surgery patient population, the patients who were studied suffered from chronic medical disorders similar, and in some instances, identical, to those encountered by patients requiring thoracic surgery. We have found the SF-36 to be a useful adjunct in the assessment and treatment of patients before and after thoracic surgery. The SF-36 has enabled us to identify patients with special physical and mental problems that have been addressed during specific treatment sessions (physical, social, or psychologic/psychiatric therapy). To

Health Status Profile — SF-36™

INSTRUCTIONS: This survey asks for your views about your health. This information will help keep track of how you feel and how well you are able to do your usual activities.

Answer every question by marking the appropriate oval. If you are unsure about how to answer a question, please give the best answer you can.

MARKING INSTRUCTIONS

- *Use a No. 2 Pencil ONLY.*
- *Make dark heavy marks that fill the oval completely*
- *Erase unwanted marks cleanly*
- *Make no stray marks on this answer sheet.*

PROPER MARK ⬭ ⬬ ⬭ IMPROPER MARKS

Before beginning this questionnaire...
Please print your ID number in the boxes to the right → and then fill in the appropriate oval next to each number. If you don't know your number, please ask the person who gave you this questionnaire.

ID NUMBER

ID										
	0	1	2	3	4	5	6	7	8	9
	0	1	2	3	4	5	6	7	8	9
	0	1	2	3	4	5	6	7	8	9
	0	1	2	3	4	5	6	7	8	9
	0	1	2	3	4	5	6	7	8	9
	0	1	2	3	4	5	6	7	8	9
	0	1	2	3	4	5	6	7	8	9
	0	1	2	3	4	5	6	7	8	9
	0	1	2	3	4	5	6	7	8	9
	0	1	2	3	4	5	6	7	8	9
	0	1	2	3	4	5	6	7	8	9

Now begin with the questions below.

1. In general, would you say your health is: (Mark only one.)

1. ① **Excellent**
2. ② **Very good**
3. ③ **Good**
4. ④ **Fair**
5. ⑤ **Poor**

2. **Compared to one year ago**, how would you rate your health in general now? (Mark only one.)

1. ① Much better now than 1 year ago
2. ② Somewhat better now than 1 year ago
3. ③ About the same as 1 year ago
4. ④ Somewhat worse now than 1 year ago
5. ⑤ Much worse now than 1 year ago

The following items are about activities you might do during a typical day. Does **your health now limit you** in these activities? If so, how much? (Mark one oval on each line.)

		Yes, Limited A Lot	Yes, Limited A Little	No, Not Limited At All
3. **Vigorous activities**, such as running, lifting heavy objects, participating in strenuous sports	3	1	2	3
4. **Moderate activities**, such as moving a table, pushing a vacuum cleaner, bowling, or playing golf	4	1	2	3
5. Lifting or carrying groceries	5	1	2	3
6. Climbing **several** flights of stairs	6	1	2	3
7. Climbing **one** flight of stairs	7	1	2	3
8. Bending, kneeling, or stooping	8	1	2	3
9. Walking **more than a mile**	9	1	2	3
10. Walking **several blocks**	10	1	2	3
11. Walking **one block**	11	1	2	3
12. Bathing or dressing yourself	12	1	2	3

During the **past 4 weeks**, have you had any of the following problems with your work or other regular daily activities **as a result of your physical health**? (Mark one oval on each line.)

13. Cut down the **amount of time** you spent on work or other activities	13	① Yes	② No
14. **Accomplished less** than you would like	14	① Yes	② No
15. Were limited in the **kind** of work or other activities	15	① Yes	② No
16. Had **difficulty** performing the work or other activities (for example, it took extra effort)	16	① Yes	② No

A ***PLEASE TURN CARD OVER TO COMPLETE QUESTIONNAIRE***

FIGURE **4–1.** *A*, *B*, The Medical Outcomes Study Short-Form Health Survey (SF-36). (Courtesy of Response Technologies, Inc., East Greenwich, RI.)

This is Side 2 of this Questionnaire.
Make sure you complete the OTHER side first.

During the **past 4 weeks**, have you had any of the following problems with your work or other regular daily activities **as a result of any emotional problems** (such as feeling depressed or anxious)? (Mark one oval on each line.)

17. Cut down the **amount of time** you spent on work or other activities	17	① Yes	② No
18. Accomplished less than you would like	18	① Yes	② No
19. Didn't do work or other activities as **carefully** as usual	19	① Yes	② No

20. During the **past 4 weeks**, to what extent has your physical health or emotional problems interfered with your normal social activities with family, friends, neighbors, or groups? (Mark one oval.)

20 ① Not at all ② Slightly ③ Moderately ④ Quite a bit ⑤ Extremely

21. How much **bodily** pain have you had during the **past 4 weeks**? (Mark one oval.)

21 ① None ② Very mild ③ Mild ④ Moderate ⑤ Severe ⑥ Very severe

22. During the **past 4 weeks**, how much did **pain** interfere with your normal work (including both work outside the home and housework)? (Mark one oval.)

22 ① Not at all ② A little bit ③ Moderately ④ Quite a bit ⑤ Extremely

These questions are about how you feel and how things have been with you **during the past 4 weeks**. For each question, please give the one answer that comes closest to the way you have been feeling. How much of the time during the **past 4 weeks . . .** (Mark one oval on each line.)

		All of the Time	Most of the Time	A Good Bit of the Time	Some of the Time	A Little of the Time	None of the Time
23. Did you feel full of pep?	23	①	②	③	④	⑤	⑤
24. Have you been a very nervous person?	24	①	②	③	④	⑤	⑤
25. Have you felt so down in the dumps that nothing could cheer you up?	25	①	②	③	④	⑤	⑤
26. Have you felt calm and peaceful?	26	①	②	③	④	⑤	⑤
27. Did you have a lot of energy?	27	①	②	③	④	⑤	⑤
28. Have you felt downhearted and blue?	28	①	②	③	④	⑤	⑤
29. Did you feel worn out?	29	①	②	③	④	⑤	⑤
30. Have you been a happy person?	30	①	②	③	④	⑤	⑤
31. Did you feel tired?	31	①	②	③	④	⑤	⑤

32. During the **past 4 weeks**, how much of the time has your **physical health or emotional problems** interfered with your social activities (like visiting with friends, relatives, etc.)? (Mark one oval.)

32 ① All of the time ② Most of the time ③ Some of the time ④ A little of the time ⑤ None of the time

How **true** or **false** is **each** of the following statements for you?

		Definitely True	Mostly True	Don't Know	Mostly False	Definitely False
33. I seem to get sick a little easier than other people	33	①	②	③	④	⑤
34. I am as healthy as anybody I know	34	①	②	③	④	⑤
35. I expect my health to get worse	35	①	②	③	④	⑤
36. My health is excellent	36	①	②	③	④	⑤

37. Are you male or female?

37 ① Male ② Female

38. How old were you on your last birthday?

38 ① less than 18 ② 18-24 ③ 25-34 ④ 35-44 ⑤ 45-54 ⑥ 55-64 ⑦ 65-74 ⑧ 75+

39. In the past year, have you had 2 weeks or more during which you felt sad, blue, or depressed; or when you lost all interest in things that you usually cared about or enjoyed?

39 ① Yes ② No

40. Have you had 2 years or more in your life when you felt depressed or sad most days, even if you felt okay sometimes?

40 ① Yes ② No

41. Have you felt depressed or sad much of the time in the past year?

41 ① Yes ② No

B ***THANK YOU FOR YOUR TIME***

FOR OFFICE USE ONLY Ⓐ Ⓑ Ⓒ Ⓓ Ⓔ

FIGURE **4–1.** *Continued*

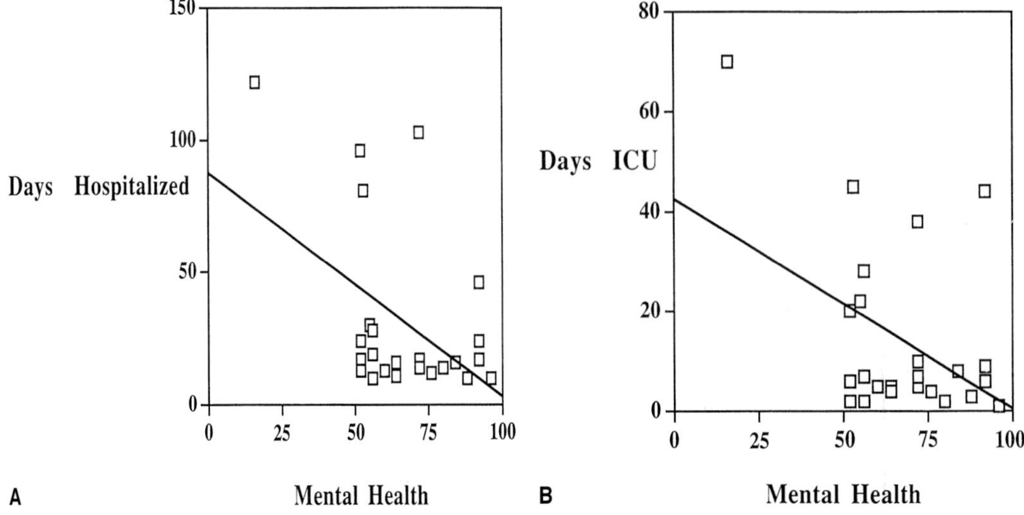

FIGURE **4–2.** Relationship of mental health to days hospitalized (*A*) and days in the ICU (*B*).

make the SF-36 more specific for the thoracic surgery patient population we have added several questions about shortness of breath during functional activities. Although the validity and reliability of these questions has not been investigated, we have found the information from them invaluable.

We have recently evaluated the relationships of mental and social health to functional status, disability, and survival in the first 25 patients to complete the SF-36 before bilateral lung volume reduction surgery.[19] Postoperative outcomes measured include days hospitalized, days in the intensive care unit (ICU), days intubated, days with chest tubes, pulmonary complications, and death. Significant univariate correlation was found between mental health and days hospitalized and days intubated (Fig. 4–2). Multivariate analysis identified social status as a significant predictor of postoperative status (Table 4–1). Measurement of patients' perceived health status may improve postoperative outcomes by identifying patients in need of mental health care or social services prior to bilateral lung volume reduction surgery. Future investigation of other thoracic surgery patient populations are needed to determine the extent of the above observations.

Methods to Administer the SF-36 Questionnaire

The SF-36 questionnaire is easy to administer (requiring only a No. 2 pencil and the answer sheet) but scoring the results can be tedious without computer analysis. The instructions to complete the SF-36 are provided directly on the answer sheet. After reading the instructions, patients choose answers to each question by marking the appropriate response on a Likert scale of 3 to 6 or answering yes-or-no questions (Fig. 4–1).

The patient responses of the SF-36 questionnaire can be tabulated manually and scores for each of the eight health profiles calculated, but computer analysis (Starting Line System—Health Care Information System, East Greenwich, RI) of the scoring sheets facilitates the analysis and can provide more ready-to-use information. A computer-generated report is shown in Figure 4–3.

TABLE **4–1**
Multivariate Predictors of Postoperative Outcomes

	Coefficient	Standard Error	*p* Value
Days hospitalized (model r = .49, r^2 = 24)			
Social functioning	.41	.21	.07
Days ICU (model r = .55, r^2 = .30)			
Social functioning	.27	.12	.04*
Days intubated (model r = .50, r^2 = .25)			
Social functioning	.25	.12	.06
Days with chest tubes (model r = .58, r^2 = .52)			
Energy/fatigue	.33	.13	.02*
Pulmonary complications (model r = .72, r^2 = .52)			
Mental health	−.03	−.009	.006*
Energy/fatigue	.02	.008	.02*

*$p < .05$.

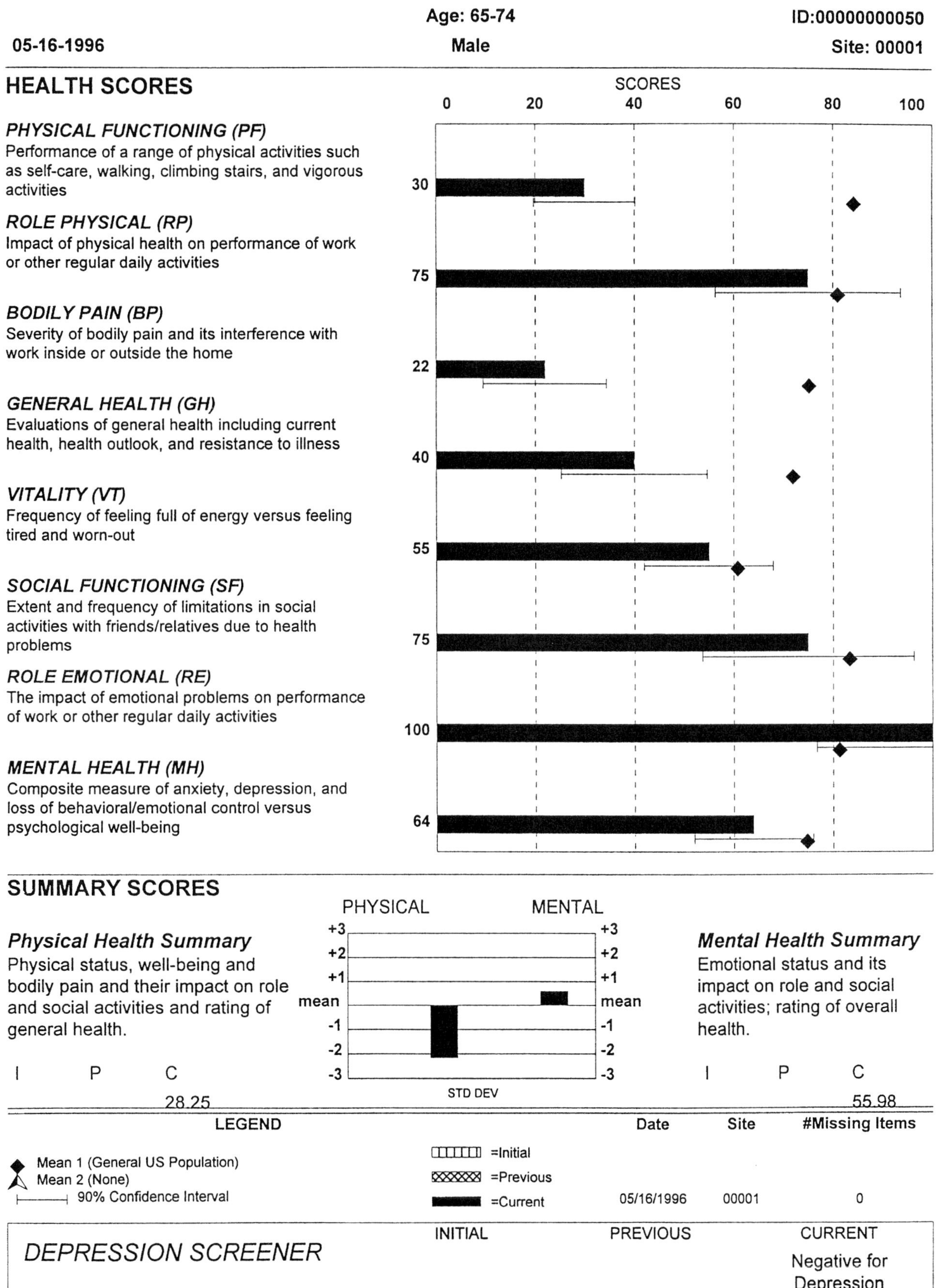

FIGURE **4–3.** Computer-generated SF-36 Health Status Profile. (Courtesy of Response Technologies, Inc., East Greenwich, RI.)

Measures of Functional and Physical Assessment

Direct and indirect measures of patient function and physical fitness have been used sporadically in evaluating patients prior to thoracic surgery.[1–4] A relatively large number of studies have been performed that have attempted to predict surgical outcome using pulmonary function tests and other resting physiologic variables (see also Chapter 3).[4,20–30] The success of resting physiologic data in predicting surgical success has been limited, except for the finding of greater success with higher forced expiratory volume in 1 second (FEV_1) levels (>2.0 L), maximal breathing capacity (>50% predicted), and DLCO.[4,20–30] However, several recent studies have used physiologic variables obtained during exercise to predict surgical outcome and these appear to be more predictive than resting data alone.[5–12] Oxygen consumption ($\dot{V}O_2$) determined during exercise stress testing has been suggested to be a useful measurement in predicting post–lung resection morbidity and mortality.[13]

Maximal Exercise Testing

The usefulness of peak $\dot{V}O_2$ has been evaluated to predict postoperative complications for a variety of surgical procedures (Table 4–2).[9–13] Eugene et al. found that in 19 patients undergoing lung resection, pulmonary function tests were not correlated to mortality, but that a peak $\dot{V}O_2$ less than 1 L/min was strongly associated with mortality.[11] Smith et al. also found resting pulmonary function tests to be unrelated to postoperative complications in 22 patients who received thoracotomy.[10] However, all six patients with a peak $\dot{V}O_2$ less than or equal to 15 ml/kg/min suffered a cardiopulmonary complication.[10]

Bechard and Wetstein also found that thoracotomy patients with a higher peak $\dot{V}O_2$ (17.0 ml/kg/min vs. 9.9 ml/kg/min; $p < .001$) had fewer complications; when the patients were further classified by peak $\dot{V}O_2$ as either high-risk (peak $\dot{V}O_2$ <10 ml/kg/min) or low-risk (peak $\dot{V}O_2$ >20 ml/kg/min) for postoperative complications, five of seven high-risk patients had complications.[9] Of particular importance in this study was the observation of greater complications in patients who demonstrated an earlier anaerobic threshold (0.61 L/min vs. 0.93 L/min; $p < .01$).[9] The use of submaximal exercise to predict outcome after thoracic surgery continues to be investigated.

Despite the above findings, several studies have found no relationship between exercise tolerance and mortality or complications in thoracotomy patients or in patients with lung resection for suspected carcinoma.[2,31–33] Coleman et al. and Markos et al. found peak $\dot{V}O_2$ to be unrelated to postoperative complications in patients undergoing lung resection for suspected lung carcinoma.[2,31] Keeley and Ussetti and their colleagues also found no relationship between peak $\dot{V}O_2$ and postoperative complications in patients undergoing thoracotomy.[32,33]

The usefulness of peak $\dot{V}O_2$ and exercise testing in predicting postoperative complications may be limited to specific diagnosis. Although Markos et al. found no relationship between peak $\dot{V}O_2$ and risk of complications after pneumonectomy, they found a relationship between peak $\dot{V}O_2$ and risk of complications in patients after lobectomy.[2] They also observed that desaturation during exercise was an important predictor of postoperative complications.

The relationship of patient age and exercise testing to predict postoperative complications was evaluated in 187 elderly patients (70 ± 7 years) undergoing major abdominal surgery.[34] Patients with a low anaerobic threshold (<11 ml/kg/min) and preoperative ischemia were observed to have a mortality rate of 42% compared

TABLE 4–2
The Relationship of Maximal Exercise Test Results Performed Prior to Thoracic Surgery to Postoperative Complications

Investigator	N	Patient Population	Measurements	Outcomes
Bechard[9]	50	Thoracotomy	Peak $\dot{V}O_2$ Peak $\dot{V}O_2$ Peak $\dot{V}O_2$	Higher peak $\dot{V}O_2$, less POC <10 ml/kg/min, high risk for POC >20 ml/kg/min, low risk for POC
Smith[10,*]	22	Thoracotomy	PFT Peak $\dot{V}O_2$	No correlation to POC ≤15 ml/kg/min, greater POC
Eugene[11,*]	19	Lung resection	PFT Peak $\dot{V}O_2$	No correlation to mortality <1 L/min, greater mortality
Epstein[12,*]	42	Lung resection	Peak $\dot{V}O_2$	<500 ml/m²/min, greater POC
Coleman[31,†]	40	Lung resection	Peak $\dot{V}O_2$	No correlation to mortality/POC
Markos[32,†]	55	Lung resection	Peak $\dot{V}O_2$	No correlation to mortality/POC
Keeley[33,†]	34	Thoracotomy	Peak $\dot{V}O_2$	No correlation to POC
Ussetti[34,†]	34	Thoracotomy	Peak $\dot{V}O_2$	No correlation to POC
Older[35,†]	187	Major abdominal surgery	$\dot{V}O_2$ & AT	At <11 ml/kg/min with M-ISCH, High mortality rate

*Studies supporting the relationship of peak $\dot{V}O_2$ to postoperative complications.
†Studies not supportive of the relationship of peak $\dot{V}O_2$ to postoperative complications.
$\dot{V}O_2$, oxygen consumption; POC, postoperative complications; PFT, pulmonary function tests; AT, anaerobic threshold; M-ISCH, myocardial ischemia.

to a mortality rate of 4% in patients with a higher anaerobic threshold (>11 ml/kg/min) and preoperative ischemia. However, the relationship between peak $\dot{V}O_2$ and postoperative complications after lung resection was recently evaluated in 42 patients with lung cancer.[12] Patients with a peak $\dot{V}O_2$ less than 500 ml/m^2/min were six times more likely to experience cardiopulmonary complications. However, multiple logistic regression analysis did not identify peak $\dot{V}O_2$ as an independent predictor of postoperative complications.[12]

Methods to Administer Maximal Exercise Tests

A variety of exercise test protocols were used in the studies discussed in the preceding section. Commonly used testing protocols are shown in Figure 4–4.[35] A review article on cardiopulmonary exercise testing prior to thoracotomy did not identify one specific protocol that is considered better than others, but suggested that an incremental test be performed that would cause exhaustion within 8 to 12 minutes.[36] Treadmill and cycle ergometry exercise testing have been used with great success but treadmill exercise typically results in higher levels of peak $\dot{V}O_2$ (8 to 10%) and greater difficulty when catheters and cardiac imaging are considerations.[36] Figure 4–5 shows a patient performing a cycle ergometry exercise test with respiratory gas analysis and cardiac imaging.

Most patients can tolerate a maximal exercise test, but several patient populations have historically not undergone maximal exercise tests. These patients include those with pulmonary hypertension, those with decompensated heart failure, and patients with frequent life-threatening dysrhythmias.[37] Several major concerns to consider during maximal exercise testing of pre–thoracic surgery patients are listed in Table 4–3. Of these, a hypoadaptive systolic blood pressure response with chronotropic incompetence and signs and symptoms of myocardial ischemia appear to be the most ominous findings from an exercise test.[35] Table 4–4 summarizes the absolute and relative contraindications to maximal exercise testing as published by the American College of Sports Medicine.

Other concerns regarding maximal exercise testing include the cost and maintenance of the necessary equipment (e.g., respiratory gas analyzers, electrocardiographic [ECG] monitors and recorders, and treadmills/cycle ergometers) and training of personnel.[35]

Finally, the person performing maximal exercise tests should be familiar with the pathophysiology of the population being tested and the normal and abnormal cardiorespiratory responses to incremental exercise.[35–37] Certification in advanced cardiac life support has been deemed imperative by several studies and organizations and occasional mock emergency sessions should be planned for most exercise testing laboratories.[38,39] Individuals performing large numbers of exercise tests appear to have greater competency and safety in exercise testing.

Nonphysician professionals have been involved with exercise testing for many years, and the safety of nonphysician exercise testing appears similar to that of physician-performed exercise testing (Table 4–5).[40–51] Assessment of competency in exercise testing via the American College of Sports Medicine Exercise Specialist Examination or independent exercise testing laboratory evaluation checks (Fig. 4–6) might further improve the safety of maximal exercise testing.

Submaximal Exercise Testing

Traditional Submaximal Exercise Testing

Many methods of submaximal exercise testing have been used in an attempt to predict surgical outcome. The traditional approach of exercise testing using treadmills and cycle ergometers at lower workloads can provide information that may be as valuable as that from maximal exercise testing. One such variable that has been extensively studied is the lactate threshold. In fact, the $\dot{V}O_2$/body surface area when the lactate level was 20 mg/dl has been used to identify survivors from nonsurvivors (471 vs. 296 ml/min/m^2) among a group of thoracotomy patients with complications.[52] Submaximal exercise (40 W/min during a bicycle ergometry exercise test) also identified survival and ventilatory dependency of 29 patients with air flow obstruction undergoing resection surgery for a lung mass. Patients with a higher mean $\dot{V}O_2$ at 40 W/min during a bicycle ergometry exercise test had greater survival rates and were extubated sooner than patients with a lower mean $\dot{V}O_2$ at the above level of submaximal exercise.[53]

Methods to Administer Submaximal Exercise Tests

Submaximal exercise tests are typically administered as low-level exercise test protocols at a low-level stage of a maximal exercise test. Submaximal exercise tests are performed (1) to attain specific information that can be obtained without maximal effort and (2) because some patients may be inappropriate for maximal exercise testing. It is interesting to note that although many believe submaximal exercise testing to be safer and to be associated with fewer complications, Stuart and Ellestad found no particular improvement in the safety of exercise testing when a submaximal exercise test was performed.[54] In fact, Stuart and Ellestad compared the safety of their exercise test study results to those of Rochmis and Blackburn and found a greater complication rate in those patients tested at submaximal levels.[54] This complication rate, however, may have been due to sicker patients with greater potential for complications during exercise.

Submaximal exercise tests are often performed in patients (1) after an acute myocardial infarction or surgical procedure, (2) with mild to moderate heart failure or valvular heart disease, and (3) with pulmonary hypertension. With such patient populations, it is apparent why Stuart and Ellestad observed greater complications dur-

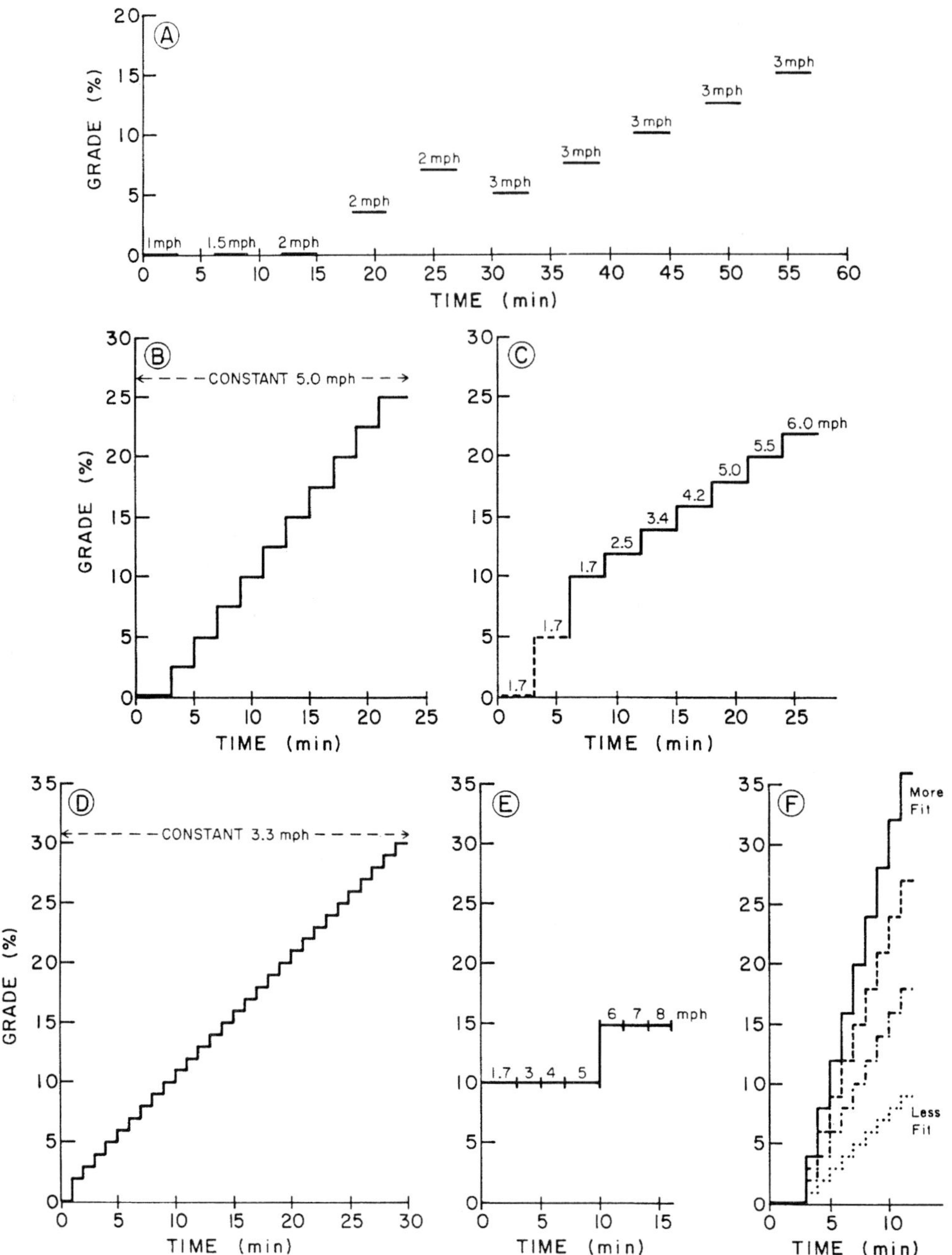

FIGURE **4–4.** Several treadmill protocols. *A*, Naughton protocol. Three-minute exercise periods of increasing work rate alternate with 3-minute rest periods. The exercise periods vary in grade and speed. *B*, Astrand protocol. The speed is constant at 5 mph. After 3 minutes at 0% grade, the grade is increased 2½% every 2 minutes. *C*, Bruce protocol. Grade and/or speed are changed every 3 minutes. The 0% and 5% grades are omitted in healthier subjects. *D*, Balke protocol. After 1 minute at 0% grade and 2 minutes at 2% grade, the grade is increased 1% per minute, all at a speed of 3.3 mph. *E*, Ellestad protocol. The initial grade is 10% and the later grade is 15% while the speed is increased every 2 or 3 minutes. *F*, Harbor protocol. After 3 minutes of walking at a comfortable speed, the grade is increased at a constant preselected amount each minute: 1%, 2%, 3%, or 4%, so that the subject reaches his maximum $\dot{V}O_2$ in approximately 10 minutes. (From Wassenman K, Hansen JE, Sue DY, Whipp BJ: Principles of Exercise Testing. Philadelphia, Lea & Febiger, 1987, p 67, with permission.)

ing submaximal exercise testing. Choosing the appropriate submaximal protocol along with extensive monitoring of the cardiorespiratory and cardiovascular response during submaximal exercise testing may increase the likelihood of safe submaximal exercise testing. End points for submaximal exercise testing can be established for the specific patient population being tested. These guidelines are not that dissimilar from the maximal exercise testing guidelines (Table 4–6) but may vary upon the primary pathology. For example, patients undergoing submaximal exercise testing after an acute surgical procedure typically exercise to a heart rate that is predetermined (e.g., 130 bpm) or a particular percentage of the patient's maximal age-predicted heart rate.

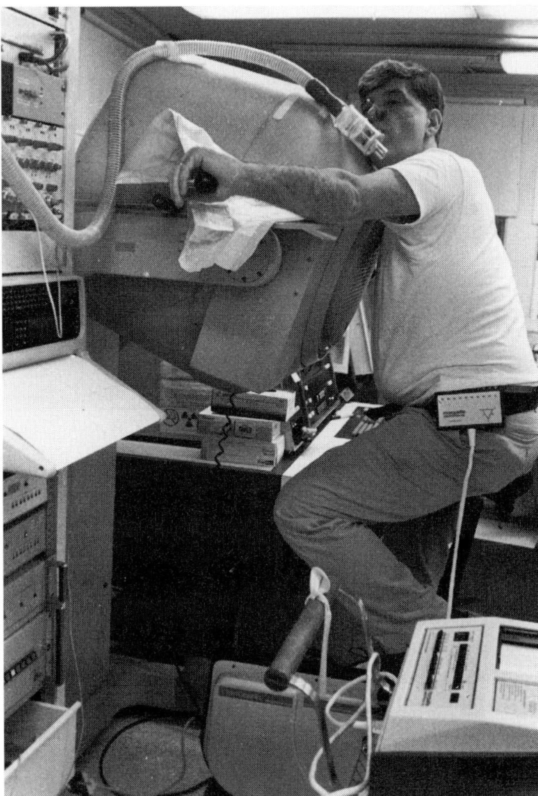

FIGURE **4–5.** Cardiopulmonary exercise testing. During such exercise testing the electrocardiogram, blood pressure, oxygen consumption, symptoms, and cardiac performance (via first-pass resting and exercise radionuclide ventriculography using a multicrystal gamma camera) are evaluated and used to establish an exercise training program.

TABLE **4–4**
Contraindications to Exercise Testing*

Absolute Contraindications
1. A recent significant change in the resting ECG suggesting infarction or other acute cardiac event
2. Recent complicated myocardial infarction (unless patient is stable and pain-free)
3. Unstable angina
4. Uncontrolled ventricular arrhythmia
5. Uncontrolled atrial arrhythmia that compromises cardiac function
6. Third-degree AV heart block without pacemaker
7. Acute congestive heart failure
8. Severe aortic stenosis
9. Suspected or known dissecting aneurysm
10. Active or suspected myocarditis or pericarditis
11. Thrombophlebitis or intracardiac thrombi
12. Recent systemic or pulmonary embolus
13. Acute infections
14. Significant emotional distress (psychosis)

Relative Contraindications
1. Resting diastolic blood pressure >115 mm Hg or resting systolic blood pressure >200 mm Hg
2. Moderate valvular heart disease
3. Known electrolyte abnormalities (hypokalemia, hypomagnesemia)
4. Fixed-rate pacemaker (rarely used)
5. Frequent or complex ventricular ectopy
6. Ventricular aneurysm
7. Uncontrolled metabolic disease (e.g., diabetes, thyrotoxicosis, or myxedema)
8. Chronic infectious disease (e.g., mononucleosis, hepatitis, AIDS)
9. Neuromuscular, musculoskeletal, or rheumatoid disorders that are exacerbated by exercise
10. Advanced or complicated pregnancy

*From American College of Sports Medicine: ACSM's Guidelines for Exercise Testing and Prescription, 5th ed. Baltimore, Williams & Wilkins, 1995, with permission.
ECG, electrocardiogram; AV, atrioventricular; AIDS, acquired immunodeficiency syndrome.

The 6- and 12-Minute Walk Tests

Other methods of submaximal exercise have been used to predict postoperative complications. The 6- and 12-minute walk tests and stair climbing tests are several such methods.

Alternative methods of submaximal exercise testing have recently received a great amount of attention because of the ease of administration, cost-savings, and relationship to postoperative outcomes (Table 4–7). Cooper was the first to evaluate the relationship of a submaximal exercise test to maximal performance.[55] He investigated the relationship of distance "walk-jogged" in 12 minutes to peak $\dot{V}O_2$ in healthy males and found a significant correlation (r = .89) between the distance "walk-jogged" in 12 minutes to peak $\dot{V}O_2$.[55] McGavin was the first to evaluate the usefulness of the 12-minute walk test in subjects who were not healthy.[56] He investigated the relationship of the 12-minute walk test to peak $\dot{V}O_2$ as well as degree of disability in 35 men with chronic bronchitis. McGavin also found a significant but less impressive correlation between distance ambulated and peak $\dot{V}O_2$ (r = .52).[56]

Bagg also utilized the 12-minute walk test, but rather than evaluate the relationship to maximal exercise performance, he investigated the usefulness of the 12-minute walk test in assessing patients with bronchial carcinoma prior to the lung resection.[57] No difference in the distance ambulated during the 12-minute walk test was observed between seven patients who suffered postoperative complications and 15 others who did not suffer postoperative complications. Even with the standardization of the 12-minute walk test distance ambulated to the Borg scale rating of perceived exertion, no significant difference in complications was found between groups.[57]

TABLE **4–3**
Major Concerns with Maximal Exercise Testing of Patients Prior to Thoracic Surgery

Early onset of dyspnea, desaturation, or fatigue which may limit the amount of useful information
Variety of symptoms requiring rapid differential diagnosis
Worsening of pulmonary hypertension
Hypoadaptive systolic blood pressure response
Exaggerated diastolic blood pressure response
Chronotropic incompetence
Myocardial ischemia and life-threatening dysrhythmias

TABLE 4–5
Complication Rates of Exercise Testing (1969–1995)*

Investigator	No. of Tests	Morbidity Rate (per 10,000)	Mortality Rate (per 10,000)	Total Complications (per 10,000)	Physician Supervised?
Rochmis & Blackburn[46]	170,000	2.4	1.0	3.4	Yes†
Stuart & Ellestad[54]	518,448	8.4	0.5	8.9	Yes†
Scherer & Kaltenbach[47]	353,638‡	0	0	0	Yes†
	712,285§	1.4	0.2	1.6	Yes†
Young et al.[48]	1,377‖	232	0	232	Yes†
Atterhog et al.[49]	50,000	5.2	0.4	5.6	Yes†
Cahalin et al.[41]/Blessey[50]	18,707	3.8	0.9	4.7	No
DeBusk[42]	>12,000	—	2.5	—	No
Gibbons et al.[51]	71,914	0.7	0.1	0.8	Yes†
Lem et al.[43]	4,050	0.3	0	0.3	No
Knight et al.[44]	28,133	3.2	0	3.2	No
Franklin et al.[45]	58,047	2.1	0.3	2.4	No

*From Franklin BA, Gordon S, Timmis GC, et al: Is direct physician supervision of exercise stress testing routinely necessary? Chest 111:262, 1997, with permission.
†>85% of these tests were directly supervised by physicians.
‡Athletes.
§Coronary patients.
‖Patients with a history of malignant ventricular arrhythmias.

The 6-Minute Walk

A more recent study compared the 6-minute walk test to conventional exercise testing and stair climbing in the evaluation of patients at high risk for pulmonary resection.[58] Peak $\dot{V}O_2$ was not significantly different between five patients who died within 90 days of surgery and 11 patients who had minor or no complications after lung resection. However, the patients with minor or no complications had significantly greater 6-minute walk tests and stair climbs. A 6-minute walk test distance of more than 1,000 ft and a stair climb of more than 44 steps were predictive of a successful surgical outcome.[58] Several other studies have also shown stair climbing to be an adequate predictor of surgical outcome in patients undergoing lung resection (see Table 4–7).[59,60] The ability of a patient to ambulate 1,000 ft or greater has been identified as not only successful predictor of surgical outcome but also of survival in patients with heart disease.[61,62]

In much the same way that McGavin et al. evaluated the relationship of the 12-minute walk test to peak $\dot{V}O_2$, we recently investigated the relationship of the 6-minute walk test to peak $\dot{V}O_2$ in 60 patients with end-stage lung disease evaluated for lung transplantation.[63] The 6-minute walk test was strongly correlated to peak $\dot{V}O_2$ ($r = .63$; $p < .0001$), and by adding several variables to the distance ambulated during the 6-minute walk test, peak $\dot{V}O_2$ could be respectably predicted ($r = .82$, $r^2 = .62$; $p < .0001$).[63] In view of the ease and economy of the 6-minute walk test, further investigation of the 6-minute walk test in predicting peak $\dot{V}O_2$, surgical outcome, and survival is warranted.

In fact, the 6-minute walk test was found to be an important univariate and multivariate predictor of complications after bilateral lung volume reduction surgery.[64] Patients ambulating more than 250 m had fewer postoperative complications.

Finally, we have also found the 6-minute walk test to be predictive of peak $\dot{V}O_2$ and survival in patients with end-stage heart disease who were being evaluated for cardiac transplantation.[62] Patients ambulating more than 300 m had a significantly improved short-term prognosis compared to patients ambulating less than 300 m (Fig. 4–7). Ambulating a distance less than 300 m has also been predictive of poor prognosis in the patients enrolled in the Studies of Left Ventricular Dysfunction (SOLVD) trial.[62]

Methods to Administer the 6-Minute Walk Test

The 6-minute walk test is a functional performance measure that is simple to administer and is well tolerated by most patients (Fig. 4–8). It involves having the patient ambulate as far as possible in 6 minutes while documenting the distance ambulated as well as other pertinent information (e.g., cardiovascular response, respiratory rate, Borg rating of perceived exertion). The instructions for the 6-minute walk test are shown in Table 4–8.

Preoperative Treatment

Value of Exercise Conditioning

The previous section has shown that subjects with greater levels of fitness appear to have better outcomes after thoracic surgery. This better outcome indicates a potentially important role exercise conditioning may play in the success of thoracic surgery. Cooper et al. conditioned patients with emphysema for 6 to 8 weeks prior to volume-reduction surgery.[65] A high degree of success was observed by Cooper et al. that in part may have been due to optimal preoperative exercise conditioning.

Nevertheless, the specific hypotheses for a positive effect of exercise conditioning upon surgical success are provided in Table 4–9. Each hypothesis is equally important and will be discussed in the following section.

	Points	Score
I. Pretest Preparation and Assessment of Patient		
A. Adequate preparation in terms of having necessary materials and information (knowledge of testing protocols/guidelines)	5	—
B. Consistently obtains *all* necessary information from patient's medical record	5	—
C. Seeks additional information directly from referring M.D. when necessary	5	—
D. Consistently completes a thorough patient interview and physical examination	5	—
E. Accurately assesses the medical data base and results from the patient interview and physical examination	21	—
F. Checks for proper calibration of testing instrumentation and correct functioning of emergency equipment	5	—
II. Test Performance		
A. Consistently makes correct judgments regarding the conducting of the test	10	—
B. Consistently obtains accurate data before, during, and after the test	30	—
C. Accurately utilizes above information to determine test end points	10	—
D. Accurately utilizes above information to determine point at which postexercise monitoring can be discontinued	5	—
E. Makes correct decision regarding need for posttest follow-up of patient	10	—
F. Adequate supervision and instruction of electrocardiograph technician during the test	5	—
III. Test Interpretation		
A. Demonstrates consistent accuracy in interpretation, assessment of physical work capacity/ functional aerobic impairment, and summary remarks/ recommendations	55	—
B. Completes test interpretation within allotted time and adequately supervises electrocardiograph technicians to ensure compliance with testing schedule	5	—
TOTAL	176	
IV. Ability to Respond to Life-Threatening Situations To test independently, the therapist must have:		
A. Clearance from the medical director of the exercise testing laboratory to take definitive action in event of an emergency		—
B. Current American Heart Association certification in Advanced Cardiac Life Support		—

FIGURE **4–6.** Independent nonphysician exercise testing competency check sheet. (From Cahalin LP, Blessey RL, Kummer D, et al: The safety of exercise testing performed independently by physical therapists. J Cardiopulm Rehabil 7:269, 1987, with permission.)

Exercise Conditioning

Aerobic and Strength Conditioning

The importance of adequate skeletal muscle performance (aerobic and strength) in maintaining physiologic homeostasis has been repeatedly demonstrated. One of the earliest trials involved a detailed evaluation of physiologic change during bed rest and after a subsequent exercise training program in five 19- to 21-year-old male college students.[66] Significant decrements in many physiologic variables were observed after a modest period of bed rest (20 days). The ability to attain pre–bed rest levels required an average of 20 days of extensive exercise training. The effects of bed rest and deconditioning upon the cardiopulmonary and muscular systems were profound, and from them, important inferences for postoperative care can be made. Primarily, earlier mobilization and better cardiorespiratory fitness should minimize the harmful effects of bed rest and enhance the recovery process.

The detrimental effects of surgery and bed rest upon cardiovascular, pulmonary, and muscular efficiency and stability have been observed by numerous investigators, many of whom found greater efficiency and stability in

TABLE 4–6
Absolute and Relative Indications for Termination of an Exercise Test*

Absolute Indications	Relative Indications
1. Acute myocardial infarction or suspicion of a myocardial infarction	1. Pronounced ECG changes from baseline (>2 mm of horizontal or down-sloping ST-segment depression, or >2 mm of ST-segment elevation [except in a VR])
2. Onset of moderate to severe angina	2. Any chest pain that is increasing
3. Drop in SBP with increasing workload accompanied by signs or symptoms or drop below standing resting pressure	3. Physical or verbal manifestations of severe fatigue or shortness of breath
4. Serious arrhythmias (e.g., second- or third-degree AV block, sustained ventricular tachycardia or increasing premature ventricular contractions, atrial fibrillation with fast ventricular response)	4. Wheezing
5. Signs of poor perfusion, including pallor, cyanosis, or cold and clammy skin	5. Leg cramps or intermittent claudication (grade 3 on 4-point scale)
6. Unusual or severe shortness of breath	6. Hypertensive response (SBP >260 mm Hg; DBP >115 mm Hg)
7. Central nervous system symptoms, including ataxia, vertigo, visual or gait problems, or confusion	7. Less serious arrhythmias such as supraventricular tachycardia
8. Technical inability to monitor the ECG	8. Exercise-induced bundle branch block that cannot be distinguished from ventricular tachycardia
9. Patient's request	

*From American College or Sports Medicine: ACSM's Guidelines for Exercise Testing and Prescription, 5th ed. Baltimore, Williams & Wilkins, 1995, with permission.
SBP, systolic blood pressure; AV, atrioventricular; ECG, electrocardiogram; DBP, diastolic blood pressure.

the above systems after exercise conditioning was implemented.[66–69] These results occur because of the exercise training stimulus, which elicits both peripheral and central physiologic adaptations. The central adaptations include improved ventilatory efficiency and cardiac performance.[70–72] Peripheral adaptations include (1) an increase in the number and size of mitochondria, (2) improved extraction of oxygen from circulating blood by the exercise muscle, (3) increased muscle strength, (4) increased mitochondrial enzymatic activity, (5) proliferation of capillaries, (6) an increase in the mean transit time of blood through muscle capillaries, (7) a lowering of peripheral vascular resistance, and (8) an increased arteriovenous oxygen difference.[73–76] Moreover, these central and peripheral adaptations produce (1) a reduction in resting and submaximal heart rate, blood pressure, respiratory rate, and rating of perceived exertion (e.g., Borg scale); (2) improved skeletal muscle and coronary blood flow; (3) increased exercise-induced lipolysis and translocation of lactate from muscle cells to the blood; and (4) improved oxygen consumption (lower levels of oxygen during submaximal exercise and higher levels at maximal exercise) and physical work capacity (Fig. 4–9).[76]

Therefore, the detrimental effects of bed rest and deconditioning affect not only peripheral physiologic processes but also central physiologic processes. Gentle, progressive exercise conditioning can improve both peripheral and central physiologic processes in anticipation of a more favorable surgical outcome. Two very impor-

TABLE 4–7
The Relationship of Submaximal Exercise Test Results Performed Prior to Thoracic Surgery and Postoperative Outcomes

Investigator	*N*	Patient Population	Measurements	Outcomes
Miyoshi et al.[52,*]	33	Thoracotomy	$\dot{V}O_2$/BSA @ 20 mg/dl LL	Greater $\dot{V}O_2$/BSA @ 20 mg/dl LL, improved survival
Olsen et al.[54,*]	29	COPD & lung resection	$\dot{V}O_2$ @ 40 W/min	Higher $\dot{V}O_2$ @ 40 W/min, greater survival & sooner extubation
Bagg[57,†]	22	BC & lung resection	12-min WT	Did not differentiate between patients with and without POC
Holden[58,†]	16	Lung resection	6-min WT Stair climbing Peak $\dot{V}O_2$	>1000 ft, less POC >44 steps, less POC Did not differentiate between patients with and without POC
Olsen et al.[59,†]	54	Thoracotomy	Stair climbing	>110 steps, fewer days hospitalized and intubated

*Traditional submaximal exercise test results.
†Nontraditional submaximal exercise test results.
$\dot{V}O_2$, oxygen consumption; BSA, body surface area; LL, lactate level; WT, walk test; POC, postoperative complications; COPD, chronic obstructive pulmonary disease.

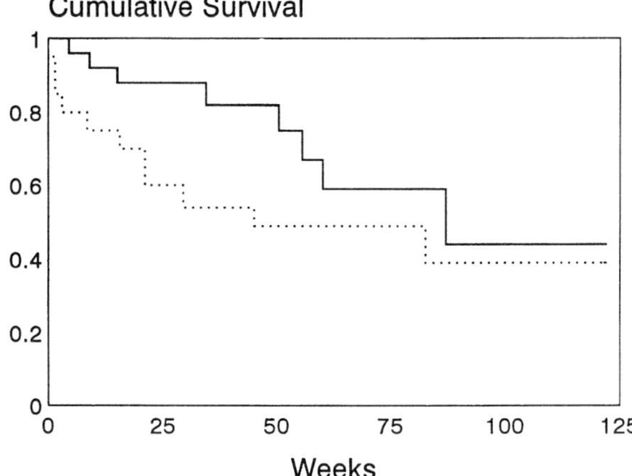

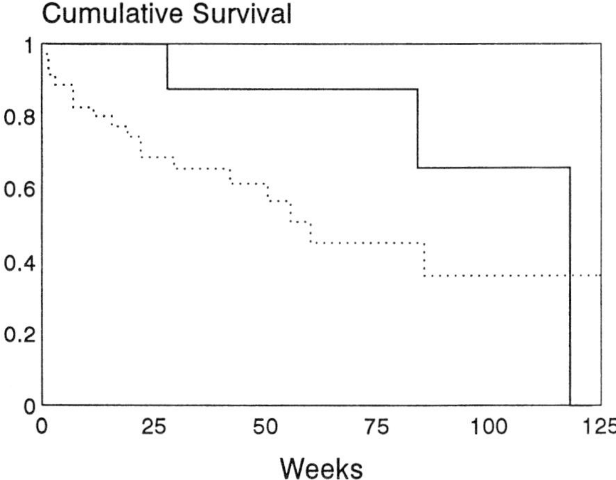

FIGURE **4–7.** *Top*, Long-term survival stratified by distance <300 m (*dotted line*) and distance >300 m (*unbroken line*) during 6-minute walk test. *Bottom*, Long-term survival stratified by peak $\dot{V}O_2$ <14 ml/kg/min (*dotted line*) and peak $\dot{V}O_2$ > 14 ml/kg/min (*unbroken line*). (From Cahalin LP, Mathier MA, Semigran MJ, et al: The six-minute walk test predicts peak oxygen uptake and survival in patients with advanced heart failure. Chest 110:325, 1996, with permission.)

tant potential exercise training adaptations for patients prior to thoracic surgery include improvements in vascular resistance and the autonomic nervous system.

Vascular Resistance (Peripheral and Pulmonary)

Both central and peripheral vascular resistance have potential to improve with properly performed long-term aerobic exercise conditioning. Patients with poor vascular response and pulmonary hypertension have a higher surgical risk in view of measurable reductions in perfusion[77,78] and exercise tolerance[79] as well as an increased incidence of cor pulmonale and death.[80–82] Although exercise has been discouraged for patients with pulmonary hypertension, a detailed review of exercise in pulmonary hypertension suggests that low- to moderate-level exercise is associated with little to no risk.[83] Only a minimal to modest rise in pulmonary artery pressure, similar to that associated with activities of daily living, was observed (Tables 4–10 and 4–11).[84] Furthermore, chronic exercise training in patients with congestive heart failure who demonstrated mild to moderate pulmonary hypertension appeared to decrease the pulmonary artery pressure slightly.[83,98] Several studies of chronic exercise training in patients with chronic obstructive pulmonary disease (COPD) and pulmonary hypertension demonstrated slightly less or equivocal changes in pulmonary artery pressure.[99–101] The exact mechanism by which the above changes occurred is unknown, but may be due to chronic vasodilatation, dampening hyperkinetic circulations, reducing sympathetic tone, or decreasing plasma insulin concentrations.[102–108]

Several studies have evaluated the pulmonary artery pressure and pulmonary artery resistance during exercise, and analyzed the exercise responses in view of postoperative complications.[109,110] In one such study by Fee et al., all patients who demonstrated a pulmonary vascular resistance greater than 2.4 Wood's units during exercise died.[109] Also of importance was the observation that the postexercise pulmonary vascular resistance of

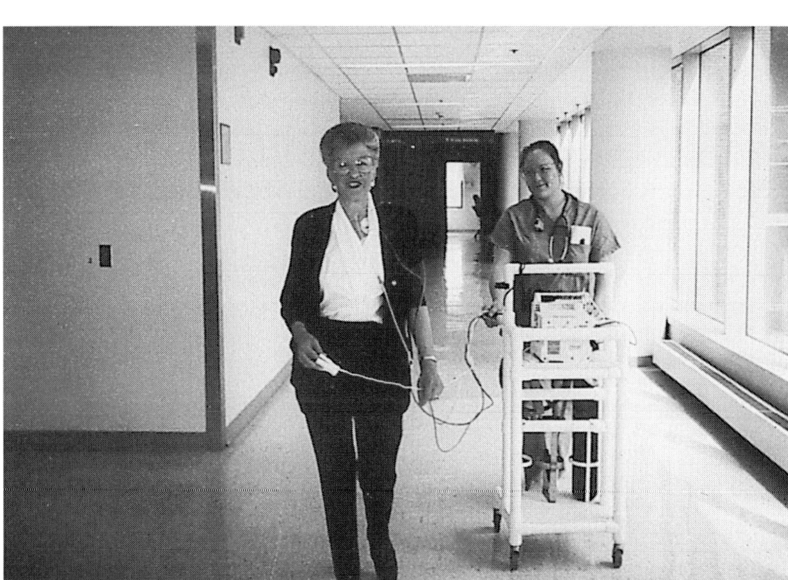

FIGURE **4–8.** Patient performing the 6-minute walk test.

TABLE 4–8
Instructions for the 6-Minute Walk Test

I. Inform patients of the purpose: The purpose of the 6-minute walk test is to attempt to quantify one's functional abilities in regard to ambulation. The total distance ambulated as well as other information obtained during the test can provide important data that will serve as a baseline measurement and allow us to compare results to document progress or deterioration.

II. Inform patients of the methods:

1. Initial 5-minute period of rest to establish a pre-exercise baseline (i.e., true resting values), and to maximize the oxygen saturation (Sao_2).
2. Monitor electrocardiogram continuously, if necessary (i.e., pulmonary hypertension, history of heart disease, irregular pulse).
3. Monitor heart rate, blood pressure, respiratory rate, Sao_2, and rating of perceived exertion before and after (minutes 2 and 4 postexercise) as well as minutes, 2, 4, and 6 of ambulation.
4. Goal: Walk as far as possible in the 6-minute period of time.
5. The walking pace will be set by the patient to achieve the greatest distance to be ambulated in 6 minutes.
6. Brief discussion of strategies to be used during the walk test:
   a. Walk at a pace to ensure continuous ambulation or walk at a pace that may require rests.
   b. Discourage patients from talking during test (use a rating of perceived exertion scale to which patients can point).
   c. Goal: Walk as far as possible.
7. Patient to walk approximately 2–3 ft in front of the tester, who will trail behind and to the side of the patient to evaluate gait and cardiopulmonary responses.

III. Responsibilities of test administrator:

1. Document distance (feet) by recording the number of completed laps on a premeasured hallway surface or by measuring the distance with a surveyor's wheel.
2. Document the cardiopulmonary responses and rating of perceived exertion before and after (minutes 2 and 4 postexercise) as well as minutes 2, 4, and 6 of ambulation.
   a. Automatic blood pressure (via Propac) and respiratory rate may be difficult to obtain at minutes 2 and 4 of exercise, but blood pressure and respiratory rate (as well as other parameters) can be obtained at minute 6 *immediately* after the patient stops walking or if the patient stops to rest.
3. Document the number of rest stops and the amount of supplemental oxygen used.
4. Offer *no* encouragement to the patient.
5. Terminate the walk if:
   a. The $Sao_2 < 80\%$ or if other signs/symptoms of significant desaturation (confusion, stupor).
   b. dizziness.
   c. Level II/IV angina.
   d. Dyspnea.
   e. Fatigue.
   f. Severe.
   g. Musculoskeletal pain, as in leg claudication.
   h. Moderate discomfort from any cause.
   i. Increasing multifocal premature contractions (PVCs), coupled PVCs, or ventricular tachycardia (three consecutive PVCs).
   j. Rapid atrial dysrhythmias.
   k. A progressive fall in systolic blood pressure of 20 mm Hg or more in the presence of an increasing heart rate and workload.
   l. An extreme hypertensive blood pressure response (i.e., systolic of 240 mm Hg or diastolic of 130 mm Hg).
   m. An uninterpretable electrocardiographic or oxygen saturation tracing.
   n. Ataxic gait.
   o. Signs of vascular insufficiency.

TABLE 4–9
Specific Hypotheses for a Positive Effect of Exercise Conditioning on Surgical Success*

1. Improvement in skeletal muscle performance: peripheral and diaphragmatic skeletal muscle fibers become more efficient and effective, decreasing the work of breathing and overall metabolic activity. This may be particularly important during the immediate postoperative period (at the time, or shortly after weaning a patient from a ventilator.)
2. Improved ability to clear secretions as a result of increased strength and endurance.
3. Increase in parasympathetic activity, which may lessen the extreme sympathetic response associated with the stress of thoracic surgery.
4. Possible decrease in total peripheral and pulmonary resistance, which may decrease the filling pressures of the heart as well as myocardial work.
5. Ability to evaluate and, if necessary, modify patient compliance and motivation. Patients observed to be noncompliant and unmotivated may be encouraged to become more compliant and motivated about an upcoming surgery, which may enable them to be better "fighters" after surgery. At the same time, postoperative teaching and instructions regarding pain control, pulmonary hygiene, and mobilization can be stressed and practiced.

*From Cahalin LP: Preoperative and postoperative conditioning for lung transplantation and volume-reduction surgery. Crit Care Nurs Clin North Am 8:305, 1996, with permission.

Central Adaptations
- Improved Ventilatory Efficiency
- Improved Cardiac Performance

Peripheral Adaptations
- Increased Number and Size of Mitochondria
- Improved Extraction Of Oxegen By Exercising Muscle
- Increased Muscle Strength
- Increased Mitochondrial Enzymatic Activity
- Proliferation of Capillaries
- Increased Mean Transit Time Of Blood Through Muscle Capillaries
- Lower Peripheral Vascular Resistance
- Increased Arteriovenous Oxegen Difference

Whole Body Adaptations
- Reduced Resting And Submaximal Heart Rate, Blood Pressure, Respiratory Rate, and Rating Of Percieved Exertion
- Improved Skeletal Muscle And Coronary Blood Flow
- Increased Exercise-Induced Lipolysis And Transloction of Lactate From Muscle Cells To The Blood
- Improved Oxegen Consumption and Physical Work Capacity

FIGURE **4–9.** Exercise conditioning adaptations. Central and peripheral adaptations occur as a result of repeated bouts of physical exercise. The central and peripheral adaptations produce whole-body adaptations that may be beneficial for a patient prior to and after thoracic surgery.

these patients remained elevated (≥190 dynes/sec/cm^{-5}).[90] However, in a more recent study, only 7% of 14 patients undergoing lung resection who had a pulmonary vascular resistance greater than 2.4 Wood's units died.[110] Lowering total peripheral resistance and pulmonary vascular resistance with aerobic exercise conditioning also improves cardiovascular and musculoskeletal performance. All of the above effects could potentially enhance surgical outcomes.

Autonomic Nervous System

Another potential central and peripheral adaptation due to chronic exercise conditioning is decreased sympathetic and increased parasympathetic nervous system stimulation. Increased parasympathetic activity is associated with chronic exercise training in normal individuals and in patients with cardiovascular disease.[70–73,111–113] Most recently, Coats et al. investigated the effects of exercise conditioning upon sympathetic and parasympathetic nervous system activity via heart rate spectral analysis and norepinephrine spillover. A significant increase in parasympathetic activity and norepinephrine spillover was observed after only 8 weeks of bicycle ergometry at 80% of maximal oxygen consumption for 20 to 30 minutes, three times per week.[113] The crossover design of this study found that 8 additional weeks of no exercise produced a nervous system profile similar to that prior to exercise training (with a greater degree of sympathetic activity). Increased sympathetic nervous system activity is associated with elevated heart rate, blood pressure, respiratory rate, oxygen consumption, and overall metabolic rate.[70–73]

Although it has never been investigated, the effects of increased parasympathetic influence (from chronic exercise training) could decrease the harmful effects of profound sympathetic stimulation preoperatively and postoperatively. This parasympathetic influence may lead to a more stable and less physiologically demanding postoperative course and subsequently decrease postoperative complications.

Aerobic and Strength Conditioning Techniques

Simple, easy-to-implement strategies can be used to begin and progress an exercise conditioning program, even in the sickest of patients. They include (1) maximizing ventilatory capacity (through proper pulmonary hygiene and supplemental oxygen); (2) maximizing ventilatory muscle performance (through ventilatory muscle training minimizing ventilatory muscle fatigue and rest); (3) appropriate pulmonary or cardiac medications; and (4) minimizing overall fatigue, cardiovascular instability, and orthopedic/neuromuscular complications (Table 4–12).

Using the proper mode of exercise can minimize the degree of fatigue, cardiovascular stress, and orthopedic/neuromuscular complications, as described in Figure 4–10. Once the proper mode of exercise is identified, exercise conditioning can be progressed by manipulating the other key elements necessary for exercise conditioning (frequency, duration, and intensity of exercise). Continual reassessment of a patient's subjective, cardiovascular, and pulmonary response during specific bouts of exercise can properly progress a patient from a basic mode of exercise (e.g., ventilatory muscle training, bicycling, walking) to the most effective combination of the key elements of conditioning. Table 4–13 also outlines the optimal patient progression for exercise conditioning. Manipulating the duration and frequency of exercise will allow for gradual increases in the intensity of exercise (the pinnacle of conditioning). This method of exercise conditioning should produce both favorable aerobic and anaerobic conditioning, which may improve surgical outcome.

AMBULATION

Hallway and treadmill ambulation can be performed as described in Table 4–14. Table 4–15 lists several types of treadmills and methods to use them for aerobic exercise conditioning before and after thoracic surgery. Note self-propelled and some motor driven treadmills can be easily transported from one patient room to another.

CYCLE ERGOMETRY

Restorator cycling, recumbent cycling, and upright stationary cycling are all modes of cycle ergometry that can produce many of the effects discussed above. Table 4–15 lists the different cycle ergometers and Table 4–16 presents the rationale and methods of progressing from one to the other.

TABLE 4–10
Acute Effects of Exercise Upon Pulmonary Hypertension*

Author	N	Methods	Results
Sietsema[89]	10	UBE (6 ft at 0–25 W) with respiratory gas analysis Mean age = 40 ± 10 Method of determining PA pressure not reported	1. Mean $\dot{V}O_2$max = 12.0 ± 3.5 ml/min/kg 2. SaO_2 response 96–91% 3. Mean PA pressure = 92/35 mm Hg 4. No complications reported
Rhodes et al.[90]	16	UBE (symptom-limited test with 20 increments every minute) without Mean age—16.9 ± 10.4 Pulmonary hypertension diagnosed by cardiac catheterization	1. Mean exercise capacity = 40 ± 36% of predicted capacity 2. Mean PA pressure = 59 ± 17 3. Mean PVR = 26 ± 17 4. Mean RA pressure = 8 ± 7 mm Hg 5. No complications reported
Morrison et al.[91]	1	SBE (protocol not described, but 2.0 L of supplemental O_2 was administered after initial test, repeated after 1 month and 8 months of O_2 therapy Age = 64-year-old male Pulmonary hypertension diagnosed by cardiac catheterization	1. Increase in workload after 8 months of O_2 therapy (100 kg-m) accompanied by an increase in PAP from 75 to 90 2. Improvement in RA pressure, arterial BP, LVEF, and PaO_2 3. No complications reported
Hebert et al.[92]	11	(7 with pulmonary hypertension) UBE (symptom-limited test with 10-W increments every 2 minutes) with respiratory gas analysis Mean age = 46 ± 16 Pulmonary hypertension diagnosed by echocardiogram	1. Mean exercise capacity range from 11–71% of predicted capacity 2. Mean $\dot{V}O_2$max = 57 ± 20% 3. No ventilatory limitations 4. No desaturation 5. No complications reported
Himelman et al.[85]	1	SBE (symptom-limited test with 10-W increments every 2 minutes) Age = 44-year-old female Pulmonary hypertension diagnosed by V/Q scans, echocardiography, pulmonary arteriogram, and PA catheterization	1. PA systolic pressure increased from 75 to 175 mm Hg during SBE 2. Excellent correlation of PA systolic pressure and Doppler echo measurement of RVSP 3. Medical therapy (O_2 and diltiazem) decreased RVSP slightly 4. Greatest decrease in RVSP occurred after PA thrombectomy 5. No complications reported
Otulana & Higginbotham[93]	8	4 minutes of supine alternate leg raising with hemodynamic and respiratory gas analysis Mean age = 32 ± 8 Pulmonary hypertension diagnosed by PA catheterization	1. Mean $\dot{V}O_2$max = 25.4 ± 75 2. Exercise produced a decrease in $P\bar{v}O_2$ and PaO_2 and an increase in PA pressure 3. No significant change in V_D/V_T or Q_S/Q_T 4. No complications reported
Adnot et al.[94]	12	SBE (symptom-limited test with 30-W increments every 5 minutes Mean age = 60 ± 7 Pulmonary hypertension diagnosed by PA catheterization	1. $\dot{V}O_2$max = 500 ml/min/m^2 2. Resting PaO_2 = 63.5 mm Hg, exercise PaO_2 = 52.5 mm Hg 3. PA pressure, PA wedge pressure, RA pressure, and mean systemic arterial pressure all increased from 29, 8.7, 4.4, & 97.6 to 55.8, 21.8, 12.2, & 135.6, respectively 4. PVR did not change 5. No complications reported
Theodore et al.[95]	16	Treadmill exercise (symptom-limited test; 7-minute workloads of varying speed and grade with 10-minute rest periods in between) Age = 22–45 $\dot{V}O_2$max was predicted Pulmonary hypertension diagnosed by PA catheterization	1. Resting PaO_2 = 59.1, exercise PaO_2 = 44.2 2. Predicted $\dot{V}O_2$max = 9.8 3. No complications reported
D'Alonzo et al.[86]	11	UBE (symptom limited test with 20-W increments each minute) with respiratory gas analysis Mean age = 42.2 ± 15.3 Pulmonary hypertension diagnosed by PA catheterization	1. Mean resting PA pressure = 56 ± 15; exercise PA pressure not measured 2. $\dot{V}O_2$max = 13.4 3. V_E, max HR, and O_2 pulse were higher in patients with pulmonary hypertension 4. Anaerobic threshold earlier 5. No complications reported

(*Table continued on opposite page*)

TABLE 4–10
Continued

Author	*N*	Methods	Results
Gibbs et al.[87]	9	Treadmill exercise test using one or two protocols based upon patient's previous exercise test results: (1) modified Bruce (1 mph, 5% grade; 1.7 mph, 10% grade; 2.4 mph, 12% grade), every 3 minutes; (2) National Heart Hospital heart failure protocol (no grade); (3) treadmill speeds of 1.0, 1.5	1. Neither symptoms nor PA pressure during max exercise was the same as during ADLs 2. Mean max systolic PA pressure = 43.5–59.4 mm Hg 3. Mean diastolic PA pressure = 20.4–27.8 mm Hg 4. No complications reported 2.0, and 2.5 mph every 3 minutes Pulmonary hypertension diagnosed by PA catheterization
Richards et al.[96]	5	UBE (submaximal test to 75% of maximum predicted heart rate) Mean age = 41 Pulmonary hypertension diagnosed by cardiac catheterization	1. Mean exercise duration = 16.6 min 2. Mean peak exercise systolic PA pressure = 49.2 mm Hg 3. Mean peak exercise diastolic PA pressure = 23.0 mm Hg 4. Range of systolic PA pressure with ADLs = 47.1–89.6 mm Hg 5. Range of diastolic PA pressure with ADLs = 21.7–37.2 mm Hg 6. No complications reported
Ashutosh & Dunsky[88]	43	UBE (system-limited test at 25–50 W) with respiratory gas analysis Mean age = 60 Pulmonary hypertension diagnosed by cardiac catheterization	1. $\dot{V}O_2max$ = 6.65–8.61 2. Resting PA pressure = 33.2–37.3 3. RVEF = 19.5–24.4% 4. LVEF = 53.3–55.4% 5. A high $\dot{V}O_2max$ (>6.5 ml/min/kg) was significantly associated with a favorable response to O_2 6. Oxygen therapy decreased pulmonary hypertension 7. 2- to 3-year survival rate for patients with pulmonary hypertension who responded to O_2 was greater than nonresponders 8. No complications reported
Himelman et al.[85]	36	SBE (symptom-limited test with 10-W increments every 2 minutes) Age = 32–80 Pulmonary hypertension diagnosed by cardiac catheterization and Doppler echo	1. Range of exercise systolic PA pressure = 40–130 mm Hg 2. Good correlation with Doppler echo (.98) 3. No complications reported

*From Cahalin L: Pulmonary hypertension and exercise. Cardiopulm Phys Ther 6:3, 1995, with permission.
UBE, upright bicycle ergometry; PA, pulmonary artery; PVR, pulmonary vascular resistance; RA, right atrial; SBE, supine bicycle ergometry; BP, blood pressure; LVEF, left ventricular ejection fraction; RVSP, right ventricular systolic pressure; HR, heart rate; ADLs, activities of daily living; RVEF, right ventricular ejection fraction.

STRENGTH TRAINING

Strength training of skeletal muscle can be performed using many methods. Most methods are simple and cost-effective to implement. Table 4–17 presents several such methods. Strength training can be directed to specific muscle groups and significantly improves the strength and endurance of weak muscle groups. One muscle group that is particularly important to train if weakness exists is the ventilatory muscles. Such training may be beneficial to the thoracic surgery patient.

Ventilatory Muscle Training

The effects of deconditioning upon ventilatory muscle strength was recently found to be strongly associated with postoperative complications.[114] Patients who were provided ventilatory muscle training significantly increased their ventilatory muscle strength and had significantly fewer postoperative complications after thoracic surgery.[114]

Finally, a recent multivariate analysis found that survival following lung transplantation evaluation was significantly related to ventilatory muscle strength.[115] Extensive data (patient characteristics, pulmonary function tests, exercise testing, and hemodynamic results) from 64 patients evaluated for lung transplantation were analyzed for their relationship to survival. Maximal inspiratory pressure (MIP), forced expiratory flow at 25 to 75% of FVC ($FEF_{25-75\%}$), patient age, and diagnosis were identified as principal determinants of survival. Significant determinants of MIP were total lung capacity (TLC), patient age, and $\dot{V}O_2max$. The authors concluded that patients with poor maximal inspiratory muscle strength are less likely to survive transplantation[115]; however, the strong association of $\dot{V}O_2max$ and ultimately exercise tolerance to MIP reinforced the importance of exercise conditioning to surgical success.

TABLE 4–11
Chronic Effects of Exercise Upon Pulmonary Hypertension*

Author	*N*	Methods	Results
Lee et al.[83]	18	Patients with heart disease (EF = 35%) Treadmill exercise (symptom-limited modified Bruce protocol) 12–24 months of walking, jogging, or bicycling at 70–85% of max HR for 20–45 minutes, 2–6 times/wk Mean age = 50 Pulmonary hypertension diagnosed by cardiac catheterization	1. Increased exercise duration 2. Resting and submaximal HR were significantly less after exercise 3. No change in cardiac performance 4. Slightly lower mean PA pressure 5. No complications reported
Sullivan et al.[98]	12	Patients with chronic CHF (EF = 24 ± 10%) Upright isokinetic bicycle ergometry (symptom-limited with 150 kg-m/min increments every 3 minutes) with respiratory gas analysis 16–24 weeks of stationary bicycling, walking, jogging, and stair climbing at 75% of $\dot{V}O_2$max for 60 minutes, 3–5 days/wk Mean age = 54 ± 10 Pulmonary hypertension diagnosed by cardiac catheterization, meeting exercise criteria for pulmonary hypertension (mean PA pressure >30 mm Hg)	1. Resting and submaximal HR were significantly less after exercise training 2. $\dot{V}O_2$max increased significantly (23%) after exercise training 3. Maximal cardiac output increased, but was not statistically significant (8.9 ± 2.7 to 3.2 L/min) 4. Resting and submaximal mean PA pressures were slightly less, but near-maximal and maximal mean PA pressures were slightly higher after exercise training 5. Maximal systemic a − vo_2 difference, leg blood flow, and leg a − vo_2 difference increased significantly after exercise training 6. No complications reported
Degre et al.[99]	11	Patients with chronic airway obstruction UBE with respiratory gas analysis (symptom-limited test with 10-W increments every minute) 6 weeks of bicycle ergometry at 75% of maximal workload for 25 minutes, 3 times/wk Mean age = 50 ± 7	1. $\dot{V}O_2$max was significantly greater after training (1.2–1.35 L/min) 2. Peak PA pressure decreased from 33 ± 18 to 31 ± 16 after training, statistically nonsignificant 3. Resting PA pressure was significantly less after exercise training (14 ± 7 vs. 18 ± 10) 4. No complications reported Pulmonary hypertension diagnosed by cardiac catheterization (meeting exercise criteria for pulmonary hypertension; PA pressure >30 mm Hg)
Chester et al.[100]	21	Male patients with COPD SBE (6 minutes at either 150 or 300 kg-m/min) 4 weeks of hospitalized treadmill ambulation at a mean HR of 125 ± bpm, as well as rowing, bicycling, and wall-mounted pulley weights to weights to "tolerance," for a variable duration, 7 days/wk Daily chest PT (breathing exercises, postural drainage, and intermittent positive-pressure breathing were also provided) Mean age = 51 ± 6 Pulmonary hypertension diagnosed by cardiac catheterization (meeting exercise criteria for pulmonary hypertension; PA pressure >30 mm Hg)	1. Resting PA increased slightly after exercise (19 ± 3 to 22 ± 5) 2. Peak PA pressure increased slightly after exercise training (30 ± 7 to 33 ± 9) 3. $\dot{V}O_2$ and minute ventilation were lower (46 ml/min/m^2 and 3.7 L/min, respectively) during this submaximal, constant workload (either 150 or 300 kg-m/min) exercise test 4. Total work performed on the treadmill increased significantly 5. All other hemodynamic, pulmonary function, and arterial blood gas values were relatively unchanged 6. No complications reported
Alpert et al.[101]	5	Patients with COPD UBE (6 minutes at constant workload; actual resistance not reported) 18 weeks of stationary bicycling at a moderate resistance (workload or exercise intensity not reported) for 20 minutes, 3 times/day, 7 days/wk Mean age not reported Pulmonary hypertension diagnosed by cardiac catheterization, meeting exercise criteria for pulmonary hypertension (mean PA pressure >30 mm Hg)	1. Exercise HRs were significantly decreased after exercise training 2. $\dot{V}O_2$ at rest and during exercise were significantly decreased after exercise training 3. Systemic a − VO_2 difference during exercise was significantly less after exercise training 4. Cardiac output, stroke work, and resistances were relatively unchanged after exercise training 5. Mean PA pressures at rest and during exercise were relatively unchanged after exercise training (22 ± 11 to 24 ± 12 and 41 + 19 to 42 ± 20 mm Hg, respectively) 6. No complications reported

*Cahalin L: Pulmonary hypertension and exercise. Cardiopulm Phys Ther 6:3, 1995, with permission.

EF, ejection fraction; HR, heart rate; PA, pulmonary artery; CHF, congestive heart failure; UBE, upright bicycle ergometry; COPD, chronic obstructive pulmonary disease; PT, physical therapy; SBE, supine bicycle ergometry.

TABLE 4–12
Methods to Minimize the Degree of Limitation to Exercise Conditioning*

Limitations	Methods
Dyspnea	Mobilization of secretions Administration of supplemental oxygen by way of nasal cannula, face mask, or noninvasive positive pressure ventilation (e.g., CPAP/BiPAP) Ventilatory muscle training if weakness or poor endurance Proper mode of exercise that enables optimal position while decreasing the biomechanical stress of exercise
Fatigue	Provide adequate nutritional support, oxygen-carrying capacity (i.e., Hgb and Hct) and rest/exercise periods
Cardiopulmonary instability	Provide optimal pharmacologic management (i.e., bronchodilators) and other methods above
Orthopedic/ neuromuscular abnormalities	Evaluate for orthopedic or neuromuscular problems (i.e., adequate range of motion, muscle strength, and coordination)
Pain	Provide adequate structural (i.e., splinting) and analgesic support

*From Cahalin LP: Preoperative and postoperative conditioning for lung transplantation and volume-reduction surgery. Crit Care Nurs Clin North Am 8:305, with permission.
CPAP, continuous positive airway pressure; BiPAP, bilevel positive airway pressure; Hgb, hemoglobin; Hct, hematocrit.

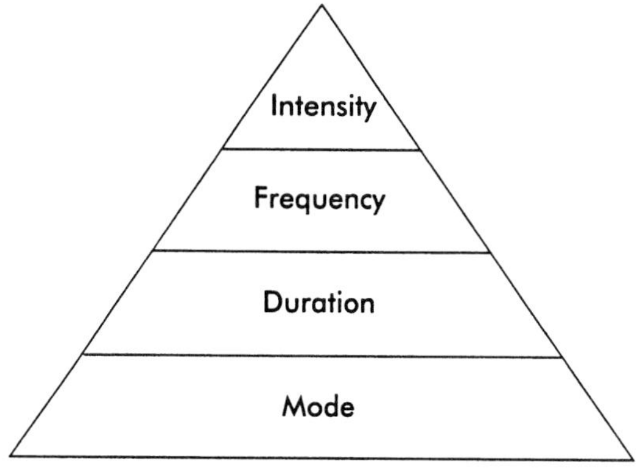

FIGURE **4–10.** Fundamentals of safe and effective exercise conditioning. (From Cahalin LP: Exercise tolerance and training for healthy persons and patients with cardiovascular disease. In Hasson SM [ed]: Clinical Exercise Physiology. St. Louis, Mosby-Yearbook, 1994, p 148, with permission.)

The effect of ventilatory muscle performance upon surgical success was recently investigated in pilot work at our institution and reinforced the importance of ventilatory muscle strength as well as ventilatory muscle endurance. Thirty-five patients with moderate to severe obstructive lung disease (FEV_1 and FVC of 24 ± 8% and 51 ± 55% of predicted, respectively) evaluated for bilateral volume reduction surgery underwent measurement of MIP, ventilatory muscle endurance (via a 2-minute incremental loading protocol), and postoperative outcomes (days hospitalized, days in the ICU, days intubated, days with chest tubes, pulmonary complications, and death). Univariate and multivariate analysis identified MIP as a significant predictor of postoperative outcomes. Significantly fewer days hospitalized, days in the ICU, days intubated, days with chest tubes, pulmonary complications, and deaths were observed with a MIP greater than 30 cm H_2O.[116] Peak workload in centimeters of water during the ventilatory muscle endurance test was a significant predictor of days with chest tubes. Finally, 11 of the 35 patients with less than optimal MIP significantly increased MIP (38 ± 12 to 54 ± 13 cm H_2O) via inspiratory muscle training, but still experienced poor postoperative outcomes.[116]

However, a recent investigation of preoperative ventilatory muscle training in 50 thoracic surgery patients found that patients demonstrating ventilatory muscle weakness after a mean of 14 days of ventilatory muscle training had significantly greater postoperative complications.[114] Postoperative complications were observed in patients with a mean MIP and maximal expiratory pressure (MEP) of 57 and 60, respectively.[114] These findings support the work of Yang, who found that lower MIP (≤40 cm H_2O) levels were associated with unsuccessful mechanical ventilatory weaning, while a lower ratio of inspiratory pressure to maximal inspiratory pressure (mean PI/PImax of 0.26) was associated with weaning success.[117]

Finally, although we did not evaluate postoperative outcomes, we found that standard inspiratory muscle training using a threshold device significantly improved ventilatory muscle strength and dyspnea in eight patients with end-stage heart failure awaiting cardiac transplantation (Fig. 4–11).[118,119] The improvements in ventilatory muscle strength and dyspnea was related to initial pulmonary function test results and level of motivation/compliance with inspiratory muscle training. Patients with the greatest compliance to inspiratory muscle training and relatively well-maintained pulmonary function prior to inspiratory muscle training made the greatest improvements in ventilatory muscle strength and dyspnea.[118,119]

Methods of Ventilatory Muscle Training

A variety of methods are available to train the ventilatory muscles. Inspiratory muscle training (IMT) has received

TABLE 4–13
Rehabilitation Program for Thoracic Surgery Patients*

Pre- and Postoperative Evaluation

1. 6-minute walk test
2. Gross assessment of muscle strength and range of motion
3. Screening for orthopedic conditions (e.g., low back pain, arthritis)
4. Respiratory muscle strength and endurance
5. Health status profile (e.g., SF-36)

Preoperative Rehabilitation

The preoperative rehabilitation program consists of approximately 6–8 weeks of exercise conditioning and education. End points for preoperative rehabilitation includes either:

1. An observable plateau of exercise (for 2–3 weeks) consisting of maximal duration of exercise that cannot be further increased at an adequate exercise training intensity (50–80% age-predicted maximal heart rate).
2. 30 minutes of continuous bicycling or walking exercise at an adequate heart rate (at least 50–80% of age-predicted maximal heart rate), oxygen saturation (at least 90% on supplemental oxygen support), or rate of perceived exertion (modified Borg scale of 3 or 4 out of 10).
3. 30–40% improvement in 6-minute walk test total distance ambulated.

Preoperative Exercise Conditioning

1. Endurance training (at an intensity of at least 50% of age-predicted maximal heart rate):
   a. Walking
   b. Cycling
   c. Arm ergometry
   d. Vertical stepping (e.g., stair stepping)
2. Strengthening:
   a. Active range of motion
   b. Weight training to the limbs via:
      - Theraband (Hygenic Corp., Akron, OH)
      - Light weights
   c. Ventilatory muscle training (if MIP <30 cm H_2O)
   d. Vertical stepping
3. Adjunct exercise:
   a. Breathing exercises/breathing retraining
   b. Stretching/chest wall mobility
4. Education:
   a. Preoperative teaching
   b. Management of dyspnea and anxiety
   c. Energy conservation

Activity Guidelines for Hospitalized Patients†

Day	Standard Activity Regimen	Gradual Activity Regimen
1	Commode/chair	Bedrest
2	Room ambulation	Bedrest/gentle active strengthening exercises
3	Hallway ambulation and cycle ergometry × 2 (1–10 min); MET level goal = 2.0–3.0	Commode/chair/bathroom/restorator cycling/room ambulation/ gentle strengthing exercises
4	Independent hallway ambulation × 3 (1–15 min); MET level goal = 3.0–4.0 Patient adequately ascends/descends two flights of stairs and is showering independently Adequate understanding of home exercise prescription Outpatient cardiac rehabilitation appointment scheduled Patient discharged	Hallway ambulation/restorator or cycle ergometry × 2 exercise duration (1–5 min); MET level goal = 1.0–2.0 Strengthening exercises
5		Hallway ambulation/restorator or cycle ergometry × 2, exercise duration (1–8 min); MET level goal = 1.5–2.5 Strengthening exercises
6		Hallway ambulation/restorator or cycle ergometry × 2, exercise duration (1–10 min); MET level goal 2.0–3.0 Strengthening exercises
7		Hallway ambulation × 2, exercise duration (1–15 min); MET level goal = 2.0–4.0 Strengthening exercises Patient adequately ascends/descends two flights of stairs and is showering independently Adequate understanding of home exercise prescription Outpatient cardiac rehabilitation appointment scheduled Patient discharged

Postoperative Rehabilitation

The postoperative rehabilitation program will contain the same components as the preoperative exercise conditioning phase with the goal of a safe and gradual progression of exercise to maximize patient function and surgical outcome. The postoperative evaluation should be performed at 3 and 6 months and should include the areas assessed during the preoperative evaluation.

*Adapted from Cahalin LP: Heart Failure. Phys Ther 76:530, 1996; and Cahalin LP: Preoperative and postoperative conditioning for lung transplantation and volume-reduction surgery. Crit Care Nurs Clin North Am 8:305, 1996. Copyright 1996, American Physical Therapy Association, with permission.

†Activity protocol is based upon risk stratification of patients (e.g., degree of ventricular dysfunction and signs/symptoms) and upon the cardiopulmonary response (heart rate not more than 20–30 bpm above resting heart rate without hypoadaptive BP response [not greater than 10–20 mm Hg decrease] and without significant dysrhythmias or dyspnea).

MIP, maximal inspiratory pressure; MET, metabolic equivalent; BP, blood pressure.

TABLE 4–14
Ambulation Methods

1. Provide patients who are deconditioned with easily provoked dyspnea handrail/arm support during ambulation (e.g., handrail of treadmill or a rolling cart as shown below).
2. Begin ambulation at the slowest possible speed after which adjustments in speed should be based upon patient comfort and establishing an optimal cadence so that the patient may ambulate to tolerance.
3. Attempt to alter the breathing pattern if a rapid respiratory rate or abnormal breathing pattern is observed (e.g., altering the pattern to be in synchrony with the ambulation cadence).
4. Gradually decrease handrail/arm support and attempt to increase the cadence and speed of ambulation.
5. Develop home ambulation goals (e.g., 25 ft of ambulation 5×/day.

much attention and controversy. The most beneficial method to administer IMT appears to be with a targeted inspiratory muscle trainer such as the Threshold inspiratory muscle trainer (Fig. 4–12). The results of several studies using such a device are presented in Table 4–18. With such a device, the patient must generate enough negative pressure to pull a spring-loaded diaphragm towards the mouth, which will allow the movement of air through the device to the patient. If the generation of negative pressure is inadequate, the diaphragm of the device will remain closed and the patient will be unable to breathe (as long as a noseclip remains on the nose and the patient keeps a tight seal around the mouthpiece of the IMT device). Because of this process, it is imperative to know the patient's MIP before IMT is initiated.

The MIP and MEP are obtained with a manometer or pressure transducer (Fig. 4–13) that measures the force a patient generates during maximal inspiration (MIP, a negative pressure) or expiration (MEP, a positive pressure) in centimeters of water. Several important methods must be employed when measuring ventilatory muscle strength (Table 4–19) of which body position and measuring at the correct time in the respiratory cycle are of paramount importance.

Once the MIP is known, the inspiratory muscle trainer can be set at a specific percentage of the MIP. This is done by placing more or less tension upon the spring by simply rotating the center stem of the inspiratory muscle trainer (Fig. 4–12). A variety of inspiratory training protocols are used but most begin with lower levels of negative pressure (e.g., 20% of MIP) and progressively increase the resistance to breathe with greater levels (e.g., 40 to 60% of MIP) after several weeks to months. Initial IMT sessions are observed for the prescribed IMT duration (e.g., 5 to 15 minutes) to ensure proper use of the

TABLE 4–15
Various Modes of Aerobic Exercise Training

Treadmills*
Self-propelled
Motor driven
Motor driven with handrail support
Motor driven with one-armed handrail support
Motor driven without handrail support

Cycle Ergometers*
Restorator (e.g., crankshaft of cycle with pedals and very rudimentary application resistance)
Recumbant ergometer
Upright ergometer
Upright ergometer with varying handrail positions

Whole-Body Exercisers (Utilizing Upper and Lower Extremities and Trunk Musculature)*
Schwinn Air-Dyne (cycle ergometry and arm exercise via moving handlebars)
Stair-steppers and elliptical exercise machines (stair-steppers with arm motion via a handlebar-like apparatus)
Gliders (upper and lower extremity and trunk exercise performed in a rowing motion)
Nordic Track cross country ski machine and other such hybrids

*The first mode of exercise in each of the three major modes of exercise is the most basic and simple, while the last mode of exercise is frequently the most sophisticated and difficult.

TABLE 4–16
Cycling Methods

1. Identify the correct seat height and handlebar height for each patient
   A. Methods to determine the correct seat height: With the patient sitting squarely on the cycle seat, extend the knee and place the heel of the foot of the extended leg upon the cycle pedal (with the pedal in the dead center bottom position). With the heel of the foot resting on the cycle pedal in this position, the optimal set height to cycle should produce a slight bend in the knee (approximately 5 degrees of flexion).
   B. Methods to determine the correct handlebar height: With the patient sitting squarely on the cycle seat, place both hands or forearms upon the handlebars. The optimal handlebar height is determined by visual assessment to minimize accessory muscular use and by patient subjective report. Some patients cycle more comfortably and for longer durations with the forearms upon relatively high handlebar settings (e.g., at the height of the acromioclavicular joint) with the trunk flexed forward slightly.
2. Begin cycling at the slowest possible cadence without resistance after which adjustments in cadence and resistance should be based upon patient comfort and establishing an optimal cadence and resistance so that the patient may cycle to their tolerance.
3. Attempt to alter the breathing pattern if a rapid respiratory rate or abnormal breathing pattern are observed (e.g., altering the pattern to be in synchrony with the cycling cadence).
4. Gradually decrease handrail/arm support and attempt to increase the cadence and resistance of cycling.
5. Develop home cycling goals (e.g., 5–15 minutes, 3×/day).

TABLE 4–17
Strength Training Methods

1. Begin strength training with active range of motion (AROM) exercises to the target muscle groups for approximately 1 week prior to the use of weights or resistance devices.
2. Initiate strength training with light weights or resistance (10–20% of maximal lifting capacity) and high repetitions (10–20 repetitions) for several weeks.
3. Gradually increase weights or resistance to a goal of approximately 60% of maximal lifting capacity for the target muscle groups and decrease the number of repetitions (5–10 repetitions).
4. Once 40–50% of maximal lifting capacity is attained, strength training can be performed every other day, rather than daily.

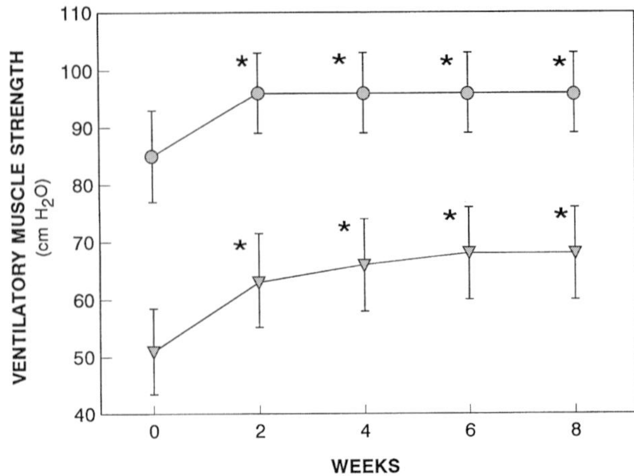

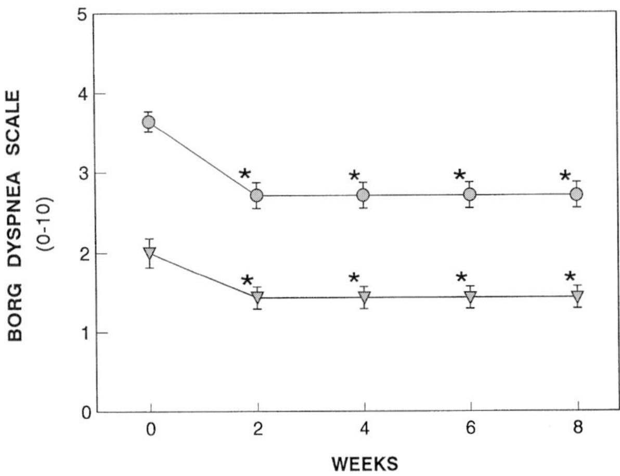

FIGURE **4–11.** (*Top*) Maximal inspiratory pressure (▽) and maximal expiratory pressure (◎) throughout the ventilatory muscle training period. (*Bottom*) Dyspnea at rest (▽) and during submaximal exercise (◎) throughout the ventilatory muscle training period. Asterisk (*) indicates value is different from baseline ($P < .05$). (From Cahalin LP, Semigran MJ, Dec GW: Inspiratory muscle training in patients with chronic heart failure awaiting cardiac transplantation: Results of a pilot clinical trial. Phys Ther 77:830, 1997. Copyright 1997, American Physical Therapy Association, with permission).

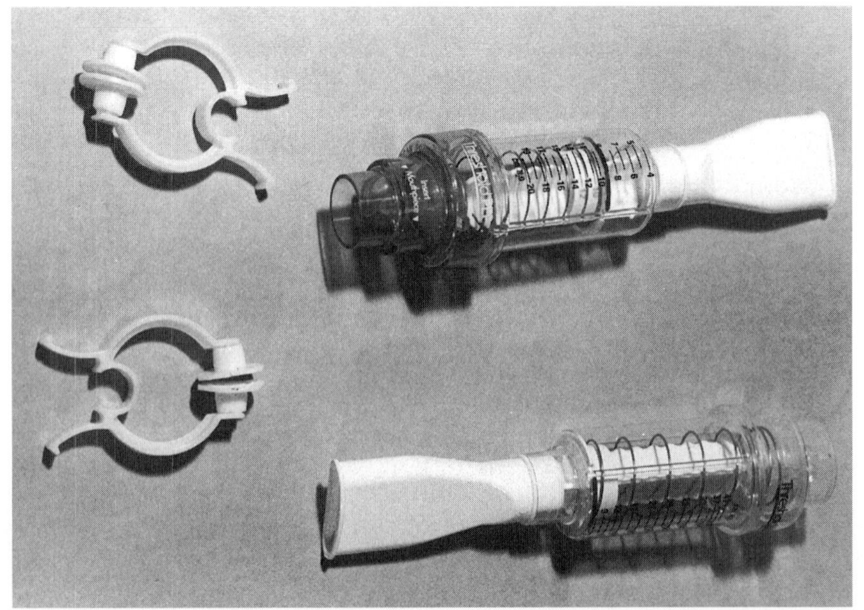

FIGURE **4–12.** Different types of ventilatory muscle training devices. *Top*, expiratory muscle trainer; *Bottom*, inspiratory muscle trainer.

TABLE 4–18
Ventilatory Muscle Training*

Author	*N*	Patient Population	Mode	Intensity	Duration	Frequency	Length of Training	Results
Chen et al.[120]	6 control 7 experimental	COPD	PFLEX-like† (nontargeted)	35% of MIP	15 min	2×/day	4 wk	Significant increase of the experimental group's strength and endurance, but no change in PFTs or exercise performance.
Larson et al.[121]	12—group 1 10—group 2	COPD	Threshold (Healthscan Products, Cedar Grove, NJ) (targeted)	Group 1 = 15% of MIP Group 2 = 30% of MIP	15–30 min	1×/day	8 wk	Significant increase in 4 weeks in inspiratory muscle strength and endurance, and 12-minute walk test in group 2, no change in functional status, mood, health status, or pulmonary symptoms.
Harver et al.[122]	9—group 1 10—group 2	COPD	Threshold-like (targeted)	Group 1 = 5 cm H_2O Group 2 = 5 to 35 cm H_2O	15 min	2×/day	8 wk	Significant improvement in inspiratory muscle strength and dyspnea in group 2.
Dekhuijzen et al.[123]	20 control 20 experimental	COPD	Threshold-like (targeted)	70% MIP	15 min	2×/day	10 wk	Significant increase in 4 weeks in inspiratory muscle strength and endurance, and 12-minute walk test that were significantly greater than those in the control group who underwent pulmonary rehabilitation alone.
Weiner et al.[124]	12 control 12 experimental—group 1 12 experimental—group 2	COPD	Threshold (targeted)	Progressed from 15% to 80% of MIP	15 min	3×/wk	24 wk	Significant increase in FVC, inspiratory muscle strength, and endurance and 12-minute walk test that were significantly greater in the VMT and pulmonary rehabilitation group versus the control of pulmonary rehabilitation group alone.
Weiner et al.[125]	15 control 15 experimental	Asthma	Threshold (targeted)	Progressed from 15% to 80% of MIP	30 min	5×/wk	24 wk	Significant improvement of the experimental group's inspiratory muscle strength and endurance, FEV, FVC, asthma symptoms, hospitalization for asthma, emergency room visits, absence from school or work, and medication consumption.
Suzuki et al.[126]	6 control 6 experimental	Healthy	Threshold (targeted)	30% of MIP	15 min	2×/day	4 wk	Significant increase of the experimental group's inspiratory muscle strength and maximal transdiaphragmatic pressure as early as 2 weeks after VMT was initiated.
Nomori et al.[114]	50 control 50 experimental	Thoracic surgery patients	Diaphragmatic breathing with 2 kg on abdomen and expiratory training‡	Inspiratory = 2 kg on abdomen Expiratory = 15 cm H_2O	10 min 10 min	3×/day 4×/day	2 wk 2 wk	Significant increase of experimental group's inspiratory and expiratory muscle strength with less postoperative complications.
Preusser et al.[127]	12—group 1 8—group 2	COPD	Threshold (targeted)	Group 1 = 52% of MIP Group 2 = 22% of MIP	Progressed from 5 to 18 min	3×/wk	12 wk	Significant increase of both group's inspiratory muscle endurance and 12-minute walk test, but only group 1 demonstrated a significant increase in inspiratory muscle strength as early as week 4 of VMT.

*From Cahalin LP: Preoperative and postoperative conditioning for lung transplantation and volume-reduction surgery. Crit Care Nurs Clin North Am 8:305, 1996, with permission.
†Mode of ventilatory muscle training was performed with a device similar to the commercially available PFLEX inspiratory muscle trainer (Healthscan Products, Cedar Grove, NJ), which creates different resistive loads by varying the hole size through which patients breathe.
‡Increased Dead Space and Expiratory Pressure Device (Kayatu Co., Tokyo, Japan).
MIP, maximal inspiratory pressure, PFT, pulmonary function tests; VMT, ventilatory muscle training.

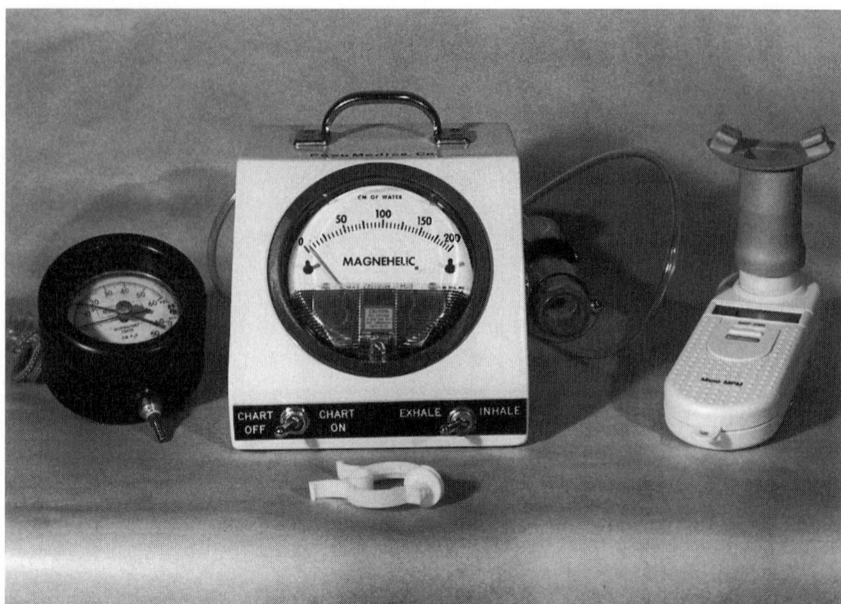

FIGURE **4–13.** Different devices used to measure ventilatory muscle strength.

TABLE **4–19**
Methods to Measure Ventilatory Muscle Performance and Administer Ventilatory Muscle Training

Measurement

Measurement Device: Several different types of devices are used to measure ventilatory muscle performance. Two types are shown in Figure 4–13. The methods to measure the positive and negative pressure (in centimeters of water) generated by the patient during such testing is by a manometer (*A*) or pressure transducer (*B*). When using a manometer a needle is deflected to the point of maximal generated pressure after which the needle may fall back to the resting level of 0. Such devices typically have poorer resolution and reliability. Newer devices such as in Figure 4–13*B* provide a digital display that remains illuminated and as a result of the transducer technology has desirable resolution and reliability.

Body Position: During the measurement of ventilatory muscle performance the patient should wear a noseclip and be seated with the trunk at a 90-degree angle.

1. Maximal inspiratory pressure (MIP):
   A. Have patient expire fully (near residual volume).
   B. Motivate patient to inspire as forcefully as possible.
   C. Document the MIP and repeat the above until a stable baseline is observed.
2. Maximal expiratory pressure (MEP):
   A. Have patient inspire fully (total lung capacity).
   B. Motivate patient to exhale as forcefully as possible.
   C. Document the MEP and repeat the above until a stable baseline is observed.

Administration of Ventilatory Muscle Training

Ventilatory muscle training should be administered by using the above results.

Inspiratory Muscle Training: Begin breathing with one of the devices shown in Figure 4–12 at 20–40% of MIP for 5–15 minutes, 2–3×/day. Increase resistance to 40–60% of MIP based upon patient tolerance.

Expiratory Muscle Training: Begin breathing with one of the devices shown in Figure 4–12 at 5–10% of MEP for 5–15 minutes, 2–3×/day. Increase resistance to 10–40% of MEP based upon patient tolerance.

device and adequate IMT with particular emphasis on monitoring for proper technique, paradoxical breathing, desaturation, and fatigue. Several other important methods to administer IMT are provided in Table 4–19, including different methods to obtain MIP and MEP.

Expiratory muscle training, or positive expiratory pressure (PEP) training, has recently been studied.[114,129,130] Nomori et al. demonstrated improved postoperative outcomes with such training and several other studies have shown that such training may be an effective adjunct to bronchial hygiene therapy[114] including ability to clear secretions through use of stronger expiratory muscles. Methods to administer PEP training include use of commercially available devices such as the device used in the Noromi study (Increased Dead Space and Expiratory Pressure Device; Kayatu Co, Tokyo, Japan) or a device manufactured by Healthscan, Inc. (Threshold Positive Expiratory Pressure Device). After a patient's MEP is obtained (see Table 4–19), the PEP device is set at a specific percentage of MEP and the patient is instructed to use the device for 5 to 15 minutes, several times per day. Other important methods to consider when administering PEP training are provided in Table 4–19. Limited data are available for PEP training, but the results of Noromi et al. warrant further investigation of PEP training in patients prior to thoracic surgery.

Limitations to Exercise Conditioning in Thoracic Surgery Patients

The primary limitations to exercise conditioning prior to thoracic surgery include dyspnea, fatigue, cardiovascular instability, orthopedic or neuromuscular abnormalities, perceived risk of exercise conditioning in an ICU setting (which is probably the ideal setting because of comprehensive monitoring), patient motivation, and acute illness requiring immediate surgery (see Table 4–12). All of these limitations, including the latter, can be approached when an exercise conditioning perspective is focused in the context that exercise conditioning may favorably affect surgical success.

Mechanical Adjuncts to Assist Exercise Conditioning

Heart Disease

Exercise conditioning for patients with heart disease has received much attention since the early 1970s. However, much of the conditioning has been in patients with mild to moderate heart disease and those after surgical intervention, all of which show favorable results. A significant literature now exists regarding exercise training in patients with severe heart disease (Table 4–20) but the effects of such training upon surgical outcome is unknown.[131–148]

A recent investigation of the safety and benefits of exercise conditioning in patients awaiting cardiac transplantation on left ventricular assist devices has confirmed many of the findings described in Table 4–20.[149] Patients on left ventricular assist devices underwent 1,173.6 hours of exercise conditioning without major complications and with only four minor complications (3.4 incidents per 1,000 patient hours). Improvement in exercise tolerance and functional capacity continued until week 6 of conditioning, after which further improvements were minimal. The authors suggested that delay in cardiac transplantation until 6 weeks of exercise conditioning have been performed may improve postoperative recovery and surgical success.[149]

Another group of patients awaiting cardiac transplantation who have received benefit from preoperative exercise conditioning are those on continuous dobutamine infusion. Although dobutamine's mechanism of action enhances cardiac inotropic function, a potential adverse effect is supraventricular and ventricular ectopy. Physical exercise performed in 40 patients on continuous dobutamine infusion at a mean dosage of 200 μg/kg/min was observed to be safe and without complication. No significant increase in ventricular ectopy from resting levels was observed during greater than 1,000 patient hours of exercise.[150]

Lung Disease

NONINVASIVE POSITIVE PRESSURE VENTILATION

Patients with lung disease awaiting thoracic surgery, who are dyspneic at rest, are frequently unable to exercise or exercise for only very short periods of time. It is possible to improve the dyspnea at rest and during exercise as well as limited exercise tolerance by using continuous positive airway pressure (CPAP) or bilevel positive airway pressure (BiPAP) ventilation during exercise conditioning.[151–154] CPAP has been used in three previous studies and has been shown to decrease the degree of dyspnea and increase the level of oxygenation and duration of exercise.[151,152,155] We have also observed an improved exercise duration and level of dyspnea and oxygenation.[153] Such exercise conditioning may improve skeletal muscle strength and endurance in a patient who otherwise would be unable to exercise and may improve surgical success. However, the effects of long-term exercise conditioning with CPAP or BiPAP upon skeletal muscle (peripheral and diaphragmatic) and surgical outcomes using noninvasive ventilatory assistance requires further investigation.

Secretion Clearance

Removal of pulmonary secretions via traditional (e.g., percussion and vibration) and nontraditional methods (e.g., autogenic drainage, flutter valves, aerobic exercise) has previously been observed to improve oxygenation and pulmonary function and positively improve compliance and atelectasis as evidenced radiographically.[154,156–161] As well, fewer pulmonary complications occur in patients receiving preoperative cardiopulmonary physical therapy.[162–164]

The patient who has excess secretion production, with adventitious breath sounds, can be put on a program of secretion clearance. This program can be done by the patient at home, with or without the assistance of a family member. Positioning, with huffing, or forced exhalation used in conjunction with positioning to put the area of the lung with retained secretions in appropriate position to allow gravity to assist in clearance, can be a very effective treatment plan that clears the retained secretions before the operative procedure. The patient should be instructed to self-clear secretions at times of particular retention, which can be when first arising in the morning. As well, many patients with excess secretions of large volumes, such as with bronchiectasis, find that drainage before retiring in the evening, as well as perhaps in the middle of the day, allows more optimal clearance. If patients are unable to clear sufficiently on their own, then either the support of a family member or a visit to the outpatient physical therapy clinic can assist in the clearance of secretion prior to the operative procedure. The optimum plan is thought to be patients clearing on their own, either through increased activity (conditioning program discussed below) or through facilitated drainage through positioning, use of the manual techniques, and coughing/huffing/forced exhalation. (Further detail regarding the efficacy and use of these techniques is in the section "Postoperative Care.")

Patient Instruction in Secretion Removal

If the patient does not have retained secretions, the benefit of short preoperative sessions focusing attention on the lungs by the therapist can further decrease postoperative complications.[162–164] This session can be very simple, direct, and time efficient. Informing the patient of the necessity to do frequent maximal inspiratory volumes postoperatively, having the patient practice briefly,

TABLE 4–20
Review of Exercise Training Studies of Patients With Congestive Heart Failure*

			Exercise Training					Mean Resting LVEF (%)		Complications	
Author	N	Type of Exercise[†]	Duration	Frequency	Intensity	Training Period	Training Effect	Before Training	After Training	Morbidity	Mortality
Lee et al.[83]	18	W, J, B	20–45 min	2–6×/wk	85% HRmax	12–42 mo	Positive	34 ± 4	35 ± 6	0	0
Williams et al.[131]	121	?	?	?	?	2–57 mo	Positive	8–26 (n = 14) 30–49 (n = 23) 51–86 (n = 84)	?	?	?
Cody et al.[132]	32	?	?	4×/wk	?	12 mo	Positive	18	?	4	0
Conn et al.[133]	10	B, W/J	35–45 min	3–5×/wk	70–80% $\dot{V}O_2$max	4–37 mo	Positive	20	?	0	0
Sullivan et al.[98]	16	B, J, B, SC	60 min	3–5×/wk	75% $\dot{V}O_2$max	4–6 mo	Positive	24 ± 10	Unchanged	4	0
Hoffman[134]	41	?	?	3–7×/wk	70–85% HRmax	4 mo	Positive	?	?	0	0
Kellerman et al.[135]	11	AE	?	2×/wk	90% HRmax	36 mo	Positive	30 ± 9.52	?	0	0
Kellerman and Shemesh[136]	11	C	?	2×/wk	2.2–7.5 kcal/min	12 mo	Positive	25.5 ± 6.8	?	0	0
Coats et al.[137§]	17	B	20 min	5×/wk	60–80% HRmax	2 mo	Positive	19	?	0	0
Belardinelli et al.[138,‡]	55	B	40 min	3×/wk	60% $\dot{V}O_2$max	2 mo	Positive	27	27	3	0
Belardinelli et al.[139]	27	B	30 min	3×/wk	40% $\dot{V}O_2$max	2 mo	Positive	31 ± 4	33 ± 4	1	0
Squires et al.[140]	20	B, W	30–40 min	4–6×/wk	50–60% $\dot{V}O_2$max	2 mo	Positive	21 ± 3	?	0	0
Baigrie et al.[141]	17	W	16 min	?	?	4 mo	Positive	21 ± 2	?	?	?
Jetté et al.[142§]	39	W, J, C, B	30–60 min 2×/day	5×/wk	70–80% HRmax	1 mo	Positive	I: 23.9 ± 3.5 II: 39.5 ± 5.7	28.2 ± 7.7 41.3 ± 8.9	3 0	0 0
Meyer et al.[143,§]	15	B	20–25 min	5×/wk	70–80% HRmax	1.5 mo	Positive	23 ± 3.2	?	1	1
Hambrecht et al.[144,§]	22	B	1st 3 wk: 10 min, 6×/day	7×/wk	70% $\dot{V}O_2$max	6 mo	Positive	26 ± 9	?	1	1
Külavuori et al.[145,§]	20	B	30 min	3×/wk	50–60% $\dot{V}O_2$max	3 mo	Positive	24 ± 6	?	0	0
Davey et al.[146,§]	22	B	20 min	5×/wk	70–80% HRmax	2 mo	Positive	22 ± 8	?	0	0
Koch et al.[147,§]	25	K	90 min	3×/wk	?	3 mo	Positive	26 ± 10	27 ± 10	0	0
Kostis et al.[148,§]	20	W, B, RW, SC	60 min	3–5×/wk	40–60% functional capacity	3 mo	Positive	35 ± 6	32 ± 6	0	0

*Adapted from Cahalin LP: Cardiac muscle dysfunction. In Hillgass E, Sadowsky HS (eds), Essentials of Cardiopulmonary Physical Therapy. Philadelphia, WB Saunders Co, 1993, p 171, with permission.
[†]W, walking; J, jogging; B, bicycling; R, running; SR, stationary running; RW, rowing; G, gymnastics; W/J, walking/jogging; SC, stair climbing; AE, arm ergometry; C, calisthenics; K, KOCH bench.
[‡]First study to evaluate the effects of exercise training in patients with diastolic dysfunction.
[§]Randomized, controlled trial.
LVEF, left ventricular ejection fraction; HRmax, maximum heart rate; $\dot{V}O_2$, maximal oxygen consumption.

asking for a strong cough to assess the patient's capability to self-clear secretions, listening to breath sounds to assess the need for future pulmonary care preoperatively, and explaining the value of position change, and potential need for manual techniques to assist in secretion clearance can be accomplished in 20 minutes. Such patient instruction and, if necessary, traditional or nontraditional methods to mobilize retained secretions might improve oxygenation and possibly decrease the pulmonary vascular resistance and work of the cardiopulmonary system.

Patient Compliance, Motivation, and Psychologic Status

Cooper has listed a noncompliant/unmotivated patient as a potential contraindication to volume-reduction surgery.[65] He states that patients unwilling to participate in a rehabilitation program will likely be unwilling to actively participate in the early postoperative period as well as later postoperative rehabilitation. The noncompliance observed preoperatively continues postoperatively and is compounded by the pain of thoracic surgery.

However, patients in whom initial noncompliance with rehabilitation was observed and who subsequently received individual counseling and behavior modification by a physical therapist, nurse, or social worker improved their compliance with preoperative rehabilitation efforts. This improvement in compliance carried over into the postoperative period and appeared to have enhanced postoperative rehabilitative efforts and appeared to decrease the length of hospitalization. The time spent in preoperative rehabilitation is helpful not only for the patient but for the whole medical-surgical team. Important patient behavior patterns can be identified and attempts made to modify them, if necessary.

Information such as that described above has been observed to be more important than was originally thought. Besides our findings of significant correlation between mental health and postoperative status after bilateral volume reduction surgery (see Fig. 4–2 and Table 4–1),[19] many other recent investigations demonstrate the importance of psychologic function with regards to morbidity and mortality.[165–169]

Postoperative Care

Postoperative pulmonary complications (PPC) remain the primary cause of morbidity and mortality for abdominal and thoracic surgical patients.[170–173] Attention to frequent position change, maximal inspiratory volume, clearance of secretions, and early mobilization greatly decrease PPC. This section will briefly comment on the major interventions available to decrease or prevent postoperative complications, some of which have greater benefit if the patient is properly instructed and educated preoperatively.

Positioning

Frequent position change, a very simple and direct approach to care, can be easily overlooked and not appreciated in relation to effects on mucus clearance and ventilation, including muscle excursion, maximizing ventilation-perfusion ($\dot{V}/\dot{Q}$) relationships, and levels of oxygenation.[174–185]

Mucus Flow/Clearance

The normal person has a mucociliary transport of 10 mm/min which decreases about 5% per decade.[175] The effects of anesthesia and intubation decrease the rate of mucociliary transport as does smoking, pre-existing chronic pulmonary disease, and acute respiratory failure requiring mechanical ventilation.[174] Excess mucus combined with low inspiratory volume, and altered mucociliary transport contributes to the pooling of secretions in gravity-dependent positions of the lungs. Frequent change in position can facilitate secretion clearance and minimize the effects of decreased mucociliary transport. Specific positioning to facilitate secretion clearance from areas with retained secretions can also prevent or minimize the secondary complication to infections.

Diaphragmatic Excursion

Positioning also affects the diaphragmatic excursion, and oxygenation, which is also often not understood or considered in relation to efficient, optimal care.[175–177] Attention to position can decrease the sense of dyspnea in the COPD patient.[178] The forward leaning position can decrease dyspnea and decrease or alleviate paradoxical breathing that is evident in other positions. We have found these same results in both the nonintubated patients, as well as in the individual who is having difficulty weaning.

Lying on the side and positioning prone can also affect diaphragmatic excursion.[175] In the nonventilated individual, the gravity-dependent position of the diaphragm has greater excursion. In the supine, the posterior portion has greater excursion, and the converse in prone.[179]

The effect of positioning on an individual's oxygenation who has unilateral or unifocal $\dot{V}/\dot{Q}$ abnormalities is most evident with the improvement in oxygenation observed with the good lung down.[181–183] As well, for the individual who is in significant respiratory failure, with poor oxygenation, the prone position can result in a significant increase in oxygenation.[183] This change is thought to occur through a counteracting of the adverse $\dot{V}/\dot{Q}$ in the gravity-dependent area of the lung, and gravity assisting with clearance of retained secretions.

Clinical concern that dramatic or significant position change will adversely affect oxygenation, cardiac response, and intracranial pressure (ICP) may, in fact, allow a detrimental hesitation to an intervention that can provide dramatic changes in oxygenation and secretion clearance, with non–medically significant changes in cardiac output and ICP.[161, 184] In acutely ill trauma patients, MacKenzie et al. found that the changes in ICP were not of a significant level to the patient; at the same time the use of dramatic positioning (Trendelenburg) and manual techniques reversed significant lung collapse, with consequent changes in lung compliance and oxygenation.[185]

Maximizing Inspiratory Volume

The basic preoperative instruction of how to inspire maximally, including a sustained inspiration, can allow a patient to understand what is expected postoperatively, as well as reverse or prevent atelectasis and retained secretions. Thoren in 1954 provided the landmark study regarding the efficacy of simple preoperative instruction followed by the simple intervention of promoting maximal inspiration, and use of other manual techniques only as needed.[162] In a population of some 400 patients who were undergoing abdominal surgery, only 12% of those who received pre- and postoperative care (focused on maximal inspiration and clearance of retained secretions) experienced PPC; as compared to 24% of those who had only postoperative intervention; and 48% in those who had usual and ordinary care, including a stir-up regimen. Similar results regarding the value of a simple, short preoperative session to educate the patient regarding maximal inspiration, positioning, and manual techniques if patients are unable to clear their own retained secretions has recently been reported by Roy, in 100 cardiac surgical patients.[164] Those patients who received preoperative education sessions had fewer postoperative therapy sessions, shorter treatment time, and a shorter average length of stay.

The individual can be instructed in how to self-monitor the maximal inspiration, attempting to get equal thoracic expansion. The temptation to hold the operative thorax stable during inspiration can result in significant decrease in lung sounds, and evidence of atelectasis on x-ray. The combination of early mobilization, sitting upright, and maximal inspirations with good thoracic motion can minimize the need for any further intervention to prevent PPC. The use of an incentive spirometer does not necessarily change or alter postoperative complications when used in conjunction with breathing exercises and other techniques or early ambulation.[186–188] The use of incentive spirometry does not necessarily alleviate the tendency to splint the operative side, and the patient must be aware that this device is only as good or beneficial as the patient's techniques in using the device. If an individual does splint the operative site, with resultant decrease in breath sounds, and atelectasis, then use of the techniques of stretch and resistance to the intercostal muscle of the operative side can result in good thoracic motion,[189] which can then be repeated by the alert patient. Judicious use of pain medications, including thoracic nerve analgesia, can also decrease or minimize thoracic splinting. A simple deep breath of reasonable volume with attention to not splint the operative side area is amazingly simple for many patients.

Use of Manual Techniques

The use of manual techniques may be necessary to dislodge thick, inspissated secretions.[190] There is some controversy over the efficacy of these techniques in the person with small amounts of retained secretions; however, Feldman et al. found significant increases in expiratory volume at low lung volumes with only 5 ml sputum produced.[191] There is a great deal of difference between the ambulatory individual who produces a relatively small amount of excess secretions, which can be cleared by activity, maximal inspirations, and forced inhalation or cough, including the use of positioning, as compared to the individual who is sedated, has undergone an operative procedure that affects mucociliary transport, and has little to no ability to self-initiate increased inspiratory volume or an effective cough.

The research regarding the efficacy of these techniques is too variable to make conclusions for vast or wide patient populations. The frequency, duration, and force of techniques such as percussion is seldom, if ever, reported.[192–194] As well, clinically defined outcomes are difficult to measure in relation to sputum amounts, changes radiographically, changes in compliance, or changes in breath sounds. Some investigators, in attempting to standardize treatment, have inappropriately controlled for the time or duration of the use of manual techniques instead of adapting treatment to patient need and response.

Our experience matches that of Maryland Shock Trauma and others, where skilled application of these techniques in the acutely ill, postsurgical patient results in reversal of atelectasis equal to that obtained by bronchoscopy, improvement in oxygenation in the marginally oxygenated patient, and dramatic changes in compliance, even with as little as 2 ml of secretions cleared.[185,195]

Clearance of Secretions

Loosened secretions must be cleared via patient's self-initiated maximal inspiratory volume. If this fails, then use of manual techniques in conjunction with maximal inspiratory volume, cough, huff, or forced exhalation in the nonintubated, alert patient should clear the secretions. Suctioning is a last resort in the nonintubated patient.

The importance of adequate inspiratory volume prior to self-initiated cough or suction, promoting spontaneous cough during suction, is often overlooked in the process of attempting to clear secretions.

The contractile capability of the diaphragm is decreased postoperatively.[196] The alert individual may find it much more effective to initiate a cough in the sitting versus the supine position.[197] To insist that the individual remain side-lying or in a drainage position to clear secretions once loosened can decrease the effect of the treatment. Supporting the surgical site during the cough and not restricting chest motion during the inspiratory phase can facilitate an effective cough.[198]

Many postoperative patients find it less threatening to huff or do a forced exhalation, especially when they are finding it difficult to actually cough. Once the individual huffs, this many times leads to a spontaneous cough, as secretions begin to mobilize.

When an individual has retained secretions, either as evidenced by breath sounds or x-ray and has other indications of collapse such as an increased temperature, poor oxygenation via O_2 oximeter or blood gases, the individual may need to be suctioned. The outcome desired is removal of secretions while maintaining good oxygenation and stable cardiac status. This chapter will not delineate the various approaches to suctioning of either the intubated or nonintubated, but these are techniques for patients who are unable to clear their own retained secretions. As well, the techniques of promoting a more effective cough during the suctioning process by instillation of small amounts of saline must not be confused in purpose. Those who have studied instillation of saline and have questioned its efficacy, as well as measured efforts on oxygenation,[199] should remember that the purpose of this saline injection is to promote a cough, and potentially provide a medium upon which the viscous secretions can travel and which can occur without deleterious effects on oxygenation.[200] As well, use of the manual techniques during suctioning have been found beneficial in patients with thick, inspissated secretions that do not clear well with just suctioning.

Mobilization/Exercise Postoperatively

The value of early position change, including sitting, standing, and ambulation is increasingly evidenced both clinically and in the literature.[73,201] If the ventilated or nonventilated patients are stable physiologically, early mobilization should be an essential and front-line intervention to their care. Even as the average length of stay decreases, preoperative endurance training and then early mobilization postoperatively can greatly facilitate the recovery of the individual. The benefits of early mobilization are many, including preventing or reversing PPC, minimizing the effects of prolonged bed rest, including deep venous thrombi, pulmonary embolism, and increasing resting heart rate. As well, potential for joint contracture, muscle atrophy, skin breakdown, and demineralization of long bones are also minimized or avoided.[73]

The concern that the patients need to recover from the effects of anesthesia before ambulating has previously delayed postoperative ambulation where physiologically stable, alert patients can be brought to sitting, standing, and even walking within hours of the operative procedure. As well, there has been a bias that the long-term ventilated patient also could not be mobilized. Mobilization can be done in the physiologically stable person, providing adequate oxygenation to allow the person to compensate for the increased energy expenditure. The dilemma of a patient on oxygen support while at bed rest, and then ambulating into the hall with the same level of oxygen support or, worse yet, with the oxygen support removed, defies logic. Ambulation requires increased energy expenditure and thus increased oxygen consumption.

The patient can be given instructions on how to maintain or increase activity, once discharged. Patients might feel safe and comfortable walking or ambulating in the hospital, since immediate assistance is available. These same patients often then limit their activity in the home if no immediate help is available, fearful of some injury or adverse response. This self-limitation can greatly affect the overall success of the procedure, and the patient and family can be motivated by being informed about the need of activity, the appropriate level, how to monitor response, and how to encourage progression in activity over time. Patients can also have a contact number to call if they have questions regarding this and other areas of concern once they go home.

Summary

Many methods have been used to evaluate successful surgical outcomes. The most important predictive variables appear to entail exercise response. Submaximal and maximal responses have been used successfully in predicting surgical success. Patients demonstrating greater levels of exercise or work, and cardiorespiratory fitness, appear to be the most successful surgical candidates.

References

1. Smith TP, Kinasewitz GT, Tucker WY, et al: Exercise capacity as a predictor of post-thoracotomy morbidity. Am Rev Respir Dis 129:730, 1984.
2. Markos J, Mullan BP, Hillman DP, et al: Preoperative assessment as a predictor of mortality and morbidity after lung resection. Am Rev Respir Dis 139:902, 1989.
3. Olsen GN: The evolving role of exercise testing prior to lung resection. Chest 95:218, 1989.
4. Olsen GN: Preoperative physiology and lung resection. Scan? Exercise? Both? (Editorial). Chest 101:300, 1992.
5. Keagy BA, Schorlemmer GR, Murray GF, et al: Correlation of preoperative pulmonary function testing and clinical course in patients after pneumonectomy. Ann Thorac Surg 36:253, 1983.
6. Zibrak JD, O'Donnell CR, Marton K: Indications for pulmonary function testing. Ann Intern Med 112:763, 1990.
7. Peters RM, Clausen JL, Tisi GM: Extending respectability for carcinoma of the lung in patients with impaired pulmonary function. Ann Thorac Surg 26:250, 1978.
8. Boysen PG, Block J, Moulder PV: Relationship between preoperative pulmonary function tests and complications after thoracotomy. Surg Gynecol Obstet 152:813, 1981.
9. Bechard D, Wetstein L: Assessment of exercise oxygen consumption as preoperative criterion for lung resection. Ann Thorac Surg 44:344, 1987.
10. Smith TP, Kinasewitz GT, Tucker AY, et al: Exercise capacity as a predictor of post-thoracotomy morbidity. Am Rev Respir Dis 129:730, 1984.
11. Eugene J, Brown SE, Light RW, et al: Maximum oxygen consumption: A physiologic guide to pulmonary resection. Surg Forum 33:260, 1982.
12. Epstein SK, Faling LJ, Daly BDT, Celli BR: Predicting complications after pulmonary resection. Preoperative exercise testing vs. a multifactorial cardiopulmonary risk index. Chest 104:694, 1993.
13. Gilbreth EM, Weisman IM: Role of exercise stress testing in preoperative evaluation of patients for lung resection. Clin Chest Med 15:389, 1994.
14. Morrone TM, Buck LA, Catanese KA, et al: Early progressive mobilization of patients with left ventricular assist devices is

safe and optimizes recovery before heart transplantation. J Heart Lung Transplant 15:423, 1996.
15. Stewart AL, Hays RD, Ware JE: The MOS Short-Form General Health Survey—reliability and validity in a patient population. Med Care 26:724, 1988.
16. McHorney CA, Ware JE, Rogers W, et al: The validity and relative precision of MOS Short- and Long-Form health status scales and Dartmouth coop charts—results from the medical outcomes study. Medical Care 30:253, 1992.
17. McHorney CA, Ware JE, Raczek AK: The MOS 36-Item Short-Form Health Survey (SF-36): Psychometric and clinical tests of validity in measuring physical and mental health constructs. Med Care 31:247, 1993.
18. Stewart AL, Hays RD, Wells KB, et al: Long-term functioning and well-being outcomes associated with physical activity and exercise in patients with chronic conditions in the medical outcomes study. J Clin Epidemiol 47:719, 1994.
19. Cahalin L, Cannan J, Cohen M, et al: Mental health and social status are related to postoperative status after bilateral lung volume reduction surgery. Chest 110:145S, 1996.
20. Gaensler EA, Cugell DW, Lindgren RL, et al: The role of pulmonary insufficiency in mortality and invalidism following surgery for pulmonary tuberculosis. J Thorac Cardiovasc Surgery 29:163, 1955.
21. Lange P, Nyboe J, Appleyard M, et al: Ventilatory function and chronic mucus hypersecretion as predictors of death from lung cancer. Am Rev Respir Dis 141:613, 1990.
22. Gass GD, Olsen GN: Preoperative pulmonary function testing to predict postoperative morbidity and mortality. Chest 89:127, 1986.
23. Ladurie ML, Ranson-Bitker B: Uncertainties in the expected value for forced expiratory volume in one second after surgery. Chest 90:222, 1986.
24. Boushy SF, Billeq DM, North LB, Helgason AH: Clinical course related to preoperative and postoperative pulmonary function in patients with bronchogenic carcinoma. Chest 59:373, 1971.
25. Lockwood P: The principles of predicting risk of post thoracotomy-function-related complications in bronchogenic carcinoma. Respiration 30:329, 1973.
26. Gracey DR, Divertie MB, Didier EP: Preoperative pulmonary preparation of patients with chronic obstructive pulmonary disease. A prospective study. Chest 76:2, 1979.
27. Tisi GM: Preoperative evaluation of pulmonary function. Am Rev Respir Dis 119:293, 1979.
28. Risser NL: Preoperative and postoperative care to prevent pulmonary complications. Heart Lung 9:57, 1980.
29. Mittman C: Assessment of operative risk in thoracic surgery. Am Rev Respir Dis 84:197, 1961.
30. Didolkar MS, Moore RH, Takita H: Evaluation of the risk in pulmonary resection for bronchogenic carcinoma. Am J Surg 127:700, 1974.
31. Colman NC, Schraufnagel DE, Rivington RN, Pardy RL: Exercise testing in evaluation of patients for lung resection. Am Rev Respir Dis 125:604, 1982.
32. Keeley RC, Pickerill RG, Ohayon JJ, et al: Resting and exercise lung function before and after thoracotomy and their relationship to perioperative complications. Am Rev Respir Dis 131:A84, 1985.
33. Ussetti P, Roca J, Agusti AGN, et al: Failure of exercise tolerance and hemodynamic studies to predict early post thoracotomy morbidity and mortality. Am Rev Respir Dis 131:A94, 1985.
34. Older P, Smith R, Courtney P, et al: Preoperative evaluation of cardiac failure and ischemia in elderly patients by cardiopulmonary exercise testing. Chest 104:701, 1983.
35. Ellestad MH: Stress Testing—Principles and Practice, 2nd ed. Philadelphia, FA Davis Co, 1980.
36. Fishman RS, Systrom DM: Preoperative cardiopulmonary exercise testing: Determining the limit to exercise and predicting outcome after thoracotomy. J Cardiothorac Vasc Anesth 5:614, 1991.
37. Fletcher GF, Balady G, Froelicher VF, et al: Exercise Standards: A statement for health professionals from the American Heart Association. Circulation 92:201, 1995.
38. Pina IL, Balady GJ, Hanson P, et al: Guidelines for clinical exercise testing laboratories: A statement for healthcare professionals from the committee on exercise and cardiac rehabilitation, American Heart Association. Circulation 91:912, 1995.
39. American College of Sports Medicine: ACSM's Guidelines for Exercise Testing and Prescription, 5th ed. Baltimore, Williams & Wilkins, 1995.
40. Franklin BA, Gordon S, Timmis GC, et al: Is direct physician supervision of exercise stress testing routinely necessary? Chest 111:262, 1997.
41. Cahalin LP, Blessey RL, Kummer D, et al: The safety of exercise testing performed independently by physical therapists. J Cardiopulm Rehabil 7:269, 1987.
42. DeBusk RF: Exercise test supervision: Time for reassessment. Exerc Standards Malpract Reporter 2:65, 1988.
43. Lem V, Krivokapich J, Child JS: A nurse-supervised exercise stress testing laboratory. Heart Lung 14:280, 1985.
44. Knight JA, Laubach CA, Butcher RJ, et al: Supervision of clinical exercise testing by exercise physiologists. Am J Cardiol 75: 390, 1995.
45. Franklin BA, Dressendorfer R, Bonzheim K, et al: Safety of exercise testing by non-physician health care providers: Eighteen year experience (Abstract). Circulation 92:1-737, 1995.
46. Rochmis P, Blackburn H: Exercise tests: A survey of procedures, safety, and litigation experience in approximately 170,000 tests. JAMA 217:1061, 1971.
47. Scherer D, Kaltenbach M: Frequency of life-threatening complications associated with exercise testing. Dtsch Med Wochenschr 33:1161, 1979.
48. Young DZ, Lambert S, Graboys TB, et al: Safety of maximal exercise testing in patients at high risk for ventricular arrhythmias. Circulation 70:184, 1984.
49. Atterhog JH, Jonsson B, Samuelsson R: Exercise testing: A prospective study of complication rates. Am Heart J 98:572, 1979.
50. Blessey RL: Exercise testing by non-physician health care professionals: Complication rates, clinical competencies and future trends. Exerc Standards Malpract Reporter 3:69, 1989.
51. Gibbons L, Blair SN, Kohl HW, et al: The safety of maximal exercise testing. Circulation 80:846, 1989.
52. Miyoshi S, Nakahara K, Ohno K, et al: Exercise tolerance test in lung cancer patients: The relationship between exercise capacity and postthoracotomy hospital mortality. Ann Thorac Surg 44:487, 1987.
53. Olsen GN, Weiman DS, Bolton JWR, et al: Submaximal invasive exercise testing and quantitative lung scanning in the evaluation for tolerance of lung resection. Chest 95:267, 1989.
54. Stuart RJ, Ellestad MH: National survey of exercise stress testing facilities. Chest 77:94, 1980.
55. Cooper KH: A means of assessing maximal oxygen intake. Correlation between field and treadmill testing. JAMA 203:201, 1968.
56. McGavin CR, Gupta SP, McHardy GJR: Twelve-minute walking test for assessing disability in chronic bronchitis. Br Med J 1: 822, 1976.
57. Bagg LR: The 12-min walking distance; its use in the preoperative assessment of patients with bronchial carcinoma before lung resection. Respiration 46:342, 1984.
58. Holden DA, Rice TW, Stelmach K, Meeker DP: Exercise testing, 6-min walk, and stair climb in the evaluation of patients at high risk for pulmonary resection. Chest 102:1774, 1992.
59. Olsen GN, Bolton JWR, Weiman DS, Horning CA: Stair climbing as an exercise test to predict perioperative complications of lung resection: Two years experience. Chest 99:587, 1991.
60. Bolton JWR, Weiman DS, Haynes JL, et al: Stair climbing as an indicator of pulmonary function. Chest 92:783, 1987.
61. Bittner V, Weiner DH, Yusuf S, et al: Prediction of mortality and morbidity with a 6-minute walk test in patients with left ventricular dysfunction. JAMA 270:1702, 1993.
62. Cahalin LP, Mathier MA, Semigran MJ, et al: The six-minute walk test predicts peak oxygen uptake and survival in patients with advanced heart failure. Chest 110:325, 1996.
63. Cahalin L, Pappagianopoulos P, Prevost S, et al: The relationship of the 6-min walk test to maximal oxygen consumption in transplant candidates with end-stage lung disease. Chest 108:452, 1995.
64. Szekely LA, Celberg DA, Wright C, et al: Preoperative predic-

tors of operative morbidity and mortality in COPD patients undergoing bilateral lung volume reduction surgery. Chest 111: 550, 1997.
65. Cooper JD, Trulock EP, Triantafillou AN, et al: Bilateral pneumectomy (volume reduction) for chronic obstructive pulmonary disease. J Thorac Cardiovasc Surg 109:106, 1995.
66. Saltin B, Blomavist G, Mitchell JH, et al: Response to exercise after bed rest and after training. A longitudinal study of adaptive changes in oxygen transport and body composition. Circulation 38:VII-1, 1968.
67. MacKenzie C (ed): Chest Physiotherapy in the Intensive Care Unit. Baltimore, Williams & Wilkins, 1981.
68. Bassey EJ, Bennett T, Birmingham AT, et al: Effects of surgical operation and bed rest on cardiovascular responses to exercise in hospital patients. Cardiovasc Res 7:588, 1973.
69. Bassey EJ, Bennett T, Birmingham AT, et al: Changes in cardiorespiratory response to exercise following bed rest in hospital patients. J Physiol 222:79, 1971.
70. Clausen JP: Circulation adjustment to dynamic exercise and effect of exercise training in normal subjects and patients with ischemic heart disease. Prog Cardiovasc Dis 18:459, 1976.
71. Clausen JP: Effect of physical training on cardiovascular adjustments to exercise in man. Physiol Rev 57:779, 1977.
72. Rowell LB: Human cardiovascular adjustments to exercise and thermal stress. Physiol Rev 54:75, 1974.
73. Astrand P, Rodahl K: Textbook of Work Physiology, 2nd ed. New York, McGraw-Hill, 1977.
74. Gollnick PD, Armstring RB, Saubert CW, et al: Enzyme activity and fiber composition in skeletal muscle of untrained and trained men. J Appl Physiol 33:312, 1972.
75. Saltin B, Nazar K, Costill DL, et al: The nature of the training response: Peripheral and central adaptations to one-legged exercise. Acta Physiol Scand 96:278, 1976.
76. Saltin B: Hemodynamic adaptation to exercise. Am J Cardiol 55:42D, 1985.
77. Hsia CCW, Carlin JI, Cassidy SS, et al: Hemodynamic changes after pneumonectomy in the exercising foxhound. J Appl Physiol 69:51, 1990.
78. DeGraff AC, Taylor HF, Ord JW, et al: Exercise limitation following extensive pulmonary resection. J Clin Invest 44:1514, 1965.
79. Harrison RW, Adams WE, Long E, et al: The clinical significance of cor pulmonale in the reduction of cardiopulmonary reserve following extensive pulmonary resection. J Thorac Surg 36:352, 1958.
80. Uggla L-G: Indications for and results of thoracic surgery with regard to respiratory and circulatory function tests. Acta Chir Scand 111:197, 1956.
81. Burrows B, Kettel LS, Niden AH, et al: Patterns of cardiovascular dysfunction in chronic obstructive lung disease. N Engl J Med 286:912, 1972.
82. Timms RM, Khaja FV, Williams GW, and the Nocturnal Oxygen Therapy Trial Group: Hemodynamic response to oxygen therapy in chronic obstructive pulmonary disease. Ann Intern Med 102: 29, 1985.
83. Lee AP, Ice R, Blessey R, Sanmarco ME: Long-term effects of physical training on coronary patients with impaired ventricular function. Circulation 60:1519, 1979.
84. Cahalin L: Pulmonary hypertension and exercise. Cardiopulm Phys Ther 6:3, 1995.
85. Himelman RB, Stulbarg M, Kircher B, et al: Noninvasive evaluation of pulmonary artery pressure during exercise by saline-enhanced Doppler echocardiography in chronic pulmonary disease. Circulation 79:863, 1989.
86. D'Alonzo GE, Pohil RL, DuRee SL, Dantzker DR: Comparison of progressive exercise performance of normal subjects and patients with primary pulmonary hypertension. Chest 92:57, 1987.
87. Gibbs JSR, Keegan J, Wright C, et al: Pulmonary artery pressure changes during exercise and daily activities in chronic heart failure. J Am Coll Cardiol 15:52, 1990.
88. Ashutosh K, Dunsky M: Noninvasive tests for responsiveness of pulmonary hypertension to oxygen. Prediction of survival in patients with chronic obstructive lung disease and cor pulmonale. Chest 92:393, 1987.
89. Sietsema KE: Oxygen uptake kinetics in response to exercise in patients with pulmonary vascular disease. Am Rev Respir Dis 145:1052, 1992.
90. Rhodes J, Barst RJ, Garofano RP, et al: Hemodynamic correlates of exercise function in patients with primary hypertension. J Am Coll Cardiol 18:1738, 1991.
91. Morrison DA, Klein C, Welsh CH: Relief of right ventricular angina and increased exercise capacity with long-term oxygen therapy. Chest 100:534, 1991.
92. Hebert CA, Byrnes TJ, Baethge BA, et al: Exercise limitation in patients with polymyositis. Chest 98:352, 1990.
93. Otulana B, Higenbottam T: The role of physiological deadspace and shunt in the gas exchange of patients with pulmonary hypertension: A study of exercise and prostacyclin infusion. Eur Respir J 1:732, 1988.
94. Adnot S, Andrivet P, Piquet J, et al: The effects of urapidil therapy on hemodynamics and gas exchange in exercising patients with chronic obstructive pulmonary disease and pulmonary hypertension. Am Rev Respir Dis 137:1068, 1988.
95. Theodore J, Morris AJ, Burke CM, et al: Cardiopulmonary function at maximum tolerable constant work rate exercise following human heart-lung transplantation. Chest 92:433, 1987.
96. Richards AM, Ikram H, Crozier IG, et al: Ambulatory pulmonary arterial pressure in primary pulmonary hypertension: Variability, relation to systemic arterial pressure, and plasma catecholamines. Br Heart J 63:103, 1990.
97. Himelman RB, Stulbarg MS, Lee E, et al: Noninvasive evaluation of pulmonary artery systolic pressures during dynamic exercise by saline-enhanced Doppler echocardiography. Am Heart J 119(3-1):685, 1990.
98. Sullivan MJ, Higginbotham MB, Cobb FR: Exercise training in patients with severe left ventricular dysfunction: Hemodynamic and metabolic effects. Circulation 78:506, 1988.
99. Degre S, Sergysels R, Messin R, et al: Hemodynamic responses to physical training in patients with chronic lung disease. Am Rev Respir Dis 110:395, 1974.
100. Chester EH, Belman MJ, Bahler RC, et al: Multidisciplinary treatment of chronic pulmonary insufficiency. Chest 72:695, 1977.
101. Alpert JS, Bass H, Szucs MM, et al: Effects of physical training on hemodynamics and pulmonary function at rest and during exercise in patients with chronic obstructive pulmonary disease. Chest 66:647, 1974.
102. Urata H, Tanabe Y, Kiyonaga A, et al: Antihypertensive and volume-depleting effects of mild exercise on essential hypertension. Hypertension 9:245, 1987.
103. National Heart, Lung, and Blood Institute: Report of the Hypertension Task Force: Current research and recommendations from the Task Force Subgroups on local and systemic hemodynamics. Bethesda, MD: Department of Health, Education, and Welfare, Public Health Service, National Institutes of Health, DHEW Publication #79-1623, 3:24 1979.
104. Bjorntorp P: Hypertension and exercise. Hypertension 4(Suppl III):56, 1982.
105. Blackburn H: Non-pharmacological treatment of hypertension: Discussion. Ann NY Acad Sci 304:236, 1978.
106. Sannerstedt R: Rehabilitation in arterial hypertension. Adv Cardiol 24:164, 1978.
107. Hagberg J, Goldring D, Ehsani A, et al: Effect of exercise training on the blood pressure and hemodynamic features of hypertensive adolescents. Am J Cardiol 52:763, 1983.
108. Krotkiewski M, Mandroukas K, Morgan L, et al: Effects of physical training on adrenergic sensitivity in obesity. J Appl Physiol 55:1811, 1983.
109. Fee HJ, Holmes EC, Gewirtz HS, et al: Role of pulmonary vascular resistance measurements in preoperative evaluation of candidates for pulmonary resection. J Thorac Cardiovasc Surg 75: 519, 1978.
110. Olsen GN, Weiman DS, Bolton JWR, et al: Submaximal invasive exercise testing and quantitative lung scanning in the evaluation for tolerance of lung resection. Chest 95:267, 1989.
111. Scheuer J, Tipton CM: Cardiovascular adaptations to physical training. Ann Rev Physiol 39:221, 1977.
112. Blomqvist CG: Cardiovascular adaptations to physical training. Ann Rev Physiol 45:169, 1983.

113. Coats AJS, Adamopoulos S, Radaelli A, et al: Controlled trial of physical training in chronic heart failure. Exercise performance, hemodynamics, ventilation, and autonomic function. Circulation 85:2119, 1992.
114. Nomori H, Kobayashi R, Fuyuno G, et al: Preoperative respiratory muscle training. Assessment in thoracic surgery patients with special reference to postoperative pulmonary complications. Chest 105:1782, 1994.
115. Scott JP, Beck KC, Peters SG, et al: Determinants of survival following lung transplant assessment. The role of respiratory muscle strength. J Heart Lung Transplant 14:S37, 1995.
116. Cahalin L, Cannan J, Szekely L, et al: Effects of ventilatory muscle performance upon outcomes after bilateral lung volume reduction surgery. J Cardiopulm Rehabil 16:316, 1996.
117. Yang KL: Inspiratory pressure/maximal inspiratory pressure ratio: A predictive index of weaning outcome. Intensive Care Med 19:204, 1993.
118. Cahalin LP, Semigran MJ, Dec GW: Ventilatory muscle training in chronic congestive heart failure. In Proceedings of the Twelfth International Congress of the World Confederation of Physical Therapy, 1995, p 445.
119. Cahalin LP, Semigran MJ, Dec GW: Inspiratory muscle training in patients with chronic heart failure awaiting cardiac transplantation: Results of a pilot clinical trial. Phys Ther 77:830, 1997.
120. Chen H, Dukes R, Martin BJ: Inspiratory muscle training in patients with chronic obstructive pulmonary disease. Am Rev Respir Dis 131:251, 1985.
121. Larson JL, Kim MJ, Sharp JT, Larson DA: Inspiratory muscle training with a pressure threshold breathing device in patients with chronic obstructive pulmonary disease. Am Rev Respir Dis 138:689, 1988.
122. Harver A, Mahler DA, Daubenspeck JA: Targeted inspiratory muscle training improves respiratory muscle function and reduces dyspnea in patients with chronic obstructive pulmonary disease. Ann Intern Med 111:117, 1989.
123. Dekhuijzen R, Folgering HTM, van Herwaarden CLA: Target-flow inspiratory muscle training during pulmonary rehabilitation in patients with COPD. Chest 99:128, 1991.
124. Weiner P, Azgad Y, Ganam R: Inspiratory muscle training combined with general exercise reconditioning in patients with COPD. Chest 102:1351, 1992.
125. Weiner P, Azgad Y, Ganam R, Weiner M: Inspiratory muscle training in patients with bronchial asthma. Chest 102:1357, 1992.
126. Suzuki S, Yoshike Y, Suzuki M, et al: Inspiratory muscle training and respiratory sensation during treadmill exercise. Chest 104: 197, 1993.
127. Preusser BA, Winningham ML, Clanton TL: High- vs. low-intensity inspiratory muscle interval training in patients with COPD. Chest 106:110, 1994.
128. Clanton TL, Diaz PT: Clinical assessment of the respiratory muscles. Phys Ther 75:983, 1995.
129. AARC Clinical Practice Guideline: Use of positive airway pressure adjuncts to bronchial hygiene therapy. Respir Care 38:516, 1993.
130. Mahlmeister MJ, Fink JB, Hoffman GL, Fifer LF: Positive-expiratory-pressure mask therapy: Theoretical and practical considerations and a review of the literature. Respir Care 36:1218, 1991.
131. Williams RS, Conn EH, Wallace AG: Enhanced exercise performance following physical training in coronary patients stratified by left ventricular ejection fraction. Circulation 64:IV-186, 1981.
132. Cody DV, Dennis AR, Ross DA, et al: Early exercise testing, physical training and mortality in patients with severe left ventricular dysfunction. J Am Coll Cardiol 1:718, 1983.
133. Conn EH, Williams RS, Wallacea AG: Exercise responses before and after physical conditioning in patients with severely depressed left ventricular function. Am J Cardiol 49:296, 1982.
134. Hoffman A: The effects of training on the physical working capacity of MI patients with left ventricular dysfunction. Eur Heart J 8(Suppl G):43, 1987.
135. Kellermann JJ, Shemesh J, Fisman E, et al: Arm exercise training in the rehabilitation of patients with impaired ventricular function and heart failure. Cardiology 77:130, 1990.
136. Kellerman JJ, Shemesh J: Exercise training of patients with severe heart failure. J Cardiovasc Pharmacol 10:S172, 1987.
137. Coats AJS, Adamopoulos S, Radaelli A, et al: Controlled trial of physical training in chronic heart failure. Exercise performance, hemodynamics, ventilation, and autonomic function. Circulation 85:2119, 1992.
138. Belardinelli R, Georgiou D, Cianci G, et al: Exercise training improves left ventricular diastolic filling in patients with dilated cardiomyopathy: Clinical and prognostic implications. Circulation 91:2775, 1995.
139. Belardinelli R, Georgiou D, Scocco V, et al: Low intensity exercise training in patients with chronic heart failure. J Am Coll Cardiol 26:975, 1995.
140. Squires RW, Lavie CJ, Brandt TR, et al: Cardiac rehabilitation in patients with severe ischemic left ventricular dysfunction. Mayo Clin Proc 62:997, 1987.
141. Baire RS, Myers MG, Kavanagh T, et al: Benefits of physical training in patients with heart failure. Can J Cardiol 8(Suppl B): 107B, 1992.
142. Jette M, Heller R, Landrey F, Blumchen G: Randomized 4-week exercise program in patients with impaired left ventricular function. Circulation 84:1561, 1991.
143. Meyer TE, Casadei B, Coats AJS, et al: Angiotension-converting enzyme inhibition and physical training in heart failure. J Intern Med 230:407, 1991.
144. Hambrecht R, Niebauer J, Fiehn E, et al: Physical training in patients with stable chronic heart failure: Effects on cardiorespiratory fitness and ultrastructural abnormalities of leg muscles. J Am Coll Cardiol 25:1239, 1995.
145. Kulavuori K, Toivonen L, Naveri H, Leinonen H: Reversal of autonomic derangements by physical training in chronic heart failure. Eur Heart J 16:490, 1995.
146. Davey P, Meyer TE, Coats AJS, et al: Ventilation in chronic heart failure: Effects of physical training. Br Heart J 68:474, 1992.
147. Koch M, Douard H, Broustet JP: The benefit of graded physical exercise in chronic heart failure. Chest 101:231S, 1992.
148. Kostis JB, Rosen RC, Cosgrove NM, et al: Nonpharmacologic therapy improves functional and emotional status in congestive heart failure. Chest 106:996, 1994.
149. Morrone T, Buck L, Catanese K, et al: Early progressive mobilization of left ventricular assist device patients is safe and optimizes recovery prior to cardiac transplant. J Cardiopulm Rehabil 15:364, 1995.
150. Cahalin LP: Heart failure. Phys Ther 76:516, 1996.
151. Henke KG, Regnis JA, Bye PTP: Benefits of continuous positive airway pressure during exercise in cystic fibrosis and relationship to disease severity. Am Rev Respir Dis 148:1272, 1993.
152. Maltais F, Reissmann H, Gottfried SB: Pressure support reduces inspiratory effort and dyspnea during exercise in chronic airflow obstruction. Am J Respir Crit Care Med 151:1027, 1995.
153. Cahalin L, Cannan J, Prevost S, et al: Exercise performance during assisted ventilation with bi-level positive airway pressure (BiPAP). J Cardiopulm Rehabil 14:323, 1994.
154. Laszlo G, Archer G, Darrell JH, et al: The diagnosis and prophylaxis of pulmonary complications of surgical operation. Br J Surg 60:129, 1973.
155. O'Donnell DE, Sanii R, Younes M: Improvement in exercise endurance in patients with chronic airflow limitation using continuous positive airway pressure. Am Rev Respir Dis 138:1510, 1988.
156. Bartlett RH, Gazzaniga AB, Geraghty TR: Respiratory maneuvers to prevent postoperative pulmonary complications. JAMA 234:1017, 1973.
157. Palmer KN, Sellick BA: The prevention of post-operative pulmonary atelectasis. Lancet 24:164, 1953.
158. Breslin EH: Prevention and treatment of pulmonary complications in patients after surgery of the upper abdomen. Heart Lung 10:411, 1981.
159. Lord G, Hiebert C, Francis D: A clinical, radiologic evaluation of chest physiotherapy. J Maine Med Assoc 63:142, 1972.
160. Wiklander O, Norlin U: Effect of physiotherapy on postoperative pulmonary complications. Acta Chir Scand 112:146, 1957.
161. Mackenzie C, Shin B, McAslan T: Chest physiotherapy: The effect on arterial oxygenation. Anesth Analg 57:28, 1978.
162. Thoren L: Postoperative pulmonary complications: Observations on their prevention by means of physiotherapy. Acta Chir Scand 107:193, 1954.

163. Vraciu JK, Vraciu RA: Effectiveness of breathing exercises in preventing pulmonary complications following open heart surgery. Phys Ther 57:1367, 1977.
164. Roy BD: Physical therapy preoperative teaching effect on postoperative treatment time and length of stay in cardiac surgical patients. 1995 (thesis).
165. Stein M, Cassara E: Preoperative evaluation and therapy for surgery patients. JAMA 211:787, 1970.
166. Frasure-Smith N, Lesperance F, Talajic M: Depression following myocardial infarction—impact on 6-month survival. JAMA 270:1819, 1993.
167. Frasure-Smith N: In-hospital symptoms of psychological stress as predictors of long-term outcome after acute myocardial infarction in men. Am J Cardiol 67:121, 1991.
168. Frasure-Smith N, Lesperance F, Talajic M: The impact of negative emotions on prognosis following myocardial infarction: Is it more than depression? Health Psychol 14:388, 1995.
169. Carney RM, Rich MW, Freeland KE, et al: Major depressive disorder predicts cardiac events in patients with coronary artery disease. Psychosom Med 50:627, 1988.
170. Gale GD, Teasdale SJ, Sanders DE, et al: Pulmonary atelectasis and other complications after cardiopulmonary bypass and investigation of etiological factors. Can Anaesth Soc J 26:15, 1979.
171. Schmidt G: Prophylaxis of pulmonary complications following abdominal surgery including atelectasis, ARDS and pulmonary embolism. JAMA 211:787, 1970.
172. Svensson LG, Hess KR, Coselli JS, et al: A prospective study of respiratory failure after high-risk surgery on the thoracoabdominal aorta. J Vasc Surg 14:271, 1991.
173. Hurford WE, Favorito F: Association of myocardial ischemia with failure to wean from mechanical ventilation. Crit Care Med 23:1475, 1975.
174. Sachner MA: Pulmonary Medicine: Tracheobronchial Toilet. Princeton, Biomedia, 1978.
175. Froese A, Bryan AC: Effects of anesthesia and paralysis on diaphragmatic mechanics in man. Anesthesiology 41:242, 1974.
176. Clauss RH, Scalabrini BY, Ray JF, Reed GE: Effects of changing body position. Circulation 37(Suppl 2):214, 1968.
177. Zack MB, Pontoppidan H, Kazemi H: The effect of lateral positions on gas exchange in pulmonary disease. Am Rev Respir Dis 110:49, 1974.
178. Sharp JT, Druz WS, Moisan T, et al: Postural relief of dyspnea in severe chronic obstructive pulmonary disease. Am Rev Respir Dis 122:201, 1980.
179. Bryan C: Comments of a devil's advocate. Am Rev Respir Dis 110:143S, 1974.
180. Prokocimer P, Garbino J, Wolff M, Regnier B: Influence of posture on gas exchange in artificially ventilated patients with focal lung disease. Intensive Care Med 9:69, 1983.
181. Remolina C, Khan AU, Santiago TV, Edelman NH: Positional hypoxemia in unilateral lung disease. N Engl J Med 304:523, 1981.
182. Seaton D, Lapp NL, Morgan WKC: Effect of body position on gas exchange after thoracotomy. Thorax 34:518, 1979.
183. Douglas WW, Rehder K, Beynen FM, et al: Improved oxygenation in patients with acute respiratory failure: The prone position. Am Rev Respir Dis 115:559, 1977.
184. Marini JJ, Tyler LM, Hudson LD, et al: Influence of head-dependent positions on lung volume and oxygen saturation in chronic airflow obstruction. Am Rev Respir Dis 129:101, 1984.
185. Mackenzie CF, Shin B, Hadi F, Imle PC: Changes in total lung/thorax compliance following chest physiotherapy. Anesth Analg 59:207, 1980.
186. Dull JC, Dull WL: Are maximal inspiratory breathing exercises or incentive spirometry better than early mobilization after cardiopulmonary bypass? Phys Ther 63:655, 1983.
187. Jenkins SC, Souter SA, Loukota JM, et al: Physiotherapy after coronary artery surgery: Are breathing exercises necessary? Thorax 44:634, 1989.
188. Crowe, Bradley CA: The effectiveness of incentive spirometry with physical therapy for high risk patients after coronary artery bypass surgery. Phys Ther 77:260, 1977.
189. Bethune DD: Neurophysiological facilitation of respiration in the unconscious adult patient. Physiother C 27:241, 1975.
190. Frownfelter DL: Chest Physical Therapy and Pulmonary Rehabilitation. Chicago, Year Book Medical Publishers, 1978.
191. Feldman J, Traver GA, Taussig LM: Maximal expiratory flows after postural drainage. Am Rev Respir Dis 119:239, 1979.
192. Flower KA, Eden RI, Lomax L, et al: New mechanical aid to physiotherapy in cystic fibrosis. Br Med J 2:630, 1979.
193. Sutton PP, Pavia D, Bateman JRM, Clarke SW: Chest physiotherapy: A review. Eur J Respir Dis 63:188, 1982.
194. Maxwell M, Redmond A: Comparative trial of manual and mechanical percussion technique with gravity assisted bronchial drainage in patients with cystic fibrosis. Arch Dis Child 54:542, 1979.
195. Marini JJ, Pierson DJ, Hudson LD: Acute labor atelectasis: A prospective comparison of fiberoptic bronchoscopy and respiratory therapy. Am Rev Respir Dis 119:971, 1979.
196. Byrd RB, Burns JR: Cough dynamics in post-thoracotomy state. Chest 67:654, 1975.
197. Curry LD, Van Edan C: The influence of posture on the effectiveness of cough. S Afr J Physiother 33:8, 1977.
198. Yamazaki S, Ogawa J, Shohzu A: Intra-pleural cough pressures in patients after thoracotomy. J Thorac Cardiovasc Surg 80:600, 1980.
199. Ackerman MH: The use of bolus normal saline instillations in artificial airways: Is it useful or necessary? Heart Lung 14:505, 1985.
200. Hudak M, Bond-Domb A: Postoperative head and neck cancer patients with artificial airways: The effect of saline lavage on tracheal mucus evacuation and oxygen saturation. ORL Head Neck Nurs 14:17, 1996.
201. Rose SD: Prophylaxis of thromboembolic disease. Med Clin North Am 63:1205, 1979.
202. Cahalin LP: Preoperative and postoperative conditioning for lung transplantation and volume-reduction surgery. Crit Care Nurs Clin North Am 8:305–322, 1996.
203. Cahalin LP: Exercise tolerance and training for healthy persons and patients with cardiovascular disease. In Hasson SM (ed): Clinical Exercise Physiology. St. Louis: Mosby-Yearbook, 1994, p 148.

CHAPTER 5

Cardiovascular Anatomy and Physiology

Carl Lynch III, M.D., Ph.D.
Carol L. Lake, M.D., M.B.A.

The Heart

The exquisitely coordinated and modulated contractile function of the heart results in ejection of blood into the vasculature, which is similarly tuned by neural, hormonal, and local mechanisms to regulate the flow of blood to various organs. Before discussing the function of the myocardium per se, it is helpful to review the biophysical basis of membrane excitability which applies to both myocardial and vascular smooth muscle cells.

Cardiac Excitation

Coordination and activation of cardiac contraction is mediated by a rapidly transmitted electrical signal. An extremely complex orchestration of events in cardiac cell membranes controls ionic flows, which in turn determine the electrophysiologic behavior. While an understanding of the membrane biophysics is not mandatory to clinical practice, it provides a molecular basis for understanding cardiac physiology and a rational framework for cardiovascular pharmacology. Cardiac electrical activity involves a coordinated entry of positive ions (Na^+ and Ca^{2+}) to depolarize the cell and activate contraction, followed by an exquisitely controlled efflux of K^+ that repolarizes the cell, all of which is determined by specialized membrane proteins, the ion channels. Each channel represents a protein that directly or indirectly controls cardiac function, as well as being a potential drug receptor. As the structure, function, and modulation of these channels are being defined, a greater understanding of the complexity of cardiac function and the potential for therapeutic intervention is occurring.

Ions and Membrane Behavior

As in all cells, the source of the membrane potential (V_m) of cardiac myocytes is the ion concentration difference that is maintained across the cell membrane. Ionic concentration differences are primarily maintained by the impermeant nature of the lipid bilayer of the cell membrane—charged particles cannot pass into and through its highly hydrophobic lipid milieu. The ions (Na^+, K^+, Ca^{2+}, Cl^-) serve as stores of electrical energy by virtue of their concentration gradients, which establish a voltage defined by the Nernst equation (Table 5–1). The equilibrium potential (E_{ion}) for any ion is that voltage generated after ions have moved down their concentration gradient to a level at which a potential is created that completely opposes further ion flow. At equilibrium the chemical gradient is counterbalanced by a voltage gradient (defined by the Nernst equation) such that no current flows. At rest the only open channels in the cell membrane conduct K^+ almost exclusively, so V_m is near E_K, the equilibrium potential for K^+.

The membrane potential depends on the ability of the membrane to separate charges. This capability is termed *capacity.* The capacity of biologic membranes is relatively constant at 1 μF (microfarad) per cm^2 of membrane surface, where a μF is 6.2×10^{12} charges per volt. For a typical cardiac myocyte the total membrane surface is about 7,000 μm^2 (7×10^{-5} cm^2) so the capacity is about 70 pF (picofarad).[1] To generate a resting potential near E_K of −90 mV, about 40 million K^+ (or about 0.003% of the cell K^+) must leave the cell before the resting membrane potential is established at E_K and the flux ceases.

At rest, the membrane is impermeant to Na^+ and Ca^{2+}, which do not contribute to the resting membrane potential. By changing the permeability from predominantly one ion (K^+) to another (Na^+ and/or Ca^{2+}) with a different E, ion fluxes will occur and alter V_m. Altered V_m, the resulting change in membrane proteins, and the ion fluxes themselves serve as mechanisms for cellular signaling. After cells begin to depolarize (because of current entering from adjacent cells), Na channels begin to open resulting in a regenerative depolarization or action potential (AP). While ion fluxes may be required to activate certain processes (e.g., Ca^{2+} to activate internal Ca^{2+} release), with regard to changing the membrane potential, a relatively small proportion of total cell ions

TABLE 5–1
Ionic Determinants of Membrane Potential

Ion	Intracellular Concentration (mM)	Extracellular Concentration (mM)	Equilibrium Potential E_{ion} (mV)	Comment
K^+	100	3.5	−90	Establishes resting potential. However, conductance decreases with decreasing $[K^+]_o$, so that membrane potential will deviate from E_K as $[K^+]_o$ decreases.
		5	−81	
	120	3.5	−95	
		5	−85	
		7	−77	
Na^+				
Quiescent	8	140	77	Normal, actively beating heart may have significantly higher $[Na^+]_i$.
Beating	12		66	
Ca^{2+}				
Diastole	0.0001	1	122	The marked change in $[Ca^{2+}]_i$ during contraction will influence I_{Ca} and I_{NaCa}.
Systole	0.003		78	
Cl^-	18	100	−46	Normally contributes little to resting conductance.

*The equilibrium potential for each ion calculated according to the Nernst equation at 37°C:

$$E_{ion} = \frac{62\text{ mV}}{n}\log\frac{[\log]_o}{[\text{ion}]_i}$$

where n is the charge on the ion and subscripts i and o designate intra- and extracellular (outside). 62 mV is calculated from RT/F × ln 10 (to convert from natural logarithms to $\log_{10}$); R = 8.314 volt/coulomb/°K/mole, a faraday (F) = 96,493 coulombs/mole of charge, and T = 310°K at 37°C. Intracellular concentrations are those based on estimates using intracellular ion selective electrodes[550–552]; values may vary depending on the tissue.[553]

must cross the membrane to discharge the cell. Using the previous example, about 55 million Na^+ must enter a myocyte to depolarize it by 120 mV to +35 mV, which increases the cell Na^+ by less than 0.025%.

Although the increase in myocyte $[Na^+]$ is small with each beat, over the 4,000 times that the heart typically beats in an hour, the K^+ and Na^+ gradients would be reduced or eliminated. In addition, the membrane bilayer and associated proteins are not totally impermeant to these ions so that some "leak" occurs. This also contributes to the rundown of the ion gradients, resulting in the loss of membrane potential as a means of cell signaling. The mechanism for maintaining normal ionic gradients in the cell is the Na^+,K^+-ATPase, or sodium pump. Using the energy supplied by hydrolyzing adenosine triphosphate (ATP) to adenosine diphosphate (ADP), three Na^+ are eliminated from the cell and two K^+ are pumped into the cell. This translocation is critical for reversing ion fluxes which generate the action potential, as well as for eliminating Na^+ entry due to "leaks" in the membrane.

Cardiac Ion Channels and Control of Ion Fluxes

In order to rapidly conduct ions through the hydrophobic milieu of the bilayer, channels must span the bilayer. Recent studies have permitted amino acid sequencing of a large number of the channel proteins themselves, revealing a similarity in structure among the major channel types, which may be ordered into superfamilies.[2–9] For example, both sodium (Na) and calcium (Ca) channels are similarly structured, with a large central conducting region of a single large protein composed of 2,000 to 2,500 amino acids. Based on the hydrophobicity of the amino acids, a proposed structure for these channels is now generally accepted in which four major domains (I to IV) are each formed from six hydrophobic transmembrane α-helical segments as shown in Figure 5–1.[10–12] In addition to the major pore forming α_1-subunit, two or three additional subunits are typically present.

The cloning of the genetic material encoding the protein structures has permitted the exploration of various structural aspects. The structural similarity of Na and Ca channel α_1-subunits is demonstrated by the fact that selective conductance of Ca^{2+} can be conferred on the Na channel by specific point mutations in the 5–6 linker region, which also determines how the ions bind as they pass through the center of the protein.[13] This similarity in structure may partially explain why a number of drugs show only partial specificity for a particular channel. For example, both the phenylalkylamines (the verapamil family of drugs) and the dihydropyridines (nifedipine, nicardipine, etc.) block Na channels as well as Ca channels, although not necessarily at clinical concentrations.[14–16] Likewise, local anesthetics as well as phenytoin can block Ca as well as Na channels.[17,18] In the Ca channel, Ca^{2+} normally binds tightly, actually preventing Na^+ from entering. Transition metal ions bind even more tightly and block the Ca channel; Mn^{2+} passes very slowly, partially blocking the channel[19]; La^{3+} or Cd^{2+} block the channel at 1 to 100 μM.[20]

Most ion channels are not continuously conducting ions, but open (activate) in response to a voltage change across the membrane or binding of an agonist molecule. When a depolarization occurs and the cell becomes more positive internally, the highly positively charged fourth α-helical segment ("voltage sensor") moves outward. This conformational change in the channel domains permits ions to flow. When a voltage change is imposed across the membrane (as with a voltage clamp), the movement of this charged region of the channel protein

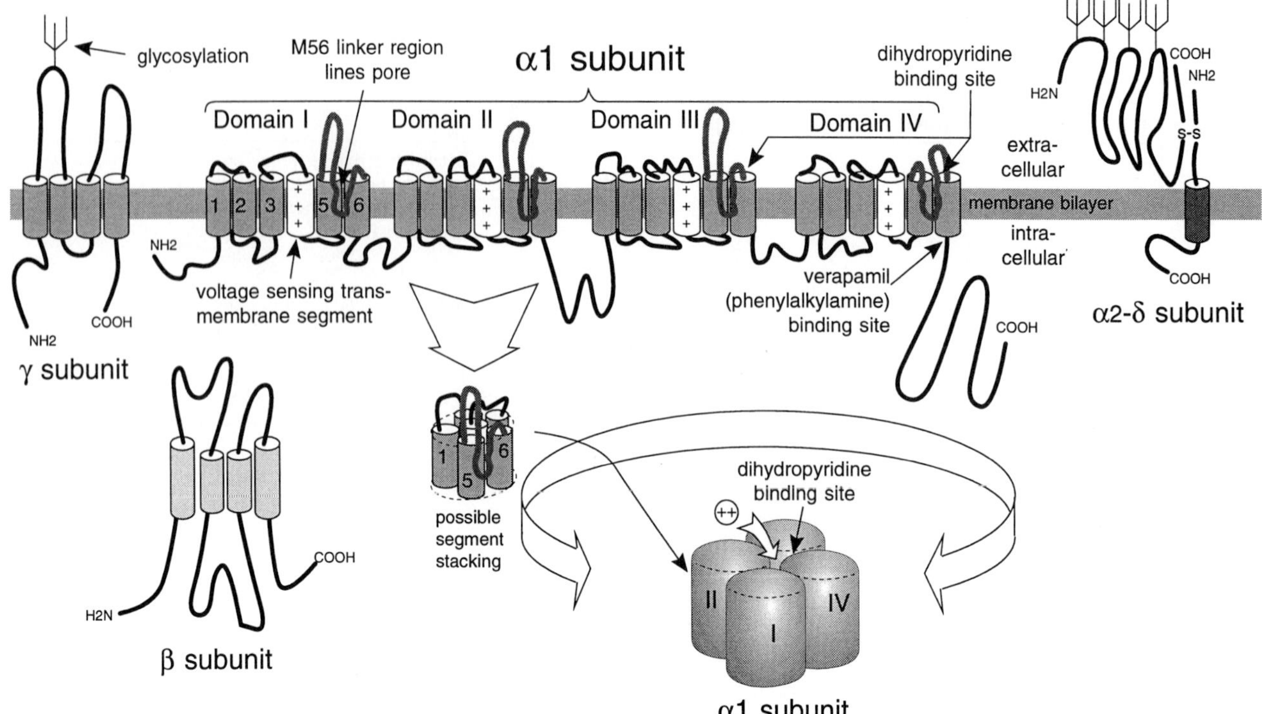

FIGURE **5–1.** Structural model of the L-type Ca channel based upon amino acid sequence analysis. The α_1-subunit is composed of 2,171 amino acids in which 24 hydrophobic regions are hypothesized to form α-helical transmembrane segments (as indicated by the small cylinders).[4] As shown for domain II, the six transmembrane segments (S1–S6) coalesce to form four domains (I–IV). The four domains gather as indicated to form a tetrameric structure with a central pore through which the ions pass. The pore itself appears to be lined by the extracellular linking segment between helix spans 5 and 6, which is thought to fold back into the pore so that the polar or negatively charged sites become available for binding by ions as they pass through the channel. The fourth transmembrane segment (S4) of each domain contains a number of positively charged amino acids (typically arginine) that can respond to the membrane voltage field, acting as a "voltage sensor" and inducing a conformational change that will permit ions to flow through the central pore.[11] It is at the junction between this region and S6 of domains III and IV that the dihydropyridines such as nifedipine appear to bind, while the diphenylalkylamines (e.g., verapamil) bind at the intracellular aspect of the α_1-subunit. Also shown in the figure are the other subunits that occur with the α_1-subunit. The β-subunit, which appears to adjoin an intracellular aspect of the α_1-subunit, appears to enhance channel opening and activation. The α_2-δ–subunit also appears to modulate channel voltage responses, while the role of the γ-subunit is unclear. (Adapted from various sources including Catterall and Striessing[547] and Jay et al.[548])

can be measured. This "gating charge" can be closely correlated with gating of the ionic currents through the specific channels.[21,22] After opening, channels remain open for a particular period of time before they close (inactivate). Voltage-gated channels may remain open until the voltage change is reversed, or may inactivate due to an ongoing conformational change in the molecule. Inactivation of the channel is sometimes mediated by an intracellular segment that binds to the inner pore mouth and "plugs" it, stopping ion flow.[6,23]

At rest, the membrane field is usually dominated by the bulk membrane potential established by the K^+ equilibrium potential (in which the loss of K^+ results in a negative charge inside the cell). However, the ion channels exist in a submicroscopic membrane environment, in which the electrical field that the channel proteins "feel" is not exactly the measured membrane potential (the potential established between the bulk intra- and extracellular solution). The electrical charges (usually negative) present on the membrane surface (on phospholipids) as well as on the protein itself (in some cases due to attached carbohydrate groups) alter the electrical field to which the "voltage sensor" responds.[24,25] In addition, these charges attract and are in part neutralized by the cations attracted to the membrane surface. When there are more ionic charges in solution, more of the negative surface charge is neutralized and the protein "feels" more of the measured potential. If these charges specifically bind particular ions (e.g., Ca^{2+}), changes in those ions may modify gating behavior. These changes may explain restoration of cardiac conduction by Ca^{2+} or Mg^{2+} administration when it is depressed by hyperkalemia (see below).[26]

SODIUM CHANNELS

Na channels expressed in various tissues have a central conducting α-subunit that contains the main pore of a complex with up to two associated subunits (β_1 and β_2). The α-subunit from heart (designated h1) is one of at least six different sodium channel α-subunits that have been cloned,[27] and has the distinction of being resistant to blockade by tetrodotoxin, a distinct feature of the cardiac Na^+ conductance.[28] Like that of skeletal muscle, the

Na channel of cardiac muscle appears to be a complex of α- and β_1-subunits.

Of critical importance for cardiac muscle function is the presence of enough working Na channels so that a large depolarizing current can spread very rapidly to adjacent cells and tissue; thus APs are conducted rapidly throughout the mass of muscle. The rate of depolarization (dV/dt) and rate of AP conduction is roughly proportional to the number of working sodium channels. The major factor affecting the availability of these channels is the membrane voltage. Negative to −80 mV, a large fraction of sodium channels are available for activation (noninactivated); rapid depolarization positive to −70 mV results in a regenerative opening and a conducted AP. Although the channels activate with a time constant of less than 1 msec, they also inactivate rapidly at a negative V_m close to threshold. In the range of V_m from −80 to −65 mV, 65 to 35% of the channels may be available, which may be enough for an abnormally slow conducted AP. When myocardial cells are partially depolarized, as occurs with hyperkalemia, fewer channels are available (not inactivated) so that conduction is impaired. This is readily apparent clinically as the widened QRS complex representing slowed conduction through the ventricle. When the potential stays positive to −65 mV, more than 75% of the channels are inactivated, and there are usually too few to open to generate a propagated AP. The extreme of the voltage-inactivation is employed clinically in the application of *cardioplegia*, in which solutions containing 20 to 30 mM K^+ depolarize the heart to −50 to −35 mV. In this potential range almost all sodium channels will be inactivated and normal APs cannot occur, resulting in plegia ("paralysis") of the heart. Fortunately, this potential is above the mechanical threshold; that is, Ca^{2+} is not released from the sarcoplasmic reticulum (SR) to activate contractions, so that energy is not consumed generating tension.

A very small fraction of cardiac Na channels appear not to inactivate rapidly, providing sustained current even during the plateau of the AP.[29,30] This subpopulation of channels provides a small "window" current that persists for the duration of depolarization and contributes to the plateau phase of the Purkinje fiber AP.[29,31] One of the actions of pure Na-channel blocking agents (tetrodotoxin and certain local anesthetics) is to decrease the AP plateau duration, presumably by blocking the sodium channel "window" current that persists in the plateau, although this effect is modest in ventricular muscle. The major mechanism by which local anesthetics inhibit Na channels is by use- (or frequency-) dependent blockade, requiring that channels be open (and possibly inactivated) before the local anesthetics bind. Once the block has occurred, the drug may unbind quickly (class Ib antiarrhythmics; e.g., lidocaine) and inhibit conduction only at high heart rates (>120 bpm), or it may stay bound more strongly, and cause some degree of tonic blockade even at normal heart rates (class Ia and Ic; e.g., quinidine, flecainide, bupivacaine).[32]

The high Na^+ current needed for rapid depolarization and action potential conduction requires a high Na channel density (4 to 50 channels/μm^2),[33] especially in the Purkinje system, yet a somewhat lower channel density of 0.3 to 5 channels/μm^2 is more typical for other myocyte ion channels. There are typically 1,500 to 25,000 units of a given channel present in a cardiac myocyte.[34,35] However, the density may not be uniform over the entire cell surface.

CALCIUM CHANNELS

L-Type Ca Channel. The major cardiac Ca channel is the cardiac L-type, responsible for 90% or more of Ca^{2+} current in ventricular myocytes. Initially termed "L" for its long-lasting single channel opening, this channel requires a depolarization of the membrane potential more positive than −40 mV to activate opening, so they are also designated high-voltage activated (HVA). The L-type channel is the best characterized of all Ca channels. In addition to the central α_1-subunit, smaller additional subunits have been cloned and structures proposed (Fig. 5–1). The β- and $\alpha_2\delta$-subunit make the α_1 channel behave in a more physiologic fashion.[36] Gene cloning has also permitted selective modification of the amino acid sequence to actually determine the regions of the L-type Ca channel that provide the highly selective binding sites for the dihydropyridines. Caterall and co-workers, in an elegant series of modifications of the channel, have demonstrated that the binding site for the dihydropyridines is in domain III at the external pore mouth.[12] In contrast, the binding site for verapamil is at the internal Ca channel pore mouth on the pore lining S5–S6 linker. This molecular evidence fits with results demonstrating that phenylalkylamines act intracellularly,[37] while dihydropyridines act extracellularly.[38] Although Mg^{2+} is frequently described as a Ca channel blocker, it actually has modest blocking action. Its ability to decrease Ca^{2+} entry into cells via Ca channels is probably related to its ability to decrease the Ca^{2+} concentration electrostatically attracted to the membrane surface, providing fewer Ca^{2+} in the vicinity of the channel mouth.

In addition to its binding within the Ca channel pore, the Ca^{2+} ion itself plays a complex role in modulating L-type channel function, causing both inactivation as well as facilitation. In many studies in which Ba^{2+} is used as the charge carrying ion or in which intracellular Ca^{2+} is heavily buffered, the currents observed do not show the prominent inactivation. While there is an inherent voltage-dependent inactivation of Ca channels, the Ca^{2+}-dependent inactivation is important,[39] and both processes contribute to normal inactivation under physiologic conditions. With repeated depolarizations and Ca^{2+} entry, peak $I_{Ca,L}$ typically increase to greater levels, and activation of Ca-calmodulin-dependent protein kinase (CaMK II) may have an important role in this Ca^{2+}-dependent facilitation.[40] An important feature contributing to Ca^{2+} regulation may be the clustering of Ca channels, since the entering Ca^{2+} can achieve higher local concentrations when a number of channels are aggregated,[41] thereby enhancing both facilitation and/or inactivation. In most channels, the intracellular regions possess serine or threonine amino acid residues, which may be phosphorylated by various regulatory kinase enzymes within the cell.[42] In the case of L-type Ca channels phosphorylation by cyclic adenosine monophosphate (cAMP) –dependent protein kinase, activated by β-adrenoceptor activation, results in enhanced voltage-dependent activation and/or a longer opening.[43]

T-Type Ca Channel. In contrast to the L-type channel, the T-type channel is activated by a smaller depolarization to less positive membrane potentials (hence low-voltage activated [LVA]).[44–47] It also has a lower conductance, and generates a more transient current (hence the T designation), more like a Na channel. T-type channel inactivation occurs even with heavy Ca^{2+} buffering, suggesting that Ca^{2+} does not contribute prominently to this process. Unlike the L-type channel, little is known regarding details of T-type channel structure and function. The channel has not yet been isolated or cloned, nor has a highly specific blocking agent or toxin been delineated. In ventricular myocytes, T-type channels are responsible for a modicum of I_{Ca}. Although Ca^{2+} entry through this channel may be sufficient to activate release of Ca^{2+} from the SR, its seems unlikely that it contributes significantly to normal activation. T-type channels constitute a greater proportion of channels in Purkinje fibers (up to 40%) and may play a role in the diastolic depolarization, as postulated in sinoatrial and atrioventricular nodes.

POTASSIUM CHANNELS

The Inward Rectifier K^+ Conductances. The cardiac electrical behavior is largely determined by the resting K^+ conductance (termed G_{K1}), which is prominent in cardiac muscle but absent in the pacemaker tissue. The amino acid sequence of this K channel subunit is composed of 428 amino acids with hydrophobic regions composing two α-helical transmembrane spans.[48] The amino acid sequence linking the transmembrane spans appears to form a pore-lining segment similar to that proposed for the larger six-segment domains present in other types of channels. The critical feature of this K channel is that it readily permits K^+ to enter the cell. Yet with increasing depolarization positive to E_K, K^+ efflux is much more difficult; with a large enough depolarization K^+ efflux ceases. This *inwardly rectifying* behavior is caused by internal cations that block the channel at more positive membrane potentials, preventing K^+ efflux. Such blockade decreases the K^+ conductance at high potentials and permits prolonged depolarization of the action potential plateau. Both intracellular Mg^{2+} and certain polyamines (e.g., spermine, putrescine),[49–51] which are present in the myocyte in micromolar concentrations, have been found to block the channel and prevent K^+ flux.

The channel underlying G_{K1} is one member (specifically, Kir2.1) of the Kir family of K channels. Two other critically important cardiac K channels of related structure are that activated by G-protein coupled receptors (GIRK, or Kir3.2 and 3.1), and that which is sensitive to intracellular ATP (K_{ATP}, or Kir6.1). Both of these channels have less inwardly rectifying character than G_{K1}, and their activation results in greater abbreviation of the cardiac AP plateau. Like Kir2.1, rectification in the former appears to be mediated by polyamines.[52] An additional K channel appears to be activated by increased intracellular $[Na^+]$, which may also modulate the electrophysiologic behavior of the heart, particularly with neuroendocrine stimulation or metabolic stress.

The Voltage-Gated Potassium Channels. In contrast to the Kir class, which establish resting membrane conductance, the voltage-gated K channels are activated with strong depolarization and are responsible for initiating repolarization. These channel subunits consist of at least 600 amino acids, each of which has at least six highly hydrophobic, α-helical transmembrane-spanning regions,[6] which coalesce into a single large transmembrane domain. Four of these individual subunits combine to form a single K channel,[53] with a quatrafoil structure similar to that for a single α_1 Ca channel subunit. Four extracellular amino acid sequences linking the fifth and sixth helices, one from each subunit or domain, line the pore as in Na, Ca, and Kir channels. Certain of the voltage-gated K channels, such as the cardiac delayed (rectifier) K^+ current (I_K), activate very slowly on depolarization, requiring 100 to 200 msec for half-maximal activation; other channels, such as the transient outward current (I_{to}), activate much more rapidly, but then inactivate. A majority of these channels are of the Kv family. The combination of K channel subunits of differing types into a single four-subunit assembly markedly increases the possible number and the behavior of the assembled channels.[23]

In addition to the Kv family, other types of voltage-gated K channels have been identified in myocardium including HERG. A mutation in this channel has been linked to long QT syndrome, in which ventricular repolarization is delayed and which is associated with sudden death.

CHLORIDE CHANNELS

While not thought to play a prominent role at the present time, influx of Cl^- through specific anion channels may contribute a repolarizing current to cardiac APs under various conditions.[54] These channels are usually blocked by a variety of negatively charged aromatic organic acids (see Table 5–2). A transient outward current (assigned I_{to2} by some) has been defined during the plateau of the AP, which may contribute to the initial repolarization of myocytes. The current appears to be activated by Ca^{2+} that is released from SR stores, and has been also designated as $I_{Cl(Ca)}$.[54–56] Normally there is only modest Cl^- conductance in atrial myocytes, mediated by an outwardly rectifying Cl channel. This channel, which has a modest basal activity, appears to be the same Cl^- conductance activated by stretch[57,58] or swelling,[59] although its precise role is unclear. While ventricular myocytes have minimal basal Cl^- conductance, a chloride channel has clearly been defined that is activated by β-adrenergic stimulation[60–64] via phosphorylation by protein kinase A (cAMP controlled). The channel is similar in many respects to the chloride channel which has been identified as the defective gene in cystic fibrosis (cystic fibrosis transmembrane regulator [CFTR]).[54] This channel is insignificant in sinoatrial and atrial cells, and is more prominent in epicardial than endocardial ventricular cells.[63]

TABLE 5–2
Cardiac Ion Channels*

Channel		Activation Kinetics	Inactivation Kinetics	Blocking Agents
Sodium ("fast")	I_{Na}	Very fast	Fast, except for a fraction that reopen	Local anesthetics & phenytoin (use-dependent), tetrodotoxin (weak)
Calcium ("slow")				
L-type (or high-voltage activated [HVA])	$I_{Ca,L}$	Fast	Variable, Ca^{2+}-dependent component	Dihydropyridines, benzothiazepines, phenylalkylamines, Cd^{2+}
T-type	$I_{Ca,T}$	Fast	Moderate	Amiloride, tetramethrin, Ni^{2+}, Cd^{2+}
Potassium				
Inward rectifier	I_{K1}	Instantaneous	Mg^{2+} & polyamine block of outward current	Cs^+, Ba^{2+} (100 μM), thiopental, zero K^+
Plateau or background	$I_{K,p(?TWIK)}$	Instantaneous or fast	None?	Ba^{2+} (1 mM)
Delayed rectifier	$I_{K,s}$	Slow	None	Tetraethylammonium
	$I_{K,r}$	Moderate	Slight	d-Sotalol, dofetilide, 1 μM La^{3+}
	I_{RAK}, I_{HK2}	Very rapid activation	None	Quinidine (HK2)
Transient outward	$I_{to\,1}$	Fast	Moderate	4-AP (1 mM), bipivacaine, quinidine
	$I_{K(Ca)}$, $I_{to\,2?}$	Fast	Moderate	4-AP (10 mM), tedisamil
ACh, adenosine, PAF-activated	$I_{K(ACh,\,Ado)}$	Instantaneous, activated via G_i protein	Mg^{2+} & polyamine block of outward current	
ATP-sensitive	$I_{K(ATP)}$	Instantaneous if active	Mg^{2+} block of outward current	Glybenclimide, amiodarone, quinidine
Na-activated	$I_{K(Na)}$	Instantaneous if active		
Fatty-acid activated	$I_{K,AA}$, $I_{K,PC}$	Instantaneous if active		
Pacemaker (nonspecific)	I_f	Slow	Slow	1–2 mM Cs^+
Chloride				
Transient outward	$I_{Cl(Ca)}$, $I_{to\,2?}$	Fast	Fast	SITS, DIDS
CFTR	$I_{Cl,cAMP}$	Instantaneous if active	None	DNDS
rest & stretch-activated				SITS, 9-AC, DNDS

*Modified from Lynch C III: Cellular electrophysiology of the heart. In Lynch C III (ed): Clinical Cardiac Electrophysiology: Perioperative Considerations. Philadelphia, JB Lippincott Co, 1994, pp 1–52, with permission.
CFTR, cystic fibrosis transmembrane regulator; DIDS, 4,4′-dithiocyanatostilbene; DNDS, 4,4′-dinitrostilbene-2,2′-disulfonic acid; PAF, platelet-activating factor; SITS, 4-acetomido-4′-isothiocyanatostilbene-2,2′-disulfonic acid; 9-AC, anthracene-9-carboxylic acid.

The membrane channels demonstrated in myocardium and responsible for its varied behavior are summarized in Table 5–2. While the number of K channels is particularly striking, it should be recalled that they all result in the same effect: an outward current that tends to stabilize the resting membrane potential, limit excitability, slow conduction, and hasten repolarization. They also represent potential sites for pharmacologic intervention.

The Na Pump

The critical role of the Na,K-ATPase (Na pump) in maintaining the K^+ and Na^+ gradients has already been noted. This heterodimer is composed of an α-subunit that contains the ion, ATP, and glycoside binding sites, and a β-subunit which has a large, heavily glycosylated extracellular domain.[65] This enzyme employs the energy obtained by hydrolyzing the terminal phosphate of ATP to transfer three Na^+ out of the cell and two K^+ in.[65] This process is therefore electrogenic, generating an outward current that creates a continuous small hyperpolarization (<1 mV) in most active myocytes. If V_m is slightly negative to E_K due to the electrogenic Na^+ extrusion, the additional K^+ (required to maintain balance) may readily enter via the inwardly rectifying G_{K1}. Pump function is enhanced by high intracellular Na^+ and/or high extracellular K^+. Such ionic changes can occur with rapid stimulation rates, and the hyperpolarizing current generated by the sodium pump following such rapid rates can cause "overdrive hyperpolarization" and transient bradycardia. In settings of ischemia and hypoxia, in which ATP becomes depleted, it is the loss of function of the sodium pump with consequent accumulation of intracellular Na^+ and extracellular K^+ that causes many of the marked abnormalities in cardiac conduction. In addition to use of the Na^+ gradient to provide a rapid depolarization, the energy generated by the entrance of Na^+ is critically important in providing energy for work by membrane proteins such as the Na-Ca exchanger, which uses Na^+ influx to extrude Ca^{2+} from the cell. Another protein that uses the Na^+ gradient is the Na^+-H^+ antiport, which is responsible in part for maintaining acid-base balance within the cell; entering Na^+ eliminates a H^+ from the cell in an electroneutral manner.[66]

The Na-Ca Exchanger

Although the bulk of the Ca^{2+} required for myofibrillar activation comes from the internal sites of the sarcoplasmic reticulum, the Ca^{2+} that enters with each depolarization must be removed from the cell to prevent Ca^{2+} overload. Although a sarcolemmal Ca^{2+}-ATPase exists that eliminates Ca^{2+} from the cell using energy derived from ATP hydrolysis, the bulk of the Ca^{2+} is removed by the Na-Ca exchanger.[67] During rest, this protein employs the energy derived from three Na^+ moving down their electrochemical gradient into the cell to eliminate one Ca^{2+} from the cell.[67] The result is a small net depolarizing current, and a flux that is sensitive to the membrane potential. During rest the "reversal" of flux may occur at −40 mV, and in the initial stage of repolarization Ca^{2+} may actually enter (and Na^+ exit) by this pathway. However, as the resting systolic level of Ca^{2+} increases, the reversal potential for the exchange becomes positive compared to the action potential plateau, and Ca^{2+} efflux occurs (with a small depolarizing current) throughout the rest of the cardiac cycle. In settings of a decreased Na^+ gradient (high intracellular or low [≤40 mM] extracellular Na^+), Ca^{2+} is retained in the cell and enhances contractions as excess Ca^{2+} accumulates in the SR. However, when ATP is depleted, the Ca^{2+} increases in the sarcoplasm and results in delayed relaxation, contracture, and ultimately, cell death.

The Mitochondria

In addition to synthesizing ATP by employing a proton gradient across the inner and outer membranes, mitochondria also carefully regulate Ca^{2+} via a Ca-H exchanger and Ca^{2+} uniport pathways. While the rate of Ca^{2+} uptake has been shown to be too slow to contribute to Ca^{2+} regulation within a contractile cycle,[68] over a time course of seconds increased myoplasmic Ca^{2+} can be assimilated by the mitochondria.[69] Likewise, during hypoxia or ischemia, the loss of the proton gradient may also result in Ca^{2+} loading of mitochondria. Sustained Ca^{2+} overload leads to mitochondrial swelling, and ultimately to disruption. However, in contrast to pathologic conditions, the increased "average" myoplasmic [Ca^{2+}] that occurs with increased heart rate of β-adrenergic activation may be reflected by a more modest increase in mitochondrial [Ca^{2+}] and a decrease in NADH.[70] A resulting increase in the activity of intramitochondrial dehydrogenases then leads to recovery of NADH levels and an appropriate increase in ATP synthesis.[69,70]

Normal Electrical Conduction through the Heart

The membrane potential changes in the heart can be viewed as a single depolarization that sweeps through the whole heart, assuming various velocities and patterns along its course. Figure 5–2 reviews the pattern of depolarization of a cardiac cycle. Except along the atrioventricular junction, the cells of the heart are intimately connected and electrically coupled so that depolarizing ionic currents entering a cell can invade adjacent cells, spreading the regenerative depolarization. The variable expression of channels in different regions of the heart (pacemaker sites, conduction tissue, ventricle, atria; see Table 5–3 and Fig. 5–3*A*) is responsible for the characteristic electrophysiologic behavior of each tissue. Modulation of these various membrane channels under the influence of various controlling molecules (G proteins) and second messengers can also dramatically alter membrane behavior. Depending upon the particular cardiac tissue, from a resting potential of −90 to −60 mV, the tissue depolarizes to +30 to +10 mV.

The Pacemaker Tissue

The Sinoatrial Node. The sequence of depolarization begins in the sinoatrial (SA) node, an aggregation of specialized cells located anterolaterally at the junction of the superior vena cava and right atrium. The most distinct cells of this region have few mitochondria, no SR or organized myofibrils, and have been termed *P cells* or *round cells*, due to their shape.[71,72] There are also slender, elongated *transitional* cells. In humans these cells conspicuously surround the sinus nodal artery, typically the largest atrial artery, derived from either the right (55%) or left circumflex (45%) coronary artery. These distinctive cells are ensheathed and separated into small groups by a rather dense collagen matrix. From birth to adulthood, there is a progressive decrease in P cells, with an increase in transitional cells and collagen. Although cholinergic innervation is present early in fetal development, adrenergic innervation occurs only some months after birth.[71]

These cells differ from the muscle tissue in having a resting potential of only around −60 mV, which is due to the critical absence of I_{K1}. Because this resting conductance is lacking, the membrane potential is not fixed near E_K, but instead can "float" or be readily altered by small amounts of current or ion flux. When not undergoing an AP the cells undergo a very gradual depolarization from approximately −60 mV (the maximum diastolic potential at the end of repolarization) at a rate of 20 to 100 mV/sec. This process is the diastolic depolarization (DD) or pacemaker potential, which is due to the action of two different ionic currents. During the AP, the delayed K^+ current (I_K) is activated, which repolarizes the cell to around −60 mV. But these K channels gradually close. In addition, a nonspecific pacemaker channel (I_f) becomes activated at more negative V_m. Thus, an increasing inward current (I_f) and decreasing outward current (I_K) lead to the gradual depolarization (Fig. 5–4*B*).[73–75] The T-type Ca^{2+} channel may also contribute inward current to the very last phase of DD (Fig. 5–3).[76] When an internal membrane potential of approximately −50 mV is reached, the depolarization rate increases to 1 to 2 V/sec, creating a slowly depolarizing AP. Although Na channels may be present, they are inactivated by the low resting potential and slow DD, and never observed physiologically. This nodal slow AP invades the zone of surrounding cells, which have more myofibrils and appear microscopically more like muscle.[72] These cells also spontaneously depolarize, but not as rapidly. As the cells become more muscle-like in character, they have a more negative resting potential, more active sodium channels, and, therefore, a more rapid AP depolarization. Once the depolarization reaches atrial muscle, which has a −85 to −90 mV resting potential, the AP spreads rapidly, with a particularly rapid anterior conduction pathway (Bachmann's bundle) toward the left atrium. Occasionally, islands of cells near the SA node may take over as dominant pacemaker with a slightly faster diastolic depolarization.[77]

Atrioventricular Node. As the borders of the atrial muscle are reached the AP stops at the nonconducting fibrous tissue that forms the annulus for each atrioventricular

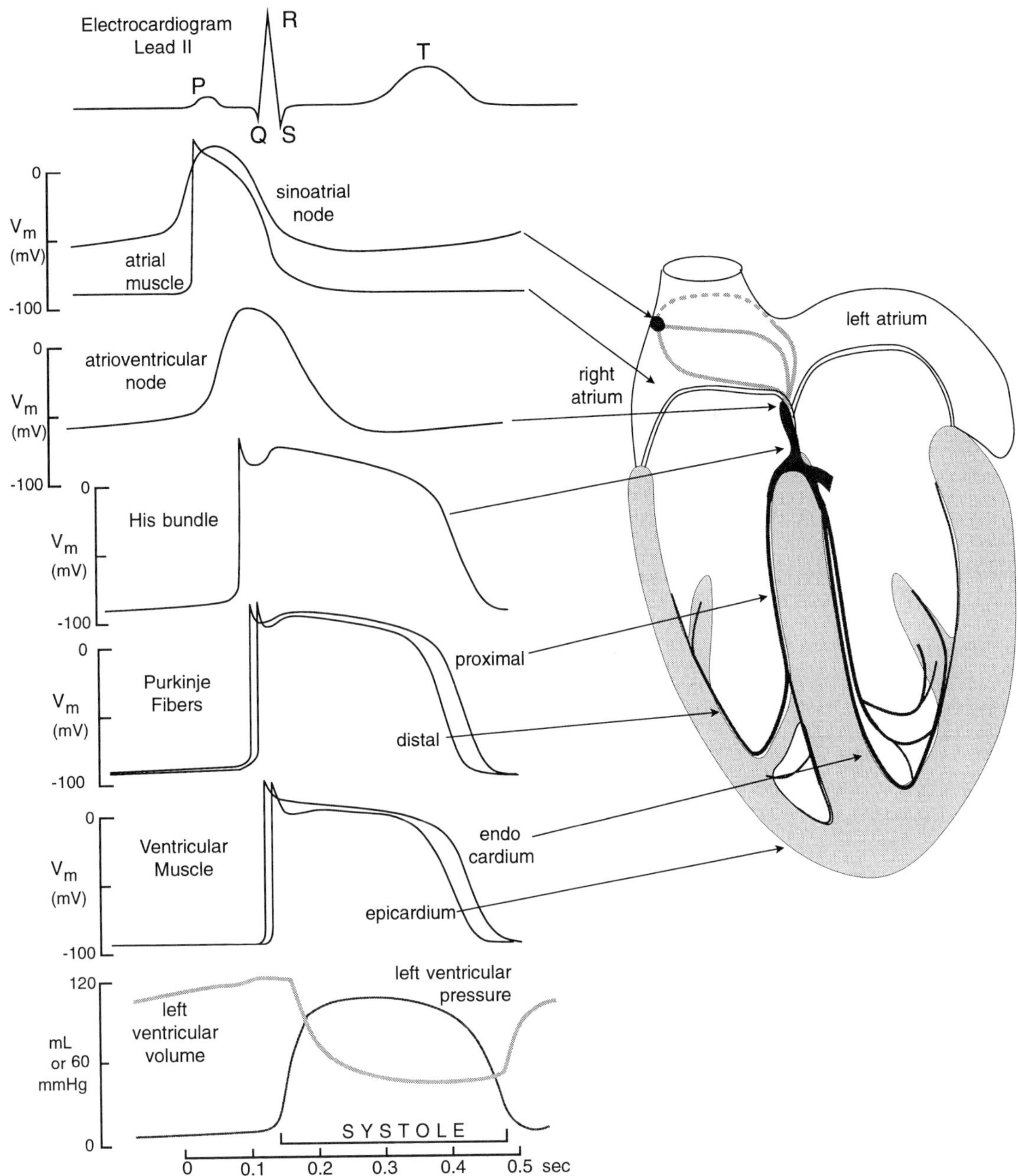

FIGURE **5–2.** Conduction of the depolarization through the heart beginning with initiation in the sinoatrial (SA) node. The action potentials (APs) observed in the various regions of the heart and their temporal relationship are shown. The delay between the P and the QRS is caused by AP conduction through the atrium and by the conduction of the Ca channel–mediated slow AP through the atrioventricular (AV) node. Although not universally accepted, three pathways (anterior, middle, and posterior) of conduction through the atrium to the AV node have been suggested.

(AV) valve. However, at a point at the junction of the atrial-ventricular septa, the arriving atrial AP passes through a zone of transitional cells (A-N zone), smaller than the normal atrial cells and separated from them by fibrous tissue. The AP is markedly slowed as it travels through the compact or N region of the node, composed of P cells or round cells similar anatomically and physiologically to the SA node cells.[71] Located on the superior right ventricular side of the ventricular septum, the AV node is similar to the SA node, except for having a slower rate of diastolic depolarization. The AP conduction velocity then increases as it travels through a second transitional zone (N-H region) to the bundle of His. The AV nodal APs appear similar to SA nodal APs, except for having a slower diastolic depolarization. It is unclear whether this is due to a higher resting conductance or lower pacemaker current. By virtue of its slow diastolic depolarization, it is a backup system of impulse initiation in case the SA node or atrial conduction fails. The delay between the atria and ventricular contraction permits bet-

TABLE 5–3
Distribution and Effects of Ion Currents in Various Tissues of the Heart*

Current	SA Node	Atrial Muscle	AV Node	Bundle of His Purkinje fibers	Ventricular muscle: Endocardial	Ventricular muscle: Epicardial
Sodium channel (I_{Na})	Inactive, if present	Prominent	Inactive	Prominent	Prominent	Prominent
Calcium channel (I_{Ca})	Contributes to late DD & provides AP	Yes	Contributes to DD & provides slow AP	Yes	Yes	Yes
Pacemaker (I_f)	DD	No (?)	DD	DD	Present, but inactive	Present, but inactive
Inward rectifier (I_{K1})	No	Yes, modest	No	Modest	Yes	Yes
Plateau current ($I_{K,p}$)	?	?	?	?	Yes	Yes
Delayed rectifier (I_K)	Yes, turn-off contributes to DD	Yes, may be modest	Yes, turn-off contributes to DD	Yes	Yes	Yes
Transient outward (I_{to})	No	Large, shortens APD	No	Yes, causes prominent "notch" in AP	Variable, minimal in many	Yes, shortens APD
ACh-induced ($I_{K(ACh)}$, $I_{K(Ado)}$)	Yes, markedly decreases rate of DD	Yes	Yes, markedly decreases rate of DD	Yes, markedly decreases rate of DD	Minimal	Modest
ATP-gated channel ($I_{K(ATP)}$)	Yes, decreases rate of DD	? Probably present	Probably similar to SA node	? Probably present	Yes, activation decreases APD	Yes, activation decreases APD

*This summary is a general pattern which may be dependent upon the particular species examined, and has been compiled from various sources.[1,73–75,561,562]
SA, sinoatrial; AV, atrioventricular; APD, action potential duration; DD, diastolic depolarizations.

ter augmentation of ventricular filling. The AV node is also a frequency gate, so that if the atria flutter (~300 bpm) or fibrillate, the ventricle will not be driven at a rate incompatible with effective pump function. This AV node represents the only electrical continuity and means of conduction between the atria and ventricles, except for individuals who have abnormal direct conduction pathways between the atria and ventricles (Wolff-Parkinson-White and Lown-Ganong-Levine syndromes).

Atrial Muscle

The transmission from the SA to the AV node depends on conduction through the atrial muscle, possibly via distinct pathways with enhanced conduction between the pacemaking regions. In comparison to ventricular muscle, the atrial AP is far more narrow, with a less prominent plateau, consistent with its brief contraction. This is true in spite of the fact that atrial muscle has a lower basal conductance (G_{K1}) than does ventricular muscle, both in animals[1] and in humans.[78] Repolarization occurs more rapidly due to the presence of one or more transient outward K currents (I_{to}; Fig. 5–3*B*).[79–81] However, the short AP duration and lower basal G_{K1} in atrial tissue permit another action potential to occur much sooner, so that very high AP frequencies are achievable (i.e., atrial flutter). In human atrial muscle, a contribution of the Na-Ca exchange has been found to contribute to a sustained late but modest depolarization. In addition to its role as a contractile muscle, the atrium also has an endocrine role by its secretion of natriuretic peptides, which modulate cardiac contractility, vascular tone, and renal function.

The Ventricular Conduction Apparatus: The His-Purkinje System

A coordinated contraction of all the ventricular myocytes is required so that all of the energy of contraction can be used to expel blood, rather than have contracting muscle stretch out other muscle that has not yet begun to contract. Yet the myocytes that make up the bulk of the heart are specialized to develop tension, not to propagate a signal. Consequently, uniform initiation of contraction is achieved by specialized myocytes or Purkinje fibers that form large-diameter (50- to 80-μm) fibers with very sparse myofibrils or sarcoplasmic reticulum. The large diameter contributes to increased conduction velocity. The bundle of His is an aggregation of these large conducting fibers that accepts the impulse from the AV node and then divides to spread the impulse through the endocardial surface via a right ventricular branch, an anterior left ventricular branch, and a large posterior left ventricular branch. While this provides a useful agreement with certain conduction defects as defined by the electrocardiogram (ECG), there is considerable anatomic variation within the left ventricle.

The APs of the Purkinje system are characterized by the most rapid rate of depolarization (400 to 800 V/sec) in the heart. The bundle of His has sufficiently high current density that it generates a discrete voltage signal. These large-diameter fibers have a conduction velocity of approximately 4 m/sec, which permits the rapid conduction of the AP from the AV node to the endocardial surface of the ventricular muscle in about 30 msec. The action potentials in the Purkinje system are also the longest in the heart, and the proximal (nearest the His bundle) are depolarized for a substantially longer time (40

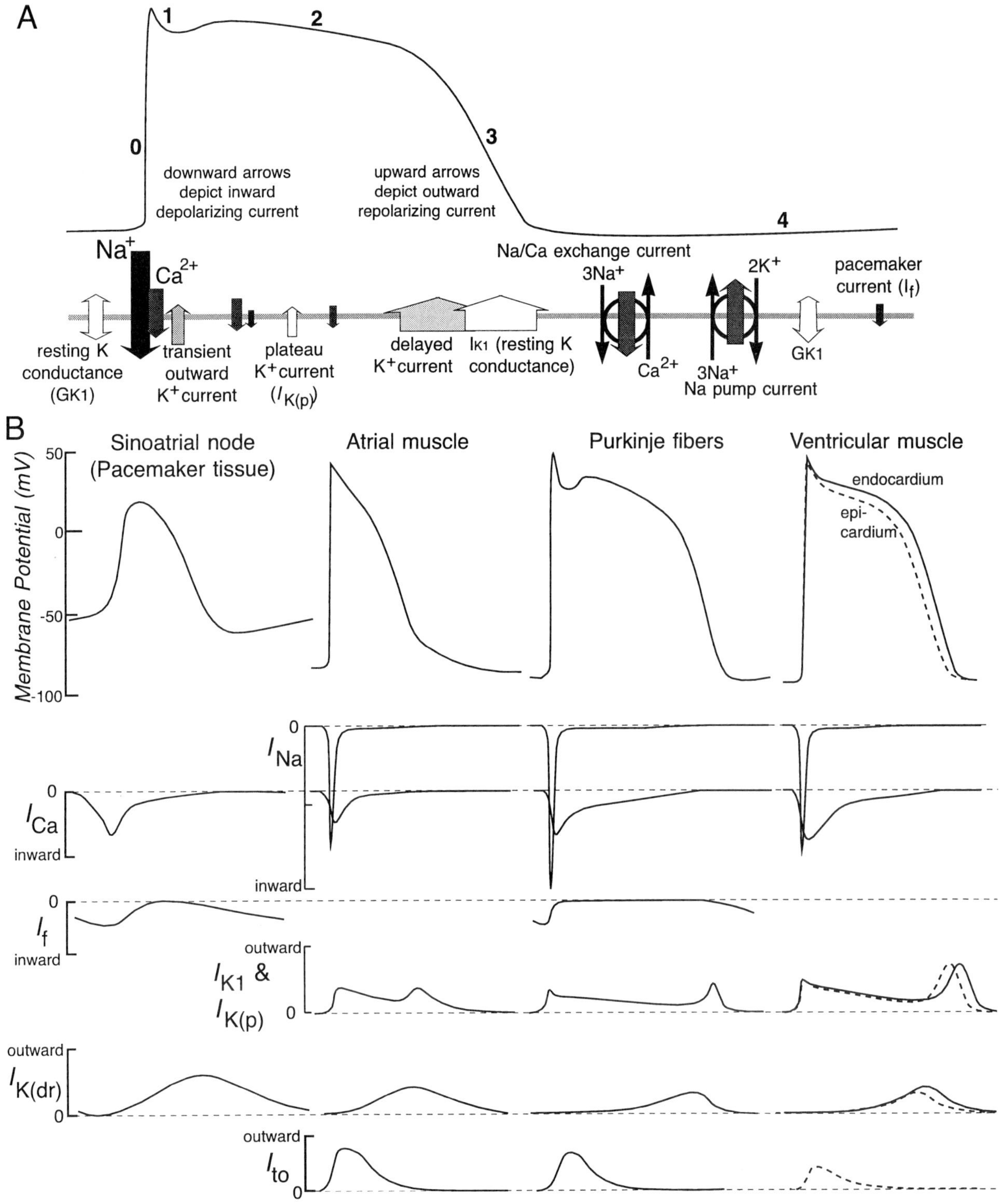

FIGURE **5–3.** *A*, Hypothetical action potential (AP) and the associated transmembrane currents as indicated by the *arrows.* The phases 0 through 4 of the action potential are indicated. *B*, Various cardiac APs with associated distinct ionic currents indicated below. The currents through the Na-Ca exchange (I_{NaCa}) and Na,K-ATPase are not indicated. In the SA and AV nodes and in Purkinje fibers, the pacemaker potential or diastolic depolarization (DD) is the result of the turn off of the delayed potassium current, $I_{K(dr)}$, as well as the hyperpolarization-induced activation of the inward pacemaker current (I_f).[75] The decline in $I_{K(dr)}$ combined with the I_f inward current results in gradual depolarization until the action potential threshold is approached and Ca channels open. The I_{Ca} probably represents T-type channels initially activated during the latter half of the DD with the L-type channels providing the major current responsible for the AP upstroke.[549] In Purkinje fibers and muscle, the depolarization is rapid due to the large Na^+ current (I_{Na}). The large depolarization initiates the more sustained I_{Ca}, although a small component of I_{Na} also persists. In epicardial ventricular muscle and atrial muscle, transient outward K^+ currents (I_{to}) are activated immediately after depolarization and are responsible for the larger phase 1 repolarization, as well as for the "notch" in Purkinje fibers. Some persistent I_{to} then results in an abbreviated plateau in atrial muscle and epicardial ventricle. Because the normal resting conductance (G_{K1}) is blocked by intracellular Mg^{2+} during depolarization, the gradual plateau repolarization relies on a small outward plateau current ($I_{K,p}$) to offset the residual I_{Ca} and I_{Na}. Initiation of the final repolarization and termination of the plateau is the result of activation of $I_{K(dr)}$ and I_{Ca} inactivation, while the more rapid final repolarization is due to outward current flowing through the resting K conductance (G_{K1}).

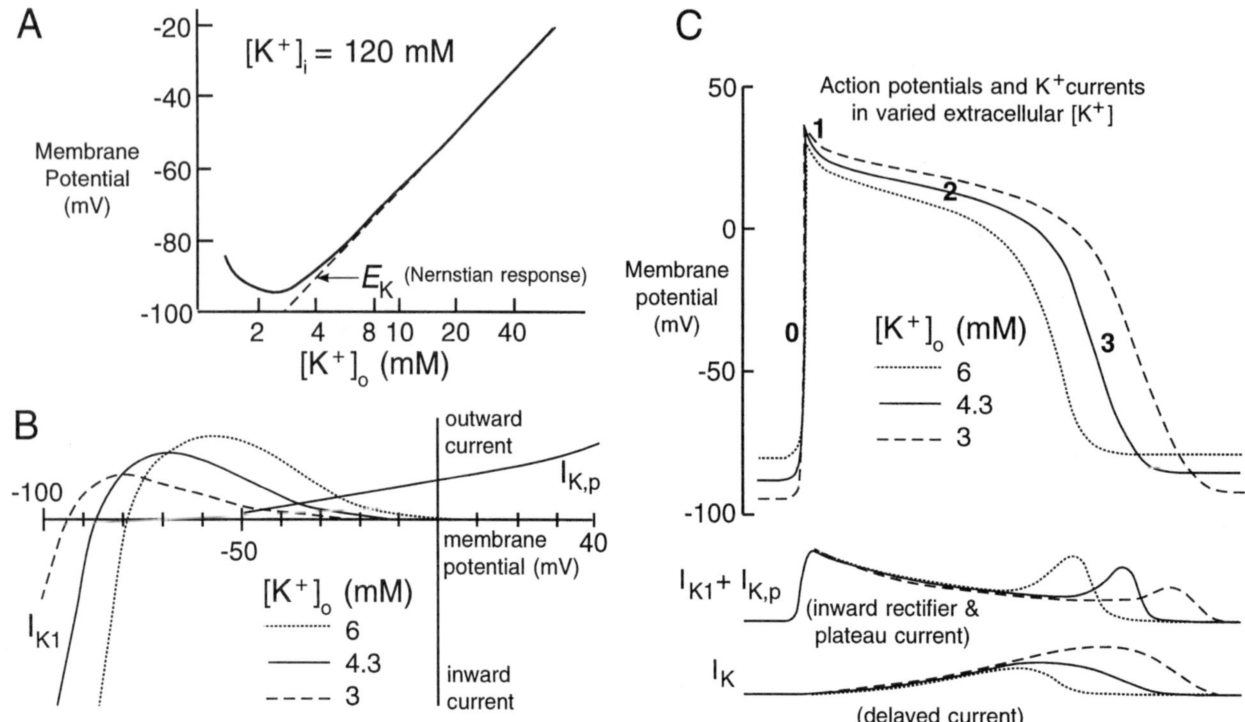

FIGURE **5–4.** Electrophysiologic effects of the inward rectifier (G_{K1}). *A*, The calculated Nernstian equilibrium potential for K^+ (E_K) and the membrane potential (V_m) recorded in myocardial tissue are shown. The intracellular K^+ ($[K^+]_i$) is based on measurements in Purkinje fibers and ventricular muscle.[550–552] Due to the dependence of the resting potassium conductance (G_{K1}, inward rectifier) on extracellular K^+ ($[K^+]_o$), as $[K^+]_o$ declines the membrane potential deviates increasingly from the E_K as G_{K1} decreases. At very low $[K^+]_o$ cells may actually depolarize.[553] *B*, Current voltage (I–V) relations of G_{K1} at various $[K^+]_o$. When $[K^+]_o$ is increased ($\geq$5 mM), there is a partial depolarization; however, G_{K1} increases so a greater depolarizing current is required to further depolarize. With decreased $[K^+]_o$ ($\leq$3 mM), the lower conductance means that less current will generate a larger depolarization. The outward current observed with positive potentials appears to be due to a separate plateau or background conductance ($I_{K,p}$).[554] *C*, Effects of varied $[K^+]_o$ on the action potential configuration. As the delayed current is activated, with increased $[K^+]_o$, G_{K1} is enhanced so that outward currents through it result in an earlier repolarization and termination of the plateau. The opposite effect is observed in low $[K^+]_o$ when G_{K1} is reduced, and the delayed current must contribute more outward current, which requires a longer period of time-dependent activation. In either case, a component of repolarizing outward current is present because of $I_{K,p}$, which is relatively insensitive to $[K^+]_o$. Inward currents are not shown. For a discussion and mathematical description, respectively, see Surawicz[555] and Luo and Rudy.[84]

to 80 msec) than those distal fibers that form electrical junctions with the myocardium. Consequently, the cardiac impulses cannot pass retrograde (back from the muscle into the depolarized conduction system) under normal conditions, protecting the heart from many erratic and premature beats that might be initiated in the distal regions. These fibers also have a very slow diastolic depolarization, which can provide pacemaking capability if the SA and AV nodes fail, albeit at very slow rates (10 to 20 bpm).

The Action Potential in Ventricular Muscle

The rapid conduction of the impulse to the endocardial surface of the heart permits a depolarization to sweep through the ventricular wall in 80 to 100 msec, so that contraction of the ventricular muscle is a unified activity. The wave of depolarizing sodium currents is normally oriented in the endocardial-epicardial direction and, when summed from the approximately 1 billion myocytes of a human heart, generates a substantial current. This current is dispersed by the extracellular fluid throughout the body, which creates vectors of electrical potential detectable as the QRS complex of the ECG. Due to the rapid and relatively uniform nature of this transmural depolarization, many of the electrical vectors (right vs. left, anterior vs. posterior) actually cancel, giving rise to the normally modest QRS complex. When depolarization is interrupted in the conduction system (e.g., left or right bundle branch block [BBB]), the depolarization must sweep through the much more slowly conducting ventricular muscle. The resulting QRS has a longer duration and frequently has a greater amplitude because the electrical vectors are not simultaneous and show less internal cancellation.

During the plateau of the AP, virtually no current is flowing, there is isoelectric behavior of the ST segment. Epicardial myocytes repolarize before those in the endocardium,[82] due at least in part to the presence of greater transient outward K^+ currents (I_{to}) in the epicardial cells (Fig. 5–3*B*).[83] Because epicardial APs are shorter than those in the endocardium, the wave of repolarization sweeps from the epicardium to the endocardium. This results in a current in the same direction as endo- to epicardial depolarization, generating the T wave of the ECG which is in the same direction as the Q wave. With the less uniform depolarization of BBB, the dispersion of the depolarization and repolarization frequently results in the QRS and T wave having opposite polarity.

EFFECTS OF ALTERED EXTRACELLULAR $[K^+]_o$

The stable behavior of the cardiac muscle is possible in part because of the high resting K^+ conductance of the inward rectifier channel (G_{K1}). Ventricular muscle contains the highest density of G_{K1} channels, providing electrical stability even in the presence of varied extracellular $[K^+]$ ($[K^+]_o$). Effects of hypo- and hyperkalemia on resting membrane conductance are shown in Figure 5–4*B*. When $[K^+]_o$ is low (2.5 mM), the conductance of G_{K1} is low so that K^+ is less able to flow out of the cell (membrane resistance is high). Although a large depolarization is required from the resting potential (−95 mV) to reach the AP threshold (−65 mV), as a consequence of the low G_{K1}, any current (from adjacent cells, or cell damage) causes a more rapid depolarization toward threshold. Since the cells are more hyperpolarized, more Na channels are available, which results in inward current and rapid AP conduction. The result may be greater excitability and a tendency for extra depolarizations (ectopy) when $[K^+]_o$ is below normal.

In contrast, when $[K^+]_o$ is increased above normal, the membrane conductance is high (membrane resistance is low) so that, ironically, G_{K1} permits more current (K^+) to escape from the cell, possibly because the higher $[K^+]_o$ decreases the blockade by intracellular Mg^{2+} and polyamines. Although the membrane is more depolarized and closer to the AP threshold, the cell is unlikely to be more excitable because current more readily passes through the membrane, and does not depolarize it. While a smaller depolarization is required to get to threshold (−65 mV) from the resting potential (−75 mV), similar or more influx of current will be necessary to depolarize the cell compared to when $[K^+]_o$ and membrane conductance is low. A major effect of hyperkalemia is slowed conduction, due to the need for increased depolarizing current to reach threshold as well as a greater number of inactivated Na channels at the more depolarized membrane potential. This anomalous behavior of G_{K1} (also called the anomalous rectifier), whereby increased $[K^+]_o$ actually increases outward current, nevertheless permits relative stability of membrane behavior over a threefold range of $[K^+]_o$.

The peculiar behavior and $[K^+]_o$ dependence of G_{K1} also influence repolarization. Once the repolarization process has been initiated by the delayed current (I_K, see below) and V_m becomes negative to −30 mV, G_{K1} increases progressively, permitting an increase in K^+ efflux and enhancing the rate of repolarization. In fact, G_{K1} is the major repolarizing current during the later half of repolarization.[84] Consequently, increases or decreases in conductance with hyper- or hypokalemia, respectively, will decrease or increase AP duration as indicated in Figure 5–4*C* (see Luo and Rudy[84]). Likewise, specific blockade of G_{K1} by 50 to 100 μM Ba^{2+} or Cs^+ or by certain barbiturates (e.g., thiopental) will prolong the AP duration by extending the later phase.[1,85] Such blockade of G_{K1} will also increase excitability and the propensity to develop arrhythmias.[86]

Myocardial Excitation-Contraction Coupling

Excitation-contraction (EC) coupling is the mechanism by which depolarization of the membrane activates contraction. The essence of the process involves Ca^{2+} delivery to and the response by the myofibrils. In contrast to skeletal muscle, in which the strength of contraction is controlled by the number of fibers activated by motor neurons, cardiac muscle is an electrical syncytium in which *all* cells are stimulated to contract under normal conditions. The strength of cardiac contractions is instead controlled by the degree of activation of the myocytes, which is determined by the length of the sarcomere and the amount of activator Ca^{2+}. The entry of Ca^{2+} and Na^+ and their interaction via the Na-Ca exchange require that electrophysiologic behavior and EC coupling are highly integrated and interdependent functions. The varied tension generation seen with changes in cardiac volume (Starling's law of the heart[87]) or rate of beating (positive frequency staircase) result from two intrinsic characteristics of the myocardium: (1) variation in the myofibril Ca^{2+} sensitivity and (2) alteration in the amount of activator Ca^{2+}. By alterations in these intrinsic determinants of cardiac contractility, a variety of extrinsic factors such as inotropic stimulation or ischemia modulate their effects.

Microscopic Structure

Unlike skeletal muscle, which is composed of long, multinucleated fibers, atrial and ventricular muscle in most mammalian species is composed of individual myocytes (mono- or binucleate), typically 80 to 150 μm in length with elliptical cross sections of 5 to 15 × 20 to 30 μm (see Fig. 5–5*A*).[88] These myocytes are connected longitudinally end-to-end, as well as end-to-side, resulting in interconnected strands. All myocytes are joined at intercalated disks, a complex interdigitation of membrane structures that permit electrical continuity via connexons (gap junctions) and mechanical continuity by means of a high concentration of cytoskeletal proteins, such as vinculin. An average cardiac myocyte will make such an electrical and mechanical connection with about seven other myocytes.[89] However, the basic functional unit of contraction in skeletal and cardiac muscle is remarkably similar, being the sarcomere, a 2.0 to 2.5 μm segment in which an array of myosin filaments (1.65 μm) is centered between and interdigitates with two arrays of actin filaments (see Fig. 5–5*B*). At the Z line, the ends of the actin filaments from adjacent sarcomeres meet; it is also the location at which the surface membrane is linked to the internal tension-generating structures by the vinculin. A variety of other cytoskeletal proteins (talin, α-actinin, integrin) and anchor fibers are also present at the Z line, while microtubules (tubulin) and longitudinally oriented

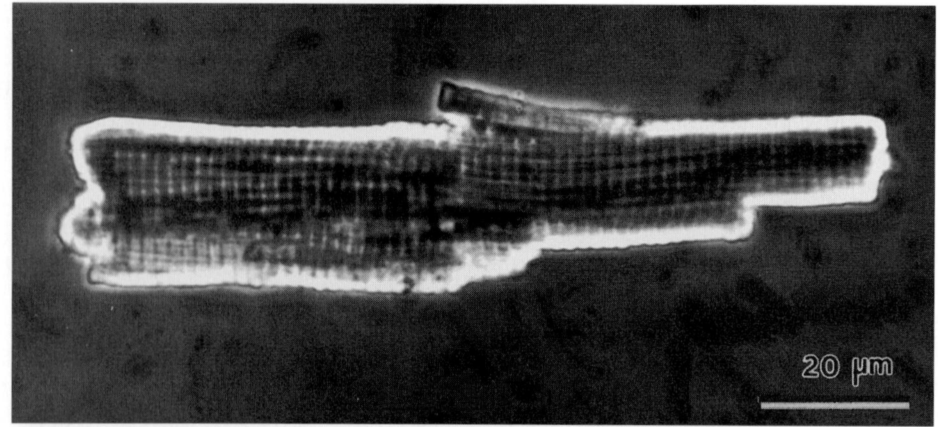

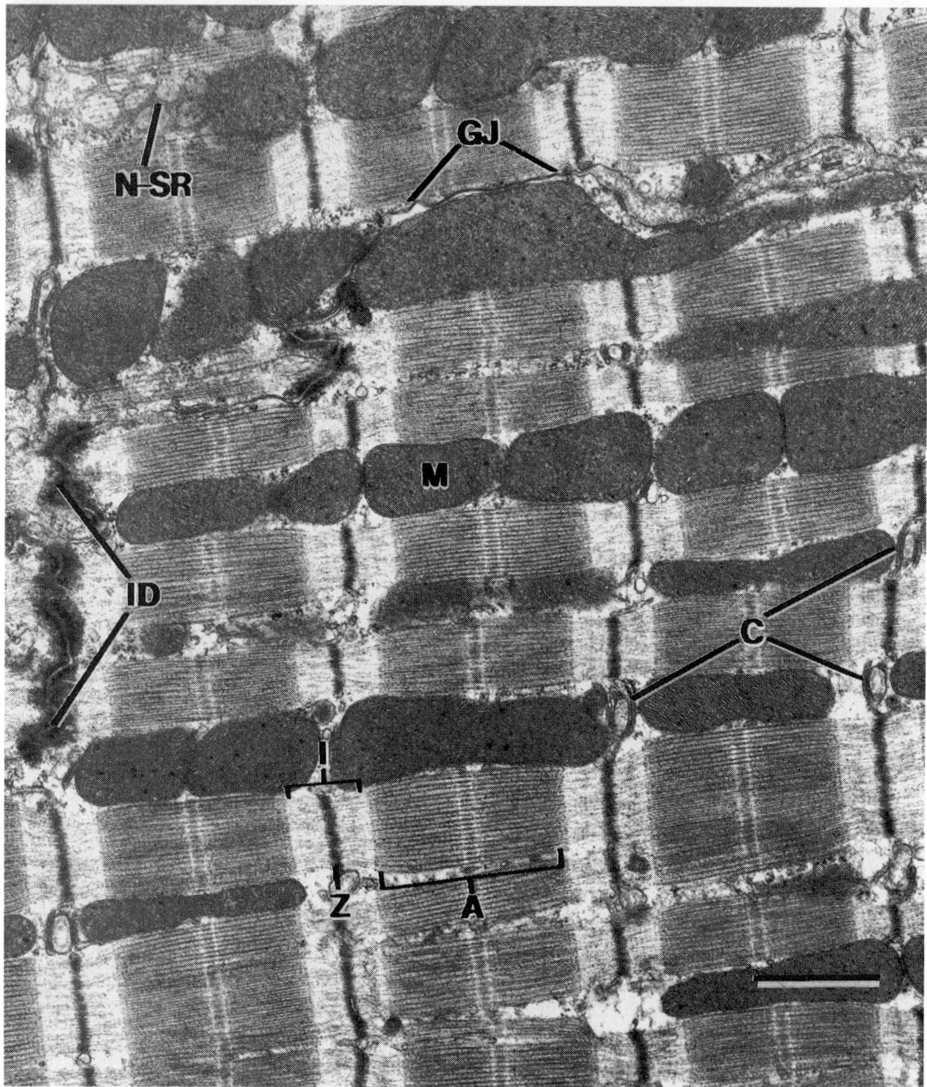

FIGURE **5–5.** *A*, Phase contrast light micrograph of enzymatically isolated rat ventricular myocardial cell. Periodic banding pattern of myofibrils is evident secondary to the sarcomeric striations of the myofibrils. The uneven contour of the cell is the result of myofibrils of different overall lengths and the formation of junctions with other myocytes along the length of the cell. *B*, Transmission electron micrograph of a longitudinal thin section through rat ventricular myocardial cells (calibration bar = 1 μm). The bulk of each cell is occupied by the myofibrils, oriented along the long axis of each cell and exhibiting the characteristic banding pattern formed by the A bands (where actin and myosin filaments overlap), I bands (consisting primarily of actin filaments), and Z lines (composed in large part of α-actinin), which bisect each I band. At the end of myofibrils, a collection of specialized junctions (the intercalated disks [ID]) connect adjacent cells at the position Z lines would occupy. Mitochondria (M) are arranged either in rows among the myofibrils or in clusters beneath the cell membrane, where they are frequently closely apposed to gap junctions (GJ), an example of which appears as a thin dark line at this magnification. The membrane systems of myocardial cells include the sarcoplasmic reticulum (SR), most of which appears in the form of tubular retes (network SR [N-SR]) on the surfaces of myofibrils. Continuous with the network SR are specialized flattened saccules of junctional SR, which are apposed either to the surface sarcolemma or its tubular extensions, the transverse tubules, forming complexes known as couplings (C), which frequently are located at the levels of the Z lines. (Courtesy of Michael Forbes.)

intermediate filaments (primarily desmin) present in myocytes partition them into quasi compartments and prevent disruption of the complex internal architecture. Adding further structure and permitting generation of macroscopic force are microfibrils and extracellular lamina, which connects the plasmalemma to the collagen matrix surrounding cell bundles. Also at the Z line, tubular invaginations of the surface membranes (0.1-μm diameter), the transverse tubules (T tubules), form a network across the myocyte.

The actin and myosin filaments that interact to generate tension are also separated into bundles 0.5 to 1 μm in diameter (myofibrils), each containing 300 to 1,000 filaments of each type. Each myofibril is surrounded by a membranous network, the SR, the lumen of which contains a high concentration of Ca^{2+}. The network of SR at the Z line is juxtaposed to the T tubules, and the SR membrane that faces the T tubules contains an array of highly specialized, very large homotetrameric protein complexes that are the Ca release channels, responsible for controlling the release of Ca^{2+}, which activates the myofibrils. This junctional SR is also characterized by a larger lumen that contains calsequestrin, a protein that binds Ca^{2+} with a low affinity and provides an extra "sink" of releasable Ca^{2+}. Unlike skeletal muscle, myocardium has a very high density of mitochondria, which are frequently present in rows between the separate myofibrils and compose 30 to 40% of cell volume. Such a high density of ATP-producing organelles is obviously critical in a continuously active tissue like the heart and may also represent a relative diffusion barrier.[90]

Within the myocardium, the interconnected strands of myocytes are enmeshed in a thin network of collagen fibers, and are gathered into small interconnecting bundles, which are also sheathed in connective tissue. This connective tissue and collagen present in the extracellular space is far greater than in skeletal muscle, being 2 to 6% of the left ventricle (LV) dry weight. While there appear to be no passive, noncontractile elements in series with the myocytes,[91] this extracellular matrix provides an important elastic component in parallel to the contractile cellular elements, which can generate considerable passive tension when myocardium is stretched. The collagen fibers and struts that attach to Z line of myocytes protect them from being overstretched and maintain the unloaded geometry of the LV.[92] Enzymatic removal of collagen results in passive stretching of the ventricle, while increases in collagen can decrease distensibility.[93]

Myofilament Response to Ca^{2+}

Actin filaments (F-actin) are composed of two intertwined strands of single actin molecules, strongly held together by noncovalent interactions (see Fig. 5–6, *right*). In the groove between the strands and overlapping seven actin monomers lies a molecule of tropomyosin. Each tropomyosin has an associated complex of troponin comprised of an inhibitory (TnI), Ca^{2+}-binding (TnC), and tropomyosin-binding (TnT) subunit. As in many cells, the myoplasmic Ca^{2+} concentration ($[Ca^{2+}]_i$) at rest (during diastole) is approximately 80 to 100 nM (~0.1 M) and no Ca^{2+} is bound to the regulatory Ca^{2+} site on troponin C (TnC). In the absence of bound Ca^{2+}, the troponin complex stabilizes the position of the tropomyosin molecule within the F-actin groove so that the sites on actin for myosin attachment are occluded. When $[Ca^{2+}]_i$ surrounding the myofibrils increases to 0.5 to 2 M, Ca^{2+} binding to TnC appears to couple TnI to TnC[94] and uncouple TnI from actin.[95,96] A conformational shift of tropomyosin in the F-actin groove occurs, revealing the active sites on actin to which the myosin head groups can bind (Fig. 5–6). By binding to TnC, this activator Ca^{2+} acts like a switch to turn on actin-myosin interaction.

Each myosin (MW ~520 kDa) is comprised of two heavy chains (MHC), each containing a globular head domain (subfragment 1, S1) with a tightly coiled, α-helical rod section or tail (S2), and a light meromyosin. In addition, a regulatory and an essential light chain are associated with each head group, and modulate its binding to actin.[97] Myosin (thick) filaments are formed by the aggregation of the individual myosins, each with its two head groups facing outward to bind to actin. It is the flexion or rotation of the head group after binding to an actin monomer (or two adjacent monomers) that generates the tension on the myosin filament, and the total tension generated within the muscle is proportional to the total number of head groups actively cycling. After head group rotation, ADP is released and the myosin and actin remain tightly bound (a rigor complex) until ATP can combine to uncouple the proteins, freeing myosin to combine again with actin (see Fig. 5–6, *left*). If other myosin head groups are generating tension and shortening has occurred, the myosin will bind to actin monomers further along the filament. If no shortening has occurred, and tropomyosin has not occluded the active site on actin, the myosin may rebind in the same location to continue tension generation (while other myosin S1s are cycling). In regard to its ability to hydrolyze an ATP and unbind from actin, two MHC isoforms exist (α and β) that can combine to form fast (V_1, αα), medium (V_2, αβ), and slow (V_3, ββ) forms of myosin.[98] Slow myosin predominates in cardiac tissue. In animal models, V_1 and V_2 isoforms are expressed in neonatal animals, or in hyperthyroidism, but their importance in human myocardium has not been demonstrated.

LENGTH- (FORCE-) DEPENDENT CONTRACTILE ACTIVATION

In a skeletal muscle fiber, the force development that results from activation is largely proportional to the amount of overlap of the sliding filaments of actin and myosin. Skeletal muscle can be stretched to the point where actin-myosin filament overlap begins to decrease and active tension decreases; unless shortening is extreme in skeletal muscle, the tension decreases only modestly with shorter sarcomere lengths of less than 1.8 μm.

In myocardium, the relationship of active force versus length has a steeper slope: when the sarcomeres are contracted and short (<1.8 μm) there is very modest active force development for a given $[Ca^{2+}]_i$, but even small

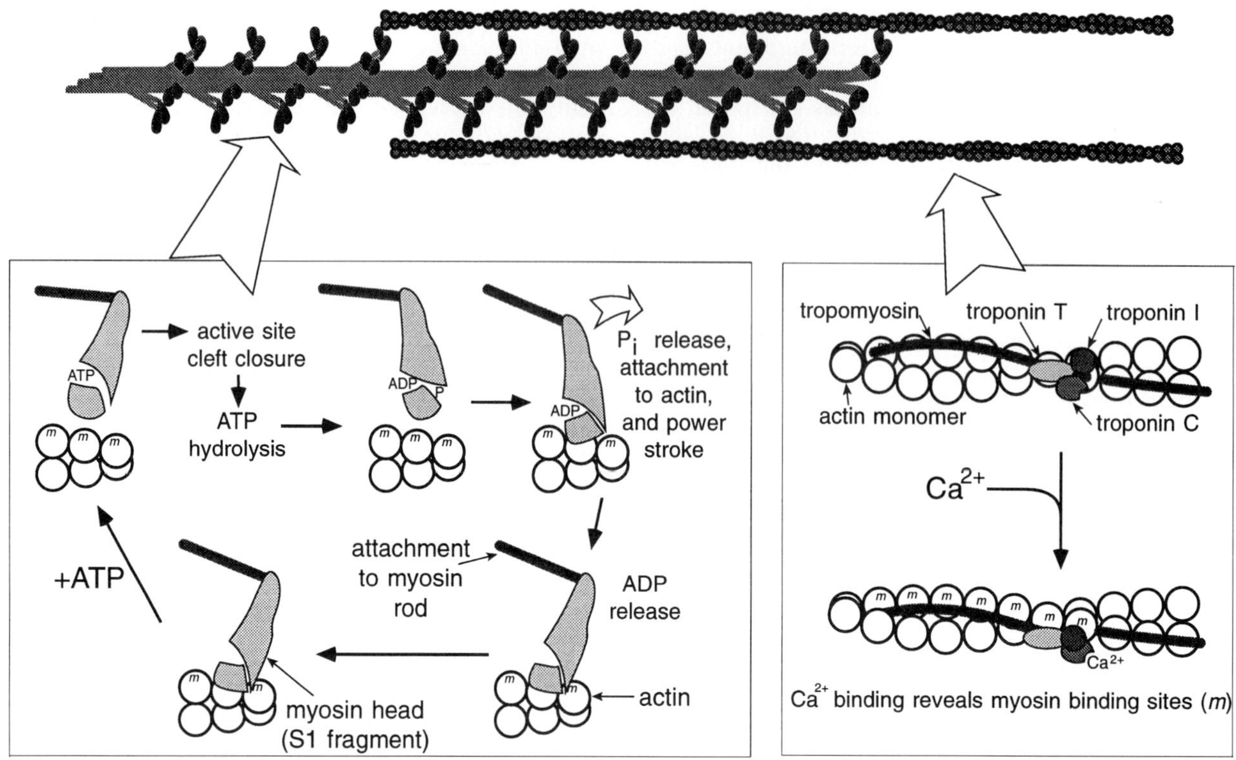

FIGURE **5–6.** Actin and myosin filaments. *Right*, Schematic enlargement of the actin filament composed of individual monomers, and the troponin-tropomyosin complex, which controls accessibility of the myosin binding site (*m*). Ca^{2+} binding to troponin C causes the inhibitory subunit (troponin I) to decrease its affinity for actin. Via tropomyosin, *m* sites on seven actin monomers become revealed. *Left*, Schematic of the cycle of the myosin head (S1) in generating tension. ATP binding dissociates the head group from actin, with a subsequent hydrolysis, P_i release, and "cocking" of the head group into a tension-generating conformation. Attachment to actin then permits the head group to apply tension to the rod portion and thus to the filament. (Adapted from Rayment I, Holden HM, Whittaker M, et al: Structure of the actin-myosin complex and implications for muscle contraction. Science 261:58, 1993. Copyright 1993, American Association for the Advancement of Science, with permission.)

amounts of stretch result in far greater force development (Fig. 5–7*A*).[99] For the same $[Ca^{2+}]_i$, more force is generated and more myofibrils appear activated when cardiac myocytes are stretched, than when contracted.[100] This effect has been attributed to the relation between activation and Ca^{2+} binding to cardiac TnC, a protein distinct from TnC of skeletal muscle. This protein may endow cardiac muscle with a far greater sensitivity to length[100] and force,[101–103] so that greater force development (or number of active cross-bridges) appears to increase the Ca^{2+} affinity of cardiac TnC, and a lower $[Ca^{2+}]_i$ is required to activate the same amount of myosin-actin binding. This effect has been attributed to differences between skeletal TnC (which requires binding of two Ca^{2+}) and cardiac TnC, since it is not seen when skeletal TnC is substituted for cardiac TnC.[104,105] However, this effect has not been universally demonstrated, and more recently it has been suggested that the major effect responsible for the decrease in tension with shortening is due to a geometric effect mediated by increased myofibril separation as myocyte cross-sectional area increases with shortening.[106] In any case, cross-bridge attachment influences TnC position and serves as a positive-feedback mechanism for tension development.[107] When myosin head groups attach to actin and generate force, less Ca^{2+} is required to be bound to TnC. Once a "tight" cross-bridge is formed, Ca^{2+} may diffuse away from TnC[108]; while the myosin is still bound to actin, Ca^{2+} may thus become available to bind to other TnC and activate other regions of the F-actin filament.

In addition to this property intrinsic to the myofibrils, enhanced SR Ca^{2+} capacity is also present when myocytes are stretched to a greater length; however, this increase in stored Ca^{2+} accounts for only about 25% of the enhanced contractility.[109] This SR effect requires a certain time to develop, whereas the more prominent myofibrillar length (or force) dependence is instantaneous.[109]

PASSIVE LENGTH-FORCE COMPONENT

The other component that sharply defines myocardial length-force relation is the passive (diastolic) behavior that is due to the large amount of connective tissue in cardiac muscle and prevents the muscle from being passively stretched beyond that point where total tension declines.[110,99] This passive length-force component increases steeply at the muscle length at which active tension development levels off. The result of the steep active length-force relation due to cardiac TnC combined with the steep passive length-force relation is a total length-force relation that is linear over the functional range (Fig. 5–7*A*). When the collagen strands that surround myocytes are enzymatically digested, the passive tension curve is shifted to the right.[92]

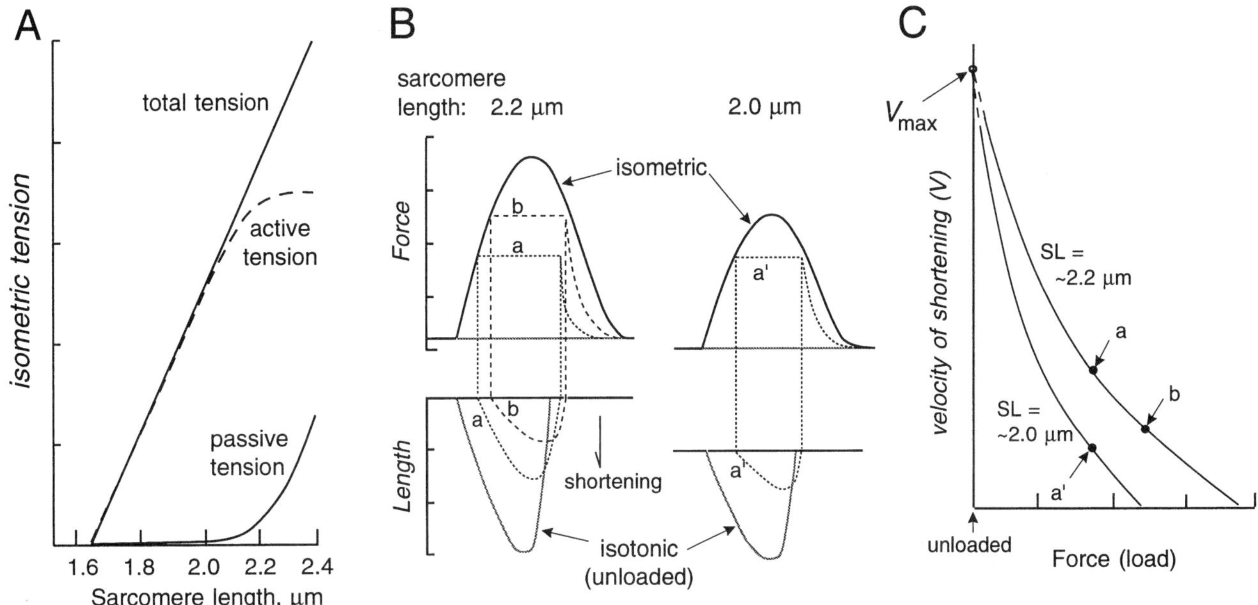

FIGURE **5–7.** The interaction of initial length and preload on force development and velocity of shortening. *A*, Dependence of active and passive force on sarcomere length (SL), which also is demonstrable in intact muscle. The difference between the total and passive tension is the active developed tension (*dotted line*). The summation of the passive and active force components create the virtually linear dependence of force on length. *B*, Simultaneous tracings of force and length from a typical papillary muscle experiment. The *left panel* shows the response of a more stretched muscle (SL ~ 2.2 μm), while the *right panel* shows the response at a shorter length (SL ~ 2.0 μm). At the shorter length, the muscle can attain less maximum tension (as plotted in *A*). Once any given force is attained, shortening is a linear function of the initial length. When more force must be generated (greater afterload), shortening is reduced and slower, as evident from the reduced initial downward slope of the length tracing. With shorter initial length and greater afterload, no shortening may occur (load a′, SL ~ 2.0 μm). *C*, According to the analysis first described by Sonnenblick, the velocity of shortening is plotted for muscles as in *B*, with SL of 2.2 or 2.0 μm. As the force generated before shortening (load) is reduced, the velocity of shortening increases and approaches a maximum rate (V_{max}) even at shorter lengths.

When a muscle is activated, there can be exclusive force or pressure development (isometric shortening or isovolemic contraction) or exclusive shortening (unloaded isotonic shortening). However, the normal physiologic situation is some combination of force and shortening. Because a greater number of myosin units are active at a longer sarcomere length, over the same time period a longer muscle will shorten more against a given resisting force or afterload. When the steep length dependence of cardiac contractility is expressed as muscle shortening instead of force development, the result is less shortening at slower velocity as the load applied to an isolated muscle is increased (Fig. 5–7*C*).[111] As the afterload is increased, more cross-bridges cycle to generate greater force, but cause a smaller degree of shortening. However, when there is no load on the muscle, the velocity of shortening is less dependent on initial muscle length, and the maximum unloaded velocity of shortening (V_{max}) is similar at various lengths. V_{max} is widely used as a measure of contractility that is relatively independent of preload (initial fiber length) and afterload.[112]

The length (or force) dependence of myofibril activation also has an important corollary with regard to relaxation, since the change in TnC Ca^{2+} affinity occurs within a single cardiac cycle. Starting from the same initial length, if a muscle is allowed to shorten instead of being maintained at a longer length and developing greater force, a decreased TnC Ca^{2+} affinity is predicted. Consequently, a muscle allowed to shorten relaxes sooner,[113–115] a phenomenon termed length- (or load-) dependent relaxation, or shortening deactivation. The decreased Ca^{2+} affinity of TnC that occurs due to shortening results in a detectably higher cytoplasmic $[Ca^{2+}]_i$, which diffuses from TnC more rapidly into the myoplasm,[101,116,117] from which it is reaccumulated into the SR. Consequently, when shortening occurs, the rate of relaxation is dependent upon the rate at which the SR can take up Ca^{2+}. When force or pressure development occurs with little shortening, the decline in $[Ca^{2+}]_i$ reflects the higher TnC Ca^{2+} affinity. Such length-dependence of relaxation is a clear demonstration of myocardial economy, since once shortening and ejection of blood has occurred, it would consume needless ATP if myosin continued to cycle. This also has important implications with regard to ventricular function, energy consumption, and perfusion. When resistance to ejection and intraventricular pressures are increased, relaxation is retarded.[118,119] Systole and ATP consumption are prolonged, by cycling of myosin with actin, while diastole is shortened. When there is considerable shortening and less force developed, Ca^{2+} diffuses off of TnC more readily and, provided that the SR can actively accumulate the Ca^{2+} (see below), systole is abbreviated. In addition, the myofilament sensitivity to Ca^{2+} and the resulting degree of activation are also modulated by receptor-mediated systems that control the TnI subunit phosphorylation as noted below.

Regulation of Intracellular Ca^{2+}

The other obvious limb of myocardial contractile control is the regulation of the amount of Ca^{2+} made available to activate each beat of the heart. The amount and source of activator Ca^{2+} in the myoplasm surrounding the myofibrils in mammalian hearts is determined by an intermixture of Ca^{2+} entering from extracellular milieu and Ca^{2+} released from the intracellular SR pool. The exact balance and mixture of activator Ca^{2+} depends upon a variety of factors such as age, species, heart rate, and temperature. As already noted, the L-type Ca channel has intrinsic Ca^{2+}-dependent feedback regulation, with both positive and negative components.[120] The clustering of channels appears to permit greater local accumulation, which activates greater current.[41] However, an inherent Ca^{2+}-dependent inactivation of Ca channels causes inherent time-dependent turn-off of current as time progresses.[39]

THE SARCOPLASMIC RETICULUM

The Ca Release Channel and Ca^{2+}-Induced Ca^{2+} Release. As in skeletal muscle, the Ca^{2+} that activates the myofibrils is primarily derived from the SR (Fig. 5–8). Unlike skeletal muscle where depolarization is more directly coupled to activate Ca release channels (CaRC), in cardiac tissue the entry of extracellular Ca^{2+} is critical for activation of Ca^{2+} release from the junctional SR (JSR). While some fraction of entering Ca^{2+} may bind to TnC to activate contractions, the Ca^{2+} entering via the plasmalemmal L-type Ca^{2+} channels is insufficient to activate the myofibrils directly. Its primary function is to activate release of the SR Ca^{2+}, a process termed Ca^{2+}-induced Ca^{2+} release (CICR).[121] Although the distinct cardiac isoform of the CaRC is structurally similar to that in skeletal muscle,[122] a portion of entering Ca^{2+} must bind to the cardiac CaRC to activate their opening in cardiomyocytes. The CaRC have very high single-channel conductance (about ten times greater than the L-type Ca channel), which permits the rapid efflux of the stored Ca^{2+} from the SR lumen into the myoplasm to bind to TnC. Since each myofibril is typically less than 1 μm in diameter, and each half sarcomere is less than 1.2 μm long, the distance over which Ca^{2+} must diffuse from the junctional SR during activation is very short, so that the time dependence of this process is not a factor. The CaRC also tightly bind the plant alkaloid ryanodine when open, hence, the name ryanodine receptor. Ryanodine binding has been used to isolate the protein and investigate the physiologic behavior of CaRC. Between the T tubule, where Ca^{2+} enters, and the opposed JSR membrane containing CaRC is a diffusion-restricted space that may be of critical importance in regulation of CIRC (contributing to a graded Ca^{2+} release with Ca^{2+} entry). The activated Ca^{2+} release is detectable as a transient increase in $[Ca^{2+}]_i$ that precedes tension development. While massive activation of release occurs during each beat, in quiescent cells, spontaneous opening of a

Calcium ion fluxes during active beating

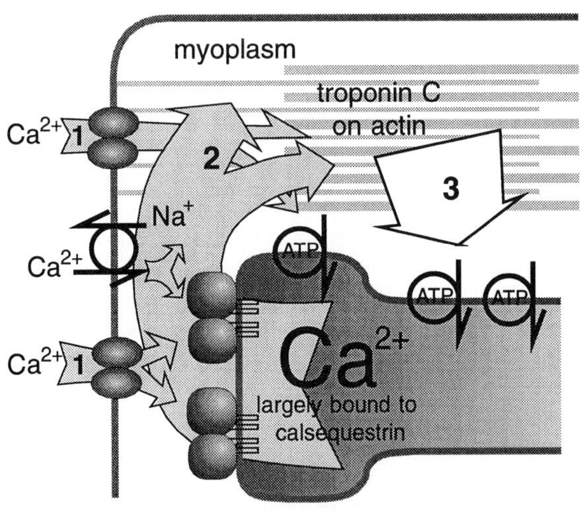

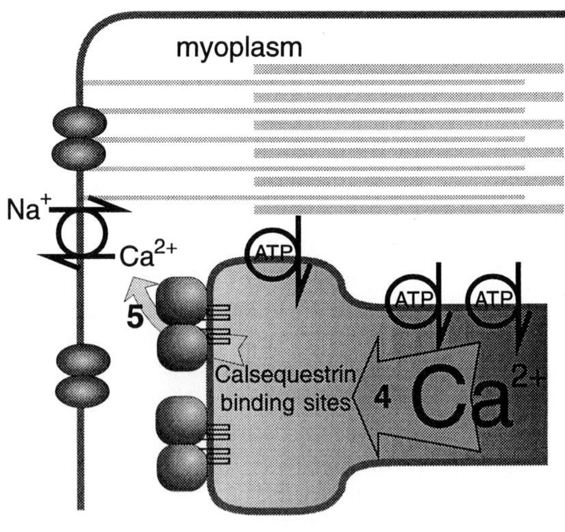

FIGURE **5–8.** Ca^{2+} cycling by myocardial sarcoplasmic reticulum (SR). *Left*, Upon depolarization, Ca^{2+} enters via L-type Ca channels and also via the Na-Ca exchanger to initiate systole (step 1). While a small fraction of entering Ca^{2+} may reach the myofibrils, the major role of Ca^{2+} entry is to bind to the Ca release channels of the junctional SR to activate release of Ca^{2+} (step 2), which represents the bulk of the activator Ca^{2+} which binds to troponin C to permit actin-myosin interaction. Following tension development, Ca^{2+} diffuses off troponin C and binds to the higher affinity binding sites on the Ca^{2+}-ATPase ("Ca pump") located on the longitudinal SR and which then transports it to the SR lumen (step 3). *Right*, During diastole, Ca^{2+} moves toward the junctional SR lumen (step 4) and the net entering Ca^{2+} is eliminated from the myocyte by the Na-Ca exchange (step 5). If diastole is not prolonged, the bulk of the Ca^{2+} is still present in the junctional SR lumen and available for release with the subsequent depolarization. With prolonged rest (>30 seconds) the SR gradually is depleted of its Ca^{2+} store.

single CaRC at the SR–T tubule junction results in localized "sparks" of Ca^{2+}.[123] During rest, such individual, uncoordinated Ca^{2+} release accounts for the depletion of Ca^{2+} from the SR.

The SR Ca^{2+}-ATPase: The Ca Pump. The SR is filled with Ca^{2+} because Ca^{2+} is accumulated by the action of the Ca^{2+}-ATPase, which "pumps" Ca^{2+}, consuming one ATP to transfer two Ca^{2+} into the SR lumen. This protein is densely distributed in the longitudinal SR (LSR) along the length of the myofibrils, and has a higher affinity for Ca^{2+} (K_M = 0.3 μM, which is the $[Ca^{2+}]$ for 50% binding) than the TnC regulatory site (K_M = 0.5 μM for TnC).[124] After the Ca^{2+} dissociates from TnC, it can either rebind (continuing to activated myofibrils), or bind to the higher affinity Ca^{2+}-binding sites on the SR ATPase from which it will be translocated into the SR lumen and become unavailable for the rest of that contraction cycle. Since in the normally beating myocardium most of the activator Ca^{2+} is derived from the SR, the bulk of Ca^{2+} removal from the myoplasm during relaxation is by reuptake into the LSR. From its location in the LSR it diffuses to the JSR, which contains the Ca release channels. The Ca-ATPase activity is modulated by phospholamban, a protein that in its unphosphorylated state binds to and inhibits the Ca-ATPase.

In addition to the troponin C, the SR also shows length-dependent behavior, so that SR Ca^{2+} stores increase following an increase in length.[109] As opposed to the immediate effect caused by length dependence of troponin and Ca^{2+}, the length dependence of the SR effect develops over a number of contractions, and it appears to account for a more modest component (15 to 25%) of length-dependent inotropism. The phenomenon is not limited to isolated muscle but is also demonstrable in intact animals.[125]

Na-Ca EXCHANGE

Although Ca^{2+} entry via Ca channels is insufficient by itself to activate a normal contraction, a substantial influx of Ca^{2+} does enter with each depolarization, which during steady-state beating must be eliminated from the myocyte to prevent overloading of Ca^{2+}. While a Ca-ATPase (Ca pump) distinct from the SR Ca-ATPase exists in the plasmalemma, it has a low capacity and does not contribute substantially to myoplasmic Ca^{2+} removal.[67,126] The system primarily responsible is the Na-Ca exchanger which, as previously noted, employs an entry of three Na^+ to eliminate one Ca^{2+}. The exchange is steeply dependent on $[Na^+]_i$,[127] so that maintenance of the normal $[Na^+]_i$ of 7 to 10 mM is critical for proper control of intracellular Ca^{2+}. During the peak of the AP (+40 to 50 mV) the driving force for Ca^{2+} current is reduced, and the Na-Ca exchange reverses its direction, so that a Ca^{2+} enters by the pathway as three Na^+ are eliminated.[128,129] This Ca^{2+} entry may be sufficient to contribute to the activation of Ca^{2+} release from the SR, and may contribute as much as 65% of the entering Ca^{2+} which triggers release from the SR,[130] and may also serve to load the SR stores.[131] While a large Na^+ gradient is required to eliminate Ca^{2+} during diastole, too large a gradient may prevent Ca^{2+} entry by this pathway during the peak of the AP.[130] For example, it is possible that this effect contributes to the decrease in contractility observed with hypertonic saline administration in normovolemic dogs.[132]

CONTINUOUS Ca^{2+} CIRCULATION AND RATE DEPENDENCE

In skeletal muscle that remains inactive, there is little change in its ability to generate tension with a depolarization because the internal store of activator Ca^{2+} remains readily available in the SR after long periods of rest. This behavior is in sharp contrast to the contractility of myocardium of most mammalian species, which shows an exponential decline with rest (rat myocardium is an important exception). Unlike skeletal muscle, in which the SR tightly retains Ca^{2+}, the Ca^{2+} that activates cardiac myofibrils undergoes much more active exchange across the sarcolemma.

Rate Effects. The most obvious example of intrinsic variation of Ca^{2+} stores occurs with variation in heart rate. During inactivity, Ca^{2+} is eliminated from cardiac SR, a process that occurs without any apparent increase in resting myoplasmic $[Ca^{2+}]$ or tension development. Perhaps mediated by such events as the spontaneous "sparks" of Ca^{2+} release from the SR in the absence of depolarization, the incrementally released Ca^{2+} is gradually eliminated by the Na-Ca exchanger. With sustained (>5 minutes) rest, Ca^{2+} is eliminated from the SR so that the resulting "rested state" contraction is minuscule compared to those at normal rates. The importance of the exchanger is evidenced by the fact that if external Na^+ is reduced, a contraction after prolonged rest is not depressed but enhanced, and the SR store remains replete with Ca^{2+}. After prolonged rest, it may require 20 to 100 beats for the myocyte SR store to be replenished with Ca^{2+} and show an unchanging contraction at any given rate. As heart rate is increased, a well-described "positive frequency staircase" or increased contraction at higher heart rates results, a phenomenon demonstrated in humans. As the diastolic rest interval is decreased, there is less time for Ca^{2+} to "leak" from the SR and be removed by the Na-Ca exchanger, so a greater SR Ca^{2+} store is available for release.

While at physiologic rates the bulk (90 to 95%) of activator Ca^{2+} is derived from loaded SR stores, the small amount of Ca^{2+} entering from outside is responsible for inducing Ca^{2+} release from the SR and contributing to 5 to 10% of Ca^{2+} for myofibrillar activation. As schematized in Figure 5–7, these two sources of Ca^{2+} are apparently intermingled, and relaxation occurs as 90 to 95% of Ca^{2+} is reaccumulated in the SR, and 5 to 10% of the Ca^{2+} (equal to the amount that entered) is eliminated from the cell during rest before depolarization stimulates the next beat. At lower rates, with more time for SR loss, the contractions are smaller and the entering Ca^{2+} now represents a higher fraction (perhaps 10 to 20%) of activator Ca^{2+}. There is evidence that a very small fraction of time (50 to 200 msec) may be required to transfer Ca^{2+} from the LSR to the JSR, so that at very high heart rates with short diastolic intervals, not all of the SR Ca^{2+} pool is at a release site. When a premature beat occurs, the contraction may be reduced because Ca^{2+} is not yet in a releasable JSR location. However, during the subsequent pause there is time for accumulation in the JSR release site of an enhanced Ca^{2+} including that from the extra beat, then there is a marked potentiation of the next beat (postextrasystolic potentiation).[133] With very high heart rates, the continued Ca^{2+} entry of each AP with reduced time between contractions for Ca^{2+} elimination can result in SR Ca^{2+} overload.

Other Effects on Ca^{2+} Stores. In rat heart, contractions after rest are sustained or increased in amplitude. Rat heart has a higher intracellular Na^+, so that the smaller Na^+ gradient produces less Na-Ca exchange-mediated Ca^{2+} elimination during rest. As a result, the rat cardiac SR pool stays filled with behavior similar to that seen with low extracellular Na^+ in other species. In frog heart, there is no SR pool and contraction depends on Ca^{2+} entry. Fetal and neonatal mammalian myocardium is similar to frog heart in having a far less developed SR structure and function, so that immature myocardium relies far more on extracellular Ca^{2+} entry, by both the Ca channel and Na-Ca exchanger, for contraction.[134] With changes in temperature, a variety of Ca^{2+}-related processes are altered, with a decrease in Ca-ATPase activity (seen as a decreased rate of relaxation) as well as a decrease in entering Ca^{2+}. The net effect is an increase in contractile strength, with a decreased dependence on SR Ca^{2+}.[135]

Myocardial Energy Substrates

The energy supply of the heart is derived primarily from lactate and fatty acids delivered by the coronary blood. Free or nonesterified fatty acids (palmitic and oleic acids) are the preferred fuel and account for 90% of myocardial oxygen consumption.[136] Myocardial uptake of fatty acids is almost linear, with the plasma concentration above the threshold of 345 μM.[137] Fatty acid uptake by the heart from either fatty acid–albumin complexes or lipoprotein triglyceride occurs by either passive diffusion or carrier-mediated transport. During fasting, free fatty acids are always used as fuel. Except for the formation of structural lipids, the heart has a limited ability to synthesize fatty acids from acetylcoenzyme A (AcCoA). The oxidation of fatty acids and ketone bodies inhibits uptake of glucose, pyruvate oxidation, and glycolysis while facilitating glycogen synthesis.[137] Fuel selection by the heart probably depends upon regulatory enzymes controlled by factors other than substrate availability and product removal. Myocardial lactate utilization is regulated by the arterial lactate concentrations and pyruvate oxidation in the Krebs tricarboxylic acid cycle. Glucose, pyruvate, acetate, and triglycerides can also be used by the heart as energy sources. As long as the entry of AcCoA into the Krebs cycle is uninhibited, the heart uses all pyruvate supplied. Glucose utilization by the myocardium depends upon the arterial glucose and insulin concentration, with some use typically occurring postprandially. Glucose use by the myocardium as the primary energy source occurs with insulin secretion and increased blood glucose, and with β-adrenergic stimulation, which can increase intracellular ATP.[138] During severe hypoxia, glucose is the only substrate used by the heart that anaerobically produces ATP by glycolysis,[137] a process which produces excess protons and may contribute to faster acidification of the cell.

Extrinsic Modulation of Cardiac Conduction and Contractility

Cardiac conduction and contraction are modulated by neurotransmitters and other agonists, which act through a variety of receptors, which in turn activate a somewhat smaller number of cell signaling pathways. While the β-adrenergic receptors (β-AR) have served as the model of cardiac signal transmission via G proteins, it is now clear that an array of metabolites, peptides, and lipid-derived compounds activate a variety of other signaling cascades involving protein kinase C and nitric oxide activation of cycle guanosine monophosphate (cGMP) synthesis. Many of these cascades interact within the cardiovascular system, frequently to variable degrees depending upon the type of tissue (atrium vs. ventricle, larger vs. smaller blood vessel) and species. The primary processes and pathways modulating cardiac function are listed in Table 5–4.

Receptor-Mediated Effects

The vast majority of receptors in the heart and peripheral cardiovascular system that modulate their function belong to a family of membrane proteins whose actions are mediated by activation of the guanine nucleotide-binding proteins, or G proteins. These molecules act as highly specialized intracellular messengers, which after activation by specific receptors, activate (or inhibit) a variety of cell effector pathways such as ion channels or second-messenger–generating enzymes.[139–141] The G protein–linked receptors are distinctive in having seven-transmembrane α-helical segments, which create a central cleft (not a channel) on the extracellular surface. When ligands (norepinephrine, histamine, etc.) bind in the cleft of these receptors, a conformational change occurs on the intracellular surface of the receptor that promotes dissociation of the heterotrimeric G protein complex. Guanosine diphosphate (GDP) and the tightly coupled βγ-subunit dissociate away from the α-subunit, which is then free to bind guanosine triphosphate (GTP). The GTP-bound α-subunit forms an activating complex which then regulates the membrane effector systems,[142] at least until the GTP is hydrolyzed. The βγ-subunit also appears to play a critical signaling role, since once it is released, it is available for direct interaction with membrane constituents such as ion channels or other modulatory subunits, until it is rebound by the GDP-bound α-subunit.[143,144]

cAMP-DEPENDENT PROTEIN KINASE–MEDIATED EFFECTS

The most widely studied G protein signal pathway, which is highly relevant to the cardiovascular system, is

TABLE 5–4
Major Modulators of Conduction and Contractility

Ligand	Membrane Receptor	Pathway	Cellular Effect	Action
Glucagon Histamine Epinephrine Norepinephrine Isoproterenol Dopamine	Glucagon H_1-Histamine β_1-Adrenergic β_2-Adrenergic	G_s protein → ↑ adenylyl cyclase→ ↑ cyclic AMP ↑ PKA activity →→	↑ I_{Ca} ↓ troponin C Ca^{2+} affinity ↓ phospholamban inhibition of SR Ca^{2+}-ATPase ?↑ Ca^{2+} release channel ↑ delayed I_K and I_{to} ↑ chloride conductance	↑ Ca^{2+} entry Faster relaxation ↑ Ca^{2+} cycling through the SR Shorter AP duration
Norepinephrine Epinephrine Angiotensin II Endothelin Bradykinin	 α_1-Adrenergic Angiotensin II Endothelin BK	G_q protein → ↑ phospholipase C activity→↑IP_3 & ↑diacyclglycerol→ ↑ PKC activity →	↑ K_{ATP} channel activity ??↑ Ca^{2+} release ↑ Na-H exchange → Alkalization of myoplasm	 Shorter AP duration ↑ myofilament Ca^{2+} sensitivity
Adenosine, ?ATP Acetylcholine	 A_1-Purinergic m_2-Muscarinic	G_i protein → ↓ adenylyl cyclase→ ↓ cAMP production, ?↑PLC→→ ↑ PKC	↑ $K_{ACh,Ado}$ channel activity ↑ K_{ATP} channel activity Effects opposite to those seen with adenylyl cyclase activation	Shorter AP duration Shorter AP duration
Nitric oxide (from the endothelium or the mycocyte itself)	→ (none) →	↑ "soluble" guanylyl cyclase activity → ↑ cGMP → ↑ PKG activity & PDE activation (?inhibition) → ↓ cAMP	Certain effects opposite to those seen with ↑ cAMP, as well as activation of Na-K-Cl ion exchange	
Natriuretic peptides	Receptor/guanylyl cyclase "particulate"	↑ cGMP → (see above)		

PDE, phosphodiesterase; PKA, cAMP-activated protein kinase; PKC, protein kinase C; PKG, cGMP-activated protein kinase.

the regulation of adenylyl cyclase (AC), which produces the second-messenger cAMP. By binding to their specific receptors, catecholamines (via the β_1- and β_2-AR), histamine (via H_2 receptor), and glucagon mediate their primary actions by activating G_s, the stimulatory G protein, which activates AC, increases intracellular [cAMP], and ultimately increases contractility and heart rate. The variety of effects on both ionic currents and Ca^{2+} regulation is extensive, as indicated in Figure 5–9.

Ca^{2+} Cycling. The cAMP-dependent protein kinase (PKA) phosphorylates various cellular proteins and enzymes that produce the positive and negative inotropic effects. Phosphorylation of the L-type Ca channel alters its gating behavior, changing its behavior to a new "mode" in which the open intervals are more sustained, so that a greater number of Ca^{2+} ions may enter the cell.[47] Because of the increase in intracellular Ca^{2+}, which can contribute to Ca^{2+}-mediated inactivation of the channel, the net effect is a marked increase in the peak current and total Ca^{2+} influx. Since entry of Ca^{2+} is not the primary regulator of activation, phosphorylation of SR proteins is also critical. Following phosphorylation, phospholamban no longer provides a brake on the SR Ca pump so that Ca^{2+} can be accumulated at a far greater rate.[145] The combination of increased Ca^{2+} entry and SR accumulation means a far greater amount of cycled Ca^{2+} with each beat. This effect may be even further increased by effects on the cardiac CaRC, whose function is enhanced by PKA phosphorylation.[146] Although the greater amount of entering Ca^{2+} results in greater SR loading, over a sustained period the greater Ca^{2+} influx must be balanced by greater Ca^{2+} efflux. The greater efflux is mediated via the Na-Ca exchanger, which obligates greater Na^+ entry. This demand is matched by phosphorylation and increased activity of the Na^+,K^+-ATPase, which provides for increased Na^+ elimination required. In Purkinje fibers, β-AR activation causes Na-K pump activation, which results in a pertussis toxin–sensitive hyperpolarization.[147]

Troponin. Phosphorylation of TnI decreases the affinity of TnC for Ca^{2+},[148] an effect that would decrease actin-myosin interaction and contractility unless Ca^{2+} had been increased. However, the decreased Ca^{2+} affinity of TnC is more than offset by actions of PKA to markedly enhance the depolarization-induced increase in myoplasmic Ca^{2+}—consequently, contractility is greatly enhanced. In addition to these actions, β-AR activation independently increases the rate of myosin cross-bridge turnover, which increases tension development.[149] The decreased Ca^{2+} affinity causes Ca^{2+} to be bound for a

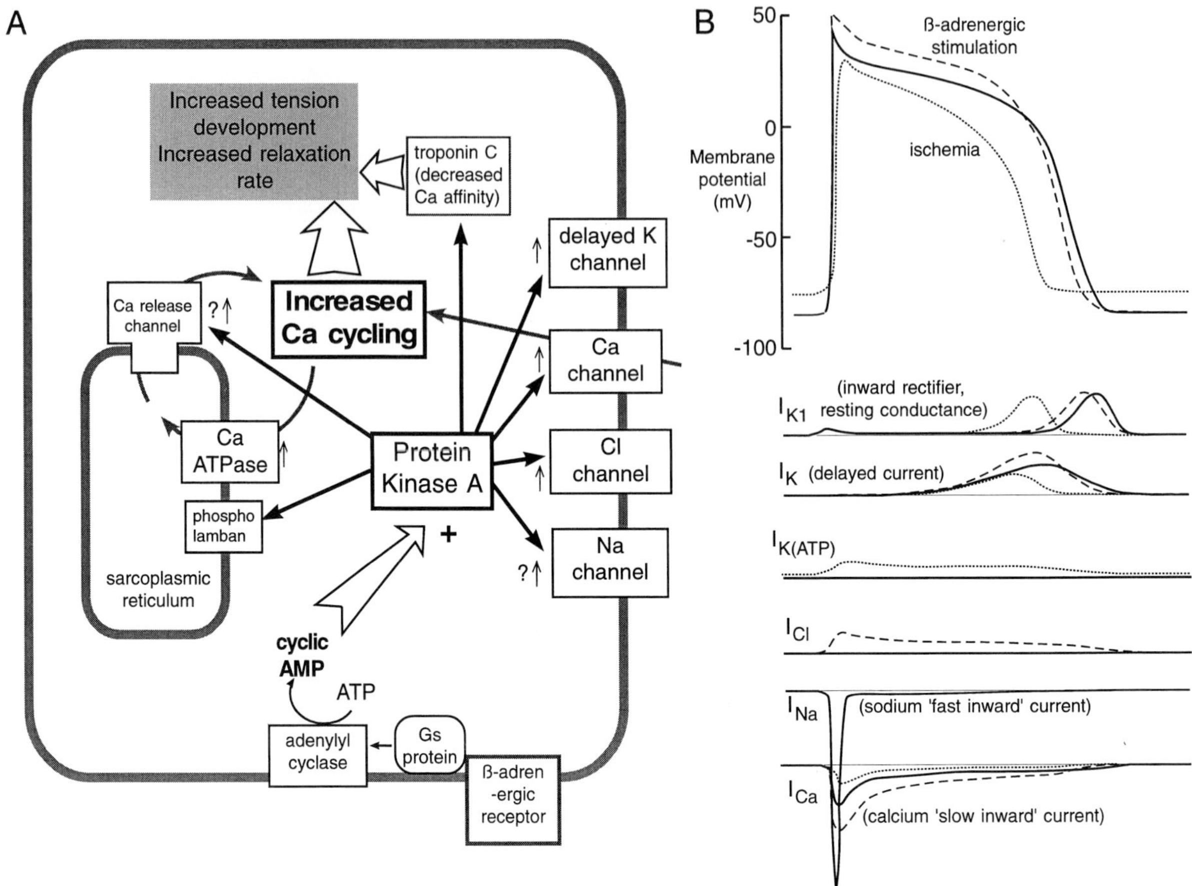

FIGURE **5–9.** Effects of adrenergic stimulation in the heart. *A*, Cellular actions of sympathetic stimulation on electrophysiologic mechanisms. Most sympathetic effects result from β-adrenergically stimulated protein phosphorylation by activation of protein kinase A activity (via increased cAMP production). The phosphorylation of multiple ion channels results in increased ion fluxes, as well as increased Ca^{2+} cycling within the cell. A direct G-protein effect activating L-type calcium channels has been described,[166,167,557] although its physiologic relevance is debated.[168,558] The decreased Ca^{2+} affinity of troponin C results in faster relaxation, but total tension development is increased because of the marked increased Ca^{2+} cycling. *B*, The effects of β-adrenergic activation of ion channels upon the cardiac action potential (AP) configuration. The increased I_{Ca} leads to a higher plateau. The activation of chloride current (I_{Cl}) and enhancement of delayed rectifier currents result in a more abbreviated plateau, while I_{Cl} may contribute to a modest depolarization (not shown). The inward rectifier appears to be little affected by adrenergic stimulation; possible enhancement of I_{Na} is not shown. With ischemia, the $I_{K(ATP)}$ activation leads to an abbreviation of the AP, while loss of K^+ from the cell will lead to increased $[K^+]_o$ and partial depolarization.

shorter time, permitting relaxation to occur more quickly. Within the context of a higher heart rate, decreased duration of contraction is critical to permit an adequate diastolic period for coronary flow and ventricular filling.

Other Ion Channels. In addition to enhancing Ca^{2+} entry and cycling, other ion channels appear to be activated by PKA. In pacemaking tissue, initial I_f is enhanced, increasing the rate of diastolic depolarization, and leading to the increased heart rate typical of β-adrenergic activation. The enhanced $I_{Ca,L}$ results in a larger and faster phase zero of the nodal APs, which will result in faster conduction of the action potential through the nodal tissue. The delayed K^+ current[150] as well as the transient outward current (I_{to})[151] are both enhanced by phosphorylation, which will serve to abbreviate the AP, an important electrophysiologic effect that ensures that the contractile state is not prolonged. In addition, a Cl^- conductance is also activated for which E_{Cl} is about −40 mV (see Table 5–1). This current will also have a repolarizing action on the plateau, but a depolarizing effect during diastole that may contribute to automaticity. In spite of the increased inward Ca^{2+} and Na^+, the repolarizing currents predominate, decreasing AP duration.

The β-AR in the myocardium are both the $β_1$-AR and $β_2$-AR subtypes. The effects noted above apply to the actions of $β_1$-AR stimulation, but not to $β_2$-AR. $β_2$-ARs appear to be present in both pacemaker tissues and myocytes, and are activated by isoproterenol and specific agonists such as zinterol,[152] but not by norepinephrine. $β_2$-AR activation does not appear to decrease myofibril Ca^{2+} sensitivity or markedly increase SR Ca^{2+}. It does enhance I_{Ca}, but the effect is distinct from that of $β_1$-AR stimulation.[152] $β_2$-AR activation is not as arrhythmogenic as $β_1$-AR stimulation, nor does it shorten the contraction.

These differential actions may depend upon different pools of AC or compartmentalized cAMP, and may have potentially important therapeutic implications.

Inhibition of Adenylyl Cyclase. The AC-inhibitory G protein G_i is activated in myocardial tissue by acetylcholine (ACh; M_2 muscarinic receptors[153]) or adenosine (A_1-adenosine receptors[154]). Such G_i activation can inhibit AC and thereby reverse the effect of β-AR stimulation, so that cAMP levels and the physiologic functions return toward nonstimulated levels.[155] In human myocardium, adenosine appears to be more efficiently coupled than ACh in this inhibitory regulatory pathway.[155] The inhibitory actions appear to be mediated in part by release of βγ subunits from $G\alpha_i$, which then bind $G\alpha_s$, resulting in the loss AC activation.[144] Within cardiac tissue, this action is most obvious in the pacemaker tissues. These tissues appear to possess a very high resting adenylyl cyclase activity resulting in a high activity of I_f and $I_{Ca,L}$, even in the absence of β-AR stimulation. Consequently, muscarinic and A_1 purinergic stimulation by adenosine will depress I_f and $I_{Ca,L}$,[156,157] slowing the diastolic depolarization and AP conduction velocity. While the isoproterenol enhancement of I_{Ca} in ventricular myocytes can be reversed by adenosine,[158] in the absence of β-adrenoceptor stimulation, the effect of adenosine on ACh or I_{Ca} and AP shortening is modest.[158,159] During aging, the β-adrenergic responsiveness declines with evidence of decreased cAMP production and decreased phosphorylation of the various proteins involved,[160] an effect that may be mediated in part by enhanced adenosine in the aged heart.[161] However, additional processes such as activation of cGMP-dependent protein kinase also appear to contribute, since decreases in contractile function can be observed in the absence of changes in [cAMP].[162]

cAMP Regulation by Phosphodiesterase. PKA activity is controlled by regulation of cAMP production and also its hydrolysis by phosphodiesterases (PDEs). The PDEs, which hydrolyze cAMP and cGMP, represent a broad class of enzymes, the activities of which are regulated by various second messengers, including cAMP and cGMP themselves.[163] Inhibition of cAMP hydrolysis by various PDE inhibitors will increase cAMP, with its consequent increase in contractile function. While the methylxanthines (e.g., caffeine, theophylline) enhance sympathetic tone by relatively nonspecific PDE inhibition, the dipyridines (e.g., amrinone, milrinone) appear to act in part by specifically inhibiting type 3 PDE, a major form present in cardiac tissue that is inhibited by cGMP. In the presence of prior cGMP inhibition of PDE3, the stimulatory actions of milrinone on Ca^{2+} current are not observed,[164] and likewise milrinone can prevent the stimulatory actions of cGMP.[165] In contrast, type 2 PDE is activated by cGMP, so that increased cGMP will result in hydrolysis of cAMP and decreased PKA-mediated effects. With high concentrations of cGMP, PDE2 activation can result, decreasing cAMP and its stimulation. Since the dipyridines increase cAMP and stimulate mammalian myocardium under most settings, the net effect of increases in cGMP on the PDEs must not be a major inhibition of PDE activity or these drugs would have minimal effect.

DIRECT ION CHANNEL EFFECTS

As well as affecting ion channels via PKA, the G proteins themselves may directly influence ion channel function.[166] G_s activation appears to directly increase Ca channel currents[167]; however, the importance and relevance of this action to physiologic function is unclear.[168] Such direct activation by β_2-adrenoceptors might explain observed behavior that differs from that seen with β_1 activation. Likewise, stimulation of P_2-purinergic receptors appears to enhance opening of L-type channels via a pathway involving a G_s pathway exclusive of cAMP production.[169]

Control of the $K_{ACh,Ado}$ Channel. The most important of the directly modulated cardiac ion currents is that carried by K^+ through a channel that is activated by ACh and adenosine—$I_{K(ACh)}$, $I_{K(Ado)}$, or $I_{K(ACh,Ado)}$. This $K_{ACh,Ado}$ channel has an inwardly rectifying character similar to G_{K1} due to blockade by intracellular Mg^{2+}[170,171] and, according to its primary structure, appears to belong to the same K channel superfamily.[172] Ligand binding to M_2 muscarinic or A_1 adenosine receptors activates G_i. When released from the $G\alpha_i$-subunit, the βγ-subunit then opens the $K_{ACh,Ado}$ channel, which causes hyperpolarization and decreases excitability due to the increase in resting K^+ conductance. The result is a profound decrease in the rate of diastolic depolarization of pacemaker tissue and a slowing of heart rate as observed with vagal stimulation or adenosine administration. Because the direct $G_{\beta\gamma}$ coupling to the channel does not require inhibition of AC or time for hydrolysis of cAMP, $I_{K(ACh)}$ can exert its action very rapidly (≤0.2 second) to depress diastolic depolarization and slow heart rate. While $I_{K(ACh,Ado)}$ is present in human ventricular myocytes, its activation by ACh is far more modest than in the atrial myocytes and it is a modest contribution to total K^+ conductance.[173] However, its activation in ventricular myocyte via adenosine can shorten ventricular AP duration, which may in turn inhibit contractility by decreasing Ca^{2+} entry.[159]

PHOSPHOLIPASE C ACTIVATION EFFECTS

Another major G protein pathway involves the activation of the phospholipases, enzymes that metabolize phospholipid components of the cell membranes.[174,175] The primary enzymes of interest in myocardium are phospholipase C (PLC) types, which are also activated by a G protein, specifically G_q, as shown in Figure 5–9 (and possibly G_i). When activated, PLC cleaves the phosphoester linkage of diphosphoinositide to produce the phosphated sugar, inositol trisphosphate (IP_3), leaving a glycerol with two fatty acids (diacylglycerol [DAG]) in the plasmalemma. Each of these agents can act alone as a second messenger. IP_3 binds to and activates Ca^{2+} flux through a specific homotetrameric protein, similar in structure to the CaRC. Several recent investigations suggest that IP_3 promotes Ca^{2+} release from cardiac SR[176–178] and this IP_3-induced Ca^{2+} release is enhanced in hypertrophic myocardium.[179] However, the IP_3 receptor that releases Ca^{2+} has a very restricted distribution in the myocardium, being located near the intercalated disks.[180] While IP_3 has a critical role in the function of smooth muscle EC coupling (see below), its role in cardiac tissue is modest and controversial.

Protein Kinase C. The classic protein kinase C (PKC) class of enzymes are activated by the combined actions of Ca^{2+} and DAG, while a number of lipophilic tumor promoters (the phorbol esters) are widely used experimentally to activate the enzyme. In its cytoplasmic state PKC has an autoinihibitory portion that binds to and inhibits the active site. In the presence of DAG (in the membrane bilayer) and Ca^{2+}, the enzyme binds to the plasmalemma with a resulting conformational change to reveal the active site (Fig. 5–10*A*).[181] In cellular homogenates the enzyme can phosphorylate a variety of the molecules activated by PKA including phospholamban and TnC.[182] However, these proteins are not in the plasmalemma and this effect is not seen in intact heart,[183] so its relevance is unclear. However, PKC also has other important actions including activation of the Na-H antiport so that H^+ are eliminated from the cell, resulting in a more alkaline intracellular milieu.[184,185] With increased pH the myofibrils become more sensitive to Ca^{2+}; that is, at a given intracellular Ca^{2+} the myofibrils will interact more and generate greater tension (Fig. 5–10*B*). Consequently, activation of the PKC can enhance tension generation in the absence of increased Ca^{2+} release or entry.

In addition to effects on the Na-H antiport, PKC also has other important actions on ion channels. PKC activation appears to blunt the stimulation by I_{Ca} of β-AR stimulation.[186] A documented PKC action also involves

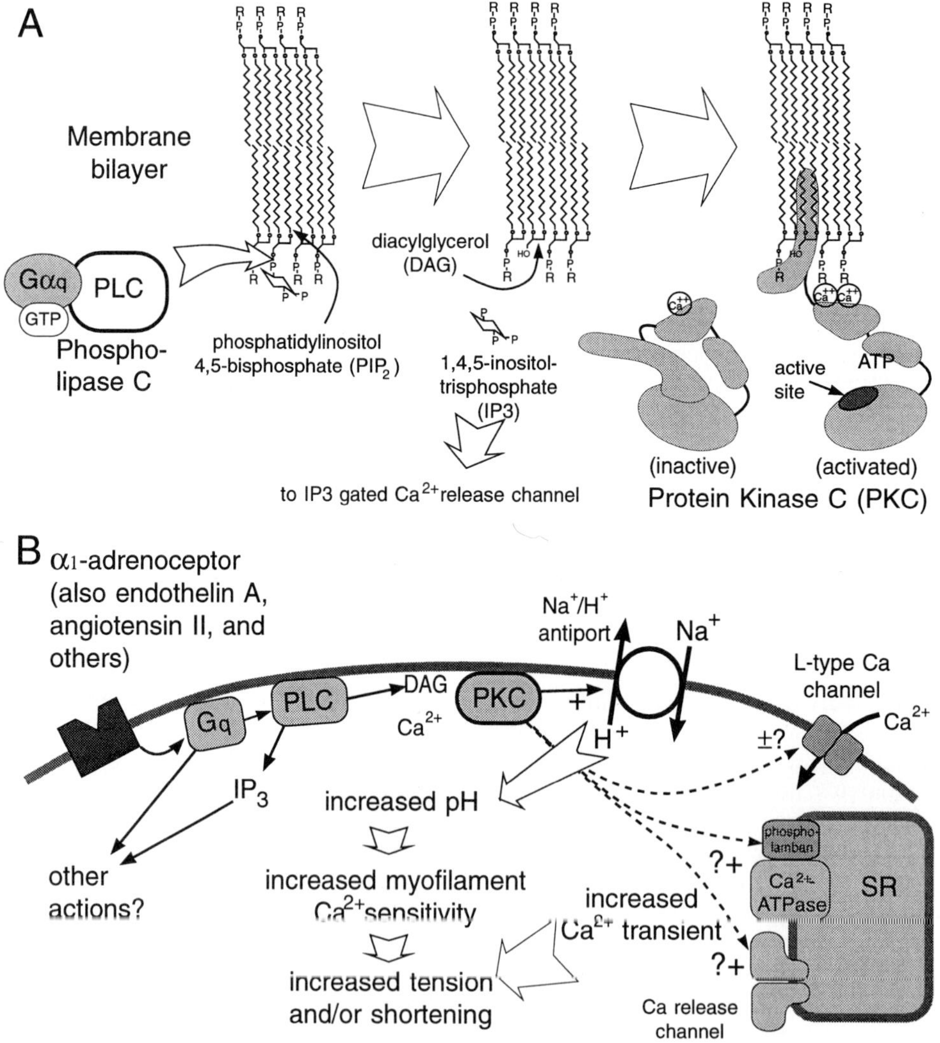

FIGURE **5–10.** Phospholipase C (PLC) and protein kinase C (PKC) cellular activation pathways. *A*, Proposed membrane molecular pathway for PLC production of diacylglycerol (DAG) and inositol 1,4,5-trisphosphate (IP_3). Activation of PKC appears to involve movement of an autoinhibitory pseudosubstrate region of the molecule to reveal the active site. This process appears to occur when there is intimate association of PKC with the membrane, as well as a requirement for Ca^{2+} (for many PKC subtypes). *B*, Proposed cardiac myocyte effects of PLC and PKC following activation by α_1-adrenoceptors (and other G_q-linked receptors).

delayed K current enhancement,[187,188] which mediates the decrease in the AP duration observed with α_1-adrenoceptor stimulation in some settings.[189] PKC has also been demonstrated to decrease L-type Ca channel currents in some systems, although its contribution remains to be defined.[190]

The inwardly rectifying K_{ATP} channel also appears to be under the regulation of PKC. Following phosphorylation by PKC, the channel shows less inhibition at higher ATP concentrations.[191] As a consequence, the channel is more likely to be activated by small changes in cellular energy supply, resulting in various energy-conserving cellular behaviors (see below). This PKC-mediated effect appears to be activated by adenosine,[192,193] as well as other receptors such as α_1-adrenoceptor, muscarinic,[194] endothelin, and bradykinin, which also activate PKC. Activation of these pathways is able to decrease infarction size with subsequent ischemic insults and to duplicate many of the protective effects of ischemic preconditioning.[195,196]

α_1-Adrenergic Effects. The importance of the PKC-mediated actions are exemplified in activation of the α_1-adrenergic receptor (α_1-AR), mediating the action of phenylephrine as well as norepinephrine. Following a transient decrease in cell shortening, contractility increased, an effect correlated with the increase in intracellular pH. The effect on both contractility and pH could be prevented by blockade of the Na^+-H^+ antiport.[185] The α_1-AR enhanced contractions do not show enhanced relaxation and shorter duration as seen with β_1-AR stimulation, and tension may in fact be prolonged.[197] It is believed that the enhanced Na^+-H^+ antiport causes protons to be eliminated from the cell, increasing intracellular pH from approximately 7.1 to 7.3. The increased Ca^{2+} affinity of TnC then results in increased tension and slower relaxation. The myocardial inotropic effect of an α_1-agonist alone may be surprising; however, the effect of the increased vascular resistance may mask this inotropic action. Nevertheless, such positive α_1-AR inotropic effects have been documented in human volunteers.[198,199] An additional effect of α_1-adrenoceptor activation includes ANP secretion by the atrium.[200]

Distinct from the action of the pure β-AR agonist isoproterenol, which shortens the duration of contractions, are the typical effects of combined β-AR and α_1-AR activation seen with epinephrine, dopamine, and norepinephrine, the major natural sympathetic agonist of the heart. The marked decrease in myofibril Ca^{2+} sensitivity seen with pure β_1-AR stimulation is far less with the mixed β-AR and α_1-AR effects, and the duration of contractions shows little reduction.[197]

Other Cellular Pathways Modulating Myocyte Function

CALMODULIN AND Ca^{2+}-DEPENDENT PHOSPHORYLATION

In addition to phosphorylation by PKA and PKC, channel and enzyme regulation can also be mediated by a multifunction calmodulin (CaM) -dependent kinase (CaM kinase II), which is activated when Ca^{2+} combines with CaM to form an activating complex. Control of the various Ca^{2+} controlling systems by this enzyme remains to be fully elucidated; however, it may explain a variety of processes. Increases in stimulation rate or extracellular Ca^{2+} (and hence peak and mean $[Ca^{2+}]_i$) appear to increase Ca^{2+} uptake and enhance Ca^{2+}-ATPase and the CaRC.[201] Such effects might well be regulated by such an enzyme that can respond to the intracellular Ca^{2+} load. Although its physiologic significance remains to be delineated, the cardiac CaRC has a site for phosphorylation not present in the skeletal muscle CaRC which, when phosphorylated by CaM kinase II, activates the channel.[202]

NITRIC OXIDE AND cGMP

While the free radical nitric oxide (NO) produced by the oxidation of arginine has received considerable attention for its role in vascular regulation (see below), NO also influences cardiac performance. One source of NO that may influence the myocytes is the endocardial endothelium (EE), which lines the ventricular cavity and trabeculae.[203] Endothelial NO synthase (eNOS, NOS3) produces NO, which can diffuse to the underlying myocytes and modulate function, but changes from baseline are usually modest (10%). However, there is intrinsic eNOS activity in myocytes themselves, and the resulting NO production appears to play an important role in mediating the normal effects of vagal stimulation and muscarinic effects in the heart.[204,205] The myocardial depressant effect of NO and NO donors such as nitroprusside have been demonstrated both in isolated cells[206,207] and in humans.[208] The myocardial depressant effect of nitroprusside may be surprising; however, the improvement in cardiac output due to decreased vascular resistance probably masks its modest depressant action. The effect of NO is most prominent in depressing the positive inotropic responsiveness to β-adrenergic stimulation.[205,209] In addition, NO production with more prominent functional importance occurs following sepsis and possibly other inflammatory states in which endotoxin and/or cytokines activate production of inducible NOS (iNOS; NOS3) both in the cardiac microvascular endothelium[210,211] and in myocytes themselves.[211–213] NO production by iNOS may more markedly alter contractile function in these settings.[210,212,213]

The effects of NO and the antiadrenergic action of muscarinic stimulation appear to be primarily mediated by activation of guanylyl cyclase activity and increased cGMP. Increased activity of cGMP-activated PDE2 results in increased hydrolysis of cAMP. Muscarinic inhibition of β-adrenergic stimulation in AV sinoatrial node appears to be mediated by such activation of PDE2 and increased cAMP degradation.[214] A second pathway involves the cGMP-activated protein kinases (PKG), which have important regulatory roles in cellular functions. The cellular signaling systems mediated by PKGs remain to be fully elucidated, but NO activation of guanylyl cyclase resulting in PKG activation appears, for example, to decrease Ca^{2+} currents in myocytes.[215,216] While many of these effects are probably mediated by activation of guanylyl cyclase, production of NO may be sufficient so that its free radical activity may play a role by itself. For example, NO and nitrosothiols appear to directly modulate activity of the L-type Ca channel in ventricular myocytes.[217]

In addition to NO-activated guanylyl cyclases ("soluble fraction"), cGMP synthesis is also mediated by the natriuretic peptide receptors,[218] transmembrane proteins whose extracellular domain binds the peptide, with an inner domain possessing guanylyl cyclase activity ("particulate fraction"). Whether the localization of cGMP synthesis by the soluble or membrane-bound guanylyl cyclases may influence its consequent actions remains to be clearly defined.

Autonomic Innervation of the Heart

While a variety of transmitters and hormones can modulate cardiac behavior by the pathways described above, the effects of norepinephrine (NE) secreted by the sympathetic nerve endings and ACh secreted by the vagal nerve endings are those that are typically predominant.

SYMPATHETIC AND PARASYMPATHETIC INNERVATION

Sympathetic nerves in the heart arise from these neurons in the middle cervical and stellate (thoracocervical) ganglia and travel to the heart via three major sympathetic cardiopulmonary nerves: stellate cardiopulmonary nerve; dorsal cardiopulmonary nerves (three on the left side); and the right dorsal lateral and dorsal medial cardiopulmonary nerves.[219] The right dorsal medial and dorsal lateral cardiac nerves frequently unite to form one large nerve that follows the course of the left main coronary artery. It further separates into branches along the anterior descending and circumflex coronary arteries. No sympathetic cardiac nerves arise from the superior cervical ganglia or the thoracic sympathetic trunks inferior to the stellate ganglia.[219] The sympathetic nerves in the heart do not typically contact specific postsynaptic areas in the myocardium, but rather the axons have thickened regions or varicosities along their course[220] which contain the NE as well as a variety of other transmitters (ATP, neuropeptide Y [NPY]) that modulate transmitter release.

These fibers enter the thorax as branches from the recurrent laryngeal nerve and thoracic vagus, located between the aortic arch and the tracheal bifurcation. The dorsal and ventral cardiopulmonary plexuses receive both parasympathetic and sympathetic branches. Three large cardiac nerves, the right and left coronary and the left lateral cardiac nerves, emerge from the plexuses. Smaller cardiac nerves also arise from the plexuses and the thoracic vagi.[219] Ganglia occur within the heart, usually close to the structures innervated by the short postganglionic neurons. Postganglionic transmission occurs from stimulation of nicotinic cholinergic receptors at the postganglionic junction by ACh. Release of ACh at the neuroeffector junction activates muscarinic M_2 receptors in the heart, particularly at the SA and AV nodes, and also on sympathetic nerve endings. After release, ACh is hydrolyzed by acetylcholinesterase, which exists in high concentration in the AV and SA nodes.[221]

SYMPATHETIC-PARASYMPATHETIC INTERACTION

The behavior of the sympathetic and parasympathetic effects cannot be simply considered as being counterbalancing forces on myocardial conduction and contraction that are centrally integrated. Both their anatomic proximity in the cardiac plexi and their physiologic and pharmacologic behavior indicate that the parasympathetic and sympathetic nerves continuously modulate each other. While ACh appears to have modest effects on the myocardium, its modulation of the outflow of the sympathetic nervous system may cause greater indirect effects on cardiac function. Vagal stimulation can markedly decrease the outflow of NE[222] and can override sympathetic stimulation,[223] an effect that is probably mediated by muscarinic receptors present on the sympathetic nerve varicosities. However, while the ATP and NPY released with NE from the sympathetic nerves may have modest effects on the electrophysiologic and mechanical behavior of the heart, these agents may have a more important role as feedback regulators of neurotransmitter release.[224] NPY mediates its actions via G_i protein–linked receptor, which decreases cAMP synthesis and inhibits or decreases further NE release. ATP and adenosine likewise depress NE release via A_1 (adenosine or P_1) receptors,[225] while NE can directly feed back via α_2-adrenoceptors to depress NE release. Sympathetic stimulation can also decrease vagal outflow also via the release of NPY.[224] While vagal depression of sympathetic nerves is usually dominant over sympathetic depression of vagal tone, sustained NPY release prior to vagal stimulation has a more profound vagolytic effect.[223] Epinephrine and, to a lesser extent, the NE itself may stimulate β_2-adrenoceptors, which may serve to augment sympathetic outflow.[226] Some of the possible interactions are indicated in Figure 5–11. While the mechanisms of these interactions are not completely delineated, there are clearly important implications. For example, when fentanyl administration increases vagal tone causing bradycardia (see "Medullary Control Centers," below), there will also be a component of sympathetic inhibition at the level of the myocardium. Depending upon the level of sympathetic outflow and presence or absence of β-adrenoceptor blockade, increased vagal tone may influence myocardial function by its modulation of sympathetic tone.

The regulation of heart rate by the vagal and sympathetic efferents results in continuous small variations in heart rate, which are frequently observed as the discrete alterations in the interval between QRS complexes (e.g., 840 msec, 900 msec, 890 msec, 850 msec). Vagal output to the sinus node causes the respiratory sinus arrhythmia (RSA) seen with normal breathing and occurs at rates of 0.3 to 0.4 Hz. This rhythmic outflow to the heart from the medullary nucleus ambiguous is generated by direct coupling to the respiratory center as well as by input from atrial and pulmonary stretch receptors. At the sinus node the vagally released ACh activates $I_{K(ACh)}$ via direct G protein coupling, with the result that the SA node rate

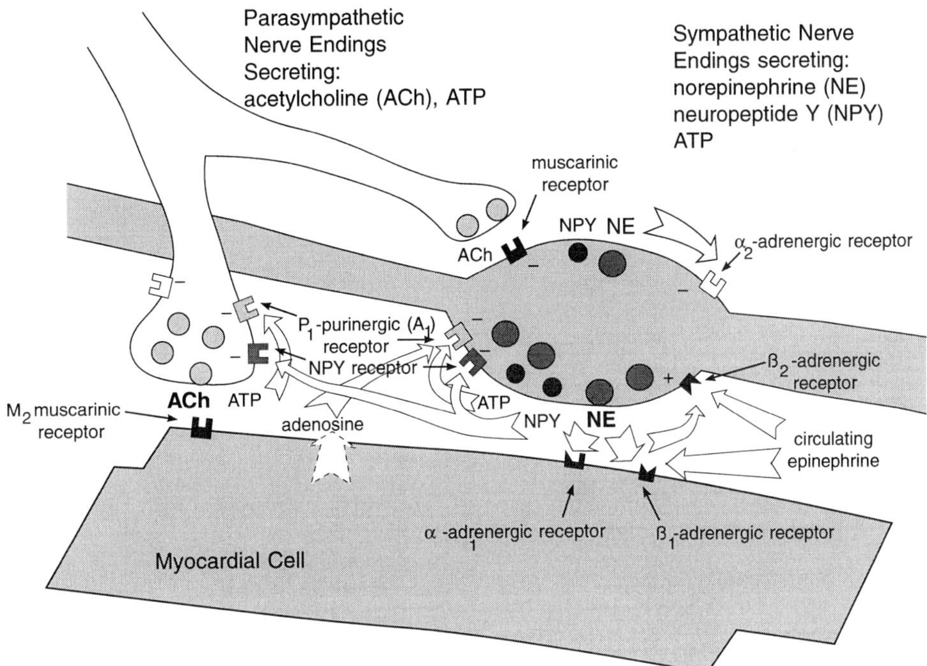

FIGURE **5–11.** Cardiac autonomic synapse. This diagram delineates the complex interaction between the parasympathetic nerve endings and the sympathetic nerve endings present in the myocardium. Acetylcholine released by the sympathetic varicosities serves to inhibit sympathetic outflow. Likewise, sympathetic stimulation with release of neuropeptide Y and ATP will then be back to inhibit the acetylcholine release by the vagal nerve endings. Stimulation of β_2-adrenergic receptors by epinephrine may also serve to enhance norepinephrine release.

can be very rapidly modulated and synchronized with breathing. In contrast, the sympathetic influence mediated by adenylyl cyclase requires a greater duration to act and accounts for variations in heart rate present at about 0.05 to 0.1 Hz (every 10 to 20 seconds). Heart rate variability (HRV) can be markedly altered in various pathologic states such as heart failure, and may serve as a predictor of cardiac sudden death following myocardial infarctions. Since anesthetics, analgesics, and hypnotics can markedly alter autonomic tone, HRV also reflects administration of such drugs.[227] There are also neurons in the SA node that secrete γ-aminobutyric acid (GABA) and thereby depress sympathetic outflow via $GABA_A$ Cl^- channel type receptors.[228] This finding suggests a potential peripheral action of benzodiazepines in modulating cardiac function.

Other Hormonal Effects

ANGIOTENSIN

The renin-angiotensin-aldosterone system plays a major role in control of blood pressure and regulation of intravascular volume. The sequential action of renin (released by the glomerular cells of the kidney) and angiotensin-converting enzyme (ACE), present on the endothelial cell membrane, on angiotensinogen produces angiotensin II (AII), which also acts via a G protein–linked receptor (AT1).[229] Binding to the AT1 receptor activates the PLC pathway outlined above for the α_1-adrenoceptor, resulting in a positive cardiac inotropic effect in which relaxation is not accelerated.[230] In the hypertrophied left ventricle of the rat, the IP_3-enhanced release of Ca^{2+}, possibly combined with any enhanced myofibrillar Ca^{2+} affinity, may contribute to impaired relaxation.[230] In addition, increased intracellular Ca^{2+} loading may occur secondary to enhanced Na channel function and Na^+ entry.[231] While these effects augment the contractile state, they may also delay relaxation and result in the impaired filling seen in pressure-overload hypertrophy. This effect may be especially prominent in the presence of concomitant myocardial ischemia.[232] Additional major actions of AII appear to involve longer term modulation, involving regulation of cardiac protein synthesis, and contributing to myocardial hypertrophy.[233] Since these actions can be inhibited by pretreatment with an ACE inhibitor, it provides an important avenue of treatment for patients with diastolic heart failure beyond the traditional use of these drugs as peripheral vasodilators.

THYROID HORMONE

Thyroid hormone has profound metabolic consequences in a variety of tissues. The primary alterations in the myocardium are usually attributed to the effects of triiodothyronine (T_3) and involve alterations in nuclear synthetic machinery. Expression of the myosin isozyme is shifted from V_3 toward the faster V_1,[234,235] while expression of SR Ca^{2+}-ATPase[235] and β-adrenergic receptors[236,237] is increased, all of which contribute to enhancing the rate of tension development, relaxation, and ATP consumption. While β-AR blockade prevents the tachycardia seen with hyperthyroid state, it does not prevent the acceleration of isovolumic relaxation, suggesting that the intracellular biochemical changes have profound importance. Nevertheless, part of the cardiac hypertrophy observed may be due in part to the generalized increase in metabolic demand and decreased peripheral vascular resistance.[238] In addition to these chronic actions, which require time for protein synthesis, T_3 has also been found to have direct actions in a variety of cellular processes that can cause a rapid increase in inotropy. T_3 has direct effects on mitochondrial respiratory rate that do not require protein synthesis[239,240] but may enhance function of adenine nucleotide translocase.[241] Mitochondria from hypothyroid rats rapidly respond to T_3 with an increase in ATP production and oxygen consumption.[240] Of relevance may also be the direct action of T_3 in increasing I_{Na},[242] since enhanced Na^+ entry would be anticipated to increase intracellular Ca^{2+} stores, by reducing its elimination by Na-Ca exchange. T_3 also directly enhances function of the sarcolemmal Ca^{2+}-ATPase,[243] an effect that might enhance relaxation. These direct effects may be clinically relevant, since cardiopulmonary bypass (CPB) causes a significant and sustained decline in T_3.[244] However, while post-CPB myocardial dysfunction can be rapidly relieved by T_3 administration in certain settings,[245] its clinical utility remains to be confirmed.[238,246]

ATRIAL NATRIURETIC PEPTIDES

Unlike the previously noted G protein–linked receptors, the atrial natriuretic peptides (ANPs) mediate their actions via a distinct class of receptors that possess guanylyl cyclase activity.[218] Binding of an ANP in the extracellular site stimulates production of cGMP from GTP by the intracellular domain. The actions of cGMP in cardiac tissue remain to be fully elucidated, although Na-Ca exchange has been demonstrated in vascular smooth muscle activation,[247] an effect expected to decrease Ca^{2+} stores and contractility. Cyclic GTP possibly activates a phosphodiesterase that degrades cAMP and curtails the stimulatory actions of PKA in the myocyte.[248] In addition, the ANPs and cGMP regulate the activation of the $Na^+/K^+/2Cl^-$ cotransporter. Increased activity of this membrane protein would be expected to decrease cell volume and reduce $[Na^+]_i$, effects that would be expected to mildly decrease contractility.[249] A cGMP downregulation of I_{Ca} has also been described that may also contribute to decreased contractility.

Endocardial Endothelium

In addition to their prominent role in modulating vascular tone (see below), endothelial cells also line the chambers of the heart, lying directly on the basal membrane and connective tissue that surrounds the endocardial myocytes. Although not as dramatic as the vascular endothelial actions on smooth muscle, this EE does modulate myocardial function.[203] Both a negative inotropic effect (myocardial relaxant factor [MRF]) as well as a stimulatory contractile effect (myocardial contractile factor, [MCF], also termed endocardin) are demonstrable. When EE is removed there is a modest decrease in contractility,[250,203] which may reflect the removal of a tonic release of low concentrations of NO that in turn activate guanylyl cyclase to produce cGMP at low levels, inhibiting PDE3. Stimulation of EE to produce more NO may result in modest depression by activation of PDE2, representing the MRF; however, release of prostacyclin may also contribute.[203] The MCF derived from EE is likely to be an endothelin, a stimulatory vasoconstricting peptide secreted by the endothelium that has been shown to have positive inotropic effects on ventricular myocytes.[251] As with α_1-agonists, endothelin receptors appear to activate the G_q-PLC-PKC cascade resulting in intracellular alkalization,[251] resulting in increased myofilament Ca^{2+} sensitivity[252] that is sufficient to reverse the effects of an imposed acidosis.[253] The full physiologic role of the EE remains to be fully realized.

Effects of Ischemia and Hypoxia

With the loss of delivery of oxygen and/or nutrients to the myocardial cells, ATP stores are rapidly depleted, and a specific sequence of mechanical and electrophysiologic events occurs.[254–257] Within 10 minutes of onset, the tension development is reduced by greater than 60% with an accompanying rise in resting tension (ischemic contracture) as $[Ca^{2+}]_i$ rises.[254] The contracture is reduced but not eliminated by rest or reduced temperature during the hypoxia.[256] In this setting, peak tension and the rate of relaxation is slowed due to impaired SR Ca^{2+} reuptake.[259] In isolated cells, hypoxia is associated with a rise of $[Ca^{2+}]_i$ to approximately 200 M and recovery with reoxygenation, while cells that do not recover show a much greater increase to approximately 400 M, in both the cytosol and mitochondria.[260] The SR appears to play an important role in postanoxic Ca^{2+} regulation upon reoxgenation.[260,261] However, global ischemia is associated with depressed SR function that persists following reoxygenation,[262,263] which may be secondary to Ca^{2+}-ATPase dysfunction[263] as well as inappropriate opening of the SR Ca release channel in certain cases.[262] Decreased Ca^{2+} responsiveness of the myofibrils also contributes to the decreased contractility (Fig. 5–12).[264]

Simultaneous with deterioration of mechanical function, the AP duration is markedly reduced and the cell typically depolarizes by 10 to 20 mV,[254,257] an effect associated with a decreased rate of depolarization, an increase in the resting conductance, and a decreased slow inward current.[265] The increase in conductance is due to the activation of a specific K channel that is inactivated by ATP, the K_{ATP} channel,[266] and blocked by lower (<1 μM) sulfonylurea drugs such as glibenclamide (glyburide).[267,268] This K_{ATP} channel appears structurally related to the inward rectifier (G_{K1}) with each subunit having only two transmembrane segments.[269] The K_{ATP} channel also inwardly rectifies due to Mg^{2+} blockade, albeit to a lesser extent than the G_{K1}.[270,49] When ATP is depleted with ongoing ischemia/hypoxia, then the channel becomes active, resulting in increased K^+ conductance, with less depolarization and decreased AP duration (see Fig. 5–8), an effect that appears to be more prominent in epicardial cells.[271] This K_{ATP} channel activation accounts for the ST-segment elevation seen during myocardial ischemia,[272] and the increased K^+ efflux and extracellular accumulation seen during hypoxia or ischemia.[273] When the K_{ATP} channel openers (KCOs) such as aprikalim[274] or pinacidil[257] are used prior to an ischemic insult, the postischemic mechanical dysfunction is reduced. This effect may be mediated in part via coronary vessel effects, but the decreased AP duration due to $I_{K(ATP)}$ combined with the intracellular acidosis[275] will decrease the duration and intensity of I_{Ca}, decreasing the rate of Ca^{2+} entry and overload. Glibenclamide attenuates the decrease in AP duration observed during ischemia and reverses the protection afforded by the KCOs. In addition, sustained (1 hour) ischemia is associated with a decrease in G_s protein and its activation of adenylyl cyclase by β-adrenergic receptors, an effect that will also decrease the response to β-AR stimulation.[276] During reperfusion, the affinity of β-adrenoceptors shows a compensatory increase in the previously ischemic region.[277]

A by-product of ischemia is the ultimate breakdown of ATP to adenosine, which has a critical regulatory role not only in coronary flow, but also on myocyte function. Activation of A_1 receptors by adenosine enhances activation of $I_{K(Ado)}$ channels, which will also abbreviate the AP. Furthermore, the K_{ATP} channel is also modulated by $G\alpha_i$, and its activation by ATP deficiency appears to be enhanced by the presence of A_1 activation,[278] so that it is activated in the presence of higher ATP concentrations.[193] While the decreased AP duration may be beneficial in decreasing metabolic demand and Ca^{2+} overload, the greater dispersion of AP duration has a potential proarrhythmic effect.[279] In addition, adenosine will have dramatic effects on the pacemaker rate via activation of $I_{K(Ado)}$ channels, which will hyperpolarize nodal tissue and depress diastolic depolarization.

During hypoxia with maintained perfusion, there is a parallel decrease in the Ca^{2+} transient and force development. In contrast, ischemia reveals apparently distinct pathophysiologic changes.[258] With complete ischemia, there is no decrement in Ca^{2+} transients, at least initially, although the basal (diastolic) $[Ca^{2+}]_i$ rises as does resting tension. As ATP stores are depleted, inorganic phosphate (P_i) rises. The increased P_i and the decreased acidosis that accompanies ischemia causes mechanical dysfunction by decreasing myofilament responsiveness to Ca^{2+}.[264,280–282] Although decreased Ca^{2+} entry may occur secondary to acidosis,[275] there is not a morbid effect immediately evident on the Ca^{2+} transient. During ischemia and the resulting acidosis, the increased intracellular H^+ is removed from the cell by the Na^+-H^+ antiport, increasing Na^+ entry and raising $[Na^+]_i$.[283,284] The native Na^+ overload and decreased Na^+ gradient will then result in less Ca^{2+} elimination and worsening Ca^{2+} overload upon reperfusion, ultimately increasing cellular dysfunction and/or death.[283,285,286] Interventions that decrease Na^+ overload prove to protect the myocyte. While there does not appear to be an increased I_{Na} with ischemia,[287] reduction of Na^+ entry by certain Na channel blockers can improve myocardial recovery[288] and prevent ventricular fibrillation.[284] A major means of protecting the cell is by blockade of the Na^+-H^+ antiport.[289,290] When ischemic damage is simulated by application of lysophosphatidylcholine to myocardium, antiport inhibitors prevent biochemical and ultrastructural changes.[291] Multiple studies document the ability of antiport blockade to prevent Na^+ and Ca^{2+} accumulation,[292,293] preserve cellular function, reduce ischemic damage,[286,293,294] and reduce reperfusion arrhythmias,[286] in spite of the fact that it causes worsening of acidosis. Previously, similar beneficial effects of acid reperfusion had been demonstrated,[295,296] presumably due to a decrease in Na^+ overload because of a decreased intra-, extracellular H^+ gradient. In contrast, interventions such as α_1-adrenergic stimulation, which increase Na^+-H^+ antiport activity, have been found to worsen reperfusion arrhythmias.[297]

Application of extracellular acidosis in the absence of ischemia or hypoxia appears relatively benign. While there is clearly a myocardial depressant effect associated with decreased I_{Ca}, it is relatively modest above pH 7.1,[280] and the intracellular acidification that results from an elevation of carbon dioxide (CO_2) shows partial recovery mediated by the Na-H^+ antiport.[298] While a decrease in myocardial sensitivity to catecholamine stimulation is frequently suggested, the magnitude of this effect above 7.0 is poorly described. In isolated tissue at pH 6.8, there is a decrease in catecholamine sensitivity; however, the maximal increase in contractility is not depressed.[299] The presence of added buffering capacity of blood does appear to ameliorate the internal acidification and delay ischemic contractures.[300]

While metabolic acidosis (pH = 6.8) and hyperkalemia (8 mM K^+) have modest and opposite effects on conduction in Purkinje fibers (PF) and ventricular muscle (VM), these changes markedly delay conduction at the junction between the PF and VM. While such PF → VM conduction was unaltered by hypoxia alone, hypoxia enhances the actions of either acidosis or increased $[K^+]_o$.[301] This may be secondary to the actions of increased $[K^+]_o$ on the rate of AP depolarization. In the SA and AV nodes, conduction is slowed by an apparent hypoxia-induced depression of slow action potentials, with inhomogeneity of impulse propagation that resulted in concealed areas of re-entry.[302]

Reperfusion. When tissue that has been totally ischemic is reperfused, a number of additional processes take place to further degrade myocyte function and viability. Upon restoration of flow, mitochondria may be sufficiently functional to permit restoration of Ca^{2+} regulation, or depending on the duration of the insult, there may be further deterioration and worsening of the Ca^{2+} overload, ultimately causing cell death.[260,303] A second major factor that causes progression of injury is production of oxygen free radicals upon reintroduction of oxygenated blood.[304,305] Xanthine dehydrogenase may be converted to xanthine oxidase in the presence of elevated cytosolic Ca^{2+}. This enzyme may produce oxygen free radicals, employing the purine derived from adenosine as added substrate. Of greater importance may be free radicals generated by polymorphonuclear leukocytes, which are activated upon re-entry into the previously ischemic vasculature.[305] Free radicals will injure not only the myocardium but its vasculature as well, so that perfusion may be further degraded. Oxidative stress and peroxidation of membrane lipids may destroy membrane integrity so that ionic gradients can no longer be maintained and unregulated Ca^{2+} entry is further increased,[306] a process that may occur in endothelial cells and myocytes as well. While cells have the capability to scavenge free radicals via reduced glutathione (GSH) and glutathione peroxidase, that capacity may be exceeded. Oxidative stress evidenced by decreases in GSH has been observed in human hearts following cardiopulmonary bypass.[307] The sequence of Ca^{2+} overload leading to free radical formulation, which than degrades membrane integrity causing further Ca^{2+} overload, clearly leads to cell death.

Stunning and Hibernation. If an episode of ischemia is not sufficient to result in cell death, the myocardium undergoes a period of recovery during which it is "stunned," exhibiting markedly depressed contractility.[308] The events that lead to this depressed function have been summarized as a gradual uncontrolled rise in cytoplasmic Ca^{2+} during ischemia, a transient worsening of Ca^{2+} overload upon reperfusion, and a persistent but ultimately reversible decrease in myofibrillar Ca^{2+} sensitivity.[309] Since Ca^{2+} regulation is largely restored, the contractile deficit appears to be caused by an alteration in the myofibrillar Ca^{2+} sensitivity. This has recently been demonstrated in permeabilized segments of stunned and normal porcine myocardium, in which a significant decrease in Ca^{2+} sensitivity was observed in myocardial biopsies (pCa shifted from 5.88 to 5.69, with no change in maximal tension).[310] Similar changes were not seen, however, in stunned rat heart.[311] The oxidative injuries caused by free radicals during reperfusion are also suggested to contribute to the phenomenon of "stunning."[304]

In contrast to the effects of stunning are those of hibernation, in which the Ca^{2+} transient is decreased, but there appears to be far less loss of myofilament sensitivity than observed with stunning (Fig. 5–12). With hibernation, which is usually produced by a moderate degree of ischemia as opposed to total loss of flow, P_i does not increase and intracellular ATP stores appear to be maintained as the Ca^{2+} transient and tension development decrease.[312] The changes ascribed to hibernation secondary to hypoperfusion are strikingly similar to those seen with hypoxic perfusion,[258] and contrast with the effects of minimal or absence of perfusion which cause Ca^{2+} overload and stunning. The decrease in Ca^{2+} and tension development that accompany hypertension appear to have a protective effect, since recovery from hypoxia is rapid (minutes), whereas the decrease in myofilament sensitivity and SR function secondary to stunning (reversible Ca^{2+} overload) requires a longer recovery period (weeks to days). In addition to the prolonged defect in EC coupling, stunning causes a similarly extended depression in myocardial fatty acid metabolism.[313] Nevertheless, some protection appears to be present during ischemic stunning, since blockade of K_{ATP} channels clearly worsens the myocardial dysfunction following ischemia.[274]

Preconditioning. If myocardium is subjected to a brief (~5 minute) episode of ischemia, the myocardium is "preconditioned," that is, it tolerates subsequent episodes of ischemia for a more sustained period before cell dysfunction and death occurs.[314,315] The protective effect includes improved recovery of contractile function following an ischemic insult and reperfusion, a decreased size of infarcted tissue, as well as protecting the heart

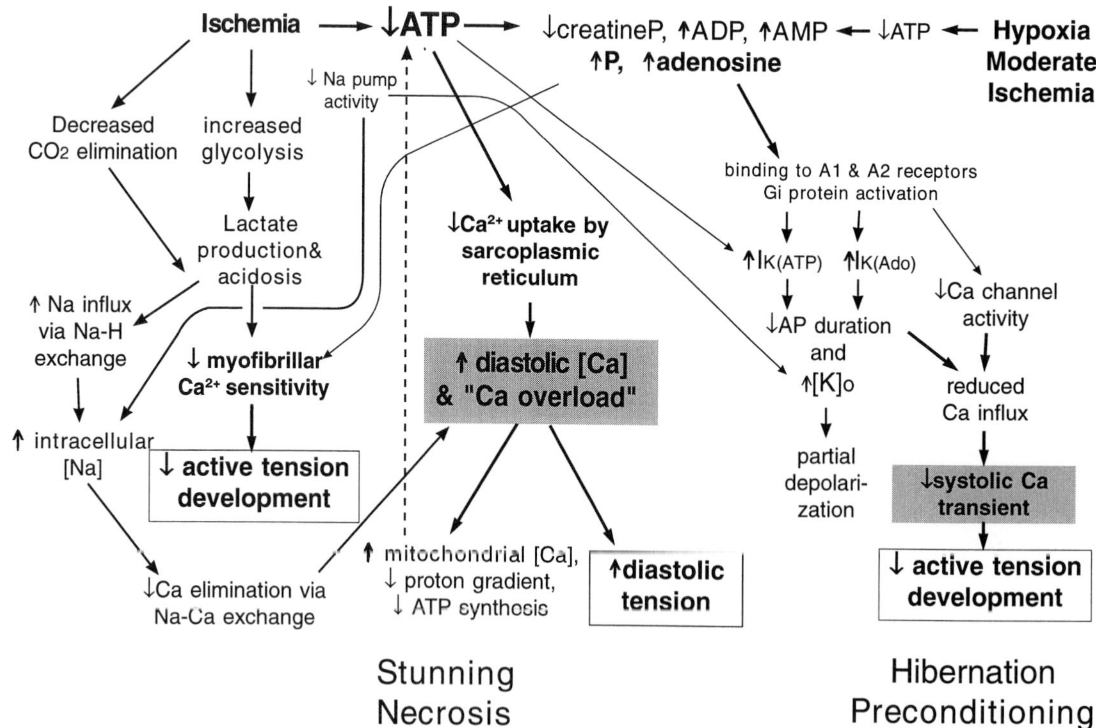

FIGURE **5–12.** Cellular metabolic interactions within the myocardium that occur with hypoxia or ischemia. The effects of hypoxia result clearly in decreased Ca^{2+} uptake and transience and the loss of contractility on this basis. In the case of ischemia, the effects of the greater acidosis would appear to predominate and intracellular Ca^{2+} does not appear to be depressed.

against ischemic arrhythmias.[316] Ischemic preconditioning (IP) lasts for a relatively brief period (<1 hour), although a long-term effect may be present.[316] The process seems to require the activity of adenosine, which not only activates $K_{Ach,Ado}$ but also modulates the function of K_{ATP} channels. Blockade of adenosine receptors blocks IP,[315,316] while enhancement of adenosine tissue levels with acadesine extends the duration of the preconditioning effect.[317] The notion that the rise in cytoplasmic Ca^{2+} is the initiating cause for stunning[309] (or is at least strongly associated with it) is supported by the observation that IP particularly inhibits the ischemic rise in cytoplasmic Ca^{2+} and attenuates the contractile dysfunction of stunning.[318] The rise in cytoplasmic Na^+ was also decreased, suggesting that it may contribute to the development of the Ca^{2+} overload as noted previously. Although IP inhibits glycolysis and H^+ production,[319] IP does not appear to involve alteration in the degree of cellular acidosis during the ischemic episode.[320]

A major effector of IP appears to be the K_{ATP} channel, since its blockade prevents IP, while activation of K_{ATP} channels by KCOs can simulate IP and protect the heart,[321–323] although some species variability is evident. Such channel activity persists into the reperfusion period and appears to contribute to the prevention of myocardial stunning.[324] While the AP duration shortening, decreased Ca^{2+} entry, and decreased myocardial energy consumption should afford some protection, it seems likely that other intracellular processes are activated during IP.[319] In addition to ischemia and KCOs, preconditioning can be activated by a variety of receptors including A_1 adenosine, α_1-adrenergic, endothelin, muscarinic, and bradykinin.[195,325–328] In addition, activation of PKC also appears to cause preconditioning.[329,330] While it seems plausible, it is unclear whether activation of the PKC signaling cascade may be the pathway for activation of K_{ATP} channels for the receptors listed, or whether direct interactions exist between certain receptors (e.g., A_1 adenosine) and the K_{ATP} channels. It is noteworthy that in addition to effects on the myocardium, K_{ATP} channel-mediated IP extends to the coronary endothelium, also maintaining vascular integrity.[331]

The various degrees of myocardial damage may be viewed as a spectrum. Depending on the duration and degree (or "dose") of ischemia, the myocardial response may be preconditioning, hibernation, stunning, or necrosis.

Anesthetic Actions

Inhalation Anesthetics. The volatile anesthetics have long been known to depress myocardial contractility in a dose-dependent fashion,[332] although at equianesthetic concentrations the amount of depression varies (halothane > isoflurane).[333,334] Isoflurane, halothane, and enflurane alter a number of specific mechanisms of cardiac EC coupling in an agent-specific fashion (see Table 5–5).[335] As determined by various investigators,[336–340] the volatile anesthetics directly depress tension development of cardiac myofibrils stimulated directly by $[Ca^{2+}]$. However, at relevant clinical levels these actions are usually modest and do not account for the greater contractile depression seen with intact plasma membranes. When equivalent depression is produced by an-

TABLE 5–5
Mechanisms of Anesthetic Actions on Myocardial Contraction*

	Ca Channel Effects	SR Ca^{2+} Stores	Relaxation (Ca^{2+} reuptake)	Contractile Proteins
Volatile Anesthetics				
Halothane	Moderate depression	Depleted due to CaRC activation	Ca^{2+}-ATPase activation	Slightly decreased Ca^{2+} sensitivity
Enflurane	Moderate depression	?CaRC activation, cooling-induced & late release depressed	Ca^{2+}-ATPase activation	No change, or slightly decreased
Isoflurane	Modest–moderate depression	No CaRC activation, cooling-induced & late release depressed	± effect	Decreased sensitivity at higher concentration
Nitrous oxide	? Modest depression	?	?	?
Intravenous Agents				
Thiopental	Moderate inhibition; AP prolongation	? Decreased release	?Slightly impaired uptake or release	?
Etomidate	None apparent	None apparent	None apparent	? Increased cross-bridge kinetics
Ketamine	Modest depression	None apparent	Slightly impaired at very high dose	None apparent
Propofol	Modest depression	None apparent	? Slightly impaired uptake	None apparent
Opiates	? Modest depression	? None apparent	? None apparent	? None apparent

*Summarized from various sources including Rusy & Komai,[334,335,363,367,563–568] Riou,[364–366] Housmans,[341,569,570] Su,[337,338,571] Bosnjak,[343,344,572] Lynch,[333,346,348,349,361,573] and others. CaRC = Ca^{2+} release channel.

esthetics and by decreased external [Ca^{2+}], the effects on the kinetic parameters of isometric and isotonic contractions are reduced to the same extent.[341] The rate of isometric relaxation is particularly increased, however, which suggests a possible decrease in affinity of TnC for Ca^{2+}.[341] A greater contribution to myocardial depression appears due to depression of the Ca^{2+} transient, which activates myofibrils. Quantitatively similar depression of tension and such Ca^{2+} transients also suggests effects are primarily related to altered activator Ca^{2+}.[342,343] A prominent action of the volatile anesthetics is depression of I_{Ca}, both via L- and T-type channels, although it is uncertain whether the degree of depression by halothane and isoflurane is similar at equianesthetic doses.[333,344] In addition, these agents also have specific effects on SR function, with a decrease in SR retention of Ca^{2+} clearly evident in skinned fibers and isolated SR vesicles.[345,346] Most prominent is the activation of CaRC specifically by halothane[347,348] and possibly enflurane,[347] resulting in depletion of the SR Ca^{2+} store; a nonspecific "leak" may also contribute.[346] The anesthetics also modify the Ca^{2+}-ATPase activity, with the major action being an enhancement of activity by enflurance,[349] while additional effects are also demonstrable on the Na-Ca exchange current.[350]

In addition to direct actions, the volatile agents also appear to influence the extrinsic modulators of contractility. The "sensitization" by halothane to catecholamines, which may generate dysrhythmias, may also enhance contractility under certain circumstances.[351] This action may be mediated by enhanced β-AR coupling, or, more likely, by interference with muscarinic receptors, which may depress contractile function.[159,352] Of considerable note is the fact that the volatile anesthetics appear to afford considerable protection against ischemia, demonstrating biochemical and functional evidence of preservation, as well as decreased incidence of ischemic arrhythmias.[353–358] While the anesthetics decrease myocardial energy utilization, which may afford a component of protection, this seems to be a specific action of the anesthetics that is reversible by glyburide,[359,360] suggesting that at least isoflurane has specific K_{ATP} channel-activating abilities.

Intravenous Anesthetics. Of the intravenous anesthetics, hypnotics, and analgesics, thiopental appears to have the most complex direct actions on the myocardium. Thiopental causes a dose-dependent depression of contractility,[361] and a major mechanism probably involves the depression of $I_{Ca,L}$,[362] which is observed in cardiac myocytes.[85] This effect on Ca channels may be counterbalanced in part by its ability to prolong the cardiac AP by inhibiting the resting K^+ conductance.[85,361] There may also be additional effects on the SR Ca^{2+} handling.[361,363]

At clinical concentrations, the depressant actions on the myocardium of other intravenous anesthetics are far less prominent. Most implications regarding subcellular sites of action have been inferred from detailed mechanical studies by Riou and co-workers on the effects of ketamine, etomidate, and propofol in rat heart.[364–366] While these agents generally have minimal effects, ketamine had a slightly positive inotropic action, with possible impairment of SR accumulation at supraclinical levels (100 μM)[364] as well as depression of I_{Ca}.[367,368] Etomidate had minimal effect, although its propylene glycol vehicle did appear to depress SR function. Propofol at high concentrations depresses the myocardium,[361,366,369] an effect that is compatible with a modest depression of $I_{Ca,L}$,[370] as well as some modest alteration in SR function at high concentrations.[361,366] Specific depression of $I_{Ca,L}$ has been seen with stimulation of opiate receptors by leu-enkephalin,[371] although the mechanism is unclear. It is unclear whether the synthetic narcotics (fentanyl and its congeners) depress I_{Ca} significantly at clinical concentrations, and whether by an opiate receptor or another mechanism.

The Anatomy of the Heart

The human heart is a parallel pump that simultaneously ejects equal volumes of blood into a lower pressure (~20 mm Hg, 0.03 atm, or 3 kPa) pulmonary circuit and a higher pressure (70 to 100 mm Hg, 0.09 to 0.13 atm, or 9 to 13 kPa) systemic circuit. These unequal pressures are generated in hollow muscular chambers compressed by the contraction of constricting muscular walls. A fibrous skeleton provides the framework for the musculature and the cardiac valves, which direct and gate the flow of blood. The framework includes the central fibrous body, which unites the mitral and tricuspid valve with the aortic root; the left fibrous trigone, which forms the annuli of the mitral and tricuspid valves; and the membranous portion of the interventricular septum. Although its weight and size vary with age, gender, and other factors, the average human heart weights 275 to 325 gm.

The Right-Sided Pulmonary Pump

Via the superior vena cava (SVC), inferior vena cava (IVC), and the coronary sinus, deoxygenated blood returns to the thin-walled (1 to 3 mm) right atrium (RA). The RA is composed of the thin-walled trabeculated portion or the right auricle, which is separated by a ridge of muscle, the crista terminalis from the smooth-walled portion into which the SVC and IVC enter. The ostium of the IVC is guarded by the eustachian valve.[372] A third opening in the RA is the coronary sinus with its ostium guarded by the thesbian valve.[373] The right and left atria are separated by the interatrial septum with its central ovoid portion, the fossa ovalis, the remnant of the fetal foramen ovale. The medial wall of the RA is slightly indented by the torus aorticus, the expanded aortic wall immediately superior to the ring of the aortic valve. In addition to functioning as reservoirs for blood entering the ventricles, the atria also serve an endocrine function, acting as the primary source outside of the brain for atrial natriuretic peptide (ANP), which is involved in control of renal function as well as vascular tone.

The right ventricle (RV) is a 5- to 7-mm thick muscular pocket or free wall wrapped around the anterior third of the conical LV. The resulting crescent-shaped cavity consists of an inferoposterior inflow (sinus) portion and a smooth-surfaced anterosuperior outflow (infundibular) portion. The inflow portion contains prominent muscle bands (moderator, septal, and parietal) and muscle bundles known as trabeculae carneae. Blood flows into the RV from the RA through the 3- to 3.5-cm-diameter tricuspid valve annulus, which is formed in part by the *crista supraventricularis*. This crest or ridge of myocardium originates at the anterior interventricular (IV) septum and passes along the superior aspect of the right ventricular free wall.[374] Retrograde flow is prevented by the tricuspid valve, which consists of anterior, posterior, and medial leaflets, comprising an area of 8 to 11 cm^2. The anterior leaflet, the largest, originates along the crista supraventricularis. The free margin of the valve is attached by thin fibrous cords (chordae tendineae) to the head of the anterior papillary muscle (APM). The APM originates on the anterolateral RV wall at the insertion of the moderator band, a cylindric muscle band that passes across the ventricular cavity from its origin on the IV septum. The septal (or medial) leaflet attaches to the junction of the interatrial and interventricular septum; the posterior leaflet originates from the diaphragmatic portion of the right ventricle. The smaller posterior and septal papillary muscles attach by chordae to the posterior and medial tricuspid valve leaflets. The coordinated contraction of the crista supraventricularis, the papillary muscles, and the ventricular wall ensure that the leaflet edges remain opposed (coapted) and do not separate or reflux back into the RA, permitting regurgitation of blood. The pumping action of the right ventricle depends in part on its being tethered to the LV wall, the contraction of which pulls the RV free wall against the normal convexity of the ventricular septum. However, the crista supraventricularis may also play a critical role in integrating RV and LV function by pulling the RV free wall toward the IV septum as well as narrowing the tricuspid orifice.[374] The traction applied by the moderator band(s) near the base of the anterior papillary muscle will also contribute to effective function.

The right ventricular contraction begins in the inflow tract and in a peristaltic manner travels to the infundibulum with a variable delay (~50 msec).[375] The right ventricular infundibulum (or conus arteriosus) directs right ventricular outflow to the main pulmonary artery (PA), which begins at the pulmonic valve. It is a trileaflet valve (right, left, and anterior cusps), normally about 4 cm^2 in area. As it originates from the anterior and superior portion of the RV, the PA passes backward and upward under the aorta before it bifurcates into right and left pulmonary arteries. The remnant of the fetal ductus arteriosus, the ligamentum arteriosum, connects the upper aspect of the bifurcation to the inferior aortic surface. Pulmonary arteries branch into arterioles and thence into capillaries, which spread over the alveolar surfaces between two alveolar endothelial layers.

The Left-Sided Systemic Pump

The blood typically returns from the lungs to the left atrium via four vessels, the left and right, superior and inferior pulmonary veins. The left atrium (LA) is divided into a smooth-walled muscular portion and a smaller, trabeculated portion (or atrial appendage) adjacent to the atrioventricular junction. The atrial appendage is relatively compliant and holds extra volume during periods of increased venous return. Leaving the LA, blood traverses the mitral valve, which consists of four cusps: a large anterior (aortic) cusp, the large posterior (mural) cusp, and two small septal or commissural cusps. Functionally, these four cusps form two major leaflets, the anteriomedial and posterolateral. The area of the mitral valve is about 6 to 8 cm^2 in adults, and valve areas of less than 1 cm^2 are considered severely stenotic. Two groups of papillary muscles and chordae tendineae loosely anchor the leaflets to the apical and mid-LV myocardium. The blood supply to the chordae and papillary muscles is often quite tenuous.[376,377] However, the mitral valve incompetence that frequently accompanies ischemic ventricular dysfunction is not usually due to papillary muscle function per se, but is probably secondary to loss of normal ventricular wall contractility.[378]

Normally, the LV has an elongated spherical shape, with a thicker (8 to 15 mm) and more densely trabeculated wall than the bellows-shaped RV. The interventricular septum with its membranous superior portion near the aortic valve and muscular inferior portion divided RV from LV. Separating the membranous and the muscular portion of the septum is the limbus marginalis. Both the shape and wall thickness permit this chamber to generate the substantially higher pressures required to eject blood into the systemic circulation. The orientation of fibers in the left ventricle varies through the thickness of the wall. In the endocardium and epicardium the fiber orientation is largely longitudinal, but the bulk of the ventricular wall contains interdigitated circumferential muscle fibers with an oblique orientation.[379] When the myocytes contract, the apex is pulled superiorly toward the base, and rotates counterclockwise, causing the ventricle to twist.

The aortic valve is adjacent to the mitral valve within the left ventricle, separated only by the fibrous tissue framework that comprises the annuli of both valves. Three pocket-like structures of similar size, the right and left (coronary) cusps, and the slightly larger posterior (noncoronary) cusps, form the aortic valve. A normal aortic valve is about 3 to 4 cm^2 in area, but the area, weight, and volume of the cusps increase with age and heart weight.[380] In the center of each aortic cusp is a small nodule, the nodule of Arantius. The free edge of the cusp is called the lunula. Coaptation of the nodules during ventricular diastole prevents regurgitation. The aorta at the level of the valve dilates to form the sinuses of Valsalva, in which the coronary ostia are located.

The Pericardium

Within the mediastinum, the heart is suspended in the pericardium, a sac that consists of thick fibrous and serous visceral layers. Although it is nonessential, it has certain anatomic functions among which are the isolation of the heart from other mediastinal structures, maintenance of the heart in optimal functional shape and position, minimization of cardiac dilatation, and prevention of adhesions.[381] Within the pericardial space are four areas: transverse sinus, oblique sinus, superior sinus, and postcaval recess into which 30 to 70 ml of pericardial fluid normally accumulates. Pericardial fluid acts as a hydrostatic system to apply a compensating hydrostatic force to the heart under conditions of acceleration and other gravitational forces.[381] The pericardium also contains vagal nerve branches.

The Cardiac Cycle

The cardiac cycle defines the behavior of the heart during one beat, with specific ordering of electrical and mechanical events as indicated in Figure 5–13.

ATRIAL CONTRACTION

The P wave of the ECG is the transmitted depolarization of the bulk of the atria, which is followed by the atrial contraction. As atrial pressure increases more blood is pushed into the filling ventricle. Atrial contraction produces the A wave on central venous pressure tracings and the soft fourth heart sound (S_4), audible in some patients. Although the atria serve primarily a reservoir function, their contraction provides an extra "kick" of blood into the ventricle, which becomes more important during tachycardia (diastole is relatively shorter), or in patients with stiff ventricles (hypertrophy, ischemia) and diseased AV valves. In these settings, atrial contraction may increase cardiac output by 40%, in contrast to the 5 to 20% increase seen in normal settings.[382] In such patients, an S_4 occurs 0.04 second after the P wave due to vibrations of left ventricular muscle and mitral valve. The Z point on the venous pressure waveform is the period when atrial and ventricular pressures are

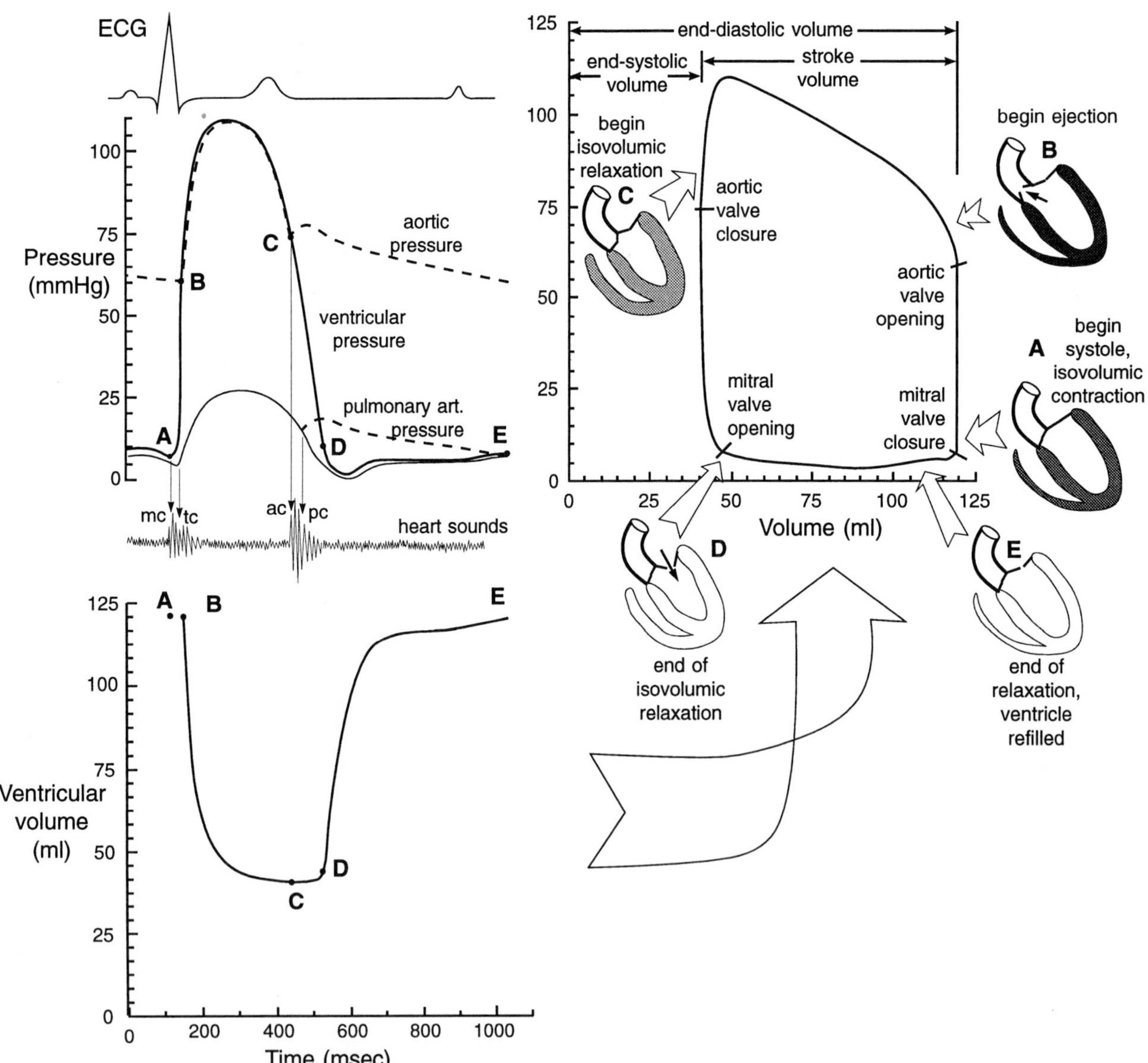

FIGURE **5–13.** Cardiac cycle as originally diagrammed by Wiggers, showing the simultaneous ECG, pressure, and volume changes within the heart. The right ventricular volume is not shown; the stroke volume is of the same magnitude as that of the left ventricle (LV), but begins from a greater end-diastolic volume (V_{ED} = 140 to 160 ml). The isochronal plot of LV volume and pressure yields the PV loop shown on the right.

essentially equal immediately preceding ventricular systole.

VENTRICULAR SYSTOLE

Isovolumic Contraction. Ventricular depolarization begins about 0.12 to 0.20 second in adults and 0.15 to 0.18 second in children after depolarization of the SA node.[383] The QRS complex marks depolarization of the ventricle and is followed closely by the onset of contraction, closure of the AV valves, and the first heart sound (S_1). (The sound is produced by vibrations resulting from the slowing of blood that occurs as a result of the closure of the AV valves as the blood is being pushed back toward the atrium.) S_1 is louder, as the AV valves are further apart and/or contractility is greater. However, some investigators suggest that S_1 results from reverberations of the left ventricular muscle, mitral valve, and left ventricular outflow tract in response to the accelerating and decelerating of blood during early systole.[384] Since right and left ventricular contraction is normally slightly asynchronous, S_1 is usually split. Early during pressure development, the AV valves bulge into the atria, increasing the atrial pressure and the c (for carotid) wave in the central venous pressure. Then atrial pressure falls, the x descent, as the ventricles are pulled away from the atria. The ventricular wall develops higher tension and increases pressure without a change in volume until the pressure exceeds the pressure (systemic diastolic pressure) on the systemic side of the semilunar valves.

Ejection. The contraction of the ventricles and ejection of blood is similar to the contraction of the isolated muscle against a set load. Blood flows through the semilunar valves, very rapidly at first, then more slowly as the ventricle empties and fiber length decreases. Later during ejection, atrial pressure rises due to incoming blood that cannot flow through the closed AV valves (the jugular wave). The amount of blood ejected by the heart depends to a very great extent on the pressure against which it is ejecting, if the resistance to ejection is very high, then the heart will use a great deal of its energy generating pressure, with less energy spent ejecting blood. The difference between the end-diastolic volume (VED) and end-systolic volume (VES) is the blood ejected by the ventricle, or stroke volume (SV). Cardiac output (CO) is the blood ejected by the heart over 1 minute, being the product of SV and heart rate (HR; in beats per minute). With initiation of relaxation, intraventricular declines and flow ceases.

The simultaneous changes in pressure and volume are of a cardiac cycle, and the associated events are indicated in Figure 5–10. Instead of plotting pressure and volume as a function of time, an isochronal plot of pressure versus volume gives rise to the pressure-volume relation or PV loop, which is valuable in the evaluation of cardiac function.

VENTRICULAR DIASTOLE

Isovolumic Relaxation. As myocardial relaxation proceeds and intraventricular pressures decline below aortic and pulmonary artery pressures, the rapid deceleration of blood and resulting vibration of the outflow tracts and great vessels, as well as closure of the semilunar valves, produces the second heart sound (S_2). As pressures are higher, S_2 has a higher pitch, and increased pressure in the aorta or pulmonary artery can increase the loudness of S_2. Pressure falls in the ventricle until the pressure falls below atrial pressure and the AV valves open.

Rapid Filling and Subsequent Diastasis. Blood that has been accumulating in the atria during ventricular ejection rapidly empties (60 to 100 msec) into the ventricles once the AV valves open, producing the y descent on the atrial pressure tracing. Peak ventricular filling in early diastole occurs at 500 to 700 ml/sec as the ventricle "sucks" blood from the atria (diastolic suction); ventricular relaxation may actually produce a negative intracavitary pressure under certain circumstances. Ventricular pressure continues to decrease because ventricular expansion exceeds filling. Thus, the elastic recoil of the heart and great vessels ~~during diastole~~ contributes to the accelerated filling phase of the ventricle, particularly during tachycardia. The third heart sound is produced by the sudden slowing of blood as it enters the ventricle, usually being heard only in disease states associated with stiff ventricles (i.e., decreased compliance), either from dilation or hypertrophy. Filling slows as atrial pressure becomes lower. During this period of diastasis, the AV valves partially close as less blood flows through them prior to atrial systole.

As originally proposed by Gorlin and Gorlin,[385] the area of the cardiac valves is estimated from the formula:

$$\text{Area} = \text{flow}/[C \cdot 44.5 \cdot (\text{pressure gradient})^{1/2}]$$

where C is an arbitrary constant, 44.5 is a derived constant for the acceleration of blood, and flow in L/min is CO divided by the applicable fraction of the cardiac cycle (diastole for the mitral valve, systole for the aortic valve). In the original report, C was 0.7 (later 0.85[386]) for the mitral valve and 1 for the aortic valve. However, an adequate estimation can be made from the simplified formula[387]:

$$\text{Area} = \text{cardiac output}/(\text{pressure gradient})^{1/2}.$$

Ventricular Function

Models of the Left Ventricle

Due to the largely circumferential orientation of the myocytes around the ventricular cavity, the primary pumping action of the ventricle is a constriction of the chamber. A 27% shortening of endocardial sarcomeres from 2.2 μm to 1.6 μm produces a 47% decrease $\{[100-(1-0.27)^2]\%\}$ in the cross-sectional area of the ventricle. Because of its finite thickness, such shortening increases wall thickness by 27%. The outer myocyte sarcomeres are required to shorten less than those of the endocardium. To decrease the disparity in epicardial versus endocardial length-tension relations, in the unloaded ventricle the epicardial sarcomeres are longer than those of endocardium.[388] As a consequence, when the myocardium is stretched during diastole (inner sarcomeres are stretched more than those of the epicardium), the sarcomeres will have a more uniform length and contractile function. Ultimately, the actual decrease in chamber volume (i.e., ejection fraction) is a cubic function of muscle fiber shortening, which reflects sarcomere length. Presuming that the sarcomere shortening is the same in all directions, the percentage volume change for any model solid can be approximated by: $[100 \times (1\text{-fractional shortening})^3]\%$. For the 27 to 30% sarcomere shortening noted above, the approximate volume decrease of 61 to 66% is very close to the estimates of ejection fraction for the normal heart.

Within the ventricular wall, the wall stress (S, or tension) during pressure development is calculated according to Laplace's law: $S = Pr/h$, where r is cardiac radius, P is interventricular pressure, and h is ventricular muscle thickness.[389] Since pressure and radius appear independently in the formula, with ventricular dilation and high P, wall stress may increase considerably. In such a setting, there will be less shortening deactivation, and the duration of tension development (and energy consumption) will be prolonged.

The ventricular chamber volume (V) has been described by ellipsoidal formulas, approximated by one or more regular solid geometric shapes, or calculated using various numbers of slices (Simpson's rule). In the normally functioning ventricle, the various models all give reasonable estimates of ventricular volume and volume changes. The ellipsoidal formulas assume a prolate ellipsoid with dimensions defined along the three spatial axes: length L and diameters $D1$ and $D2$.

$$V = (4\pi/3)(0.5*L/2)(0.5*D1)(0.5*D2).$$

This method seems to underestimate the volume of smaller hearts and overestimate the volume of larger ventricles.[390] Angiographically, it has been assumed that the anterior oblique transverse left ventricular inner diameter (LVID) equals both $D1$ and $D2$ and one half the length. Substituting into the above equation yields the "D^3" rule or $V = (\text{LVID})^3$.

Under a variety of circumstances, most notably regional ischemia, the regional shortening may not be equal. In this setting, the ventricular volume may be approximated by longitudinal slices of set width, for which the cross-sectional area can be estimated echocardiographically, as well as by other means.

Starling's Law of the Heart

Of considerable importance is the fact that the linear relation between length and total force of isolated myocardium is well maintained when translated into three dimensions, so that there is a linear relation between pressure and volume when the heart is maximally contracted, near the end of systole (Fig. 5–14*A*). The PV relation further amplifies the particularly steep linear length-force relation that characterizes cardiac muscle (Fig. 5–7). Consequently, when ventricular outflow is occluded, the pressure developed in the ventricle is a steep linear function of LV VED. In contrast, if instead of developing pressure the heart ejects blood, SV is also a linear function of the starting rest volume, which is determined by the amount of cardiac fiber shortening that can occur. However, the condition that applies in the normal physiologic situation is ejection of blood against pressure. After achieving a given pressure, the SV of the heart is in direct proportion to the initial diastolic volume. The greater SV and CO seen with greater VED is indicated in Figure 5–14*B*. If greater pressure must be developed before ejection, SV maintains the same linear relation to VED. This was first defined by Starling's law of the heart: "within physiological limits the larger the volume of the heart, the greater are the energy of its contraction and the amount of chemical change at each contraction."[87,391] As anticipated by this statement, the Frank-Starling relation is really the whole-organ expression of molecular behavior: the length-dependent cardiac TnC Ca^{2+} binding, combined with passive length-force relation of the extensive collagen matrix around the myofibrils, determines how much work is accomplished and energy consumed. As classically formulated, Starling's law employs readily measurable quantities of CO versus end-diastolic pressure (PED), permitting rapid assessment of increased or decreased contractility by the shift in the relation. Because of the curvilinear VED:PED relation, a nonlinear relation results when SV is expressed as a function of PED (Fig. 5–14*C*).

Since appropriate comparison of CO requires a constant HR and ejection pressure (conventionally called "afterload"), the relation is better expressed for each beat by the "ventricular function curve" (VFC) introduced by Sarnoff, in which the external work performed by the ventricle (LV stroke work or SW) in moving the SV with each heart beat is estimated and plotted versus the LV PED.[392] By employing SW instead of SV, Sarnoff's VFC accounts for changes in ventricular ejection due to changes in afterload. When there is a decrease in ejected volume due to increased afterload, the increased blood pressure against which the heart pumps maintains the value of SW (i.e., volume work is replaced by pressure work). SW may be estimated by $K \cdot \text{SV} \cdot (\text{MEP-PED})$, where MEP is mean ejection pressure (in mm Hg) and volume is expressed in milliliters. Clinically, PED is estimated by the pulmonary capillary occlusion ("wedge") pressure. For units of $\text{gm} \cdot \text{m/m}^{-2}$, K equals 1.36×10^{-2}; for units of joules, K equals 1.33×10^{-4}.

Pressure-Volume Loops and the End-Systolic Pressure-Volume Relation

However, the work performed by the heart may be readily expressed in a graphic analysis. If a mass is lifted against the force of gravity, the work accomplished is defined by the force generated over the distance moved, with the end point falling on the linear length-force relation of maximally active muscle (Fig. 5–15 *top*). In the same fashion, the work performed by the heart pumping a volume of blood against pressure accomplishes work, and the area of the resulting PV loop is a graphical representation of the SW, the external work of pumping blood in a single beat (Fig. 5–15 *bottom*).

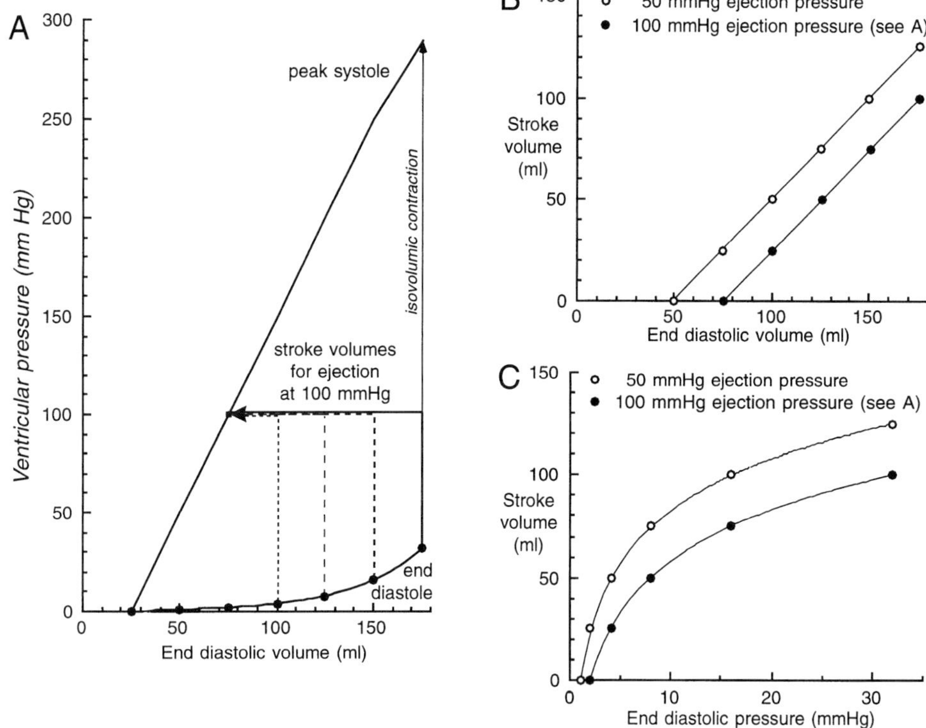

FIGURE **5–14.** Cardiac performance. *A*, Pressure-volume (PV) relation of the left ventricle at rest (end diastole [ED]) due to passive connective tissue elements of the ventricle, and at the peak of systole (ES) due to active force and passive elements. From any initial end-diastolic volume (VED), the peak isovolumic pressure developed is a linear function defined by the slope of the ESPV relation (*thick solid line*). This slope can be also be considered the maximum elastance (E_{max}) developed by the ventricle. *B*, Stroke volume (SV) as a function of VED. The *filled circles* indicate the linear increase in stroke volume with VED at an afterload of 50 and 100 mm Hg (latter shown in *A*). *C*, SV as a function of end-diastolic pressure (PED), the typical Starling curve. Due to the curvilinear relation of PED and VED, the SV-PED is curved.

When the heart ejects blood into the elastic compliance of the aorta, there is an increase in pressure against which ejection is occurring. Near the end of systole the heart is maximally contracted, having generated pressure (PES) and ejected its SV down to end-systolic volume (VES). This particular PV combination falls on the linear PV relation previously noted, and is the end-systolic pressure volume (ESPV) relation of the LV. When preload (i.e., VED) is varied, a family of PV loops is created and the upper left corner defines the maximal cardiac contraction. However, afterload can also be varied so that from a given VED various PV points are generated. The end-systolic PV relation observed with these variations in preload and/or afterload remain linear and reproducible over a wide range. While the initial definitions of ESPV relation were first done in isolated hearts with tight control of experimental variables,[393] such studies have subsequently been performed in vitro. Typically such studies are done by decreasing preload or altering afterload (pharmacologically or with partial aortic occlusion); thus the ESPV point of a PV loop is shifted down (and leftward) or up (and rightward) in order to define the full relation (Fig. 5–16*A* and *B*). In animals, preload is typically decreased by inflation of a vena caval balloon to decrease venous return. In patients preload can be manipulated by infusion of a venodilator.

Elastance is the linear relationship between length and force. The slope of the PV relation can be defined as elastance (in three dimensions), in which the change in pressure results from a change in volume, as originally described in isolated hearts.[393] The contraction is assumed to occur because the elastance of the ventricular wall suddenly increases when activated, as if a stretched spring were suddenly made out of thicker, stiffer wire. This concept of time-varying elastance, $E_{(t)}$, increasing from a minimum during diastole and having its steepest slope (E_{max}) near the end of systolic ejection, is a useful description of ventricular function. Because the cardiac muscle length-force relation is linear over physiologic sarcomere lengths, the concept of elastance can be simplified to $P_{ES} = E_{max} (V_{ES} - V_0)$, where V_0 is the volume of the empty heart with no distending pressure.

The linearity of the relation required for elastance is not always present in the intact heart, however, which places certain restrictions on its application. With increased shortening, the period of high elastance will be briefer. Rather than decreasing VED to define the relation, if afterload is increased, the ESPV relation is also concave downward (Fig. 5–16*B*).[394] Part of this effect is due to geometric factors. At large end-systolic volumes, small changes in wall stress result in large changes in end-systolic pressure. The slope of the ESPV relation

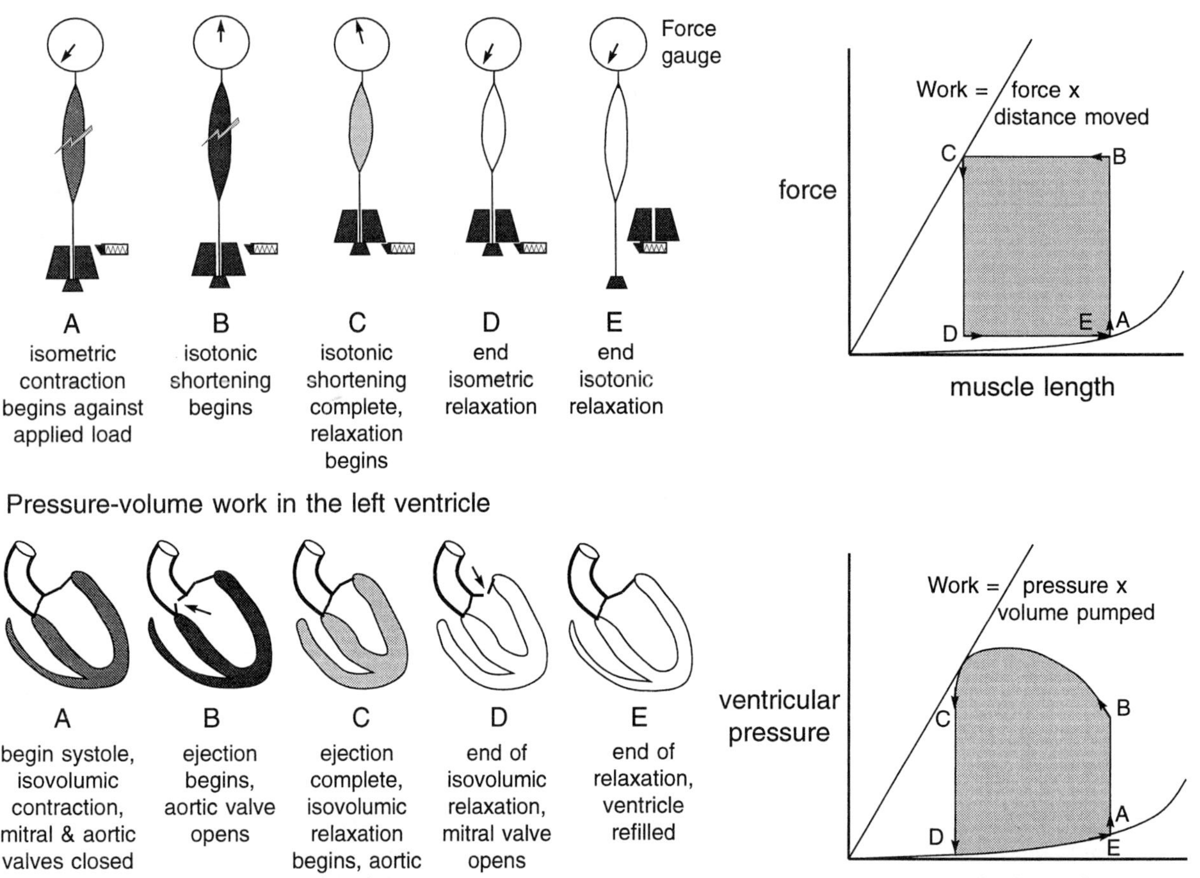

FIGURE **5–15.** Work performed in isolated muscle and in left ventricle. In isolated muscle (*top*) the lifting of a weight, whose height is then fixed, permits work to be accomplished. The work is defined by the force exerted times the distance moved, and is represented by the area indicated in the force-length plot. In the same way (*bottom*), work is accomplished by the heart when it pumps blood which is gated by the closure of the aortic valve following ejection. The work in that setting is defined by the pressure times volume area, or PV loop.

becomes steeper and more convex with inotropic stimulation (Fig. 5–16*C*).[394] This latter effect may result from the fact that the active force-length component in myocardium is increased by inotropic stimulation, while passive force is not, which tends to make the total force-length relation (Fig. 5–7*A*) less linear.

CORRELATION WITH OXYGEN CONSUMPTION

The PV loop and ESPV relation provide a framework to relate contractile behavior to ventricular oxygen consumption (MVO_2) under conditions of differing pressure and ejection, incorporating variations in mechanics and vascular compliance. As Sagawa and colleagues have elegantly demonstrated,[391,395] various combinations of pressure and SV may give the same estimate of SW, but MVO_2 may vary profoundly. While initially defined in isolated hearts, the relation between oxygen consumption and myocardial PV work has been demonstrated in conscious animals and humans. When from the same VED a ventricle does the same SW by generating twice the ejection pressure and ejecting half the stroke volume, the ejecting ventricle consumes considerably more oxygen. The greater cost of "pressure work" than "volume work" in terms of oxygen can be neatly quantitated by a graphic analysis that employs the linear relation of E_{max} (Fig. 5–17*A* and *B*). Myocardial oxygen consumption can be approximated by assuming that it is proportional to the pressure-volume area (PVA), which is the SW area plus the area between the E_{max} line and the PV loop (termed the "potential energy"). Suga and colleagues[391] rejected the term "internal work" for this component of energy consumption; the term "pressure generation energy" may be more appropriate than "potential energy." In addition to the PVA component of oxygen consumption, which represents ATP hydrolysis associated with actin-myosin interactions, oxygen consumption is associated with "basal metabolism" and "activation energy," the latter representing the ATP consumed in the cycling of the Ca^{2+} to control tension development (Fig. 5–16*C*). Both of these processes consume a significant fraction of ATP even in the working heart.

The neat linear relation between PVA and oxygen consumption is possible due to the linear behavior of E_{max},

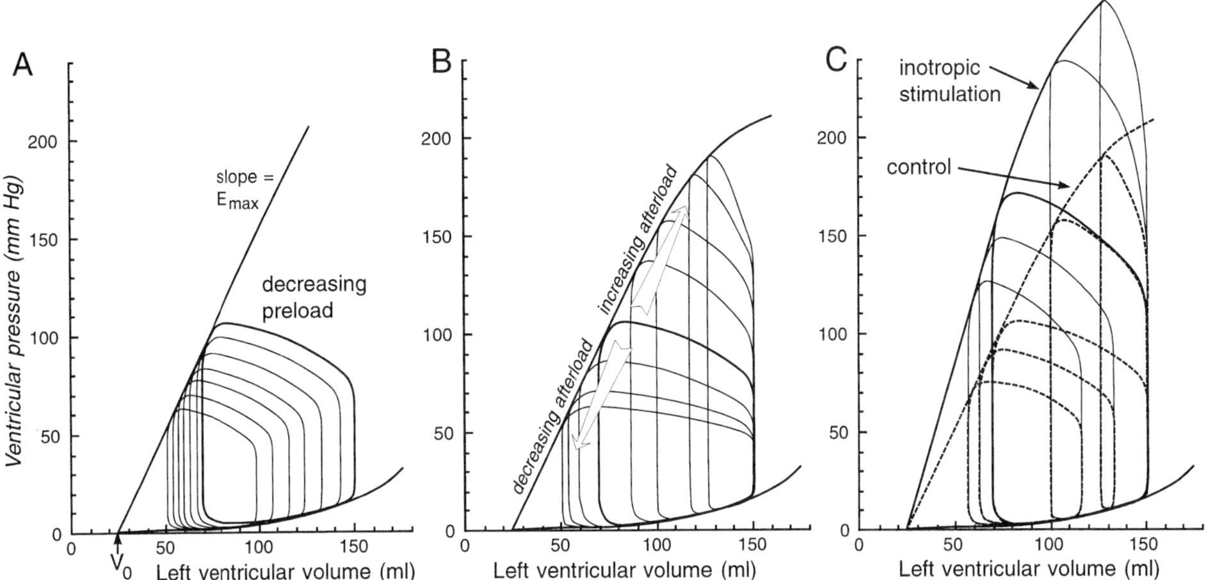

FIGURE **5–16.** Definition of the end-systolic pressure-volume (ESPV) relation, which represents maximum elastance (E_{max}) of the ventricle. *A*, Determination of ESPV relation by use of decreased preload. *B*, Determination of ESPV by alteration in afterload. *C*, Effect of enhanced inotropy of the PV relation. The nonlinearity of the ESPV is enhanced when contractility is enhanced by inotropic stimulation.

which is in turn due to predominantly linear length-force of myocardium. The greater oxygen consumption observed with "pressure work" (excessive "potential energy") probably arises from two major cardiac micromechanical behaviors. When myofilaments are sliding past each other during shortening, myosin head groups may form fewer cross-bridges, which require less ATP consumption to break. In contrast, when pressure is developed there are a greater number of cross-bridges cycling to generate pressure and consume oxygen. In addition, because of shortening deactivation (load-dependent relaxation), greater ejection results in a shorter systole,[119] which consumes less ATP. Recent evidence indicates that if active unloading of the ventricle occurs during ejection (even after the same peak pressure is developed), oxygen consumption is decreased in proportion to the decrease in PVA, and attributable to shortening deactivation.[396] In contrast, if filling is enhanced during diastole after cross-bridges are already dissociated, there is no effect on oxygen consumption.[397] The PV loop-PVA does not incorporate such time-dependent components of myocardial function and oxygen consumption, and it remains a surprisingly useful tool to understand and approximate myocardial work and oxygen consumption.

If the heart rate is increased by an increase in pacing rate, no greater oxygen is consumed on a per-beat basis for the same amount of work performed.[391] It has already been noted that at a high heart rate, greater amounts of Ca^{2+} are cycled, which should in and of itself increase oxygen consumption. However, due to the intrinsic regulation of the cells, higher heart rates result in a shorter systolic period, so the greater Ca^{2+} cycling may be counterbalanced by a shorter duration of contraction, so there is no net increase in energy requirement and oxygen consumption. Physiologically, increased heart rates are usually achieved by an increase in sympathetic tone, which has important consequences.

Inotropic stimulation by catecholamines markedly increases Ca^{2+} consumption. In this setting there is no alteration in myofibrillar efficiency with each beat; that is, to generate the same combination of tension and shortening, the same amount of ATP is consumed. However, because of the decreased TnC Ca^{2+} affinity and enhancement of Ca^{2+} entry, uptake, and release, the far greater amount of Ca^{2+} cycled with each beat consumes more ATP, as does the Na^+,K^+-ATPase turnover, which supports the requirement for greater Ca-Na exchange. This results in an upward shift in the O_2 consumption–PVA relation (Fig. 5–17*B*). These actions may almost double the amount of "activation" energy. Oxygen consumption is further increased by tachycardia.

REGIONAL PRESSURE–SEGMENT LENGTH RELATIONS

The assessment of LV function by PV relations assumes uniform ventricular function in all dimensions. While the typical PV loop describes global LV function, a similar plot can be made for the segments of the ventricular wall, similar to the length-force relation (Fig. 5–15). Using sonomicrometric methods, the shortening of different regions of the ventricle can be determined. While such techniques can be employed using the various ventricular volume models mentioned above to determine global function, these methods can be employed to determine differential contractile function of different regions. When there is normal ventricular function, a pressure–segment length (P-SL) loop may be generated similar in shape to the pressure-volume loop. It is clear,

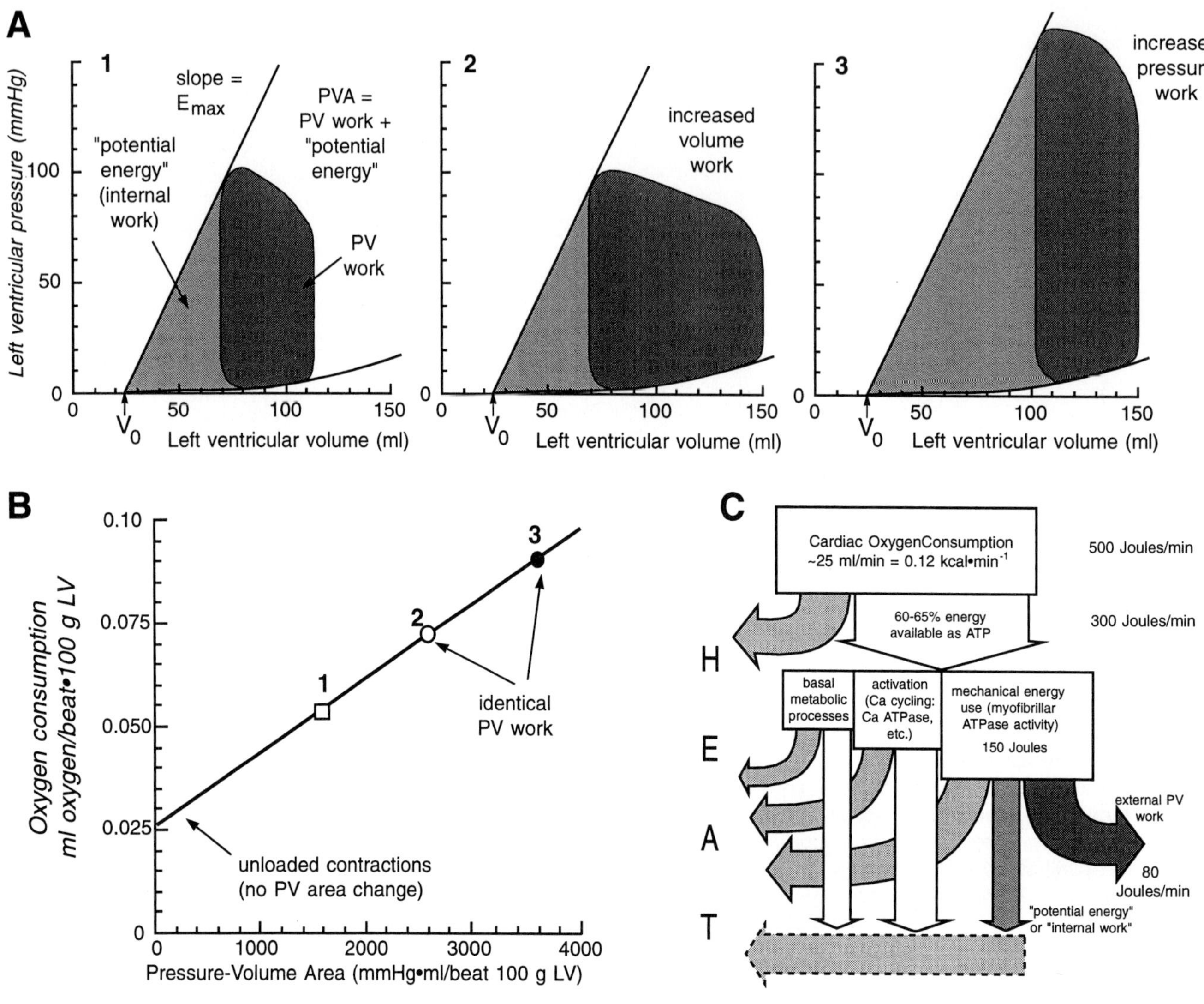

FIGURE **5–17.** Relationship of pressure-volume area to oxygen consumption. *A*, When the heart pumps blood, the oxygen consumed depends upon both the amount of work performed against the environment, that is, the blood pumped, which is the pressure-volume (PV) work, as well as upon a component of potential energy, which represents energy expended by the cardiac muscle in generating pressure. In panel *A-1*, the PV work and the potential energy are of similar magnitude. When the end-diastolic volume is increased with a resulting increase only in the stroke volume, the "potential energy" remains the same. In *A-3*, the increase in afterload and the resulting increase in pressure result in a PV loop that is equivalent to that in *A-2* (the same external work), but with a marked increase in the "potential energy." *B*, The relation between oxygen consumption and the pressure-volume area. The points from part *A* as well as the oxygen consumption for an unloaded isotonic contraction and for an isometric contraction are indicated. Note that in the case of *A-3*, greater oxygen is consumed, although the PV work is the same. (Adapted from Sagawa K, Maughan L, Suga H, Sunagawa K: Cardiac Contraction and the Pressure-Volume Relationship. New York, Oxford University Press, 1988, with permission.) 1,000 mm Hg·ml = 0.133 joules. *C*, The breakdown of distribution of oxygen consumption into the various metabolic processes of a 250-gm working left ventricle beating approximately 90 bpm. The area of the *rectangles* and *arrows* roughly approximates the proportion of energy consumed by the process. Depending upon afterload and diastolic dimensions, the distribution between external work and potential energy or internal work may vary considerably.

however, that while certain regions of the myocardium may function normally, in other regions, typically those areas subject to inadequate coronary perfusion, contractile function may be impaired or absent. When there is ischemic dysfunction of a particular segment, the segment lengthens instead of shortening during systole and functional segments stretch the nonfunctional segment even during isovolemic contractile phase. The ischemic P-SL loop is consequently tilted to the right, while the hyperfunctioning segment shows opposite changes. In an excellent review, Foëx and Leone[398] summarize many of these considerations.

In addition to the immediate dysfunction, compensatory segmental hypertrophic processes can occur in the surviving segments of myocardium over a sustained period of time. A combination of pressure- and volume-like overload hypertrophy occurs because noninfarcted myocardium is exposed to increased systolic and diastolic wall stress. Late congestive heart failure may develop after extensive myocardial infarction solely as a result of decompensation of regionally hypertrophic myocardium, despite an absence of further ischemic insult.[399] Histologically, remodeled myocardium may resemble that observed in patients with end-stage pressure or volume overload.[400] Although the underlying etiology of the complex process of ventricular remodeling is incompletely understood, activation of the renin-angiotensin axis and sympathetic nervous system appears to play important roles.[399,401]

PRESSURE VOLUME LOOPS UNDER VARIOUS CONDITIONS

Effects of Systolic and Diastolic Dysfunction. Myocardial failure may occur due to deterioration in the ability of the heart muscle to (1) generate pressure and shorten (decreased inotropy); or (2) relax and lengthen rapidly during diastole (decreased lusitropy); or (3) some combination of these. A pure decrease in inotropy (decreased E_{max}), which occurs with a decrease in myofibrillar Ca^{2+} sensitivity and/or a decrease in the amount of activator Ca^{2+} cycled per beat, causes an acute decrease in SV at the same LV end diastolic volume (LVEDV). The heart rapidly compensates by increasing LVEDV and end diastolic pressure (EDP), so that SV is increased toward normal. Figure 5–18*A* shows the effect on the PV relation. Physiologically, this process usually is likely accomplished by a component of vasoconstriction, venoconstriction that increases the diastolic pressure,[402] while arteriolar constriction maintains blood pressure when cardiac output is not totally restored. While SV may be normalized, measures of contractile function may not be fully restored.

Decreased lusitropy ("diastolic dysfunction") may occur secondary to myocardial hypertrophy involving either the contractile component (myocytes) or connective tissue. Alternatively, a decreased ability of Ca^{2+} reaccumulation within or elimination from the myocyte will depress lusitropy, frequently the first mechanical evidence of ischemia.[403] In either case ventricular compliance will be reduced, requiring a greater distending pressure to achieve the same LVEDV. The effect of such decreased compliance will be reduced LVEDV at any given LVEDP, which means that stroke volume will be reduced (Fig. 5–18*B*). If the LVEDV is restored by an increase in LVEDP, SV is restored. Frequently, a combination of both inotropic and lusitropic dysfunction is present in cardiac failure, resulting in markedly reduced SV. Therapeutic interventions to improve SV include attempts to decrease afterload (vasodilation), decrease compliance, and increase inotropy.

Hypertrophic Cardiomyopathy. Hypertrophic changes of the LV typically occur with both excess preload (volume overload) or excess afterload (pressure overload), resulting in both cellular hypertrophy and extensive remodeling of the ventricular architecture. Typical examples of such overload are aortic stenosis (AS) resulting in marked pressure overload, and mitral regurgitation (MR) resulting in diastolic volume overload. In both cases, there is a dramatic increase in SW of the ventricle, as indicated in Figure 5–18*C*. While pressure overload results in a marked increase in ventricular mass, the response to chronic volume overload has been noted to be far more variable. In a carefully controlled study in dogs, AS was found to cause increases in LV mass that par-

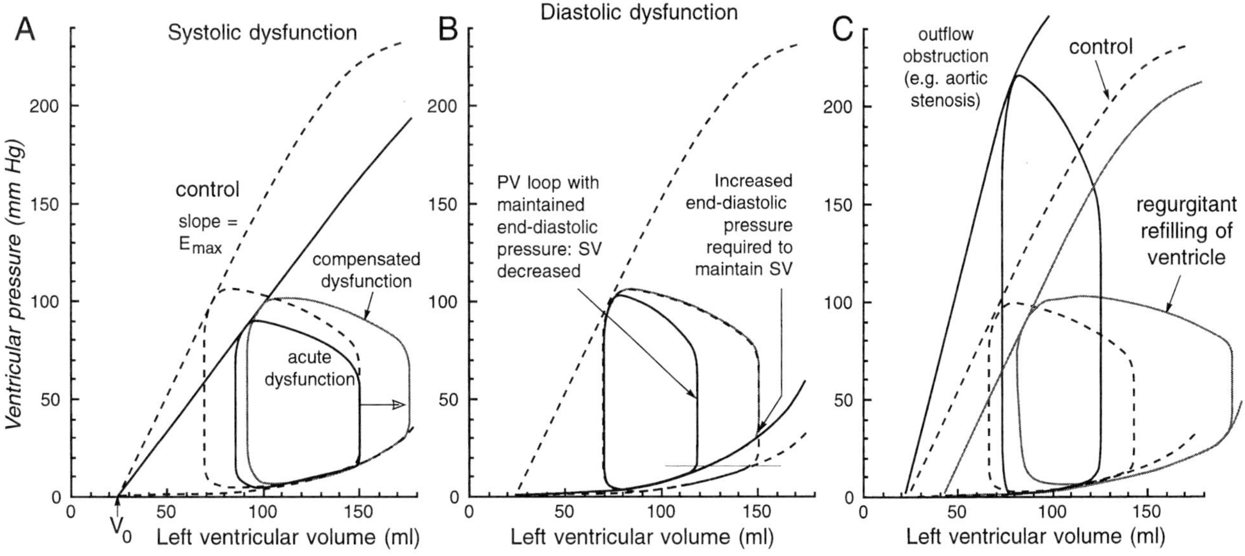

FIGURE **5–18.** Pressure-volume relationships in various settings. *A*, Systolic dysfunction results in a depression of the E_{max} and a decrease in stroke volume until compensation occurs and end-diastolic volume increases to restore stroke volume. *B*, When diastolic dysfunction occurs at the same filling pressure (indicated by the *fine horizontal line*) there will be less stroke volume that can be ejected. However, when end-diastolic pressure is increased to restore end-diastolic volume, then the stroke volume will be restored. *C*, Aortic stenosis. The systolic function is enhanced by the hypertrophy, but diastolic dysfunction will also be present. The increased afterload in diastolic dysfunction will then decrease stroke volume, although ventricular work will be markedly increased, as evident from the increased pressure-volume area. When there is regurgitant refilling of the ventricle, there is eventual compensation and an increase in stroke volume to permit ejection of the regurgitant blood.

alleled the SW, while a similar increase in SW caused by MR did not elicit LV hypertrophy comparable to that seen with AS.[404] The MR hypertrophy was associated with a decrease in circumferential shortening velocity and a decreased LV mass-volume ratio. The response to MR seems inappropriate compared to AS; an analysis of the PVA suggests that for the same SW, oxygen consumption would likely be greater in the AS group, which may constitute a greater hypertrophic stimulus.

Other Measures of Ventricular Function

Preload Recruitable Stroke Work. Since both SV and pressure are linear functions of LVEDV, their product, SW, will also be a linear function of LVEDV. Consequently, the ventricular function curve of Sarnoff will be linearized if LVSW is plotted against LVEDV instead of LVEDP, as predicted by Sarnoff.[392] Since the SW will increase when VED is greater (i.e., increased preload), and decrease with unloading, the SW-VED relation has been formalized as "preload recruitable stroke work" (PRSW).[405] The PRSW can be determined by a plot of the SW from successive PV loops obtained while preload (VED) is being altered. In a comparative study, Little and co-workers[406] examined the sensitivity of the ESPVR and the PRSW as measures of LV function. In addition, they compared the relation between maximum rate of pressure development (dP/dt) and VED (dP/dt_{max} − VED), another frequently employed isovolumic measure of LV performance.[394,407] The slope of the PRSW was the least variable at a constant inotropic state, while increased afterload caused a shift or greater variation in E_{max} of the ESPV relation and slope of the dP/dt_{max} − VED relations. In contrast, dP/dt_{max} − VED relation was the most sensitive measure of changes in contractility.[394,406] While ESPVR and PRSW are excellent measures of LV function, difficulty in assessing ventricular dimensions as opposed to pressure has prevented more widespread application, at least until the more widespread recent application of transesophageal echocardiography. As a consequence, ventricular workload and oxygen consumption have been estimated by other means such as the ventricular function curve.

Analysis of ventricular contractility is often separated into isovolumic (pre-ejection) and ejection phases of function. A variety of other measures used to describe ventricular function are listed in Table 5–6. Using an estimate of myocardial elastance, pre-ejection pressure measurements have been employed to estimate the maximum velocity of shortening (V_{max}) in the clinical setting.[112] However, V_{max} did not identify depressed ventricular function. Ejection phase indices, such as the mean velocity of circumferential shortening (V_{cf}), seem to be more accurate assessments of LV function.[408] Of the available measures, one of the most simply obtainable by ventriculography or echocardiography is the ejection fraction (i.e., 100% × SV/VED). Although sensitive to afterload, the ejection fraction is a practical and useful assessment of the ability of the heart to pump blood.

TABLE 5–6
Measurements of Myocardial Contractility*

Measures†	Comment
Isovolumic Phase Indices (IPI)	
(dP/dt)/P at 40 mm Hg pressure	Useful in acute changes of contractility. Not useful in evaluating basal contractility.
Maximum dP/dt	Dependent on timing of aortic valve opening. Useful in acute changes of contractility.
V_{max} (based on total pressure)	Decreases with increased preload or afterload. Not as useful as (dP/dt)/P(40) in acute changes. Useful in evaluating basal contractility.
V_{pm} [point of maximum (dP/dt)/P]	Most reliable IPI for evaluating basal contractility; dependent on preload and afterload at high levels of either.
V_{max} (based on developed pressure)	Useful in acute changes but little advantage over (dP/dt)/DP(40) or max dP/dt. Not useful in evaluating basal contractility.
Ejection Phase Indices (EPI)	
Stroke volume versus EDP Ventricular function curve (stroke work vs EDP)	Useful in acute changes of contractility if ventricular function curve obtained, but afterload sensitive. May not be useful in evaluating basal contractility.
Maximum acceleration of aortic blood flow	Dependent on afterload.
Ejection fraction	Dependent on afterload; useful in evaluating basal contractility when EDV is known.
Mean velocity of circumferential fiber shortening (V_{cf})	Afterload-dependent, and more sensitive than ejection fraction in evaluating basal contractility.
Mean normalized systolic ejection rate	Afterload-dependent. Less useful than mean V_{cf}.
Maximum chamber elastance (E_{max})	Useful in acute changes, but not nonlinear behavior; may complicate interpretation.

*Data from Strobeck JE, Sonnenblick EH: Pathophysiology of heart failure: Deficiency in cardiac contraction. In Cohn JN (ed): Drug Treatment in Heart Failure. Secaucus, NJ, Advanced Therapeutics Communications International, 1988, p 13.

†P is intraventricular pressure. *V* represents the velocity of shortening of the contractile elements (*V*CE), which in the case of the isovolumic indices of contraction is calculated using an estimate of stiffness (or series elastic modulus, the change in wall tension for a change in length) of ventricular muscle and dP/dt.[112]

Effects of Abnormal Conduction on Ventricular Function

The coordinated depolarization of the myocardium is important for the efficient mechanical function of the heart. Segmental wall motion abnormalities are observed with left bundle branch block (LBBB),[409] and rate-dependent LBBB reduces ejection fraction.[410] Ventricular pacing markedly alters the pattern of regional contraction causing reciprocal interaction of opposing myocardial regions, with volume sequestration and pressure dissipation in relatively inactive segments that are out of phase with the bulk of contracting myocardium, ultimately degrading global ventricular function.[411] If ventricular electrical activation is by right ventricular epicardial leads, instead of by the normal His-Purkinje pathway, the resulting contractions eject less blood[412] and have a decreased maximum LV dP/dt, but require increased oxygen consumption.[413]

Right Ventricular Function and Interventricular Interaction

The heart obviously operates as two side-by-side simultaneous (as opposed to reciprocating) pumps. While transient differences can exist, the outputs of the two pumps must be equal over more than a few beats, or congestion of either the pulmonary or systemic vascular beds will result. The right ventricle operates as a very-low-pressure pump, since the pulmonary circuit is a very-low-pressure system. In fact, over half of the RV free wall can be totally nonfunctional, and pulmonary flow and cardiac output are altered very little, although a greater initial ventricular volume (filling pressure) is needed. The RV does only about 11 to 17% of the work done by the LV, since it is pumping the same cardiac output against far lower pressures. In some ways, the septum primarily functions as part of the left ventricle and the adjacent low-pressure RV has little effect upon the LV. However, both clinically and experimentally when the RV is overloaded by elevation of pulmonary vascular resistance, the septum actually shifts leftward, decreasing LV function.[414,415]

Ventricular interdependence is augmented by the presence of the pericardium, which has important physiologic functions in the maintenance of normal biventricular filling.[416] RV filling and SV are particularly augmented by pericardiectomy.[417] However, Mangano et al.[418] noted that neither LV systolic function nor compliance are normally affected by its presence. As dilatation of the LV occurs, intrapericardial pressure limits RV filling and reduces forward flow to the lungs, possibly preventing pulmonary edema.[419] Shifts of the LV diastolic pressure-volume relationship are equal to changes in pericardial pressure and volume.[420] Thus, the role of the pericardium in the maintenance of normal ventricular systolic and diastolic function appears to be limited.[419] During pathologic conditions, the pericardium assumes more physiologic importance. Increased intrapericardial fluid (cardiac tamponade) decreases ventricular compliance and filling resulting in hypotension, decreased cardiac output, myocardial ischemia, and tachycardia. However, a vagally mediated depressive reflex is also operative, contributing further to the decreased cardiac output resulting from the presence of pericardial fluid.[421] Increased intrapericardial pressure results in an underfilled ventricle, which operates on the ascending limb of Starling's curve.

Effects of Intrathoracic Pressure

Changes in intrathoracic pressure (ITP) have multiple effects. Negative ITP increases the gradient for venous return, increases pulmonary vascular capacitance and decreases resistance, and increases the gradient against which the heart pumps blood systematically ("afterload").[422] Consequently, during normal spontaneous ventilation, the SV typically decreases ~20% from the mean with inspiration,[423] which may be explained by (1) pulmonary venous capacitance increases during inspiration to a greater extent than the increase in right heart venous return; (2) an effective increase in right ventricular filling pressure not present on the left side, which causes a slight shift in the septum which further reduces left ventricular filling; and (3) the additional increase in left ventricular afterload results in the significant decrease in LVSV. Due largely to the change in SV, arterial pressure varies with the respiratory cycle, typically decreasing approximately 6 mm Hg during inspiration. With passive expiration, SV is increased approximately 10% above the mean,[423] as the accumulated pulmonary blood fills the LV against a normal gradient. These changes are exaggerated with hypovolemia or in the presence of pericardial tamponade, causing pulsus paradoxus. The Müller maneuver is a maintained inspiratory effort against a closed airway. During such sustained negative ITP, LVEDV and ESV are both increased, with a net decrease in ejection fraction. When LV "afterload" is corrected for the negative ITP, the resulting increased LV transmural pressure correlates closely with LV function.[424] In patients with coronary artery disease, ventricular akinesis may be seen during the Müller maneuver. This finding may be due to increased wall stress increasing myocardial oxygen demand or increased LV transmural pressure decreasing motion in nonfunctional ventricular myocardium.[424] The net effect of these changes on LV function depends upon ventricular interdependence, heart rate, and contractility (position of heart on diastolic pressure-volume curve).

With positive ITP, the opposite changes occur. The initial increase in ITP augments LV ejection by decreasing the thoracic-systemic pressure gradient ("afterload"), while pulmonary venous return is briefly enhanced. However, with quiet positive-pressure ventilation at a normal rate (~15 breaths/min) in mask-ventilated volunteers, changes in LVSV with the respiratory cycle are small (<5%) compared to the much larger changes observed with spontaneous ventilation at the same rate.[423] The relatively rapid cycle of normal respiration prevents the hemodynamic consequences from becoming so large that major neural compensatory mechanisms are activated, although neural modulation of the cardiovascular system linked to respiratory rate is certainly present.[425] With sustained positive ITP the changes in hemodynamics are far greater and conspicuous as demonstrated by voluntary closing of the glottis during a forced expiration (the Valsalva maneuver). After the transient increase in LVSV and pulse pressure as blood is shifted from the pulmonary vessels (phase 1), the increased ITP reduces venous return to the right side of the heart, increases venous pressure in the head and extremities, and increases pulmonary vascular resistance, reducing RV ejection. LVEDV is thus reduced by both a septal shift and decreased filling pressure, reducing SV (phase 2). Compensatory reflex changes intervene, however, in the presence of total autonomic blockade, mean blood pressure (BP) and pulse pressure decrease by 30% and almost 50%, respectively.[426]

The cardiovascular changes observed with sustained positive-pressure ventilation employed clinically may be more profound. Perhaps due in part to underlying changes in lung compliance that alter pulmonary vascular behavior, positive-pressure ventilation has far greater effects on LVSV.[423] It is clear that positive end-expiratory pressure (PEEP) has marked consequences on LV function, decreasing SV and cardiac output. Although decreased myocardial contractility may contribute, the most prominent effect of PEEP is an increase in RVEDV and V_{ES}, with a decrease in LV distensibility and LVEDV and SV.[427] The increased RVEDV shifts the septum leftward, impinging on LV volume.[414]

Abnormalities in Cardiac Conduction

Arrhythmias represent abnormal behavior of the ion channel fluxes, which result in abnormal impulse conduction (conduction block, re-entry, reflection) or abnormal impulse initiation (abnormal automaticity or triggered rhythms), or possibly both (parasystole, phase 4 block).[428] The major categories, each with their own particular membrane micropathology and mechanism, are re-entry, triggered activity, and automaticity.[429]

Abnormal Automaticity

While the SA and AV nodes are typically automatic, any cardiac tissue has the potential to spontaneously depolarize to threshold at a regular rate. Automaticity may in many cases represent the appearance of the dormant pacemaker current (I_f). Due to partial depolarization because of damage or drug/hormonal stimulation, other cardiac tissue may achieve a rate superseding the normal pacemaking tissue, particularly in settings where the normal pacemaker is depressed. Normally the depolarizing current is insufficient to bring the tissue to the AP threshold, at least in ventricular tissue. However, similar to early afterdepolarizations, in situations of reduced resting conductance, the inward I_f current may be sufficient to induce ectopic beats.

Triggered Activity

Abnormal potentials, termed *afterdepolarizations*, follow closely on a previous normal AP, occurring either with phase 3 repolarization (early afterdepolarizations [EADs]) or after complete repolarization (late or delayed afterdepolarizations [DADs]). In contractile tissue, these depolarizations may be accompanied by a small amount of tension development or aftercontractions. However, the mechanisms of these two forms of triggered activity differ markedly.

EARLY AFTERDEPOLARIZATIONS

EADs arise during the late plateau or early phase 3 of AP depolarization.[428] They appear to occur under circumstances in which the resting K^+ conductance is blocked and in which Ca channels are not fully inactivated.[429] Circumstances in which this activity is observed include low or K^+-free medium, which inactivates G_{K1}, or blockade of G_{K1} by other means.[429–431] Slowly conducted APs arise that conduct to more fully repolarized regions and can then lead to a propagated ectopic beat. Such a decrease in K^+ conductance may explain the repolarization abnormality that occurs in the long QT interval syndrome, which is associated with torsades de pointes ventricular arrhythmia and sudden death.[430,432] Increasing K^+ conductance with potassium channel activators may prove to be beneficial in these circumstances.[433] While blockade of G_{K1} can be responsible, it seems likely that blockade of other K^+ currents can contribute to EADs. For example, the torsades de pointes rhythm observed with quinidine, sotalol, and bupivacaine overdose appear to be due to inhibition of I_K or I_{to}.[434,435] Furthermore, a window current of L-type calcium current has been recently identified, which may contribute.

DELAYED AFTERDEPOLARIZATIONS

The best present explanation for DADs involves "overload" of the sarcoplasmic reticulum (SR) with Ca^{2+}.[428,429] Situations involving DADs usually include increased Ca^{2+} entry and or increased SR Ca^{2+} uptake as occurs with very rapid beating rates or β-adrenergic stimulation. Ca^{2+} overload and DADs also occur with excessive cardiac glycosides poisoning the sodium pump, so that a decreased Na^+ gradient is no longer able to eliminate Ca^{2+} from the cell. The SR accumulates the Ca^{2+} until it can store no more. Once overloaded, the SR spontaneously releases Ca^{2+} into the myoplasm. The pattern of Ca^{2+} release in DADs is associated with a wave-like release of Ca^{2+} in the cell, while in the case of EADs the second Ca^{2+} transient occurs uniformly throughout the cell.[436] The released Ca^{2+} is then eliminated by the Na-Ca exchanger, which in turn results in a net inward depolarizing current (three Na^+ in for one Ca^{2+} out).[437–439] If the inward current causes sufficient depolarization to reach threshold, activation of an AP occurs. Such APs can result in a vicious cycle of continued rapid rhythms and continuing Ca^{2+} entry and overload. Such triggered tachyarrhythmias are thought to account for many ventricular tachycardias associated with acute myocardial infarction, right ventricular outflow tract tachycardias, and certain atrial tachycardias.[428,440] Obviously, prevention of such tachycardias must be ultimately directed at prevention of Ca^{2+} overload. In this regard, the activation of K_{ATP} channels appears to have antiarrhythmic activity, which may involve attenuation of late afterdepolarization, as well as early afterdepolarizations and abnormal automaticity.[279]

Re-entry

Since the myocardium, either atrial or ventricular, is an electrical syncytium, any mass of the tissue, microscopic or its whole, represents a potential circular path in which membrane potentials may be conducted. Normally, this tissue is depolarized rapidly and uniformly, and then repolarizes with relative uniformity. Usually, after sustained cardiac depolarization, it is difficult to initiate another propagated depolarization. Re-entry is a phenomenon of recurring and self-perpetuating depolarization around a circuit (also termed a "circus" movement). Re-entry requires an area of one-way conduction or unidirectional block and a circumscribed conduction path around the block, so that the AP can be reintroduced and propagate retrograde through the blocked area. Although normal conduction velocity in a long circuit may support re-entry, an area of slowed conduction (due to damaged tissue, K^+ accumulation, ischemia) is typically present.[428]

Unidirectional block arises when a nonuniform injury exists in a conducting pathway, such as with graduated injury in one direction and an abrupt injury in the other. Conduction (from the "forward" direction) will fail when the depolarization enters an area of increasing injury or damage in which the depolarizing current dissipates before it reaches healthy tissue from which an AP can propagate. Conduction may succeed (from the "reverse" direction) when depolarization enters an abrupt region of injury, because the high density of depolarizing current does not have a region of partially injured tissue in which to dissipate before it depolarizes tissue from which an AP will propagate.[429]

Re-entry can exist with circuits of variable size. Clinical settings thought to involve re-entry are[428]: (1) atrial tachycardias, flutter, and fibrillation, with circuits several centimeters in diameter; (2) sinus node and AV node re-entrant tachycardias, which may involve microscopic circuits within the nodal tissue itself; (3) AV re-entry tachycardia due to an accessory AV pathway; (4) bundle branch re-entrant tachycardia; and (5) ventricular tachycardia, which is thought to involve small (mm) circuits in damaged portions of the Purkinje system, endocardium, or ventricular wall.

Slowed Conduction. Because almost all the sodium channels inactivate with depolarization, a brief period of at least partial repolarization (negative to ~ -50 mV) is necessary before they return to their activatible form. The period during which a second propagated AP cannot be elicited is the absolute (or effective) refractory period (ARP). Once repolarization is negative to -50 or -60 mV, a second AP may be elicited, but due to limited availability of working Na channels, dV/dt and conduction velocity will be low. This period of time is the relative refractory period. Following repolarization, sufficient numbers of noninactivated (or activatible) Na channels only gradually accumulate with phase 3 repolarization, so that 10 to 50 msec are required before the normal density of working sodium channels is available to support normal conduction. In the presence of ischemia, hypoxia, and pericellular hyperkalemia, the increased conductance (due to K_{ATP} and Na^+-activated K channels) and partial depolarization will lead to most Na channels being inactivated. However, if sufficient active Ca channels are present, they may contribute to depolarization at more positive membrane potentials. If depolarizing current arrives during repolarization, a few activatible Na channels can combine with Ca channels and a slowly conducted AP can occur through the tissue, which may contribute to re-entry circuits and dysrhythmias. Even in the early stages of ventricular fibrillation, Na^{2+} currents still[441] appear to contribute depolarizing current. In the presence of hypoxia, ischemia, and/or hyperkalemia, the effect of β-adrenergic stimulation may be significant in terms of its ability to restore APs by generating a larger number of activatible Ca channels.

Normally the various K^+ currents ensure that depolarization and repolarization occur in a coordinated and temporally unified fashion, and provide considerable electrophysiologic stability so that it is difficult to induce sustained tachycardia in a normal heart. When APs in one region of the heart are shortened, leaving others unaltered, this creates greater temporal dispersion in AP duration. When such temporal dispersion is produced experimentally in ventricular tissue, tachycardia can be induced by an appropriate single stimulation.[442] When ischemia or hypoxia results in AP shortening due to activation of K_{ATP} channels, portions of myocardium may be repolarized at times when other areas may remain depolarized.[443] In hypertrophied myocardium, greater dispersion of refractory periods can be demonstrated and is associated with greater VF vulnerability.[444] An additional change that can increase the dispersion of AP duration is hypothermia.[445] If an adequate electrical pathway exists, then depolarizing current may flow to the more repolarized region and initiate an AP. When this occurs, a depolarization cyclical pattern can result.

To prevent such temporal dispersion of AP duration, the use of K channel–blocking agents has been suggested,[446] and has proven to have beneficial effects in certain models.[279,444,447,448] However, the specific potassium channel to be blocked is important. It is clear that under certain conditions, reduced K^+ conductance can lead to increased excitability and triggered dysrhythmias,[429–431] so that decreasing G_{K1}, which may lengthen the terminal aspect of the AP, may have proarrhythmic effects. Likewise, while blockade of K_{ATP} channels may have antiarrhythmic actions by decreasing AP dispersion, but by preventing the metabolic sparing that occurs with K_{ATP} channel activation, K_{ATP} channel blockade may worsen Ca^{2+} overload and be proarrhythmic.

The Vasculature

The vasculature constitutes that tissue which directs and controls the flow of blood ejected from the heart to all the organs of the body, including the heart itself. The cardiac output in the human body at rest is typically distributed as follows: brain, 12%; coronary, 4%; liver, 24%; kidneys, 20%; muscle, 23%; skin, 6%; and intestines, 8%. In contrast to the variety of organs and vasculatures supplied by systemic circulation, the pulmonary circulation is a far more uniform but distinctly controlled vascular path.

The Arteries

The wall of all arteries and arterioles possess similar constituents. From the inside out, there is the endothelium, which rests on a basement membrane; the media, which is comprised largely of vascular smooth muscle (VSM) but also includes a major component of the elastin and collagen fibers; and the adventitia or loose connective tissue outer layer, which merges with the surrounding tissue. Although muscle constitutes the greater proportion of vessel mass in most vessels, the elastin content of the aorta and major arteries has led to their classification as elastic arteries, as opposed to the more distal muscular arteries. The major arterial conductance vessels absorb and store part of the energy of the ejected blood, so that the energy can be redistributed over time as maintained perfusion pressure during diastole. The response of vascular tissue depends upon its diameter and its organ of origin. Consequently, experiments in aortic rings may not necessarily apply to the microvasculature.

By carefully controlling the circumferential tension, and thus circumference, smaller arteries and particularly the arterioles (100- to 25-μm diameter) control the amount of blood that flows from the larger arteries into the various organs. The flow within the organ, the microcirculation, is controlled by the precapillary sphincters (<30-μm diameter), which control the microscopic distribution from the arterioles into the various capillaries that permeate an organ. The total tissue blood flow in a given vascular bed is a function of the effective perfusion pressure and vascular resistance. Effective perfusion pressure is the difference between arterial and venous pressure across the vascular bed. Organs that autoregulate to keep blood flow constant in the face of changes in perfusion pressure include the cerebral, renal, coronary, hepatic arterial, intestinal, and muscle circulation. The total peripheral resistance is the sum of the reciprocal resistance (conductance) of all of the organs. That is:

$$(R_{total})^{-1} = (R_{brain})^{-1} + (R_{heart})^{-1} + R_{skin})^{-1}$$
$$+ (R_{intestine})^{-1} + (R_{muscle})^{-1} + \text{etc.},$$

where $(R_{organ})^{-1}$ is the vascular conductance.

Capillaries

While the arteries and veins serve as conduits for the blood, it is at the capillaries that the actual exchange of oxygen, nutrients, and waste products takes place. The capillaries are tubes of basement membrane lined with endothelial cells 0.1 to 0.3 μm in thickness, having an average diameter of 5 to 8 μm and highly variable lengths from 10 to 100 μm. Depending upon the tissue, the capillary wall may show considerable variability, with either continuous, fenestrated, or discontinuous architecture. Fenestrated capillaries, which are typical of the gastrointestinal mucosa, have a relatively high permeability to water and small molecules. Discontinuous capillaries, which permit transit of cells with relative ease, are located in such tissues as the bone marrow, spleen, and liver sinusoids. Transit of larger molecules may occur either directly or by active transport through endothelial cell vesicles. The typical density of capillaries is approximately 1,000/mm^2; however, it may be extremely variable, again depending upon the tissue. The average intercapillary distance in skeletal muscle, heart, and brain is 10 to 15 μm.[389]

Due to their high density, blood flow through the capillaries is in the range of 0.5 to 1.5 mm/sec, considerably slower than in the major vessels. The blood flowing through capillaries typically has a hematocrit of as little as half that of normal blood because the plasma is preferentially segregated to the edges of arterioles, and a greater portion of this is skimmed off to flow through the capillaries, providing for a dilution of the red blood cells. The mean pressure in the capillaries is typically 26 to 38 mm Hg but varies considerably depending upon the tissue and on the distance along its length. The lower pressure in the pulmonary circulation means that the average pulmonary capillary pressure is approximately 9 mm Hg. The transfer of fluid across the capillary wall is defined by the Starling hypothesis, which states that the efflux of fluid from or influx into the capillary is based on the net difference between the perfusion pressure and the osmotic pressure of plasma. In the proximal end of the capillary, which has a somewhat higher perfusion pressure, fluid enters the interstitium. At the distal end of the capillary, where perfusion pressure may typically be 10 mm Hg lower, fluid is resorbed into the capillary. This is aided by the fact that the capillary permeability appears to be higher at the distal end.[389]

The Veins

Venules and veins of increasingly larger dimensions return blood to the heart. Since the veins do not have to sustain a substantial pressure gradient, their requirement for an elastic component is small. However, VSM is present and important in providing the capacitance role provided by these vessels. Normally, the small and large veins contain about two thirds of the total blood volume. Contractile function in these vessels permits large volumes of blood to be shifted to the heart when needed.[389]

The Lymphatics

As noted, of the blood that passes through a tissue capillary network, a small fraction is filtered through the capillary endothelium into tissue. About 90% is resorbed into the capillary; the remaining 10% remains in the interstitium of the tissue. This colorless fluid of low protein content, the lymph, is transported back into the circulation via a system of fine vessels composed of only a single layer of endothelial cells on a basement membrane. The lymphatic capillaries are permeable to molecules of various sizes, and are also able to admit particles as large as 25 μm in diameter, such as chylomicrons from the intestinal tract, as well as bacteria. These lymph capillaries come together to form larger trunks, which transport the fluid to the lymph nodes through which it flows in a plexus of channels, being filtered and monitored for the presence of immunologically active material. The larger efferent lymph vessels unite and ultimately enter the thoracic and right lymphatic ducts, which then empty into the innominate veins. The total lymphatic flow in humans is approximately 2 to 4 L/day, roughly the amount of total plasma present in the vascular space, but representing only about 0.04% of the daily cardiac output. In settings of increased muscular activity, increased venous pressure, or inflammatory reactions the flow will increase. Normally, approximately 25 to 50% of the total lymphatic flow comes from the liver, while the renal, cardiac, and pulmonary lymphatics each contribute approximately 3 to 10% of total lymph duct drainage.[389] Lymphatic drainage in the lungs is particularly important, since with high pulmonary capillary pressures excessive fluid loss into interstitium results in pulmonary edema when the pressure exceeds 20 to 25 mg Hg.

Vascular Smooth Muscle Stimulation-Contraction Coupling

Unlike skeletal muscle, in which a nerve ending releases ACh onto closely juxtaposed postsynaptic receptors to cause an immediate (<1 msec) depolarization and twitch, VSM has an array of receptors that respond to ligands from various sources with a much slower time course (>0.5 second). Depending upon whether a specific receptor is present on the cell and facing the appropriate surface, the particular VSM will respond by an increase or decrease in tone to thereby control vessel diameter, resistance to blood flow, and nutrient delivery to the tissue. A wide variety of neural and hormonal transmitters are known to activate contraction of VSM. While each of these various agents appears to be binding to distinct receptors, the structure of which is known in many cases by cloning of the responsible genetic material, the mechanism of activation is largely identical. Binding of transmitter to its respective receptor typically initiates contraction by activation of a cascade mediated by G_q protein. As indicated for the myocardium in Figure 5–10, G_q activates phospholipase C, which in turn hydrolyzes the membrane phospholipid PIP_2 to IP_3 and DAG. IP_3 controls Ca^{2+} release.

Regulation of Vascular Smooth Muscle $[Ca^{2+}]_i$

While Ca^{2+} also activates tension development in VSM, it does so by a process distinct from that previously described for striated muscle (see Fig. 5–19). Although APs can be elicited when K^+ conductance is decreased, transmitted APs are not a prominent feature of VSM activation.[449] While many of the electrophysiologic and cellular control mechanisms described for the heart apply to the VSM, different mechanisms assume prominence. Unlike cardiac muscle in which Ca^{2+} entry serves to activate Ca^{2+} release from the SR, intracellular $[Ca^{2+}]$ is determined far more by entry of extracellular Ca^{2+} and by intracellular messenger control of Ca^{2+} stores.

The IP_3 Receptor. Following receptor binding, the IP_3 produced by PLC plays a critical role as an intracellular second messenger, which binds to its own specific receptor.[450] Similar in structure to the ryanodine receptor, the IP_3 receptor is a quatrefoil channel molecule present on the sarcoplasmic reticulum of VSM. Upon the binding of IP_3, Ca^{2+} passes through the IP_3 receptor channel from the intercellular stores into the myoplasm. In addition, this channel is modulated by Ca^{2+}, as well as by phosphorylation by a variety of intercellular protein kinases. In smooth muscle, it represents a major pathway by which Ca^{2+} is released to activate tension development.[451] Ca release channels (ryanodine receptors) are also present in vascular smooth muscle; however, their role is incompletely understood. In certain studies the Ca^{2+} store, which is controlled by IP_3 receptors and ryanodine receptors, appears to overlap; however, this has not been a consistent finding. As in cardiac SR, a Ca^{2+}-ATPase is present on the SR of VSM and is responsible for reaccumulating Ca^{2+}.

Voltage-Operated Ca Channels. While the representation and regulation of the ion channels in VSM is in many ways similar to that of heart, VSM does not have a prominent resting K^+ conductance or inward rectifier current. Consequently, cells are typically less polarized (resting V_m ~50 mV) and do not demonstrate physiologically relevant Na channels or fast action potentials. Furthermore, unlike taenia coli of the intestine, which undergoes rhythmic contractions, VSM does not usually exhibit action potentials except with specific pharmacologic stimulation.[449] As in cardiac cells, although T-type channels are present, dihydropyridine-sensitive L-type channels represent the predominant type. With stimulation of specific receptors, depolarization may occur and activate L-type Ca channels, which may provide additional depolarizing current in addition to Ca^{2+} entry into the cell. Since the membrane potential determines the number of open Ca channels, its regulation is of critical importance to modulate Ca^{2+} entry.[452] Such carefully regulated Ca^{2+} entry appears to play a prominent role in maintaining vascular tone. The dihydropyridine compounds (e.g., nifedipine) are remarkably active in VSM, since these drugs bind to and down-regulate the L-type Ca channels more strongly at more positive membrane potentials.

By virtue of their prominent role in regulating the membrane potential, K channels have a critical role in regulating the entry and removal of Ca^{2+} from the vascular myocyte. The resting K^+ conductance of VSM is very small so that Ca^{2+}-activated K ("big" K_{Ca} [BK]) and K_{ATP} channels play a more significant role. When hyperpolarization occurs secondary to K_{ATP} and/or BK channel activation, the Ca channels will inactivate and less Ca^{2+} will enter. Conversely, when K channels are less active or nonspecific cation channels are activated,

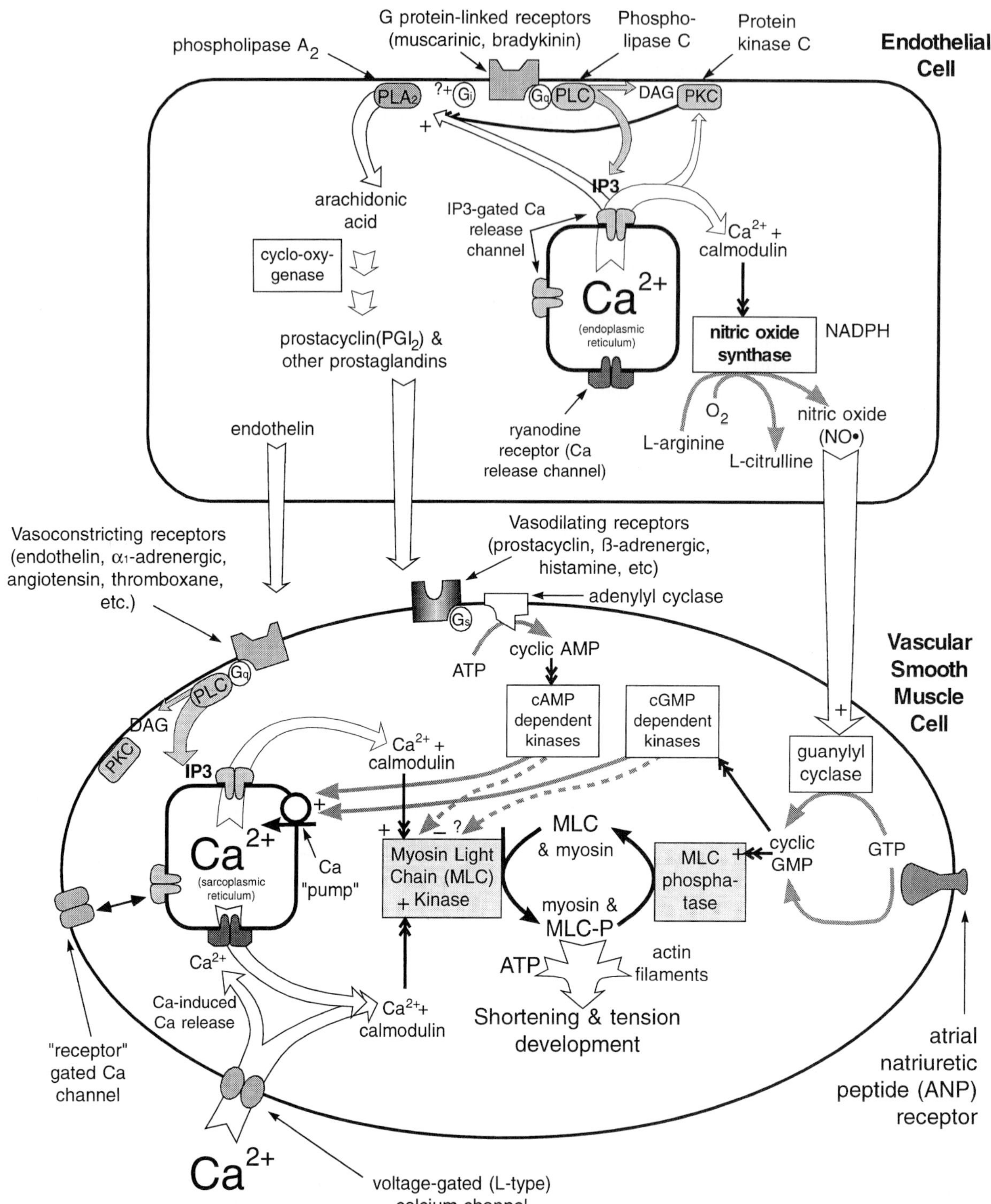

FIGURE **5–19.** Endothelial and vascular smooth muscle function. Both cells have internal stores of Ca^{2+} whose release is gated by production of inositol trisphosphate (IP_3). In each case binding of agonist to specific receptors activate phospholipase C (PLC) via the guanine nucleotide protein G_q (alpha). In the endothelial cell Ca^{2+} then binds to calmodulin to activate nitric oxide (NO) synthase. NO can diffuse to the vascular smooth muscle and modulate its behavior by activating guanylyl cyclase. In addition to NO, phospholipase A_2 may also be activated either by a G-protein–linked pathway, or by the action of Ca^{2+} and phosphokinase C (PKC). Production of arachidonic acid results in reproduction of prostacyclin, which may also cause relaxation of vascular smooth muscle. In addition, endothelial cell activation may cause release of the vasoconstriction peptide endothelin. In the vascular smooth muscle cell, activation of PLC results in IP_3 formation, which activates release of intracellular Ca^{2+} stores. Ca^{2+} then binds to calmodulin, which activates myosin light chain (MLC) kinase, which in turn phosphorylates MLC, so that myosin interacts with actin to generate tension and/or shortening. Modulation of the phosphorylation state of MLC may be decreased by activation of MLC phosphatase, as well as by inhibition of MLC kinase by the cyclic nucleotide–dependent kinases as indicated. The cyclic nucleotide–dependent kinases may also activate the Ca^{2+} pump, which will decrease free Ca^{2+} in the cell and thereby depress MLC kinase. Depolarization of the cell may result in direct entry of Ca^{2+}, which may then activate release of Ca^{2+} from the sarcoplasmic reticulum (SR) by ryanodine receptors (Ca^{2+} release channels located also in these cells). IP_3-gated channels in the SR may also feedback and may be responsible for the phenomenon of "receptor-gated" Ca^{2+} entry described in vascular smooth muscle.

then partial depolarization will open L-type channels and enhance Ca^{2+} entry. As oxygen delivery to an area is decreased and ATP in the vascular myocyte decreases, decreased concentration may permit the channel to open, hyperpolarizing the cell and resulting in relaxation. In addition, this channel and the stoichiometry of ATP regulation may be strongly modified by various cellular modulatory systems, particularly G proteins and the PKCs, which can change the responsiveness of the system. For example, the vasoconstricting action of neuropeptide Y, α-adrenergic, serotonergic, and histaminergic stimulation can inhibit arteriolar K_{ATP} channels via a PKC pathway.[453] Activators of K_{ATP} channels, in contrast, have distinct vasodilating actions.[454] However, since most of these studies defining the K_{ATP} channel make use of the sulfonylurea compound glibenclamide, which has been shown to be imperfectly selective at higher concentrations,[455] such results should be interpreted with caution. Similarly, a K_{ATP}-activated channel that is relatively insensitive to glibenclamide has recently been described in portal vein,[456] and its role remains to be completely defined.

"Receptor-Operated" Ca Channels. It has long been recognized that Ca^{2+} entry appears to be activated by receptor activation in the absence of distinct depolarization, and "receptor-operated" Ca channels (ROCs) have been postulated. The case has been made strongly by some that many characteristics attributed to ROC in VSM may be explained by modulation of the voltage-operated Ca channels (VOCs).[452] For example, protein kinase has been demonstrated to increase the current through L-type Ca channels,[457] although this has yet to be documented in VSM per se. However, it appears that the state of Ca^{2+} loading of the internal stores can modulate Ca^{2+} entry. When the intracellular Ca^{2+} stores are depleted, Ca^{2+} entry via this pathway is enhanced.[458,459] Although the exact mechanism remains to be elucidated, there clearly appears to be Ca^{2+} entry that becomes activated once the internal stores have been activated by IP_3. While IP_3 does not itself appear to be the activator, its metabolite, IP_4, has been suggested as a candidate to gate Ca^{2+} entry.[458] Nevertheless, this Ca^{2+}-store–modulated entry fulfills many of the characteristics of ROC, and certainly plays a critical role in maintaining VSM activation.

VARIATIONS IN EC COUPLING

It is clear that both Ca^{2+} entry and release of intracellular Ca^{2+} stores can provide a major component of activator Ca^{2+} in VSM. Indeed, depending on the tissue and the size of the vessel, the VSM may use primarily released internal stores, or may be activated by Ca^{2+} entry from outside of the cell. Major vessels such as the aorta appear to be much more reliant on internal stores, while certain smaller peripheral vessels are much more sensitive to Ca^{2+} entry. The latter have much greater sensitivity to calcium entry blockers, which may be the reason these agents are so effective in decreasing vascular resistance.[460]

Regulation of Myosin Activity

Unlike striated muscle in which Ca^{2+} binding to troponin C seems to act very much like a switch to turn on tension development, the interaction of VSM myofibrils involves a modulated enzyme system controlling myosin activity. Activation of myosin interaction occurs when a small myosin-associated protein subunit, the myosin regulatory light chain (MRLC), is phosphorylated, which then permits myosin interaction with actin. The degree of phosphorylation of MRLC is controlled in part by MLC kinase (MLCK). When myoplasmic Ca^{2+} is increased, it complexes with the Ca^{2+}-binding protein calmodulin (CaM), and the Ca^{2+}–CaM complex activates MLCK. MLCK is itself regulated, with phosphorylation by cAMP-dependent kinase and CaMK II causing decreased Ca^{2+}-CaM affinity and thereby decreasing Ca^{2+} sensitivity.

MECHANISMS OF SUSTAINED CONTRACTION

An important characteristic of VSM is its ability to maintain a high level of force, but with a decreased rate of cross-bridge cycling and consequently less ATP consumption. In order to attain rapid onset and offset of tension, skeletal and cardiac muscle consume considerable ATP, cycling large quantities of Ca^{2+} to activate a rapidly responsive but energy-expensive mechanism. In contrast, VSM can operate with a far slower response time, which permits cellular economy by utilizing far less energy. At least two mechanisms permit this sustained activity.

Phosphatase Inhibition. In addition, the degree of MLC phosphorylation and myosin activity is also controlled "downstream" by phosphatases that dephosphorylate MLC. If such phosphatases are inactivated, as appears to be the case with certain α_1-adrenoreceptor stimulations, then even if myoplasmic Ca^{2+} levels decline to near normal, the MLC will remain phosphorylated and permit ongoing tension generation. This separate G-protein–controlled process has been termed "calcium sensitization," and may play a prominent role in ongoing physiologic activation and maintenance of vascular tone.

The Latch Mechanism. One mechanism to sustain tension at a given length is for cross-bridges to remain intact. Murphy and associates have proposed that if MRLC is dephosphorylated while attached, the detachment rate of myosin from actin is greatly decreased.[461] As a consequence, tone can be maintained in the absence of the continuous cross-bridge cycling, but at the expense of rapid shortening. Such an explanation accounts for the markedly lower energy consumption of smooth muscle in comparison to striated muscle.

Control of Vascular Tone

The blood flow within any particular organ of the body is a function of the perfusion pressure within the vascular system, divided by the vascular resistance within that organ. The vascular resistance will be determined by the degree of VSM activation, which is the result of five major mechanisms: (1) intrinsic response to stretch, (2) transmitter or autocoid substances released by adjacent endothelial cells, (3) transmitters released from neuronal fibers at the adventitial surface or intramurally, (4) substances released from the surrounding tissue, and (5) circulating factors. These various controlling mechanisms provide sometimes synergistic and sometimes antagonistic influences on the vascular tone, which controls blood flow. While it would be tempting to delineate these agents as either vasoconstrictors or vasodilators, this is not always possible. For example, ACh applied to smooth muscle directly elicits a contractile response, while when given in the circulation, the response will be vasodilation, because of its activation of NO synthesis by endothelium and its action on the VSM. It is clear that depending upon the density of receptors for a particular ligand present on VSM versus EC and the source of the ligand, the *net* response to a particular stimulus may be constriction (α_1-adrenoceptors) or dilation (M_2 muscarinic) of the vessel.

Control by the Endothelium

Over the last decade the critical role of the endothelium in regulating the tone of vascular smooth muscle has been recognized, as illustrated in Figure 5–19. The role of endothelium-derived relaxing factor (EDRF), now identified as NO,[462,463] as well as endothelins and arachidonic acid derivatives (eicosanoids) in modulating the response of VSM has been the subject of intense investigation.

NITRIC OXIDE PRODUCTION

Perhaps surprising is that many of the subcellular processes that regulate Ca^{2+} in VSM to control tension also apply to the largely Ca^{2+}-mediated regulation of NO production in the EC. Since NO initiates relaxation, activation of Ca^{2+} elevation in VSM and EC initiates counteracting mechanisms, but it is unlikely that such counteracting measures are activated simultaneously by the same receptors on each cell.[464]

NO is synthesized from the free amino acid L-arginine[465] by a heme-containing enzyme called NO synthase (NOS), which normally exists in the cytoplasm of EC.[466] NOS requires a variety of cofactors, but the major physiologic control mechanism appears to be its activation by a rise in $[Ca^{2+}]_i$, caused by extracellular Ca^{2+} entry and/or intracellular Ca^{2+} release.[463] The major release of Ca^{2+} stores appears to be mediated by the receptor G_q protein-PLC-PKC-IP_3 pathway. The Ca^{2+} entry appears to be mediated by Ca channels that are regulated by internal stores. When internal stores are emptied, Ca^{2+} entry is activated,[467] similar to effects seen in VSM. Because such entry is not via voltage-dependent channels, such Ca^{2+} entry is actually enhanced by maintaining the cell in a polarized state by activation of K channels. By maintaining more hyperpolarized cells, a larger gradient is maintained to drive Ca^{2+} entry and NOS activation.[468] Recently, the molecular[469] and functional[470] presence of a ryanodine receptor–gated Ca^{2+} pool has also been demonstrated in endothelium. Clearly, such a CICR pathway could also amplify increases in $[Ca^{2+}]_i$ and presumably increase NO production, but its exact role remains to be defined. Regulation and modulation of NOS is critical to control of vascular tone by NO and remains to be fully elucidated. However, NOS appears to exhibit negative feedback control by NO itself, which serves to depress its ongoing activity.[471]

A number of receptor types and responses that cause relaxation have been localized to the endothelium and found to be mediated by Ca^{2+}-CaM–dependent activation of NOS. In addition to the classically studied ACh-induced relaxation, bradykinin and ATP also vasodilate via specific G_q-linked BK and P_{2Y} receptors, respectively. The vasocilating action of isoproterenol via β-ARs also appears to be mediated, at least in part, via NO production.[472] Furthermore, stimulation of adenylate cyclase in EC and subsequent production of cAMP may amplify the Ca^{2+} signal and enhance synthesis of NO.[473] Such mechanisms provide pathways in which different ligands and receptors (or one ligand and multiple receptors) might generate a potent vasodilating response. As with the other aspects of VSM regulation, there is considerable heterogeneity in expression of NO-mediated regulation, with certain vascular beds demonstrating far greater blockade of relaxation in the presence of NOS inhibition.[474] Volatile anesthetics may also influence this process, since they are able to depress the intracellular rise in Ca^{2+} activated by such agents as bradykinin.[475]

Guanylyl Cyclase Regulation. Most of the effects of NO appear to be mediated by its diffusion into the VSM cell and, as previously noted for cardiocytes, activation of a cytosolic (soluble) heterodimeric heme-containing enzyme (guanylyl cyclase) that converts GTP to cGMP. The regulation of cGMP production controls a variety of cell process via cGMP-dependent protein kinases (PKGs), PDEs, and ion channel proteins. For example, GMP appears to mediate activation of the Na-Ca exchange in VSM cells, which will result in decreased Ca^{2+} stores to activate contraction.[247] Phospholamban of VSM is phosphorylated by PKG, resulting in disinhibition of the SR Ca^{2+}-ATPase and accumulation of Ca^{2+} into the SR of the VSM.[248] PKG-mediated phosphorylation of IP_3 receptors also appears to result in decreased Ca^{2+} release, while additional effects may be mediated by actions on PLC, G proteins, and contractile proteins.

cGMP-Independent Actions. NO is a reactive free radical and as such may have a variety of potential sites of action, some of which may be by virtue of its ability to form Fe-NO complexes with both heme and nonheme iron-containing proteins. Recently, it has been shown to directly activate Ca-activated K channels, an effect that would hyperpolarize VSM and thereby decrease Ca^{2+} entry through voltage-gated channels, thereby reducing vascular tone.[476] In addition to relaxation and K channel activation mediated by NO, another distinct hyperpolarization has been shown to accompany endothelial activation. Even in the presence of NOS blockade by L-arginine analogs, a transmitter that can activate hyperpolarized VSM has been described, termed endothelium-derived hyperpolarizing factor (EDHF).

Flow-Dependent Regulation. Increases in flow of fluid through a vessel cause dilation, and such flow-dependent decreases in vascular tone appear to be mediated by NO. The increased shear stress caused by increased flow along the endothelial membrane appears to activate EC K channels.[477] Such activation maintains a more negative intracellular potential so that the gradient for Ca^{2+} to enter the cells is maintained. Since the Ca^{2+} channels of endothelial cells are not of the voltage-gated type, more Ca^{2+} enters to activate NOS and increase NO production.

PROSTACYCLIN

Products of arachidonic acid metabolism also have a prominent role in controlling vascular tone. While there are a number of active arachidonate metabolites, the most prominent in endothelium is PGI_2 or prostacyclin, which via G_s protein activates adenylate cyclase and induces relaxation, at least in part by activation of the SR Ca^{2+}-ATPase.

ENDOTHELINS

In addition to its potent vasodilating modulation of VSM, endothelial cells also secrete the endothelins. These four 21-amino-acid peptides (ET-1, ET-2, ET-3, and ET-β or vasoactive intestinal contractor) represent a family of potent vasoconstricting agents, with additional mitogenic and neuroendocrine functions.[478] These peptides are synthesized from large precursors (e.g., preproET-1, 203 aa), but have a very similar hairpin loop with polar amino acids. These peptides bind to specific G_q-linked receptors that mediate their effects by activating release of IP_3-receptor–gated Ca^{2+} stores. Attenuation of VSM responses to endothelin may have considerable therapeutic potential. A new endothelin inhibitor (Ro 46-2005) has been demonstrated to inhibit ischemia-induced renal vasoconstriction on reperfusion, as well as cerebral vasoconstriction in a model of subarachnoid hemorrhage.[479]

Myogenic Control

The myogenic response of VSM represents a tendency to develop tension and increase $[Ca^{2+}]_i$ in response to stretch and increased intravascular pressure.[480] Recently, this response has been found to be mediated by depolarization activating Ca channel–mediated Ca^{2+} entry into VSM.

Autonomic Regulation of the Vasculature

Beyond local regulation, the primary short-term control of vascular tone in the entire body is mediated by the sympathetic nervous system (see below). Sympathetic outflow to the periphery originates in the sympathetic motor neurons most prominent in the intermediolateral (IML) column of the spinal cord. As previously indicated for the sympathetic nerve endings in the heart (Fig. 5–11), release of norepinephrine and other co-transmitters (such as ATP) of the sympathetic nervous system is a complicated metabolic pathway.[225] Within the sympathetic nerve ending there are a number of negative and positive feedback pathways (see Fig. 5–11 and 5–20). ATP co-released by the sympathetic nerve endings enhances entry of synaptic $[Ca^{2+}]_i$ and thereby increases neurotransmitter release,[481,482] an effect mediated by P_{2Y} receptors. NPY, galanin, neurotensin, and a variety of other vasoactive peptides are also released that not only influence VSM behavior but provide feedback to the nerve ending itself.

Other Modulators of Vascular Tone

A variety of transmitters that modulate vascular tone are listed in Table 5–7. These substances are derived from various locations, and some have both direct and indirect (via endothelium) actions.

THE RENIN-ANGIOTENSIN SYSTEM

The renin-angiotensin system (RAS) is classically regulated by secretion of the proteolytic enzyme renin from the juxtaglomerular cells of the kidney nephron. Renin secretion is activated by decreases in blood pressure in the proximal glomerular arterioles; however, its secretion is modulated by the sympathetic nervous system as well as by other circulating transmitters. Renin cleaves four amino acids from angiotensinogen, a 14-amino-acid protein secreted by the liver into the circulation, producing the decapeptide angiotensin I. This protein is then converted by ACE to AII. ACE is localized primarily on the surface membrane of the vascular endothelium, and production of AII at this site makes it readily available to activate VSM. Although three major AII receptors have been cloned (AT_1, AT_2, and AT_3), the receptor distributed on the vasculature is AT_1. This belongs to the class of G-protein–linked receptors such as the α_1-AR and ET-1, which activate the G_q-PLC-IP_3 cascade.[483] As indicated in Figure 5–20, AII may be localized and released from the EC and activate VSM, as well as activating NO release.

PROSTANOIDS AND LEUKOTRIENES

As noted, metabolites of arachidonic acid (AA) play a prominent role in cardiovascular control.[484] Following activation in platelets, phospholipase A_2 action on phospholipid substrates generates AA. Cyclo-oxygenase action on AA yields the prostanoid PGH_2, the precursor for thromboxane A_2 (TXA_2). Binding to a distinct G_q-protein–linked receptor activates the PLC-IP_3-PKC cascade, leading to tension development,[485] akin to the action of α_1-adrenergic class. A similar cellular action is mediated by prostaglandin F_2 alpha ($PGF_{2\alpha}$). In mast cells, AA is converted via 5-lipoxygenase to 5-hydroperoxyeicosatetraenoic acid (5-HPETE), which is subsequently converted to leukotrienes. The leukotriene receptors also activate the PLC-IP_3-PKC cascade,[485] leading to tracheal constriction as well as to the adverse effects on myocardium.[486]

NATRIURETIC PEPTIDES

Atrial natriuretic peptide (ANP, also ANF) is stored in the perinuclear granules of human atrial myocytes, with

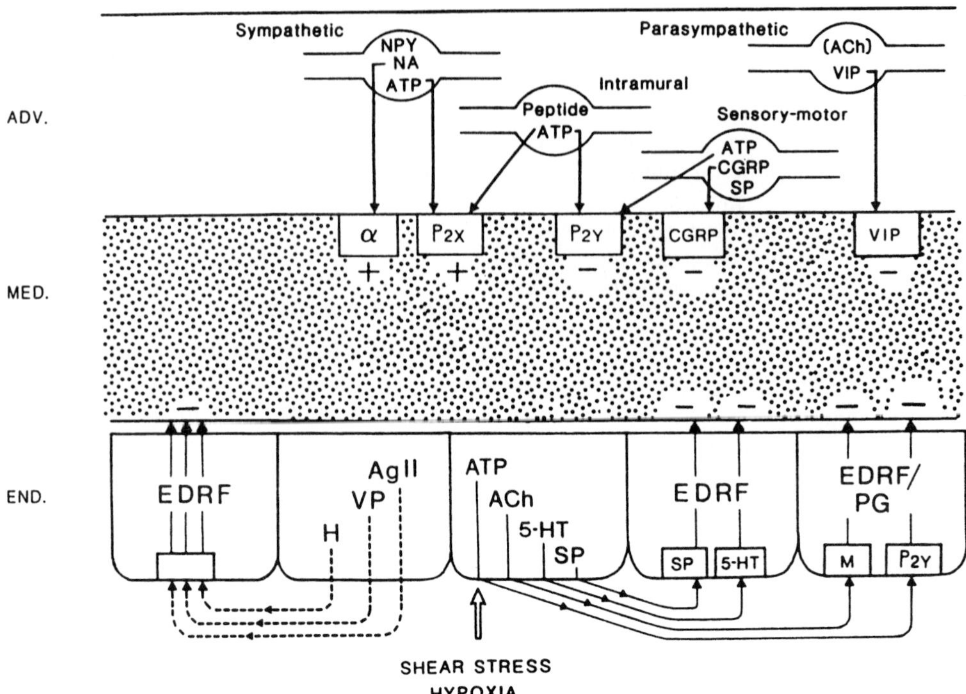

FIGURE **5–20.** Regulation of vascular tone by perivascular nerves and endothelial cells. Neuropeptide Y (NPY), noradrenaline (NA), adenosine 5′-triphosphate (ATP), calcitonin gene-related peptide (CGRP), substance P (SP), and vasoactive intestinal polypeptide (VIP) can be released from nerve varicosities in the adventitia (ADV) to act on receptors in the media (MED), causing vasoconstriction or vasodilation. ATP, ACh, 5-hydroxytryptamine (5-HT), and SP, released from endothelial cells (END) by shear stress or hypoxia, act on their receptors on endothelial cells to cause a release of EDRF or prostaglandins (PG), which, in turn, act on the smooth muscle to cause relaxation. Angiotensin II (AgII), vasopressin (VP), and histamine (H) are also contained in, and may be released from, subpopulations of endothelial cells. In areas denuded of endothelial cells, opposite effects may be produced by receptors on the smooth muscle cells; for example, via P_{2X}- and P_{2Y}-purinoceptors and muscarinic receptors (M). (From Burnstock G: Integration of factors controlling vascular tone: Overview. Anesthesiology 79:1368, 1993, with permission.)

greater amounts in the right versus the left atrium.[487] Secretion of ANP is limited to cells specialized for mechanical rather than conductive activity, and release is mediated by a Ca^{2+}-dependent process.[200] ANP begins as a 150- to 152-amino-acid precursor, prepro-ANP, which is cleaved to a 126-amino-acid prohormone, pro-ANP, the predominant storage form that is released intact from atria.[487] After release from the granules, cleavage by a serum protease occurs to form the 28-amino-acid C-terminal hormone, atriopeptin I circulating in the plasma.[488] ANP release is activated by atrial distention due to increased vascular volume, as well as by epinephrine, vasopressin (or antidiuretic hormone [ADH]), morphine, and increased myocardial (atrial) pressure.[487] In addition, brain natriuretic peptide (BNP), also present in heart, has also been defined whose active form is a 32-amino-acid peptide.[218]

The primary effects of ANP and BNP are direct peripheral vasodilation; suppression of ADH release when elevated by hemorrhage or dehydration; inhibition of aldosterone release; and direct renal effects such as increased glomerular filtration, natriuresis, and diuresis. Like NO, the major vasodilating action of ANP appears to be mediated by production of cGMP.[488] However, this action relies on the fact that the ANP receptors possess an intracellular portion with guanylyl cyclase activity (''particulate'' guanylyl cyclase). When an ANP binds to either of two specific receptors, the signal is transmitted via a single transmembrane domain to the intracellular portion and results in the synthesis of cGMP from GTP.[218] Once activated, the increased cGMP has cardiovascular effects similar to those described previously. A renal tubular site of action mediated by guanylyl

TABLE 5–7
Transmitters and Modulators of Vascular Tone

Endothelium-derived	Perivascular nerves
Nitric oxide (NO)	Norepinephrine (NE)
Endothelin(s) (ET-1, ET-2, ET-3)	Acetylcholine (ACh)
Prostacyclin (PGI_2)	ATP
Substance P (SP)	Neuropeptide Y (NPY)
Vasopressin (VP)	Serotonin (5-hydroxytryptamine)
Histamine	Dopamine
Angiotensin II	Calcitonin gene–related peptide (CGRP)
Serotonin (5-hydroxytryptamine)	Enkephalin-dynorphin
	Vasoactive intestinal peptide (VIP)
	Galanin
Humoral	Somatostatin
Leukotrienes (LTA_4, LTB_4, LTC_4, LTD_4)	Neurotensin (NT)
Thromboxane (TXA_2)	Tissue-derived
Angiotensin II	Adenosine
Vasopressin (VP)	Kallidin
	Bradykinin

cyclase appears likely.[489] Factors such as renal perfusion pressure and renal sympathetic nerve activity in conjunction with physiologic plasma concentrations of ANP produce natriuresis, but kaliuresis does not occur.[489] ANP affects not only blood pressure (by decreasing cardiac output and vascular resistance) but also water and electrolyte balance, and blood volume. It has no direct inotropic or chronotropic properties. In normal volunteers, administration of ANP does not cause significant changes in renin, aldosterone, cortisol, norepinephrine, or ADH at doses that increase urinary output, decrease blood pressure, and reduce forearm vascular resistance.[490] Disease states such as congestive heart failure and atrial tachyarrhythmias increase circulating ANP levels.

Special Considerations in the Coronary Vasculature

The heart has one of the highest metabolic rates of any organ. MVO_2 is typically 8 to 10 ml of O_2 per 100 gm of myocardium per minute. To supply the high metabolic demands of the continuously active muscle mass, presuming a normal hematocrit and oxygen-carrying capacity, a blood flow of 70 to 120 ml/min per 100 gm of tissue is typical at a resting heart rate, with 50 to 75% of oxygen being extracted.[491] This figure may increase dramatically with increases in heart rate, wall tension, and myocardial contractility. The subendocardium requires about 20% more oxygen than the epicardium, and in part for this reason the subendocardium is more vulnerable to ischemia.

The Coronary Arterial Anatomy

Two main coronary arteries, right and left, originating from the sinuses of Valsalva in the aortic valve supply arterial blood to the myocardium (Table 5–8). A uniform inflow into these vessels is aided by the turbulent flow characteristics of the sinuses of Valsalva. The ventricular mass supplied by these vessels may be divided into five walls (Fig. 5–21): the intraventricular septum, the left lateral and left posterior (inferior or diaphragmatic) walls comprising the LV, and the right anterior and right posterior (inferior) walls, comprising the RV. The junction of the posterior interventricular groove and the posterior atrioventricular sulcus represents the crux of the heart. The major branches of these arteries are listed in Table 5–8. The left coronary artery usually has a short common or left main coronary (LMC) artery before bifurcation into left anterior descending (LAD) and left cir-

TABLE **5–8**
The Coronary Arteries and their Branches*

Vessel	Comment
Right coronary artery (RCA)	Courses in the right atrioventricular sulcus.
Conus branch	Arises just after the RCA origin or may arise from the aorta directly; supplies right side of the infundibulum.
Sinus node branch	Present in 60% of cases, in 40% it is derived from the LCx, rarely the sinus note is supplied by both.
Anterior right ventricular and atrial branches	Usually small branches arising variably along the length anterior segment of the RCA.
Acute marginal branch	A major branch and the main artery of the RV wall.
Posterior right ventricular and atrial branches	Highly variable in size and number.
AV-nodal branch	Arising near the origin of the PD artery, in 10% of cases it is supplied by the LCx.
Posterior descending branch	The largest and most important branch of the RCA in 90% of hearts.
Posterior left ventricular and atrial branches	Varying in size and precise origin, these are present in 70% of hearts.
Left (main) coronary artery (LMCA)	A short (0.5–2 cm) vessel that typically bifurcates.
Left anterior descending artery (LAD)	Courses along the anterior interventricular septum, reaching the apex to supply a portion of the posterior wall or form collaterals with the RCA.
Conus branch	Fairly constant, supplies the left side of the infundibulum.
Septal branches	Variable with at least one or two large branches that course straight into the septum.
Diagonal branches	Large and variable in number.
Apical branches	The terminus of the LAD, these small branches course into the thickness of the apex, and often into the posterior ventricular walls.
Circumflex artery (LCxA)	In 10% of cases it is the sole supply of the PD artery; it may also be short, not passing beyond the left margin.
Obtuse marginal branch	A large constant branch, which may rarely be the terminal branch of the LCx.
Lateral left ventricular and atrial branches	Highly variable in size and number, since these regions are supplied primarily by the LAD diagonal branches.
Posterior left ventricular and atrial branches	Variable in size and extent, they typically combine with RCA branches to supply the posterior wall.
Medial diagonal artery	Present if the first diagonal arises at an LMCA trifurcation, although more than one vessel may arise in this fashion.

*Data from Zamir M: Flow strategy and functional design of the coronary network. In Kajiya F, Klassen GA, Spaan JAE, Hoffman JIE (eds): Coronary Circulation: Basic Mechanism and Clinical Relevance. Tokyo, Springer-Verlag, 1990, p 15.

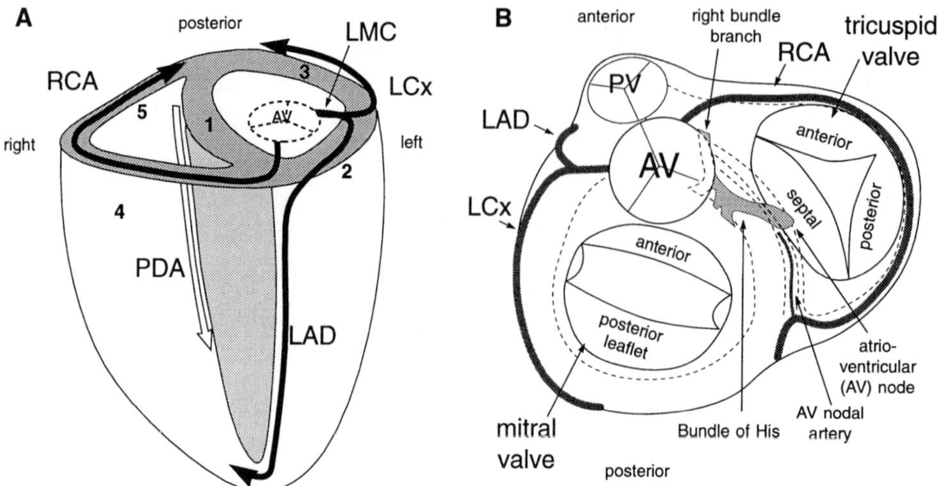

FIGURE **5–21.** Coronary anatomy. *A*, The usual arrangement of the coronary vessels. The right coronary artery (RCA) distributes blood to the anterior and posterior right ventricular wall and in 90% of cases to the posterior descending artery (PDA), which then supplies the posterior septum. The left main coronary (LMC) divides into the left circumflex (LCx), which then supplies the posterior ventricular wall and in 10% goes on to the PDA. In 70% of cases part of the posterior left ventricular wall is supplied by the RCA. The left anterior descending artery supplies the anterior left ventricular wall as well as the anterior half to two thirds of the ventricular septum. *B*, Superior view of the base of the heart, indicating the position of the valves as well as the conduction system. In 90% of cases the AV nodal artery is derived from the RCA, while in 10% of cases the LCx supplies this artery (not shown).

cumflex (LCx) branches, although additional branches frequently originate with the LAD and LCx. The LAD artery courses downward near the anterior interventricular groove, supplying the anterior half to two thirds of the septum through its septal perforator branches, the lateral free wall via diagonal branches, and the ventricular apex. The circumflex branch follows the atrioventricular groove posteriorly, frequently being hidden by the overhanging left atrial appendage, and gives rise to the obtuse marginal branch(es), which to varying degrees supplies the posterior LV wall.[492] The right coronary (RC) artery flows deep into the right atrioventricular sulcus, in a fold of the crista supraventricularis, supplying the anterior and posterior RV free wall, with smaller branches that ascend to supply the right atrium.

CORONARY DOMINANCE

Beginning at the crux, the posterior descending (PD) artery courses along the posterior interventricular groove, supplying blood to the posterior interventricular septum as well as the artery to the AV node. The source of its blood flow shows considerable variation. In 10% of human hearts the PD arises from the LCx artery, and this circulation is termed ''left dominant.'' In 70% of individual hearts, the RCA supplies the PD artery, and a branch continues to supply part of the posterior LV wall, a situation termed ''right dominant.'' In the remaining 20% the PD artery is supplied by the termination of RCA giving a ''balanced'' pattern. Even though PD artery flow is derived from the RCA in 90% of cases, in most cases the flow in the LMC artery exceeds that in the RCA, due to the greater mass and metabolic demands of the thicker LV walls supplied by the LMC artery. Zamir suggests that the concept of *dependence* be applied to the LV blood supply, and suggests the terms ''totally left-dependent,'' ''mostly left-dependent,'' and ''balanced,'' the latter describing the approximately 70% of cases in which a large portion of posterior LV wall and septum are supplied by the RCA.[493]

Anastomoses between the branches of the coronary arteries are evident both within the circulation of the same coronary artery (''homocoronary anastomoses'') and between branches of different coronary arteries (''heterocoronary anastomoses'').[494] Such collaterals may exist both epicardially as well as within the myocardial wall. Such native vessels are usually small (20 μm to 1 mm), but they may increase dramatically in size in response to the gradual occlusion of one parent vessel, becoming sufficiently large to carry the bulk of coronary flow. While human, primate, and canine hearts have such collaterals, they are lacking in swine.

CORONARY MICROVASCULATURE

From these large epicardial arteries, smaller transmural vessels branch off and penetrate the ventricular wall. Although there is regularity in the pattern of branching down to vessels of 400-μm diameter, a consistent branching pattern is not present in vessels of diameters ranging from 400 to 10 μm. Thus a terminal arteriole (≤30-μm diameter) from which capillaries arise may be preceded by several generations of smaller vessels, or instead it may branch directly from an artery (≥250-μm diameter).[491,494] Perfusion pressure decreases by less than 10% out to the level of the arteriole (200- to 250-μm diameter), and then decreases steeply as vessel diameter decreases to 50 μm.[495,496] The density of capillaries (4- to 6-μm diameter, depending on contractile phase of the heart) in myocardium is extremely high, estimated to be

3,000 to 3,500 per mm^2. Thus, each capillary supplies an area about 16 to 20 μm in diameter, which is the same diameter of a typical myocyte, giving a 1:1 capillary-myocyte ratio. At normal heart rates, there may be flow through only 50% of capillaries, although they may undergo rapid recruitment and closure.[494]

An important regulatory mechanism of the coronary vessels involves both NO as well as K_{ATP} channel, processes that may interact in modulating vascular tone. Recently, it has been demonstrated that K_{ATP} channels may be activated by NO[497]; however, such regulation may vary with the size and location of the vessels. Coronary microvessels show differential regulation by NO and K_{ATP} channels, depending upon their size. Whereas K_{ATP} in a channel blockade with glibenclamide caused constriction of all microvessels, inhibition of the NO pathway appeared to involve only larger microvessels (>130-μm diameter).[498] K_{ATP} channels appear to play a more prominent role in regulating tone in subepicardial than in subendocardial regions.[499] When vascular myocytes have been stimulated by endotoxin, the inducible NOS that is induced in the VSM cells themselves may provide endogenous NO to activate the relaxant action cGMP synthesis and K_{ATP} channels.[497] Anesthetics are notable for their ability to dilate coronary vasculature, an effect that may in part be mediated by activation of K_{ATP} channels, since K_{ATP} channel blockade is able to reduce that vasodilating action.[500,501]

Venous Drainage of the Myocardium

The capillary outflow enters venules that consolidate flow into veins of increasing size. Although a higher density of venules than arterioles is reported for the dog, this may not be present in man. Transmural veins, often with frequent small (100 μm) anastomotic connections, drain into epicardial veins, which also have frequent anastomoses. The epicardial veins converge and drain into anterior and posterior descending vessels, which follow their respective arteries; an obtuse marginal (or middle) branch runs parallel to the posterior vein. These three vessels flow into the great cardiac vein, which circles the left side of the heart posteriorly along the atrioventricular sulcus and flows into a posterior aspect of the right atrium at the coronary sinus.[493] The posterior and anterior veins have an anastomotic network at the apex of the heart, which with the other interconnections provide for alternative drainage if obstruction occurs in this low-pressure system. Near the orifice of the great cardiac vein, the oblique vein of Marshall (vein of the left atrium) enters the coronary sinus. Anterior cardiac veins and small cardiac veins that drain the RV wall frequently enter the right atrium directly, independent of the coronary sinus.[491] Consequently, retrograde perfusion of the myocardium via the coronary sinus will usually not include the RV. The deep venous system drains a very small fraction (~2%) of coronary flow.[502] *Thebesian veins* extend from some capillaries and small vessels and drain directly into various cardiac chambers.[503] Arterioluminal vessels communicate between small coronary arteries and cardiac chambers, and arteriosinusoidal channels result from arterioles that lead into irregular, 50- to 200-μm endothelium-lined spaces. Thebesian venous flow, coupled with bronchial and pleural venous flow, contributes the normal 1 to 3% arteriovenous shunt.

LYMPHATICS

The myocardium has a system of lymphatic vessels that drain fluid from the interstitium of the myocardium, which normally occupies about 20% of the tissue volume. Lymph capillaries are much larger (45-μm diameter) and far less common than capillaries, although transcapillary water transport is significant and may constitute 3% of blood flow (3 ml/min per 100 gm of tissue). However, under normal conditions most of that volume must be reabsorbed by the blood, since lymph flow as measured in the dog (0.05 ml/min per 100 gm of tissue) is only 1 to 2% of the filtered fluid. Nevertheless, the flow of lymph, which is increased by elevation in coronary sinus pressure or anoxia, may be important in preventing myocardial edema that may in turn increase the inherent stiffness of the tissues.[504] Lymph, from interstitial myocardial lymphatics, collects on the epicardial surfaces and in the pericardial space before drainage into the lymphatic system via pericardial lymphatic vessels.[505]

Control of Coronary Flow

MYOCARDIAL SUPPLY-DEMAND RATIO

Of all the major organs of the body the heart is the most energy consuming and extracts the greatest amount of oxygen and nutrients from its blood supply. A balance must always exist between oxygen consumption (demand) and myocardial oxygen supply if ischemia is to be avoided. Myocardial oxygen supply is dependent upon the diameter of the coronary arteries, left ventricular end-diastolic pressure (LVEDP), aortic diastolic pressure, and arterial oxygen content. Myocardial blood flow is determined by the blood pressure at the coronary ostia, arteriolar tone, intramyocardial pressure or extravascular resistance, coronary occlusive disease, heart rate, coronary collateral development, and blood viscosity.

In the normal heart, the coronary perfusion pressure may be approximated by the difference between the aortic diastolic pressure and the left ventricular end-diastolic pressure. Due to the intracavitary and intramural tension in the left ventricle during systole that will equal or exceed blood pressure in the coronary lumen, systolic blood flow is largely restricted to the atria and right ventricle. During systole as the ventricular intramural pressure increases, blood is expelled from the capillaries and intramural vessels into the cardiac veins and retrograde into the surface coronary arteries. There is also significant forward flow from the aorta into the compliant superficial coronary arteries. The compliance of the coronary vessels permits detectable phasic systolic blood flow in the larger vessels, in spite of the cessation of left intramyocardial flow during systole (see Fig. 5–22). Blood flow through the vessels that run on the surface or within the muscle mass of the heart may be

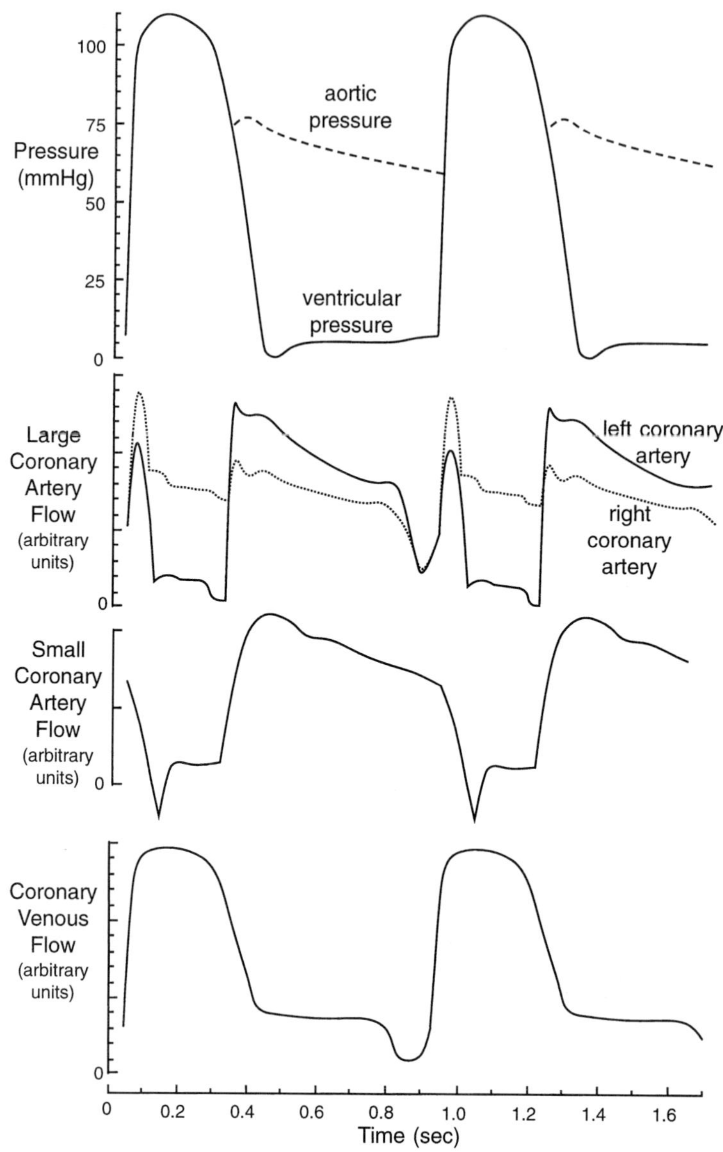

FIGURE **5–22.** Coronary flow. The coordination of the flow in the great vessels of the heart shows a complex pattern. In spite of the substantial pressure developed in the ventricular wall, there is still substantial flow to the left coronary artery initially, due to the distention of the epicardial coronary vessels, with a small amount of ongoing perfusion during systole into the epicardium. After relaxation of the ventricle there is substantial increase in flow through the left coronary artery, and the substantial flow indicated through the small coronary arteries. In contrast, the coronary venous flow occurs primarily during systole, when the increase in ventricular wall tension extrudes desaturated blood into the larger veins. (Data from Wilson RF, Laughlin DE, Ackell PH, et al: Transluminal, subselective measurement of coronary artery blood flow velocity and vasodilator reserve in man. Circulation 72:82, 1985, and Chilean WM, Marcus ML: Phasic coronary blood flow velocity in intramural and epicardial coronary arteries. Circ Res 50:775, 1982.)

markedly affected by the contraction and high tissue pressures within the ventricular wall. When the pressure outside the vessels exceeds the pressure at the downstream ends, the vessels behave as Starling resistors or vascular waterfalls.[506] There is compelling evidence that in extramural coronary veins and in collateral vessels, such waterfall behavior occurs. While high systolic tissue pressures develop, particularly in the subendocardial left ventricular wall, it remains to be proven that waterfall effects limit flow intramurally.[506] In the right ventricular wall and left ventricular epicardium some flow may persist during systole, assuming that the tissue pressures are lower than in the bulk of the left ventricle.

Because the pressure distal to a coronary stenosis will be lower than aortic diastolic pressure, the prior consideration may not apply in coronary occlusive disease. In these cases, myocardial blood flow may be particularly sensitive to decreases in aortic diastolic pressure. Tachycardia, which shortens diastole, reduces the duration of blood flow. Increasing preload and thus P_{ED} increases wall tension and oxygen demand, while decreasing subendocardial perfusion. Myocardial oxygen supply is also affected by the level of arterial oxygenation. Oxygen content, resulting from PaO_2, hemoglobin, 2,3-diphosphoglycerate (DPG), and pH, PCO_2 or temperature effects on the oxyhemoglobin dissociation curve, can be an important factor in patients with obstructive lung disease or severe anemia.

In addition to its nutritive function, the distention of the coronary vessels during diastole provides a slight "stretch" of surrounding myocytes, which via the length-tension relation enhances contractions. With loss of coronary perfusion, there is an immediate decrease in mechanical function that precedes measurable biochemical changes and which has been attributed to this "garden hose" effect.[507]

AUTOREGULATION AND ADENOSINE

An increase in oxygen extraction and coronary vasodilation constitute the metabolic reserve of the heart to increased demand. Normal oxygen extraction by the heart is 50 to 70% and changes very little with increased cardiac work because coronary vascular resistance decreases, permitting an increase in flow. Because of the autoregulatory mechanisms, there is little change in arteriovenous oxygen difference across the coronary bed with moderate increases in heart rate. Coronary flow can increase over threefold with extreme exercise. At extreme tachycardia, the arteriovenous oxygen difference increases. Because tachycardia shortens diastole more than systole and increases myocardial contractility, the autoregulatory increases in blood flow are exceeded, and oxygen extraction increases. However, if the coronary vascular resistance response is limited, oxygen extraction can be increased to more than 90%.[508]

Berne in 1962 suggested the critical role that adenosine, as a by-product of ATP consumption, might play in regulation of the coronary vasculature. Since that initial suggestion, the definition of adenosine receptors has been described, and the mechanism of adenosine-mediated actions has been elucidated (see above). While adenosine plays a critical role in modulating coronary tone, hypoxic dilation of coronary arteries may not involve hyperpolarization secondary to activation of K_{Ado} channels. Instead, modulation of basal tone[509] and normal autoregulation[510] of the coronary vessels, as well as hyperemic responses to hypoxia,[511,512] appear to be mediated by glibenclamide-sensitive K_{ATP} channels. However, since the K_{ATP} channel is enhanced by adenosine receptor activation,[278] modulation of K^+ conductance by adenosine is still a component of the control pathway. Furthermore, the response to ischemia[512] or adenosine[513] was not completely inhibited by glibenclamide, suggesting involvement of additional pathways. Prostacyclin also appears to cause vasodilation via enhanced activation of K_{ATP} channels.[514] As in the other vascular beds, increases in coronary flow alone can decrease vascular tone, associated with increased production of NO, endothelin, and $PGF_{1\alpha}$.[515]

In addition to feedback control by adenosine and other metabolites to control coronary tone, there is also evidence for feed-forward control in which decreases in flow appear to decrease oxygen demand.[516] It is possible that this represents an early form of preconditioning or hibernation in which adenosine or other mediators decrease myocardial contractility to decrease oxygen consumption, prior to the onset of frank ischemic changes.

Integration of the Heart and Vasculature

Autonomic Regulation of the Cardiovascular System

While many hormones and neurotransmitters influence the behavior of the cardiovascular system via the pathways described, the autonomic nervous system is primarily responsible for mediating the second-by-second control of the circulation. Although influenced by the patient's consciousness of external surroundings, this largely autonomous system regulates the conduction of the cardiac impulse and the excitability of the cardiac membrane, contractility of the heart, delivery of oxygen and nutrients by the blood to the body, as well as controlling temperature and influencing conscious behavior. It is important to recognize that both sympathetic and parasympathetic arms are normally active and influence each other. Likewise, it is important to remember that the "depression" of the myocardium or the cardiovascular system described in intact animals or patients may not be a direct effect but rather the alteration of some component of autonomic tone.

Medullary Control Centers

Sympathetic nervous system activation of the heart and vasculature originates in medullary brain stem centers, particularly the rostral ventrolateral medulla (RVL), ventromedial rostral medulla, and the parvocellular region of the paraventricular nucleus. Neurons in the RVL appear to serve as modulated "pacemakers" driving sympathetic output, and receive multiple inputs from various sources including the respiratory center and other medullary nuclei, as well as from the cerebellum and cerebral centers (Fig. 5–23).[517] Impulses are transmitted monosynaptically to sympathetic preganglionic neurons (SPGNs) located in the interemediolateral (IML) cell column along the entire length of the spinal cord. For the heart, SPGNs are usually in thoracic segments 1 through 4. Axons from the SPGNs in the spinal cord traverse cephalad in the sympathetic chain to form excitatory nicotinic synapses with interneurons in the caudal half of the cervical sympathetic trunk bilaterally.

Parasympathetic preganglionic fibers arise from neurons in the dorsal motor nucleus of the vagus and the nucleus ambiguous (NucA) of the medulla oblongata, which receives modulating input from the nucleus tractus solitarius (NTS). The parasympathetic aspect of cardiovascular control is mediated primarily via alteration in cardiac function. A typical action of the opioids is significant bradycardia.[518] Intravenous fentanyl selectively activates cardioinhibitory vagal fibers to produce bradycardia.[519] Application of fentanyl in the fourth cerebral ventricle duplicates this effect.[520] More specifically, iontophoretic injection of fentanyl or metenkephalinamide at the NucA produces a dramatic bradycardia similar to that caused by NucA stimulation.[521] Since in most settings the narcotics are inhibitory, one might speculate that the opioids are inhibiting neurons

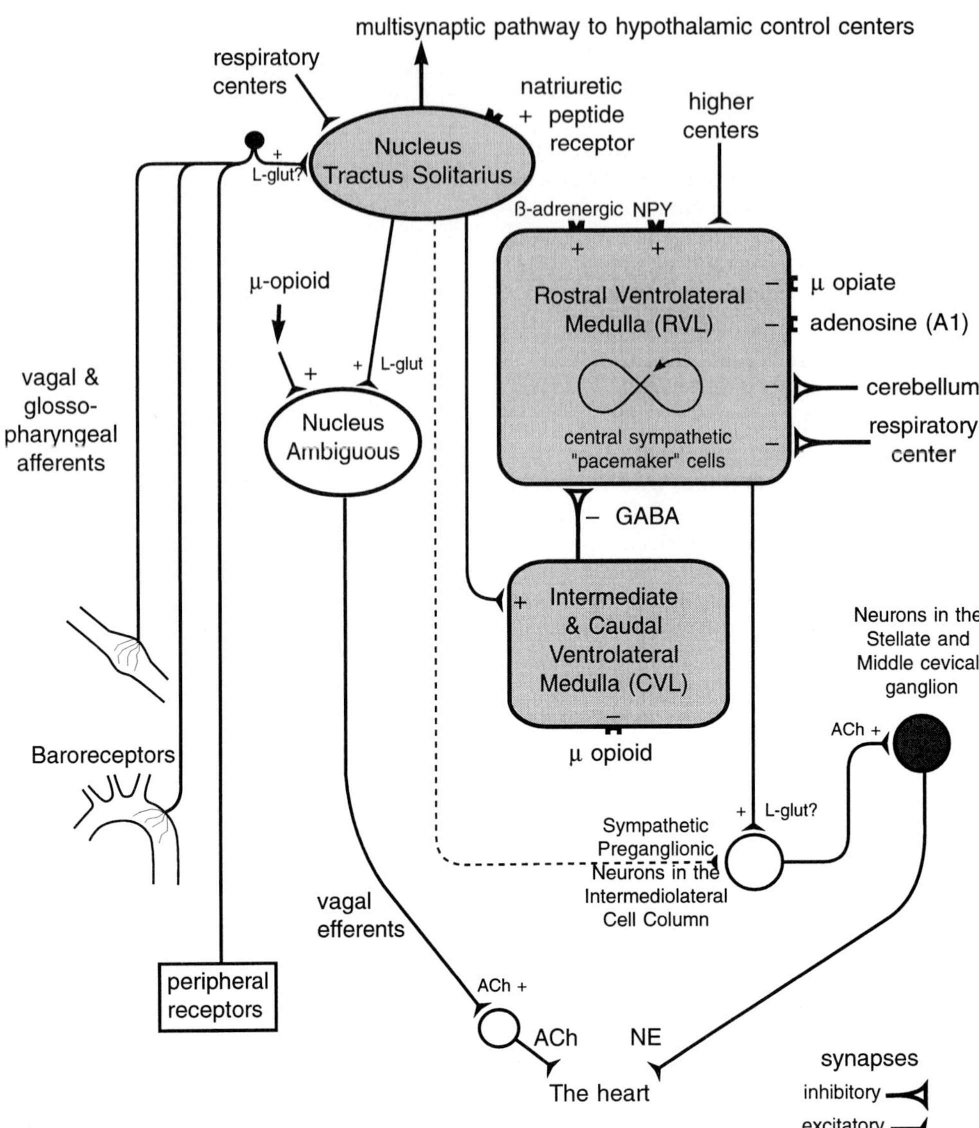

FIGURE **5–23.** Diagram of central nervous system control of autonomic output to the heart. The primary features of the central sympathetic drive and the baroreceptor reflex arcs are indicated. Neurons in the rostral lateral medulla (RVL) appear to have a continuing pacemaker function providing regular output to sympathetic preganglionic neurons. Input from the baroreceptor arcs activate neurons in the nucleus tractus solitarius that relay in the nucleus ambiguous and provide parasympathetic input in response to baroreceptor activation. In contrast, activation of the caudal ventrolateral medulla (CVL) depresses via GABAergic input, the central sympathetic drive at the RVL. Opioids have an antagonistic effect by decreasing CVL depression of the RVL neurons, while at the same time depressing them directly.

that provide an inhibitory input to the NucA. By itself, fentanyl blunted the heart rate but not the pressor response of the baroreceptor reflex.[522] Although a modest bradycardia (5% slowing) following high-dose fentanyl can be detected in the denervated heart, the centrally mediated action is far greater.[523]

As in the heart, sympathetic nerve endings to the vasculature do not typically have specific contacts on VSM, but rather have thickened varicosities at which transmitter is released to affect small areas of a vessel.

Cardiovascular Afferent Nerves

Sensory innervation of the heart is carried by afferents in both the sympathetic and vagal fibers. The atria have three types of parasympathetic receptors; type A, type B, and receptors innervated by group C fibers that are less responsive than types A and B. The primary location of types A and B are the cavoatrial junction, pulmonary venous-atrial junction, atrial appendage, and atrial body.[524] Atrial receptors usually reflexively alter intravascular volume or heart rate. Atrial receptor types A and B are innervated by myelinated vagal afferent fibers. Type A receptors discharge at the time of the A wave of the atrial pressure waveform. They may actually respond to heart rate rather than atrial pressure, since they are unaffected by the amplitude of the A wave or the rate of atrial pressure increase.[524] Type B receptors are stretch receptors that discharge during late systole, during the v wave of the atrial pressure waveform. Their discharge is closely related to atrial volume and varies with the rate of increase of atrial pressure. Type B receptors, inactive during normal atrial contraction, increase their rate of discharge during tachyarrhythmias, which increase atrial volume.[524]

Of greatest importance to reflex control are the baroreceptors in the carotid sinus and aortic arch, which are sensitive to distending pressure. The carotid sinus represents a highly innervated dilated region of the common carotid located just proximal to the artery's bifurcation into its external and internal branches. Its relatively thin-walled and aneurysmal structure may make it sensitive to pressure and distention. Two distinct types of receptors encode pressure sensed in the carotid sinus,[525] and resulting impulses are transmitted along the afferent nerve of Hering[526] to the glossopharyngeal nerve and subsequently to the NTS. Descending inputs from more rostral structures also converge in the NTS, and modulate the baroreceptor signals that are subsequently relayed to the subsequent cardiovascular control centers.[527] The output of NTS neurons regulates output from the NucA to vagus, and the RVL to sympathetic nerves (see Fig. 5–23). Increasing pressure and stimulation of these baroreceptors activates vagal tone and depresses sympathetic outflow. The vagal afferents appear to carry responses of both pain and mechanoreceptors, the latter contributing to baroreceptor reflexes when there is considerable distention.[389] In addition to mechanical stimuli, chemical and metabolic stimuli can activate receptors located in the ventricular wall.[528]

Peripheral chemoreceptors sensitive to decreasing oxygen tension or increased hydrogen ion concentrations in the blood are located in the carotid and aortic bodies.[529] The chemoreceptive cells in these organs mediate their action by releasing dopamine to activate the surrounding nerves. Although exquisitely sensitive to Po_2 and proton concentration, sensitivity is modulated by other substances, perhaps most notably $[K^+]$, an elevation of which an markedly increase output. Nerve fibers from the chemoreceptors pass through the nerve of Hering and the vagus to the medullary vasomotor centers. Ischemia, caused by coronary occlusion, triggers sympathetic fibers and neurons in the spinothalamic and spinoreticular tracts.[530]

Reflex Modulation of the Cardiovascular System

While control of cardiac function and the vasculature of various organs may be individually regulated, a variety of reflex responses with generalized characteristics are well defined. It is important to recognize the coordinated action of the autonomic nervous system in response to various stimuli. Within the medullary preganglionic control centers, sympathetic drive by the RVL, and parasympathetic drive by the NucA usually are coordinated so that activation of one includes inhibition of the other.

Baroreceptor Reflex. This reflex (also termed the pressoreceptor) is a classic example of a negative feedback loop with dual effector pathways. When an increase in blood pressure stretches pressure receptors in the carotid sinus or arch of the aorta, their frequency of discharge increases. After relay in the NTS, this signal depresses the sympathetic "pacemaking" of the RVL, which drives the SPGNs in the IML, thereby decreasing vascular tone and cardiac stimulation. NucA parasympathetic activity increases, resulting in decreased heart rate, cardiac contractility, and vascular tone. Furthermore, the peripheral interaction of the vagus and sympathetic neurons in the heart (see above) will also contribute to the final effect. As the arterial pressure decreases as a result of these alterations, there are fewer afferent impulses from peripheral pressure sensors to the cardiovascular center, so that sympathetic tone is partially restored and vagal tone decreases. The baroreceptor reflex reduces changes in arterial pressure to about one third of expected. The threshold of the reflex is about 60 mm Hg and its limits are pressures of 175 to 300 mm Hg,[531] while its gain is determined by the pulse pressure.[532] Although this reflex has also been termed the "carotid sinus reflex," the aortic receptors also appear to contribute to the response. In fact, while the hypertension resulting from carotid sinus denervation is transient, aortic denervation results in prolonged hypertension.[533]

The circulatory response to the Valsalva maneuver demonstrates the effects of the baroreceptor reflex. As a consequence of the sustained increase in ITP, cardiac output and BP decrease, resulting in a reflex inhibition of vagal outflow and an increase in heart rate (phase 2). After the initial decrease, BP stabilizes as sympathetic outflow also increases and causes vasoconstriction. With glottic opening and decreased ITP, venous return refills the right heart and pulmonary vessels, causing a transient reduction in LV outflow and BP (phase 3). The arrival of the enhanced venous return to the sympathetically stimulated LV results in a forceful ejection and an "overshoot" in BP (phase 4). The increase in blood pressure then elicits the baroreceptor response to produce vagally mediated bradycardia.[426] Consequently, this maneuver is effective in elucidating autonomic dysfunction, as well as ventricular dysfunction.[534]

Reflex Responses to Intramyocardial Stimuli. The Bezold-Jarisch reflex results when noxious chemical, mechanical, or metabolic stimuli in the ventricular wall activate left ventricular receptors. The result is a vagally mediated reflex with bradycardia, accompanied by hypotension and parasympathetically induced coronary vasodilation.[528] The afferent pathway is nonmyelinated vagal C fibers located primarily in the inferoposterior ventricular wall. Reperfusion of previously ischemic tissue, particularly the right coronary artery,[535] also appears to elicit the reflex.[536]

Atrial Reflexes. Bainbridge described a reflex increase in heart rate when vagal tone was high and the right atrium or central veins were distended. The response of heart to atrial distention depends upon the pre-existing heart rate. There is no effect with pre-existing tachycardia, but volume loading at slow heart rate causes progressive tachycardia.[524] Although the Bainbridge reflex is primarily mediated through vagal myelinated afferent fibers, activation of sympathetic afferent fibers may also occur.[524] Increased right atrial pressure directly stretches the SA node and enhances its automaticity increasing the heart rate, making the existence of this reflex questionable. Experimental distention of the cavoatrial junctions or other small portions of the atria increases heart rate, but clinical conditions such as heart failure usually do not produce such locally increased atrial pressure.[537] Global atrial distention to high pressures causes bradycardia, hypotension, and decreased systemic vascular resistance.[538]

Chemoreceptor Reflexes. Normally, the peripheral chemoreceptors are minimally active. However, occlusion of the carotid artery decreases their oxygen supply and activates the reflex to increase pulmonary ventilation and blood pressure while decreasing heart rate. Stimulation of the aortic bodies causes tachycardia. The cardiogenic hypertensive chemoreflex described by James appears to be mediated by chemoreceptors located between the aorta and pulmonary artery and supplied by the left coronary artery.[539] The afferent reflex pathway is intrathoracic vagal branches and the efferent path is via phrenic, vagal, and sympathetic routes. In response to serotonin, arterial pressure increases markedly in 4 to 6 seconds due to increased inotropy and peripheral vasoconstriction. This reflex may be responsible for hypertension during angina and myocardial infarction, and after coronary bypass grafting. It is abolished by vagotomy, atropine, local anesthesia of the intertruncal space, or cyproheptadine.[539]

Cushing's Reflex. Increased cerebrospinal fluid pressure compresses cerebral arteries, causing cerebral ischemia. The response to cerebral ischemia is an increase in arterial pressure sufficient to reperfuse the brain. Intense sympathetic activity causes severe peripheral vasoconstriction as a result of this reflex, while the increase in blood pressure results in increased vagal tone and a decrease in heart rate.

Oculocardiac and Celiac Reflex. Traction on the extraocular muscles or pressure on the globe causes bradycardia and hypotension as a consequence of this reflex. Traction on the medial rectus, rather than the lateral rectus, is likely to elicit the reflex. Afferent fibers run with the short or long ciliary nerves to the ciliary ganglion and then with the ophthalmic division of the trigeminal nerve to the gasserian ganglion. Likewise, traction on the mesentery or gallbladder, stimulation of vagal nerve fibers in the respiratory tract, or rectal distention may stimulate afferent vagal nerve endings to cause bradycardia, apnea, and hypotension (vagovagal reflex). Manipulation around the celiac plexus decreases systolic pressure, narrows pulse pressure, and slightly decreases heart rate.

Coupling of Ventricular Function and Vascular Tone

Distribution of Blood

Approximately 15% of the blood volume resides in the heart and pulmonary circulation, the remainder being distributed in the systemic circulation. Typically only 20% of that blood volume is in the arterial vessels and capillaries, so that two thirds of the blood resides in the venous system.[389] Just as the cardiac output can be determined as a function of "filling pressure" or LVEDP, similarly a venous return curve can be plotted as a function of right atrial pressure (CVP), as first described by Guyton and associates.[540] For any level of vascular volume in the intact circulation, as CVP is increased venous return decreases. In the absence of pulmonary vascular pathology, and cardiac valvular or contractile dysfunction, CVP approximates LVEDP. As a consequence, since in the steady state the venous return must equal cardiac output, a single RAP and cardiac output describes the circulatory state, represented by the crossing point between the venous return and Starling relation (Fig. 5–24). When vascular volume is decreased, the decreased blood volume on the venous side decreases cardiac output so that a new lower balance of between atrial pressure and cardiac output is achieved. However, as cardiac contractility is increased, the blood is pumped from the venous side to the arterial side of the circulation, so that there is a decrease in CVP and a modest increase in the blood within the arterial side of the circuit. With depressed contractility, more blood will accumulate on the venous side. Since flow from the arterial to the venous side depends upon the vascular resistance, alteration in resistance by reflex compensatory changes or pharmacologic intervention may alter the cardiac output and effective vascular volume.

Pulsatile Flow and Pressure Waveforms

While the relation of perfusion pressure and flow in individual organs is expressed in terms of resistance, the relationship between the pulsatile pressure and flow into the vascular tree when generated by the ventricle is more accurately described by impedance. Unlike resistance, with which it is sometimes used synonymously, impedance includes energy that is lost or gained by the dynamics of the pressure waves within the closed vascular system. As with electrical or acoustic impedance, vascular impedance is a complex relation between arterial pressure and flow that involves the continuously changing dynamics of pulsatile flow. The arterial pulse is a wave of vascular distention resulting from the impact of the stroke volume of each beat being ejected into the closed system of the central and peripheral vasculature. The wave of distention begins at the base of the aorta and passes over the entire arterial system with each heartbeat. The pressure waves generated by the heart travel at considerable velocities within the vascular bed (6 to 15 m/sec), considerably faster than the velocity of blood flow (typically maximum of 0.1 to 0.2 m/sec in the aorta). The velocity of the pulse wave depends on the elasticity of the vessel, traveling fastest in the least distensible vessels. In the aortic arch, the pulse wave travels 3 to 5 m/sec; in large distensible arteries such as the subclavian, 7 to 10 m/sec; while in the small nondistensible peripheral arteries it travels about 15 to 30 m/sec. Atherosclerotic and aging changes in the great vessels will also markedly alter the rate, increasing it from 5 to 15 m/sec in the aorta. As a consequence, while

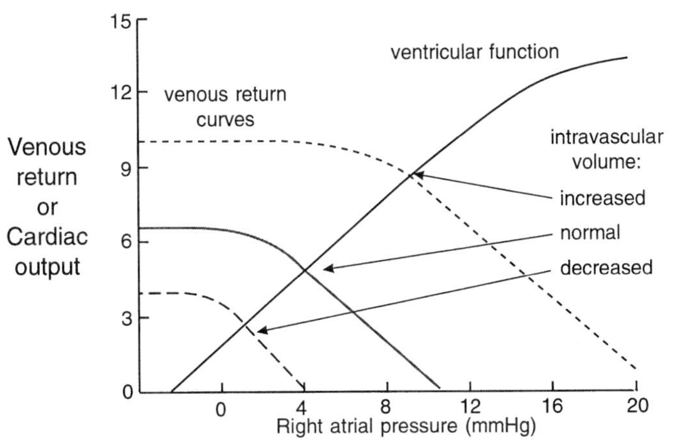

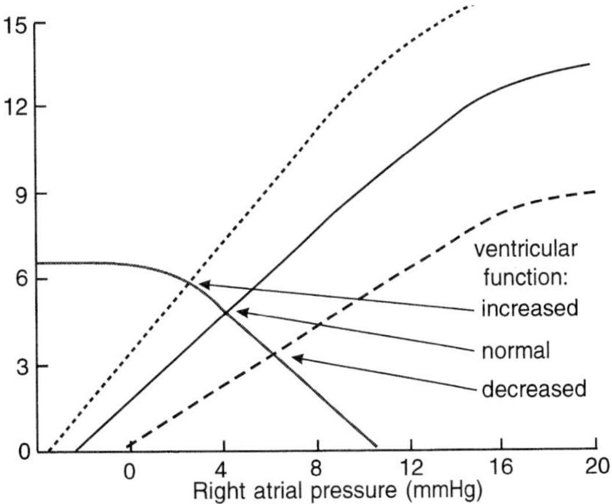

FIGURE **5–24.** The balance between venous return and cardiac output. In the steady state, venous return must equal cardiac output, the point represented by the point where the venous return line crosses the ventricular function curve. *Left*, When intravascular volume is decreased, the blood volume on both the venous and arterial sides of the circulation is decreased; venous return and cardiac output decrease, with a decrease in the right atrial pressure. With increases in intravascular volume the opposite changes take place. *Right*, When inotropy increases, the heart can pump more blood into the arterial side of the circulation, depleting slightly the venous store, thus decreasing right atrial pressure, although venous return is increased. When contractility is depressed, more blood accumulates on the venous side as the heart pumps less to the arterial side.

the aortic pulse waveform may precede the brachial waveform by 0.05 second, the delay may vary depending upon the vascular status. Such differences become important when timing the counterpulsation of an intra-aortic balloon.

Most of the energy of the pressure wave does not travel the entire distance down the vascular tree, but is reflected. Wave reflection may occur in high-resistance arterioles, branching points, or sites of changes in arterial distensibility, but the major source is the arteriole.[541] As a consequence, the pulse pressure wave that results is not due to the passage of the blood itself, but rather the combined effects of the forward-propagating pressure wave and its reflectance back toward the heart from various parts of the vasculature. With regard to wave transmission, the vascular bed can be considered as an asymmetric T tube with closed ends into which a pressure wave is applied.[542] A short end of the tube represents the head and upper extremities and a longer tube is the descending aorta and its derivative vessels. The reflections within the system give rise to the large but variable dicrotic notch observed in most arterial pressure waves. It is important to distinguish the dicrotic notch from the smaller deflection of the incisura during the declining pressure, which represents aortic valve closure and is seen in central aortic pressure tracings, but is seldom transmitted to the periphery.

Peripheral pulse waveforms have a delay in rise due to transmission (Fig. 5–25), and due to a resistive loss of power the diastolic and mean pressures are slightly lower. However, their peak amplitude is typically increased as the pressure wave being transmitted down increasingly narrow vessels meets the wave reflected from the arterioles. Peripheral peak pressures may exceed central pressures by 50%.[542] While pressure waves increase progressively in the periphery, the amplitude of flow actually decreases. This may in part be due to pressure wave reflections in the upper extremity contributing to flow down the descending aorta, with the reversal of flow when the lower body pressure wave reflection arrives, suggesting that "during diastole blood sloshes back and forth between the upper and lower body."[542] The velocity and exact contour of the pressure wave depends upon the distensibility of the vessels, which defines the velocity of the pressure wave; peripheral resistance, which defines the effective length of the tube; and the volume and pressure of the blood ejected.[541] In more distensible vessels, as in children and adolescents, wave transmission is slowed and the primary reflection in the central aorta may come after aortic valve closure, augmenting diastolic pressure. The secondary reflection back to the periphery then causes a large secondary wave and prominent dicrotic notch (Fig. 5–25*A*). When the vessels are less distensible, as in the elderly, wave velocity is faster and the primary reflection may actually enhance central systolic pressure waves (Fig. 5–25*B*).

Effects of Arterial Compliance on Ventricular Function

Pulsatile flow incurs a burden of external work that is about 10% of the total work performed in pumping blood.[543] However, depending upon the compliance of the system and the reflections that may be induced, the added component of external work entailed by pulsatile flow may be considerably increased when the impedence of the system increases. The ratio of pulsatile to steady work is increased in settings of decreased arterial compliance. When compliance is decreased cardiac ejection and work performed by the heart is decreased, although oxygen consumption is unchanged. In hearts in which function is decreased by ischemia or lidocaine administration, the decrease in cardiac performance is further impaired by decreased arterial compliance.[544] In the setting of high arterial compliance, more of the energy of ejection distends the vascular volume, which can then

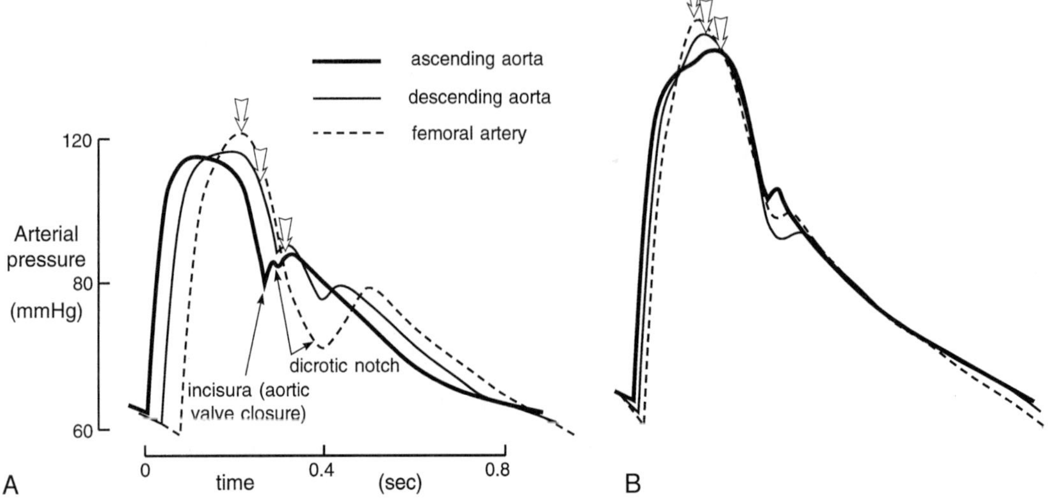

FIGURE **5–25.** Alterations in arterial pressure waves in a compliant vasculature (*A*) and in a stiffer vascular system (*B*). Note the greater interval between pressure waves in *A*, which is caused by the slower velocity of wave transmission compared to the less compliant vascular bed (*B*). The first reflection of the pressure wave causes the enhancement indicated by the *open arrows*. Due to the slower wave reflection in *A*, the augmentation occurs in late systole in the descending aorta and after aortic valve closure in the ascending aorta. In *B*, the wave reflections arrive during systole. (Data from O'Rourke MF: Vascular impedance in studies of arterial and cardiac function. Physiol Rev 62:570, 1982.)

"run off" during diastole. When arterial compliance is low, as in the elderly or in vasoconstricted patients, more of the pressure wave is rapidly transmitted and reflected back toward the heart, where it may retard ejection, if it arrives prior to aortic valve closure. Administration of vasodilators can decrease left ventricular loading by decreasing arterial compliance and reducing the burden of peripheral wave reflections. Employing trinitroglycerin (TNG) as a vasodilator, wave transmission was slowed and reflections delayed, an effect that appeared to not involve the proximal aorta but more distal aspects of the arterial bed.[545]

Ejection volume also markedly influences the pressure waveforms. When ejection volume is decreased during a Valsalva maneuver, the reflection is greatly decreased and appears to have little influence on aortic flow.[546] Pulse waveforms vary in atrial fibrillation, with beats with short systolic duration demonstrating diastolic waves and those with long durations having accentuated systolic peaks. Patients with hypertrophic cardiomyopathy have double systolic pulse waveforms because the initial systolic wave of ventricular ejection occurs during the first half of systole and the reflected wave returns during the same systole, increasing myocardial loading.[541]

References

1. Giles WR, Imaizumi Y: Comparison of potassium currents in rabbit atrial and ventricular cells. J Physiol (Lond) 405:123, 1988.
2. Catterall WA: Molecular properties of voltage-sensitive sodium channels. Annu Rev Biochem 55:953, 1986.
3. Catterall WA, Seagar MJ, Takahashi M: Molecular properties of dihydropyridine-sensitive calcium channels in skeletal muscle. J Biol Chem 263:3535, 1988.
4. Mikami A, Imoto K, Tanabe T, et al: Primary structure and functional expression of the cardiac dihydropyridine-sensitive calcium channel. Nature 340:230, 1989.
5. Brehm P, Okamura Y, Mandel G: Ion channel evolution. Semin Neurosci 3:355, 1991.
6. Miller C: 1990: Annus mirabilis of potassium channels. Science 252:1092, 1991.
7. Tamkun MM, Knoth KM, Walbridge JA, et al: Molecular cloning and characterization of two voltage-gated K^+ channel CDNAs from human ventricle. FASEB J 5:331, 1991.
8. Tsien RW, Ellinor PT, Horne WA: Molecular diversity of voltage-dependent Ca^{2+} channels. Trends Pharmacol Sci 12:349, 1991.
9. Katz AM: Cardiac ion channels. N Engl J Med 328:1244, 1993.
10. Noda M, Shimizu S, Tanabe T, et al: Primary structure of *Electrophorus electricus* sodium channel deduced from cDNA sequence. Nature 312:121, 1984.
11. Noda M, Ikeda T, Kayano T, et al: Existence of distinct sodium channel messenger RNAs in rat brain. Nature 320:188, 1986.
12. Catterall WA: Molecular properties of voltage-gated ion channels in the heart. In Fozzard HA, Haber E, Jennings RB, et al (eds): The Heart and Cardiovascular System: Scientific Foundations, 2nd ed. New York, Raven Press, 1991, p 945.
13. Heinemann SH, Terlau H, Stuhmer W, et al: Calcium channel characteristics conferred on the sodium channel by single mutations. Nature 356:441, 1992.
14. Bayer R, Kalusche D, Kaufmann R, Mannhold R: Inotropic and electrophysiological actions of verapamil and D600 in mammalian myocardium. III. Effects of optical isomers on transmembrane action potentials. Naunyn-Schmiedebergs Arch Pharmacol 290:87, 1975.
15. Yatani A, Brown AM: The calcium channel blocker nitrendipine blocks sodium channels in neonatal rat cardiac myocytes. Circ Res 56:868, 1985.
16. Gilliam FR III, Rivas PA, Wendt DJ, et al: Extracellular pH modulates block of both sodium and calcium channels by nicardipine. Am J Physiol 259:H1178, 1990.
17. Scheuer T, Kass RS: Phenytoin reduces calcium current in the cardiac Purkinje fiber. Circ Res 53:16, 1983.
18. Scamps F, Undrovinas A, Vassort G: Inhibition of I_{Ca} in single frog cardiac cells by quinidine, flecainide, ethmozin, and ethacizin. Am J Physiol 25:C549, 1989.
19. Kohlhardt M, Bauer B, Krause H, Fleckenstein A: Selective inhibition of the transmembrane Ca conductivity of mammalian myocardial fibres. Pflugers Arch 338:115, 1973.
20. Lee KS, Tsien RW: Reversal of current through calcium channels in dialysed single heart cells. Nature 297:498, 1982.

21. Field AC, Hill C, Lamb GD: Asymmetric charge movement and calcium currents in ventricular myocytes of neonatal rat. J Physiol (Lond) 406:277, 1988.
22. Bean BP, Ríos E: Nonlinear charge movement in mammalian cardiac ventricular cells. J Gen Physiol 94:65, 1989.
23. Po S, Roberds S, Snyders DJ, et al: Heteromultimeric assembly of human potassium channels: Molecular basis of a transient outward current? Circ Res 72:1326, 1993.
24. McLaughlin S, Szabo G, Eisenman G: Divalent ions and the surface potential of charged phospholipid membrane. J Gen Physiol 58:667, 1971.
25. Ji S, Weiss JN, Langer GA: Modulation of voltage-dependent sodium and potassium currents by charged amphiphiles in cardiac ventricular myocytes. Effects via modification of surface potential. J Gen Physiol 101:355, 1993.
26. Kraft LF, Katholi RE, Woods WT, James TN: Attenuation by magnesium of the electrophysiologic effects of hyperkalemia on human and canine heart cells. Am J Cardiol 45:1191, 1980.
27. Rogart RB, Cribbs LL, Muglia LK, et al: Molecular cloning of a putative tetrodotoxin-resistant rat heart Na^+ channel isoform. Proc Natl Acad Sci USA 86:8170, 1989.
28. Baer M, Best PM, Reuter H: Voltage-dependent action of tetrodotoxin in mammalian cardiac muscle. Nature 263:344, 1976.
29. Atwell D, Cohen I, Eisner D, et al: The steady state TTX sensitive ("window") sodium current in cardiac Purkinje fibers. Pflugers Arch 379:147, 1979.
30. Grant AO, Starmer CF: Mechanisms of closure of cardiac sodium channels in rabbit ventricular myocytes: Single-channel analysis. Circ Res 60:897, 1987.
31. Coraboeuf E, Deroubaix E, Colombe A: Effect of tetrodotoxin on the action potentials of the conducting system in the dog heart. Am J Physiol 236:H561, 1979.
32. Barber MJ: Class I antiarrhythmic agents. In Lynch C III (ed): Clinical Cardiac Electrophysiology: Perioperative Considerations. Philadelphia, JB Lippincott Co, 1994, p 85.
33. Fozzard HA, Hanck DA: Sodium channels. In Fozzard HA, Haber E, Jennings RB, et al (eds): The Heart and Cardiovascular System: Scientific Foundations, 2nd ed. New York, Raven Press, 1991, p 1091.
34. Kameyama M, Kiyosue T, Soejima M: Single channel analysis of the inward rectifier K current in the rabbit ventricular cells. Jpn J Physiol 33:1039, 1983.
35. Veldkamp MW, Ginneken ACGV, Bouman LN: Single delayed rectifier channels in the membrane of rabbit ventricular myocytes. Circ Res 72:865, 1993.
36. Lacerda AE, Kim HS, Ruth O, et al: Normalization of current kinetics by interaction between the α_1 and β subunits of the skeletal muscle dihydropyridine-sensitive Ca^{2+} channel. Nature 352:527, 1991.
37. Hescheler J, Pelzer D, Trube G, Trautwein W: Does the organic channel blocker D600 act from inside or outside on the cardiac cell membrane. Pflugers Arch 393:287, 1982.
38. Kass RS, Arena JP, Chin S: Block of L-type calcium channels by charged dihydropyridines. Sensitivity to side of application and calcium. J Gen Physiol 98:63, 1991.
39. Hadley RW, Lederer WJ: Ca^{2+} and voltage inactivate Ca^{2+} channels in guinea-pig ventricular myocytes through independent mechanisms. J Physiol (Lond) 444:257, 1991.
40. Yuan W, Bers DM: Ca-dependent facilitation of cardiac Ca current is due to Ca-calmodulin-dependent protein kinase. Am J Physiol 267:H982, 1994.
41. DeFelice LJ: Molecular and biophysical view of the Ca channel: A hypothesis regarding oligomeric structure, channel clustering, and macroscopic current. J Membr Biol 133:191, 1993.
42. Shenolikar S: Protein phosphorylation: Hormones, drugs, and bioregulation. FASEB J 2:2753, 1988.
43. Yue DT, Herzig S, Marban E: β-Adrenergic stimulation of calcium channels occurs by potentiation of high-activity gating modes. Proc Natl Acad Sci USA 87:753, 1990.
44. Bean BP: Two kinds of calcium channels in canine atrial cells: Differences in kinetics, selectivity, and pharmacology. J Gen Physiol 86:1, 1985.
45. Nilius B, Hess P, Lansman JB, Tsien RW: A novel type of cardiac calcium channel in ventricular cells. Nature 316:443, 1985.
46. Mitra R, Morad M: Two types of Ca^{2+} in guinea pig ventricular myocytes. Proc Natl Acad Sci USA 83:5340, 1986.
47. McDonald TF, Pelzer S, Trautwein W, Pelzer DJ: Regulation and modulation of calcium channels in cardiac, skeletal, and smooth muscle cells. Physiol Rev 74:365, 1994.
48. Kubo Y, Baldwin TJ, Jan YN, Jan LY: Primary structure and functional expression of a mouse inward rectifier potassium channel. Nature 362:127, 1993.
49. Matsuda H: Magnesium gating of the inwardly rectifying K^+ channel. Annu Rev Physiol 53:289, 1991.
50. Ficker E, Taglialatela M, Wible BA, et al: Spermine and spermidine as gating molecules for inward rectifier K^+ channels. Science 266:1068, 1994.
51. Lopatin AN, Makhina EN, Nichols CG: Potassium channel block by cytoplasmic polyamines as the mechanism of intrinsic rectification. Nature 372:366, 1994.
52. Yamada M, Kurachi Y: Spermine gates inward-rectifying muscarinic but not ATP-sensitive K^+ channels in rabbit atrial myocytes. J Biol Chem 270:9289, 1995.
53. Tomaselli GF, Backx PH, Marban E: Molecular basis of permeation in voltage-gated ion channels. Circ Res 72:491, 1993.
54. Ackerman MJ, Clapham DE: Cardiac chloride channels. Trends Cardiovasc Med 3:23, 1993.
55. Zygmunt AC, Gibbons WR: Calcium-activated chloride current in rabbit ventricular myocytes. Circ Res 68:424, 1991.
56. Zygmunt AC, Gibbons WR: Properties of the calcium-activated chloride current in heart. J Gen Physiol 99:391, 1992.
57. Hagiwara N, Masuda H, Shoda M, Irisawa H: Stretch-activated anion currents of rabbit cardiac myocytes. J Physiol (Lond) 456: 285, 1992.
58. Duan D, Hume JR, Nattel S: Evidence that outwardly rectifying Cl^- channels underlie volume-regulated Cl^- currents in heart. Circ Res 80:103, 1997.
59. Sorota S: Swelling-induced chloride-sensitive current in canine atrial cells revealed by whole-cell patch clamp. Circ Res 70:679, 1992.
60. Bahinski A, Nairn AC, Greengard P, Gadsby DC: Chloride conductance regulated by cyclic AMP-dependent protein kinase in cardiac myocytes. Nature 340:718, 1989.
61. Harvey RD, Hume JR: Autonomic regulation of a chloride current in heart. Science 244:983, 1989.
62. Harvey RD, Clark CD, Hume JR: Chloride current in mammalian cardiac myocytes—novel mechanism for autonomic regulation of action potential duration and resting membrane potential. J Gen Physiol 95:1077, 1990.
63. Takano M, Noma A: Distribution of the isoprenaline-induced chloride current in rabbit heart. Pflugers Arch 420:223, 1992.
64. Ehara T, Matsuura H: Single-channel study of the cyclic AMP-regulated chloride current in guinea-pig ventricular myocytes. J Physiol (Lond) 464:307, 1993.
65. Horisberger J-D, Lemas V, Kraehenbuhl J-P, Rossier B: Structure-function relationship of Na,K-ATPase, Annu Rev Physiol 53:565, 1991.
66. Cairns SP, Westerblad H, Allen DG: Changes in myoplasmic pH and calcium concentration during exposure to lactate in isolated rat ventricular myocytes. J Physiol (Lond) 464:561, 1993.
67. Langer GA: Calcium and the heart: Exchange at the tissue, cell, and organelle levels. FASEB J 6:893, 1992.
68. Scarpa A, Graziotti P: Mechanisms for intracellular calcium regulation in heart. I. Stopped-flow measurements of Ca uptake by cardiac mitochondria. J Gen Physiol 62:756, 1973.
69. Bassani JWM, Bassani RA, Bers DM: Ca^{2+} cycling between sarcoplasmic reticulum and mitochondria in rabbit cardiac myocytes. J Physiol (Lond) 460:603, 1993.
70. Brandes R, Bers DM: Intracellular Ca^{2+} increases the mitochondrial NADH concentration during elevated work in intact cardiac muscle. Circ Res 80:82, 1997.
71. James TN: Cardiac conduction system: Fetal and postnatal development. Am J Cardiol 6:1083, 1970.
72. Bleeker WK, McKaay AJC, Masson-Pevot M, et al: The functional and morphological organization of the rabbit sinus node. Circ Res 46:11, 1980.
73. Campbell DL, Rasmusson RL, Strauss HC: Ionic current mechanisms generating vertebrate primary cardiac pacemaker activity at the single cell level: An integrative view. Annu Rev Physiol 54:279, 1992.
74. DiFrancesco D: Pacemaker mechanisms in cardiac tissue. Annu Rev Physiol 55:455, 1993.

75. Irisawa H, Brown HF, Giles W: Cardiac pacemaking in the sinoatrial node. Physiol Rev 73:197, 1993.
76. Doerr T, Denger R, Trautwein W: Calcium currents in single SA nodal cells of the rabbit heart studied with action potential clamp. Pflugers Arch 413:599, 1989.
77. Woehlck HJ, Vicenzi MN, Bosnjak ZJ, Atlee JL III: Anesthetics and automaticity of dominant and latent pacemakers in chronically instrumented dogs. I. Methodology, conscious state, and halothane anesthesia: Comparison with and without muscarinic blockade during exposure to epinephrine. Anesthesiology 79: 1304, 1993.
78. Nánási PP, Varró A, Lathrop DA: Isolation of human ventricular and atrial cardiomyocytes: Technical note. Cardioscience 4:111, 1993.
79. Escande D, Coulombe A, Faivre J-F, et al: Two types of transient outward currents in adult human atrial cells. Am J Physiol 249: H142, 1987.
80. Clark RB, Giles WR, Imaizumi Y: Properties of the transient outward currents in rabbit atrial cells. J Physiol (Lond) 405:147, 1988.
81. Beuckelmann DJ, Näbauer M, Erdmann E: Alterations of K^+ currents in isolated human ventricular myocytes from patients with terminal heart failure. Circ Res 73:379, 1993.
82. Franz MR, Bargheer K, Rafflenbeul W, et al: Monophasic action potential mapping in human subjects with normal electrocardiograms: Direct evidence for the genesis of the T wave. Circulation 75:379, 1987.
83. Litovsky SH, Antzelevitch C: Transient outward current prominent in canine ventricular epicardium but not endocardium. Circ Res 62:116, 1988.
84. Luo C, Rudy Y: A model of the ventricular cardiac action potential: Depolarization, repolarization, and their interaction. Circ Res 68:1501, 1991.
85. Pancrazio JJ, Frazer MJ, Lynch C III: Barbiturate anesthetics depress the resting K^+ conductance of myocardium. J Pharmacol Exp Ther 265:358, 1993.
86. Lynch C III: Cellular electrophysiology of the heart. In Lynch C III (ed): Clinical Cardiac Electrophysiology: Perioperative Considerations. Philadelphia, JB Lippincott Co, 1994, p 1.
87. Starling EH: The Linacre Lecture of the Law of the Heart. London, Longmans Green & Co Ltd, 1918.
88. Forbes MS, Sperelakis N: Ultrastructure of Mammalian Cardiac Muscle. In Sperelakis N (ed): Physiology and Pathophysiology of the Heart. Boston, Martinus Nijhoff Publishing, 1984, p 3.
89. Sommer JR, Jennings RB: Ultrastructure of Cardiac Muscle. In Fozzard HA, Haber E, Jennings RB, et al: (eds): The Heart and Cardiovascular System: Scientific Foundations, 2nd ed. New York, Raven Press, 1991, p 3.
90. Engel J, Fechner M, Sowerby AJ, et al: Anisotropic propagation of Ca^{2+} waves in isolated cardiomyocytes. Biophys J 66:1756, 1994.
91. Campbell KB, Kirkpatrick RD, Tobias AH, et al: Series coupled non-contractile elements are functionally unimportant in the isolated heart. Cardiovasc Res 28:242, 1994.
92. MacKenna D, Omens J, McCulloch AM, Covell J: Contribution of collagen matrix to passive left ventricular mechanics in isolated rat hearts. Am J Physiol 266:H1007, 1994.
93. Omens J, Rockman H, Covell J: Passive ventricular mechanics in tight-skin mice. Am J Physiol 266:H1169, 1994.
94. Wang Z, Gergely J, Tao T: Characterization of the Ca^{2+}-triggered conformational transition in troponin C. Proc Natl Acad Sci USA 89:11814, 1992.
95. Potter JD, Gergely J: Troponin, tropomyosin, and actin interactions in the Ca^{2+} regulation of muscle contraction. Biochemistry 13:2697, 1974.
96. Tao T, Gong BJ, Leavis P: Calcium-induced movement of troponin-I relative to actin in skeletal muscle thin filaments. Science 247:1339, 1990.
97. Rayment I, Rypniewski WR, Schmidt-Bäse K, et al: Three-dimensional structure of myosin subfragment-1: A molecular motor. Science 261:50, 1993.
98. Pagani E, Julian F: Rabbit papillary muscle myosic isozymes and the velocity of muscle shortening. Circ Res 54:586, 1984.
99. ter Keurs HEDJ, Rijnsburger WH, van Heuningen R, Nagelsmit MJ: Tension development and sarcomere length in rat cardiac trabeculae. Evidence of length dependent activation. Circ Res 46:703, 1980.
100. Kentish JC, ter Keurs HEDJ, Ricciardi L, et al: Comparison between the sarcomere length-force relations of intact and skinned trabeculae from rat right ventricle: Influence of calcium concentrations on these relations. Circ Res 58:755, 1986.
101. Allen DG, Eisner DA, Pirolo JS, Smith GL: The relationship between intracellular calcium concentration and contraction in calcium-overloaded ferret papillary muscles. J Physiol (Lond) 364:169, 1985.
102. Hofmann P, Fuchs F: Evidence for a force-dependent component of calcium binding to cardiac troponin C. Am J Physiol 22:C541, 1987.
103. Saeki Y, Kurihara S, Hongo K, Tanaka E: Alterations in intracellular calcium and tension of activated ferret papillary muscle in response to step length changes. J Physiol (Lond) 463:291, 1993.
104. Babu A, Sonnenblick E, Gulati J: Molecular basis for the influence of muscle length on myocardial performance. Science 240: 74, 1988.
105. Gulati J, Sonnenblick E, Babu A: The role of troponin C in the length dependence of Ca^{2+}-sensitive force of mammalian skeletal and cardiac muscle fibers. J Physiol (Lond) 444:305, 1990.
106. Fuchs F: Mechanical modulation of the Ca^{2+} regulatory protein complex in cardiac muscle. News Physiol Sci 10:6, 1995.
107. Hannon JD, Martyn DA, Gordon AM: Effects of cycling and rigor crossbridges on the conformation of cardiac troponin C. Circ Res 71:984, 1992.
108. Landesberg A, Sideman S: Coupling calcium binding to troponin C and cross-bridge in skinned cardiac cells. Am J Physiol 266: H1260, 1994.
109. Allen DG, Kurihara S: The effects of muscle length on intracellular calcium transients in mammalian cardiac muscle. J Physiol (Lond) 327:79, 1982.
110. Julian FJ, Sollins MR: Sarcomere length-tension relations in living rat papillary muscle. Circ Res 37:299, 1975.
111. Sonnenblick EH: Determinants of active state in heart muscle; force, velocity, instantaneous muscle length, time. Fed Proc 24: 1396, 1964.
112. Mason DT, Spann Jr JF, Zelis R: Quantification of the contractile state of the intact human heart. Am J Cardiol 26:248, 1970.
113. Brutsaert DL, De Clerck NM, Goethals MA, Housmans PR: Relaxation of ventricular cardiac muscle. J Physiol (Lond) 283:469, 1978.
114. Brutsaert DL, Housmans PR, Goethals MA: Dual control of relaxation: Its role in the ventricular function in the mammalian heart. Circ Res 47:637, 1980.
115. Pery-man N, Chemla D, Coirault C, et al: A comparison of cyclopiazonic acid and ryanodine effects on cardiac muscle relaxation. Am J Physiol 265:H1364, 1993.
116. Housmans PR, Lee NKM, Blinks JR: Active shortening retards the decline of the intracellular calcium transient in mammalian heart muscle. Science 221:159, 1983.
117. Lab MJ, Allen DG, Orchard CH: The effects of shortening on myoplasmic calcium concentration and on the action potential in mammalian ventricular muscle. Circ Res 55:825, 1984.
118. Zile MR, Blaustein AS, Gaasch WH: The effect of acute alterations in left ventricular afterload and β-adrenergic tone on indices of early diastolic filling rate. Circ Res 65:406, 1989.
119. Burkhoff D, de Tombe PP, Hunter WC: Impact of ejection on magnitude and time course of ventricular pressure-generating capacity. Am J Physiol 265:H899, 1993.
120. Bates SE, Gurney AM: Ca^{2+}-dependent block and potentiation of L-type calcium current in guinea-pig ventricular myocytes. J Physiol (Lond) 466:345, 1993.
121. Fabiato A: Calcium-induced release of calcium from the cardiac sarcoplasmic reticulum. Am J Physiol 245:C1, 1983.
122. Otsu K, Willard HF, Khanna VK, et al: Molecular cloning of cDNA encoding of the Ca^{2+} release channel (ryanodine receptor) of rabbit cardiac muscle sarcoplasmic reticulum. J Biol Chem 265:13472, 1990.
123. Shacklock PS, Wier WG, Balke CW: Local Ca^{2+} transients (Ca^{2+} sparks) originate at the transverse tubules in rat heart cells. J Physiol (Lond) 487:601, 1995.
124. Balke CW, Egan TM, Wier WG: Processes that remove calcium from the cytoplasm during excitation-contraction coupling in intact rat heart cells. J Physiol (Lond) 474:447, 1994.

125. Lew WYW: Mechanisms of volume-induced increase in left ventricular contractility. Am J Physiol 265:H1778, 1993.
126. Langer GA, Peskoff A, Post JA: How does the Na^+-Ca^{2+} exchanger working the intact cardiac cells? J Mol Cell Cardiol 25: 637, 1993.
127. Wier WG: Cytoplasmic [Ca^{2+}] in mammalian ventricle: Dynamic control by cellular processes. Annu Rev Physiol 52:467, 1990.
128. Mullins LJ: The generation of electric currents in cardiac fibers by Na/Ca exchange. Am J Physiol 236:C103, 1979.
129. Blaustein MP: Sodium/calcium exchange and the control of contractility in cardiac muscle and vascular smooth muscle. J Cardiovasc Pharmacol 12(Suppl 5):S56, 1988.
130. Levi AJ, Brooksby P, Hancox JC: One hump or two? The triggering of calcium release from the sarcoplasmic reticulum and the voltage dependence of contraction in mammalian cardiac muscle. Cardiovasc Res 27:1743, 1993.
131. Nuss HB, Houser SR: Sodium-calcium exchange-mediated contractions in feline ventricular myocytes. Am J Physiol 263: H1161, 1992.
132. Constable PD, Muir WW, Binkley PF: Hypertonic saline is a negative inotropic agent in normovolumic dogs. Am J Physiol 267:H677, 1994.
133. Yue DT, Burkhoff D, Franz MR, et al: Postextrasystolic potentiation of the isolated canine left ventricle. Circ Res 56:340, 1985.
134. Baum VC, Klitzner TS: Excitation-contraction coupling in neonatal myocardium: Effects of halothane and isoflurane. Dev Pharmacol Ther 16:99, 1991.
135. Miao N, Lynch C III: Effect of temperature on volatile anesthetic depression of myocardial contractions. Anesth Analg 76:366, 1993.
136. Opie LH: Metabolism of the heart in health and disease. Am Heart J 77:100, 1969.
137. Randle PJ, Tubbs PK: Carbohydrate and fatty acid metabolism. In Berne RM (ed): Handbook of Physiology. The Cardiovascular System. Bethesda, MD, American Physiological Society, 1979, p 805.
138. Collins-Nakai RL, Noseworthy D, Lopaschuck GD: Epinephrine increases ATP production in hearts by preferentially increasing glucose metabolism. Am J Physiol 36:H1862, 1994.
139. Birnbaumer L: G Proteins in signal transduction. Annu Rev Pharmacol Toxicol 30:675, 1990.
140. Holmer SR, Homcy CJ: G proteins in the heart: A redundant and diverse transmembrane signaling network. Circulation 84: 1891, 1991.
141. Lynch C III, Jaeger JM: The G protein cell signalling system. In Lake C (ed): Advances in Anesthesia. Chicago, Mosby-Year Book, 1994, p 65.
142. Hepler JR, Gilman AG: G proteins. Trends Biochem Sci 17:383, 1992.
143. Iñiguez-Lluhi J, Kleuss C, Gilman AG: The importance of G-protein $\beta\gamma$ subunits. Trends Cell Biol 3:230, 1993.
144. Iyengar R: Molecular and functional diversity of mammalian Gs-stimulated adenylyl cyclases. FASEB J 7:768, 1993.
145. Kim HW, Steenart NAE, Ferguson DG, Kranias EG: Functional reconstitution of the cardiac sarcoplasmic reticulum Ca^{2+}-ATPase with phospholamban in phospholipid vesicles. J Biol Chem 265:1702, 1990.
146. Takasago T, Imagawa T, Shigekawa M: Phosphorylation of the cardiac ryanodine receptor by cAMP-dependent kinase. J Biochem 106:872, 1989.
147. Charpentier F, Legato MJ, Steinberg SF, et al: β-Adrenergic modulation of Na-K pump activity in young and adult canine cardiac Purkinje fibers. Am J Physiol 40:H706, 1996.
148. Robertson S, Johnson J, Holroyde M, et al: The effect of troponin I phosphorylation on the Ca^{2+}-binding properties of the Ca^{2+}-regulatory site of bovine cardiac troponin. J Biol Chem 257:260, 1982.
149. Hoh J, Rossmanith G, Kwan L, Hamilton A: Adrenaline increases the rate of cycling of crossbridges in rat cardiac muscle as measured by pseudo-random binary noise-modulated perturbation analysis. Circ Res 62:452, 1988.
150. Walsh KB, Begenisich TB, Kass RS: β-Adrenergic modulation in the heart: Independent regulation of K and Ca channels. Pflugers Arch 411:232, 1988.
151. Nakayama T, Fozzard HA: Adrenergic modulation of the transient outward current in isolated canine Purkinje cells. Circ Res 62:162, 1988.
152. Xiao P-P, Lakatta EG: β_1-Adrenoceptor stimulation and β_2-adrenoceptor stimulation differ in their effects on contraction, cytosolic Ca^{2+}, and Ca^{2+} current in single rat ventricular cells. Circ Res 73:286, 1993.
153. Barnard EA: Separating receptor subtypes from their shadows. Nature 335:301, 1988.
154. Shryock J, Song Y, Wang D, et al: Selective A_2-adenosine receptor agonists do not alter action potential duration, twitch shortening, or cAMP accumulation in guinea pig, rat, or rabbit isolated ventricular myocytes. Circ Res 72:194, 1993.
155. Böhm M, Gierschik P, Schwinger RHG, et al: Coupling of M-cholinoceptors and A_1 adenosine receptors in human myocardium. Am J Physiol 266:H1951, 1994.
156. DiFrancesco D, Ducouret P, Robinson RB: Muscarinic modulation of cardiac rate at low acetylcholine concentrations. Science 243:669, 1989.
157. Petit-Jacques J, Bescond J, Bois P, Lenfant J: Particular sensitivity of the mammalian heart sinus node cells. News Physiol Sci 9:77, 1994.
158. Isenberg G, Belardinelli L: Ionic basic for the antagonism between adenosine and isoproterenol on isolated mammalian ventricular myocytes. Circ Res 55:309, 1984.
159. Boyett MR, Kirby MS, Orchard CH, Roberts A: The negative inotropic effect of acetylcholine on ferret ventricular myocardium. J Physiol (Lond) 404:613, 1988.
160. Jiang M, Moffat M, Narayanan N: Age-related alterations in the phosphorylation of sarcoplasmic reticulum and myofibrillar proteins and diminished contractile response to isoproterenol in intact rat ventricle. Circ Res 72:102, 1993.
161. Dobson JG, Fenton RA: Adenosine inhibition of β-adrenergic induced responses in aged hearts. Am J Physiol 265:H494, 1993.
162. Zhang JZ, MacLeod KM: Dissociation of negative inotropic effect of carbachol from changes in cAMP and PKA in perfused rat hearts. Am J Physiol 40:H404, 1996.
163. Beavo JA: Cyclic nucleotide phosphodiesterases: Functional implications of multiple isoforms. Physiol Rev 75:725, 1995.
164. Ono K, Trautwein W: Potentiation by cyclic GMP of β-adrenergic effect on Ca^{2+} current in guinea-pig ventricular cells. J Physiol (Lond) 443:387, 1991.
165. Méry P-F, Pavoine C, Belhassen L, et al: Nitric oxide regulates cardiac Ca^{2+} current. Involvement of cGMP-inhibited and cGMP-stimulated phosphodiesterases through guanylyl cyclase activation. J Biol Chem 268:26286, 1993.
166. Brown AM, Birnbaumer L: Ion channels and their regulation by G protein subunits. Ann Rev Physiol 52:197, 1990.
167. Yatani A, Brown AM: Rapid β-adrenergic modulation of cardiac calcium channel currents by a fast G protein pathway. Science 245:71, 1989.
168. Hartzell HC, Fischmeister R: Direct regulation of cardiac Ca^{2+} channels by G proteins: Neither proven nor necessary? Trends Pharmacol Sci 13:380, 1992.
169. Scamps F, Nilius B, Alvarez J, Vassort G: Modulation of L-type Ca channel activity by P_2-purinergic agonist in cardiac cells. Pflugers Arch 422:465, 1993.
170. Horie M, Irisawa H: Rectification of muscarinic K^+ current by magnesium ion in guinea pig atrial cells. Am J Physiol 253:10, 1987.
171. Agus ZS, Morad M: Modulation of cardiac ion channels by magnesium. Annu Rev Physiol 53:299, 1991.
172. Kubo Y, Reuveny E, Slesinger PA, et al: Primary structure and functional expression of a rat G-protein-coupled muscarinic potassium channel. Nature 364:802, 1993.
173. Koumi S-I, Wasserstrom JA: Acetylcholine-sensitive muscarinic K^+ channels in mammalian ventricular myocytes. Am J Physiol 266:H1812, 1994.
174. Smrcka AV, Hepler JR, Brown KO, Sternweiss PC: Regulation of polyphosphoinositide-specific phospholipase C activity by purified G_q. Science 251:804, 1991.
175. Sternweis PC, Smrcka AV: Regulation of phospholipase C by G proteins. Trends Biochem Sci 17:502, 1992.
176. Nosek TM, Williams MF, Zeigler ST, Godt RE: Inositol triphosphate enhances calcium release in skinned cardiac and skeletal muscle. Am J Physiol 250:C807, 1986.

177. Dösemeci A, Dhallan RS, Cohen NM, et al: Phorbol ester increases calcium current and simulates the effects of angiotensin II on cultured neonatal rat heart myocytes. Circ Res 62:347, 1988.
178. Baker KM, Aceto JA: Characterization of avian angiotensin II cardiac receptors: Coupling to mechanical activity and phosphoinositide metabolism. J Mol Cell Cardiol 21:375, 1989.
179. Kawaguchi H, Shoki M, Sano H, et al: Phospholipid metabolism in cardiomyopathic hamster heart cells. Circ Res 69:1015, 1991.
180. Kijima Y, Saito A, Jetton TL, et al: Different intracellular localization of inositol 1,4,5-triphosphate and ryanodine receptors in cardiomyocytes. J Biol Chem 268:3499, 1993.
181. Sando JJ, Maurer MC, Bolen EJ, Grisham CM: Role of cofactors in protein kinase C activation. Cell Signal 4:595, 1992.
182. Noland TA Jr, Kuo JF: Protein kinase C phosphorylation of cardiac troponin I and troponin T inhibits Ca^{2+}-stimulated Mg-ATPase activity in reconstituted actomyosin and isolated myofibrils, and decreases actin-myosin interactions. J Mol Cell Cardiol 25:53, 1993.
183. Edes I, Kranias E: Phospholamban and troponin I are substrates for protein kinase C in vitro but not in intact beating guinea pig hearts. Circ Res 67:394, 1990.
184. Gambassi G, Spurgeon HA, Lakatta EG, et al: Different effects of α- and β-adrenergic stimulation on cytosolic pH and myofilament responsiveness to Ca^{2+} in cardiac myocytes. Circ Res 71:870, 1992.
185. Terzic A, Pucéat M, Clément O, et al: α_1-Adrenergic effects on intracellular pH and calcium and on myofilaments in single rat cardiac cells. J Physiol (Lond) 447:275, 1992.
186. Zheng J-S, Christie A, Levy M, Scarpa A: Ca^{2+} mobilization by extracellular ATP in rat cardiac myocytes: Regulation by protein kinase C and A. Am J Physiol 263:C933, 1992.
187. Walsh KB, Kass RS: Regulation of a heart potassium channel by protein kinase A and C. Science 242:67, 1988.
188. Tohse N, Kameyama M, Sekiguchi K, et al: Protein kinase C activation enhances the delayed rectifier potassium current in guinea-pig heart cells. J Mol Cell Cardiol 22:725, 1990.
189. Tohse N, Nakaya H, Kanno M: α_1-Adrenoceptor stimulation enhances the delayed rectifier K^+ current of guinea pig ventricular cells through the activation of protein kinase C. Circ Res 71: 1441, 1992.
190. Boutjdir M, Restivo M, Wei Y, El-Sherif N: α_1-β-Adrenergic interactions on L-type calcium current in cardiac myocytes. Pflugers Arch 421:397, 1992.
191. Light PE, Sabir AA, Allen BG, et al: Protein kinase C-induced changes in the stoichiometry of ATP binding activate cardiac ATP-sensitive K^+ channels. Circ Res 79:399, 1996.
192. Lester JW, Gannaway KF, Reardon RA, et al: Effects of adenosine and protein kinase C stimulation on mechanical properties of rat cardiac myocytes. Am J Physiol 40:H1778, 1996.
193. Kim E, Han J, Ho W, Earm YE: Modulation of ATP-sensitive K^+ channels in rabbit ventricular myocytes by adenosine A_1 receptor activation. Am J Physiol 272:H325, 1997.
194. Brown JH, Buxton IL, Brunton LL: Alpha$_1$-adrenergic and muscarinic cholinergic stimulation of phosphoinositide hydrolysis in adult rat cardiomyocytes. Circ Res 57:532, 1985.
195. Goto M, Liu Y, Yang X-M, et al: Role of bradykinin in protection of ischemic preconditioning in rabbit hearts. Circ Res 77: 611, 1995.
196. Bugge E, Ytrehus K: Endothelin-1 can reduce infarct size through protein kinase C and K_{ATP} channels in the isolated rat heart. Cardiovasc Res 32:920, 1996.
197. Endoh M, Blinks JM: Actions of sympathomimetic amines on the Ca^{2+} transients and contractions of rabbit myocardium: Reciprocal changes in myofibrillar responsiveness to Ca^{2+} mediated through α- and β-receptors. Circ Res 62:247, 1988.
198. Curiel R, Pérez-González J, Brito N, et al: Positive inotropic effects mediated by α_1 adrenoceptors in intact human subjects. J Cardiovasc Pharmacol 14:603, 1989.
199. Landzberg JS, Parker JD, Gauthier DF, Colucci WS: Effects of myocardial α_1-adrenergic receptor stimulation and blockade on contractility in humans. Circulation 84:1608, 1991.
200. Doubell A, Thibault G: Calcium is involved in both positive and negative modulation of the secretory system for ANP. Am J Physiol 266:H1854, 1994.
201. Abdelmeguid AE, Feher JJ: Effect of perfusate [Ca^{2+}] on cardiac sarcoplasmic Ca^{2+} release channel in isolated hearts. Circ Res 71:1049, 1992.
202. Witcher DR, Kovacs RJ, Schulman H, et al: Unique phosphorylation site on the cardiac ryanodine receptor regulates calcium channel activity. J Biol Chem 266:11114, 1991.
203. De Hert SG, Gillebert TC, Andries LJ, Brutseart DL: Role of the endocardial endothelium in the regulation of myocardial function. Physiologic and pathophysiologic implications. Anesthesiology 79:1354, 1993.
204. Han X, Shimoni Y, Giles WR: An obligatory role for nitric oxide in autonomic control of mammalian heart rate. J Physiol (Lond) 476:309, 1994.
205. Hare JM, Keaney JF Jr, Balligand J-L, et al: Role of nitric oxide in parasympathetic modulation of b-adrenergic myocardial contractility in normal dogs. J Clin Invest 95:360, 1995.
206. Balligand J-L, Kelly RA, Marsden PA, et al: Control of cardiac muscle cell function by an endogenous nitric oxide signaling system. Proc Natl Acad Sci USA 90:347, 1993.
207. Brady AJB, Warren JB, Poole-Wilson PA, et al: Nitric oxide attenuates cardiac myocyte contraction. Am J Physiol 265:H176, 1993.
208. Paulus WJ, Vantrimpont PJ, Shah AM: Acute effects of nitric oxide on left ventricular relaxation and diastolic distensibility in humans: Assessment by bicoronary sodium nitroprusside infusion. Circulation 89:2070, 1994.
209. Keaney JF Jr, Hare JM, Balligand J-L, et al: Inhibition of nitric oxide synthase augments myocardial contractile responses to β-adrenergic stimulation. Am J Physiol 271:H2646, 1996.
210. Ungureanu-Longrois D, Balligand J-L, Okada I, et al: Contractile responsiveness of ventricular myocytes to isoproterenol is regulated by induction of nitric oxide synthase activity in cardiac microvascular endothelial cells in heterotypic primary culture. Circ Res 77:486, 1995.
211. Singh K, Balligand J-L, Fischer TA, et al: Regulation of cytokine-inducible nitric oxide synthase in cardiac myocytes and microvascular endothelial cells. J Biol Chem 271:1111, 1996.
212. Brady AJB, Poole-Wilson PA, Harding SE, Warren JB: Nitric oxide production within cardiac myocytes reduces their contractility in endotoxemia. Am J Physiol 263:H1963, 1992.
213. Kinugawa K-I, Kohmoto O, Yao A, et al: Cardiac inducible nitric oxide synthase negatively modulates myocardial function in cultured rat myocytes. Am J Physiol 272:H35, 1997.
214. Han X, Shimoni Y, Giles WR: A cellular mechanism for nitric oxide-mediated cholinergic control of mammalian heart rate. J Gen Physiol 106:45, 1995.
215. Méry P-F, Lohmann SM, Walter U, Fischmeister R: Ca^{2+} current is regulated by cGMP-dependent protein kinase in mammalian cardiac myocytes. Proc Natl Acad Sci USA 88:1197, 1991.
216. Wahler GM, Dollinger SJ: Nitric oxide donor SIN-1 inhibits mammalian cardiac calcium current through cGMP-dependent protein kinase. Am J Physiol 268:C45, 1995.
217. Campbell DL, Stamler JS, Strauss HC: Redox modulation of L-type calcium channels in ferret ventricular myocytes. J Gen Physiol 108:277, 1996.
218. Garbers DL: Guanylyl cyclase-linked receptors. Pharmacol Ther 50:337, 1991.
219. Janes RD, Brandys JC, Hopkins DA, et al: Anatomy of human extrinsic cardiac nerves and ganglia. Am J Cardiol 57:299, 1986.
220. Bennett MR: Quantal release at visualized sympathetic nerve varicosities. News Physiol Sci 8:199, 1993.
221. Massing GK, James JN: Anatomic configuration of the His bundle and bundle branches in the human heart. Circulation 53:609, 1976.
222. Vanhoutte PM, Levy MN: Prejunctional cholinergic modulation of neurotransmission in the cardiovascular system. Am J Physiol 238:H275, 1980.
223. Yang T, Levy MN: Sequence of excitation as a factor in sympathetic-parasympathetic interactions in the heart. Circ Res 71:898, 1992.
224. Yang T, Levy MN: Effects of intense antecedent sympathetic stimulation on sympathetic neurotransmission in the heart. Circ Res 72:137, 1993.
225. Burnstock G: Overview: Purinergic mechanisms. Ann N Y Acad Sci 603:1, 1990.

226. Boudreau G, Péronnet F, de Champlain J, Nadeau R: Presynaptic effects of epinephrine on norepinephrine release from cardiac sympathetic nerves in dogs. Am J Physiol 265:H205, 1993.
227. Latson TW: Principles and applications of heart rate variability analysis. In Lynch C III (ed): Clinical Cardiac Electrophysiology: Perioperative Considerations. Philadelphia, JB Lippincott Co, 1994, p 307.
228. Matsuyama S, Saito N, Shuntoh H, et al: GABA modulates neurotransmission in sinus node via stimulation of $GABA_A$ receptor. Am J Physiol 264:H1057, 1993.
229. Baker KM, Singer HA: Identification and characterization of guinea pig angiotensin II ventricular and atrial receptors: Coupling to inositol phosphate production. Circ Res 62:896, 1988.
230. Moravec CS, Schluchter MD, Paranandi L, et al: Inotropic effects of angiotensin II on human cardiac muscle in vitro. Circulation 82:1990, 1990.
231. Moorman JR, Kirsch GE, Lacerda AE, Brown AM: Angiotensin II modulates cardiac N^+ channels in neonatal rat. Circ Res 65: 1804, 1989.
232. Eberli FR, Apstein CS, Ngoy S, Lorell BH: Exacerbation of left ventricular ischemic diastolic dysfunction by pressure-overload hypertrophy: Modification by specific inhibition of cardiac angiotensin converting enzyme. Circ Res 70:931, 1992.
233. Unger T, Gohlke P: Converting enzyme inhibitors in cardiovascular therapy: Current status and future potential. Cardiovasc Res 28:146, 1994.
234. Litten RZ, Martin BJ, Low RB, Alpert NR: Altered myosin isozyme patterns from pressure-overloaded and thyrotoxic hypertrophied rabbit hearts. Circ Res 50:856, 1982.
235. Dillman WH: Biochemical basis of thyroid hormone action in heart. Am J Med 88:626, 1990.
236. Williams TL, Lefkowitz RJ: Thyroid hormone regulation of β-adrenergic receptors number. J Biol Chem 252:2787, 1977.
237. Disatnik MH, Shainberg A: Regulation of beta-adrenoceptors by thyroid hormone and amiodarone in rat myocardial cells in culture. Biochem Pharmacol 41:1039, 1991.
238. Polikar R, Burger AG, Scherrer U, Nicod P: The thyroid and the heart. Circulation 87:1435, 1993.
239. Sterling K, Lazarus JH, Milch PO, et al: Mitochondrial thyroid hormone receptor: Localization and physiological significance. Science 201:1126, 1978.
240. Sterling K, Brenner MA, Sakurada T: Rapid effect of triiodothyronine on the mitochondrial pathway in rat liver in vivo. Science 210:340, 1980.
241. Sterling K: Direct thyroid hormone activation of mitochondria: The role of adenine nucleotide translocase. Endocrinology 119: 292, 1986.
242. Dudley SC Jr, Baumgarten CM: Bursting of cardiac sodium channels after acute exposure to 3,5,3′-triiodo-L-thyronine. Circ Res 73:301, 1993.
243. Rudinger A, Mylotte KM, Davis PJ, et al: Rabbit myocardial membrane Ca^{2+}-adenosine triphosphatase activity: Stimulation *in vitro* by thyroid. Arch Biochem Biophys 229:379, 1984.
244. Bremner W, Taylor K, Baird S: Hypothalamo-pituitary-thyroid axis function during cardiopulmonary bypass. J Thorac Cardiovasc Surg 75:392, 1978.
245. Novitsky D, Human PA, Cooper DKC: Inotropic effect of triiodothyronine following myocardial ischemia and cardiopulmonary bypass: An experimental study in pigs. Ann Thorac Surg 45:500, 1988.
246. Teiger E, Menasche P, Mansier P, et al: Triiodothyronine therapy in open heart surgery: From hope to disappointment. Eur Heart J 14:629, 1993.
247. Furukawa K-I, Ohshima N, Tawada-Iwata Y, Shigekawa M: Cyclic GMP stimulates Na^+/Ca^{2+} exchange in vascular smooth muscle cells in primary culture. J Biol Chem 266:12337, 1991.
248. Lincoln TM, Cornwell TL: Intracellular cyclic GMP receptor proteins. FASEB J 7:328, 1993.
249. Clemo HF, Feher JJ, Baumgarten CM: Modulation of rabbit ventricular cell volume and $Na^+/K^+/2Cl^-$ cotransport by cGMP and atrial natriuretic factor. J Gen Physiol 100:89, 1992.
250. Smith JA, Shah AM, Lewis MJ: Factors released from endocardium of the ferret and pig modulate myocardial contraction. J Physiol (Lond) 439:1, 1991.
251. Kohmoto O, Ikenouchi H, Hirata Y, et al: Variable effects of endothelin-1 on $[Ca^{2+}]_i$ transients, pH_i, and contraction in ventricular myocytes. Am J Physiol 265:H793, 1993.
252. Wang J, Morgan JP: Endothelin reverses the effects of acidosis on the intracellular Ca^{2+} transient and contractility in ferret myocardium. Circ Res 71:631, 1992.
253. Wang J, Paik G, Morgan JP: Endothelin 1 enhances myofilament Ca^{2+} responsiveness in aequorin-loaded ferret myocardium. Circ Res 69:582, 1991.
254. Brooks WW, Struckow B, Bing OHL: Myocardial hypoxia and reoxygenation: Electrophysiologic and mechanical correlates. Am J Physiol 226:523, 1974.
255. Carmeliet E: Cardiac transmembrane potentials and metabolism. Circ Res 42:577, 1978.
256. Lewis MJ, Grey AC, Henderson AH: Determinants of hypoxic contracture in isolated heart muscle preparations. Cardiovasc Res 13:86, 1979.
257. Cole W, McPherson CD, Sontag D: ATP-regulated K^+ channels protect the myocardium against ischemia/reperfusion damage. Circ Res 69:571, 1991.
258. Kihara Y, Grossman W, Morgan JP: Direct measurement of changes in intracellular calcium transients during hypoxia, ischemia, and reperfusion of the intact mammalian heart. Circ Res 65:1029, 1989.
259. Sys SU, Housmans PR, Van Ocken ER, Brutsaert DL: Mechanisms of hypoxia-induced decrease of load dependence of relaxation in cat papillary muscle. Pflugers Arch 401:368, 1984.
260. Miyata H, Lakatta EG, Stern MD, Silverman HS: Relation of mitochondrial and cytosolic free calcium to cardiac myocyte recovery after exposure to anoxia. Circ Res 71:605, 1992.
261. Siegmund B, Zude R, Piper HM: Recovery of anoxic-reoxygenated cardiomyocytes from severe Ca^{2+} overload. Am J Physiol 263:H1262, 1992.
262. Davis MD, Lebolt W, Feher JJ: Reversibility of the effects of normothermic global ischemia on the ryanodine-sensitive and ryanodine-insensitive calcium uptake of cardiac sarcoplasmic reticulum. Circ Res 70:163, 1992.
263. Kaplan P, Hendrikx M, Mattheussen M, et al: Effect of ischemia and reperfusion on sarcoplasmic reticulum calcium uptake. Circ Res 71:1123, 1992.
264. Hajjar R, Gwathmey J: Direct evidence of changes in myofilament responsiveness to Ca^{2+} during hypoxia and reoxygenation in myocardium. Am J Physiol 259:H784, 1990.
265. Vleugels A, Vereeke J, Carmeliet E: Ionic currents during hypoxia in voltage-clamped cat ventricular muscle. Circ Res 47: 501, 1980.
266. Noma A: ATP-regulated K^+ channels in cardiac muscle. Nature 305:147, 1983.
267. de Weille JR: Modulation of ATP sensitive potassium channels. Cardiovasc Res 26:1017, 1992.
268. Edwards G, Weston AH: The pharmacology of ATP-sensitive potassium channels. Annu Rev Pharmacol Toxicol 33:597, 1993.
269. Ho K, Nichols CG, Lederer WJ, et al: Cloning and expression of an inwardly rectifying ATP-regulated potassium channel. Nature 362:31, 1993.
270. Horie M, Irisawa H, Noma A: Voltage-dependent magnesium blockade of adenosine-triphosphate-sensitive potassium channel in single guinea-pig ventricular cells. J Physiol (Lond) 287:251, 1987.
271. Furukawa T, Kimura S, Furukawa N, et al: Role of cardiac ATP-regulated potassium channels in differential responses of endocardial and epicardial cells to ischemia. Circ Res 68:1693, 1991.
272. Kubota I, Yamaki M, Shibata T, et al: Role of ATP-sensitive K^+ channel on ECG ST segment elevation during a bout of myocardial ischemia: A study on epicardial mapping in dogs. Circulation 88:1845, 1993.
273. Weiss JN, Vankatesh N, Lamp ST: ATP-sensitive K^+ channels and cellular K^+ loss in hypoxic and ischaemic mammalian ventricle. J Physiol (Lond) 447:649, 1992.
274. Auchampach JA, Maruyama M, Cavero I, Gross GJ: Pharmacological evidence for a role of ATP-dependent potassium channels in myocardial stunning. Circulation 86:311, 1992.
275. Vogel S, Sperelakis N: Blockade of myocardial slow inward current at low pH. Am J Physiol 233:C99, 1977.
276. Susanni EE, Manders WT, Vatner DE, et al: One hour of myocardial ischemia decreases the activity of the stimulatory

guanine-nucleotide regulatory protein G_s. Circ Res 65:1145, 1989.
277. Vatner D, Kiuchi K, Manders W, Vatner S: Effects of coronary arterial reperfusion on β-adrenergic receptor-adenylyl cyclase coupling. Am J Physiol 264:H196, 1993.
278. Kirsch GE, Codina J, Birnbaumer L, Brown AM: Coupling of ATP-sensitive K^+ channels to A_1 receptors by G proteins in rat ventricular myocytes. Am J Physiol 28:H820, 1990.
279. Wilde AAM, Janse MJ: Electrophysiological effects of ATP sensitive potassium channel modulation: Implications for arrhythmogenesis. Cardiovasc Res 28:16, 1994.
280. Fry CH, Poole-Wilson PA: Effects of acid-base changes on excitation-contraction coupling in guinea-pig and rabbit cardiac ventricular muscle. J Physiol (Lond) 313:141, 1981.
281. Klöckner U, Isenberg G: Calcium channel current of vascular smooth muscle cells: Extracellular protons modulate gating and single channel conductance. J Gen Physiol 103:665, 1994.
282. Klöckner U, Isenberg G: Intracellular pH modulates the availability of vascular L-type Ca^{2+} channels. J Gen Physiol 103:647, 1994.
283. Tani M, Neely JR: Role of intracellular Na^+ in Ca^{2+} overload and depressed recovery of ventricular function of reperfused ischemic rat hearts: Possible involvement of H^+-Na^+ and Na^+-Ca^{2+} exchange. Circ Res 65:1045, 1989.
284. Neubauer S, Newell JB, Ingwall JS: Metabolic consequences and predictability of ventricular fibrillation in hypoxia: A ^{31}P- and ^{23}Na-magnetic resonance study of the isolated rat heart. Circulation 86:302, 1992.
285. Haigney MCP, Miyata H, Lakatta EG, et al: Dependence of hypoxic cellular calcium loading on Na^+-Ca^{2+} exchange. Circ Res 71:547, 1992.
286. Scholz W, Albus U, Linz W, et al: Effects of Na^+/H^+ exchange inhibitors in cardiac ischemia. J Mol Cell Cardiol 24:731, 1992.
287. Mejía-Alvarez R, Marban E: Mechanism of the increase in intracellular sodium during metabolic inhibition—direct evidence against mediation by voltage-dependent sodium channels. J Mol Cell Cardiol 24:1307, 1992.
288. Ver Donck L, Borgers M, Verdonck F: Inhibition of sodium and calcium overload pathology in the myocardium: A new cytoprotective principle. Cardiovasc Res 27:349, 1993.
289. Karmazyn M, Moffat MP: Role of Na^+/H^+ exchange in cardiac physiology and pathophysiology: Mediation of myocardial reperfusion injury by the pH paradox. Cardiovasc Res 27:915, 1993.
290. Scholz W, Albus A: Potential of selective sodium-hydrogen exchange inhibitors in cardiovascular therapy. Cardiovasc Res 29:184, 1995.
291. Hoque ANE, Haist JV, Karmazyn M: Na^+-H^+ exchange inhibition protects against mechanical, ultrastructural, and biochemical impairment induced by low concentrations of lysophosphatidylcholine in isolated rat hearts. Circ Res 80:95, 1997.
292. Anderson SE, Murphy E, Steenbergen C, et al: Na-H exchange in myocardium: Effects of hypoxia and acidification on Na and Ca. Am J Physiol 259:C940, 1990.
293. Meng H, Pierce GN: Involvement of sodium in the protective effect of 5-(N,N-dimethyl)-amiloride on ischemia-reperfusion injury in isolated rat ventricular wall. J Pharmacol Exp Ther 256:1094, 1991.
294. Myers ML, Mathur S, Li G-H, Karmazyn M: Sodium-hydrogen exchange inhibitors improve postischaemic recovery of function in the perfused rabbit heart. Cardiovasc Res 29:209, 1995.
295. Panagiotopoulos S, Daly MJ, Nayler WG: Effect of acidosis and alkalosis on postischemic Ca gain in isolated rat heart. Am J Physiol 258:H821, 1990.
296. Ibuki C, Hearse DJ, Avkiran M: Mechanisms of antifibrillatory effect of acidic reperfusion: Role of perfusate bicarbonate concentration. Am J Physiol 264:H783, 1993.
297. Yasutake M, Avkiran M: Exacerbation of reperfusion arrhythmias by α_1 adrenergic stimulation: A potential role for receptor mediated activation of sarcolemmal sodium-hydrogen exchange. Cardiovasc Res 29:222, 1995.
298. Cingolani H, Koretsune Y, Marban E: Recovery of contractility and pH_i during respiratory acidosis in ferret hearts: Role of Na^+-H^+ exchange. Am J Physiol 259:H843, 1990.
299. Than H, Orchard CH: The effect of acidosis and hypoxia on the response of cardiac muscle isolated from ferret hearts to noradrenaline. J Physiol (Lond) 435:98P, 1991.
300. Yan G-X, Kléber AG: Changes in extracellular and intracellular pH in ischemic rabbit papillary muscle. Circ Res 71:460, 1992.
301. Veenstra RD, Joyner RW, Wiedman RT, et al: Effects of hypoxia, hyperkalemia, and metabolic acidosis on canine subendocardial action potential conduction. Circ Res 60:93, 1987.
302. Senges J, Mizutani T, Pelzer D, et al: Effect of hypoxia on the sinoatrial node, atrium and atrioventricular node in the rabbit heart. Circ Res 44:856, 1979.
303. Piper H, Noll T, Siegmund B: Mitochondrial function in the oxygen depleted and reoxygenated myocardial cell. Cardiovasc Res 28:1, 1994.
304. Bolli R, Patel BS, Jeroudi MO, et al: Demonstration of free radical generation in "stunned" myocardium of intact dogs with the use of the spin trap α-phenyl N-tert-butyl nitrone. J Clin Invest 82:476, 1988.
305. Kukreja RC, Hess ML: The oxygen free radical system: From equations through membrane-protein interactions to cardiovascular injury and protection. Cardiovasc Res 26:641, 1992.
306. Nakaya H, Tohse N, Kanno M: Electrophysiological derangements induced by lipid peroxidation in cardiac tissue. Am J Physiol 253:H1089, 1987.
307. Ferrari R, Alfieri O, Curello S, et al: Occurrence of oxidative stress during reperfusion of the human heart. Circulation 81:201, 1990.
308. Braunwald E, Kloner RA: The stunned myocardium: Prolonged, postischemic ventricular dysfunction. Circulation 66:1146, 1982.
309. Kusuoka H, Marban E: Cellular mechanisms of myocardial stunning. Annu Rev Physiol 54:243, 1992.
310. Hofmann PA, Miller WP, Moss RL: Altered calcium sensitivity of isometric tension in myocyte-sized preparations of porcine postischemic stunned myocardium. Circ Res 72:50, 1993.
311. Dietrich DLL, van Leeuwen GR, Stienen GJM, Elzinga G: Stunning does not change the relation between calcium and force in skinned rat trabeculae. J Mol Cell Cardiol 25:541, 1993.
312. Marban E: Myocardial stunning and hibernation—the physiology behind the colloquialisms. Circulation 83:681, 1991.
313. Heyndrickx GR, Wijns W, Vogelaers D, et al: Recovery of regional contractile function and oxidative metabolism in stunned myocardium induced by 1-hour circumflex coronary artery stenosis in chronically instrumented dogs. Circ Res 72:901, 1993.
314. Murry CE, Jennings RB, Reimer KA: Preconditioning with ischemia: A delay of lethal cell injury in ischemic myocardium. Circulation 74:1124, 1986.
315. Lawson CS, Downey JM: Preconditioning: State of the art myocardial protection. Cardiovasc Res 27:542, 1993.
316. Parratt JR: Protection of the heart by preconditioning: Mechanisms and possibilities for pharmacologic exploitation. Trends Pharmacol Sci 15:19, 1994.
317. Tsuchida A, Yang X-M, Burckhartt B, et al: Acadesine extends the window of protection afforded by ischemic preconditioning. Cardiovasc Res 28:379, 1994.
318. Steenbergen C, Perlman ME, London RE, Murphy E: Mechanism of preconditioning—ionic alterations. Circ Res 72:112, 1993.
319. Finegan BA, Lopaschuk GD, Gandhi M, Clanachan AS: Ischemic preconditioning inhibits glycolysis and proton production in isolated working rat hearts. Am J Physiol 269:H1767, 1995.
320. Cave AC, Garlick PB: Ischemic preconditioning and intracellular pH: A ^{31}P NMR study in the isolated rat heart. Am J Physiol 272:H544, 1997.
321. Grover GJ, McCullough JR, Henry DE: Anti-ischemic effects of the potassium channel activators pinacidil and cromakalim and the reversal of these effects with the potassium channel blocker glyburide. J Pharmacol Exp Ther 251:98, 1989.
322. Rohmann S, Weygandt H, Schelling P, et al: Involvement of ATP-sensitive potassium channels in preconditioning protection. Basic Res Cardiol 89:563, 1994.
323. Van Winkle DM, Chien GL, Wolff RA, et al: Cardioprotection provided by adenosine receptor activation is abolished by blockade of the K_{ATP} channel. Am J Physiol 266:H829, 1994.
324. Shigematsu S, Sato T, Abe T, et al: Pharmacological evidence for the persistent activation of ATP-sensitive K^+ channels in early phase of reperfusion and its protective role against myocardial stunning. Circulation 92:2266, 1995.
325. Speechly-Dick ME, Mocanu MM, Yellon DM: Protein kinase C:

Its role in ischemic preconditioning in the rat. Circ Res 75:586, 1994.
326. Tsuchida A, Liu Y, Liu GS, et al: α_1-Adrenergic agonists precondition rabbit ischemic myocardium independent of adenosine by direct activation of protein kinase C. Circ Res 75:576, 1994.
327. Bugge E, Ytrehus K: Bradykinin protects against infarction but does not mediate ischemic preconditioning in the isolated rat heart. J Mol Cell Cardiol 28:2333, 1996.
328. Cleveland JC Jr, Wollmering MM, Meldrum DR, et al: Ischemic preconditioning in human and rat ventricle. Am J Physiol 271: H1786, 1996.
329. Ytrehus K, Liu Y, Downey J: Preconditioning protects ischemic rabbit heart by protein kinase C activation. Am J Physiol 266: H1145, 1994.
330. Speechly-Dick ME, Grover GJ, Yellon DM: Does ischemic preconditioning in the human involve protein kinase C and the ATP-dependent K^+ channel. Circ Res 77:1030, 1995.
331. Bouchard J-F, Lamontagne D: Mechanisms of protection afforded by preconditioning to endothelial function against ischemic injury. Am J Physiol 271:H1801, 1996.
332. Brown BR, Crout JR: A comparative study of the effects of five general anesthetics on myocardial contractility: Isometric conditions. Anesthesiology 34:236, 1971.
333. Lynch C III: Differential depression of myocardial contractility by halothane and isoflurane *in vitro*. Anesthesiology 64:620, 1986.
334. DeTraglia MC, Komai H, Rusy BF: Differential effects of inhalational anesthetics on myocardial potentiated-state contractions *in vitro*. Anesthesiology 68:534, 1988.
335. Rusy BF, Komai H: Anesthetic depression of myocardial contractility: A review of possible mechanisms. Anesthesiology 67: 745, 1987.
336. Su JY, Kerrick WGL: Effects of halothane on Ca^{2+}-activated tension development in mechanically disrupted rabbit myocardial fibers. Pflugers Arch 375:111, 1978.
337. Su JY, Kerrick WGL: Effects of enflurane on functionally skinned myocardial fibers from rabbits. Anesthesiology 52:385, 1980.
338. Su JY, Bell JG: Intracellular mechanism of action of isoflurane and halothane on striated muscle of the rabbit. Anesth Analg 65: 457, 1986.
339. Murat I, Ventura-Clapier R, Vassort G: Halothane, enflurane, and isoflurane decrease calcium sensitivity and maximal force in detergent-treated rat cardiac fibers. Anesthesiology 69:892, 1988.
340. Herland JS, Julian FJ, Stephenson DG: Effects of halothane, enflurane, and isoflurane on skinned rat myocardium activated by Ca^{2+}. Am J Physiol 264:H224, 1993.
341. Housmans PR: Negative inotropy of halogenated anesthetics in ferret ventricular myocardium. Am J Physiol 259:H827, 1990.
342. Bosnjak ZJ, Kampine JP: Effects of halothane, enflurane and isoflurane on the SA node. Anesthesiology 58:314, 1983.
343. Bosnjak ZJ, Aggarwal A, Turner LA, et al: Differential effects of halothane, enflurane, and isoflurane on Ca^{2+} transients and papillary muscle tension in guinea pigs. Anesthesiology 76:123, 1992.
344. Bosnjak ZJ, Supan FD, Rusch NJ: The effects of halothane, enflurane and isoflurance on calcium currents in isolated canine ventricular cells. Anesthesiology 74:340, 1991.
345. Casella ES, Suite DA, Fisher YI, Blanck TJJ: The effect of volatile anesthetics on the pH dependence of calcium uptake by cardiac sarcoplasmic reticulum. Anesthesiology 67:386, 1987.
346. Frazer MJ, Lynch C III: Halothane and isoflurane effects on Ca^{2+} fluxes of isolated myocardial sarcoplasmic reticulum. Anesthesiology 77:316, 1992.
347. Connelly TJ, Coronado R: Activation of the Ca^{2+} release channel of cardiac sarcoplasmic reticulum by volatile anesthetics. Anesthesiology 81:459, 1994.
348. Lynch C III, Frazer MJ: Anesthetic alteration of ryanodine binding by cardiac calcium release channels. Biochim Biophys Acta 1194:109, 1994.
349. Miao N, Frazer MJ, Lynch C III: Anesthetic actions on Ca^{2+} uptake and Ca-ATPase activity of cardiac sarcoplasmic reticulum. Adv Pharmacol 31:145, 1994.
350. Baum VC, Wetzel GT: Sodium-calcium exchange in neonatal myocardium: Reversible inhibition by halothane. Anesth Analg 78:1105, 1994.
351. Böhm M, Schmidt U, Schwinger RHG, et al: Effects of halothane on β-adrenoceptors and M-cholinoceptors in human myocardium: Radioligand binding and functional studies. J Cardiovasc Pharmacol 21:296, 1993.
352. Durieux ME: Halothane inhibits signalling through m1 muscarinic acetylcholine receptors expressed in *Xenopus* oocytes. Anesthesiology 82:174, 1995.
353. Davis RF, DeBoer LWV, Rude RE, et al: The effect of halothane anesthesia on myocardial necrosis, hemodynamic performance, and regional myocardial blood flow in dogs following coronary artery occlusion. Anesthesiology 59:402, 1983.
354. Warltier DC Jr, Al-Wathiqui MH, Kampine JP, Schmeling WT: Recovery of contractile function of stunned myocardium in chronically instrumented dogs is enhanced by halothane or isoflurane. Anesthesiology 69:552, 1988.
355. Davis RF, Sidi A: Effect of isoflurane on the extent of myocardial necrosis and on systemic hemodynamics, regional myocardial blood flow, and regional myocardial metabolism in dogs after coronary artery occlusion. Anesth Analg 69:575, 1989.
356. Buljubasic N, Marijic J, Stowe DF, et al: Halothane reduces dysrhythmias and improves contractile function after global hypoperfusion in isolated hearts. Anesth Analg 74:384, 1992.
357. Buljubasic N, Stowe DF, Marijic J, et al: Halothane reduces release of adenosine, inosine, and lactate with ischemia and reperfusion in isolated hearts. Anesth Analg 76:54, 1993.
358. Oguchi T, Kashimoto S, Yamaguchi T, et al: Comparative effects of halothane, enflurane, isoflurane and sevoflurane on function and metabolism in the ischaemic rat heart. Br J Anaesth 74:569, 1995.
359. Kersten JR, Lowe D, Hettrick DA, et al: Glyburide, a K_{ATP} channel antagonist, attenuates the cardioprotective effects of isoflurane in stunned myocardium. Anesth Analg 83:27, 1996.
360. Kersten JR, Schmeling TJ, Hettrick DA, et al: Mechanism of myocardial protection by isoflurane. Role of adenosine triphosphate-regulated potassium (K_{ATP}) channels. Anesthesiology 85:794, 1996.
361. Park WK, Lynch C III: Propofol and thiopental depression of myocardial contractility—a comparative study of mechanical and electrophysiologic effects in isolated guinea pig ventricular muscle. Anesth Analg 74:395, 1992.
362. Ikemoto Y: Reduction by thiopental of the slow-channel-mediated action potential of canine papillary muscle. Pflugers Arch 372:285, 1977.
363. Komai H, Redon D, Rusy BF: Effects of thiopental and halothane on spontaneous contractile activity induced in isolated ventricular muscles of the rabbit. Acta Anaesthesiol Scand 35: 373, 1991.
364. Riou B, Lecarpentier Y, Chemla D, Viars P: Inotropic effect of ketamine on rat cardiac papillary muscle. Anesthesiology 71: 116, 1989.
365. Riou B, Lecarpentier Y, Chemla D, Viars P: *In vitro* effects of etomidate on intrinsic myocardial contractility in rat. Anesthesiology 72:330, 1990.
366. Riou B, Besse S, Lecarpentier Y, Viars P: *In vitro* effects of propofol on rat myocardium. Anesthesiology 76:609, 1992.
367. Rusy BF, Amuzu JK, Bosscher HA, et al: Negative inotropic effect of ketamine in rabbit ventricular muscle. Anesth Analg 71:275, 1990.
368. Baum VC, Tecson ME: Ketamine inhibits transsarcolemmal calcium entry in guinea pig myocardium: Direct evidence by single cell voltage clamp. Anesth Analg 73:804, 1991.
369. Cook DJ, Housmans PR: Mechanism of the negative inotropic effect of propofol in isolated ferret ventricular myocardium. Anesthesiology 80:859, 1994.
370. Olcese R, Usai C, Maestrone E, Nobile M: The general anesthetic propofol inhibits transmembrane calcium current in chick sensory neurons. Anesth Analg 78:955, 1994.
371. Xiao R-P, Spurgeon HA, Capogrossi MC, Lakatta EG: Stimulation of opioid receptors on cardiac ventricular myocytes reduces L type Ca^{2+} channel current. J Mol Cell Cardiol 25:661, 1993.

372. Powell EDU, Mullaney JM: The Chiari network and the valve of the inferior vena cava. Br Heart J 579, 1960.
373. Silver MA, Rowley NE: The functional anatomy of the human coronary sinus. Am Heart J 115:1080, 1988.
374. James TN: Anatomy of the crista supraventricularis: Its importance for understanding right ventricular function, right ventricular infarction and related conditions. J Am Coll Cardiol 6:1083, 1985.
375. Raines RA, LeWinter MM, Cowell JW: Regional shortening patterns in the canine right ventricle. Am J Physiol 231:1395, 1976.
376. Estes EH, Dalton FM, Entman ML, et al: The anatomy and blood supply of the papillary muscles of the left ventricle. Am Heart J 71:356, 1966.
377. Lam JHS, Ranganathan N, Wigle ED, Silver MD: Morphology of the human mitral valve. I. Chordae tendineae. Circulation 41: 449, 1970.
378. Kaul S, Spotnitz WD, Glasheen WP, Touchstone DA: Mechanism of ischemic mitral regurgitation—an experimental evaluation. Circulation 84:2167, 1991.
379. Streeter DD Jr, Spotnitz HM, Patel DJ, et al: Fiber orientation in the canine left ventricle during diastole and systole. Circ Res 24:339, 1969.
380. Silver MA, Roberts WC: Detailed anatomy of the normally functioning aortic valve in hearts of normal or increased weight. Am J Cardiol 55:454, 1985.
381. Spodick DH: The normal and diseased pericardium: Current concepts of pericardial physiology, diagnosis and treatment. J Am Coll Cardiol 1:240, 1983.
382. White CW, Holida MD, Marcus ML: Effects of acute atrial fibrillation on the vasodilator reserve of the canine atrium. Cardiovasc Res 20:683, 1986.
383. Hoffman BF, Moore EN, Stuckey JH, Cranefield PF: Functional properties of the atrioventricular conduction system. Circ Res 13:308, 1963.
384. Abrams J: Current concepts of the genesis of heart sounds. I. First and second sounds. II. Third and fourth sounds. JAMA 239: 2787, 1978.
385. Gorlin R, Gorlin SG: Hydralic formula for calculation of the area of the stenotic mitral valve, other cardiac valves, and central circulatory shunts. Am Heart J 41:1, 1951.
386. Cohen MV, Gorlin S: Modified orifice equation for the calculation of mitral valve area. Am Heart J 84:839, 1972.
387. Hakki A-H, Iskandrian AS, Bemis CE, et al: A simplified valve formula for the calculation of stenotic cardiac valve areas. Circulation 63:1050, 1981.
388. Rodriguez EK, Omens JH, Waldman LK, McCulloch AD: Effect of residual stress on transmural sarcomere length distributions in rat left ventricle. Am J Physiol 264:H1048, 1993.
389. Milnor WR: Cardiovascular Physiology. New York, Oxford University Press, 1990.
390. Marshall SA, Levine RA, Weyman AE: Echocardiography in cardiac research. In Fozzard HA, Haber E, Jennings RB, et al (eds): The Heart and Cardiovascular System: Scientific Foundations, 2nd ed. New York, Raven Press, 1991, p 745.
391. Sagawa K, Maughan L, Suga H, Sunagawa K: Cardiac Contraction and the Pressure-Volume Relationship. New York, Oxford University Press, 1988.
392. Sarnoff SJ, Mitchell JH: The regulation of the performance of the heart. Am J Med 30:747, 1961.
393. Suga H, Sagawa K: Instantaneous pressure-volume relationships and their ratio in the excised, supported canine left ventricle. Circ Res 35:117, 1974.
394. Noda T, Cheng C-P, de Tombe PP, Little WC: Curvilinearity of LV end-systolic pressure-volume and dP/dt_{max}-end-diastolic volume relations. Am J Physiol 265:H910, 1993.
395. Suga H: Ventricular energetics. Physiol Rev 70:247, 1990.
396. Kawaguchi O, Goto Y, Futaki S, et al: Ejecting deactivation does not affect O_2 consumption-pressure-volume area relation in dog hearts. Am J Physiol 265:H934, 1993.
397. Suga H, Goto Y, Yamada O, Igarashi Y: Independence of myocardial oxygen consumption from pressure-volume trajectory during diastole in canine left ventricle. Circ Res 55:734, 1984.
398. Foëx P, Leone BJ: Pressure-volume loops: A dynamic approach to the assessment of ventricular function. J Cardiothorac Vasc Anesth 8:84, 1994.
399. Pfeffer MA, Braunwald E: Ventricular remodeling after myocardial infarction: Experimental observations and clinical implications. Circulation 81:1161, 1990.
400. Olivetti G, Capasso JM, Meggs LG, et al: Cellular basis of chronic ventricular remodeling after myocardial infarction in rats. Circ Res 68:856, 1991.
401. Lamas GA, Pfeffer MA: Left ventricular remodeling after acute myocardial infarction: Clinical course and beneficial effects of angiotensin-converting enzyme inhibition. Am Heart J 121:1194, 1991.
402. Burkhoff D, Tyberg JV: Why does pulmonary venous pressure rise after onset of LV dysfunction: A theoretical analysis. Am J Physiol 265:H1819, 1993.
403. Shintani H, Glantz SA: Influence of filling on left ventricular diastolic pressure-volume relation during pacing ischemia in dogs. Am J Physiol 266:H1373, 1994.
404. Carabello B, Zile M, Tanaka R, Cooper G: Left ventricular hypertrophy due to volume overload versus pressure overload. Am J Physiol 263:H1137, 1992.
405. Glower DD, Spratt JA, Snow ND, et al: Linearity of the Frank-Starling relationship in the intact heart: The concept of preload recruitable stroke work. Circulation 71:994, 1985.
406. Little WC: Comparison of measures of left ventricular contractile performance derived from pressure-volume loops in conscious dogs. Circulation 80:1378, 1989.
407. Little WC: The left ventricular dP/dt_{max}-end-diastolic volume relation in closed-chest dogs. Circ Res 56:808, 1985.
408. Peterson KL, Skloven S, Ludbrook P, et al: Comparison of isovolumic and ejection phase indices of myocardial performance in man. Circulation 49:1088, 1974.
409. Williams RS, Behar VS, Peter RH: Left bundle branch block: Angiographic segmental wall motion abnormalities. Am J Cardiol 44:1046, 1979.
410. Bramlet D, Morris KG, Coleman RE, et al: Effects of rate-dependent left bundle branch block on global and regional left ventricular function. Circulation 67:1059, 1983.
411. Badke FR, Boinay P, Covell JW: Effects of ventricular pacing on regional left ventricular performance in the dog. Am J Physiol 238:H858, 1980.
412. Grover M, Glantz SA: Endocardial pacing site affects left ventricular end-diastolic volume and performance in the intact anesthetized dog. Circ Res 53:72, 1983.
413. Heyndrickx GR, Vilaine J-P, Knight DR, Vatner SF: Effects of altered site of electrical activation on myocardial performance during inotropic stimulation. Circulation 71:1010, 1985.
414. Jardin F, Farcot J-C, Boisante L, et al: Influence of positive end-expiratory pressure on left ventricular performance. N Engl J Med 304:387, 1981.
415. Visner MS, Arentzen CE, O'Connor MJ, et al: Alterations in left ventricular three-dimensional dynamic geometry and systolic function during acute right ventricular hypertension in the conscious dog. Circulation 67:353, 1983.
416. Hoit BD, Dalton N, Bhargava V, Shabetai R: Pericardial influences on right and left ventricular filling dynamics. Circ Res 68: 197, 1991.
417. Reich DL, Konstadt SN, Thys DM: The pericardium exerts constraint on the right ventricle during cardiac surgery. Acta Anaesthesiol Scand 34:530, 1990.
418. Mangano DT, Van Dyke DC, Hickey RF, Ellis RJ: Significance of the pericardium in human subjects: Effects on left ventricular volume, pressure, and ejection. J Am Coll Cardiol 6:290, 1985.
419. Santamore WP, Li KS, Nakamoto T, Johnston WE: Effects of increased pericardial pressure on the coupling between the ventricles. Cardiovasc Res 24:768, 1990.
420. Refsum H, Junemann M, Lipton MJ, et al: Ventricular diastolic pressure volume relation and the pericardium. Effects of changes in blood volume and pericardial effusion in dogs. Circulation 64:997, 1981.
421. Friedman HS, Lajam F, Gomes JA, et al: Demonstration of a depressor reflex in acute cardiac tamponade. J Thorac Cardiovasc Surg 73:278, 1977.
422. McGregor M: Pulsus paradoxus. N Engl J Med 301:480, 1979.
423. Innes JA, De Cort SC, Kox W, Guz A: Within-breath modulation of left ventricular function during normal breathing and positive-pressure ventilation in man. J Physiol (Lond) 460:487, 1993.

424. Buda AJ, Pinsky MR, Ingels NB Jr, et al: Effects of intrathoracic pressure on left ventricular performance. N Engl J Med 301:453, 1979.
425. Malliani A, Pagani M, Lombardi F, Cerutti S: Cardiovascular neural regulation explored in the frequency domain. Circulation 84:482, 1991.
426. Korner PI, Tonkin AM, Uther JB: Reflex and mechanical circulatory effects of graded Valsalva maneuvers in normal man. J Appl Physiol 40:434, 1976.
427. Dorinsky PM, Whitcomb ME: The effect of PEEP on cardiac output. Chest 84:210, 1983.
428. Waldo AL, Wit AL: Mechanisms of cardiac arrhythmias. Lancet 341:1189, 1993.
429. Janse M: The premature beat. Cardiovasc Res 26:89, 1992.
430. Levine JH, Morganroth J, Kadish AH: Mechanisms and risk factors for proarrhythmia with type Ia compared with Ic antiarrhythmic drug therapy. Circulation 80:1063, 1989.
431. Gilat E, Nordin CW, Aronson RS: The role of reduced potassium conductance in generating triggered activity in guinea-pig ventricular muscle. J Mol Cell Cardiol 22:619, 1990.
432. Zipes DP: The long QT interval syndrome: A rosetta stone for sympathetic related ventricular tachyarrhythmias. Circulation 84:1414, 1991.
433. Fish FA, Prakash C, Roden DM: Suppression of repolarization-related arrhythmias in vitro and in vivo by low-dose potassium channel activator. Circulation 82:1362, 1990.
434. Imaizumi Y, Giles WR: Quinidine-induced inhibition of a transient outward current in rabbit heart. Am J Physiol 253:H704, 1987.
435. Castle NA: Bupivacaine inhibits the transient outward K^+ current but not the inward rectifier in rat ventricular myocytes. J Pharmacol Exp Ther 255:1038, 1990.
436. Miura M, Ishide N, Oda H, et al: Spatial features of calcium transients during early and delayed afterdepolarizations. Am J Physiol 265:H439, 1993.
437. Karagueuzian HS, Katzung BG: Voltage-clamp studies of transient inward current and mechanical oscillations induced by ouabain in ferret papillary muscle. J Physiol (Lond) 327:255, 1982.
438. Lakatta EG, Capogrossi MC, Kort AA, Stern MD: Spontaneous myocardial calcium oscillations: Overview with emphasis on ryanodine and caffeine. Fed Proc 44:2977, 1985.
439. Lakatta EG: Functional implications of spontaneous sarcoplasmic reticulum Ca^{2+} release in the heart. Cardiovasc Res 26:193, 1992.
440. Campbell RWF: Ventricular ectopic beats and non-sustained ventricular tachycardia. Lancet 341:1454, 1993.
441. Zhou X, Guse P, Wolf PD, et al: Existence of both fast and slow channel activity during the early stages of ventricular fibrillation. Circ Res 70:773, 1992.
442. Kuo C-S, Munakata K, Reddy CP, Surawicz B: Characteristics and possible mechanism of ventricular arrhythmia dependent on the dispersion of action potential durations. Circulation 67:1356, 1983.
443. Rosenbaum DS, Kaplan DT, Kanai A, et al: Repolarization inhomogeneities in ventricular myocardium change dynamically with abrupt cycle length shortening. Circulation 84:1333, 1991.
444. Kowey PR, Friehling TD, Sewter J, et al: Electrophysiological effects of left ventricular hypertrophy: Effect of calcium and potassium channel blockade. Circ Res 83:2067, 1991.
445. Bjørnstad H, Lathrop DA, Refsum H: Prevention of some hypothermia induced electromechanical changes by calcium channel blockade. Cardiovasc Res 28:55, 1994.
446. Lynch JJ Jr, Sanguinetti MC, Kimura S, Bassett AL: Therapeutic potential of modulating potassium currents in the diseased myocardium. FASEB J 6:2952, 1992.
447. Bacaner MB, Clay JR, Shrier A, Brochu RM: Potassium channel blockade: A mechanism for suppressing ventricular fibrillation. Proc Natl Acad Sci USA 83:2223, 1986.
448. Gross GJ, Auchampach JA: Role of ATP dependent potassium channels in myocardial ischaemia. Cardiovasc Res 26:1011, 1992.
449. Harder DR, Sperelakis N: Membrane electrical properties of vascular smooth muscle from the guinea pig superior mesenteric artery. Pflugers Arch 378:111, 1978.
450. Berridge MJ: Inositol trisphosphate and calcium signalling. Nature 361:315, 1993.
451. Johns A, Leijten P, Yamamoto H, et al: Calcium regulation in vascular smooth muscle contractility. Am J Cardiol 59:18A, 1987.
452. Nelson MT, Patlak JB, Worley JF, Standen NB: Calcium channels, potassium channels, and voltage dependence of arterial smooth muscle tone. Am J Physiol 259:C3, 1990.
453. Bonev AD, Nelson MT: Vasoconstrictors inhibit ATP-sensitive K^+ channels in arterial smooth muscle through protein kinase C. J Gen Physiol 108:315, 1996.
454. Faraci F, Heistad D: Role of ATP-sensitive potassium channels in the basilar artery. Am J Physiol 264:H8, 1993.
455. Song Y, Srinivas M, Belardinelli L: Nonspecific inhibition of adenosine-activated K^+ current by glibenclamide in guinea pig atrial myocytes. Am J Physiol 271:H2430, 1996.
456. Zhang H-L, Bolton TB: Two types of ATP-sensitive potassium channels in rat portal vein smooth muscle cells. Br J Pharmacol 118:105, 1996.
457. Bourinet F, Fournier F, Lory P, et al: Protein kinase C regulation of cardiac calcium channels expressed in *Xenopus* oocytes. Pflugers Arch 421:247, 1992.
458. Irvine RF: Inositol phosphates and Ca^{2+} entry: Toward a proliferation or a simplification? FASEB J 6:3085, 1992.
459. Vaca L, Kunze DL: Depletion and refilling of intracellular Ca^{2+} stores induce oscillations of Ca^{2+} current. Am J Physiol 264: H1319, 1993.
460. Cauvin C, Lukeman S, Cameron J, et al: Differences in norepinephrine activation and diltiazem inhibition of calcium channels in isolated rabbit aorta and mesenteric resistance vessels. Circ Res 56:822, 1985.
461. Murphy RA: What is special about smooth muscle? The significance of covalent crossbridge regulation. FASEB J 8:311, 1994.
462. Moncada S, Palmer RMJ, Higgs EA: Nitric oxide: Physiology, pathophysiology and pharmacology. Pharmacol Rev 43:109, 1991.
463. Johns RA: Endothelium, anesthetics, and vascular control. Anesthesiology 79:1381, 1993.
464. Burnstock G: Integration of factors controlling vascular tone: Overview. Anesthesiology 79:1368, 1993.
465. Palmer RMJ, Ashton DS, Moncada S: Vascular endothelial cells synthesize nitric oxide from L-arginine. Nature 333:664, 1988.
466. Bredt DS, Hwang PM, Glatt CE, et al: Cloned and expressed nitric oxide synthase structurally resembles cytochrome P-450 reductase. Nature 351:714, 1991.
467. Thuringer D, Sauvé R: A patch clamp study of the Ca^{2+} mobilization from internal stores in bovine aortic endothelial cells. II. Effects of thapsigargin on the cellular Ca^{2+} homeostasis. J Memb Biol 130:138, 1992.
468. Himmel HM, Whorton AR, Strauss HC: Intracellular calcium, currents, and stimulus-response coupling in endothelial cells. Hypertension 21:112, 1993.
469. Lesh RE, Marks AR, Somlyo AV, et al: Anti-ryanodine receptor antibody binding sites in vascular and endocardial endothelium. Circ Res 72:481, 1993.
470. Ziegelstein RC, Spurgeon HA, Pili R, et al: A functional ryanodine-sensitive intracellular Ca^{2+} store is present in vascular endothelial cells. Circ Res 74:151, 1994.
471. Rengasamy A, Johns RA: Regulation of nitric oxide synthase by nitric oxide. Mol Pharmacol 44:124, 1993.
472. Gray DW, Marshall I: Novel signal transduction pathway mediating endothelium-dependent β-adrenoceptor vasorelaxation in rat thoracic aorta. Br J Pharmacol 107:684, 1992.
473. Graier WF, Groschner K, Schmidt K, Kukovetz WR: Increases in endothelial cyclic AMP levels amplify agonist-induced formation of endothelium-derived relaxing factor (EDRF). Biochem J 288:345, 1992.
474. Nagao T, Illiano S, VanHoutte P: Heterogeneous distribution of endothelium-dependent relaxations resistant to N^G-nitro-L-arginine in rats. Am J Physiol 263:H1090, 1992.
475. Pajewski TN, Miao N, Lynch C III, Johns RA: Volatile anesthetics affect calcium mobilization in bovine endothelial cells. Anesthesiology 85:1147, 1996.
476. Bolotina VM, Najibi S, Palacino JJ, et al: Nitric oxide directly activates calcium-dependent potassium channels in vascular smooth muscle. Nature 368:850, 1994.
477. Cooke JP, Rossitch Jr E, Andon NA, et al: Flow activates an

endothelial potassium channel to release an endogenous nitrovasodilator. J Clin Invest 88:1663, 1991.
478. Ghandi CR, Berkowitz DE, Watkins WD: Endothelins: Biochemistry and pathophysiologic actions. Anesthesiology 80:892, 1994.
479. Clozel M, Breu V, Burri K, et al: Pathophysiologic role of endothelin revealed by the first orally active endothelin receptor antagonist. Nature 365:759, 1993.
480. Davis MJ, Meininger GA, Zawieja DC: Stretch-induced increases in intracellular calcium of isolated vascular smooth muscle cells. Am J Physiol 263:H1292, 1992.
481. Haass M, Forster C, Richardt G, et al: Role of calcium channels and protein kinase C for release of norepinephrine and neuropeptide Y. Am J Physiol 259:R925, 1990.
482. Yang J, Tsien RW: Enhancement of N- and L-type calcium currents by protein kinase C in frog sympathetic neurons. Neuron 10:127, 1993.
483. Inagami T, Iwai N, Sasaki K, et al: Angiotensin II receptors: Cloning and regulation. Arzneim-Forsch/Drug Res 43:226, 1993.
484. Johns RA, Peach MJ: Metabolism of arachidonic acid and release of endothelium-derived relaxing factors. In Vanhoute PM (ed): Clifton, NJ, Humana, 1988, p 65.
485. Watson S, Girdlestone D: TiPS receptor nomenclature supplement 1993. Trends Pharmacol Sci 1993.
486. Burke JA, Levi R, Guo Z-G, Corey EJ: Leukotrienes C_4, D_4 and E_4: Effects on human and guinea-pig cardiac preparations *in vitro.* J Pharmacol Exp Ther 221:235, 1982.
487. Ferrari R, Agnoletti G: Atrial natriuretic peptide: Its mechanism of release from the atrium. Int J Cardiol 25:S3, 1989.
488. Needleman P, Greenwald JE: Atriopeptin: A cardiac hormone intimately involved in fluid, electrolyte, and blood-pressure homeostasis. N Engl J Med 314:828, 1986.
489. Blaine EH: Atrial natriuretic factor plays a significant role in body fluid homeostasis. Hypertension 15:2, 1990.
490. Richards AM, Nicholls MG, Ikram H, et al: Renal, hemodynamic, and hormonal effects of human alpha atrial natriuretic peptide in healthy volunteers. Lancet 1:545, 1985.
491. Spaan JAE: Coronary Blood Flow: Mechanics, Distribution, and Control. Dordrecht, Kluwer Academic Publishers, 1991.
492. James TN: Blood supply of the human interventricular septum. Circulation 17:391, 1958.
493. Zamir M: Flow strategy and functional design of the coronary network. In Kajiya F, Klassen GA, Spaan JAE, Hoffman JIE (eds): Coronary Circulation: Basic Mechanism and Clinical Relevance. Tokyo, Springer-Verlag, 1990, p 15.
494. Tomanek RJ: Anatomical principles of the coronary circulation. In Kajiya F, Klassen GA, Spaan JAE, Hoffman JIE (eds): Coronary Circulation: Basic Mechanism and Clinical Relevance. Tokyo, Springer-Verlag, 1990, p 3.
495. Chilean WM, Eastham CL, Marcus ML: Microvascular distribution of coronary vascular resistance in beating left ventricle. Am J Physiol 251:H779, 1986.
496. Chilean WM, Layne SM, Nellis SH: Microvascular pressure profiles in the left and right coronary circulations. In Kajiya F, Klassen GA, Spaan JAE, Hoffman JIE (eds): Coronary Circulation: Basic Mechanism and Clinical Relevance. Tokyo, Springer-Verlag, 1990, p 56.
497. Miyoshi H, Nakaya Y, Moritoki H: Nonendothelial-derived nitric oxide activates the ATP-sensitive K^+ channel of vascular smooth muscle cells. FEBS Lett 345:47, 1994.
498. Komaru T, Tanikawa T, Sugimura A, et al: Mechanisms of coronary microvascular dilation induced by the activation of pertussis toxin-sensitive G proteins are vessel-size dependent. Circ Res 80:1, 1997.
499. Mori H, Chujo M, Tanaka E, et al: Modulation of adrenergic coronary vasoconstriction via ATP-sensitive potassium channel. Am J Physiol 268:H1077, 1995.
500. Larach DR, Schuler HG: Potassium channel blockade and halothane vasodilation in conducting and resistance coronary arteries. J Pharmacol Exp Ther 267:72, 1993.
501. Cason BA, Shubayev I, Hickey RF: Blockade of adenosine triphosphate-sensitive potassium channels eliminates isoflurane-induced coronary artery vasodilation. Anesthesiology 81:1245, 1994.
502. Moir TW, Driscol TE, Eckstein RW: Thebesian drainage in the left heart of the dog. Circ Res 14:245, 1964.
503. Wearn JT, Mettier SR, Klumpp TG, Zschiesche L: The nature of the vascular communications between the coronary arteries and the chambers of the heart. Am Heart J 9:143, 1933.
504. Vergoesen I, Han Y, Dankelman J, Spaan JAE: Water balance within the myocardium. In Spaan JAE (ed): Coronary Blood Flow: Mechanics, Distribution, and Control. Dordrecht, Kluwer Academic Publishers, 1991.
505. Miller AJ, Pick R, Johnson PJ: The production of acute pericardial effusion: The effects of various degrees of interference with venous blood and lymph drainage from the heart muscle of the dog. Am J Cardiol 28:463, 1971.
506. Hoffman JE, Spaan JAE: Pressure-flow relations in coronary circulation. Physiol Rev 70:331, 1990.
507. Vogel WM, Apstein CS, Briggs LL, et al: Acute alterations in left ventricular diastolic chamber stiffness. Role of the "erectile" effect of coronary arterial pressure and flow in normal and damaged hearts. Circ Res 51:465, 1982.
508. Weber KT, Janicki JS: The metabolic demand and oxygen supply of the heart: Physiologic and clinical considerations. Am J Cardiol 44:722, 1979.
509. Samaha FF, Heineman W, Ince C, et al: ATP-sensitive potassium channel is essential to maintain basal coronary vascular tone in vivo. Am J Physiol 31:C1220, 1992.
510. Narishige T, Egashira K, Akatsuka Y, et al: Glibenclamide, a putative ATP-sensitive K^+ channel blocker, inhibits coronary autoregulation in anesthetized dogs. Circ Res 73:771, 1993.
511. Daut J, Maier-Rudolph W, von Beckerath N, et al: Hypoxic dilation of coronary arteries is mediated by ATP-sensitive potassium channels. Science 247:1341, 1990.
512. Aversano T, Ouyang P, Silverman H: Blockade of the ATP-sensitive potassium channel modulates reactive hyperemia in the canine coronary circulation. Circ Res 69:618, 1991.
513. Orito K, Satoh K, Taira N: Involvement of ATP-sensitive K^+ channels in the sustained coronary vasodilator response to adenosine in dogs. Eur J Pharmacol 231:183, 1993.
514. Jackson WF, Konig A, Dambacher T, Busse R: Prostacyclin-induced vasodilation in rabbit heart is mediated by ATP-sensitive potassium channels. Am J Physiol 264:H238, 1993.
515. Wennmalm Å, Benthin G, Karawatowska-Prokopczuk E, et al: Release of endothelial mediators and sympathetic transmitters at different coronary flow rates in rabbit hearts. J Physiol (Lond) 435:163, 1991.
516. Balaban RS, Heineman FW: Interaction of oxidative phosphorylation and work in the heart, in vivo. News Physiol Sci 4:215, 1989.
517. Brown DL, Guyenet PG: Electrophysiological study of cardiovascular neurons in the rostral ventrolateral medulla in rats. Circ Res 56:359, 1985.
518. Marta JA, Davis HS, Eisele JH: Vagomimetic effects of morphine and Innovar® in man. Anesth Analg 52:817, 1973.
519. Inoue K, Samodelov LF, Arndt JO: Fentanyl activates a particular population of vagal efferents which are cardioinhibitory. Naunyn Schmiedebergs Arch Pharmacol 312:57, 1980.
520. Freye E, Arndt JO: Perfusion of the fourth cerebral ventricle with fentanyl induces naloxone-reversible bradycardia, hypotension, and EEG synchronization in conscious dogs. Naunyn Schmiedebergs Arch Pharmacol 307:123, 1979.
521. Laubie M, Schmitt H, Vincent M: Vagal bradycardia produced by microinjection of morphine-like drugs into the nucleus ambigous in anaesthetized dogs. Eur J Pharmacol 59:287, 1979.
522. Freye E, Arndt JO: Perfusion of fentanyl through the fourth cerebral ventricle and its cardiovascular effects in awake and halothane anesthetized dogs. Anaesthetist 29:208, 1980.
523. Alvarez L, Escudero C, Carmona JA, et al: Effect of fentanyl on cardiac automaticity and conduction: Direct or mediated action? Eur Heart J 13:1277, 1992.
524. Longhurst JC: Cardiac receptors: Their function in health and disease. Prog Cardiovasc Dis 27:201, 1984.
525. Seagard JL, Van Brederode JFM, Dean C, et al: Firing characteristics of single-fiber carotid sinus baroreceptors. Circ Res 66:1499, 1990.
526. Hering HE: Der karotisdruckversuch. Munch Med Wochenschr 70:1287, 1923.
527. Mifflin S, Felder R: Synaptic mechanisms regulating cardiovascular afferent inputs to solitary tract nucleus. Am J Physiol 259:H653, 1990.

528. Mark AL: The Bezold Jarisch reflex revisited: Clinical implications of inhibitory reflexes originating in the heart. J Am Coll Cardiol 1:90, 1983.
529. Marshall JM: Peripheral chemoreceptors and cardiovascular function. Physiol Rev 74:543, 1994.
530. Blair RW, Ammons WS, Foreman RD: Response of thoracic spinothalamic and spinoreticular cells to coronary artery occlusion. J Neurophysiol 51:636, 1984.
531. Aviado DM, Schmidt CF: Reflexes from stretch receptors on blood vessels, heart and lungs. Physiol Rev 35:247, 1955.
532. Schmidt RM, Kumada M, Sagawa K: Cardiovascular responses to various pulsatile pressures in the carotid sinus. Am J Physiol 223:1, 1972.
533. Ito CS, Scher AM: Hypertension following denervation of aortic baroreceptors in unanesthetized dogs. Circ Res 45:26, 1979.
534. Nishimura RA, Tajik AJ: The Valsalva maneuver and response revisited. Mayo Clin Proc 61:211, 1986.
535. Esente P, Giambartolomei A, Gensini GG, Dator C: Coronary reperfusion and the Bezold-Jarisch reflex (bradycardia and hypotension). Am J Cardiol 52:221, 1983.
536. Koren G, Weiss AT, Ben-David Y, et al: Bradycardia and hypotension following reperfusion with streptokinase (Bezold-Jarisch reflex): A sign of coronary thrombolysis and myocardial salvage. Am Heart J 112:468, 1986.
537. Ledsome JR, Linden RJ: A reflex increase in heart rate from distention of the pulmonary vein-atrial junction. J Physiol (Lond) 170:456, 1964.
538. Lloyd TC Jr: Control of systemic vascular resistance by pulmonary and left heart baroreflexes. Am J Physiol 225:1511, 1972.
539. James TN: A cardiogenic hypertensive chemoreflex. Anesth Analg 69:633, 1989.
540. Guyton AC, Douglas BH, Langston JB, Richardson TQ: Instantaneous increase in mean circulatory pressure and cardiac output at onset of muscular activity. Circ Res 11:431, 1962.
541. O'Rourke MF, Yaginuma T: Wave reflections and the arterial pulse. Arch Intern Med 144:366, 1984.
542. O'Rourke MF: Vascular impedance in studies of arterial and cardiac function. Physiol Rev 62:570, 1982.
543. O'Rourke MF: Steady and pulsatile energy losses in the systemic circulation under normal conditions and in simulated arterial disease. Cardiovasc Res 1:313, 1966.
544. Maruyama Y, Nishioka O, Nozaki E, et al: Effects of arterial distensibility on left ventricular ejection in the depressed contractile state. Cardiovasc Res 27:182, 1993.
545. Latson T, Hunter W, Katoh N, Sagawa K: Effect of nitroglycerin on aortic impedance, diameter, and pulse-wave velocity. Circ Res 62:884, 1988.
546. Murgo JP, Westerhof N, Giolma JP, Altobelli SA: Manipulation of ascending aortic pressure and flow wave reflections with the Valsalva maneuver: Relationship to input impedance. Circulation 63:122, 1981.
547. Catterall WA, Striessnig J: Receptor sites for Ca^{2+} channel antagonists. Trends Pharmacol Sci 13:256, 1992.
548. Jay SD, Sharp AH, Kahl SD, et al: Structural characterization of the dihydropyridine-sensitive calcium channel α-2 subunit and the associated δ peptides. J Biol Chem 266:3287, 1991.
549. Hagiwara N, Irisawa H, Kameyama M: Contribution of two types of calcium currents to the pacemaker potentials of rabbit sino-atrial node cells. J Physiol (Lond) 395:233, 1988.
550. Miura DS, Hoffman BF, Rosen MR: The effect of extracellular potassium on the intracellular potassium ion activity and transmembrane potential of beating canine cardiac Purkinje fibers. J Gen Physiol 69:463, 1977.
551. Lee CO, Fozzard HA: Membrane permeability during low potassium depolarization in sheep cardiac Purkinje fibers. Am J Physiol 237:C156, 1979.
552. Cohen CJ, Fozzard HA, Sheu SS: Increase in intracellular sodium activity during stimulation in mammalian cardiac muscle. Circ Res 50:651, 1982.
553. Baumgarten CM, Singer DH, Fozzard HA: Intra- and extracellular potassium activities, acetylcholine and resting potential in guinea pig atria. Circ Res 54:65, 1984.
554. Backx PH, Marban E: Background potassium current active during the plateau of the action potential in guinea pig ventricular myocytes. Circ Res 72:890, 1993.
555. Surawicz B: Role of potassium channels in cycle length dependent regulation of action potential duration in mammalian cardiac Purkinje and ventricular muscle fibres. Cardiovasc Res 26: 1021, 1992.
556. Rayment I, Holden HM, Whittaker M, et al: Structure of the actin-myosin complex and implications for muscle contraction. Science 261:58, 1993.
557. Yatani A, Codina J, Imoto Y, et al: A G protein directly regulates mammalian cardiac calcium channels. Science 238:1288, 1987.
558. Hartzell HC, Méry PF, Fischmeister R, Szabo G: Sympathetic regulation of cardiac calcium current is due exclusively to cAMP-dependent phosphorylation. Nature 351:573, 1991.
559. Wilson RF, Laughlin DE, Ackell PH, et al: Transluminal, subselective measurement of coronary artery blood flow velocity and vasodilator reserve in man. Circulation 72:82, 1985.
560. Chilean WM, Marcus ML: Phasic coronary blood flow velocity in intramural and epicardial coronary arteries. Circ Res 50:775, 1982.
561. Gadsby DC, Wit AL, Cranefield PF: The effects of acetylcholine on the electrical activity of canine cardiac Purkinje fibers. Circ Res 43:29, 1978.
562. Giles WR, Van Ginneken ACG: A transient outward current in isolated cells from the crista terminalis of rabbit heart. J Physiol (Lond) 368:243, 1985.
563. Komai H, Rusy BF: Effect of halothane on rested-state and potentiated state contraction in rabbit papillary muscle relationship to negative inotropic effect. Anesth Analg 61:403, 1982.
564. Komai H, Rusy BF: Differences in the myocardial depressant action of thiopental and halothane. Anesth Analg 63:313, 1984.
565. Komai H, Rusy BF: Negative inotropic effects of isoflurane and halothane in rabbit papillary muscles. Anesth Analg 66:29, 1987.
566. Komai H, Redon D, Rusy BF: Effects of isoflurane and halothane on rapid cooling contractures in myocardial tissue. Am J Physiol 257:H1804, 1989.
567. Komai H, Rusy BF: Direct effect of halothane and isoflurane on the function of the sarcoplasmic reticulum in intact rabbit atria. Anesthesiology 72:694, 1990.
568. Rusy BF, Thomas-King PY, King GP, Komai H: Effects of propofol on the contractile state of isolated rabbit papillary rabbit muscles under various stimulation conditions. Anesthesiology 73:A559, 1990.
569. Housmans PR, Murat I: Comparative effects of halothane, enflurane, and isoflurane at equipotent anesthetic concentrations on isolated ventricular myocardium of the ferret. II. Relaxation. Anesthesiology 69:464, 1988.
570. Housmans PR, Murat I: Comparative effects of halothane, enflurane, and isoflurane at equipotent anesthetic concentrations on isolated ventricular myocardium of the ferret. I. Contractility. Anesthesiology 69:451, 1988.
571. Su JY, Kerrick WGL: Effects of halothane on caffeine-induced tension transients in functionally skinned myocardial fibers. Pflugers Arch 380:29, 1979.
572. Bosnjak ZJ, Kampine JP: Effects of halothane on transmembrane potentials, Ca^{++} transients, and papillary muscle tension. Am J Physiol 251:H374, 1986.
573. Lynch C III: Differential depression of myocardial contractility by volatile anesthetics *in vitro*: Comparison with uncouplers of excitation-contraction coupling. J Cardiovasc Pharmacol 15:655, 1990.
574. Strobeck JE, Sonnenblick EH: Pathophysiology of heart failure: Deficiency in cardiac contraction. In Cohn JN (ed): Drug Treatment in Heart Failure. Secaucus, NJ, Advanced Therapeutics Communications International, 1988, p 13.

CHAPTER 6

Pulmonary Anatomy and Physiology

Thomas J. Gal, M.D.

Of all the body systems, none is more intimately related to the interventions of anesthesiologists than the respiratory system. Therefore, familiarity with its anatomy and physiology form an essential groundwork for the safe and rational practice of anesthesiology. The respiratory system is as complex as it is unique. Its major component, the lung, for example, must accept the entire cardiac output as it functions to maintain gas exchange as well as to regulate other metabolic processes. This chapter will attempt to focus on three principal areas whose behavior is affected during anesthesia: (1) functional anatomy of the respiratory system, (2) respiratory mechanics, and (3) alterations imposed by general anesthesia on respiratory mechanics and gas exchange.

Functional Anatomy of the Respiratory System

Upper Airway Structure and Function

Nose

The normal airway begins functionally at the nares. As air passes through the nose, the very important functions of warming and humidification occur. The nose is the primary pathway for normal breathing unless obstruction by polyps or upper respiratory infection is present. During quiet breathing the resistance to airflow through the nasal passages accounts for nearly two thirds of the total airway resistance.[1] The resistance through the nose is nearly twice that associated with mouth breathing. This explains why mouth breathing is utilized when high flow rates are necessary, as with exercise.

The sensory innervation of the nasal mucosa arises from two divisions of the trigeminal nerve. The anterior ethmoidal nerve supplies the anterior septum and lateral wall, and the posterior areas are innervated by nasopalatine nerves from the sphenopalatine ganglion. Local anesthesia can be produced by blocking anterior ethmoidal and maxillary nerves bilaterally; however, simple topical anesthesia is usually quite effective.

Pharynx

The pharyngeal airway extends from the posterior aspect of the nose down to the cricoid cartilage where the passage continues as the esophagus. An upper area, the nasopharynx, is separated from the lower oropharynx by the tissue of the soft palate. The principal impediments to air passage through the nasopharynx are the prominent tonsillar lymphoid structures. The tongue is the principal source of oropharyngeal obstruction, usually because of decreased tone of the genioglossus muscle. The latter contracts to move the tongue forward during inspiration and thus acts as a pharyngeal dilator.

Larynx

The larynx, which lies at the level of the third through sixth cervical vertebrae, serves as the organ of phonation and as a valve to protect the lower airways from the contents of the alimentary tract. The structure consists of muscles, ligaments, and a framework of cartilages. These include the thyroid, cricoid, arytenoids, corniculates, and epiglottis. The latter, a fibrous cartilage, has a mucous membrane covering that reflects as the glossoepiglottic fold onto the pharyngeal surface of the tongue. On either side of this fold are depressions called valleculae. These areas provide the site for placement of the curved Macintosh laryngoscope blade. The epiglottis projects into the pharynx and overhangs the laryngeal inlet. However, it is not absolutely essential for sealing off the airway during swallowing.[2]

The laryngeal cavity extends from the epiglottis to the lower level of the cricoid cartilage. The inlet is formed by the epiglottis, which joins to the apex of the arytenoid cartilages on each side by the aryepiglottic folds. Inside the laryngeal cavity one first encounters the vestibular folds, which are narrow bands of fibrous tissue on each side. These extend from the anterolateral surface of each arytenoid to the angle of the thyroid where the latter attaches to the epiglottis. These folds are referred to as the false vocal cords and are separated from the true vocal cords by the laryngeal sinus or ventricle. The true vocal cords are pale white ligamentous structures that attach to the angles of the thyroid anteriorly and to the arytenoids posteriorly. The triangular fissure between these vocal cords is termed the glottic opening; it represents the narrowest segment of the laryngeal opening in adults. In small children (<10 years old) the narrowest segment lies just below the cords at the level of the cricoid ring. The mean length of the relaxed open glottis is about 23 mm in males and 17 mm in females. The glottic width is 6 to 9 mm but can be stretched to 12 mm. Thus the cross-sectional area of the relaxed glottis may be 60 to 100 mm^2.

The scope of this chapter does not permit a detailed description of the actions of the laryngeal muscles; however, these muscles may be classified into three basic groups on the basis of their actions on the vocal cords: (1) abductors, (2) adductors, and (3) regulators of tension. The entire motor innervation to these muscles as well as the sensory supply to the larynx are supplied by two branches of the vagus nerve, the superior and recurrent laryngeal nerves. The latter supplies motor function to all but one of the laryngeal muscles and some sensory innervation to the subglottic mucosa. The superior laryngeal nerve provides most of the sensory innervation of the laryngeal area and innervates a single muscle, the cricothyroid, which serves largely as a tensor of the vocal cords.

Trachea

The trachea is a tubular structure that begins opposite the sixth cervical vertebra at the level of the thyroid cartilage. It is flattened posteriorly and supported along its 10- to 15-cm length by 16 to 20 horseshoe-shaped cartilaginous rings until bifurcating into right and left main bronchi at the level of the fifth thoracic vertebra. The cross-sectional area of the trachea is considerably larger than that of the glottis and may be more than 150 mm^2 and as high as 300 mm^2.

There are a number of receptors in the trachea that are sensitive to mechanical and chemical stimuli. Slowly adapting stretch receptors are located in the trachealis muscle of the posterior tracheal wall. These are involved in regulating the rate and depth of breathing but also produce dilation of upper airways and the bronchi by decreasing vagal efferent activity. Other rapidly adapting irritant receptors lie all around the tracheal circumference. These are usually considered to be cough receptors, although their other reflex actions consist of bronchoconstriction. Studies of topical anesthesia in dogs suggest that the latter receptors are more readily blocked by local anesthetics than the slowly adapting stretch receptors.[3]

It is physiologically important to note that the upper half of the trachea is extrathoracic, while the lower half resides within the thoracic cavity. This creates differences in behavior during inspiration and expiration. The extrathoracic trachea, which is subject to the surrounding influence of atmospheric pressure, undergoes a slight decrease in caliber during inspiration and an increase during expiration. The intrathoracic trachea, on the other hand, undergoes expansion during inspiration as the surrounding pleural pressure becomes more subambient (i.e., more negative). During expiration, however, the surrounding pleural pressure may diminish the tracheal caliber especially in the face of increased expiratory effort as with obstruction.

Upper Airway Protection

The pharynx, epiglottis, and vocal cords play a role in protecting the lower airway from aspiration of foreign bodies and secretions. Although the epiglottis covers the laryngeal inlet, it is not absolutely essential for airway protection.[2] Most vital in this protective function is the glottic closure reflex, which produces protective laryngeal closure during deglutition. The physiologic exaggeration of this reflex, laryngospasm, is counterproductive to respiration. Laryngospasm consists of prolonged intense glottic closure in response to direct glottic or supraglottic stimulation from inhaled agents, secretions, or foreign bodies. Stimulation from the periosteum, celiac plexus, or dilation of the rectum may also precipitate the problem on a reflex basis.

An indispensable mechanism for expelling secretions and foreign bodies from the respiratory tract is the act of coughing. The major stages of a cough are characterized by three events. First of all there is a deep inspiration to attain a high lung volume, which allows attainment of maximum expiratory flow rates. Next a tight closure of glottis occurs along with the contraction of the expiratory muscles. Intrapleural pressure rises to above 100 cm H_2O such that during the final or expiratory phase, a sudden expulsion of air occurs as the glottis opens. Glottic opening at the onset of the phase is associated with oscillation of tissue and gas, which results in the characteristic noise of a cough. Various physiologic aspects of cough have been observed with radiologic and endoscopic techniques. None is more important than the dramatic narrowing of the airway lumen that occurs. The physiologic significance of this reduced airway caliber is that the decreased cross-sectional area increases linear velocity of gas flow and improves cough effectiveness. Various estimates suggest that this dynamic compression decreases the cross-sectional area of the trachea and main bronchi to about 40% of their caliber during normal breathing and thus increases linear velocity two and a half times.[4]

Glottic closure is the one phase of cough that differentiates it from the other forced expiratory maneuvers and allows for greater development of pressures. Closure of the glottis is not crucial, however, to the development of high pressures and flow rates of a normal cough. This is well illustrated in patients who have undergone tracheal intubation or tracheostomy. The presence of the endotracheal tube, for example, does not lessen the buildup of peak pressure during coughing. However, by preventing normal glottic closure, the tube allows flow to begin as soon as pressure begins to increase, and in most cases, the tube allows flow to continue between cough bursts.[5] The normal timing of pressure and flow is altered such that cough resembles a normal forced expiration. Also, since the tube is noncollapsible, it does not permit the high velocities through the tracheal segment that it occupies. Secretions, therefore, are likely to accumulate in the area at the end of the tube unless subsequent coughs are begun from high lung volumes that allow high flow rates to be achieved.

Upper Airway Obstruction

Airway obstruction may be total or partial. Total obstruction is characterized by the lack of any air movement or breath sounds. In the face of ineffective breathing efforts, it is important that inexperienced persons not interpret any retractive movements of the rib cage and the diaphragmatic tugging motions as respiration. Actual air movements must be perceived by feeling with the hand or placing the ear over the mouth. Recognition of obstruction depends on close observation and a high index of suspicion.

In the presence of partial obstruction there is usually diminished tidal exchange, which is associated with retraction of the upper chest and accompanied by a snoring sound if the obstruction is nasopharyngeal or inspiratory stridor if obstruction is near the area of the larynx. If inspiratory efforts are severe, the upper airway may undergo a dynamic inspiratory compression because of the marked pressure gradient in the upper airway.

Treatment of upper airway obstruction depends for the most part on whether it is due to soft tissue obstruction, tumor, foreign body, or laryngospasm. Most often upper airway obstruction is due to reduction of the space between the pharyngeal wall and the base of the tongue by relaxation of the tongue and jaw. The same picture of obstruction may occur with foreign bodies or even dentures. In the absence of a foreign body, airflow may be restored by preventing the mandible from falling back. Forward motion is applied by placing the forefinger and second finger behind the angle of the mandible. The patient's neck can also be slightly extended to provide an optimal airway. The resultant changes in head position have been shown to modify upper airway resistance significantly.[6]

Oropharyngeal obstruction can also be overcome to some extent by increased oropharyngeal pressure from manual inflations with a breathing bag. One of the major concerns with such manual inflation of the lungs without tracheal intubation is the potential for gastric insufflation with high inflation pressures. The relationship between pressure and gas entry into the stomach has been examined in unconscious paralyzed patients.[7] The authors reported that gastric inflation rarely occurred when pressures less than 15 to 20 cm H_2O were utilized. In general, pressures above such values were associated with excessively large delivered tidal volumes (>1 L).

Lower Airway Structure and Function

Conducting Airways

The trachea bifurcates at the sternal angle, which usually lies at the level of the fourth thoracic vertebra. The two mainstem bronchi that arise from the trachea each have a diameter approximately two thirds that of the trachea but differ markedly in length. The right bronchus is about 2.5 cm long, whereas the left extends about twice that length before branching into the next generation of airways, the lobar bronchi. The left bronchus also leaves the trachea at an angle of about 45 degrees from the latter's axis while the right forms an angle of about one half that with the trachea.

The lobar bronchi divide into segmental and then into subsegmental bronchi; with each airway generation, cartillagenous support diminishes progressively while total cross-sectional area increases. After 15 or more generations the bronchioles are reached. These very small airways (<1-mm diameter) have no cartilage but a great deal of smooth muscle. The smallest of the three or four generations of bronchioles are designated as the terminal bronchioles. These are the last component of the conducting airways (i.e., the portion of the tracheobronchial tree not directly involved in gas exchange).

Respiratory Airways

The first portions of the tracheobronchial tree that allow direct gas exchange with the pulmonary circulation are the respiratory bronchioles. These have intermittent sac-like outpouchings. The next airway generation consists of the alveolar ducts, which have multiple sac-like openings whose final divisions terminate into alveolar clusters. The actual alveoli themselves are 100 to 300 μm in diameter. The interface with pulmonary capillaries facilitates exchange of oxygen (O_2) and carbon dioxide (CO_2) and consists of thin capillary epithelial layers, basement membrane, capillary endothelium, and a surfactant lining. The flat type I alveolar cells provide the surface for gas exchange while the interspersed type II cells produce surfactant. Both of these epithelial cells form tight junctions that markedly restrict transport of fluids across them.

Respiratory Muscles

Air moves in and out of the lungs as the thoracic cavity expands and decreases in size. This volume change is accomplished by the contraction of the respiratory muscles. Functionally, these are skeletal muscles whose prime task is to displace the chest wall rhythmically. There are three major muscle groups responsible for ventilation. These are the diaphragm, the intercostal muscles, and the accessory muscles. Although the functions of these muscles will be considered individually, it is most important to remember that they actually must work together in a coordinated fashion.[8]

Diaphragm

The diaphragm is a dome-shaped muscle that separates the thoracic cavity from the abdomen. The muscle is somewhat unique in that its fibers radiate from a central tendon to insert peripherally on the anterolateral aspects of the upper lumbar vertebrae (crural portion) and on the xiphoid and upper margins of the lower ribs (costal portion). The motor innervation originates from the phrenic nerve, which is formed by the combination of cervical roots III, IV, and V. Contraction of the diaphragm causes its dome to descend, thereby expanding the chest longitudinally. The attachments to costal margins also cause the lower ribs to rise and the chest to widen. This action of the diaphragm is responsible for about two thirds of quiet resting ventilation. The normal excursion of the diaphragm during such quiet breathing is about 1.5 cm. As the dome descends to expand the thorax, the abdominal contents are displaced caudally. Thus the fall in pleural pressure and accompanying lung expansion produces an increase in abdominal pressure and some outward protrusion of the abdominal wall.

Intercostal Muscles

The intercostal muscles are composed of two sheet-like layers that run between the ribs and receive their innervation from nerves that exit from the spinal cord at levels from the 1st to 11th thoracic segments. The external intercostals and the parasternal portion of the internal intercostals produce an inspiratory action. Their contraction elevates the upper ribs to increase the anteroposterior dimensions of the chest (pump-handle motion). The lower ribs are also raised to increase the transverse diameter of the thorax (bucket-handle motion). Although these actions of the intercostals do not play a major role in normal resting ventilation, they are important in maintaining high levels of ventilation such as required by exercise.

Accessory Muscles

The accessory muscles contribute to inspiration by elevating and stabilizing the rib cage. The principal accessory muscles are the scalenes and sternocleidomastoids. The scalenes originate from the transverse processes of the lower five cervical vertebrae and receive innervation from the same spinal segments. The muscles slope caudally to insert on the first two ribs such that contraction elevates and fixes the rib cage. While this plays only a minor role in quiet breathing, the enlargement of the upper chest is important at high levels of ventilation. The second group of accessory muscles, the sternocleidomastoids, elevates the sternum and increases the longitudinal dimensions of the thorax. They also are only active at high levels of ventilation and assume great importance in disease states such as severe airway obstruction.

Expiratory Muscles

In contrast to the active phase of inspiration, expiration is passive during quiet breathing and occurs because of the elastic recoil of the respiratory system. However, when high levels of ventilation are required or if air movement is impeded by airway obstruction, expiration must involve active muscle contraction. This is achieved in part by the internal intercostal muscles, which depress the ribs, but the major participants in active expiration are the abdominal muscles. These muscles, which comprise the ventrolateral abdominal wall, are innervated by the lower six thoracic and first lumbar nerves. They consist of the midline rectus abdominus and the internal and external oblique and transversus abdominus laterally. These muscles act to displace the rib cage by pulling the lower ribs downward and inward. They also pull the abdominal wall inward and thus increase intra-abdominal pressure. This displaces the diaphragm cranially into the thorax with a resultant increase in pleural pressure and decrease in lung volume at end-expiration. In addition to their role as powerful muscles of expiration, the abdominal muscles are also important contributors to other respiratory activities such as forced expiration and coughing and the nonrespiratory functions of defecation and parturition.

All measurements of pulmonary function that require patient effort are influenced by respiratory muscle strength. This can be evaluated specifically by measurements of maximal forced effort and can be measured with simple aneroid gauges.[9] The inspiratory muscles are at their optimal length near residual volume. Thus, maximal inspiratory pressure (PImax) is usually measured after a forced exhalation. Similarly, maximum expiratory pressure (PEmax) is measured at total lung capacity where expiratory muscles are stretched to their optimum length by a full inspiration. Typical values for PImax in healthy young males are approximately -125 cm H_2O, while PEmax may be as high as $+200$ cm H_2O.

Values for PEmax less than $+40$ cm H_2O suggest impaired coughing ability, whereas PImax values of -25 cm H_2O or less indicate severe inability to take a deep breath. The latter value is often used as a criterion for extubation; however, observations in healthy volunteers during partial curarization suggest that this level of ventilatory ability does not ensure adequate upper airway integrity.[10]

Respiratory Mechanics

Static Lung Volumes

In order to study the behavior of the respiratory system it is useful to define its various dimensions. These are the subdivisions of gas volumes contained within the lungs during various breathing maneuvers. Although not the first to measure ventilatory volume, John Hutchinson is credited with inventing the spirometer, coining the term "vital capacity," and defining the functional subdivisions of lung volumes.[11] The four major subdivisions of lung volume are residual volume (RV), tidal volume (VT), expiratory reserve volume (ERV), and inspiratory reserve volume (IRV). These four volumes can in turn be combined to form four capacities: total lung capacity (TLC), vital capacity (VC), inspiratory capacity (IC), and functional residual capacity (FRC). The relationships between these various lung volumes and capacities are defined in Table 6–1.

Physiologic Determinants of Lung Volume

A young adult male of average height would be likely to have a TLC of about 6.5 L, of which 1.5 L is residual volume. Therefore, vital capacity is about 5 L. Differences in lung volumes among individuals are largely a function of differences in body size; in particular height. Other determinants of TLC include the strength of the

TABLE 6–1
Lung Volume Subdivisions

Tidal volume (VT)—Air volume inspired and expired during quiet breathing.

Residual volume (RV)—Volume remaining in the lungs after a maximal expiration.

Expiratory reserve volume (ERV)—The volume of air that can be forcibly exhaled between the resting end-expiratory position and RV.

Inspiratory reserve volume (IRV)—The volume of air that can be inspired with maximal effort over and above the normal resting end-inspiratory position of a tidal volume.

Vital capacity (VC)—The amount of air that can be exhaled from the point of maximal inspiration to the point of maximal expiration.

Total lung capacity (TLC)—Total volume of air in the lungs after a maximal inspiration. It is the sum of all subdivisions of lung volume.

Functional residual capacity (FRC)—Amount of air in the lung at the end of a quiet exhalation. It is the sum of RV + ERV.

inspiratory muscles and elastic recoil properties of lung and chest wall. The magnitude of RV is influenced primarily by expiratory muscle strength and the outward recoil of the chest wall. The limits of expiration may also be affected by dynamic airway closure, particularly with advancing age.[12] The volume at the end of a spontaneous exhalation during quiet breathing, the FRC, corresponds to the resting volume of the respiratory system. At this volume airway pressure is zero, as a reflection of the balance between the opposing recoil pressures of the lung and chest wall.

The respiratory system and its component lung and chest wall are elastic structures. That is, they tend to regain their original size and configuration following deformation when deforming forces are removed. Both lung and chest wall have their own positions of equilibrium. These are the volumes that they tend to assume in the absence of external forces acting upon them, and the volumes to which they continuously attempt to return when displaced. The equilibrium position of the lung is at or near RV (Fig. 6–1*A*). To sustain any volume in the lung above this, force must be applied to the lung and the lung will recoil with an equal and opposite force. At all volumes above RV, the lung tends to recoil inward. The equilibrium position of the chest wall is at a relatively large volume, about 60% of vital capacity (Fig. 6–1*B*). To sustain any volume in the chest wall above this point, the chest wall must be actively enlarged by inspiratory muscle contraction, and at such large volumes will tend to recoil inward in concert with the lung.

In the intact respiratory system, the lung and chest wall are coupled and work together. Behavior of the respiratory system is determined by the individual properties of the lung and chest wall. The equilibrium position of the respiratory system will be at that volume where the tendency of the lung to recoil inward is balanced by the tendency of the chest wall to recoil outward. To sustain any volume in the respiratory system other than this resting volume, a force must be applied to displace both lung and chest wall. The recoil pressure of the respiratory system (Prs) which develops is the algebraic sum of the individual recoil pressure of the lung (PL) and the chest wall (Pcw). Thus Prs = PL + Pcw. The volume at which Prs is zero is termed the resting or relaxation volume (Vrx) of the respiratory sys-

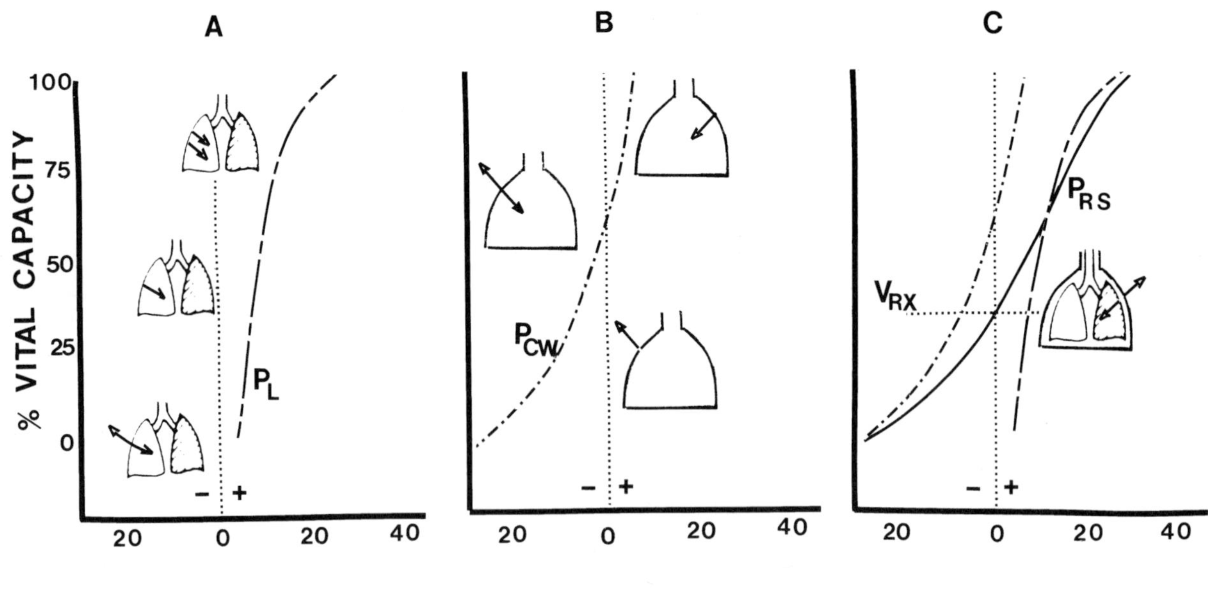

FIGURE 6–1. Pressure-volume relationships of the total respiratory system (*C*) and its components, the lung (*A*) and chest wall (*B*). Vrx, relaxation volume of the respiratory system (i.e., resting equilibrium volume); PL, recoil pressure of the lung; Pcw, chest wall recoil pressure; Prs, recoil pressure for the total respiratory system. (From Gal TJ: Respiratory Physiology in Anesthetic Practice. Baltimore, Williams & Wilkins, 1991, with permission.)

tem (Fig. 6–1*C*). In normal persons during quiet breathing the volume of the lung at end-expiration (FRC) approximates this Vrx. Under certain circumstances, however, FRC may differ from Vrx. Static factors such as respiratory muscle tone, posture, and external forces may reduce end-expiratory lung volume, while dynamic mechanisms may increase it.

Postural alterations in the pressure-volume relationships of the respiratory system are largely accounted for by the influence of gravity on the abdomen, which behaves mechanically like a fluid-filled container. In the erect posture the downward pull of gravity on the abdominal contents exerts an inspiratory action on the diaphragm. In contrast, the action on the rib cage is more expiratory in nature. In the supine posture gravity also exerts a small expiratory action on the rib cage by pulling the ribs down and in but has a marked expiratory action on the diaphragm and abdomen. The pressure-volume curve for the chest wall is thus shifted to the right (i.e., it produces less opposition to the inward recoil of the lung). As a result FRC in normals decreases from about 50% to about 40% TLC in the supine position, and even further to about 30% of TLC in Trendelenburg position. Interestingly, these striking changes with posture do not appear to be manifest in patients with pulmonary emphysema. The enlarged FRC volume in such patients is relatively unaffected by body position.[13]

Adult humans and most of the larger terrestrial mammals with relatively stiff chest walls breathe near their Vrx, and FRC is approximately equal to Vrx or about 50% TLC. The single exception to this is the horse, which appears to breathe around its Vrx with active inspiratory and expiratory phases such that FRC is less than Vrx. This respiratory pattern is believed to minimize the high elastic work of breathing, associated with the horse's low chest wall compliance.[14]

During quiet breathing, ample time exists for passive emptying of the lungs. When ventilation must be increased (as with exercise) or emptying is delayed because of obstruction to flow, the end-expiratory lung volume may be determined by a dynamic rather than static equilibrium. In obstructive lung disease, for example, FRC is commonly increased. Although an increase in Vrx may result from decreased lung elastic recoil, factors such as expiratory flow limitation may result in an even higher dynamically determined FRC.

The human newborn provides a particularly important example of a dynamically determined end-expiratory lung volume. The chest wall of infants and neonates is highly compliant (i.e., its outward recoil is exceedingly small). Although the inward recoil of the lungs is slightly less than in the adult, the lungs are relatively stiff compared to the chest wall. The static balance of forces would predict an FRC at a very low lung volume (as low as 10% of TLC).[15] Since such a low lung volume seems incompatible with airway stability and adequate gas exchange, there is reason to suspect that the infant's dynamically determined FRC is substantially above the passive static Vrx. Indeed, it has been observed that the lung volume during apnea was lower than the usual end-expiratory level in neonates.[16]

Dynamic FRC is determined by the balance between two factors. The time available for expiration (TE) and the rate of lung emptying. The expiratory time (TE) is highly influenced by respiratory rates. In the neonate, the rapid breathing frequency results in a relatively short TE. The rate of lung emptying is governed by the expiratory time constant (τ), which can be most simply viewed as the product of resistance (R) and compliance (C). Neonates, because of the small size of the airways, have an increased R and because of the mechanical properties of the rib cage have a highly compliant chest wall (increased C). Thus τ, which equals R $\times$ C is relatively prolonged. Whenever the ratio TEτ is less than 3, dynamic FRC exceeds Vrx and airway pressure at end-expiration does not reach zero. Such appears to be the case in the human neonate. The transition from this dynamically maintained FRC appears to occur at about 1 year of age.[17] At this point, the end-expiratory level approximates Vrx, presumably because of changes in the mechanical properties of the lungs and chest wall as well as increases in TE.

Forces Producing Airflow

Air flows in and out of the respiratory system because of differences in pressure. Flow occurs from a region of higher pressure to one of lower pressure. Basically there are two pressure differences in the lung and another across the chest wall. The force driving airflow is the pressure differential between the airway opening or mouth (Pm) and the pressure in the alveoli (Palv). This is termed the transairway pressure (Table 6–2). The lung distends and collapses because of a pressure gradient between the alveoli (Palv) and the pleural space (Ppl). This difference is termed transpulmonary pressure (PL) (i.e., the pressure across the lung). The pressure across the chest wall (Pcw) is reflected by the difference between the pleural pressure (Ppl) and the atmospheric or body surface pressure (Pbs).

Forces Opposing Airflow

Within the respiratory system certain elements oppose airflow and thus result in pressure drops. These forces opposing airflow result from the elastic, flow resistive, and inertial properties of the respiratory system. They are thus termed elastance, resistance, and inertance. Inertance deals with the mass of the lung and the acceleration of these tissues and the linear acceleration of gas

TABLE 6–2
Pressure Differences Across the Respiratory System

Airway (Paw)	Palv − Pm
Lung (PL)	Palv − Ppl
Chest wall (Pcw)	Ppl − Pbs
Total respiratory system (Prs)	Palv − Pbs

Palv, pressure in airspaces (alveoli); Pbs, pressure at body surface (atmospheric); Ppl, intrapleural pressure (estimated as esophageal pressure); Pm, mouth pressure (airway opening).

in the lung. It is analogous to inductance in an electrical circuit. Thus pressure losses due to inertial forces increase progressively as respiratory frequency increases. These pressure losses are quite small and negligible during quiet breathing and in most clinical situations. However, inertance may assume some importance during very rapid breathing such as in exercise and other physiologic testing. Elastance and its reciprocal, compliance, are reflections of the relationships of pressure to volume when there is no airflow. Hence such measurements are referred to as static. Resistance, on the other hand, is highly dependent on the rate of changes of lung volume (i.e., flow). Such measurements during active breathing are referred to as dynamic.

Statics

The lung is a distensible elastic body enclosed in an elastic container, the thoracic cavity. Just as a spring is described by the force required to stretch it to a certain length, so can the respiratory system be described by the static pressure required to change its volume. This relation between changes in volume and changes in pressure is termed compliance ($\Delta V/\Delta P$) and is the reciprocal of elastance. For the various components of the respiratory system, compliance is determined by relating the change in volume to a given pressure difference as listed in Table 6–2.

Because the pressure-volume curves for the respiratory system are somewhat curvilinear (Fig. 6–1), compliance will vary from one portion of the curve to another depending on the range of lung volume. Values therefore are usually obtained in the range of 1 L above FRC where the pressure-volume relationships are most linear.

It is important to make the distinction between the terms static and dynamic compliance. When no gas flow occurs and pressure and volume are kept constant, the measurement is termed static compliance. Such would be the case if the patient's lungs were inflated by a device, such as a super syringe, and then held. Dynamic compliance, on the other hand, relates pressure and tidal volume at the moment inspiration changes to expiration and flow ceases only momentarily. Ideally these two compliance measurements are similar. However, if flow is impeded for some reason, for instance, by bronchoconstriction or a kink in the endotracheal tube, dynamic compliance is influenced by resistance to flow and does not reflect the true static compliance. They differ by an amount related to flow resistance at end-inspiration. The difference between the peak dynamic pressures and a quasi-static pressure (plateau) can be readily appreciated in circuits utilizing a ventilator equipped with an inspiratory hold or pause, or by interrupting flow by merely clamping the expiratory line. The relation of volume and the plateau pressure during this pause is often referred to as the "quasi-static" or "effective" compliance, while dynamic compliance relates to the relationship between delivered volume and peak dynamic pressure before the pause.

There is one final area of respiratory statics that deserves special comment. This concerns the relationship of the pressure in the alveoli (Palv) in relation to alveolar size. According to Laplace's equation, the pressure within an alveolus (P) should exceed ambient pressure by an amount determined by the surface tension (T) and the radius of curvature (r) of the alveolus. Thus $P = 2T/r$. According to the equation, the pressure inside small alveoli should exceed that in larger ones if surface tension were the same. Thus one might expect the small alveoli to empty into larger ones. This problem is resolved by the fact that surface tension of the fluid lining alveoli varies by decreasing as an alveolus decreases in size. The surface tension actually decreases to a greater extent than alveolar size (r). Therefore, the recoil pressure (P) of the small alveoli is less than that of the large ones. The lipoprotein substance responsible for this reduction of alveolar surface tension (surfactant) is secreted by type II pneumocytes and floats on the surface of the alveolar lining. As the lining surface decreases in area, surfactant concentration in the area increases and functions to decrease the surface tension of the lining fluid.

Dynamics

This deals with conditions of airflow and describes the relationships between pressure and flow in the respiratory system. Resistance therefore is computed from pressure differences responsible for flow and the simultaneous measurement of airflow ($R = \Delta P/\Delta \dot{V}$).

Various components of the respiratory system contribute to the total resistance to airflow. These include an elastic component, the chest wall, and a nonelastic component termed "pulmonary resistance." Approximately 40% of total respiratory resistance is accounted for by the chest wall. It is important to note that the "chest wall" in physiologic terms includes not only the bony thorax but the diaphragm and abdominal contents as well. Therefore, changes in muscle tone may affect measurements of total respiratory system resistance.

The remaining 60% of total respiratory resistance is pulmonary resistance, which was assumed to be essentially the same as airway resistance and thus a reflection of airway caliber. Recent studies in dogs, however, have shown that lung tissue contributes a significant component of pulmonary resistance during constriction[18] or bronchodilation.[19]

Perhaps the most important factor to consider about airway resistance (Raw) is the fact that resistance to airflow is determined by the size of the airways. Airways are largest at high lung volumes and smallest at low volumes, such as residual volume. Passive changes in Raw can thus occur with changes in the lung volume in the absence of bronchodilation or constriction. Since the relationship of Raw to lung volume is not linear (Fig. 6–2), the reciprocal of Raw, conductance (Gaw) is related to lung volume in linear fashion and is utilized to identify presence of bronchoconstriction or bronchodilation. Such determinants of Raw and Gaw are by convention made at FRC. The quotient of Gaw/FRC is designated as specific conductance (sGaw).

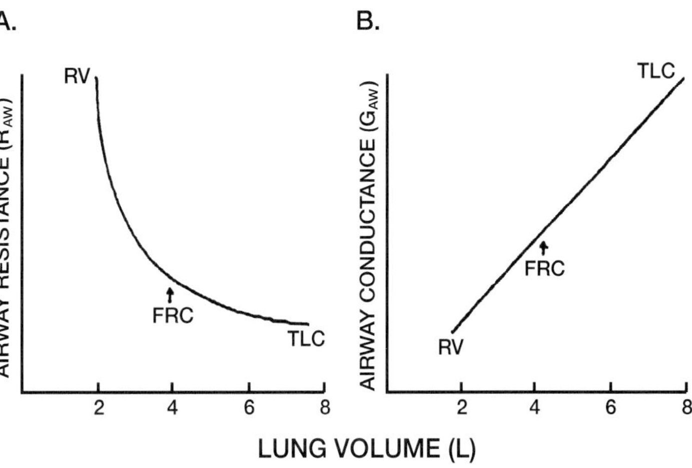

FIGURE **6–2.** The hyperbolic relationship of airway resistance (Raw) to lung volume (*A*) is contrasted with the linear relationship (*B*) of its reciprocal airway conductance (Gaw). RV, residual volume; TLC, total lung capacity; FRC, functional residual capacity. (From Gal TJ: Pulmonary function testing. In Miller RD [ed]: Anesthesia, 4th ed. New York, Churchill Livingstone, 1994, with permission.)

Respiratory Mechanics and Gas Exchange During Anesthesia

Alterations in Respiratory Mechanics

General anesthesia affects the static (pressure-volume) and the dynamic (pressure-flow) behavior of the respiratory system. These mechanical effects have interested clinicians and investigators because of their potential contribution to the impaired gas exchange so characteristic in anesthetized patients. Perhaps no facet of respiratory system behavior has received as much attention as the change in FRC. A decrease in FRC with induction of general anesthesia was first noted by Bergman.[20] Subsequent observations in supine anesthetized humans indicate that FRC is reduced an average of about 500 ml or 15 to 20% of the awake value.[21] The decreased volume is similar in magnitude to that observed when subjects go from the erect to the recumbent position. The magnitude of FRC reduction also appears to be related to age and body habitus (i.e., weight-height ratio). In fact, morbidly obese patients demonstrate a much larger decrease in FRC, to about 50% of the preanesthetic values.[22]

The changes in FRC occur within a minute after induction of anesthesia,[23] do not appear to progress with time,[24] and are not further affected by addition of muscle paralysis.[25] A number of factors may contribute to the FRC reduction but the underlying mechanisms are complex and as yet not totally clear. Some of these possibilities include atelectasis, increased expiratory muscle activity, trapping of gas in distal airways, cephalad displacement of the diaphragm, decreased outward chest wall recoil, increased lung recoil, and increases in thoracic blood volume.

Atelectasis may contribute to or result from the reduction of FRC. The rapid appearance of densities on computed tomography (CT) support this possibility.[26] The prompt development of the densities and their lack of dependence on high inspired oxygen concentrations suggest that they may be due to compression of gas rather than resorption as initially suggested by Dery et al.[27]

Trapping of gas behind closed distal airways does not appear to be a major contributor to the decreased FRC because measurements of thoracic gas volume have demonstrated the FRC changes.[28] Furthermore, measurement of nitrogen washout, which measures only gas in contact with the open airways, gave similar results to those that measured total thoracic gas volume by body plethysmography.[25]

During rapid-eye-movement sleep and with halothane anesthesia the tonic activity of the diaphragm decreases. Muller et al.[29] postulated that this reduced diaphragmatic tone was responsible for the FRC reduction with anesthesia. The intercostal muscles appear to be even more sensitive to depression by volatile agents such as halothane.[30] This would make it attractive to hypothesize that the reduced tone of diaphragm and intercostals results in a reduced outward recoil of the chest wall. This process does not appear to progress further, since addition of neuromuscular blockade, which would be expected to diminish muscle tone further, produces no additional changes in FRC. The absence of any additional effect with paralysis also argues against any role of increased tone of the expiratory (abdominal) muscles in determining the end-expiratory lung volume.

Although the changes in FRC could reflect increased elastic recoil of the lungs, most favor the hypothesis that the initial effect is a reduction of outward recoil of the chest wall. The changes in the lung are probably secondary to breathing at low lung volumes. Changes similar to those induced by anesthesia have been demonstrated with chest strapping.[31]

Another possible mechanism contributing to reduction of FRC may involve a shift of blood from the limbs to the lung and abdomen. The blood in the lungs may have a twofold effect. First, lung congestion may decrease lung compliance and thus increase lung recoil. Second, the blood competes with air for intrathoracic volume. At the same time an increase in abdominal blood volume can act to displace the diaphragm upward or the abdominal wall outward. A report by Hedensteirna et al.[32] suggested that the diaphragm was displaced cranially and that the decrease in thoracic volume of FRC is associated with a shift of blood from thorax to the abdomen. Others noted that changes in volume of the rib cage share a position of the diaphragm, and intrathoracic fluid (blood) and gas contribute in varying amounts to reducing FRC in different subjects.[33] In the latter study thoracic gas volume was reduced considerably more than thoracic volume. This suggests that there is some increase in thoracic blood volume with induction of anesthesia.

Reduction in functional residual capacity with intravenous agents differs from the more dramatic effect of inhalation anesthetics. Thiopental[23] and methohexital[34] produced changes in nonintubated subjects that were similar to those associated with normal sleep.[35] In most cases the decrement in FRC was less than 200 ml. The relatively small magnitude of change was attributed to maintenance of rib cage activity in contrast to the marked depression seen with agents such as halothane.[30] Another intravenous agent, ketamine, also appears to have a sparing action on intercostal muscle activity and is associated with a maintenance of FRC at awake levels in adults[36] and in children.[37] In the latter group the increased respiratory rates and prolonged passive lung emptying as illustrated by the τ were associated with an FRC greater than the static relaxation volume.[38] The authors speculated that the prolonged τ with ketamine anesthesia was the result of increases in respiratory system compliance (thus τ, the product of $R \times C$ is increased). With halothane, on the other hand, τ is shortened, presumably because respiratory system compliance decreases.

In supine subjects the induction of general anesthesia reduces FRC such that end-expiratory volume decreases close to residual volume. This FRC may lie below the closing capacity (i.e., the volume associated with dependent airway closure, or more precisely, dynamic flow limitation).[39] Early observations with halothane anesthesia suggested a correlation between the degree of impaired oxygenation and the reduction in FRC[40] and led to the hypothesis that airway closure and atelectasis were the consequences of a reduced FRC.

The degree of intrapulmonary shunting does appear to correlate with the reduction in FRC[41] and with the degree of atelectasis demonstrated with CT in dependent lung regions.[42] It is thus tempting to attribute such atelectasis simply to the reduced FRC. However, a study in awake supine subjects with thoracoabdominal restriction argues against this simple mechanism.[43] The restriction in these subjects reduced lung volume and altered pulmonary mechanics in a fashion similar to that seen with general anesthesia. The FRC decreased by more than 20% and was matched by a reduction of CC as measured by the resident gas (N_2) technique. No atelectasis was noted with CT scanning and $\dot{V}A/\dot{Q}$ distribution, and arterial blood gases were unchanged from the control state. Thus, gas exchange in these awake subjects with chest restriction differed from anesthetized subjects, although they both had some relative decrement in FRC. The authors concluded that the development of compression atelectasis in the anesthetized patients cannot be ascribed solely to a decrease in FRC, nor can the changes in pulmonary mechanics with restriction be attributed solely to the development of atelectasis.

The atelectasis that develops in the dependent lung regions of anesthetized subjects was seen to a similar extent whether patients were anesthetized with inhalation agents (halothane, enflurane, or isoflurane) or with intravenous agents such as thiopental or propofol.[44] Quite interestingly, ketamine which, unlike the other agents, did not reduce muscle tone or FRC, did not produce such atelectasis unless neuromuscular blockade was instituted.

Impairment of Pulmonary Gas Exchange During Anesthesia

Abnormalities of pulmonary gas exchange with general anesthesia have long been recognized. Impaired oxygenation and, to some extent, CO_2 elimination appear to be a reflection of increased $\dot{V}A/\dot{Q}$ mismatch, right-to-left intrapulmonary shunting, and an increase in dead space. A number of theories have been proposed to account for these changes. Foremost among these is the reduction in lung volume (FRC), which has been discussed. Other theories that have been proposed to account for the change include inhibition of hypoxic pulmonary vasoconstriction and alterations in the normal distribution of ventilation.

Inhibition of Hypoxic Pulmonary Vasoconstriction

In the systemic vascular beds, hypoxia produces vasodilation in order to aid oxygen delivery and CO_2 removal. The pulmonary vessels, on the other hand, respond to acute hypoxia by constricting. This unique behavior in response to hypoxia is called hypoxic pulmonary vasoconstriction (HPV). The HPV response is an important compensatory mechanism that serves to divert flow away from hypoxic alveoli. Blood flow thus shifts from poorly ventilated alveoli to better ventilated ones in order to match ventilation and perfusion and minimize arterial hypoxemia.

The physiologic manifestations of HPV depend heavily on the size of the lung area that is hypoxic. If the segment of hypoxic lung is small, HPV will result in diversion of flow away from the hypoxic area in an attempt to limit hypoxemia. Little or no change in pulmonary artery pressure occurs (Fig. 6–3*A*). If, on the other hand, the hypoxic area is very large or more so if the alveolar hypoxia is diffuse and generalized, flow cannot be diverted and the vasoconstriction results in an increased pulmonary artery pressure (Fig. 6–3*B*). Thus, for flow diversion to occur the hypoxic segment must comprise a relatively small fraction of the total lung, and flow diversion is inversely related to the size of the hypoxic segment. The increases in pulmonary artery pressure, on the other hand, are directly related to the fraction of total lung that is hypoxic. Thus, the proportion of flow diversion to pressure change decreases as the size of the hypoxic lung segment increases. This distinction between localized and more generalized or diffuse hypoxia is essential to understanding the nature of HPV.

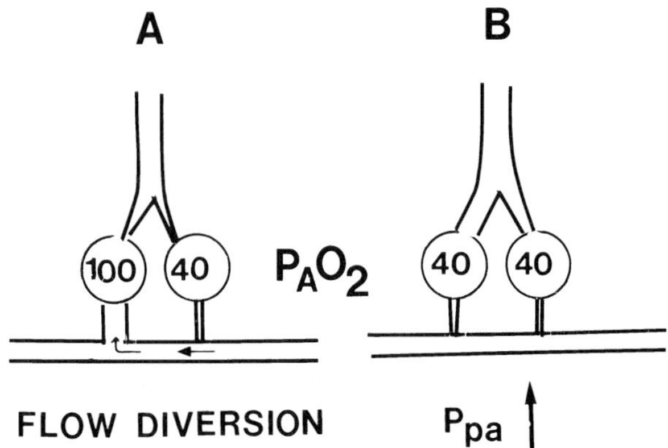

FIGURE **6–3.** Change in pulmonary artery pressure (Ppa) and diversion of blood flow are depicted to illustrate difference with local or regional lung hypoxia (*A*) and diffuse or generalized hypoxia (*B*). With the latter flow diversion cannot occur and Ppa increases. (From Gal TJ: Respiratory Physiology in Anesthetic Practice. Baltimore, Williams & Wilkins, 1991, with permission.)

The major segment of the vascular system at which HPV occurs appears to be at the level of the precapillary arterioles (30 to 50 μm).[45] These small muscular vessels are closely related to alveoli and are in an ideal position to respond to changes in alveolar oxygen concentration. Indeed, the most important stimulus to HPV appears to be the alveolar oxygen tension (PAO_2). Constriction occurs as PAO_2 decreases below normal, and the response reaches a maximum at about 30 mm Hg. The oxygen tension in the mixed venous blood ($P\bar{v}O_2$) also plays a role in the HPV response. The $P\bar{v}O_2$ becomes increasingly important at very low levels of PAO_2 and in an atelectatic lung may be the only stimulus for HPV. At alveolar oxygen tensions of about 60 mm Hg or greater, $P\bar{v}O_2$ appears to have only a minor constrictive effect.[46]

The HPV response is attenuated in a number of diverse clinical situations and by many classes of drug (Table 6–3), the most notable of which are the anesthetic drugs. Intravenous drugs of most classes utilized in anesthesia (opioids, barbiturates, benzodiazepines, ketamine) do not appear to have a detectable effect on the HPV response. In vitro and in vivo experiments have shown that the pulmonary vasoconstrictive response to hypoxia is maintained at blood concentrations of these drugs sufficient to produce analgesia and anesthesia.[47,48]

In vitro experiments utilizing isolated perfused lungs have generally shown that the current halogenated inhalation agents halothane, enflurane, and isoflurane all inhibit HPV in a dose-related manner. In vitro observations with nitrous oxide also suggest that it produces little or no effect on HPV.[47] Studies in intact animals, however, suggest that 70% nitrous oxide moderately diminishes the HPV response.[48,49] The halogenated anesthetics also appear to antagonize the HPV response in intact animals and humans, but widely divergent results have been reported. The Marshals[50] have provided a unifying concept for these findings based on the proportion of the lung that is made hypoxic. They suggest that the differences in most studies arose from the size of the lung segment used: The larger the hypoxic segment studied, the less effective the vasoconstriction and flow diversion away from the hypoxic site. They have also suggested that the antagonism of HPV by inhalation anesthetics may be obscured by other hemodynamic effects. The anesthetics depress myocardial function and produce a decrease in cardiac output. The latter is associated with decreased $P\bar{v}O_2$ and pulmonary artery pressures, both of which tend to intensify HPV. Thus, unless such effects are considered, the anesthetic actions on HPV may be subtle or misinterpreted.

The hypothesis that antagonism of HPV by inhalation anesthetics is important in the etiology of abnormal gas exchange during anesthesia is indeed an attractive one. However, blunting of the HPV response does not appear to sufficiently account for the impaired oxygenation observed. Inappropriately low PaO_2 values are often seen in patients breathing hyperoxic mixtures that would be expected to provide most if not all alveolar units with an oxygen tension far above that at which HPV comes into play. Therefore, other factors such as altered lung mechanics may play a more significant role in the impaired gas exchange.[51]

TABLE **6–3**
Hypoxic Pulmonary Vasoconstriction (HPV) with Drugs

Increased HPV	Decreased HPV
Almitrine bimesylate	β-Adrenergic agonists
Cyclo-oxygenase inhibitors	Calcium channel blockers
Propranolol	Inhalation anesthetics
	Minoxidil
	Nitroglycerin
	Nitroprusside
	Theophylline

Altered Distribution of Ventilation

Ventilation is not normally uniform throughout the lung. The effects of gravity on the lung and the forces necessary to allow it to conform to the shape of the thorax result in a vertical gradient of pleural pressure. The pleural pressure acting on the upper (nondependent) areas of the lung is more subatmospheric (negative) than that acting on the lower (dependent) portions. As a result, the nondependent areas are more inflated than the dependent ones. The gradient of pleural pressure up and down the lung changes about 0.4 cm H_2O per each centimeter of lung height. Thus, in a lung 30 cm high, a 7.5-cm H_2O pressure difference exists from apex to base. In the supine position, the dorsal areas become dependent. The height of the lungs is reduced by nearly one third, and thus the gravitational effect is diminished somewhat.

Although the nondependent lung areas are more distended at FRC, a given transpulmonary pressure generated during a normal breath produces a greater volume change or ventilation to the dependent areas. This is because of the rather sigmoid shape of the lung's pressure-volume curve (Fig. 6–1*A*). The larger nondependent areas have a lower regional compliance (i.e., they lie on a less steep portion of the pressure-volume curve).

These regional differences in ventilation are important in matching ventilation to perfusion. The dependent or basal areas tend to be better perfused because of gravitational effects. Since the bases are also better ventilated, there is good matching of ventilation and perfusion (Fig. 6–4). Higher ventilation and blood flow are delivered to the bases. In supine anesthetized paralyzed humans, the ventilation or distribution of inspired gas becomes more uniform from top to bottom lung areas (Fig. 6–4), largely because basal lung units undergo further reduction in size to a point that reduces their regional compliance. Anesthetics, meanwhile, produce a decrease in pulmonary artery pressure, which impedes perfusion of nondependent lung regions. Increased alveolar pressures with mechanical ventilation further interfere with perfusion of nondependent areas. Thus, dependent lung areas are well perfused but rather poorly ventilated. In contrast, nondependent areas receive more ventilation but considerably less perfusion.

In addition to changes in static lung mechanics, the overall $\dot{V}_A/\dot{Q}$ inhomogeneity may also be increased during anesthesia because of changes in dynamics (i.e., the pressure-flow relationships in the airways). The smooth muscle relaxation associated with anesthetics may be useful in preventing the increased bronchial tone associated with bronchospasm. However, reductions in normal bronchomotor tone may interfere with the normal $\dot{V}_A/\dot{Q}$ matching and thus impair gas exchange.[52]

Local decreases in alveolar CO_2 tension also tend to improve the normal $\dot{V}_A/\dot{Q}$ matching by producing local increases in bronchomotor tone. In a sense, this hypocapneic bronchoconstriction is analogous to hypoxic pulmonary vasoconstriction. Whether the inhalation anesthetics as a group block this bronchoconstriction induced by hypocapnia is not known. Thus far, only halothane has been shown to reduce this bronchoconstrictive effect of hypocapnia.[53,54]

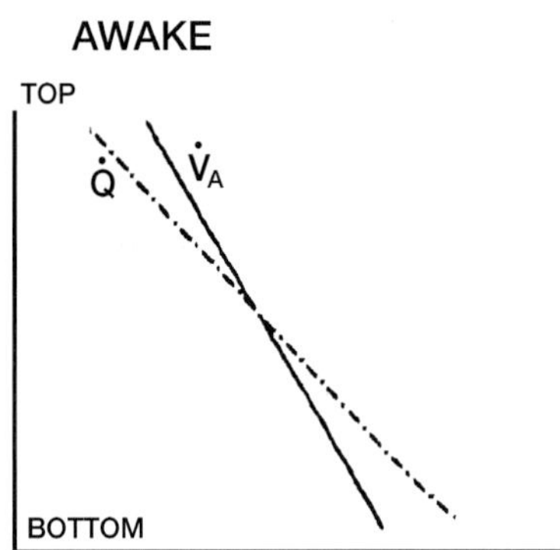

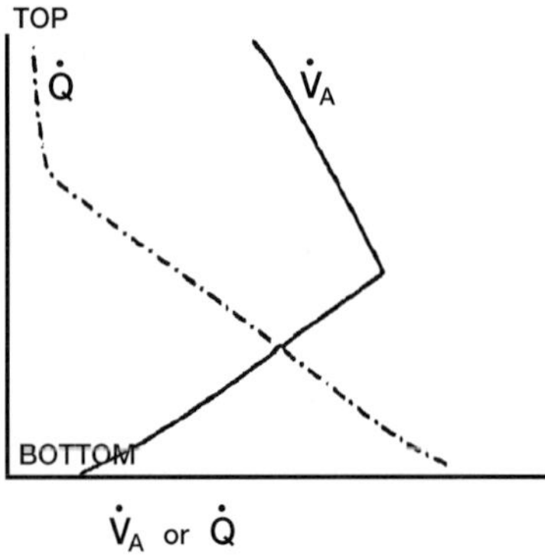

FIGURE **6–4.** Diagramatic representation of the distribution of ventilation (VA) and perfusion (Q) between nondependent (*top*) lung areas and dependent (*bottom*) areas. Note that VA tends to be distributed more uniformly from top to bottom in the anesthetized paralyzed state. (From Gal TJ: Respiratory physiology during anesthesia. In Kaplan JA [ed]: Thoracic Anesthesia, 2nd ed. New York, Churchill Livingstone, 1990, with permission.)

Distribution of Ventilation in the Lateral Position

Subjects while lying in the lateral decubitus position exhibit a greater blood flow to the dependent lung, largely because of gravitational effects. In the awake state, the normal vertical gradient of pleural pressure also allows for greater ventilation of the same dependent lung and maintenance of normal $\dot{V}_A/\dot{Q}$ distribution. This is more true in the case of the larger right lung, which is not subject to compression by an enlarged heart. In fact, in relatively normal persons with unilateral lung disease, respiratory gas exchange is optimal if the good lung is dependent.[55,56] Exceptions to this appear to occur in infants and in patients with chronic obstructive pulmonary disease. In these groups, the nondependent lung appears to be better ventilated.[57,58]

Radiographic and bronchospirometric studies show that the dependent lung normally receives a greater ventilation and has a higher O_2 uptake in the lateral position. Although its FRC is lower than the nondependent lung, N_2 washout is also more rapid.[59] When patients are anesthetized in the lateral position, as for thoracic surgery, distribution of the pulmonary blood flow is similar to the awake state (i.e., the dependent lung receives greater perfusion). The greater portion of ventilation, however, is switched from the dependent to the nondependent lung. In a sense, the ventilation is more uniform, and this is reflected in more equal N_2 clearance for each lung.[59] This shift in distribution of ventilation results from a loss of lung volume (decreased FRC) that is shared but unequally by both lungs. The dependent lung, which undergoes a greater decrease in FRC, moves to a less steep portion near the bottom of the pressure-volume curve, while the nondependent lung moves from a relatively flat portion to a steeper one. The abdominal contents, as well as the mediastinum, also impede dependent lung expansion. Thus, the anesthetized patient in the lateral position has a nondependent lung that is well ventilated but poorly perfused. In contrast, the well-perfused dependent lung is poorly ventilated. Opening the chest may only serve to increase the overventilation of the nondependent lung.

In summary, the increased $\dot{V}_A/\dot{Q}$ mismatching that accompanies anesthesia and paralysis whether in the supine or lateral position appears to be largely a result of altered distribution of ventilation with a relative failure of intrapulmonary perfusion to adjust.[60] Although some of this failure of blood flow to adjust for the altered ventilation may relate to inhibition of hypoxic pulmonary vasoconstriction by the inhalation anesthetics, the altered pattern of expansion of the lung with anesthesia and paralysis may also affect the distribution of blood flow along with the ventilation.

References

1. Ferris BG, Mead J, Odie LH: Partitioning of respiratory flow resistance in man. J Appl Physiol 19:653, 1964.
2. Proctor DF: The upper airway. II: Larynx and trachea. Am Rev Respir Dis 115:315, 1977.
3. Camporesi EM, Mortola JP, SantAmbrogia F, SantAmbrogio B: Topical anesthesia of tracheal receptors. J Appl Physiol 47:1123, 1979.
4. Macklem PT, Wilson NJ: Measurement of intrabronchial pressure in man. J Appl Physiol 20:653, 1965.
5. Gal TJ: Effects of endotracheal intubation on normal cough performance. Anesthesiology 52:324, 1980.
6. Liistro G, Stanescu D, Dooms G, et al: Head position modifies upper airway resistance in men. J Appl Physiol 64:1285, 1988.
7. Lawes EG, Campbell I, Mercer D: Inflation pressure, gastric insufflation and rapid sequence induction. Br J Anaesth 59:315, 1987.
8. Detroyer A, Estenne M: Functional anatomy of the respiratory muscles. Clin Chest Med 9:175, 1988.
9. Black LF, Hyatt RE: Maximal respiratory pressures. Normal values and relationship to age and sex. Am Rev Respir Dis 103:641, 1971.
10. Pavlin EG, Holle RH, Schoene RB: Recovery of airway protection compared with ventilation in humans after paralysis with curare. Anesthesiology 70:381, 1989.
11. Hess D: History of pulmonary function testing. Respir Care 34: 427, 1989.
12. Leith DE, Mead JL: Mechanisms determining residual volume of the lungs in normal subjects. J Appl Physiol 23:221, 1967.
13. Tucker DH, Sieker HO: The effect of change in body position on lung volumes and intrapulmonary gas mixing in patients with obesity, heart failure and emphysema. Am Rev Respir Dis 85: 787, 1960.
14. Koterba AM, Kosch PC, Beech J, Whitlock T: Breathing strategy of the adult horse (*Equus caballus*) at rest. J Appl Physiol 64: 337, 1988.
15. Bryan AC, Wohl ME: Respiratory mechanics in children. In Macklem PT, Mead J (eds): Handbook of Physiology. The Respiratory System. Bethesda MD, American Physiological Society, 1986, p 180.
16. Olinsky A, Bryan MH, Bryan AC: Influence of lung inflation on respiratory control in neonates. J Appl Physiol 36:426, 1974.
17. Colin AA, Wohl MEB, Mead J, et al: Transition from dynamically maintained to relaxed end expiratory volume in human infants. J Appl Physiol 67:2107, 1989.
18. Ludwig MS, Dreshas O, Solway J, et al: Partitioning of pulmonary resistance during constriction in the dog: Effect of volume history. J Appl Physiol 62:807, 1987.
19. Warner DO, Bettermann J, Brusasco V, Rehder K: Pulmonary resistance during halothane anesthesia is not determined only by airway caliber. Anesthesiology 70:453, 1989.
20. Bergman NA: Distribution of inspired gas during anesthesia and artificial ventilation. J Appl Physiol 18:1085, 1963.
21. Render K, Marsh HM: Respiratory mechanics during anesthesia and mechanical ventilation. In Macklem PT, Mead J (eds): Handbook of Physiology. The Respiratory System. Mechanics of Breathing. Bethesda, MD, American Physiological Society, 1986, p 737.
22. Damia G, Mascheroni D, Croci M, Tarenzi L: Perioperative changes in functional residual capacity in morbidly obese patients. Br J Anaesth 60:574, 1988.
23. Bergman NA: Reduction in resting end-expiratory position of the respiratory system with induction of anesthesia and neuromuscular paralysis. Anesthesiology 57:14, 1982.
24. Hewlett AM, Hulands GH, Nunn JF, Millwdge JS: Functional residual capacity during anesthesia. II. Spontaneous respiration. Br J Anaesth 46:486, 1974.
25. Westbrook PR, Stubbs, SE, Sesler AD, et al: Effects of anesthesia and muscle paralysis on respiratory mechanics in normal man. J Appl Physiol 34:81, 1973.
26. Brismar B, Hedenstierna G, Lundquist H, et al: Pulmonary densities during anesthesia with muscular relaxation. A proposal of atelectasis. Anesthesiology 62:422, 1985.
27. Dery R, Pelletier J, Jaques A, et al: Alveolar collapse induced by nitrogenation. Can Anaesth Soc J 12:531, 1965.
28. Hedenstierna G, Lofstrom B, Lundh R: Thoracic gas volume and chest abdomen dimensions during anesthesia and muscle paralysis. Anesthesiology 55:499, 1981.
29. Muller N, Volgyesi G, Becker L, et al: Diaphragmatic muscle tone. J Appl Physiol 47:279, 1979.
30. Tusiewicz K, Bryan AC, Froese AB: Contributions of changing rib cage-diaphragm interactions to the ventilatory depression of halothane and anesthesia. Anesthesiology 47:327, 1977.
31. Scheidt M, Hyatt RE, Rehder K: Effect of rib cage or abdominal restriction on lung mechanics. J Appl Physiol 51:1115, 1981.
32. Hedenstierna G, Strandberg A, Brismar B, et al: Functional residual capacity, thoracoabdominal dimensions, and central blood volume during general anesthesia with muscle paralysis and mechanical ventilation. Anesthesiology 62:247, 1985.
33. Krayer S, Render K, Beck KC, et al: Quantification of thoracic volumes by three-dimensional imaging. J Appl Physiol 62:591, 1987.
34. Bickler PE, Dueck R, Prutow R: Effects of barbiturate anesthesia and functional residual capacity and rib cage/diaphragm contributions to ventilation. Anesthesiology 60:147, 1987.
35. Hudgel DQ, Devadatta P: Decrease in functional residual capacity during sleep in normal humans. J Appl Physiol 57:1319, 1984.
36. Mankikian B, Cantineau JP, Sartene R, et al: Ventilatory pattern and chest wall mechanics during ketamine anesthesia in humans. Anesthesiology 65:492, 1986.
37. Shulman D, Bearsmore CS, Aronson HG, Bodrey S: The effect of ketamine on functional residual capacity in young children. Anesthesiology 62:551, 1985.
38. Shuman D, Bar-yishay E, Beardsmore C, Godfrey S: Determinants of end-expiratory lung volume in young children during ketamine or halothane. Anesthesia 66:636, 1987.
39. Render K, Marsh HM, Rodarte JR, Hyatt RE: Airway closure. Anesthesiology 47:40, 1977.
40. Hickey RF, Visick WD, Fairley HB, Fourcade HE: Effects of halothane anesthesia on functional residual capacity and alveolar-arterial oxygen tension difference. Anesthesiology 38:20, 1973.
41. Dueck R, Prutow RJ, Davies NHJ, et al: The lung volume at which shunting occurs with inhalation anesthesia. Anesthesiology 69:854, 1988.
42. Hedenstierna G, Tokics L, Strandberg A, et al: Correlation of gas exchange impairment to development of atelectasis during anesthesia and muscle paralysis. Acta Anaesthesiol Scand 30:183, 1986.
43. Tokics L, Hedenstierna G, Brismar BO, et al: Thoracoabdominal restriction in supine men: CT and lung function measurements. J Appl Physiol 64:599, 1988.
44. Hedenstierna G: Gas exchange during anaesthesia. Br J Anaesth 64:507, 1990.
45. Nagasaka Y, Bhattacharya J, Nanjo S, et al: Micropuncture measurements of lung microvascular pressure profile during hypoxia in cats. Circ Res 54:90, 1984.
46. Marshall C, Marshall B: Influence of perfusate PO_2 on hypoxic pulmonary vasoconstriction in rats. Circ Res 52:691, 1983.
47. Bjertaines LJ: Hypoxia-induced vasoconstriction in isolated perfused lungs exposed to injectable or intravenous anesthetics. Acta Anaesthesiol Scand 21:133, 1977.
48. Benumof JL, Wahrenbrock EA: Local effects of anesthetics on regional hypoxic pulmonary vasoconstriction. Anesthesiology 43: 525, 1975.
49. Mathers J, Benumof JL, Wahrenbrock EA: General anesthetics and regional hypoxic pulmonary vasoconstriction. Anesthesiology 46:111, 1977.
50. Marshall BE, Marshall C: Continuity of response to hypoxic pulmonary vasoconstriction. J Appl Physiol 49:189, 1980.
51. Marshall BE, Marshall C: Anesthesia and the pulmonary circulation. In Covino BG, Fozzard HA, Render K, Stricharz GR (eds): Effects of Anesthesia. Bethesda, MD, American Physiological Society, 1985, p 121.

52. Crawford ABH, Makowska M, Engel LA: Effect of bronchomotor tone on static mechanical properties of lung and ventilation distribution. J Appl Physiol 63:2278, 1987.
53. McAslan C, Mima M, Norden I, Norlander O: Effects of halothane and methoxyflurane on pulmonary resistance gas flow during lung bypass. Scand J Thorac Cardiovasc Surg 5:193, 1971.
54. Coon RL, Kampine JP: Hypocapnic bronchoconstriction and inhalation anesthetics. Anesthesiology 43:635, 1975.
55. Remolina C, Kahn AU, Santiago TV, Edelman NH: Positional hypoxemia in unilateral lung disease. N Engl J Med 304:523, 1981.
56. Fishman AF: Down with the good lung. N Engl J Med 304:537, 1981.
57. Davies H, Kitchman R, Gordon I, Helms P: Regional ventilation in infancy. Reversal of adult pattern. N Engl J Med 313:1626, 1985.
58. Shim C, Chun K, Williams MH, Blaufox MD: Positional effects on distribution of ventilation in chronic obstructive pulmonary disease. Ann Intern Med 105:346, 1986.
59. Rehder K, Katch DJ, Sessler AD, Fowler WS: The function of each lung of anesthetized and paralyzed man during mechanical ventilation. Anesthesiology 37:16, 1972.
60. Landmark SJ, Knopp TJ, Render K, Sessler AD: Regional pulmonary perfusion and V/Q in awake and anesthetized paralyzed man. J Appl Physiol 43:993, 1977.

CHAPTER 7

Organ System Effects of Anesthetics

David Kramer, M.D.
Mark F. Newman, M. D.

Anesthesia affects the cardiac, central nervous, pulmonary, renal and hepatic systems in a variety of ways. The pharmacologic effects of the anesthetic drugs may also depend upon the pathophysiology present in a patient undergoing cardiac, thoracic, or vascular surgery.

Effects of Anesthetic Agents on the Cardiovascular System

Cardiac Electrophysiology

Action Potential

The normal cardiac action potential results from the transmembrane potential that occurs following spontaneous depolarization to threshold potential or from external excitation in those cells not exhibiting automaticity. Depolarization of the cardiac cell is due to net inward movement of positive charges. The entire action potential results from synchronized changes in permeability to sodium (Na^+), potassium (K^+), calcium (Ca^{2+}), and chloride ions (Cl^-) during the five action potential phases illustrated in Figure 7–1.

Depolarization

Phase 0 of the action potential is primarily dependent on the brief intense movement of Na^+ in atrial and ventricular muscle fibers and Purkinje fibers. Phase 0 in slower response fibers in the sinoatrial (SA) and atrioventricular (AV) nodes is dependent on Na^+ movement and slow inward current of Ca^{2+}. Repolarization occurs in phase 1, 2, and 3 of the action potential. Phase 1, rapid repolarization, is primarily due to an inward movement of Na^+ and an outward movement of K^+ producing the early rapid change. In phase 2, the plateau phase, the inward movement of Ca^{2+} through the slow Ca^{2+} channels balances the outward K^+ movement, producing little change in membrane potential during phase 2. Phase 3, final rapid repolarization, is due primarily to the rapid efflux of K^+ from the cell. The ionic movement for the cardiac action potential is shown in Figure 7–1.

In phase 4, electrical diastole, the cell is very permeable to K^+ but relatively impermeable to other ions. In nonpacemaker contractile atrial and ventricular cells, the Na^+-K^+ exchange pump maintains the intracellular Na^+ low and the intracellular K^+ high and the cells remain at rest until activated by a propagated impulse or other stimulus. The inside of the cell remains negative in relation to the outside of the cell, with the Na^+-Ca^+ exchange mechanism also playing a role in maintenance of membrane potential depending on membrane voltage and ionic concentrations.

Automaticity

Automaticity in cardiac cells results from net reduction in the outward movement of positive charges during phase 4 of the action potential. This can obviously occur by a decrease in the outward current or an increase in the inward current or both. In the sinoatrial node this net reduction in outward movement of positive charge occurs due to a delay in the outward movement of potassium, along with slowly recovering Ca^{2+} inward currents. Regardless of the ionic mechanism for the changing membrane potential, the rate of automaticity is determined by (1) maximum diastolic potential, (2) threshold potential, and (3) the rate of spontaneous phase 4 depolarization. This is schematically represented in Figure 7–2.

Anesthetic Effects

Anesthetic agents alter electrophysiology through direct and indirect mechanisms. The classic inhalational anesthetics slow the rate of SA node automaticity.[1,2] Clinically, the actions of the anesthetic agents must be separated from those of other drugs or the effects of autonomic compensation.[1–3] Using an isolated perfused canine right atrial preparation, it was determined that epinephrine or norepinephrine augment the automaticity of atrial pacemakers more than the SA node. Most im-

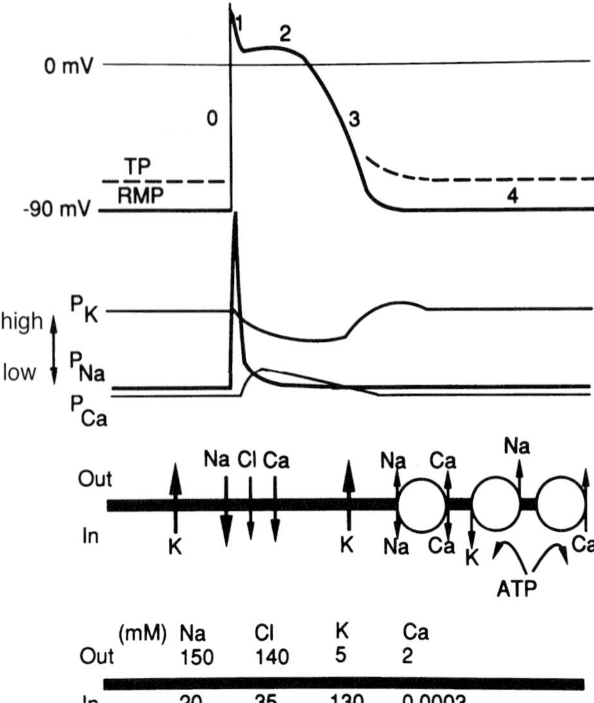

FIGURE 7–1. Schematic representation of different phases of cardiac Purkinje action potential. Action potential is shown in relation to ion permeability (P) across the membrane, along with ionic exchange mechanisms and ionic concentrations outside (out) and inside (in) the cell. TP, threshold potential; RMP, resting membrane potential (From Atlee JL, Bosnjak ZJ: Mechanisms for cardiac dysrhythmias during anesthesia. Anesthesiology 72:347, 1990, with permission.)

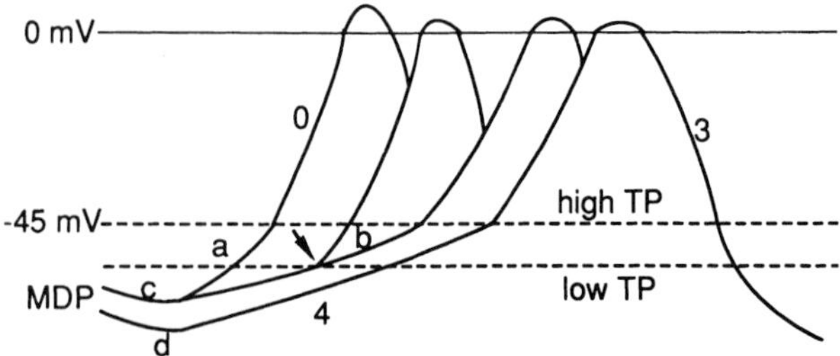

FIGURE 7–2. Schematic representation of the mechanisms that can alter automaticity of the sinoatrial (SA) node. A decrease in slope of the phase 4 depolarization from *a* to *b* slows the rate of automatic discharge by increasing the time to reach threshold potential (TP). An increase in TP from high to low level of membrane potential (more negative) increases the rate of discharge (*arrow*) by decreasing the time to reach the TP. In addition, automatic discharge can be slowed by an increase in maximum diastolic potential from *c* to *d*. (From Atlee JL, Bosnjak ZJ: Mechanisms for cardiac dysrhythmias during anesthesia. Anesthesiology 72:347, 1990, with permission.)

portantly, ectopic atrial rhythms require epinephrine or norepinephrine.

Inhalational Anesthetics

All commonly used inhalational anesthetics slow the rate of SA node pacemaker discharge by both direct and indirect effects on SA node automaticity (Fig. 7–3).[1,2] In addition to their effects on the SA node, halothane and enflurane produce dose-dependent prolongation of AV node conduction and refractoriness, while isoflurane was shown not to effect AV node conduction time.[4] Although AV nodal conduction time is prolonged in dogs, there is no evidence that currently used inhalational anesthetics are likely to cause second- or third-degree heart block in the absence of pre-existing cardiac conditions or drugs that prolonged AV node conduction. In addition, the autonomic response to the anesthetic agents in humans makes a significant AV nodal block even less likely.

Enflurane and halothane produce prolongation of the His-Purkinje and ventricular conduction time in dogs.[5,6] In addition, halothane shortens action potential duration and refractoriness in normal Purkinje fibers.[7,8] Most importantly, it appears that the inhaled anesthetics produce greater effects in proximal rather than distal Purkinje fibers, indicating a potential for dysrhythmias due to the disparity in regional refractoriness.

Current data on the inhaled anesthetics suggest they have both dysrhythmic and antidysrhythmic action.[9] All anesthetic agents appear to reduce the potential for ventricular fibrillation after acute left anterior descending (LAD) coronary artery occlusion in rats.[10,11] However, halothane appears to increase the range of premature responses conducted into the ischemic (distal) region slowly enough to produce unstimulated responses that could re-excite the nonischemic region facilitating reentrant dysrhythmias.[12] Halothane's effects may be mediated by its action on Ca^{2+} slow inward current,[13,14] although more recent data would point to alteration in Na^+ window current producing the regional differences in action potential duration that could contribute to re-entry.[15]

To summarize the effect of volatile anesthetics on cardiac rhythm[16]: (1) the volatile anesthetics are conducive to bradycardia and AV conduction disturbances; (2) in depressed fibers (ischemia or infarction) halothane, and most likely the other agents as well, is conducive to reentrant excitation. However, halothane and possibly other agents oppose abnormal automaticity and delay after depolarization-induced sustained rhythm activity, possibly explaining their effectiveness against ouabain-induced dysrhythmias.[17]

Intravenous Anesthetics

OPIOIDS

Opioids, including morphine, do not sensitize the heart to catecholamines. Opioids tend to reduce heart rate (HR) or induce bradycardia primarily through vagal mediation, which probably reflects stimulation of the vagal nucleus of the medulla, which has a high density of opioid receptors. Opioids may also exert a direct depressant effect on the sinoatrial node and slow conduction of cardiac impulses through the AV node. In addition, the opioids depress baroreceptor reflexes, which may contribute to their hemodynamic and electrophysiologic effects.

Fentanyl and sufentanil have been shown to enhance the calcium current that occurs during phase 2 (the plateau phase) of the action potential and depress the outward potassium current responsible for terminal depolarization, resulting in significant prolongation of the

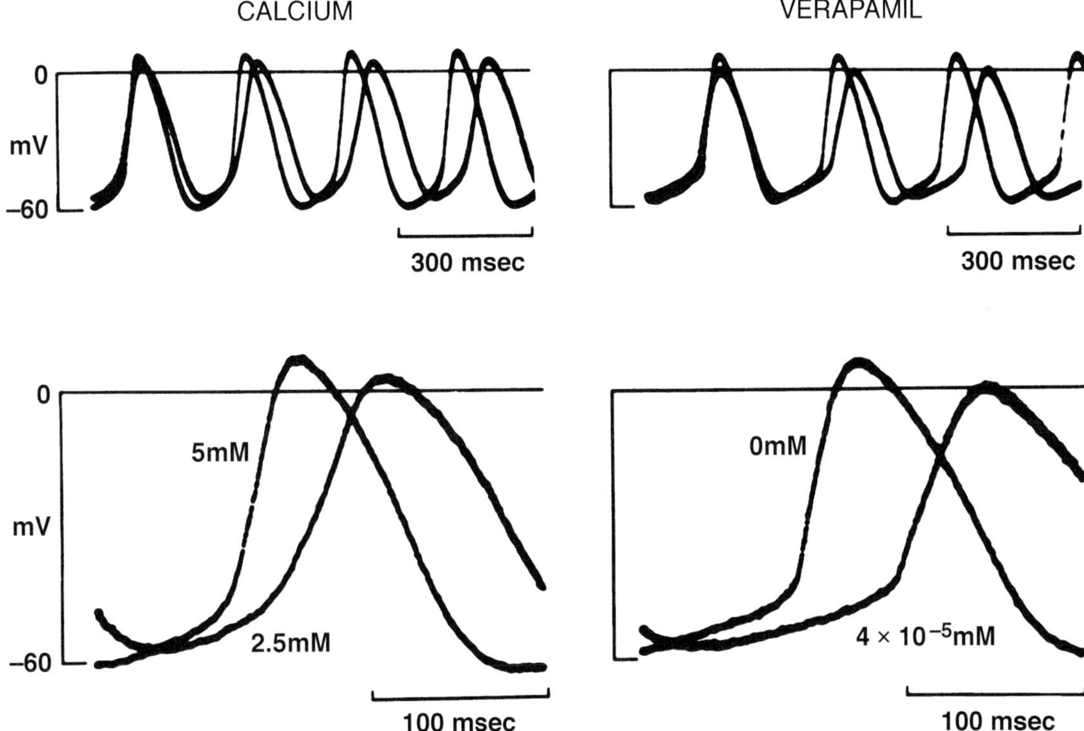

FIGURE **7–3.** The effects of halothane, enflurane, and isoflurane on the action potential of spontaneously active fibers in the guinea pig sinoatrial nodal region. The action potential tracings of the control and after 5 minutes of exposure to anesthetics (2 MAC) are superimposed at two different speeds and magnifications. (From Bosnjak ZK, Kampine JP: Effects of halothane, enflurane and isoflurane on the SA node. Anesthesiology 58:314, 1983, with permission.)

duration of the action potential (Fig. 7–4).[18] The same group of investigators noted that fentanyl and sufentanil produced a direct membrane effect similar to class III antiarrhythmic drugs.[19] Large doses of opioids prolong the QT interval, possibly explaining the reported antiarrhythmic effects of the opioids in the presence of myocardial ischemia.[20,21] This finding appears to be in contradiction to the reported antiarrhythmic effect of naloxone in coronary artery ligation models in isolated heart preparations and in intact animals.[22,23] This discrepancy appears due to difference in the μ- and κ-receptors, with the κ-receptor being most likely associated with arrhythmogenesis during myocardial ischemia.[24] Sufentanil and fentanyl are primarily μ-agonists, possibly explaining the discrepancy that opioid agonists and antagonists produce antiarrhythmic effects.

Nonopioid Intravenous Agents

Barbiturates produce differing results on the cardiac action potential.[25,26] Thiopental has been most extensively studied and is known to produce increased action potential duration consistent with decreased potassium conductance, and depressed dV/dt_{max}, consistent with decreased calcium channel ion flux.[25] This is in agreement with data on sodium pentobarbital showing reduction of the slow inward potassium current but contrasts with the results of methohexital on cardiac ionic current.[27] Baum showed that the delayed rectifier and inward rectifier potassium currents were unaffected by methohexital, indicating an interesting contrast with the other barbiturates.[27] Baum contrasted the effects of methohexital with those of propofol and ketamine. The results showed a specific pattern for each agent, with ketamine producing a significant reduction in inward rectifier potassium current in guinea pig ventricular myocyte preparations, while propofol produced a significant reduction in delayed rectifier potassium current with no effect on the inward rectifier.[27] These data suggest that the intravenous anesthetics as a group have more specific actions than would be implied by a generalized membrane effect.

Cardiac Contractility and Hemodynamic Effects

The effects of anesthetic agents on myocardial contractility are even more complex than their effects on electrophysiology. The "supporting" effect of diethyl ether and cyclopropane is an excellent example of the complex effects of anesthetic agents in the intact animal. Diethyl ether and cyclopropane maintained or supported cardiovascular function, but it was not until many years after their introduction that it was discovered that this occurred by sympathetic activation that overcame their direct myocardial depression.[28] Current anesthetic agents are often as complex as our original agents, with confounding direct and indirect effects (Fig. 7–5). This section attempts to evaluate the direct effects of these agents, where possible, and contrast these with the re-

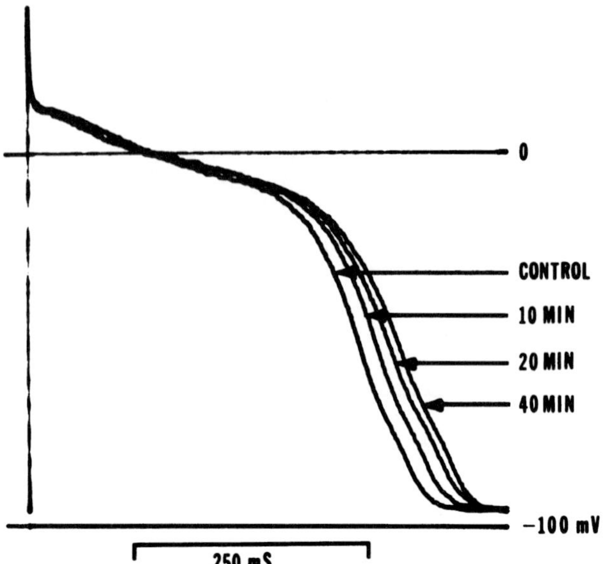

FIGURE 7–4. Superimposed action potentials recorded from Purkinje fiber during control and after exposure to 0.17 μmol of sufentanil for 10, 20, and 40 minutes. (From Blair JR, Pruett JK, Introna RPS, et al: Cardiac electrophysiologic effects of fentanyl and sufentanil in canine cardiac Purkinje fibers. Anesthesiology 71:565, 1989, with permission.)

sponse expected in the whole animal or patients. The overall hemodynamic effects produced by changes in cardiac electrophysiology, myocardial contractility, peripheral blood vessels, baroreflexes, the autonomic nervous system as well as local metabolic and neurohumoral factors at the tissue level will be included.

Inhalational Anesthetics

Inhalational anesthetic agents have received the most intensive study into their direct and indirect effects on cardiac contractility. Merin noted that all inhalational anesthetics (isoflurane, halothane, and enflurane) produce a dose-dependent decrease in the peak rate of the ventricular pressure rise (dP/dt), but felt that the lack of elevated filling pressures of isoflurane indicated less myocardial depression.[29] This finding was confirmed by VanTrigt et al. in animals and humans showing that equipotent doses of halothane and enflurane produced similar myocardial depressant effects.[30] Concerns remained that the lesser effects of isoflurane were due to reflex-mediated outcomes (i.e., nervous system activity) until Pagel et al. compared equipotent dosages of halothane and isoflurane in chronically instrumented dogs with pharmacologic autonomic nervous system blockade.[31] Even with autonomic blockade, isoflurane produced significantly less myocardial depression.[31] Recent studies from the same group comparing isoflurane with the newer inhaled agent, desflurane, in the dog model of "preload recruitable stroke work" (PRSW), showed similar depression of contractility by these two agents.[32] All inhalational anesthetics produce myocardial depression, with halothane and enflurane producing similar more significant depression than isoflurane and desflurane (halothane ≅ enflurane > isoflurane ≅ desflurane).

The hemodynamic effects produced by these changes in contractility and the associated compensatory mechanisms produce the now well-appreciated differences in clinical responses to inhalation anesthetics. Halothane produces minimal changes in systemic vascular resistance (SVR) and HR, while there is a dose-dependent

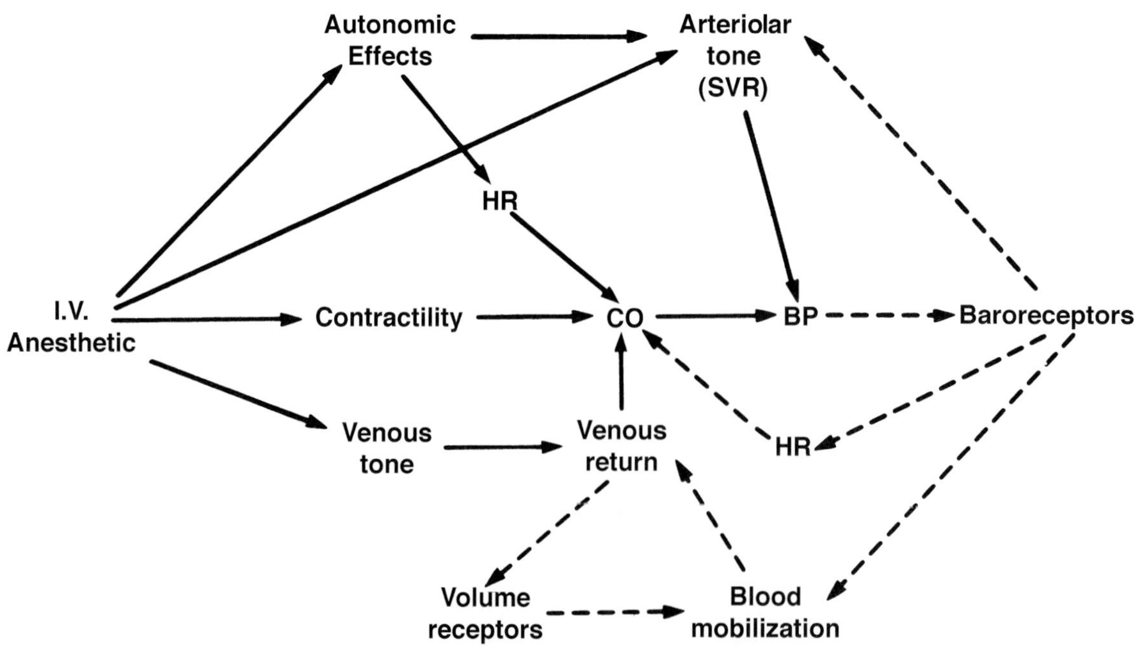

FIGURE 7–5. Direct (*solid arrows*) and indirect (*broken arrows*) effects of intravenous anesthetics on cardiovascular function. CO, cardiac output; HR, heart rate; BP, blood pressure; SVR, systemic vascular resistance. (From Reves JG, Gelman S: Cardiovascular effects of the intravenous anesthetic drugs. In Effects of Anesthesia. Bethesda, MD, American Physiological Society, 1985, p 179, with permission.)

decrease in mean arterial pressure (MAP) due to decreasing cardiac output (CO) and decreased stroke volume (SV) in the face of increased filling pressures (Fig. 7–6).[33,34] This is well delineated in the accompanying figure from Weiskopf et al. showing that halothane produces its hemodynamic effects through the depression of myocardial contractility. Enflurane also produces a dose-dependent decrease in MAP similar to halothane, with the exception that enflurane produces a decrease in SVR with compensatory increases in HR.[35,36] The heart rate

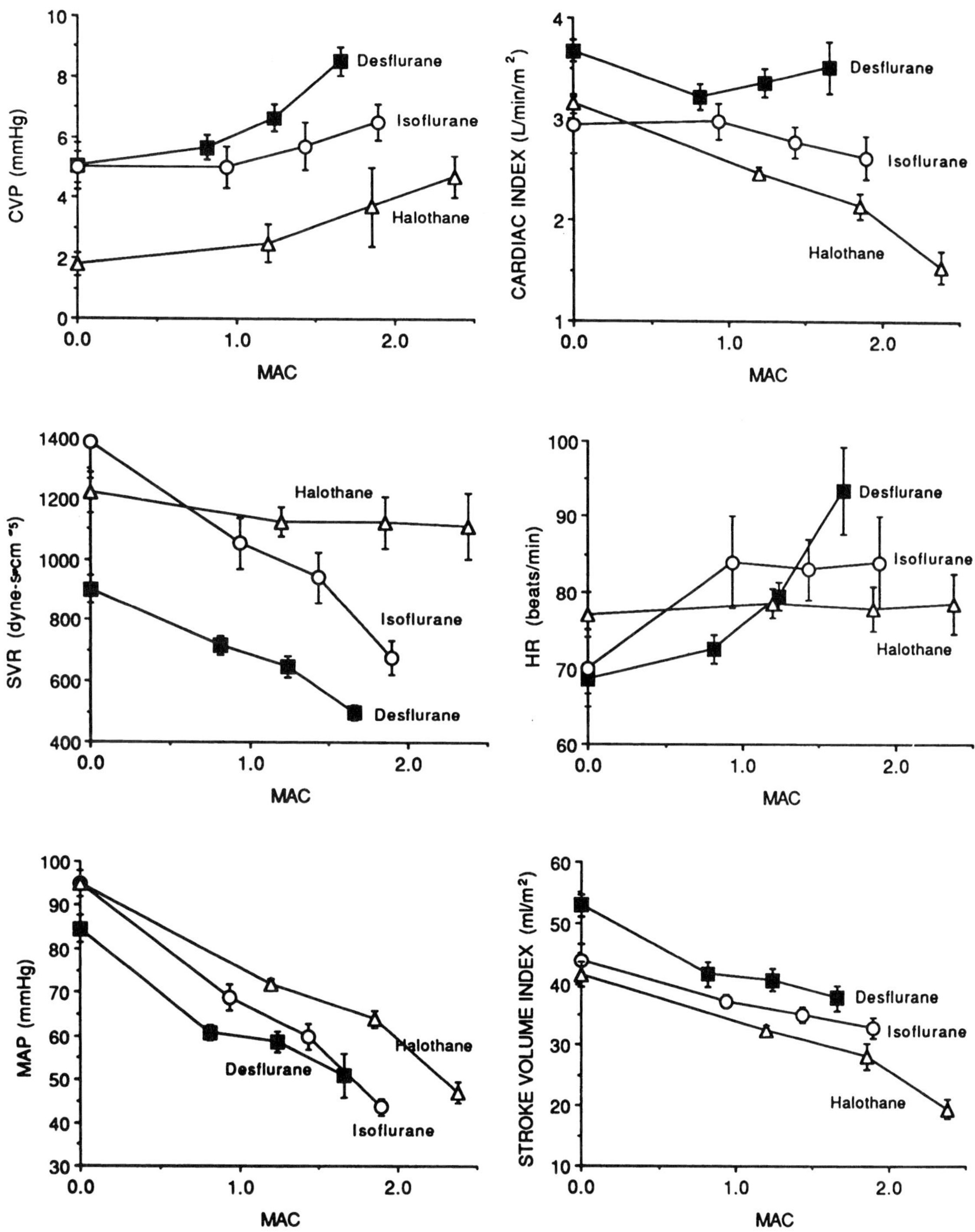

FIGURE 7–6. Comparison of the cardiovascular effects of desflurane with those of isoflurane and halothane. Note that, at light levels of desflurane anesthesia, there is no significant increase in HR, and there is much better maintenance of cardiac function with desflurane than with isoflurane or halothane, especially at deeper levels of anesthesia. (From Weiskopf RB, Cahalan MK, Eger EI, et al: Cardiovascular actions of desflurane in normocarbic volunteers. Anesth Analg 73:143, 1991, with permission.)

increase is not enough to maintain CO in these patients. The increase in filling pressures associated with enflurane is less than that produced with halothane.

In contrast to halothane and enflurane, isoflurane produces a dose-dependent decrease in blood pressure (BP) primarily through the reduction of SVR with minimal to no change in CO at lower doses.[37–40] Cardiac output is maintained secondary to mild increases in heart rate to compensate for decreased stroke volume. Filling pressures do increase with increasing doses of isoflurane demonstrating its depressive effect on myocardial contractility that was previously described.[34,39]

The hemodynamic effects of desflurane are similar to those described for isoflurane (Fig. 7–6). In contrast to isoflurane, induction of anesthesia with desflurane in patients with coronary artery disease (CAD) produced worse tachycardia when desflurane was utilized as the primary agent, resulting in significant concern for the use of this agent in high-risk cardiac patients.[41] This tachycardia appears related to release of catecholamines at higher doses, an effect recently demonstrated for isoflurane as well. The cardiovascular effects of desflurane, halothane, and isoflurane in healthy volunteers are contrasted in Figure 7–6 from Weiskopf.[34]

The effect of nitrous oxide (N_2O) on cardiac contractility remained controversial for many years.[42,43] The majority of current data points to nitrous oxide as a mild myocardial depressant, but this is complicated by N_2O stimulation of the sympathetic nervous system producing confounding results in the intact animal.[44–48] Pagel et al. evaluated the effect of N_2O on PRSW in chronically instrumented dogs with pharmacologic blockade of the autonomic nervous system (ANS) and found mild dose-dependent depression of contractility by N_2O[45] that in the intact animal or patient is counterbalanced by sympathetic activation resulting in minimal myocardial depression or hemodynamic consequences.

Opioids

Opioids are extensively used in cardiac surgery because of their lack of myocardial depression. Although morphine and meperidine anesthesia was fraught with many complications, use of fentanyl for cardiac anesthesia, first reported in 1978, produced striking stability.[49] Isolated heart muscle preparations have demonstrated dose-related negative inotropy of morphine, meperidine, fentanyl, and alfentanil.[50–53] This depression occurred at doses that were hundreds to thousands of times greater than those found even during high-dose narcotic anesthesia. At concentrations similar to those produced by narcotic anesthesia, fentanyl, morphine, and the other potent narcotics produced little or no change in myocardial contractility.[51,54]

Since myocardial depression by opioids in minimal, hemodynamic consequence of these agents must relate to their alteration of sympathetic outflow from the central nervous system (CNS), specific vagal effects, or in the case of morphine and meperidine, histamine release.[55,56] Depression of baroreceptor reflexes by opioids may also contribute to the overall hemodynamic profile.[57,58]

The hemodynamic stability of the different potent opioids appears to vary depending on the study. Fentanyl and sufentanil appeared superior to alfentanil during cardiac anesthesia, with more stable hemodynamics and less myocardial ischemia.[59] It appears that alfentanil may be less effective than sufentanil and fentanyl in suppressing reflex sympathetic and hemodynamic responses to stimuli.[60] The hemodynamic response to large doses of fentanyl and sufentanil are minimally different. Sufentanil produced slightly greater reduction in HR and SVR than fentanyl, and possesses an improved context-sensitive half-time projecting an undocumented improvement in reliability of awakening, an advantage in cost-sensitive times.[61,62] Although profound overdoses of sufentanil and fentanyl produce minimal hemodynamic effects, they also fail to reliably prevent BP and hormonal responses to painful stimuli such as median sternotomy, indicating that the term "narcotic anesthesia" is really a misnomer.[63,64] Adjuvant anesthetics are necessary to provide complete anesthesia in patients undergoing cardiac surgery.

Nonopioid Intravenous Agents

BENZODIAZEPINES

Benzodiazepines produce similar minimal hemodynamic changes when used for induction of anesthesia in patients with coronary artery or valvular heart disease.[65–73] The summary of these hemodynamics is shown in Table 7–1. Diazepam and midazolam produce small decreases in cardiac contractility in isolated heart and intact canine models, with dose-related decreases in dP/dt_{max}.[74,75] In humans given midazolam, the reduction in left ventricular stroke work index (LVSWI) may reflect decreases in cardiac contractility or in pulmonary capillary wedge pressure (PCWP).[65,71] The minimal hemodynamic effects of midazolam are confirmed by the stability provided

TABLE 7–1
Hemodynamic Changes After Benzodiazepine Induction*

	Diazepam	Lorazepam	Midazolam
HR	−9 to + 13%	Unchanged	−14 to +21%
MBP	0 to −19%	−7 to −20%	−12 to −26%
SVR	−22 to +13%	−10 to −35%	0 to −20%
PAP	0 to −10%		Unchanged
PVR	0 to −19%	Unchanged	Unchanged
LA/PAO	Unchanged		0 to −25%
RAP	Unchanged		Unchanged
CI	Unchanged	0 to +16%	0 to −25%
SV	0 to −8%		0 to −18%
LVSWI	0 to −36%		−28 to 42%
RVSWI	0 to −21%		−41 to 57%
dP/dt	Unchanged		0 to −12%

*From Reves JG, Berkowitz DE: Pharmacology of the intravenous induction drugs. In Kaplan JA (ed): Cardiac Anesthesia, 3rd ed. Philadelphia, WB Saunders Co, 1993, p 512, with permission.

HR, heart rate; MBP, mean blood pressure; SVR, systemic vascular resistance; PAP, mean pulmonary artery pressure; PVR, pulmonary vascular resistance; LA/PAO, left atrial pressure/pulmonary artery occluded pressure; RAP, right atrial pressure; CI, cardiac index; SV, stroke volume; LVSWI, left ventricular stroke work index; RVSWI, right ventricular stroke work index; dP/dt, ventricular pressure rise.

even with a 40-fold increase in dose in the intact animal model.[75]

The major hemodynamic consequence of benzodiazepines, particularly midazolam or diazepam, is the decrease in MAP and CO that can occur with the combination of these drugs with potent opioids.[76,77] The exact mechanism of this interaction is unknown but may be associated with the ability of diazepam or midazolam to ablate normal sympathetic tone.[77,78] Regardless of the mechanism, the change in MAP is easily compensated with phenylephrine in small boluses, indicating the role that venous pooling and SVR may play in this decrease in BP.

BARBITURATES

Thiopental and methohexital both produce greater depression of cardiac contractility than described for the benzodiazepines,[78–80] and early claims of less myocardial depression with methohexital have not been supported.[81] Reduction in contractility associated with the barbiturates is believed due to decreased availability of calcium to myofibrils.[82] Although thiopental's propensity for myocardial depression is well documented, this primarily occurs with larger doses given rapidly. Smaller doses of thiopental given slowly or by infusion seem to be well tolerated even in patients with coronary artery disease.[83] The minimal changes in hemodynamics usually produced by thiopental induction indicate the compensatory increase in HR and other sympathetic nervous system–mediated mechanisms to maintain hemodynamic stability (Table 7–2). The marked reductions in CO (69%) and MAP with thiopental in hypovolemic patients indicate the need for extra care in hypovolemic patients or patients with minimal cardiovascular reserve.[84]

ETOMIDATE

Etomidate, a carboxylated imidazole derivative, produces a small dose-dependent direct negative inotropic effect in dogs, that at equianesthetic doses was half as pronounced as that produced by thiopental.[85] Riou et al., studying the effects of etomidate on intrinsic myocardial contractility using isolated left ventricular papillary muscle, demonstrated that etomidate induced a slightly positive inotropic effect as manifested by increased maximum shortening velocity.[86] It appears, however, that propylene glycol, the solvent in which etomidate is available, may result in sarcoplasmic reticulum (SR) dysfunction, with a slight negative inotropic effect in some clinical conditions.

Despite the controversy over its action in the isolated heart, etomidate (0.3 mg/kg) produced no significant hemodynamic changes even in patients with acute myocardial infarction.[87] In addition to its stable profile when used alone, the simultaneous use of other agents such as N_2O often results in the maintenance of stable hemodynamics compared to other anesthetic agents.[88] The hemodynamics of induction doses of etomidate propofol and ketamine are listed in Table 7–3.[89] Emergency situations requiring rapid induction and control of the airway in patients with decreased cardiac reserve has become the primary indication for the use of etomidate.

TABLE 7–2
Hemodynamic Changes After Barbiturate Induction*

	Thiopental	Methohexital
HR	0 to +36%	+40 to +50%
MBP	−18 to +8%	0 to −10%
SVR	0 to +19%	NR
PAP	Unchanged	NR
PVR	Unchanged	NR
LA/PAO	Unchanged	NR
RAP	0 to +33%	0 to +5%
CI	0 to −24%	0 to −12%
SV	−12 to −35%	NR
LVSWI	0 to −26%	NR
RVSWI	NR	NR
dP/dt	−14%	NR

*From Reves JG, Berkowitz DE: Pharmacology of the intravenous induction drugs. In Kaplan JA (ed): Cardiac Anesthesia, 3rd ed. Philadelphia, WB Saunders Co, 1993, p 512, with permission.

HR, heart rate; MBP, mean blood pressure; SVR, systemic vascular resistance; PAP, mean pulmonary artery pressure; PVR, pulmonary vascular resistance; LA/PAO, left atrial pressure/pulmonary artery occluded pressure; RAP, right atrial pressure; CI, cardiac index; SV, stroke volume; LVSWI, left ventricular stroke work index; RVSWI, right ventricular stroke work index; dP/dt, ventricular pressure rise; NR, not reported.

KETAMINE

Ketamine produces markedly different effects on contractility in the isolated heart preparation than in the intact animal. Ketamine produces direct myocardial depression in isolated rabbit heart and isolated dog heart preparations.[90–92] In the intact animal or human, ketamine stimulates the CNS and blocks the reuptake of norepinephrine resulting in sympathetic nervous system (SNS) output producing increases in HR, cardiac index (CI), SVR, BP, and pulmonary artery pressure (PAP).[93,94] The hemodynamic changes produced in normal patients appear similar to changes produced in patients with VHD or CAD.[95] This interaction is well illustrated by

TABLE 7–3
Hemodynamic Changes After Induction with Nonbarbiturate Hypnotics*

	Etomidate	Propofol	Ketamine
HR	0 to +22%	−6 to +12%	0 to +59%
MBP	0 to −20%	0 to −47%	0 to +40%
SVR	0 to −17%	−9 to −25%	0 to +33%
PAP	0 to −17%	−4 to +8%	+44 to +47%
PVR	0 to +27%		0 to +33%
LVEDP/PAO	0 to −11%	+13%	Unchanged
RAP	Unchanged	−8 to −21%	+15 to +33%
CI	0 to +14%	−6 to −26%	0 to +42%
SV	0 to −15%	−8 to −18%	0 to −21%
LVSWI	0 to −27%	−15 to −40%	0 to 27%
dP/dt	0 to −18%		Unchanged
STI	Unchanged		NR

*From Reves JG, Berkowitz DE: Pharmacology of the intravenous induction drugs. In Kaplan JA (ed): Cardiac Anesthesia, 3rd ed. Philadelphia, WB Saunders Co, 1993, p 512, with permission.

HR, heart rate; MBP, mean blood pressure; SVR, systemic vascular resistance; PAP, mean pulmonary artery pressure; PVR, pulmonary vascular resistance; LVEDP/PAO, left ventricular end-diastolic pressure/pulmonary artery occluded pressure; RAP, right atrial pressure; CI, cardiac index; SV, stroke volume; LVSWI, left ventricular stroke work index; dP/dt, ventricular pressure rise; STI, systolic time interval; NR, unreported.

the difference in response to ketamine in the denervated heart (heart transplant recipient) versus other patients with intact cardiac innervation illustrated in Figure 7–7.[96] The combination of other anesthetic agents, such as the benzodiazepines, with ketamine reduces the hemodynamic changes seen on induction.[97,98] The use of these adjuvant agents appears to block the increase in catecholamines produced by ketamine; however, the role that ketamine's cocaine-like neuronal inhibition of reuptake of norepinephrine may have during cardiopulmonary bypass (CPB) or other high-stress procedures has not been evaluated.[99–108]

PROPOFOL

Propofol, an alkylphenol derivative, has been shown to produce direct dose-dependent myocardial depression in multiple animal models.[109–111] Coetzee et al. measured regional myocardial contractility in an open-chested pig model using piezoelectric crystals to measure segmental length shortening and demonstrated a significant correlation between propofol plasma concentration and decrease in myocardial contractility.[109] Similar work in dogs showed a significant reduction in LV force generated by force probes in the myocardium with increasing propofol doses.[111] In a clinical study evaluating the effects of propofol on cardiac contractility in humans utilizing transesophageal echocardiography and systolic blood pressure to construct the end-systolic pressure-volume relationship (ESPVR) as an index of global ventricular contractility induction doses or 1.5 mg/kg, or 2.5 mg/kg, produced significant depression of myocardial contractility.[112] Despite its negative inotropic effects, propofol has been used successfully in patients with CAD, but the additive or synergistic effect in producing decreases in MAP when combined with potent opioids must be remembered in its use.[113] Low-dose continuous-infusion propofol is used to allow rapid controlled awakening, earlier extubation, and decreased intensive care unit (ICU) stay in "fast-track" coronary artery bypass graft (CABG) programs targeted at reducing hospital stay and cost.[113]

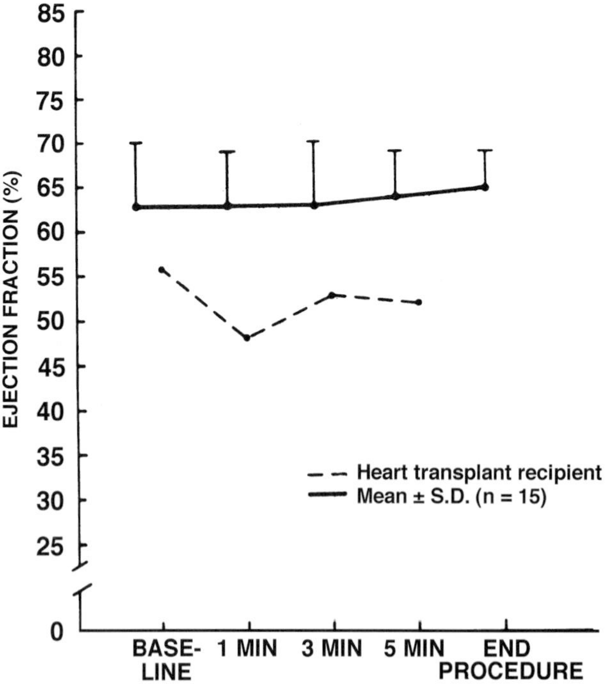

FIGURE **7–7.** Effect of cardiac autonomic system denervation on response to ketamine (2 mg/kg). Patient with transplanted (denervated) heart had a 10% reduction in ejection fraction after ketamine induction, whereas patients with normally innervated heart had no effect. (From Reves JG, Gelman S: Cardiac effects of the intravenous anesthetic drugs. In Effects of Anesthesia. Bethesda, MD, American Physiological Society, 1985, p 179, with permission.)

The Coronary Circulation

Coronary blood flow is dependent on many global and local factors. Maintenance of necessary available oxygen (O_2) is accomplished in the myocardial circulation by increasing coronary blood flow, because the heart at baseline extracts the majority of available oxygen in the delivered blood. Although systemic hemodynamics including aortic diastolic pressure, left ventricular end-diastolic pressure, and heart rate do affect coronary blood flow, predominant control is via alteration in coronary vascular resistance. In normal coronaries the coronary blood flow and oxygen delivery generally vary with changes in myocardial oxygen demand.

Inhalational anesthetics, but not intravenous anesthetics, have been found to significantly alter coronary vascular resistance and thus increase overall coronary blood flow (Fig. 7–8).[114] In patients with normal coronaries this is not a problem, but in patients with significant coronary artery disease and particularly with anatomy dependent on collateral circulation, inappropriate coronary vasodilation may be associated with a coexistence of luxury perfusion and potential for coronary steal.[115]

Isoflurane's effect on the coronary circulation has been extensively studied. Controversy exists because isoflurane is a more potent coronary dilator than the other older inhalational anesthetics, although desflurane and sevoflurane may be similar, with some studies indicating that isoflurane produced myocardial ischemia in patients with ischemic heart disease.[116] Many of these initial reports were complicated by methodologic problems including significant reductions in MAP or tachycardia with the institution of isoflurane producing conditions where ischemia was possible (i.e., increased demand and decreased perfusion pressure in pressure-dependent coronary collaterals). Newer studies with strict hemodynamic controls have confirmed that the coronary vasodilation of isoflurane is dose dependent and that concentrations of 1.0 minimal alveolar concentration (MAC) or greater are necessary to produce significant coronary vasodilation under clinical conditions.[117] The vast majority of outcome studies have not shown any significant correlation between isoflurane, or any anesthetic, and outcome after cardiac surgery.[118–123] This indicates that with adjuvant anesthetic agents allowing reduction of isoflurane dosage, little coronary vasodilation occurs and, therefore, coronary steal is unlikely to produce myocardial ischemia and significantly affect myo-

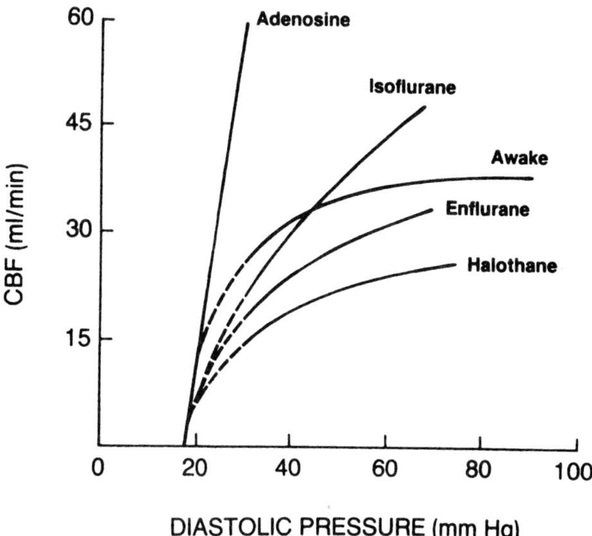

FIGURE **7–8.** Schematic presentation of pressure–coronary blood flow (CBF) relationships during awake state, during various inhalational anesthetics, and during adenosine-induced maximum coronary vasodilatation (which did not differ between awake and anesthetized animals). *Dashed lines* represent the nonlinear portions of the curves and are estimates. From this diagram it would appear that isoflurane anesthesia shifts the "autoregulated" flow curve upward, and that coronary vascular reserve becomes progressively less with increasing diastolic pressures when compared to awake, halothane-anesthetized and enflurane-anesthetized states. (From Hickey RF, Sybert PE, Verrier ED, Cason BA: Effect of halothane, enflurane and isoflurane on coronary blood flow autoregulation and coronary vascular reserve in the canine heart. Anesthesiology 68:21, 1988, with permission.)

cardial outcome after cardiac or noncardiac vascular surgery.

Desflurane appears to produce similar coronary hemodynamic changes to those of isoflurane in animal studies.[124–126] Studies have not been performed on coronary blood flow in humans, but clinical studies comparing ischemia on induction in CABG patients anesthetized with thiopental and vecuronium followed by either desflurane or sufentanil reported significantly greater ischemia associated with abnormal hemodynamics in the desflurane group.[41] This is not an indication of coronary steal with desflurane, but may indicate that desflurane is not an optimal agent at higher concentrations in patients with coronary artery disease.

Effects of the Anesthetics on the CNS

Despite significant advances in CPB technology, surgical techniques, and anesthetic management, CNS complications occur in a high percentage of patients undergoing surgery requiring CPB. Although the relative percentage of death due to cardiac causes has decreased, deaths due to neurologic deficits have increased from 7.2% to 19.6%.[127] Recent outcome studies have shown that stroke rate reached a low of 0.6% in 1979 and had increased fourfold by 1983 presumably secondary to the higher risk elderly population now undergoing cardiac surgery.[128] In addition to frank stroke, approximately 27 to 60% of patients develop neuropsychologic dysfunction after CPB.[129,130] This relative risk of CNS dysfunction after cardiac or major vascular surgery confirms the significance of CNS dysfunction on overall morbidity and mortality of cardiovascular surgery. This section will discuss effects of anesthetics on the CNS.

The CNS is a complex neural network processing immense sensory input, maintaining subcortical automatic responses and coordinating complex motor output. Anatomic divisions of the brain reflect distribution of brain functions. The cerebral cortex is the largest division of the brain, where sensory, motor, and other information is processed and controlled. The cerebral cortex sends and receives input through the thalamocortical system. Other than olfactory input, all sensory signals pass through the thalamocortical system, which also controls the activity level at the cerebral cortex.

The automatic activities of the body are controlled or mediated in the brain stem. Regulation of blood pressure, breathing, as well as input to the cerebral cortex occur here. The brain stem includes the medulla, pons, thalamus, reticular activating system (RAS), limbic system, basal ganglia, and cerebellum. The RAS plays a significant role in the electrical activity of the cerebral cortex. Neurons of this system are both inhibitory and excitatory. The RAS controls much cortical activity, including sleep and wakefulness, and is critical in coordinating the specific activity of the cerebral cortex. Although the mechanism is controversial, it is believed that many clinical inhaled or injected anesthetics exert depressant effects on the RAS as part of their mechanisms of inducing unconsciousness.

Anesthetic agents produce profound CNS depression resulting in loss of consciousness and, it is hoped, accompanied by lack of awareness or recall. The mechanism is complex and controversial. This section will concentrate on the effects of anesthetic agents on cerebral metabolic activity, cerebral blood flow, electrical activity, intracranial pressure (ICP), and the known receptors mediating the action of these agents.

CNS Electrophysiology

The electroencephalogram (EEG) is a recording of brain waves resulting from CNS spontaneous activity. The character of the wave (amplitude and frequency) is primarily dependent on the level of cortical activity and degree of wakefulness. There is a complex relationship between degree of wakefulness and EEG frequencies. Brain waves are classified as alpha, beta, theta, and delta depending on frequency and amplitude (Table 7–4).[233] Anesthetic agents have characteristic effects on EEG activity depending on dose or concentration (Table 7–5).

Inhaled Anesthetics

Low concentrations of inhaled anesthetics (<0.2 MAC) produce increases in EEG frequency (excitement).[131] As concentrations increase, this excitement or high-frequency activity disappears, but at this point individual

TABLE 7–4
Characteristics of Fundamental EEG Rhythms*

Rhythm	Frequency	Predominant Amplitude	Predominant Location	Associated Physiologic State
Alpha	8–13 Hz	Medium	Occiput	Relaxed, awake
Beta	13–30 Hz	Low	Frontal	Alert, awake
Theta	4–8 Hz	High	Diffuse	Sleeping infant, child
Delta	0–4 Hz	High	Diffuse	Metabolic coma, cerebral ischemia, normal deep sleep, deep anesthesia

*From Wickey GS, Hickey PR: In Hensley FA, Martin DE (eds): The Practice of Cardiac Anesthesia. Boston, Little, Brown & Co, 1990, with permission.
EEG, electroencephalograph.

agents diverge in their actions. Isoflurane suppresses high-frequency activity, eventually progressing to burst suppression and isoelectricity at concentrations greater than 2.0 MAC.[132] Halothane also produces suppression of high-frequency activity with increasing concentrations, although burst suppression or isoelectric EEG are not achieved unless concentrations greater than 4 MAC are utilized.[133] Enflurane produces similar effects at lower concentrations, but is known to produce seizure activity at high doses when combined with moderate hyperventilation.[127,134,135] High-dose inhalational anesthetics make interpretation or evaluation of EEG ischemia difficult due to profound effects on frequency and amplitude.

TABLE 7–5
EEG Changes Associated with Drugs and Altered Psychology*

Increased frequency
Hyperoxia
Hypercarbia: mild
Hypoxia: initial
Seizure
Barbiturates: small dose
Diazepam: ambulatory dose
N_2O: 30–70%
Inhalation agents: <1 MAC
Ketamine
Decreased frequency, increased amplitude
Hypoxia: mild
Hypocarbia: moderate to extreme
Hypothermia
Barbiturates: moderate dose
Etomidate
Narcotics
Inhalation agents: >1 MAC
Decreased frequency, decreased amplitude
Hypoxia: marked
Hypocarbia: severe
Barbiturates: large dose
Electrical silence
Brain death
Hypoxia: severe
Hypothermia: profound
Barbiturates: coma dose
Isoflurane: 2 MAC

*From Donegan JH: In Blitt CD (ed): Monitoring in Anesthesia and Critical Care Medicine. New York, Churchill Livingstone 1985, with permission.
EEG, electroencephalograph; N_2O, nitrous oxide; MAC, minimal alveolar concentration.

Opioids

Opioids also produce characteristic EEG changes at high doses. Potent narcotics such as sufentanil and fentanyl decrease high-frequency activity and increase low-frequency relative delta power.[136,137] The activity of alfentanil appears similar to that with fentanyl and sufentanil.[138]

Nonopioid Intravenous Agents

BENZODIAZEPINES

At low doses, benzodiazepines produce activation of EEG with increased high-frequency activity.[139] Unlike barbiturates, increasing dosages of benzodiazepines do not produce the same marked slowing of the EEG.[140] In addition to its ceiling effect in depressing EEG activity, midazolam decreases cerebral oxygen utilization and cerebral blood flow in a dose-related fashion, with peaks at a dose of 10 mg/kg with no additional EEG, cerebral metabolic rate of oxygen ($CMRO_2$), or cerebral blood flow (CBF) changes produced with higher doses.[141]

BARBITURATES

Small intravenous doses of barbiturates increase low-voltage, fast-wave activity similar to the excitement or activation described for inhaled anesthetics.[127,142] As the dosage of barbiturates is increased, this activation is replaced by high-voltage, slow-wave activity (low-frequency, high-amplitude activity) accompanied by unconsciousness. Continued escalation of the dose produces burst suppression and eventually electrical silence. The reduction in cerebral metabolic rate associated with this marked reduction in EEG is about 50%, reflecting decreased neuronal but not metabolic needs for oxygen.

ETOMIDATE AND PROPOFOL

Etomidate and propofol produce similar EEG effects to those described for the barbiturates, also producing decreases in CBF and $CMRO_2$.[143–145] Etomidate, like methohexital, may activate seizure foci, with fast activity on the EEG.[146] Caution is recommended with etomidate in patients with focal epilepsy. Etomidate has also been shown to augment somatosensory evoked potentials.[147]

KETAMINE

Ketamine EEG effects are characterized by decreasing high-frequency alpha and predominance of theta activity.[148] Ketamine produces excitatory activity in the thalamus and limbic system that does not spread to cortical regions.[149] Ketamine does not appear to alter seizure threshold in epileptic patients.[150]

Cerebral Physiology and Intracranial Pressure

Changes in neuronal activity or electrophysiology are accompanied by changes in cerebral metabolic rate (CMR). CBF is typically coupled to CMR both globally and regionally. Studies have demonstrated that localized brain activities produce localized increases in CMR (rCMR) that are associated with changes in CBF (rCBF).[151,152] The exact mechanisms by which these localized changes occur is a matter of debate.[153] CMR and the coupling of CMR to CBF are affected by many factors including temperature and anesthetic agents, which will be discussed in the following sections.

Inhalational Anesthetics

Inhalational anesthetics produce reductions in CMR similar to other anesthetic agents, but their confounding effect is their cerebral vasodilating characteristics. With cerebral vasodilation CBF increases and, secondarily, increases in cerebral blood volume (CBV) and ICP may occur. The combination of CMR reduction and vasodilation is in marked contrast to the intravenous anesthetic agents, which produce parallel changes in CMR and CBF. All the volatile anesthetics produce dose-related reductions in CMR while causing variable increases in CBF.[154-157] It is appropriate to conclude that the CBF-CMR ratio is altered by inhalational anesthetics but not completely uncoupled. Studies on the cerebral physiologic effects of isoflurane during CPB show reduction of CMR and CBF.

Inhalational anesthetics produce different CBF responses at different doses. Comparison of the agents reveals that when MAP is maintained at 80 mm Hg, equipotent 1.1 MAC levels of halothane, enflurane, and isoflurane cause CBF increases of 191, 37, and 18%, respectively (Fig. 7–9).[158] The CMR response of the inhalational agents is nonlinear, with the majority of reductions occurring precipitously with induction of anesthesia (Fig. 7–10).[159] The reduction in CMR is greater with isoflurane and enflurane than halothane at similar MAC concentrations.[160] Of the three commonly used inhalational anesthetics, only isoflurane produces EEG electrical silence at clinically applicable concentrations (<2.0 MAC).[161]

In summary, the inhalational agents' effect on CMR is nonlinear reduction that is greatest with isoflurane and enflurane. Cerebral vasodilation also occurs with these agents, but can reliably be overcome with induction of hypocapnia.[162] Regardless of the protection afforded by hypocapnia, care should be taken with inhalational anesthetics in patients with impaired intracranial compliance.

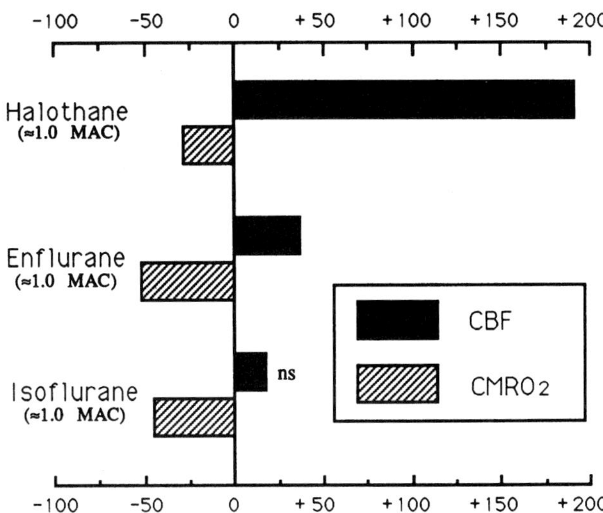

FIGURE 7–9. Percent changes in cerebral blood flow (CBF) and $CMRO_2$ caused by volatile anesthetics. The CBF data were obtained during 1.1 MAC anesthesia (with blood pressure support) in humans and are expressed as percent change from awake control values. The $CMRO_2$ data were obtained in animals, and are expressed as percent change from N_2O-sedated control values. (From Drummond JC, Shapiro HM: In Miller RD [ed]: Anesthesia, 3rd ed. New York, Churchill Livingstone, 1990, p 635, with permission.)

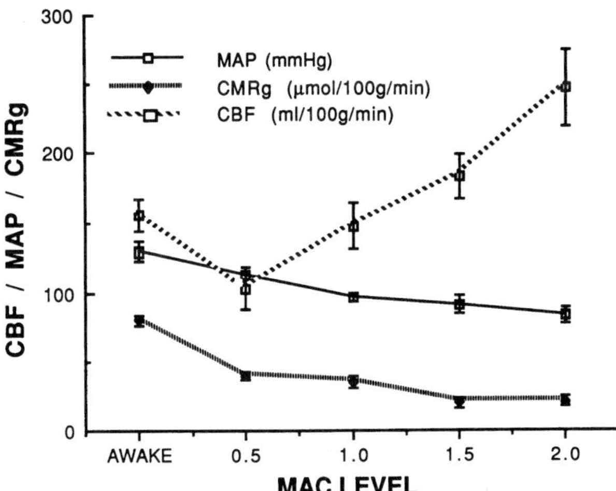

FIGURE 7–10. Relationship between changes in 1-CMRg and 1-CBF in the motor-sensory cortex in rats during isoflurane anesthesia. The majority of the CMR suppression caused by isoflurane has occurred by 1.0 MAC and in this concentration range CBF is not increased. Thereafter, additional isoflurane causes little further CMR reduction and cerebral vasodilatation occurs. These data suggest the importance of metabolic coupling determining the CBF effects of isoflurane. (From Drummond JC, Shapiro HM: Cerebral physiology. In Miller RD [ed]: Anesthesia, 3rd ed. New York, Churchill Livingstone, 1990, p 636, with permission. Data originally from Maekawa T, Tommasino C, Shapiro HM, et al: Local cerebral blood flow and glucose utilization during isoflurane anesthesia in a rat. Anesthesiology 65: 144, 1986, with permission.)

Opioids

Data on the CMR and CBF effects of the opioids are inconsistent and vary from agent to agent. Most data indicate that moderate doses of opioids produce mild reductions in CMR and CBF. Many of the inconsistencies in available data may relate to the confounding effects of nitrous oxide or other adjuvant anesthetics, which also produce significant changes in CMR and CBF. The following sections will describe the effects of each of the commonly used narcotics.

Human data on the effect of morphine on CBF and CMR are extremely varied. An early study by Moyer et al. showed that 1 mg/kg of morphine as sole anesthetic produced a 41% reduction in CMR without affecting CBF.[163] This finding would indicate uncoupling of CBF and CMR, inconsistent with other data, and may point to uncontrolled effects of morphine on P_{CO_2} in the experiment. In further human studies Jobes et al. evaluated 1 to 3 mg/kg of morphine and 70% nitrous oxide, observing no significant changes in either CMR or CBF.[164] Balancing for the expected minimal increases in CBF and CMR from nitrous oxide, it appears that if any significant change in cerebral physiology is produced by morphine it is a small reduction in CBF and CMR, which is shown in the accompanying figure from Drummond and Shapiro (Fig. 7–11). As a result, if ventilation is maintained, little or no change in ICP would be expected when morphine is used in patients with decreased intracranial compliance.

From the sparse human data available, it appears that fentanyl also produces a modest reduction in CMR and CBF when given to awake humans.[165] In previously sedated patients the data are less consistent. Murkin et al. reported 25% reductions in CBF in patients anesthetized with high-dose fentanyl (100 μg/kg) and diazepam (0.4 mg/kg).[166] This reduction is consistent with use of diazepam alone and it is difficult to detect the effects of fentanyl. Other studies with moderate doses of fentanyl in sedated animals and humans have found minimal effects on cerebral physiology.[167] Although the data are somewhat inconclusive, the majority points to modest reduction in CMR and CBF when fentanyl is given to awake or mildly sedated patients, with less response seen in those patients or animals given previous heavy sedation.

Sufentanil (10 μg/kg) produced a 25% reduction in CBF and a 21% reduction in $CMRO_2$ when used for induction of anesthesia in minimally sedated patients undergoing cardiac surgery.[168] Based on these data and additional animal and human studies of sufentanil and cerebral hemodynamics, no change or a minimal reduction in ICP would be expected when sufentanil was in increased intracranial compliance.[161,169] This expectation was not supported by data from Marx et al., who reported a significant increase in lumbar cerebrospinal fluid pressure (L-CSFP) after sufentanil and alfentanil, with fentanyl producing no significant changes.[170] In a dog venous outflow model, Milde and Milde also reported increases in CBF and ICP following sufentanil administration.[171,172] The changes were transient, possibly explaining differences with previously described studies. Additional data are necessary to determine if this potential transient vasodilation by sufentanil holds any significance in clinical practice. Several human clinical studies evaluating surgical conditions during craniotomies performed with sufentanil have found no adverse effects.[173,174]

Few data are available on the effects of alfentanil on CMR and CBF in humans. Alfentanil produced similar increases in L-CSFP to those of sufentanil with greater reductions in cerebral perfusion pressure secondary to greater decreases in MAP.[166]

Nonopioid Intravenous Agents

BENZODIAZEPINES

Benzodiazepines produce similar reductions in CMR and CBF in both animals and humans. Many studies evaluating diazepam, lorazepam, and midazolam have shown moderate decreases in CMR and CBF indicating that the

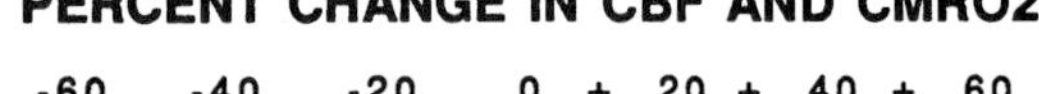

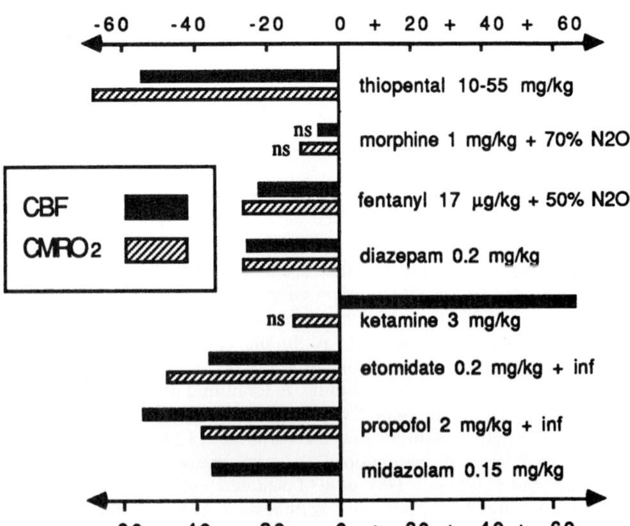

FIGURE 7–11. Changes in CBF and $CMRO_2$ caused by intravenous anesthetics. The data are derived from multiple human investigations and are presented as percent change from control values. No data on CNS effects of midazolam are available. (From Drummond JC, Shapiro HM: Cerebral physiology. In Miller RD [ed]: Anesthesia, 3rd ed. New York, Churchill Livingstone, 1990, p 631, with permission.)

CBF effect seems metabolically coupled.[175–178] The reduction of CMR and CBF appears greater and more consistent than that produced by the opioids, but less than the substantial reduction produced by the barbiturates. ICP is likely reduced in patients with decreased intracranial compliance when benzodiazepines are administered unless respiratory depression and accompanying increases in Pa_{CO_2} occur.

BARBITURATES

Barbiturates produce dose-dependent reductions in CBF and CMR. Induction doses of barbiturates produce 30% reductions in both CMR and CBF.[179,180] Burst suppression doses of thiopental reduce CMR and CBF by approximately 50%, further increases in dose having less effect.[181,182] Tolerance to cerebral physiologic responses produced by barbiturates develop quickly. Blood levels required to maintain isoelectric silence on EEG increase after 24 hours and continue to increase thereafter.[183] Despite increasing doses at similar EEG suppression levels, CBF and $CMRO_2$ increased over a period of 24 hours in dogs.[184]

Thiopental has been reported as a protective agent in patients undergoing valvular heart surgery, reducing the incidence of significant persistent CNS events.[185] Subsequent studies by Zaidan et al. in patients undergoing CABG showed no trend toward improvement in CNS outcome.[186] Studies evaluating the effects of thiopental on cerebral physiology during rewarming from hypothermic CPB indicate a propensity for greater reductions in CBF than $CMRO_2$ resulting in increasing cerebral arterial-venous oxygen content difference $[C(a-\bar{v})O_2]$.[143] This does not indicate that thiopental does not provide cerebral protection, but does indicate that if protective, it is by a mechanism other than improvement in global cerebral oxygen supply and demand.

ETOMIDATE

Etomidate appears to produce similar reductions in CMR and CBF to barbiturates.[187,188] The reductions of CMR and CBF are profound, with the ceiling effect at isoelectricity seen with barbiturates also present with etomidate in animals.[189] The absolute reduction of CMR with etomidate compared with thiopental and isoflurane is less profound. This may be explained by the observations of Davis et al. showing that CMR suppression with etomidate is regionally variable, occurring predominantly in forebrain structures.[190] Etomidate's primary advantage compared to barbiturates for reduction in ICP is improved maintenance of cerebral perfusion pressure (CPP) in head-injured patients due to minimal effects on cardiac contractility and hemodynamics.[191] Concerns of adrenocortical suppression with long-term infusions have limited its use.

KETAMINE

Ketamine is unique in its cerebral physiologic effects among the intravenous anesthetics. Studies evaluating effects of ketamine on CMR are variable, but most data indicate that ketamine causes mild to moderate increases in CMR.[192] Ketamine produces substantial increases in CBF that have been correlated with accompanying increases in ICP.[192,193] Conflicting data in humans showing large increases in CBF with little change in CMR indicate much of the increased CBF with ketamine relates to direct cerebral vasodilation rather than metabolic activation.[194] Ketamine produces increased CBF through both direct vasodilation and indirect metabolic activation mechanisms. Regardless of the etiology, ketamine can potentially increase CBF and secondarily ICP in patients with decreased intracranial compliance. Ketamine has been evaluated as a potential cerebral protection agent secondary to its noncompetitive inhibition at the *N*-methyl-D-aspartate (NMDA) receptor.[195] It psychomimetic side effects and concerns over CBF and ICP changes have limited its consideration.

PROPOFOL

Studies on the cerebral physiologic effects of propofol have indicated substantial reductions in both CBF and CMR.[196,197] Stephan et al. showed that after bolus administration and continuous infusion of propofol, CBF and CMR decreased by 51 and 36%, respectively.[197] This would be expected to produce reduction in ICP in patients with reduced intracranial compliance. Ravussin et al. reported a 32% reduction in L-CSFP with a slow bolus of propofol (1.5 mg/kg).[198] Studies of cerebral physiologic effects of burst suppression doses of propofol during CPB have found significant reductions in CMR and CBF even at moderate degrees of hypothermia (28° to 30°C).[199]

Effects of Anesthetics on the Pulmonary System

Surgery on the thorax, lungs, heart, and great vessels impose unique challenges to the practitioners of cardiac, vascular, and thoracic anesthesiology. Conventional mechanical ventilation, one-lung ventilation, cardiopulmonary bypass, muscle relaxants, and all anesthetic agents alter normal lung physiology. A comprehensive survey of pulmonary physiology and the perturbations during one-lung ventilation and cardiopulmonary bypass are beyond the scope of this chapter.

Basic Pulmonary Physiology

The lungs, of course, provide oxygen for cellular respiration and dispose of carbon dioxide. During each minute of normal tidal breathing, 2 to 3 ml/kg/min of oxygen are exchanged. This amount may be increased to 60 ml/kg/min during periods of heavy exercise. The human lung can move upwards of 4½ L of gas per minute, while it transfers gases to and from the blood. This transfer is achieved through the 50 to 150 m^2 of surface area divided among the 300 million alveoli. Through progressive division into sequentially smaller and thinner walled units, the final barrier of diffusion in the human alveoli is 0.2 μm. In clinical anesthetic practice, abnormalities in diffusion of gases at the alveoli are rarely responsible for abnormal blood gases.

Widening alveolar-arterial oxygen gradient and increases in arterial carbon dioxide are possible if common perturbations in lung physiology are left unattended during anesthesia. In awake erect humans one would expect the force opposing expansion of alveoli located at the lung base to be greater at end-expiration than for those at the top of the lung. At end-expiration alveolar units at the base are smaller than those at the top lung fields, and more compliant. With inspiration, basal alveoli expand more (i.e., assume a larger portion of total ventilation) than less distensible units at the top of the lung, producing a ventilation gradient from the lung base to the top. Perfusion of lung segments also occurs along segmental gradients. Since the heart pumps blood against a hydrostatic gradient, determined by height of the lung and weight of blood, segments at the uppermost portion of the lung (ribs two and three) receive less blood flow than those near the base (i.e., perfusion is greatest at the base). The relative effects of each of these semi-independent variables result in the fact that ventilation to perfusion ($\dot{V}/\dot{Q}$) is greatest at the lung apex and lowest at the base. In the normal erect individual, $\dot{V}/\dot{Q}$ varies from 0.6 to 3.0 from base to apex, averaging approximately 1 for all lung segments. Conditions or medications that increase segmental $\dot{V}/\dot{Q}$ inhomogeneity will increase alveolar-arterial oxygen differences [$P(A-a)O_2$]. As we will discuss, many of the effects on oxygenation seen during general anesthesia result from abnormalities in global ventilation or perfusion, regional $\dot{V}/\dot{Q}$ abnormalities, or alterations in adaptive mechanisms that normally maintain regional ventilation to perfusion (hypoxic vasoconstriction).

All inhalational anesthetics cause derangements in oxygenation; if left unattended, these derangements will produce widening of the alveolar-arterial oxygen gradient. By proper control of ventilation and increased concentrations of inspired oxygen, the anesthesiologist can often ameliorate these abnormalities in oxygenation. Derangements in oxygenation seen during inhalational anesthetics are predominantly the result of four factors: (1) increased dead space; (2) increased intrapulmonary shunt; (3) worsened heterogeneity of ventilation to perfusion ($\dot{V}/\dot{Q}$ mismatching), and (4) reduced minute volume of ventilation.[200]

Physiologic Dead Space

Dead space (V_{DS}) is the volume of inspired gas during each breath which is not in proximity with alveolar units; this portion of ventilation is wasted and not of use for alveolar gas exchange. The normal dead space for a conscious 70-kg subject is 150 ml (about 2 ml/kg) or approximately one third the total tidal volume (V_T). This ratio of dead space to tidal volume (V_{DS}/V_T) is useful to understanding impaired oxygenation during anesthesia. Normal V_{DS}/V_T in a young, conscious 70-kg individual is about 0.32. Anesthetizing and intubating a patient does not materially affect V_{DS} or V_{DS}/V_T. Since tracheal intubation bypasses upper airway dead space, maintenance of V_{DS} with changes during inhalational anesthesia with tracheal intubation implies that dead space below the carina has increased by 150 ml. Connecting the patient to a mechanical ventilator increases V_{DS}/V_T to approximately 0.50; most of this increase in V_{DS} is comprised of increased apparatus dead space of the ventilator and connection tubing. Anesthetizing and mechanically ventilating by mask increases V_{DS}/V_T to approximately 0.66. This is because overventilation of underperfused alveolar segments during anesthesia results in inhomogeneity of ventilation to perfusion.[197] Increased apparatus dead space also contributes to overall V_{DS}. Bronchodilatation contributes to increased physiologic dead space during inhalational or ketamine anesthesia.[201]

Intrapulmonary Shunt

In normal spontaneously breathing awake individuals, the typical intrapulmonary shunt is 1 to 2% of cardiac output. During anesthesia, intrapulmonary shunt increases to 10 to 15%,[202] but the etiology of this decrease remains controversial. This phenomenon may by explained by decreased lung volumes during anesthesia resulting in a segmental overperfusion to areas of relative underventilation.[203] Inhibition of hypoxic vasoconstriction by inhalational agents and increased closing volumes are other sources of increased intrapulmonary shunt during general anesthesia (see "Hypoxic Vasoconstriction," below).

$\dot{V}/\dot{Q}$ Mismatch

Anesthesia generally increases $\dot{V}/\dot{Q}$ mismatch by increasing intrapulmonary shunt.[204] This worsens $\dot{V}/\dot{Q}$ after induction, and correlates with decreasing functional residual capacity (FRC) and with loss of lung volume.[205,206] Elderly patients have greater derangements in oxygenation and this is, in part, the result of worsened $\dot{V}/\dot{Q}$ mismatching with advanced age[200,207,208] (Fig. 7–12). This increased $\dot{V}/\dot{Q}$ mismatching with general anesthesia is due to increases in areas of low $\dot{V}/\dot{Q}$ (intrapulmonary shunt), rather than increased dead space ventilation.[209] Application of positive end-expiratory pressure (PEEP) reduces intrapulmonary shunt, but may or may not improve oxygenation. Although PEEP does decrease shunt, it may also decrease cardiac output, which causes redistribution of blood flow toward dependent atelectatic regions.[199,201]

Although worsening of $\dot{V}/\dot{Q}$ mismatch is ubiquitous with all inhalational anesthetics, the magnitude of this derangement is somewhat agent specific. Even in healthy young individuals, intrapulmonary shunts on the order of 10% are common during halothane anesthesia. Nitrous oxide–halothane anesthesia increases intrapulmonary shunt to 13.9 ± 5.3%.[210] Thiopental-methoxyflurane anesthesia with muscle relaxant and mechanical ventilation did not appreciably increase shunt (0.9 ± 0.4%).[211] Intravenous thiopental, when used alone, also did not increase intrapulmonary shunt (1.1 ± 1.2%). Although anesthesia with ketamine alone did not produce atelectasis or shunt, paralysis of patients anesthe-

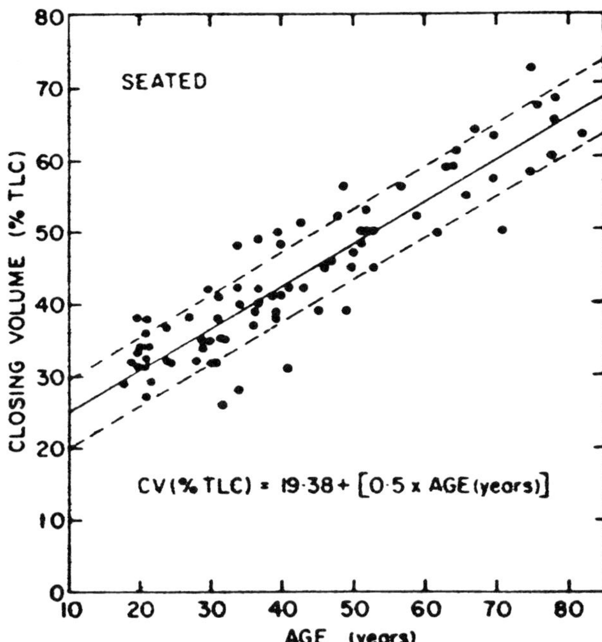

FIGURE 7–12. Individual values for "closing volume" (CV), expressed as percentage of TLC as a function of age. (From LeBlanc P, Ruff F, Milic-Emili J: Effects of age and body position on "airway closure" in man. J Appl Physiol 28:448, 1970, with permission.)

tized with ketamine increases intrapulmonary shunt substantially.[212]

Hypoxic Vasoconstriction

The reduction of PaO_2 during anesthesia is multifactorial. Derangements in oxygenation result from changes in lung mechanics as well as from perturbations in regional $\dot{V}/\dot{Q}$ relationships. Nunn et al. was the first to show that intrapulmonary shunt increases from 1% in normal awake controls to 10 to 14% in spontaneously breathing subjects with halothane anesthesia.[213] He and other workers showed that increasing shunt was caused by changes in regional perfusion of unventilated lung segments.[201,214] Inhalational anesthetics worsen $\dot{V}/\dot{Q}$ mismatching, atelectasis, and segmental dependent ventilation after changes in position, but these factors do not account for all changes in oxygenation that occur under inhalational anesthesia. Intravenous agents result in many perturbations in lung mechanics but do not produce the same degree of hypoxia as do the inhalational agents.[215]

Inhibition of hypoxic pulmonary vasoconstriction (HPV) may worsen hypoxia during inhalational anesthesia. During HPV, the blood supply to relatively underventilated lung segments is decreased relative to areas of greater ventilation.[216] Inhalation of hypoxic mixtures of inspired gas, in an intact whole-lung cat model, was shown to increase pulmonary artery resistance.[213] Regional delivery of hypoxic gas mixtures to specific lung segments, while maintaining delivery of 100% O_2 to the remainder of the lung, results in flow diversion from the hypoxic segments and increases pulmonary pressure in hypoxic segments.[217] HPV is clearly protective. During periods of subtotal hypoxia, arterial constriction of underperfused segments diverts flow to better perfused segments and returns $\dot{V}/\dot{Q}$ matching, and subsequently total oxygenation, toward normal.

Conditions that interfere with diversion of blood from underperfused segments (inhibition of HPV) worsen arterial oxygenation. Buckley et al. demonstrated that 0.5% halothane anesthesia inhibited HPV and worsened $\dot{V}/\dot{Q}$ matching without significantly affecting cardiac output.[218] Numerous studies have demonstrated that inhalational agents both in vitro and in vivo uniformly inhibit HPV.[219–221] The mechanism of inhibition of HPV is unknown. Inhibition of HPV has been shown to occur on the arterial side close to the alveoli.[212]

HPV is of most physiologic significance when intermediate portions of the lung (30 to 70%) are underventilated or hypoxic. When most of the lung is hypoxic, as in the case of delivery of hypoxic mixtures of inspired gas to all lung segments or in diffuse lung disease, perfusion cannot be shunted to normal segments. During such instances, pulmonary perfusion pressure will increase with little change in arterial oxygenation. When only small segments of the lung are underperfused, as in regional dependent atelectasis, HPV will also have little effect on total arterial oxygenation[212] (Fig. 7–13). Intravenous agents including fentanyl, ketamine, pentazocine, propofol, droperidol, diazepam, pentobarbital, and thiopental do not interfere with HPV.[222–224] To the cardiothoracic anesthesiologist, inhibition of HPV is of most clinical importance in patients with pre-existing lung disease in which HPV may be important in normalizing arterial oxygenation even at rest, awake and during one-lung ventilation, when perfusion to the unventilated lung may exacerbate hypoxemia.[225] Whether there are differences in degree of inhibition of HPV among the inhalational agents is controversial. Some studies have shown that isoflurane may not inhibit HPV,[226] but others have disagreed.[227] It is unclear if there is an advantage of isoflurane over halothane.[228] The consensus is that use of inhalational anesthesia is *not contraindicated* in most patients during one-lung ventilation or with pre-existing lung disease. Administration of high inspired fractions of oxygen will compensate for the theoretical risk of worsening $\dot{V}/\dot{Q}$ by blockade of HPV in most patients.[212,221,229]

Lung Volumes

Sixty to 90% of patients undergoing cardiac surgery requiring cardiopulmonary bypass have evidence of postoperative atelectasis on chest x-ray. Postoperative pulmonary tests in patients undergoing cardiac surgery are consistent with a restrictive pattern.[230,231] Vital capacity, FRC, and total lung volumes are decreased, while residual volume is unchanged or increased.[232,235] These abnormalities are greatest at 24 to 72 hours and may last up to 10 to 14 days.[223]

Normal FRC for a 40-year-old, 70-kg man is approximately 3,400 ml, decreasing to approximately 2,500 ml in the supine position. Additionally, induction of anesthesia decreases FRC about 450 ml with generally on the order of 20% of baseline lung volumes occurring

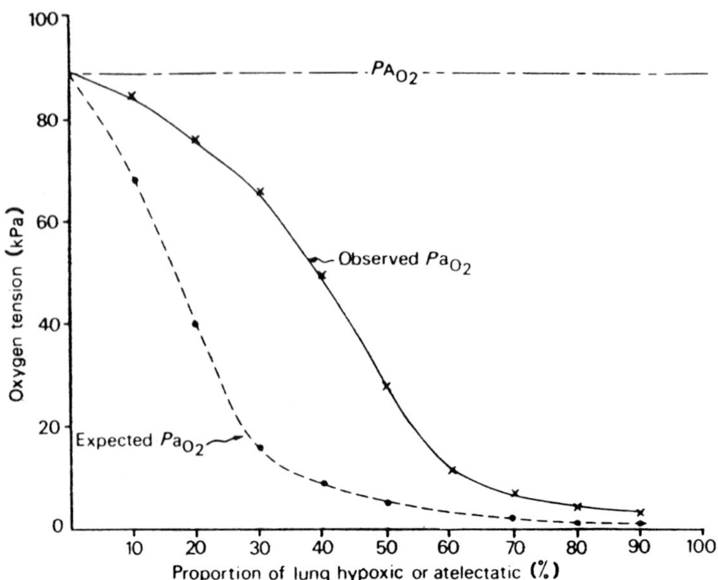

FIGURE **7–13.** Role of hypoxic pulmonary vasoconstriction (HPV) in preserving arterial oxygen tension. (From Eisenkraft JB: Effects of anaesthetics on the pulmonary circulation. Br J Anaesthesia 65:63, 1990. Copyright 1990, BMJ Publishing Group, with permission.)

with all anesthetic agents, inhalational or intravenous.[199] Decreases in FRC occur within minutes of onset of anesthesia and usually do not progress throughout anesthesia.

Decreases in lung volumes, specifically FRC, during general anesthesia relate to (1) relaxation of the diaphragm with cephalad movement, due to abdominal contents, which decreases total lung capacity (TLC) by about 500 ml in the adult; (2) relaxation of chest wall musculature, which decreases transverse thoracic volume by 250 ml; and (3) decreases in total lung compliance.

Although atelectasis of dependent lung areas may be demonstrated on chest computed tomography (CT) in anesthetized patients, this phenomenon is not simply related to resorption atelectasis because (1) the degree of atelectasis is independent of the carrier gas used with inhalational anesthetics (nitrous oxide, pure oxygen, or nitrous oxide/oxygen mixtures result in the same degree of atelectasis); (2) intraoperative administration of PEEP or hyperinflation of the lungs do not influence pulmonary shunt fraction; and (3) once anesthetized, changes in position do not influence pulmonary shunt fraction. The explanation for atelectasis that is unresponsive to conventional treatment during anesthesia may be anesthetic-induced inhibition of hypoxic vasoconstriction (see "Hypoxic Vasoconstriction," above). Because of this lack of inhibition of blood flow to existing atelectatic (underventilated) segments, $\dot{V}/\dot{Q}$ mismatching and intrapulmonary shunting are worsened during inhalational anesthesia.

Anesthetics not only diminish FRC but also worsen the relationship between FRC and closing volume. With inhalational anesthetics, small airway closure begins to occur at lung volumes that are greater than the FRC plus the tidal volume.[234] This implies that there is a great degree of air trapping with anesthetic agents, which contributes to worsening blood gases and $\dot{V}/\dot{Q}$ mismatching. This phenomenon is age related and occurs uniformly over the age of 45 (Fig. 7–14).

Compliance

General anesthesia may cause a general reduction in total lung compliance (the change in volume per unit change in pressure expressed as L/kPa or ml/cm H_2O).[235] During general anesthesia the entire lung chest wall system appears stiffer. Total lung compliance is not changed by muscle relaxants and is predominantly the result of decreased lung parenchymal compliance[226] (Fig. 7–15). Chest wall compliance is increased under anesthesia with or without paralysis.[226] Changes in compliance (as do changes in lung volumes) occur early after induction of anesthesia and do not usually progress. Inhalational anesthetics decrease pulmonary compliance by (1) inhibition or alteration in surfactant production,[236] or (2) as a consequence of decreases in lung volumes secondary to atelectasis and decreased FRC.[237] Decreased total

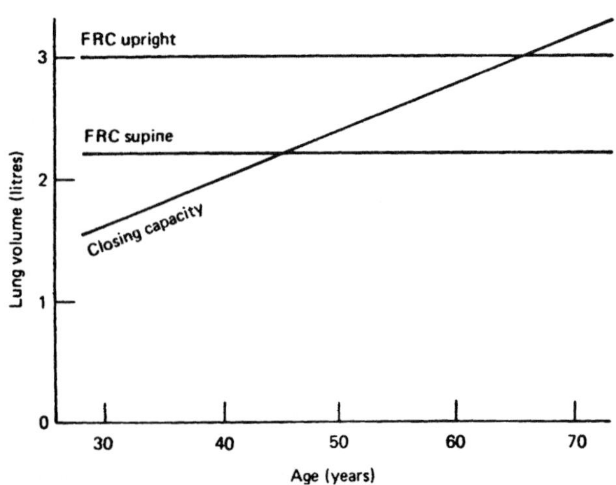

FIGURE **7–14.** Functional residual capacity (FRC) and closing capacity as a function of age. (From Nunn JF: Respiratory aspects of anaesthesia, In Nunn JF [ed]: Applied Respiratory Physiology, (3rd ed. London, Butterworth's, 1987, p 41, with permission.)

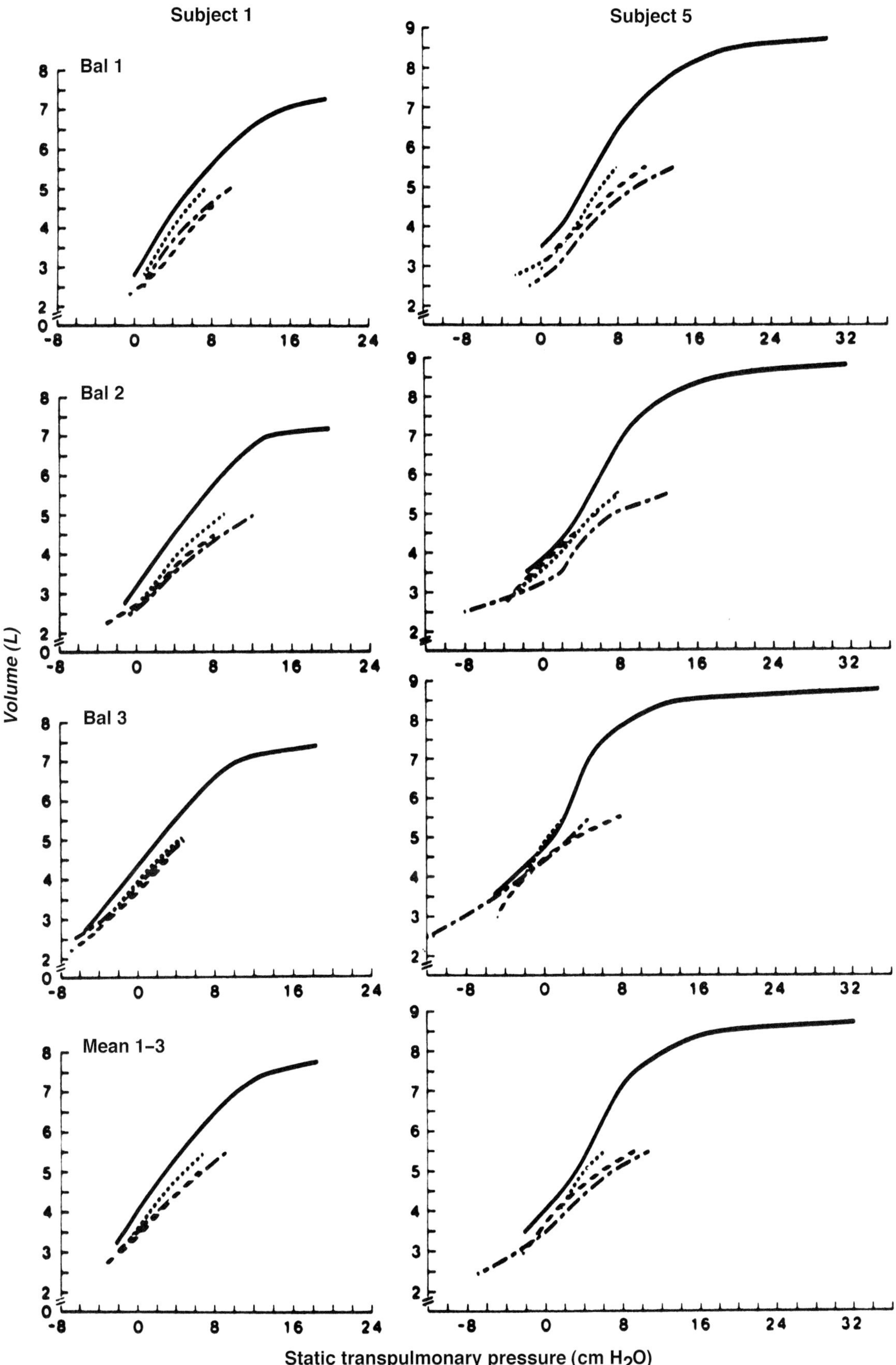

FIGURE 7–15. Static deflation pressure-volume curves of two representative subjects at three different sites in esophagus (Bal 1, 2, and 3 and Mean) during control rib cage restriction and abdominal restriction, illustrating effects of chest wall and pleura on overall lung compliance. (From Scheidt M, Hyatt RE, Rehder K: Effects of rib cage or abdominal restriction on lung mechanics. J Appl Physiol 51:1115, 1981, with permission.)

compliance is not a direct result of anesthetics on lung parenchyema.[199]

Chest wall rigidity after administration of narcotics may be associated with decreased total thoracic compliance and FRC.[238–240] Rigidity may be readily treated with neuromuscular blocking agents and is distinct from changes in pulmonary compliance associated with inhalational anesthetics.[241,242] Delayed or postoperative muscular rigidity may occur as opioid levels peak postoperatively.[243] Intravenous agents other than narcotics do not significantly affect chest wall rigidity.[244]

Reduced Minute Volume of Ventilation

Anesthesia changes the pattern of respiration and the minute ventilation (volume of inspired gas per minute). Inhalational anesthetics initially produce increased respiratory rate, initially irregular, progressing to regular rhythmic patterns. Breath holding is frequently observed with light planes of anesthesia. As inhalational anesthesia is deepened, respiration becomes faster, more regular, with diminished tidal volumes. This pattern of breathing eventually resembles panting. Narcotic-based anesthesia produces slower breathing, with increased tidal volumes, compared to inhalational-based techniques.

Although respiratory rate may increase with inhalational anesthetics, minute volume of ventilation decreases. As discussed in the section on ventilatory control (below), respiratory response to arterial CO_2 is decreased. Of the traditionally used inhalational agents, enflurane causes the most respiratory depression, with isoflurane causing less and halothane the least.

Ventilatory Drive

After reviewing the normal ventilatory response to carbon dioxide and oxygen we can discuss the effects of anesthetics on ventilatory drive. Ventilation is under control of central medullary chemoreceptors and peripheral chemoreceptors (i.e., the carotid bodies).[245] Aortic chemoreceptors have minimal effects on ventilation. The central and peripheral chemoreceptors appear complementary. Within 1 to 3 seconds, the peripheral chemoreceptors can respond to changes in arterial gas and acid composition.[246] The central receptors are slower to respond, but may be responsible for 80% of changes in ventilation in response to carbon dioxide.[238]

If one graphs the Pa_{CO_2} on the x axis (ordinate) and respiratory minute ventilation (as expressed in liters per minute) on the y axis (abscissa), the P_{CO_2}/ventilation response curve is defined.[238] This relationship is linear up to a Pa_{CO_2} of 80 mm Hg. The normal resting P_{CO_2} and ventilation are defined by the intersection of the curve at normal arterial concentration (Fig. 7–16). The P_{CO_2}/ventilation response curve represents the *overall* response of the respiratory system; as such, it may reveal diminished thoracic muscular/pulmonary response (as in the case of severe parenchymal lung disease or neuromuscular disease) despite increased chemoreceptor stimulation.

Several important facts may be obtained from analysis of the P_{CO_2}/ventilation response curve. First, the x intercept is "the apnea threshold to CO_2" and defines the point at which respiratory drive ceases as arterial CO_2 is lowered. Concurrent physiologic conditions, such as metabolic acidosis or alkalosis, presence of anesthetics, or intensity of surgical stimuli, may shift this point. A shift to the right indicates that apnea will occur at higher Pa_{CO_2}. The slope of the curve (expressed as min/kPa or min/mm Hg) predicts changes in ventilation under a given physiologic condition. This slope may vary widely among normal individuals, and is sensitive to changes in arterial O_2.

All inhalational anesthetics are marked respiratory depressants and therefore shift the P_{CO_2}/ventilatory response curve to the right and, in dose-dependent fashion, depress its slope. The degree to which respiratory depression occurs is somewhat agent specific (i.e., least-to-most, halothane, isoflurane, enflurane.[247] Apnea occurs

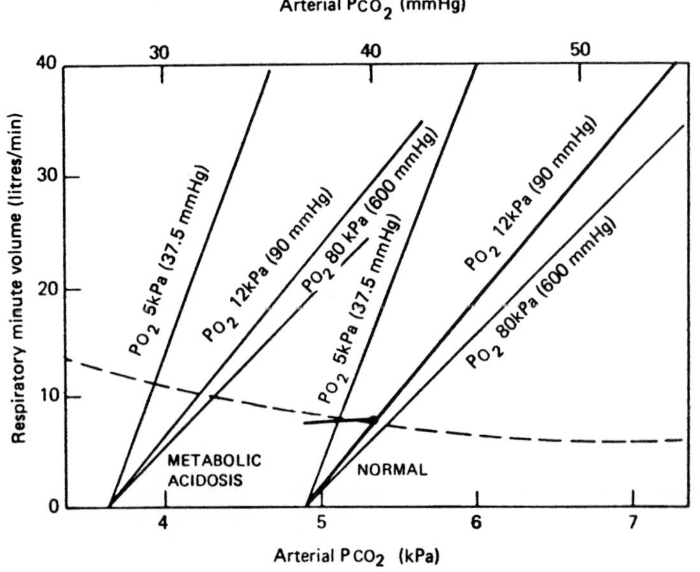

FIGURE **7–16.** Two fans of P_{CO_2}/ventilation curves at different values of Pa_{O_2}. The *right-hand fan* is at normal metabolic acid-base. The *left-hand fan* represents metabolic acidosis. The *broken line* represents the P_{CO_2} produced by the indicated ventilation for zero inspired P_{CO_2} at basal metabolic rate. The intersection of the *broken curve* and any response indicates the resting P_{CO_2} and ventilation for the relevant metabolic acid-base state and P_{O_2}. The *heavy curve* is the normal curve. (From Nunn JF: Respiratory aspects of anaesthesia. In Nunn JF [ed]: Applied Respiratory Physiology, 3rd ed. 1987, p 90, with permission.)

with all inhalational agents at MAC levels greater than 2[248,249] (Fig. 7–17).

Duration of anesthesia appears to affect response to CO_2; respiratory depression decreases over time, as measured by slope of the CO_2 response curve and resting $Paco_2$. After 5 to 6 hours of anesthesia the magnitude of ventilatory depression is reduced. After 6 hours of anesthesia with halothane, isoflurane, or enflurane, the magnitude of the respiratory depression is less than after 3 hours.[250]

All inhalational anesthetic agents, including N_2O, depress respiratory drive to increasing CO_2. N_2O is less respiratory depressant than halogenated inhalational anesthetics. When used with volatile agents and compared to the same equipotent dose of volatile agent alone, $Paco_2$ is lower than with volatile agents alone.[251] This phenomenon is dubbed "the sparing effect of N_2O."[252,253]

The intravenous anesthetic agents have variable effects on ventilatory drive. Ketamine has minimal effect on the Pco_2/ventilatory response curve.[254] Barbiturates, in doses to provide a surgical plane of anesthesia, depress respiration to a similar degree as inhalational agents. In doses that facilitate mild sedation, barbiturates have little effect on ventilatory response to CO_2.[197] Propofol depresses ventilatory drive to the same or lesser extent than does thiopental.[255] Induction doses will produce apnea[256] and lower doses will depress response to CO_2.[257] Etomidate is a lesser respiratory depressant than thiopental[258] or propofol.[259] Benzodiazepines such as valium and midazolam produce somewhat less respiratory depression than thiopental, etomidate, opiates, or propofol, at similar levels of sedation.

Opiates (via μ-receptor binding) depress respiration and shift the Pco_2/ventilatory response curve to the right. Other factors such as age, surgical stimulation, arousal state, and presence of other respiratory depressants will affect degree of opioid-induced respiratory depression.[252]

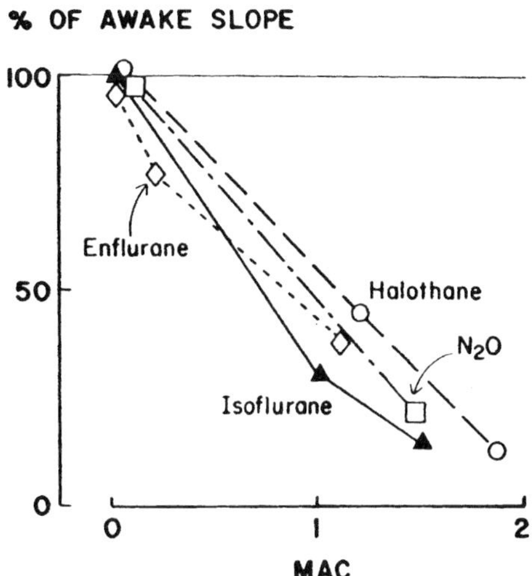

FIGURE 7–17. Ventilatory response to increases in $Paco_2$ in subjects anesthetized with enflurane, halothane, isoflurane, or nitrous oxide. Note that response progressively decreases as anesthetic concentration approaches 2 MAC. (From Eger EI II: Isoflurane: A review. Anesthesiology 55:559, 1981, with permission.)

Opiates may produce respiratory depression to the point of apnea, even after an apparent "safe" level of arousal postoperatively. Respiratory depression is seen with meperidine, fentanyl, and sufentanil and is more likely in patients with acidosis or renal failure. This delayed respiratory depression has been explained by several factors. Fentanyl binding to plasma protein is a pH-dependent phenomenon. As blood pH becomes progressively acidotic, less protein binding occurs,[260] and free opiate blood levels increase, worsening respiratory depression; the latter will in turn worsen the respiratory acidosis and this can spiral to apnea.[261]

Another explanation for the postoperative, "late," respiratory depression of opiates relates to the skeletal muscle as a pool for opiate stores.[262] Postoperatively, when the patient begins to move, the skeletal stores of opioids are released and plasma opiate levels increase. Lack of surgical stimuli in the postanesthesia care unit or the surgical care unit may also exacerbate opiate-associated respiratory depression.

In summary, the respiratory depressive effects of the inhalational anesthetics may be summarized as enflurane > isoflurane > halothane >> N_2O.[241] For the intravenous anesthetics this may be summarized as thiopental = methohexital > propofol > etomidate > midazolam >> ketamine.[241]

Response to Hypoxia

The ventilatory response to hypoxia is hyperbolic with maximal ventilation occurring when Pao_2 is reduced to 32 mm Hg.[197] Hypercapnia shifts this curve to the right and upward, without changing the overall shape. As might be anticipated, changes in oxygen content without changes in Pao_2 (such as induced by anemia or methemoglobinemia) have no effect on ventilation. Anesthetics blunt the effect of hypoxia on ventilatory drive, probably at carotid bodies. All inhalational agents including nitrous oxide inhibit the ventilatory drive to hypoxia.[263,264]

Response to Metabolic Acidemia

Inhalational anesthetics blunt the normal ventilatory drive to acidemia, and this effect may occur at subanesthetic inhalational doses, which may cause more physiologic derangements in ventilatory drive than do perturbations in hypoxic hyperventilation.[265]

Bronchomotor Tone and Airway Caliber

All inhalational agents, in experimental models, have been shown to increase airway caliber by decreasing bronchomotor tone through direct actions on smooth muscle, inhibition of airway innervation, inhibition of prostaglandins, and possibly through augmentation of β-adrenergic tone.[266] All inhalation agents cause bronchodilation in the setting of increased bronchomotor tone (such as during asthma). Enflurane and halothane unquestionably decrease vasomotor tone at rest. There is controversy regarding the effect of isoflurane on *baseline* bronchomotor tone; some studies with isoflurane report decreased bronchomotor tone, whereas others show increased bronchomotor tone at rest.[266]

Nunn et al. have questioned the effects of inhalational agents on airway resistance in clinical settings.[197] Although all inhalational agents bronchodilate via inhibition of airway reflexes, some investigators believe loss of lung volume during inhalational anesthesia actually increases airway resistance. Although large individual variation exists, the net effect seen with all inhalational agents is no effect or moderate *increases* in airway resistance when changes in lung volumes are taken into account[197] (Fig. 7–18). Specific intravenous anesthetic agents may have variable effects on airway caliber. Ketamine is a well-known bronchodilator that directly bronchodilates and inhibits neural reflexes.[267] Ketamine bronchodilates by inhibition of vagal pathways, by direct relaxation of airway smooth muscle, and by decreasing bronchomotor tone by increasing circulating catecholamines. Ketamine's indirect effect on β_2-adrenergic receptors appears to be of most clinical importance.[259] In patients with asthma and reactive airways, ketamine facilitates anesthetic induction and maintenance without precipitation of bronchospasm.[268,269]

The effect of barbiturate on bronchomotor tone is controversial. Because thiobarbiturates are capable of releasing histamine from mast cells, thiopental has been implicated in bronchospasm.[270] Thiobarbiturate-induced bronchospasm is of less clinical relevance than formerly taught because of the following three reasons:

1. Whereas light anesthesia with barbiturates produces little depression of airway reflex,[259] deep anesthesia with induction doses produces suppression.[271,272]
2. Although thiobarbiturates can result in degranulation of skin mast cells, pulmonary mast cells are not degranulated by thiobarbiturate administration.[259]
3. Although thiobarbiturates can cause constriction of bronchiolar smooth muscle in vitro, when used in doses for anesthesia induction, inhibitory effects on the parasympathetic nervous system may override these effects.[265] Oxybarbiturates (such as methohexital) do not cause histamine release from mast cells.[263]

Opioids may increase airway resistance, by direct effects on smooth muscle[273] or, indirectly, through histamine release.[274] These effects may be of little clinical consequence. Diazepam,[275] midazolam, etomidate, and propofol do not affect bronchomotor tone.[241]

Immunologic and Pulmonary Defense Mechanisms

Inhalational agents inhibit various components of the immune system including ciliary movement and velocity of movement in tracheal mucosa in the upper respiratory tract; cell-mediated immunity; neutrophil, lymphocyte and macrophage chemotaxis; and neutrophil superoxide peroxide production.[276,277]

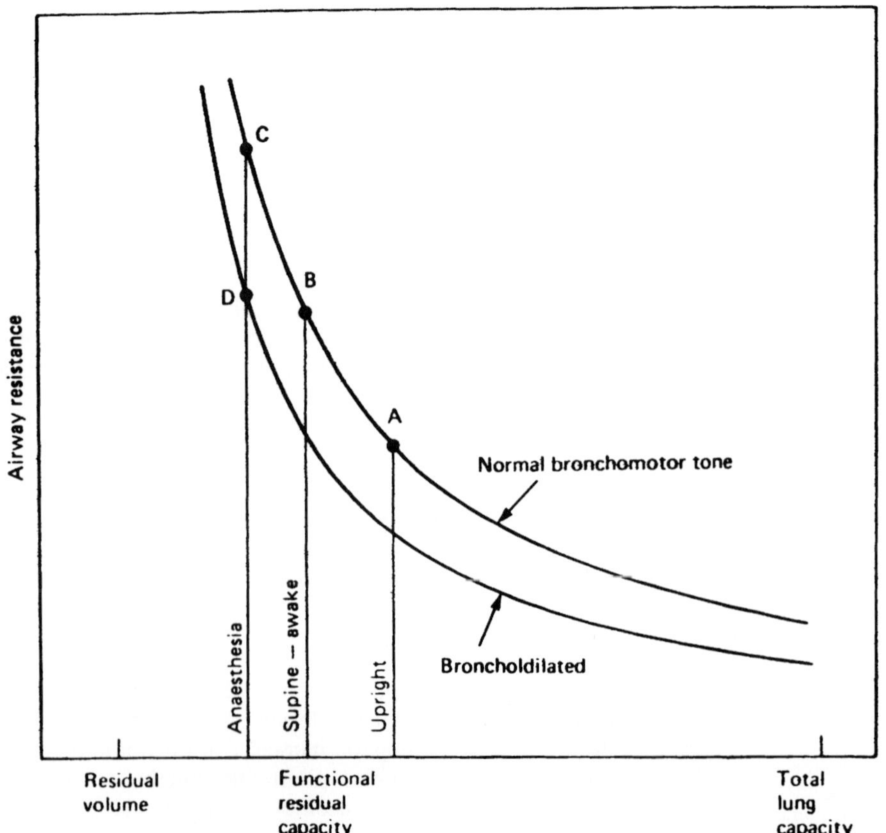

FIGURE **7–18.** Airway resistance as a function of lung volume with normal bronchomotor tone and vasodilated. (From Nunn JF: Respiratory aspects of anaesthesia. In Nunn JF [ed]: Applied Respiratory Physiology, 3rd ed. 1987, p 362, with permission.)

Ciliary Effects

The cilia of the upper airway are important as a defense mechanism and in helping prevent atelectasis secondary to mucous plugging and obstruction. It is well established experimentally that inhalational anesthetics impair tracheal ciliary movement.[278-282] Nitrous oxide has more variable effects on ciliary clearance than do halogenated inhalational agents.[272,273,275] This inhibition is dose related and may last 2 to 6 days after anesthesia.[283] The etiology of the inhibition of ciliary movement may be multifactorial, and involves relatively dry inspired gases, positive-pressure ventilation, and tracheal intubation.[241] In addition to direct effects on upper airway ciliary cells, anesthetics increase mucus viscosity in the upper respiratory tract.[284] Although most intravenous anesthetic agents in clinical doses appear not to effect ciliary movement, opioids inhibit ciliary function in a dose-dependent fashion.[267]

Neutrophil Function

Inhalational agents inhibit leukocyte function and mobility, and decrease the expression of leukocyte glycoprotein receptors,[285] neutrophil superoxide production,[286] and general bactericidal activity.[287,288] Propofol has also been associated with decreased leukocyte motility,[289] whereas etomidate does not affect leukocyte motility but may decrease leukocyte function.[290] Phenobarbital and thiopental do not affect leukocyte motility or function.[291,283]

Macrophage Function

Inhalational agents impair chemotaxis of macrophages[269] as well as macrophage microbicidal oxidative activity[292,293] and the ability of alveolar macrophages to generate ATP.[294]

Lymphocyte Function

There are scant and conflicting data on the effects of anesthesia on pulmonary lymphocyte function.[270] Postoperative T-lymphocyte impairment correlates more with degree of surgical trauma than to anesthetics used intraoperatively.[270] Anesthesia is not believed to influence β-lymphocyte proliferative capacity,[295] although postoperative patients consistently show decreased numbers of β lymphocytes.

In summary, although there is much published information regarding in vivo and in vitro effects of anesthesia and surgery on individual components of the immune system, one should approach these results with caution when extrapolating individual laboratory experiments to the clinical arena.[270]

Effects of the Anesthetics on the Renal System

The kidneys reabsorb 180 L of ultrafiltered plasma and 20,000 mEq of sodium per day.[296] Although they comprise less than one half of 1% of total body mass, they receive 10 to 20% of the cardiac output.[297] Development of renal insufficiency is not always clinically apparent. It is not until 50 to 60% of renal mass is physiologically compromised that characteristic changes in blood urea nitrogen (BUN) and creatinine occur; overt renal failure may go undetected until end-stage renal disease in imminent.[298]

Renal insufficiency has a profound impact on perioperative outcome. The first to emphasize this point was Butler, who in 1930 reported a threefold increase in the mortality of patients with "nephritis" who underwent surgery.[299,300] More recent studies have indicated that preoperative renal insufficiency is an independent risk factor for morbidity and mortality following either cardiac or noncardiac surgery.[292,301-303] Renal insufficiency also serves as a possible predictor of *intraoperative sudden death*.[302] Chronic hemodialysis adds marked risk to cardiac surgery with 7.7% operative mortality in elective cases and emergent valvular replacement having a 57.1% mortality in one study.[304]

Renal dysfunction following cardiac surgery is not uncommon and is devastating. Up to 40% of cardiac operations are complicated by acute renal insufficiency and 2 to 5% percent of all cardiac patients develop severe acute renal failure (defined as serum creatinine value >5 mg/dl). The perioperative mortality for patients with severe acute renal failure (ARF) approaches 90%.[305-307] Patients with milder elevations of serum creatinine (serum creatinine value 1.5 to 2.0 mg/dl) have a five-fold increase in perioperative mortality.[305] The prognosis for the pediatric patient who develops ARF is poor, with mortality following cardiac surgery approaching 50 to 67%.[308] As renal dysfunction progresses along a continuum from mild renal dysfunction to nonoliguric renal failure to oliguria, perioperative mortality climbs substantially.[309]

Renal Microanatomy and Physiology

Adverse renal effects of anesthetic agents may result from nephrotoxic effects of their metabolites on the kidney or derangements in mechanisms responsible for regulation of renal ultrafiltrate and the maintenance of normal segmental renal perfusion.[310] Prior to a discussion of the potential adverse effects of these agents on the kidneys, renal microanatomy and physiology will be reviewed.

Blood enters the kidney via *afferent arteries*, which originate from the arcuate arteries. The arcuate arteries are branches of larger intralobular arteries, which in turn arise from one of two trunks of the renal artery. These afferent arteries divide within the microtubular system of the kidney, *the nephron* (Fig. 7–19), to form individual networks of capillaries, *Bowman's capsule* (Fig. 7–20).

Each kidney contains up of 1,200,000 nephrons. The structural unit of Bowman's capsule and the surrounding endothelial cells, mesangial cells, epithelial cells, and basement membrane are termed the *glomerulus*. Blood does not enter the renal venous circulation without first passing through a glomerulus. Once filtered by the glo-

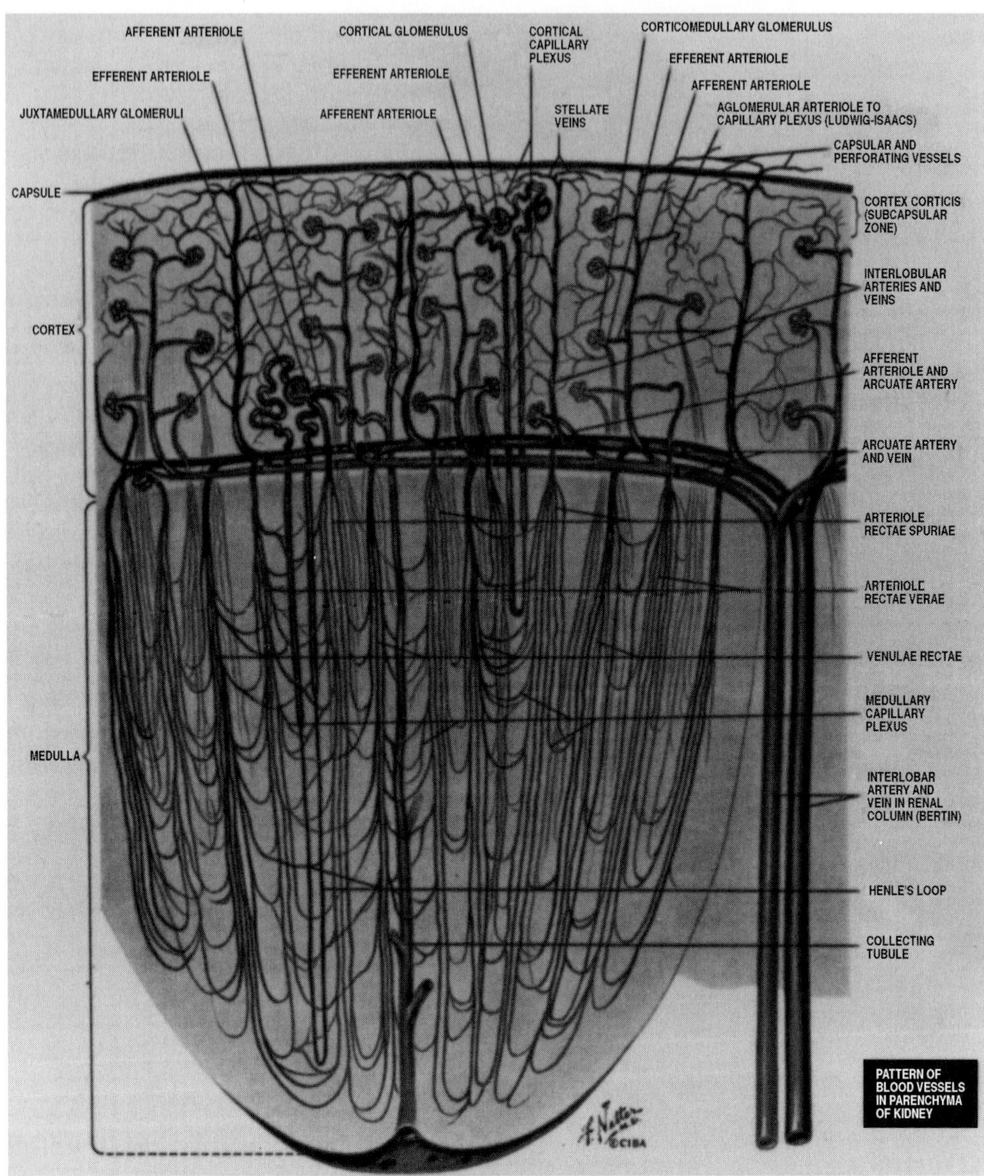

FIGURE **7–19.** Pattern of blood vessels in parenchyma of the kidney. (From Netter F: The CIBA Collection of Medical Illustration 6:18, 1973, with permission.)

merulus, the remaining serum and cellular portion of blood enters the *efferent arteriole*.

The glomerular mesangium has been shown to contain contractile elements, which respond to vasoactive substances, of which angiotensin II is most important. Through mesangial contractility, numerous hormones and vasoactive substances regulate the degree of ultrafiltrate delivered to the nephron. These mesangial contractile elements are important in development of angiotensin II–related hypertension and atrial natriuretic factor–related hypotension.[310]

Regional Renal Perfusion

Excellent reviews of laboratory and clinical measurements of glomerular filtration, renal blood flow, and renal plasma flows are available.[290,303,311] Through these measurements, it has been determined that blood flow decreases from the outer to the inner cortex of the kidney.[304] The outer receives twice the blood flow of the inner.[312,313] Total medullary blood flow is estimated to be only 3% of total renal blood flow[314] (Fig. 7–21). Redistribution of regional renal blood flow is important in the pathogenesis of renal injury during periods of severe global renal hypoperfusion. During hemorrhage, suprarenal cross-clamping, and periods of cardiogenic shock, medullary hypoperfusion results from blood selectively shunted from the renal medulla. Changes in regional perfusion in the face of global ischemia have been shown to occur, although the exact mechanism by which this transpires remains speculative. Regional differentiation of segmental blood flow and the ischemic/toxic injury based on it is termed *heterogeneity*.[315]

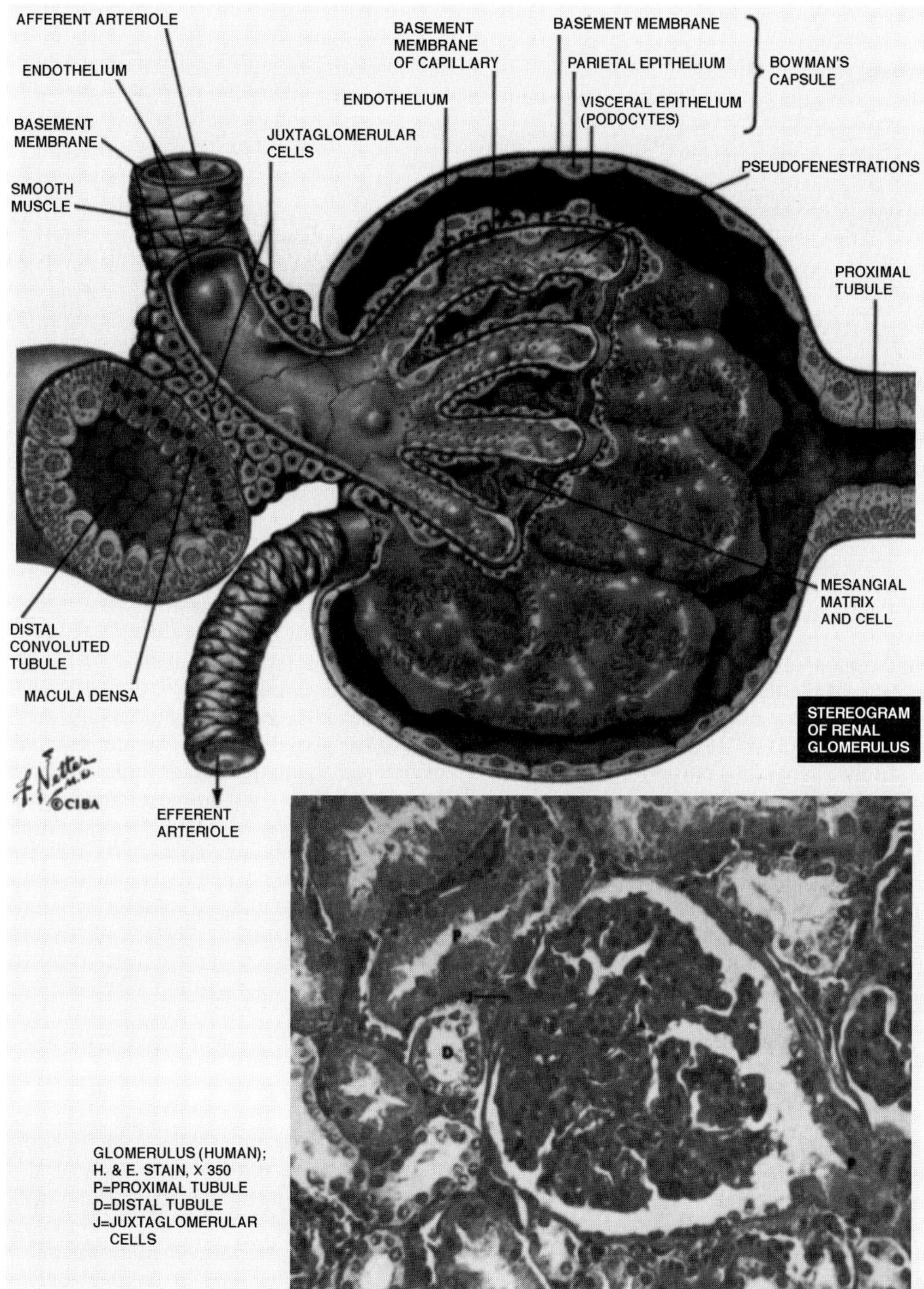

FIGURE **7–20.** The structure of the glomerulus. (From Netter F: The CIBA Collection of Medical Illustration 6:7, 1973, with permission.)

Heterogeneity of renal perfusion appears important to the mechanism of anesthetic-induced renal dysfunction. Some have emphasized cortical hypoperfusion in acute renal failure,[316] although most have observed impaired outer medullary perfusion during acute renal failure.[305,306] Following periods of renal ischemia, juxtamedullary flow is significantly compromised, while flow to cortical segments is preserved.[307,317] The renal medulla is especially susceptible to reperfusion injury following ischemic compromise.[318] A dark zone in the red medullary is often seen in human pathologic specimens of ischemic ARF. Pathologic changes of the outer medulla are also prominent features in toxic renal injury.[314,318]

With global hypoperfusion, there is often regional heterogeneity in the pathology of nephrotic injury. Severe selective damage to the medullary thick ascending limb (partially in the juxtamedullary region) is probably related to regional hypoxia imposed by deranged medullary blood flow. The medullary thick ascending loop is much more dependent on oxygen delivery and has lower

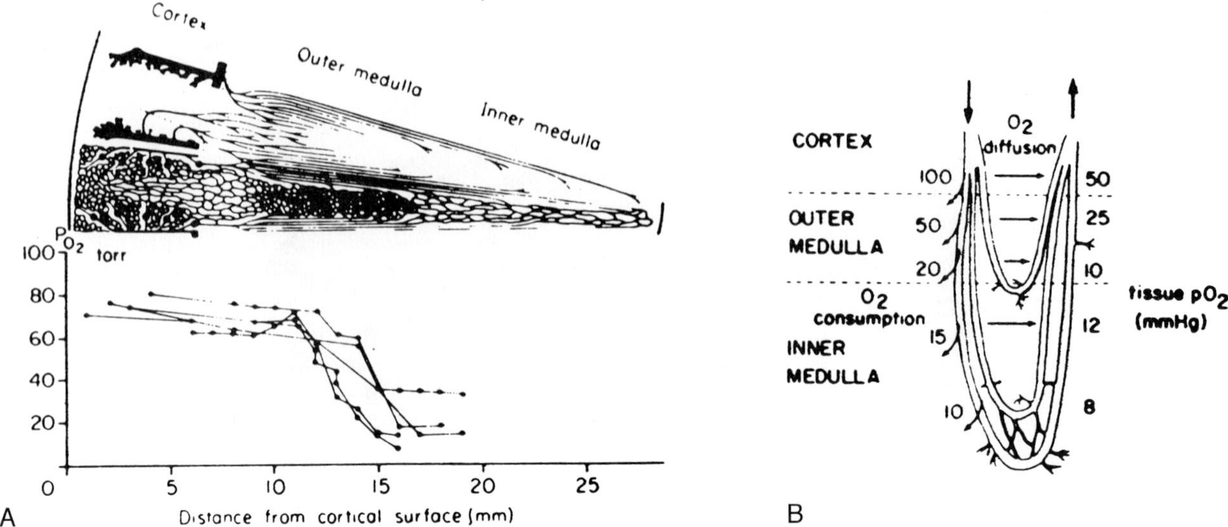

FIGURE 7–21. Tissue PCO_2 as a function of distance from cortical surface. (From Brezis M, Rosen S, Epstein F: Acute Renal Failure. In Brenner BM, Rector FG [eds]. The Kidney. Philadelphia, Ardmore Medical Books, 1986, p 735, with permission.)

regional oxygen content than in the cortical segments. The extraction ratio of the renal medulla is 0.79 and for the renal cortex is 0.18; Po_2 in the medulla is 8 mm Hg versus 50 mm Hg in the cortex[314] (Table 7–6). This may explain why the thick ascending portion of the loop of Henle is particularly susceptible to the nephrotoxic effects of fluorinated anesthetic agents.

The particular susceptibility of the outer medullary region may be further explained by its specialized function in concentrating urine.[314] The tubules and the vascular supply of the renal medulla are arranged in a hairpin, allowing countercurrent exchange of solute and efficient concentration of urine.[314,319] The thick ascending portion of Henle's loop is involved in active transport of sodium and in the creation of an osmotic gradient. The combination of a high metabolic load, imposed by active electrolyte transport, and the unique architecture of the vasa recta limit blood flow to the renal medulla and prevent washout of solute gradient. Renal medullary susceptibility to hypoxia appears to be an inevitable trade-off for the effective concentrating ability of the kidney.[314] The outer medullary zone of the kidney is particularly susceptible to ischemic and toxic insults such as nephropathy associated with methoxyflurane and analgesics, nephrosclerosis, diabetes mellitus, and chronic urinary tract infection.[320–322] Polyuric ARF is associated with marked heterogeneity of injury on pathologic examination of the kidney. Oliguric renal failure is associated with homogeneity of injury: All nephrons are injured, whereas in polyuric renal failure there is segmental sparing of renal segments. After toxic nephropathies or renal failure associated with hypotensive hemorrhage, pathologic heterogeneity is often a prominent feature. Heterogeneity of renal injury in development of acute tubular necrosis (ATN) is of interest to anesthesiologists because renal failure associated with fluorinated anesthetic agents most often clinically presents as polyuric renal failure.[323–325]

TABLE 7–6
Differential Perfusion of Renal Cortex and Medulla*

	Cortex	Medulla
% of RBF (RBF)	94%	6%
Blood flow (ml/min/gm)	5.0	0.03
O_2 extraction ratio ($\dot{V}o_2/\dot{D}o_2$)	0.18	0.79
Po_2 (mm Hg)	50	8

*From Sladen RN: Perioperative Renal Protection. 1992 Annual Refresher Course Lectures. American Society of Anesthesiologists, 1992 and data obtained from Brezis M, Rosen S, Epstein F: Am J Kidney Dis 1989:13, 253, with permission.
RBF, renal blood flow.

In daily practice, the precise causative agent of renal failure is not always readily apparent. Often, more than one potential risk factor is responsible for initiation of renal failure, such as long cross-clamp time, prolonged positive-pressure ventilation, and nephrotoxic antibiotics. Considering the multifactorial causality of ATN, the synergistic relationship of the various etiologic agents in the development of ARF becomes more apparent. Toxic agents, for example, often manifest nephrotoxic potential in the setting of global or regional hypoperfusion.[314,317] Thus renal failure develops in postoperative cardiac patients with left ventricular contractile abnormalities, low cardiac output, and decreased global renal perfusion.[298,299,326–328]

This synergy between global or regional ischemia and nephrotoxic agents may be explained by several factors:

1. Reduced renal perfusion results in decreased urine flow and increased transit time through the tubules, and prolongs the time toxic substances are in physical contact with tubular structures.
2. Toxic metabolites may trigger release of local mediators (e.g., prostaglandin synthesis inhibitors) that interfere with renal autoregulation and segmental blood flow.

3. Cellular and mitochondrial damage may exacerbate inefficient metabolic demands, and uncouple the cellular oxidative process, potentiating anoxic injury.
4. Impaired membrane integrity leads to increased cytosolic calcium, which leads to vasoconstriction and impaired tubular metabolism.[329]
5. Toxic substances and O_2 deprivation can in turn lead to adenosine triphosphate (ATP) deprivation.[313,317]

The mechanism proposed above probably accounts for the nephrotoxicity of the fluorinated anesthetic agents (i.e., methoxyflurane); most renal effects of anesthetic agents are believed to be the result of perturbations of neuronal and hormonal supplies to the kidney. These effects on segmental blood flow are mediated through hormonal changes in regional renal blood flow.

Renal Humoral Homeostasis

The renal microcirculation is controlled via the homeostatic balance of two opposing hormonal systems: The renin-angiotensin-aldosterone/antidiuretic hormone system and the prostaglandin-bradykinin–atrial natriuretic peptide (ANP) system.[303,330] The renin-angiotensin-aldosterone/antidiuretic system is prominent during hypovolemia and low systemic blood pressure; the prostaglandin-bradykinin-ANP system during periods of elevated systemic blood pressure and hypervolemia. Many of the effects of anesthetic agents on renal function are secondary to changes in the extrarenal perfusion rather than to their direct effects on the kidney.[303] The decreased urine output and sodium retention seen in the acute postoperative period are mediated through the renin-angiotensin-aldosterone/antidiuretic hormone system.

The Renin-Angiotensin-Aldosterone/ Antidiuretic Hormone System

The renin-angiotensin-aldosterone system integrates components of the hepatic, pulmonary, and renal systems to maintain systemic perfusion pressure and volume status. The juxtaglomerular (JG) apparatus, which consists of the afferent and efferent arterioles as well as the modified epithelial cells of the afferent arterioles and the JG cells, is crucial to this process. The JG cells produce and store renin,[325] a proteolytic enzyme with a molecular weight of 40,000.[325] Renin enzymatically cleaves angiotensin I from angiotensinogen. This process is the rate-limiting step in the formation of angiotensin II.[325] Angiotensinogen is derived from α_2-globulins, produced in the liver. Angiotensin I is converted to angiotensin II by angiotensin-converting enzyme, which is present in the lungs, kidneys, and to a lesser extent in vascular endothelium (Fig. 7–22).

Renin

Release of renin is affected by numerous factors, and is extensively covered by Keeton and Campbell.[330] Renin is released in response to decreased renal perfusion pressure sensed by baroreceptors in the afferent arteriole, decreased sodium delivery to the macula densa, and β-adrenergic stimulation of receptors in the JG apparatus. Aldosterone facilitates renin release. Prostaglandins and angiotensin II antagonize release of renin.[331] Renin catalyzes conversion of angiotensin I from angiotensinogen.

Angiotensin II

Angiotensin II stimulates vasoconstriction of peripheral vascular smooth muscles. It is responsible for CNS stimulation, which increases peripheral sympathetic outflow, which then increases myocardial contractility and potentiates norepinephrine release from cardioaccelerator nerves. It also potentiates sodium reabsorption in the proximal tubule. Angiotensin II increases systemic blood pressure by increasing cardiac output and systemic vascular resistance. Angiotensin II stimulates the steroidogenesis and release of the mineralocorticoid *aldosterone*. Angiotensin II inhibits the release of renin from JG cells.

Aldosterone

Aldosterone is a salt-retaining mineralocorticoid steroid produced by adrenal cortex,[332] and secreted in response to angiotensin II, hyperkalemia, adrenocorticotropic hormone (ACTH), and hyponatremia. Angiotensin II and K^+ are the predominant mediators of aldosterone release. Surgery is an important stimulus for elevation in serum aldosterone. Aldosterone binds to specific (type I) mineralocorticoid receptors,[333] and ultimately results in increased transcription of mRNA for the Na^+-K^+ transport systems in the kidney, although, to date, no aldosterone-responsive or type I–specific receptor-regulated gene has been reported.[327] In addition to renal type I mineralocorticoid receptors, cerebral and cardiac type I mineralocorticoid receptors have been identified. The increase in aldosterone-induced Na^+-K^+ ATPase activity in the distal tubule results in Na^+ retention, expanded blood volume, and K^+ and H^+ elimination. Through these actions it is the major determinant of plasma sodium regulation.

Antidiuretic Hormone

Antidiuretic hormone (ADH) stimulates reabsorption of water from renal collecting ducts. It is released in response to (1) increased osmolarity, as sensed by neurons in the supraoptic nuclei; (2) in response to decreased volume, as sensed by atrial stretch receptors; and (3) nonvolumetric or osmotic release as stimulated by pain, emesis, hypoxia, or emotional stress. This last effect is probably modulated by neuronal input from the higher cortical areas. The effects of ADH are potentiated by aldosterone. ADH stimulates secretion of renal prostaglandins.

Sympathorenal Axis

Sympathetic innervation to the kidney is mediated by release of norepinephrine from fibers arising predomi-

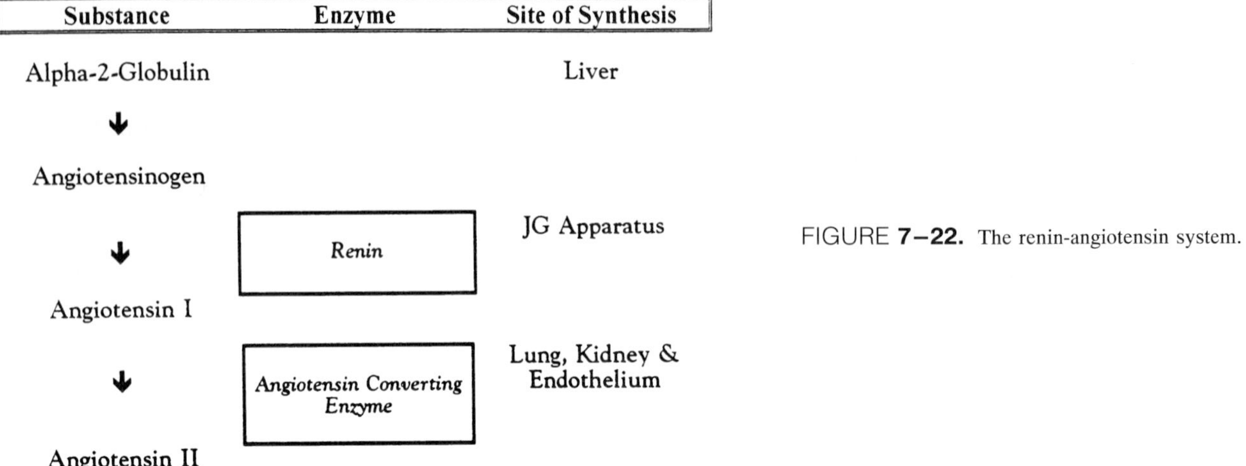

FIGURE **7–22.** The renin-angiotensin system.

nantly from T12–L4 spinal segments and via the effects of circulating catecholamines. Low-intensity α-adrenergic stimulation results in efferent arteriolar constriction, which increases hydrostatic perfusion pressure across Bowman's capsule, and maintains glomerular filtration rate (GFR) (Fig. 7–23). With increased α-sympathetic stimulation, afferent and efferent arterioles are constricted, impeding GFR and renal blood flow (RBF). β-Adrenergic stimulation results in release of renin from the juxtamedullary apparatus and promotes proximal tubular sodium reabsorption. β-Blockade inhibits same.

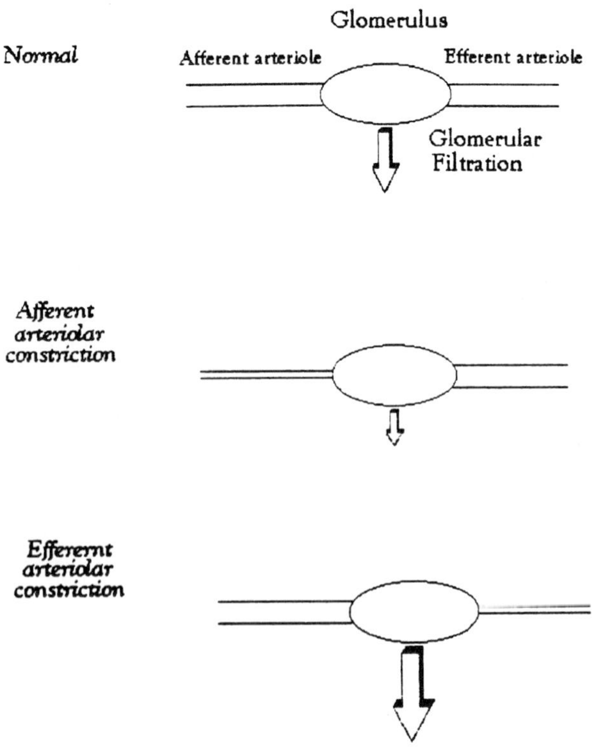

FIGURE **7–23.** Effect of afferent and efferent arteriolar constriction on glomerular filtration. Afferent arteriolar constriction leads to decreased glomerular filtration pressure and decreased glomerular filtration. Efferent arteriolar constriction leads to increased glomerular filtration pressure and increased glomerular filtration.

Prostaglandin-Kinin–ANP System

The prostaglandin-kinin–ANP system facilitates decreasing circulating blood volume, systemic blood pressure, and serum sodium during periods of hypertension, relative hypervolemia, or hypernatremia.

Prostaglandins

Renal prostaglandins are generally not of much importance during basal conditions.[334,335] Prostaglandins help preserve renal function during periods of ischemic insult and counteract the medullary cortical shunting of blood during surgery and trauma. Prostaglandin F_2 (PGF_2), PGE_2,[336,337] and PGI_2 (prostacyclin) are important to renal physiology.[338] PGE_2, PGF_2, and PGI_2 are renal vasodilators and site-specific antagonists of the renal effects of ADH and aldosterone[329]; they augment RBF. PGE_2 and PGF_2 are synthesized predominantly in the renal medulla, while PGI_2 is synthesized in the cortex.[339] Renal prostaglandin secretion is stimulated by ischemia, hypotension, norepinephrine, angiotensin II, ADH, and bradykinin. Although they do not appear to be of physiologic importance during basal states, numerous conditions result in prostaglandin-mediated vasodilatation (Table 7–7). Inhibitors of prostaglandin synthesis (nonsteroidal anti-inflammatory drugs) cause deterioration of renal function in patients with decreased effective arterial blood volume, such as those with congestive heart failure (CHF), cirrhosis, volume depletion, sepsis, and following general anesthesia. Juxtamedullary ischemia is ameliorated by intrarenal infusion of PGE_2, PGI_2, and PGD_2, which augment juxtamedullary flow relative to cortical flow.[307,329,340] PGE_2 reduces transport-related oxygen consumption in this portion of the kidney.[307,341] Indomethacin, an inhibitor of prostaglandin synthesis, preferentially diminishes juxtamedullary blood flow.[307]

Atrial Natriuretic Peptide

ANP is one of several substances excreted by myocardial tissue that regulate renal circulation and sodium excretion.[303,342] ANP is released in response to local atrial wall stretch (e.g., during periods of elevated atrial pressure).[343]

TABLE 7–7
Renal Vasoconstrictors and Vasodilators*

Effective circulating volume contraction
Diuretic administration
Excessive gastrointestinal salt losses
Heat exhaustion
Severe sodium deprivation
Reduced cardiac output (congestive heart failure, myocardial infarction, constrictive pericarditis, cardiac tamponade)
Nephrotic syndrome
Hepatic cirrhosis with ascites
Hemorrhage
Septic shock
Hypotension
Renal ischemia
Renal arterial constriction or occlusion
Urinary tract obstruction
Renal parenchymal diseases, especially glomerulonephritides
Acute and chronic renal insufficiency or failure
Cellular dehydration (hyperosmolality—hypernatremia, hyperglycemia, mannitol, dextran, glycerol)
Hypercalcemia
Hypoxemia
Mechanical trauma
Anesthesia
Surgery
Stress

*From Norris SH: Renal eicosanoids. Semin Nephrol 10:64, 1990, with permission.

ANP causes rapid increases in GFR[344] by selective efferent arteriolar constriction and afferent arteriolar dilation.[345,346] ANP promotes sodium and water excretion, counteracts norepinephrine- and angiotensin II–induced vasoconstriction, decreases renin secretion, blocks angiotensin II–stimulated aldosterone release, and blocks the salt-retaining action of aldosterone[347–349] (Table 7–8). The net effect of ANP secretion is a decrease in blood pressure; an increase in sodium and water excretion; and an inhibition of angiotensin II, aldosterone, endothelin, renin, and ADH[343] (Fig. 7–24). These actions are mediated through ANP-dependent cyclic guanosine monophosphate (cGMP).[343]

Vasodilatory renal prostaglandins have beneficial effects in preserving GFR in experimental models of acute[350] and established ischemic acute renal failure,[351] as well as in catecholamine-induced acute renal failure[352] and radiocontrast-induced nephropathy.[353,347] ANP may help prevent renal ischemia and toxic nephrotoxicity by augmenting the medullary circulation and redistributing blood flow from the cortical to the medullary segments.[354]

The Renal Humoral Effect of Specific Anesthetic Agents

Anesthetic Agents and Renin Release

All anesthetic agents, in doses that produce surgical anesthesia, stimulate renin release in human.[355] The mechanism of this release is specific to the class of anesthetic agent.[330] Inhalational agents (halothane, enflurane, and methoxyflurane) in doses of 0.5% to 2.5% increase plasma renin.[356] Halothane stimulates renin release in a β-adrenergic–independent fashion.[330] The magnitude of this effect is dependent on the hydrational status of the patient.[330,356] Nitrous oxide increases plasma renin levels in humans when given with 50% oxygen and 1 mg/kg morphine.[357,358]

Both morphine (1 mg/kg) and Innovar (droperidol/fentanyl) have been shown to increase serum renin levels 1.5- to 3.5-fold in humans.[330,357] When pentobarbital is administered in doses that decrease MAP by 5 to 50%, RBF and renal sodium excretion can decrease substantially, 26 and 33%, respectively.[330] Infusion of Pentothal can reduce RBF by 35 to 40% without a change in MAP.[330,359] These changes are associated with elevated renin. Pentobarbital may stimulate renin secretion through activation of baroreceptors or via decreased sodium load at the macula densa. Both mechanisms may or may not be temporally linked.[330] The mechanism of pentobarbital-stimulated renin release appears independent of β-adrenergic or prostaglandin stimulation.[330,360] Increases in plasma renin promoted by barbiturate are short lived, and once a level plane of anesthesia is reached, renin levels return to normal.

Ketamine causes an initial increase of plasma renin in animals 20 minutes after injection. This increase is related to β-adrenergic stimulation. This increase in serum renin is short lived, and subsequently serum renin levels decline. Although animal studies appear to show consistent acute increases in serum renin, not all human studies have documented this effect.

Anesthetic Agents and ADH Release

Most anesthetics, with the exception of ketamine, cause release of ADH.[361,362] Opiates have a bimodal effect on

TABLE 7–8
Hemodynamic Effects of ANP

Effect of ANP	Result on Hemodynamics
Increased vagal afferent activity	Decreased heart rate, cardiac contractility
Increased coronary vasoconstriction	? Decreased cardiac contractility
Increased capillary leak	Decreased intravascular volume
Relaxation of resistance arterioles	Decreased peripheral vascular resistance
Decreased renin release	Decreased angiotensin II & decreased peripheral vascular resistance
Renal effects	Decreased peripheral vascular resistance
Increased diuresis	
Increased natriuresis	

ANP, atrial natriuretic peptides.

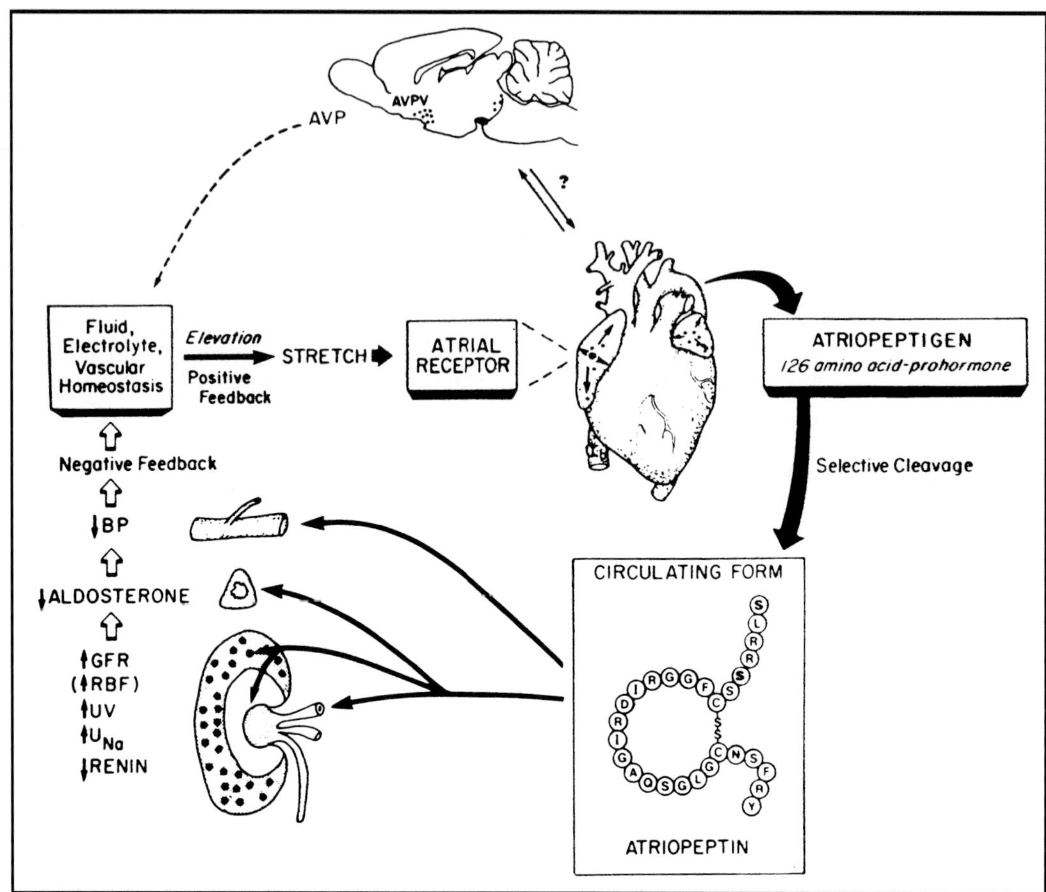

FIGURE **7–24.** Schematic diagram of the atriopeptin hormonal system. The 126-amino-acid prohormone, atriopeptigen, is stored in granules in perinuclear atrial cardiocytes. Elevated vascular volume results in the release of atriopeptin, which acts on the kidney (glomeruli and papilla) to increase the glomerular filtration rate (GFR), renal blood flow (RBF), urine volume (UV), and sodium excretion (U_{Na}), and to decrease plasma renin activity. Natriuresis and diuresis are also facilitated by the suppression of aldosterone and the release of arginine vasopressin (AVP). Diminution of vascular volume provides a negative feedback that suppresses circulating levels of atriopeptin. (From Needleman P, Greenwald JE: Atriopeptin: a cardiac hormone intimately involved in fluid, electrolyte, and blood-pressure homeostasis. N Engl J Med 314:828, 1986. Copyright 1986, Massachusetts Medical Society, with permission.)

ADH release: low-dose opiates (oxilophran, butophanol, morphine, fentanyl, sufentanil, and alfentanil) antagonize release of ADH[363–367]; high-dose opiates (apomorphine and morphine) stimulate ADH release. Naloxone appears to antagonize ADH release.[334,367] Surgical stimulation further increases circulating ADH,[362,368,369] but this transient increase may be attenuated by preoperative hydration and is readily reversible with termination of surgery and anesthesia.[356,362]

Anesthetic Agents and Aldosterone Release

Aldosterone secretion is markedly increased following surgery, and may remain elevated for several days postoperatively.[370,371] Etomidate suppresses cortisol, 17-hydroprogesterone, and cortisone production, and inhibits aldosterone production and release.[372,373] Etomidate suppresses 17-hydroxylase and 11-hydroxylase activity.[373] This effect following induction doses may last for up to 5 to 8 hours,[374] and infusion may inhibit aldosterone production for up to 20 hours.[375] Propofol and thiopental appear to stimulate aldosterone secretion[376,377] at two distinct sites in the biochemical pathway of its production.[378] Midazolam does not affect aldosterone production,[375] and there is no in vivo evidence to suggest that aldosterone production is suppressed by other intravenous agents.[248,379,380]

Inhalational anesthetics produce increased serum aldosterone, but[324,361] the mechanism (i.e., direct steroidogenesis vs. secondary response to atrial and systemic baroreceptors) is unresolved. Although serum aldosterone levels are elevated by inhalational anesthetics, serum sodium is usually decreased postoperatively. This is secondary to dilutional hyponatremia, the predominant effect of increased serum ADH levels following surgery and anesthesia.[324,361]

Anesthetic Agents and ANP Release

Halothane can increase ANP release.[381] Ketamine increases plasma ANP, and pentobarbital may decrease it slightly.[382,383]

Intravenous opioids can increase ANP levels[343] with μ-agonists increasing ANP,[382,383] whereas K-receptor agonists have no effect on plasma ANP.[384,385] Studies with high-dose narcotics failed to show consistent increases in ANP during anesthesia.[382] This may be related to mechanism of action because at low doses μ-agonists directly stimulate atrial ANP release and at high doses opiates mediate predominantly through hemodynamic changes.[343]

Cardiac surgery and CPB do not consistently alter plasma ANP,[386–388] although rewarming from hypothermia may increase ANP.[389]

Most anesthetic agents and surgical stimuli increase circulating renin, aldosterone, and ADH, accompanied by increased renal water resorption and decreased renal sodium excretion. These hormonal changes result in a general vasoconstrictive renal state. For most patients, these hormonal changes and their concomitant decreases in GFR and RBF are well tolerated, or manifest simply as fluid retention or transient oliguria. The changes in the hormonal milieu when compounded with the insults of such frequent perioperative occurrences as CPB and mechanical ventilation,[323,390] especially with PEEP ventilation,[391–396] can be of significant consequence for the patient with underlying renal dysfunction.[363] Such changes may be detrimental in the dehydrated, elderly, or hemorrhaging patient, or in those with decreased left ventricular contractile function.[305,306,326–328] Patients who develop postoperative renal failure have a tendency to have had longer coronary pulmonary bypass times and appear not to tolerate the bypass procedure as well as patients without postoperative renal dysfunction.[323]

Direct Renal Effects of Anesthetic Agents

Inhalational anesthetic agents depress renal function, although the specific effects of anesthetic agents upon RBF, GFR, and renal vascular resistance (RVR) vary.[297] The effects have been studied most intensively with halothane, which decreases GFR and urine output.[310,325,397,398] Halothane is a direct renal vasodilator decreasing RVR.[310,323,391,399] RBF is maintained in chronically instrumented dogs undergoing induced hypotension with halothane or isoflurane.[400] Preservation of RBF with halothane or isoflurane has been confirmed[310,401,402] and represents preservation of autoregulation of blood flow.[310,403] Enflurane at doses greater than or equal to 1.6 MAC resulted in a significant decrease in RBF[400] and RVR.[404,405] As with halothane and isoflurane, enflurane decreases GFR and urine output in a dose-related fashion.[404,406]

Desflurane preserves RBF and decreases RVR[407] and may maintain RBF to a greater extent than either isoflurane or halothane. Although halothane, isoflurane, and desflurane decrease cortical blood flow, desflurane may preserve cortical blood flow better by decreasing cortical vascular resistance to a greater extent than the other volatile agents.[408] Barbiturates decrease or have no effect on RBF and uniformly lower GFR. Urine output during barbiturate anesthesia is lowered, with barbiturates having variable effects on autoregulation depending on the type of barbiturate used (oxybarbiturates vs. thiobarbiturates).[356]

Ketamine increases both RBR and RVR. Urine output is decreased with ketamine as it is with other anesthetic agents[409]; even with hemorrhagic hypovolemia, ketamine maintains RBF.[310,410] Although propofol maintains RBF, its use has been associated with decreased renal clearance of organic anions.[411,412] Diazepam administration results in a slight decrease in RBF.[409]

High-dose morphine has minimal effect on renal hemodynamics in patients with normal renal function.[413] When administered in doses associated with systemic hypotension, morphine is found not to affect RBF.[414] Although the effects of fentanyl on RBF are variable, urine output and GFR have been shown to uniformly decrease.[410] Renal hemodynamics are markedly altered when nitrous oxide is added to opiate anesthesia.[413]

Direct Nephrotoxic Effects of Anesthetic Agents

Some inhalational anesthetics, in addition to producing hormonal and regional flow perturbations, have been associated with direct nephrotoxicity. The direct nephrotoxic effects of anesthetic agents are the result of biotransformation of these agents into toxic metabolites.[415] Increased biotransformation, as seen in obese patients[404] and after enzyme induction, may increase the nephrotoxic potential of anesthetic agents. The nephrotoxic potential of any anesthetic agent may be increased when used in conjunction with other nephrotoxic agents.[416] Pre-existing renal disease also increases nephrotoxicity of inhalational agents.[248,417]

The toxicity of fluoride-containing volatile agents was first reported with methoxyflurane in 1966.[418] The fluoride ion produces a heterogenetic, ADH-resistant, polyuric renal failure.[324,419] The nephrotoxicity of methoxyflurane is by far the greatest of the inhalational agents because (1) it is metabolized to fluoride in toxic quantities; (2) its metabolism produces a second potential nephrotoxin, oxalate; and (3) methoxyflurane is ten times more lipid soluble then enflurane or isoflurane, and thus remains in the body for days, with continued production of fluoride ion[415] (Fig. 7–25). The nephrotoxic potential of methoxyflurane has led to its disappearance from clinical use.[248,415]

Of the five commonly used inhalational agents, sevoflurane is defluorinated most extensively. Fluoride levels after 1 MAC-hour of anesthesia with sevoflurane are almost 30 times that of desflurane. Serum fluoride levels with sevoflurane anesthesia are typically 20 μmol but can range up to 70 μmol. The degree of biometabolism of currently used volatile anesthetic agents are: sevoflurane > halothane > enflurane > isoflurane > desflurane.[248] The serum fluoride levels after 1 MAC-hour of their use are: sevoflurane > enflurane > isoflurane > desflurane > halothane.[420]

Enflurane is not generally considered nephrotoxic, although significant amounts of fluoride are released during its metabolism.[421] In mild to moderate renal insuffi-

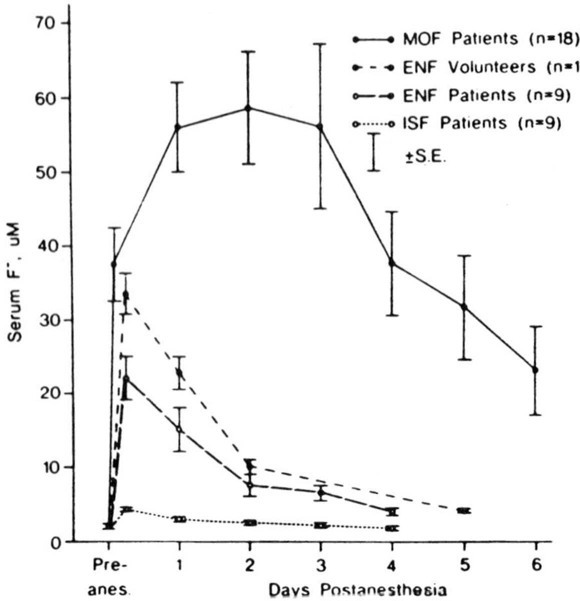

FIGURE 7–25. Serum inorganic fluoride (F^-) concentration prior to and following enflurane, isoflurane and methoxyflurane anesthesia. (From Mazze RI: Fluorinated anaesthetic nephrotoxicity: An update. Can Anaesth Soc J 31:S16, 1984, with permission.)

ciency (serum creatinine, 1.5 to 3.0 mg/dl), both enflurane and halothane are associated with, if anything, a small improvement in renal function postoperatively.[422] Enflurane increases nephrotoxicity of aminoglycoside antibiotics.[423]

Halothane is metabolized to a much greater extent than enflurane, yet undergoes little defluorination and is not considered nephrotoxic.[248,415] Isoflurane is also considered devoid of nephrotoxic potential.[415] Isoflurane has been used for up to 24 hours,[424] and in patients with pre-existing renal dysfunction,[425] without adverse outcome.

Desflurane is the least defluorinated of the inhalational agents and negligible increases in serum fluoride are observed after 1 MAC-hour of anesthesia.[426] It is devoid of renal toxicity in normal volunteers.[427] Desflurane has been used in patients with pre-existing renal dysfunction without deterioration in renal function.[425] Intravenous anesthetic agents have not been reported to be directly nephrotoxic.[248]

Effects of Anesthetic Agents on the Hepatic System

Hepatic Blood Flow

The liver is unique in that it receives nutrients and oxygen from a dual circulation: one arterial and one venous. Approximately 30% of the total cardiac output (1,450 ml of blood per minute) is directed to the liver. Under normal physiologic circumstances, the portal vein delivers 75% of total hepatic blood flow (THBF) and the hepatic artery provides 25%. Prior to entry into the portal circulation, blood leaving the preportal system—the gastrointestinal tract, spleen, and pancreas—has been partially deoxygenated. Portal vein flow supplies 50 to 55% of total hepatic oxygen (Fig. 7–26).

The hepatic circulation is different from that of other vital circulatory beds, such as the cerebral, coronary, and renal circulatory beds, in that both hepatic arterial and portal venous flow exhibit minimal autoregulation (Fig. 7–27).[428–431] Hepatic artery flow is regulated by the arterioles of the liver. Normally, hepatic artery resistance is high (i.e., there is a greater than 100-mm Hg pressure drop through the hepatic circulation).[431] Portal flow is not markedly affected by changes in the intrahepatic portal system and is regulated by the preportal system.[431] When portal vein flow is compromised, increases in hepatic artery blood flow can offset decreased total hepatic oxygen delivery even though total increase in hepatic artery blood flow is only a fraction of the deficient portal vein flow. This phenomenon has been termed the "hepatic arterial buffer response."[432,433] Increases in hepatic

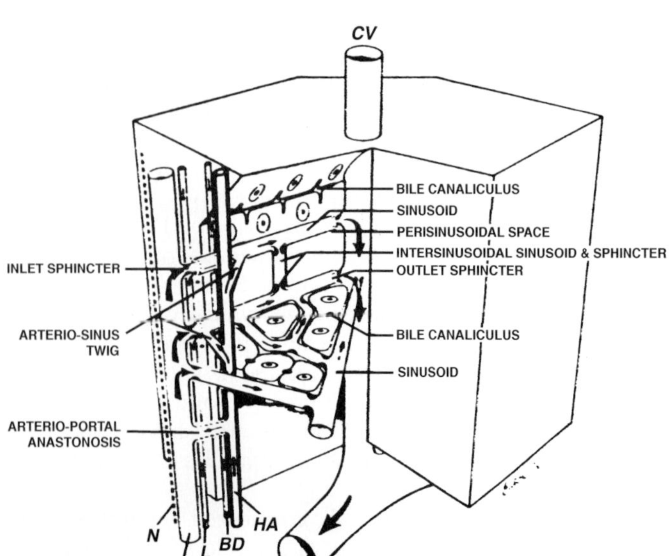

FIGURE 7–26. Diagram of the hepatic microvasculature. PV, portal venule; HA, hepatic arteriole; L, lymphatic; B, bile ductule; N, nerve; CV, central venule; SLV, sublobular hepatic venule. (From Ballet F: Hepatic circulation: Potential for therapeutic intervention. Pharmacol Ther 47:281, 1990. Copyright 1990, Elsevier Science, with permission.)

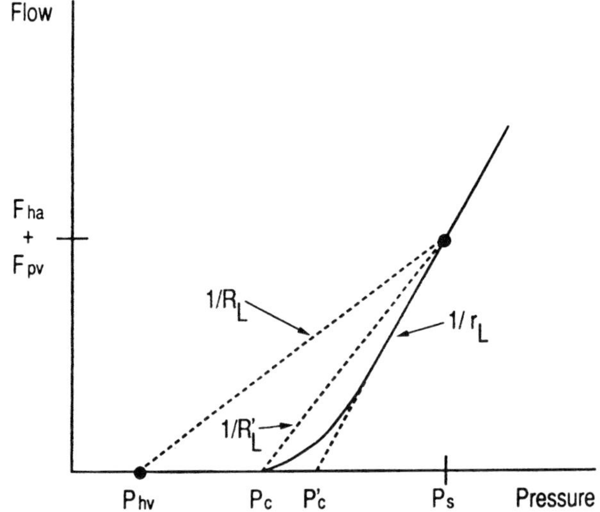

FIGURE 7–27. Idealized pressure-flow characteristic of hepatic resistance showing calculation and interpretation of pertinent resistances and pressures. F_{ha} + F_{pv}, hepatic + portal vein flow; F_L, total liver blood flow at normal sinusoid pressure (P_S); Phv, hepatic venous pressure; P_c, closing pressure; P'_c, weighted arithmetic mean of all closing pressures; R_L, outflow resistance, R'_L, liver resistance taking into account the existence of closing pressures; r_L, incremental resistance. (From Ballet F: Hepatic circulation: Potential for therapeutic intervention. Pharmacol Ther 47:281, 1990. Copyright 1990 Elsevier Science, with permission.)

arterial flow can also ameliorate deficiencies in hepatic clearance of endogenous and exogenous compounds. Factors that affect preportal circulation, such as vasoconstrictive state of the preportal circulation, cardiac output, arterial blood pressure, and blood volume, can greatly influence portal vein blood flow.[434]

Hepatic artery flow, relative to that of the portal vein, is regulated by neural, hormonal, and myogenic factors, in addition to mediators derived from portal vein blood and hepatic metabolism.[435,436] α-Adrenergic stimulation is predominately responsible for governing flow to and from the liver by regulating intrahepatic flow,[437] through increases in hepatic artery and portal resistance and portal vein pressure. Cholinergic stimulation appears to play a minimal role in the regulation of total hepatic flow.[438,439]

Various vasoactive substances (adenosine, serotonin, prostaglandins, leukotrienes, neuropeptides, free radicals, endothelin, and nitric oxide) have been suggested to regulate sinusoidal pressure.[440] Of these local mediators, adenosine may have a particularly important position in increasing portal vein flow during periods of decreased hepatic perfusion.[445] Selective adenosine antagonism has been shown to markedly inhibit the hepatic arterial buffer response. There appears to be much intralobar heterogeneity of the liver's response to these various vasoactive substances.

Adrenergic stimulation and local vasoactive substances are intimately involved in regulating the exchange of nutrients across sinusoids. This regulation involves alterations in capillary hydrostatic pressure, permeability coefficients of the sinusoidal capillaries, and presinusoidal capillary sphincters.

Effects of Laparotomy and Surgery on Hepatic Blood Flow

Surgical procedures such as laparotomy may significantly reduce hepatic and splanchnic blood flow.[436,441–444] Peripheral procedures cause minor changes in THBF; major abdominal procedures result in sizable decreases in THBF.[445] THBF decreases 30% following the stress of laparotomy,[446] primarily from decreased portal vein flow despite secondary increases in hepatic artery flow.[436,443] It has been emphasized that: "(1) surgical intervention, rather than anesthesia, is the main determinate of alterations in splanchnic circulation, and that (2) anesthesia can play a modifying role for circulatory disturbances during surgical stress."[436]

Traction and manipulation of splanchnic organs during surgery decreases THBF and explains in part why peripheral procedures and procedures distal to the liver have smaller perturbations in THBF.[447] Catecholamine release and activation of the renin-angiotensin system may also significantly alter THBF.[448,449]

Effects of Physiologic Factors on Hepatic Blood Flow

Positive-pressure ventilation is associated with decreased splanchnic and hepatic blood flow.[450] Large tidal volumes and positive end-expiratory pressure further decrease splanchnic and hepatic blood flows.[434,451–453] Changes in hepatic flow with positive-pressure ventilation may be related to compression of splanchnic organs and to effects of positive-pressure ventilation[454] on venous return and cardiac output.[436,455]

Hypercarbia increases preportal circulation[456–458] via dilation of mesenteric artery flow[459] and also enhances portal vein flow.[460] Hypercarbia either decreases or does not affect hepatic artery flow.

Hypocarbia decreases THBF and increases splanchnic vascular resistance; while portal vein flow decreases, hepatic arterial flow increases, and hepatic arterial resistance decreases. Hypocarbia also increases arteriovenous shunting within preportal organs.[436,461]

The relationship between plasma CO_2 and hepatic blood flow is complex. Hypercapnia has a more profound effect on hepatic blood flow than does hypocapnia.[434]

Discrepancies in the reported effect of plasma CO_2 on directional changes in hepatic artery, portal vein, and total hepatic flood flow may be related to alterations in systemic hemodynamics specific to experimental design. Most studies have been in general agreement about these directional changes.[434,460]

Hypoxia has been reported to have conflicting effects on the hepatic circulation. *Hypoxia* has been shown to increase hepatic flow,[462] predominantly via increases in hepatic artery flow,[463] or have no effect on THBF.[456]

Hemodilution is uniformly used today during cardiopulmonary bypass. It has been shown to decrease portal vein oxygen content and increase portal vein blood flow. Lesser increases in hepatic artery blood flow have also been reported. Whether total oxygen delivery to the liver is significantly impaired by hemodilution is unknown.[436]

Decreased hepatic oxygen delivery secondary to hemodilution may, in fact, be important in the etiology of hepatic damage and dysfunction following cardiopulmonary bypass.[464]

Effects of Anesthetics on Hepatic Blood Flow

Most agents decrease total splanchnic blood flow.[436] Inhalational anesthetics influence THBF, hepatic artery, and portal vein flows via their effects on systemic and regional hemodynamics and through the modulation of the body's neural and hormonal response to surgery. Many effects of inhalational agents are believed specifically related to anesthetic effects on the preportal circulation.

HALOTHANE

Preportal blood flow is reduced by halothane. This reduction in preportal blood flow parallels changes in cardiac output and blood pressure. During halothane anesthesia, cardiac output is the main determinant of portal vein flow and, to a lesser extent, a determinant of hepatic artery flow. Although halothane is a hepatic artery vasoconstrictor, its major effect on hepatic artery flow is related to changes in systemic hemodynamics. Halothane inhibits the hepatic arterial buffer response, so decreases in portal blood flow are not met with compensatory increases in hepatic artery flow. Halothane anesthesia can exacerbate hepatic hypoxia by decreasing portal oxygen delivery and increasing oxygen extraction in the preportal circulatory system. Halothane interferes with hypercarbia-induced splanchnic vasoconstriction[436,465] and, therefore, is a particularly poor agent to use in situations in which hypoventilation and hypoxia are likely to occur.

Through its effect on hepatic blood flow, halothane can prolong the half-life of certain drugs, and possibly alter protein binding. This is particularly true for propofol, ketamine, morphine, fentanyl, sufentanil, midazolam, β-blockers and lidocaine, which have high extraction ratios.[466] The metabolism of low-extraction-ratio drugs, such as barbiturates and diazepam, is primarily unaffected by halothane (Fig. 7–28).

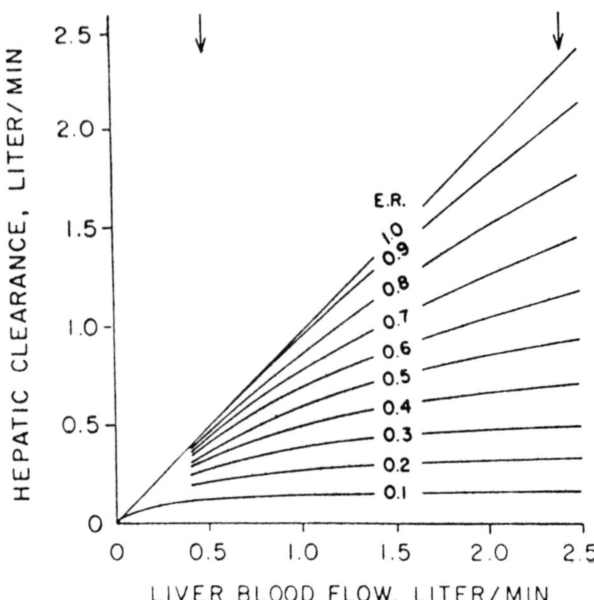

FIGURE **7–28.** Effect of increasing liver blood flow on the hepatic clearance of drugs with varying extraction ratios. For drugs with low extraction ratios, increases in liver blood flow produce little change in hepatic clearance. For drugs with high extraction ratios, increasing liver blood flow greatly increases hepatic clearance. (From Wood AJJ: Drug disposition and pharmacokinetics. In Wood M, Wood AJJ (eds): Drugs and Anesthesia: Pharmacology for Anesthesiologists, 2nd ed. 1990, p 27, with permission.)

ENFLURANE

Enflurane use is associated with decreased portal blood flow, which parallels changes in cardiac output. The ratio of hepatic artery flow to systemic cardiac output is increased, although this increase in hepatic artery flow does not compensate for decreased portal vein flow and oxygen delivery, hence THBF decreases. Although enflurane decreases portal vein flow, it does so to a lesser extent than halothane; enflurane preserves splanchnic blood flow and liver oxygen supply better than halothane in equipotent doses.

ISOFLURANE

Isoflurane decreases blood flow through the preportal circulation, as described for the other inhalational anesthetics. This decrease in THBF is related to decreased cardiac output. Perturbations in the preportal circulation occur to a lesser extent with isoflurane than with enflurane or halothane. Hepatic arterial blood flow increases with isoflurane, which probably represents better preservation of the hepatic arterial buffer response. The net result of isoflurane use is a decrease in portal vein flow and an increase in hepatic artery flow[467]; net THBF is unchanged or slightly increased during isoflurane. Following ischemic episodes, reperfusion and hepatic lactate uptake is supranormal in animals anesthetized with fentanyl or isoflurane, but remains subnormal in animals anesthetized with enflurane, halothane, or barbiturates. In patients undergoing surgery involving interruption of hepatic flow, such as thoracic aortic surgery, surgery following hepatic trauma, liver transplantation, or cardiac procedures requiring total circulatory arrest, isoflurane or fentanyl are preferable to halothane or enflurane.[468,469]

DESFLURANE

Desflurane maintains hepatic artery blood flow and hepatic vascular resistance. At high concentrations, desflurane decreases total hepatic blood flow, predominantly through a decrease in portal vein flow.[406,470]

SEVOFLURANE

Sevoflurane reduces portal vein blood flow at 1.5 and 2 MAC, although to a lesser extent than does halothane or enflurane. Total hepatic artery flow and total hepatic oxygen delivery are maintained with sevoflurane. Total hepatic blood flow is preserved to a similar extent with sevoflurane and isoflurane, although the hepatic arterial buffer response is not preserved as well with sevoflurane as it is with isoflurane.[471]

NITROUS OXIDE

Nitrous oxide, without inhalational agents, has minimal effects on the splanchnic and hepatic circulations.[402,436] Prolonged use of N_2O may result in accumulation of intestinal gas, which may reduce flow through the preportal circulation and decrease portal vein flow by compressing intestinal capillaries.[436]

In summary, isoflurane and sevoflurane preserve THBF better than desflurane and much better than enflurane and halothane. The hepatic arterial buffer response is better preserved with isoflurane than desflurane and sevoflurane, less well with enflurane, and least well with halothane. Of all the inhalational agents, halothane is particularly poor in allowing increased hepatic artery flow to compensate for decreased portal vein flow.

Halothane Hepatitis

Postoperative hepatic dysfunction has been associated with inhalational agents since the era of diethyl ether anesthesia,[472,473] with halothane the most commonly implicated agent.[474] The first reports of unexplained jaundice following halothane anesthesia appeared in 1957.[475,476] With an incidence of between 1 in 6,000 and 1 in 20,000 anesthetics, halothane-associated hepatitis is an uncommon occurrence; however, it is a potentially serious complication of halothane use, which can progress to fulminant hepatic failure and death.[447–479] The mortality for halothane hepatitis is as high as 50%,[480] with patients who proceed to fulminant hepatic failure having a greater than 75% mortality.[481]

In 1969, the National Institutes of Health formulated the U.S. National Halothane Study to investigate reports of halothane-associated hepatitis.[482] This retrospective study examined 856,000 general anesthetics and identified 82 cases of fatal hepatic necrosis. Of 255,000 patients who received halothane, 7 deaths could not be attributed to other causes,[248] and in four of these seven cases, patients had received halothane on more than one occasion. The incidence of fatal hepatopathy associated with halothane use from these data is 1 death in 35,000 anesthetics.[479] The main conclusion to emerge from this study, nevertheless, was that halothane is generally safe and is only rarely associated with fatal hepatopathy.[248,479] This study has been criticized because of its retrospective nature, and because pathologic examination of the liver was obtained in only 40% of patients deaths.[479]

The U.S. National Halothane Study reported a 10 to 20% increase in serum transaminases following repeated exposure to halothane.[480,482] Halothane use is associated with an increase in sensitive serum markers of hepatic damage (such as glutathione S-transferase). Increase in these markers has not been witnessed with isoflurane use.[483,484] Halothane also may cause ultrastructural, electromicrographic, hepatic changes that are not seen with isoflurane.[485] Results from several small prospective studies investigating changes in liver function tests in patients undergoing minor surgery have yielded varying results[486–492]; however, most conclude that, although halothane is associated with alterations in liver biochemistries and possibly ultrastructural changes, its use does not usually manifest as full-blown "halothane hepatitis."[479]

There are many causes of postoperative jaundice and abnormalities in liver biochemistries, including viral hepatitis, septicemia, hepatopathies from other hepatotoxins, intra- and postoperative hypoxia and hypotension, as well as surgical trauma to liver, and pre-existing or coexisting liver disease.[473] Anesthetic-related hepatitis is a diagnosis of exclusion; these causes should be excluded before this diagnosis is given to a patient with postoperative hepatic dysfunction.

Risk Factors for Developing Halothane Hepatitis

Over the almost four decades since halothane hepatitis was first described, several risk factors which place the patient at jeopardy of developing this disease have been identified (Table 7–9).

GENETIC PREDISPOSITION

Patients who develop halothane hepatitis have different frequencies of specific HLA antigen than control groups. Halothane hepatitis may occur within family groups.[493] In rat and guinea pig models of halothane hepatitis, there is a genetic variation in susceptibility,[494] with the possible patter of transmission for nonsusceptibility to halothane hepatitis sex-linked and of variable penetrance.

REPEATED HALOTHANE ANESTHESIA

The risk of halothane hepatitis increases with repeated exposure, especially over short intervals of time.[477–479,495] More than 80% of patients who develop hepatic necrosis have had multiple exposures to halothane.[495] Hepatic dysfunction after multiple exposure to halothane is associated with a higher mortality rate than after a single exposure.[479] Short intervals between exposures are associated with more severe cases of hepatic necrosis.[497] Explanations for more severe hepatic necrosis with repeated exposures over short intervals of time include:

TABLE 7–9
Possible Risk Factors for Halothane Hepatitis*

Genetic predisposition
Repeated halothane anesthesia
Obesity
Middle age or older
Female sex
Enzyme induction

*From Husser AJ, Aldridge LM, Paul D, et al: Plasma glutathione-S-transferase concentration as a measure of hepatocellular integrity following a single general anaesthetics with halothane, enflurane, and isoflurane. Br J Anaesth 60:130, 1988. Copyright 1988, BMJ Publishing Group, with permission.

(1) halothane's metabolites may act as haptens for subsequent antibody formation; (2) halothane may induce its own metabolism, resulting in larger amounts of toxic metabolites; and (3) if halothane causes liver injury on the first exposure, injured liver may respond differently on repeated exposures.[486]

OBESITY

Halothane hepatitis is more common in obese patients.[498,499] Obese patients may metabolize halothane more extensively than the nonobese.[500] There is a higher incidence of fatty liver in these patients preoperatively, and these patients may have different regional hepatic oxygenation and blood flow than their nonobese counterparts.[481]

MIDDLE AGE OR OLDER

Middle-aged patients have the highest incidence of halothane hepatitis.[479,481,499] The incidence in children appears to be much lower than that of adults, between 1 in 82,000 and 1 in 200,000.[501,502] Peak incidence occurs over the age of 40, with most occurring between 50 and 60 years of age.[481] This differential incidence of halothane-related hepatic dysfunction has also been noted in a guinea pig model of the disease.[503]

FEMALE SEX

Females have twice the incidence of halothane hepatitis than do their male counterparts, although males may have a worse prognosis.[499] In animal models, females have more extensive metabolism of halothane than males. This fact may explain the increased incidence in females,[481] although it has not been conclusively determined if clinically significant gender differences exist in the rate of metabolism of halothane in human.[481] Due to differences in total body fat composition from males, females may store more halothane and its metabolites in the perioperative period. Some of these gender dissimilarities in the incidence of halothane hepatitis are attributed to differences in the rate of metabolism of halothane in each gender group.[481]

ENZYME INDUCTION

Halothane may induce its own metabolism by increasing the activity of microsomal enzymes, such as the cytochrome P-450 system. Induction of enzymes involved in reductive metabolism appears to be more crucial to the pathogenesis of halothane-related hepatopathy than induction of oxidative metabolism.[248,492,500,504,505] Animal models in which subjects are pretreated with barbiturates, an inducer of microsomal enzymes, have increased hepatic injury.[506] Patients undergoing neurosurgical procedures who have been taking barbiturates for seizure disorders also appear to have slightly more frequent and extensive hepatic injury postoperatively.[507]

A general cause-and-effect relationship between induction of microsomal enzymes and halothane-related hepatotoxicity cannot be stated. Inhibition of microsomal enzymes with the H_2-blocker cimetidine does not decrease hepatic damage following exposure to halothane.[508] In animal studies, induction of microsomal enzymes with phenytoin or isoniazid does not affect halothane metabolism or hepatotoxicity.[504,505]

It has been generally advised that halothane should be avoided in patients with pre-existing liver disease.[481] There is no conclusive evidence that patients with pre-existing liver disease are at greater risk of halothane hepatitis than those in the general patient population.[479,509] Similarly, duration and site of surgery do not necessarily correlate with incidence of halothane hepatitis.[510]

Pathology of Halothane Hepatitis

By light microscopy, halothane hepatitis is similar to viral hepatitis. The most predominant feature of halothane hepatitis is centrilobular necrosis. Other pathologic features include balloon degradation of hepatocytes, fatty infiltration, inflammatory cell infiltration, and stromal fibrosis.[479,510–515] Electromicrographic features include mitochondrial membrane abnormalities and an increase in the number of hepatic cellular lysozymes.[485,512]

Proposed Mechanisms of Hepatic Injury

There are three proposed mechanisms of hepatic injury from halothane: (1) direct hepatic toxicity from reductive metabolites of halothane biotransformation, (2) hepatic cellular deprivation, and (3) immunologic-mediated hepatopathy.

Twenty per cent of halothane undergoes biotransformation via the microsomal cytochrome P-450 system of the liver.[516] There are two metabolic pathways of halothane biotransformation: *oxidative* and *reductive*.[479] The oxidative pathway is predominant in times of high hepatic oxygen content and high redox states. The reductive pathway predominates during periods of low oxygen delivery and low redox states. Substrates such as volatile anesthetic agents accept electrons from microsomal cytochromes. *Oxidative* metabolism results in the production of trifluroacetic acid (TFA-halide) and bromide, while *reductive* metabolism produces 1-chloro2,2,2-trifluroethyl radical, 2-chloro-1,1,1, trifluroenthane, 2-chloro-1-1,-trifluroethane, and fluroide ion[506] (Fig. 7–29).

The *metabolic theory of halothane hepatopathy* states that metabolic products or intermediaries of reductive oxidation are directly toxic to hepatocytes. Free radicals are potential hepatotoxins produced during reductive metabolism. The metabolic theory of halothane hepatopathy is supported by evidence that products of reductive metabolism covalently bind to hepatocytes.[517] This binding is enhanced by barbiturate induction, occurs in the microsomal portion of the liver, and depends on the cytochrome P-450 system. Covalent bonding is enhanced during periods of hypoxia.[479]

Although this theory is often used to explain the mechanism of halothane hepatitis, there are certain clinical and experimental data that are not consistent with the theory:

1. No end product of halothane metabolism has been shown to be directly hepatotoxic. This finding, how-

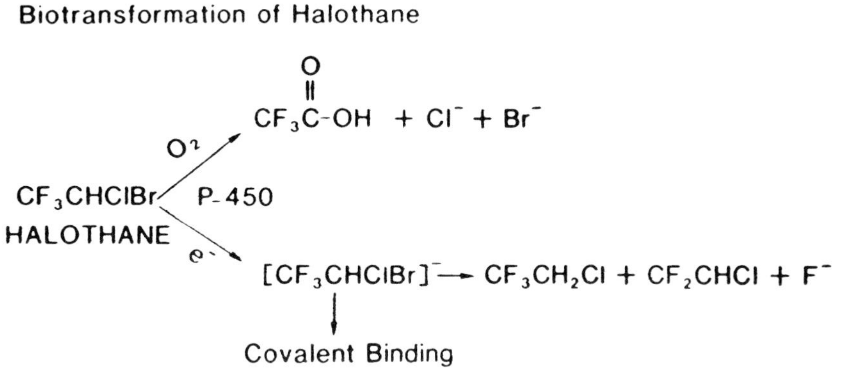

Biotransformation of Halothane

$$CF_3CHClBr \text{ (HALOTHANE)} \xrightarrow[P\text{-}450]{O_2} CF_3\overset{O}{\overset{\|}{C}}\text{-}OH + Cl^- + Br^-$$

$$CF_3CHClBr \xrightarrow[P\text{-}450]{e^-} [CF_3CHClBr]^- \longrightarrow CF_3CH_2Cl + CF_2CHCl + F^-$$

$$[CF_3CHClBr]^- \downarrow \text{Covalent Binding}$$

FIGURE **7–29.** Proposed pathways for the oxidative and reductive biotransformation of halothane by hepatic cytochrome. (From Lind RC, Gandolfi AJ, Sipes IG: Oxygen concentrations required for reductive defluorination of halothane by rat hepatic microsomes. Anesth Analg 65:835, 1986, with permission.)

ever, does not mean that intermediaries of halothane metabolism are not hepatotoxic.
2. Halothane hepatopathy is not usually associated with systemic hypoxia.
3. Free radical formation occurs only in a narrow window of oxygen tensions, which rarely occur in clinical practice.
4. Fasting increases hepatotoxicity; however, it does not appear to affect halothane metabolism.
5. Guinea pigs have minimal reductive metabolism of halothane; however, they develop hepatotoxicity after halothane exposure.[473]

There is an abundance of evidence from animal experimentation to support the role of *hypoxia in the pathogenesis of halothane hepatopathy*. The outer portion of the hepatic acinar, centrilobular region (zone 3) appears particularly susceptible to oxygen deprivation injury. Centrilobular necrosis may be produced experimentally by the induction of hypoxia following barbiturate exposure, even in the absence of inhalation agents.[518,519] All volatile agents decrease hepatic perfusion.[436] With respect to hepatic perfusion and oxygen consumption, isoflurane has certain theoretical advantages over enflurane and halothane. The order of hepatotoxicity parallels degree of perturbations in hepatic circulation[436] (see "Hepatic Blood Flow," above).

Arguments against the hypoxic/hypoperfusional etiology of halothane hepatopathy are: (1) halothane hepatopathy is not usually associated with *systemic* hypoxia; and (2) although there is a theoretical argument that surgical stimulation may lead to sympathetic-mediated vasoconstriction of splanchnic circulation, this has not been found evident in placebo-controlled studies using epidural catheters to abolish sympathetic (T8–T12) stimulation of these circulatory beds.[481,520]

Decreased hepatic perfusion and regional hypoxia do not appear to be primary pathophysiologic factors in the etiology of halothane hepatopathy; the role of derangements in hepatic circulation in the setting of other primary insults (immunologic or direct hepatotoxic) remains to be determined.

IMMUNOLOGIC-MEDIATED HEPATOPATHY

A role for immunologic-mediated injury in halothane-related hepatopathy has been postulated. Halothane hepatopathy is dose independent, associated with peripheral eosinophilia and circulating antibodies, and is often associated with rash and fever. Halothane metabolism produces metabolites that covalently bind to heptocytes and act as haptens.[248] (see Table 7–10).

In 1978, Vergani reported that white cells from patients with halothane hepatitis were sensitized to homogenates of liver from halothane-anesthetized rabbits. Sera from patients with halothane hepatitis contain antibodies to antigens present on specimens of liver from rabbits anesthetized with halothane. These sera do not react with hepatocytes from rabbits anesthetized with ether. These antibodies are found only in patients with halothane hepatitis and not in patients with other hepatopathies.[521,522]

Oxidative metabolism results in production of TFA-halide. Antibodies from patients with halothane hepatitis appear to be reactive against liver microsomal polypeptides conjugated with TFA-halide (TFA-adducts). Five specific antigen species have been identified and distinguished based on molecular weight of the specific antigen (100, 76, 59, 57, and 54 kDa). Specimens from patients with halothane hepatitis contain these antigens. Similar antigens have been detected in rabbits and rats treated with halothane. Furthermore, it has been shown that removal of TFA hapten from rat liver microsomes by treating it with 1 mol piperidine removes all reactivity with sera from patients with halothane hepatitis. Halothane hepatitis patients contain cytotoxic lymphocytes against these antigens.

Halothane hepatitis usually occurs about 5 days after exposure, or re-exposure, to halothane, although intraoperative liver biopsies from patients undergoing halo-

TABLE **7–10**
Clinical Markers of Halothane Hepatitis*

Gender (female)	70%
Obesity	63%
Repeated exposure	78%
Fever	75%
Eosinophilia	30%
Rash	10%
Autoantibodies	29%

*Modified from Neuberger J, Williams R: Halothane hepatitis. Dig Dig 6:52, 1988.
Based on Brown BR Jr, Gandolfi AJ: Adverse effects of volatile anaesthetics. Br J Anaesth 59:14, 1987. Copyright 1987, BMJ Publishing Group, with permission.

thane anesthesia revealed TFA-adduct antibodies at the time of initial exposure.

Recently, several laboratories have developed enzyme-linked immunosorbent assay (ELISA)–based assays for the presence of these antibodies in patients suspected of having halothane hepatitis. Liver biopsies may also be tested for TFA-adduct antigens.

Hepatotoxicity of Other Inhalational Agents

ENFLURANE

Enflurane has been associated with postoperative hepatic dysfunction.[523] Some of the earlier reports of enflurane hepatitis have been criticized.[473,524] A more thorough review of 88 suspected cases of enflurane-associated hepatic dysfunction revealed 15 cases that were related to enflurane administration.[525] Unlike halothane, repeated exposure to enflurane does not appear to increase hepatotoxicity.[486] Enflurane has similar effects to halothane on hepatic artery and portal vein flow; it differs in that enflurane preserves global hepatic perfusion better than halothane.[436,461,479]

Enflurane lies between halothane and isoflurane in its degree of biometabolism and perhaps its potential for hepatotoxicity. Enflurane does not undergo extensive biotransformation (e.g., 2.4% of inhaled dose). Metabolism does not produce significant free radicals[525,526] (Fig. 7–30). Enflurane metabolites may be able to form adducts that bind to hepatocyte microsomes. Enflurane metabolites may covalently bind cellular macromolecules.[527]

The incidence of enflurane-associated hepatitis is low, estimated at 1 in 800,000 patients exposed to enflurane, and is controversial if this entity exists at all.[248,491]

ISOFLURANE

Isoflurane is generally felt to be devoid of hepatotoxic potential. This has been attributed to limited metabolism of the drug, namely, 0.17% of absorbed isoflurane is recovered in the form of urinary metabolites.[528] Isoflurane does not undergo reductive metabolism,[529,530] nor is it metabolized to free radicals.[531,532] Isoflurane tends to maintain hepatic blood flow better than halothane or enflurane.[530] It decreases portal vein flow but increases hepatic artery flow, with little net change in hepatic perfusion.[436,461,479]

Forty-five instances of hepatic dysfunction after isoflurane anesthesia were reviewed by a subcommittee of the Food and Drug Administration's Anesthesia and Life Support Drug Advisory Committee. The subcommittee concluded that it was unlikely that isoflurane was responsible for the occurrence of postoperative hepatic dysfunction.[531] Histologic changes within the liver do not occur after prolonged anesthetic and subanesthetic exposure.[525]

DESFLURANE AND SEVOFLURANE

Desflurane does not appear to cause hepatic dysfunction. In healthy volunteers, inhalation of up to 2.1 MAC-hours

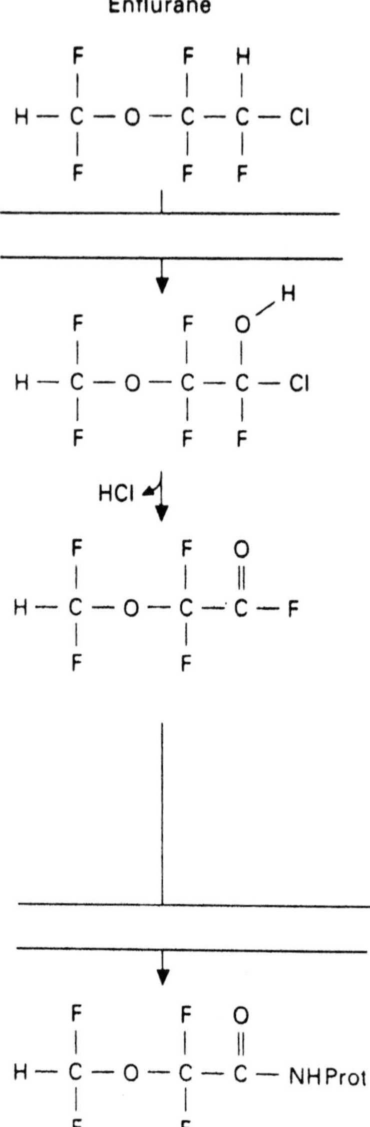

FIGURE **7–30.** Biotransformation of enflurane via oxidative metabolism and subsequent generation of TFA molecule. (From Elliott RH, Strunin L: Hepatotoxicity of volatile anesthetics. Br J Anaesth 70:339, 1993. Copyright 1993, BMJ Publishing Group, with permission.)

of desflurane does not produce increases in serum liver biochemistries.[426,427] Desflurane is identical to isoflurane except for a substitution of a methyl group for a fluoride on the α carbon.[426] Desflurane undergoes little biotransformation; only 0.02% of the drug undergoes biotransformation, making it the least metabolized of the currently used halogenated inhalational agents[427] (Fig. 7–31). The potential for free radical formation or oxidative metabolic haptens is minimal.[533,534] This lack of hepatopathic potential with desflurane has been substantiated in animal models with prolonged exposure.[535] In patients with chronic hepatic dysfunction, anesthesia with desflurane or isoflurane does not adversely effect serum liver biochemistries.[425]

Sevoflurane is a fluoridated derivative of ethyl isopropyl ether that appears to undergo extensive defluorina-

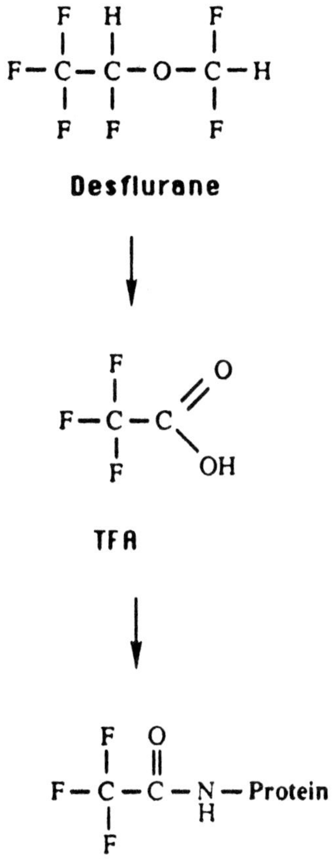

Desflurane

TFA

FIGURE 7–31. Theoretical production of trifluoroacetyl protein hapten (antigen) after hepatic degradation of desflurane to trifluoroacetic acid (TFA). (From Koblin DD: Characteristics and implications of desflurane metabolism and toxicity. Anesth Analg 75:510, 1992, with permission.)

tion[528] (Fig. 7–32). Prolonged anesthesia with greater than an average of 4.7 MAC-hours produces serum fluoride levels of greater than 50 μmol/L.[471] Defluorination has been shown to increase pretreatment with isoniazid or phenobarbital.[536,537] Although serum transaminases do not increase with sevoflurane administration, indirect bilirubin rises.[471] Sevoflurane undergoes extensive metabolism, yet this is unlikely to result in immunogenic hepatotoxic metabolites.[473] To date there are no reports of clinical cases of fulminant hepatic failure causally linked with sevoflurane usage.[473]

NITROUS OXIDE

Nitrous oxide inhibits hepatic methionine synthetase activity.[533] Nitrous oxide does not increase liver serum biochemistries one or three days postoperative. The safety of nitrous oxide with relation to hepatotoxicity is evident in both young and old patients. One study in the literature[538] indicates that patients anesthetized with halothane and oxygen have less of an increase in serum transaminases than those anesthetized with halothane and nitrous oxide; as long as hypoxia is avoided, the use of nitrous oxide should be considered safe, even in patients with hepatic dysfunction.[539]

Hepatic Effects of Intravenous Anesthetic Agents

Effects on Hepatic Blood Flow (Table 7–11)

KETAMINE

In vitro ketamine is a direct vasodilator[540]; however, in an intestinal loop preparation[541] an in intact animals[542–544] it produces hepatic artery and splanchnic circulatory vasoconstriction. This discrepancy is probably secondary to ketamine's in vivo effect of sympathetic release.[545] Ketamine has been reported to have no effect on,[546] or increases by approximately 30%, portal vein blood flow.[543,547] Total hepatic blood flow decrease under ketamine anesthesia,[542] and preportal AV shunting increases, as with halothane.[436]

ETOMIDATE

Etomidate is generally considered devoid of systemic hemodynamic effects, yet its administration may significantly influence the hepatic circulation, by decreasing hepatic artery blood flow.[458] It produces a greater change in hepatic arterial resistance and decreases in hepatic artery blood flow than barbiturates.[458] This effect is

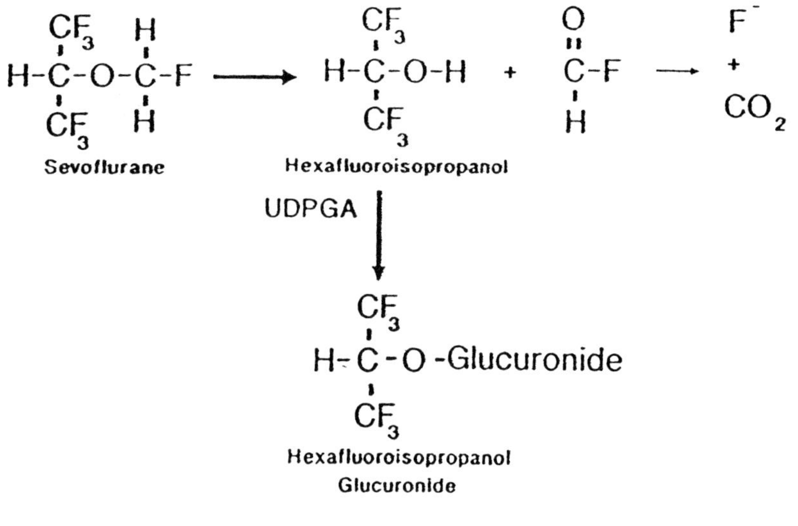

Sevoflurane

Hexafluoroisopropanol

UDPGA

Hexafluoroisopropanol Glucuronide

FIGURE 7–32. Proposed biotransformation of sevoflurane. UDPGA, uridine diphosphate glucuronic acid. (From Frink EJ, Ghantous H, Malan TP, et al: Plasma inorganic fluoride with sevoflurane anesthesia: Correlation with indices of hepatic and renal function. Anesth Analg 74:231, 1992, with permission.)

TABLE 7–11
Summary of Effects of IV Anesthetic Agents on Hepatic Circulation

Agent	Splanchnic Flow	Hepatic Artery Flow	Portal Vein Flow	Total Hepatic Blood Flow	Hepatic Oxygen Consumption
Ketamine	⇓	⇓	⇔ or ⇑	⇓	
Etomidate	⇓	⇓	⇓	⇓	⇔
Low-dose	⇓				
High-dose	⇑	⇑	⇓		
Barbiturates					
Low-dose	⇔ or ⇓	⇓	⇓	⇓	⇓
High-dose	⇑			⇓	
Opiates					
Morphine					
Low-dose	⇑	⇑	⇑	⇑	⇔
Intermediate-dose	⇑	⇑	⇑	⇑	⇔
High-dose	⇓			⇓	⇔
Fentanyl	⇑	⇔ or ⇑	⇑	⇔ or ⇑	⇔ or ⇑
Sufentanil	?	?	?	⇓	
Alfentanil	?	⇓	?	?	
Propofol				⇔ or ⇑	⇔

⇑, Increased; ⇓, Decreased; ⇔, no change; ?, unknown or not well researched.

thought to result from hepatic artery vasoconstriction. Low-dose etomidate produces increased mesenteric artery resistance. At higher infusion rates mesenteric resistance drops and portal vein flow is decreased. Hepatic oxygen consumption is maintained by increased oxygen extraction and a mild increase in hepatic artery flow. Administration of etomidate blunts the hepatic buffer response.[458,548]

BARBITURATES

The hepatic circulation is generally assumed to be not dramatically affected by barbiturates. Effects of barbiturates on the splanchnic circulation have yielded contradictory results.[436] Some investigators have not found dramatic effects of barbiturates on splanchnic blood flow,[445,549] while others have demonstrated dramatically decreased splanchnic blood flow.[550,551] Bolus doses of barbiturates dilate preportal vessels and increase splanchnic blood flow,[552] transiently mirroring the time course of the cerebral effect of barbiturates.

At low infusion doses (205 μg/kg/min) barbiturates are vasoconstrictors of the splanchnic circulation. Hepatic artery, portal vein, and THBF decrease at low dosages of barbiturates at which cardiac output and systemic vascular resistance remain unchanged.[553] Hepatic and mesenteric arteries vasoconstrict at low dosages, decreasing hepatic blood flow. At higher infusion doses, barbiturates decrease hepatic flow through effects on systemic hemodynamics, even though at these doses thiopentone is a hepatic artery vasodilator. During barbiturate infusion hepatic oxygen consumption is maintained, although hepatic oxygen delivery may decrease. This effect is mediated by increased oxygen extraction by hepatic cells and increased hepatic artery blood flow relative to hepatic vein flow. The hepatic buffer response is not maintained with barbiturates.[458,548]

OPIATES

Morphine in low dosages (0.2 mg/kg) is an intestinal vasodilator and at massive dosages (3 to 5 mg/kg) is an intestinal vasoconstrictor.[554–557] The administration of intermediate dosages of morphine (2 mg/kg) results in splanchnic vasodilation; at this dose morphine increases hepatic artery and portal vein blood flow.[555] The mediator of the physiologic response at lower doses appears to be histamine release and a possible decrease in central sympathetic activity. At higher morphine dosages catecholamine-mediated α-adrenergic response predominates.[448,554] *Fentanyl* produces dose-related splanchnic vasodilation.[468,554] Fentanyl administration maintains or increases THBF without changing systemic hemodynamics by increasing portal vein flow and maintaining hepatic artery blood flow.[446,554,558] Hepatic circulatory parameters do not correlate with systemic hemodynamics during fentanyl infusion[446]; this implies that the effect of fentanyl on hepatic circulation is independent of systemic hemodynamic changes and is predicated on preportal circulatory changes. Fentanyl increases portal vein oxygen content while maintaining the hepatic oxygen supply/uptake relationship; this should help maintain hepatic oxygen delivery during times of decreased hepatic blood flow during fentanyl use.[446,468,469,554]

Sufentanil decreases total hepatic blood flow by 24% after induction doses of 0.1 mg/kg in association with parallel decreases in cardiac output (26%) and MAP (20%). During this period, the hepatic demand/delivery relationship remained unchanged.[559]

Alfentanil, in doses associated with systemic hypotension, reduces hepatic artery blood flow. A bolus dose of 3 μg/kg followed by an infusion (45 μg/kg/min) produces a decrease in hepatic arterial flow by 60%. Whether this is a consequence of global decreases in THBF or a consequence of reciprocal changes resulting from increased preportal and portal vein flow remains to be determined.[436]

PROPOFOL

Propofol has been reported to have variable effects on hepatic blood flow.[560,561] After a bolus dosage, THBF decreases as much as 40% then blood flow returns rapidly to baseline. Hepatic oxygen consumption is unaltered by a bolus dose of propofol.[466]

Effects on Liver Function Test

No significant or consistent change in liver biochemistries occurs after use of most intravenous agents. Studies with barbiturates, propofol, etomidate, fentanyl, and midazolam have not revealed adverse effects of intravenous agent on liver biochemistries.[248,555] Neuroleptanesthesia is also without adverse effect on liver biochemistries.[562,563] Ketamine has been associated with increased serum glutamate pyruvate transaminase (SGPT) and γ-glutamyltransferase (GGT) in 40% of patients after ketamine anesthesia.[564] The hypnotic/sedative agents have not been thoroughly investigated after repeated exposures.[555]

Effects on Hepatic Drug Metabolism and Hepatic Enzyme Activity

Of all the intravenous anesthetic agents, chronic administration of barbiturates is the only one consistently associated with *increased* hepatic cytochrome P-450 system activity.[565] Enzyme induction does not occur after a single exposure to thiopental.[566]

Propofol administration has been associated with *decreases* in cytochrome P-450 system activity.[567,568,569] Propofol has been shown to interfere with alfentanil and sufentanil metabolism in pigs and in humans[570]; however, it is not considered to affect the metabolism of inhalational agents.[568]

Etomidate *inhibits* cytochrome P-450 system activity in humans. Drugs with low hepatic clearance (such as diazepam, barbiturates, and theophylline) are most likely to be affected by propofol or etomidate inhibition of the cytochrome P-450 system.[571] Halothane has been shown

TABLE 7–12
Use of Anesthetic Agents in Patients with Porphyria

Class of Agents	Clinical Summary	Laboratory Assay
Barbiturates	Unsafe	Increases activity of ALA synthetase rat liver model and DCC-primed rat models
Benzodiazepines	Diazepam; clonazepam; chlorodiazepoxide, oxazepam probably unsafe; lorazepam safe; others unknown	Diazepam, clonazepam, chlorodiazepoxide, oxazepam probably unsafe; lorazepam safe
Opiates	Most opiates safe; morphine, methadone, merperidine sufentanil, codeine; fentanyl laboratory results questionable; however, probably clinically safe	Fentanyl stimulates heme biosynthesis in rats, used safely in human porphyrics; other opiates safe
Ketamine	Probably safe; rare reports of clinical exacerbations	ALA and DCC-primed rat model safe; increased ALA activity in chicken embryo assay
Etomidate	Probably safe	Increased ALA and DCC-primed rat activity
Propofol	Probably safe	Safe
Muscle relaxation	Safe: succinylcholine, d-tubocurarine, gallamine, and atracurium; pancuronium the most questionable of the muscle relaxants	Safe
Reversal agents	Neostigmine, prostigmine safe	Safe
Droperidol/diphenhydramine	Safe	Safe
Inhalational agents	Enflurane and isoflurane have been clinically safe; questionable results with halothane; clinical reports of exacerbation with methoxyflurane	Halothane: questionable results; enflurane and methoxyflurane intermediate ALA assay; sevoflurane and desflurane unknown
N_2O	Safe	Safe

ALA, 5-aminolevulinate synthase.

to inhibit the metabolism of intravenous agents such as fentanyl and ketamine.[565]

Effects of Intravenous Agents on Expression of Porphyria

Porphyria is a group of genetic and inherited diseases related to defects in the biosynthesis of heme with resultant increases in porphyrins and porphyrin precursors.[572,573] The incidence of porphyria varies from 1 in 1,000 to 1 in 80,000 depending on geographical location.[555] Intravenous anesthetic agents have long been implicated in precipitation of acute porphyria (Table 7–12). The majority of drugs that precipitate attacks of porphyria are lipid soluble, and induce cytochrome P-450 enzymes and 5-aminolevulinate synthetase (ALA).[576] Results of the porphyrinogenicity of various anesthetic agents have differed depending on the animal model used; however, barbiturates have been uniformly shown to be porphyrinogenic. The two most commonly used animal models to test porphyrinogenicity are: (1) the effect of the anesthetic agent on hepatic ALA activity in rat liver homogenate and (2) the DCC-primed rat model.[555] Results of these tests vary. Barbiturate, pentazocine, and etomidate increase ALA activity, while morphine, ketamine, morphine, diazepam, and nitrous oxide do not use.[555] Using this model, enflurane and methoxyflurane had intermediate response in ALA activity in rat liver homogenates. According to the DCC-primed rate model, ketamine is not porphyrinogenetic in rat liver assays, whereas etomidate is.[575] Ketamine has been shown to be porphyrinogenic in a chick embryo liver assay of ALA and, therefore, the use of ketamine for patients with porphyria is controversial.[576,577] Propofol does not increase ALA activity.[578,579] Despite the results of assays cited above, ketamine, etomidate, and propofol have been used safely in patients with porphyria.[580,581]

Diazepam has been associated clinically with precipitation of porphyria.[573,575] Fentanyl has been listed as a drug that might precipitate porphyria, but has been used safely in patients with known porphyria undergoing coronary bypass and valve replacement.[575,582,583] Morphine and meperidine are generally considered safe.[574,575] Sufentanil has not been widely investigated in patients with asymptomatic porphyria, although a recent report of sufentanil for aortic valve replacement in a patient with acute intermittent porphyria (AIP) has been reported. Muscle relaxation with succinylcholine, d-turbocurarine, gallamine, and atracurium is safe.[575,574] Halothane has been associated with precipitation of porphyria.[575] Its use must be viewed as controversial. Isoflurane has not been extensively studied, but there are data supporting its clinical use. No data on sevoflurane and desflurane are available. Diphenhydramine and droperidol are safe. Barbiturates must be considered contraindicated in patients with document or suspected porphyria.

References

1. Atlee JL, Brownlee SW, Burstrom RE: Conscious-state comparisons of the effects of inhalation anesthetics on specialized atrioventricular conduction times in dogs. Anesthesiology 64:703, 1986.
2. Bosnjak ZJ, Kampine JP: Effects of halothane, enflurane and isoflurane on the SA node. Anesthesiology 58:314, 1983.
3. Seagard JL, Bosnjak ZJ, Hopp FA Jr, et al: Cardiovascular effects of general anesthesia. In Covino BJ, Fozzard HA, Rheder K, Strichartz G (ed): Effect of Anesthesia. Baltimore, American Physiological Society, 1985.
4. Blitt CD, Raessler KI, Wightman MA, et al: Atrioventricular conduction in dogs during anesthesia with isoflurane. Anesthesiology 50:210, 1979.
5. Atlee JL, Rusy BF: Halothane depression of A-V conduction studied by electrograms of the bundle of His in dogs. Anesthesiology 36:112, 1972.
6. Atlee JL, Rusy BF, Kreul JF: Supraventricular excitability in dogs during anesthesia with halothane and enflurane. Anesthesiology 49:407, 1978.
7. Reynolds AK, Chiz JF, Pasquet AF: Halothane and methoxyflurane: A comparison of their effects on cardiac pacemaker fibers. Anesthesiology 33:602, 1970.
8. Hauswirth O: Effects of halothane on single atrial ventricular and Purkinje fibers. Circ Res 24:745, 1969.
9. Atlee JL, Bosnjak ZJ: Mechanisms for cardiac dysrhythmias during anesthesia. Anesthesiology 72:347, 1990.
10. Jang TL, MacLeod BA, Walker MJ: Effects of halogenated hydrocarbon anesthetic on responses to ligation of a coronary artery in chronically prepared rats. Anesthesiology 59:309, 1983.
11. MacLeod BA, Augereau P, Walker MJA: Effects of halothane anesthesia compared with fentanyl anesthesia and no anesthesia during coronary ligation in rats. Anesthesiology 58:44, 1983.
12. Wit AL, Bigger, JT: Possible electrophysiological mechanisms for lethal arrhythmias accompanying myocardial ischemia and infarction. Circulation 96(Suppl 3):51, 1975.
13. Bosnjak ZJ, Supan FD, Rusch NJ: The effects of halothane, enflurane and isoflurane on calcium current in isolated canine ventricular cells. Anesthesiology 74:340, 1991.
14. Eskinder H, Rusch NJ, Supan FD, et al: The effects of volatile anesthetics on L- and T-type calcium channel currents in canine cardiac Purkinje cells. Anesthesiology 74:919, 1991.
15. Turner LA, Marijic J, Kampine JP, et al: A comparison of the effects of halothane and tetrodotoxin on the regional repolarization characteristics of canine Purkinje fibers. Anesthesiology 73:1158, 1990.
16. Boznjal ZJ, Kampine JP: Physiology of the heart. In Estafanous, Barash, Reves (eds): Cardiac Anesthesia: Principles and Clinical Practice. Philadelphia, JB Lippincott Co, 1994, p 3.
17. Gallagher JD, Bianchi JJ, Gessman IJ: Halothane antagonizes ouabain toxicity in isolated canine Purkinje fibers. Anesthesiology 71:1989.
18. Pruett JK, Blair JR, Adams RJ: Cellular and subcellular actions of opioids in the heart. In Estafanous FG (ed): Opioids in Anesthesia II. Boston, Butterworth-Heinemann, 1991, pp 61–71.
19. Blair JR, Pruett JK, Introna RP, et al: Cardiac electrophysiologic effects of fentanyl and sufentanil in canine cardiac Purkinje fibers. Anesthesiology 71:565, 1989.
20. Saini V, Carr DB, Hagestad EI, et al: Antifibrillatory action of the narcotic agonist fentanyl. Am Heart J 115:598, 1988.
21. Saini V, Carr DB, Verrier RL: Comparative effects of the opioids fentanyl and buprenorphine on ventricular vulnerability during acute coronary artery occlusion. Cardiovasc Res 23:1001, 1989.
22. Zhan CY, Lee A YS, Wong TM: Naloxone blocks the cardiac effects of myocardial ischemia and reperfusion in the rat isolated heart. Clin Exp Pharmacol Physiol 12:373, 1985.
23. Lee AYS, Wong TM: Effects of dynorphin 1-13 on cardiac rhythm and cyclic adenosine monophosphate (cAMP) levels in the isolated perfused rat heart. Neurosci Lett 80:289, 1987.
24. Wong TM, Lee AY, Tai KK: Effects of drugs interacting with opioid receptors during normal perfusion or ischemia and reperfusion in the isolated rat heart—an attempt to identify cardiac opioid receptor subtype(s) involved in arrhythmogenesis. J Mol Cell Cardiol 22:1167, 1990.
25. Park WK, Lynch C: Propofol and thiopental depression of myocardial contractility. A comparative study of mechanical and electrophysiologic effects in isolated guinea pig ventricular muscle. Anesth Analg 74:395, 1992.
26. Gilat E, Rubinstein I, Binah O: Effect of sodium pentobarbital on the transmembrane action potential and the slow inward cur-

rent of guinea pig ventricular myocytes. J Cardiovasc Pharmacol 10:485, 1987.

27. Baum VC: Distinctive effects of three intravenous anesthetics on the inward rectifier (IK1) and the delayed rectifier (IK) potassium currents in myocardium: Implications for the mechanism of action. Anesth Analg 76:18, 1993.
28. Brewster WR Jr, Isaacs JP, Waino-Andersen T: Depressant effect of ether on myocardium of the dog and its modification by reflex release of epinephrine and norepinephrine. Am J Physiol 175: 399, 1953.
29. Merin RG: Are the myocardial functional and metabolic effects of isoflurane really different from those of halothane and enflurane? Anesthesiology 55:398, 1981.
30. VanTrigt P, Christian CC, Fragraeus L, et al: Myocardial depression by anesthetic agents (halothane, enflurane and nitrous oxide): Quantitation based on end-systolic pressure-dimension relations. Am J Cardiol 53:243, 1984.
31. Pagel PS, Kampine JP, Schmeling WT, et al: Comparison of end-systolic pressure-length relations and preload recruitable stroke work at indices of myocardial contractility in the conscious and anesthetized, chronically instrumented dog. Anesthesiology 73: 278, 1990.
32. Pagel PS, Kampine JP, Schmeling WT, et al: Influence of volatile anesthetics on myocardial contractility in vivo: Desflurane versus isoflurane. Anesthesiology 74:900, 1991.
33. Eger EI II, Smith NT, Stoelting RK, et al: Cardiovascular effects of halothane in man. Anesthesiology 32:396, 1970.
34. Weiskopf RB, Calahan MK, Eger EI II, et al: Cardiovascular actions of desflurane in normocarbic volunteers. Anesth Analg 73:143, 1991.
35. Calverley RK, Smith NT, Prys-Roberts C, et al: Cardiovascular effects of enflurane anesthesia during controlled ventilation in man. Anaesth Analg 57:619, 1978.
36. Pagel PS, Pampine JP, Schmeling WT, et al: Comparison of the systemic and coronary hemodynamic actions of desflurane, isoflurane, halothane and enflurane in the chronically instrumented dot. Anesthesiology 74:539, 1991.
37. Stevens WC, Cromwell TH, Halsey MJ, et al: The cardiovascular effects of a new inhalation anesthetic, forane, in human volunteers at constant arterial carbon dioxide tension. Anesthesiology 35:8, 1971.
38. Wolf WJ, Neal MB, Peterson MD: The hemodynamic and cardiovascular effects of isoflurane and halothane anesthesia in children. Anesthesiology 64:328, 1986.
39. Weiskopf RB, Holmes MA, Eger EI II, et al: Cardiovascular effects of 1653 in swine. Anesthesiology 69:303, 1988.
40. Merin RG, Bernard JM, Doursout MF, et al: Comparison of the effects of isoflurane and desflurane on cardiovascular dynamics and regional blood flow in the chronically instrumented dog. Anesthesiology 74:568, 1991.
41. Helman J, Bellows W, Leung J, et al: Anesthetic induction of high-risk patients: Effects of desflurane on hemodynamics and echocardiographic measures of ischemia. Anesthesiology 75: A152, 1991.
42. Price HL: Myocardial depression by nitrous oxide and its reversal by Ca^{++}. Anesthesiology 44:211, 1976.
43. Lunn JK, Stanley TH, Eisele J, et al: High-dose fentanyl anesthesia for coronary artery surgery: Plasma fentanyl concentrations and influence of nitrous oxide on cardiovascular responses. Anesth Analg 58:390, 1979.
44. Lawson D, Frazer M, Lunch C III: Is nitrous oxide a myocardial depressant? A reexamination in vitro. Anesthesiology 71:A504, 1989.
45. Pagel PS, Kampine JP, Schmeling WT, et al: Effects of nitrous oxide on myocardial contractility as evaluated by the preload recruitable stroke work relationship in chronically instrumented dogs. Anesthesiology 73:1148, 1990.
46. Eisele JH, Reitan JA, Massumi RA, et al: Myocardial performance and N_2O analgesia in coronary artery disease. Anesthesiology 44:16, 1976.
47. Wynne J, Mann T, Alpert S, et al: Hemodynamic effects of nitrous oxide administered during cardiac catheterization. JAMA 243:1440, 1980.
48. Sellgren J, Ponten J, Wallin BG: Percutaneous recordings of muscle nerve sympathetic activity during propofol, nitrous oxide and isoflurane anesthesia in humans. Anesthesiology 73:20, 1990.
49. Stanley TH, Webster LR: Anesthetic requirements and cardiovascular effects of fentanyl-oxygen and fentanyl-diazepam-oxygen anesthesia in man. Anesth Analg 57:411, 1978.
50. Goldberg AH, Padget CH: Comparative effects of morphine and fentanyl on isolated heart muscle. Anesth Analg 48:978, 1969.
51. Strauer B: Contractile responses to morphine, piritramide, meperidine and fentanyl: A comparative study of effects on the isolated ventricular myocardium. Anesthesiology 37:304, 1972.
52. Sullivan DC, Wong KC: The effects of morphine on the isolated heart during normothermia and hypothermia. Anesthesiology 38: 550, 1973.
53. Chen Zhang C, Su JY, Calkins D: Effects of alfentanil on isolated cardiac tissues of the rabbit. Anesth Analg 71:268, 1990.
54. Blaise GA, Witzeling TM, Sill Vinay P, et al: Fentanyl is devoid of major effects on coronary vasoreactivity and myocardial metabolism in experimental animals. Anesthesiology 72:535, 1990.
55. Flacke JW, Flacke WE, Bloor BC, et al: Histamine release by four narcotics: A double-blind study in humans. Anesth Analg 66:723, 1987.
56. Rosow CE, Philbin DM, Keegan CR, et al: Hemodynamics and histamine release during induction with sufentanil or fentanyl. Anesthesiology 60:489, 1984.
57. Carr DB, Saini V, Verrier RL: Opioids and cardiovascular function: Neuromodulation of ventricular ectopy. In Kulbertus HE, Franck G (ed): Neurocardiology. New York, Ventura, 1988, pp 223–245.
58. Murat I, Levron JC, Berg A, Saint-Maurice C: Effects of fentanyl on baroreceptor reflex control of heart rate in newborn infants. Anesthesiology 68:717, 1988.
59. Miller DR, Wellwood M, Teasdale SJ, et al: Effects of anesthetic induction on myocardial function and metabolism: A comparison of fentanyl, sufentanil and alfentanil. Can J Anaesth 35:219, 1988.
60. Swenzen GO, Chakrabarti MK, Sapsed-Byrne S, et al: Selective depression by alfentanil of group III and IV somatosympathetic reflexes in the dog. Br J Anaesth 61:441, 1988.
61. Gravlee GP, Ramsey FM, Roy RC, et al: Rapid administration of narcotic and neuromuscular blocker: A hemodynamic comparison of fentanyl, sufentanil, pancuronium and vecuronium. Anesth Analg 67:39, 1988.
62. Hughes MA, Glass PSA, Jacobs, JR: Context-sensitive half-time in multi-compartment pharmacokinetic models for intravenous anesthetic drugs. Anesthesiology 66:334, 1992.
63. Philbin DM, Rosow CE, Schneider RC, et al: Fentanyl and sufentanil anesthesia revisited: How much is enough: Anesthesiology 73:5, 1990.
64. Hug CC Jr: Does opioid "anesthesia" exist? Anesthesiology 73: 1, 1990.
65. Samuelson PN, Reves JG, Kouchoukos NT, et al: Hemodynamic responses to anesthetic induction with midazolam or diazepam in patients with ischemic heart disease. Anesth Analg 60:802, 1981.
66. Lebowitz PW, Cote ME, Daniels AL, et al: Cardiovascular effects of midazolam and thiopentone for induction of anaesthesia in ill surgical patients. Can Anaesth Soc J 30:19, 1983.
67. Massaut J, d'Hollander A, Barvais L, et al: Haemodynamic effects of midazolam in the anaesthetized patient with coronary artery disease. Acta Anaesthesiol Scand 27:299, 1983.
68. Schulte-Sasse U, Hess W, Tarnow J: Haemodynamic responses to induction of anaesthesia using midazolam in cardiac surgical patients. Br J Anaesth 54:1053, 1982.
69. Marty J, Nitenberg A, Blancet F, et al: Effects of midazolam on the coronary circulation in patients with coronary artery disease. Anesthesiology 64:206, 1986.
70. Kwar P, Carson IW, Clarke RSJ, et al: Haemodynamic changes during induction of anaesthesia with midazolam and diazepam (Valium) in patients undergoing coronary artery bypass surgery. Anaesthesia 40:767, 1985.
71. Reves JG, Samuelson PN, Lewis S: Midazolam maleate induction in patients with ischemic heart disease. Haemodynamic observations. Can Anaesth Soc J 26:402, 1979.
72. Reves JG, Samuelson PN, Linnan M: Effects of midazolam maleate in patients with elevated pulmonary artery occluded pressure. In Aldrete JA, Stanley TH (ed): Trends in Intravenous An-

esthesia. Chicago, Year Book Medical Publishers, 1980, pp 253–275.
73. Fragen RJ, Meyers SN, Barresi V, et al: Hemodynamic effects of midazolam in cardiac patients. Anesthesiology 51:S103, 1979.
74. Adams P, Gleman S, Reves JG, et al: Midazolam pharmacodynamics and pharmacokinetics during acute hypovolemia. Anesthesiology 63:140, 1985.
75. Jones DJ, Stehling LC, Zauder HL, et al: Cardiovascular responses to diazepam and midazolam maleate in the dog. Anesthesiology 51:430, 1979.
76. Stanley TH, Webster LR: Anesthetic requirements and cardiovascular effects of fentanyl-oxygen and fentanyl-diazepam-oxygen anesthesia in man. Anesth Analg 57:411, 1978.
77. Tomichek RC, Rosow CE, Schneider RC, et al: Cardiovascular effects of diazepam-fentanyl anesthesia in patients with coronary artery disease. Anesth Analg 61:217, 1982.
78. Seltzer JL, Gerson JI, Allen FB: Comparison of the cardiovascular effects of bolus v. incremental administration of thiopentone. Br J Anaesth 52:527, 1980.
79. Sonntag H, Hellberg K, Schenk HD, et al: Effects of thiopental (Trapanal) on coronary blood flow and myocardial metabolism in man. Acta Anaesthesiol Scand 19:69, 1975.
80. Toner W, Howard PJ, McGowan WAW, et al: Another look at acute tolerance to thiopentone. Br J Anaesth 52:1005, 1980.
81. Dundee JW, Moore J: Thiopentone and methohexital. A comparison as main anesthetic agents for a standard operation. Anaesthesia 16:50, 1961.
82. Frankl WS, Poole-Wilson PA: Effects of thiopental on tension development, action potential, and exchange of calcium and potassium in rabbit ventricular myocardium. J Cardiovasc Pharmacol 3:554, 1981.
83. Reiz S, Balfors E, Friedman A, et al: Effects of thiopentone on cardiac performance, coronary hemodynamics and myocardial oxygen consumption in chronic ischemic heart disease. Acta Anaesthesiol Scand 25:103, 1981.
84. Pedersen T, Engbaek J, Klausen NO, et al: Effects of low-dose ketamine and thiopentone on cardiac performance and myocardial oxygen balance in high-risk patients. Acta Anaesthesiol Scand 26:235, 1982.
85. Kissan I, Motomura S, Aultman DF, et al: Inotropic and anesthetic potencies of etomidate and thiopental in dogs. Anesth Analg 62:961, 1983.
86. Riou B, Lecarpentier Y, Chemla D, et al: In vitro effects of etomidate on intrinsic myocardial contractility in the rat. Anesthesiology 72:330, 1990.
87. Kates RA, Stack RS, Hill RF, et al: General anesthesia for patients undergoing percutaneous transluminal coronary angioplasty during acute myocardial infarction. Anesth Analg 65:815, 1986.
88. Firestone S, Kleinman CS, Jaffe CC, et al: Human research and noninvasive measurement of ventricular performance. An echocardiographic evaluation of etomidate and thiopental. Anesthesiology 51:S22, 1979.
89. Reves JG, Berkowitz DE: Pharmacology of the intravenous induction drugs. In Kaplan JA (ed): Cardiac Anesthesia, 3rd ed. Philadelphia, WB Saunders Co, 1993, p 512.
90. Dowdy EG, Kaya K: Studies of the mechanism of cardiovascular responses to CI-581. Anesthesiology 29:931, 1968.
91. Valicenti JF, Newman WH, Bagwell EE, et al: Myocardial contractility during induction and steady-state ketamine anesthesia. Anesth Analg 52:190, 1973.
92. Urthaler F, Walker AA, James TN: Comparison of the inotropic action of morphine and ketamine studied in canine cardiac muscle. J Thorac Cardiovasc Surg 72:142, 1976.
93. Sonntag H, Heiss HW, Knoll D, et al: Coronary blood flow and myocardial oxygen consumption in patients during induction of anesthesia and droperidol/fentanyl or ketamine. Z Kreislaufforsch 61:1092, 1972.
94. Balfors E, Haggmark S, Nyhman H, et al: Droperidol inhibits the effects of intravenous ketamine on central hemodynamics and myocardial oxygen consumption in patients with generalized atherosclerotic disease. Anesth Analg 62:193, 1983.
95. Tweed WA, Mymin D: Myocardial force-velocity relations during ketamine anesthesia at constant heart rate. Anesthesiology 41:49, 1974.
96. Reves JG, Gelman S: Cardiovascular effects of the intravenous anesthetic drugs. In Effects of Anesthesia. Bethesda, Md, American Physiological Society, 1985, p 179.
97. Hatano S, Keane DM, Boggs RE, et al: Diazepam-ketamine anaesthesia for open heart surgery: A "micro-mini" drip administration technique. Can Anaesth Soc J 23:648, 1976.
98. Tuman KJ, Keane DM, Spiess BD, et al: Effects of high-dose fentanyl on fluid and vasopressor requirements after cardiac surgery. J Cardiothorac Anesth 2:419, 1988.
99. Slogoff S, Allen GW: The role of baroreceptors in the cardiovascular response to ketamine. Anesth Analg 53:704, 1974.
100. Clanachan AS, McGrath JC, Mackenzie JE: Cardiovascular effects of ketamine in the pithed rat, rabbit and cat. Br J Anaesth 48:935, 1976.
101. Traber DL, Wilson RD, Priano LL: Differentiation of the cardiovascular effects of CI-581. Anesth Analg 47:769, 1968.
102. Traber DL, Wilson RD: Involvement of the sympathetic nervous system in the pressor response to ketamine. Anesth Analg 48:248, 1969.
103. Traber DL, Wilson RD, Priano LL: Blockade of the hypertensive response to ketamine. Anesth Analg 49:420, 1970.
104. Traber DL, Wilson RD, Priano LL: The effect of beta-adrenergic blockade on the cardiopulmonary response to ketamine. Anesth Analg 49:604, 1970.
105. Traber DL, Wilson RD, Priano LL: A detailed study of the cardiopulmonary response to ketamine and its blockade by atropine. South Med J 63:1077, 1970.
106. Traber DL, Wilson RD, Priano LL: The effect of beta-adrenergic blockade on the cardiopulmonary response to ketamine. Anesth Analg 50:737, 1971.
107. Hill GE, Wong KC, Shaw CL, et al: Interactions of ketamine with vasoactive amines at normothermia and hypothermia in the isolated rabbit heart. Anesthesiology 48:315, 1978.
108. Miletich DJ, Ivankovich AD, Albrecht RF, et al: The effect of ketamine on catecholamine metabolism in the isolated perfused rat heart. Anesthesiology 39:271, 1973.
109. Coetzee A, Fourie P, Coetzee D, et al: Effects of various propofol plasma concentrations on regional myocardial contractility and left ventricular afterload. Anesth Analg 69:473, 1989.
110. De Hert SG, Vermeyen KM, Adriensen HF: Influence of thiopental, etomidate and propofol on regional myocardial function in the normal and acute ischemic heart segments. Anesth Analg 70:600, 1990.
111. Brussel T, Theissen JL, Vigfusson G, et al: Hemodynamic and cardiodynamic effects of propofol and etomidate: Negative inotropic properties of propofol. Anesth Analg 69:35, 1989.
112. Heinrich H, Fosel TH, Fontaine I, et al: Assessment of contractility changes in humans by transesophageal echocardiography: The peak-systolic pressure end-systolic diameter relationship. Int J Clin Monit Comput 4:243, 1987.
113. Mora CT, Dudek C, Epstein R, et al: Comparison of fentanyl to thiopental and propofol for maintenance of anesthesia during cardiac surgery. Anesthesiology 69:A59, 1988.
114. Hickey RF, Subert PE, Verrier ED, et al: Effects of halothane, enflurane and isoflurane on coronary blood flow autoregulation and coronary vascular reserve in the canine heart. Anesthesiology 68:21, 1988.
115. Becker LC: Conditions of vasodilator-induced coronary steal in experimental myocardial ischemia. Circulation 57:1103, 1978.
116. Reiz S, Balfors E, Sorensen MB, Ariola S Jr, et al: Isoflurane: A powerful coronary vasodilator in patients with coronary artery disease. Anesthesiology 59:91, 1983.
117. Hohner P, Nancarrow C, Backman C, et al: Anaesthesia for abdominal vascular surgery in patients with coronary artery disease (CAD), Part I: Isoflurance produces dose-dependent coronary vasodilation. Acta Anaesthesiol Scand 38:780, 1994.
118. Forrest JB, Cahalan MK, Rehder K, et al: Multicenter study of general anesthesia. II. Results. Anesthesiology 72:262, 1990.
119. Slogoff S, Keats AS: Randomized trial of primary anesthetic agent on outcome of coronary artery bypass operations. Anesthesiology 70:179, 1989.
120. Tuman KJ, McCarthy RJ, Spiess BD, et al: Does choice of anesthetic agent significantly affect outcome after coronary artery surgery? Anesthesiology 70:189, 1989.
121. Leung JM, Goehner P, O'Kelly BF, et al: Isoflurane anesthesia

and myocardial ischemia: Comparative risk versus sufentanil anesthesia in patients undergoing coronary artery bypass graft surgery. Anesthesiology 74:838, 1991.
122. Inoue K, Reichelt W, El-Banayosy A, et al: Does isoflurane lead to a higher incidence of myocardial infarction and perioperative death than enflurane in coronary artery surgery? A clinical study of 1178 patients. Anesth Analg 71:469, 1990.
123. Slogoff S, Keats AS, Dear WE, et al: Steal-prone coronary anatomy and myocardial ischemia associated with four primary anesthetic agents in humans. Anesth Analg 72:22, 1991.
124. Pagel PS, Kampine JP, Schmeling WT, et al: Comparison of the systemic and coronary hemodynamic actions of desflurane, isoflurane, halothane, and enflurane in the chronically instrumented dog. Anesthesiology 74:539, 1991.
125. Weiskopf RB, Holmes MA, Eger EI II, et al: Cardiovascular effects of 1653 in swine. Anesthesiology 69:303, 1988.
126. Merin RG, Bernard JM, Doursout MF, et al: Comparison of the effects of isoflurane and desflurane on cardiovascular dynamics and regional blood flow in the chronically instrumented dog. Anesthesiology 74:568, 1991.
127. Cosgrove DM, Loop FD, Lytle BW, et al: Primary myocardial revascularization, J Thorac Cardiovasc Surg 88:673, 1984.
128. Gardner TJ, Horneffer PJ, Manolio TA, et al: Stroke following coronary artery bypass grafting. A ten year study. Ann Thorac Surg 40:574, 1985.
129. Nussmeier NA, Arlund C, Slogoff S: Neuropsychiatric complications after cardiopulmonary bypass: Cerebral protection by a barbiturate. Anes 64:165, 1988.
130. Shaw PJ, Bates R, Cautlidge NE, et al: Early neurologic complications of coronary bypass surgery. Br Med J 291:1384, 1985.
131. Clark DL, Rosner BS: Neurophysiologic effects of general anesthetics. I. The electroencephalogram and sensory evoked responses in man. Anesthesiology 38:564, 1973.
132. Schwilden H, Stoeckel H: Quantitative EEG analysis during anaesthesia with isoflurane in nitrous oxide at 1.3 and 1.5 MAC. Br J Anaesth 59:738, 1987.
133. Galla SJ, Olmeda AK, Kretchmer HE, et al: Correlation of EEG patterns with arterial concentrations and clinical signs during halothane anesthesia. Anesthesiology 23:147, 1962.
134. Burchiel KJ, Stockard JJ, Calverley RK, et al: Relationships of pre- and post-anesthetic EEG abnormalities to enflurane-induced seizure activity. Anesth Analg 56:509, 1977.
135. Julien RM, Kavan EM: Electrographic studies of a new volatile anesthetic agent: Enflurane (Ethrane). J Pharmacol Exp Ther 183:393, 1972.
136. Sebel PS, Bovill JG, Wauquier A, et al: Effects of high-dose fentanyl anesthesia on the electrocephalogram. Anesthesiology 55:203, 1981.
137. Bovill JG, Sebel PS, Wauquier A, et al: Electroencephalographic effects of sufentanil anaesthesia in man. Br J Anaesth 54:45, 1982.
138. Bovill JG, Sebel PS, Wauquier A, et al: Influence of high-dose alfentanil anaesthesia on the electroencephalogram: Correlation with plasma concentrations. Br J Anaesth 55:199S, 1983.
139. Fink M: Cerebral electrometry-quantitative EEG applied to human psychopharmacology. In Dolce G, Kunkel H (ed): Computerized EEG Analysis. Stuttgart, Gustav Fischer Verlag, 1975, p 271.
140. Marrosu F, Marchi A, De Martino, et al: Aminophylline antagonizes diazepam-induced anesthesia and EEG changes in humans. Psychopharmacology 85:69, 1985.
141. Fleischer JE, Milde JH, Moyer TP, Michenfelder JD: Cerebral effects of high-dose midazolam and subsequent reversal with Ro 15-1788 in dogs. Anesthesiology 68:234, 1988.
142. Brechner VL, Walter RD, Dillon JB: Practical electroencephalography for the anesthesiologist. Springfield, IL, Charles C Thomas, 1962.
143. Newman M, Croughwell N, Baldwin B, et al: Effects of thiopental and isoflurane on jugular bulb desaturation during nonpulsatile cardiopulmonary bypass. Anesthesiology 77:A53, 1992.
144. Milde LN, Milde JH, Michenfelder JD: Cerebral functional, metabolic and hemodynamic effects of etomidate in dogs. Anesthesiology 63:371, 1985.
145. Pinaud M, Leusque JN, Chetanneau A, et al: Effects of propofol on cerebral hemodynamics and metabolism in patients with brain trauma. Anesthesiology 73:404, 1990.
146. Ebrahim ZY, DeBoer GE, Luders H, et al: Effect of etomidate on the electroencephalogram of patients with epilepsy. Anesth Analg 65:1004, 1986.
147. Sloan TB, Ronai AK, Toleikis R, et al: Improvement of intraoperative somatosensory evoked potentials by etomidate, Anesth Analg 67:582, 1988.
148. Pichmayr I, Lips U, Kunkel H: Intravenous anesthetics. In The Electroencephalogram in Anesthesia, Fundamentals, Practical Applications, Examples. Berlin, Springer Verlag, 1984, p 90.
149. Ferrer-Allado T, Brechner VI, Diamond A, et al: Ketamine induced electroconvulsive phenomena in the human limbic and thalamic regions. Anesthesiology 38:333, 1973.
150. Celesia GG, Chen RC, Bamfort BJ: Effects of ketamine in epilepsy. Neurology 25:169, 1975.
151. Miyaoka M, Shinohara M, Batipps M, et al: The relationship between the intensity of the stimulus and the metabolic response in the visual system of the rat. Acta Neurol Scand 60(Suppl 72): 16, 1979.
152. Greenberg J, Hand P, Sylverstro A, et al: Localized metabolic flow couple during functional activity. Acta Neurol Scand 60(Suppl 72):12, 1979.
153. Lou HC, Edvinsson L, MacKenzie ET: The concept of coupling blood flow to brain function: Revision required? Ann Neurol 22: 289, 1987.
154. Newburg LA, Milde JH, Michenfelder JD: The cerebral metabolic effects of isoflurane at and above concentrations that suppress cortical electrical activity. Anesthesiology 59:23, 1983.
155. Michenfelder JD, Theye RA: In vivo toxic effects of halothane on canine cerebral metabolism pathways. Am J Physiol 229: 1050, 1975.
156. Michenfelder JD, Cucchiara RF: Canine cerebral oxygen consumption during enflurane anesthesia and its modification during induced seizures. Anesthesiology 40:575, 1974.
157. Todd MM, Drummond JC: A comparison of the cerebrovascular and metabolic effects of halothane and isoflurane in the cat. Anesthesiology 60:276, 1984.
158. Murphy FL, Kennell EM, Johnstone RE, et al: The effects of enflurane, isoflurane and halothane on cerebral blood flow and metabolism in man. Abstracts of Scientific Papers, 61 ASA Meeting, 1974.
159. Stulken EH, Milde JH, Michenfelder JD, et al: The non-linear response of cerebral metabolism to low concentrations of halothane, enflurane, isoflurane and thiopental. Anesthesiology 46: 28, 1977.
160. Todd MM, Drummond JC, Shapiro HM: Comparative cerebrovascular and metabolic effects of halothane, enflurane and isoflurane. Anesthesiology 57:A332, 1982.
161. Eger EI, Stevens WC, Cromwell TH: The electroencephalogram in man anesthetized with forane. Anesthesiology 35:504, 1971.
162. Grosslight K, Foster R, Colohan AR, et al: Isoflurane for neuroanesthesia: Risk factors for increases in intracranial pressure. Anesthesiology 63:533, 1985.
163. Moyer JH, Pontius R, Morris G, et al: Effect of morphine and N-allylnormorphine on cerebral hemodynamics and oxygen metabolism. Circulation 15:379, 1957.
164. Jobes DR, Kennell EM, Bush GL, et al: Cerebral blood flow and metabolism during morphine-nitrous oxide anesthesia in man. Anesthesiology 47:16, 1977.
165. Vernhiet J, Marcez P, Renou AM, et al: Effets des fortes doses de morphinomimetiques (fentanyl et fentathienyl) sur la circulation cerebrale du sujet normal. Ann Anesthesiol Fr 18:803, 1977.
166. Murkin JM, Farrar JK, Tweed WA, et al: Relationship between cerebral blood flow and O_2 consumption during high dose narcotic anesthesia for cardiac surgery. Anesthesiology 63:A44, 1985.
167. McPherson RW, Traystman RJ: Fentanyl and cerebral vascular responsivity in dogs. Anesthesiology 60:180, 1984.
168. Murkin JM, Farrar JK, Tweed WA: Sufentanil anaesthesia reduces cerebral blood flow and cerebral oxygen consumption. Can J Anaesth 35:S131, 1988.
169. Young WL, Prohovnik I, Correll JW, et al: The effect of sufentanil on cerebral hemodynamics during carotid endarterectomy. Anesthesiology 69:A591, 1988.

170. Marx W, Shah N, Long C, et al: Sufentanil, alfentanil and fentanyl: Impact on cerebrospinal fluid pressure in patients with brain tumors. J Neurosurg Anesth 1:3, 1989.
171. Milde LN, Milde JH: The cerebral hemodynamic and metabolic effects of sufentanil in dogs. Anesthesiology 67:A570, 1987.
172. Milde LN, Milde JH: Cerebral effects of sufentanil in dogs with reduced intracranial compliance. Anesth Analg 68:S196, 1989.
173. Shupak RC, Harp JR: Comparison between high-dose sufentanil-oxygen and high-dose fentanyl-oxygen for neuroanesthesia. Br J Anaesth 57:375, 1985.
174. Bristow A, Shalev D, Rice B, et al: Low-dose synthetic narcotic infusions for cerebral relaxation during craniotomies. Anesth Analg 66:413, 1987.
175. Cotev S, Shalit MN: Effects of diazepam on cerebral blood flow and oxygen uptake after head injury. Anesthesiology 43:117, 1975.
176. Rockoff MA, Naughton KVH, Ingvar M, et al: Cerebral circulatory and metabolic responses to intravenously administered lorazepam. Anesthesiology 53:215, 1980.
177. Forster A, Juge O, Morel D: Effects of midazolam on cerebral blood flow. Anesthesiology 56:453, 1982.
178. Forster A, Juge O, Louis M, et al: Effects of a specific benzodiazepine antagonist (RO 15-1788) on cerebral blood flow. Anesth Analg 66:309, 1987.
179. Stulken EH, Milde JH, Michenfelder JD, et al: The non-linear response of cerebral metabolism to low concentrations of halothane, enflurane, isoflurane and thiopental. Anesthesiology 46: 28, 1977.
180. Albrecht RF, Miletich DJ, Rosenberg R, et al: Cerebral blood flow and metabolic changes from induction to onset of anesthesia with halothane or pentobarbital. Anesthesiology 47:252, 1977.
181. Michenfelder JD: The interdependency of cerebral function and metabolic effects following massive doses of thiopental in the dog. Anesthesiology 41:231, 1974.
182. Pierce EC, Lambertsen CJ, Deutch S, et al: Cerebral circulation and metabolism during thiopental anesthesia and hyperventilation in man. J Clin Invest 41:1664, 1962.
183. Sawada Y, Sugimoto H, Kobayashi H, et al: Acute tolerance to high-dose barbiturate in patients with severe head injuries. Anesthesiology 56:53, 1982.
184. Gronert GA, Michenfelder JD, Sharbrough FW, et al: Canine cerebral metabolic tolerance during 24 hours deep pentobarbital anesthesia. Anesthesiology 55:110, 1981.
185. Nussmeir NA, Arlund C, Slogoff S: Neuropsychiatric complications after cardiopulmonary bypass: Cerebral protection by a barbiturate. Anesthesiology 64:165, 1986.
186. Zaidan JR, Martin W, Klochany A: Preservation of CNS function with thiopental after coronary artery surgery. Anesthesiology 71: A283, 1989.
187. Renou AM, Vernhiet J, Macrez P, et al: Cerebral blood flow and metabolism during etomidate anaesthesia in man. Br J Anaesth 50:1047, 1978.
188. Cold GE, Eskesen V, Eriksen H, et al: CBF and $CMRO_2$ during continuous etomidate infusion supplemented with N_2O and fentanyl in patients with supratentorial cerebral tumour. A dose-response study. Acta Anaesthesiol Scand 29:490, 1985.
189. Milde LN, Milde JH, Michelfelder JD: Cerebral functional, metabolic and hemodynamic effects of etomidate in dogs. Anesthesiology 63:371, 1985.
190. Davis DW, Mans AM, Biebuyck JR, et al: Regional brain glucose utilization in rats during etomidate anesthesia. Anesthesiology 64:751, 1986.
191. Dearden NM, McDowall DG: Comparison of etomidate and althesin in the reduction of increased intracranial pressure after head injury. Br J Anaesth 57:361, 1985.
192. Cavazutti M, Porro CA, Biral GP, et al: Ketamine effects on local cerebral blood flow and metabolism in the rat. J Cereb Blood Flow Metab 7:806, 1987.
193. Crosby G, Crane AM, Sokoloff L: Local changes in cerebral glucose utilization during ketamine anesthesia. Anesthesiology 56:437, 1982.
194. Takeshita H, Okuda Y, Sari A: The effects of ketamine on cerebral circulation and metabolism in man. Anesthesiology 36:69, 1972.
195. Church J, Zeman S, Lodge D: The neuroprotective action of ketamine and MK-801 after transient cerebral ischemia in rats. Anesthesiology 69:702, 1988.
196. Vandesteene A, Trempont V, Engleman E, et al: Effect of propofol on cerebral blood flow and metabolism in man, Anaesthesia 43:42, 1988.
197. Stephan H, Sonntag H, Schenk HD, et al: Effects of Diprovan on cerebral blood flow, cerebral oxygen consumption and cerebral vascular reactivity. Anaesthetist 36:60, 1987.
198. Ravussin P, Guinard JP, Ralley F, et al: Effects of propofol on cerebrospinal fluid pressure and cerebral perfusion pressure in patients undergoing craniotomy. Anaesthesia 43:37, 1988.
199. Newman M, Murkin J, Roach G, et al: Cerebral physiologic effects of burst suppression doses of propofol during nonpulsatile cardiopulmonary bypass. Anesth Analg 81:452, 1995.
200. Nunn JF: Respiratory aspects of anaesthesia. In Nunn JF (ed): Applied Respiratory Physiology, 3rd ed. London, Butterworth's, 1987.
201. Fletcher R: Deadspace during anaesthesia. Acta Anaesthesiol Scand 34(Suppl 94):46, 1990.
202. Nunn JF: Effects of anaesthesia on respiration. Br J Anaesth 65: 54, 1990.
203. Dueck R, Prutow RJ, Davies JH, et al: The lung volume at which shunting occurs with inhalation anesthesia. Anesthesiology 69: 854, 1988.
204. Hedenstierna G: Gas exchange during anaesthesia. Acta Anaesthesiol Scand 34(Suppl 94):27, 1990.
205. Hedenstierna G, Strandberg A, Tokics L, et al: Correlation of gas exchange impairment to development of atelectasis during anaesthesia and muscle paralysis. Acta Anaesthesiol Scand 30: 183, 1986.
206. Tokics L, Hedenstierna G, Strandberg A, et al: Lung collapse and gas exchange during general anesthesia: Effects of spontaneous breathing, muscle paralysis and positive end-expiratory pressure. Anesthesiology 66:157, 1987.
207. Bindslev L, Santesson J, Hedenstierna G: Distribution of inspired gas to each lung in anesthetized human subjects. Acta Anaesthesiol Scand 25:297, 1981.
208. Rehder K: Mechanics of the lung and chest wall. Acta Anaesthesiol Scand 34(Suppl 94):32, 1990.
209. Dueck R, Young I, Clausen J, Wagner PD: Altered distribution of pulmonary ventilation and blood flow following induction of inhalational anesthesia. Anesthesiology 52:113, 1985.
210. Dueck R, Rathbun M, Greenburg G: Lung volume and VA/Q distribution response to intravenous versus inhalational anesthesia in sheep. Anesthesiology 61:55, 1984.
211. Rehder K, Knopp TJ, Sessler AD, Didier EP: Ventilation-perfusion relationship in young healthy awake and anesthetized-paralyzed man. J Appl Physiol 47:745, 1979.
212. Tokics L, Strandberg A, Brismar B, et al: Computerized tomography of the chest and gas exchange during ketamine anaesthesia. Acta Anaesthesiol Scand 31:684, 1987.
213. Nunn JF: Factors influencing the arterial oxygen tension during halothane anesthesia with spontaneous respiration. Br J Anaesth 36:327, 1964.
214. Marshall BE, Hoffman DA, Neufeld GR, Colton ET: Influence of induction agent on pulmonary venous admixture during halothane-oxygen anesthesia with controlled respiration in man. Can Anaesth Soc J 21:461, 1974.
215. Eisenkraft JB: Hypoxic pulmonary vasoconstriction and anesthetic drugs. Mount Sinai J Med 54:290, 1985.
216. Von Euler US, Liljestrand G: Observations on the pulmonary arterial blood pressure in the cat. Acta Physiol Scand 12:301, 1946.
217. Marshall BE, Marshall C, Benumof JL, Saidman LJ: Hypoxic pulmonary vasoconstriction in dogs: Effects of lung segment size and oxygen tension. J. Appl Physiol 51:1543, 1981.
218. Buckley MJ, McLaughlin JS, Fort L, et al: Effects of anesthetic agents on pulmonary vascular resistance during hypoxia. Surg Forum 15:189, 1964.
219. Benumorf JL, Wahrenbrock EA: Local effects of anesthetics on regional hypoxic pulmonary vasoconstriction. Anesthesiology 46:111, 1977.
220. Bjertnaes LJ: Hypoxia-induced pulmonary vasoconstriction in man: Inhibition due to diethyl ether and halothane anesthesia. Acta Anaesthesiol Scand 22:57, 1978.

221. Domino KB, Borowec L, Alexander CM, et al: Influence of isoflurane on hypoxic pulmonary vasoconstriction in dogs. Anesthesiology 64:423, 1986.
222. Bjertnaes LJ: Hypoxia-induced vasoconstriction in isolated perfused lungs exposed to injectable or inhalational anesthetics. Acta Anaesthesiol Scand 21:133, 1977.
223. Carlsson J, Hendenstierna G, Bindslev L: Hypoxia-induced vasoconstriction in human lung exposed to enflurane anaesthesia. Acta Anaesthesiol Scand 31:57, 1987.
224. Mendoza CV, Suarez M, Castaneda R, et al: Comparative study between the effects of total intravenous anesthesia with propofol and balanced anesthesia with halothane on the alveolar-arterial oxygen tension difference and on the pulmonary shunt. Arch Med Res 23:139, 1992.
225. Benumof JL: One-lung ventilation and hypoxic pulmonary vasoconstriction: Implications for anesthetic management. Anesth Analg 64:821, 1985.
226. Carlsson AJ, Bindsle VL, Hedenstierna G: Hypoxia-induced pulmonary vasoconstriction in the human lung. Anesthesiology 66: 312, 1987.
227. Domino KB, Borowec L, Alexander CM, et al: Influence of isoflurane on hypoxic pulmonary vasoconstriction in dogs. Anesthesiology 64:423, 1986.
228. Rogers SN, Benumof JL: Halothane and isoflurane do not decrease PaO2 during one-lung ventilation in intravenously anesthetized patients. Anesth Analg 64:946, 1985.
229. Sykes LA, Bowe EA: Cardiorespiratory effect of anesthesia. Clin Chest Med 14:211, 1993.
230. Henling CE: Respiratory management of the cardiovascular surgical patient. Int Anesth Clin 24:115, 1986.
231. Turnbull KW, Miyagishima RT, Coerein AN: Pulmonary complications and cardiopulmonary bypass: A clinical study in adults. Can Anaesth J 21:181, 1974.
232. Howatt WF, Talner NS, Sloan H, et al: Pulmonary function changes following repair of heart lesions with the aid of extracorporeal circulation. J Thorac Cardiovasc Surg 43:649, 1962.
233. Wickey GS, Hickey PR: In Hensley FA, Martin DE (eds): The Practice of Cardiac Anesthesia. Boston, Little, Brown & Co, 1990.
234. Hedenstierna G: New aspects of atelectasis formation and gas exchange impairment during anaesthesia. Clin Physiol 64:507, 1989.
235. Westbrook PR, Stubbs SE, Sessler AD, et al: Effects of anesthesia and muscle paralysis on respiratory mechanics in normal man. J Appl Physiol 34:81, 1973.
236. Stanley TH, Zikria BA, Sullivan SF: The surface tension of tracheobronchial secretions during general anesthesia. Anesthesiology 37:445, 1972.
237. Schmidt ER, Rehder K: General anesthesia and the chest wall. Anesthesiology 55:668, 1981.
238. Kallos T, Wyche MQ, Garman JK: The effects of innovar on functional residual capacity and total chest wall compliance in man. Anesthesiology 39:558, 1975.
239. Scamman FL: Fentanyl-O2-N2O rigidity and pulmonary compliance. Anesth Analgesia 62:332, 1983.
240. Comstock MK, Carter JG, Moyers JR, Stevens WC: Rigidity and hypercapnia associated with high-dose fentanyl induction of anesthesia (Letter). Anesth Analg 60:362, 1981.
241. Bailey PL, Wilbrink J, Zwanikken P, et al: Anesthetic induction with fentanyl. Anesth Analg 64:48, 1985.
242. Hill AB, Narhrwold ML, de Rosayro M, et al: Prevention of rigidity during fentanyl-oxygen induction of anesthesia. Anesthesiology 55:452, 1981.
243. Golgberg M, Ishak S, Garcia F, McKenna J: Postoperative rigidity following sufentanil administration. Anesthesiology 63: 199, 1985.
244. Morel DR, Forster A, Bachmann M, Suter PM: Effect of intravenous midazolam on breathing pattern and chest wall mechanics in humans. J Appl Physiol 57:1104, 1984.
245. Nunn JF: Control of breathing. In Nunn JF (ed): Applied Respiratory Physiology, 3rd ed. London, Butterworth's, 1987.
246. Ponte J, Purves MJ: Frequency response of carotid body chemoreceptors in the cat to changes of PaO2, PaO2, and pHa. J Appl Physiol 37:635, 1974.
247. Eger EI: The pharmacology of isoflurane. Br J Anaesthesia 56: 71S, 1984.
248. Berthoud MC, Reilly CS: Adverse effects of general anaesthetics. Drug Safety 7:434, 1992.
249. Fourcade HE, Stevens WC, Larson CP, et al: The ventilatory effects of Forane, a new inhaled anesthetic. Anesthesiology 35: 26, 1971.
250. Fourcade HE, Larson CP, Hickey RF, et al: Effect of time on ventilation during halothane and cyclopropane anesthesia. Anesthesiology 36:83, 1972.
251. Drummond GB: Factors influencing the control of breathing. Int Anesth Clin 22:59, 1984.
252. France CJ, Plummer MH, Eger, EI, et al: Ventilatory effects of isoflurane (Forane) or halothane when combined with morphine, nitrous oxide and surgery. Br J Anaesth 46:117, 1974.
253. Lam AM, Clements JL, Chung DC, Knill RL: Respiratory effects of nitrous oxide during enflurane anesthesia in humans. Anesthesiology 56:298, 1982.
254. Soliman MG, Brinale GF, Kuski G: Response to hypercapnia under ketamine anaesthesia. Can Anaesth Soc J 22:486, 1975.
255. Taylor MB, Ground RM, Mulrooney PD, Morgan M: Ventilatory effects of propofol during induction of anaesthesia. Comparison with thiopentone. Anaesthesia 41:816, 1986.
256. Taylor MB, Grounds, Dulrooney PD, et al: Ventilatory effects of propofol during induction of anesthesia. Comparison with thiopentone. Anaesthesia 41:816, 1986.
257. Goodman NW, Black AMS, Carter: Some ventilatory effects of propofol as sole anesthetic agent. Br J Anaesth 59:1497, 1987.
258. Chui HH, Van WK: Clinical evaluation of ethomidate as an induction agent. Anaesth Intensive Care 6:129, 1978.
259. Wells JKG: Comparison of ICI 35868, etomidate and methohexitone for day-care anaesthesia. Br J Anaesth 57:732, 1985.
260. McClain DA, Hug CC: Intravenous fentanyl kinetics. Clin Pharmacol Ther 28:106, 1980.
261. Stoeckel H, Schuttler J, Magnussen H, et al: Plasma fentanyl concentration and the occurrence of respiratory depression in volunteers. Br J Anaesth 54:1087, 1982.
262. Hug CC, Murphy MR: Tissue redistribution of fentanyl and termination of its effects in rats. Anesthesiology 55:369, 1981.
263. Yacoub O, Doell D, Kryger MH, Anthonisen NR: Depression of hypoxic ventilatory response by nitrous oxide. Anesthesiology 45:385, 1976.
264. Knill RL, Clement JL: Variable effects of anaesthetics on the ventilatory response to hypoxaemia in man. Can Anaesth Soc J 29:93, 1982.
265. Knill RL, Clement JL: Ventilatory responses to acute metabolic acidemia in human awake, sedated and anesthetized with halothane. Anesthesiology 62:745, 1985.
266. Hirschman CA, Bergman NA: Factors influencing intrapulmonary airway calibre during anaesthesia. Br J Anaesth 65:30, 1990.
267. White PF, Way WL, Trevor AJ: Ketamine—its pharmacology and therapeutic uses. Anesthesiology 56:119, 1982.
268. Strube PJ, Hallam PL: Ketamine by continuous infusion in status asthmaticus. Anaesthesia 41:1017, 1986.
269. Rock MJ, De al Rocha S, L'Hommedieu CS, Truemper E: Use of ketamine in asthmatic children to treat respiratory failure refractory to conventional therapy. Crit Care Med 14:514, 1986.
270. Hirschman CA, Edelstein RA, Ebertz JM, Hanifin JM: Thiobarbiturate-induced histamine release in human skin mast cells. Anesthesiology 63:353, 1985.
271. Adriani J, Rovenstein EA: The effect of anesthetic drugs upon bronchi and bronchioles of excised lung tissue. Anesthesiology 4:253, 1943.
272. Jackson DM, Richards IM: The effect of pentobarbitone and chloralose anaesthesia on the vagal component of bronchoconstriction produced by histamine aerosol in the anesthetized dog. Br J Pharm 61:251, 1977.
273. Toda N, Hatano Y: Contractile responses of canine tracheal muscle during exposure to fentanyl and morphine. Anesthesiology 53:93, 1980.
274. Stoelting RK: Opioid agonists and antagonists. In Stoelting RK (ed): Pharmacology & Physiology in Anesthetic Practice, 2nd ed. Philadelphia, JB Lippincott Co, 1991.
275. Heinonen J, Muittari A: The effect of diazepam on airway resistance in asthmatics. Anaesthesia 27:37, 1972.
276. Tait AR, Davidson BA, Johnson KJ, et al: Halothane inhibits the intralveolar recruitment of neutrophils, lymphocytes, and

macrophages in response to influenza virus infection in mice. Anesth Analg 76:1106, 1993.
277. Stevenson GW, Hall SC, Rudnick S, et al: The effect of anesthetic agents on the human immune response. Anesthesiology 72:542, 1990.
278. Forbes AR: Halothane depresses mucociliary flow in the trachea. Anesthesiology 45:59, 1976.
279. Forbes AR, Horrigan RW: Mucociliary flow in the trachea during anesthesia with enflurane, ether, nitrous oxide and morphine. Anesthesiology 46:319, 1977.
280. Lee KS, Park SS: Effect of halothane, enflurane, and nitrous oxide on tracheal ciliary activity in vitro. Anesth Analg 59:426, 1980.
281. Manawadu BR, Mostow SR, LaForce FM: Impairment of tracheal ring ciliary activity by halothane. Anesth Analg 58:500, 1979.
282. Forbes AR, Gamsu G: Mucociliary clearance in the canine lung during and after general anesthesia. Anesthesiology 50:26, 1979.
283. Gamsu G, Singer MM, Vincent HH, et al: Postoperative impairment of muscous transport in the lung. Am Rev Respir Dis 114:673, 1979.
284. Pizov R, Takahashi M, Hirshman CA, Croxton TI: Halothane inhibition of ion transport of the tracheal epithelium. A possible mechanism for anesthetic-induced impairment of mucociliary clearance. Anesthesiology 76:985, 1992.
285. Bardosi L, Bardosi A, Gabius HJ: Changes of expression of endogenous sugar receptors by polymorphonuclear leukocytes after prolonged anaesthesia and surgery. Can J Anaesth 39:143, 1992.
286. Nakagawara M, Takeshige K, Takamatsu J, et al: Inhibition of superoxide production and Ca^{2+} mobilization in human neutrophils by halothane, enflurane, and isoflurane. Anesthesiology 64: 4, 1986.
287. Welch WD: Inhibition of neutrophil cidal activity by volatile anesthetics. Anesthesiology 64:1, 1986.
288. Welch WD: Effect of enflurane, isoflurane, and nitrous oxide on the microbicidal activity of human polymorphonuclear leukocytes. Anesthesiology 61:188, 1984.
289. Jensen AG, Dahlgren C, Eintrei C: Propofol decreases random and chemotactic stimulated locomotion of human neutrophils in vitro. Br J Anaesth 70:99, 1993.
290. Knudsen F, Klausen NO, Ferguson AH, Pedersen JO: In vitro effect of etomidate and thiopental on granulocyte migration. Acta Anesthesiol Scand 31:93, 1987.
291. Yang KD, Liou WY, Lee CS, et al: Effect of phenobarbital on leukocyte activation: Membrane potential, actin polymerization, chemotaxis, respiratory burst, cytokine production, and lymphocyte proliferation, J Leukocyte Biol 52:151, 1992.
292. Welch W: Halothane inhibits the microbicidal oxidative activity of pulmonary alveolar macrophages. Anesthesiology 5:456, 1983.
293. Welch WD: Enflurane and isoflurane inhibit the oxidative activity of pulmonary alveolar macrophages. Respiration 47:24, 1985.
294. Viosin C, Scherpereel PA, Aerts C, Lepot D: In vitro toxicity of halogenated anaesthetics on guinea pig alveolar macrophages, surviving in gas phase. Br J Anaesth 56:415, 1984.
295. Stevenson GW, Hall SC, Miller PJ, et al: The effect of anesthetic agents on human immune system function. I. Design of a system to deliver inhalational anesthetic agents to leukocyte culture in vitro. J Immunol Methods 88:277, 1986.
296. Fernandez P, Cox M: Basic concepts of renal physiology. Int Anesth Clin 22(1):1, 1984.
297. Margolis BL, Stein JH: The renal circulation. Int Anesth Clin 22(1):35, 1984.
298. Madden PJ: Anaesthesia for the patient with impaired renal function. Anaesth Intensive Care 11:321, 1983.
299. Ross AF, Tinker JH: Cardiovascular disease. In David Brown (ed): Risk & Outcome in Anesthesia, 2nd ed. Philadelphia, JB Lippincott Co, 1992, p 39.
300. Butler S, Feeney N, Levine SA: The patient with heart disease as surgical risk. JAMA 95:85, 1930.
301. Goldman L, Caldera DL, Nussbaum SR, et al: Multifactorial index of cardiac risk in noncardiac surgical procedures. N Engl J Med 297:845, 1977.
302. Duncan PG, Cohen MM: Postoperative complications: Factors of significance to anesthetic practice. Can J Anaesth 34:2, 1987.
303. Mangano DT, Browner WS, Hollenberger M, et al: Association of perioperative myocardial ischemia with cardiac morbidity and mortality in men undergoing surgery. N Engl J Med 323:1781, 1990.
304. Miller CF: Evaluation of the patient with renal disease. In Rogers MC, Tinker JH, Covino BG, Longnecker (eds): Principles and Practice of Anesthesiology. St Louis, Mosby Year Book, 1993, p 310.
305. Corwin HL, Sprague SS, DeLaria GA, et al: Acute renal failure associated with cardiac operations: A case-control study. J Thorac Cardiovasc Surg 98:1107, 1989.
306. Paganini EP, Bosworth CR: Acute renal failure after open heart surgery: Newer concepts and current therapy. Semin Thorac Cardiovasc Surg 3:63, 1991.
307. Leurs PB, Mulder WA, Fiers HA, Hoorntje SJ: Acute renal failure after cardiac surgery. Current concepts in pathophysiology, prevention, and treatment. Eur Heart J 10(Suppl H):38, 1989.
308. Giuffre RM, Tam KH, Williams WW, et al: Acute renal failure complicating pediatric cardiac surgery: A comparison of survivors and nonsurvivors following peritoneal dialysis. Pediatr Cardiol 13:208, 1992.
309. Anderson RJ, Linas SL, Berns AS, et al: Non-oliguric acute renal failure. N Engl J Med 296:1134, 1977.
310. Sladen RN: Effect of anesthesia and surgery on renal function. Crit Care Clin 3:373, 1987.
311. Brenner BM, Zatz Roberto, Lekuni Ichikawa: The renal circulations. In Brenner BM, Retor FG (eds): The Kidney. Philadelphia, WB Saunders Co, 1986, p 93.
312. Rush GF, Smith JH, Newton JF, et al: Chemically induced nephrotoxicity: Role of metabolic activation. Crit Rev Toxicol 13: 99, 1984.
313. Hook JB, Smith JH: Biochemical mechanisms of nephrotoxicity. Transplant Proc 17(Suppl):41, 1985.
314. Brezis M, Rosen S, Epstein F: The pathophysiology of medullary hypoxia. Am J Kidney Dis 13:252, 1989.
315. Finn WF: Nephron heterogeneity in polyuric acute renal failure. J Lab Clin Med 98:21, 1981.
316. Hollenberg NK, Solomon HS, Adams DF: Renal vascular response to angiotensin and norepinephrine in normal man. Circ Res 31:750, 1972.
317. Brezis M, Rosen S, Epstein F: Acute renal failure. In Brenner BM, Rector FG (eds): The Kidney. Philadelphia, WB Saunders Co, 1986, p 735.
318. Lennon GM, Ryan PC, Gaffney EF, et al: Changes in regional renal perfusion following ischemia/reperfusion injury to the rat kidney. Urol Res 19:259, 1991.
319. Chou SY, Poroush JG, Faubert PF: Hormonal control of medullary circulation. Kidney Int 37:1, 1990.
320. Burry A, Axelsen RA, Troloce P, et al: Calcification in the renal medulla. A calcification based on a prospective study of 2261 necropsies. Hum Pathol 7:435, 1976.
321. Burry A, Cross R, Axelsen RA: Analgesic nephropathy and renal concentrating mechanism. In Sommers SC, Rosen PP (eds): Pathology Annual, Part 2. New York, Appleton-Century-Crofts, 1977, p 1.
322. Hagitt RC, Pitcock JA, Muirhead EE: Renal medullary fibrosis in hypertension. Hum Pathol 2:587, 1971.
323. Halperin BD, Feeley TW: The effects of anesthesia and surgery on renal function. Int Anesth Clin 22:157, 1984.
324. Cousins MJ, Mazze RI: Methoxyflurane nephrotoxicity. JAMA 225:1611, 1973.
325. Deutsch S: Effects of anesthetics on the kidney. Surg Clin North Am 55:775, 1975.
326. Abel RM, Buckley MJ, Austen GW: Etiology, incidence, and prognosis of renal failure following cardiac operations: Results of a prospective analysis of 500 consecutive patients. J Thorac Cardiovasc Surg 71:323, 1976.
327. Hilberman M, Meyers B, Carrie B, et al: Acute renal failure following cardiac surgery. J Thorac Cardiovasc Surg 77:880, 1979.
328. Bhat JG, Gluck M, Lowenstein J, et al: Renal failure after open heart surgery. Ann Intern Med 84:677, 1976.
329. De Torrente A: Acute renal failure. Int Anesth Clin 2:83, 1984.

330. Keeton TK, Campbell: The pharmacologic alteration of renin release. Pharmacol Rev 31:81, 1981.
331. Patrono C, Pugliese F, Ciabattoni G: Evidence for a direct stimulatory effect of prostacyclin and renin release in man. J Clin Invest. 69:231, 1982.
332. Funder JW: Aldosterone action. Ann Rev Physiol 55:115, 1993.
333. Funder JW, Feldman D, Edelman IS: Specific aldosterone binding in rat kidney and parotid. J Steroid Biochem 3:209, 1972.
334. Norris SH: Renal eicosanoids. Semin Nephrol 10:64, 1990.
335. Stein JH: 1990 Regulation of the renal circulation. Kidney Int 38:571, 1990.
336. Hassid A, Dunn MJ: Microsomal prostaglandin biosynthesis of human kidneys. J Biol Chem 255:2472, 1980.
337. Argent NB, Wilkinson R, Baylis PH: Local hormones in the kidney: Protectors of the kidney against the body? J Endocrinol 126:351, 1990.
338. Whorton AR, Smigel M, Oates JA, Frolich JC: Regional differences in prostaglandin formation by the kidney: Prostacyclin is a major prostaglandin of the renal cortex. Biochem Biophys Acta 529:176, 1978.
339. Friesinger CC, Olez O, Sweetman BJ, et al: Prostaglandin D_2, another renal prostaglandin. Prostaglandins 15:969, 1978.
340. Chang LCT, Splawinski JA, Oates JA, et al: Enhanced renal prostaglandin production in the dog. II: Effects on intrarenal hemodynamics. Circ Res 36:204, 1975.
341. Lear S, Silva P, Epstein FH: Adenosine and PGE2 modulate transport by thick ascending limb cells. Clin Res 33:586A, 1985.
342. Forssmann WG, Nokihara K, Gagelman M, et al: The heart is the center of a new endocrine, paracrine, and neuroendocrine system. Arch Histol Cytol 52 (Suppl):293, 1989.
343. Ruskoaho H: Atrial natriuretic peptide: Synthesis, release, and metabolism. Pharmacol Rev 44:479, 1992.
344. Cogan MG: Nephrology forum: Atrial natriuretic peptide. Kidney Int 37:1148, 1990.
345. Harris PJ, Skinner SL: 1990 Intra-renal interactions between angiotensin and norepinephrine in normal man. Circ Res 31:750, 1972.
346. Marin Grey M, Fleming JT, Steinhausen M: Atrial natriuretic peptide causes pre-glomerular vasodilation and post-glomerular vasoconstriction in rat kidney. Nature 324:473, 1986.
347. Awazu M, Ichikawa I: Biological significance of atrial natriuretic peptide in the kidney (Editorial). Nephron 63:1, 1993.
348. Johnston CI, Hodsman PG, Kohzuki M, et al: Interaction between atrial natriuretic peptide and renin angiotensin aldosterone system. Endogenous antagonists. Am J Med 87(6B):24S, 1989.
349. Johnston CI, Phillips PA, Ardolda L, et al: Modulation of renin-angiotensin system by atrial natriuretic peptide. J Cardiovasc Pharmacol 16(Suppl 7):43, 1990.
350. Shaw SG, Weidmann P, Hodler J, et al: Atrial natriuretic peptide protects against acute ischemic renal failure in the rat. J Clin Invest 80:1232, 1987.
351. Conger JD, Falk SA, Hammond WS: Atrial natriuretic peptide and dopamine in established acute renal failure in the rat. Kidney Int 40:21, 1991.
352. Schafferhans K, Heidbreder E, Grimm D, et al: Norepinephrine-induced acute renal failure: Beneficial effects of atrial natriuretic factor. Nephron 14:240, 1986.
353. Margulies KB, McKinley LJ, Cavero PG, et al: Induction and prevention of radiocontrast-induced nephropathy in dogs with heart failure. Kidney Int 38:1101, 1990.
354. Takezawa K, Cowley AW, Skeleton M, et al: Atriopeptin II alters renal medullary hemodynamics and pressure-diuresis response in rats. Am J. Physiol 252:F992, 1987.
355. Pettinger WA: Anesthetics and renin-angiotensin-aldesterone axis. Anesthesiology 48:393, 1978.
356. Mujais SK: Transport and renal effects of general anesthesia. Semin Nephrol 6:251, 1986.
357. Bailey DB, Miller ED, Kaplan JA, et al: The renin-angiotensin-aldosterone system during cardiac surgery with morphine-nitrous oxide anesthesia. Anesthesiology 42:538, 1975.
358. Barry KG, Mazze RI, Schwartz FD: Prevention of surgical oliguria and renal hemodynamics suppression by sustained hydration. N Engl J Med 270:1371, 1964.
359. Burger BM, Hopkins T, Tulloch A, Hollenberg NK: The role of angiotensin in canine renal vascular response to barbiturate anesthesia. Circ Res 38:196, 1976.
360. Yun JC, Kelly GD, Bratter FC, Tate JE: Mechanism for the increase in plasma renin activity by pentobarbital anesthesia. Life Sci 22:1545, 1978.
361. Cousins MJ, Skowronski G, Plummer JL: Anaesthesia and the kidney. Anaesth Intensive Care 11:292, 1983.
362. Ishihara H, Ishida K, Oyrma T, et al: Effects of general anaesthesia and surgery on renal function and plasma ADH levels. Can Anaesth Soc J. 25:312, 1978.
363. Stanley TH, Philbin DM, Coggins CH: Fentanyl-oxygen anesthesia for coronary artery surgery: Cardiovascular and antidiuretic hormone responses. Can Anaesth Soc J 26:168, 1979.
364. Kono K, Philbin DM, Coggins CH, et al: Renal function and stress response during halothane or fentanyl anesthesia. Anesth Analg 61:552, 1981.
365. DeLange S, Boscoe MJ, Stanley TH, et al: Antidiuretic and growth hormone responses during coronary artery surgery with sufentanil-oxygen and alfentanil-oxygen anesthesia in man. Anesth Analg 61:434, 1982.
366. Philbin DM, Coggins CH: Plasma antidiuretic hormone levels in cardiac surgical patients during morphine and halothane anesthesia. Anesthesiology 49:95, 1978.
367. Lehtinen A, Fyhrquist F, Kivalo I: The effect of fentanyl on arginine vasopressin and cortisol secretion during anesthesia. Anesth Analg 63:25, 1984.
368. Bormann BV, Weidler B, Dennhardt R, et al: Influence of epidural fentanyl on stress-induced elevation of plasma vasopressin (ADH) after surgery. Anesth Analg 62:727, 1983.
369. Cochrane JPS, Forsling ML, Gow NM, et al: Arginine vasopressin following surgical operations. Br J Surg 68:209, 1981.
370. Casey JH, Bickel EY, Zimmerman B: The pattern and significance of aldosterone secretion in the postoperative patient. Surg Gynecol Obstet 105:179, 1957.
371. Breslow MJ: Clinical implications of the stress response to surgery. In Rogers MC (eds): Principles and Practices of Anesthesiology. St. Louis, Mosby-Yearbook, 1993, p 103.
372. Duthie DR, Fraser R, Nimmo WS: Effect of induction anaesthesia with etomidate on corticosteroid synthesis in man. Br J Anaesth 57:156, 1985.
373. Wagner RL, White PP, Kan PB, et al: Inhibition of adrenal steroidogenesis by the anesthetic etomidate. N Engl J Med 310: 1415, 1984.
374. Fragen RJ, Shanks CA, Molteni A, et al: Effects of etomidate on hormonal response to surgical stress. Anesthesiology 61:652, 1984.
375. Crozier TA, Beck D, Schlaeger M, et al: Endocrinological changes following etomidate, midazolam, or methohexital for minor surgery. Anesthesiology 66:628, 1987.
376. Lambert A, Mitchell R, Robertson WR: Effects of etomidate, thiopentone, and etomidate on adrenal steroidogenesis in vitro. Br J Anaesth 57:505, 1985.
377. Kenyon CJ, McNeil LM, Fraser R: Comparison of the effects of etomidate, thiopentone and propofol on cortisol synthesis. Br J Anaesth 57:505, 1985.
378. Robertson WR, Reader SCJ, Davidson B, et al: On the biopotency and site of action of drugs affecting endocrine tissue with specific reference to antisteroidogenic effects of anesthetic agents. Postgrad Med J 61(Suppl 3):145, 1985.
379. Lacoumenta S, Walsh ES, Waterman, et al: Effects of ketamine on the metabolic response of pelvic surgery. Br J Anaesth 57: 493, 1984.
380. Sear JW, Uppington J, Kay NH: Haematological and biochemical changes during anaesthesia with propofol. Postgrad Med J 6 (Suppl 3):165, 1985.
381. Eskay R, Zukowska GZ, Hass M, et al: Circulating atrial natriuretic peptides in conscious rats: Regulation of release by multiple factors. Science 232:636, 1982.
382. McIntyre RW, Schwinn DA: Atrial natriuretic peptide. J Cardiothorac Anesth 3(1):91, 1989.
383. Horky K, Gutkowska, Garcia R, et al: Effect of different anesthetics on immunoreactive atrial natriuretic factor concentrations in rat plasma. Biochem Biophys Res Commun 129:651, 1985.
384. Vollmar AM, Arendt RM, Schultz R: The effect of opioids on rat plasma atrial natriuretic peptide. Eur J Pharmacol 143:315, 1987.
385. Gutkowska J, Raczk, Garcia R, et al: The morphine effect on plasma ANF. Eur J Pharmacol 131:91, 1986.

386. Schaff HV, Mashburn JP, McCarthy PM, et al: Natriuresis during and early after cardiopulmonary bypass: Relationship to atrial natriuretic factor, aldosterone, and antidiuretic hormone. J Thorac Cardiovasc Surg 98:979, 1989.
387. Dewar ML, Walsh G, Chiu CJ, et al: Atrial natriuretic factor: Response to cardiac operation. J Thorac Cardiovasc Surg 96: 266, 1988.
388. Girardin EP, Berner ME, Favre HR: Atrial natriuretic factor after heart operations in children. J Thorac Cardiovasc Surg 102:526, 1991.
389. Flezzani P, McIntyre RW, Xuan YT, et al: Atrial natriuretic peptide plasma peptide levels during cardiac surgery. J Cardiothorac Anesth 2:274, 1988.
390. Berry A: Respiratory support and renal function. Anesthesiology 55:655, 1981.
391. Baratz RA, Philbin DM, Patterson RW: Urinary output and plasma levels of ADH during intermittent positive pressure breathing in dog. Anesthesiology 34:510, 1971.
392. Jarnberg PO, Dominquez de Villota E, Eklund J, et al: Effects of positive end expiratory pressure on renal function. Acta Anaesthesiol Scand 22:508, 1978.
393. Marquez JM, Douglas ME, Downs, Wu WH, et al: Renal function and cardiovascular response during positive airway pressure. Anesthesiology 50:393, 1979.
394. Kharasch ED, Yeo KT, Kenny MA, et al: Atrial natriuretic factor may mediate the renal effects of PEEP ventilation. Anesthesiology 69:862, 1988.
395. Andrivet P, Adnot S, Brun-Buisson C, et al: Involvement of ANF in the acute antidiuresis during PEEP ventilation. J Appl Physiol 65:1967, 1988.
396. Rossaint R, Jorres D, Nienhaus M, et al: Positive end-expiratory pressure reduces renal excretion without horizontal activation after volume expansion in dogs. Anesthesiology 77:700, 1992.
397. Mazze RI, Schwartz FD, Slocum HC, et al: Renal function during anesthesia and surgery. The effects of halothane anesthesia. Anesthesiology 24:279, 1963.
398. Deutsch S, Goldberg M, Stephen GM: Effects of halothane anesthesia on renal function in normal man. Anesthesiology 27: 793, 1966.
399. Bastron RD, Pyne JL, Inagaki M: Halothane-induced renal vasodilation. Anesthesiology 50:126, 1979.
400. Hysing ES, Chelly JE, Doursout MF, Merin RG: Comparative effects of halothane, enflurane, isoflurane at equihypotensive doses on cardiac performance and coronary and RBFs in chronically instrumented dogs. Anesthesiology 76:979, 1972.
401. Gelman S, Fowler KC, Smith LR: Regional blood flow during isoflurane and halothane anesthesia. Anesth Analg 63:557, 1984.
402. Lundeen G, Manohar M, Parks C: Systemic distribution of blood flow in swine while awake and during 1.0 and 1.5 MAC isoflurane anesthesia with and without 50% nitrous oxide. Anesth Analg 62:499, 1983.
403. Leighton KM, MacLeod BA, Bruce C: RBF: Differences in autoregulation during anesthesia with halothane, methoxyflurane, or alphaprodine in the dog. Anesth Analg 57:389, 1978.
404. Cousins MJ, Greenstein LR, Hitt BA, Mazze RI: Metabolism and renal effects of enflurane in man. Anesthesiology 44:44, 1976.
405. Tranquilli WJ, Manohar M, Parks CM, et al: Systemic and regional blood flow distribution in unanesthetized swine and swine anesthetized with halothane + nitrous oxide, halothane, or enflurane. Anesthesiology 56:369, 1982.
406. Jarnberg PO, Marrone B, Priano LL: Enflurane preserves RBF (Abstract). Anesthesiology 73:A572, 1990.
407. Merin RG, Bernard JM, Doursout MF, et al: Comparison of the effects of isoflurane and desflurane on cardiovascular dynamics and regional blood flow in the chronically instrumented dog. Anesthesiology 74:568, 1991.
408. Hartman JC, Pagel PS, Proctor LT, et al: Influence of desflurane, isoflurane and halothane on regional tissue perfusion in dogs. Can J Anaesth 39:877, 1992.
409. Priano LL: Alterations of renal hemodynamics by thiopental, diazepam, and ketamine in conscious dogs. Anesth Analg 61: 853, 1982.
410. Priano LL: Renal hemodynamic alterations following administration of thiopental, diazepam, or ketamine to conscious, hypovolemic dogs. Adv Shock Res 9:173, 1983.
411. Mather LE, Shelby DG, Runciman WB: Effects of propofol and of thiopentone anaesthesia on the regional kinetics of penthidine in the sheep. Br J Anaesth 65:365, 1990.
412. Shelby DG, Mather LE, Runciman WB: Effects of propofol and of thiopentone anaesthesia on the renal clearance of cefoxitin in the sheep. Br J Anaesth 65:360, 1990.
413. Stanley TH, Gray NH, Bidawai AV, et al: The effects of high dose morphine and morphine plus N_2O on urinary output in man. Can Anaesth Soc J 21:379, 1974.
414. Bidwai AV, Stanley TH, Bloomer HA, Blatnick RA: Effects of anesthetic doses of morphine on renal function in the dog. Anesth Analg 54:357, 1975.
415. Mazze RI: Fluorinated anaesthetic nephrotoxicity: An update. Can Anaesth Soc J 31:S16, 1984.
416. Mazze RI, Woodruff, Heerdt MEC: Isoniazid-induced enflurane defluorination in humans. Anesthesiology 57:5, 1977.
417. Fish KJ, Sievenpiper TJ, Rice SA, et al: Enflurane and gentamicin in chronic renal failure. Anesthesiology 51(Suppl 35): S262, 1979.
418. Crandell WB, Pappas SG, MacDonald A: Nephrotoxicity associated with methoxyflurane anesthesia. Anesthesiology 27:591, 1966.
419. Mazze RI, Shue GL, Jackson SH: Renal dysfunction associated with methoxyflurane anesthesia. A randomized prospective clinical evaluation. JAMA 216:278, 1971.
420. Shiraishi Y, Ideka K: Uptake and biotransformation of sevoflurane in humans: A comparative study of sevoflurane with halothane, enflurane and isoflurane. J Clin Anesth 2:381, 1990.
421. Barr GA, Cousins MJ, Mazze RI: A comparison of the renal effects and metabolism of enflurane and methoxyflurane in Fischer 344 rats. J Pharmacol Exp Ther 188:257, 1974.
422. Mazze RI, Sievenpiper TS, Stevenson J: Renal effects of enflurane and halothane in patients with abnormal renal function. Anesthesiology 60:161, 1984.
423. Motuz DJ, Watson WA, Barlow JC, et al: The increase in urinary alanine aminopeptidase excretion associated with enflurane anesthesia is increased further by aminoglucocides. Anesth Analg 67:770, 1988.
424. Kong KL, Tyler JE, Willatts SM, et al: Isoflurane sedation for patients undergoing mechanical ventilation: Metabolism to inorganic fluride and renal effects. Br J Anaesthesia 64:159, 1990.
425. Zaleski L, Abello D, Gold MI: Desflurane versus isoflurane in patients with chronic hepatic and renal disease. Anesth Analg 76:353, 1993.
426. Jones RM, Koblin DD, Cashman EI, et al: Biotransformation and hepato-renal function in volunteers after exposure to desflurane (I-653). Br J Anaesth 64:482, 1990.
427. Weiskopf RB, Eger EI, Ionescu P et al: Desflurane does not produce hepatic or renal injury in human volunteers. Anesth Analg 74:570, 1992.
428. Condon RE, Chapman ND, Nyhus LM, et al: Hepatic arterial and portal venous pressure-flow relationship in isolated, perfused liver. Am J Physiol 202:1090, 1962.
429. Richardson PDI, Withrington PG: Pressure-flow relationships and effects of noradrenaline and isoprenaline on the hepatic arterial and portal venous vascular beds of the dog. Am J Physiol 282:451, 1978.
430. Mitzner W: Hepatic overflow resistance, sinusoid pressure, and vascular waterfall. Am J Physiol 227:513, 1974.
431. Ballet F: Hepatic circulation: Potential for therapeutic intervention. Pharmacol Ther 47:281, 1990.
432. Lautt WW: Hepatic vasculature: Conceptual review. Gastroenterology 73:1163, 1977.
433. Lautt WW: Role and control of the hepatic artery. In Lautt WW (ed): Hepatic Circulation in Health and Disease. New York, Raven Press, 1981, p 203.
434. Gelman S: Carbon dioxide and hepatic circulation (Editorial). Anesth Analg 69:149, 1989.
435. Lautt WW: Relationship between hepatic blood flow and overall metabolism: The hepatic arterial buffer response. Fed Proc 42: 1662, 1983.
436. Gelman S: General anesthesia and hepatic circulation. Can J Physiol Pharmacol 65:1762, 1987.
437. McCuskey RS, Reilly FD: Hepatic microvasculature: Dynamic structure and its regulation. Semin Liver Dis 13:1, 1993.

438. Koo A, Liang IYS, Cheng KK: Adrenergic mechanisms in the hepatic microcirculation in the rat. Q J Exp Physiol 62:199, 1977.
439. Reilly CS, Wood AJJ, Koshakji RP, et al: The effects of halothane on drug disposition: Contribution of changes in intrinsic drug metabolizing capacity and hepatic blood flow. Anesthesiology 63:70, 1985.
440. Whittle BJR: Nitric oxide: The elusive mediator of the hyperdynamic circulation of cirrhosis. Hepatology 16:1089, 1992.
441. Bond JH, Prentiss RA, Levitt MD: The effect of anesthesia and laparotomy on blood flow to the stomach, small bowel, and the colon of the dog. Surgery 87:313, 1980.
442. Granger DN, Bulkley GB: Measurement of Blood Flow: Application To The Splanchnic Circulation. Baltimore, Williams & Williams, 1981.
443. Bohrer SL, Rogers EL, Koehler RC, et al: Effects of hypovolemic hypotension and laparotomy on splanchnic and hepatic arterial blood flow in dogs. Curr Surg 38:325, 1981.
444. Gelman S: Use of microspheres for gut blood flow determinations. Surgery 89:526, 1981.
445. Gelman S: Disturbances in hepatic blood flow during anesthesia and surgery. Arch Surg 111:881, 1976.
446. Gelman S, Dillard E, Bradley EL: Hepatic circulation during surgical stress and anesthesia with halothane, isoflurane, or fentanyl, Anesth Analg 66:936, 1987.
447. Seltzer JL, Ritter DE, Starnic MA, et al: The hemodynamic response to traction on the abdominal mesentery. Anesthesiology 63:96, 1985.
448. Donald DE: Splanchnic circulation. In Sheperd JT, Abboud FM, Geiger ST (eds): Handbook of Physiology, Vol III. American Physiological Society, Bethesda, MD, 1983, p 219.
449. McNeill JR, Pang CC: Effect of pentobarbital anesthesia and surgery on the control of arterial pressure and mesenteric resistance in cats: Role of vasopressin and angiotensin. Can J Physiol Pharmacol 60:363, 1982.
450. DeCastro MTBB, Downey HF, Crystal GJ, et al: Effect of controlled ventilation on renal and splanchnic blood flows during nicotine. Am J Physiol 248:H360, 1985.
451. Johnson EE: Splanchnic hemodynamic response to passive hyperventilation. J Appl Physiol 38:156, 1975.
452. Manny J, Justice R, Hechtman HB: Abnormalities in organ blood flow and its distribution during positive end-expiratory pressure. Surgery 85:245, 1979.
453. Halden E, Jakobson S, Janeras L, et al: Effects of positive end-expiratory pressure on cardiac output distribution in the pig. Acta Anaesthesiol Scand 26:403, 1982.
454. Moreno AH, Burchell AR: Respiratory regulation of the splanchnic and systemic venous return in normal subjects and in patients with hepatic cirrhosis. Surg Gynecol Obstet 154:257, 1982.
455. Brendenberg CE, Paskanik A, Fromm D: Portal hemodynamics in dogs during mechanical ventilation with positive end-expiratory pressure. Surgery 90:817, 1981.
456. Dutton R, Levitzky M, Berkman R: Carbon dioxide and liver flow. Bull Eur Physiopathol Respir 12:265, 1976.
457. Hughes RL, Mathie RT, Campbell D, et al: Effects of hypercapnia on hepatic blood flow and oxygen consumption in the grey hound. Br J Anaesth 51:289, 1979.
458. Thomson IA, Fitch W, Hughes RL, et al: Effect of increased concentrations of carbon dioxide during halothane anaesthesia on liver blood flow and hepatic oxygen consumption. Br J Anaesth 55:1231, 1983.
459. Gelman S, Ernst E: Role of pH, pCO_2 and O_2 content of portal blood in hepatic circulatory autoregulation. Am J Physiol 233: E255, 1977.
460. Frujita Y, Sakai T, Ohsumi A, et al: Effects of hypocapnia and hypercapnia on splanchnic circulation and hepatic function in the beagle. Anesth Analg 69:152, 1989.
461. Gelman S, Fowler KC, Bishop SP, et al: Cardiac output distribution and regional flow during hypocarbia in monkeys. J Appl Physiol 58:1225, 1985.
462. Adachi H, Strauss W, Ochi H, et al: The effect of hypoxia on the regional distribution of cardiac output in the dog. Circ Res 39:314, 1976.
463. Meyers KT, Berkman RA, Dutton RE: Gas exchange in the liver and intestines during hypoxia. Bull Eur Physiopathol Respir 13: 541, 1977.
464. Biernat S, Kulig A, Lepert R, et al: Pathomorphologic and histochemical changes in the liver during hemodilution. Am J Surg 128:24, 1974.
465. Epstein RM, Deutsch S, Cooperman LH, et al: Splanchnic circulation during halothane anesthesia and hypercapnia in normal man. Anesthesiology 27:654, 1966.
466. Lange H, Stephan H, Rieke H, et al: Hepatic and extrahepatic disposition of propofol in patients undergoing coronary bypass surgery. Br J Anaesth 64:563, 1990.
467. Gelman S, Fowler KC, Smith LR: Regional circulation and function during isoflurane and halothane anesthesia. Anesthesiology 61:726, 1984.
468. Nagano K, Gelman S, Parks D, et al: Hepatic circulation and oxygen supply-uptake relationship after ischemic insult during anesthesia with volatile anesthetics and fentanyl in miniature pigs. Anesth Analg 70:53, 1990.
469. Nagano K, Gelman S, Parks D, et al: Hepatic oxygen supply-uptake relationship and metabolism during anesthesia in miniature pigs. Anesthesiology 72:902, 1990.
470. Warltier DC, Pagel PS: Cardiovascular and respiratory actions of desflurane: Is desflurane different from isoflurane? Anesth Analg 75(4 Suppl):S17, 1992.
471. Frink EJ, Ghantous H, Malan P, et al: Plasma inorganic fluoride with sevoflurane anesthesia: Correlation with indices of hepatic and renal function. Anesth Analg 74:231, 1992.
472. Little DM, Barbour CM, Given JB: The effects of flurothane, cyclopropane and ether on liver function. Surg Gynecol Obst 107:712, 1958.
473. Elliot RH, Strunin L: Hepatotoxicity of volatile anesthetics. Br J Anaesth 70:339, 1993.
474. Stock JGL, Strunin L: Unexplained hepatitis following halothane. Anesthesiology 63:424, 1985.
475. Robson JG, Sheridan CA: Preliminary investigation with flurothane. Anesth Analg 36:62, 1957.
476. Virtue RW, Payne KW: Postoperative death after flurothane. Anesthesiology 19:562, 1958.
477. Bottiger LE, Dalen E, Hallen B, et al: Halothane induced liver damage: An analysis of the material reported to the Swedish Adverse Drug Reaction Committee 1966–1973. Acta Anaesthesiol Scand 20:40, 1976.
478. Inman WHW, Mushin WW: Jaundice after repeated exposure to halothane: An analysis of reports to the Committee on Safety of Medicines. Br Med J 1:5, 1974.
479. Ray DC, Drummond GB: Halothane hepatitis. Br J Anaesth 67: 84, 1991.
480. Farrel GC: The hepatic side-effects of drugs. Med J Aust 145: 600, 1986.
481. Cousins MJ, Plummer JL, Hall P: Risk factors for halothane hepatitis. Aust NZ J Surg 59:5, 1989.
482. Bunker JP, Forrest WH, Mosteller F, et al: National Halothane Study. A study of possible association between halothane anesthesia and post operative hepatic necrosis. Washington, DC: US Government Printing Office, 1969.
483. Allan LG, Howie J, Smith AF, et al: Hepatic glutathione-S-transferase release after halothane anesthesia: Open randomized comparison with isoflurane. Lancet 1:771, 1987.
484. Husser AJ, Aldridge LM, Paul D, et al: Plasma glutathione-S-transferase concentration as a measure of hepatocellular integrity following a single general anaesthetics with halothane, enflurane, and isoflurane. Br J Anaesth 60:130, 1988.
485. Goldfarb G, Rogier E, Gebauer C, et al: Comparative effects of halothane and isoflurane anesthesia on the ultrastructure of human hepatic cells. Anesth Analg 69:491, 1989.
486. Fee JPH, Black GW, Dundee JW, et al: A prospective study of liver enzyme and other changes following repeat administration of halothane and enflurane. Br J Anaesth 51:1133, 1979.
487. Trowell J, Peto R, Crampton-Smith A: Controlled trials of repeated halothane anaesthetics in patients with carcinoma of the cervix treated with radium. Lancet 1:821, 1975.
488. Wright R, Chisholm M, Lloyd B: A controlled prospective study of the effects of liver function of multiple exposures to halothane. Lancet 1:817, 1975.
489. Allen PJ, Downing JW: A prospective study of hepatocellular function after repeated exposures to halothane or enflurane in women undergoing radium therapy for cervical cancer. Br J Anaesth 49:1035, 1977.

490. McEwan J: Liver function tests following anaesthesia. Br J Anaesth 48:1065, 1979.
491. Brown BR Jr. Gandolfi AJ: Adverse effects of volatile anaesthetics. Br J Anaesth 59:14, 1987.
492. Cousins MJ, Gourlay GK, Knights KM, et al: A randomized prospective controlled study of the metabolism and hepatopathy of halothane in humans. Anesth Analg 66:299, 1987.
493. Hoft H, Bunker JP, Goodman HI, et al: Halothane hepatitis in three pairs of closely related women. N Engl J Med 304:1023, 1981.
494. Gourlay GK, Adams JF, Cousins MJ, et al: Genetic differences in reductive metabolism and hepatotoxicity of halothane in three rat strains. Anesthesiology 55:96, 1981.
495. Moult PJA, Sherlock S: Halothane related hepatitis. Q J Med 44:99, 1975.
496. Touloukian J, Kaplowitz N: Halothane-induced hepatic disease. Semin Liver Dis 1:134, 1986.
497. Neuberger J, Williams R: Halothane anesthesia and liver damage. Br J Med 289:1136, 1984.
498. Peters RL, Edmondson HA, Reynolds TB, et al: Hepatic necrosis associated with halothane anesthesia. Am J Med 47:748, 1969.
499. Carney FMT, VanDyke R: Halothane hepatitis: A critical review, Anesth Analg 51:135, 1972.
500. Bentley JB, Vaughan RW, Cork RC, et al: Does evidence of reductive halothane biotransformation correlate with hepatic binding of metabolites in obese patients? Anesth Analg 60:548, 1981.
501. Wark HJ: Postoperative jaundice in children: Influence of halothane. Anaesthesia 38:237, 1983.
502. Warner LO, Beach TP, Garvin JP, et al: Halothane and children: The first quarter century. Anesth Analg 63:838, 1984.
503. Lind RC, Gandolfi AJ, Sipes JG, et al: Oxygen concentrations required for reductive defluorination of halothane by rat hepatic microsomes. Anesth Analg 65:835, 1986.
504. Jenner MA, Plummer JL, Cousins MJ: Differential induction of pathways of halothane metabolism. Clin Exp Pharmacol Physiol Suppl 9:24, 1985.
505. Jenner MA, Plummer JL, Cousins MJ: Influences of phenytoin and pregenolone-16 alpha-carbonitrile on halothane metabolism and hepatotoxicity. Clin Exp Pharmacol Physiol Suppl 10:14, 1987.
506. Schlieble TM, Costa AK, Heffel DF, et al: Comparative toxicity of halothane, isoflurane and phenobarbital induction in monolayer culture of rate hepatocytes. Anesthesiology 68:485, 1988.
507. Normura F, Hatano H, Ohnishi K, et al: Effects of anticonvulsant drugs on halothane-induced liver injury in human subjects and experimental animals. Hepatology 6:952, 1986.
508. Ray DC, Howie AF, Beckett GJ, et al: Preoperative cimetidine does not prevent subclinical halothane hepatotoxicity in man. Br J Anesth 63:531, 1989.
509. Brown BR JR: halothane hepatitis revisited. N Engl J Med 313: 1374, 1985.
510. Benjamine SB, Goodman ZD, Ishak KG, et al: The morphologic spectrum of halothane induced hepatic injury: An analysis of 77 cases. Hepatology 5:1163, 1985.
511. Blackburn WR, Ngai SH, Lindenbaum J: Morphologic changes in hepatic necrosis following halothane anesthesia in man. Anesthesiology 25:270, 1964.
512. Klion FM, Schaffnier F, Poper H: Hepatitis after exposure to halothane. Ann Intern Med 71:467, 1969.
513. Slater EM, Gibson JM, Dykes MHM, et al: Postoperative hepatic necrosis: Its incidence and diagnostic value in association with the administration of halothane. N Engl J Med 270:983, 1964.
514. Willis EJ, Walton B: A morphologic study of unexplained hepatitis following halothane anesthesia. Am J Pathol 91:11, 1978.
515. Uzunalimoglu B, Yarkely JH, Boitnott JK: The liver in mild halothane hepatitis: Light and electron microscopic findings with special reference to mononuclear cell infiltrate. Am J Pathol 61: 457, 1970.
516. Rehder K, Forbes J, Alter H, et al: Halothane biotransformation in man: A quantitative study. Anesthesiology 28:711, 1967.
517. Cohen EN: Metabolism of halothane-2-14C in the mouse. Anesthesiology 31:560, 1969.
518. Shingu KI, Eger EI II, Johson BH, et al: Hepatic injury induced by anesthetic agents in rats. Anesth Analg 61:820, 1982.
519. Shingu KI, Eger EI II, Johnston BH: Hypoxia per se can produce hepatic damage without death in rats. Anesth Analg 61:820, 1983.
520. Nancarrow C, Plummer JL, Ilsley AH, et al: Effects of combined extradural blockage and general anesthesia on indocyanine green clearance and halothane metabolism. Br J Anaesth 58:29, 1986.
521. Vergani D, Mieli-Vergani G, Alberti A, et al: Antibodies to the surface of halothane altered rabbit hepatocytes in patients with severe halothane associated hepatitis. N Engl J Med 303:66, 1980.
522. Martin JL, Kenna JG, Pohl LR: Antibody assays for the detection of patients sensitized to halothane. Anesth Analg 70:154, 1990.
523. Lewis JH, Zimmerman HJ, Ishak KG, et al: Enflurane hepatotoxicity. A clinicopathologic study of 24 cases. Ann Intern Med 98:984, 1983.
524. Dykes MHM: Is enflurane hepatotoxic? Anesthesiology 61:235, 1984.
525. Eger EI II: Pharmacology of isoflurane. Br J Anaesth 56:71S, 1984.
526. Carpenter RL, Eger RL, Johnson BH, et al: The extent of metabolism of inhaled anesthetics in humans. Anesthesiology 65: 201, 1986.
527. Christ DD, Satoh H, Kenna JG, et al: Potential metabolic basis for enflurane hepatitis and apparent cross-sensitivity between enflurane and halothane. Drug Metab Dispos 16:135, 1988.
528. Holaday DA, Smith FR: Clinical characteristics and biotransformation of sevoflurane in healthy human volunteers. Anesthesiology 54:100, 1981.
529. Ross WT Jr: Plasma fluoride concentration during halogenated anesthetic administration with normoxia and hypoxia. Anesthesiology 57:A217, 1982.
530. Stoelting RK, Blitt CD, Cohen PJ, et al: Hepatic dysfunction after isoflurane anesthesia. Anesth Analg 66:147, 1987.
531. Massion WH, Poyer JL, Downs P, et al: Comparative study of halogenated hydrocarbon toxicity and free radical formation in rat liver. Anesthesiology 61:A274, 1984.
532. Plummer JL, Beckwith AL, Bastin FN, et al: Free radical formation in vivo and hepatotoxicity due to anesthesia with halothane. Anesthesiology 57:160,1982.
533. Koblin DD, Waskell L, Watson JE, et al: Nitrous oxide activates methionine synthetase in human liver. Anesth Analg 61:75, 1978.
534. Sutton TS, Koblin DD, Gruenke LD: Fluoride metabolites after prolonged exposure of volunteers and patients to desflurane. Anesth Analg 73:180, 1991.
535. Holmes MA, Weisfkopf RB, Eger EI II, et al: Hepatocellular integrity in swine after prolonged desflurane I-163 and isoflurane anesthesia: Evaluation of plasma alanine aminotransferase activity. Anesth Analg 71:249, 1990.
536. Cook TL, Beppu WJ, Hitt BA, et al: Renal effects and metabolism of sevoflurane in Fischer 344 rats: An in-vivo and in-vitro comparison with methoxyflurane. Anesthesiology 43:70, 1975.
537. Rice SA, Sbordone L, Mazze RI: Metabolism by rat hepatic microsomes of fluorinated ether anesthetics following isoniazid administration. Anesthesiology 53:489, 1980.
538. Pratilas V, Pratilas MG, Bramis J, et al: The hepatoprotective effect of oxygen during halothane anesthesia. Anesth Analg 57: 481, 1978.
539. Lampe GH, Wauk LA, Whitendale P, et al: Nitrous oxide does not impair hepatic function in young or old surgical patients. Anesth Analg 71:606, 1990.
540. Fukuda S, Murakawa T, Takeshita H, et al: Direct effects of ketamine on isolated canine cerebral and mesenteric arteries. Anesth Analg 62:553, 1983.
541. Tverskoy M, Gelman S, Fowler KC, et al: Effects of anaesthesia induction drugs on circulation in denervated intestinal loop preparation. Can Anaesth Soc J 32:516, 1985.
542. Debaene B, Goldfarb G, Braillon A, et al: Effects of ketamine, halothane, enflurane, and isoflurane on systemic and splanchnic hemodynamics in normovolemic and hypovolemic cirrhotic rats. Anesthesiology 73:118, 1990.
543. Seyde WC, Longnecker DE: Anesthetic influences on regional hemodynamics in normal and hemorrhaged rats. Anesthesiology 61:686, 1984.

544. Idvall J: Influences of ketamine anesthesia on cardiac output and tissue perfusion in rats subjected to hemorrhage. Anesthesiology 55:297, 1981.
545. Wong DH, Jenkins LC: An experimental study of the mechanism of action of ketamine on the central nervous system. Can Anaesth Soc J 21:57, 1974.
546. Dhasmana KM, Sexena PR, Prakash O, et al: A study on the influence of ketamine on systemic and regional hemodynamics in conscious rabbits. Arch Int Pharmacodyn Ther 269:323, 1984.
547. Idvall J, Aronsen KF, Sternberg P: Tissue perfusion and distribution of cardiac output during ketamine anesthesia in normovolemic rats. Acta Anaesthiol Scand 24:257, 1980.
548. Sears JW: Toxicity of IV anaesthetics. Br J Anaesth 59:24, 1987.
549. Galindo: Hepatic circulation and hepatic function during anaesthesia and surgery. II. The effect of various anaesthetic agents. Can Anaesth Soc J 12:337, 1965.
550. Larson CP Jr, Mazze RI, Cooperman LH, et al: Effects of anesthetics on cerebral, renal, and splanchnic circulations: recent developments. Anesthesiology 41:169, 1974.
551. Svanik J, Lundgren O: Gastrointestinal circulation. Int Rev Physiol 12:1, 1977.
552. Kawaue Y, Iriuchijima J: Changes in cardiac output and peripheral flows on pentobarbital anesthesia in the rat. Jpn J Physiol 34:283, 1984.
553. Ahlgren I, Aronsen F, Bjorkman I, et al: Hemodynamics during superficial thiopental anesthesia in the dog. Acta Anaesthesiol Scand 22:76, 1978.
554. Tverskoy M, Gelman S, Fowler KC, et al: Influence of fentanyl and morphine on intestinal circulation. Anesth Analg 64:577, 1985.
555. Leaman DM, Levenson L, Zelis, R, et al: Effect of morphine on splanchnic blood flow. Br Heart J 40:569, 1978.
556. Miller RI, Forsyth RP, Melon KL: Morphine-induced redistribution of cardiac output in the unanesthetized monkey. Pharmacology 7:138, 1972.
557. Priano LL: Morphine effects on cardiac output and regional blood flow distribution in conscious dogs. 55:236, 1981.
558. Dhasmana KM, Prakash O, Saxena PR: Effects of fentanyl and antagonism by naloxone, on regional blood flow and biochemical variables in conscious rabbits. Arch Int Pharmacodyn Ther 260:115, 1982.
559. Lange H, Stephan H, Zielmann S, et al: Hepatic disposition of sufentanil in patients undergoing coronary bypass surgery. Acta Anesthesiol Scand 37:154, 1993.
560. Murray JM, Trinick TR: Hepatic function and idocyanine green clearance during and after prolonged anaesthesia with propofol. Br J Anaesth 69:643, 1992.
561. Mathers LE, Selby DG, Runciman WB: Effects of propofol and of thiopentone anaesthesia on the regional kinetics of pethidine in the sheep. Br J Anaesth 65:365, 1990.
562. Duvaldestein P, Mazze RI, Nivoche Y, et al: Effect of induction following surgery with halothane and neurolept anesthesia. Anesth Analg 6:319, 1981.
563. Nimmo G, Thompson PG, Prescott LF: Microsomal enzyme induction after halothane anaesthesia. Br J Clin Pharmacol 12:433, 1981.
564. Dundee JW, Fee JPH, Moore J, et al: Changes in serum enzyme levels following ketamine infusions. Anaesthesia 35:12, 1980.
565. Morio M, Osafumi Y, Fujii K: Biotransformation and toxicity of inhalational anaesthetics. Can J Anaesth 37:Scxvi, 1990.
566. Fee JPH, Dundee JW: Antipyrine elimination is not increased by a single induction dose of thiopentone. Br J Clin Pharmacol 22:224, 1986.
567. Ward SA, Walle T, Walle UK, et al: Propranolol's metabolism is determined by both mephenytoin and debrisoquin hydroxylase activities. Clin Pharmacol Ther 45:72, 1989.
568. Baker MT, Chadam MV, Ronnenberg C: Inhibitory effects of propofol on cytochrome p450 activities in rat hepatic microsomes. Anesth Analg 76:817, 1993.
569. Mouton Perry S, Whelan E, Shay S, et al: Effect of IV anesthesia with propofol on drug distribution and metabolism in the dog. Br J Anaesth 66:66, 1991.
570. Janicki PK, James MFM, Erskine WAR: Propofol inhibits enzyme degradation of alfentanil and sufentanil by isolated liver microsomes in vitro. Br J Anaesth 68:311, 1992.
571. Atiba JO, Horai Y, White PF, et al: Effect of etomidate on hepatic drug metabolism in humans. Anesthesiology 68:920, 1988.
572. Mees DE, Fredrickson EL: Anaesthesia and the porphyrias. South Med J 69:29, 1975.
573. Bloomer JR, Bonkosky HL: The porphyrias. Dis Month 35:1, 1989.
574. Campos JH, Stein DK, Michel MK, et al: Anesthesia of aortic valve replacement in a patient with acute intermittent porphyria. J Cardiac Vasc Anesth 5:258, 1991.
575. Harrison GG, Moore MR, Meissner PN: Porphyrinogenicity of etomidate and ketamine as continuous infusions. Screening in the DCC-primed rat model. Br J Anaesth 57:420, 1985.
576. Capouet V, Dernovoi B, Azagra JS: Induction of anaesthesia with ketamine during an acute crisis of hereditary coproporphyria. Can J Anaesth 34:388, 1987.
577. Kostrzewska E, Gregor A, Lipinska D: Ketamine in acute intermittent porphyria—dangerous or safe? Anesthesiology 49:376, 1978.
578. Mitterschiffhaler G, Theiner A, Hetzel H, et al: Safe use of propofol in a patient with acute intermittent porphyria. Br J Anaesth 60:109, 1988.
579. Meissner PN, Harrison GG, Hift RJ: Propofol as an induction agent in variegate porphyria. Br J Anaesth 66:60, 1991.
580. Risk SF, Jacobson JH Jr, Silvay G: Ketamine as an induction agent for acute intermittent porphyria. Anesthesiology 46:305, 1977.
581. Bancoft GH, Lauria JI: Ketamine induction for cesarean section in a patient with acute intermittent porphyria and achondroplastic dwarfism. Anesthesiology 59:143, 1983.
582. Roby HP, Harrison GA: Anaesthesia for coronary artery bypass in a patient with porphyria variegata. Anaesth Intensive Care 10: 276, 1982.
583. Shipton EA, Roelofse JA: Anaesthesia in a patient with variegate porphyria undergoing bypass surgery. S Afr Med J 61:656, 1984.

SECTION II

MONITORING

CHAPTER 8

Monitoring Cardiac Electrical Activity

Eric Jacobsohn, M.B.Ch.B., F.R.C.P.C.
Hans J. Wilke, II, M.D.
John E. Ellis, M.D.

The monitoring of cardiac electrical activity by electrocardiography (ECG) is one of the important responsibilities of the anesthesiologist or intensivist. The aim of this chapter is to review the key concepts of electrocardiography and their application to the practice of cardiac, thoracic, and vascular anesthesia.

In 1924, the Dutch physician and physiologist Willem Einthoven received the Nobel prize for his groundbreaking systematic description and analysis of cardiac electrical activity.[1] Refining and elaborating on earlier work done by Waller and Clement, Einthoven utilized a simple string galvanometer to record the electrical activity of the heart. He assigned the now universally used P-QRS-T notation to the electrical signal. Through careful study of patients at the University Hospital of Leiden, Einthoven was the first to describe basic clinical abnormalities such as bundle branch blocks and ischemic ST-T changes. In the early 1930s, Einthoven's string galvanometer was replaced by a more practical cathode ray oscilloscope. However, routine clinical use of electrocardiography did not occur until after the Second World War when direct-writing ECG machines became available. Another 20 years passed before the first analog to digital conversion systems for the ECG were introduced. The currently used monitoring devices, which use computerized signal processing and interpretation, did not become readily available until the 1980s.

Cardiac Electrophysiology

In their resting state, cardiac cells are electrically polarized, the inside of the cells being negatively charged with respect to the outside. This polarity is maintained by membrane pumps, which require a constant supply of energy to function. Cardiac cells lose their internal negativity in a process called depolarization. Depolarization is propagated from one cardiac cell to another, producing a flow of electrical current that may be recorded by electrodes placed on the surface of the body. The restoration of the cell's resting electrical negativity (i.e., the process of repolarization) can be similarly recorded. All ECG signals are manifestations of these two fundamental processes (Fig. 8–1).[2]

Initiation and Conduction of the Cardiac Electrical Impulse

The cardiac impulse originates in the sinoatrial (SA) node, a group of specialized pacemaker cells at the junction of the right atrium with the superior vena cava. The membranes of these cells allow a constant, slow influx of sodium and calcium that results in a less negative resting membrane potential (Fig. 8–2). In these cells, the fast sodium channels are inactivated and the action potential is primarily due to ion movement across the slow calcium channels. The SA node cells are capable of regular spontaneous depolarizations. Initially, influx of sodium causes the cell membrane to become progressively less negative; when threshold potential is reached, calcium channels open, potassium permeability decreases, and an action potential develops. Restoration of normal potassium permeability returns the cells in the SA node to their normal resting membrane potential. The impulse generated at the SA node is rapidly conducted via specialized atrial fibers across the atria to the atrioventricular (AV) node, which is located in the septal wall of the right atrium (Fig. 8–3). The AV node consists of three distinct areas: an upper junctional area, a lower junctional area, and a middle nodal area. Both junctional areas are capable of intrinsic spontaneous activity, but the middle nodal area is not. Since the rate of spontaneous depolarizations in the AV node is normally slower than the depolarization rate of the SA node, the SA node controls the heart rate. However, when the rate of SA node depolarizations is decreased or the automaticity of the AV node is increased, the AV node can take over the pacemaker function for the heart. An electrical impulse from the SA node normally reaches the AV node in about 0.04 second. The propagation of the impulse through the

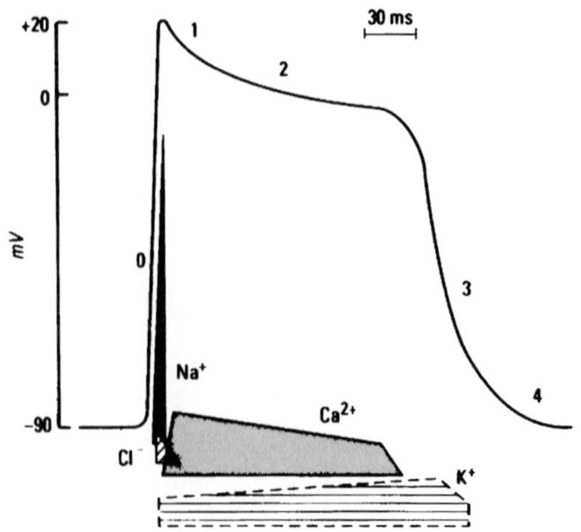

FIGURE **8–1.** Phases of the action potential of cardiac muscle fiber and the corresponding changes in ionic conductance across the muscle membrane. 0, depolarization; 1, rapid repolarization; 2, plateau phase; 3, late rapid depolarization; 4, baseline; Na, sodium; Ca, calcium; K, potassium; Cl, chloride. (From Ganong WF: Origin of the heartbeat and the electrical activity of the heart. In Review of Medical Physiology, 16th ed. Stamford, CT, Appleton & Lange, 1993, p 492, with permission.)

AV node itself is considerably slower and takes approximately 0.1 second. The impulse is then conducted down the bundle of His. It enters the interventricular septum and divides into the left and right bundle branches. They in turn separate into the complex network of the Purkinje fibers, which depolarize the ventricles. The His-Purkinje fibers conduct the electrical impulse rapidly, and within 0.03 second the endocardium of both ventricles is depolarized. Ionic movement for myocyte depolarization is represented in Figure 8–1. The spread of the impulse from the endocardium to the epicardium of the ventricles requires another 0.03 second. Thus, an impulse from the SA node requires less than 0.2 second to depolarize the entire heart.

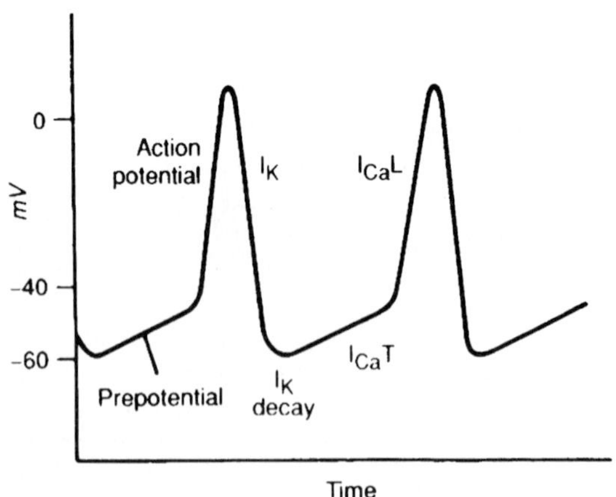

FIGURE **8–2.** Diagram of the membrane potential of the pacemaker cells in the SA node. Note that the resting potential is less than that of the cardiac myocyte. I_K, potassium current; $I_{Ca}L$, L-type slow calcium channel; $I_{Ca}T$, T-type slow calcium channel. (From Ganong WF: Origin of the heartbeat and the electrical activity of the heart. In Review of Medical Physiology, 16th ed. Stamford, CT, Appleton & Lange, 1993, p 492, with permission.)

Relationship of the Cardiac Excitation Process to the ECG Curve

The ECG reflects these electrical events with separate atrial and ventricular components (Fig. 8–3). The atrial component begins with the P wave and represents spread of the depolarization over the two atria. During the subsequent PQ interval, the atria as a whole are depolarized. The ventricular component begins with the first deflection after the PQ segment and extends to the end of the T wave. The QRS complex represents spread of the depolarization over both ventricles. The ST segment and T wave reflect ventricular repolarization. The PQ interval represents the time elapsed from the onset of atrial excitation to the onset of ventricular excitation and is normally less than 0.20 second. A longer PQ interval represents a disturbance in conduction in the region of the AV node or the bundle of His. In contrast, a QRS complex greater than 0.12 second indicates a disturbance in the spread of excitation over the ventricles. The duration of the QT interval depends on heart rate, and is represented by Qtc (QT interval corrected for heart rate); for example, when the heart rate increases from 40 to 180 bpm, the QT duration decreases from about 0.4 to 0.2 second.

Practical Electrocardiography

The Lead Systems

Since the heart is a three-dimensional organ, the electrical activity must be analyzed in those dimensions as well. The fact that recordings from a single pair of electrodes were insufficient was recognized by Einthoven when he devised the classical three-lead system. Today's standard 12-lead ECG records the heart's electrical activity in the frontal and horizontal planes. The six limb leads—that is, the three standard "Einthoven" leads (I, II, III) and the three augmented "Goldberger" leads (aVR, aVL, aVF)—view the heart in the frontal plane (Fig. 8–4),[3] and the six precordial or chest leads (V_1 through V_6) view the heart in the horizontal plane (Fig. 8–5). The three standard leads are termed bipolar leads because they measure differences in electrical potential between pairs of electrodes. They are obtained by placing electrodes on the right arm, the left arm, and the left leg (Fig. 8–6). Since lead II maximizes P-wave morphology, it is the preferred lead for the differential diagnosis of dysrhythmias. The three augmented limb leads are unipolar and are created by choosing a single positive lead and making all the others negative, with their average serving as the negative electrode or common ground. The unipolar leads provide additional information about the lateral (lead aVL), inferior, and diaphragmatic (lead aVF) portions of the left ventricle. In the unipolar chest lead system, the exploring electrode is placed on the chest wall in six defined positions (Fig. 8–7). Lead V_5 is highly sensitive to ischemic changes of the anterior wall.[4]

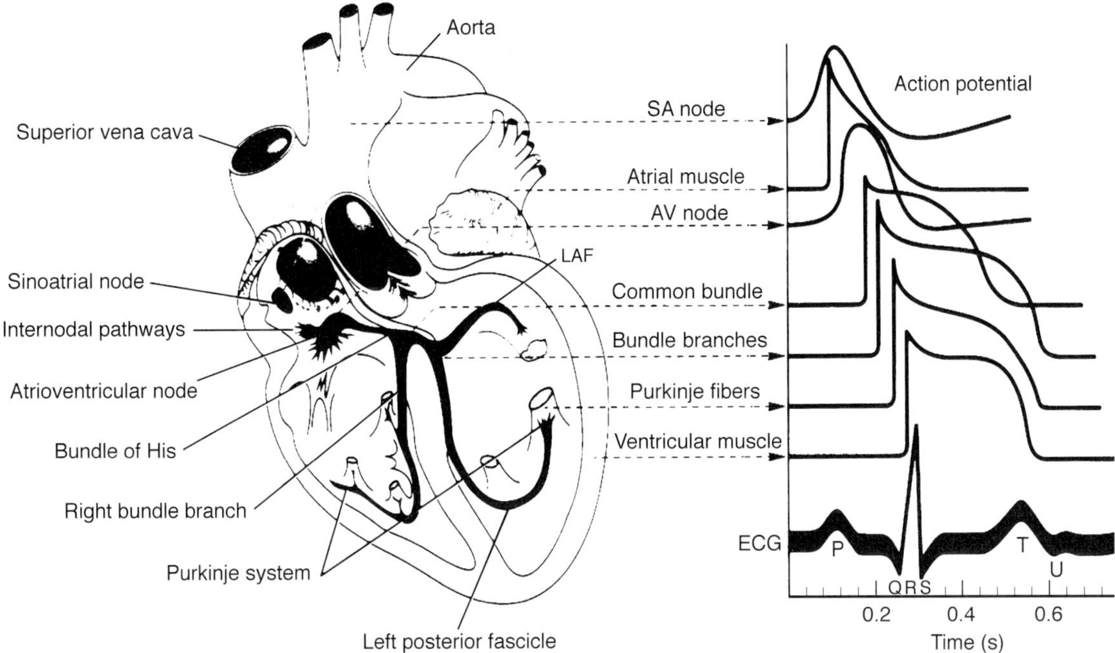

FIGURE **8–3.** The conducting system of the heart. Typical transmembrane potentials for the SA, AV nodes, and other parts of the conducting system are shown, with the corresponding ECG. The action potentials and the ECG are plotted on the same axis but with different zero points on the vertical scale. (From Ganong WF: Origin of the heartbeat and the electrical activity of the heart. In Review of Medical Physiology, 16th ed. Stamford, CT, Appleton & Lange, 1993, p 492, as adapted from Shepherd JT, Vanhoutte M: The Human Cardiovascular System: Facts and Concepts. New York, Raven Press, 1979, with permission.)

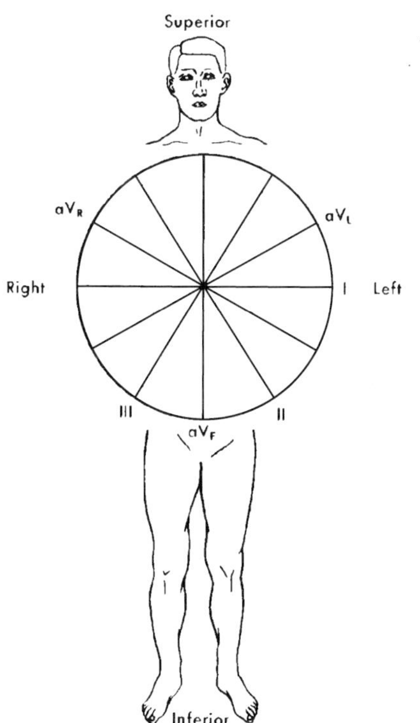

FIGURE **8–4.** Spatial relationships of the six frontal plane leads. (From Goldberger AL, Goldberger E: Clinical Electrocardiography: A Simplified Approach, 5th ed, St Louis, Mosby Year Book, 1994, with permission.)

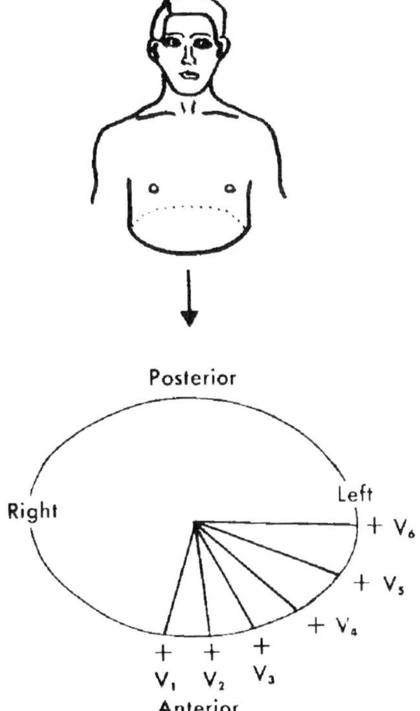

FIGURE **8–5.** Spatial relationships of the six horizontal plane leads. (From Goldberger AL, Goldberger E: Clinical Electrocardiography: A Simplified Approach, 5th ed, St Louis, Mosby Year Book, 1994, with permission.)

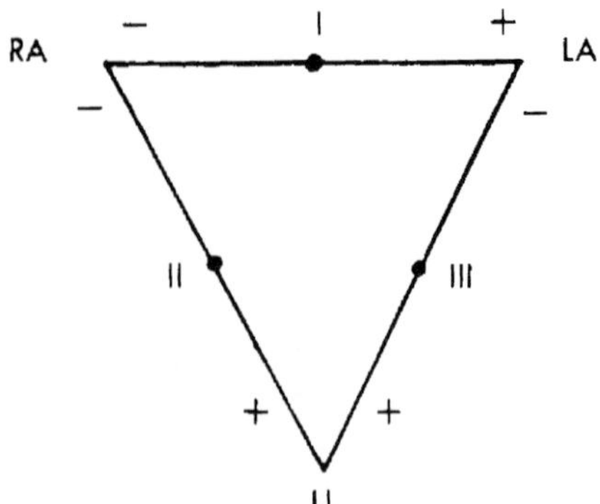

FIGURE 8–6. Orientation of leads I, II, and III. Lead I records the difference in electrical potentials between the left arm and the right arm. Lead II records it between the left leg (LL) and the right arm (RA). Lead III records it between the left leg and left arm. (From Goldberger AL, Goldberger E: Clinical Electrocardiography: A Simplified Approach, 5th ed, St Louis, Mosby Year Book, 1994, with permission.)

For maximum intraoperative data retrieval, the use of a continuous 12-lead ECG would be ideal. However, at the present time this is neither feasible nor practical. Three-lead, modified three-lead, or five-lead systems are used for intraoperative monitoring. In certain instances, nonsurface, invasive electrocardiographic monitoring is employed.

Three-Electrode Systems

The standard limb leads I, II, and III are recorded by means of appropriate placement of three electrodes as described (Fig. 8–5). A selector switch on the ECG machine allows for sequential but not simultaneous viewing of either leads I, II, or III. This simple lead system is generally sufficient for dysrhythmia diagnosis, but its limited view of the left ventricular wall makes it inadequate for myocardial ischemia monitoring.

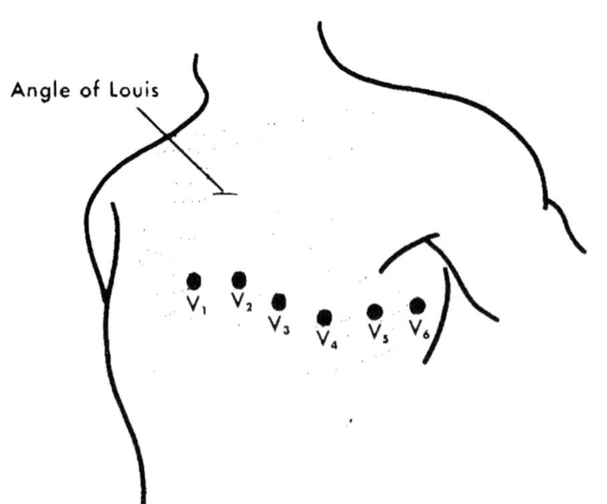

FIGURE 8–7. Location of the electrodes for the chest (precordial or V) leads. (From Goldberger AL, Goldberger E: Clinical Electrocardiography: A Simplified Approach, 5th ed, St Louis, Mosby Year Book, 1994, with permission.)

Modified Three-Electrode Systems

These systems are used if precordial electrode positions are not accessible (for surgical reasons) or to look at one aspect of the heart more closely. The nomenclature of the modified three-electrode system can be confusing, as it has evolved over time. Figure 8–8 and Table 8–1 represent the common, modified three-lead systems.[5] Studies have shown that the central subclavian (CS_5) lead is as sensitive for the detection of ischemic changes in the anterior wall as lead V_5.[6] Similarly, the control back (CB_5) lead was determined to be as good as V_5 in ischemia detection.[7] Moreover, it was superior to lead V_5 for dysrhythmia diagnosis because of a better (P-wave) representation.

Five-Electrode System

By adding two electrodes to the classic three-electrode system, leads I, II, III, aVR, aVL, aVF, and any one of the six precordial leads can be displayed. The five-electrode ECG system normally consists of four electrodes on the extremities and a fifth electrode in the V_5 position. In their classic study, London et al. showed that the greatest sensitivity for the detection of myocardial ischemia was achieved by intraoperative monitoring of either lead V_5 (sensitivity 75%) or lead V_4 (sensitivity 61%)[8] in patients with significant coronary artery disease (Fig. 8–9).[9] Simultaneous monitoring of leads V_4 and V_5 had a sensitivity of 90%, compared to a sensitivity of 80% for the combination of leads II and V_5. Simultaneous monitoring of leads II, V_4, and V_5 resulted in a sensitivity of almost 100%. However, the routine intraoperative monitoring of three leads is not yet routinely available.

Holter Monitoring

Ambulatory ECG monitoring was first introduced by N.J. Holter in 1961.[10] During a standard Holter study, data are gathered for 24 to 48 hours from one or two bipolar ECG leads. The earlier Holter units were either frequency or amplitude modulated and used analog tape and playback recorders. It soon became evident that the amplitude modulated units had a tendency to distort the low-frequency spectrum, including the ST segment, making ST-segment monitoring unreliable.[11] The data gathered also had to be converted from analog to digital and this involved a great deal of operator time and interaction. As a result, bias could often be introduced into the tabulation and interpretation of the results.

Improvements in technology have made Holter monitoring reliable. Modern Holter units have large memory capabilities and can store large numbers of ECG signals in digital form. Some Holter monitors even offer ECG surveillance, making information such as ST-segment depression immediately available to both physician and patient. Tzivoni et al. compared the detection of ST-segment depression by simultaneous two-channel Holter monitoring and 12-lead ECG during exercise testing.[12] The concordance of these methods was found to be 96%.

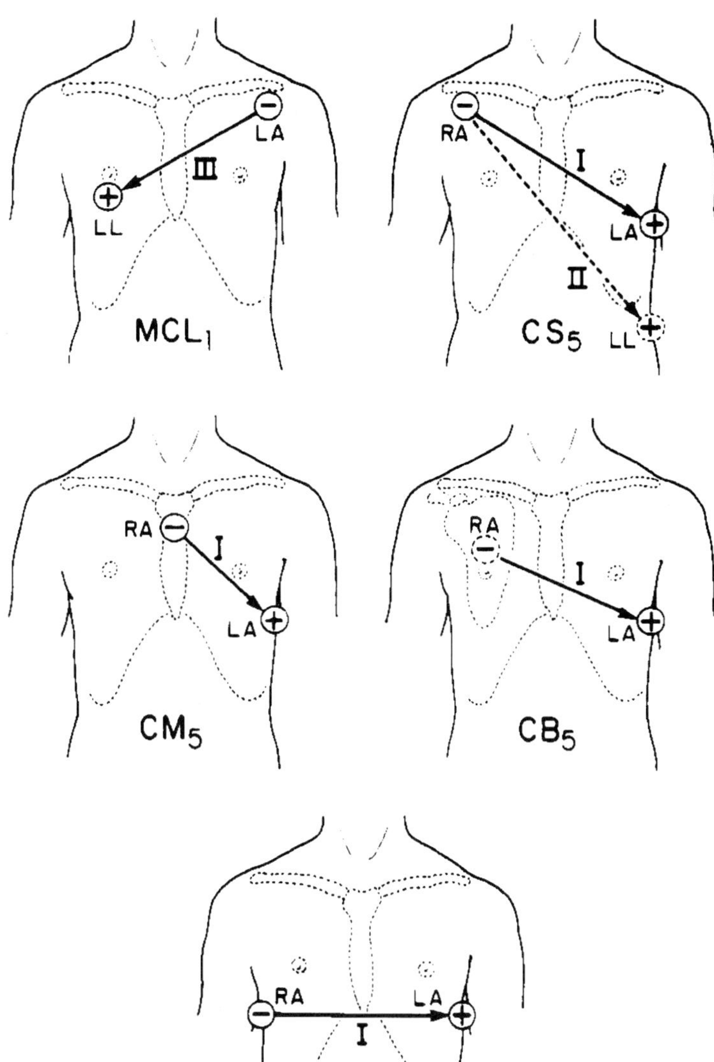

FIGURE 8–8. The modified three-lead systems. MCL, midclavicular line; CS_5, central subclavicular; CB_5, central back; CC_5, right anterior axillary line; CM_5, central manubrium. (From Kaplan J, Thys DM: Electrocardiography. In Miller RD [ed]: Anesthesia, 3rd ed, New York, Churchill Livingstone, 1990, p 1101, with permission.)

TABLE 8–1
Bipolar Leads for Use with Three Electrodes*

Lead System	MCL_1	CS_5	CM_5	CB_5	CC_5
Right arm electrode	Ground	Under right clavicle (−) (subclavicular)	Manubrium sternum (−)	Center of right scapula (−)	Right anterior axillary line (V_{5R}) (−)
Left arm electrode	Under left clavicle (−)	V_5 (+)	V_5 (+)	V_5 (+)	V_5 (+)
Left leg electrode	V_1 (+)	Ground	Ground	Ground	Ground
Lead selected	III	I	I	I	I
Advantages and indications	Good P-wave and QRS complex; useful for diagnosis of arrhythmias	Monitoring for anterior ischemia	Monitoring for anterior ischemia	Monitoring for anterior ischemia; good P wave for diagnosis of arrhythmias	Monitoring for ischemia

*From Kaplan J, Thys DM: Electrocardiography. In Miller RD (ed): Anesthesia, 3rd ed. New York, Churchill Livingstone, 1990, p 1101, with permission.
+, positive electrode; −, negative electrode.

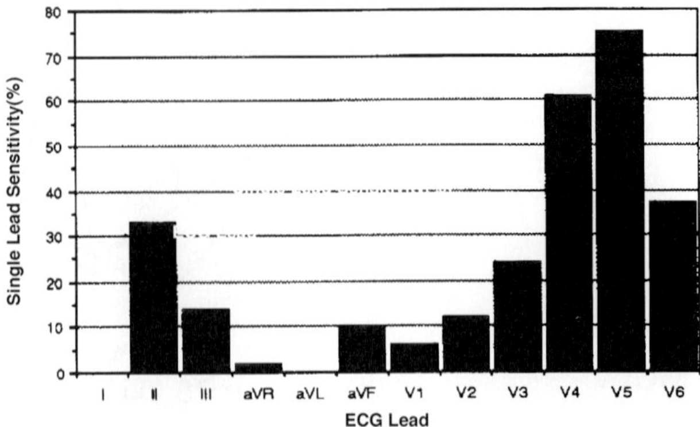

FIGURE **8–9.** Single-lead sensitivity for detection of myocardial ischemia during noncardiac surgery. (From London MJ, Hollenberg M, Wong MG, et al: Intraoperative myocardial ischemia: Localization by continuous 12-lead electrocardiography. Anesthesiology 69:232, 1988, with permission.)

The sensitivities were similar—81% for Holter and 84% for the 12-lead ECG. The specificity of both Holter and the 12-lead ECG was 85%.

Nonsurface, Invasive Electrocardiographic Monitoring

It is possible to monitor the heart invasively from the esophagus, trachea, or heart itself. Kates et al. studied the value of esophageal leads by comparing them to intra-atrial leads.[13] Using the intra-atrial ECG as the reference standard, they found that esophageal leads were 100% sensitive for the detection and analysis of dysrythmias. Due to the proximity of the electrodes to the atria, distinct P waves were recorded that were helpful in establishing the temporal relationship between atrial and ventricular electrical activity (Fig. 8–10). The proximity of the electrodes to the posterior wall of the heart made the detection of ischemic changes in this area of the heart more practical (Fig. 8–11).[14] Other investigators have used the esophageal electrodes for atrial pacing, and they can also be useful in patients with emphysema or in critically ill patients in whom a satisfactory surface ECG cannot be obtained.[15–17] Alternatively, a standard endotracheal tube with embedded electrodes can be used in a manner similar to the esophageal electrodes.[18] Other investigators have evaluated electrode-equipped pulmonary artery catheters and found them to be useful for diagnostic and therapeutic interventions. These catheters allow the recording of large-voltage, intracavitary ECGs, which greatly facilitate the diagnosis of atrial, ventricular, and AV nodal dysrhythmias.[19] Intravascular electrocardiography may be utilized in the operating room to accurately place long multiorifice central venous pressure (CVP) catheters prior to neurosurgical procedures. The proper positioning of these catheters is crucial for attempts at treating large venous air emboli. Proper positioning of these catheters can be determined by monitoring the intravenous ECG as the catheter is being advanced past the cavoatrial junction (Fig. 8–12).[20] Finally, the coronary guidewire used during coronary angioplasty has been used to record what was termed an intracoronary ECG. In one study, intracoronary ECG monitoring during coronary angioplasty detected ischemia in 83% of patients, whereas only 67% of patients had ischemia detected by conventional ECG.[21]

Technical Aspects of ECG Acquisition

When recording an ECG, it is important to be aware of the major causes of poor signal quality and artifacts. Some of these include incorrect lead application, interference from other electrical equipment in the operating room, and incorrect use of frequency filters.

Problems with Lead Application

Broken or out-of-date electrodes should not be used, as they may mimic every major electrocardiographic abnormality.[22] Similarly, inadequately insulated electrode cables will pick up other electric fields in the operating room.

To obtain the best ECG signal, it is important to prepare the patient's skin. Hair should be removed and the skin should be cleaned with alcohol. Hair oil and dirt may contribute to increased impedance, resulting in sig-

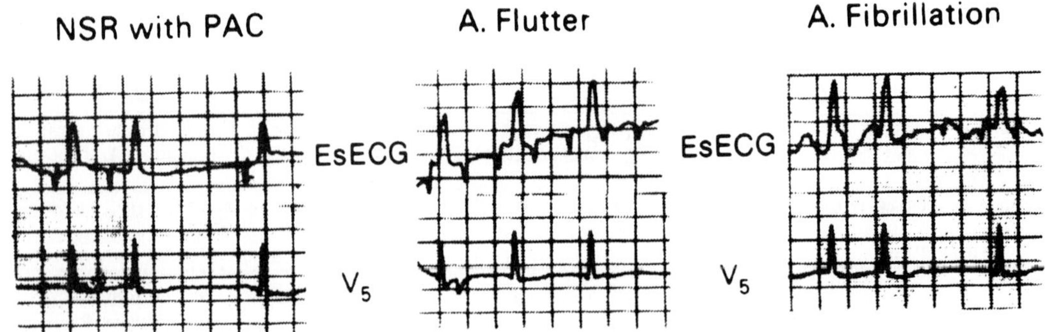

FIGURE **8–10.** Enhanced detection of atrial electrical activity using the esophageal ECG (EsECG). EsECG demonstrates arrhythmia progression from normal sinus rhythm (NSR) with one premature contraction (PAC) to atrial flutter (A Flutter) and atrial fibrillation (A Fibrillation). (From Kaplan J, Thys DM: Electrocardiography. In Miller RD [ed]: Anesthesia, 3rd ed, New York, Churchill Livingstone, 1990, p 1101, with permission.)

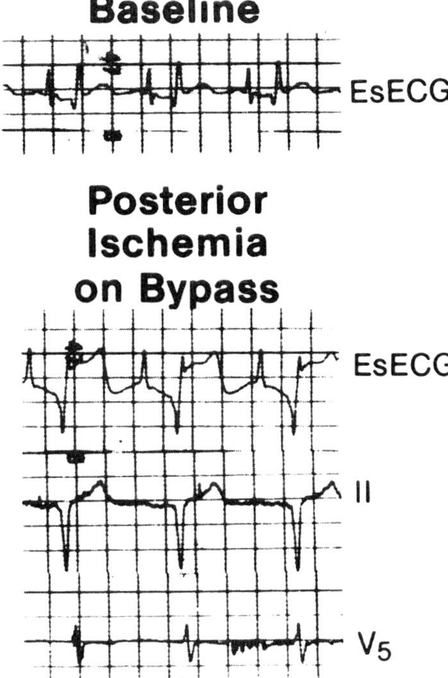

FIGURE 8–11. Tracing of esophageal ECG (EsECG), II, V_5 showing posterior ischemia. (From Kates RA, Zaidan JR, Kaplan JA: Esophageal lead for intraoperative electrocardiographic monitoring. Anesth Analg 61:781, 1982, with permission.)

nal attenuation. Mild superficial abrasion of the skin will reduce the thickness of the stratum corneum and thus reduce the resistance. The electrodes should adhere firmly to prevent movement artifacts.[23]

Artifacts Caused by Other Electrical Equipment in the Operating Room

Even with properly insulated electrodes, interference still occurs from electrical fields generated by 60-Hz operating room lights, electrocautery units, and cardiopulmonary bypass equipment. The most common cause of ECG signal distortion is the use of electrocautery. The ECG tracing is usually completed obliterated. Presently there is no reliable method to suppress this interference More unusual sources of interference include the use of a percutaneous lumbar diskectomy nucleotomes, fluid drops in the drip chamber of a warming unit, and the intraoperative recording of somatosensory evoked potentials.[24–26]

Artifacts Due to Improper Use of Filtering Mechanisms

In order to reduce recording artifacts, all modern ECG monitors use filters to narrow the range of recorded frequencies. The high-frequency filter reduces electrical interference caused by lights and electrocautery equipment. The low-frequency filter leads to a more stable baseline by reducing respiratory and body movement artifacts. The American Heart Association recommends that a flat frequency response be obtained at a bandwidth of 0.05 to 100 Hz.[27] The 100-Hz high-frequency limit ensures the adequate display of rapid electrocardiographic events such as atrial dysrhythmias and the 0.05-Hz frequency limit allows the accurate representation of slow events such as ST-segment and T-wave changes.

Most modern operating room and intensive care unit ECG monitors make allowance for the fact that monitoring needs vary among different patients and therefore enable the user to manipulate the filter setting of the ECG. If a careful analysis of the ST segment is necessary, the diagnostic mode with a bandwidth of 0.05 to 130 Hz should be selected. The low-frequency filter setting of 0.05 Hz ensures high-fidelity reproduction of the ST segment. If the main concern is dysrhythmia detection, the monitoring mode with a bandwidth of 0.5 to 40 Hz should be selected. Assessment of the P-wave and QRS morphology is facilitated in the monitoring mode. The correct choice of filter settings has important clinical consequences. Slogoff et al. showed that if ischemia detection was done in the monitoring mode with filter limits from 0.5 to 30 Hz, both the incidence and severity of observed intraoperative ischemic events (ST-segment depression and ST-segment elevation) nearly doubled compared to the diagnostic mode.[28] For this reason, most ECG monitors automatically select the appropriate filter when the automatic ST-segment analyzer is activated.

Significance of ECG Abnormalities

Resting Electrocardiogram

A standard 12-lead resting electrocardiogram is easily and inexpensively obtained in most patients and the basic results can be interpreted by most physicians. It provides an invaluable reference point for intraoperative and postoperative ECG tracings. Moorman et al. studied routine admission ECGs in medical patients.[29] They showed that they were cost effective and that the incidence of abnormalities increased with patient age and the presence of a clinically evident cardiac disease. Resting ECG abnormalities have the potential to alter anesthetic management and may be useful in predicting perioperative risk. Such abnormalities include premature atrial or ventricular contractions, atrial flutter or filbrillation, shortened PR intervals, conduction system blocks, myocardial ischemia or infarction, ventricular hypertrophy, electrolyte abnormalities, pulmonary disease, prolonged QT interval, and evidence of drug toxicity.

Premature Atrial or Ventricular Contractions

Goldman et al. determined that a nonsinus rhythm and more than five premature ventricular contractions on the resting ECG were independent predictors of increased perioperative risk after noncardiac surgery. While isolated premature ventricular contractions do occur in perfectly healthy individuals (Fig. 8–13),[30] more than five

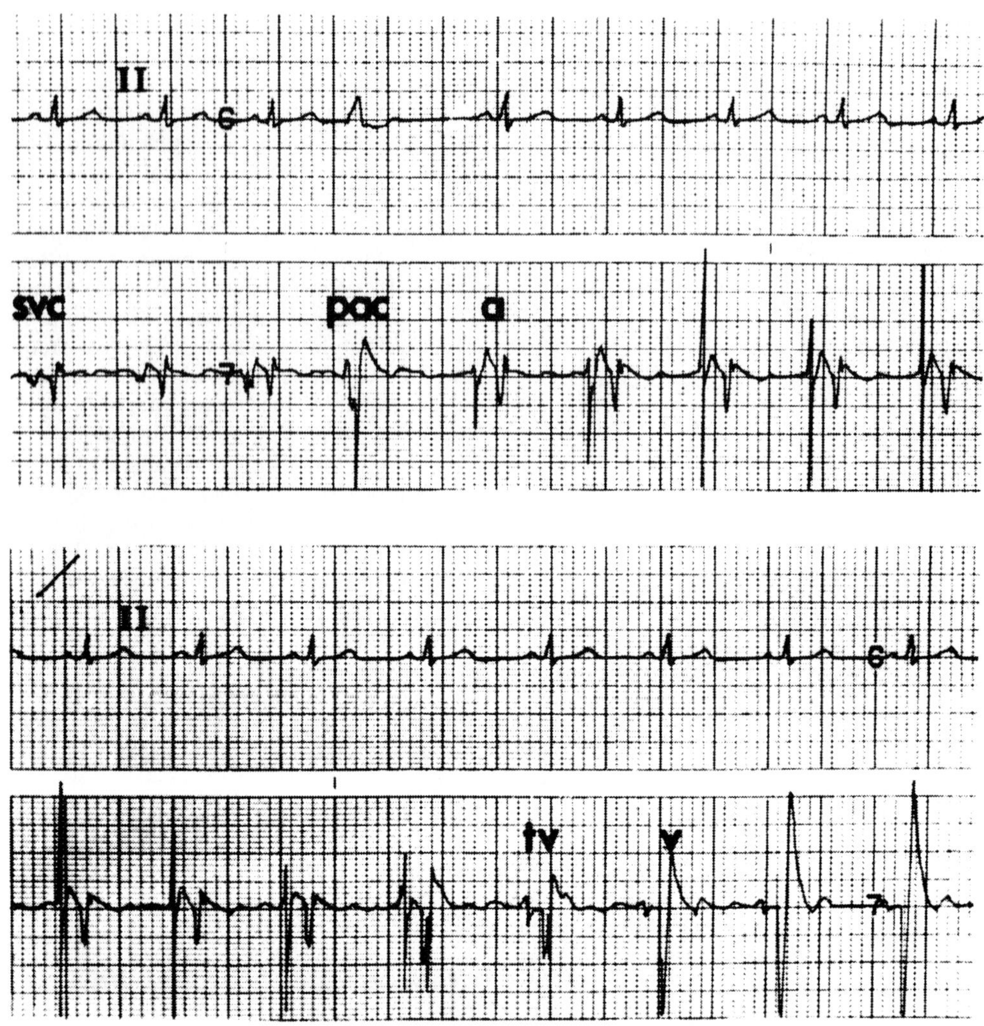

FIGURE **8–12.** Change in P-wave morphology on intravascular ECG as a catheter is advanced from the SVC to the RV. SVC, superior vena cava; PAC, premature atrial contraction; a, atrium; tv, tricuspid value; v, ventricle. (From Zaidan JR: Electrocardiography. In Barash PG, Cullen BF, Stoelting RK [eds]: Clinical Anesthesia, 2nd ed. Philadelphia, JB Lippincott Co, 1992, p 771, with permission.)

premature ventricular contractions per minute, multifocal ventricular ectopy, salvos, and runs of premature ventricular beats may all be indicators of serious underlying cardiac disease.[31] The position of a premature ventricular contraction in relation to the preceding T wave is important. Premature ventricular contractions occurring near the apex of a T wave can trigger ventricular fibrillation (R on T phenomenon). Premature atrial contractions also represent a higher than normal perioperative risk in patients who are elderly, face major surgery, or who are characterized as medically or surgically unstable. More recent investigations of perioperative risk by Detsky et al., Gerson et al., Cooperman et al., and Eagle et al. support Goldman's original findings.[32–38]

Atrial Flutter and Fibrillation

Atrial flutter occurs when a nonsinus, atrial pacemaker discharges at a rate of approximately 300 bpm. The normal P waves are replaced by the classic sawtooth flutter waves (Fig. 8–14). The resulting ventricular rhythm is often regular, since there is usually a fixed 2:1 or 3:1 AV block (ventricular rate 150 and 100, respectively). The ventricular response may be irregular if the block is variable and may mimic atrial fibrillation. The QRS complex configuration is normal. The T waves are lost in the flutter waves. Atrial flutter is always associated with organic heart disease such as coronary artery disease, valvular heart disease, myocarditis, or longstanding pulmonary disease. Treatment depends on the clinical situation and includes rate control and cardioversion (medical or electrical).

Like atrial flutter, atrial fibrillation is usually associated with the underlying heart disease. Sustained atrial fibrillation is present in approximately 10% of the population over 60 years. The ECG reveals chaotic atrial activity or absent atrial activity (Fig. 8–15). The ventricular rhythm is irregularly irregular and the ventricular response rate may be slow or fast. The QRS complexes are normal unless there is aberrant ventricular conduction. Since there is no effective atrial contraction, there is a loss of active ventricular filling and cardiac output

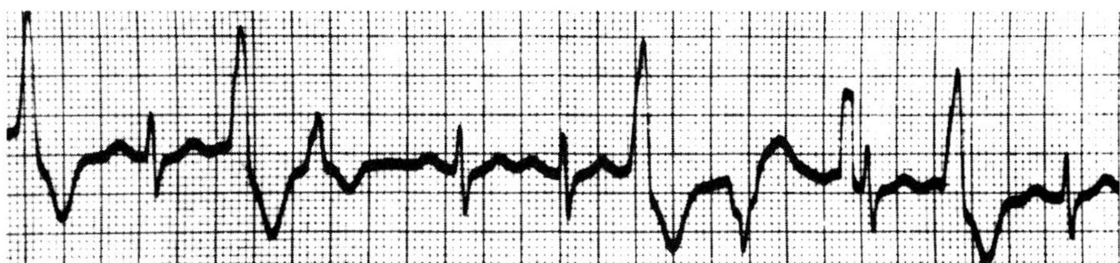

FIGURE **8–13.** Multifocal PVCs. (From Phibbs B: Cardiac Arrhythmias, 2nd ed. St Louis, CV Mosby Co, 1973, p 26, with permission.)

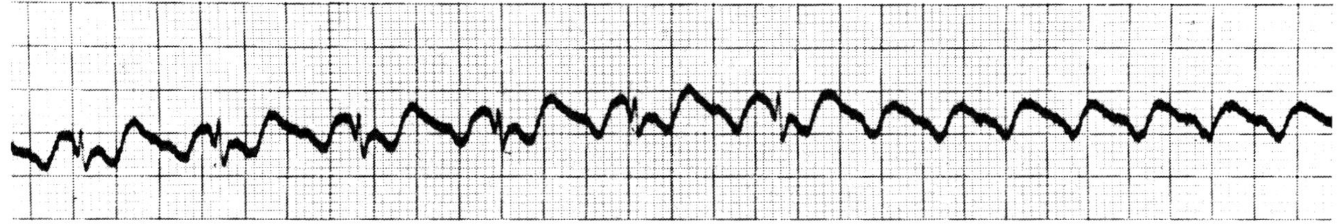

FIGURE **8–14.** Atrial flutter. Carotid sinus massage is applied after the sixth ventricular beat. (From Phibbs B: Cardiac Arrhythmias, 2nd ed. St Louis, CV Mosby, 1973, p 26, with permission.)

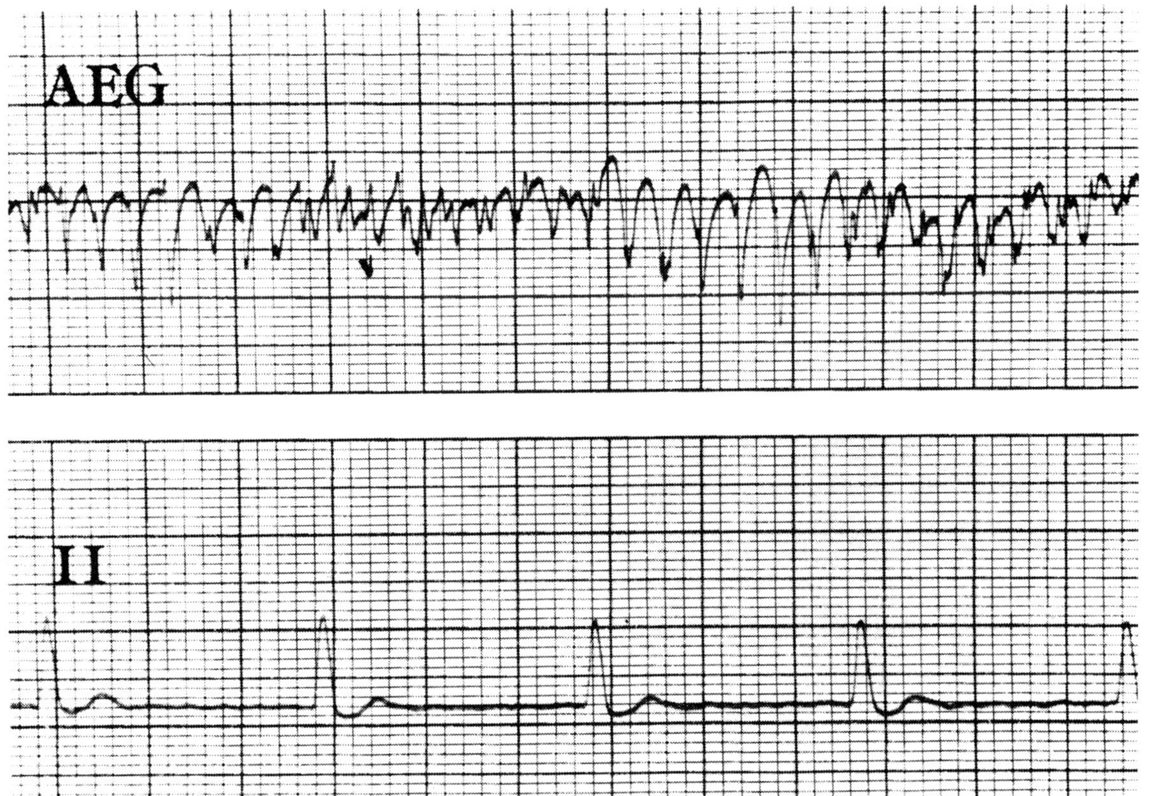

FIGURE **8–15.** Atrial fibrillation on the atrial electrocardiogram (AEG) and in lead II. (From Zaidan JR: Electrocardiography. In Barash PG, Cullen BF, Stoelting RK [eds]: Clinical Anesthesia, 2nd ed. Philadelphia, JB Lippincott Co, 1992, p 771, with permission.)

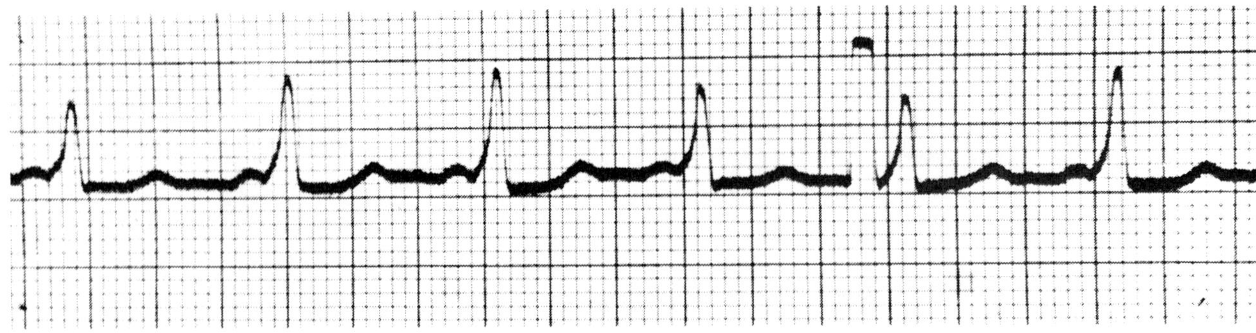

FIGURE **8–16.** Wolff-Parkinson-White syndrome. The PR interval is shortened and there is a delta wave. (From Phibbs B: Cardiac Arrhythmias, 2nd ed. St Louis, CV Mosby, 1973, p 26, with permission.)

will decrease. This is particularly so in patients with noncompliant ventricles. In patients undergoing coronary artery bypass surgery, the incidence of atrial fibrillation is 20 to 30%. The peak incidence is on the second or third postoperative day and the risk factors include increasing patient age, presence of chronic obstructive pulmonary disease (COPD), preoperative digoxin use, and aortic cross-clamp time.[39,40] The development of atrial fibrillation after coronary artery bypass surgery increases both morbidity (cerebrovascular accidents and ventricular arrhythmias) as well as hospital costs.[39] Treatment depends on the clinical situation and the hemodynamic status of the patient. Principles of treatment include rate control and cardioversion.

Shortened PR Intervals (Pre-excitation Syndromes)

Premature activation of the ventricles through anomalous pathways that bypass the AV node manifest as a shortened PR interval (<0.1 second). In the Wolff-Parkinson-White syndrome, the QRS is abnormal (Fig. 8–16). In the Lown-Ganong-Levine syndrome, the QRS complex is normal. Pre-excitation is present in 0.1 to 0.3% of the population.[41] In 50 to 70% of the patients with pre-excitation syndromes, there are self-limited, sporadic attacks of supraventricular tachycardia. These include atrial flutter, atrial fibrillation, and paroxysmal atrial tachycardia. While these arrhythmias are usually benign, malignant dysrhythmias such as ventricular tachycardia or ventricular fibrillation may occur and sudden death is possible.[42]

Conduction System Blocks

FIRST-DEGREE AV BLOCK

First degree AV block is recognized as a PR interval greater than 0.2 second (Fig. 8–17). Since the PR interval is determined by the atrial, AV node, and His-Purkinje activation, delay in any one of these levels can cause first-degree AV block. In the presence of a normal QRS, the delay is almost always at the level of the AV node. If the QRS is prolonged, the delay may be at any of the levels. Causes include enhanced parasympathetic tone, drugs, inferior myocardial infarction, and aging of the cardiac conduction system. First-degree AV block does not require treatment.

SECOND-DEGREE AV BLOCK

There are two forms of second-degree AV block—Mobitz type I block (Wenckebach block) and Mobitz type II block. Mobitz type I block is due to pathology at the level of the AV node. There is a progressive prolongation of the PR interval until an atrial beat is dropped (Fig. 8–18). After the dropped beat there is a pause that is not fully compensatory (i.e., less than two normal sinus intervals). Mobitz type I is associated with a normal QRS complex. The causes of Mobitz type I block include inferior myocardial infarction and drugs (digitalis, calcium channel blockers, β-blockers), and can be seen in individuals with increased vagal tone. Mobitz type I rarely progresses to complete heart block and, therefore, does not mandate therapy. In rare cases where Mobitz type I progresses to complete heart block, the escape rhythm is usually in the His bundle and is therefore stable.[43] In contrast, Mobitz type II block represents infranodal disease, usually of the His-Purkinje system. The PR interval is normal and dropped beats occur without any progressive lengthening of the PR interval (Fig. 8–19). The

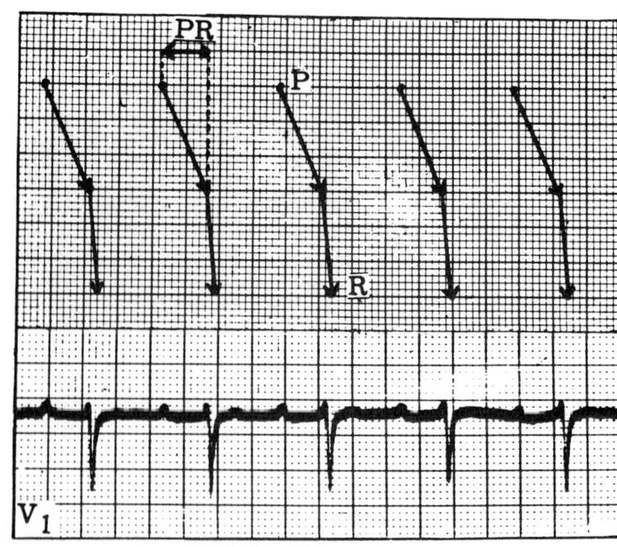

FIGURE **8–17.** First-degree AV block. PR = 0.28 second.

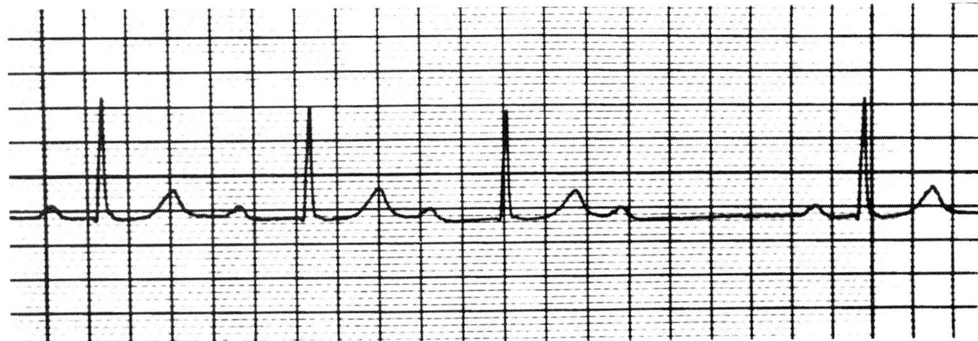

FIGURE **8–18.** Mobitz type I block (Wenckebach). (From Zaidan JR: Electrocardiography. In Barash PG, Cullen BF, Stoelting RK [eds]: Clinical Anesthesia, 2nd ed. Philadelphia, JB Lippincott Co, 1992, p 771, with permission.)

QRS interval is often prolonged. This type of block is always associated with significant cardiac disease and frequently progresses to complete heart block. It can occur as a result of sclerodegeneration and calcification of the conducting system and may complicate anteroseptal myocardial infarction. The escape rhythm is lower and slower and, therefore, unstable. Placement of a pacemaker is indicated, even in asymptomatic patients.[44]

It is important to remember that in patients who have had a heart transplant, the presence of two P waves before each QRS complex has a different significance. When a cardiac transplant is performed, the recipient sinoatrial node and part of the right atrium remains. They are attached to the right atrium of the donor heart. Consequently, the native P wave is followed by a second P wave resulting from depolarization of the transplanted right atrium.

RIGHT AND LEFT BUNDLE BRANCH BLOCK

Right bundle branch block (RBBB) manifests as a prolonged QRS complex (>0.12 second) with a typical RSR[1] configuration in precordial leads V_1 and V_2 (Fig. 8–20). This results from the delayed activation of the right ventricle. The initial forces of septal depolarization are not delayed and the ability to diagnose infarction is therefore not affected. The activation of the right ventricle is represented by the terminal anteriorly directed forces. RBBB is usually accompanied by ST-segment depression and T-wave inversion in leads V_1 through V_3. Isolated RBBB can be a normal finding, although it is frequently associated with chronic lung disease and atrial septal defects.[45]

In contrast, the presence of left bundle branch block (LBBB) is associated with organic heart disease. The QRS is greater than 0.12 second and the ECG shows a generalized disturbance reflecting abnormal septal depolarization (Fig. 8–21). Septal Q waves in leads I, aVL, and V_6 are lost and the anterior forces in V_1 are lost. Secondary ST- and T-wave changes occur in V_4 through V_6. The axis may be normal or leftward. A leftward axis implies more extensive conduction system disease and left ventricular dysfunction. Pre-existing LBBB pattern can effectively hide the electrocardiographic signs of infarction and ischemia. LBBB also masks the electrocardiographic signs of severe ventricular hypertrophy. A patient with a new LBBB may have had a recent myocardial infarction. This may also be the case in patients with existing LBBB who have increased symptoms of ischemia or heart failure. The clinician should therefore always attempt to locate the old ECG when confronted with a LBBB pattern. During anesthesia, the appearance of a LBBB during episodes of tachycardia or hypertension is an ominous sign and may signal an impending myocardial infarct.[46–48] The presence of LBBB may complicate the insertion of a pulmonary artery catheter (PAC). Progression of LBBB to complete heart block has been described.[49] Fortunately, the incidence is low and the use of a PAC in patients with LBBB is not contraindicated.[50] When inserting a PAC in a patient with LBBB, equipment for immediate cardiac pacing should be available. Often, pacing is accomplished

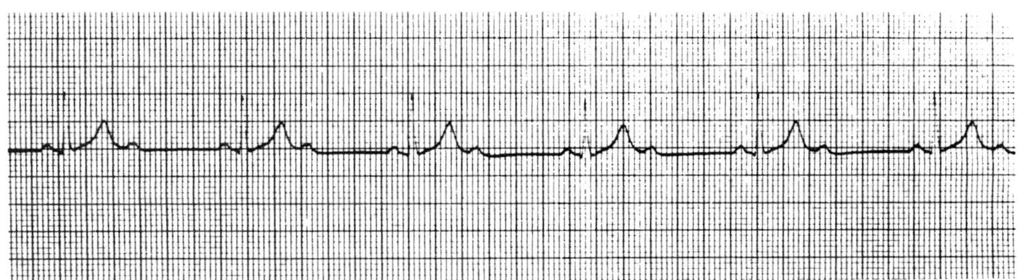

FIGURE **8–19.** Mobitz type II block. (From Zaidan JR, Curling PE: Cardiac dysrhythmias: Recognition and management. In Stoelting RK, Barash PG, Gallagher TH [eds]: Advances in Anesthesia, vol 2. Chicago, Year Book Medical, 1985, with permission.)

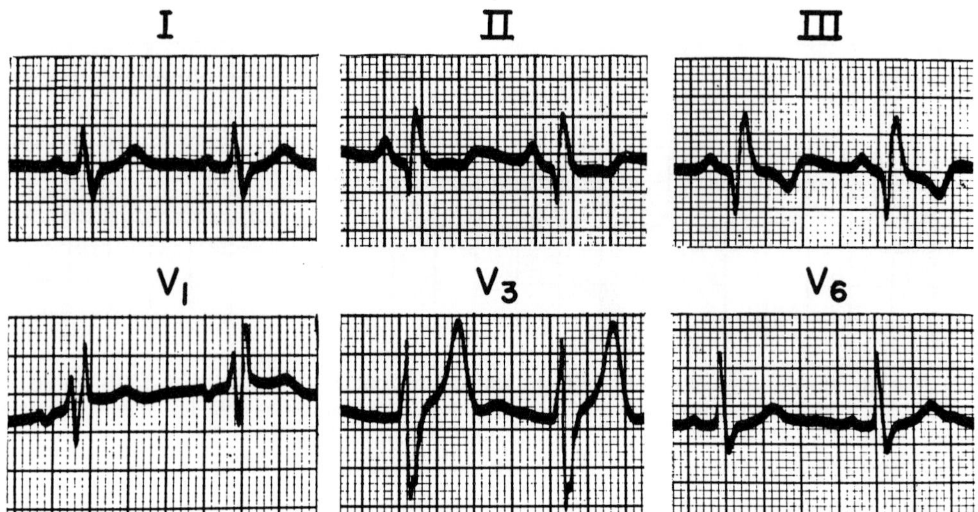

FIGURE **8–20.** Right bundle branch block. (From Goldberger AL, Goldberger E: Clinical Electrocardiography: A Simplified Approach, 5th ed, St Louis, Mosby Year Book, 1994, with permission.)

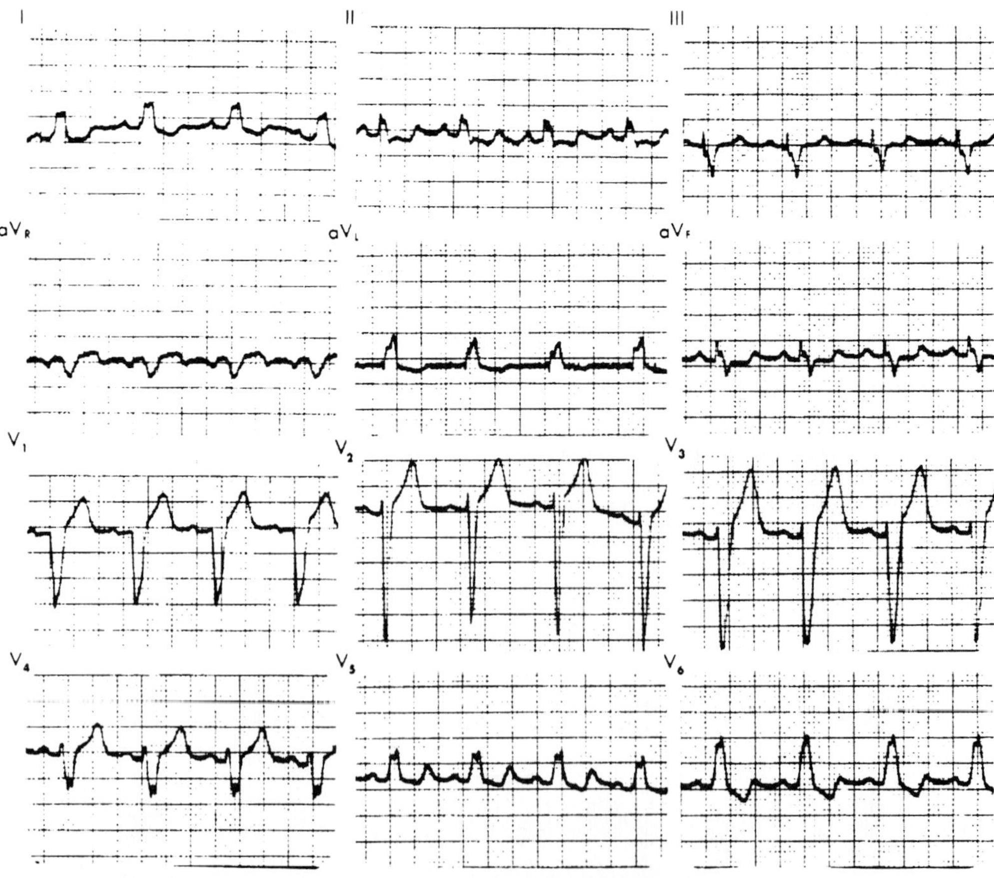

FIGURE **8–21.** Left bundle branch block. (From Goldberger AL, Goldberger E: Clinical Electrocardiography: A Simplified Approach, 5th ed, St Louis, Mosby Year Book, 1994, with permission.)

with a wire through a pacing PAC or via percutaneous pacing pads.

BIFASCICULAR AND TRIFASCICULAR BLOCK

RBBB in combination with a block of one of the fascicles of the left bundle branch is termed bifascicular block. The commonest cause is advanced coronary artery disease. Bifascicular block manifests as RBBB in combination with either a left- or a right-axis deviation. If the anterior fascicle of the left bundle is blocked, the ECG shows RBBB and left-axis deviation (Fig. 8–22); if the posterior fascicle of the left bundle is blocked, there is RBBB and right-axis deviation (Fig. 8–23). Bifascicular block is found on about 1% of adult ECGs.[51] The combination of RBBB and left posterior hemiblock is less common than RBBB and left anterior hemiblock, but the development of complete heart block occurs more frequently. Overall, 2% of patients per year with bifascicular block progress to complete heart block.[37] The presence of a bifascicular block per se does not require the prophylactic placement of a temporary pacemaker prior to surgery. However, it may be indicated if massive fluid shifts or physiologic derangements are expected or there is any suggestion of syncope.[52,53]

Trifascicular block is diagnosed when a bifascicular block pattern exists and the PR interval is also prolonged (Fig. 8–24). There is a high incidence of progression to complete heart block. Perioperative temporary pacemaker insertion is indicated.

THIRD-DEGREE AV HEART BLOCK

Third-degree heart block occurs when no atrial impulses reach the ventricles (Fig. 8–25). Cardiac activity is maintained by an escape pacemaker. If the QRS is normal, has a rate of 40 to 55, and increases with exercise or atropine, AV nodal block is likely. If the block is lower than the AV node, the escape rhythm is usually less than 40, the QRS is widened, and there is no response to exercise or atropine. This is an unreliable escape rhythm and mandates a permanent pacemaker.

Evidence of Myocardial Ischemia or Infarction

The resting ECG is normal in 25 to 50% of patients with coronary artery disease who have not had a prior myocardial infarct (MI).[54] Carliner et al. showed that patients undergoing noncardiac surgery who have ischemic ST-T changes on the preoperative ECG, had a three times higher risk of sustaining a perioperative adverse cardiac event (unstable angina, MI, significant dysrhythmia, congestive heart failure, or death) than those with no changes.[55] A normal preoperative ECG does not rule out a prior, non–Q-wave MI. However, the presence of pathologic Q waves (Q waves with a duration of >0.04 second and/or an amplitude of >25% of the associated R-wave amplitude) always represents a significant finding. Pathologic Q waves in leads V_1 through V_4 represent anterior infarction; those in I, aVL, V_5, and V_6 lateral

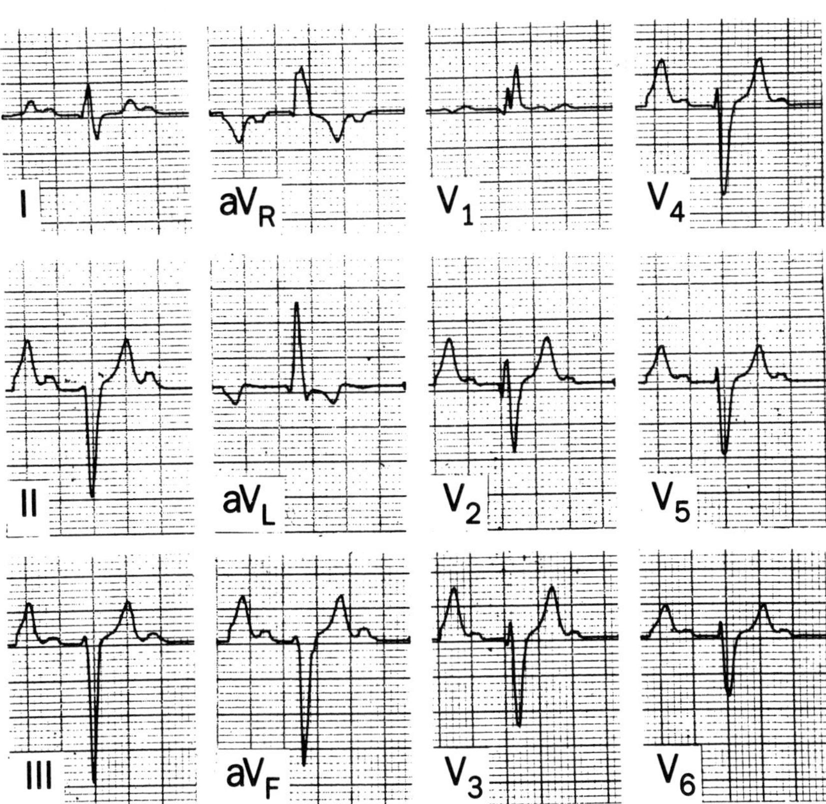

FIGURE **8–22.** RBBB and left anterior hemiblock. (From Kaplan J, Thys DM: Electrocardiography. In Miller RD [ed]: Anesthesia, 3rd ed, New York, Churchill Livingstone, 1990, p 1101, with permission.)

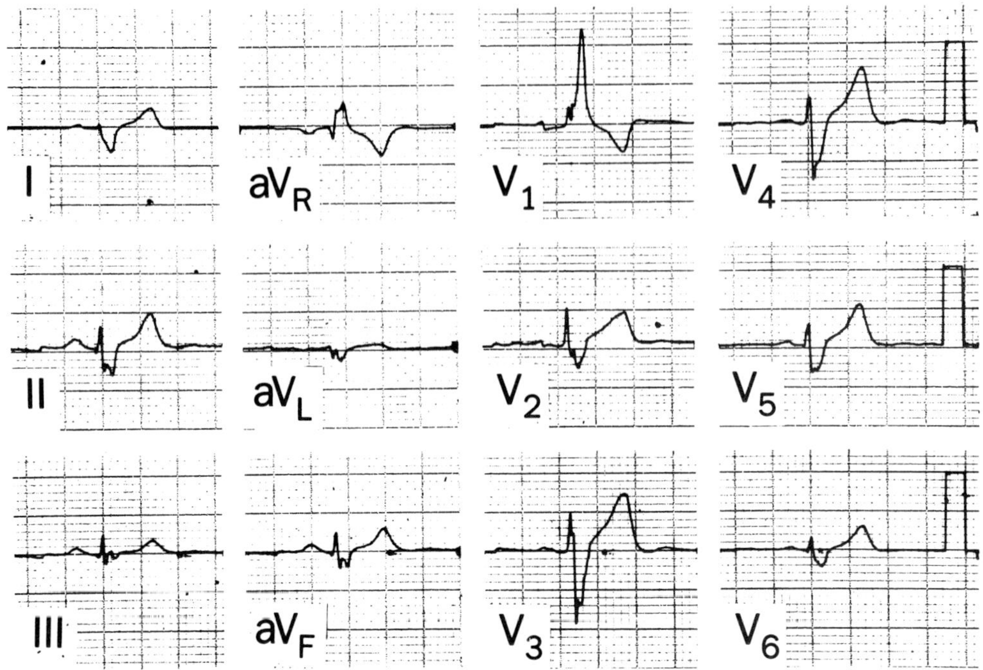

FIGURE **8–23.** RBBB and left posterior hemiblock. (From Kaplan J, Thys DM: Electrocardiography. In Miller RD [ed]: Anesthesia, 3rd ed, New York, Churchill Livingstone, 1990, p 1101, with permission.)

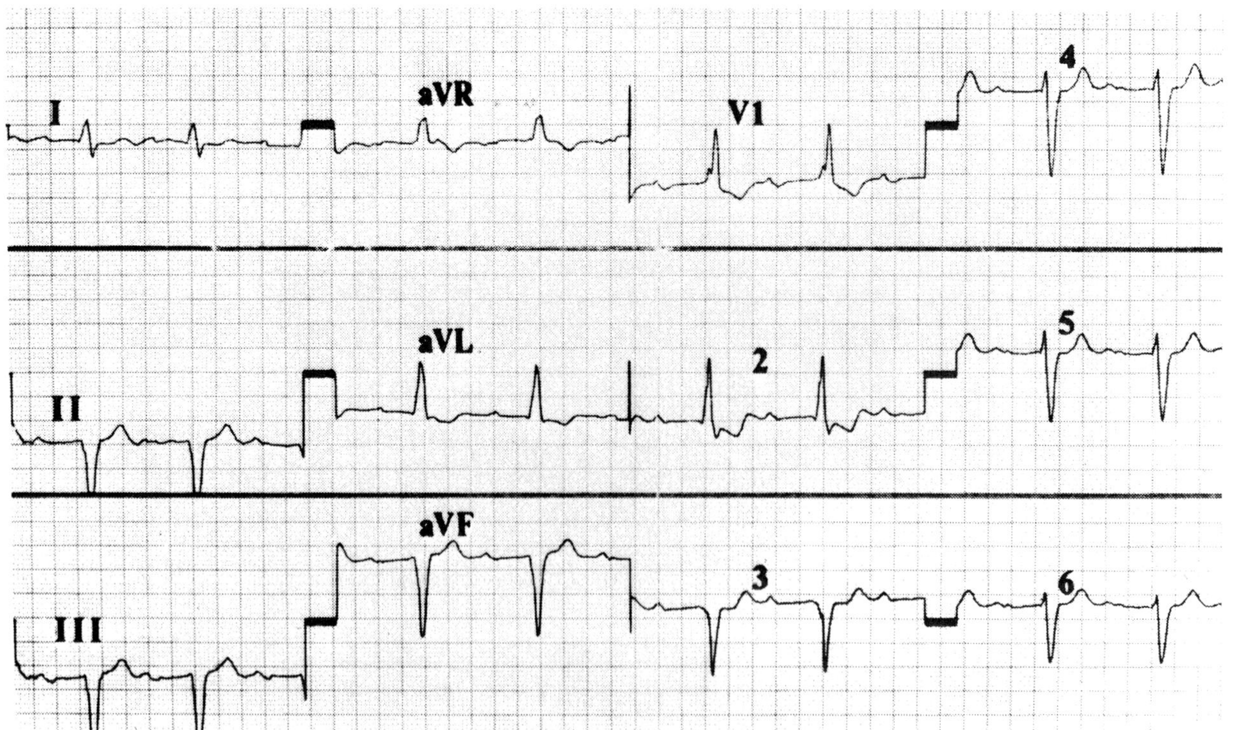

FIGURE **8–24.** Trifasicular block—RBBB, left-axis deviation, and prolonged PR interval. (From Zaidan JR, Curling PE: Cardiac dysrhythmias: Recognition and management. In Stoelting RK, Barash PG, Gallagher TH [eds]: Advances in Anesthesia, vol 2. Chicago, Year Book Medical, 1985, with permission.)

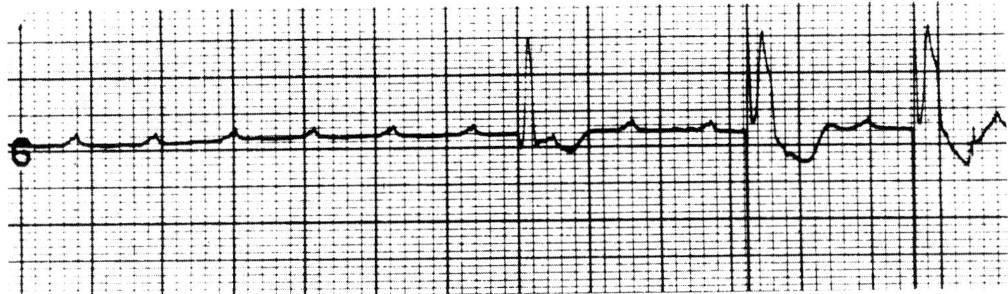

FIGURE **8–25.** Complete heart block. (From Zaidan JR: Electrocardiography. In Barash PG, Cullen BF, Stoelting RK [eds]: Clinical Anesthesia, 2nd ed. Philadelphia, JB Lippincott Co, 1992, p 771, with permission.)

infarction; and those in II, III, and a VF inferior infarction. Isolated posterior myocardial infarction can easily be missed, as none of the classic ECG leads lie over the posterior myocardium. The only sign of posterior infarction may be an R wave in lead V_1 that is larger than the associated S wave. While a similar pattern may be seen in right ventricular hypertrophy, right ventricular hypertrophy is always associated with right-axis deviation.

Patients with a history of prior myocardial infarction are at 50 times greater risk of having a perioperative MI (during major, noncardiac surgery) than patients without a previous MI (0.1% vs. 5%). An infarct within a 3-month period before surgery is associated with a 5.7 to 30% incidence of reinfarction.[56–60] When surgery occurs between 3 and 6 months after MI, the incidence of reinfarction varies from 2.3 to 15%. An infarct more than 6 months before surgery is associated with a 1.9 to 6% incidence of reinfarction. The mortality of perioperative myocardial infarction is reported to be about 50%, with little difference between studies. Lower rates of infarction in each of the time categories were reported by Rao et al.[50] Aggressive hemodynamic monitoring and intensive postoperative care were employed for all their patients. To date, other investigators have not been able to duplicate their results.

Ventricular Hypertrophy

Hollenberg et al. found that electrocardiographic evidence of ventricular hypertrophy was an independent predictor of increased perioperative risk after noncardiac surgery.[61] Left ventricular hypertrophy (LVH) appears as tall R waves in V_5 and V_6 (>2.5 mV) and deep S waves (>2.5 mV) in V_1 and V_2 (Fig. 8–26). If the T waves are normal, the voltage criteria must be interpreted in relation to the body habitus. Thin-chested individuals may exceed the voltage criteria for LVH despite having normal left ventricular mass. In LVH, the axis is usually leftward (between 0 and −30 degrees). It is unusual for LVH alone to deviate the axis more than −30 degrees in the absence of left anterior hemiblock. Severe left ventricular hypertrophy results in episodes of subendocardial ischemia, appearing as the strain pattern (ST-segment depression and T-wave inversion). Left ventricle strain often heralds the onset of ventricular dilatation and failure.

Right ventricular hypertrophy appears as tall R waves in V_1 (>0.5 mV) and deep S waves (>0.7 mV) in V_5 and V_6 (Fig. 8–27). The frontal QRS axis shifts rightward, usually greater than 110 degrees. This is always a significant finding on ECG and should prompt an investigation for the underlying cause.

Electrolyte Abnormalities

Electrolyte abnormalities can alter the ECG and cause numerous perioperative cardiac dysrhythmias. Abnormalities of potassium, calcium, and magnesium can lead to specific and nonspecific ECG changes.

POTASSIUM

Serum potassium levels below 2.5 to 3.0 mEq/L can either cause or potentiate dysrhythmias due to re-entry or increased automaticity. Although not specific for hypokalemia, the ECG may initially show a U wave without significant QT prolongation. There may also be ST-segment depression, T-wave flattening, or T-wave inversion. Prolongation of the QT interval (actually the QU intervals) often precedes the occurrence of serious ventricular dysrhythmias.

Hyperkalemia (serum potassium level 6.5 to 7 mEq/L) results in the appearance of tall, slender "tented" T waves on the ECG. As the severity of hyperkalemia increases (K +8.0), the QRS widens and blends with the tall peak T waves. The PR interval prolongs and the P waves may disappear. The classic changes of hyperkalemia are not seen in all patients with hyperkalemia.

CALCIUM AND MAGNESIUM

The ECG change caused by both hypercalcemia and hypermagnesemia is shortening of the QT interval. Conversely, both hypocalcemia and hypomagnesemia cause prolongation of the QT interval. Increased QT interval is accompanied by an increased incidence of a variant of ventricular tachycardia known as torsades de pointes.[62,63]

Pulmonary Disorders

The ECG in chronic obstructive pulmonary disease may show low-voltage, right-axis deviation and poor R-wave

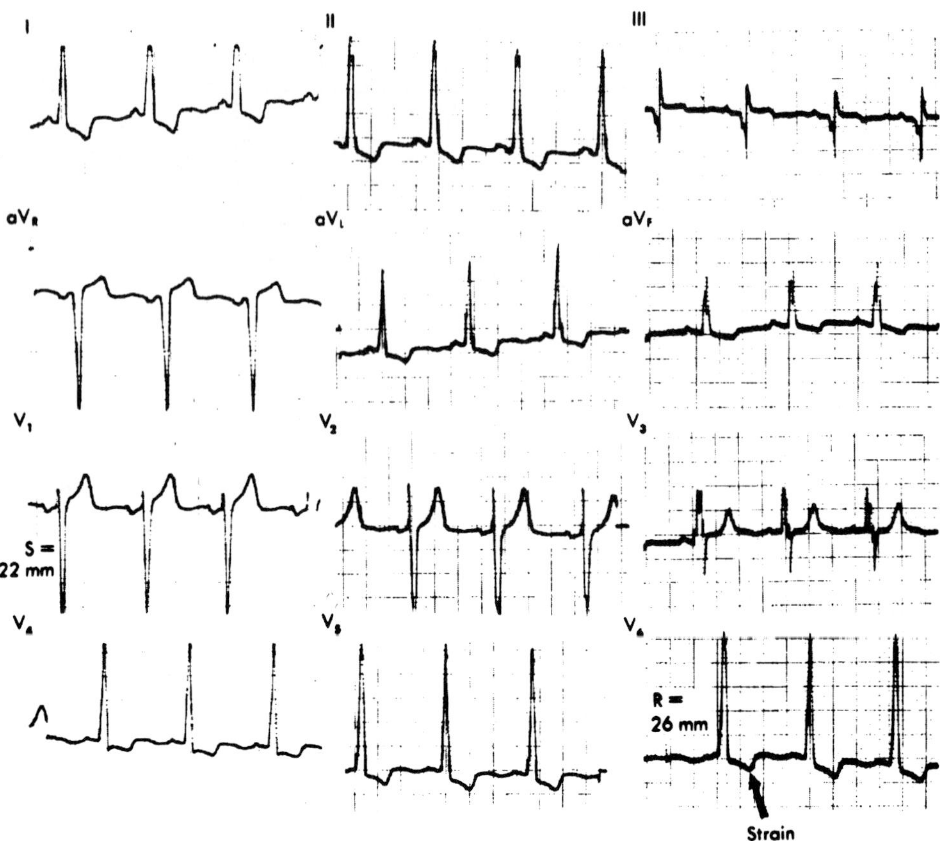

FIGURE **8–26.** Left ventricular hypertrophy with strain. (From Goldberger AL, Goldberger E: Clinical Electrocardiography: A Simplified Approach, 5th ed, St Louis, Mosby Year Book, 1994, with permission.)

progression in the precordial leads (Fig. 8–28). The R-wave loss and the low voltage are caused by the dampening effects of the hyperinflated lungs, and the axis deviation is caused by hyperinflated lungs forcing the heart into a vertical or rightward position. The associated right ventricular hypertrophy also causes right-axis deviation. There are also signs of right atrial enlargement.

Sudden massive pulmonary embolism may cause ECG changes including right bundle branch block, right ventricular strain, a large S wave in lead I, deep Q waves and inverted T waves in lead III, sinus tachycardia, and atrial fibrillation. However, none of the ECG changes of pulmonary embolism are very sensitive or specific (Fig. 8–29).

Prolonged QT Interval

A rate-corrected QT interval (QTc) greater than 0.44 second is associated with an increased susceptibility for development of life-threatening ventricular dysrhythmias, especially torsades de pointes (Fig. 8–30).[64] A prolonged QT interval can be caused by congenital syndromes (Jervell-Lange-Nielsen and Romano-Ward syndromes), electrolyte abnormalities, and drugs (quinidine-like drugs, tricyclic antidepressants, and many others).

Drug Toxicity

Analysis of the preoperative resting ECG may alert the anesthesiologist to possible toxic levels of some commonly administered drugs.

DIGITALIS

Digitalis effect refers to the shortening of the QT interval and sagging of the ST-T complex produced by therapeutic doses of digitalis. Digitalis toxicity manifests as either dysrhythmias or conduction blocks. These may be benign or malignant ventricular ectopy, nodal rhythms, sinus bradycardia, episodes of sinus arrest, paroxysmal atrial tachycardia, or the various degrees of AV block. A variety of factors including renal failure, hypokalemia, hypercalcemia, hypomagnesemia, hypoxemia, old age, acute myocardial infarction, and the concomitant administration of many drugs predispose to digitalis toxicity.

PSYCHOACTIVE DRUGS

The tricyclic antidepressants have negative inotropic effects and impair AV conduction. These drugs may prolong the PR interval, the QRS complex, and the QT interval. They may also alter the ST segment and T wave and can induce both atrial and ventricular dysrhythmias.[65] Therapeutic levels of lithium may cause nonspe-

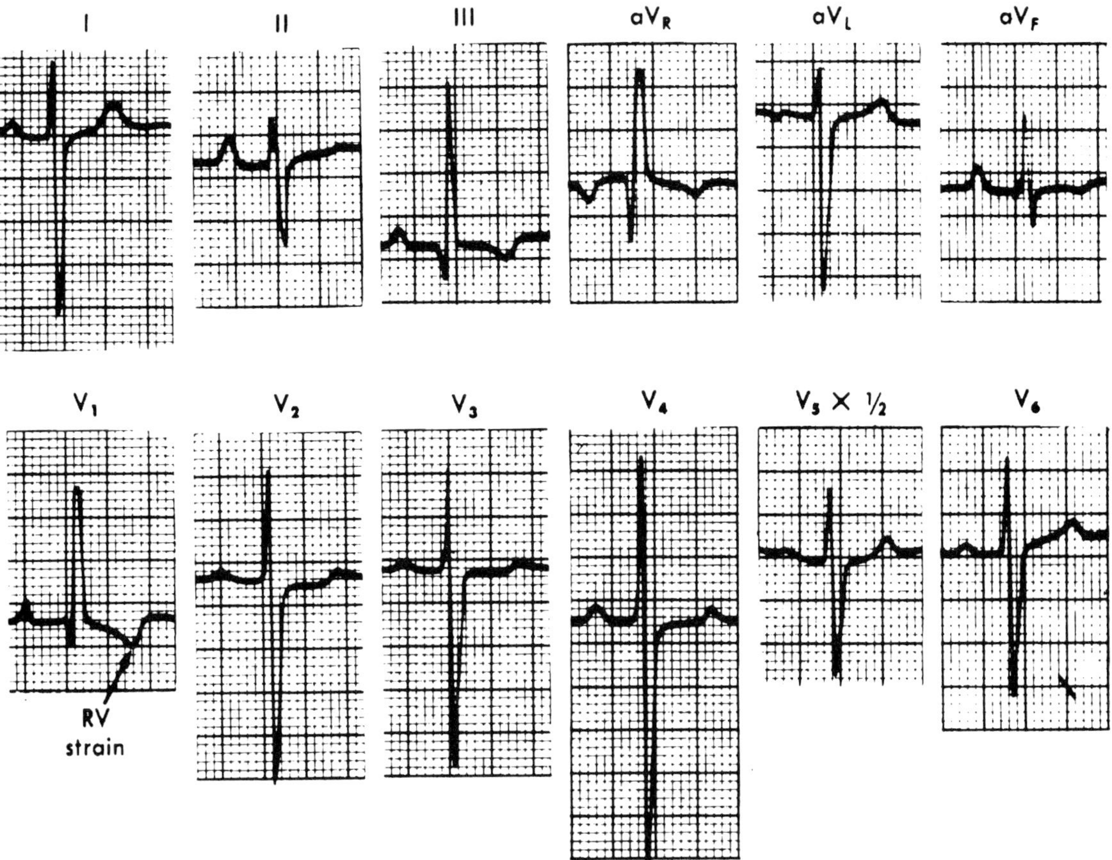

FIGURE **8–27.** Right ventricular hypertrophy. (From Goldberger AL, Goldberger E: Clinical Electrocardiography: A Simplified Approach, 5th ed, St Louis, Mosby Year Book, 1994, with permission.)

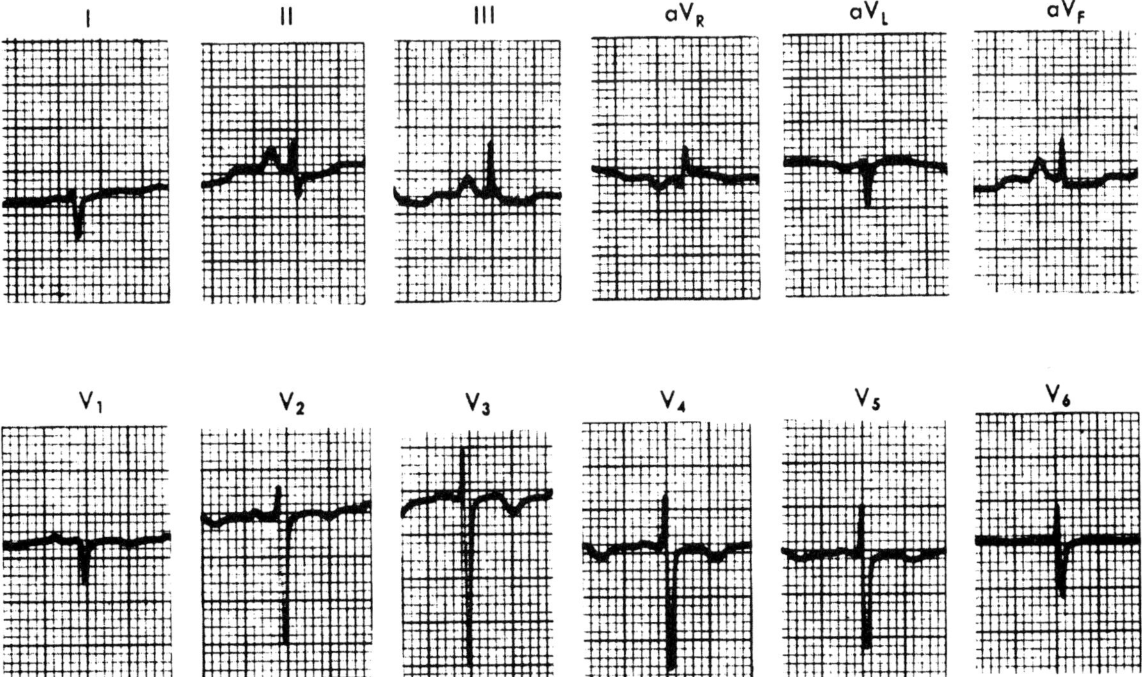

FIGURE **8–28.** Notice the characteristic low voltages in the limb leads, right-axis deviation, P pulmonale, and poor R-wave progression. T-wave inversions (V_1 through V_4) due to right ventricular strain. (From Goldberger AL, Goldberger E: Clinical Electrocardiography: A Simplified Approach, 5th ed, St Louis, Mosby Year Book, 1994, with permission.)

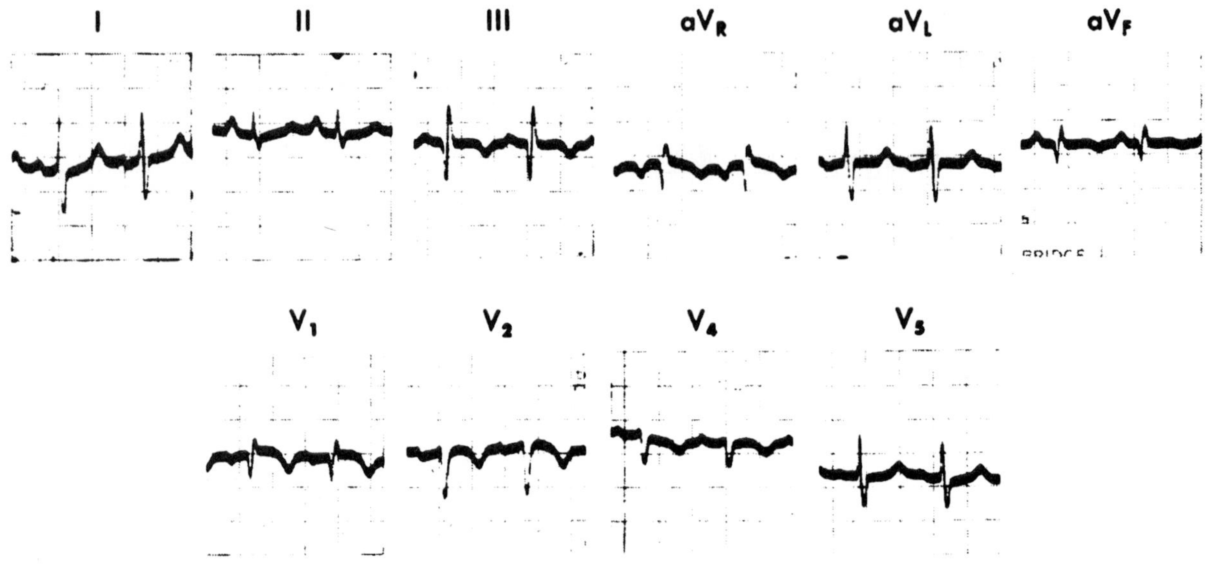

FIGURE 8–29. Features that may be seen with pulmonary embolism include sinus tachycardia, S waves in lead I, Q waves and T wave inversion in lead III, and right ventricular strain. (From Goldberger AL, Goldberger E: Clinical Electrocardiography: A Simplified Approach, 5th ed, St Louis, Mosby Year Book, 1994, with permission.)

cific ST-segment and T-wave changes; toxic levels may cause severe bradyarrhythmias.

Prognostic Value of the Preoperative ECG

Standard 12-Lead ECG

The prognostic value of the standard 12-lead preoperative ECG has been discussed previously.

Holter Monitoring

Continuous ambulatory electrocardiographic monitoring is useful for monitoring dysrhythmias and the severity and/or frequency of ischemic episodes. The detection of Mobitz type II or complete AV block may indicate the need for a permanent pacing. Patients with evidence of impaired ventricular function may show frequent premature ventricular beats, R on T phenomenon, or sustained periods of ventricular tachycardia. In patients with coronary artery disease, Holter monitoring may reveal episodes of silent ischemia. Ischemic episodes on Holter monitoring correlate well with both intra- and postoperative ischemia. Raby et al. showed that 33% of vascular surgery patients with preoperative ischemia on Holter monitoring had intra- and postoperative cardiac complications, whereas only 1% of patients without preoperative ischemia had cardiac complications.[66] A recent meta-analysis showed that intraoperative Holter monitoring was effective in predicting postoperative adverse cardiac events.[67]

Exercise Electrocardiography

The overall sensitivity and specificity of exercise electrocardiography for ischemia detection is 65% and 90%, respectively.[68] The sensitivity increases to about 85% in patients with three-vessel or left main coronary artery disease. A normal test does not exclude coronary artery disease but suggests that severe disease is unlikely. The time of onset to ST-segment depression, the severity of the ST depression, and the time to resolution are valuable guides to perioperative anesthetic management by setting limits to the hemodynamic stresses that the patient can safely tolerate. Exercise-induced ventricular ectopy is frequently associated with severe coronary artery disease and impaired ventricular function. Additional findings associated with severe multivessel disease include greater than 2 mm horizontal or down-sloping ST-

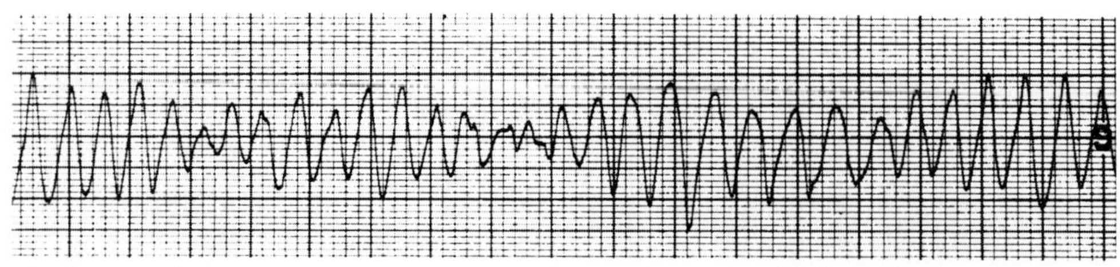

FIGURE 8–30. Torsades de pointes. (From Zaidan JR, Curling PE: Cardiac dysrhythmias: Recognition and management. In Stoelting RK, Barash PG, Gallagher TH [eds]: Advances in Anesthesia, vol 2. Chicago, Year Book Medical, 1985, with permission.)

segment depression, persistent ST-segment depression for more than 5 minutes after exercise, decrease (≥15 mm Hg) in systolic blood pressure, and failure to reach a maximal heart rate greater than 70% of predicted. The utility of exercise electrocardiography is limited in patients with baseline ST-segment abnormalities (LBBB or ventricular hypertrophy). The test cannot be used in patients who are unable to increase their heart rate due to claudication, fatigue, dyspnea, or drug therapy.

Intraoperative ECG Monitoring for Dysrhythmias

The occurrence of dysrhythmias during surgery is common. Using continuous electrocardiographic monitoring, Bertrand et al. reported an 84% incidence of ventricular or supraventricular dysrhythmias.[69] Another study has reported an incidence of about 65%.[70] The incidence is higher in patients with heart disease, and regional anesthesia does not reduce the incidence of perioperative dysrhythmias.[71] The incidence of perioperative cardiac dysrhythmias with life-threatening hemodynamic consequences is rare.

An in-depth discussion of all aspects of perioperative dysrhythmias is beyond the scope of this section, and the reader is referred to Chapter 32. This section focuses on the prerequisites for good electrocardiographic dysrhythmia monitoring and reviews the electrophysiologic basis of the development of dysrhythmias.

Prerequisites for Dysrhythmia Monitoring

Since it is critical to establish the relation between atrial and ventricular depolarization to correctly diagnose dysrhythmias, the leads selected must maximize P-wave morphology. Most operating rooms and critical care units use either five- or three-lead ECG systems. If a five-lead system is available, P waves should be monitored in leads II, III, aVF, and V_1. If a three-lead system is used, the modified bipolar leads MCL_1 and CB_5 are most suitable.[72–75]

Electrophysiologic Basis of Dysrhythmias

Cardiac dysrhythmias can be explained electrophysiologically in two ways—abnormal cardiac impulse conduction (re-entry) and abnormal impulse formation.[76] For re-entry to occur, there must be two pathways through which cardiac impulses are conducted at different velocities. Antegrade conduction occurs through one pathway and retrograde conduction through the other. When a state of suitable conduction velocities and refractory periods coincide, a re-entry circuit can be established with rapid, repeated generation of electrical impulses. Automatic (ectopic) cardiac dysrhythmias are due to enhanced automaticity of a focus that is capable of undergoing spontaneous depolarization. The slope of phase 4 depolarization of the cell is increased, which results in irritability of the cell. This irritability is manifested as isolated premature beats or episodes of tachycardia.

Supraventricular Dysrhythmias

Sinus Bradycardia

In sinus bradycardia, the sinus node pacemaker is discharging at a rate of less than 60 bpm. The rhythm is regular, and there is a 1:1 relationship between the normally shaped P wave and the QRS complex. The PR interval and QRS complex is normal. Treatment is not indicated unless the bradycardia is profound and hemodynamic compromise exists.

Sinus Tachycardia

The heart rate is greater than 100 bpm and may be as high as 200 bpm. Sinus tachycardia is the most common perioperative dysrhythmia and the causes are numerous. Treatment will depend on the clinical situation. A search for the underlying cause is crucial.

AV Junctional Rhythm Disturbances

In AV junctional rhythm, the heart rate is regular and varies from 40 to 180 bpm. There may be one P wave for every QRS complex, but the PR interval is usually less than 0.1 second. The P-wave morphology is abnormal. The P waves may either precede, follow, or be embedded in the QRS complex. Junctional rhythms are common during anesthesia and frequently occur when halogenated anesthetics are used. Treatment is not usually required. However, junctional rhythms may not be well tolerated in patients with noncompliant ventricles.

Paroxysmal Supraventricular Tachycardias

Paroxysmal supraventricular tachycardia (PSVT) is defined as a run of three or more supraventricular premature beats. There are three major types of PSVTs: (1) paroxysmal atrial tachycardia (PAT), (2) AV nodal re-entrant tachycardia, and (3) bypass tract tachycardia (e.g., Wolff-Parkinson-White syndrome). In PAT, an ectopic atrial pacemaker fires at a rate of up to 200 bpm. The rhythm is regular and the relationship of the P waves to the QRS is 1:1. The P waves are usually superimposed on the preceding T waves (Fig. 8–31).

AV nodal re-entrant tachycardia presents as a rapid, regular rhythm with rates ranging from 140 to 250 bpm. It is caused by a re-entrant impulse in the AV node. The P waves are usually absent, since atria and ventricles are depolarized simultaneously, effectively hiding the P waves in the QRS complex.

In a bypass tract tachycardia, the electrical impulse travels down the normal conduction system (AV node and bundle of His) into the ventricles (antegrade conduction), and recycles to the atria via an anomalous by-

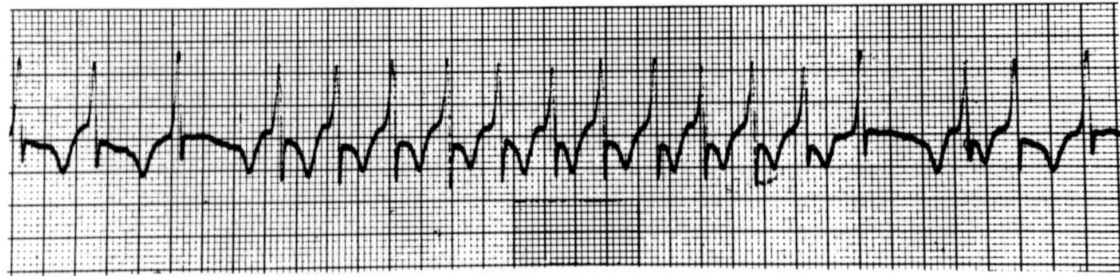

FIGURE 8–31. Paroxysmal atrial tachycardia. (From Kaplan J, Thys DM: Electrocardiography. In Miller RD [ed]: Anesthesia, 3rd ed. New York, Churchill Livingstone, 1990, p 1101, with permission.)

pass tract (retrograde conduction). A re-entrant tachyarrhythmia is therefore established, with rates up to 200 bpm.

Ventricular Dysrhythmias

Ventricular Extrasystoles

Ventricular extrasystoles present as bizarre QRS complexes with no associated P waves. However, whether frequent or complex intraoperative ventricular extrasystoles can trigger potentially lethal ventricular tachycardia (VT) or ventricular fibrillation is controversial. While this occurs in the presence of an acute myocardial infarct, there is no definitive proof in the anesthesia setting (Fig. 8–13).[77,78]

Ventricular Tachycardia and Ventricular Fibrillation

Any tachycardia with wide or bizarre looking QRS complexes should be presumed to be ventricular in origin, although it could represent a PSVT with aberrant conduction (Fig. 8–32). The differential diagnosis of PSVT versus VT is summarized in Table 8–2.[79] If VT is sustained, treatment is always indicated because of the high incidence of degeneration of ventricular tachycardia into ventricular fibrillation. Ventricular fibrillation is characterized by irregular undulations in the baseline with no recognizable QRS complexes, ST segments, or T waves (Fig. 8–33).

ECG Monitoring for Myocardial Ischemia

Lead Selection

The V_5 lead is the best single lead for detecting ischemia, with a sensitivity of 75%. If lead II is also monitored, sensitivity increases to 80%. If leads II, V_4, and V_5 are monitored concurrently, sensitivity increases to 96% (Fig. 8–9). In the absence of a five-lead system, the modified bipolar limb leads CS_5 and CM_5 are good alternatives.[80]

Leads II, III, and aVF reveal ischemia in the inferior (diaphragmatic) portion of the left ventricle, which is normally supplied by the right coronary artery. The right coronary artery also supplies the SA node, the AV node, the proximal part of the bundle of His, the posterior fascicle of the left bundle branch, the right atrium, and the posterior portion of the interventricular septum. The posterior wall of the left ventricle and the greater part of the right ventricle are also supplied by the right coronary artery. They can be monitored indirectly by observing reciprocal changes in leads V_1 and V_2. There are no standard ECG leads that directly face the posterior wall. In patients with both left and right coronary artery disease, the standard leads may, therefore, be inadequate for ischemia monitoring. DeHert et al. evaluated the use of a specialized V_{4R} lead in patients with both right and left coronary artery disease.[81] They found that monitoring of V_{4R} allowed the detection of 20% more ischemic episodes than monitoring only leads I, II, V_5, and/or CB_5.

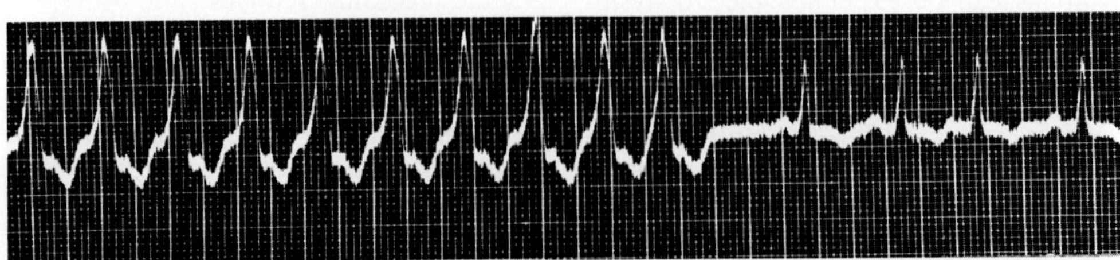

FIGURE 8–32. Ventricular tachycardia and resumption of sinus rhythm after lidocaine. (From Phibbs B: Cardiac Arrhythmias, 2nd ed. St Louis, CV Mosby, 1973, p 26, with permission.)

TABLE 8–2
The Differential Diagnosis of Broad Complex Tachycardias Using the 12-Lead ECG

Feature	Comments
Regularity (RR interval variability <40 msec)	Ventricular origin likely
Independent atrial activity	Diagnostic of VT
Capture or fusion beats	Diagnostic of VT, if present
QRS width of more than 0.14 sec	VT likely
Left-axis deviation	VT likely
Rsr complex in lead V_1	VT likely
rsR complex in lead V_1	SVT with aberrant conduction likely

VT, ventricular tachycardia; SVT, supraventricular tachycardia.

Lead V_{4R} is the most sensitive and specific lead for detecting right ventricular ischemia and infarction.[82,83]

Blood supply to the anterior wall of the left ventricle, anterior portions of the interventricular system, the distal part of the bundle of His, the right bundle, the main stem of the left bundle branch, and the left anterior fascicle are supplied by the left anterior descending branch of the left coronary artery. Ischemic changes in these areas appear in leads V_1 through V_4. The circumflex branch of the left coronary artery supplies the lateral wall of the left ventricle. Leads V_5, V_6, I, and aVL monitor ischemia of the lateral wall. Myocardial ischemia causes delayed and abnormal repolarization of the cardiac myocytes, causing changes in the ST segment and T wave.

ECG Manifestations

ST-Segment Changes

Myocardial ischemia is defined as greater than 1 mm horizontal or down-sloping ST-segment depression at a point of 60 to 80 msec after the J point (Fig. 8–34).[84] The degree of ST-segment depression correlates with the severity of the ischemia. When compared with horizontal ST-segment depression, down-sloping ST-segment depression is associated with an increased number of diseased coronary arteries and an increased mortality.[85,86] In contrast, up-sloping ST-segment depression of less than 2 mm usually represents a benign occurrence and is not associated with myocardial ischemia. However, greater than 2 mm of up-sloping ST segment is associated with the same incidence of two- and three-vessel coronary artery disease as horizontal ST-segment depression. As myocardial ischemia progresses in severity from subendocardial to transmural, ST segments may progress from up-sloping to horizontal or down-sloping (Fig. 8–35). ST-segment elevation represents acute myocardial injury (i.e., preinfarction). It may also represent coronary vasospasm and epicardial ischemia.

T-Wave Changes

Like ST-segment changes, T-wave changes may indicate myocardial ischemia. Inversion of the T waves may be the earliest electrocardiographic evidence of subendocardial ischemia. The combination of T-wave inversion and ST-segment depression in patients with unstable angina may be a sign of severe disease. Sclarovsky et al. found these patients had a high incidence of left main coronary artery stenosis and in-hospital death.[87] Similarly, Renkin et al. showed that these patients often had left anterior descending (LAD) coronary artery disease.[88]

However, in about 10 to 30% of patients, pre-existing electrocardiographic changes make analysis of ischemia impossible. These abnormalities include LBBB, preexcitation syndromes, ventricular pacemakers, and ventricular hypertrophy with strain. In these patients, other diagnostic modalities such as transesophageal echocardiography (TEE) may be considered for intraoperative ischemia monitoring.

Other Electrocardiographic Changes Associated with Ischemia

The appearance of new perioperative dysrhythmias or conduction system disturbances may be the only sign of myocardial ischemia.[89] Perioperative "normalization" of a pre-existing ST-segment depression or T-wave inversion may also be indicative of ischemia.

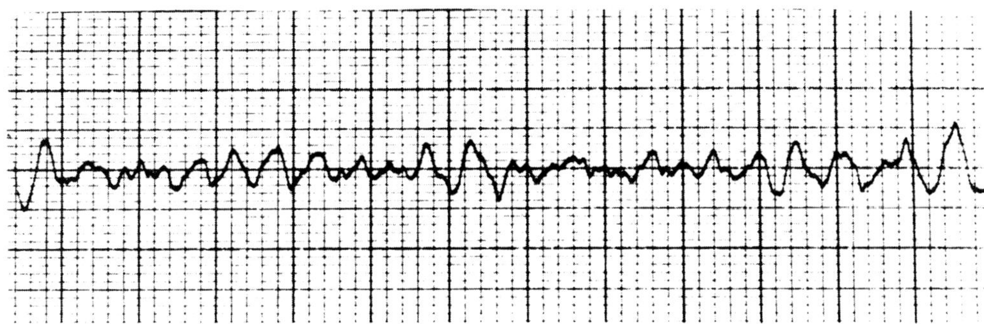

FIGURE 8–33. Ventricular fibrillation. (From Zaidan JR: Electrocardiography. In Barash PG, Cullen BF, Stoelting RK [eds]: Clinical Anesthesia, 2nd ed. Philadelphia, JB Lippincott Co, 1992, p 771, with permission.)

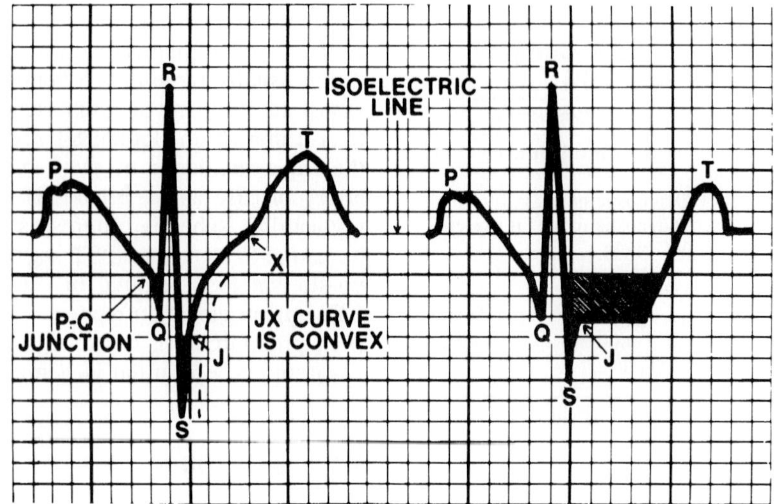

FIGURE **8–34.** The left represents a normal QRS complex. The right shows 2-mm ST-segment depression at the J point. (From Ellestad MH: Stress Testing, Principles and Practice, 3rd ed. Philadelphia, FA Davis Co, 1986, p 233, with permission.)

Comparison of the ECG to Other Modalities for Intraoperative Ischemia Detection

The ECG changes of ischemia occur relatively late in the ischemic process.[90,91] When a coronary artery is occluded, the first changes are biochemical. Oxygen deficit results in an intracellular acidosis and increased intracellular calcium.[92] The cells become anaerobic and lactate production increases. The next changes are mechanical. Ventricular wall motion abnormalities appear and initially manifest as hypokinesis (decreased movement). These progress to akinesis (no movement) and eventually dyskinesis (unproductive or counterproductive movements) results. Simultaneously, there is an increase in end-diastolic pressure and the ejection fraction decreases. Only after all these changes have occurred does the ECG manifest ischemic changes.[93]

The intraoperative assay of myocardial lactate production is impractical. However, wall motion abnormalities can be detected by echocardiography and increased end-diastolic pressure can be estimated by pulmonary capillary wedge pressure (PCWP). These techniques are invasive and impractical for the majority of patients. However, they may be useful when there are pre-existing ECG abnormalities in high-risk patients.

Transesophageal Echocardiography

A 25% decrease in coronary blood flow produces regional wall motion abnormalities (RWMAs) without ECG changes, whereas a 50% decrease is required to cause ECG signs of ischemia.[81] DeBruijn and Clements showed that in patients with coronary artery disease, RWMAs occurred within 30 seconds of exercise, while ECG changes did not occur until 90 seconds.[94] Smith et al. also found that RWMAs were more sensitive than ST-segment changes for detecting intraoperative ischemia. They showed that RWMAs developed in 24 of 50 patients with coronary artery disease undergoing major vascular or cardiac surgery. There were three perioperative myocardial infarctions; only one of these patients

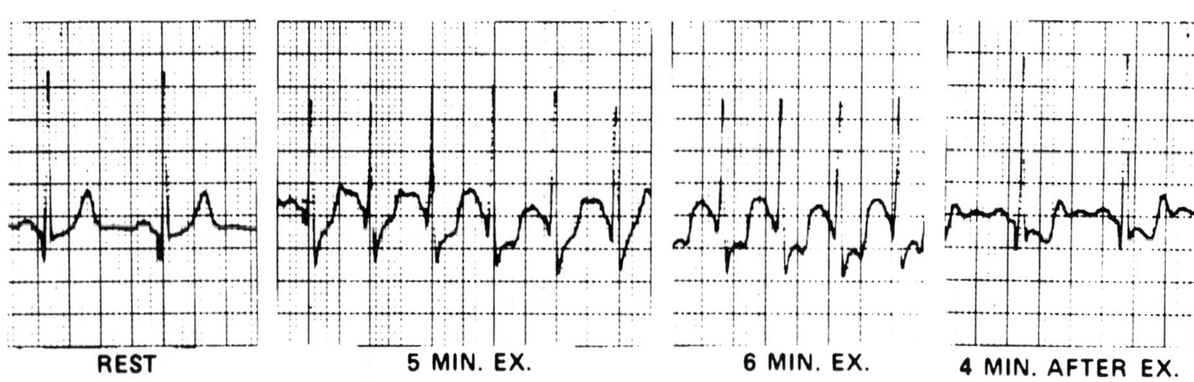

FIGURE **8–35.** The ECG of a 50-year-old man with severe disease of the right and left anterior descending coronary arteries. Note J-point changes, which evolve horizontal and finally down-sloping ST-segment depression. (From Ellestad MH: Stress Testing: Principles and Practice, 3rd ed. Philadelphia, FA Davis Co, 1986, with permission.)

had intraoperative ST-segment changes, but all had exhibited new RWMAs.[95] Leung et al. compared ECG and TEE monitoring in 50 patients undergoing coronary artery bypass grafting (CABG). They demonstrated that no patients had adverse cardiac outcomes without new RWMAs. In contrast, ST-segment changes had no predictive value at any point during surgery. Ellis et al. compared automated ST-segment analysis, electrocardiography, and TEE for detecting myocardial ischemia during noncardiac surgery.[96] The sensitivities of automated ST-segment monitoring (Hewlett Packard) were 40% for TEE-diagnosed ischemia and 75% for ECG-diagnosed ischemia. Comparing the printed ECG with TEE revealed that the ST-segment changes in the printed ECG, as analyzed by a cardiologist, were 25% specific and 6% sensitive for the detection of TEE-diagnosed myocardial ischemia. When T-wave inversions were added to ST-segment depression as a criterion for the diagnosis of myocardial ischemia by the printed ECG, the sensitivity of ECG for the detection of TEE-determined myocardial ischemia was 40% and the specificity was 58%. There is good evidence that TEE is a sensitive indicator of ischemia, but other investigators have not been able to establish an association between intraoperative RWMAs and postoperative adverse cardiac events.[97,98] The cost, skill level required, and invasiveness of TEE make it an impractical monitor in many patients.

Pulmonary Capillary Wedge Pressure

In 1981, Kaplan et al. compared abnormal wedge pressure waveforms to ECGs in patients undergoing CABG surgery. They concluded that PCWP could be more sensitive than the ECG in the detection of ischemia.[99] Although acute increases in PCWP or the development of V waves may reflect ischemia, the absence of these changes does not exclude ischemia. Haggmark et al. found that both the sensitivity and specificity of PCWP for detecting ischemia were only 40%.[100] Similarly, Leung et al. found that 60% of new RWMAs during CABG occurred without significant changes in PCWP.[101] Roizen et al. found that 90% of patients developed TEE wall motion abnormalities on supraceliac aortic clamping and that the PCWP remained normal in more than 80% of episodes.[102] Pulmonary capillary wedge pressure, therefore, does not appear to be a sensitive indicator of myocardial ischemia.

Prognostic Value of Perioperative Ischemic ECG Changes

Preoperative Ischemia

Sixty to 80% of patients with stable angina experience between five and ten episodes of ischemia per week. The average duration of these ischemic events is 17 minutes. Seventy to 85% of these ischemic episodes are painless.[103-105] The majority of ischemic episodes occur with minimal physical activity and occur between 6:00 and 10:00 AM.[106,107] The predictive value of preoperative ischemia for perioperative cardiac morbidity and mortality is not clear. Pasternack et al. showed that preoperative silent ischemia was predictive of perioperative myocardial infarction in patients undergoing vascular surgery.[108] Raby et al. studied patients undergoing elective peripheral vascular surgery.[109] He showed that 40% of the patients with preoperative ischemia developed a postoperative ischemic complication. In contrast, of 144 patients without preoperative ischemia, only 1 developed a postoperative cardiac complication. Mangano et al. using ambulatory ECG monitoring in 474 patients with or at risk for coronary artery disease undergoing noncardiac surgery were unable to show an association between preoperative ischemia and perioperative cardiac events.[110]

Intraoperative Ischemia

Slogoff et al. showed that intraoperative ischemia during CABG is predictive of adverse perioperative cardiac events.[111] In their study of more than 1,000 CABG patients, intraoperative ischemia occurred in 40% of all patients. Patients with intraoperative ischemia had an infarction rate of 6.9% versus 2.5% in patients without ischemia. In a recent study, Raby et al. also showed an association between intraoperative ECG-detected ischemia and postoperative cardiac events in vascular surgery.[109]

Postoperative Ischemia

Most investigators have been able to document a strong association between postoperative ischemia and an increased incidence of adverse cardiac events. Table 8–3[112-114] summarizes the most important studies. Mangano et al. showed a ninefold increase and Raby et al. a 16-fold increase in risk of an adverse cardiac event with postoperative ischemia.[109,110] However, the positive predictive value remains low. Landesberg showed a 14% incidence of adverse cardiac events in the presence of postoperative ischemia versus none in the absence of ischemia.[115] Breslow et al. confirmed the significance of postoperative ischemia for adverse cardiac outcomes, but showed that isolated T-wave changes without ST-segment changes were not associated with adverse outcomes. They noted that this was a common occurrence in the postanesthesia care unit.[116]

Special Considerations for Vascular, Thoracic, and Cardiac Surgery

Vascular Surgery

Ischemic heart disease is common in patients with peripheral vascular disease.[117,118] Significant coronary artery stenosis (>70%) is present in up to 80% of these patients.[119] The long-term prognosis of patients with peripheral vascular disease depends on extent of the ischemic heart disease and the degree of ventricular dysfunction.[120] Patients with peripheral vascular disease un-

TABLE 8–3
Incidence of Postoperative Myocardial Ischemia Detected by Continuous ECG Monitoring and its Complications

Study	No. of Patients	Patient Characteristics	Incidence of Postoperative Ischemia	Incidence of Ischemic Complications (MI, UA, and Cardiac Death in Those with Postoperative Ischemia)
Mangano et al., 1990[110]	474	Noncardiac surgery with CAD or with CAD risk factors	194 of 474 = 41%	15 of 194 = 8% (2 deaths, 8 MI, 5 UA)
Ouyang et al., 1989[112]	24	Vascular surgery and CAD	15 of 24 = 62%	17 of 15 = 47% (2 MI, 5 UA)
McCann, 1989[113]	50	Vascular surgery—lower extremity	19 of 50 = 38%	4 of 19 = 21% (2 deaths, 2 MI)
Pasternack et al., 1989[114]	200	Vascular surgery	57 of 200 = 28%	11 of 57 = 19% (9 MI, 2 deaths)
Raby, et al., 1992[109]	35	Peripheral vascular surgery	10 of 30 = 30%	8 of 35 = 22% (3 deaths, 2 MI, 3 UA)
Landesberg et al., 1993[115]	151	Vascular surgery	88 of 151 = 58%	8 of 88 = 9% (6 MI, 2 UA)

MI, myocardial infarction; UA, unstable angina; CAD, coronary artery disease.

dergoing vascular surgery have a 50% incidence of perioperative dysrhythmias; ischemia can occur in up to 60% of patients and myocardial infarction in up to 15% of patients.[121] The high perioperative morbidity and mortality is related to a combination of the stresses of surgery and the presence of coronary artery disease.[122]

Thoracic Surgery

The lateral decubitus position may make accurate lead placement difficult. It may also affect the ECG by shifting the heart within the chest, thereby altering the electrical axis. Mechanical stimulation of the heart may cause dysrhythmias and ischemia changes. Surgical complications of thoracotomies or pneumonectomies such as a tension pneumothorax and herniation of the heart, shift the electrical axis and can cause dysrhythmias and ischemia.[123] In left-sided cardiac herniation, the ECG changes may precede clinical symptoms by several hours.[124]

Myocardial Ischemia and Infarction

Von Knorrig et al. reported a 3.8% incidence of ischemic events and a 1.2% incidence of myocardial infarction in patients undergoing noncardiac thoracic operations.[125] The majority of the ischemic episodes and dysrhythmias occurred on the second postoperative day. This coincides with the time of maximum decrease in postoperative pulmonary function. There appears to be a direct relationship between the degree of Spo_2 decrease and the degree of ST-segment depression, and sinus tachycardia is often present during these episodes of hypoxemia.[126]

Dysrhythmias

Supraventricular dysrhythmias occur commonly after major thoracic procedures (especially after pneumonectomies). This applies even to patients without coexisting cardiac disease.[127] Table 8–4 summarizes the results of several studies. Supraventricular dysrhythmias occur in approximately 25% of patients and atrial fibrillation ac-

TABLE 8–4
Incidence and Prognosis of Postoperative SVT in Patients Following Pneumonectomy

Study	No. of Patients	No. of Patients with SVT	Incidence of A-Fib. in Patients with SVT	Perioperative Morbidity and Mortality in Patients without SVT	Perioperative Morbidity and Mortality in Patients with SVT
Von Knorring et al., 1992[125]	598	16%	78%	2.4%	17%
Wahi et al., 1989[128]	213	28%	77%	7%	25%
Krowke et al., 1987[127]	187	22%	89%	2%	7%
Beck-Nielsen et al., 1973[129]	300	20%	85%	3%	9%
Mowry et al., 1964[130]	215	22%	81%	4%	12%

SVT, Supraventricular tachycardia (atrial tachycardia, atrial flutter, atrial fibrillation; A-Fib, atrial fibrillation.

counts for 80% of these.[128–130] These dysrhythmias are caused by mechanical factors and trauma to the heart, increase in right-sided afterload, pre-existing cardiac disease, and perioperative sympathetic stimulation. Dysrhythmias are more common after intrapericardial dissection and in patients undergoing a pneumonectomy.[113] Postoperative perihilar infiltrates and interstitial pulmonary edema are also associated with a higher incidence of dysrhythmias. The acute increase in right ventricular afterload due to the surgical resection contributes to dysrhythmia development. The increased afterload may cause dilatation/strain of the right ventricle and atrium, triggering the dysrhythmias. In patients with coexisting cardiac disease, the incidence of dysrhythmias is increased. The perioperative sympathetic stimulation that accompanies surgery also plays a significant role. These dysrhythmias are associated with an increased perioperative morbidity and mortality.[131] Wahi et al. reported a higher mortality rate in patients undergoing pneumonectomy who developed atrial fibrillation than those who did not.[128] Patients with recurrent dysrhythmias have a significantly higher mortality than those with a single episode only (see Table 8–4).

Cardiac Surgery

Electrocardiographic monitoring may be problematic. Surgical equipment and technique may interfere with monitoring by causing artifacts. Induction of anesthesia, hypothermia, and reperfusion cause many ECG changes. Specialized electrocardiographic monitoring techniques may be useful in the perioperative period.

ECG Artifacts During Cardiac Surgery

The tubing of the extracorporeal circuit may be the cause of ECG artifacts. It is postulated that the artifact is either caused by a piezoelectric effect due to deformation of the tubing or the build-up of static electricity between the tubing and the roller-pump. The artifact is more common at an operating room temperature below 20°C and a humidity below 50%.[132] The artifacts cause high- and low-amplitude irregularities on the ECG. The artifacts can often be corrected by applying a ground wire to the pump. This procedure dissipates the accumulated electrical charges to ground.[133] The low-amplitude irregularity of the baseline may simulate continued electrical activity of the heart. During rewarming, the reappearance of normal QRS complexes may be completely obliterated by high-amplitude artifacts. Another common artifact simulates atrial flutter during CPB. It occurs when the ECG leads are not properly applied, causing the ECG to track the frequency of the roller-pump head.[134]

Artifacts may also be introduced by the lead systems that are chosen to monitor ischemic changes. The modified limb leads such as CS_5 show a greater R-wave amplitude and a correspondingly magnified ST segment. Bipolar leads may therefore exaggerate the severity of ischemia. By incorporating an R-wave gain factor, the diagnosis of ischemia can become more accurate.[135,136] Similarly, sudden change in R-wave amplitude (either an increase or a decrease) may be a subtle but important sign of myocardial ischemia. However, intraoperative R-wave amplitude analysis is difficult, and many intraoperative R-wave changes occur due to positional changes and sternal retraction. Mark et al. demonstrated that the placement of a Canadian sternal retractor was associated with a reduction in both R-wave amplitude and ST-segment depression.[135]

ECG Changes During Cardiac Surgery

PREBYPASS PERIOD

The prebypass period is associated with several stressful events during which myocardial ischemia can occur. These include tracheal intubation, skin incision, sternotomy, cannulation, and initiation of bypass.[137]

APPLICATION OF AORTIC CROSS-CLAMP

Application of the aortic cross-clamp is inevitably associated with a degree of myocardial ischemia. As cross-clamp time increases, so does the potential for ischemic injury and subsequent infarction. Unfortunately, the electrical and mechanical quiescence during cardioplegia makes electrocardiographic ischemia monitoring impossible.

REMOVAL OF AORTIC CROSS-CLAMP

ST-segment elevation is indicative of transmural ischemia. It may be encountered at any time during cardiac surgery, but it is most common during cardiac reperfusion. This ST-segment elevation usually occurs in the distribution of the right coronary artery and is detected in the leads I, III, and aVF. The causes include coronary vasospasm, intracoronary air or atheromatous emboli, and kinking or mechanical occlusion of coronary grafts. Persistent ST-segment elevation refractory to treatment indicates evolving transmural infarction.[138] To determine the incidence of postbypass ST-segment elevation, Lockerman et al. studied 50 patients. They used continuous Holter monitoring for 24 hours after pericardial closure. They found an 8% incidence of ST-segment elevation (>2 mm and lasting at least 30 seconds).[139] Although none of the episodes were accompanied by hemodynamic deterioration, the incidence was much higher than that of earlier reports. These earlier studies had used intermittent monitoring only and had described ST-segment elevation as being rare.[140] Two other studies have confirmed Lockerman's findings.[138,141] They reported incidences of 14% and 12%, respectively. These reversible episodes of ST-segment elevation may herald serious postoperative events. Smith et al. showed that 50% of patients undergoing coronary revascularization with adverse cardiac outcomes had prior reversible ST-segment elevation.[141] Patients without adverse outcomes had a 7% incidence of ST elevation. Thomson et al. found that postoperative release of CK-MB isoenzyme was significantly higher in patients with ST-segment elevation that in those without.[138]

ECG Detection of Myocardial Ischemia in Patients without Coronary Artery Disease

Electrocardiographic monitoring for ischemia during cardiac procedures in children and young adults may alert the clinician to potential problems. One study showed that the use of topical pericardial hypothermia in pediatric cardiac surgery temporarily caused post-bypass ST-segment elevation.[142] This finding was thought to result from hypothermic and osmotic injury caused by the ice. Whitten et al. showed that in patients without coronary artery disease undergoing cardiac electrophysiologic surgery, the use of local hypothermia and mechanical stimulation may cause potentially dangerous coronary vasospasm with ST-segment elevation.[143]

Value of Specialized Electrocardiographic Devices

Both preoperative left ventricular hypertrophy and low ejection fraction are associated with an increased incidence of atrial fibrillation after cardiac surgery.[144] The signal-averaged electrocardiograph allows accurate detection of atrial conduction delays and can be used to predict the development of postoperative atrial fibrillation. In a study of 130 patients undergoing cardiac surgery, Steinberg et al. found that a prolonged atrial conduction time resulted in a fourfold increase in the incidence of atrial fibrillation.[144]

Epicardial pacing wires may be connected to the right and left upper limb leads of a standard ECG machine

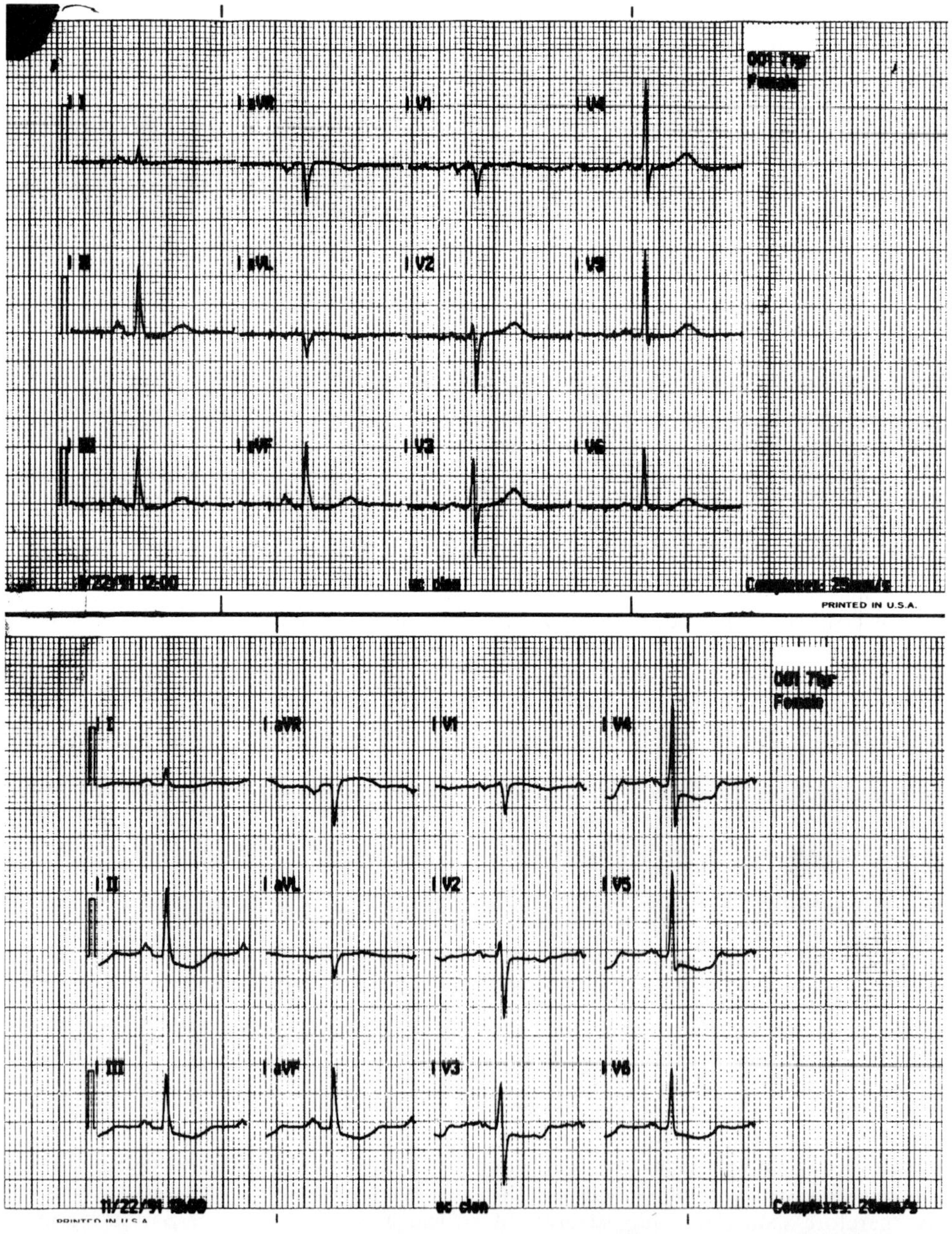

FIGURE **8–36.** Continuous 12-lead ECGs in a patient undergoing abdominal aortic reconstruction. The baseline ECG is normal, but bleeding after opening the aorta was associated with ischemic changes in leads II, III, aVF, and V_3 through V_6.

(which is electrically safe) to obtain an atrial ECG. This arrangement facilitates the diagnosis of many dysrhythmias by improved visualization of atrial electrical activity.

Automated ST-Segment Analysis and Routine Postoperative Ischemia Monitoring

The poor prognostic implications of perioperative ischemia and dysrhythmias and the low rate of detection by clinicians has fostered the development of automated ST-segment monitoring. An example of intraoperative myocardial ischemia detected by continuous 12-lead ECG analysis during vascular surgery is shown in Figure 8–36.

Using an automated ST-segment detection device, Kotter et al. studied the incidence of ischemic ECG changes in 125 patients before initiation of cardiopulmonary bypass. Patients presenting for their first coronary revascularization had a lower incidence of ischemia than patients for repeat surgery (8 vs. 24%) and patients presenting for combined coronary/valve operations had an incidence of 36%.[145] Roy et al. found that anesthesiologists observing the ECG detected only 15% of episodes of ST-segment depression recorded during the same time period by Holter monitoring.[146] Many current intraoperative and intensive care ECG monitoring system have computerized ST-segment analyzers. When activated, these analyzers automatically switch to the diagnostic mode for accurate measurement of the ST segment. These systems exclude abnormal ECG signals by sampling, comparing, and averaging several incoming QRS-ST complexes to form a baseline or "dominant template" for each ECG lead being monitored. This template is then used by the computer as a reference to analyze normal or abnormal ECG signals. An adjustable alarm alerts the physician to the onset of ST changes. London tested one of these analyzers by assessing its ability to accurately respond to simulated horizontal ST-segment depression, ST-segment elevation, and downsloping ST-segment depression.[147] He found that 80% of all cases of ST-segment elevation and 95% of downsloping ST-segment depression were measured with an accuracy of ±0.5 mm. In contrast, only 10% of horizontal ST-segment depression samples were accurate to within ±0.5 mm. Our own group has compared two commercially available ST-segment analyzers to a printed eight-lead ECG. The ECG was assessed by a blinded cardiologist. One analyzer detected 75% and the other 100% of the ischemic episodes reported by the cardiologist.[148]

Another problem in accurate automated ST-segment analysis occurs with the initial construction of the reference template by the computer. Burns et al. showed that occasionally the computer does not reject a subtle pathologic ECG signal.[149] The incorporation of this signal in the reference template will taint the subsequent analysis by introducing a systematic error. Automated ST-segment monitoring represents an improvement over visual inspection, but presently there is no evidence that the use of these systems improves outcome. However, Kotrly et al. reported that an ST-segment analyzer was often the first monitor to warn clinicians of impending ischemic complications.[150] They believe that the primary benefit of ST-segment analyzers is to increase the clinician's awareness of subtle ST-segment changes, resulting in more frequent and timely interventions.[151]

Postoperative myocardial ischemia is associated with an increased risk of adverse outcomes and often precedes the cardiac event by a day. Continuous postoperative ST-segment monitoring may make clinicians aware of an impending cardiac event and prophylactic therapy could then be instituted. Current microprocessor ECG monitoring systems permit continuous storage of 12-lead ECGs and are small enough to enable patients to wear them during the critical days after surgery. Will aggressive postoperative monitoring and treatment decrease ischemic complications? A very large randomized study would be necessary to study this outcome. If the rate of postoperative ischemia is 40% and careful perioperative management results in a rate of ischemic complications of only 3%, approximately 3,000 patients would be required in both the control and treatment groups to demonstrate a 33% reduction in the incidence of ischemic complications (with a power of 0.80). For this reason, future studies of aggressive therapy will likely focus on ischemia reduction rather than decreasing ischemic complications.

References

1. Fye WB: A history of the origin, evolution and impact of electrocardiography. Am J Cardiol 73:937, 1994.
2. Ganong WF: Origin of the heartbeat and the electrical activity of the heart. In Review of Medical Physiology. Stamford, CT, Appleton & Lange, 1993, p 492.
3. Goldberger AL, Goldberger, E: Clinical Electrocardiography: A Simplified Approach, 5th ed, St Louis, Mosby Year Book, 1994.
4. Kaplan JA, King SB: The precordial electrocardiographic lead V_5 in patients who have coronary artery disease. Anesthesiology 45:570, 1976.
5. Kaplan J, Thys DM: Electrocardiography. In Miller RD (ed): Anesthesia, 3rd ed, New York, Churchill Livingstone, 1990, p 1101.
6. Griffin RM, Kaplan JA: Comparison of ECG V_5, CS_5, CB_5 and II by computerized ST-segment analysis. Anesth Analg 65:S1, 1986.
7. Bazaral MG, Norfleet EA: Comparison of CB_5 and V_5 leads for intraoperative electrocardiographic monitoring. Anesth Analg 60:849, 1981.
8. London MJ, Hollenberg M, Wong MG, et al: Intraoperative myocardial ischemia: Localization by continuous 12-lead electrocardiography. Anesthesiology 69:232, 1988.
9. London MJ: Anesthesiology 69:236, 1988.
10. Holter NJ: New methods for heart studies. Science 134:1214, 1961.
11. Balasubramania V, Lahiri A, Green HL, et al: Ambulatory ST-segment monitoring. Problems, pitfalls, solutions and clinical applications. Br Heart J 44:419, 1980.
12. Tzivoni D, Benhorin J, Gavish A, et al: Holter recording during treadmill testing in assessing myocardial ischemic changes. Am J Cardiol 55:1200, 1985.
13. Kates RA, Zaidan JR, Kaplan JA: Esophageal lead for intraoperative electrocardiographic monitoring. Anesth Analg 61:781, 1982.
14. Brown DL, Greenberg, DJ: A simple device for monitoring the esophageal electrocardiogram. Anesthesiology 59:482, 1983.

15. Heinke M, Volkmann H: Balloon electrode catheter for transesophageal atrial pacing and transesophageal ECG recording. PACE 15:1953, 1992.
16. Srivastara P, Mittal SR, Srivastara N: Role of esophageal electrocardiograms in differentiation of old anteroseptal myocardial infarction from emphysema in cases with poor R-wave progression in precordial leads. J Assoc Phys India 39:249, 1991.
17. Katz A, Guetta V, Ousyshcher IA: Transesophageal electrocardiography using a temporary pacing balloon-tipped electrode in acute cardiac care. Ann Emerg Med 20:961, 1991.
18. Mylrea KC, Calkins JM, Carlson J, et al: ECG lead with the endotracheal tube. Crit Care Med 11:199, 1983.
19. Lichtenthal PR: Multipurpose pulmonary artery catheter. Ann Thorac Surg 3:493, 1983.
20. Zaidan JR: Electrocardiography. In Barash PG, Cullen BF, Stoelting RK (eds): Clinical Anesthesia, 2nd ed. Philadelphia, JB Lippincott Co, 1992, p 771.
21. Pande AK, Meier B, Urban P, et al: Intracoronary electrocardiogram during coronary angioplasty. Am Heart J 124:337, 1992.
22. Mirvis DM, Berson AS, Goldberger AL: Instrumentation and practice standards for electrocardiographic monitoring in special care units. Circulation 79:464, 1989.
23. Herman MV, Ingram DA, Levy JA, et al: Variability of electrocardiographic precordial lead placement: A method to improve accuracy and reliability. Clin Cardiol 14:469, 1991.
24. Lampert BA, Sundstrom ED: ECG artifacts simulating supraventricular tachycardia during automated percutaneous lumbar discectomy. Anesth Analg 67:1096, 1988.
25. Paulsen AW, Pritchard DG: ECG artifact produced by crystalloid administration through blood/fluid warmer sets. Anesthesiology 69:803, 1988.
26. Legatt AD, Frost EAM: ECG artifacts during intraoperative evoked potential monitoring. Anesthesiology 70:559, 1989.
27. Pipberger HV, Arzbaecher RC, Berson AS, et al: Recommendations for standardization of leads and of specifications for instruments in electrocardiography and vectorcardiography. Report of the Committee on Electrocardiography, American Heart Association. Circulation 52:11, 1975.
28. Slogoff S, Keats AS, David T, et al: Incidence of perioperative myocardial ischemia detected by different electrocardiographic systems. Anesthesiology 73:1074, 1990.
29. Moorman JR, Hlatky MA, Eddy DM, et al: The yield of the routine admission electrocardiogram—a study in a general medical service. Ann Intern Med 103:590, 1985.
30. Phibbs B: Cardiac Arrhythmias, 2nd ed. St Louis, C V Mosby Co, 1973, p 26.
31. Goldman L, Caldera DL, Nussbaum SR, et al: Multifactorial index of cardiac risk in noncardiac surgical procedures. N Engl J Med. 297:845, 1977.
32. Detsky AS, Abrams HB, Forbath N, et al: Cardiac assessment for patients undergoing noncardiac surgery: A multifactorial clinical risk index. Arch Intern Med 146:2131, 1986.
33. Detsky AS, Abrams HB, McLaughlin JR, et al: Predicting cardiac complications in patients undergoing noncardiac surgery. J Gen Intern Med 1:211, 1986.
34. Gerson MC, Hurst JM, Hertzberg VS, et al: Cardiac prognosis in noncardiac geriatric surgery. Ann Intern Med 103:832, 1985.
35. Gerson MC, Hurst JM, Hertzberg VS, et al: Prediction of cardiac and pulmonary complications related to elective and noncardiac thoracic surgery in geriatric patients. Am J Med 88:101, 1990.
36. Cooperman M, Plug B, Martin EW, et al: Cardiovascular risk factors in patients with peripheral vascular disease. Surgery 84: 505, 1978.
37. Eagle KA, Singer DE, Brewster DC, et al: Dipyridamole-thallium scanning in patients undergoing vascular surgery. JAMA 257:2185, 1987.
38. Eagle KA, Coley CM, Newell JB, et al: Combining preoperative assessment of cardiac risk before major vascular surgery. Ann Intern Med 110:859, 1989.
39. Creswell LL, Schuessler B, Rosenbloom M, et al: Hazards of postoperative atrial arrhythmias. Ann Thorac Surg 56:539, 1993.
40. Frost L, Molgaard H, Christiansen EH, et al: Atrial fibrillation and flutter after coronary artery bypass surgery: Epidemiology, risk factors and preventive trials. Int J Cardiol 36:253, 1992.
41. Wellens HJJ, Brugada P, Penn OC: The management of preexcitation syndromes. JAMA 257:2325, 1987.
42. Klein GJ, Basore TM, Sellers TD, et al: Ventricular fibrillation in the Wolff-Parkinson-White-syndrome. N Engl J Med 301: 1080, 1979.
43. Kastor JA: Atrioventricular block. N Engl J Med 292:462, 1976.
44. Phibbs B, Friedman HS, Graboys TB, et al: Indications for pacing in the treatment of bradyarrhythmias. Report of an independent study group. JAMA 252:1307, 1984.
45. Hecht HH, Kossman EC, Childers WR, et al: Atrioventricular and intraventricular conduction: Revised nomenclature and concepts. Am J Cardiol 31:232, 1973.
46. Rorie DK, Muldoon SM, Krabill DR: Transient bundle branch block occurring during anesthesia, Anesth Analg 51:633, 1972.
47. Pratila M, Pratilas V, Dimich I: Transient left bundle branch block during anesthesia. Anesthesiology 51:461, 1979.
48. Edelman JD, Hurlbert BJ: Intermittent left bundle branch block during anesthesia. Anesth Analg 59:628, 1981.
49. Thomson IR, Dalton BC, Lappas DG, et al: Right bundle-branch block and complete heart block caused by the Swan-Ganz catheter. Anesthesiology 51:359, 1979.
50. Morris D, Mulrihill D, Wilbur YWL: Risk of developing complete heart block during bedside pulmonary artery catheterization in patients with left bundle branch block. Arch Intern Med 147:2005, 1987.
51. Rooney SM, Goldiner PL, Muss E: Relationship of right bundle-branch block and marked left axis deviation to complete heart block during general anesthesia. Anesthesiology 44:64, 1976.
52. Venkataraman K, Madias JE, Hood WB: Indications for prophylactic preoperative insertion of pacemakers in patients with right bundle block and left anterior hemiblock. Chest 68:501, 1975.
53. Coriat P, Harari A, Ducardonet A, et al: Risk of advanced heart block during extradural anesthesia in patients with right bundle branch block and left anterior hemiblock. Br J Anaesth 53:545, 1981.
54. Ellestad MH: Stress Testing: Principles and Practice, 3rd ed. Philadelphia, FA Davis Co, 1986.
55. Carliner NH, Fisher ML, Plotnick GD, et al: The preoperative electrocardiogram as an indicator of risk in major noncardiac surgery. Can J Cardiol 2:134, 1986.
56. Goldberger AL, O'Konski M: Utility of the routine electrocardiogram before surgery and on general hospital admission. Ann Intern Med 105:552, 1986.
57. Tarhan S, Moffitt EA, Taylor WE, et al: Myocardial infarction after general anesthesia. JAMA 220:1451, 1972.
58. Steen PA, Tinker JH, Tarhan S: Myocardial reinfarction after anesthesia and surgery. An update: Incidence, mortality and predisposing factors. JAMA 239:2566, 1978.
59. Rao TK, Jacobs EH, El-Etr AA: Reinfarction following anesthesia in patients with myocardial infarction. Anesthesiology 59: 499, 1983.
60. Shah KB, Kleinman BS, Sami H, et al: Reevaluation of perioperative myocardial infarction in patients with prior myocardial infarction undergoing non-cardiac operations. Anesth Analg 71: 231, 1991.
61. Hollenberg M, Mangano DT, Browner WS, et al: Predictors of postoperative myocardial ischemia in patients undergoing noncardiac surgery. JAMA 268:205, 1992.
62. Moss AJ: Prolonged QT interval syndromes. JAMA 256:2985, 1986.
63. Galloway PA, Glass PSA: Anesthetic implications of prolonged QT interval syndromes. Anesth Analg 64:612, 1985.
64. Adu-Gyamfi Y, Said A, Chowdhardy LM, et al: Anesthetic induced ventricular tachyarrhythmia in Jervell and Lange-Nielsen syndrome. Can J Anesth 38:345, 1991.
65. Borganelli M, Forman M: Simulation of acute myocardial infarction by desipramine hydrochloride. Am Heart J 119:14134, 1990.
66. Raby KE, Goldman L, Creagher M, et al: Correlation between preoperative ischemia and major cardiac events after peripheral vascular surgery. N Engl J Med 321:1296, 1989.
67. Mantha S, Roizen MF, Bernard J, et al: Relative effectiveness of four preoperative tests for predicting adverse cardiac outcome after vascular surgery. A meta analysis. Anesth Analg 79:422, 1994.
68. Froelicher VF: Exercise and the Heart—Clinical Concepts, 2nd ed. Chicago, Year Book Medical Publishers, 1987.

69. Bertrand CA, Steiner NV, Jameson AG, et al: Disturbances of cardiac rhythm during anesthesia and surgery. JAMA 216:1615, 1971.
70. Kuner J, Enescu V, Utsu F, et al: Cardiac arrhythmias during anesthesia. Dis Chest S2:580, 1967.
71. Vanik PE, Davis HS: Cardiac arrhythmias during halothane anesthesia. Anesth Analg 47:299, 1968.
72. Atlee JL, Rusy BF: Ventricular conduction times and AV nodal conductivity during enflurane anesthesia in dogs. Anesthesiology 47:498, 1977.
73. Edwards R, Winnie AP, Ramamurthy S, et al: Acute hypocapneic hypokalemia: An iatrogenic anesthetic complication. Anesth Analg 56:786, 1977.
74. Angelini L, Feldman MI, Lufscholnowski R, et al: Cardiac arrhythmias during and after heart surgery. Diagnosis and management. Prog Cardiovasc Dis 16:469, 1974.
75. Damen J: Ventricular arrhythmias during insertion and removal of pulmonary artery catheters. Chest 88:190, 1985.
76. Atlee JL, Bosnjak ZJ: Mechanisms for cardiac dysrhythmias during anesthesia. Anesthesiology 72:347, 1990.
77. Myerburg RJ, Kessler KM, Luceri RM: Classification of ventricular arrhythmias based on parallel hierarchies of frequency and form. Am J Cardiol 54:1355, 1984.
78. Bethge KP: Classification of arrhythmias. J Cardiovasc Pharmacol 17:13, 1991.
79. Stokes DN: Monitoring the electrical activity of the heart. In Hutton P, Prys-Roberts (eds): Monitoring in Anaesthesia and Intensive Care. London, WB Saunders Ltd, 1994, p 82.
80. Robertson D, Kostok WJ, Atuja SP: The localization of coronary artery stenosis by 12-lead ECG response to graded exercise test. Am Hart J 91:437, 1976.
81. DeHert SG, Moens M, Vermeyen KM, et al: Use of the right-sided precordial lead V_4R in the detection of intraoperative myocardial ischemia. J Cardiothorac Vasc Anesth 7:659, 1993.
82. Dell'Italia LJ: Right ventricular infarction: Identification by hemodynamic measurements before and after volume loading and correlation with noninvasive techniques. J Am Coll Cardiol 4: 931, 1984.
83. Dell'Italia LJ: Comparative effects of volume loading, dobutamine and nitroprusside in patients with predominant right ventricular infarction. Circulation 2:1327, 1985.
84. Ellestad MH: Stress Testing, Principles and Practice, 3rd ed. Philadelphia, FA Davis Co, 1986, p 233.
85. Robb GP, Marks H: Post-exercise electrocardiogram in arteriosclerotic heart disease. JAMA 200:918, 1967.
86. Goldschlager N, Selzer A, Cohn K, et al: Treadmill stress tests as indicators of presence and severity of coronary artery disease. Ann Intern Med 85:277, 1986.
87. Sclarovsky S, Rechavia E, Straserg B, et al: Unstable angina: ST-segment depression with positive versus negative T-wave deflections—clinical course, ECG evolution and angiographic correlation. Am Heart J 116:933, 1988.
88. Renkin J, Wijns W, Ladha Z, et al: Reversal of segmental hypokinesis by coronary angioplasty in patients with unstable angina, persistent T-wave inversion, and left anterior descending coronary artery stenosis. Additional evidence for myocardial stunning in humans. Circulation 82:913, 1990.
89. Bonoris PE: Evaluation of R-wave changes vs ST-segment depression in stress testing. Circulation 57:904, 1978.
90. Waters DD, daLuz P, Wyatt HL, et al: Early changes in regional and global left ventricular function induced by graded reductions in regional coronary perfusion. Am J Cardiol 39:537, 1977.
91. Tomoiki H, Franklin D, Ross JJ: Detection of myocardial ischemia by regional dysfunction during and after rapid pacing in conscious dogs. Circulation 58:48, 1978.
92. Tennant R, Wiggers CJ: The effect of coronary occlusion on myocardial contraction. Am J Physiol 112:351, 1935.
93. Barash PG: Monitoring myocardial oxygen balance: Physiologic basis and clinical application. ASA Refresher Courses in Anesthesiology 13:21, 1985.
94. Clements FM, deBruijn NP: Temporal relationships between acute coronary constriction and onset of ECG and regional wall motion abnormalities. Anesth Analg 66:249, 1987.
95. Smith JS, Calahan MK, Benefiel DJ, et al: Intraoperative detection of myocardial ischemia in high risk patients: Electrocardiography vs two-dimensional transesophageal echocardiography. Circulation 75:1015, 1985.
96. Ellis JE, Shah MN, Briller JE, et al: A comparison of methods for the detection of myocardial ischemia during noncardiac surgery: Automated ST-segment analysis systems, electrocardiography, and transesophageal echocardiography. Anesth Analg 75: 764, 1992.
97. London MJ, Tubau JF, Wong MG, et al: The "natural history" of segmental wall motion abnormalities in patients undergoing noncardiac surgery. Anesthesiology 73:644, 1990.
98. Eisenberg MJ, London MJ, Leung JM: Monitoring for myocardial ischemia during noncardiac surgery. A technology assessment of transesophageal echocardiography and 12-lead electrocardiography. JAMA 268:210, 1992.
99. Kaplan JA, Wells PH: Early diagnosis of myocardial ischemia using the pulmonary artery catheter. Anesth Analg 60:789, 1981.
100. Haggmark S, Hohner P, Ostman M, et al: Comparison of hemodynamic, electrocardiographic, mechanical and metabolic indicators of intraoperative myocardial ischemia in vascular surgical patients with coronary artery disease. Anesthesiology 70: 19, 1989.
101. Leung J, O'Kelley B, Browner W, et al: Prognostic importance of postbypass regional wall-motion abnormalities in patients undergoing noncardiac surgery. Anesthesiology 71:16, 1989.
102. Roizen MF, Beaupre PN, Alpert RA, et al: Monitoring with two-dimensional transesophageal echocardiography: Comparison of myocardial function in patients undergoing supraceliac, suprarenal infraceliac, or infrarenal aortic occlusion. J Vasc Surg 1: 300, 1984.
103. Deanfield JE, Selwyn AP, Chierchia S, et al: Myocardial ischemia during daily life in patients with stable angina: Its relation to symptoms and heart rate changes. Lancet 2:753, 1983.
104. Deanfield JE, Kensett M, Wilson RA, et al: Silent myocardial ischemia due to mental stress. Lancet 2:1001, 1984.
105. Deanfield JE, Ribliro P, Oakley K, et al: Analysis of ST-segment changes in normal subjects: Implications for ambulatory monitoring in angina pectoris. Am J Cardiol 54:1321, 1984.
106. Mullen JE, Stone PH, Turi ZG, et al: Circadian variations in the frequency of the onset of acute myocardial infarction. N Engl J Med 313:1315, 1985.
107. Stern S, Tzivoni D: Dynamic changes in the ST-T segment during sleep in ischemic heart disease. Am J Cardiol 32:17, 1973.
108. Pasternak PF, Grossi EA, Baumann FG, et al: The value of silent myocardial ischemia monitoring in the prediction of perioperative myocardial infarction in patients undergoing peripheral vascular surgery. J Vasc Surg 10:617, 1989.
109. Raby KE, Barry J, Creagher MA, et al: Detection and significance of intraoperative and postoperative myocardial ischemia in peripheral vascular surgery. JAMA 268:222, 1992.
110. Mangano DT, Browner W, Hollenberg M, et al: Prediction of cardiac morbidity and mortality in patients undergoing noncardiac surgery. N Engl J Med 323:1787, 1990.
111. Slogoff S, Keats AS: Does perioperative myocardial ischemia lead to postoperative myocardial infarction. Anesthesiology 62: 107, 1985.
112. Ouyang P, Gerstenblith G, Furman WR, et al: Frequency and significance of early postoperative silent myocardial ischemia in patients having peripheral vascular surgery. Am J Cardiol 64: 1113, 1989.
113. McCann RL, Clements FM: Silent myocardial ischemia in patients undergoing peripheral vascular surgery: Incidence and association with perioperative cardiac morbidity and mortality. J Vasc Surg 9:583, 1989.
114. Pasternack PF, Grossi EA, Baumann FG, et al: Beta blockade to decrease silent myocardial ischemia during peripheral vascular surgery. Am J Surg 158:113, 1989.
115. Landesberg F, Luria MH, Cotev S, et al: Importance of long-duration postoperative ST-segment depression in cardiac morbidity after vascular surgery. Lancet 341:715, 1993.
116. Breslow MJ, Miller CF, Parker SD, et al: Changes in T-wave morphology following anesthesia and surgery: A common recovery room phenomenon. Anesthesiology 64:398, 1986.
117. Brown OW, Hollier LH, Pairolero PC, et al: Abdominal aortic aneurysm and coronary artery disease. Arch Surg 116:1484, 1981.

118. Rokey R, Rolak LA, Harati Y, et al: Coronary artery disease in patients with cerebrovascular disease: A prospective study. Ann Neurol 16:50, 1984.
119. Tomatis LA, Fierens EE, Verbrugge GP: Evaluation of surgical risk in peripheral vascular disease by coronary arteriography: A series of 100 cases. Surgery 71:429, 1972.
120. Pasternack PF, Imparato AM, Bear G, et al: The value of radionuclide angiography as a predictor of perioperative myocardial infarction in patients undergoing abdominal aortic aneurysm resection. J Vasc Surg 1:320, 1984.
121. Hertzer NR: Myocardial ischemia. Surgery 93:97, 1983.
122. Schoeppel LS, Wilkinson C, Waters J, et al: Effects of myocardial infarction on perioperative cardiac complications. Anesth Analg 62:493, 1983.
123. Ruo W, Rupani G: Left tension pneumothorax mimicking myocardial ischemia after percutaneous central venous cannulation. Anesthesiology 76:306, 1992.
124. Baaijens PFJ, Hasenbos AWM, Lacquet LK, et al: Cardiac herniation after pneumonectomy. Acta Anaesthesiol Scand 36:842, 1992.
125. Von Knorring J, Lepantalo M, Lindgen L, et al: Cardiac arrhythmias and myocardial ischemia after thoracotomy for lung cancer. Ann Thorac Surg 53:642, 1992.
126. Reeder MK, Muir AD, Foex P, et al: Postoperative myocardial ischemia: Temporal association with nocturnal hypoxemia. Br J Anaesth 67:626, 1991.
127. Krowke MJ, Pairolera PC, Trastek VF, et al: Cardiac dysrhythmia following pneumonectomy. Clinical correlates and prognostic significance. Chest 91:490, 1987.
128. Wahi R, McMurtney MJ, DeCaro LF, et al: Determinants of perioperative morbidity and mortality after pneumonectomy. Ann Thorac Surg 48:33, 1989.
129. Beck-Nielsen J, Sorenson HR, Astroup P: Atrial fibrillation following thoracotomy for noncardiac disease; in particular cancer of the lung. Acta Med Scand 193:425, 1973.
130. Mowry F, Reynolds E: Cardiac rhythm disturbances complicating resectional surgery of the lung. Ann Intern Med 61:688, 1964.
131. Shields TW, Ujiki G: Digitalization for prevention of arrhythmias following pulmonary surgery. Surg Gynecol Obstet 126: 743, 1968.
132. Khambatta HJ, Stone JG, Wald A, et al: Electrocardiographic artifacts during cardiopulmonary bypass. Anesth Analg 71:88, 1990.
133. Metz S: ECG artifacts during cardiopulmonary bypass—an alternative method (Letter). Anesth Analg 72:715, 1991.
134. Kleinman B, Shak K, Belusko R, et al: Electrocardiographic artifact caused by extracorporeal roller pump (Letter). J Clin Monit 6:258, 1990.
135. Mark JB, Chien GL, Steinbrook RA, et al: Electrocardiographic R-wave changes during cardiac surgery. Anesth Analg 74:26, 1992.
136. Hakki AH, Iskandrian AS, Kutalek S, et al: R-wave amplitude: A new determinant of failure of patients with coronary heart disease to manifest ST-segment depression during exercise. J Am Coll Cardiol 3:1155, 1984.
137. Slogoff S, Keats AS: Does perioperative myocardial ischemia lead to postoperative myocardial infarction. Anesthesiology 62: 107, 1985.
138. Thomson H, Franklin D, Ross JJ: Electrocardiographic ST-segment elevation after myocardial reperfusion during coronary artery surgery. Anesth Analg 66:1183, 1987.
139. Lockerman Z, Rose DM, Cunningham JN, et al: Postoperative ST-segment elevation in coronary artery bypass surgery. Chest 89:647, 1986.
140. Buxton AE, Goldberg S, Harken A, et al: Coronary artery spasm immediately after myocardial revascularization: Recognition and management. N Engl J Med 304:1249, 1981.
141. Smith RC, Leung JM, Mangano DT, et al: Postoperative myocardial ischemia in patients undergoing coronary bypass graft surgery. Anesthesiology 74:464, 1991.
142. Corno A, Zoia E, Santoro E, et al: Epicardial damage induced by topical cooling during pediatric cardiac surgery. Br Heart J 67:174, 1992.
143. Whitten CW, Latson TW, Cochran RP, et al: ST-segment elevation during cardiac electrophysiologic surgery. Anesthesiology 75:161, 1991.
144. Steinberg JS, Zelenkoske S, Wong SC, et al: Value of the P-wave signal averaged ECG for predicting atrial fibrillation after cardiac surgery. Circulation 88:2618, 1993.
145. Kotter GS, Kotrly KJ, Kalbfleisch JH, et al: Myocardial ischemia during cardiovascular surgery as detected by an ST-segment trend monitoring systems. Cardiothorac Anesth 1:190, 1987.
146. Roy WL, Edelist G, Gilbert B: Myocardial ischemia during noncardiac surgical procedures in patients with coronary artery disease. Anesthesiology 51:393, 1979.
147. London MJ: Validation testing of commercially available ST-segment simulator (Abstract). Presented at the Society of Cardiovascular Anesthesiologists 15th Annual Meeting, San Diego, 1993, p 273.
148. Ellis JE, Shah MN, Briller JE, et al: A comparison of methods for the detection of myocardial ischemia during non-cardiac surgery: Automated ST-segment analysis systems, electrocardiography and transesophageal echocardiography. Anesth Analg 75: 764, 1992.
149. Burns PM, Downs WG: Clinical evaluation of a bedside ST-segment monitor. Proc Comput Cardiol 1:97, 1988.
150. Kotrly KJ, Kotter GS, Mortara D, et al: Intraoperative detection of myocardial ischemia with an ST-segment trend monitoring system. Anesth Analg 63:343, 1984.
151. Kotter GS, Kotrly KJ, Kalbfleisch JH, et al: Myocardial ischemia during cardiovascular surgery as detected by an ST-segment trend monitoring system. Cardiothorac Anesth 1:190, 1987.

CHAPTER 9

Monitoring Ventricular Function

Raymond Hasel, M.D.
Roberta L. Hines, M.D.

Systolic and Diastolic Function

When thinking about monitoring ventricular function, one usually thinks of technology that aids in the qualitative or quantitative assessment of left and right performance. Ventricular failure is classified as either systolic or diastolic. Diastolic dysfunction as a cause of "heart failure" is a relatively new concept, and has recently been reviewed.[1,2] Diastolic dysfunction, due to failure of the ventricle to relax, is frequently an early manifestation of ventricular dysfunction due to coronary artery disease. In order to fill this stiff, noncompliant left ventricle (LV), filling pressures are increased. Pulmonary pressures increase, as pressure is transmitted retrograde to the pulmonary vasculature. Systolic dysfunction is characterized by an inability of the left ventricle to increase cardiac output in proportion to metabolic demands.

One way of conceptualizing the cardiovascular system is to think of the heart as two separate pumps, in series. When insufficiency of one or both pumps develops, this is referred to clinically as "failure," either "forward failure," "left ventricular failure," or "right ventricular failure."

Forward Failure

Forward failure can be thought of as hypoperfusion, when the forward cardiac output or perfusion is insufficient to meet metabolic demands. This situation produces the physical symptoms and signs demonstrated in Table 9–1. Hypoperfusion of the central nervous system (CNS) produces the classic symptoms of presyncope (lightheadedness, faintness, postural dizziness), and eventually syncope. Coronary artery hypoperfusion leads to angina. Renal hypoperfusion leads to oliguria, and finally, anuria. Generalized organ hypoperfusion may also be manifested by a metabolic acidosis ("lactic acidosis"), due to the cellular use of anaerobic metabolism in the face of generalized organ hypoperfusion.

Left Ventricular Failure or "Backward Failure"

As left ventricular failure develops, left atrial pressure increases, culminating in pulmonary congestion. The severity of left ventricular failure can be easily quantified by using the New York Heart Association Functional Classification (Table 9–2). This index of left ventricular function is useful preoperatively, to guide decision making regarding both preoperative testing and the selection of intraoperative monitoring modalities.

Right Ventricular Failure

The most common cause of right ventricular failure is left ventricular failure. In addition, right ventricular failure is frequently associated with pulmonary hypertension. As a result, an often overlooked measurement to assess the severity and duration of right ventricular dysfunction is testing of hepatic function. With chronic hepatic congestion, ascites and eventually, anasarca, develop due to profound loss of albumin and total proteins. Moreover, the developing vitamin K deficiency reduces vitamin K–dependent coagulation factors, beginning with factor VII deficiency (seen as an elevated prothrombin time [PT] only), but eventually leading to deficiency of factors II, VII, IX, and X (seen as an elevated PT and activated partial thromboplastin time [aPTT]). Therefore, albumin and total protein levels, as well as PT/aPTT, are quick screening tests to determine the clinical impact of right ventricular *dysfunction.*

Determinants of Ventricular Performance

Mathematically the determinants of cardiac output are:

$$CO = BP \times SVR$$

$$CO = SV \times HR$$

where CO = cardiac output, BP = blood pressure, sys-

TABLE 9–1
Physical Symptoms and Signs of Forward Failure

Organ System	Symptom	Sign
Central nervous system	*Presyncope → syncope* Mental confusion Light headedness Faintness	Signs of dilirium Loss of consciousness
Cardiovascular system	Angina	Orthostatic hypotension Hypotension, decreased pulse pressure, shock
Renal Skin	Oliguria → anuria	Oliguria → anuria Cold clammy skin Peripheral cyanosis Mottling Delayed capillary refill
Metabolic		Metabolic (lactic) acidosis
Left ventricular failure	Dyspnea PND Orthopnea	Tachypnea Left sided S_3, S_4 gallop Rales Wheezing (cardiac asthma) Functional MR murmur Pulsus alternans
Right ventricular failure	Peripheral edema Nocturia RUQ pain/abdominal Fullness	JVD, HJR Hepatosplenomegaly Ascites/anasarca Right sided S_3, S_4 gallop TR (pulsatile liver, elevated jugular v wave) Signs of pulmonary hypertension

PND, paroxysmal nocturnal dyspnea; JVD, jugular venous distention; HJR, hepatojugular reflux; TR, tricuspid regurgitation; MR, mitral regurgitation; RUQ, right upper quadrant.

temic vascular resistance (SVR) = mean arterial pressure (MAP) − central venous pressure (CVP), SV = stroke volume, and HR = heart rate.

The determinants of stroke volume are preload, afterload, and contractility.

Preload is the end-diastolic stress or end-diastolic fiber length on the ventricular myocardium and is accurately measured as end-diastolic volume (EDV) intraoperatively. End-diastolic *pressure* is often taken to approximate end-diastolic *volume* or ventricular preload, but does not correlate linearly with true preload as will be discussed later. True ventricular preload is determined by blood volume, ventricular compliance, ventricular afterload, venous tone, and myocardial contractility.

Afterload is the ventricular contraction against the resistance of the peripheral vasculature and refers to the wall stress or tension faced by the myocardium during ventricular ejection. True ventricular afterload is the force opposing ventricular fiber shortening during systole. Left ventricular afterload is dependent on ventricular shape, size, radius, and wall thickness. The principal determinants of afterload are the radius of the left ventricle (related to preload or ventricular volume) and aortic impedance (controlled by atrial compliance and systemic vascular resistance). Furthermore, afterload is also affected by aortic wall stiffness, blood viscosity, and the mass blood in the aorta, but these are of lesser importance clinically. Systemic vascular resistance is a poor index of left ventricular afterload, as SVR reflects peripheral arteriolar tone, and not left ventricular systolic wall tension. SVR can be calculated mathematically if blood pressure and cardiac output are known, and therefore, although easy to obtain clinically, SVR is an imperfect estimate of ventricular afterload.

In the evaluation of ventricular performance, ventricular inotropy may be studied using either ejection phase indices or isovolemic phase indices. Ejection phase indices, by definition, characterize left ventricular contractile state by the ejection phase of the cardiac cycle, and hence, are afterload dependent (e.g., increased afterload would reduce ventricular ejection fraction, as myocardial work is used for pressure generation as opposed to ejec-

TABLE 9–2
New York Heart Association Functional Classification

Class I	No limitation	Ordinary physical activity does not cause symptoms
Class II	Slight limitation	Comfortable at rest Ordinary physical activity causes symptoms
Class III	Marked limitation	Comfortable at rest Less than ordinary activity causes symptoms
Class IV	Inability to carry on any physical activity	Symptoms present at rest

tion ventricular volume). Ejection phase indices include mean velocity of circumferential fiber shortening, peak velocity of circumferential fiber shortening, mean systolic ejection rate, mean normalized systolic ejection rate, ejection fraction, fractional shortening, cardiac output, left ventricular ejection time, pressure-length loops, pressure-volume loops, and the end-systolic pressure-volume relationship.

Isovolemic phase indexes are measurements made during the period of isovolemic contraction, *prior to* the opening of the aortic valve, and include Peak dP/dt, dP/dt_{max}, dP/dt_{40}, peak velocity of shortening of contractile element, velocity of shortening of the unloaded contractile element, force-velocity curves, and pre-ejection period. Isovolemic phase indexes tend to be more preload dependent. A detailed discussion of these indexes is beyond the scope of this chapter.

Ventricular performance is, therefore, determined by these various techniques, and integrated into the hemodynamic database for diagnostic purposes. Of the above-mentioned indexes of contractility, cardiac output is the only commonly used measure of ventricular inotropy, and is determined intraoperatively by thermodilution or echocardiography.

Heart rate is an important determinant of ventricular function, particularly in the rate-dependent heart of the neonate or in the "failing heart" (e.g., cardiomyopathies). In the patient with a fixed stroke volume, cardiac output is "rate-dependent" as decreased heart rate proportionately reduces the cardiac output.

Cardiac rhythm, although not expressed mathematically in the indices above also affects the loading conditions of the myocardium, particularly preload. The normal ventricle is dependent on a 15% atrial contribution to ventricular filling. In the patient with a noncompliant left ventricle (aortic stenosis, ischemic heart disease, or left ventricular hypertrophy), the atrial contribution may account for up to 40% of ventricular preload. Loss of sinus rhythm in these patients reduces ventricular filling by 40%, and hence, ventricular output. In these potentially life-threatening situations, rhythm is restored emergently with a consultation to the local power company (i.e., cardioversion).

The primary determinants of stroke volume, therefore, are preload, afterload, contractility, and heart rate. This hemodynamic information is then integrated for both diagnostic ad therapeutic decisions about ventricular function. A convenient form of expressing most of this information is the pressure-volume loop. Figures 9–1 and 9–2*A* represent the ventricular pressure versus volume during the cardiac cycle. During diastole, the mitral valve opens and EDV increases as a curvilinear function until the mitral valve closes, the end-diastolic volume. The brisk upstroke or rise in pressure is the isovolumetric contraction phase, ending with the opening of the aortic valve. During the subsequent phase, ventricular ejection occurs, seen as a diminishing LV volume and rising pressure, ending with the end-systolic volume as the aortic valve closes. Finally isovolemic relaxation occurs as the pressure declines in the LV, terminating with mitral valve opening. After having mastered the volume and pressure changes in this idealized cardiac cycle (Fig. 9–1), pathology of the ventricles and pharmacologic treatments are better understood (Fig. 9–2*B–F*).

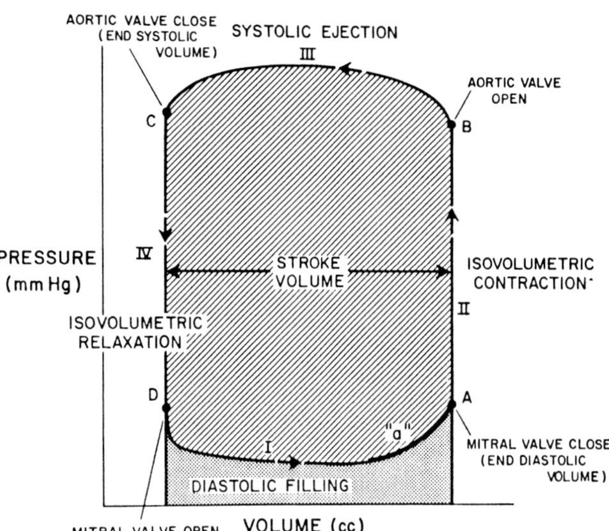

FIGURE **9–1.** Pressure-volume loop of the idealized heart, depicting ventricular pressure versus ventricular volume over the entire cardiac cycle. The cycle begins at the bottom left-hand side with opening of the mitral valve and filling of the ventricle to end-diastolic volume (*bottom right*). Isovolumetric contraction begins at the lower right-hand portion with closure of the mitral valve and rising ventricular pressure (isovolumetric phase). The aortic valve opens at the upper right-hand portion of the curve, as ventricular ejection begins (ejection phase). At the upper left-hand border, the aortic valve closes (end-systolic volume), and isovolumetric relaxation begins, as the ventricular pressure declines. Stroke volume is the difference between the ventricular volume at end-systole and end-diastole.

Figure 9–3*A* shows the normal pressure-volume loop (shaded area), and superimposed upon this loop is a loop of aortic stenosis. Assuming end-diastolic volume to be the same as a normal ventricle, end-diastolic pressure is elevated, consistent with the diastolic dysfunction seen in aortic stenosis due to the noncompliant LV with severe concentric left ventricular hypertrophy. During isovolemic contraction, a much larger pressure is required to allow blood to be ejected through the stenotic valve, causing the pressure-volume loop to appear taller. Once open, the aortic valve allows ejection of the normal stroke volume and once again, the ventricle begins another cycle. The area in the pressure-volume loop is larger, reflecting greater myocardial work. This ventricular work (pressure × volume) has been shown to be linearly related to myocardial oxygen consumption under various hemodynamic conditions (Fig. 9–2*A*).[3] In this case, there is a greater myocardial oxygen consumption due to greater "pressure work" by the left ventricle. The end-systolic volume occurs at a markedly higher pressure, and if the slope is taken from this point, the end-systolic pressure-volume relationship (ESPVR) would suggest an increased contractility. If the loop is replotted with wall stress, which normalizes the pressure for increased wall thickness, the ESPVR is unchanged, indicating normal contractility (Fig. 9–2*B*). Similarly, the end-diastolic pressure-volume relationship is shifted upward and to the left, indicating diminished ventricular compliance. The stroke volume and ejection fraction are

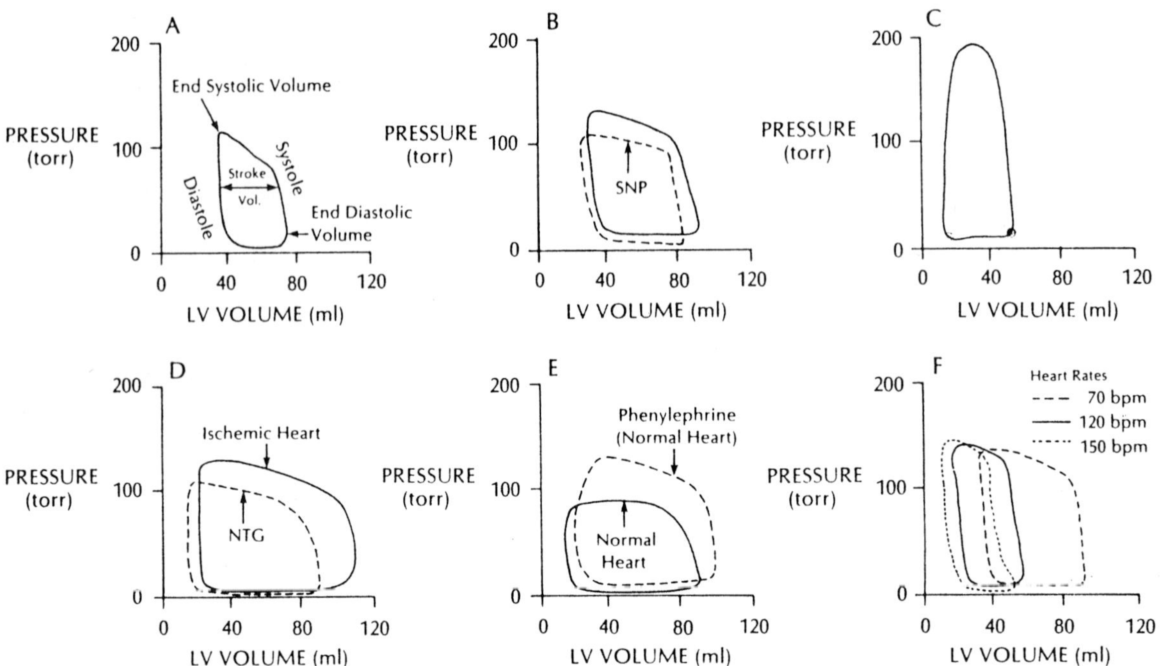

FIGURE **9–2.** *A*, Ventricular pressure-volume loop of the normal heart. *B*, Effect of reduced afterload on the heart with the administration of sodium nitroprusside, whereas *E* shows the effect of increased afterload on the heart produced by phenylephrine. *C*, Changes in the pressure-volume loop in a patient with aortic stenosis, with high peak ventricular pressure. *D*, Effect of venodilation and coronary vasodilation produced by nitroglycerin on the ischemic heart. Nitroglycerin reduces end-diastolic volume or ventricular compliance, as well as improving systolic contractility. *F*, Effect of heart rate on filling volume, as LV volume *decreases* as heart rate *increases*. (From Lake CL: Cardiovascular anatomy and physiology. In Barash PG, Cullen BF, Stoelting RK [eds]: Clinical Anesthesia, 3rd ed. Philadelphia, JB Lippincott Co, 1997, p 822, with permission.)

preserved in this example of aortic stenosis. The pressure-volume loop allows for a pictorial description of the loading conditions of the heart (preload as volume, afterload implied by pressure) as well as contractility (stroke volume, ESPVR). It still does not add new hemodynamic information that is clinically useful to the practicing anesthesiologist, but provides a model to better understand the pathology and therapeutic interventions aimed at improving pump function (Fig. 9–2*B*, *D*, and *E*).

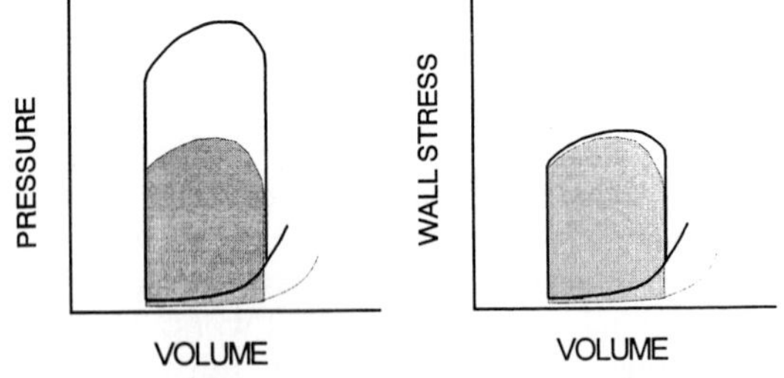

FIGURE **9–3.** A pressure-volume (PV) loop of the normal heart (*shaded area*) with the PV loop of the heart with aortic stenosis superimposed on the normal loop. Note that the end-diastolic pressure-volume relationship (EDPVR) is shifted upward and to the left, suggesting diminished ventricular compliance of "filling" despite a normal stroke volume and ejection fraction. Intraventricular (systolic) pressure is markedly elevated, giving a larger PV area, suggesting higher myocardial work. ESPVR is shifted upward and to the left, suggesting increased contractility of the ventricle. However, if loop *A* is replotted with wall stress (which normalizes pressure for increased wall thickness) on the y axis, the ESPVR is unchanged, indicating normal contractility as seen in loop *B*. (Modified from Ross J Jr: Cardiac function and myocardial contractility: A perspective. J Am Coll Cardiol 1:52, 1983 with permission of Elsevier Science *and* Jackson JM: Valvular heart disease. In Thomas SJ, Kramer JL [eds]: Manual of Cardiac Anesthesia, 2nd ed. New York, Churchill Livingstone, 1993, p 83, with permission.)

Monitoring Modalities

Electrocardiographic Monitoring of Ventricular Function

The primary use of echocardiographic (ECG) monitoring as a monitor of ventricular function is in the monitoring of ischemia. Coronary artery ligation results in biochemical abnormalities such as a reduction in oxygen availability, reduction in adenosine triphosphate (ATP) production, development of intracellular acidosis, and increase in intracellular calcium stores. Although evidence of biochemical dysfunction occurs first, mechanical dysfunction follows with a concomitant reduction in wall thickening and wall motion abnormalities (hypokinesis proceeding to akinesis, proceeding to dyskinesis). Following biochemical and mechanical dysfunction are electrocardiographic signs of abnormalities, with endocardial ECG ST-segment changes followed by surface ECG ST changes. Therefore, clinically electrocardiographic monitoring as a monitor of ischemia is a late marker, as shown in Figure 9–4*B*.

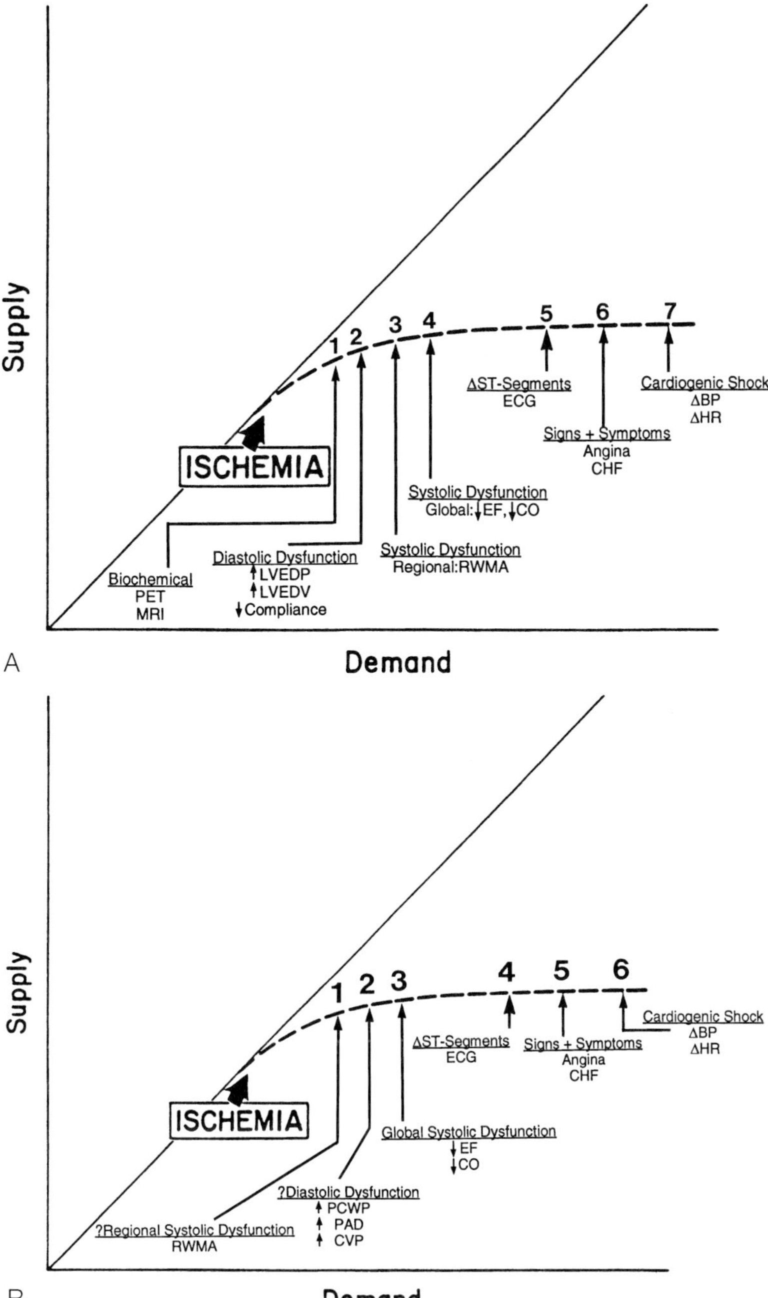

FIGURE **9–4.** *A*, Myocardial oxygen demand versus supply. When supply is insufficient to meet demands, ventricular ischemia develops. Numbers 1 to 7 represent the monitoring modalities used *experimentally* to detect ventricular ischemia. Experimentally (1) biochemical evidence of ventricular ischemia can be detected by MRI or PET scanning as the earliest markers of ischemia, followed by evidence of (2) diminished ventricular compliance (↑LVEDP, ↑LVEDV). Systolic dysfunction occurs later, seen as (3) regional ventricular dysfunction (RWMA) followed by (4) global ventricular dysfunction (EF, CO). (5) Electrocardiographic evidence of ischemia (ST-segment changes) occur later, prior to (6) symptoms (angina, dyspnea). Signs of (7) cardiogenic shock (↓ BP, ↑HR) are very late findings in monitoring. MRI, magnetic resonance imaging; PET, positron emission tomography. (Modified from Barash PG: Monitoring myocardial oxygen balance: Physiologic basis and clinical application. ASA Annual Refresher Course Lectures, 1985, p 24, with permission.) *B*, Myocardial oxygen demand versus supply. When supply is insufficient to meet metabolic demands, ventricular ischemia develops. Numbers 1 to 6 represent the monitoring modalities used *intraoperatively* to detect ventricular ischemia. *Clinically*, regional systolic dysfunction is first detected by (1) RWMA on TEE, prior to evidence of (2) diastolic dysfunction noted on a PAC. (3) Global systolic dysfunction (↓CO, ↓EF) is seen later intraoperatively, followed by electrocardiographic evidence of ischemia. (5) Clinical symptoms of coronary insufficiency (angina, dyspnea) and (6) signs of cardiogenic shock (↓BP, ↑HR) are late events in monitoring of ventricular ischemia. (Modified from Barash PG: Monitoring myocardial oxygen balance: Physiologic basis and clinical application. ASA Annual Refresher Course Lectures, 1985, p 24, with permission.)

After acute coronary artery occlusion, ST-segment elevation is seen on epicardial ECG in animals,[4,5] analogous to that seen with a transmural myocardial infarction in humans in the precordial or limb leads of a 12-lead ECG. This ST-segment change is associated with a loss of systolic myocardial wall thickening or contraction, reaching a maximum in 5 to 7 minutes, and is believed to be due to the loss of intracellular potassium. Therefore, the failure of ischemic areas to depolarize normally leads to abnormal current flows during electrical systole. ECG monitoring is, therefore, a monitor of the flow of electrical currents.

Coronary anatomy is localized by using multiple leads, for instance, the standard ECG with 12 leads: three frontal, three augmented, and six precordial leads. This has been validated in humans during angioplasty,[6,7] where ST-segment *elevation* correlates with regional myocardial ventricular dysfunction. The difficulty arises due to the fact that not all ischemia is transmural or "supply side" ischemia as described above with a complete coronary artery occlusion. Secondly, not all ischemia is reflected by ST-segment elevation. Subendocardial ischemia is usually diffuse and poorly localized, and is reflected as ST-segment depression. The ability to detect ischemia by electrocardiography grossly (i.e., the sensitivity and specificity) is influenced by lead selection. Lead V_5,[8] in particular, may overlap the distribution of both the left anterior descending coronary artery and the circumflex coronary artery. Therefore, subendocardial ischemia in V_5 is a poor indicator of coronary artery distribution or true regional ventricular ischemia.

Intraoperatively, ischemic ST-segment changes are infrequently (30%) associated with hemodynamic changes (heart rate, systolic blood pressure, diastolic blood pressure, or pulmonary artery diastolic pressure [PADP]).[9] This finding is expected, as perioperatively most major hemodynamic changes are associated with acute changes in systemic vascular resistance, such as those during induction or emergence, as opposed to the heart rate or cardiac output changes associated with treadmill testing. Furthermore, localization of ST-segment changes is affected by the variability in coronary anatomy, lead selection (type and number of leads, lead placement), and type of ECG monitor used.[10] Other factors such as ventricular hypertrophy, electrolyte abnormalities (potassium), drugs (digoxin), ventilation (positive-pressure ventilation vs. spontaneous), temperature, stray electrical currents (electrical cautery devices), and neurologic changes (stellate ganglion stimulation or stellate ganglion block, head trauma) can all impact on ST-segment morphology. In summary, then, the quantification of ischemia is affected by both the criteria used to define ischemia, and the type of ischemia. Which leads are most useful intraoperatively? Again, leads II and V_5 when used together are most accurate in patients with or at risk for coronary artery disease in noncardiac surgery, with an 80% sensitivity.[11] Using a three-lead system, II, V_4, V_5, 96% of intraoperative ischemic episodes can be detected[12] (see also Chapter 8).

In patients undergoing cardiac surgery, changes in ST-segment morphology can also be affected by hemodynamic variations (i.e., blood pressure and heart rate). The impact of these hemodynamic changes remains a source of controversy. Slogoff et al. have shown that only 50% of ECG changes are temporally related to a change in heart rate of blood pressure alone.[12–14] Leung et al.[11] have demonstrated that only 25% of ischemic episodes are related to changes in heart rate or blood pressure. These studies suggest that changes in heart rate and blood pressure are not sensitive indicators of variances in myocardial oxygen supply and demand. This observation has been validated by angioplasty studies where peak negative dP/dt during coronary artery occlusion is followed by diminished systolic fractional shortening and increase in left ventricular end-diastolic pressure with no change in heart rate or blood pressure.[15]

Other nonhemodynamically related causes of ECG evidence of ischemia include reductions in oxygen supply seen in animals and humans,[16,17] showing ischemic regional dysfunction occurs frequently despite normal left ventricular function and stable hemodynamics. This is evidence for silent ischemia.[18–20] Mechanisms to explain these findings include localized coronary artery spasm and thrombosis formation in the presence of stenotic coronary arteries leading to myocardial ischemia.[15,21,22] Prinzmetal's angina or classic coronary artery spasm may also occur in patients with coronary artery disease.

Arterial Blood Pressure Monitoring

The most frequently monitored variable of left ventricular function is arterial blood pressure. The difficulty with using arterial blood pressure arises due to the fact that blood pressure per se, is an indirect measure of ventricular function, providing only part of the information required to make a useful assessment. Cardiac output is derived from both blood pressure and systemic vascular resistance ($BP = CO \times SVR$). The cardiac index is, therefore, a more physiologic measurement of true left ventricular output or function than blood pressure measurement alone. For example, a systolic blood pressure of 90 mm Hg can be achieved with a cardiac index of less than 2 L/min/m^2, 2 to 3 L/min/m^2, or 10 L/min/m^2. More importantly, alterations of blood pressure are usually a late finding of ventricular dysfunction, as shown in Figure 9–4. Changes in blood pressure alone are not sufficient to connote left ventricular dysfunction. In addition, changes in arterial pressure are a very late event in the process of ventricular dysfunction.

When monitoring blood pressure, it is often useful to determine the clinical significance of the measurement. Myocardial oxygen requirements have been shown to correlate with changes in systolic blood pressure.[23] However, errors in measuring systolic blood pressure are common.[24] This fact, coupled with the uncertainty of the clinical significance of changes in systolic blood pressure, has limited its application as a sole indication of ventricular performance.

Diastolic blood pressure is an important determinant of coronary perfusion pressure, defined simplistically as aortic diastolic blood pressure minus left ventricular end-diastolic pressure.[25] Unfortunately, diastolic blood pressure measurements are the most inaccurate measurements to be obtained, particularly from the automated noninvasive blood pressure and direct blood pressure monitoring devices.[26,27] Therefore, although diastolic blood pressure is important to define coronary perfusion pressure, due to the inaccuracies of obtaining diastolic blood pressure, it is rarely used clinically to make decisions about ventricular dysfunction. However, in patients with aortic insufficiency, diastolic blood pressure monitoring is helpful to ensure adequate coronary perfusion pressure.[28]

Clinically, the most appropriate blood pressure to monitor is the mean blood pressure. Mean pressure is the integrated mean of the arterial pressure wave, which represents "the hydrostatic force" that powers diffusion and filtration functions of the pressure wave. Fortunately, the mean pressure is also the most clinically reproducible arterial blood pressure. Compared to systolic or diastolic pressures, mean blood pressure determinations are more accurately measured with either indirect, noninvasive[29,30] or direct, invasive monitoring modalities.[31] Moreover, mean blood pressure is most useful clinically, as all "organ perfusion pressures" (cerebral perfusion pressure, coronary perfusion pressure, renal perfusion pressure, hepatic blood pressure, uterine perfusion pressure) are dependent upon mean blood pressure.

If the mean blood pressure can be determined, and the resistance is known, then the cardiac output (as a measure of left ventricular performance) can be obtained (as cardiac output equals blood pressure divided by systemic vascular resistance). Clinically, the reverse is performed: CO is determined and MAP and SVR are derived mathematically; SVR = (MAP − RAP) × 80/CO, normal SVR = 800 to 1,200 dynes. However, clinically we use the adequacy of arterial blood pressure as an indirect assessment of sufficient ventricular function and tissue organ perfusion (Fig. 9–5).[32]

Noninvasive Blood Pressure Monitoring

Noninvasive blood pressure measurement devices presently in clinical use are all occlusive cuff devices that measure blood pressure *indirectly*, based on the Riva-Rocci sphygmomanometer.[33] This measurement may be done intermittently and manually, with the auscultation of Korotkoff sounds, or intermittently and automatically with an automated noninvasive blood pressure (ANIBP) device.[34] Methods to continuously measure blood pressure noninvasively have been developed,[35] but unfortunately are not sufficiently reliable to be used commonly during cardiothoracic or major vascular surgeries.[36] For

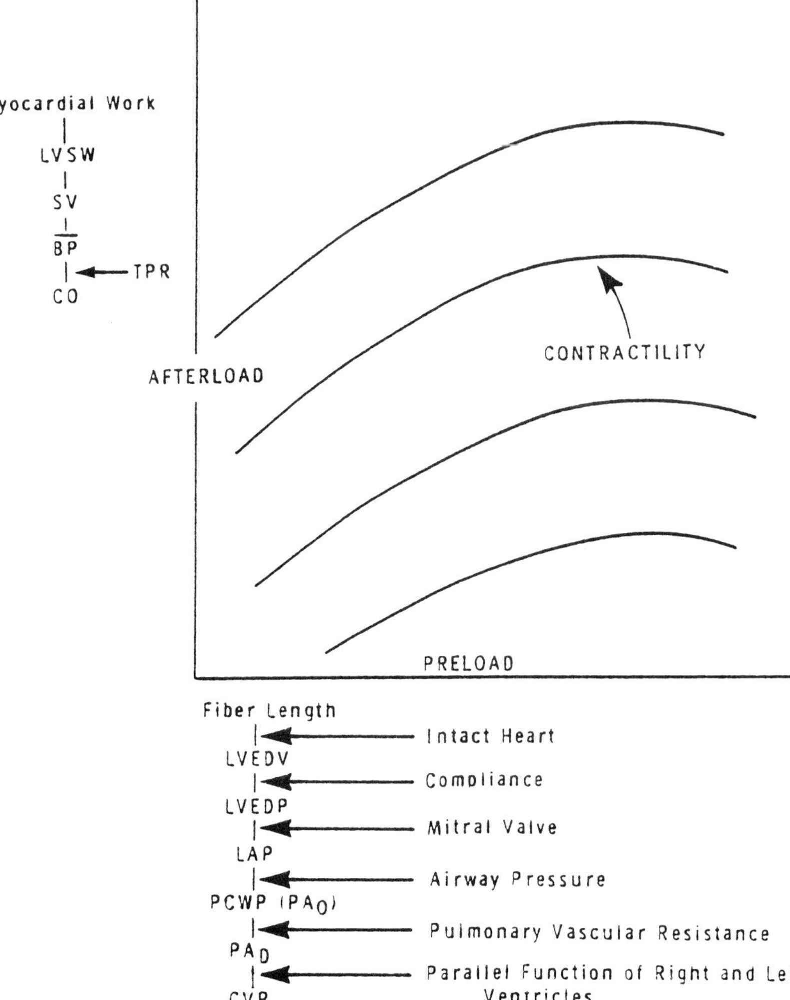

FIGURE **9–5.** The ventricular function curve can be constructed by using various different estimates of preload versus performance. The horizontal axis represents preload of the ventricle, and can be assessed by these various factors (central venous pressure, pulmonary artery diastolic pressure, pulmonary capillary wedge pressure, left atrial pressure, left ventricular end-diastolic pressure, left ventricular end-diastolic volume, fiber length). To the right of these variables are factors known to influence the accuracy of the estimates of ventricular preload. The vertical axis represents myocardial work or ventricular performance, and is affected by afterload. Variables used to assess ventricular performance include cardiac output, blood pressure, stroke volume, left ventricular stroke work, and myocardial work. (From Thys DM, Kaplan JA: Cardiovascular Physiology. In Miller RD [ed]: Anesthesia, 3rd ed. New York, Churchill Livingstone, 1990, p 557, with permission.)

descriptions of these various technologies and their limitations, the reader is referred to the reviews of Stanley and Bedford.[34,37]

The indications of noninvasive blood pressure monitoring (NIBP) are clearly defined by the American Society of Anesthesiologists (ASA) standards.[39] There are relatively few contraindications to NIBP monitoring, but sickle cell disease is one such disease where care must be taken to avoid overzealous use of occlusive blood pressure cuffs. The complications associated with NIBP are few, but isolated events have been described.[40,41] In essence, repetitive cycling of blood pressure measurements leads to inadequate perfusion of the monitored limb. Paraesthesia from nerve injury[41] and compartment syndrome[40] from arterial insufficiency have also been described. Therefore, as few complications have been ascribed to NIBP monitoring, it has a very low risk-benefit ratio.

Invasive (Direct) Arterial Pressure Monitoring

The principle involved in this technology is the transduction of the arterial pressure wave (from the monitored artery) via an electrical signal that can be visually displayed. In-depth discussions of the physics and specific methodologies are beyond the scope of this chapter.

There are large variations involved in monitoring various invasive waveforms. This is seen in the cardiac surgical operating room where after discontinuing cardiopulmonary bypass, aortic root and radial artery pressures are often monitored simultaneously to assess the similarity or differences in blood pressure measurements. These discrepancies are due to, among other things, wave reflection (Fig. 9–5).[42] Theoretically, one would anticipate a higher systolic blood pressure in the radial artery than in the ascending aorta (Fig. 9–6), but in fact, the reverse is usually true immediately following cardiopulmonary bypass (Fig. 9–7).[43] The physiologic basis for this has been suggested to be related to vasodilation of the hand or vasodilation of the forearm and redistribution of flow away from the wrist, similar to that observed in an arterial venous fistula.[43,44] Similar to the NIBP determination, absolute blood pressure measurement via the invasive technique is dependent on multiple variables including measuring technique, site, and intrinsic physiologic state of the individual. Three principal indications for direct arterial blood pressure monitoring have been previously well described[45]: to monitor beat-to-beat changes in arterial pressure, for intra-arterial access for repetitive blood analysis, and prolonged duration of the procedure.

There are no absolute contraindications to invasive blood pressure monitoring; among the few relative contraindications are Raynaud's disease, anticoagulation, and inadequate collateral circulation to the cannulated artery. The most frequent complication seen with invasive arterial pressure monitoring is thrombosis.[37] This is thought to be due to platelet aggregation as a result of catheter-induced vessel injury.[37] Other complications associated with arterial catheterization are related to cannulation misadventures, such as hematomas and damage

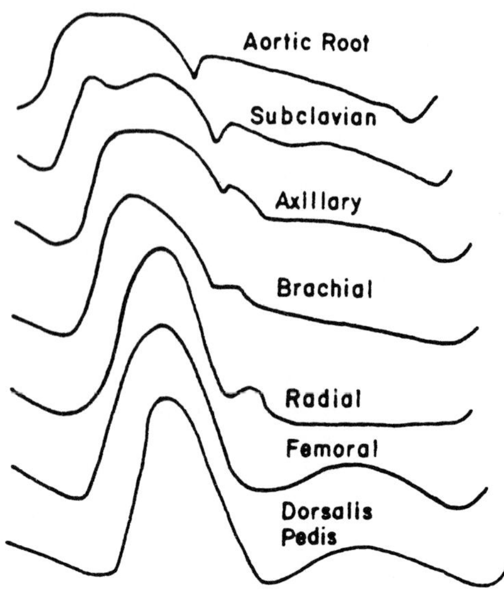

FIGURE **9–6.** The configuration of the arterial pressure wave at various sites in the arterial tree. (From Bedford FR, Shah NK: Blood pressure monitoring: Invasive and noninvasive. In Blitt CD, Hines RL [eds]: Monitoring in Anesthesia and Critical Care Medicine, 3rd ed. New York, Churchill Livingstone, 1995, p 100, with permission.)

to adjacent structures (e.g., nerve injuries), as well as ischemia to the distal extremity.[37,38] Ischemia may be due to inadequate flow due to the obstruction by the catheter, or due to thrombosis at the site of cannulation, during or after removal of the cannula.[46]

Central Venous Pressure Monitoring

Right atrial pressure, often used interchangeably with central venous pressure, is used clinically to determine right ventricular function and the intravascular volume status. This is a paradox, as central venous pressure influences ventricular function via preload of the ventricle, and ventricular function affects the central venous pressure via the compliance of the ventricles.

The clinical utility of CVP measurement is as an indirect assessment of ventricular performance and an aid in the construction of ventricular function or Frank-Starling curves (Fig. 9–5). Ventricular performance is dependent on venous return or "preload"[47] so that with increasing filling pressure (defined here as right atrial pressure), ventricular output is improved, assuming normal contractility of the ventricle. Alternatively, by maintaining constant filling pressures, changes in ventricular performance are denoted by changes in the slope of the ventricular function curve. As can be clearly seen, measuring CVP in and of itself provides only one half of the information required to construct this curve. Furthermore, the assumption that central venous pressure correlates linearly with end-diastolic volume of the ventricle is inaccurate, particularly in the perioperative setting or in the critically ill patient. Table 9–3 is a list of factors commonly affecting the accuracy of central venous pressure measurement.[48]

As a result of the interrelationship of central venous pressure not only to cardiac performance but also to the

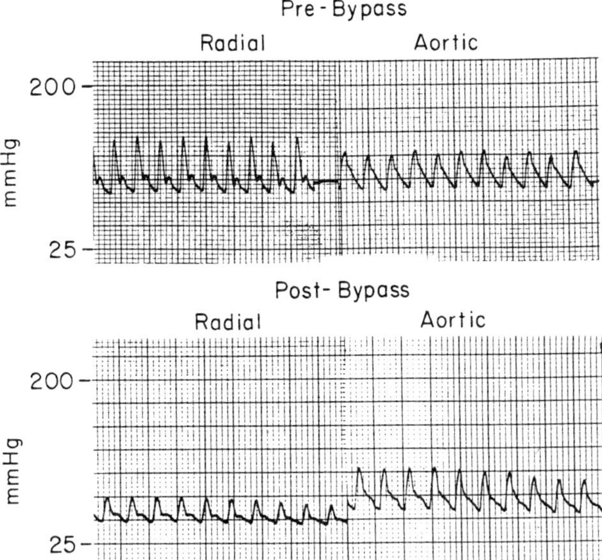

FIGURE **9–7.** Photograph of data showing the reversal of the relationship between radial and aortic blood pressure measurements immediately following cardiopulmonary bypass in a single patient. (From Stern DH, et al: Can we trust the direct radial artery pressure immediately following cardiopulmonary bypass? Anesthesiology 62: 557, 1985, with permission.)

factors cited in Table 9–4, it is clear that a single, absolute, central venous pressure measurement is of little clinical utility. Clinically, it is more relevant to use the "trend," rather than isolated central venous pressure measurements, to indicate intravascular volume status.

The presence of normal atrioventricular coordination or discoordination (as noted by wave morphology) can also be obtained from CVP measurements. The usual CVP waveform, when coupled to a rhythm strip, provides useful information regarding ventricular conduction (normal rhythm vs. arrhythmias) (Fig. 9–8). In atrial fibrillation, no a waves are noted, whereas with atrioventricular dissociation, a characteristic cannon a wave is noted. Analysis of x and y descents may also be useful to assess right ventricular compliance, and hence, right ventricular dysfunction.[49] Patients with right ventricular ischemia or infarction may develop tricuspid regurgitation with exaggerated v waves on a right atrial pressure tracing. Also, increased absolute right atrial pressure has been used as a marker of right ventricular dysfunction, particularly in the presence of systemic hypotension or deterioration in global ventricular function.[50]

TABLE **9–3**
Factors that Affect CVP (RAP)

Left heart function
Pulmonary vascular resistance
Right ventricular function
Tricuspid valve function
Venous return
Intravascular volume/venous return
Paricardial disease
Intrathoracic pressure

TABLE **9–4**
Conditions Resulting in Discrepancy Between PAOP and LVEDP*

Mean PAOP > LVEDP
Positive-pressure ventilation
PEEP
Increased intrathoracic pressure
Non–zone III PAC placement
Chronic obstructive lung disease
Tachycardia, sepsis
Increased pulmonary vascular resistance
Noncompliant left atrium
Mitral valve obstruction (stenosis, myxoma, clot)
Pulmonary venous compression (tumor, fibrosis)
Mitral regurgitation
Left-to-right intracardiac shunt
Mean PAOP < LVEDP
Large a wave
Pressure recorded before a wave
Falsely ↓ PAOP
Noncompliant left ventricle → aortic stenosis
Aortic regurgitation → premature mitral valve closure → LAEDP
Reduced pulmonary arterial tree (pneumonectomy, pulmonary embolus) → pulmonary vascular bed
Right bundle branch block

*Modified from Tuman KJ, Carroll GC, Ivankovich AD: Pitfalls in interpretation of pulmonary artery catheter data. J Cardiothorac Anesth 3(5):625, 1989, with permission.

PAOP, pulmonary artery occlusion pressure; LVEDP, left ventricular end-diastolic pressure; PEEP, positive end-expiratory pressure; PAC, pulmonary artery catheter; LAEDP, left atrial end-diastolic pressure.

The single most limiting factor in using central venous pressure measurement during the perioperative setting is the application of positive-pressure ventilation. Mechanical ventilation leads to elevated intrathoracic pressure, which is partly transmitted to the right atrium, elevating right atrial pressure. However, transmural pressure (true filling pressure) is actually decreased, as this airway pressure is transmitted to all the intrathoracic structures.[51] In this situation, due to a reduction in true preload, cardiac output is reduced by the Frank-Starling mechanism. Taken together, an increasing central venous pressure and decreasing cardiac output or systemic blood

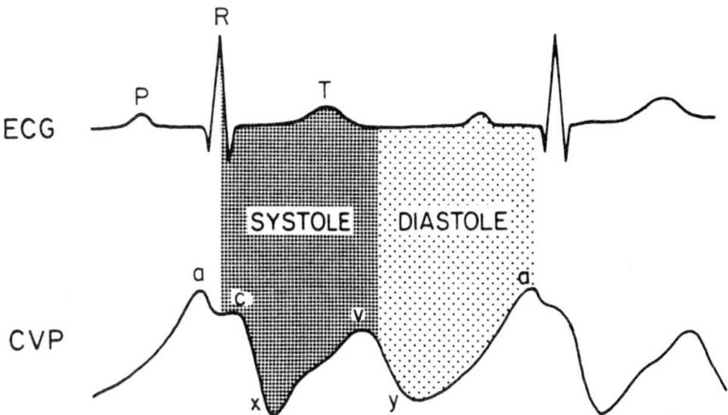

FIGURE **9–8.** The normal central venous pressure tracing (mechanical event), with the corresponding electrocardiographic tracing above (electrical event), used to ascertain the timing of the hemodynamic wave for interpretation. (From Mark JB: Central venous pressure monitoring: Clinical insights beyond the numbers. J Cardiothorac Anesth 5:163, 1991, with permission.)

pressure suggest right ventricular failure as opposed to hypovolemia.[52]

Indications for central venous pressure monitoring have been previously described.[52] Briefly, the indications for CVP monitoring in the perioperative period are: monitoring right atrial filling pressure or wave morphology, to secure central venous access for drug delivery or volume resuscitation, and for the aspiration of air emboli. There are no absolute contraindications to central venous pressure monitoring, but relative contraindications do exist. These include systemic anticoagulation or coagulopathy, sepsis, or skin infection at the site, etc. The complications of central venous access have been well documented,[53] but can be generalized as complications related to cannulation, complications of catheter or guidewire insertion, and complications of the catheter in situ. In perioperative settings cannulation of the internal jugular vein is commonly performed. An increase in successful cannulation of the internal jugular vein and a decrease in cannulation-related complications has been reported using ultrasonographic guidance.[54]

Pulmonary Artery Catheterization

The balloon-tipped pulmonary artery flotation catheter (PAC) was originally developed by Swan and Ganz as a research tool for the study of the sequelae of myocardial infarction.[55] Since the first clinical description in 1970, its use and complexity have grown exponentially. Presently, PACs are routinely used to monitor myriad variables, including right atrial pressure, right ventricular pressure, pulmonary artery pressure, pulmonary capillary wedge pressure (PCWP), cardiac output by thermodilution, intravascular temperature, mixed venous oxygen saturation, and continuous cardiac output. Furthermore, the PAC allows infusion of drugs and performance of angiography, intracavitary electrograms, atrial and/or ventricular pacing, lung water calculation, and the calculation of ejection fraction.[56–65] For catheter design and review of basic principles, see Barash and Hines.[66]

Pressure Measurements

The theoretical basis for monitoring ventricular function with a pulmonary artery catheter is similar to that of central venous pressure monitoring. However, the PAC provides information regarding both right and left ventricular function via a single "right heart catheterization," reducing the need for a more invasive "left heart catheterization" to obtain left ventricular end-diastolic pressure (LVEDP) measurements.

The conceptual basis for right heart catheterization is diagrammatically illustrated in Figure 9–9. Use of a PAC assumes that when the balloon is inflated in the wedge position, the pulmonary artery occlusion pressure is in equilibrium with the pulmonary venous pressure, which is in equilibrium with the left atrial pressure and sequentially with the LVEDP, before closure of the mitral valve. An uninterrupted column of blood must be present from the tip of the pulmonary artery catheter to the left ventricle (i.e., that no pressure gradients exist between the distal tip of the pulmonary artery catheter pressure transducer and the LVEDP). Furthermore, it is *assumed* that LVEDP correlates linearly with left ventricular end-diastolic volume (Fig. 9–10), allowing for the calculation of ventricular function curves or pressure-volume loops.

In certain clinical instances, this is true, as the PCWP correlates with a left atrial pressure over a wide range of filling pressures.[67–71] In these situations, the PCWP is used to assess ventricular preload and *assumed* to parallel end-diastolic volume of the ventricle, end-diastolic dimension, or end-diastolic fiber length of the myocardium.[72] Traditionally, all pressures are measured at end-expiration in both spontaneously breathing and mechanically ventilated patients.[73]

In the normal patient population or in the absence of any risk factors that would alter pressure measurement between the distal tip of the pulmonary artery catheter and LVEDP, the PADP may be used as a surrogate of PCWP or LVEDP (Table 9–4). The usual gradient between PADP and PCWP is approximately 1 to 4 mm Hg.[74–77] Use of the PADP avoids repetitive wedging of the pulmonary artery catheter and its inherent complications, most notably, pulmonary artery rupture.

Unfortunately, these assumptions are incorrect in a variety of clinical settings (Table 9–4).[72] Hansen et al.[78] have demonstrated the poor correlation between PCWP and left ventricular end-diastolic volume (LVEDV) following cardiopulmonary bypass (Fig. 9–11). Ellis et al.[79] and Raper et al.[72] have shown poor correlation between changes in PCWP and end-diastolic volume after myo-

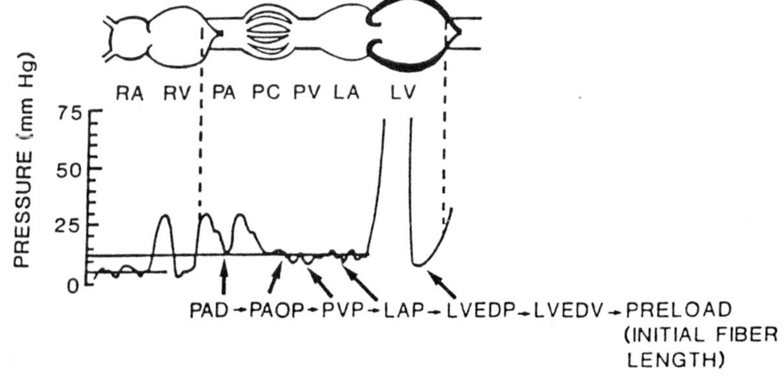

FIGURE **9–9**. Theoretical common chamber from the tip of the PAC to the aortic valve, when the mitral valve is open (*top*). Below this is a typical pressure tracing found from the various chambers, with absolute pressure given on the vertical axis. The assumption is that all pressures from PAD to LVEDP correlate with LVEDV and hence, "preload." (From Tuman KJ, Carroll GC, Ivankovich AD: Pitfalls in interpretation of pulmonary artery catheter data. J Cardiothorac Anesth 3[5]:625, 1989, with permission.)

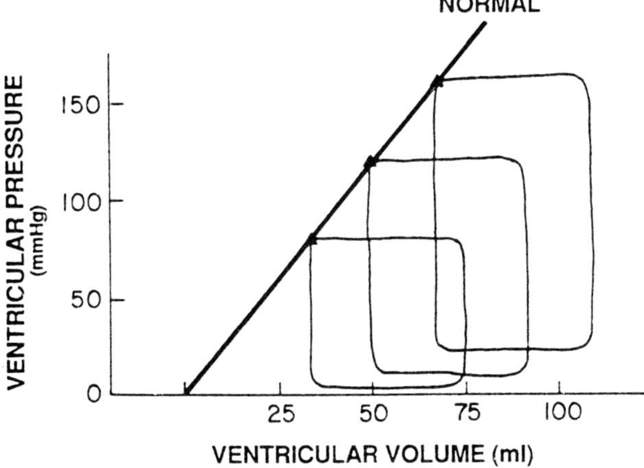

FIGURE **9–10.** The assumed relationship of ventricular filling pressure (*vertical axis*) to ventricular filling volume (*horizontal axis*) in the "normal" heart. (From LaMantia KR, Hines RL, Barash PG: Cardiac performance. In Scurr C, Feldman S, Soni N [eds]: Scientific Foundations of Anesthesia, 4th ed. Chicago, Year Book Medical Publishers, 1990, p 147, with permission.)

cardial revascularization and in critically ill patients with acute respiratory insufficiency and varying degrees of pulmonary hypertension (Fig. 9–12). Therefore, Figure 9–10 shows graphically the correlation of filling pressure to ventricular volume of the normal or ideal heart, whereas Figures 9–11 and 9–12 show the lack of correlation of filling pressure to preload in the diseased heart. For example, in a patient with aortic stenosis, what would a wedge pressure of 20 mm Hg mean? The pressure could signify hypovolemia, a normal filling pressure for this patient, or early left ventricular failure or diastolic dysfunction. As with CVP measurements, absolute filling pressure obtained from the pulmonary artery catheter, per se, may be of limited clinical utility. Trends in pulmonary capillary wedge measurements are used clinically to assess left ventricular preload.

Although PCWP or PADP may not provide absolute indices of ventricular preload, in theory the PCWP tracing itself may be useful in detecting global left ventricular ischemia by the presence of a contoured change, a new v wave.

Kaul et al.[80] demonstrated in a dog model that ischemic mitral regurgitation (MR) occurs only in the presence of significant *global* LV dysfunction, produced by either regional or global *ischemia*. This is due to incomplete mitral leaflet closure (IMLC), and the severity of mitral regurgitation correlated linearly with the degree of IMLC ($r = .98$). MR was never associated with mitral valve prolapse when either the papillary muscles or the immediately adjacent LV myocardium was rendered ischemic. Hence, a new v wave on the intraoperative PCWP tracing (or pulmonary artery pressure [PAP] tracing, often noted by the diastolic component of PAP wave larger than the systolic component) may herald the onset of new global LV dysfunction and functional MR. The global LV dysfunction may be due to global LV ischemia or regional LV ischemia, if remaining areas of myocardium were previously dysfunctional. An example of this is shown in Figure 9–13 demonstrating ischemic MR intraoperatively, diagnosed by transesophageal echocardiography (TEE). Note that the mitral leaflets are not prolapsing, as the origin of the regurgitant jet of MR is at the coaptation points of the mitral valve, and the jet is centrally oriented, consistent with IMLC. MR jets due to mitral valve prolapse are usually eccentric, and take a course posterior to the normally functioning valve.

Acute papillary muscle dysfunction (clinically seen as a rare complication of acute myocardial infarction with papillary muscle rupture, or ruptured chordae) may also be heralded by the new onset of a v wave on the pulmonary capillary wedge tracing.[81,82] In this situation, the v wave is due to flail mitral valve leaflet, as opposed to IMLC explained above. Furthermore, it has been suggested that in selected patients, abnormalities of the a–c wave component may be an early indicator of myo-

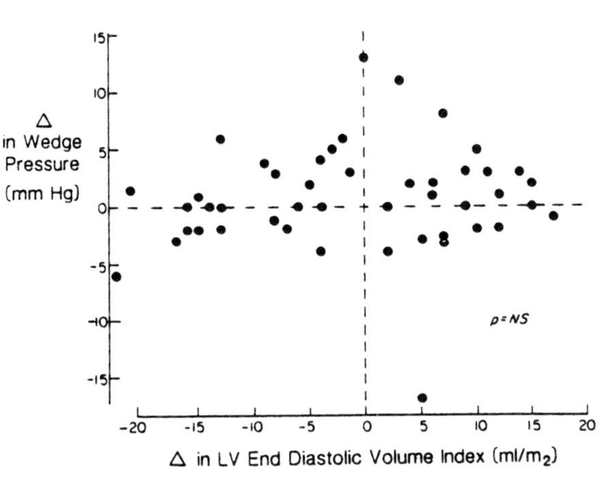

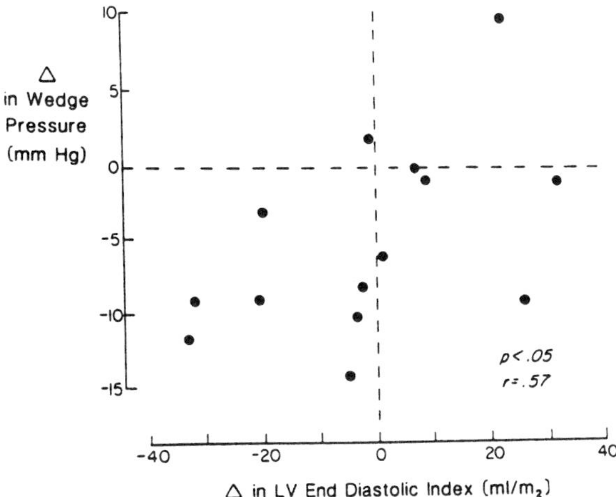

FIGURE **9–11.** The relationship of pulmonary wedge pressure (as an approximation of LVEDP) to LVEDV. Note in *A* that the relation is random in 12 patients following coronary artery bypass graft surgery. *B* shows the same poor correlation in patients treated with vasodilators for congestive heart failure in the coronary care unit. (From Hansen RM, Viquerat CE, Matthay MA, et al: Poor correlation between pulmonary arterial pressure and left ventricular end-diastolic volume after coronary artery bypass heart surgery. Anesthesiology 64:764, 1986, with permission.)

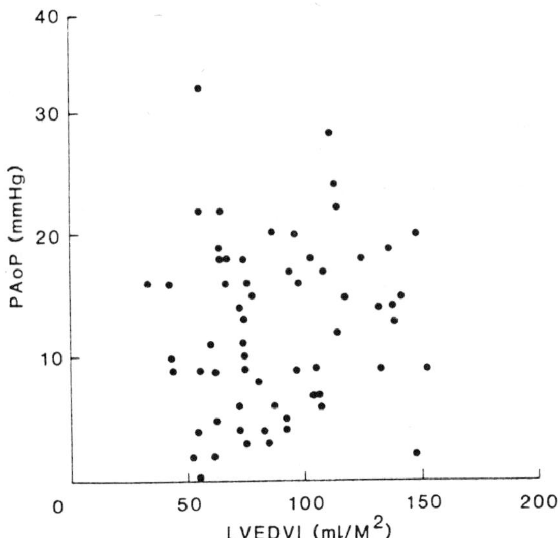

FIGURE **9–12.** Poor correlation between pulmonary artery occlusion pressure (PAOP) and left ventricular end-diastolic volume index (LVEDVI) in patients with acute respiratory failure and varying degrees of pulmonary hypertension. (From Raper R, Sibbald WJ: Misled by the wedge? The Swan-Ganz catheter and left ventricular preload. Chest 89:427, 1986, with permission.)

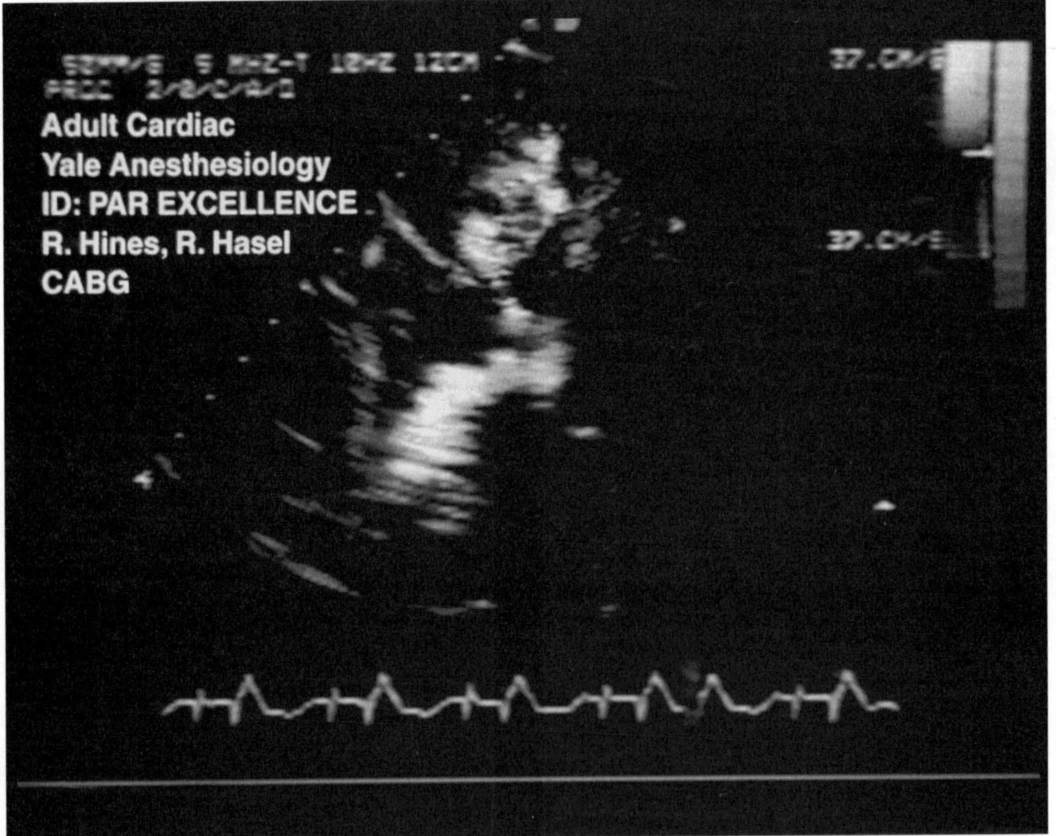

FIGURE **9–13.** 2D TEE image of the mitral valve with color flow Doppler showing mitral regurgitation as a bright, multicolored "mosaic" jet from mitral valve into left atrium. Apex of sector fan (*top*) is left atrium, base of fan (*bottom*) is left ventricle, and on the right of the image is the left ventricular outflow tract. This image was obtained intraoperatively and confirmed global ischemia of the left ventricle before bypass, which responded to high-dose nitroglycerin (5 μg/kg/min). *See Color Plate.*

cardial ischemia.[83] Unfortunately, not all episodes of ventricular ischemia are associated with the new onset of v waves, and therefore, this is another area of controversy surrounding the use of the pulmonary artery catheter for monitoring ventricular ischemia. The ability of the PAC to aid in ischemia detection is severely limited.

Indications, Contraindications, and Complications

Recently, the perioperative recommendations for pulmonary catheterization have been described[84] in cardiac surgical patients[66] (Table 9–5), as well as in noncardiac operations in patients with significant cardiac disease,[85–88] abdominal aortic procedures,[89–94] neurosurgical operations,[95,96] obstetric and gynecologic procedures,[97–102] and pediatric patients.[103–105] In view of the sparsity of data documenting favorable outcomes with the use of pulmonary catheters,[89–94] and the well-documented complications associated with the use of these catheters, some authors have suggested restraint in the use of the PAC.[84,106–110] The final decision on the use of the PAC rests, therefore, with the practitioner who assesses the risk-benefit ratio in each individual patient. It is the opinion of the authors that a PAC is clinically useful and warranted in noncardiac surgery for the patient with significant cardiac and/or respiratory disease coming for a prolonged procedure (i.e., craniotomies), extensive blood loss (e.g., vascular surgery), or in the presence of other significant medical illnesses (e.g., chronic renal failure). Filling pressure is useful as a guide to intravascular volume status, whereas cardiac output measurement is an index of ventricular function.

The potential complications associated with PAC are best described by dividing them into complications of venous cannulation,[113–116] complications of catheter passage (or removal!), and complications of the catheter in situ[45] (Table 9–6). The most dreaded complication is pulmonary artery perforation.[117] When wedging a PAC that is too distally located, balloon inflation can distend the vessel wall and cause rupture. With slow balloon inflation, an overwedged tracing is often seen (Fig. 9–14).[118] By careful withdrawal and reinflation, a true wedge tracing is identified. When unsure of the waveform, it is safest to withdraw the PAC into the main pulmonary artery and use the PADP as an indirect assessment of LVEDP, as previously discussed, to avoid this complication. Guidelines for the safe insertion of PAC have been described (Table 9–7).

TABLE **9–5**
Recommendations for Pulmonary Artery Catheterization in Patients Undergoing Cardiac Surgery*

Poor ventricular function (EF <0.4, LVEDP >16 mm Hg, CI <2 L/min/m²)
Noncompliant ventricle
Left main coronary lesion (or equivalent)
Aortic stenosis/aortic insufficiency
Mitral stenosis/mitral insufficiency
Acute ventricular septal defect
Acute papillary muscle dysfunction
Combined lesions (coronary + valvular)
Recent infarct (<6 mo)
Intra-aortic balloon counterpulsation
Hemodynamic instability

*From Hines RL, Barash PG: Pulmonary artery catheterization. In Blitt CD, Hines RL (eds): Monitoring in Anesthesia and Critical Care Medicine, 3rd ed. New York, Churchill Livingstone, 1995, p 213, with permission.
EF, ejection fraction; LVEDP, left ventricular end-diastolic pressure; CI, cardiac index.

TABLE **9–6**
Reported Incidence of Adverse Effects*

Complication	Reported Incidence (%)
Central Venous Access	
Arterial puncture	1.1–13
Bleeding at cut-down site (children)	5.3
Postoperative neuropathy	0.3–1.1
Pneumothorax	0.3–4.5
Air embolism	0.5
Catheterization	
Minor dysrhythmias†	4.7–68.9
Severe dysrhythmias (ventricular tachycardia or fibrillation)†	0.3–62.7
Right bundle branch block†	0.1–4.3
Complete heart block (in patients with prior LBBB)†	8–8.5
Catheter Residence	
Pulmonary artery rupture†	0.1–1.5
Positive catheter tip cultures	1.4–34.8
Catheter-related sepsis	0.7–11.4
Thrombophlebitis	6.5
Venous thrombosis	0.5–66.7
Pulmonary infarction†	0.1–5.8
Mural thrombus†	28–61
Valvular/endocardial vegetations or endocarditis†	2.2–100
Deaths (attributed to PA catheter)†	0.02–1.5

*From Zion MM, Balkin J, Rosenmann D, et al: Use of pulmonary artery catheters in patients with acute myocardial infarction: Analysis of experience in 5,841 patients in the SPRINT registry. Chest 98:1331, 1990, with permission.
LBBB, left bundle branch block; PA, pulmonary artery.

Cardiac Output and Derived Cardiovascular Variables

One of the most useful aspects of the pulmonary catheter is the ability to rapidly and repetitively assess cardiac output and to integrate this flow information to the pressure measurements to better understand the meaning of the pressure per se. For guidelines for the performance of thermodilution cardiac outputs, we refer the reader to a standard text.[66]

Cardiac output determination may be performed by numerous techniques. Echocardiographic determinations are described in Chapter 10.

Three techniques, the Fick oxygen technique, the indicator dilution technique, and thermodilution, performed and based on the Fick principle, are described here.[119]

Cardiac outputs can be determined by the Fick oxygen method as follows:

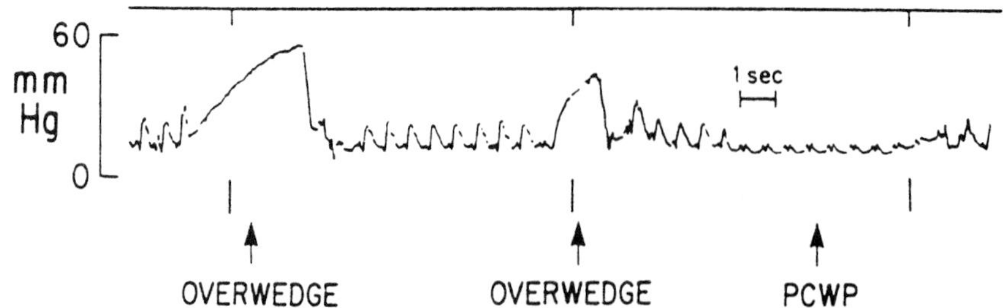

FIGURE **9–14.** Intraoperative pulmonary artery pressure waveform demonstrating overwedging with balloon inflation (*left*). Catheter is pulled back, and balloon reinflation again demonstrates an overwedge waveform. Further withdrawal and reinflation shows normal transition from pulmonary artery to pulmonary capillary wedge pressure waveform. (From Barash PG, et al: Catheter induced pulmonary artery perforation: Mechanisms, management and modifications. J Thorac Cardiovasc Surg 82:5, 1981, with permission.)

$$CO = \frac{\dot{V}O_2}{C(a - v)O_2}$$

where CO = cardiac output, $\dot{V}O_2$ = minute O_2 consumption, and $C(a - v)O_2$ = arteriovenous O_2 content differences.

The assumptions made with this technique are that the pulmonary blood flow is equal to systemic blood flow, and hence, cardiac output. This is not entirely true due to bronchial venous and thebesian venous drainage, and is inaccurate in the presence of intracardiac or intrapulmonary shunts. Nevertheless, it is a reliable technique clinically.

Oxygen consumption or uptake by the lungs is measured by either the polarographic method or the Douglas bag method. The reader should consult a standard text for a description of this technique.[120] The arteriovenous oxygen content difference across the lungs can be determined by using a mixed venous blood gas obtained from the distal part of the PAC, and arterial blood-gas analysis, as described in Table 9–5. The equation is then solved to derive cardiac output. Under steady-state conditions, the oxygen saturation of mixed venous blood ($S\bar{v}O_2$) varies proportionately with the cardiac output, assuming constant oxygen uptake ($\dot{V}O_2$), hemoglobin concentration (Hgb), and temperature. Hypoperfusion or low cardiac output cause increased arteriovenous oxygen content difference because of increased oxygen uptake by the tissues. This situation is reflected by mixed venous oxygen desaturation. It is precisely these assumptions which make the Fick oxygen method *invalid* intraoperatively, as patients have tremendous fluctuations in oxygen consumption, hemoglobin levels, and temperature. Furthermore, it is difficult and impractical to measure oxygen consumption intraoperatively. Finally, the Fick oxygen method is more inaccurate at high inspired oxygen tensions, as the arteriovenous oxygen content difference declines.[120] Parenthetically, the Fick oxygen method is most accurate in patients with low cardiac output where the arteriovenous oxygen content difference is increased.

The indicator dilution method is a modification of the Fick principle, where the indicator is usually indocyanine green dye (as opposed to oxygen in the Fick oxygen method). The interested reader should consult a standard text for further details.[120] Briefly, in the single-injection method, a known concentration of indicator (I) is injected into the pulmonary artery and the blood concentration versus time, $C(t)$, is continuously assessed in the arterial circulation (e.g., radial artery).

$$I = CO\int_0^\infty C(t)\,dt$$

By rearranging this equation, cardiac output can be determined.

$$CO = \frac{I}{\int_0^\infty C(t)\,dt}$$

Many sources of error have been described with this technique.[120] In particular, severe valvular regurgi-

TABLE **9–7**
Guidelines for Safe Insertion of Pulmonary Artery Flow-Guided Catheters*

Balance risk versus benefit.
Slowly inflate balloon while continuously monitoring the PA waveform.
Upon transition from the pulmonary artery to the PCWP trace, immediately stop inflation.
If an overwedge pattern is observed, the balloon should be immediately deflated, and the catheter immediately withdrawn 1–2 cm (Fig. 9–9). The balloon is slowly reinflated and a normal wedge pressure waveform is noted.
Minimize duration of PCWP measurements.
If balloon inflates with <1.5 ml of gas, the catheter should be withdrawn at least 1–2 cm.
Spontaneous tip migration may occur; therefore continuously monitor the PA trace for "spontaneous wedging." If this occurs withdraw the catheter 1–2 cm or until a normal PA tracing reappears.
Minimize number of PCWP measurements in patients who are elderly, anticoagulated, or have pulmonary hypertension.
If pulmonary artery diastolic pressure is <18 mm Hg use pulmonary artery diastolic pressure rather than PCWP as an index of left ventricular filling pressure.

*From Hines RL, Barash PG: Pulmonary artery catheterization. In Blitt CD, Hines RL (eds): Monitoring in Anesthesia and Critical Care Medicine, 3rd ed. New York, Churchill Livingstone, 1995, p 213, with permission.
PA, pulmonary artery; PCWP, pulmonary capillary wedge pressure.

tation and very-low-output states will prolong the concentration-versus-time curve and lead to recirculation of the dye before the "first-pass" curve is completed, giving spurious results. In low-output states, the indicator dilution method is inaccurate, but in high-output states, it is the most accurate method. Due to the above-mentioned limitations as well as the labor-intensive set-up required to perform these calculations, the indicator dilution method is rarely used for clinical measurements of cardiac outputs intraoperatively.

Thermodilution cardiac outputs are performed as a variant of the indicator dilution technique where cold is used as the indicator. Cooling of blood is accomplished by the injection of cold fluid in the proximal port of the PAC and noting the changes in the blood temperature of the downstream sampling site, located 4 cm from the distal tip of the PAC. The computer creates a thermodilution time-versus-temperature curve, and the area under the curve is proportional to the cardiac output, as described by the Stewart-Hamilton equation.

$$Q = \frac{V_I(T_B - T_I)K_I K_2}{T_B(t)\ \mathrm{dt}}$$

where Q = cardiac output, V_I = injectate volume, T_B = blood temperature, T_I = injectate temperature, K_I = density factor (specific heat)(specific gravity) injectate/(specific heat)(specific gravity) blood, and K_2 = computation constant.

Thermodilution cardiac output measurements have been shown to correlate accurately with other techniques, including the Fick method, the Doppler method, and radionuclear and electromagnetic flow meters.[121–132] Pitfalls in thermodilution cardiac output measurements can be most easily determined by analyzing the various factors in the Stewart-Hamilton equation.

The volume of injectate in standard cardiac output measurements is usually 2.5, 5, or 10 ml. If attention is paid to filling of the syringe, the error introduced by refilling is on the order of 1%. An error of 0.5 ml in a 5-ml injectate would give a 10% error. Finally, if a separate injectate catheter is used, it should have the same volume as the proximal port of the PAC,[133,134] or the computation constant (K_2) should be changed to avoid error.

Blood temperature (T_B) should be stable during performance of thermodilution COs. Baseline blood temperature varies little with the phase of the normal respiratory cycle (0.001° to 0.02°C), but varies more in dyspneic patients or mechanically ventilated patients. This error can be eliminated by standardizing each injection at the same point in the respiratory cycle.[135] Injectate temperatures range from 0°C to room temperature (19° to 24°C). Iced solutions increase the signal-to-noise ratio by a factor of 2:3, due to the larger temperature changes. Theoretically, this may lead to better reproducibility of measurements. Unfortunately, in vitro studies have failed to show any difference in accuracy or reproducibility between iced injectate or room temperature injectate.[74] Furthermore, Nishikawa and Dohi[136] have described transient bradycardia following the injection of 10 ml of iced D_5W. Therefore, most cardiac output measurements are performed with room temperature injectate. These warmer solutions require larger injectate volumes and higher thermistor sensitivities than do iced solutions,[137] as the injectate-to-blood temperature difference is less. Finally, the time between withdrawal of the injectate and injection should be minimized, as significant warming of the solution may occur. A 1°C increase in temperature of the injectate is associated with a 3% error in cardiac output. Most computation constants assume injection to have been made in less than 4 seconds, to minimize this error. The choice of injectate solution does not significantly alter the computation of density factor (K_I), (NS/blood, K_I = 1.08, D_5W/blood K_I = 1.10).

The computation constant, K_2, combines several components of the Stewart-Hamilton equation, and adjusts the units to liters per minute. K_2 is based on temperature change of injectate in transit, injection rate, and the dead space of the injection port. Altering the injection port requires a change in computation constant, unless it has the same volume as the proximal port of the PAC.[130,137] Therefore, the appropriate computation constant must be entered into the computer based on the volume and temperature of injectate, as well as the manufacturer's assumptions for the specific injection port and catheter used. Therefore, injection through the side port of the catheter introducer as opposed to the right atrial port on a PAC will give different results unless the computation constant is altered.

The bolus of cold thermal indicator into the warm bloodstream creates a time-temperature plot when temperature change is plotted versus time. The computer can be used to integrate the area under the curve, $T_B(t)$ dt. The distal portion of the curve is an exponential decay to baseline temperature and, therefore, various mathematical algorithms are used to terminate the curve. A high-amplitude curve would be associated with a low cardiac output, as the thermistor in the PAC records a prolonged decrease in temperature as the "cooled blood" passes slowly through the pulmonary artery. Similarly, with tricuspid regurgitation or pulmonary insufficiency,[124] there is recirculation of the cold injectate, and hence the thermodilution curve is strung out, giving a large area under the curve and hence falsely low cardiac output. In high-output states, a low-amplitude curve is seen. These can also be created erroneously with low-volume injectates, inadequate temperature differential between injectate and blood, or an improperly positioned thermistor.[138] Irregular curves may result from poor mixing, contact between thermistor and vessel wall (described below), or changes in heart rate or blood pressure (arrhythmias, intraoperatively during surgical manipulation of the heart). Irregular curves should be discarded.

The location of the thermistor was initially at the tip of the PAC. When the tip impinges upon the pulmonary vessel, irregular thermodilution curves were obtained with a prolonged up-slope, a reduced peak deflection, and an increased down-slope. The PAC has now been modified with the thermistor placed 4 cm from the catheter tip, resulting in less abnormalities of thermodilution cardiac outputs.[139]

Integrating cardiac output with filling pressure measurements, the various observed cardiovascular variables can then be obtained and interpreted (Table 9–8). The various hemodynamic subsets can usually be determined in terms of pump failure, hypovolemia, and high- or low-resistance states. The nature of ventricular dysfunction can usually be determined by the hemodynamic subset identified, whether left ventricular dysfunction, right ventricular dysfunction, or biventricular dysfunction.[140] Algorithms for the diagnosis and treatment of each category of ventricular failure have been described.[34,141] Figure 9–15 is a graphic illustration of ventricular function curves obtained by plotting filling pressure or filling volume versus cardiac performance.

Continuous Cardiac Output Monitoring

As an alternative to intermittent bolus injections of iced or room temperature solutions to measure cardiac output intermittently, a system providing semicontinuous cardiac output values every 30 to 60 seconds is now available. This system includes a pulmonary artery catheter that is inserted and positioned with its tip in the pulmonary artery and a monitor. The catheter has a low-power thermal filament that infuses 7.5 W of heat into the right ventricular blood and is cycled on an off in a pseudorandom sequence. The surface of the catheter remains less than 44°C and the temperature is constantly measured and adjusted to ensure safe temperatures. Thermal contact with blood is brief and limited by blood flow at the filament-blood interface. The monitor calculates cardiac output using a cross-correlation algorithm that combines the pseudorandom sequence of filament activation and the downstream pulmonary artery temperature. Cardiac output is determined from the area under the thermal curve. Signal processing enhancement is required because of the thermal noise caused by changes in venous return associated with patient movement, respiration, or hemodynamic changes. The thermal filament is located in the right ventricle and the temperature change is measured by a rapid-response thermistor located 4 cm from the distal catheter tip. In the stat mode, the cardiac output value is updated every 54 seconds based upon an averaged sequence of determinations.

Yelderman et al. suggested use of such a catheter to monitor volume infusion, titration of vasoactive drugs, and early detection of adverse trends.[142] In critical care unit patients, the semicontinuous method demonstrated correlation coefficients of .94 with bolus injection of room temperature solutions.[143] However, Siegel and coworkers recently reported that the time response of this system demonstrates a clinically important delay.[144] The longest delay in response to changing output was seen with rapid volume infusions (an 80% change required 14.5 ± 4.1 minutes) while changes in output resulting from dobutamine were measured within 3.1 ± 2.1 minutes.

Monitoring Right Ventricular Ejection Fraction

The importance of right ventricular function in the success of many cardiac procedures has been recognized in the past decade. The function of the right ventricle (RV) is difficult to evaluate because of its complex geometry and functional anatomy. Because hemodynamic variables such as right atrial or central venous pressure may not fully assess right ventricular performance, the measurement of the right ventricular ejection fraction is helpful in the management of patients with right ventricular infarctions, increased pulmonary vascular resistance, inadequate myocardial protection during cardiac surgery, or right coronary arterial sufficiency.

The technique is based upon indicator dilution theory and requires a rapid-response (50 msec) pulmonary artery catheter.[145] The thermal washout curve generated by injection of cold solution in the right atrium includes successive diastolic plateaus from which the ejection fraction can be calculated. Normal RV ejection fraction is about 40%. Right ventricular stroke, end-systolic, and end-diastolic volumes can also be calculated (RV stroke volume = cardiac output/heart rate; RV end-diastolic volume = RV stroke volume/RV ejection fraction; RV end-systolic volume = end-diastolic volume − RV stroke volume).

Catheter measurements of right ventricular ejection fraction are accurate in patients with normal right ventricular function, minimal tricuspid regurgitation, and sinus rhythm.[146] However, their accuracy may be compromised by significant tricuspid or pulmonic regurgitation or atrial fibrillation or other nonsinus rhythms. The problem caused by arrhythmias is overcome by averaging the thermal curves obtained over several beats. Location of the injection site within the RV also reduces accuracy as compared to right atrial injection. Overall, determinations of RV ejection fraction vary about 12%[147] but correlate well with nuclear radiographic and echocardiographic measurements.

Mixed Venous Blood Gas Determination

Mixed venous oxygen tension ($P\bar{v}O_2$) can be used diagnostically as well as prognostically.[148–153] Mixed venous desaturation can be used to determine systemic hypoperfusion due to poor cardiac performance, whereas high mixed venous oxygen tension and/or saturation is characteristic of patients with left-to-right shunts or sepsis. Again, single measurements of mixed venous oxygenation are less useful than repetitive or continuous measurements. Continuous $S\bar{v}O_2$ monitoring can be performed with an oximeter pulmonary artery catheter, using reflectance spectrophotometry.

The theoretical basis of mixed venous oximetry is that by maintaining oxygen content and oxygen consumption constant, changes in mixed venous oxygen determination vary directly with cardiac output. If this were correct, then mixed venous oxygen tension could serve as a marker of adequate systemic perfusion or ventricular performance in relation to the global tissue oxygen requirement.[154]

The normal mixed venous oxygen tension is 40 mm Hg, associated with a mixed venous oxygen saturation of 75%. Factors that have been shown to be associated

TABLE 9–8
Hemodynamic Variables Obtained from the PAC*

Pressure
RAP (CVP—mean)
RVP (systolic, mean, diastolic)
PAP (systolic, mean, diastolic)
PCWP (mean)

Flow
CO (by thermodilution)

Temperature
Intravascular or core temperature

Blood Gas
Mixed venous blood gas from PA (distal) port: ($P\bar{v}O_2$, $S\bar{v}O_2$, $P\bar{v}CO_2$)
PA, RV, and RA blood-gas analyses for intracardiac shunt detection

Derived Hemodynamic Variables
CI = CO/BSA
SV = CO/HR
SVR = MAP − RAP/CO
PVR = PAP − PCWP/CO
LVSWI = MAP − PCWP × SVI × 0.0136
CO = BP/SVR = SV/HR
SVI = CI/HR
SVRI = MAP − RAP/CI
PVRI = PAP − PCWP/CI

Derived Indices of Respiratory Function

$Qs/Qt = Cco_2 - Cao_2/Cco_2 - C\bar{v}o_2$	(normal, 7%)
$A - ao_2 = PAo_2 - Pao_2$	(normal, 9 mm Hg if FIo_2 = 0.21, 34 mm Hg if FIo_2 = 1.0)
$\dot{V}o_2 = CO \times C(a - v)o_2$	(normal, 240 ml/min in 70-kg patient)
$O_2T = CO(CaO_2)$	(normal, 1,000 ml/min in 70-kg patient)
$C(a - v)o_2 = Cao_2 - C\bar{v}o_2$	(normal, 4–6 ml/100 ml)

*Modified from Hines RL, Barash PG: Pulmonary artery catheterization. In Blitt CD, Hines RL (eds): Monitoring in Anesthesia and Critical Care Medicine, 3rd ed. New York, Churchill Livingstone, 1995, p 213, with permission.
†Assumes FIo_2 .35 (Sao_2 = 100%).
‡Assumes PB = 760 mm Hg.
§Assumes $PACO_2 = PaCO_2$.
‖Assumes respiratory quotient (RQ) = 0.8.
MAP, mean arterial pressure; RAP, right atrial pressure; RVP, right ventricular pressure; PAP, pulmonary artery pressure; PCWP, pulmonary capillary wedge pressure; CO, cardiac output; CI, cardiac index; SV, stroke volume; SVI, stroke volume index; SVR, systemic vascular resistance; SVRI, systemic vascular resistance index; PVR, pulmonary vascular resistance, PVRI, pulmonary vascular resistance index; LVSWI, left ventricular stroke work index; Qs/Qt, intrapulmonary shunt; Cco_2, capillary O_2 content (Hgb × 1.39†) + [FIo_2 × 713) − (Pao_2] × .0031; Cao_2, arterial O_2 content (Hgb × 1.39 × Sao_2) + (Pao_2 × .0031); $C\bar{v}o_2$, mixed venous O_2 content (Hgb × 1.30 × $S\bar{v}o_2$) + ($P\bar{v}o_2$ × .0031); $A - ao_2$, alveolar–arterial O_2 gradient; PAo_2, alveolar O_2 tension PAo_2 = (PB‡ − 47)FIo_2 − $Paco_2$§/RQ‖; Pao_2, arterial O_2 tension; $\dot{V}o_2$, minute O_2 consumption; CO, cardiac output; O_2T, tissue oxygen transport; $C(a - v)o_2$, arteriovenous O_2 content difference.

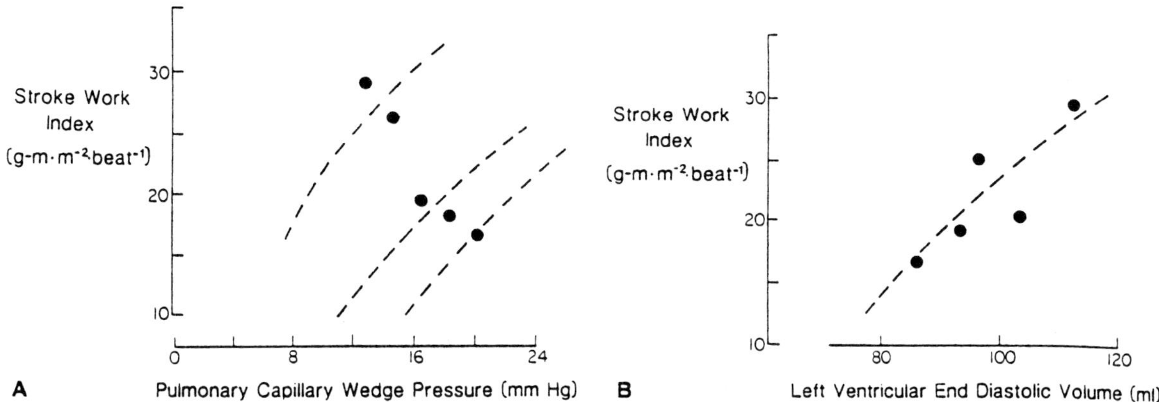

FIGURE 9–15. *A*, Poor correlation of stroke work index (ventricular performance) to pulmonary capillary wedge pressure (ventricular preload) in a single patient. Note that the slope is in fact negative. *B*, When SWI is plotted against LVEDV (true preload), a normal ventricular function curve is obtained. (From Hansen RM, Viquerat CE, Matthay MA, et al: Poor correlation between pulmonary arterial pressure and left ventricular end-diastolic volume after coronary artery bypass heart surgery. Anesthesiology 64:764, 1986, with permission.)

with a decreased $P\bar{v}O_2$ include diminished oxygen delivery, diminished oxygen content, diminished atrial oxygen tension, diminished hemoglobin, or increased tissue requirements, such as seen with hypermetabolic states (malignant hyperthermia), fever, or endocrinopathies. Alternatively, elevated $P\bar{v}O_2$ may be seen with left-to-right cardiac shunts,[103,155] impaired cellular respiration with sepsis, or cyanide poisoning as seen with prolonged nitroprusside infusions. Elevation of mixed venous oxygen tension can also occur as the result of errors in measurement (i.e., from the rapid aspiration of mixed venous blood gases).[156] Rapid aspiration causes oxygenated blood to be withdrawn retrograde across the pulmonary capillaries.

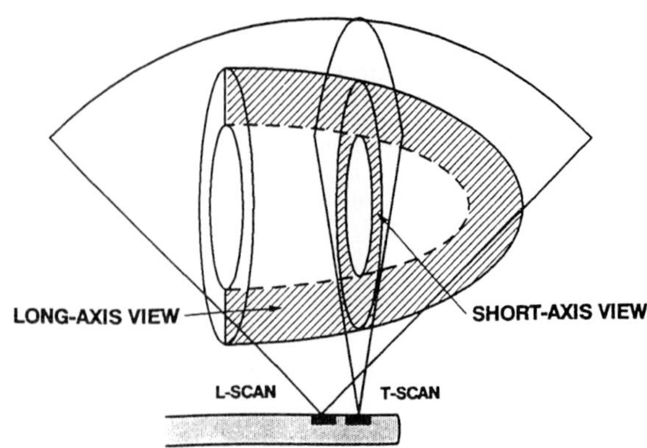

FIGURE **9–16.** Transverse plane (T-SCAN) or horizontal plane imaging transects the left ventricle in the short axis, giving an image of a circle. Orthogonal scanning at 90 degrees give the long-axis view of the left ventricle, known as longitudinal scan (L-SCAN) or vertical plane imaging. (From Mauer G [ed]: Transesophageal Echocardiography. New York, McGraw-Hill, 1994, p 259, with permission.)

Transesophageal Echocardiographic Monitoring of Ventricular Function

TEE evaluates not only cardiac anatomy but also cardiac performance and intravascular volume status. From its inception, cardiac anesthesiologists have been at the forefront of TEE use in critically ill patients. As with all technologies, there are limitations, including the daunting task for the practicing anesthesiologist to both perform and integrate TEE data while concurrently managing the patient. For description of the physics of TEE, the reader is referred to standard texts and Chapter 10.[157–159]

Monitoring Myocardial Function

The primary use of two-dimensional TEE (2D-TEE) has been in the assessment of biventricular, systolic, and diastolic function. During coronary angioplasty, TEE is used to delineate the time sequence of ventricular dysfunction from complete coronary occlusion. Segmental or regional wall motion changes are the earliest abnormality seen clinically, preceding electrocardiographic changes or other hemodynamic variables[6,160,161] (Fig. 9–4*B*). It is interesting to note that although diastolic dysfunction is known to occur prior to systolic dysfunction in experimentally induced ventricular ischemia[1,2] (Fig. 9–4*A*), the reverse is likely when monitoring for ventricular ischemia intraoperatively with present monitoring capabilities (Fig. 9–4*B*). Using 2D echocardiography, left ventricular function is customarily assessed by the transgastric, transverse (horizontal) short axis view of the left ventricle at the midpapillary muscle level (Fig. 9–16). This view was selected, as it contains portions of the left ventricle supplied by all three coronary arteries (Fig. 9–17). The image is divided into four segments, representing anterior, lateral, posterior, and septal walls. The regional wall motion of each segment is assessed via a grading system—0 = normal, 1 = hypokinetic, 2 = akinetic, and 3 = dyskinetic[162]—and a wall motion score is obtained. Higher scores connote a more dysfunctional ventricle. Alternatively, regional wall thickening may be assessed, from epicardium to endocardium. Normal systolic wall thickening is 40 to 80% by ultrasound.[163] TEE, therefore, allows not only identification but also quantification of the dysfunctional quadrants of the left ventricle, helping to delineate the specific coronary vessel involved in the ischemic process.

In addition to regional ventricular function, global assessment of ventricular performance can be obtained from TEE. Using the midpapillary level, transgastric short axis view of the left ventricle, ejection fraction measurements are obtained by measuring the fractional area of change.[164] These fractional area changes have been shown to correlate well with radionuclide- and angiography-derived ejection fraction assessments. Alternatively, wall motion scores, as previously mentioned may be used as a means of assessing ventricular performance.[165,166] A higher score correlates with more severe ventricular *dysfunction*. These scoring systems allow for the early identification of patients at risk for ventricular dysfunction. Rafferty et al.[166] have stated that a minimum of two moving quadrants are essential for perioperative

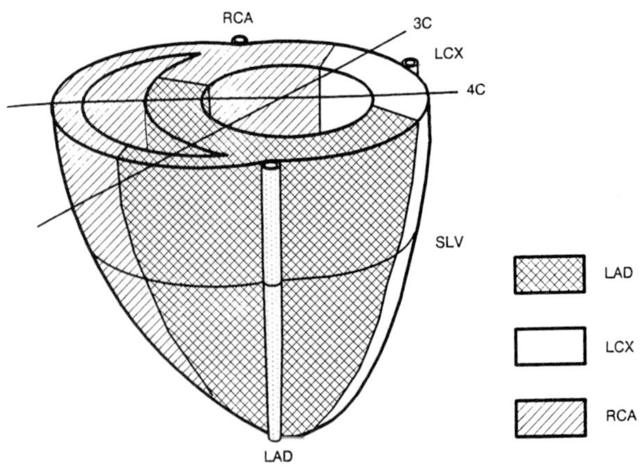

FIGURE **9–17.** As shown in the transgastric short-axis view of the left ventricle, the right coronary artery (RCA) supplies the posteroseptal region, the left circumflex (LCX) supplies the lateral wall, and the left anterior descending artery (LAD) supplies the anteroseptal areas. (From Hong YW, Oka Y: Left and right ventricles. In Oka Y, Goldiner P [eds]: Transesophageal Echocardiography. Philadelphia, JB Lippincott Co, 1992, p 69, with permission.)

survival following cardiac surgery. This remains to be proven prospectively, but demonstrates the useful information obtainable with TEE monitoring of left ventricular function. Clearly, global as well as regional left ventricular function can be continuously monitored, providing not only an accurate assessment of left ventricular contractility but also the anatomic areas of dysfunction. Also, as previously mentioned, the addition of Doppler technology to 2D increases the diagnostic and monitoring capabilities for intraoperative ischemia monitoring (Fig. 9–13).

In addition to the *left* ventricular performance monitoring, TEE can be used to assess *right* ventricular performance. The geometry of the right ventricular chamber is dynamic, changing its shape with changes in loading conditions. These changes limit the usefulness of continuous echocardiography to monitor right ventricular volume status or loading conditions. Therefore, in the right ventricle, global ejection fraction measurements would only be accurate under conditions of homogeneity of regional shape and performance.

Kaul et al.[167] first proposed the term tricuspid annular plane systolic excursion (TAPSE) as a transthoracic (not TEE) determination of right ventricular systolic performance. This technique showed a close correlation with right ventricular ejection fraction measurements by radionuclide angiography. This method has been validated by Rafferty et al. using TEE.[168] The amplitude of the excursion of the tricuspid annulus can be expressed in absolute terms or as a function of the measured baseline (diastolic) dimensions. In clinical practice, the underlying right ventricular dimensions are integrated into the judgment of absolute TAPSE, making this a more subjective clinical judgment.

Integral to the monitoring of ventricular function is the assessment of intravascular volume status or ventricular preload. Several investigators have compared 2D-TEE measurements of LVEDV with various "gold standards." Smith et al.[169] compared ventriculography data obtained using cardiac catheterization to TEE data (r = .84 to .88). For their analysis these authors used left ventricular short axis and long axis measurements in a modified Simpson's rule formula, as well as area-length and diameter-length formulae. Clements et al.[170] compared TEE assessments of LVEDV to first-pass radionuclide angiography during abdominal aortic aneurysmectomy, and obtained similar correlations (r = .85). In coronary artery bypass graft patients, Urbanowitz et al.[171] compared papillary muscle level short axis planimetered area measurements of blood-pool scintigraphic measurements of ejection fraction and thermodilution cardiac outputs. Left ventricular end-diastolic area measurements had a correlation of .74. The ability of TEE to assess left ventricular volume status is particularly useful intraoperatively, due to the low specificity of other invasive monitoring measurements. Currently, the accuracy of echocardiographic assessments of left ventricular volume status is being debated. Some clinicians state that 2D-TEE–derived volumes should only be used to determine large differences or extremes of intravascular volume status.[171] Others, including the authors, feel that with clinical experience, continuous real-time assessment of LVEDV provides useful information to optimize ventricular function.[168]

Although TEE is considered a noninvasive form of monitoring, complications have been reported with its use.[172] Of particular concern to the echocardiographer is esophageal disease, such as diverticula, tumors, or bleeding varices.[173] In these circumstances, TEE is usually avoided unless benefit of the exam is felt to outweigh the risks involved. Finally, full systemic anticoagulation has not been demonstrated to be of major concern when using TEE in the cardiac surgical operating room. However, restraint should be exercised when manipulating the probe during periods of anticoagulation.

TEE, like any other modality of ventricular function monitored intraoperatively, has limitations as well as benefits. The single most limiting factor of TEE is the cost involved in establishing an intraoperative TEE service. Costs include the purchase and service of equipment, but, more importantly, the time required for the practicing anesthesiologist to acquire the technical and cognitive skills to perform and interpret TEE findings.

Summary

It is the impression of the authors (shared by many of the referenced authors in this text)[166,173,174] that no single monitor is ideal for clearly delineating ventricular function in all clinical settings. Rather, most monitoring devices complement one another, providing more useful information to the clinician. When the monitors are properly integrated, patient care should be improved. The future will certainly bring forth many new monitors of ventricular dysfunction. One example of such new technology for monitoring regional ventricular function perioperatively are epicardial pulsed Doppler transducers developed and tested in the early 1980s.[175,176] These transducers, capable of providing continuous on-line measurement of systolic myocardial wall thickening, have now been tested and validated in coronary artery bypass graft patients.[177] This "sonomicrometry" technology gives left ventricular systolic wall thickening measurements of roughly 25 to 35%. These catheters are sewn onto the epicardium preoperatively, and therefore can be used as a guide to regional left ventricular dysfunction as ischemia reduces wall thickening. This transducer is left in place for a few days postoperatively and is removed when the patient is ambulating or out of intensive care. Variations of this theme include implantable Doppler flow sensors that are wrapped onto a blood vessel and secured with releasable ties.[178] These sensors provide continuous on-line blood flow through the targeted vessel. Although of unquestionable possible benefit the future of these and many other technologies remains in question due to need for cost containment in health care.

References

1. Pagel PS, et al: Left ventricular diastolic function in the normal and diseased heart: Perspectives for the anesthesiologist (first of two parts). Anesthesiology 79:836, 1993.

2. Pagel PS, et al: Left ventricular diastolic function in the normal and diseased heart: Perspectives for the anesthesiologist (second of two parts). Anesthesiology 79:1104, 1993.
3. Chung N, Wu X, Bailey KR, Ritman EL: LV pressure-volume area and oxygen consumption, evaluation by intact dog by fast CT. Am J Physiol 258:H1208, 1990.
4. Ekmekci A, Toyoshima H, Kwoczynski JK, et al: Angina pectoris. IV. Clinical and experimental difference between ischemia with S-T elevation and ischemia with S-T depression. Am J Cardiol 7:412, 1961.
5. Rakita L, Borduas JL, Rothman S, Prinzmetal M: Studies on the mechanism of ventricular activity. XII. Early changes in the RS-T segment of QRS complex following acute coronary artery occlusion in experimental study and clinical applications. Am Heart J 48:351, 1954.
6. Wohlgelernter D, Cleman M, Highman HA, et al: Regional myocardial dysfunction during coronary angioplasty: Evaluation by two-dimensional echocardiography and 12 lead electrocardiography. J Am Coll Cardiol 7:1245, 1986.
7. Alam M, Khaja F, Brymer J, et al: Echocardiographic evaluation of left ventricular function during coronary artery angioplasty. Am J Cardiol 57:20, 1986.
8. Blackburn H, Taylor H, Okamata N: Standardization of the exercise electrocardiogram: A systemic comparison of chest lead configuration employed for monitoring during exercise. In Maroven M, Barry AJ (eds): Physical Activity and the Heart. Springfield, IL, Charles C Thomas, 1967, p 101.
9. Leung JM, O'Kelly BF, Mangano DT: The SPI Research Group: Relationship of regional wall motion abnormalities to hemodynamic indices of myocardial oxygen supply and demand in patients undergoing CABG surgery. Anesthesiology 73:802, 1990.
10. Chaitman BR, Bourassa MG, Wagniart P, et al: Improved efficiency of treadmill exercise testing using a multiple lead ECG system and basic hemodynamic exercise response. Circulation 57:71, 1978.
11. London JM, Hollenberg M, Wong M, et al: Intraoperative myocardial ischemia: Localization by continuous 12-lead electrocardiography. Anesthesiology 69:232, 1988.
12. Slogoff S, Keats AS: Does perioperative myocardial ischemia lead to postoperative myocardial infarction? Anesthesiology 62: 107, 1985.
13. Slogoff S, Keats AS: Further observations on perioperative myocardial ischemia. Anesthesiology 65:539, 1986.
14. Slogoff S, Keats AS: Does chronic treatment with calcium entry blocking drugs reduce perioperative myocardial ischemia? Anesthesiology 68:676, 1988.
15. Sigwart U, Grbic M, Payot M, et al: Ischemic events during coronary artery balloon obstruction. In Rutishauser WRH (ed): Silent Myocardial Ischemia. Berlin, Springer-Verlag, 1984, p 29.
16. Lowenstein E, Foex P, Francis CM, et al: Regional ischemic ventricular dysfunction in myocardium supplied by a narrowed coronary artery with increasing halothane concentration in the dog. Anesthesiology 55:349, 1981.
17. Distante A, Picano E, Moscarelli E, et al: Echocardiographic versus hemodynamic monitoring during attacks of variant angina pectoris. Am J Cardiol 55:1319, 1985.
18. Maseri A: Role of coronary artery spasm in symptomatic and silent myocardial ischemia. J Am Coll Cardiol 9:249, 1987.
19. Brown BG, Lee AB, Bolson EL, Dodge HT: Reflex constriction of significant coronary stenosis as a mechanism contributing to ischemic left ventricular dysfunction during isometric exercise. Circulation 70:18, 1984.
20. Brown B, Bolson E, Dodge H: Dynamic mechanisms in human coronary stenosis. Circulation 70:917, 1984.
21. Willerson JT, Campbell WB, Winniford MD, et al: Conversion from chronic to acute coronary artery disease: Speculation regarding mechanisms (Editorial). Am J Cardiol 54:1349, 1984.
22. Willerson JT, Hillis D, Winniford M, Buja M: Speculation regarding mechanisms responsible for acute ischemic heart disease syndromes (Editorial). J Am Coll Cardiol 8:245, 1986.
23. Braunwald E: Control of myocardial oxygen consumption: Physiologic and clinical considerations. Am J Cardiol 27:416, 1971.
24. Bedford FR, Shah NK: Blood pressure monitoring: Invasive and noninvasive. In Blitt CD, Hines RL (eds): Monitoring in Anesthesia and Critical Care Medicine, 3rd ed. New York, Churchill Livingstone, 1995.
25. Barash PG, Cullen BF, Stoelting RK (eds): Clinical Anesthesia, 3rd ed. Philadelphia, JB Lippincott Co, 1997, p 836.
26. Rutten AJ, et al: A comparative study of the measurement of mean arterial blood pressure using automatic oscillometers, arterial cannulation and auscultation. Anesth Intensive Care 14:58, 1986.
27. Quill TJ: Blood pressure monitoring. In Ehrenwerth J, Eisencraft JB (eds): Anesthesia Equipment Principles and Practice. St Louis, Mosby Year Book, Inc, 1993.
28. Braunwald E: Valvular heart disease. In Braunwald E (ed): Heart Disease: A Textbook of Cardiovascular Medicine, 4th ed. Philadelphia, WB Saunders Co, 1992, p 1084.
29. Miller RD (ed): Anesthesia, 4th ed. New York, Churchill Livingstone, 1994, p 1164.
30. Ramsey M: Blood pressure monitoring: Automated oscillometric devices. J Clin Monit 7:56, 1991.
31. Gorback MS: Considerations in the interpretation of systemic pressure monitoring. In Lumb PD, Bryan-Brown CW (eds): Complications in Critical Care Medicine. Chicago, Year Book Medical Publishers, 1988.
32. Milnor WR: Hemodynamics. Baltimore, Williams & Wilkins, 1982.
33. Riva-Rocci S: Un nuovo sfigmomanometro. Gaca Med Torino 47:981, 1896.
34. Stanley TE, Newman MF: Monitoring of the cardiac surgical patient. In Estafanous FG, Barash PG, Reves JG (eds): Cardiac Anesthesia Principles and Clinical Practice. Philadelphia, JB Lippincott Co, 1994, p 185.
35. Petersen MEV, Williams TR, Sutton R: A comparison on noninvasive continuous finger blood pressure measurement (Finapres) with intra-arterial pressure during prolonged head-up tilt. Eur Heart J 16:1647, 1995.
36. Weiss BM, Spahn DR, Rahmig H, et al: Radial artery tonometry: Moderately accurate but unpredictable technique of continuous non-invasive arterial pressure measurement. Br J Anaesth 76: 405, 1996.
37. Bedford FR, Shah NK: Blood pressure monitoring: Invasive and noninvasive. In: Blitt CD, Hines RL (eds): Monitoring in Anesthesia and Critical Care Medicine, 3rd ed. New York, Churchill Livingstone, 1995, p 100.
38. Qvist J, Peterfreund RA, Perlmutter GS: Transient compartment syndrome of the forearm after attempted radial artery cannulation. Anesth Analg 83:180, 1996.
39. American Society of Anesthesiologists: Standards for Basic Anesthetic Monitoring. Park Ridge, IL, Directory of Members, 1995, p 384.
40. Celoria G, Dawson JA, Teres D: Compartment syndrome in a patient monitored with an automated blood pressure cuff. J Clin Monit 3:139, 1987.
41. Sy WP: Ulnar nerve palsy related to use of automatically cycled blood pressure cuff. Anesth Analg 60:687, 1981.
42. Bedford FR, Shah NK: Blood pressure monitoring: Invasive and noninvasive. In Blitt CD, Hines RL (eds): Monitoring in Anesthesia and Critical Care Medicine, 3rd ed. New York, Churchill Livingstone, 1995, p 95.
43. Stern DH, et al: Can we trust the direct radial artery pressure immediately following cardiopulmonary bypass? Anesthesiology 62:557, 1985.
44. Pauca AL, Meredith JW: Possibility of A-V shunting upon cardiopulmonary bypass discontinuation. Anesthesiology 67:91, 1987.
45. Miller RD: Anesthesia, 4th ed. New York, Churchill Livingstone, 1994, p 1166.
46. Stanley TE, Newman MF: Monitoring of the cardiac surgical patient. In Estanfanous FG, Barash PG, Reves JG (eds): Cardiac Anesthesia Principles and Clinical Practice. Philadelphia, JB Lippincott Co, 1994, p 189.
47. LaMantia KR, Hines RL, Barash PG: Cardiac performance. In Scurr C, Feldman S, Soni N (eds): Scientific Foundations of Anesthesia, 4th ed. Chicago, Year Book Medical Publishers, 1990, p 147.
48. Tuman KJ, Carroll GC, Ivankovich AD: Pitfalls in interpretation of pulmonary artery catheter data. J Cardiothorac Anesth 3:625, 1989.

49. Sharkey SW: Beyond the wedge: Clinical physiology and the Swan-Ganz catheter. Am J Med 83:111, 1987.
50. Hines R, Barash PG: Intraoperative right ventricular dysfunction detected with a right ventricular ejection fraction catheter. J Clin Monit 2:206, 1986.
51. Qvist J, Pontoppidan H, Wilson RS, et al: Hemodynamic response to mechanical ventilation with PEEP: The effect of hypervolemia. Anesthesiology 42:45, 1975.
52. Otto CW: Central venous pressure monitoring. In Blitt CD, Hines RL (eds): Monitoring in Anesthesia and Critical Care Medicine, 3rd ed. New York, Churchill Livingstone, 1995, p 179.
53. Miller RD (ed): Anesthesia, 4th ed. New York, Churchill Livingstone, 1994, p 1177.
54. Troianos CA, Kuwik RJ, Pasqual JR, et al: Internal jugular vein and carotid artery anatomic relation as determined by ultrasonography. Anesthesiology 85:43, 1996.
55. Swan HJC, Ganz W, Forrester J, et al: Catheterization of the heart in man with use of a flow directed balloon tipped catheter. N Engl J Med 283:447, 1970.
56. Applefeld JJ, Caruthers TE, Reno DJ, et al: Assessment of the sterility of long-term cardiac catheterization using thermodilution Swan-Ganz catheter. Chest 74:377, 1978.
57. Beique F, Ramsay J: The pulmonary artery catheter: A new look. Semin Anesth 13:14, 1994.
58. Berryhill RE, Benumof JL: PEEP-induced discrepancy between pulmonary arterial wedge pressure and left atrial pressure: The effects of controlled vs. spontaneous ventilation and compliant vs noncompliant lungs in the dog. Anesthesiology 51:303, 1979.
59. Chun GM, Ellestad MH: Perforation of the pulmonary artery by a Swan Ganz catheter. N Engl J Med 284, 1971.
60. Keefer JR, Barash PG: Pulmonary artery catheterization: A disease of clinical progress? (Editorial). Chest 84:241, 1983.
61. Lopez-Sendon J, Coma-Canella I, Gamallo C: Sensitivity and specificity of hemodynamic criteria in the diagnosis of acute right ventricular infarction. Circulation 64:515, 1981.
62. Nehme AE: Swan Ganz catheter: Comparison of insertion techniques. Arch Surg 115:1194, 1980.
63. Page DW, Teres D, Hartshorn JW: Fatal hemorrhage from Swan Ganz catheter (Letter). N Engl J Med 291:260, 1974.
64. Tarhan S, Moffitt EA, Taylor WF, et al: Myocardial infarction after general anesthesia. JAMA 220:1451, 1972.
65. Zion MM, Balkin J, Rosenmann D, et al: Use of pulmonary artery catheters in patients with acute myocardial infarction: Analysis of experience in 5,841 patients in the SPRINT registry. Chest 98:1331, 1990.
66. Hines RL, Barash PG: Pulmonary artery catheterization. In Blitt CD, Hines RL (eds): Monitoring in Anesthesia and Critical Care Medicine, 3rd ed. New York, Churchill Livingstone, 1995, p 213.
67. Woods M, Scott RN, Harken AH: Practical considerations for the use of a pulmonary artery thermodilution catheter. Surgery 79:469, 1976.
68. Hobelmann CF Jr, Smith DE, Vergilio RW, et al: Left atrial and pulmonary artery wedge pressure difference with positive end-expiratory pressure. Surg Forum 25:232, 1974.
69. Jardin F, Farcot JC, Boisante L, et al: Influence of positive end-expiratory pressure on left ventricular performance. N Engl J Med 304:387, 1981.
70. Kane PB, Askanazi J, Neville JF Jr et al: Artifacts in the measurement of pulmonary artery wedge pressure. Crit Care Med 6:36, 1978.
71. Manjuran RS, Agarwal JB, Roy SB: Relationship of pulmonary artery diastolic and pulmonary artery wedge pressures in mitral stenosis. Am Heart J 89:207, 1975.
72. Raper R, Sibbald WJ: Misled by the wedge? The Swan-Ganz catheter and left ventricular preload. Chest 89:427, 1986.
73. Downs JB: A technique for direct measurement of intrapleural pressure. Crit Care Med 4:207, 1976.
74. Boyd KD, Thomas SJ, Gold J, et al: A prospective study of complications of pulmonary artery catheterizations in 500 consecutive patients. Chest 84:245, 1983.
75. Bouchard RJ, Gault JH, Ross J Jr: Evaluation of pulmonary arterial end-diastolic pressure as an estimate of left ventricular end-diastolic pressure in patients with normal and abnormal left ventricular performance. Circulation 44:1072, 1971.
76. Braunwald E: On the difference between the heart's output and its contractile state. Circulation 43:171, 1971.
77. Shah DM, Browner BD, Dutton RE, et al: Cardiac output and pulmonary wedge pressure. Arch Surg 112:1161, 1977.
78. Hansen RM, Viquerat CE, Matthay MA, et al: Poor correlation between pulmonary arterial pressure and left ventricular end-diastolic volume after coronary artery bypass heart surgery. Anesthesiology 64:764, 1986.
79. Ellis RJ, Mangano DT, VanDyke DC: Relationship of wedge pressure to end-diastolic volume in patients undergoing myocardial revascularization. J Thorac Cardiovasc Surg 78:605, 1979.
80. Kaul S, Spotnitz WD, Glasheen WP, et al: Mechanism of ischemic mitral regurgitation: An experimental evaluation. Circulation 84:2167, 1991.
81. Carlon GC, Kahn RC, Bertoni G, et al: Unexpected giant "V" waves during pulmonary artery catheterization. Intensive Care Med 5:55, 1979.
82. Edwards JE: Mitral regurgitation resulting from "overshooting" of leaflets. Circulation 43:606, 1971.
83. Kaplan JA, Wells PH: Early diagnosis of myocardial ischemia using the pulmonary artery catheter. Anesth Analg 60(II):789, 1981.
84. American Society of Anesthesiologists Task Force on Pulmonary Artery Catheterization: Practice Guidelines for pulmonary artery catheterization. Anesthesiology 78:380, 1993.
85. Goldman L, Caldera DL, Nussbaum SR, et al: Multifactorial index of cardiac risk in noncardiac surgical procedures. N Engl J Med 297:845, 1977.
86. Larsen SF, Ilesen KH, Jacobson R, et al: Prediction of cardiac risk in noncardiac surgery. Eur Heart J 8:179, 1987.
87. Rao TLK, El-Etr AA: Myocardial reinfarction following anesthesia in patients with recent infarction. Anesth Analg 60:271, 1981.
88. Rao TL, Jacobs KH, El-Etr AA: Reinfarction following anesthesia in patients with myocardial infarction. Anesthesiology 59: 499, 1983.
89. Russell JA, Ronco JJ, Lockhat D, et al: Oxygen delivery and consumption and ventricular preload are greater in survivors than in nonsurvivors of the adult respiratory distress syndrome. Am Rev Respir Dis 141:659, 1990.
90. Isaacson IJ, Lowden JD, Berry AJ, et al: The value of pulmonary artery and central venous monitoring in patients undergoing abdominal aortic reconstructive surgery: A comparative study of two selected, randomized groups. J Vasc Surg 12:754, 1990.
91. Joyce WP, Provan JL, Ameili FM, et al: The role of central hemodynamic monitoring in abdominal aortic surgery; a prospective randomized study. Eur J Vasc Surg 4:633, 1990.
92. Hesdorffer CS, Milne JF, Meyers AM, et al: The value of Swan Ganz catheterization and volume loading in preventing renal failure in patients undergoing abdominal aneurysmectomy. Clin Nephrol 28:272, 1987.
93. Quinn K, Quebberman EJ: Pulmonary artery pressure monitoring in the surgical intensive care unit. Arch Surg 116:872, 1981.
94. Quintin L, Whalley DG, Wynands JE, Morin JE: The effects of vascular catheterizations upon heart rate and blood pressure before aorto-coronary bypass surgery. Can Anaesth Soc J 28:244, 1981.
95. Bedford RF, Marshall WK, Butler A, et al: Cardiac catheters for diagnosis and treatment of venous air embolism. J Neurosurg 55:610, 1981.
96. Noel TA: Air embolism removal from both pulmonary artery and right atrium during sitting craniotomy using a new catheter: Report of a case. Anesthesiology 70:709, 1989.
97. Berkowitz RL, Rafferty TD: Invasive hemodynamic monitoring in critically ill pregnant patients: Role of Swan Ganz catheterization. Am J Obstet Gynecol 137:127, 1980.
98. Hjertberg R, Belfrage P, Hagnevick K: Hemodynamic measurements with Swan-Ganz catheter in women with severe proteinuric gestational hypertension (pre-eclampsia). Acta Obstet Gynecol Scand 70:193, 1991.
99. Clark SL, Cotton, DB: Clinical indications for pulmonary artery catheterization in the patient with severe preeclampsia. Am J Obstet Gynecol 158:453, 1988.
100. Cohn JD, Engler PE, Timpawat C, et al: Physiologic profiles in circulatory support and management of the critically ill. JACEP 6:479, 1977.

101. Spapen HD, Umbrain V, Brakemans P, Hughens L: Use of the Swan Ganz catheter in amniotic fluid embolism (Letter). Intensive Care Med 14:678, 1988.
102. Orr JW Jr, Shingleton HM, Soong SJ, et al: Hemodynamic parameters following pelvic exenteration. Am J Obstet Gynecol 146:882, 1983.
103. Todres ID, Crone RK, Rogers MC, Shannon DC: Swan Ganz catheterization in the critically ill newborn. Crit Care Med 7: 330, 1979.
104. Katz RW, Pollack MM, Weibley RE: Pulmonary artery catheterization in pediatric intensive care. Adv Pediatr 30:169, 1983.
105. Neches WH, Park SC, Lenox CC, et al: Pulmonary artery wedge pressure in congenital heart disease. Cathet Cardiovasc Diagn 3: 11, 1977.
106. Shoemaker WC, Appel PL, Kram HB: Prospective trial of supranormal values of survivors as therapeutic goals in high-risk surgical patients. Chest 94:1176, 1988.
107. American College of Physicians/American College of Cardiology/American Heart Association Task Force on Clinical Privileges in Cardiology: Clinical competence in hemodynamic monitoring. J Am Coll Cardiol 15:1460, 1990.
108. Technology Subcommittee of the Working Group on Critical Care, Ontario Ministry of Health: Hemodynamic monitoring: A technology assessment. Can Med Assoc J 145:114, 1991.
109. European Society of Intensive Care Medicine, Expert Panel: The use of the pulmonary artery catheter. Intensive Care Med 17:I, 1991.
110. Robin E, et al: Death by pulmonary artery flow directed catheter (Editorial). Time for a moratorium? Chest 92:727, 1987.
111. Connors AF, Speroff T, Dawson NV, et al: The effectiveness of right heart catheterization in the initial care of critically ill patients. JAMA 276:889, 1996.
112. Dalen JE, Bone RC: Is it time to pull the pulmonary artery catheter? JAMA 276:916, 1996.
113. Lyew MA, Bacon DR, Nesarajah MS: Right ventricular perforation by a pulmonary artery catheter during coronary artery bypass surgery. Anesth Analg 82:1089, 1996.
114. Kainuma M, Yamada M, Miyake T: Pulmonary artery catheter passing between the chordae tendineae of the tricuspid valve. Anesthesiology 83:1130, 1995.
115. Gilbert TB, Scherlis ML, Fiocco M, Lowinger TA: Pulmonary artery catheter migration causing venous cannula obstruction during cardiopulmonary bypass. Anesthesiology 82:596, 1995.
116. Grosgnach M, Bourel LM, Ducart A, et al: Pulmonary artery catheter balloon: An unusual cause of severe anaphylactic reaction. Anesthesiology 83:220, 1995.
117. Kearney TJ, Shabot MM: Pulmonary artery rupture associated with the Swan Ganz catheter. Chest 198:1349, 1995.
118. Barash PG, et al: Catheter induced pulmonary artery perforation: Mechanisms, management and modifications. J Thorac Cardiovasc Surg 82:5, 1981.
119. Fick A: Uber Die Messung Des Blutquantums in Herzventrikeln Sitz Der Physik-Med Ges Wurtzberg, 1870, p 16.
120. Grossman W: Cardiac Catheterization and Angiography, 3rd ed. Philadelphia, Lea & Febiger, 1986.
121. Bing R, Heimbecker R, Falholt W: An estimation of the residual volume of blood in the right ventricle and diseased hearts in vivo. Am Heart J 42:483, 1951.
122. Bilfinger TV, Lin CY, Anagnostopoulos CE: In vitro determination of accuracy of cardiac output measurements by thermal dilution. J Surg Res 33:409, 1983.
123. Branthwaite MA, Bradley RD: Measurement of cardiac output by thermal dilution in man. J Appl Physiol 24:434, 1968.
124. Fischer AP, Benis AM, Jurado RA, et al: Analysis of errors in measurement of cardiac output by simultaneous dye and thermal dilution in cardiothoracic surgical patients. Cardiovasc Res 12: 190, 1978.
125. Hendriks FF, Schipperheyn JJ, Quanjer PH: Thermal dilution measurement of cardiac output in dogs using an analog computer. Basic Res Cardiol 73:459, 1978.
126. Hoel BL: Some aspects of the clinical use of thermodilution in measuring cardiac output. Scand J Clin Lab Invest 38:383, 1978.
127. Jansen JR, Schreuder JJ, Bogaard JM, et al: Thermodilution techniques for measurement of cardiac output during artificial ventilation. J Appl Physiol 51:584, 1981.
128. Merjavy JP, Hahn JW, Barner HB: Comparison of thermodilution cardiac output and electromagnetic flowmeter. Surg Forum 25:145, 1974.
129. Nelson LD, Houtchens BA: Automatic vs manual injections for thermodilution cardiac output determinations. Crit Care Med 10: 190, 1982.
130. Olsson SB, Wassen R, Varnauskas E, et al: A simple analogue computer for cardiac output determination by thermodilution. Cardiovasc Res 6:303, 1972.
131. Olsson B, Pool J, Vandermoten P, et al: Validity and reproducibility of determination of cardiac output by thermodilution in man. Cardiology 55:136, 1970.
132. Sottile FD, Durbin CG, Hoyt JW, et al: Evaluation of pulmonary artery oximetry as a predictor of cardiac output. Anesthesiology 57:A127, 1982.
133. Maruschak GF, Potter AM, Schauble JF, et al: Overestimation of pediatric cardiac output by thermal indicator loss. Circulation 65:380, 1982.
134. Mattea EJ, Paruta AN, Worthen LR: Sterility of prefilled syringes for thermal dilution cardiac output measurements (Letter). Am J Hosp Pharm 36:1156, 1979.
135. Armengol J, Man GC, Balsys AJ, et al: Effects of the respiratory cycle on cardiac output measurements: Reproducibility of data enhanced by timing the thermodilution injections in dogs. Crit Care Med 9:852, 1981.
136. Nishikawa T, Dohi S: Slowing of heart rate during cardiac output measurement by thermodilution. Anesthesiology 57:538, 1982.
137. Nelson LD, Anderson HB: Patient selection for iced versus room temperature injectate for thermodilution cardiac output determinations. Crit Care Med 13:182, 1985.
138. Levett JM, Replogle RL: Thermodilution cardiac output: A critical analysis and review of the literature. J Surg Res 27:392, 1979.
139. American Edwards Laboratories: Swan-Ganz flow directed thermodilution catheters. Product Information Bulletin 093-4/82.
140. Forrester JS, et al: Medical therapy of acute myocardial infarction by application of hemodynamic subsets I. N Engl J Med 295:1356, 1976.
141. Miller RD (ed): Anesthesia, 4th ed. New York, Churchill Livingstone, 1994, p 1797.
142. Yelderman ML, Ramsay MA, Quinn MD, et al: Continuous thermodilution cardiac output measurement in intensive care unit patients. J Cardiothorac Vasc Anesth 6:270, 1992.
143. Yelderman M, Quinn MD, McKeown RC: Thermal safety of a filamented pulmonary artery catheter. J Clin Monit 8:147, 1992.
144. Seigel LC, Hennessy MM, Pearl RG: Delayed time response of the continuous cardiac output pulmonary artery catheter. Anesth Analg 83:1173, 1996.
145. Bing R, Heimbecker R, Falholt W: An estimation of the residual volume of blood in the right ventricle of normal and disease human hearts in vivo. Am Heart J 42:483, 1951.
146. Kay H, Afshari M, Barash PG, et al: Measurement of ejection fraction by thermal dilution techniques. J Surg Res 34:337, 1983.
147. Urban P, Scheidegger D, Gabathuler J, Rutishauser W: Thermodilution determination of right ventricular volume and ejection fraction: A comparison with biplane angiography. Crit Care Med 15:652, 1987.
148. Armstrong RF, St Andrew D, Cohen SL, et al: Continuous monitoring of mixed venous oxygen tension (P_vO_2) in cardiorespiratory disorders. Lancet 1:632, 1978.
149. Armstrong RF, Moxham J, Cohen SL, Vallis CJ: Intravascular mixed venous oxygen tension monitoring. Br J Anaesth 53:89, 1981.
150. Kasnitz P, Druger GL, Yorrs F, et al: Mixed venous oxygen tension and hyperlactatemia. JAMA 236:570, 1976.
151. Krauss XH, Verdouw PD, Hugenholtz PG, Nauta J: On line monitoring of mixed venous oxygen saturation after cardiothoracic surgery. Thorax 30:636, 1975.
152. Muir AL, Kirby BJ, King AJ, et al: Mixed venous oxygen saturation in relation to cardiac output in myocardial infarction. Br Med J 4:276, 1970.
153. Prakash O, Meij SH, Van Der Borden SG, et al: Cardiovascular monitoring with special emphasis on mixed venous oxygen measurements. Acta Anaesthesiol Belg 29:253, 1978.

154. Armstrong RF, St Andrew D, Cohen SL, et al: Continuous monitoring of mixed venous oxygen tension (P_vO_2) in cardiorespiratory disorders. Lancet 1:632, 1978.
155. Meister SG, Helfant RH: Rapid bedside differentiation of ruptured interventricular septum from acute mitral insufficiency. N Engl J Med 287:1024, 1972.
156. Shapiro HM, Smith G, Pribble AH, et al: Errors in sampling pulmonary arterial blood with a Swan-Ganz catheter. Anesthesiology 40:291, 1974.
157. Weyman AE (ed): In Principles and Practice of Echocardiography, 2nd ed. Philadelphia, Lea & Febiger, 1994.
158. Hong YW, Oka Y: Left and right ventricles. In Oka Y, Goldiner P (eds): Transesophageal Echocardiography. Philadelphia, JB Lippincott Co, 1992, p 69.
159. Watanabe H, Panopoulos J, Oka Y: TEE assessment of left ventricular function for intraoperative monitoring. In Mauer G (ed): Transesophageal Echocardiography. New York, McGraw-Hill, 1994, p 259.
160. Wohlgelernter D, Jaffe CC, Cabin HS, et al: Silent ischemia during coronary occlusion produced by balloon inflation: Relation to regional myocardial dysfunction. J Am Coll Cardiol 10: 491, 1987.
161. Hauser AM, Gangadharan V, Ramos RG, et al: Sequence of mechanical, electrocardiographic and clinical effects of repeated coronary artery occlusion in human beings: Echocardiographic observations during coronary angioplasty. J Am Coll Cardiol 5: 193, 1985.
162. Hong YW, Orihashi K, Oka Y: Intraoperative monitoring of regional wall motion abnormalities for detecting myocardial ischemia by TEE. Echocardiography 7:323, 1992.
163. McDonald IG, Feigenbaum H, Chang S: Analysis of left ventricular wall motion by reflected ultrasound. Circulation 46:14, 1972.
164. Konstadt SN, Thys D, Mindich BP, et al: Validation of quantitative intraoperative transesophageal echocardiography. Anesthesiology 65:418, 1986.
165. Stamm RB, Carabello BA, Mayers DL, et al: Two-dimensional echocardiographic measurement of left ventricular ejection fraction: Prospective analysis of what constitutes an adequate determination. Am Heart J 104:136, 1982.
166. Rafferty T, Hines RL: Transesophageal single-plane two-dimensional echocardiography: A clinical approach. Semin Anesth 13: 26, 1994.
167. Kaul S, Tei C, Hopkins JM, et al: Assessment of right ventricular function using two dimensional echocardiography. Am Heart J 107:526, 1984.
168. Rafferty T, Durkin M, Harris S, et al: Transesophageal two-dimensional echocardiographic analysis of right ventricular systolic performance indices during coronary artery bypass grafting. J Cardiothorac Vasc Anesth 7:160, 1993.
169. Smith MD, MacPhail B, Harrison MR, et al: Value and limitations of transesophageal echocardiography in determination of left ventricular volumes and ejection fraction. J Am Coll Cardiol 19:1213, 1992.
170. Clements FM, Harpole DH, Quill T, et al: Estimation of left ventricular volume and ejection fraction by two-dimensional transesophageal echocardiography: Comparison of short axis imaging and simultaneous radionuclide angiography. Br J Anaesth 64:331, 1990.
171. Urbanowitz J, Shaaban J, Cohen N, et al: Comparison of transesophageal echocardiographic and scintigraphic estimates of left ventricular end-diastolic volume index and ejection fraction in patients following coronary artery bypass grafting. Anesthesiology 72:607, 1990.
172. Lighty GW, et al: Training in transesophageal echocardiography: Esophageal disease: Considerations for the uninitiated echocardiographer. Video J Echocardiogr 1:9, 1991.
173. Leung JM, O'Kelly B, Browner WS, et al: Prognostic importance of postbypass regional wall motion abnormalities in patients undergoing coronary artery bypass graft surgery. Anesthesiology 71:16, 1989.
174. Smith JS, Cahalan MK, Benefiel DJ, et al: Intraoperative detection of myocardial ischemia in high-risk patients: Electrocardiography vs two dimensional transesophageal echocardiography. Circulation 72:1015, 1985.
175. Hartley CJ, et al: Doppler measurement of myocardial thickening with a single epicardial transducer. Am J Physiol 245:H1066, 1983.
176. Zhu W-X, et al: Validation of a single crystal for measurement of transmural and epicardial thickening. Am J Physiol 251: H1045, 1986.
177. Bolli R, et al: An accurate, nontraumatic ultrasound method to monitor myocardial wall thickening in patients undergoing cardiac surgery. J Am Coll Cardiol 15:1055, 1990.
178. Rabinovitz RS, et al: Implantable sensor for intraoperative and postoperative monitoring of blood flow: A preliminary report. J Vasc Surg 12:148, 1990.

CHAPTER 10

Transesophageal Echocardiography for the Anesthesiologist

Michael K. Cahalan, M.D.
Elyse Foster, M.D.

Transesophageal echocardiography continuously and simultaneously depicts cardiovascular anatomy and blood flow, providing more direct and rapid assessment of cardiovascular pathology than any other perioperative technique.

History and Overview

Dr. Leon Frazin is generally credited with the introduction of transesophageal echocardiography (TEE) in 1976 when he published the results of his studies using a steerable transesophageal M-mode transducer.[1] Subsequently, Matsumoto et al. demonstrated the feasibility of using the M-mode TEE to monitor left ventricular (LV) function during cardiovascular surgery.[2] Unfortunately, M-mode echocardiograms provide an extremely limited view of spatial relationships, and as a result have little practical value for intraoperative monitoring. Thus, TEE contributed little in practical terms until Dr. Peter Hanrath, then at the University of Hamburg Eppendorf, introduced a two-dimensional (2D), phased-array transducer mounted on the tip of a flexible gastroscope.[3] One of Hanrath's colleagues, Dr. Peter Kremer, brought this technique to the University of California, San Francisco, where the Chief of Echocardiography, Dr. Nelson Schiller, and colleagues in the Department of Anesthesia, recognized the potential use for this technique in the operating room.[4,5] Enthusiasm for intraoperative TEE spread quickly through the anesthesia community, while most cardiologists were relatively slow to embrace it because of its somewhat invasive nature.

In the mid 1980s, two additional technical advances fundamentally changed the view of the cardiology community. First, researchers at the Thorax Center of Erasmus University in Rotterdam developed an even higher resolution TEE probe.[6] Now, 64 piezoelectric elements (double the original number in Hanrath's probe) produced echocardiographic images so vivid that even the most reluctant cardiologist could envision powerful applications for this new technique. Second, a number of major manufacturers introduced color flow Doppler for their commercially available ultrasonographs (echo machines). Suddenly, TEE could provide not only high-resolution images of cardiac structure and function but also simultaneously superimposed maps of intracardiac blood flow. At last the stage was set for the myriad of TEE applications utilized today. This chapter reviews the current intraoperative applications and their supporting studies.

Anesthesiologists have embraced TEE because of the direct look it provides at cardiac structures and function. Since the start of their specialty, anesthesiologists have been charged with assessing the adequacy of cardiac filling and ejection. TEE provides a more direct and rapid method for this assessment than any other technique. Second, intraoperative TEE allows immediate assessment of surgical results. Advancements in valvular repairs, congenital repairs, and other cardiovascular interventions have been greatly facilitated by the immediate feedback TEE provides the surgical team. A new partnership has developed in many centers among surgeons, anesthesiologists, and cardiologists with TEE forming the common ground[7] employed to launch innovative surgical repairs such as mitral valvuloplasty and revise them if needed prior to leaving the operating room. Third, anesthesiologists are called upon in the operating rooms and in the intensive care units to help rescue patients with dangerously inadequate hemodynamics. When traditional and presumed appropriate measures fail, TEE offers an extremely rapid and comprehensive method to determine the etiology of hypotension and low cardiac output states. Clearly, passage of a TEE probe into an already intubated, anesthetized, and ventilated patient in an emergency may prove faster, safer, and more informative than passage of a pulmonary artery catheter. Finally, anesthesiologists directly benefit from TEE individually and collectively because their role as consultants is enhanced through the increased expertise TEE allows in detecting intraoperative events that affect a patient's prognosis and treatment. Thus, TEE and the specialties of anesthesiology and cardiology (echocardiography) form a natural and necessary partnership.

Finally the reader is cautioned to appreciate that this chapter is not an adequate substitute for a textbook in echocardiography. Many, but not all, TEE references are provided, and the reader should understand that the growth of publications in TEE has become exponential. No textbook can provide the latest references in such a rapidly growing field. A number of fine texts are available which provide comprehensive treatment of the underlying principles of ultrasound and its diagnostic applications. For the practitioner who plans extensive use of TEE, one or more of these textbooks should prove invaluable.[8–10]

Ultrasound Imaging Modalities

Physical Principles

Piezoelectric crystals are the transmitters and receivers of the sound waves used in echocardiography. These quartz crystals vibrate when electrically stimulated to produce ultrasound—sound at frequencies above the level detectable by the human ear. Conversely, when struck by ultrasound, the crystals produce an electrical signal. Typically, an echocardiographic study involves intermittent pulses of ultrasound at 2.5 to 7.5 MHz. When ultrasound strikes the interface of tissues of different densities—for example, the pericardium and the heart—a portion of it is reflected. The greater the difference in densities, the greater the portion of ultrasound reflected. For example, air in the LV reflects a much greater portion of the transmitted ultrasound than blood, and is translated as a brighter signal on the display screen. The longer the sound wave takes to bounce back to the transducer, the greater its distance from the transducer. This provides information on the location of the tissue. (Sound is assumed to travel at 1,540 m/sec in all tissues of the body at 37°C.) No ionizing radiation of any type is used in echocardiography, and no adverse effects of ultrasound have been demonstrated in humans.

M-Mode and 2D Echocardiography

The first echocardiograms were single-plane, "ice-pick" views of cardiac structures traced on moving photosensitive paper, and were called "motion" or "M-mode" studies. Today, M-mode echocardiograms are still used for viewing rapidly moving structures such as valve leaflets, because M-mode transducers can produce up to 1,000 images per second. However, M-mode echocardiograms reveal only a small portion of the heart at one time, making orientation and interpretation of spatial relationships difficult (Fig. 10–1). By using multiple crystals (linear or phased-array transducers) or rapidly moving a single crystal (mechanical transducer), multiple views can be obtained and collated into a 2D image. Although 2D techniques produce only about 30 images per second, definition in two dimensions provides an enormous advantage in recognizing anatomic and pathologic landmarks. Images are displayed in "real time" on a monitor screen and recorded on videotape or digital format for later review. By altering the position or angle of the ultrasound beam, the operator produces multiple cross-sectional (tomographic) images that together reveal the external and internal anatomy and function of the heart and great vessels.

Pulsed-Wave Doppler

Although 2D echocardiography exquisitely defines anatomic structures, it does not provide information about intracardiac blood flow velocity or volume. By measuring the Doppler shift, modern ultrasonographs produce quantitative analysis of blood flow while simultaneously displaying 2D echocardiograms. The Doppler shift is the shift in frequency of a wave when the source of the wave (in this case, the reflected wave) is moving in relation to a stationary listener or observer. The classic example is the change in pitch of a train whistle as the train approaches and then passes the observer. When the ultrasound beam strikes a moving object, the reflected sound returns to the transducer with a slightly altered frequency. This shift in frequency is proportional to the speed of the moving object, for instance, a red blood cell. When pulses of sound are used (pulsed wave [PW] Doppler), the operator defines a small area (termed "sample volume") anywhere in the 2D sector scan, and the ultrasonograph automatically converts the Doppler data to a display of the instantaneous blood flow velocities in that sample volume (Fig. 10–2). Thus, PW Doppler defines blood flow velocities and their location within the heart.

However, two important limitations apply. First, the Doppler shift is proportional to the cosine of the angle between the ultrasound beam and the direction of the blood cells. Thus, if the cells are moving directly parallel to the ultrasound beam, the angle is 0 and the cosine of 0 is 1. At all other angles, the cosine is less than 1, and the Doppler shift will be less, resulting in underestimation of the blood flow velocity. For practical purposes, angles of less than 20 degrees are considered insignificant (the cosine is almost 1). At angles of greater than 20 degrees, the Doppler shift is markedly attenuated and caution must be used when interpreting such data. Second, with PW Doppler, an inherent limit (termed "Nyquist limit") exists for the maximum velocity of blood flow that can be unambiguously measured. The Nyquist limit is determined by the pulse repetition frequency, which in turn depends directly on the depth of the ultrasound scan and inversely on the ultrasound frequency. If the Nyquist limit is exceeded, sudden apparent flow reversal will be depicted. This apparent flow reversal is called "aliasing" and is analogous to the sudden apparent reversal of direction of wagon wheels in old western movies when the velocity of the spokes of the wheels exceeded the frame rate of the movie camera. Typically, aliasing of PW Doppler occurs at blood flow velocities of 0.4 to 0.6 m/sec. Unfortunately, normal flow within the heart may reach 1.4 m/sec and pathologic flows up to 6 m/sec.

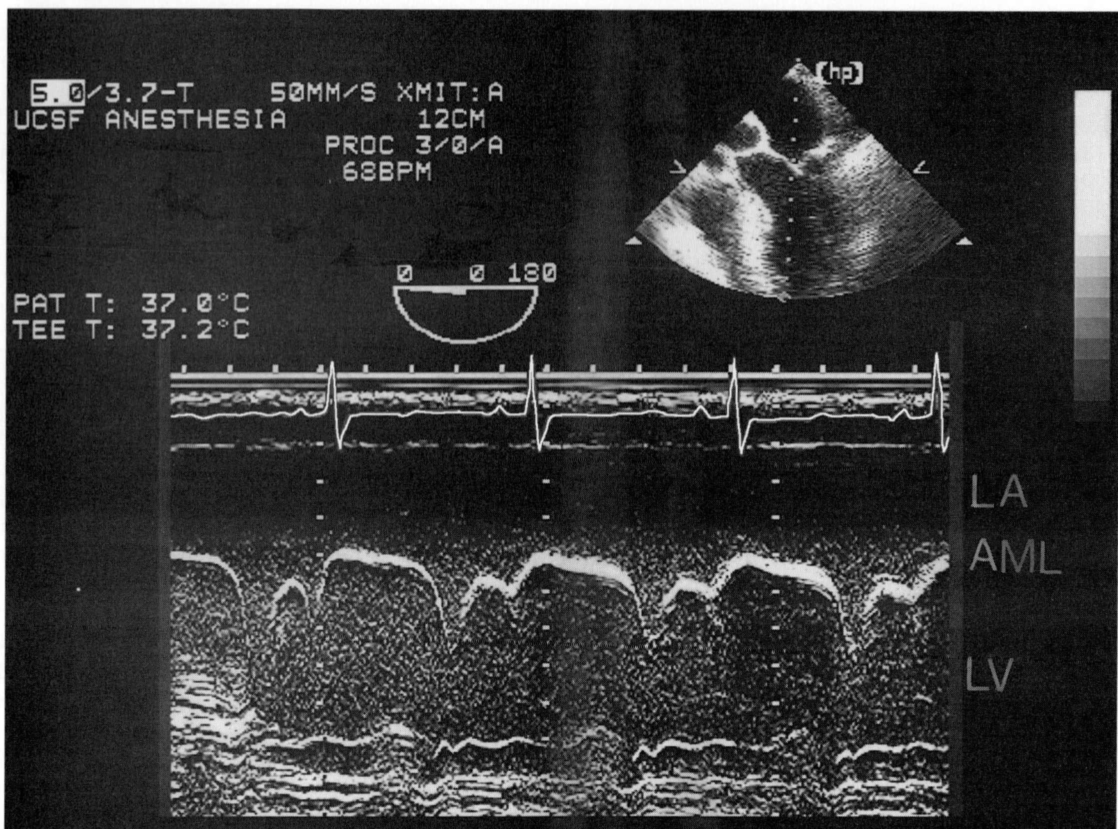

FIGURE **10–1.** M-mode transesophageal echocardiogram. For orientation purposes, the corresponding two-dimensional image is shown at upper right. The M-mode cursor in this five-chamber two-dimensional view is represented by the *vertical dotted line* (please see Fig. 10–2 for description of five-chamber view). The M-mode tracing (shown in the lower half of the figure) is produced by the movement over time of the cardiac structures that intersect the M-mode cursor. The electrocardiogram is superimposed across the top of the M-mode tracing for timing purposes. The *bright line* (labeled AML) undulating through the center of the tracing is produced by the recurrent movements of the anterior mitral leaflet during four cardiac cycles. LA, left atrium; LV, left ventricle; AML, anterior mitral leaflet.

Continuous Wave Doppler

To measure these velocities, continuous wave (CW) Doppler is needed. CW Doppler uses two separate crystals: one to continuously emit ultrasound, and one to continuously receive it. The reader might think of CW Doppler as PW Doppler with an infinite pulse repetition frequency, and by this logic understand how the problem of aliasing has been eliminated (Fig. 10–3). However, with CW Doppler, this infinite pulse repetition rate allows insufficient time for the first pulse of sound to return to the transducer before the next pulse is emitted. When a Doppler shift is detected with CW Doppler, the ultrasonograph cannot determine which pulse of sound was frequency shifted, and therefore cannot define the location of the moving target. Nevertheless, the maximum velocity can prove to be vital information. By simplification of the Bernoulli equation, Holen et al. and Hatle et al. have proven that the peak gradient across a stenotic valve equals $4V^2$, where V is the CW Doppler determined velocity.[11,12] Thus, CW Doppler defines higher blood flow velocities than PW, but unlike PW Doppler, CW cannot precisely define the location of the velocities.

Color Doppler

Frequently, point-by-point determination of blood flow velocities is too time consuming, and does not reveal the instantaneous distribution of flow velocities throughout the cross-sectional image that is needed for diagnostic decisions. For these reasons, color-coded Doppler flow imaging was developed. This technique is a form of PW Doppler in which many areas of the sector scan are simultaneously sampled for their Doppler shifts. A color code is used to depict flow toward (red) and away (blue) from the transducer. Lighter and darker shades of red and blue are used for relatively faster and slower velocities, but color Doppler is generally a semiquantitative technique (see also Figs. 10–21 and 10–22). Nevertheless, it is remarkably revealing: continuous color maps of flow superimposed on monochromatic cross-sectional echocardiograms. However, like PW Doppler, color

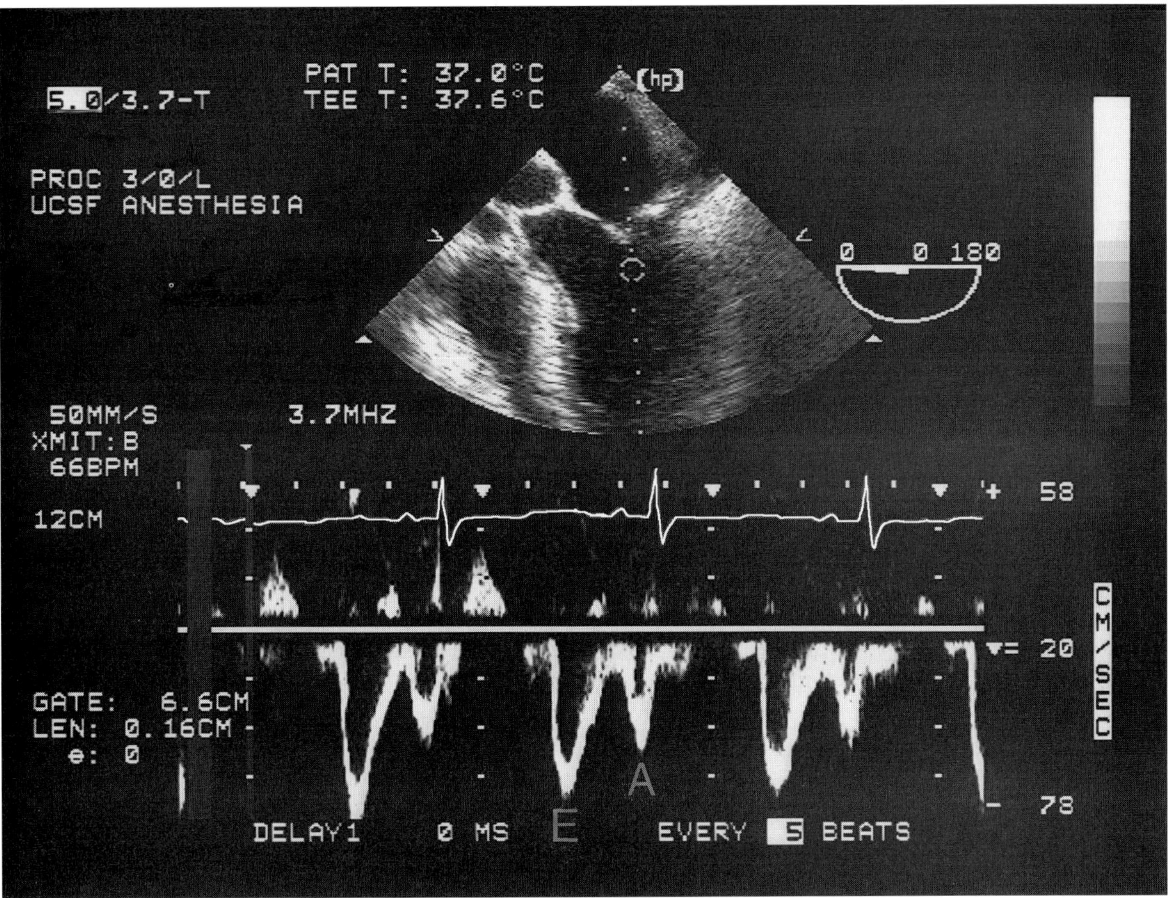

FIGURE **10–2.** Pulsed wave Doppler transesophageal echocardiogram. For orientation purposes, the corresponding two-dimensional image is shown at upper right. The Doppler sample volume in this five-chamber two-dimensional view is represented by the *dashed circle* positioned just below the leaflets of the mitral valve (please see Fig. 10–5 for description of five-chamber view). The Doppler tracing (shown in the lower half of the figure) depicts the instantaneous velocity of blood in that sample volume during three cardiac cycles. The electrocardiogram is superimposed across the top of the Doppler tracing for timing purposes. The *solid horizontal line* through the middle of the Doppler tracing is baseline or zero velocity. Flow toward the transducer is represented by an upward deflection from the baseline; flow away from the transducer, a downward deflection. Normal left ventricular inflow is seen in this tracing as downward deflections with an early component (labeled E) and a late component due to atrial contraction (labeled A). The velocity scale (from −78 to +58 cm/sec) is shown on the right of the tracing.

Doppler will alias (color reversal) when the Nyquist limit is exceeded, and two aliasing patterns are easily recognized. The first is "normal" aliasing in which the area of apparent flow reversal forms one or more smooth color surfaces. Blood flow velocities within a normal heart frequently produce this type of aliasing, because normal velocities (0.6 to 1.4 m/sec) frequently exceed the Nyquist limit for color Doppler (0.4 to 0.6 m/sec). The second type of aliasing results from disturbed or turbulent flow within the heart (e.g., mitral regurgitation) and is never normal (see Fig. 10–22). When the ultrasonograph detects two different velocities within the same small sample volume (due to disturbed flow), it displays a mixture or mosaic of colors. These mosaics often form jet-like configurations and are commonly called "color jets" (see Figs. 10–21 and 10–22). Because color Doppler presents the spatial relationships between structure and blood flow, it greatly enhances the recognition of valvular abnormalities and intracardiac shunts.

Equipment Design and Operation

TEE Probes

TEE probes are a marvel of engineering. Typically, the simplest TEE probe ("monoplane") has one phased-array transducer with 64 piezoelectric elements. The transducer is about 40 mm long, 13 mm wide, 11 mm thick, operates at 5 or 7.5 MHz, and is mounted on the tip of a 9-mm-diameter gastroscope. The ultrasound beam is oriented at right angles to the gastroscope to produce transverse imaging planes of the heart. Like standard gastroscopes, two rotary knobs ("wheels")

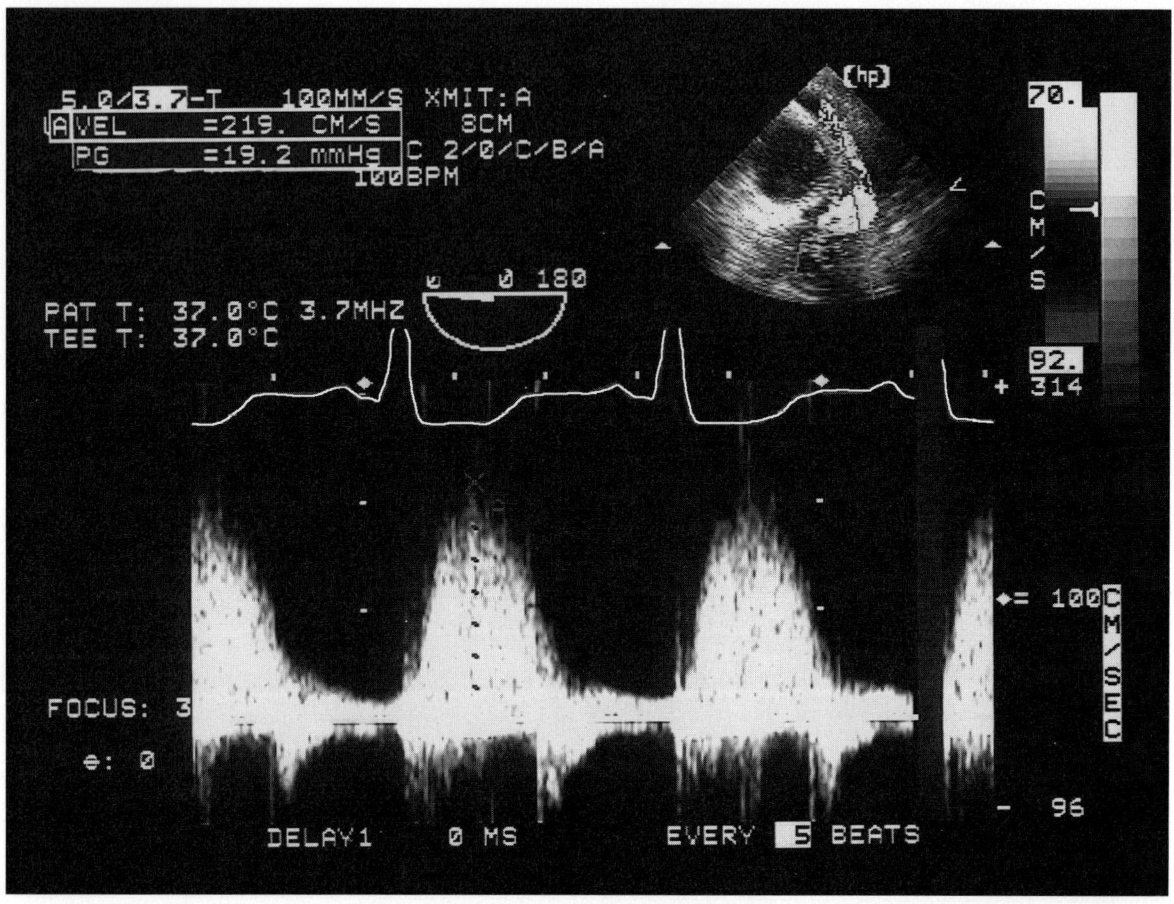

FIGURE **10–3.** Continuous wave Doppler transesophageal echocardiogram. For orientation purposes, the corresponding two-dimensional image is shown at upper right. The Doppler cursor in this two-dimensional pulmonary artery bifurcation view is represented by the nearly vertical *solid line* (please see Fig. 10–13 for description of pulmonary artery bifurcation view). Color Doppler reveals aliasing (a mosaic-like mixture of colors) in the main pulmonary artery (due to mild pulmonary artery stenosis). However, the continuous wave Doppler tracing (shown in the lower half of the figure) unambiguously depicts the instantaneous velocity of blood in that sample volume during three cardiac cycles. The electrocardiogram is superimposed across the top of the Doppler tracing for timing purposes. The *solid horizontal line* through the middle of the Doppler tracing is baseline or zero velocity. Flow toward the transducer is represented by an upward deflection from the baseline; flow away from the transducer, a downward deflection. The peak velocity toward the transducer is measured at point A (also marked with an X) to be 219 cm/sec corresponding to a gradient of 19.2 mm Hg (see text for additional details). The velocity scale (from −96 to +314 cm/sec) is shown on the right of the tracing. *See Color Plate.*

control the movement of the tip of the scope. One of the wheels moves the transducer anterior or toward the heart (usually called flexion) and posterior or away from the heart (retroflexion). The other wheel moves the transducer to the right and left. One step up in price and complexity is the "biplane" transducer, which incorporates a second transducer mounted immediately proximal and at right angles to the first to add a longitudinal imaging plane. Biplane probes have a significantly longer inflexible tip than the single-transducer probes, but rarely does this prevent esophageal passage in the unconscious patient. Most complex is the "multiplane" transducer. It uses a single 64-element transducer mounted on a rotating (Lazy Susan–like) device that allows the transducer to spin on its axis from 0 to 180 degrees. Multiplane transducers are a few millimeters wider and thicker than single-plane transducers, but again this doesn't prevent easy passage in the unconscious patient. Because cardiac structures and blood flow are not always aligned precisely with the transverse or longitudinal plane, multiplane transducers are a significant refinement in imaging capability. Biplane and multiplane probes use the same gastroscopic controls as single-plane probes. By reducing the number of crystals and further miniaturization of the transducer, manufacturers have produced single-plane and biplane transducers small enough (6- to 7-mm-diameter gastroscopes) for use in infants and neonates.

Ultrasonographs

Ultrasonographs contain high-powered computers capable of initiating the ultrasound signal and processing the returning data. A series of electronic transforms (some are guarded commercial secrets) produce the real-time images displayed on the video screen. Although all ultrasonographs share common technical features, they are distinct enough that few generalizations are appropriate.

Fortunately, ultrasonographs come with detailed manuals that should be read prior to use. Cardiac sonographers are technicians trained to operate ultrasonographs to obtain precordial echocardiograms, and often they are the best source of instruction in the operation of ultrasonographs.

Image Orientation

Image orientation remains a controversial area that deserves special mention. Adult and pediatric echocardiographers (cardiologists specially trained in cardiac ultrasound) do not agree on this topic for precordial echocardiograms. The former displays the apex of the sector scan (i.e., the location of the transducer) at the top of the screen and the latter at the bottom. Thus, both groups can claim the other group displays their images upside down! Similarly, no final accord has been reached with TEE images. Some advocate the simplest approach, which uses the same orientation throughout the examination; others advocate an "anatomic orientation," which requires that the orientation be inverted for certain views. In this chapter, the apex of the sector scan will always be oriented at the top of the image.

Basic Examination Technique and Imaging Cross Sections

Justification

Frequently, intraoperative TEE is performed by an anesthesiologist unless specific diagnostic questions require the assistance of a cardiologist. Because of time constraints and limited diagnostic goals, the anesthesiologist performs a more limited examination than often described in the cardiology literature. However, an absolute minimum of four cross sections should be attempted even when only a single-plane transducer is available. Without these views, common cardiac pathology may be missed, and correct interpretation of subsequent hemodynamic alterations may be impossible. Therefore, the following standardized intraoperative examination is recommended as a foundation for monitoring and for more detailed diagnostic imaging when indicated.

Probe Introduction

Once the patient is unconscious and the trachea securely intubated, the contents of the stomach are suctioned. Gentle massage of the stomach area during suctioning may help remove air, which otherwise can degrade imaging. Then, the patient's neck is extended, and the well-lubricated TEE probe is introduced into the midline of the hypopharynx with the transducer side facing anteriorly. Usually, the probe will pass with minimal force blindly into the esophagus. However, if it does not, a laryngoscope is used to lift the larynx anteriorly, and the probe is placed into the esophagus under direct vision. Whenever the transducer is inserted or withdrawn in the esophagus, the controls of the gastroscope should be in the neutral or relaxed positions. In so doing, the transducer is allowed to follow the natural course of the esophagus, and the risk of injury is theoretically minimized.

Basic Transverse Plane Examination

With the transducer at 28 to 32 cm (measured at the upper incisors), the basal short-axis view of the aortic valve is easily obtained by turning the shaft of the gastroscope and adjusting its depth in the esophagus until the ultrasound beam is directly behind the aortic valve (Fig. 10–4). "Basal" refers to the position of the transducer behind the base of the heart. This cross section is ideal for detection of aortic valve abnormalities including aortic stenosis. The transducer is advanced another few millimeters, turned slightly leftward (by rotating the shaft of the gastroscope), and retroflexed (with the appropriate wheel of the gastroscope) to direct the ultrasound beam downward (10 to 30 degrees caudal) and obtain the LV outflow tract or "five-chamber view": left atrium and ventricle, right atrium and ventricle, and LV outflow tract (Fig. 10–5). This cross section (using color Doppler) is ideal for detection of mitral stenosis, mitral regurgitation, and aortic insufficiency. Next, the transducer is advanced 0.5 to 1 cm deeper into the esophagus, the beam again angled downward 10 to 30 degrees, and the four-chamber view can be seen (Fig. 10–6). This view is best for evaluation of relative left and right ventricular size and function as well as color Doppler evaluation of tricuspid regurgitation. When the right ventricle is normal, it will appear smaller than the left (intracavitary area roughly two thirds of the LV cavity area), because it is crescent shaped and partially wraps around the left ventricle. Then, the transducer is advanced another 2 to 7 cm and flexed (angled upward 10 to 30 degrees) to obtain the short-axis cross section of the left ventricle at the level of the papillary muscles (Fig. 10–7). This view is often obtained with the transducer in the stomach and is ideal for monitoring LV filling and ejection for three reasons.

First, all major coronary arteries supply myocardium viewed in this cross section. The right coronary supplies the inferior wall and part of the septum. The left anterior descending supplies part of the septum and anterior wall, while the circumflex artery usually supplies the remainder of the anterior and lateral wall of the left ventricle at this midpapillary muscle level. Thus, if a single monitoring position is to be used during surgery (the usual situation given the many other tasks of the anesthesiologist), the short-axis cross section at the midpapillary muscle level is probably best for detection of myocardial ischemia. Second, changes in preload cause larger changes in the short-axis dimension than in the long-axis dimension of the left ventricle. Thus, changes in filling are more easily appreciated by viewing the short-axis cross section. Third, movement of the probe from its

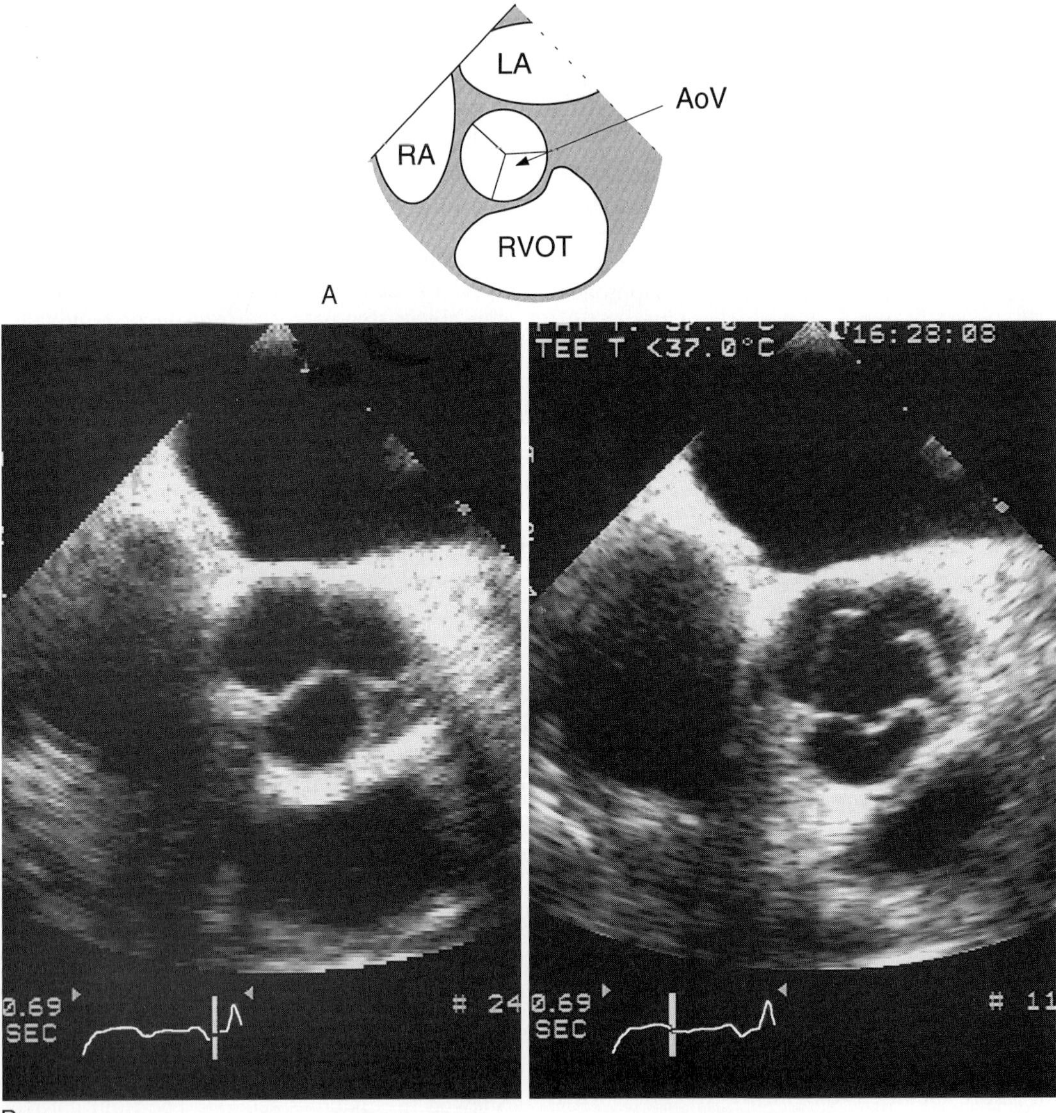

FIGURE **10–4.** Transverse plane, aortic valve, short-axis, transesophageal echocardiogram. *A*, Line drawing of the structures seen in this view. LA, left atrium; RA, right atrium; RVOT, right ventricular outflow tract; AoV, aortic valve. *B*, Corresponding echocardiograms with the valve leaflets captured in the closed (*left* a) and opened (*right* b) positions.

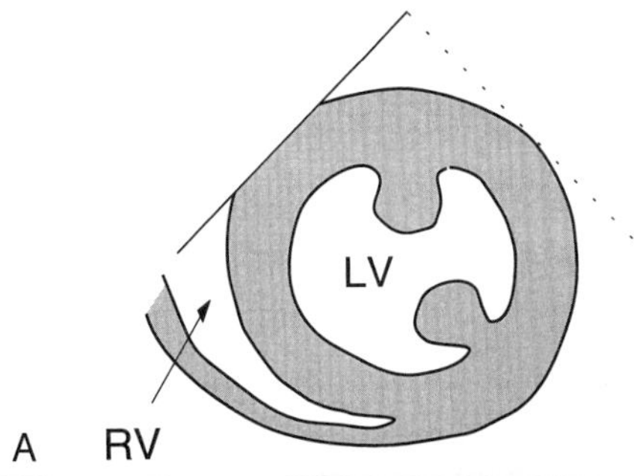

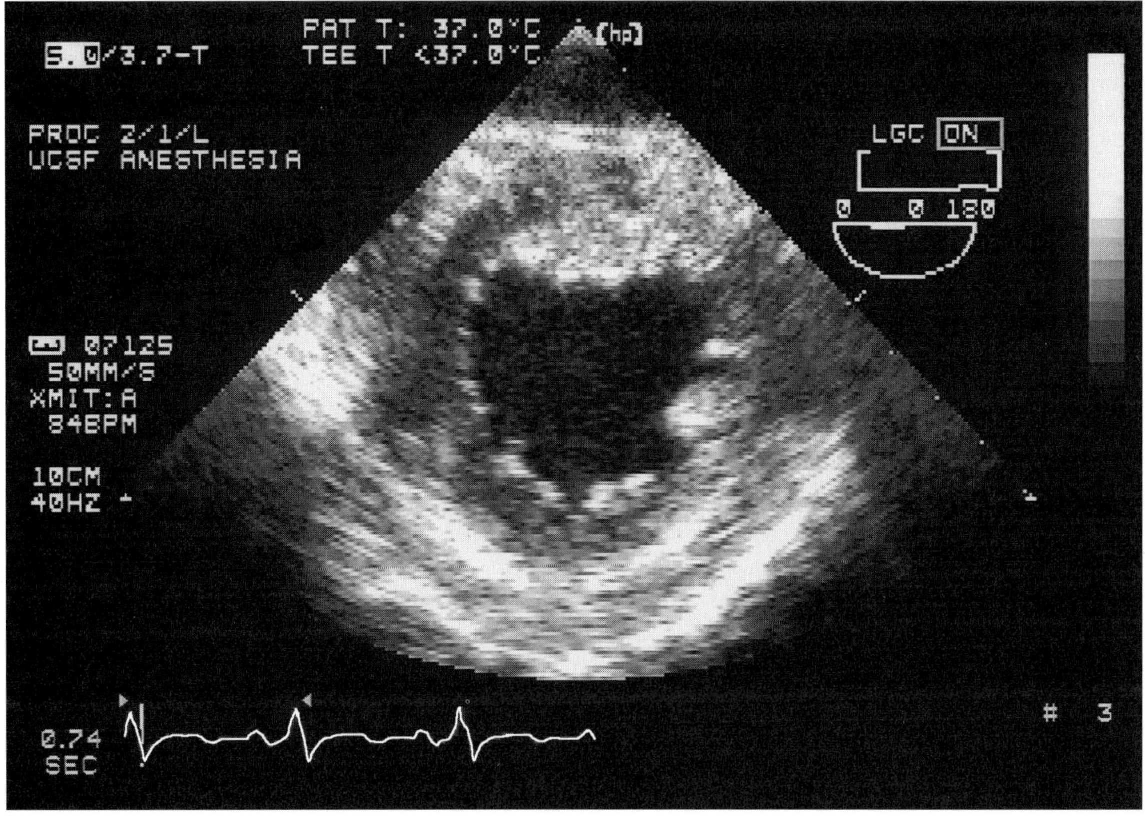

FIGURE **10–7.** Transverse plane, midpapillary, short-axis, transesophageal echocardiogram. *A*, Line drawing of the structures seen in this view. LV, left ventricle; RV, right ventricle. Two papillary muscles are also depicted (but not labeled) as rounded protrusions into the LV at approximately 12 and 5 o'clock. *B*, Corresponding echocardiogram captured at end-diastole.

monitoring position at the short-axis, midpapillary muscle level is immediately apparent, because the morphology of the papillary muscles changes as they extend from their origins in the wall of the ventricle to their insertions into the chordae. Relative changes in filling and ejection are assessed during surgery, and to make such evaluations valid the same cross section must be viewed. The work of Cohen and co-workers provides reference values for normal adult transesophageal echocardiographic measurements using a single-plane probe.[13]

Biplane and Multiplane Examination

If a biplane or multiplane probe is available, five additional longitudinal cross sections are added to the basic examination: three basal views obtained at the aortic valve level, one midesophageal view at the mitral valve level, and one transgastric view at LV level. However, some 3D conceptualization is required to appreciate the relationship between transverse and longitudinal cross sections. At the aortic valve level, transverse plane, short-axis view, one needs to imagine the ascending aorta coming out of the video screen and the LV outflow tract behind it. When the transducer is reoriented at right angles (accomplished by activating the second transducer in a biplane system or rotating the transducer in a multiplane system to 90 degrees), one should imagine the heart rotating 90 degrees so that the ascending aorta is positioned on the right side of the screen and the LV outflow tract on the left (Fig. 10–8). This view is excellent for detection of ascending aortic abnormal-

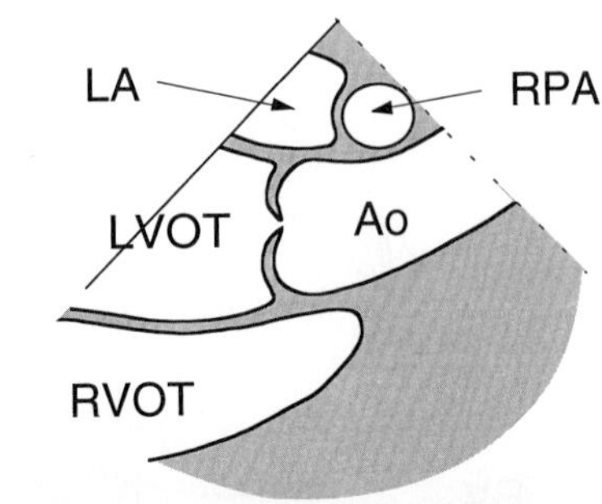

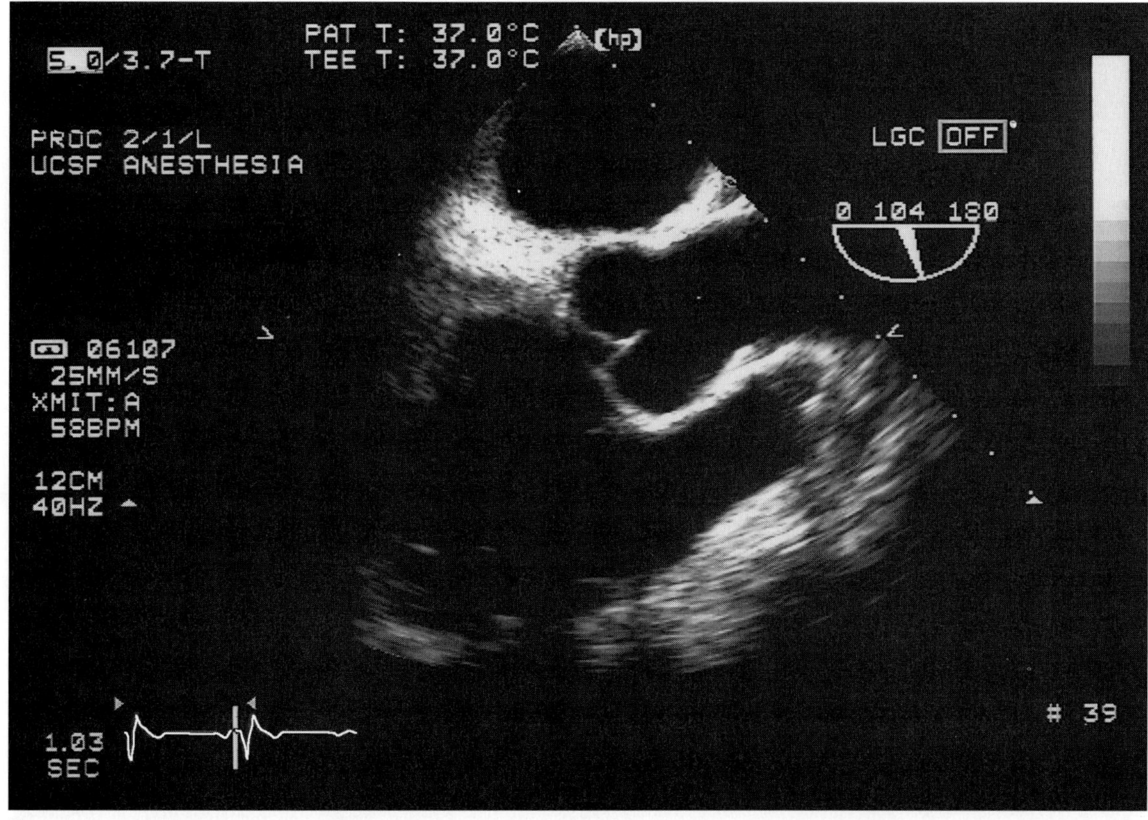

FIGURE **10–8.** Longitudinal plane, ascending aorta, long-axis, transesophageal echocardiogram. *A*, Line drawing of the structures seen in this view. LA, left atrium; RPA, pulmonary artery; Ao, ascending aorta; LVOT, left ventricular output; RVOT, right ventricular outflow tract. Aortic valve leaflets are also depicted (but not labeled) between the LVOT and Ao. *B*, Corresponding echocardiogram captured at end-diastole with the aortic leaflets closed. The half-circle–shaped icon to the left of the Ao signifies the position of the multiplane transducer at 104 degrees (see text for additional details).

ities. Next, the gastroscope is rotated slightly to the patient's left to align the longitudinally oriented beam with the right ventricular outflow tract and pulmonary artery (Fig. 10–9). This view is ideal for locating the tip of a pulmonary artery catheter and some ventricular septal defects. Finally at this level, the gastroscope is rotated rightward past the ascending aortic view until it is aligned with the superior vena cava and right atrium. This view is ideal for locating central venous catheters and certain types of atrial septal defects (Fig. 10–10).

Next, at the midesophageal, mitral valve level, transverse plane, four-chamber view, one needs to imagine the anterior wall of the left ventricle coming out of the video screen and the inferior wall behind it. When the transducer is reoriented at right angles (accomplished by activating the second transducer in a biplane system or rotating the transducer in a multiplane system to 90 degrees), one should imagine the heart rotating 90 degrees so that the anterior wall of the left ventricle is on the right side of the screen and the inferior wall on the left side (two-chamber view; Fig. 10–11). Frequently, this view provides the best look at the apical portion of the left ventricle obtainable with TEE. Last, with the probe

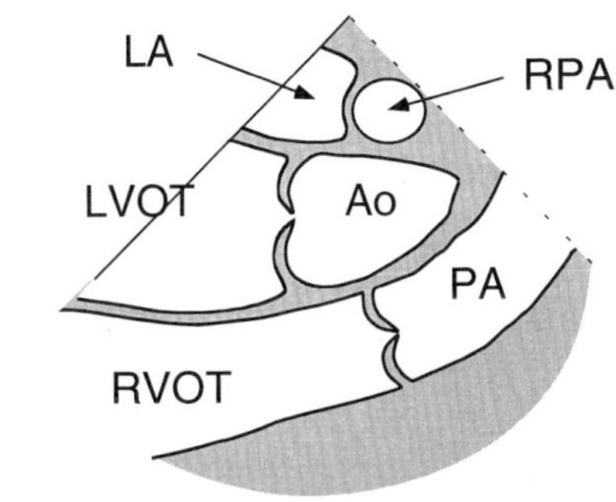

A

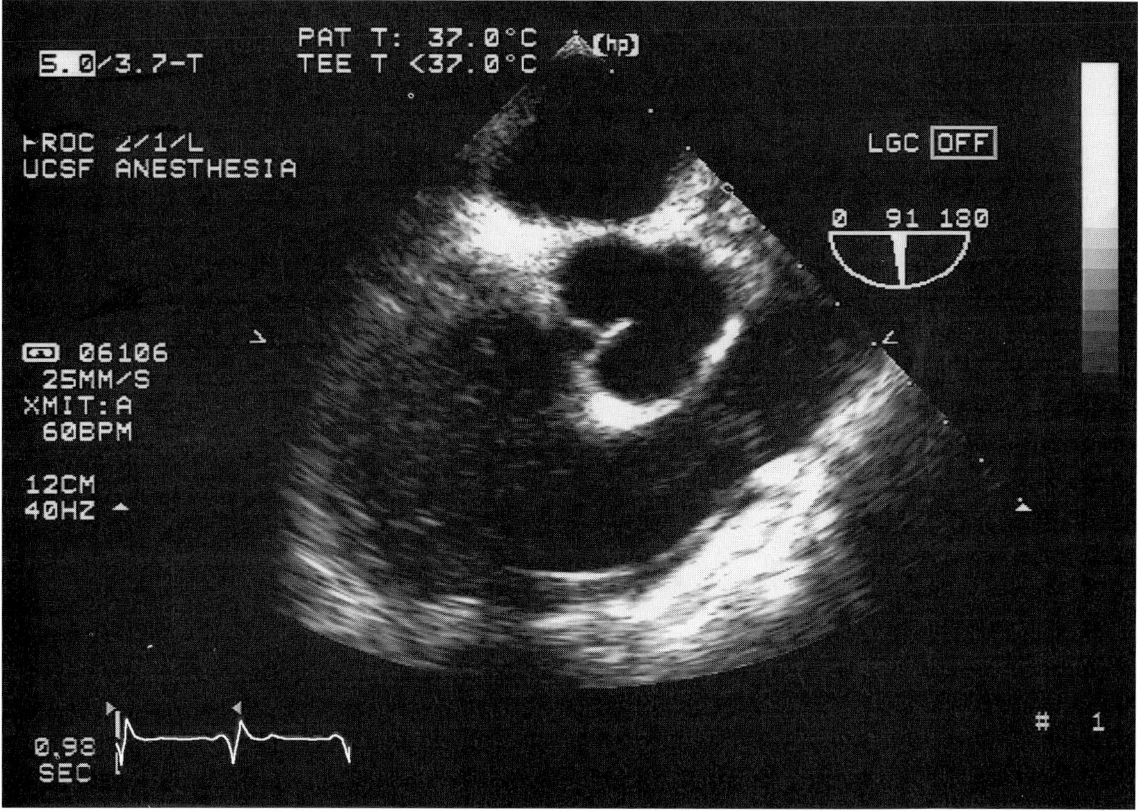

B

FIGURE **10–9.** Longitudinal plane, right ventricular outflow tract, long-axis, transesophageal echocardiogram. *A*, Line drawing of the structures seen in this view. LA, left atrium; RPA, right pulmonary artery; Ao, ascending aorta; LVOT, left ventricular output; PA, pulmonary artery; RVOT, right ventricular outflow tract. Pulmonary valve leaflets are also depicted (but not labeled) between the RVOT and PA. *B*, Corresponding echocardiogram captured at end-diastole with the pulmonary leaflets closed (but not well seen). The half-circle–shaped icon to the left of the Ao signifies the position of the multiplane transducer at 91 degrees (see text for additional details).

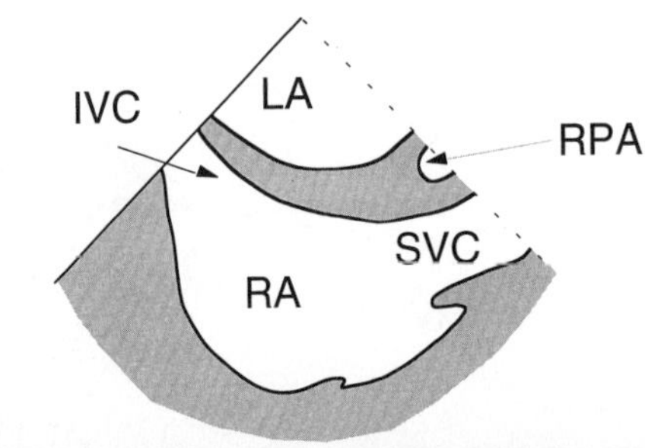

A

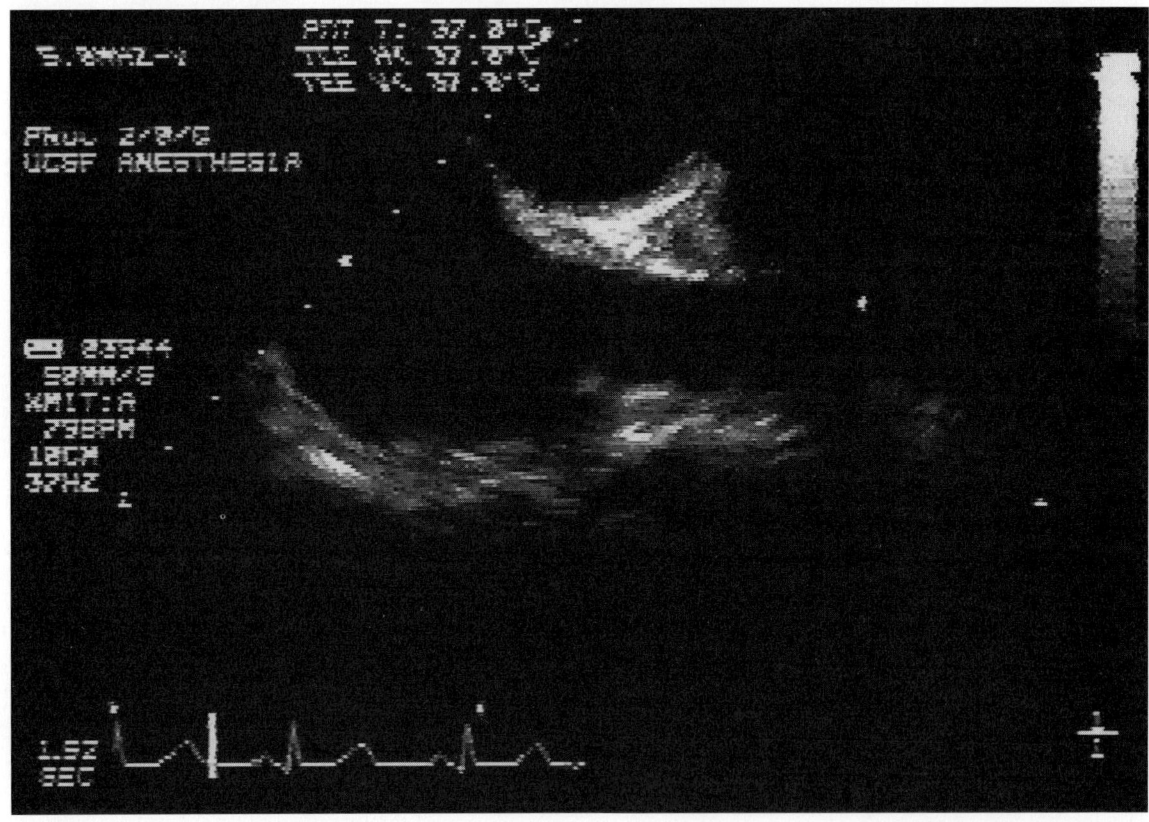

B

FIGURE **10–10.** Longitudinal plane, superior vena cava, long-axis, transesophageal echocardiogram. *A*, Line drawing of the structures seen in this view. LA, left atrium; RPA, right pulmonary artery; RA, right atrium; SVC, superior vena cava; IVC, inferior vena cava. *B*, Corresponding echocardiogram. The IVC is not seen in this example. The longitudinally oriented transducer of a biplane probe was used to capture this image (see text for additional details).

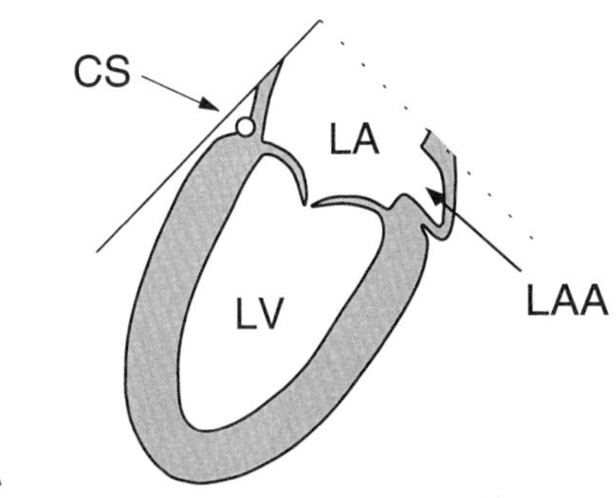

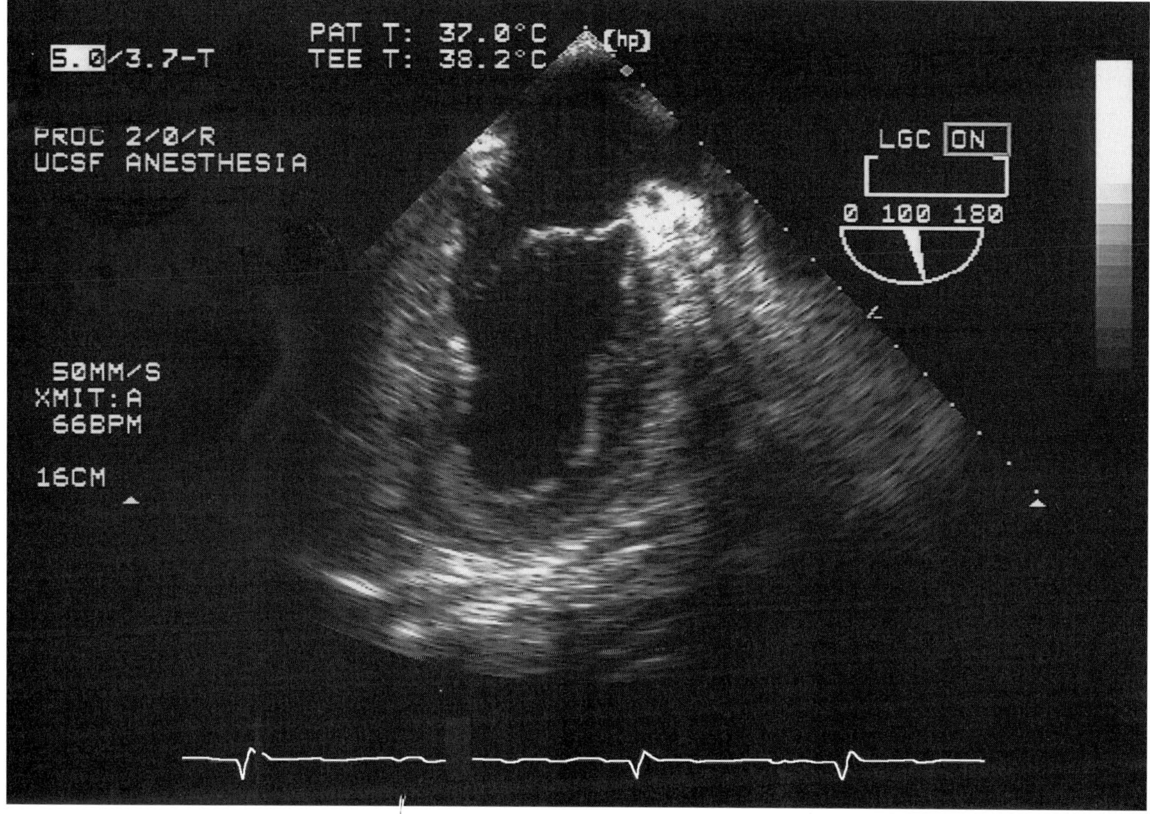

B

FIGURE **10–11.** Longitudinal plane, two-chamber, long-axis, transesophageal echocardiogram. *A*, Line drawing of the structures seen in this view. LA, left atrium; LV, left ventricle; LAA, left atrial appendage; CS, coronary sinus. *B*, Corresponding echocardiogram. The CS is not seen in this example. The half-circle–shaped icon to the left of the LAA signifies the position of the multiplane transducer at 100 degrees (see text for additional details).

in the transgastric, transverse plane, midpapillary short-axis view, imagine the mitral valve in front of the video screen and the LV apex behind it. When the transducer is reoriented at right angles, the mitral valve is seen on the right and part of the apex on the left (midpapillary long-axis view; Fig. 10–12). This view shows less of the apex than the two-chamber view, but does not require repositioning of the probe (just a flip of a switch) from its usual monitoring position in the midpapillary short-axis view (where changes in LV filling and ejection are most easily appreciated). Thus, nine cross sections make up the basic examination whenever biplane or multiplane technology is available.

Inserting the TEE probe and recording this basic examination usually requires less than 5 minutes. Thereafter, the short-axis view of the left ventricle at the level of the papillary muscles is monitored and additional recordings are made of it prior to surgical incision, at conclusion of surgery, and at strategic intervals during surgery: for instance, during unclamping of the abdominal aorta or whenever hemodynamic or cardiac problems develop. The real-time interpretations ("preliminary TEE note") are placed in the patient's chart by the anesthesiologist or consulting cardiologist after completion of surgery. The videotape is subsequently evaluated ("over read") by an echocardiographer who issues a formal report for the patient's chart with a copy to the anesthesiologist.

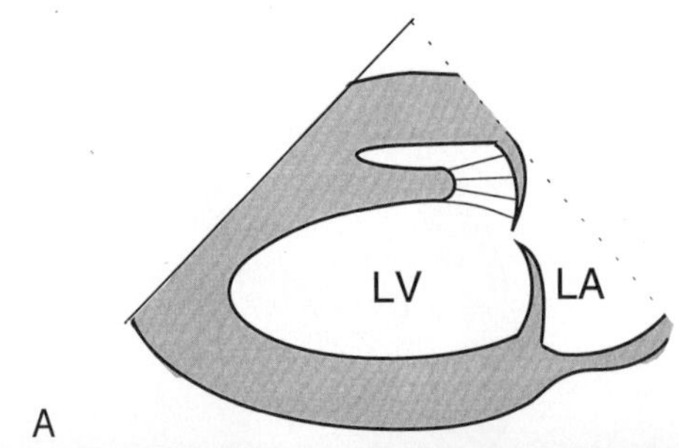

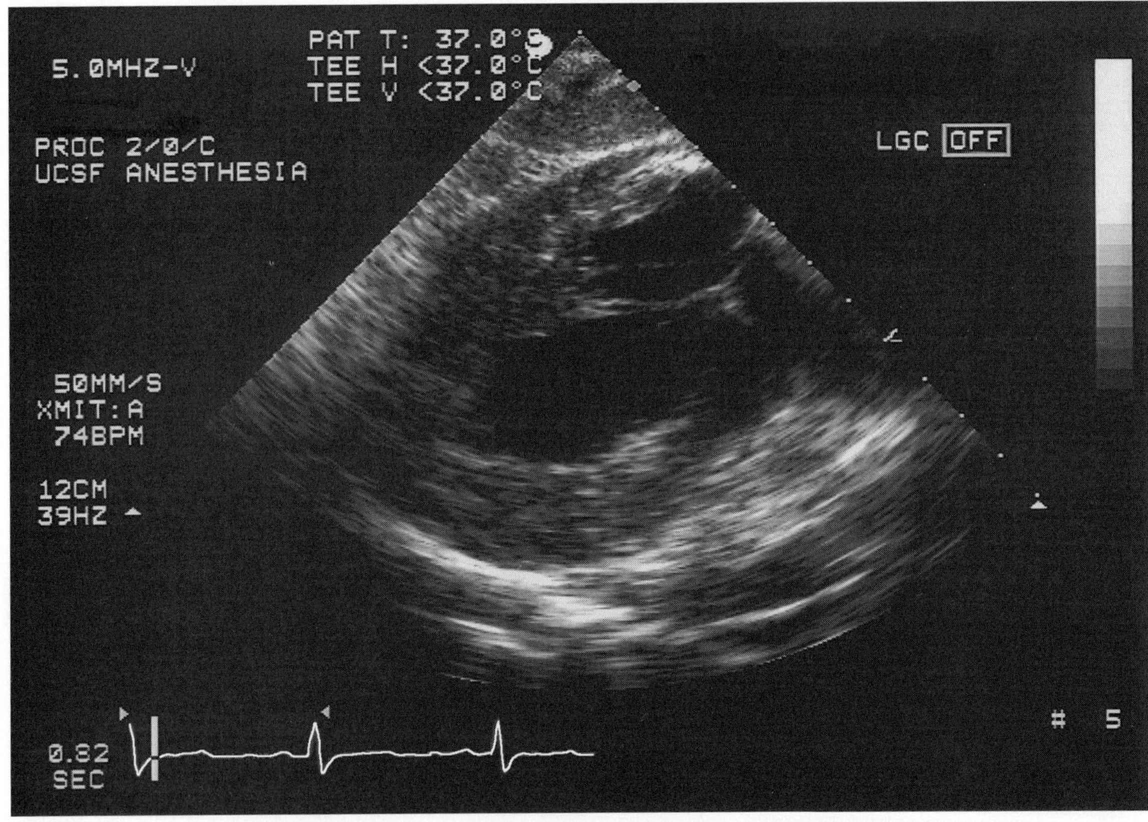

FIGURE **10–12.** Longitudinal plane, midpapillary, long-axis, transesophageal echocardiogram. *A*, Line drawing of the structures seen in this view. LA, left atrium; LV, left ventricle. Mitral valve leaflets, cordae tendinea (attached to the anterior mitral leaflet), and the posteriomedial papillary muscle (giving rise to the cordae tendinea) are also depicted (but not labeled). *B*, Corresponding echocardiogram. The mitral leaflets are incompletely seen in this example. The longitudinally oriented transducer of a biplane probe was used to capture this image (see text for additional details).

Additional Cross Sections Frequently Required

Pulmonary Artery, Pulmonary Vein, and Left Atrial Appendage

Although the basic exam reveals most of the essential information available from TEE, a few other cross sections are frequently needed to resolve specific issues. For instance, with the transverse plane transducer, withdrawing the probe about 1 cm above the aortic valve level reveals the main pulmonary artery and its bifurcation (Fig. 10–13). At this level, pulmonary artery flow is almost directly parallel to the ultrasound beam, and therefore Doppler measurements provide true blood flow velocity estimates for calculation of cardiac output (see below). Midway between this view and the aortic valve short-axis view are two more transverse imaging planes of special interest. First, by rotating the probe about 45 degrees leftward, the left superior pulmonary vein's entrance into the left atrium can be imaged (Fig. 10–14). PW Doppler measurements of blood flow velocities in this vein provide estimates of left atrial filling pressure or the severity of mitral regurgitation (see below). Searching for this structure is often facilitated by activation of color Doppler (Fig. 10–15). Rotating the probe about 20 degrees back toward the midline reveals the

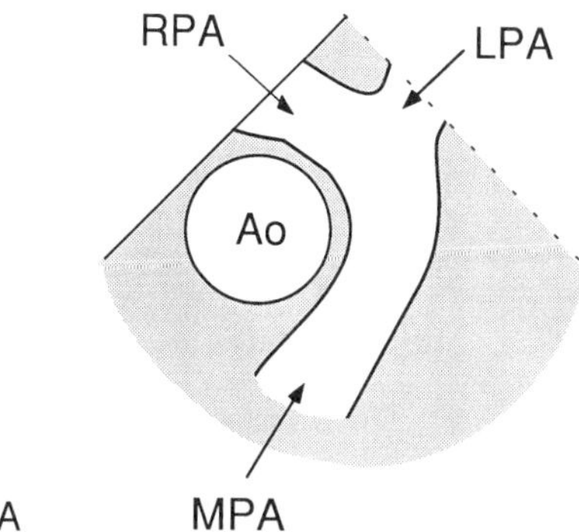

A

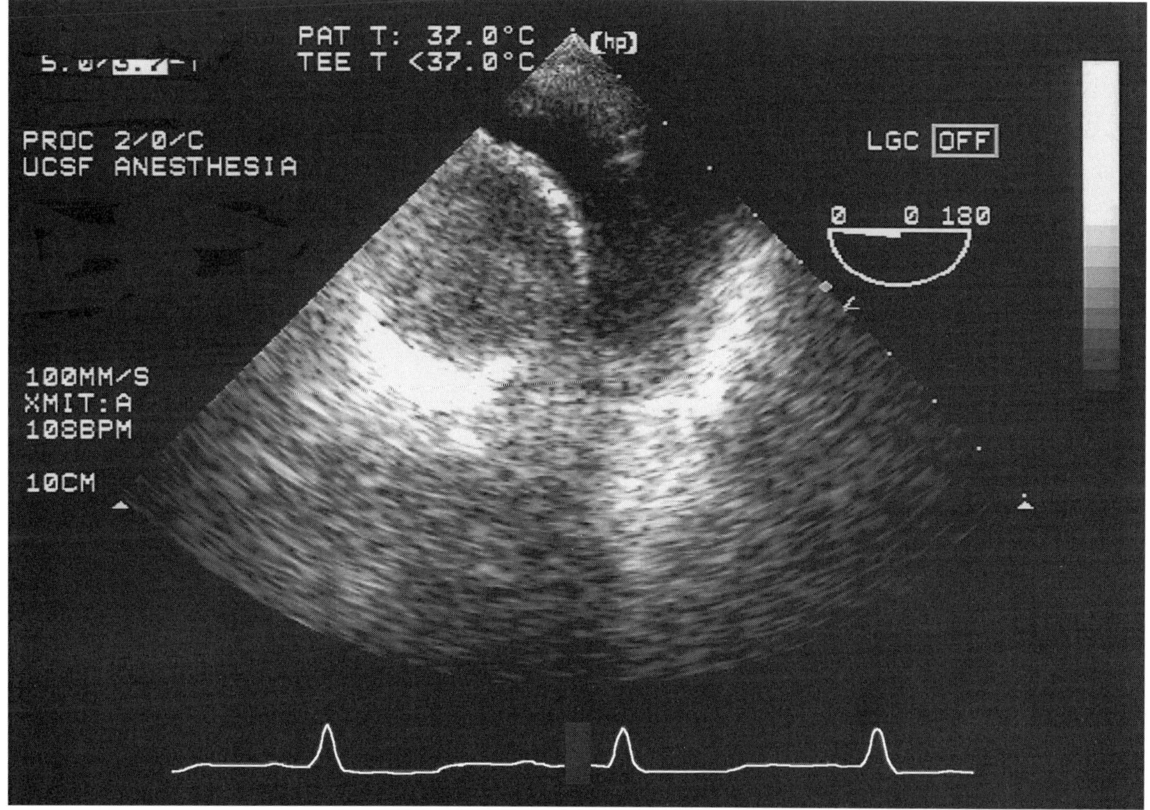

B

FIGURE **10–13.** Transverse plane, pulmonary artery bifurcation, transesophageal echocardiogram. *A*, Line drawing of the structures seen in this view. RPA, right pulmonary artery; LPA, left pulmonary artery; MPA, main pulmonary artery; Ao, ascending aorta. *B*, Corresponding echocardiogram. The main pulmonary artery is incompletely seen in this example. The half-circle–shaped icon to the left of the LPA signifies the position of the multiplane transducer at 0 degrees (see text for additional details).

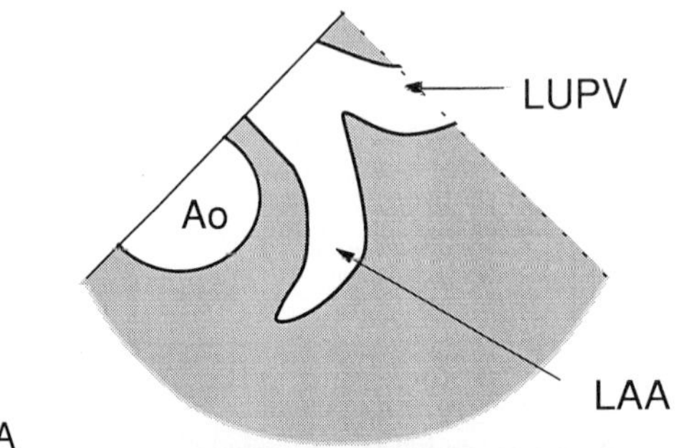

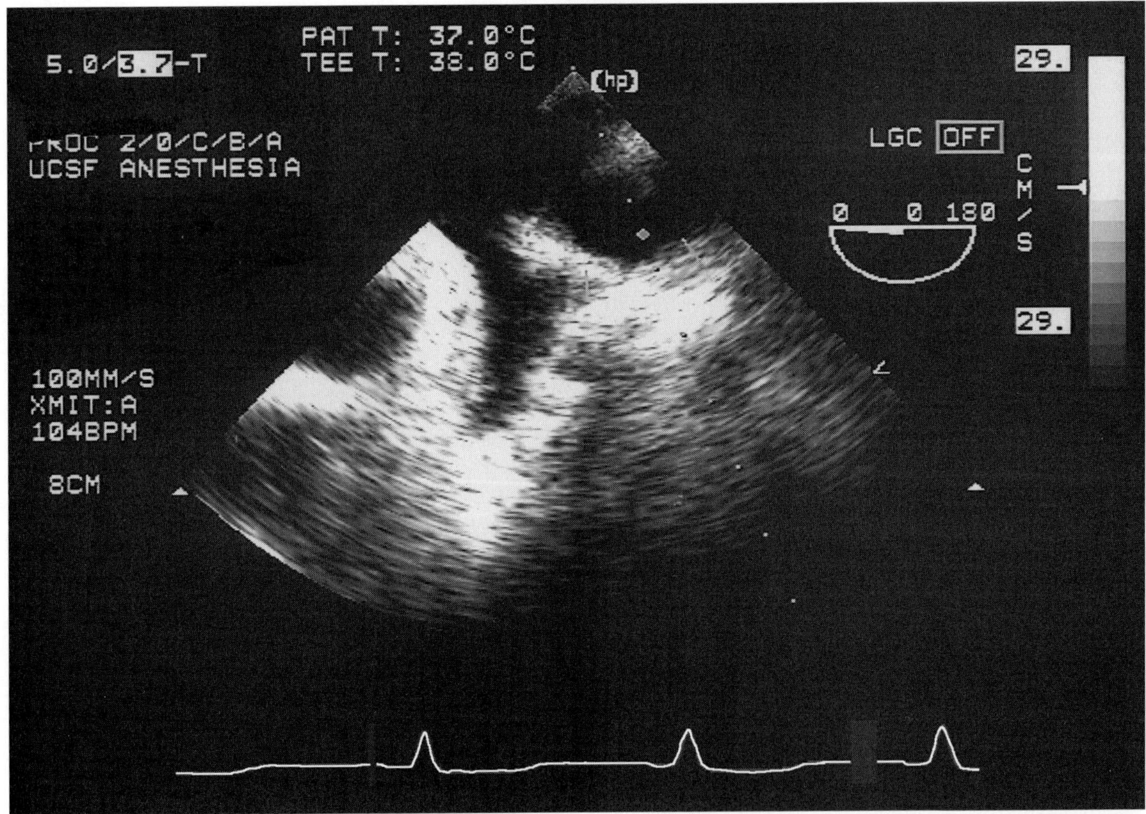

B

FIGURE **10–14.** Transverse plane, pulmonary vein, and left atrial appendage transesophageal echocardiogram. *A*, Line drawing of the structures seen in this view. LUPV, left upper pulmonary vein; LAA, left atrial appendage; Ao, ascending aorta. *B*, Corresponding echocardiogram. The half-circle–shaped icon to the left of the LAA signifies the position of the multiplane transducer at 0 degrees (see text for additional details).

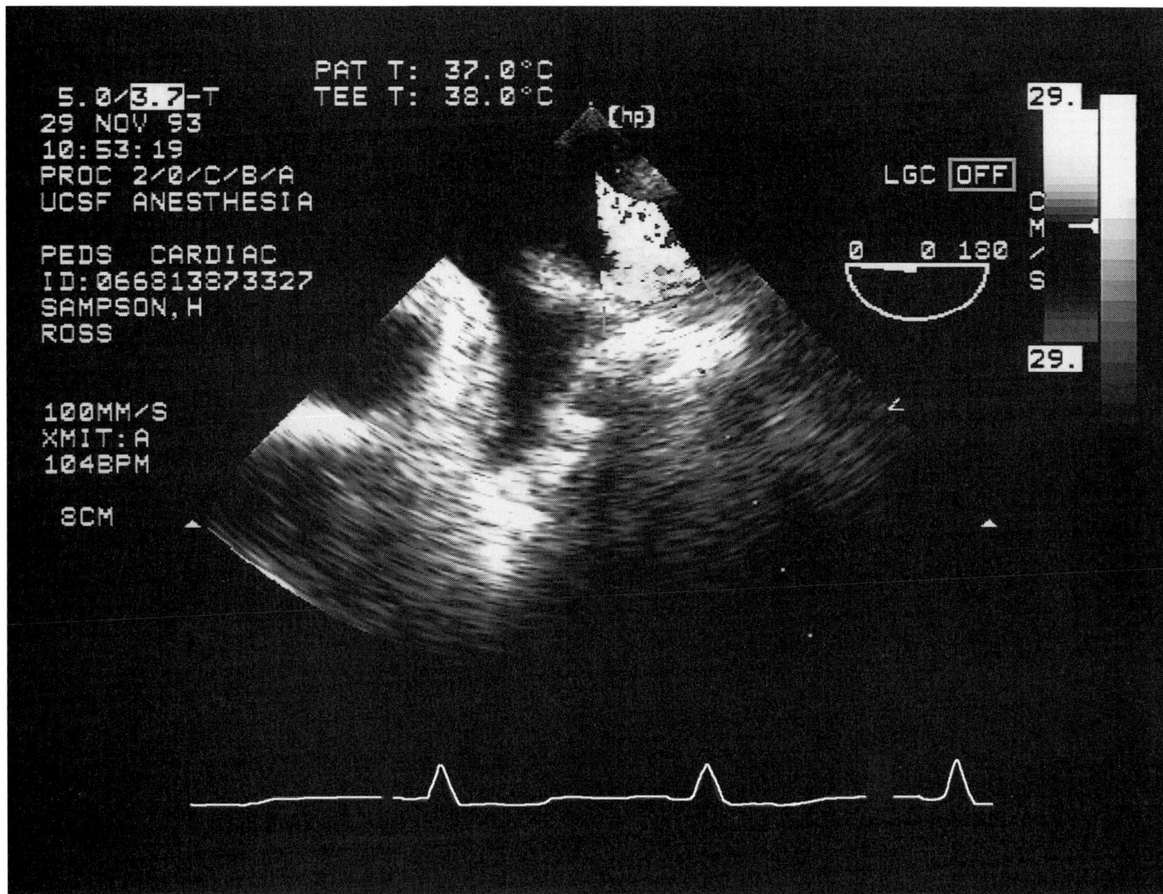

FIGURE **10–15.** Transverse plane, pulmonary vein, and left atrial appendage transesophageal echocardiogram with color Doppler. See Figure 10–14 for orientation. *See Color Plate.*

left atrial appendage where clots commonly occur in patients with left atrial enlargement and atrial fibrillation.

Transverse and Descending Aorta

At the aortic valve level, 90 degrees of leftward probe rotation reveals the descending aorta. By insertion and withdrawal of the probe, the descending aorta (Figs. 10–16 and 10–17) and parts of the transverse arch (Figs. 10–18 and 10–19) can be imaged using both transverse and longitudinal transducer orientations. The presence and extent of dissection, atheroma, and thrombi in the descending aorta are reliably evaluated.

Transgastric Five-Chamber

Finally, if the transversely oriented transducer is advanced well into the stomach, flexed maximally, and then gently withdrawn until it meets resistance at the gastroesophageal junction, an inverted five-chamber view is obtained. From this vantage, the ultrasound beam may be well aligned with the LV outflow tract and aortic valve. Thus, CW Doppler estimates sometimes reveal true blood flow velocities across the valve and valid estimates of the severity of aortic stenosis (see below).

LV Preload, Ejection, Afterload, and Contractility

Preload

Like precordial echocardiography, TEE provides valid estimates of LV filling and ejection. In 30 patients undergoing cardiac surgery, Cheung and co-workers removed 15% of the blood volume in six equal aliquots prior to cardiopulmonary bypass.[14] A significant decrease in end-diastolic heart size after removal of the first aliquot was seen using TEE. Removal of subsequent aliquots produced a linear decrease in size so that at the end of volume removal, end-diastolic heart size decreased 27% in patients with normal LV function and 21% in patients with depressed LV function. Although pulmonary artery and central venous pressures decreased, they correlated poorly with end-diastolic area.

In settings in which LV compliance changes, TEE may be the only practical way to assess preload. For instance, Clements et al. studied 14 patients during resection of abdominal aortic aneurysm.[15] At multiple times during surgery, echocardiograms and first-pass radionuclide studies were recorded simultaneously. The correlation between echocardiographic and radionuclide

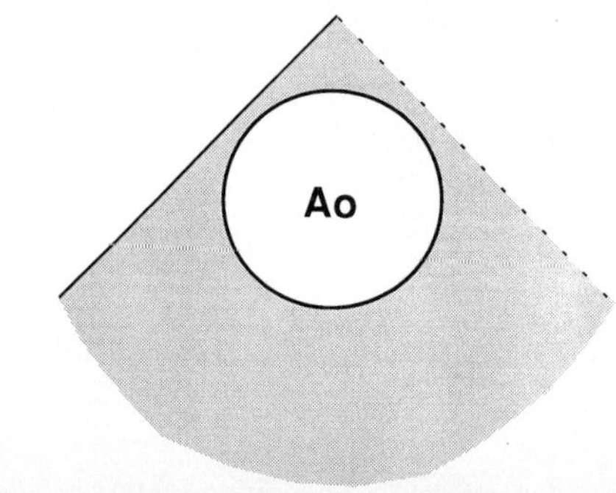

A

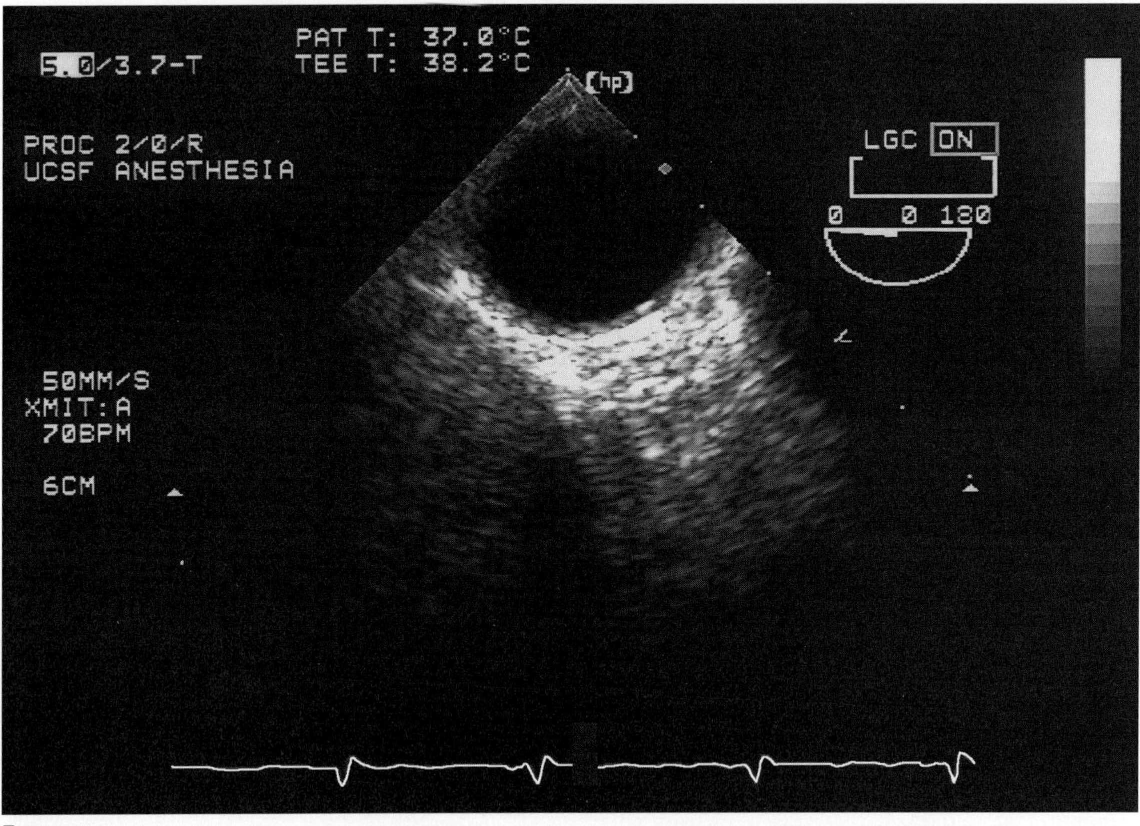

B

FIGURE **10–16.** Transverse plane, descending aorta, short-axis, transesophageal echocardiogram. *A*, Line drawing of the structure seen in this view. Ao is descending aorta. *B*, Corresponding echocardiogram. The half-circle–shaped icon to the left of the Ao signifies the position of the multiplane transducer at 0 degrees (see text for additional details).

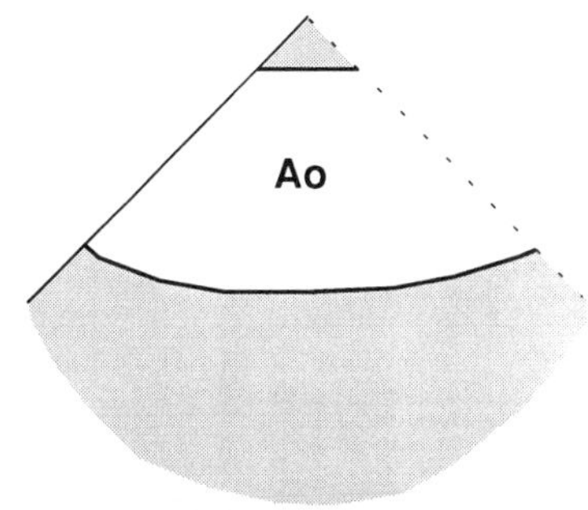

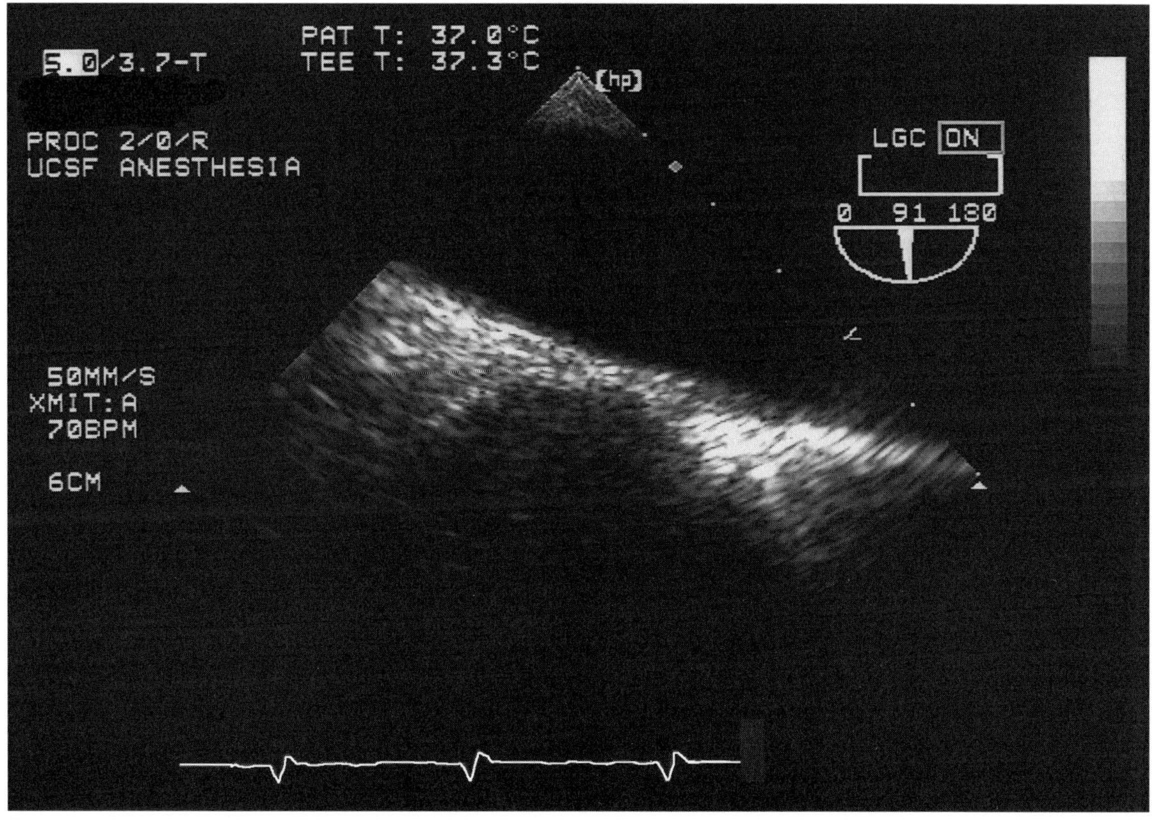

FIGURE **10–17.** Longitudinal plane, descending aorta, long-axis transesophageal echocardiogram. *A*, Line drawing of the structure seen in this view. Ao, descending aorta. *B*, Corresponding echocardiogram. The half-circle–shaped icon to the left of the Ao signifies the position of the multiplane transducer at 91 degrees (see text for additional details).

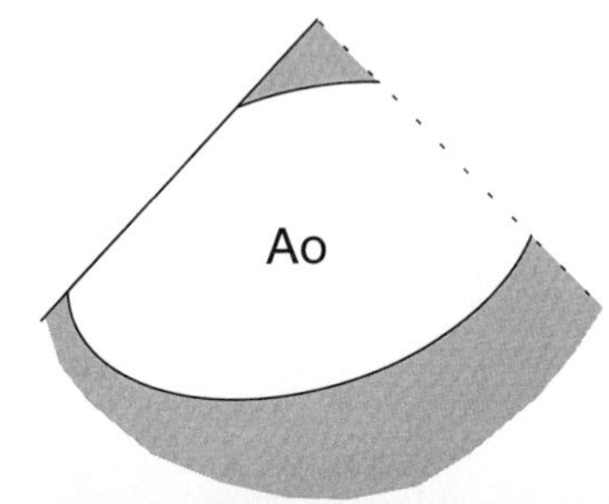

A

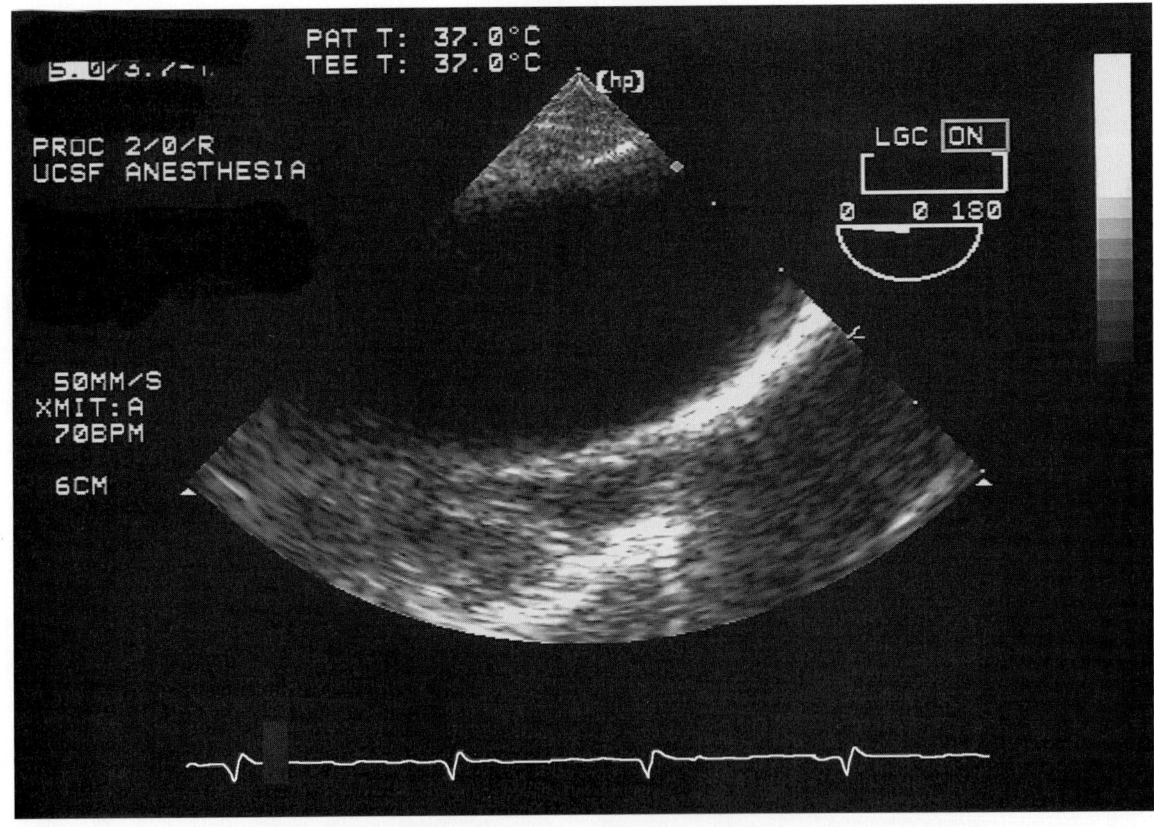

B

FIGURE **10–18.** Transverse plane, distal aortic arch, transesophageal echocardiogram. *A*, Line drawing of the structure seen in this view. Ao, distal aortic arch. *B*, Corresponding echocardiogram. The half-circle–shaped icon to the left of the Ao signifies the position of the multiplane transducer at 0 degrees (see text for additional details).

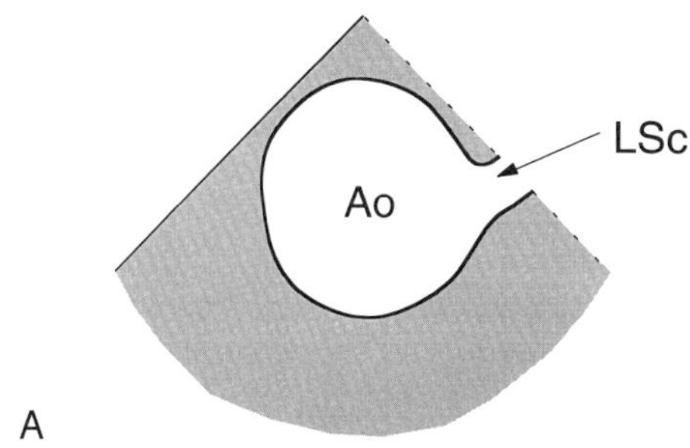

A

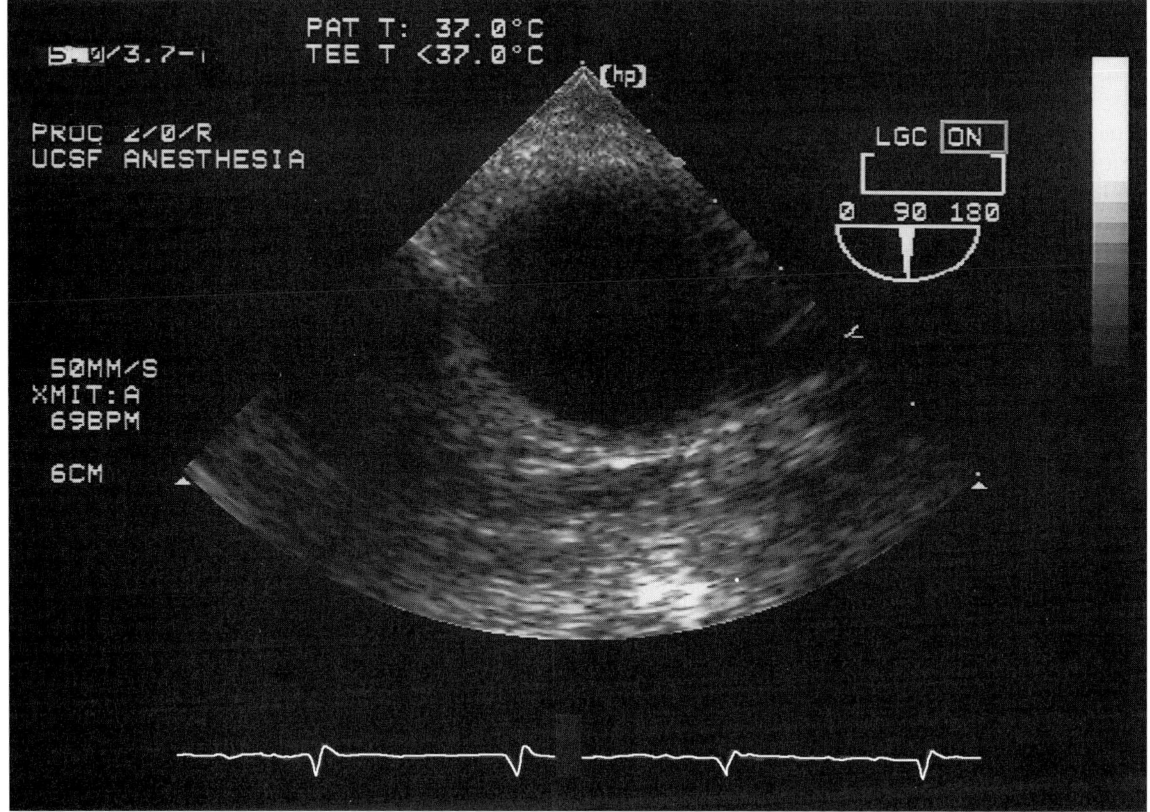

B

FIGURE **10–19.** Longitudinal plane, distal aortic arch, transesophageal echocardiogram. *A*, Line drawing of the structures seen in this view. Ao, descending aorta; LSc, left subclavian artery. *B*, Corresponding echocardiogram. The half-circle–shaped icon to the left of the LSc signifies the position of the multiplane transducer at 90 degrees (see text for additional details).

estimates was excellent; however, virtually no correlation was seen between estimates from either of these techniques and pulmonary artery pressures. Thus, TEE (but not the pulmonary artery catheter) provides a direct, quantitative method to assess LV preload and ejection.

Automated Assessment of Preload and Ejection

Quantitative analysis of TEE used in research settings is now available in the operating room using an automated analysis system (automated border detection [ABD]), which continuously tracks the endocardial borders and computes the cross-sectional area of the LV cavity. The automated estimates of LV end-diastolic area (EDA) and end-systolic area (ESA) are, for all practical purposes, identical to the laboratory measurements made independently by an expert, provided the echocardiographic images are of good or excellent quality (87% of the data sets at end-diastole and 74% at end-systole).[16] The operator dependency and technical pitfalls of acquiring optimal images for ABD are discussed by Bednarz and colleagues.[17] Unfortunately, the automated system slightly underestimates EDA and overestimates ESA, resulting in a significant underestimation of the area ejection fraction. With further computer processing, ventricular volume can be calculated but animal studies confirm the underestimation of volume by the automated technique.[18]

TABLE 10–1
TEE and the Etiology of Hypotension

	LV Filling	LV Ejection
Hypovolemia	⇓⇓	⇑⇑
Cardiac depression	⇑⇑	⇓⇓
Arterial vasodilatation	Adequate	⇑⇑

Hypotension

With a sudden, severe change in hemodynamics, qualitative estimates of LV filling and ejection serve as a practical guide for administration of fluids and inotropes. In some ultrasonographs, computer technology converts the echocardiographic images from one cardiac cycle into digital code and then plays the cycle over and over again for side-by-side comparison with other cardiac cycles captured at other times during surgery. This juxtapositioning of images greatly facilitates the qualitative evaluation of changes in LV performance and the prompt diagnosis of the etiology of hypotension (Table 10–1). When arterial vasodilatation is considered the apparent cause of hypotension and vasoconstrictor therapy is planned, severe aortic regurgitation, mitral regurgitation, and ventricular septal defect should be ruled out first, because they can produce exactly the same LV filling and ejection pattern as severe arterial vasodilatation, but they require different therapy.

Cardiac Output

Although viewing the real-time images of LV filling and ejection gives one an excellent and immediate sense of the adequacy of cardiac output, substantial research has been conducted to establish that TEE can actually measure it by determining the velocity of blood flow through a valve or great vessel and the cross-sectional area of that valve or great vessel. Investigators have studied flows in the main pulmonary artery and across the mitral valve. Although initial results were somewhat disappointing,[19] more recent studies excluding patients with tricuspid regurgitation (known to confound thermodilution) suggest that TEE should have a bias of near zero and limits of agreement of less than 1 L/min when compared with thermodilution.[20–23]

LV Filling Pressure

Surprisingly, TEE provides two practical ways to estimate LV filling pressure. By placing the Doppler cursor at the junction of the left atrium and left superior pulmonary vein, Kuecherer et al. demonstrated that the systolic fraction of pulmonary venous flow into the left atrium was inversely correlated with left atrial pressure.[24] The proximity of the TEE transducer to the pulmonary veins permits excellent Doppler recordings of their flow, which is biphasic (systolic and diastolic). A systolic fraction of flow of less than 55% was a specific and sensitive marker of left atrial pressure greater than 15 mm Hg. This can be easily recognized in real time as predominance of flow during diastole. When the peak pulmonary flow velocity is greater during systole than diastole, left atrial pressure is normal or low; when the peak flow velocity is higher during diastole, left atrial pressure is high.[25] Unfortunately, significant mitral regurgitation, nonsinus rhythms, and marked changes in LV contractility affect pulmonary venous flow also. In a separate study, Kusumoto et al. noted that at low or normal left atrial pressures, the interatrial septum transiently reverses its normal rightward curvature during the exhalation phase of positive-pressure ventilation (because for just this moment the right atrial pressure exceeds the left atrial pressure).[26] Absence of this reversal has a positive predictive value of 0.97 for a left atrial pressure of greater than 15 mm Hg.[26] Therefore, TEE cannot precisely estimate left atrial pressure, but it appears able to reliably identify a clinically significantly increased left atrial pressure.

LV Contractility

Measuring LV contractility is much more difficult. The LV fractional area change ([EDA-ESA]/EDA) measured at the midpapillary short-axis view is a reasonable approximation of LV ejection fraction, but the ejection fraction is clearly afterload dependent and should be viewed cautiously as an index of overall ventricular performance. However, it is an excellent predictor of survival in patients with coronary artery disease, and is widely used in preoperative assessment of high-risk patients. Preliminary studies suggest that TEE may be used to estimate pressure-volume–derived indices of contractility that are independent of loading conditions.[27]

LV Afterload

In contrast, TEE provides a better estimate of LV afterload and end-systolic wall stress (which incorporates LV systolic dimension, pressure, and wall thickness) than is possible with other intraoperative monitors. For instance, Smith et al. showed a strong association of TEE-determined wall stress and intraoperative myocardial ischemia in a study of patients undergoing carotid endarterectomy.[28] Systolic blood pressure and heart rate were maintained at the patient's ward level in both groups, using phenylephrine in one group and "light" anesthesia in the other. A 40% higher wall stress and a 2.5-fold higher incidence of ischemia were found in the group receiving phenylephrine (because of LV distention and wall thinning), indicating the importance of afterload as a determinant of oxygen demand and myocardial ischemia.

Detecting Myocardial Ischemia

Intraoperative Studies

Since Tennant and Wiggers first described the association of segmental wall motion abnormalities (SWMAs) and ischemia, many other investigators have proven that ischemic segments of human and animal heart do not exhibit normal inward wall motion or thickening during systole.[29] During acute myocardial ischemia, subsequent experimental and clinical studies have confirmed that SWMAs precede and may occur in the absence of ECG changes.[30–32] With the advent of TEE, anesthesiologists began to directly observe SWMAs. For instance, Smith et al. utilized TEE in 50 patients undergoing coronary artery or major vascular surgery.[33] At predetermined intervals, echocardiograms and seven-lead ECG (three limb leads, three augmented leads, and V_5) were recorded, both of which were evaluated by "blinded" observers. Intraoperatively, six patients had ST-segment changes diagnostic of myocardial ischemia (≥0.1 mV deviation), while 24 had new SWMAs diagnostic of myocardial ischemia (marked decrement in LV segmental motion and thickening). No patient experienced an ST-segment change before or in the absence of a new SWMA. In three of the six patients who experienced ST-segment change, the SWMA occurred minutes before the ECG change. Three of the 50 patients suffered intraoperative myocardial infarctions, and all had an SWMA develop and persist until the end of surgery in the corresponding area of myocardium. Only one of these patients had intraoperative ST-segment change diagnostic of ischemia. Four of five patients with double-vessel disease had new SWMAs, and these changes were in regions of myocardium supplied by the diseased coronary arteries and never in the "risk-free" myocardium. Ten patients without coronary disease were also studied and none of these patients had ST-segment changes or SWMA.

Two subsequent studies confirmed these initial results. Leung et al. used continuous TEE and two-lead Holter recordings in 50 patients undergoing coronary artery surgery: 56 new SWMAs occurred, of which 8 (14%) were accompanied by ST-segment change; 18 ST-segment changes occurred, of which 8 (44%) were accompanied by SWMAs, 4 (22%) by equivocal SWMAs, and 6 (33%) by no change in segmental wall motion.[34] All of the six patients with major adverse outcomes (two deaths from cardiac causes, three myocardial infarctions, and one ventricular failure) had new SWMAs detected after cardiopulmonary bypass that persisted to the conclusion of surgery. Van Daele et al. compared 12-lead ECG and TEE in 98 anesthetized patients with severe ischemic heart disease.[35] They detected myocardial ischemia in 14 patients by TEE, 10 of whom had concomitant ST-segment change. One other patient had ST-segment change but no TEE evidence of ischemia. Thus, based on these three studies, one can conclude that TEE is a more sensitive method to detect myocardial ischemia than ECG—even continuous two-lead Holter or standard 12-lead ECG in patients with coronary artery disease.

In contrast to these studies, Eisenberg et al. have recently published a comparison of TEE, two-lead Holter, and 12-lead continuous ECG monitoring in noncardiac surgical patients judged to be at risk for coronary artery disease.[36] They found very poor concordance in the diagnosis of myocardial ischemia: only 17 of 174 (10%) of the total episodes of ischemia were detected by all three monitors. The concordance between TEE and two-lead Holter or 12-lead ECG was 16%, and between two-lead Holter and 12-lead ECG only 37%, with the two-lead Holter actually detecting almost twice as many episodes of ischemia as either the 12-lead system or TEE (122 vs. 74 vs. 72 episodes, respectively).

The authors offered no adequate explanation for this striking lack of concordance or the apparent superior sensitivity of two-lead Holter. However, on careful scrutiny, their results may not be so surprising. First, the electrocardiograms (two-lead Holter and 12-lead ECG) were monitored continuously while TEE was evaluated only intermittently. Second, TEE images were analyzed by review of videotape recordings and not by cineloop analysis. With the latter technique, now standard for stress echocardiography studies, individual cardiac cycles can be viewed side by side on the same video screen (for instance, a baseline recording juxtaposed to a subsequent recording). In this way, diagnostic changes in segmental wall motion and thickening are more reliably identified.[37] Third, the authors evaluated only one TEE cross section. Shah et al. have proven that in addition to the short-axis cross section monitored by Eisenberg, monitoring a long-axis cross section will increase detection of ischemia by approximately 40%.[38] Thus, TEE evaluation was performed for only a fraction of the time ECG evaluation was performed, with a relatively insensitive technique, and in only one cross section.

An additional explanation is that just over half of Eisenberg's patients had proven coronary artery disease. This observation is critical, because as the prevalence of a disease decreases in a population, the risk of false-positive findings increases unless the diagnostic test has perfect specificity. The two-lead Holter is far from a perfectly specific monitor of myocardial ischemia because it reveals ST changes diagnostic of ischemia in 7% of healthy young adults[39] and can be confounded by a variety of metabolic and medicinal factors. For instance, when healthy young adults are given digitalis, 26% of them will exhibit ST changes diagnostic of ischemia during 24 hours of Holter monitoring.[40] In Eisenberg's study, 13% of patients were receiving digitalis. Thus, in healthy patients (who have no coronary artery disease), two-lead Holter monitoring will reveal more apparent episodes of myocardial ischemia (false-positives) than monitors with greater specificity and equal or even greater sensitivity!

Sensitivity and Specificity of ST Change and SWMAs

No studies are available that directly compare TEE to two-lead Holter and independently confirm the actual presence or absence of ischemia. However, four different laboratories have directly compared TEE and 12-lead ECG for the detection of myocardial ischemia during stress testing, and independently confirmed the presence or absence of coronary disease with arteriography.[41–44] In all four studies, TEE proved more sensitive than 12-lead ECG (mean sensitivity 90%, range 83 to 93%, vs.

mean 52%, range 43 to 63%) for the diagnosis of significant coronary artery disease. In three out of four of these studies, TEE proved more specific than 12-lead ECG (mean 97%, range 93 to 100%, vs. 84%, range 67 to 100%; data from all four studies included).

Studies conducted during angioplasty offer another chance to compare echocardiography (not TEE, but transthoracic in these studies) and ECG sensitivity during myocardial ischemia. Hauser et al. showed that interruption of coronary blood flow produced a new SWMA in the distribution of the occluded coronary artery in 86% of the dilations, but did not alter wall motion when highly collateralized areas of myocardium were involved or when baseline wall motion was absent.[31] The onset of the SWMA began approximately 19 seconds after coronary occlusion, and began to resolve 17 seconds after reperfusion. Seven ECG leads were monitored (three limb leads, three augmented leads, and V_5). ST-segment change occurred in 30% of the dilations approximately 30 seconds after coronary artery occlusion. ST changes invariably followed the onset of SWMA. However, only seven ECG leads were used in this study. In contrast, Wohlgelernter et al. utilized the standard 12-lead ECG in 30 patients undergoing angioplasty.[32] All patients in this study had a positive exercise treadmill test, an isolated obstructive lesion of the left anterior descending coronary artery without collateral blood supply, normal baseline LV function, and no conduction disturbances or ST-segment abnormalities on the ECG that would preclude assessment of ischemia. All patients developed SWMA at 10 seconds (on the average) after coronary artery occlusion, and 27 of 30 (90%) developed ST-segment change at 22 seconds. Thus, in patients who experienced 45 to 90 seconds of complete coronary occlusion, SWMAs are an earlier and more sensitive indicator of myocardial ischemia than the ECG, even the 12-lead ECG.

However, if a coronary artery is compromised for longer than 90 seconds, would the ECG reveal diagnostic changes eventually? For ethical reasons, this question can't be answered with studies in humans. Therefore, Battler et al. used sonomicrometers (miniature ultrasound transducers) to measure myocardial thickening in dogs during progressive constriction of a coronary artery.[30] With mild constriction (producing <25% decrease in wall thickening), epicardial and endocardial but not the surface electrocardiogram (11-lead vector system) revealed ST change. With more severe constriction, the surface electrocardiogram changed but always minutes after the onset of wall thickening changes. Thus, during mild coronary stenosis, SWMAs can occur in the absence of surface ECG changes, and during moderate to severe stenosis, they may precede ECG changes by several minutes.

TEE Limitations

However, a number of general limitations of TEE in the diagnosis of ischemia should be mentioned. Even when an area of myocardium is clearly in view, its segmental contraction can be difficult to evaluate if the entire heart rotates or translates markedly during systole, or if discoordinated contraction occurs due to bundle branch block or ventricular pacing. Consequently, a valid system for assessing SWMAs must first compensate for global motion of the heart (usually done by a "floating" frame of reference), and then evaluate both regional endocardial motion and myocardial thickening. At least a two-class worsening of segmental wall motion and thickening is required (in the absence of similar global changes) to make the diagnosis of ischemia (Table 10–2) because less pronounced changes are not consistently interpreted, even by experts.

Unfortunately, no currently available automated wall motion analysis system has proven adequate for TEE images. Interpretation of septal motion is most often confounded by discoordinated contraction. When the septum is viable and nonischemic, it will appreciably thicken during systole, although its inward motion may begin slightly before or after inward motion of the other ventricular segments. Thus, new SWMAs can be detected during bundle branch block, ventricular pacing, and marked global movements of the heart, but not by assessment of endocardial motion alone.

Moreover, all SWMAs are not indicative of myocardial ischemia. Owing to biologic differences in normal patients, not all hearts contract normally, and not all parts of the same heart contract to the same degree.[45] Myocardial infarction and myocarditis can cause SWMAs, but an acute decrease or cessation of segmental contraction (e.g., a new SWMA during surgery) is almost certainly due to myocardial ischemia.

One exception to this rule is myocardial stunning, or prolonged, postischemic ventricular dysfunction.[46] When ischemia has been prolonged, full restoration of blood flow may occur minutes to hours before return of normal segmental contraction. Does a new SWMA detected immediately after bypass represent inadequate revascularization and ongoing ischemia, or stunned myocardium from inadequate cooling during bypass? Inadequate revascularization may require placement of additional grafts, while stunned myocardium requires only supportive measures until its function returns. Echocardiographic contrast agents, capable of readily delineating myocardial blood flow, are described later but are still undergoing refinement.[47] Therefore, when faced with this clinical dilemma, graft status should be re-evaluated and the new SWMA watched for signs of improvement. If worsening occurs, if graft status is questionable, or if

TABLE 10–2
TEE and the Diagnosis of Ischemia

	Wall Thickening	Δ in Radius*
Normal	Marked	>30%⇓
Mild hypokinesis	Moderate	10–30%⇓
Severe hypokinesis	Minimal	<10, >0%⇓
Akinesis	None	no Δ
Dyskinesis	Thinning	⇑

*Percentage change during systole in the radius from the endocardium to the imaginary center of the LV as seen in the midpapillary short-axis view. A two-class worsening of segmental function is required for the diagnosis of ischemia.

hemodynamics are tenuous, then additional revascularization should be provided if possible.

Another conceivable cause of acute SWMAs is unmasking areas of scarring by changes in LV afterload. For instance, a marked increase in blood pressure might retard contraction in an already damaged segment of myocardium more than in a normal segment. Three observations make this an unlikely explanation for the acute SWMAs reported in the studies above. First, only marked changes in segmental contraction were taken as indicative of ischemia. It is hard to imagine that a sudden increase in afterload would cause one segment to cease or nearly cease contracting in the absence of changes in the other segments. Buffington and Coyle used an animal model to test the effects of extreme increases in afterload and could demonstrate changes so minimal that they are unlikely to be detected with TEE.[48,49] Second, with one exception (see Smith et al.,[28] above) none of the intraoperative studies to date have found any consistent correlation between hemodynamics and new SWMAs. In general, anesthesiologists prevent marked changes in loading conditions. Third, the vast majority of new SWMAs occurred in segments of myocardium with normal contraction at baseline (after induction of anesthesia).

In contrast, one preliminary report suggests that tachycardia and marked decreases in preload can induce acute SWMAs in the absence of myocardial ischemia. Seeberger et al. noted the immediate recovery (within one beat) of severe SWMAs, when rapid atrial pacing was abruptly stopped and simultaneously preload recovered to the prepacing baseline.[50] They reasoned that myocardial ischemia could not possibly recover so quickly. Therefore, because marked alterations in LV loading can cause myocardial ischemia and perhaps confound the analysis of LV segmental motion, such loading abnormalities should be corrected before the anesthesiologist's attention is diverted to a detailed evaluation of segmental LV function.

Tethering or systolic dysfunction of nonischemic myocardium adjacent to ischemic or infarcted myocardium is also commonly mentioned as another cause of "artifactual" SWMAs. Tethering probably accounts for the consistent overestimation of infarct size by echocardiography when compared to postmortem studies. However, Force et al. used an improved analysis system, and found that segmental contraction is normal to within 1 cm of the ischemic area.[51] Thus, tethering may actually help the intraoperative detection of myocardial ischemia by making a new SWMA involve an area of myocardium slightly larger than the true area of ischemia. However, tethering does not create new SWMAs in the absence of acute myocardial ischemia.

Finally, changes in wall thickening, rather than wall motion, have been suggested as a more useful indicator of ischemia.[52] However, such measurements showed high variability between observers, owing to the inability to accurately visualize the endocardial border.[52] In subsequent work, the importance of measurements in multiple planes, on multiple occasions, and with careful standardization of location and edge definition was emphasized to limit interobserver variability.[53]

Evaluation of Valvular Function

Overview

Echocardiography so clearly reveals the extent and severity of valvular heart disease that many patients can be spared cardiac catheterization prior to surgery. For some valvular lesions, TEE is the procedure of choice even in the outpatient setting. In the operating room, TEE occasionally detects unsuspected valvular lesions, but more often is called upon to confirm the adequacy of a valvular procedure. Thus, one can view intraoperative valvular assessment performed at two levels. The first is recognition of severe valvular abnormalities that threaten hemodynamic stability; the second, detailed assessment of valvular function required for evaluation of valvular repairs and replacements. With a modest degree of training (see below), TEE practitioners master the first level, as color Doppler and 2D imaging are usually all that are required. The second level is much more difficult and can frequently challenge even the most experienced echocardiographers. In the setting of a questionably adequate valve repair or replacement, the surgical team should insist on the most expert echocardiographic evaluation possible.

Aortic Stenosis

The degree of aortic stenosis is easily appreciated in the transverse plane, aortic valve short-axis view (Fig. 10–20). When the ultrasound beam can be positioned exactly perpendicular to the aortic valve opening (most easily accomplished with the multiplane transducer rotated to 20 to 30 degrees), the extent of leaflet opening can often be directly measured with planimetry.[54–56] Doppler studies in this view reveal turbulence above the valve and in the sinuses of Valsalva, but they provide no quantitative measure of severity because blood flow is perpendicular to the ultrasound beam. In contrast, the transgastric five-chamber view sometimes allows excellent alignment of the beam with blood flow resulting in valid determination of blood flow velocity across the valve. Additional information on the morphology of the valve and aortic root abnormalities is often gained in the longitudinal plane, ascending aorta view.

Aortic Regurgitation

Even modest degrees of aortic regurgitation may have clinical significance during cardiac surgery, because they may result in LV distention during cardiopulmonary bypass and may diminish the effectiveness of antegrade cardioplegia. Fortunately, aortic regurgitation is easily recognized using color Doppler in the transverse plane, five-chamber view and longitudinal plane, ascending aorta view (Fig. 10–21). In these views, mild regurgitation is characterized by a narrow-based, diastolic color jet (<2 mm at its origin in the valve) that occupies less than a third of the cross-sectional area of the LV outflow

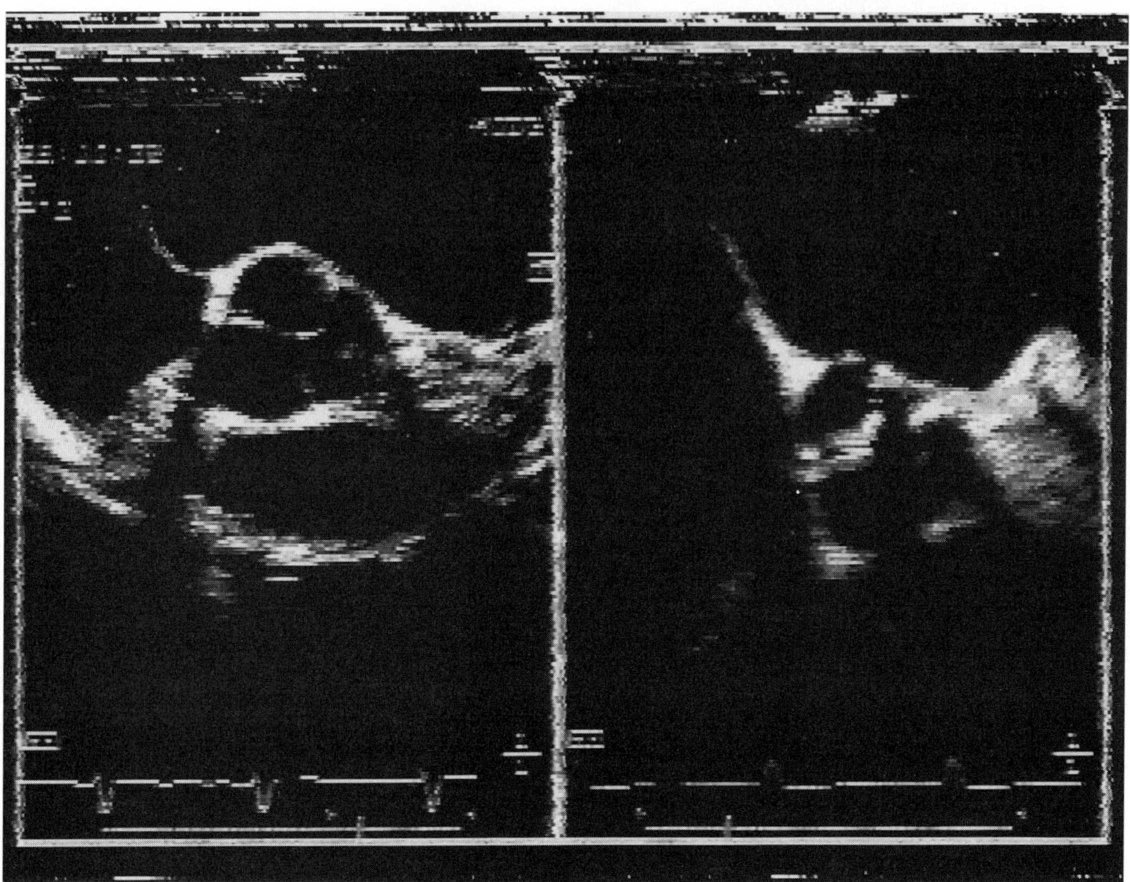

FIGURE **10–20.** Transverse plane, aortic valve, short-axis, transesophageal echocardiograms: normal aortic valve (*left*) and stenotic (*right*). (Please see Fig. 10–4 for orientation.) Note thickening of the leaflets on the left and acoustic shadowing distal to these thickened leaflets.

tract and extends minimally into the left ventricle (1 to 2 cm). Moderate regurgitation is characterized by a broader-based, diastolic color jet (3 to 5 mm) that occupies less than two thirds of the cross-sectional area of the LV outflow tract and extends moderately into the left ventricle (3 to 5 cm). Severe regurgitation is characterized by a broad-based, diastolic color jet (>5 mm) that occupies all of the LV outflow tract and extends well into the left ventricle.

Mitral Stenosis

The presence and severity of mitral stenosis are easily determined with TEE using the transverse plane, four- or five-chamber views and the longitudinal plane, two-chamber and midpapillary long-axis views. 2D imaging reveals thickened leaflets that dome toward the left ventricle while their tips open poorly. Color Doppler reveals laminar flow acceleration into the stenotic orifice and a turbulent jet emerging into the ventricle. Severe stenosis is easily recognized as an exceedingly narrow valve opening (<2 mm at its maximum). However, severity is best measured with CW Doppler, which reliably yields the pressure gradient across the valve (from the mean velocity determination and the equation $4V^2$) and pressure half-time estimates of valve area.[11,12,57] Significant mitral stenosis always causes left atrial enlargement, and frequently spontaneous contrast can be visualized in the enlarged left atrium. Spontaneous contrast is a swirling, smoke-like appearance of 1- to 2-mm densities that are not due to exogenously administered contrast agents. Instead, they are due to aggregation of red cells in areas of low flow. Whenever left atrial enlargement and spontaneous contrast are noted, a careful search for thrombus should be performed in the left atrium and, in particular, in the left atrial appendage.[58]

Mitral Regurgitation

TEE is the ideal technique for evaluation of mitral regurgitation. Its presence and severity are evaluated in the save views used for evaluation of mitral regurgitation and with the same grading strategy used for aortic regurgitation (Fig. 10–22). Mild regurgitation is characterized by a narrow-based, systolic color jet (<2 mm at its origin in the valve) that occupies less than 25% of the left atrial cross-sectional area and extends less than half of the distance to the posterior wall of the left atrium. Moderate regurgitation is characterized by a broader-based, systolic color jet (3 to 5 mm at its origin in the valve) that occupies less than 50% of the left atrial cross-sectional area and extends 50 to 90% of the dis-

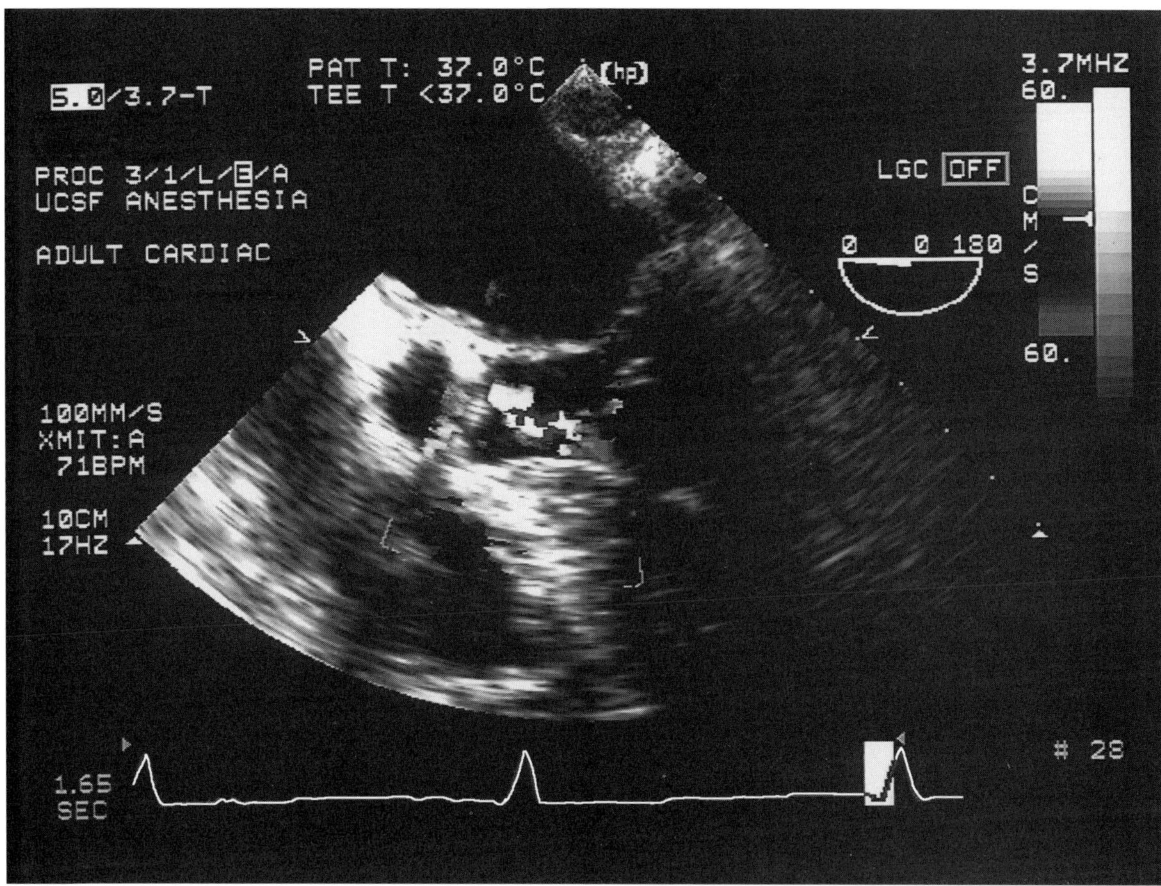

FIGURE **10–21.** Transverse plane, five-chamber, long-axis, transesophageal echocardiogram: mild aortic regurgitation. See Figure 10–5 for orientation and text for grading criteria. *See Color Plate.*

tance to the posterior wall of the left atrium. Severe regurgitation is characterized by a broad-based, diastolic color jet (>5 mm) that occupies most of the left atrium and extends into the pulmonary veins and left atrial appendage. Eccentrically directed jets that hug the wall of the atrium are generally associated with more severe valvular regurgitation than their cross-sectional area might suggest.[59] Moreover, eccentrically directed jets usually point away from the defective leaflet (i.e., laterally directed jets are usually associated with anterior leaflet defects and medially directed jets with posterior leaflet defects). These general guidelines are widely used, but at least 20 more criteria have been described.[60] Most importantly, the degree of regurgitation may be exquisitely dependent on LV loading conditions and myocardial perfusion status.

Tricuspid Stenosis and Regurgitation

These valvular abnormalities are evaluated using the transverse plane, four-chamber view and longitudinal plane, right ventricular outflow tract view. The same principles apply here as discussed for mitral valve evaluations. Tricuspid stenosis is quite uncommon in the adult population, while mild tricuspid regurgitation is seen commonly when a pulmonary artery catheter is in place. In this setting and in the absence of right ventricular and right atrial enlargement, mild tricuspid regurgitation has no clinical significance.

Pulmonary Stenosis and Regurgitation

These valvular abnormalities are evaluated using the transverse plane, pulmonary artery view and longitudinal plane, right ventricular outflow tract view (the latter view is usually required for adequate evaluation). As for aortic valve evaluation, the same principles apply to the pulmonary valve. Serious pulmonary valve dysfunction is uncommon in adults but is a major concern in congenital heart surgery. When a Doppler estimate is needed of the gradient across the right ventricular outflow tract or pulmonary valve, the operator can sometimes optimally align the ultrasound beam from the transgastric approach. First, the transgastric five-chamber view is obtained, and then the gastroscope is rotated leftward until the pulmonary valve and artery come into view.

Prosthetic Valves

Although TEE is the method of choice in many patients with prosthetic valve dysfunction, there are two major

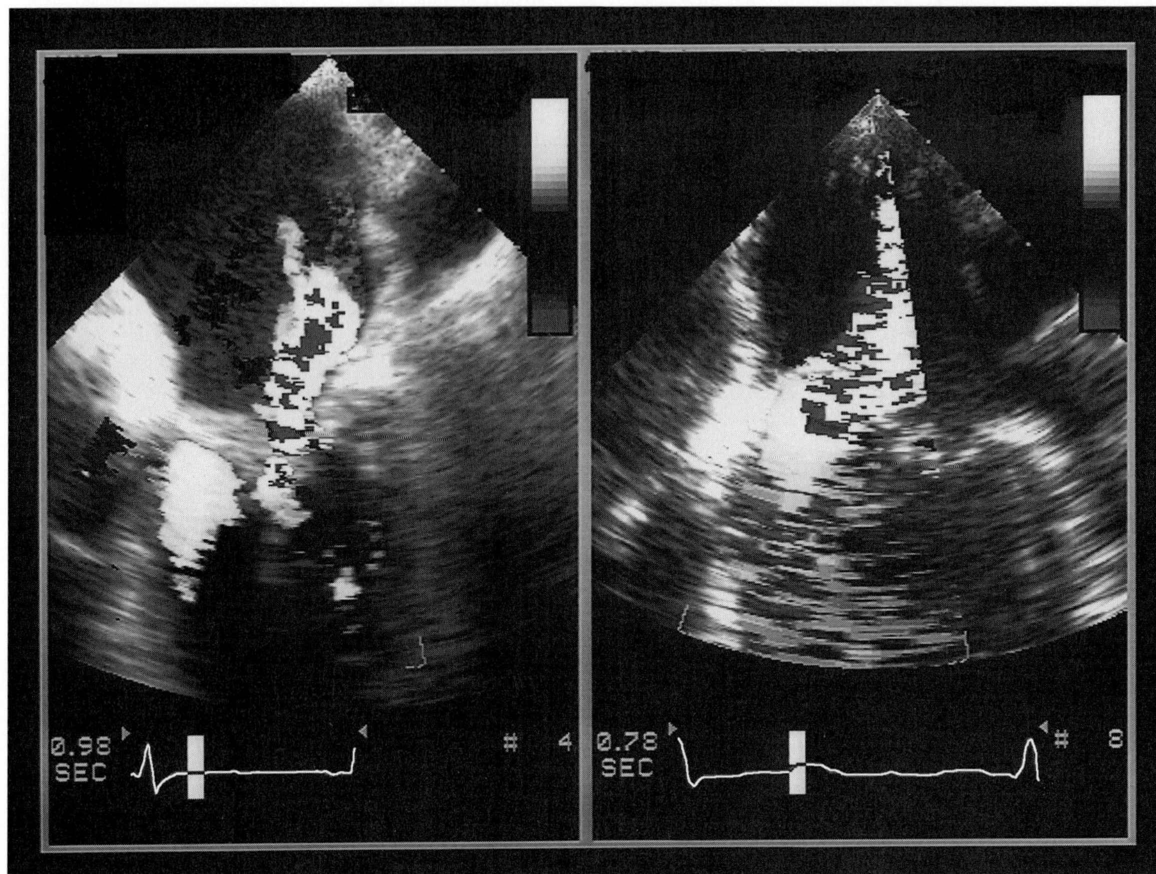

FIGURE **10–22.** Transverse plane, five-chamber, long-axis, transesophageal echocardiogram showing moderate mitral regurgitation (*left*) and transverse plane, four-chamber, long-axis, transesophageal echocardiogram showing severe mitral regurgitation (*right*). See Figure 10–5 for orientation and text for grading criteria. *See Color Plate.*

problems in this use. First, the prosthetic material may be impenetrable with ultrasound, resulting in "acoustic shadowing." Thus, structures located behind the prosthesis (relative to the esophagus) are sometimes rendered invisible to TEE. For instance, the LV outflow tract is difficult to image in the five-chamber view when a mechanical valve is seated in the mitral position. Second, all prostheses have one or more leaks (regurgitant jets) that are distinct to the design. Unless the operator knows the normal pattern for the prosthesis under study, he or she will be unable to determine whether its function is acceptable. Standard echocardiographic textbooks detail these patterns. However, two generalizations are useful.

First, although a well-seated prosthesis will move in concert with cardiac movements (e.g., a mitral prosthesis descends as the base of the heart descends during systole), only dehiscent valves rock to and fro in the annulus during cardiac contraction. Once this movement has been seen, it is not easy to forget. Second, normal prosthetic leaks occur within the sewing ring (prosthetic annulus) not outside it (perivalvular regurgitation). Even a relatively small perivalvular color jet may be important. Although it represents a small fraction of the cardiac output, if high shear forces are involved, severe hemolysis can result. Unfortunately, no definitive studies are currently available to reliably say which perivalvular leaks require reoperation, when seen immediately after cardiopulmonary bypass. The surgical team should insist on the most expert echocardiographic evaluation possible and weigh this advice against the perceived risk of an additional period of cardiopulmonary bypass.

Assessing Surgical Repairs

Valve Surgery

TEE has profoundly affected cardiac valvuloplasty because it provides the surgical team with a definitive evaluation of the repair immediately after cardiopulmonary bypass, so that if the repair is flawed, it can be corrected before leaving the operating room. Morbidity and mortality are reduced if the patient leaves the operating room with a properly functioning repair. For instance, Sheikh et al. studied 154 patients undergoing valve surgery.[61] TEE revealed unsatisfactory repairs after bypass in ten patients (6%) resulting in immediate further surgery. At the conclusion of surgery, TEE revealed adequate valvular function in 123 patients: 18 of these patients (15%)

suffered a major postoperative complication and 6 died (5%). In contrast, TEE revealed moderate valve dysfunction in seven patients: six of these patients suffered major complications and three died. Similar results have been reported by Freeman et al. in 154 patients who underwent mitral valve repair. Eleven patients (7%) were found to have 3+ mitral regurgitation after the first attempt at repair, and 13 patients (9%) had severe systolic anterior motion of the mitral leaflet. "Systolic anterior motion of the mitral leaflet" refers to an abnormal, septally directed motion of the anterior mitral leaflet during systole (best seen in the five-chamber view) that partially pulls open the mitral valve and obstructs the LV outflow tract. TEE verified that the systolic anterior motion resolved with restoration of normal hemodynamics in 8 of the 13 patients without surgical intervention. Although traditional methods of assessing mitral function during surgery may detect some failed repairs,[62,63] they are not highly reliable and do not reveal the mechanism of failure—a key issue in the decision to rerepair or replace. TEE, on the other hand, reliably detects prosthetic malfunction and periprosthetic leaks.[64] While moderate or severe periprosthetic leaks should almost always undergo immediate repair, the treatment of small periprosthetic leaks is controversial.[65] Recent data suggest that TEE may allow determination of which of the small periprosthetic leaks has sufficient shearing forces to produce hemolysis and require reoperation on that basis.[66]

Pediatric TEE

There is convincing evidence that perioperative TEE in pediatric patients provides diagnostic information comparable to epicardial echocardiography.[67,68] For instance, Gussenhoven et al. studied 195 patients with epicardial echocardiography and found new information before cardiopulmonary bypass that significantly altered the planned surgery in four patients, and new information after bypass that resulted in immediate revision of the repair in six patients.[69] Thus 10 of 195 (5%) of the patients had their surgical course fundamentally altered (improved?) by intraoperative epicardial echocardiography. Similarly, Ungerleider et al. used epicardial echocardiography in 328 patients during congenital heart surgery.[70] Twenty-two patients (7%) underwent immediate revision of their repair based on the postbypass imaging. The authors noted that without epicardial imaging these residual defects would have been missed and likely resulted in increased morbidity.

Coronary Artery Surgery

TEE may change the course of coronary artery surgery at four points. First, some patients will have acute graft problems detected by TEE (as new SWMAs noted after bypass), and this finding prompts additional graft placement. For instance, Deutsch et al. studied 50 consecutive patients undergoing coronary artery surgery.[71] In three of these patients, a new SWMA together with other clinical signs of ischemia prompted graft thrombectomy or additional medical therapy. In two other patients, a new SWMA led to the discovery of unsuspected graft occlusions and prompted graft revisions. Thus, TEE information had a significant impact on the care of five patients (10%) including two patients (4%) in whom it provided the only immediate sign of acute graft occlusion. Second, some patients scheduled for coronary surgery are unexpectedly discovered to need mitral valvuloplasty as well. For instance, of 182 patients scheduled for coronary surgery, Sheikh et al. found five patients with unsuspected mitral regurgitation so severe that unscheduled mitral valve repair was performed in addition to coronary surgery.[72] Interestingly, these authors also found that 22 of 51 patients scheduled for combined coronary artery and mitral valve surgery had so little mitral valve dysfunction revealed by TEE prior to bypass that the mitral procedure was omitted.

Third, TEE may provide information needed to decrease the incidence of stroke associated with coronary artery surgery. Katz et al. studied 130 patients over 65 years of age undergoing this surgery. Five of these patients suffered strokes. Using logistic regression analysis, the authors identified only protruding atheroma of the ascending aorta (revealed by TEE) as an independent predictor of these strokes—not age, previous stroke, carotid bruit, transient ischemic attacks, or surgical palpation of the ascending aorta.[73] The sensitivity and specificity of TEE in the detection of ascending aortic atherosclerosis was compared with an epicardial approach by Konstadt and co-workers in patients undergoing cardiac surgery.[74] They found that TEE was very sensitive but only mildly specific in determining the presence of ascending aortic atherosclerosis. In an associated study, Ribakove used TEE to reveal mobile atheroma of the ascending aorta in ten patients.[75] Six of these patients underwent the customary cardiopulmonary bypass, and three had strokes. Four of these ten patients were treated with circulatory arrest and aortic débridement prior to coronary surgery, and none had strokes.

Myocardial Contrast Echocardiography

Another use of echocardiography in the patient with coronary artery disease is to assess coronary perfusion. While myocardial ischemia can be detected by changes in ventricular wall thickening, such information does not directly assess perfusion. Myocardial contrast echocardiography is based upon the combination of echocardiographic contrast agents acting as tracers and ultrasonic scanners acting as detectors of contrast concentration. Both integrated backscatter analysis of radiofrequency signals and quantitative assessments by videodensitometry have been used to detect the changes in myocardial acoustic properties with the former providing superior enhancement.[76] Detection of changes in myocardial echocardiographic appearance after injection of one of the contrast agents, sonicated human serum albumin (Albunex), has been difficult except when using right atrial injections of highly concentrated microspheres during dipyridamole-induced coronary hyperemia and epicardial ultrasonography in animals.[77] While myocardial contrast agents are usually injected into the aortic root or left atrium, Monaghan and co-workers successfully administered them intravenously to determine time intensity curves from myocardial integrated backscatter to indicate coronary perfusion in humans.[78] Despite these successes, it is still unclear whether the echocardiographic contrast changes seen reflect alterations in coronary blood flow in terms of flow reserve, changes in coronary blood volume resulting from coronary recruitment, or both.[79] Continuing refinements of the technique are likely before it becomes a frequently used intraoperative tool.

Evaluation of Aortic Pathology

TEE has become the preoperative test of choice in suspected traumatic aortic injuries and aortic dissection. In such situations in which patients may be hemodynamically unstable, TEE can be performed more easily, in less time, and at less expense than aortography, computed tomography (CT), or magnetic resonance imaging (MRI). In 160 patients with blunt chest trauma, Buckmaster and co-workers reported that TEE correctly identified aortic injury in 14 patients and suggested it in two others but produced no false-positive diagnoses.[80] Aortography required more time and produced one false-positive and four false-negative diagnoses in Buckmaster's series. Transesophageal echocardiography reliably differentiates two distinct patterns of aortic injury: (1) subadventitial disruptions requiring emergent surgery; and (2) intimal tears not requiring immediate surgery.[81] Transesophageal echocardiography is superior to aortography and CT and marginally less specific for aortic dissections originating in the aortic arch.[82–84] Because TEE can be performed at the bedside in the critical care unit or emergency room, it minimizes delays in treatment for potentially fatal aortic lesions.

Organizing the Intraoperative TEE Service

Personnel

Neither anesthesiologists alone nor echocardiographers alone can properly run an intraoperative TEE service. Without the expert consultation of an echocardiographer, anesthesiologists will face diagnostic dilemmas for which they are unprepared. Echocardiographers, of course, are unprepared to be present throughout surgery to assist in monitoring LV function. Therefore, at least one anesthesiologist committed to learning TEE and one echocardiographer committed to supporting an intraoperative TEE service are required. The partnership of these two specialties is the foundation upon which the service is built.

A properly trained anesthesia technician is usually responsible for the cleaning and set-up of the TEE equipment in the operating room. Following each study, he or she fills in the accounting forms and transports the video tape to the echocardiography laboratory. Although echocardiography technicians are extremely well qualified to operate the ultrasonograph, they are rarely available in the operating room when needed.

Equipment

An intraoperative service can begin with equipment borrowed from the echocardiography laboratory. However, as intraoperative demand increases, the laboratory's function may be compromised. Ultimately, an intraoperative TEE service needs dedicated equipment, because efficient use of operating room and laboratory time is more cost-advantageous than sharing a TEE system. The difficult question is how much of a system to buy? Most manufacturers offer machines with a variety of options or upgrades which, if all are selected, can quintuple the price of the machine (from $50,000 to $250,000). Most echocardiographers recommend every option. However, an ultrasonograph primarily needed for intraoperative monitoring can function adequately in some patients with just 2D imaging and a video recorder (truly the "bare bones" monitoring package). However, without color Doppler (essential for assessment of valvular function) and a dual or quad screen video review system (essential for assessment of changes in global and regional LV function), the machine will prove inadequate in many clinical situations. Next, PW Doppler (for estimating left atrial pressure), CW Doppler (for estimating peak gradients across valves), and image processing software (for quantifying the images) should be considered. Last, specialized recording devices such as color printers, thermal strip charts, and digital storage units can be considered, especially if the machine is to serve a teaching environment.

Choosing the best echo probes is a little easier. First, the bare bones package should include a single plane (transverse) TEE probe and a high-resolution, near-field focused precordial type probe suitable for epicardial imaging. However, other more expensive options are available. For instance, biplane and multiplane probes offer numerous diagnostic advantages over single-plane probes, but for monitoring purposes the practical advantages may be more limited. Pediatric-sized probes are now widely available and are essential for the assessment of congenital heart repairs.

Training

The single most difficult task in organizing an intraoperative TEE service is to make sure the physicians participating are adequately trained. Savage and co-workers at the Cleveland Clinic have defined training objectives, cognitive skills, and technical skills needed to perform intraoperative echocardiography.[85] At the University of California, San Francisco, three different TEE training programs have been created for anesthesiology residents and fellows: a 1- or 2-month (full-time) introduction to TEE for senior residents (includes 25 to 50 supervised TEE examinations and daily 2-hour echocardiography interpretation sessions with an echocardiographer), a 6-month fellowship (full-time) in adult intraoperative echocardiography (includes 200 to 300 TEE examinations and daily interpretation sessions), and a 1-year fellowship (full-time) in adult and pediatric intraoperative echocardiography (includes extensive training in TEE and epicardial techniques and interpretations). In the 1 month of full-time training, senior residents acquire the technical and interpretative skills necessary for a basic TEE examination and LV monitoring. However, they still require frequent consultation with more experienced practitioners. Moreover, none of these programs is designed to produce independent echocardiographers, and perhaps the single most important aspect of this training is how and when to recognize that the assistance of an echocardiographer is necessary. Training faculty is usually accomplished by a variety of individualized programs of study and supervised participation to accomplish an adequate level of expertise. This approach takes much longer than concentrated training over 1 to 12 months, but eventually it works.

The American Society of Echocardiography has published guidelines for physician training in TEE.[86] They suggest that formal training (or equivalent experience) in 300 precordial studies, 50 TEE studies, and a yearly experience of 50 to 75 TEE studies together with a broad-based knowledge of the field should be required for the independent practice of TEE. However, these guidelines are the result of expert opinion only; no objective data are available to support them. Moreover, these guidelines tacitly acknowledge that a more limited amount of training (not specified) may be appropriate for an anesthesiologist who uses TEE primarily as a monitoring tool, but they clearly state that expert consultation must be immediately available in this setting. The American Society of Anesthesiologists and the Society of Cardiovascular Anesthesiologists have published guidelines for intraoperative TEE and the training required to practice it.[87]

Formal certification in echocardiography is now available, as the American Society of Echocardiography gave its first qualifying examination in May 1996. The Society of Cardiovascular Anesthesiologists has developed a content outline for perioperative TEE and plans to administer an annual examination for certification in perioperative TEE under the direction of the National Board of Echocardiography. Local practices and standards of hospital credentials committees are also relevant. When a mechanism is in place to review the appropriateness of the indications for TEE, the validity of the examinations, and the accuracy of interpretations, TEE is likely to have a positive effect on patients. The American Society of Echocardiography published recommendations for continuous quality improvement in echocardiography in 1995.[88] Interdepartmental cooperation greatly facilitates proper TEE utilization; indeed, it has been the hallmark of most really successful TEE services.

Indications and Complications

Indications

In 2 to 10% of patients undergoing cardiac surgery, information provided by TEE will fundamentally alter the course of clinical care.[61,71,72,75,89–97] Because the patients who will benefit from TEE cannot always be identified in advance of surgery, TEE is an exceedingly low-risk procedure (see below), and surgical complications and reoperations are very expensive, TEE is likely to become routine in all patients undergoing cardiac surgery.

In other patient populations, the indications for TEE are less clear. If a pulmonary artery catheter is planned principally for intraoperative monitoring, TEE should be considered as a potentially more informative and lower risk alternative. Whenever marked intraoperative changes in hemodynamics are anticipated in patients in whom those changes are not likely to be well tolerated, TEE should be considered. Moreover, in persistently hypotensive patients and patients with low-output syndromes who fail to respond to apparently appropriate therapy, TEE should be used because the presumed diagnosis may be wrong. For instance, Reichert et al. have shown that in persistently hypotensive patients following cardiac surgery, TEE corrected erroneous diagnoses (based on standard hemodynamic measurements) in half the patients.[98] In neurosurgical patients at special risk for air embolism, TEE should be considered because it is more sensitive than alternative monitors to detect intravascular air, and because it readily reveals paradoxical transit of air.[99–101] Finally, TEE should be considered whenever it is likely to reveal information that will alter care in a significant way, and comparable information cannot be obtained with less costly or less invasive procedures.

Complications

Most of the reported complications of TEE have occurred in outpatients and have been associated with the stress response that awake or minimally sedated patients experience while swallowing the probe. However, a low incidence of oral and pharyngeal injuries (0.1 to 0.3%) has been reported,[102] but controlled studies have not shown a significant increase in this incidence or postoperative gastrointestinal complaints when compared to the incidence in comparable patients who did not undergo TEE.[103–105] One early report describes two patients who suffered temporary unilateral vocal cord paralysis after TEE monitoring during "sitting" craniotomies.[99] Both of these patients were positioned with nearly full neck flexion. In this position, the recurrent laryngeal nerve may be injured when the larynx, endotracheal tube, and shaft of the gastroscope are compressed between the chin and vertebral column. Subsequent, uncontrolled studies have reported a 0.1 to 12% incidence of transient hoarseness after TEE.[106] Serious hypopharyngeal, esophageal, and gastroesophageal junction injury following TEE have been reported but are rare.[107–111] The

European, multicenter study recorded 1 esophageal perforation in 10,218 patients undergoing TEE (mostly outpatients).[112] As a result, the patient died and autopsy revealed a malignant tumor invading the esophagus. Endocarditis from TEE-induced bacteremia has been reported, but not in the intraoperative setting where prophylactic antibiotics are commonly given.[113,114] In infants, even an appropriate-size TEE probe may occasionally obstruct the airway distal to the endotracheal tube, compress the descending aorta,[115,116] or be associated with inadvertent extubation (personal experience).

Summary and Conclusions

2D TEE provides continuous, vivid images of cardiac anatomy and function without interrupting surgery. Anesthesiologists use these images for earlier and more reliable detection of myocardial ischemia, cardiac depression, inadequate preload, valvular dysfunction, and air embolism than is possible with current alternatives. In addition, TEE may critically influence surgical and anesthetic management by revealing information that results in the avoidance of unnecessary reoperations and the salvage of viable myocardium.

Finally, however, a cost-benefit analysis is appropriate. While data on the use of TEE for noncardiac surgical procedures are insufficient to permit a definitive cost-benefit analysis, data are available for patients undergoing congenital, valvular, or coronary surgery. Assuming at least 300 TEE studies per year, patients undergoing surgery for congenital heart disease derive the greatest overall benefits—approximately a $600 savings per case. Patients receiving coronary bypass grafts derive the next greatest benefit—ranging from $100 to $300 per case depending upon assumptions regarding the role of TEE in the prevention of intraoperative strokes.[73–75] In contrast, patients having valve replacement have an increased cost of about $150 per case.[117]

References

1. Frazin L, Talano JV, Stephanides L, et al: Esophageal echocardiography. Circulation 54:102, 1976.
2. Matsumoto M, Oka Y, Strom J, et al: Application of transesophageal echocardiography to continuous intraoperative monitoring of left ventricular performance. Am J Cardiol 46:95, 1980.
3. Schluter M, Langenstein BA, Polster J, et al: Transoesophageal cross-sectional echocardiography with a phased array transducer system. Technique and initial clinical results. Br Heart J 48:67, 1982.
4. Roizen MF, Beaupre PN, Alpert RA, et al: Monitoring with two-dimensional transesophageal echocardiography. Comparison of myocardial function in patients undergoing supraceliac, suprarenal-infraceliac, or infrarenal aortic occlusion. J Vasc Surg 1: 300, 1984.
5. Beaupre PN, Roizen MF, Cahalan MK, et al: Hemodynamic and two-dimensional transesophageal echocardiographic analysis of an anaphylactic reaction in a human. Anesthesiology 60:482, 1984.
6. Lancee CT, de JN, Bom N: Design and construction of an esophageal phased array probe. Med Prog Technol 13:139, 1988.
7. Hodgins L, Kisslo JA, Mark JB: Perioperative transesophageal echocardiography: The anesthesiologist as cardiac diagnostician. Anesth Analg 80:4, 1995.
8. Missri J: Transesophageal Echocardiography. Clinical and Intraoperative Applications. New York, Churchill Livingstone, 1993.
9. Stumper O, Sutherland GR: Transesophageal Echocardiography in Congenital Heart Disease. London, Edward Arnold, 1994.
10. Kolev N, Huemer G, Zimpfer M: Transesophageal echocardiography. New York, Springer-Verlag, 1995.
11. Hatle L, Brubakk A, Tromsdal A, Angelsen B: Noninvasive assessment of pressure drop in mitral stenosis by Doppler ultrasound. Br Heart J 40:131, 1978.
12. Holen J, Simonsen S: Determination of pressure gradient in mitral stenosis with Doppler echocardiography. Br Heart J 41:529, 1979.
13. Cohen GI, White M, Sochowski RA, et al: Reference values for normal adult transesophageal echocardiographic measurements. J Am Soc Echocardiogr 8:221, 1995.
14. Cheung AT, Savino JS, Weiss SJ, et al: Echocardiographic and hemodynamic indexes of left ventricular preload in patients with normal and abnormal ventricular function. Anesthesiology 81: 376, 1994.
15. Clements FM, Harpole DH, Quill T, et al: Estimation of left ventricular volume and ejection fraction by two-dimensional transoesophageal echocardiography: Comparison of short axis imaging and simultaneous radionuclide angiography. Br J Anaesth 64:331, 1990.
16. Cahalan MK, Ionescu P, Melton HJ, et al: Automated real-time analysis of intraoperative transesophageal echocardiograms. Anesthesiology 78:477, 1993.
17. Bednarz JE, Marcus RH, Lang RM: Technical guidelines for performing automated border detection studies. J Am Soc Echocardiogr 8:293, 1995.
18. Morrissey RL, Siu SC, Guerrero JL, et al: Automated assessment of ventricular volume and function echocardiography: Validation of automated border detection. J Am Soc Echocardiogr 7:107, 1994.
19. Muhiudeen IA, Kuecherer HF, Lee E, et al: Intraoperative estimation of cardiac output by transesophageal pulsed Doppler echocardiography. Anesthesiology 74:9, 1991.
20. Savino JS, Troianos CA, Aukburg S, et al: Measurement of pulmonary blood flow with transesophageal two-dimensional and Doppler echocardiography. Anesthesiology 75:445, 1991.
21. Darmon P-L, Hillel Z, Mogtader A, et al: Cardiac output by transesophageal echocardiography using continuous-wave Doppler across the aortic valve. Anesthesiology 80:796, 1994.
22. Pu M, Griffin BP, Vanderwoort PM, et al: Intraoperative validation of mitral inflow determination by transesophageal echocardiography: Comparison of single-plane, biplane and thermodilution. J Am Coll Cardiol 26:1047, 1995.
23. Feinberg MS, et al: Multiplane transesophageal echocardiographic Doppler imaging accurately determines cardiac output measurements in critically ill patients. Chest 107:769, 1995.
24. Kuecherer HF, Muhiudeen IA, Kusumoto FM, et al: Estimation of mean left atrial pressure from transesophageal pulsed Doppler echocardiography of pulmonary venous flow. Circulation 82: 1127, 1990.
25. Hofmann T, Keck A, van Ingen G, et al: Simultaneous measurement of pulmonary venous flow by intravascular catheter Doppler velocimetry and transesophageal Doppler echocardiography: Relation to left atrial pressure and left atrial and left ventricular function. J Am Coll Cardiol 26:239, 1995.
26. Kusumoto FM, Muhiudeen IA, Kuecherer HF, et al: Response of the interatrial septum to transatrial pressure gradients and its potential for predicting pulmonary capillary wedge pressure: An intraoperative study using transesophageal echocardiography in patients during mechanical ventilation. J Am Coll Cardiol 21: 721, 1993.
27. Gorcsan J, Gasior TA, Mandarino WA, et al: Assessment of the immediate effects of cardiopulmonary bypass on left ventricular performance by on-line pressure-area relations. Circulation 89: 180, 1994.
28. Smith JS, Roizen MF, Cahalan MK, et al: Does anesthetic technique make a difference? Augmentation of systolic blood pressure during carotid endarterectomy: Effects of phenylephrine versus light anesthesia and of isoflurane versus halothane on the incidence of myocardial ischemia. Anesthesiology 69:846, 1988.
29. Tennant R, Wiggers C: The effect of coronary occlusion on myocardial contraction. Am J Physiol 112:351, 1935.

30. Battler A, Froelicher VF, Gallagher KP, et al: Dissociation between regional myocardial dysfunction and ECG changes during ischemia in the conscious dog. Circulation 62:735, 1980.
31. Hauser AM, Gangadharan V, Ramos RG, et al: Sequence of mechanical, electrocardiographic and clinical effects of repeated coronary artery occlusion in human beings: Echocardiographic observations during coronary angioplasty. J Am Coll Cardiol 5: 193, 1985.
32. Wohlgelernter D, Jaffe CC, Cabin HS, et al: Silent ischemia during coronary occlusion produced by balloon inflation: Relation to regional myocardial dysfunction. J Am Coll Cardiol 10: 491, 1987.
33. Smith JS, Cahalan MK, Benefiel DJ, et al: Intraoperative detection of myocardial ischemia in high-risk patients: Electrocardiography versus two-dimensional transesophageal echocardiography. Circulation 72:1015, 1985.
34. Leung JM, OKelly B, Browner WS, et al: Prognostic importance of postbypass regional wall-motion abnormalities in patients undergoing coronary artery bypass graft surgery. Anesthesiology 71:16, 1989.
35. van Daele ME, Sutherland GR, Mitchell MM, et al: Do changes in pulmonary capillary wedge pressure adequately reflect myocardial ischemia during anesthesia? A correlative preoperative hemodynamic, electrocardiographic, and transesophageal echocardiographic study. Circulation 81:865, 1990.
36. Eisenberg MJ, London MJ, Leung JM, et al: Monitoring for myocardial ischemia during noncardiac surgery. A technology assessment of transesophageal echocardiography and 12-lead electrocardiography. The Study of Perioperative Ischemia Research Group. JAMA 268:210, 1992.
37. Saada M, Cahalan M, Lee E, et al: Echocardiographic evaluation in real time of ischemia and filling problems during surgery [in French]. Ann Fr Anesth Reanim 1989.
38. Shah PM, Kyo S, Matsumura M, Omoto R: Utility of biplane transesophageal echocardiography in left ventricular wall motion analysis. J Cardiothorac Vasc Anesth 5:316, 1991.
39. Voller H, Andresen D, Bruggemann T, et al: Transient ST segment depression during Holter monitoring: How to avoid false positive findings. Am Heart J 124:622, 1992.
40. Mooss AN, Prevedel JA, Mohiuddin SM, et al: Effect of digoxin on ST-segment changes detected by ambulatory electrocardiographic monitoring in healthy subjects. Am J Cardiol 68:1503, 1991.
41. Agati L, Renzi M, Sciomer S, et al: Transesophageal dipyridamole echocardiography for diagnosis of coronary artery disease. J Am Coll Cardiol 19:765, 1992.
42. Zabalgoitia M, Gandhi DK, Abi MP, et al: Transesophageal stress echocardiography: Detection of coronary artery disease in patients with normal resting left ventricular contractility. Am Heart J 122:1456, 1991.
43. Lambertz H, Kreis A, Trumper H, Hanrath P: Simultaneous transesophageal atrial pacing and transesophageal two-dimensional echocardiography: A new method of stress echocardiography. J Am Coll Cardiol 16:1143, 1990.
44. Kamp O, De CC, Kupper AJ, et al: Simultaneous transesophageal two-dimensional echocardiography and atrial pacing for detecting coronary artery disease. Am J Cardiol 69:1412, 1992.
45. Pandian NG, Skorton DJ, Collins SM, et al: Heterogeneity of left ventricular segmental wall thickening and excursion in 2-dimensional echocardiograms of normal human subjects. Am J Cardiol 51:1667, 1983.
46. Braunwald E, Kloner RA: The stunned myocardium: Prolonged, postischemic ventricular dysfunction. Circulation 66:1146, 1982.
47. Aronson S, Lee BK, Wiencek JG, et al: Assessment of myocardial perfusion during CABG surgery with two-dimensional transesophageal contrast echocardiography. Anesthesiology 75: 433, 1991.
48. Buffington CW, Coyle RJ: Altered load dependence of postischemic myocardium. Anesthesiology 75:464, 1991.
49. Lowenstein E, Haering JM, Douglas PS: Acute ventricular wall motion heterogeneity. A valuable but imperfect index of myocardial ischemia. Anesthesiology 75:385, 1991.
50. Seeberger MD, Cahalan MK, Chu E, et al: Sensitivity of intraoperative stress testing for the detection of coronary artery disease (Abstract). Anesthesiology 79:A64, 1993.
51. Force T, Kemper A, Perkins L, et al: Overestimation of infarct size by quantitative two-dimensional echocardiography: The role of tethering and of analytic procedures. Circulation 73:1360, 1986.
52. Abel MD, Nishimura RA, Cahalan MJ, et al: Evaluation of intraoperative transesophageal two-dimensional echocardiography. Anesthesiology 66:64, 1987.
53. Konstadt SN, Abrahams HP, Nejat M, Reich DL: Are wall thickening measurements reproducible? Anesth Analg 78:619, 1994.
54. Stoddard MF, Arce J, Liddell NE, et al: Two-dimensional transesophageal echocardiographic determination of aortic valve area in adults with aortic stenosis. Am Heart J 122:1415, 1991.
55. Hoffmann R, Flachskampf FA, Hanrath P: Planimetry of orifice area in aortic stenosis using multiplane transesophageal echocardiography. J Am Coll Cardiol 22:529, 1993.
56. Hofmann T, Kasper W, Meinertz T, et al: Determination of aortic valve orifice area in aortic valve stenosis by two-dimensional transesophageal echocardiography. Am J Cardiol 59:330, 1987.
57. Stamm RB, Martin RP: Quantification of pressure gradients across stenotic valves by Doppler ultrasound. J Am Coll Cardiol 2:707, 1983.
58. Black IW, Hopkins AP, Lee LC, Walsh WF: Left atrial spontaneous echo contrast: A clinical and echocardiographic analysis. J Am Coll Cardiol 18:398, 1991.
59. Thomas JD, Liu CM, Flachskampf FA, et al: Quantification of jet flow by momentum analysis. An in vitro color Doppler flow study. Circulation 81:247, 1990.
60. Schiller NB, Foster E, Redberg RF: Transesophageal echocardiography in the evaluation of mitral regurgitation. Cardiol Clin 11:339, 1993.
61. Sheikh KH, de Bruijn NP, Rankin JS, et al: The utility of transesophageal echocardiography and Doppler color flow imaging in patients undergoing cardiac valve surgery. J Am Coll Cardiol 15:363, 1990.
62. Risk SC, D'Ambra MN, Griffin B, et al: Left atrial V waves following mitral valve replacement are not specific for significant mitral regurgitation. J Cardiothorac Vasc Anesth 6:3, 1992.
63. Moulijn AC, Smulders YM, Koolen JJ, et al: Intraoperative assessment of the mitral valve: Transesophageal Doppler echocardiography vs. left ventricular filling of the flaccid heart. Eur J Cardiothorac Surg 6:122, 1992.
64. Meloni L, et al: Regurgitant flow of mitral valve prostheses: An intraoperative transesophageal echocardiographic study. J Am Soc Echocardiogr 7:36, 1994.
65. Movsowitz HD, et al: Long-term followup of mitral paraprosthetic regurgitation by transesophageal echocardiography. J Am Soc Echocardiogr 7:488, 1994.
66. Garcia MJ, Vandervoort P, Stewart WJ, et al: Mechanisms of hemolysis with mitral prosthetic regurgitation. J Am Coll Cardiol 27:399, 1996.
67. Muhiudeen IA, Roberson DA, Silverman NH, et al: Intraoperative echocardiography in infants and children with congenital cardiac shunt lesions: Transesophageal versus epicardial echocardiography. J Am Coll Cardiol 16:1687, 1990.
68. Muhiudeen IA, Roberson DA, Silverman NH, et al: Intraoperative echocardiography for evaluation of congenital heart defects in infants and children. Anesthesiology 76:165, 1992.
69. Gussenhoven EJ, van HL, Roelandt J, et al: Intraoperative two-dimensional echocardiography in congenital heart disease. J Am Coll Cardiol 9:565, 1987.
70. Ungerleider RM, Greeley WJ, Sheikh KH, et al: Routine use of intraoperative epicardial echocardiography and Doppler color flow imaging to guide and evaluate repair of congenital heart lesions. A prospective study. J Thorac Cardiovasc Surg 100:297, 1990.
71. Deutsch HJ, Curtius JM, Leischik R, et al: Diagnostic value of transesophageal echocardiography in cardiac surgery. Thorac Cardiovasc Surg 39:199, 1991.
72. Sheikh KH, Bengtson JR, Rankin JS, et al: Intraoperative transesophageal Doppler color flow imaging used to guide patient selection and operative treatment of ischemic mitral regurgitation. Circulation 84:594, 1991.
73. Katz ES, Tunick PA, Rusinek H, et al: Protruding aortic atheromas predict stroke in elderly patients undergoing cardiopulmonary bypass: Experience with intraoperative transesophageal echocardiography. J Am Coll Cardiol 20:70, 1992.

74. Konstadt SN, Reich DL, Kahn R, Viggiani RF: Transesophageal echocardiography can be used to screen for ascending aortic atherosclerosis. Anesth Analg 81:225, 1995.
75. Ribakove GH, Katz ES, Galloway AC, et al: Surgical implications of transesophageal echocardiography to grade the atheromatous aortic arch. Ann Thorac Surg 53:758, 1992.
76. Angermann CE, Kruger TM, Junge R, et al: Intravenous Albunex during transesophageal echocardiography. Quantitative assessment by videodensitometry and integrated backscatter analysis from unprocessed radiofrequency signals. J Am Soc Echocardiogr 8:839, 1995.
77. Villanueva FS, Glasheen WP, Sklenar J, et al: Successful and reproducible myocardial opacification during two dimensional echocardiography from right heart injection of contrast. Circulation 4:1557, 1992.
78. Monaghan MJ, Metcalfe JM, Odunlami S, et al: Digital radiofrequency echocardiography in the detection of myocardial contrast following intravenous administration of Albunex®. Eur Heart J 14:1200, 1993.
79. Rovai D, Ferdeghini EM, Mazzarisi A, et al: Quantitative aspects in myocardial contrast echocardiography. Eur Heart J 16(Suppl J):42, 1995.
80. Buckmaster MJ, et al: Further experience with transesophageal echocardiography in the evaluation of thoracic aortic injury. J Trauma 37:989, 1994.
81. Vignon P, Gueret P, Vedrinne J-M, et al: Role of transesophageal echocardiography in the diagnosis and management of traumatic aortic disruption. Circulation 92:2959, 1995.
82. Bansal RC, Chandrasekaran K, Ayala K, Smith DC: Frequency and explanation of false negative diagnosis of aortic dissection by aortography and transesophageal echocardiography. J Am Coll Cardiol 25:1393, 1995.
83. Nienaber CA, von Kodolitsch Y, Nicolas V, et al: The diagnosis of thoracic aortic dissection by noninvasive imaging procedures. N Engl J Med 328:1, 1993.
84. Blanchard DG, Kimura BJ, Dittrich HC, DeMaria AN: Transesophageal echocardiography of the aorta. JAMA 272:546, 1994.
85. Savage RM, Llana MG, Koch CG, et al: Educational program for intraoperative transesophageal echocardiography. Anesth Analg 81:399, 1995.
86. Pearlman AS, Gardin JM, Martin RP, et al: Guidelines for physician training in transesophageal echocardiography: Recommendations of the American Society of Echocardiography Committee for Physician Training in Echocardiography. J Am Soc Echocardiogr 5:187, 1992.
87. ASA/SCA Task Force on Perioperative TEE: Guidelines for perioperative transesophageal echocardiography. Anesthesiology 84: 986, 1996.
88. American Society of Echocardiography: Recommendations for continuous quality improvement in echocardiography. J Am Soc Echocardiogr 8:S1, 1995.
89. de Simone R, Lange R, Saggau W, et al: Intraoperative transesophageal echocardiography for the evaluation of mitral, aortic and tricuspid valve repair. A tool to optimize surgical outcome. Eur J Cardiothorac Surg 6:665, 1992.
90. de Simone R, Lange R, Tanzeem A, et al: Adjustable tricuspid valve annuloplasty assisted by intraoperative transesophageal color Doppler echocardiography. Am J Cardiol 71:926, 1993.
91. Dan M, Bonato R, Mazzucco A, et al: Value of transesophageal echocardiography during repair of congenital heart defects. Ann Thorac Surg 50:637, 1990.
92. Fyfe DA, Kline CH, Sade RM, et al: The utility of transesophageal echocardiography during and after Fontan operations in small children. Am Heart J 122:1403, 1991.
93. Guyton SW, Paull DL, Anderson RP: Mitral valve reconstruction. Am J Surg 163:497, 1992.
94. Stumper O, Kaulitz R, Elzenga NJ, et al: The value of transesophageal echocardiography in children with congenital heart disease. J Am Soc Echocardiogr 4:164, 1991.
95. Freeman WK, Schaff HV, Khandheria BK, et al: Intraoperative evaluation of mitral valve regurgitation and repair by transesophageal echocardiography: Incidence and significance of systolic anterior motion. J Am Coll Cardiol 20:599, 1992.
96. Roberson DA, Muhiudeen IA, Silverman NH, et al: Intraoperative transesophageal echocardiography of atrioventricular septal defect. J Am Coll Cardiol 18:537, 1991.
97. Dahm M, Iversen S, Schmid FX, et al: Intraoperative evaluation of reconstruction of the atrioventricular valves by transesophageal echocardiography. Thorac Cardiovasc Surg 2:140, 1987.
98. Reichert CL, Visser CA, Koolen JJ, et al: Transesophageal echocardiography in hypotensive patients after cardiac operations. Comparison with hemodynamic parameters. J Thorac Cardiovasc Surg 104:321, 1992.
99. Cucchiara RF, Nugent M, Seward JB, Messick JM: Air embolism in upright neurosurgical patients: Detection and localization by two-dimensional transesophageal echocardiography. Anesthesiology 60:353, 1984.
100. Cucchiara RF, Seward JB, Nishimura RA, et al: Identification of patent foramen ovale during sitting position craniotomy by transesophageal echocardiography with positive airway pressure. Anesthesiology 63:107, 1985.
101. Glenski JA, Cucchiara RF, Michenfelder JD: Transesophageal echocardiography and transcutaneous O2 and CO2 monitoring for detection of venous air embolism. Anesthesiology 64:541, 1986.
102. Rafferty T, LaMantia KR, Davis E, et al: Quality assurance for intraoperative transesophageal echocardiography monitoring: A report of 846 procedures. Anesth Analg 76:228, 1993.
103. Owall A, Stahl L, Settergren G: Incidence of sore throat and patient complaints after intraoperative transesophageal echocardiography during cardiac surgery. J Cardiothorac Vasc Anesth 6: 15, 1992.
104. Messina AG, Paranicas M, Fiamengo S, et al: Risk of dysphagia after transesophageal echocardiography. Am J Cardiol 67:313, 1991.
105. Hulyalkar AR, Ayd JD: Low risk of gastroesophageal injury associated with transesophageal echocardiography during cardiac surgery. J Cardiothorac Vasc Anesth 7:175, 1993.
106. Shintani H, Nakano S, Matsuda H, et al: Efficacy of transesophageal echocardiography as a perioperative monitor in patients undergoing cardiovascular surgery. Analysis of 149 consecutive studies. J Cardiovasc Surg (Torino) 31:564, 1990.
107. Latham P, Hodgins LR: A gastric laceration after transesophageal echocardiography in a patient undergoing aortic valve replacement. Anesth Analg 81:638, 1995.
108. Kharasch ED, Sivarajan M: Gastroesophageal perforation after intraoperative transesophageal echocardiography. Anesthesiology 85:426, 1996.
109. Spahn DR, Schmid S, Carrel T, et al: Hypopharynx perforation by a transesophageal echocardiography probe. Anesthesiology 82:581, 1995.
110. Dewhirst WE, Stragand JJ, Fleming BM: Mallory-Weiss tear complicating intraoperative transesophageal echocardiography in a patient undergoing aortic valve replacement. Anesthesiology 73:777, 1990.
111. Polhamus CD, Werth TE, Clement DJ, et al: Gastrointestinal bleeding complicating transesophageal echocardiography. Endoscopy 25:198, 1993.
112. Daniel WG, Erbel R, Kasper W, et al: Safety of transesophageal echocardiography. A multicenter survey of 10,419 examinations. Circulation 83:817, 1991.
113. Foster E, Schiller NB: The role of transesophageal echocardiography in critical care: UCSF experience. J Am Soc Echocardiogr 5:368, 1992.
114. Read RC, Finch RG, Donald FE, et al: Infective endocarditis after transesophageal echocardiography. Circulation 87:1426, 1993.
115. Lunn RJ, Oliver WJ, Hagler DJ, Danielson GK: Aortic compression by transesophageal echocardiographic probe in infants and children undergoing cardiac surgery. Anesthesiology 77:587, 1992.
116. Gilbert TB, Panico FG, McGill WA, et al: Bronchial obstruction by transesophageal echocardiography probe in a pediatric cardiac patient. Anesth Analg 74:156, 1992.
117. Benson M, Cahalan MK: Cost effectiveness of transesophageal echocardiography during cardiac surgery. Echocardiography 12: 171, 1995.

CHAPTER 11

Monitoring Oxygenation and Ventilation

James B. Eisenkraft, M.D.
Steven J. Barker, M.D., Ph.D.

Monitoring oxygenation and ventilation is fundamental to the care of all anesthetized patients. It is especially important in those undergoing major surgery of the heart, lungs, or major vessels because the surgical procedures may well involve the vital organs responsible for maintaining gas exchange and perfusion.

The basic physiology of oxygen and carbon dioxide transfer are extensively described elsewhere[1] and will therefore be only reviewed briefly in this chapter. Similarly, monitoring technology is the subject of several major texts[2–4] and so it too will be reviewed only briefly. The intent of this chapter will be to discuss each of the commonly used clinical monitors in relation to its application during cardiac, thoracic, and vascular surgery.

Oxygen and Oxygenation

Oxygen

Cascade

Oxygen flows from the environment, down a partial pressure gradient, to the mitochondria of the cells where it is used to maintain aerobic metabolism. The partial pressure of oxygen in dry room air is 159 mm Hg (21% of 760 mm Hg). The critical oxygen tension for aerobic metabolism in the mitochondria of cells is about 2 mm Hg; at lower Po_2's oxidative phosphorylation stops and aerobic metabolism ensues. Movement of oxygen between the atmosphere and the cells involves several steps, at each of which the oxygen tension decreases. These steps, which constitute the *oxygen cascade*, have been nicely described by Nunn,[1] and include:

Inspired oxygen tension dry (P_{IO_2})
Inspired oxygen tension humidified (at 37°C)
End-expiratory oxygen tension ($P_{E'O_2}$)
Ideal alveolar oxygen tension (P_{AO_2})
Arterial oxygen tension (Pa_{O_2})
Mean capillary blood oxygen tension (Pc'_{O_2})
Cytoplasmic oxygen tension
Mitochondrial oxygen tension

Oxygen Transport

The first part of the oxygen cascade involves delivery of oxygen to the alveoli whence it is transported in the arterial blood to the tissues. The amount of oxygen brought to the tissues depends upon the oxygen content of the blood and the blood flow to the tissues. The main determinant of oxygen transport is therefore the arterial blood oxygen *content* (Ca_{O_2}), which is expressed in milliliters of oxygen per 100 ml of blood. Thus

$$Ca_{O_2} = Hb \times 1.34 \times HbO_2\% + 0.003 \times Pa_{O_2} \quad (11-1)$$

where Ca_{O_2} = ml O_2/dl blood, Hb = total hemoglobin concentration (gm/dl), 1.34 = ml O_2 carried by 1 gm of fully saturated Hb, $HbO_2\%$ = fractional saturation of total hemoglobin, and 0.003 = solubility coefficient of oxygen in plasma (ml O_2/dl plasma per mm Hg O_2 tension). Thus oxygen is carried in combination with hemoglobin and as dissolved oxygen in the plasma.

Hemoglobin Saturation

Oxygen combines reversibly with normal adult hemoglobin. This reversible combination depends upon several factors, but most important is the Pa_{O_2}; the higher the Pa_{O_2}, the more O_2 is combined with hemoglobin. The ratio of the amount of oxygen actually combined with hemoglobin to the amount that could be bound if the hemoglobin carried all the oxygen that it possibly could is termed the hemoglobin saturation, which is normally expressed as a percentage ($HbO_2\%$). The normal relationship between HbO_2 and Pa_{O_2} is sigmoid (Fig. 11–1). The position of the oxygen-hemoglobin dissociation curve is often defined by the P_{50} (i.e., the Po_2 at which the hemoglobin is 50% saturated with oxygen). This is normally 26.5 mm Hg. Changes in 2,3-diphos-

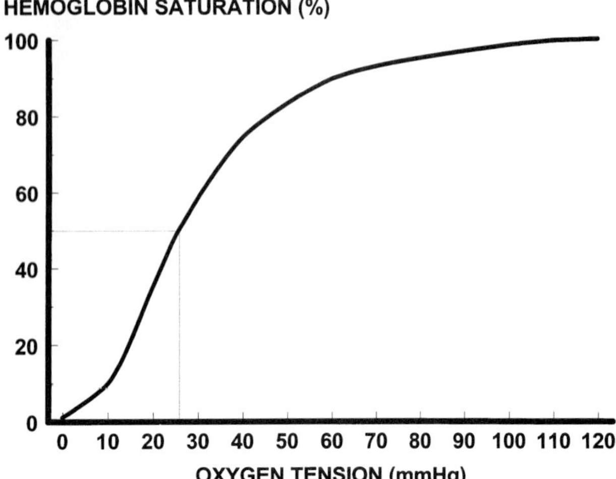

FIGURE **11–1.** Oxygen hemoglobin dissociation curve. The *dotted line* shows the P_{50}. This is the Po_2 at which the hemoglobin is 50% saturated with oxygen. It is normally 26.5 mm Hg.

phoglycerate (2,3-DPG), temperature and acid-base balance result in a shift of the curve and a change in the P_{50}. At Pao_2's greater than 100 mm Hg, $HbO_2\%$ is normally 100 and becomes independent of the Pao_2.

In Equation 11–1 above, Hb is defined as the *total* hemoglobin concentration. Total hemoglobin comprises all species of hemoglobin that may be present in the blood sample, including oxygenated (HbO_2) and deoxygenated (loosely termed "reduced") hemoglobin (RHb), methemoglobin (MetHb), and carboxyhemoglobin (COHb). The latter two are termed dyshemoglobins and do not combine with oxygen. It is therefore necessary to further qualify the definitions of saturation as being either fractional or functional.

Fractional saturation ($HbO_2\%$)

$$= \frac{\text{oxygenated hemoglobin}}{\text{total hemoglobin}}$$

$$\text{i.e., } HbO_2\% = \frac{HbO_2}{HbO_2 + RHb + COHb + MetHb} \times 100$$

Functional saturation ($Sao_2\%$)

$$= \frac{\text{oxygenated hemoglobin}}{\text{hemoglobin capable of } O_2 \text{ carriage}} \times 100$$

$$\text{i.e., } Sao_2\% = \frac{HbO_2}{RHb + HbO_2} \times 100$$

Note that dyshemoglobins are not part of the denominator in the determination of functional hemoglobin.

Fractional and functional saturation are usually measured in a laboratory co-oximeter. This is a spectrophotometric instrument that uses four or more different wavelengths of light to measure the hemoglobin species present and to quantify each. Thus if a co-oximeter analysis of a sample of arterial blood showed HbO_2 = 96%, RHb = 0%, COHb = 2%, and MetHb = 2%, the $HbO_2\%$ would be 96 (96/100), while the Sao_2 would be 100% (96/96).

In calculating Cao_2, it is important to multiply *total Hb* by the *fractional* hemoglobin oxygen saturation. Thus if the Pao_2 = 100 mm Hg, $HbO_2\%$ = 96 (dyshemoglobins = 4%), and total Hb = 15 gm/dl, the quantity of oxygen carried in combination with hemoglobin would be

$$15 \times 0.96 \times 1.34 = 19.3 \text{ ml/dl blood}$$

Dissolved Oxygen

Oxygen is also transported in solution (i.e., dissolved) in the plasma. The quantity of oxygen dissolved in plasma is directly proportional to Po_2, but also varies with temperature, being greater at lower temperatures. At 37°C the solubility of oxygen is 0.003 ml/dl/mm Hg Po_2. Thus at a Po_2 of 100 mm Hg the dissolved oxygen is 0.3 ml/dl plasma.

The volume of oxygen carried in solution is normally much less than that carried in combination with hemoglobin (0.3 ml/dl vs. 19.3 ml/dl). Thus the Cao_2 is normally most dependent upon *total* hemoglobin and *fractional* saturation. In the above example, Cao_2 = (19.3 + 0.3) = 19.6 ml/dl blood.

In certain circumstances (e.g., in a hyperbaric chamber), the Po_2 can be increased substantially, in which case dissolved oxygen can become a significant quantity.[5] Thus at 3 atmospheres absolute pressure breathing 100% O_2 the $PIo_2 = 3 \times 760 = 2{,}280$ mm Hg. Arterial blood equilibrated at a Po_2 of 2,200 mm Hg would dissolve $0.003 \times 2{,}200 = 6.6$ ml/dl oxygen.

Oxygen Delivery/Oxygen Flux

The total flow rate of oxygen to the tissues is the product of the arterial blood oxygen content (Cao_2) and the cardiac output (CO). This is termed the oxygen delivery ($\dot{D}o_2$) or oxygen flux.

If CO is 5,000 ml/min, using the Cao_2 of 19.6 ml/dl derived above, $\dot{D}o_2 = 19.6 \times 50 = 980$ ml/min or approximately 1 L/min. The oxygen flux represents the quantity of oxygen leaving the left side of the heart per minute.

Arteriovenous Oxygen Content Difference

In a 70-kg man the oxygen consumption is approximately 250 ml/min. If CO is 5,000 ml/min, this oxygen consumption represents an oxygen removal of 250/5,000 or 5 ml oxygen per deciliter of arterial blood. Thus the arteriovenous blood oxygen content difference is 5 ml/dl. Since Cao_2 is normally about 20 ml/dl, mixed venous blood oxygen content ($C\bar{v}o_2$) is 15 ml/dl. The hemoglobin saturation of mixed venous blood is 75% (15/20 × 100%), and this corresponds to a Po_2 of about 40 mm Hg (Fig. 11–1).

Oxygen consumption ($\dot{V}O_2$) may be derived as follows:

$$\dot{V}O_2 = (CaO_2 - C\bar{v}O_2) \times CO \qquad (11-2)$$

This is an adaptation of the Fick principle. Solution of the equation requires analysis of an arterial blood sample to measure Hb, $HbO_2\%$, and PaO_2. $C\bar{v}O_2$ requires analysis of a mixed venous blood sample, which is drawn from the pulmonary artery via a pulmonary artery catheter and represents a mixture of venous blood from the drainage areas of both the superior and inferior venae cavae. The blood is sampled when the balloon on the catheter tip is deflated. If the sampling is performed with the balloon inflated (i.e., catheter in wedged position), an arterialized blood sample would be obtained, which would result in erroneous values for the $C\bar{v}O_2$ term. CO is also measured using the pulmonary artery catheter.

Patient Appearance: Clinical Diagnosis of Hypoxemia

The clinical assessment of a patient's oxygenation ("blueness" or "pinkness") is unreliable. Comroe and Botelho[6] studied the ability of observers to detect cyanosis by comparing their estimations of patient color with hemoglobin-oxygen saturation, which were at that time measured using a Millikan ear oximeter (accuracy ±3%). Most of the 127 observers failed to detect the presence of definite cyanosis until hemoglobin-oxygen saturation fell to approximately 80%. Twenty-five per cent of the observers did not recognize saturation levels of 71 to 75%. Kelman and Nunn[7] pointed out that the type of lamp used affected recognition of cyanosis and that the hospital lighting should be standardized. More recent studies using modern pulse oximeters have shown that major desaturations (defined as <85%) often pass undetected by the clinician if a pulse oximeter is not used.[8,9] Thus, while an astute clinician is important for patient care, certain aspects of clinical observation are greatly enhanced by use of modern technology.

Monitors of Oxygen and Oxygenation

Anesthesia Delivery System

ANESTHESIA MACHINE

Oxygen is usually delivered to the patient from an anesthesia delivery system.[10] Such systems are supplied with compressed oxygen either via the pipeline or from oxygen tanks. The anesthesia delivery system incorporates various safeguards to ensure that a hypoxic gas mixture is not delivered from the machine's common gas outlet to the anesthesia circuit. Such safeguards include the medical gas pin index system and the diameter indexed safety system which ensure, respectively, that only an oxygen tank can hang in an oxygen hanger yoke on the machine, and that the oxygen pipeline hose connects specifically with the oxygen inlet of the machine. An oxygen low-pressure alarm is activated if the oxygen supply pressure to the machine decreases below a threshold of 30 pounds per square inch gauge (psig), and the pressure sensor shut-off ("fail-safe") valve interrupts the flow of all gases other than oxygen if the oxygen supply pressure decreases to lower levels. Despite these features, delivery of a hypoxic mixture from the machine can still occur (e.g., pipeline crossover), thus one of the most important monitors is the oxygen analyzer in the anesthesia circuit.

CIRCUIT OXYGEN ANALYZER

The oxygen analyzer is generally located in the vicinity of the inspiratory unidirectional valve of the circle system, where it measures the oxygen concentration in the gas mixture flowing to the inspiratory limb. These analyzers are usually fuel cells that are essentially oxygen batteries in which a voltage is developed in response to the PO_2. They are described in more detail elsewhere.[11] These analyzers have a slow response time and, therefore, measure the average concentration of oxygen. For example, the North American Dräger O_2 Med oxygen analyzer has a 90% response time of 20 seconds.[12] They are, however, simple, reliable, inexpensive, and readily calibrated to 21% using room air as the freely available calibration standard. They are also specific for oxygen and may provide an early warning of an undesired oxygen concentration in the inspired gas when analyzers using other technologies (e.g., mass spectrometry) provide erroneous readings. Thus, a helium-oxygen mixture would result in an erroneously high oxygen concentration reading from a mass spectrometer that was not configured for helium. An excessively high concentration of desflurane may be noted as an unexpectedly low reading on the circuit oxygen analyzer.

In contemporary anesthesia delivery systems the oxygen analyzer is equipped with a low-oxygen-concentration alarm that is enabled whenever the machine is capable of delivering an anesthetic gas mixture.[13] A high-oxygen-alarm limit may also be set for situations in which the administered oxygen concentration should be limited, such as during the use of a helium-oxygen (70:30) mixture for laser surgery of the airway. If the helium tank were to become exhausted, the delivered oxygen concentration would increase to 100% and might result in an airway fire.

SIDESTREAM-SAMPLING: BREATH-BY-BREATH OXYGEN ANALYSIS

Monitoring of respired gases on a breath-by-breath basis is now possible with sidestream sampling (diverting) gas sampling and analysis systems. Using technologies that permit rapid (i.e., very short response times) analysis of all respired gases, and oxygen in particular, a continuous measure of oxygen concentration can be obtained. A display of oxygen concentration on the y axis against time on the x axis is termed the oxygram (analogous to the capnogram for carbon dioxide) and from it can be determined the inspired (FIO_2) as well as end-expiratory or end-tidal oxygen ($FE'O_2$) (Fig. 11–2). The normal oxygram is almost a mirror image of the normal capnogram; that is, during inspiration oxygen increases (while CO_2

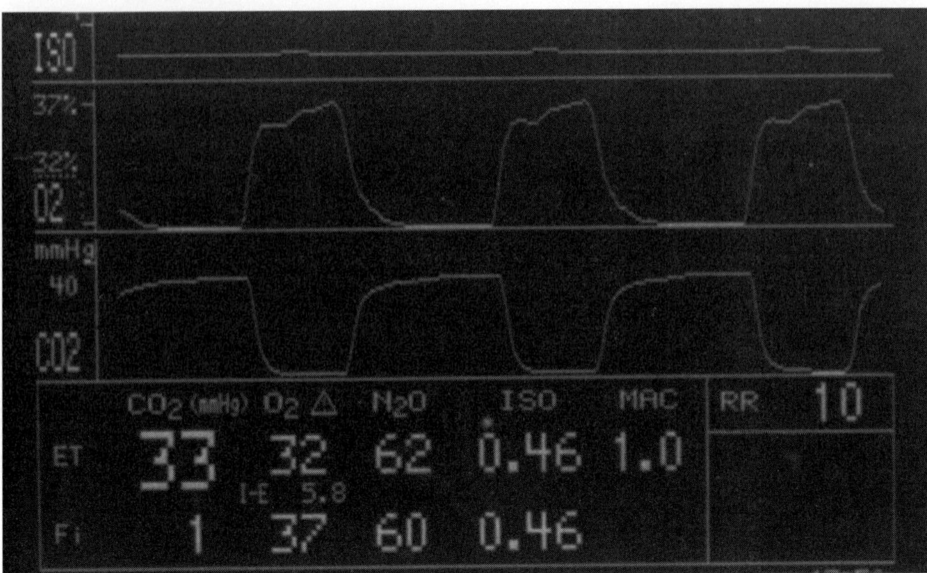

FIGURE **11–2.** Oxygram (plot of exhaled oxygen concentration vs. time) and simultaneous capnogram from a patient during mechanical ventilation as displayed by a Datex Capnomac Ultima Respiratory Gas Analyzer (Datex, Tewksbury, MA). The oxygram is almost a mirror image of the capnogram. The inspired-to-end-tidal oxygen gradient (Δ) is 5.8%.

decreases) and during exhalation oxygen concentration decreases while CO_2 increases.

The technologies that are used to measure oxygen in such monitoring systems are mass spectrometry (e.g., Marquette Advantage, Marquette Random Access Mass Spectrometer System), Raman Spectroscopy (used in the Ohmeda Rascal II monitor), paramagnetic analysis (used in the Datex AS/3, Criticare, and certain Marquette monitors), and magnetoacoustic analysis, a variant of the paramagnetic system (used in the Brüel & Kjäer and the Hewlett Packard gas monitors). These technologies are described in detail elsewhere but each provide readings of inspired and end-expired oxygen, and most will display an oxygram.[11] Certain monitors (e.g., Datex AS/3) also display the "delta" or difference between inspired and end-tidal oxygen measurements (Fig. 11–2), and this measure has been touted as an indicator of metabolic status and oxygen consumption.

Monitoring oxygen by the patient's airway offers certain advantages over the fuel cell discussed in the previous section. In this sampling location one can double-check that the FIO_2 is as desired and all recent models of monitors have audible and visual low-oxygen-concentration alarms.

A rapidly responding oxygen analyzer measuring oxygen concentration at the patient's airway may be used to monitor preoxygenation of the patient prior to induction of anesthesia.[14–16] The usual period recommended for preoxygenation is 3 to 5 minutes, during which time nitrogen is washed out of the functional residual capacity of the lungs and oxygen is washed in. Thus, during preoxygenation the inspired oxygen concentration should be 100% and, as wash-in occurs, the $FE'O_2$ approaches 95%, since the normal delta for oxygen is about 5%. Using this technology, a study of 40 volunteers found that at 60, 120, and 180 seconds of oxygen breathing mean $FE'O_2$ was 0.78, 0.87, and 0.89, respectively —alveolar denitrogenation was approximately 83% complete at 60 seconds (allowing for 5% CO_2).[16] This was increased by a further 9% at 2 minutes. After an additional 60 seconds, only a further 2% denitrogenation was achieved.[16] Prolonging preoxygenation does, however, improve oxygen stores in various compartments of the body, from 1.2 L before oxygenation, to 3.2 L at 1 minute, to 4.8 L at 3 minutes.[16]

Monitoring of $FE'O_2$ can be used to improve the anesthesiologist's preoxygenation technique. One study found that even among experienced practitioners, more than 20% of volunteers who were being preoxygenated did not achieve an $FE'O_2$ of 0.90 by 3 minutes.[16] This is often due to leakage between mask and face because effective denitrogenation cannot occur if room air is being entrained during preoxygenation. Monitoring $FE'O_2$ during preoxygenation is recommended in all patients who require optimal oxygen reserve prior to the induction of anesthesia, and the rapid-response oxygen analyzers provide the means to accomplish this.[15]

Monitoring the difference between inspired and end-tidal oxygen has also been suggested as a means to estimate the patient's oxygen consumption ($\dot{V}O_2$), and that $\dot{V}O_2 = \dot{V}_{exp} \times (FIO_2 - FE'O_2)$, where $\dot{V}_{exp}$ is the expired minute volume read from the spirometer in the expiratory limb of the anesthesia circle, and FIO_2 and $FE'O_2$ are read from the rapid response oxygen analyzer.[17,18] Such an approach does not provide an accurate estimate of $\dot{V}O_2$ for the following reasons. The rate of oxygen uptake by the lungs per minute ($\dot{V}O_2$) is given by the following equation:

$$\dot{V}O_2 = (\dot{V}_{insp} \times FIO_2) - (\dot{V}_{exp} \times F\bar{E}O_2), \quad (11\text{–}3)$$

where $\dot{V}_{insp}$ = inspired minute volume; FIO_2 = inspired oxygen fraction, therefore $(\dot{V}_{insp} \times FIO_2)$ = total amount of oxygen entering the lungs per minute; $\dot{V}_{exp}$ = expired minute volume; and $F\bar{E}O_2$ = mixed expired oxygen fraction, therefore $(\dot{V}_{exp} \times F\bar{E}O_2)$ = total amount of oxygen leaving the lungs per minute. The volumes $\dot{V}_{insp}$ and $\dot{V}_{exp}$ are not identical, and $F\bar{E}O_2$ is not the same as $FE'O_2$. $FE'O_2$ is less than $F\bar{E}O_2$. The simplified formula $\dot{V}O_2 = \dot{V}_{exp} \times (FIO_2 - FE'O_2)$, therefore, provides an overestimate of the oxygen consumption. This was confirmed in a study in which $\dot{V}O_2$ calculated using the formula in

Equation 11–3 was compared with $\dot{V}O_2$ derived via the Fick equation (Equation 11–3): $\dot{V}O_2 = (CaO_2 - C\bar{v}O_2) \times CO$.[19]

Arterial Blood Oxygen Monitoring

Oxygen Tension, Saturation, and Content

As mentioned previously, amount of oxygen in the blood can be characterized in three ways: oxygen tension (PO_2), hemoglobin saturation, and oxygen content. Oxygen tension, measured in millimeters of mercury (mm Hg), is the partial pressure exerted by oxygen in a gas phase that is in thermodynamic equilibrium with the blood. At 1 atmosphere total gas pressure, the possible range for blood oxygen tension is 0 to 760 mm Hg. Hemoglobin saturation is the percentage of the blood hemoglobin that is in the oxyhemoglobin form. This percentage can be described in two ways: The "fractional" and "functional" hemoglobin saturation as defined above. The oxygen content of the blood is usually measured in milliliters of oxygen per deciliter of blood, or vol%. The CaO_2 depends upon both oxygen tension and *fractional* hemoglobin saturation according to Equation 11–1 above.

Monitoring of Oxygen Tension

Intra-arterial Blood-Gas Sensors

The polarographic oxygen tension electrode, invented by Clark in 1956, was combined with the Severinghaus-Stowe carbon dioxide electrode and the glass pH electrode to produce the first in vitro blood-gas analyzer in 1958.[20] Although these laboratory analyzers have been the "gold standard" of blood-gas analysis for more than 30 years, they suffer two serious shortcomings for use as an intraoperative monitor. First, they provide only intermittent data, making it difficult to predict trends and immediately evaluate the effects of treatment. Second, the data are not available in "real-time"; that is, there is considerable delay between the decision to obtain blood-gas analysis and the availability of results. The need for continuous and real-time data during cardiovascular anesthesia led to several attempts to miniaturize the Clark electrode for insertion through an arterial cannula.[21,22] Although some clinical studies were promising, the miniature Clark electrodes were beset with calibration drift problems that prevented their widespread acceptance.

Another technology for oxygen tension measurement is based upon the phenomenon of photoluminescence quenching. In some chemicals, electrons can be excited to higher energy states by the absorbance of light of a specific wavelength. These excited electrons may then decay to a lower energy level by emitting light of a wavelength different from that of the excitation. This process is called photoluminescence. In some photoluminescent dyes, the emission of light can be inhibited or "quenched" by the presence of specific molecules. During photoluminescence quenching, the inhibitor molecules absorb the energy that would otherwise have been radiated as light.

Some dyes, such as pyrene-butyric acid, are specifically quenched by oxygen. The luminescent light intensity from these dyes is related to their PO_2 by an empiric formula called the Stern-Volmer equation:

$$1/I = 1/I_0 + K(PO_2) \qquad (11\text{–}4)$$

where I = intensity of luminescent light from the dye at PO_2, I_0 = intensity of luminescent light in the absence of oxygen, PO_2 = oxygen tension in the dye, and K = quenching constant.

This principle was first used to measure oxygen tension by Lubbers,[23] who coined the term "optode" to describe his sensor. After the first intra-arterial optode measurements were reported in 1984,[24] the technology underwent a period of refinement, further miniaturization; and finally the incorporation of pH, PO_2, and PCO_2 optodes into one fiberoptic sensor. Figure 11–3 shows a recent three-component optode sensor that is approximately 0.6 mm in diameter and passes easily through a

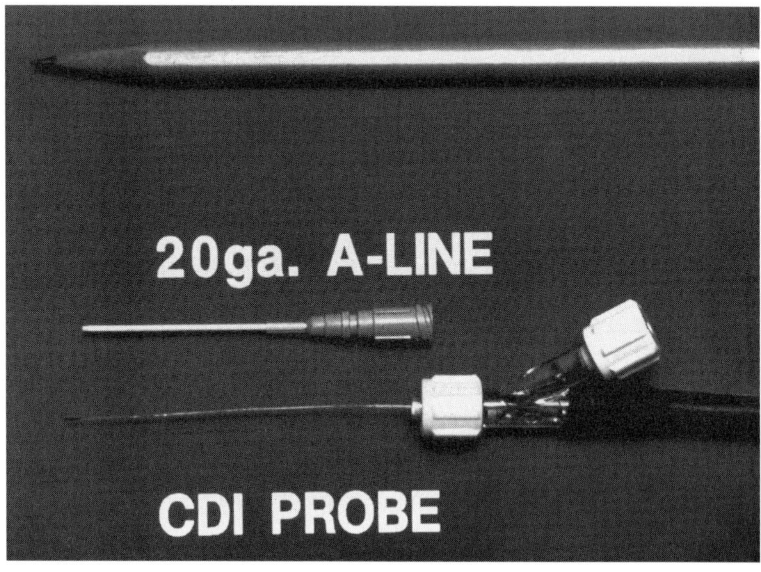

FIGURE **11–3.** Photograph of a three-component fiberoptic intra-arterial blood-gas sensor. The sensor diameter is 0.6 mm. It will fit easily through a 20-gauge arterial cannula without interfering with continuous pressure measurement and blood sampling.

20-gauge arterial cannula. The sensing dyes are encapsulated in the tips of optical fibers that transmit both the excitation light to the sensor and the luminescent light from the sensor. The luminescent light is analyzed by the instrument using a calibration based upon Equation 11–4 above. Since this equation contains two constants (I_0 and K), optodes generally require a two-point calibration prior to use. The patient data display provides continuous values of all three variables, calculated either at patient temperature or at 37°C. The sensor tip also contains a thermocouple or thermistor for measurement of blood temperature.

In vitro studies of optodes in anticoagulated, tonometered blood have demonstrated accuracy comparable to that of a commercial laboratory blood-gas analyzer.[25] The sensors also show excellent repeatability and reliability characteristics in this setting. However, when inserted into the vasculature, the optode's performance has been somewhat inconsistent. Early studies in critical care patients encountered a "down-up-down" (DUD) phenomenon, in which the optode pH values were erroneously low, P_{CO_2} was high, and P_{O_2} was low. Several explanations of this artifact have been proposed, including clot formation on the sensor, arterial wall effects, and longitudinal gradients of blood-gas values.[26] Recent development efforts have focused upon reduction of these in vivo artifacts.

Despite the technical problems in these intra-arterial sensors, some encouraging clinical results have been obtained. Figure 11–4 shows a scatter plot of intra-arterial optode oxygen tension (P_{OO_2}) versus simultaneous values of Pa_{O_2} from an in vitro analyzer.[27] These data were obtained in 14 patients undergoing various surgical procedures under general anesthesia. Figure 11–5 is a plot of P_{OO_2} and P_{OCO_2} versus time for a patient undergoing one-lung ventilation during thoracotomy. Note that the episode of hypoxemia and hypercarbia that occurred at 12:30 PM was essentially missed by the intermittent arterial blood-gas analyses, shown as + symbols. In another case report, a sudden change in P_{OO_2} alerted the anesthesiologist that a massive venous air embolism had occurred during a suboccipital craniectomy.[28] A laboratory study in dogs found that the optode was the fastest and most reliable detector of accidental endobronchial intubation (EBI) when compared with transcutaneous oxygen, blood-gas analysis, and pulse oximetry.[29] Pulse oximetry is not a reliable detector of EBI, because when F_{IO_2} is greater than 0.3 the Pa_{O_2} value may not decrease below 80 mm Hg after the event, resulting in negligible arterial desaturation. Intra-arterial optodes have also been studied in the intensive care unit (ICU), with results that encourage further development.[30]

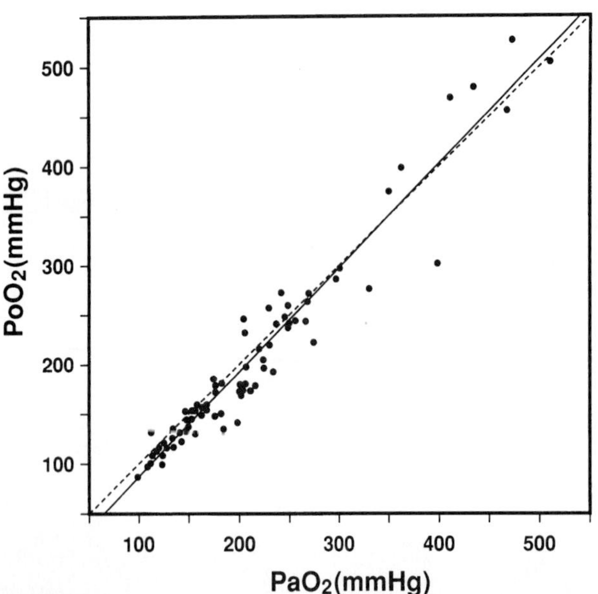

FIGURE 11–4. Scatter plot showing optode values of intra-arterial oxygen tension (P_{OO_2}) versus simultaneous values from in vitro blood gas analyzer (P_{OO_2}) (14 patients, n = 87). ----, line of identity; ——, linear regression.

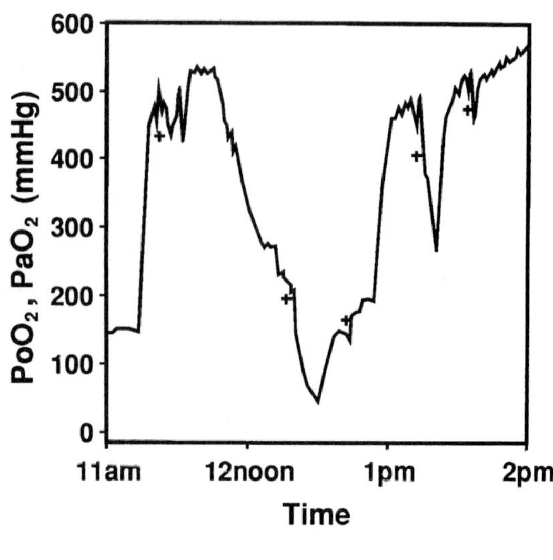

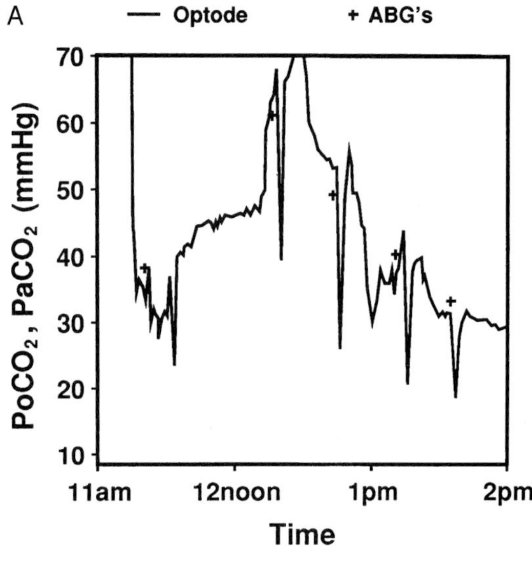

FIGURE 11–5. Continuous tracings of P_{OO_2} (*A*) and P_{OCO_2} (*B*) versus time during a thoracotomy requiring one-lung ventilation. Sequential in vitro blood-gas values are shown by + signs. Episode of hypoxemia and hypercarbia at 12:20 PM is shown in detail in optode tracing (*solid line*), but is missed by sequential blood-gas analyses (+). Trend of falling P_{OO_2} and rising P_{OCO_2} is seen well before hypoxemia or any changes in Sp_{O_2} occurred.

Intra-arterial blood-gas sensors are not in widespread use today because the above-mentioned problems of accuracy and reliability are not yet adequately solved. However, an ex vivo optode system that measures blood-gas values in a cardiopulmonary bypass circuit is commercially available and exhibits acceptable accuracy and reliability.[31] The sensors in this system are larger than the intravascular probes and are exposed to anticoagulated blood. Other applications of optode technology are under investigation, including sensors in major organs such as the brain.

Pulse Oximetry

Pulse oximetry is the technology whereby the monitor provides a noninvasive estimate of arterial hemoglobin saturation with oxygen. The ASA Standards for Basic Intraoperative Monitoring (last amended October 21, 1998) state (Standard II, Oxygenation Methods 2) that, "Blood oxygenation: During all anesthetics a quantitative method of assessing oxygenation such as pulse oximetry shall be employed."[32]

Principles of Pulse Oximetry

Pulse oximetry is a combination of two technologies: (1) spectrophotometry, whereby hemoglobin-oxygen saturation is measured; and (2) optical plethysmography, whereby the pulsatile changes in blood volume (arterial) are detected at the sensor site. While the technology is described in some detail elsewhere,[33,34] it bears a brief review here.

SPECTROPHOTOMETRY

Consider a glass chamber of fixed dimensions containing a solution of deoxygenated (loosely termed "reduced") hemoglobin (RHb). On one side of the chamber is a source of monochromatic (single wavelength) light of intensity I_{in}. On the other side of the chamber is a photodetector that detects the intensity of the light emerging. The intensity of the light emerging (I_{out}) is related to I_{in} according to the Lambert-Beer law such that

$$I_{out} = I_{in} * e^{(-\beta\lambda * C * X)} \qquad (11-5)$$

where $\beta\lambda$ is the molecular extinction coefficient for deoxygenated hemoglobin (RHb) at wavelength λ, C is the concentration of RHb, and X is the path length of the light. From this equation it can be appreciated that I_{out}/I_{in} will be small when the extinction coefficient at the wavelength chosen ($\beta\lambda$) is large (i.e., each hemoglobin molecule absorbs a lot of incident light), if C is high (i.e., there are a lot of molecules of hemoglobin per unit volume), and if X is long (i.e., long path length exposes the light to more molecules of hemoglobin). Assume for this experiment that only RHb is present, C and X remain constant, and that wavelength λ is varied. This results in the extinction curve for RHb where extinction (opacity of a unit concentration and path length of a given substance) is plotted on the y axis against wavelength λ on the x axis. Let us now keep the concentration of hemoglobin the same but fully oxygenate it so that it is now fully saturated with oxygen (i.e., RHb → HbO_2). The above experiment is repeated and provides the extinction curve for oxygenated hemoglobin (HbO_2). The curves cross at wavelength 805 nm, which is termed the isobestic point for hemoglobin (Fig. 11–6).

Pulse oximeter probes use two light-emitting diodes (LEDs), one of which emits light at 660 nm and the other at 940 nm. Reference to the extinction curves shows that at 660 nm, if all of the hemoglobin is desaturated (RHb), the absorbance of light is high, whereas if it is fully saturated the absorbance at 660 nm is low. Intermediate saturations give intermediate values for absorbance at 660 nm (Fig. 11–6).

At 940 nm, the extinction curve shows that if all of the hemoglobin is oxygenated (i.e., HbO_2), absorbance is high; whereas if it is deoxygenated (RHb), absorbance is low (Fig. 11–6). This is the opposite of what was seen at 660 nm. Intermediate saturations result in intermediate absorbencies. If the "curve" for 660 nm is divided by that for 940 nm, the result is a plot of hemoglobin saturation on the y axis, against the ratio of the absorbencies at wavelength 660 nm to that at 940 nm on the x axis. Thus, if the ratio of absorbencies 660/940 is known, the hemoglobin saturation with oxygen can be predicted. The plot of saturation against the ratio of absorbencies 660/940 is the basis for the calibration algorithm of the pulse oximeter (Fig. 11–7). In the pulse oximeter probe the LED 660 nm and LED 940 nm cycle on and off on one side of the fingertip and the single photodetector detects the intensity of the light transmitted through the finger, which is inversely related to absorbance. This cycling occurs 480 times per second (480 Hz) in the Ohmeda Biox pulse oximeter.

OPTICAL PLETHYSMOGRAPHY

Let us assume that the probe is on a fingertip and consider only LED 660 nm cycling on. The emitted light passes through skin, bone, subcutaneous tissue, venous blood, and arterial blood, any and all of which can absorb the 660-nm light. However, as a pulse of arterial (oxygenated) blood passes into the digital vessels, the path length for the light increases as the arterial bed expands to accept the extra volume of blood. An increase in absorbance (decrease in I_{out}) of light therefore occurs due to the pulse of arterial blood. This increase in absorbance is termed the "pulse-added absorbance." Similarly, there is an increase in pulse-added absorbance at wavelength 940 nm. As the LEDs cycle on and off, the resulting signals from the photodetector facilitate a continuous plot of absorbance at 660 nm and at 940 nm. The computer effectively subtracts out the constant absorbance (termed the "DC component") at each wavelength and separates out the pulse-added signal (termed the "alternating" or "AC component"). Thus from these two absorbance signals, 660 nm and 940 nm, the ratio (R) of pulse-added absorbencies is calculated and the saturation reading obtained via the algorithm discussed above and shown in Figure 11–7:

$$R = \frac{AC_{660}/DC_{660}}{AC_{940}/DC_{940}}$$

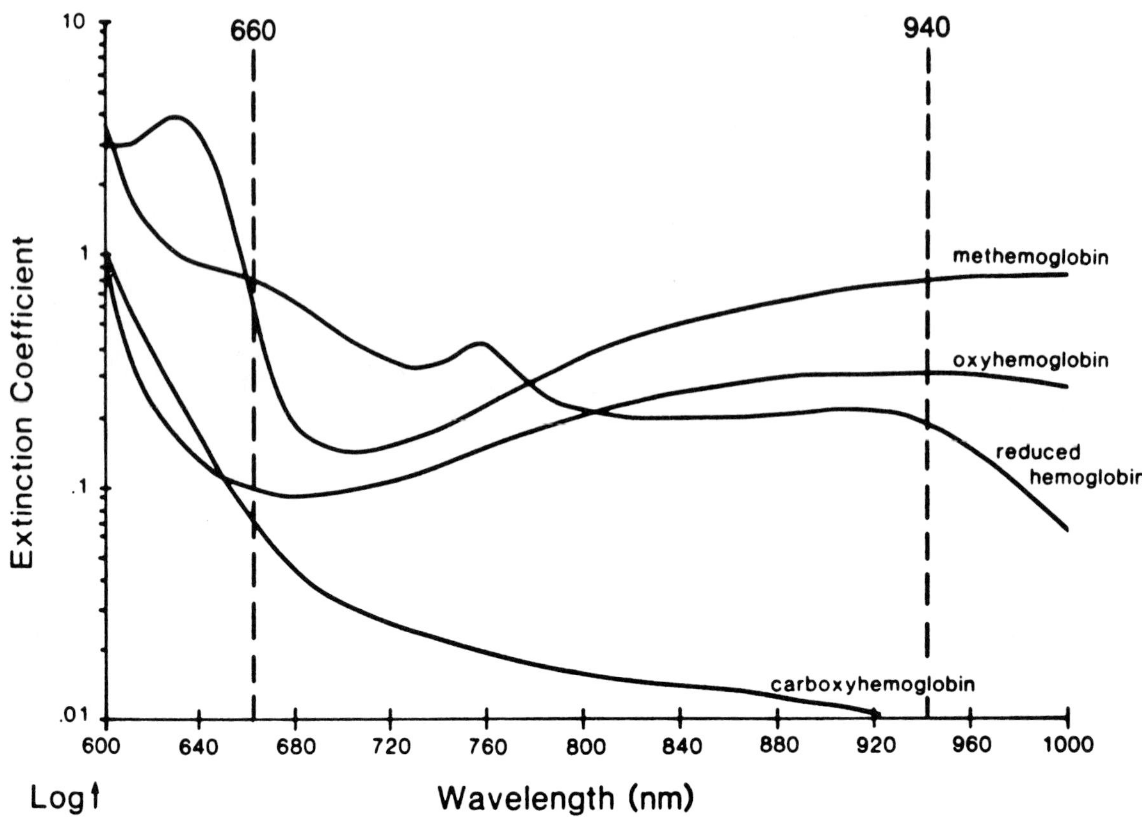

FIGURE **11–6.** Absorbance spectra for four species of hemoglobin: oxyhemoglobin; deoxygenated ("reduced") hemoglobin; carboxyhemoglobin; and methemoglobin. The *vertical dotted lines* at 660 and 940 nm indicate the wavelengths used in pulse oximetry. (From Barker SJ, Tremper KK: Pulse oximetry: Applications and limitations. Int Anesth Clin 25:155, 1987, with permission.)

Because the oximeter relies on pulsatile blood flow, it can also provide a read out of heart rate as well as (in some models, e.g., Ohmeda Biox 3700) a graphic display of the processed optical plethysmographic signal.

Calibration of the Pulse Oximeter

Pulse oximeters are calibrated empirically by the manufacturer. In the case of the Ohmeda pulse oximeter, the empiric algorithm was generated as follows. Healthy volunteers had a pulse oximeter probe attached to each finger and each ear lobe making a total of 12 probes per subject, each probe being connected to an oximeter. Each volunteer also had an artery cannulated for the withdrawal of arterial blood samples. The volunteers were then given varying concentrations of inspired oxygen to breathe (and therefore had different hemoglobin oxygen saturations), and at each steady state the average of the 12 *R* values (ratios of pulse-added absorbencies, i.e., one from each oximeter) was computed and simultaneously an arterial blood sample was drawn and analyzed for hemoglobin oxygen saturation in a laboratory co-oximeter. This process was repeated at different $F\text{IO}_2$'s (and therefore different arterial hemoglobin oxygen saturations) and the results averaged among the volunteers to develop the empiric algorithm (Fig. 11–7). This empiric algorithm is made part of the oximeter's software so that when the probe is placed on a patient, the oximeter can relate the 660/940 absorbance ratio directly to an empiric saturation reading. It should be noted that, in the case of the Ohmeda Biox 3700 algorithm, the volunteers upon whom the calibration algorithm is based had dyshemoglobin concentrations of 2% or less.

Definitions of Saturation

The definitions of saturation have been stated previously but are the cause of much confusion. Laboratory co-oximeters (e.g., Instrumentation Laboratory IL 282, IL 482; Corning; Radiometer) use multiple wavelengths of light and separately measure RHb, HbO_2, and dyshemoglobins MetHb and COHb. From these can be calculated the fractional ($HbO_2\%$) and functional ($Sa\text{O}_2\%$) saturations.

Which value ($HbO_2\%$ or $Sa\text{O}_2$) should be used in the calibration algorithm of the pulse oximeter remains controversial.[36] Most manufacturers (e.g., Nellcor) use $Sa\text{O}_2$ in the algorithm, while Ohmeda uses $HbO_2\%$. Thus if probes connected to two different brands of pulse oximeter are placed on the same patient, differences in readings between the oximeters may be due to differences in the software calibration algorithm. As saturation decreases, however, any such differences become smaller.[36] This phenomenon may also be noted in reports evaluating pulse oximeters (i.e., the pulse oximeter reading is compared with simultaneously obtained $Sa\text{O}_2$ or

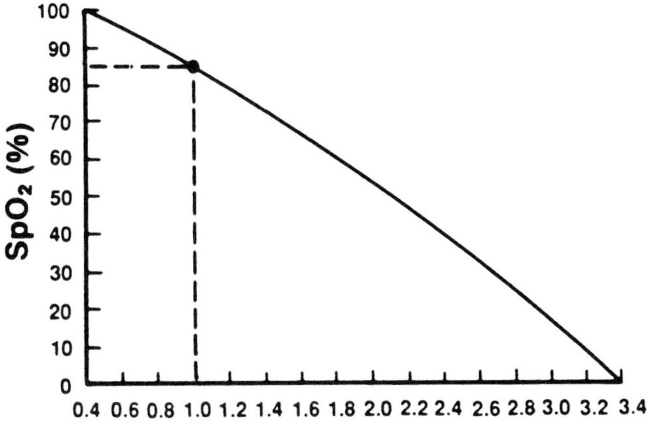

$$R = \frac{AC_{660}/DC_{660}}{AC_{940}/DC_{940}}$$

FIGURE **11–7.** Pulse oximeter calibration algorithm. The pulse oximeter reading (Spo_2) is estimated from the ratio (R) of the pulse-added absorbencies at 660 and 940 nm. Note that when $R = 1.0$, Spo_2 reads 85%. (From Tremper KK, Barker SJ: Pulse oximetry. Anesthesiology 70:98, 1989, with permission.)

HbO_2% values measured from an arterial blood sample). Clearly, pulse oximeters will be most accurate when the conditions of clinical use are most like the conditions under which the calibration algorithm was developed.

Limitations of Pulse Oximetry

1. A pulsatile arterial bed is needed. In order to measure pulse-added absorbance, arterial pulsations are required. Readings may not be obtainable when pulsatile flow is lost, such as during intense vasoconstriction, hypothermia, severe peripheral vascular disease, hypovolemia, or cardiopulmonary bypass.
2. Motion artifact. Patient or probe movement may interfere with oximeter function, since motion causes changes in optical path length. The oximeter may then fail to recognize actual pulsatile flow (see "Motion Artifact," later). The C-LOCK electrocardiogram (ECG) synchronization system is used in certain models of Nellcor pulse oximeter to overcome the above limitations. In this patented system, hemoglobin oxygen saturation is measured from a composite pulse signal obtained by timing the optical signal with the QRS complex of the ECG.[37]
3. Pulse oximetry requires a nonpulsatile venous bed. Venous pulsations (e.g., due to tricuspid regurgitation) are not distinguishable from arterial. Venous pulsations will contribute to the pulse-added absorbance signal causing a spuriously low saturation reading.
4. Pulse oximetry requires hemoglobin as the dominant color species present in the blood. Intravascular dyes, if present, may interfere with function. Similarly, certain colors of nail polish may cause spurious readings.[39]
5. The saturation reading is based upon absence of significant amounts of dyshemoglobins (e.g., MetHb, COHb). Their presence may result in spurious readings.[35,40]
6. Sensitivity to interference by electrocautery, intense ambient light, and infrared radiation.
7. Errors in pulse oximetry reading produced by improperly positioned sensors.[41,42]

DYSHEMOGLOBINS

Dyshemoglobins are hemoglobins in which the heme moiety has been changed in some way. Changes in the heme moiety affect absorbance of radiation (absorbance spectra) and may result in spurious oximeter readings. Dyshemoglobins do not combine with oxygen and can, if present in sufficient amount, produce a functional anemia.

METHEMOGLOBIN

In normal hemoglobin, iron is in the ferrous (Fe^{2+}) form; if it is oxidized to the ferric state (Fe^{3+}) methemoglobin (MetHb) results.[34,35,43,44] At wavelength 660 nm MetHb absorbs similar to RHb and at 940 nm the absorbance is similar to that at 660 nm. Thus, as the amount of MetHb increases, so the ratio of absorbencies 660/940 approaches unity. Reference to the calibration algorithm (Fig. 11–7) shows that when $R = 1.0$, the saturation reading is approximately 85%. If functional saturation (Sao_2) is high, say 100%, then increasing amounts of MetHb tend to lower the pulse oximeter saturation reading (Spo_2) towards 85%. If Sao_2 is low (e.g., 60%), increasing amounts of MetHb cause a spuriously high reading, tending towards a value of 85%.[35] If MetHb is suspected, an arterial blood sample should be drawn for analysis in a laboratory co-oximeter.[44]

Drugs causing methemoglobinemia include dapsone (used recently in prophylactic treatment of *Pneumocystis carinii* in patients infected with human immunodeficiency virus [HIV]), prilocaine, benzocaine (Hurricaine spray), nitrates, sodium nitroprusside, sulfonamides, and antimalarials.[43–45]

CARBOXYHEMOGLOBIN

Smoke inhalation and cigarette smoking result in carbon monoxide binding to hemoglobin and prevent it from carrying oxygen. Reference to the absorbance spectrum for COHb (Fig. 11–6) shows that at 660 nm it resembles HbO_2, while at 940 nm the absorbance is virtually 0. The effect on the pulse oximeter reading is such that at increasing concentrations of COHb, the reading (Spo_2) is erroneously high[40] (thus functional saturation is underestimated and fractional saturation is overestimated). If the presence of COHb is suspected, an analysis of arterial blood in a laboratory co-oximeter will provide a more accurate assessment of saturation.

PULSE OXIMETER SATURATION READING (Spo_2)

From the foregoing, it is apparent that the pulse oximeter measures neither fractional (HbO_2%) nor functional (Sao_2) saturation. For this reason the pulse oximeter estimate of saturation is designated Spo_2%. A laboratory co-oximeter uses one wavelength of light for each hemoglobin species analyzed (i.e., it would need at least four wavelengths to measure four hemoglobin species). Thus, because the pulse oximeter uses only two wavelengths, it will read inaccurately in the presence of significant amounts of dyshemoglobins.

FETAL HEMOGLOBIN AND HEMOGLOBINOPATHIES

In fetal hemoglobin (HbF) and hemoglobinopathies (e.g., HbS) the heme moiety is unaffected, the changes being in the globin chains of hemoglobin. Such changes do not produce clinically significant alterations in Spo_2 reading (i.e., any changes are well within the stated ±2% error of the pulse oximeter reading). When used in neonates or in patients with sickle cell disease or sickle cell trait the Spo_2 may be considered accurate. When used in a neonate who has a patent ductus arteriosus, however, the Spo_2 will be affected by the location of the sensor, depending upon whether the site chosen is pre- or postductal.

INTRAVENOUS DYES

The dyes most commonly used intravenously are methylene blue, indocyanine green, and indigo carmine. The first two dyes show an absorbance peak at 660 nm. Absorbance at 940 nm can be discounted for all three dyes. An intravenous bolus of methylene blue or indocyanine green causes an increase in the pulse-added absorbance ratio 660/940, resulting in a spuriously low Spo_2 reading. The reading remains low until the dye becomes sufficiently diluted in the blood.[38] At low concentrations of dye the effect on Spo_2 is not significant. From the absorbance curves it can be predicted, and clinical studies have shown, that methylene blue and indocyanine green cause spurious desaturation, while indigo carmine has little or no effect on the Spo_2 reading.[38]

It should be noted that if true Sao_2 is high, MetHb causes a spuriously low Spo_2 reading. The treatment of clinically significant methemoglobinemia is methylene blue (usually 1 mg/kg) intravenously (IV), which will produce a further spuriously low reading of Spo_2. Once the MetHb has been converted back to normal hemoglobin and the methylene blue dye has become diluted and/or excreted, the Spo_2 reading will return to normal.

NAIL POLISH

The pulse oximeter probe is usually placed so that light is transmitted across a nail bed. Certain nail polishes can affect the Spo_2 reading, causing it to be spuriously low. Coté et al.[39] found that blue and green colors caused the greatest error, while red and purple caused essentially no error in their study. They also found that error could not be predicted simply by looking at nail polish color.[39]

In order to avoid errors due to nail polish colors, polish should be removed from the nail of the finger on which the probe is to be placed. Alternatively, if the nails are polished or so thick that the intensity of transmitted light at the photodetector is too weak, the probe may be turned through 90 degrees so that light passes through the nail bed from side to side, thus avoiding the finger nail color or thickness problem.

OTHER LIMITATIONS OF PULSE OXIMETRY

From the plot of hemoglobin saturation against Po_2 (Fig. 11–1), it is apparent that at Pao_2's above about 120 mm Hg, hemoglobin oxygen saturation is 100%. The pulse oximeter is thus a poor predictor of Pao_2 until the saturation falls below 100%. A patient receiving an Fio_2 of 1.0 may have a large shunt yet still show an Spo_2 of 100%. For this reason, the pulse oximeter is a poor indicator of endobronchial intubation, especially if the Fio_2 is greater than 0.5.[29]

Standards for Monitoring

As stated above, monitoring of oxygenation is included in the ASA Standards for Basic Anesthetic Monitoring of all patients undergoing anesthesia.[32] The ASA Standards do state, however, that under extenuating circumstances the responsible anesthesiologist may waive this requirement, but they recommend that when this is done it should be so stated, with the reasons, in a note in the patient's medical record. Certain states, including New York and New Jersey, have regulations *requiring* use of pulse oximetry or superior technology for monitoring oxygenation of all patients undergoing anesthesia.[46,47]

Failure Rate of Pulse Oximeters

Recognizing that monitoring standards and regulations exist, it is important to appreciate that although the pulse oximeter probe may be applied to a patient, the pulse oximeter may not always provide a reading of saturation. This may be because of patient problems (poor circulation, hypothermia) or other technical problems. At the University of Washington Hospitals, investigators studied the failure rate of pulse oximeters.[48] In these hospitals the Spo_2 reading is normally recorded on the chart every 15 minutes. If it was *n*ot *o*btainable, "N.O." was written on the anesthesia record. Failure of the pulse oximeter was considered to be present if N.O. was recorded for two consecutive 15-minute periods. Using these criteria, the failure of pulse oximeters in the operating rooms was found in 124 of 11,046 cases (1.12%).[48] The failure rate was highest at the VA Medical Center. ASA Physical Status 3 patients accounted for 72% of the failures, the mean duration of which was 1 hour 15 minutes (mean anesthesia time 3 hours 47 minutes). In the postanesthesia care unit (PACU), the overall failure rate was 0.64% (note that high-risk patients were sent to the surgical ICU not the PACU).[49] Reich et al.[50] theorized that because previous studies of pulse oximetry failure were based upon handwritten records, the failure rates reported may be underestimates. They therefore reviewed the case files of more than 9,000 computerized anesthesia records. Pulse oximetry data failure was defined as presence of at least one continuous gap in data of 10 minutes or longer duration in a case. The overall incidence of cases with such a gap was 9.18%. Independent preoperative predictions of data failure were ASA physical status 3, 4, or 5, and orthopedic, vascular, and cardiac surgery. Thus, pulse oximetry data failure rates based upon review of computerized records were much greater than those previously reported for handwritten records. The authors recommended that regulations and expectations regarding pulse oximetry monitoring should reflect the limitations of the technology.

Special Considerations in Cardiac, Thoracic, and Vascular Anesthesia

Pulse oximetry has been proven useful in the management of patients during one-lung ventilation (OLV). Brodsky et al.[51] showed how the Spo_2 can be used to effectively monitor the improvement in oxygenation when positive end-expiratory pressure (PEEP) and continuous positive airway pressure (CPAP) are applied during OLV and that, "we no longer are dependent on frequent arterial blood gas samples to follow arterial oxygenation during OLV." These authors compared Spo_2 readings with those obtained from laboratory co-oximeter analysis of arterial blood samples on a total of 120 occasions in 19 patients (Sao_2 range, 79 to 100%). A plot of Brodsky et al.'s results is shown in Figure 11–8. Note that in most cases the percentage difference between pulse oximeter and laboratory co-oximeter reading is zero; the differences that were found have the appearance of a normal distribution (i.e., bell-shaped curve). Because pulse oximeters use an empiric algorithm to generate a saturation reading, they tend to be most accurate (zero difference) when the conditions of clinical use are most like those under which the algorithm was created. Pulse oximeters are reported by their manufacturers to have an accuracy of ±2% (1 standard deviation [SD]) for Spo_2 values between 70 and 100%. The SD increases to 3% for Spo_2 values from 50 to 70%.[34]

Review of Brodsky et al.'s data (Fig. 11–8) illustrates the SD of 2% for the Nellcor pulse oximeter used in their study. The Spo_2 reading should therefore be used as a guide to the actual saturation: that is, for Spo_2 readings greater than 70%, the Spo_2 value should be within 2% (1 SD) of the actual saturation 68% of the time, and within 4% (2 SD) of the actual saturation 95% of the time.[34]

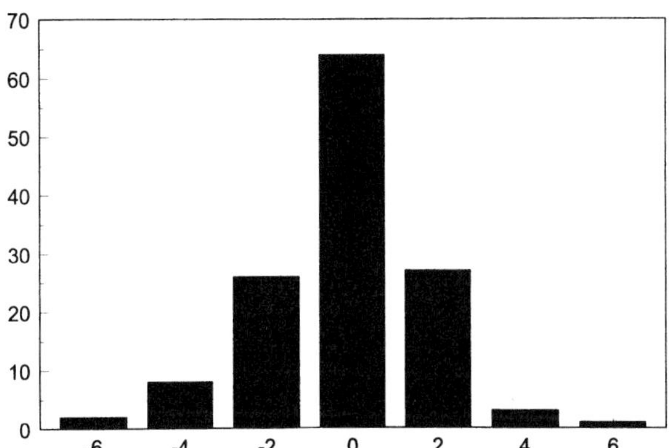

FIGURE **11–8.** The range of differences between Sao_2 obtained by laboratory co-oximeter and pulse oximeter (Spo_2) in 19 patients undergoing one-lung ventilation (From Brodsky JB, Shulman MS, Swan M, Mark JBD: Pulse oximetry during OLV. Anesthesiology 63: 212, 1985, with permission.)

Other studies have found the pulse oximeter to be less accurate during thoracic surgical procedures. Some of these studies suffer from methodologic flaws. Thus one study found that during OLV, Spo_2 values were significantly higher than the measured (laboratory co-oximeter) values and that Spo_2 alone should not be used as a substitute for frequent arterial blood-gas determination.[52] In this study, however, it was not stated whether the Spo_2 was compared with fractional (HbO_2%) or functional (Sao_2) saturation values from the co-oximeter. If Spo_2 values from a Nellcor or Novametrix monitor (in which the calibration algorithm uses Sao_2 rather than HbO_2%) are compared with HbO_2% values from a laboratory co-oximeter, the findings of this study are not unexpected. Another study of pulse oximetry during thoracic surgery compared Spo_2 with saturations that were *calculated* from measured Pao_2 readings from a blood-gas analyzer.[53] Both of these studies[52,53] used regression analysis to compare two measurements, while the preferred statistic for studies comparing methods is Bland-Altman analysis, which assesses bias and precision.[54]

Other Sources of Pulse Oximeter Error during Cardiac, Thoracic and Vascular Surgery

VENOUS PULSATIONS

The pulse oximeter assumes that pulsations in light absorbance are due to changes in arterial blood volume only. Venous blood may also pulsate, the extent of the pulsations varying in different parts of the body. In one study of human volunteers, mean Spo_2 measured using a fingertip probe decreased by 1.6% when the arm was moved from an elevated to a dependent position. When the probe was located on the hypothenar eminence during the same change in limb position, Spo_2 fell by 7 to 8%.[55] If a patient is in the lateral decubitus position, a higher Spo_2 reading is to be expected from a probe on the upper limb compared to one on the lower limb. Similarly, venous pulsations due to tricuspid incompetence (regurgitation) could result in a decreased Spo_2 reading.

THRESHOLD DURING LOW PERFUSION STATES

During low perfusion states, pulsations at the pulse oximeter probe site may decrease and there may be insufficient signal to permit the monitor to function. Lawson et al.[56] induced gradual occlusion of limb blood flow using a blood pressure cuff as a tourniquet, while monitoring perfusion at the fingertip using a laser Doppler flow probe. In healthy volunteers, the pulse oximeter signal was lost when flow decreased to 8.6% of its baseline value. This occurred at a cuff pressure that was 96% of systolic pressure. When the blood pressure cuff was deflated, the signal returned at a blood flow of only 4% of baseline.

Pälve and Vuori[57] studied the lowest pulse pressure and peripheral temperature values associated with a reliable Spo_2 reading during partial cardiopulmonary bypass, as well as the ability of the pulse oximeter to work immediately before and after total cardiopulmonary bypass. The lowest mean pulse pressure with a reliable Spo_2 reading was 13 mm Hg, and the lowest mean peripheral temperature was 23.6°C. The lowest value of pulse pressure needed for a reliable reading before total cardiopulmonary bypass did not differ significantly from that needed after total bypass.

SENSOR MALPOSITION (PENUMBRA EFFECT)

Kelleher and Ruff[41] reported that a pulse oximeter could yield a spuriously low Spo_2 value in a normoxic subject if the clip-on finger sensor was malpositioned. As the sensor was gradually withdrawn from the finger, the Spo_2 values decreased to between 86% and 95% before a loss-of-signal alarm was annunciated. The cause of this error is that light passes through the fingertip at a grazing incidence so that R [where $R = (AC_{660}/DC_{660})/(AC_{940}/DC_{940})$] approaches 1.0, at which value Spo_2 is read as 85%. This is the penumbra effect.

Barker et al.[42] studied the effect of sensor malpositioning on accuracy of Spo_2 readings during hypoxemia. They found that sensor malpositioning changed the calibration curves greatly but in an unpredictable direction and that at low Sao_2 values, these changes could cause the oximeter to indicate that a patient was only mildly hypoxemic when the hypoxemia was, in fact, profound. They recommended that sensor position be checked frequently and that inaccessible locations for the sensor be avoided whenever possible.[42]

MOTION ARTIFACT

Motion artifact is a common cause of pulse oximetry failure and loss of accuracy, particularly in the PACU. Masimo Corporation (Mission Viejo, CA) has developed a new Signal Extraction Technology (SET) designed to minimize motion artifact. This system uses adaptive digital signal processing to cancel the noise signal that is common to the two wavelengths used in pulse oximeters (i.e., 660 and 940 nm). In a study comparing a prototype Masimo SET pulse oximeter with other standard oximeters, the new system was superior and considered to represent a significant advance in low signal-to-noise performance.[58,59]

Transcutaneous Oxygen and Carbon Dioxide Measurement. Both oxygen and carbon dioxide tensions can be measured through the skin using noninvasive, heated electrodes. Transcutaneous oxygen tension ($Ptco_2$) was first measured by a heated Clark electrode in neonates in 1972.[60,61] The transcutaneous measurement of carbon dioxide tension ($Ptcco_2$) was developed more recently, using the Severinghaus electrode.[62,63] Neither method provides a direct determination of arterial blood-gas values, and hence both require an understanding of the underlying physiology for their interpretation. This physiology is briefly reviewed below, along with the advantages and limitations of transcutaneous techniques.

Transcutaneous gas sensors measure the oxygen and carbon dioxide that diffuse to the skin surface from the dermal capillary bed beneath (Fig. 11–9). To obtain meaningful values with an adequate time response, the skin must be heated to about 43°C. The stratum corneum layer, which is normally an effective barrier to gas transport, undergoes reversible changes as the temperature increases above 41°C. The lipid component of this layer essentially melts, greatly increasing the diffusion constant and allowing gases to reach the surface.[64] At the same time, heating causes hyperemia of the dermal capillary bed, thus "arterializing" the capillary blood. Heating also shifts the oxyhemoglobin dissociation curve of the capillary blood to the right, thereby increasing oxygen tension for a given oxygen content (Fig. 11–1). These effects, which tend to increase $Ptco_2$, are opposed by factors that tend to decrease it: diffusion gradients through the skin layers and metabolic oxygen consumption in the living cells. (Note that metabolism tends to decrease $Ptco_2$ but increase $Ptcco_2$.)

In the skin of healthy neonates these conflicting influences fortuitously balance, so that $Ptco_2$ very nearly equals Pao_2. This led to an initial enthusiasm for $Ptco_2$ as a noninvasive monitor of Pao_2, and the technique became routine in the care of premature infants.[65] Then, in the mid 1970s, several investigators reported that $Ptco_2$ values were much lower than Pao_2 values in hemodynamically unstable patients,[66–68] which led to the discovery that $Ptco_2$ depends upon skin perfusion as well as upon Pao_2. This behavior was shown quantitatively in several laboratory studies, as illustrated in Figure 11–10.[69] In this experiment, animals monitored by $Ptco_2$

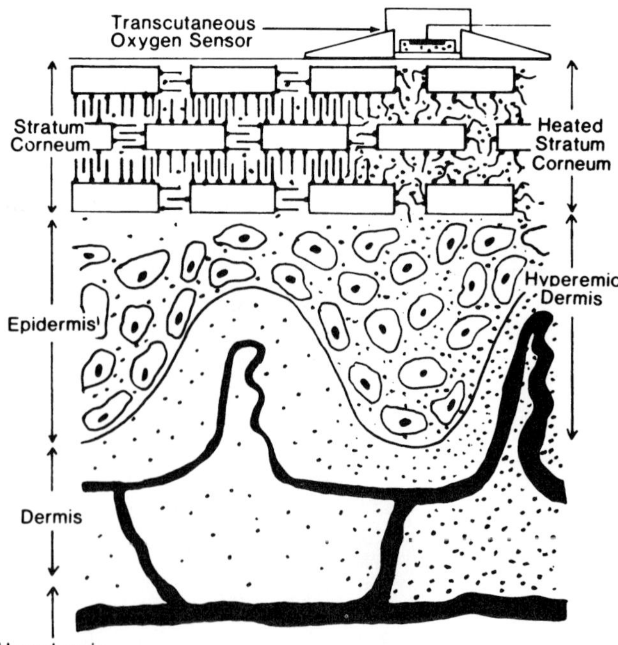

FIGURE 11–9. Cross section of the heated skin and transcutaneous gas sensor. Heating of the skin "melts" the lipid component of the stratum corneum and produces hyperemia of the dermal capillaries. (From Tremper KK, Waxman K, Shoemaker WC: Effects of hypoxia and shock on transcutaneous Po_2 values in dogs. Crit Care Med 7:526, 1979, with permission.)

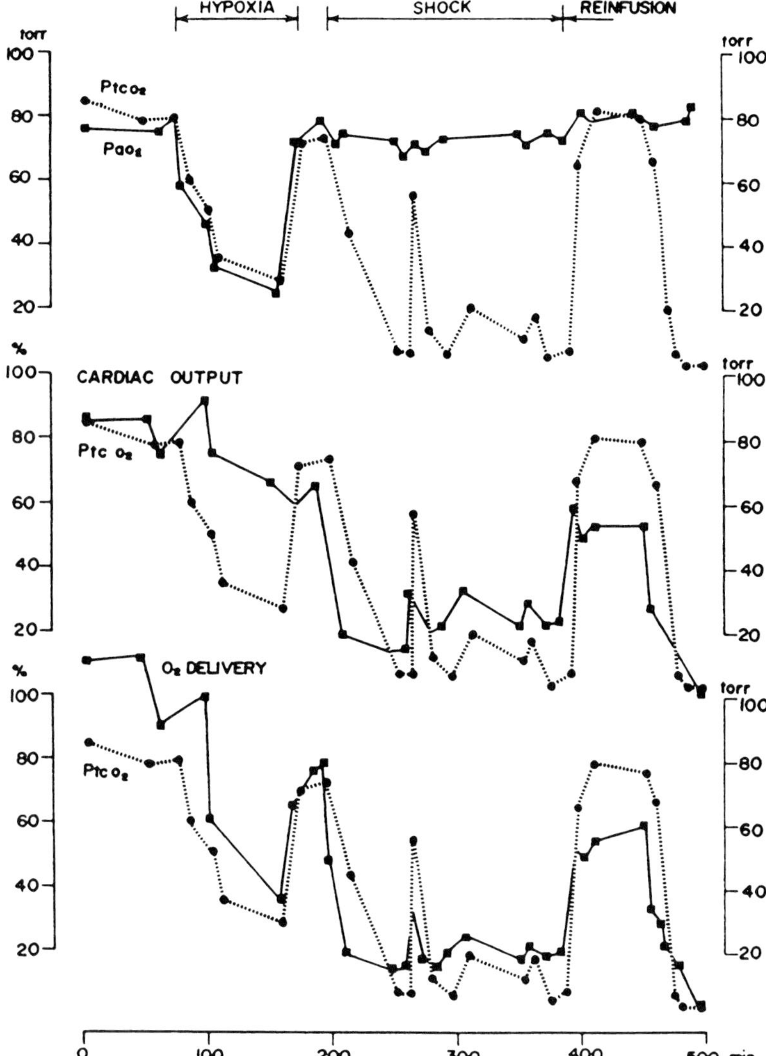

FIGURE **11–10.** Values of $Ptco_2$, Pao_2, cardiac output, and oxygen delivery (CO × Cao_2) plotted versus time during an experiment. In the first phase, Fio_2 is reduced to produce hypoxemia and then returned to normal. In the second phase, the animal is hemorrhaged until cardiac output reaches 20% of control value. Hemorrhaged blood is then reinfused, followed finally by cardiac arrest. $Ptco_2$ follows trends in PaO_2 during hypoxemia, it follows trends in cardiac output during shock, and it follows trends in oxygen delivery during both processes. (From Tremper KK, Waxman K, Shoemaker WC: Effects of hypoxia and shock on transcutaneous Po_2 values in dogs. Crit Care Med 7:526, 1979, with permission.)

were first subjected to hypoxia (reduced Fio_2), then hemorrhagic hypovolemic shock, followed by resuscitation by reinfusion of lost blood. The three sections of the figure show that $Ptco_2$ values follow Pao_2 trends during hypoxia, cardiac output trends during shock, and trends in oxygen delivery during both insults.

A study of patients in an ICU showed a similar phenomenon.[68] A series of 1,073 data sets from 106 patients was divided into three groups according to cardiac index (CI). The transcutaneous index (TCI), defined as the ratio $Ptco_2/Pao_2$, was determined for each data set. In the hemodynamically stable group (CI = 4.1 ± 1.0 L/min/m^2), the transcutaneous index was 0.79 ± 0.12, which is considered a normal value for adults. In the moderate hypoperfusion group (CI = 2.0 ± 0.2 L/min/m^2), the TCI was 0.48 ± 0.07. In the hypotensive shock group (CI = 0.9 ± 0.2), the TCI was 0.12 ± 0.12. In the latter group, $Ptco_2$ values showed no correlation with Pao_2, but correlated well with CI (r = .86). Transcutaneous oxygen is a measure of the oxygen delivery to vascular tissue, and as such it responds to changes in tissue perfusion as well as arterial blood oxygenation. Reductions in cardiac index will thus reduce $Ptco_2$ and TCI. Hyperventilation is another phenomenon that reduces blood flow to the skin, and thereby reduces $Ptco_2$ independently of Pao_2. Figure 11–11 shows the variation of the transcutaneous index with $Paco_2$ during progressive hyperventilation in pigs.[70] This study reported similar reductions in human volunteers, and simultaneous laser velocimetry showed that skin blood flow diminished by up to 50% during hyperventilation.

Since transcutaneous oxygen depends upon local skin characteristics, it is not surprising that the "normal" value of TCI is a function of age. As shown in Table 11–1, the average TCI for hemodynamically stable individuals ranges from 1.1 in premature newborns to 0.7 in the elderly. The decrease in TCI with advancing age is primarily a result of thickening of the skin, particularly the stratum corneum, which is practically absent in neonates.

In addition to the questions of interpretation described above, there are a few technical problems with transcutaneous O_2 and CO_2 measurements. The sensors must be calibrated by the user prior to being applied to the skin,

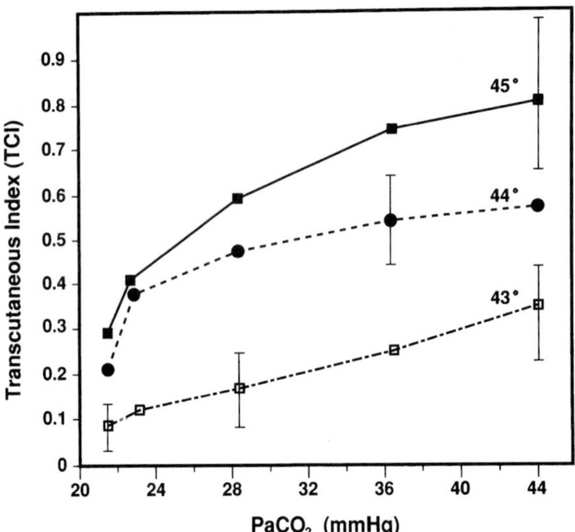

FIGURE **11–11.** Transcutaneous index (TCI) versus Pa_{CO_2} for F_{IO_2} = 1.0. Each point is an average (± SD) of data from five animals. Three transcutaneous electrode temperatures are shown: 43°, 44°, and 45°C. Hyperventilation (Pa_{CO_2} = 21 mm Hg) reduces TCI to 35% of its normocapnic control value at 45°, and 20% of its control value at 43°C.

and they require a 10- to 15-minute warm-up period after they are applied. Transcutaneous CO_2 exhibits a faster warm-up than Ptc_{O_2} and in children will provide stable readings within 5 minutes of application. This makes it particularly useful in very small premature infants in whom capnography is technically difficult.

Halothane is reduced at the cathode of the Clark electrode, raising the concern that sensor accuracy may be affected by the presence of potent inhaled volatile anesthetic agents. A clinical study has shown that halothane-induced calibration drift is measurable but not significant to Ptc_{O_2} sensors covered by 25-μm Teflon membranes.[71] However, in combination transcutaneous P_{O_2}/P_{CO_2} sensors covered by 12.5-μm membranes, the upward calibration drift is much more significant. Isoflurane and enflurane have negligible effect, and no data are presently available for desflurane or sevoflurane.

Although small skin burns and blister formation have been reported in the past, this problem can usually be avoided by using the following guidelines. For premature infants, an electrode temperature of 43° to 43.5°C and a change of sensor site every 2 to 3 hours are recommended. For older children and adults, a temperature of 44°C can be used, and the sensor can be safely left in one location for 4 to 6 hours.

Transcutaneous gas measurements are subject to difficulties both in measurement and in interpretation of data. Nevertheless, they are presently the only noninvasive techniques for measuring oxygen and carbon dioxide *tensions* in blood or tissue. Pulse oximetry measures arterial hemoglobin saturation, which does not provide the same information as oxygen tension. Capnography measures CO_2 tension in expired gas, which is not equivalent to CO_2 tension in blood or tissue. Transcutaneous gas measurements, when interpreted in the context of other variables such as Sp_{O_2} and end-expired CO_2 ($P_{E'CO_2}$), can yield helpful indications of oxygen and carbon dioxide transport to and from the tissues.

TABLE **11–1**
The Most Common Causes of Increased or Decreased Values of $S\bar{v}_{O_2}$*

Causes	Clinical Condition
Causes of decreased $S\bar{v}_{O_2}$	
Decreased Hb_{O_2}%	Hypoxemia
Decreased Hb	Anemia
Decreased CO	Hypovolemic shock
	Cardiogenic shock
	Pericardial tamponade
Increased $\dot{V}_{O_2}$	Fever
	Malignant hyperthermia
	Thyrotoxicosis
	Exercise; shivering
	Light anesthesia
Causes of increased $S\bar{v}_{O_2}$	
CO higher than needed for $\dot{V}_{O_2}$	Sepsis
	Peripheral L-R shunt (Paget's disease)
	Inotropic drugs
	Hypothermia
	Cell poisoning (cyanide)
Artifact (PA oximetry)	Wedged PA catheter

*Values outside of the normal range of 67 to 77% often indicate one of the conditions listed here. Trends in $S\bar{v}_{O_2}$ may provide earlier warning than do absolute values.

Hb_{O_2}%, arterial hemoglobin oxygen saturation; Hb, hemoglobin; CO, cardiac output; $\dot{V}_{O_2}$, oxygen consumption; $S\bar{v}_{O_2}$, mixed venous oxygen saturation; PA, pulmonary artery; L-R, left-to-right.

Mixed Venous Oximetry

The oxygen content of the mixed venous blood reflects the "reserves" left at the end of the oxygen transport process, and as such it is a useful indicator of oxygen homeostasis. The Fick equation (Equation 11–2) can be solved for either the oxygen consumption or the mixed venous oxygen saturation to yield:

$$\dot{V}_{O_2} = 13.8 \times Hb \times CO \times (Hb_{O_2}) - S\bar{v}_{O_2})/100, \quad (11–5)$$

$$(S\bar{v}_{O_2}/100) = (Hb_{O_2}/100) - \dot{V}_{O_2}/(13.8 \times Hb \times CO) \quad (11–6)$$

where $S\bar{v}_{O_2}$ = mixed venous oxygen saturation (%), Hb_{O_2} = fractional arterial oxygen saturation (%), $\dot{V}_{O_2}$ = oxygen consumption (ml/min), Hb = hemoglobin concentration (gm/dl), and CO = cardiac output (L/min).

If we substitute "normal" values of Hb = 15 gm/dl, CO = 5 L/min, Hb_{O_2} = 100%, and $S\bar{v}_{O_2}$ = 75% into Equation 11–5, we obtain $\dot{V}_{O_2}$ = 259 ml/min as a normal value for oxygen consumption. Assuming that a maximally stressed individual can increase CO to 15 L/min and decrease $S\bar{v}_{O_2}$ to 32%, we obtain a maximum steady-state oxygen consumption of $\dot{V}_{O_2}$ = 2,111 ml/min. The healthy subject can invoke these reserves of increased CO and decreased $S\bar{v}_{O_2}$ within seconds to either increase $\dot{V}_{O_2}$ or maintain normal $\dot{V}_{O_2}$ values in the face of other stresses. For example, Equation 11–5 predicts that a subject with a hemoglobin of 1.7 gm/dl (Hct = 5.1%) can maintain normal oxygen consumption with CO = 15 and $S\bar{v}O_2$ = 32%. A hypoxic subject having HbO_2 = 40% (PaO_2 = 23 mm Hg) can also maintain normal $\dot{V}O_2$.

In anemia and hypoxia, reserves in both CO and $S\bar{v}O_2$ can be quickly recruited to compensate for the primary insult. In low output shock, on the other hand, one of the two reserves (CO) has been eliminated by the primary insult itself. Thus the cardiac output can decrease only to 1.7 L/min (a threefold change) while maintaining normal $\dot{V}O_2$ by decreasing $S\bar{v}O_2$. In all three of these examples, a decrease in $S\bar{v}O_2$ signals the utilization of reserves in order to maintain normal oxygen consumption. The lower limit of $S\bar{v}O_2$ = 32% is a theoretical extreme, and we must recognize that most patients will not tolerate values this low for extended periods. Nevertheless, these examples illustrate that significant oxygen transport reserves are available for short-term compensation.

Although the normal value of $S\bar{v}O_2$ is usually stated as 75%, the normal range actually extends from 67 to 77%. Values below 60% indicate stressing of the oxygen transport system; that is, a supply-versus-demand imbalance. Lactic acidosis usually occurs if $S\bar{v}O_2$ is less than 50% for a prolonged period. Unconsciousness ensues at roughly 30%, and permanent cellular damage is associated with values near 20%.[72]

Trends of $S\bar{v}O_2$ can be more significant than the absolute value, thus a continuous plot of $S\bar{v}O_2$ versus time is particularly useful. As shown by Equation 11–6, $S\bar{v}O_2$ will decrease during decreases in HbO_2 (hypoxemia), Hb (anemia), or CO (low-output shock), and during increases in $\dot{V}O_2$. The latter may be indications of light anesthesia, fever, malignant hyperthermia, or other hypermetabolic states (e.g., thyrotoxicosis). An $S\bar{v}O_2$ value above the normal range generally signifies a cardiac output that is inappropriately high for metabolic demands. Prominent causes include sepsis, hypothermia, peripheral left-to-right shunt (e.g., Paget's disease of bone), cellular poisoning (e.g., cyanide), and inappropriate use of inotropic drugs. When $S\bar{v}O_2$ is measured by pulmonary artery oximetry, a wedged pulmonary artery (PA) catheter will cause a high value of $S\bar{v}O_2$, usually greater than 90%. This artifact can actually alert the user to the presence of an accidentally wedged PA catheter. Table 11–1 summarizes the most common causes of increased or decreased $S\bar{v}O_2$.

Mixed venous oxygen saturation has long been recognized as an indicator of oxygen transport homeostasis. Mixed venous blood samples obtained through a pulmonary artery catheter can be analyzed by a laboratory in vitro co-oximeter to provide $S\bar{v}O_2$ data. Although this method can yield accurate values, the data are neither continuous nor immediately available. As noted above, much of the diagnostic value of $S\bar{v}O_2$ lies in continuous trend information; that is, in which direction and how fast is the value changing.

Continuous in vivo intravascular and intracardiac oximetry was reported as early as 1962,[73] and a fiberoptic pulmonary artery oximetry catheter was reported in 1973.[74] Using optical fibers to transmit light to and from the tip of the PA catheter, this device measured the light reflected from red cells in the mixed venous blood at two wavelengths. Since the reflectance properties of HbO_2 and RHb are very different, light measurements at two wavelengths theoretically determine the relative proportions of HbO_2 and RHb. This oximetric principle is the same as that upon which pulse oximetry is based, except that here reflected rather than transmitted light is used.

For the two-wavelength system, the relationship between $S\bar{v}O_2$ and light intensities depends upon the total Hb as well as blood flow velocity and pH. To eliminate the dependence upon Hb, a three-wavelength reflectance catheter was developed by Oximetrix, Inc. This system was used in an umbilical artery catheter for neonates in 1978,[75] and it was incorporated into a 7.5-Fr PA catheter in 1981.[72] Clinical studies suggest that the three-wavelength system is reasonably accurate over a wide range of hemoglobin values, whereas the user must input the current Hb value into the processor of any two-wavelength system.[76] In the presence of significant levels of the dyshemoglobins COHb and MetHb, neither the two- nor three-wavelength system can be expected to provide accurate data. As shown in Figure 11–12, increasing levels of MetHb cause progressively larger overestimates of $S\bar{v}O_2$ by a three-wavelength pulmonary artery oximeter.[77]

Continuous measurements of $S\bar{v}O_2$ can detect stresses upon the oxygen transport system that may not be shown by other monitors, yet may eventually lead to decompensation. For example, Figure 11–13 shows a continuous tracing of $S\bar{v}O_2$ versus time in a patient who began

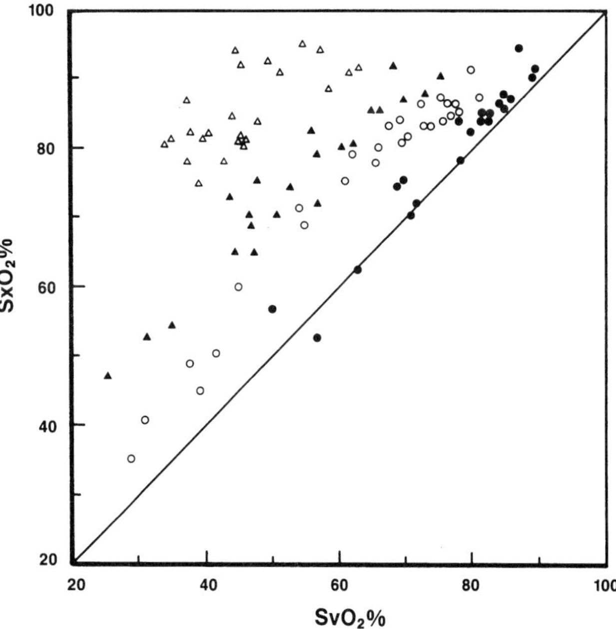

FIGURE **11–12.** Three-wavelength pulmonary artery oximeter saturation values (SxO_2) plotted versus simultaneous values from an IL-282 in vitro co-oximeter ($S\bar{v}O_2$) in dogs at various FIO_2 and MetHb values. *Filled circles*, MetHb < 10%; *open circles*, 10% < MetHb < 20%; *filled triangles*, 20% < MetHb < 40%; *open triangles*, MetHb > 40%. (From Barker SJ, Tremper KK, Hyatt SJ: Effects of methemoglobinemia on pulse oximetry and mixed venous oximetry. Anesthesiology 70:112, 1989, with permission.)

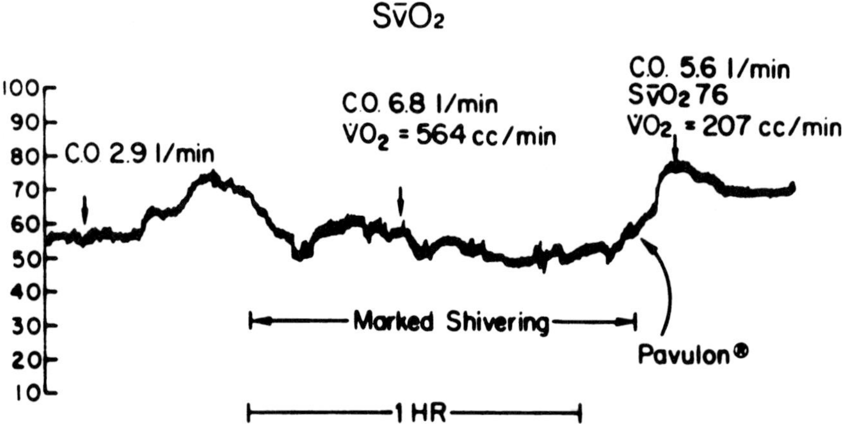

FIGURE **11–13.** A continuous tracing of $S\bar{v}O_2$ versus time in a postoperative patient, showing the effect of shivering. During the shivering period, $S\bar{v}O_2$ decreased from 70% to less than 50% despite a cardiac output of 6.8 L/min. Intravenous pancuronium quickly terminated the shivering, and $S\bar{v}O_2$ promptly returned to 76% with a cardiac output of 5.6 L/min. $\dot{V}O_2$ was decreased by 63% from the prepancuronium value. (From Hoyt JW, et al: Continuous measurement of blood oxygen saturation in the high risk patient. In Schweiss JF [ed]: Beach International, Inc, Vol 1, 1982, p 54, with permission.)

intense shivering in the PACU. During the shivering period, the $S\bar{v}O_2$ value is well below normal (near 50%) despite a cardiac output of 6.8 L/min. The $\dot{V}O_2$ was increased to 564 ml/min, which is typical of a shivering patient. After one dose of pancuronium, the shivering ceased, CO decreased to 5.6 L/min, and $S\bar{v}O_2$ rapidly increased to 76%. These changes reflect a decrease in $\dot{V}O_2$ to 207 ml/min, or 63% less than the prepancuronium value.

Continuous $S\bar{v}O_2$ tracings can be helpful in monitoring the effects of various cardiovascular interventions. Figure 11–14 shows the tracing of a patient whose $S\bar{v}O_2$ value decreased to less than 40% due to low cardiac output. Afterload reduction with sodium nitroprusside led to a rapid increase in $S\bar{v}O_2$, accompanied by a corresponding increase in CO.

Although there remains a controversy regarding the indications for PA catheterization, there is no doubt that anesthesiologists will continue to employ invasive monitoring in the operating room. A recent task force report has attempted to develop general guidelines based upon an analysis of risks versus documented outcome benefits.[78] Although there are today no prospective studies demonstrating improved patient outcome from pulmonary oximetry, there are data that suggest that continuous $S\bar{v}O_2$ monitoring can reduce the number of cardiac output and blood-gas determinations in ICU patients.[79] Furthermore, recent studies suggest that in critically ill patients the relationship between oxygen delivery ("flux") ($\dot{D}O_2$ = CO × CaO_2) and oxygen consumption may be abnormal. The "plateau" in the $\dot{V}O_2$-versus-$\dot{D}O_2$ curve, above which $\dot{V}O_2$ normally becomes independent of $\dot{D}O_2$, may be displaced or may not even exist.[80,81] Prospective, randomized studies of high-risk patients imply that maintaining supranormal values of $\dot{D}O_2$ by increasing cardiac output may lead to improved patient outcome.[82–84] To determine the relationship of $\dot{D}O_2$ and $\dot{V}O_2$, frequent measurements of cardiac output as well as $S\bar{v}O_2$ (see Equa-

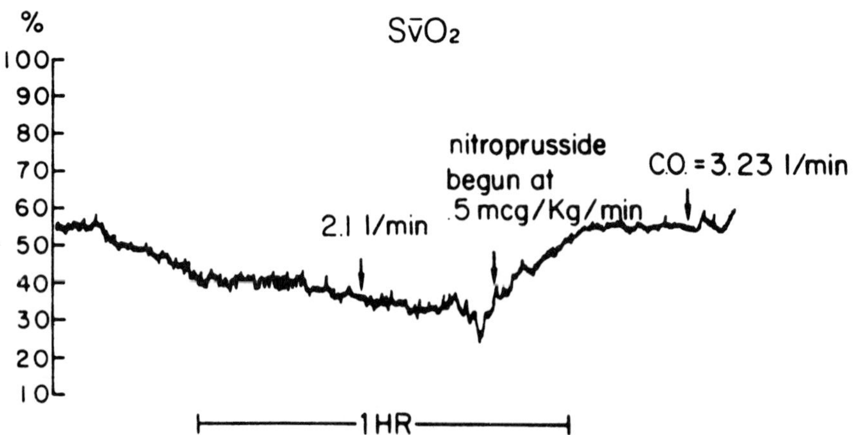

FIGURE **11–14.** A tracing of $S\bar{v}O_2$ versus time in a patient with falling cardiac output. Afterload reduction with sodium nitroprusside caused a rapid increase in $S\bar{v}O_2$, accompanied by an increase in CO from 2.1 L/min to 3.2 L/min. (From Hoyt JW, et al: Continuous measurement of blood oxygen saturation in the high risk patient. In Schweiss JF [ed]: Beach International, Inc, Vol 1, 1982, p 50, with permission.)

tion 11–5) are required. Pulmonary artery oximetry thus provides a means to continuously monitor this relationship.

Mixed venous oxygen saturation is a useful variable in monitoring the well-being of the oxygen transport system, particularly in high-risk and critically ill patients. Pulmonary artery catheterization is a well-established monitoring modality that will continue to be used by anesthesiologists despite its concomitant risks. In patients for whom invasive monitoring is deemed appropriate, one should consider the potential benefits of continuous $S\bar{v}O_2$ monitoring, which adds no further risks to those of pulmonary artery catheterization.

Thys et al.[85] studied how lung collapse during thoracic anesthesia changes $S\bar{v}O_2$ and determined whether these changes correlate with changes in SaO_2 and/or cardiac index. They found that changes in $S\bar{v}O_2$ are determined primarily by changes in oxygenation (SaO_2) rather than by changes in cardiac output.

Zaune et al.[86] assessed the value of dual oximetry (SpO_2 and $S\bar{v}O_2$) during pulmonary resections. Like Thys et al.,[85] they also found that $S\bar{v}O_2$ is determined primarily by oxygenation rather than cardiac index. Since the oxygen delivery index increased during one-lung ventilation to maintain the oxygen supply-demand balance, they concluded that $S\bar{v}O_2$ monitoring might be useful as an early indicator in identifying high-risk patients with compromised oxygen delivery resulting from decreased cardiac index.

Carbon Dioxide

Carbon dioxide is produced in the cells, mainly in the mitochondria. It reaches the bloodstream by molecular diffusion down a concentration gradient, and from here it diffuses into red cell cytoplasm where most is converted to bicarbonate by carbonic anhydrase. Carbonic anhydrase is found only in cell cytoplasm, not in plasma. Some CO_2 is bound to hemoglobin to form carbamino compounds. Thus CO_2 may be transported in the blood in four ways: in solution (dissolved); as bicarbonate; as carbonic acid; and as carbamino compounds. The arterial CO_2 tension is normally 40 mm Hg and the CO_2 content 48 vol%. The venous CO_2 tension is 44 mm Hg and the venous blood CO_2 content 52 vol%. The arteriovenous CO_2 content difference is therefore 4 vol%. Comparing this with the arteriovenous oxygen content difference of 5 vol% gives a respiratory exchange ratio (respiratory quotient: CO_2 produced/O_2 consumed) of 0.8.[1]

Monitoring of Carbon Dioxide

Blood

The values of PCO_2 and bicarbonate in blood are obtained by drawing the appropriate blood sample (arterial, mixed venous) and analyzing it in a blood-gas analyzer (e.g., Radiometer, Copenhagen). These instruments also measure PO_2 and pH, and calculate other values such as base excess. The measurement of PCO_2 using transcutaneous electrodes and intravascular optodes has been described in the section "Arterial Blood Oxygen Monitoring," above.

Exhaled Gas

The measurement of CO_2 in exhaled gas (capnometry) and its graphic display over time (capnography) are valuable monitors of patient well-being. A number of physical methods are available for the measurement of CO_2 in respired gas. These methods, which are described in detail elsewhere and which therefore will not be discussed here, include infrared and acoustic spectroscopy, Raman spectroscopy, and mass spectroscopy.[11] These methods all have short response times (90% response in 50 to 100 msec) and permit breath-by-breath CO_2 measurement. As with any monitor, it is important to ensure that the system is calibrated and used correctly, since erroneous readings may otherwise occur.[87]

Most CO_2 analyzers display CO_2 concentration (mm Hg or vol%) as ordinate against time as abscissa. A normal capnogram obtained during mechanical ventilation is shown in Figure 11–15. It can be divided into four phases: (I) inspiratory baseline; (II) expiratory upstroke; (III) expiratory plateau; and (IV) inspiratory downstroke. The inspired ($PICO_2$) and end-expired ($PE'CO_2$) values are usually also displayed digitally.[88]

Fundamental to the production of a capnogram is that the patient be producing CO_2 and that there be adequate circulation of blood to carry it to the lungs. Once technical problems have been excluded, absence of a capnogram waveform may indicate an esophageal intubation, or tracheal intubation with no cardiac output.

Phase I of the capnogram (exhalation of apparatus and anatomic dead space) should be a flat line near the x axis (i.e., PCO_2 = 0 mm Hg), since dead space gas is the same as inspired gas and should not contain any CO_2. If the baseline is not zero, one should check the calibration of the instrument. If correctly calibrated, the cause of rebreathing or other source of CO_2 should be sought.

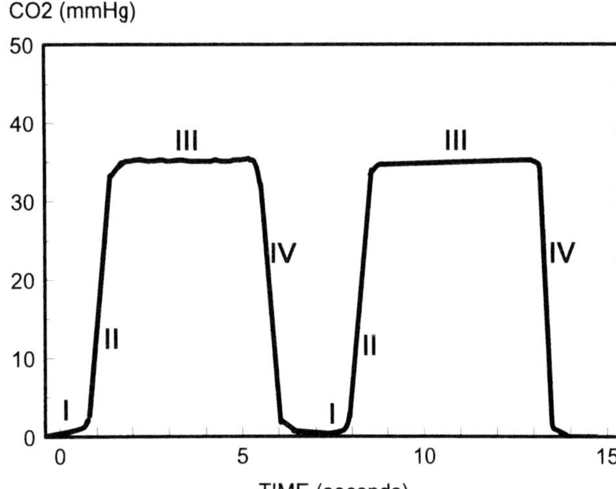

FIGURE **11–15.** Normal capnogram, showing the four phases. For details, see text.

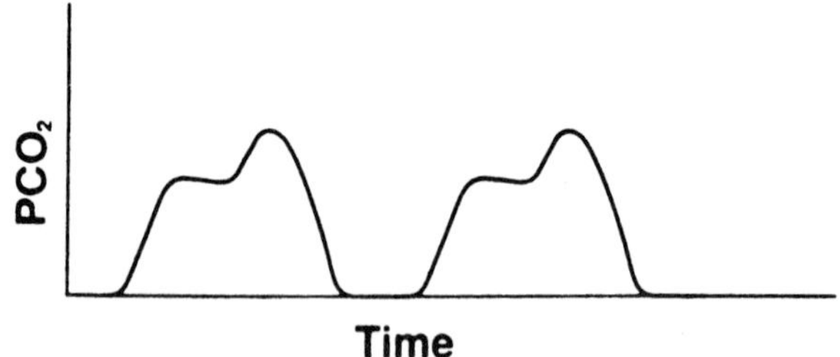

FIGURE **11–16.** Camel capnogram, showing the "hump" during phase III. For details, see text.

Phase II, the rapid steep upstroke, will show a decreased slope if there are problems affecting expiratory flow. Such problems include bronchospastic disease (increased airways resistance) and emphysema (gas trapping). The decrease in phase II slope is caused by a mixing of dead space gas with ideal alveolar gas (see next section). If the airway resistance is very high, a plateau (phase III) may never be reached and the end-tidal CO_2 may be much lower than the true alveolar CO_2.

A patient in the lateral decubitus position may exhibit a camel-shaped capnogram (Fig. 11–16). In this position the nondependent lung receives more ventilation and less perfusion than the dependent lung and therefore contains more alveolar dead space. During exhalation the nondependent lung empties first and gives rise to the lower phase III plateau. As the dependent lung (more perfusion, less alveolar dead space) empties later, it gives rise to the later, higher phase III plateau. While the camel capnogram should be observed most often in association with the patient's lateral decubitus position, it is probably more commonly due to artifact.[89]

Dead Space

The noninvasively obtained end-tidal CO_2 measurement is often used as a guide to the arterial (invasively obtained) CO_2 tension. In the normal patient the arterial-to-alveolar (end-tidal) gradient is usually approximately 4 mm Hg (range, 2 to 8 mm Hg). This is not always the case, however, and an understanding of the interrelationships, and of dead space in particular, is in order.

Dead space is that part of the respiratory tract in which no gas exchange occurs and therefore represents wasted ventilation.[1] When a patient's lungs are being ventilated from a circle anesthesia system, during inspiration the tidal volume flows first from the inspiratory limb into the apparatus dead space. This comprises those parts of the breathing system that are distal to the y-piece and may include a "goose-neck" extension tube, sidestream gas analyzer sampling connector, elbow, and tracheal tube or face mask. Gas then enters the anatomic dead space, which includes the oropharynx and nasopharynx, the trachea, major bronchi, and other large airways in which there is no gas exchange. In the average adult, anatomic dead space ($V_{D_{anat}}$) is approximately 2 ml/kg. The apparatus or "mechanical" dead space together with the anatomic dead space form "series dead space" because the tidal volume must flow through these to reach the alveoli where gas exchange occurs.

Having flowed through the series dead space, some of the tidal volume (V_T) enters the alveoli and constitutes alveolar ventilation ($V_T - V_{D_{anat}}$). Not all alveoli are well perfused, however, so that for purposes of modeling, alveoli can be considered either as "ideal" (i.e., those that are well perfused and ventilated), and "alveolar dead space" (i.e., those that are ventilated but not perfused). The alveolar dead space is therefore in parallel with the ideal alveoli. In the ideal alveoli, because CO_2 diffuses so rapidly, the CO_2 tension (P_{ACO_2}) is equal to that of pulmonary capillary blood, which becomes systemic arterial blood (Pa_{CO_2}). In the dead space alveoli, because there is no perfusion the P_{CO_2} is that of inspired gas (i.e., P_{ICO_2}).

During exhalation, the first gas to be exhaled is the apparatus and anatomic dead space gas (end of phase I, beginning of phase II; Fig. 11–15), followed by anatomic dead space plus alveolar gas (phase II). As the alveoli continue to empty, phase III is observed and represents a mixture of ideal and dead space alveolar gas. The difference between the end-expired ($P_{E'CO_2}$) and Pa_{CO_2} thus depends upon how much of the alveolar ventilation was "wasted" in alveolar dead space. If all of the exhaled gas volume (i.e., mechanical dead space, anatomic dead space, and alveolar gas) is collected in a bag over time, it is termed mixed expired gas, and the CO_2 tension of the mixture is termed mixed expired CO_2 ($P\bar{E}_{CO_2}$).

Using these definitions, the following aspects of dead space and dead space/tidal volume (V_D/V_T) ratio can be established: Physiologic dead space ($V_{D_{phys}}$) = apparatus ("mechanical") dead space + anatomic dead space ($V_{D_{anat}}$) + alveolar dead space ($V_{D_{alv}}$).

$$\frac{V_{D_{phys}}}{V_T} = \frac{Pa_{CO_2} - P\bar{E}_{CO_2}}{Pa_{CO_2}}$$

$$\frac{V_{D_{anat}}}{V_T} = \frac{P_{E'CO_2} - P\bar{E}_{CO_2}}{P_{E'CO_2}}$$

$$\frac{V_{D_{alv}}}{V_A} = \frac{Pa_{CO_2} - P_{E'CO_2}}{Pa_{CO_2}}$$

where V_T = tidal ventilation and V_A = alveolar ventilation. If Pa_{CO_2} = 40 mm Hg, $P_{E'CO_2}$ = 36 mm Hg and $P\bar{E}_{CO_2}$ = 24 mm Hg; then $V_{D_{phys}}/V_T = (40 - 24)/40 = 16/40 = 0.40$; $V_{D_{anat}}/V_T = (36 - 24)/36 = 12/36 = 0.33$; and $V_{D_{alv}}/V_T = (40 - 36)/40 = 0.10$. Let us use these numbers and assume that a patient has a delivered tidal volume (V_T) of 600 ml. Of this 600 ml, $600 \times 0.33 = 200$ ml is wasted in the (anatomic + "mechanical") dead space ($V_{D_{anat}}$). The remaining 400 ml flows beyond this "series dead space" to enter the alveoli (V_A), where $(400 \times 0.10) = 40$ ml is wasted in unperfused alveoli ($V_{D_{alv}}$) and 360 ml takes place in gas exchange. The physiologic (total) dead space is (mechanical + anatomic) + alveolar, or $(200 + 40) = 240$ ml. The $V_{D_{phys}}/V_T$ is $240/600 = 0.40$. It is important to realize that the $V_{D_{alv}}/V_A$ ratio is applied to the *alveolar* ventilation (V_A), not to the total ventilation (V_T).

In these simple calculations and relationships it is also important to recognize that end-expired ($P_{E'CO_2}$), is considered to be the same as alveolar (PA)CO_2; that any increase in VD_{alv} will cause an increase in the gradient of end-expired-to-arterial CO_2; and that end-expired CO_2 is not the same as mixed-expired ($P\bar{E}CO_2$). Capnometers display inspired and *end-expired* CO_2, not mixed expired CO_2.

Applications of CO_2 Monitoring During Cardiothoracic and Vascular Anesthesia

The maintenance of a normal $PaCO_2$ (i.e., adequacy of ventilation) is not usually a problem during anesthesia, even during one-lung ventilation for thoracic surgery. In the latter situation, if the same tidal volume is used as during two-lung ventilation, more CO_2 is removed from the one ventilated lung, offsetting the higher CO_2 content of blood returning to the left side of the heart from the nonventilated lung, so that $PaCO_2$ is maintained. Thus during one-lung ventilation, removal of CO_2 is usually less of a problem than maintaining an adequate oxygenation (PaO_2).

During thoracic surgery, capnography may be useful in placing a double-lumen endobronchial tube and in detecting endobronchial intubation. Shafieha et al.[90] used two capnographs, one connected to each lumen of a double-lumen tube, and found that the correct position of the double-lumen tube could be identified "by simultaneous and synchronous needle movement of the two analyzers" (their capnometers had a needle analog gauge). Clamping of each lumen of the double-lumen tube would result in absence of needle oscillation of the appropriate analyzer. Most operating room suites would likely not have two such analyzers available, however.

Werner et al.[91] studied CO_2 elimination from each lung separately during endobronchial anesthesia. They found that variations in pulmonary arterial pressure during surgical stimulation may significantly affect the pattern of CO_2 elimination in the lungs but that there was no evidence that these effects were important clinically.

Since end-expired (PE′) CO_2 can be monitored noninvasively and continuously, while arterial blood sampling for $PaCO_2$ is invasive and intermittent, it is important to consider how the gradient of end-expired to arterial CO_2 or D(a-E′)CO_2, may be affected during anesthesia. As stated previously, the D(a-E′)CO_2 is normally 2 to 8 mm Hg in an awake subject. The gradient may be increased by the following:

1. A decrease in pulmonary arterial pressure. This increases the size of West zone I in the lung and, with more unperfused alveoli, there is increased alveolar dead space.
2. Upright posture increases West zone I.
3. Pulmonary embolism due to air, thrombus, or fat decreases lung perfusion.
4. Chronic obstructive pulmonary disease causes more nonvascular air space (e.g., bullae) and nonalveolar parallel dead space.
5. Mechanical obstruction of, and hence decreased flow in, the pulmonary arteries.
6. Ventilation gas leaving the normal gas passages (e.g., bronchopleural fistula, tracheal disruption, cuff leak).

Fletcher[92] has reviewed the topic of the D(a-E′)CO_2 during cardiothoracic surgery and found that it increases during thoracotomy and one-lung ventilation. Pansard et al.[93] found a significant increase in D(a-E′)CO_2 after patients were placed in the lateral decubitus position.

In a recent study, Yam et al.[94] investigated how closely end-expired PCO_2 values reflect changes in arterial PCO_2 in patients undergoing thoractomy for pulmonary resection during one-lung ventilation. They found a wide variation (1.5 to 18 mm Hg) in the D(a-E′)CO_2 during one-lung ventilation and concluded that the accuracy of estimation of $PaCO_2$ by monitoring PE′CO_2 remains questionable during one-lung ventilation.

Raemer et al.[95] studied the D(a-E′)CO_2 in patients undergoing cardiac surgery and also found large variations in this difference. Thus, monitoring of PE′CO_2, while possibly useful for gross changes or trends, does not accurately predict $PaCO_2$ in patients undergoing cardiothoracic surgery.

References

1. Nunn JF: Nunn's Applied Respiratory Physiology, 4th ed. Boston, Butterworth-Heinemann, 1993.
2. Saidman LJ, Smith NT (eds): Monitoring in Anesthesia, 3rd ed. Boston, Butterworth-Heinemann, 1993.
3. Lake CL (ed): Clinical Monitoring in Anesthesia and Critical Care, 2nd ed. Philadelphia, WB Saunders Co, 1994.
4. Blitt CD, Hines RL (eds): Monitoring in Anesthesia and Critical Care Medicine, 3rd ed. New York, Churchill Livingstone, 1994.
5. Atlas G, Camporesi EM: Hyperbaric oxygen therapy. Eisenkraft JB (ed): In Progress in Anesthesiology. San Antonio, TX, Dannemiller Memorial Educational Foundation, 1994, p 395.
6. Comroe JH, Botelho S: The unreliability of cyanosis in the recognition of arterial hypoxemia. Am J Med Sci 214:1, 1947.
7. Kelman GR, Nunn JF: Clinical recognition of hypoxaemia under fluorescent lamps. Lancet 1:1400, 1966.
8. Raemer DB, Warren DL, Morris R, et al: Hypoxemia during ambulatory gynecologic surgery as evaluated by the pulse oximeter. J Clin Monit 3:244, 1987.
9. Coté CJ, Goldstein EA, Coté MA, et al: A single blind study of pulse oximetry in children. Anesthesiology 68:184, 1988.
10. Eisenkraft JB: Anesthesia machine. In Ehrenwerth J, Eisenkraft JB (eds): Anesthesia Equipment, Principles and Applications. St. Louis, Mosby Year Book, Inc, 1993, p 27.
11. Eisenkraft JB, Raemer DB: Monitoring gases in the anesthesia delivery system. In Ehrenwerth J, Eisenkraft JB (eds): Anesthesia Equipment: Principles and Applications. St Louis, Mosby Year Book, Inc, 1993.
12. Operator's Manual, O_2 Med. Telford, PA, North American Dräger, Inc.
13. Standard specification for minimum performance and safety requirements for components and systems of anesthesia gas machines. ASTM F1161-88. West Conshohocken, PA, 1989. American Society for Testing and Materials.
14. Meriläinen PT: A differential paramagnetic sensor for breath-by-breath oximetry. J Clin Monit 6:65, 1990.
15. Campbell IT, Beatty PCW: Monitoring preoxygenation (Editorial). Br J Anaesth 72:3, 1994.
16. Berry CB, Myles PS: Preoxygenation in healthy volunteers: A graph of oxygen "washin" using end-tidal oxygraphy. Br J Anaesth 72:116, 1994.
17. Jameson LC: Applications of mass spectrometry. Park Ridge, IL. American Society of Anesthesiologists ASA Refresher Course Lecture #226, 1986.
18. Gronert GA: Calculation of O_2 consumption and CO_2 production during anesthesia (Letter). Anesth Analg 79:1018, 1994.
19. Eisenkraft JB, Neustein SM, et al: Estimation of VO_2 during aortic cross-clamping. Mass spectrometry vs. Fick (Abstract). Presented at Society Cardiovascular Anesthesiologists Annual Meeting, May 1991.

20. Severinghaus JW, Bradley AF: Electrodes for blood PO_2 and PCO_2 determination. J Appl Physiol 13:515, 1958.
21. Harris TR, Nugent M: Continuous arterial oxygen tension monitoring in the newborn infant. J Pediatr 82:929, 1973.
22. Bratanow N, Polk K, Bland R, et al: Continuous polarographic monitoring of intraarterial oxygen in the perioperative period. Crit Care Med 13:859, 1985.
23. Lubbers DW, Opitz N: Die pCO2/pO2-Optode: eine neue pCO2 bzw. pO2-Messonde zur Messung des pCO2 oder pO2 von Gasen und Flussigkeiten. Z Naturforsch [C] 30:532, 1975.
24. Peterson J, Fitzgerald R, Buckhold D: Fiberoptic probe *in vivo* measurement of oxygen partial pressure. Anal Chem 56:62, 1984.
25. Gehrich JL, Lubbers DW, Opitz N, et al: Optical fluorescence and its application to an intravascular blood-gas monitoring system. IEEE Trans Biomed Eng 33:117, 1986.
26. Mahutte CK, Sassoon CS, Muro JR, et al: Progress in the development of a fluorescent intravascular blood-gas system in man. J Clin Monit 6:147, 1990.
27. Barker SJ, Hyatt J: Continuous measurement of intraarterial pHa, PaCO2, and PaO2 in the operating room. Anesth Analg 73:43, 1991.
28. Greenblott GB, Barker SJ, Tremper KK, et al: Detection of venous air embolism by continuous intraarterial oxygen monitoring. J Clin Monit 6:53, 1990.
29. Barker SJ, Tremper KK, Heitzmann H: Comparison of three oxygen monitors in detecting endobronchial intubation. J Clin Monit 4:240, 1988.
30. Shapiro BA, Cane RD, Chomka CM, et al: Preliminary evaluation of an intraarterial blood-gas system in dogs and humans. Crit Care Med 17:455, 1989.
31. Bashein G, Pino JA, Nessly ML, et al: Clinical assessment of a flow-through fluorometric blood-gas monitor. J Clin Monit 4:195, 1988.
32. Standards for Basic Anesthetic Monitoring. ASA 1996 Directory of Members, ASA Park Ridge, IL, 1999, p 463.
33. Pologe JA: Pulse oximetry technical aspects of machine design. Int Anesth Clin 25:137, 1987.
34. Barker SJ, Tremper KK: Pulse oximetry. In Ehrenwerth J, Eisenkraft JB (eds): Anesthesia Equipment: Principles and Applications. St Louis, Mosby Year Book, 1993, p 249.
35. Eisenkraft JB: Pulse oximeter desaturation due to methemoglobinemia. Anesthesiology 68:279, 1988.
36. Pologe JA: Functional saturation vs. fractional saturation: Which does pulse oximetry read? (Abstract). J Clin Monit 5:298, 1989.
37. Swedlow DB, Irving SM: Monitoring and patient safety. In Blitt CD (ed): Monitoring in Anesthesia and Critical Care Medicine. New York, Churchill Livingstone, 1990, p 43.
38. Scheller MS, Unger RJ, Kelner MJ: Effects of intravenously administered dyes on pulse oximetry readings. Anesthesiology 65: 550, 1986.
39. Coté CJ, Goldstein EA, Fuchsman WH, Hoaglin DC: Effects of nail polish on pulse oximetry. Anesthesiology 67:683, 1988.
40. Barker SJ, Tremper KK: The effect of carbon monoxide inhalation on pulse oximeter signal detection. Anesthesiology 66:677, 1987.
41. Kelleher JF, Ruff RH: The penumbra effect. Vasomotion dependent pulse oximeter artifact to due to probe malposition. Anesthesiology 71:787, 1989.
42. Barker SJ, Hyatt J, Shah NK, Kao YJ: The effect of sensor malpositioning on pulse oximeter accuracy during hypoxemia. Anesthesiology 79:248, 1993.
43. Trillo RA, Aukberg SJ: Dapsone-induced methemoglobinemia and pulse oximetry. Anesthesiology 77:594, 1992.
44. Barker SJ, Tremper KK, Hyatt SJ: Effects of methemoglobinemia on pulse oximetry and mixed venous oximetry. Anesthesiology 70:112, 1989.
45. Anderson TA, Hajduczek J, Barker SJ: Benzocaine-induced pulse oximetry with methemoglobinemia. Anesth Analg 67:1099, 1988.
46. New York State Hospital Code Section XII: 405.13, p 33, May 1990.
47. New Jersey Register: 21 NJR 504, Feb 21, 1989.
48. Freund PR, Overand PT, Cooper J, et al: A prospective study of intraoperative pulse oximetry failure. J Clin Monit 7:253, 1991.
49. Gillies B, Posner K, Freund P, Cheney F: Failure rate of pulse oximetry in the post-anesthesia care unit. J Clin Monit 9:326, 1993.
50. Reich DL, Timcenko A, Bodian A, et al: Predictors of pulse oximetry data failure. Anesthesiology 84:859, 1996.
51. Brodsky JB, Shulman MS, Swan M, Mark JBD: Pulse oximetry during OLV. Anesthesiology 63:212, 1985.
52. Desiderio DP, Wong G, Shah K, et al: A clinical evaluation of pulse oximetry during thoracic surgery. J Cardiothorac Anesth 4: 30, 1990.
53. Thys DM, Cohen E, Girard D, et al: The pulse oximeter: A noninvasive monitor of oxygenation during thoracic surgery. Thorac Cardiovasc Surg 34:380, 1986.
54. Altman DG, Bland JM: Measurement in medicine: The analysis of method comparison studies. Statistician 32:307, 1983.
55. Kim JM, Arakawa K, Benson KT, et al: Pulse oximetry and circulatory kinetics associated with pulse volume amplitude measured by photoelectric plethysmograph. Anesth Analg 65:1333, 1986.
56. Lawson D, Norley I, Korbon G, et al: Blood flow limits and pulse oximeter signal detection. Anesthesiology 67:599, 1987.
57. Pälve H, Vuori A: Minimum pulse pressure and peripheral temperature needed for pulse oximetry during cardiac surgery with cardiopulmonary bypass. J Cardiothorac Vasc Anesth 5:372, 1991.
58. Barker SJ, Shah NK: Effects of motion on the performance of pulse oximeters. Anesthesiology 85:774, 1996.
59. Dumas C, Wahr JA, Tremper KK: Clinical evaluation of a prototype motion artifact resistant pulse oximeter in the recovery room. Anesth Analg 83:269, 1996.
60. Eberhard P, Hammacher K, Mindt W: Methods zur kutanen Messung des sauerstoffpartialdrukkes [Method for cutaneous measurement of the oxygen partial pressure]. Biomed Tech 18:212, 1973.
61. Huch A, Huch R, Meinzer K, et al: Eine schuelle, behizte Ptoberflachenelektrode zur kontinuierlichen Uberwachung des PO_2 beim Menschen. Elcktrodenaufbau and Eigenschaften (Abstract). Stuttgart, Proc Medizin-Technik, 1972, p 26.
62. Severinghaus JW, Stafford M, Bradley AF: $tcPcO_2$ electrode design, calibration and temperature gradient problems. Acta Anaesthesiol Scand Suppl 68:118, 1978.
63. Severinghaus JW: A combined transcutaneous PO_2-PCO_2 electrode with electrochemical HCO_3 stabilization. J Appl Physiol Respir Environ Exercise Physiol 51:1027, 1981.
64. Van Duzee BF: Thermal analysis of human stratum corneum. J Invest Dermatol 65:404, 1975.
65. Huch R, Huch A, Lubbers DE: Transcutaneous measurement of blood PO2 (tcPO2): Method and application in perinatal medicine. J Perinat Med 1:183, 1973.
66. Row MI, Weinberg G: Transcutaneous oxygen monitoring in shock and resuscitation. J Pediatr Surg 14:773, 1979.
67. Rooth G, Hedstrand U, Tyden H, Ogren C: The validity of transcutaneous oxygen tension method in adults. Crit Care Med 4:162, 1976.
68. Tremper KK, Shoemaker WC: Transcutaneous oxygen monitoring of critically ill adults, with and without low flow shock. Crit Care Med 9:706, 1981.
69. Tremper KK, Waxman K, Shoemaker WC: Effects of hypoxia and shock on transcutaneous PO_2 values in dogs. Crit Care Med 7:526, 1979.
70. Barker SJ, Hyatt J, Clarke C, Tremper KK: Hyperventilation reduces transcutaneous oxygen tension and skin blood flow. Anesthesiology 75:619, 1991.
71. Tremper KK, Barker SJ, Blatt DH, Wender RH: Effects of anesthetic agents on the drift of a transcutaneous PO_2 sensor. J Clin Monit 2:234, 1986.
72. Baele PL, McMichan JC, Marsh HM, et al: Continuous monitoring of mixed venous oxygen saturation in critically ill patients. Anesth Analg 61:513, 1982.
73. Enson Y, Briscoe WA, Polanyi MI, Cournand A: In vivo studies with an intravascular and intracardiac reflection oximeter. J Appl Physiol 17:552, 1962.
74. Martin WE, Cheung PW, Johnson CC, Wong KC: Continuous monitoring of mixed venous oxygenation saturation in man. Anesth Analg 52:784, 1973.
75. Wilkinson AR, Phibbs RH, Gregory GA: Continuous measurement of oxygen saturation in sick newborn infants. J Pediatr 93: 1016, 1978.

76. Gettinger A, Detraglia MC, Glass DD: In vivo comparison of two mixed venous saturation catheters. Anesthesiology 66:373, 1987.
77. Barker SJ, Tremper KK, Hyatt J, Zaccari J: Effects of methemoglobinemia on pulse oximetry and mixed venous oximetry. Anesthesiology 70:112, 1989.
78. ASA Task Force on Pulmonary Artery Catheterization: Practice guidelines for pulmonary artery catheterization. Anesthesiology 78:380, 1993.
79. Cernaianu AC, DelRossi AJ, Boatman GA, et al: Continuous venous oximetry for hemodynamic and oxygen transport stability post cardiac surgery. J Cardiovasc Surg 33:14, 1992.
80. Clarke C, Edwards JD, Nightingale P, et al: Persistence of supply dependency of oxygen uptake at high levels of delivery in adult respiratory distress syndrome. Crit Care Med 19:497, 1991.
81. Shoemaker WC, Appel PL, Kram HB: Hemodynamic and oxygen transport responses in survivors and nonsurvivors of high-risk surgery. Crit Care Med 21:977, 1993.
82. Boyd O, Grounds RM, Bennett D: A randomized clinical trial of the effect of deliberate perioperative increase of oxygen delivery on mortality in high-risk surgical patients. JAMA 270:2699, 1993.
83. Yu M, Levy MM, Smith P, et al: Effect of minimizing oxygen delivery on morbidity and mortality rates in critically ill patients: A prospective, randomized, controlled study. Crit Care Med 21: 830, 1993.
84. Fleming A, Bishop M, Shoemaker WC, et al: Prospective trial of supranormal values as goals of resuscitation in severe trauma. Arch Surg 127:1175, 1992.
85. Thys DM, Cohen E, Eisenkraft JB: Mixed venous oxygen saturation during thoracic anesthesia. Anesthesiology 69:1005, 1988.
86. Zaune U, Knarr C, Krüselmann M, et al: Value and accuracy of dual oximetry during pulmonary resections. J Cardiothorac Anesth 4:441, 1990.
87. Eisenkraft JB: Respiratory Gas Monitoring. ASA Refresher Course Lecture #263, 1995. ASA Park Ridge, IL, 1995.
88. Good ML, Gravenstein N: Capnography. In Ehrenwerth J, Eisenkraft JB (eds): Anesthesia Equipment: Principles and Applications. St Louis, Mosby Year Book, Inc, 1993, p 237.
89. Zupan J, Martin M, Benumof JL: End-tidal CO_2 excretion waveform and error with gas sampling line leak. Anesth Analg 67:579, 1988.
90. Shafieha MJ, Sit J, Kartha R, et al: End-tidal CO_2 analyzers in proper positioning of the double-lumen tubes. Anesthesiology 64: 844, 1986.
91. Werner O, Malmkvist G, Beckman A, et al: Carbon dioxide elimination from each lung during endobronchial anesthesia. Br J Anaesth 56:995, 1984.
92. Fletcher R: The arterial-end tidal CO_2 difference during cardiothoracic surgery. J Cardiothorac Anesth 4:105, 1990.
93. Pansard JL, Cholley B, Devilliers C, et al: Variation in arterial to end-tidal CO_2 tension differences during anesthesia in the "kidney rest" lateral decubitus position. Anesth Analg 75:506, 1992.
94. Yam PCI, Innes PA, Jackson M, et al: Variation in the arterial to end-tidal pCO_2 difference during one-lung thoracic anaesthesia. Br J Anaesth 72:21, 1994.
95. Raemer DB, Francis DM, Philip JH, Gabel RA: Variation in PCO_2 between arterial blood and peak expired gas during anesthesia. Anesth Analg 62:1065, 1983.

CHAPTER 12

Monitoring Central and Peripheral Nervous System Function

Maria K. Sturaitis, M.D.
Robert W. McPherson, M.D.

Several monitors of cerebral hemodynamics, brain electrical function, and brain metabolic function are available for intraoperative use. A detailed description of the techniques and equipment used to monitor the central and peripheral nervous system is beyond the scope of this chapter and the reader is referred to a standard textbook on monitoring. Monitoring the adequacy of cerebral blood flow (CBF) is of particular importance during major vascular and cardiac procedures because coexisting neurologic disease and drastically changing hemodynamic conditions occur in a setting where clinical examination for diagnosis of cerebral ischemia is usually impossible. Changes in brain electrical or metabolic function can reflect the neuronal alterations associated with regional hypoperfusion. Assessment of cerebral physiology by transcranial Doppler (TCD; blood velocity in large cerebral arteries) and jugular bulb catheter (JBC; cerebral venous oxygen content, an indirect assessment of brain oxygen utilization) or computerized assessment of the electroencephalogram (EEG) and evoked potentials (EP), contribute to understanding the pathophysiology of neurologic injury. These monitoring techniques provide the opportunity to prevent cerebral, spinal cord, or peripheral nerve damage by identifying neural tissue at risk sufficiently early to prevent permanent injury. Aggressive intraoperative monitoring of neurologic status, however, does not guarantee prevention of neurologic injury, since not all parts of the brain (or spinal cord or peripheral nervous system) are assessed given currently available monitoring.

Monitoring the nervous system under anesthesia differs from monitoring of the respiratory or cardiovascular systems in several important ways. First, there may be no physical correlates for changes in neurologic function suggested by the monitors, and other monitors are not likely available to confirm or refute physiologic changes suggestive of injury. For example, changes in ST segments with electrocardiographic (ECG) monitoring suggesting myocardial ischemia may be associated with hypotension and hemodynamic instability, and may be correlated with changes in pulmonary artery occlusion pressure. In contrast, EEG changes suggestive of injury to part of the nervous system that could lead to permanent disability would otherwise be confirmed only at the end of a surgical procedure. Validation of the changes seen in monitors of brain electrical activity may be possible by recent advances in technology and understanding. For instance, EEG changes with carotid artery cross-clamp can now be correlated with changes in blood velocity by transcranial Doppler.

Monitoring of central nervous system (CNS) electrical function (EEG, evoked potentials) gives information concerning instantaneous adequacy of oxygen delivery but does not give information concerning reserve capacity (i.e., what would happen if blood pressure [and CBF] were to decrease slightly). Thus TCD, near-infrared spectroscopy (NIRS; amount of oxygen and deoxygenation hemoglobin near the surface of the brain), and jugular bulb catheters give complementary information because they suggest conditions of risk, such as embolic phenomenon or hypoperfusion prior to changes in neurologic function.

Whether measures of cerebral hemodynamics and perfusion or measures of nervous system function are considered, the clinical significance of these monitoring indices hinges on correlation with ischemia, the limitation of substrates to neural tissue, and the tolerance of the nervous system to such insults.

The nervous system is particularly resistant to injury. In a study of profound hypotension that caused death due to cardiovascular collapse (40% of animals), in survivors, recovery of severely depressed brain electrical activity (electroencephalogram and somatosensory evoked potential [SSEP]) occurs with restoration of blood pressure, without apparent neurologic injury.[1]

Normal values of CBF and other cerebral physiologic values, in the absence of anesthesia are shown in Table 12–1. These values indicate that in the normal state, oxygen delivery to neural tissue is well in excess of that needed for normal function because oxygen extraction is relatively low. The brain response to oxygen deprivation (hypoxia, anemia) is either an increase in CBF or an increase in oxygen extraction if the ability to increase CBF if limited. Cerebral oxygen consumption ($CMRO_2$)

TABLE 12–1
Normal Values of Cerebral Physiologic Function

Cerebral blood flow	50 ml/min/100 gm
Gray matter	80 ml/min/100 gm
White matter	20 ml/min/100 gm
Cerebral oxygen consumption	3.5 ml/min/100 gm
Jugular venous Po_2	38–42 mm Hg
Jugular venous oxygen saturation	60–70%

is maintained at baseline level, when CBF decreases below the lower limit of autoregulation, by increased oxygen extraction until CBF declines to less than 60% of baseline flow. Since monitors of neurologic function (EEG, EPs) do not change until $CMRO_2$ is decreased, changes in those monitors indicate failure of all compensatory mechanisms (Fig. 12–1).

Transient changes in CNS function that reverse either due to therapeutic interventions or spontaneously complicate the issue of true- or false-positives or true- or false-negatives for intraoperative monitoring. Changes or lack of changes that correlate with postoperative neurologic status are "true-positives" or "true-negatives," respectively. Transient changes reflecting intraoperative events that reverse spontaneously or by altering clinical techniques (e.g., elevation of systemic blood pressure, unclamping of a major vessel, change in limb position) are equivocal. Strictly speaking, these transient changes are "false-positive," since intraoperative changes occurred without changes in postoperative neurologic function. Similarly, there are "false-negatives" where a postoperative neurologic change is discovered without there having been a change detected by the monitoring modality.

Although monitoring of electrical function is the most direct monitor of brain function, a major disadvantage is lack of signal change until all compensatory mechanisms have been exhausted. Monitors of cerebral hemodynamic function such as TCD or metabolic function such as JBC or NIRS may suggest changes in compensatory mechanisms prior to the level that produces dysfunction of the nervous system because of oxygen deprivation. For instance, an increase in JBC oxygen extraction may suggest a decrease in CBF prior to a level that decreases $CMRO_2$ and brain electrical activity.

Anesthetic Agents and Cerebral Blood Flow (Spinal Cord Responds Like Brain)

Anesthetic agents may directly affect nervous system function and the monitors of nervous system function such as EEG and SSEP. Opposing effects may make interpretation difficult. For example, isoflurane increases CBF and decreases cerebral metabolic rate, perhaps decreasing the risk of ischemia; however, isoflurane also causes a dose-dependent decrease in EEG frequency and SSEP amplitude (wave size). Decreased EEG frequency and decreased SSEP amplitude superficially resemble changes caused by cerebral oxygen deprivation, and depressed wave amplitudes may make diagnosis of cerebral oxygen deprivation difficult.

Volatile anesthetic agents increase CBF in a dose-dependent manner. Intravenous hypnotic agents such as thiopental, etomidate, and propofol all decrease CBF (Table 12–2). Both volatile and intravenous agents decrease cerebral metabolic rate.

The effect of ketamine on both CBF and $CMRO_2$ is controversial. Ketamine has been reported to increase CBF, although probably associated with increased $Paco_2$.[2] In mechanically ventilated normocarbic animals, intravenous ketamine had no effect on CBF, but decreased $CMRO_2$ by 14%, whereas in spontaneously breathing animals, a similar dose of ketamine increased CBF by 40% (associated with a 7-mm Hg increase in $Paco_2$).[3] A delayed increase in $CMRO_2$ (42%) occurred 10 minutes after ketamine administration and was associated with an increase in intermediate EEG frequency and voltage of 97%.[4] Narcotics and neuromuscular blocking drugs generally have little effect on CBF.

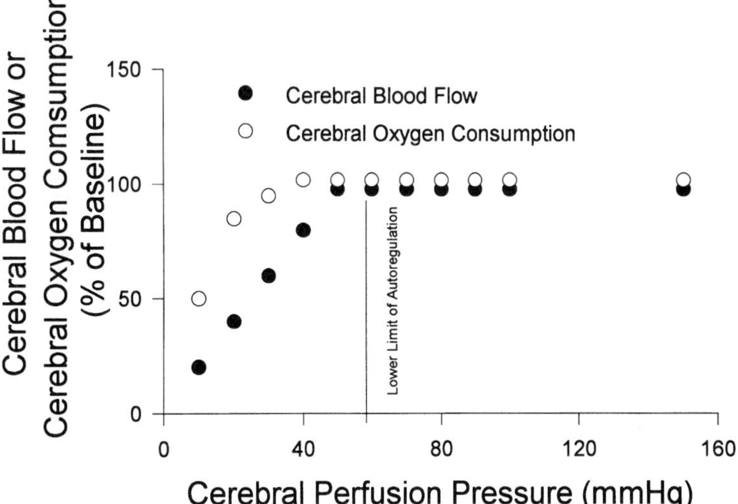

FIGURE 12–1. The relationship between cerebral blood flow and cerebral oxygen consumption as cerebral perfusion pressure is decreased is shown. Note that cerebral oxygen consumption is maintained at a normal level even after cerebral blood flow decreases. Increased oxygen extraction maintains cerebral oxygen consumption and can be demonstrated by a decrease in jugular bulb oxygen saturation.

TABLE 12–2
Cerebral Blood Flow and Intracranial Pressure

	MAC/IV Dose	Cerebral Blood Flow	Intracranial Pressure
Halothane	0.75%	↑	↑
Enflurane	1.7%	↑	↑
Isoflurane	1.2%	↑	↑
Desflurane	6.0%	↑	↑
Sevoflurane	2.1%	↑	↑
Nitrous oxide	105%	↑	↑
Thiopental	4 mg/kg	↓	↓
Fentanyl	25 μg/kg	↓→	↓
Etomidate	0.4 mg/kg	↓	↓
Propofol	2 mg/kg	↓	↓
Ketamine	2–4 mg/kg	↑→*	↑→

*No change in CBF unless associated with an increase in $PaCO_2$.[2–4]
MAC, alveolar concentration necessary to prevent movement in 50% of subjects.

Monitors of Cerebral Hemodynamics

Transcranial Doppler Ultrasonography

TCD ultrasonography is a noninvasive measure of continuous blood flow velocity in major cerebral vessels. The ultrasonic probe can be placed on the skin at regions of the skull where the bone is relatively thin and directed at an intracranial artery. The middle, anterior, and posterior cerebral arteries, posterior communicating artery, and distal internal carotid arteries can be monitored via the temporal bone "ultrasonic window." The carotid siphon, anterior communicating artery, and ophthalmic arteries can be studied via the transorbital approach, and the posterior circulation, including basilar and distal vertebral arteries, may be monitored through the foramen magnum.

Pulses of ultrasound are reflected by moving blood and a change in energy level occurs, with a shift in frequency of the reflected wave proportional to blood velocity. TCD displays velocity versus time, and by analysis of signals received within a specific interval of time, velocities within small sample volumes along a vessel can be measured.

Factors that determine blood velocity are: (1) pressure gradient along a vessel, (2) vessel length, (3) cross-sectional area, and (4) blood viscosity. Inferences regarding changes in CBF are made with an assumption of constant vascular caliber and blood viscosity (hematocrit). Under conditions of hypothermia with increasing blood viscosity, or hemodilution, therefore, the assessment of CBF by TCD must be modified, or at least comparisons with values obtained under other conditions must be made carefully.

The measurement of mean velocity (MV) is strongly influenced by arterial vessel diameter and its significance has been questioned.[5] However, most vascular reactivity occurs in precapillary arterioles rather than the larger cerebral arteries, which behave as "stiff pipes," and except for unusual situations of middle cerebral artery or carotid siphon stenosis or vasospasm (subarachnoid hemorrhage), MV changes should reflect blood flow changes.[6] Moderate changes in blood pressures and $PaCO_2$ cause only slight changes in middle cerebral artery diameter.[7] Changes in middle cerebral artery velocity correlate well with changes in CBF measured by standard techniques such as xenon-133 (^{133}Xe) clearance, radioactive microspheres, and single photon emission computed tomography (SPECT).[8–10] Van DerLinden et al.[11] compared TCD and thermodilution venous cerebral blood flow in seven adult patients undergoing hypothermia CPB and found a correlation between TCD middle cerebral artery velocity and cerebral venous flow of 0.77 ($p < .001$).

With each cardiac cycle, blood is pushed along the arterial tree, and the more resistance the blood encounters along an artery, the less bounding the velocity tracing appears. When blood passes through a narrowed region, or region of collateral flow, increased resistance can be seen. Systolic and diastolic velocities slow at different rates, and the pulsatility index reflects these changes, as it is calculated by the difference between the systolic and diastolic velocities divided by the mean velocity.

Air and solid emboli produce distinctive TCD patterns. In a swine model, internal carotid injection of air (0.1 to 5 ml) produced characteristic signals of very high velocity that exceeded the maximum systolic peak velocity, and a simultaneous equal velocity signal away from the probe, suggesting bubble expansion. The associated audible signal was variable. Characteristic signals due to atherosclerotic plaque fragments (0.075 to 0.1 mm) included a uniform single discreet spectra that was always within the limits of the velocity waveform, and which had a consistent duration related to plaque size. The audible signal has a reproducible high pitch[12,13] (Fig. 12–2).

Constancy of TCD probe angle with an insonation angle nearly parallel to the vessel is required to obtain valid data.[14] During perioperative monitoring minor alterations in patient head position can result in small changes in insonation angle with significant consequent changes in the TCD waveform.

Anatomic differences in temporal bone window may interfere with producing an adequate waveform signal.

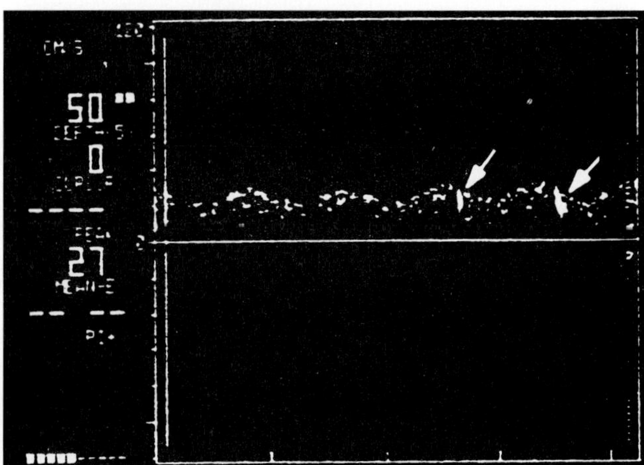

FIGURE **12–2.** Characteristic transcranial Doppler pattern of emboli (*arrows*).

Transtemporal window quality deteriorates progressively with age due to hyperostosis, more severe in women than men and more severe in African-Americans than Caucasians[15] Several studies suggest that both age and gender play an important role in determining normal blood flow velocities.[16,17]

In normal volunteers, presyncopal symptoms (presumably due to decreased CBF) appeared at a MV of 33 (normal 52), and symptoms increased in severity at MV of 25, suggesting a further decrease in CBF. Arterial collapse was observed (diastolic velocity of zero) in one subject at a brain diastolic blood pressure of 21 mm Hg (with severe presyncopal symptoms).[18]

TCD flow velocities do not distinguish patients who develop neurologic symptoms with cerebral vasospasm following subarachnoid hemorrhage. High flow velocities (suggesting low CBF) do not necessarily mean impending neurologic deficits: 8 of 66 patients tolerated flow velocities over 200 cm/sec.[19]

TCD may be useful in determining cerebral distribution of paradoxical emboli. Agitated saline contrast injection was used to determine preferential distribution of the contrast into the anterior or posterior intracranial circulation of patients with a acute stroke or transient ischemic attack. Microcavitations were detected in the proximal right middle cerebral artery in 12 of 49 patients (24% with patent foramen ovale). Of those 12 patients, microcavitations were also detected in the proximal basilar artery in 9 patients.[20]

Finally, TCD measurements of MV during anesthesia parallel anesthetic effects on CBF.

Table 12–3 displays effects of anesthetics on middle cerebral artery MV.

Laser Doppler Flowmetry

TCD measurements give information concerning changes in cerebral perfusion within the region supplied by major cerebral arteries. Laser Doppler flowmetry (LDF) measures local cerebral blood flow but must be placed after craniectomy. LDF measures local CBF in a small area by measuring red blood cell movement through a sampled volume of the microcirculation. This technique is based on the Doppler principle. Infrared light emitted from a laser probe directed to the tissue interacts with moving red blood cells, and the frequencies of the photons undergo a Doppler shift related to the velocity of the red cells. A photodetector collects the reflected light, which is amplified and processed, with generation of a signal proportional to blood flow.[37] The sampled volume of brain microvascular network, which includes arterioles, capillaries, and venules, is usually about 1 mm^3.[38] Although different laser sources will provide different dimensions for the sampled volume, vessels in the sampled volume range in diameter from 5 to 500 μm.[39,40]

Attempts have been made to derive conversion factors for LDF arbitrary flow units (AU), to absolute flow units (i.e., from millivolts to milliliters per 100 gm per minute). This is currently unreliable, since sampled volume varies due to changes in hemoglobin content, which affects laser light tissue absorption. Interpretation of arbitrary units based on continuous monitoring in patients has led to description of a range for LDF values that suggests cerebral ischemia if below 50 AU or 500 MV, and cerebral hyperemia if above 150 AU or 1500 MV.[37] The validity of these ischemic or hyperemic values has been questioned, and further studies are needed to assess whether the relative changes in flow, accurately measured by LDF, can be used to define the presence of cerebral ischemia.[41]

Several technical limitations of LDF, such as the requirement for placement of the probe adjacent to cortical tissue, the impact of hematocrit on sample volume (and consequent blood flow measurement), sensitivity of the probe to positional changes and movement artifacts, need to be addressed before this monitoring technique can achieve reliable intraoperative applicability.

Monitors of Cerebral Metabolic Function

Near Infrared Spectroscopy

NIRS is a noninvasive method of measuring brain hemoglobin oxygen saturation and, thus, a means of measuring brain function by obtaining data about oxygen utilization. The cerebral microvasculature consists of 20% arterial, 5% capillary, and 75% venous blood. A sensor is placed just lateral to the midline of the forehead and emits near infrared light at 2 to 3 wavelengths between 650 and 1,100 nm. The infrared light penetrates scalp, skull, and brain and is reflected and refracted

TABLE 12–3
Anesthetic Effects of TCD

Drug	Blood Flow Velocity	Pulsatility Index	References
Thiopental	Decrease	No change?	21, 22
Etomidate	Decrease	Increase	23
Ketamine	Increase	Decrease	24
Propofol	Decrease	Increase	25, 26
Midazolam	Decrease	Increase	27
Narcotics	Decrease with sufentanil, slight decrease with alfentanil	Increase	28, 29, 30
Volatile anesthetics	Increased with isoflurane, N_2O; no change in children for halothane and isoflurane, and slight change for N_2O		31, 32; 33, 34, 35, 36

TCD, transcranial Doppler; N_2O, nitrous oxide.

before return to the sensor. The light is attenuated by the light-absorbing iron-porphyrin in oxyhemoglobin or deoxyhemoglobin, and copper in cytochrome-*c* oxidase.[42]

Normal cerebral oxygen saturation in awake humans is about 70%. Hampson and co-workers demonstrated decreased oxyhemoglobin and oxidized cytochrome and increased deoxyhemoglobin during induced hypoxia in normal adult volunteers.[43] Pollard and co-workers confirmed the findings of Hampson and colleagues, but noted the importance of maintaining a constant patient position during monitoring.[44,45]

The sensitivity of NIRS is enhanced because the dominant pigment for light absorption in brain tissue is hemoglobin, cytochrome oxidase absorbs only partly in this region of the spectrum at a factor of approximately 20 nm less than hemoglobin, and melanin interferes little with measurements. The specificity of the technique is a reflection of how measures of hemoglobin oxygenation correlate with cerebral ischemia. Owen-Reece and co-workers have used NIRS to determine cerebral blood flow in conscious and anesthetized adults.[46] They noted that cerebral blood flow values measured from the scalp underestimated the true flow measured by invasive techniques. However, the technique may eventually be used to assess cerebral perfusion at the bedside.

Cerebral oximetry and spectroscopy have been performed in animals, children, and adults in various situations of hypoxia, hyperventilation, cardiopulmonary bypass, drug-induced vascular changes (indomethacin, aminophylline), and during reduced cerebral blood flow (carotid ligation or endarterectomy). Ferrari et al.[47] assessed noninvasive determination of hemoglobin saturation in dogs with NIRS and found that the standard deviation for the difference between sagittal sinus O_2 saturation (reflecting brain O_2 extraction) and that predicted by NIRS was 3.2% and the correlation coefficient was .97 (Fig. 12–3). In adults, Levy and co-workers found a mean cerebral saturation of 56.5% during general anesthesia with hyperventilation.[42] Ausman et al.[48] studied seven patients with NIRS undergoing hypothermic circulatory arrest (10 to 65 minutes) and found a negative correlation between arrest time and oxygen saturation. Five patients had O_2 saturation greater than 35% and had no neurologic injury. One patient with O_2 saturation less than 35% had global injury (Fig. 12–4). During induced ventricular fibrillation, cerebral saturation decreased and a threshold of 47% correlated with signs of cerebral ischemia.[42] During cardiopulmonary bypass in adults, Nollert et al. found that cerebral cellular oxygenation depended upon temperature, pH, and hemoglobin while cerebral oxygenated hemoglobin depended solely upon P_{CO_2}.[49]

Confirming the earlier work of Greeley et al.,[50] Kurth and co-workers followed changes in cerebral hemoglobin oxygenation during hypothermic circulatory arrest in neonates, infants, and children.[51] They noted that the cerebral hemoglobin oxygen saturation had a half-life of 9 ± 1 minutes in neonates following onset of circulatory arrest and was shorter in infants and children. In pediatric patients in whom the usual increase in cerebral hemoglobin oxygen saturation during hypothermic cardiopulmonary bypass was impaired, postoperative neurologic status was abnormal.[50]

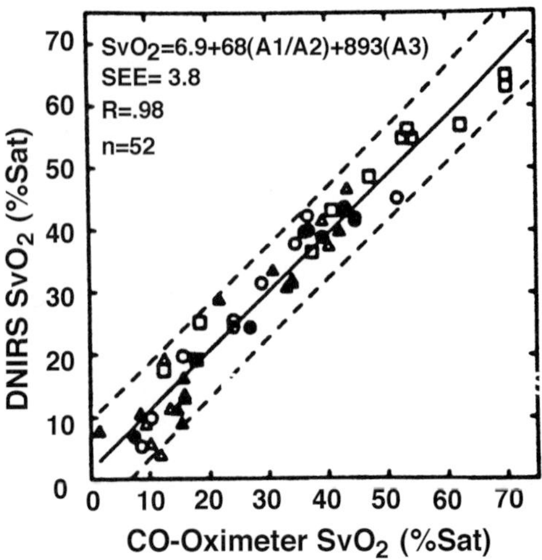

FIGURE **12–3.** The correlation of near infrared spectroscopy (NIRS) with saturation in the superior sagittal sinus. Relationships in five dogs are shown, each represented by a different symbol, between venous O_2 saturation (S_{VO_2}) calculated from a linear algorithm using first derivative at three wavelengths and value measured in superior sagittal sinus (A1, A2, A3: derivatives calculated at 818, 728, and 879 nm). Each *data point* represents a different hypoxic hypoxia level. *Line* represents first-order regression that fits all data points. *Dashed lines* represents 95% prediction confidence intervals. Note that there is a very good correlation over a wide range of oxygen saturation. *Inset*: Multiple regression slope and intercept, correlation coefficient (*r*), standard error of estimation (SEE), and number of data points represented (*n*). DNIRS, derivative near-infrared spectroscopy. (From Ferrari M, Wilson DA, Hanley F, et al: Noninvasive determination of hemoglobin saturation in dogs by derivative near infrared spectroscopy. Am J Physiol 256:H1493, 1989, with permission.)

The utility of NIRS during carotid endarterectomy has been reported by Samra, Kirkpatrick, Mason and co-workers.[52–54] A decrease in the ipsilateral cerebral hemoglobin oxygen saturation was demonstrated during carotid clamping but varied widely among patients and could not be correlated with clinically detectable neurologic dysfunction.[52] Similar NIRS findings during carotid clamping, which correlated with flow velocity changes demonstrated by transcranial Doppler, were reported by Kirkpatrick[53] and Mason.[54]

Jugular Bulb Catheter

In man, drainage of the jugular vein is essentially uncontaminated cerebral venous blood and forms the basis of the classic Kety-Schmidt method of determination of CBF. Advantage can be taken of the relationship between CBF and cerebral oxygen consumption to obtain important information concerning cerebral physiology from blood drawn from the jugular bulb.

$$\text{Cerebral oxygen consumption}$$
$$= \text{cerebral blood flow (CBF)} \times O_2 \text{ extraction}$$
$$= \text{CBF} \times (\text{arterial-jugular venous } O_2 \text{ content difference})$$

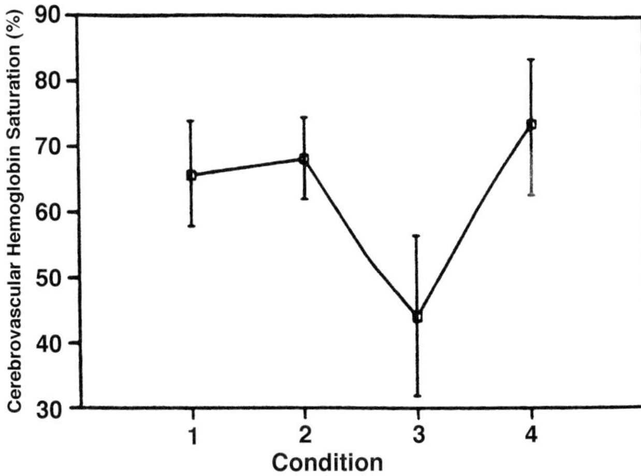

FIGURE 12–4. NIRS. Graph illustrating cerebrovascular saturation at four conditions: (1) the end of passive cooling; (2) the end of active cooling; (3) the end of circulatory arrest; and (4) immediately following reperfusion. A significant ($p < .01$) desaturation of residual cerebral hemoglobin is demonstrated during condition 3. There is no significant difference between conditions 1, 2, and 4. *Vertical bars* represent standard error of the mean. (From Ausman JI, McCormick PW, Stewart M, et al: Cerebral oxygen metabolism during hypothermic circulatory arrest in humans. J Neurosurg 79:810, 1993, with permission.)

Since arterial oxygen content is constant (over short periods of time) and it is usually safe to assume that $CMRO_2$ is also constant (over short periods of time and constant brain temperature), venous oxygen content is directly related to CBF. A decrease in CBF should increase O_2 extraction (and lower jugular venous oxygen content) and vice versa.

Jugular O_2 saturation is greater than 60% in awake man (Pvo_2 38 to 42 mm Hg). During isoflurane anesthesia in dogs, Pvo_2 is 50 to 56 mm Hg due to increased CBF and lower $CMRO_2$.[55] The ability to increase CBF and to increase oxygen extraction is maintained during isoflurane anesthesia. During hypoxic hypoxia, cerebral venous O_2 decreased to 19 to 21 mm Hg (O_2 content of 6.6 to 8.0 ml/dl) when Pao_2 was 24 to 26 mm Hg.[55]

In animal studies of decreased cerebral perfusion pressure (CPP), brain energy failure occurs at an average arteriovenous oxygen content difference ($AVDO_2$) of 8.4 vol%. The venous oxygen content (Vo_2) at energy failure was 1.45 vol% and the range was relatively small (1.0 to 2.9 vol%).[56]

Jugular venous bulb saturations can be determined with intermittent measurements from a catheter or continuously using a fiberoptic catheter. During cardiopulmonary bypass, both methods demonstrate decreases in oxygen saturation during the rewarming phase.[57,58] More recent work, however, raises questions regarding the accuracy of fiberoptic catheter measurements.[59] Trubiano and colleagues found a correlation of only .44 on linear regression of catheter and co-oximeter values.[59] They noted particular difficulties with low-amplitude signals obtained when the catheter tip touched the vessel wall as it faced venous blood flow.

Goetting and Preston[60] assessed JBC placement in 123 pediatric patients and found catheter insertion time was about 16 minutes with a median number of two skin punctures. They found a carotid puncture rate of 3%. In 28 pediatric patients they found that the maximum increase in ICP with JBC insertion was 2 mm Hg.[61] Under special circumstances (newborn on extracorporeal membrane oxygenation), a jugular bulb catheter may significantly decrease superior sagittal sinus flow and may be associated with a higher incidence of cerebrovascular injury.[62]

Monitors of Nervous System Electrical Function

EEG reliably assesses only cortical function, although subcortical structures are involved in wave generation. SSEP assesses the neural axis from peripheral nerve through brain stem to contralateral cerebral cortex. Brain stem auditory evoked response (BAER) assesses only brain stem (waves occurring <10 msec), although long-latency cortical waves (>20 msec after stimuli) can be assessed to evaluate cortical function. The motor evoked potential (MEP) assesses function of the motor cortex and descending motor tracts with the peripheral response assessed by compound muscle action potential. All modalities of brain function, EEG (unprocessed EEG; computer-processed EEG), and evoked potentials (auditory, somatosensory) and motor evoked potentials may be monitored intraoperatively, depending upon the neural tissue at risk.

Visual evoked responses (VER) have been used to assess function of the visual apparatus, including the occipital cortex in unanesthetized patients. Intraoperative instability of VER waves during intracranial procedures has limited its intraoperative use.[63]

Intraoperative monitoring occurs over a prolonged period, and data should be presented so that significant blocks of time can be evaluated for trends. Although there is an obvious need to quickly correct abnormalities caused by cerebral ischemia, such abnormalities may be self-limited.[64]

Electrical activity of the nervous system, both spontaneous and evoked, is measured using a reference electrode system that records and amplifies voltage changes over time at an active electrode compared to a reference electrode (electrically quiet). With both EEG and evoked potential monitoring, the international 10 to 20 system of electrode placement normalizes electrode placement for variability in skull shape and size.

Electroencephalogram

The EEG may be monitored to determine anesthetic level or to assess adequacy of brain oxygenation. Global or localized cerebral oxygen deprivation may occur and the monitoring system should detect either type of event. The EEG is evaluated for wave amplitude and frequency and patterns of brain waves with specific amplitude and frequency characteristics previously validated in normal individuals or pathologic circumstances.

Intraoperative EEG monitoring requires recognition of characteristic EEG patterns that occur normally or represent changes in the EEG due to anesthetic agents or cerebral oxygen deprivation. Characteristic rhythms are defined according to frequency, amplitude, and location. *Alpha rhythm* has a frequency between 8 and 12 Hz and a variable amplitude of less than 50 μV with rounded or sinusoidal waves. This rhythm is best seen when eyes are closed and the subject is relaxed and blocked or attenuated by attention. Maximum alpha rhythm voltage is found over the occipital region. *Beta rhythm* (13 to 40 Hz) is found chiefly over the frontal and central regions with amplitude less than 30 μV. *Theta waves* (4 to 7.5 Hz) have amplitude of greater than 50 μV. Theta rhythm is usually found in infants and children but may persist to 25 to 30 years of age. *Delta waves* (0.1 to 3.5 Hz, >75 μV) occur during normal sleep. There is always a small amount of theta activity in a normal EEG. In the awake individual, the EEG consists of mainly beta activity with small amounts of delta and theta activity. If the individual is relaxed with eyes closed, alpha activity may be present.

Burst suppression is a dramatic EEG pattern in which there are short periods of electrocortical silence alternating with low-frequency, high-voltage activity (Fig. 12–5). Whether drug-induced burst suppression is a valid neuroprotective maneuver for episodes of potential ischemia (e.g., temporary vessel occlusion), remains controversial. This pattern may be produced by high doses of hypnotic drugs (barbiturates, etomidate, and propofol), by high inspired concentrations of isoflurane, and by hypothermia to the degree seen during cardiopulmonary bypass. Heart rate changes are associated with burst suppression during isoflurane anesthesia. At the onset of an EEG burst, the heart rate starts to accelerate and at the onset of suppression starts to decelerate.[65] At least in the rat, a burst suppression pattern during isoflurane anesthesia does not ensure lack of purposeful response to stimuli.[66]

Depending on patient age and temperature, the dose of thiopental required to produce a greater than 60-second burst suppression in patients on CPB varies from 8 mg/kg[67] to 15 mg/kg.[68] Etomidate (0.2 mg/kg plus infusion of 20 mg/min) also causes burst suppression.[69]

Mild ischemia decreases high-frequency EEG activity, whereas a decrease in high-frequency and an increase in the low-frequency activity occurs with moderate ischemia. Severe ischemia decreases activity of all frequencies. Burst suppression may also be seen as the brain is deprived of oxygen and during reoxygenation as the metabolic status of the brain is repaired. The decrease in activity is usually bilateral if ischemia is caused by hypotension, and the changes seen are almost always unilateral on the side of the cross-clamp, if due to carotid cross-clamping.

Intraoperative EEG monitoring requires data reduction to allow timely evaluation and therapeutic decisions. EEG in the operating room may be contaminated by rhythmic artifacts produced by pumps and other machines that may be incorporated by computer-processed EEG and presented as normal EEG due to frequency or amplitude characteristics resembling brain waves. Thus,

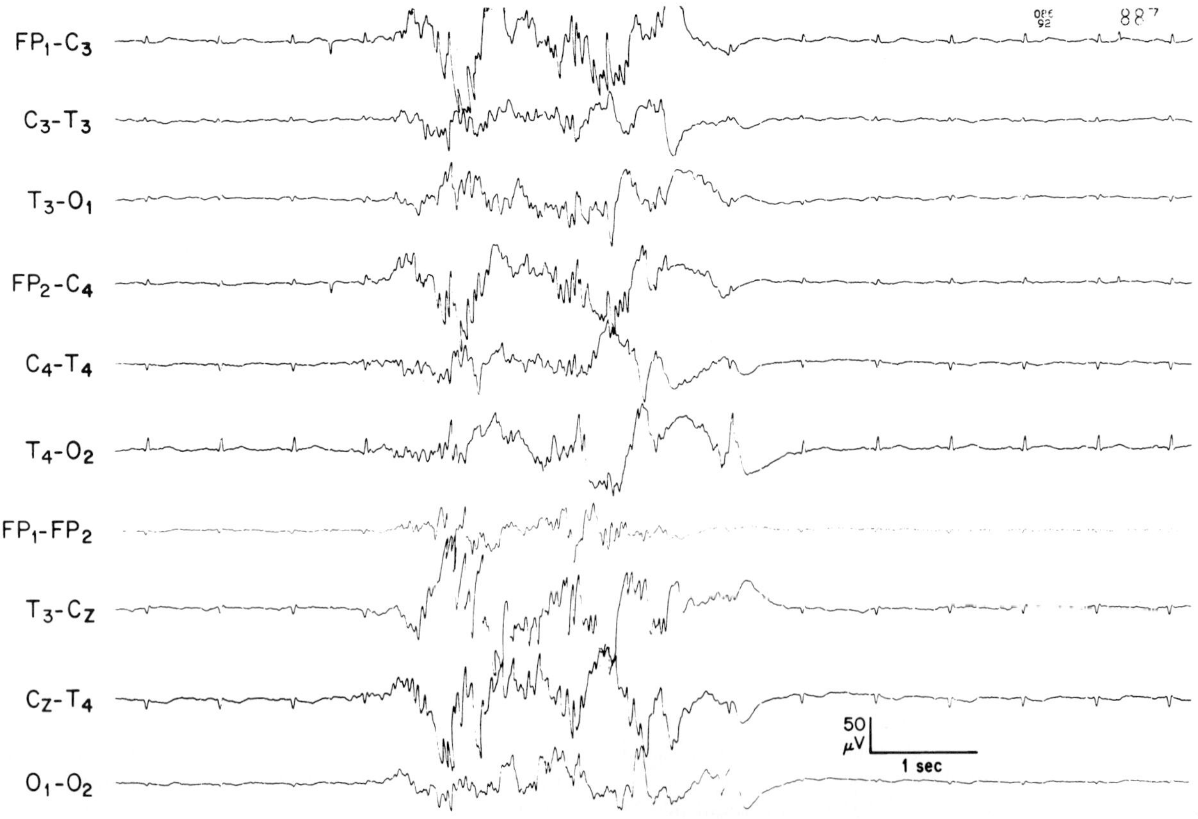

FIGURE **12–5.** Drug-induced burst suppression is shown. Burst suppression due to cerebral oxygen deprivation is similar in appearance.

all computer-processed EEG should provide easy access to the unprocessed data for visual evaluation.

Multiple methods of computer EEG analysis are available,[70] all of which use analysis of amplitude, frequency, or both, or some mathematical derivation of one or both to represent brain activity. Fast-Fourier transform (FFT) allows rapid evaluation of amplitude and latency and allows data to be displayed in compressed spectral array (CSA) or density spectral array (DSA). Band spectral analysis (BSA) is another display method in which power in bands (delta, theta, alpha, and beta) are displayed.

Assessment of spectral edge frequency (SEF) is an attempt to simplify EEG interpretation. SEF is the highest frequency present. During cardiopulmonary bypass there is correlation with spectral edge frequency and tympanic membrane temperature. Transient bilateral slowing (decrease in SEF) occurs in 50% of patients after removal of aortic clamp (no neurologic deficits).[71] Changes in EEG power are more sensitive than spectral edge frequency variation for detection of cerebral ischemia during carotid endarterectomy.[72]

Changes in SEF correlate with hemodynamic response to laryngoscopy and intubation.[73] However, Ghouri et al.[74] found that spectral edge analysis is not useful in predicting hypertensive response to surgical stimulation. EEG descriptors for awakening such as SEF are more accurate during isoflurane anesthesia than fentanyl-based anesthesia.[75]

EEG changes due to hypothermia on CPB, particularly loss of higher frequencies, require specialized methods of analysis such as the augmented delta quotient (increased emphasis on delta band).[76] This quotient emphasizes detection of changes in low-frequency components.

Sensory Evoked Potentials

Evoked potentials are computer averages of the brain's response to repetitive peripheral stimuli. These waves are small (1 to 2 μV) compared to the average EEG voltage (50 to 100 μV). Averaging reinforces electrical activity that occurs at the same time and polarity following each stimulation. Random electrical activity is eventually averaged to zero. The number of averages (and hence the time) required to produce a stable waveform is inversely proportional to the amplitude of the wave, so that anesthetic depression of waves may substantially increase the time for waveform evaluation.

Waveforms are evaluated for latency (delay after stimulus) or size (amplitude) of characteristic waves. Waveforms are designated for polarity, negative (N) or positive (P), plus nominal latency following stimulation for SSEP. BAER waves occurring within 10 msec of stimulation are designated in order of appearance by consecutive roman numerals (I through VII), whereas later waves are designated similar to SSEP waves by polarity and nominal latency. Characteristic waves originate in brachial plexus (Erb's point) and from the cervical spine (C2), and so injury can be localized centrally versus peripherally.

Brain electrical activity may be classified as either near-field or far-field waves. Near-field waves are generated near the recording electrode, for example, scalp-recorded SSEP waves. Far-field waves are recorded by electrodes distant from the neural generators. BAER waves are generated in the brain stem but recorded over the vertex of the skull and, thus, are far-field waves.

Somatosensory Evoked Potentials

SSEPs are the response of the neural axis from peripheral nerve to contralateral somatosensory cortex to repetitive peripheral nerve stimulation. Function of peripheral nerve, spinal cord (posterior columns), and brain (brain stem, medial lemniscus, internal capsule, contralateral somatosensory cortex) can be assessed with this monitoring modality. SSEPs can be used to detect localized injury to specific areas of the neural axis or as a nonspecific indicator of adequacy of cerebral oxygen delivery by assessing cortically generated waves. Thus, processes that produce major changes in SSEPs due to lower extremity stimulation indicate injury to the posterior columns of the spinal cord.

Although anesthetics produce direct effects on monitored SSEP waveforms, suppression of muscle artifact by neuromuscular blocking agents and the ability to use a much higher stimulus intensity in the anesthetized patient allows rapid production of waves, which are reproducible but differ moderately from those found in the awake patient. Increased stimulus intensity increases wave amplitude and tends to reverse anesthesia-related depression.

Diagnostic criteria to evaluate intraoperative waveform changes have been difficult to establish. Using conventional averaging techniques, latency changes of 7 to 15% and amplitude decreases of 45 to 50% may occur without changes in postoperative neurologic function during spinal surgery.[77,78] The exact causes of amplitude variability in those studies is unclear. However, during stable barbiturate anesthesia in an animal study, SSEP amplitude is directly related to cerebral oxygen available during hypoxia and also directly correlated with the brain's ability to utilize oxygen following an insult.[79] Use of the amplitude ratio of median nerve to posterior tibial nerve SSEP has been suggested as a method to evaluate systemic effects on the posterior tibial waveform. Such adjustments might be helpful during monitoring of intra-abdominal vascular procedures.

Brain Stem Auditory Evoked Responses

Auditory nerve stimulation produces both brain stem components and cortical components, although the latter have received only modest interest in intraoperative monitoring. The BAER is the response of the auditory apparatus to stimulation of the auditory nerve. Widespread use has occurred despite the extremely small amount of neural tissue involved and the resistance of BAER to oxygen deprivation compared to other neural monitors such as EEG or cortical SSEP waves.[80]

The origin of the waves are wave I (auditory nerve), wave II (pontomedullary junction), wave III (caudal pons), wave IV (rostral pons), wave V (midbrain), and wave VI (thalamus). The BAER is generated by delivering pure tone clicks individually to each ear. The characteristic peaks are labeled with roman numerals. Interpeak latencies can be used to assess brain stem injury, and calculation of I through V interpeak latency assesses transmission from the eighth cranial nerve to the inferior colliculi.

Motor Evoked Potentials

The limitation in SSEP monitoring of the spinal cord (i.e., monitoring of posterior columns rather than motor pathways) has focused interest on directly monitoring the motor system. The motor cortex has been stimulated using transcranial electrical stimulation (E-MEP) and, more recently, by magnetic stimulation (M-MEP). Corticospinal response to direct stimulation of the motor cortex can be recorded from the lateral columns of the spinal cord or spinal epidural space using percutaneous needles.[81] Monitoring of MEPs is difficult because of the efficiency of the CNS in conducting impulses via the spinal cord and peripheral nerves to muscle groups. These extremely small electrical impulses are difficult to record over the spinal cord or peripheral nerves. The muscle response to stimulation of the motor cortex is much larger than the neural response and therefore much easier to record. The majority of understanding of MEPs is based on compound muscle action potential responses despite the fact that both volatile anesthetic and neuromuscular blocking agents obtund those responses. Latency is increased with magnetic compared to electrical generation of the MEPs. Less stimulus artifact is produced with magnetic stimulation than with electrical stimulation because stimulus artifact ceases at termination of stimulus, whereas with electrical stimulation artifact persists for a short time after stimulation.[82]

Magnetic MEPs are produced by discharging an electromagnet near the skull over the motor cortex, which is easily tolerated in awake humans. Coil characteristics and orientation for stimulation are currently under intensive investigation. Electrical stimulation theoretically can cause seizures. Stimuli typically necessary to cause seizures are of greater duration than those required for MEPs and kindling is not produced at a stimulus rate less than 3 per second. Implanted metallic devices such as aneurysm clips pose increased risk with magnetic stimulation because of movement potential.

Pathophysiologic Anesthesia Effects

Electroencephalogram

Thiopental causes a biphasic effect on EEG with an initial increase in fast activity (beta rhythm) with slowing, burst suppression, and electrocortical silence occurring with higher doses.[83] Etomidate causes a sustained theta activity with underlying fast activity that is similar to barbiturates but with two- to threefold higher power.[84] With higher doses of etomidate, high-amplitude theta activity and then burst suppression occurs[84] with EEG frequency inversely related to the serum etomidate level.[85]

Fentanyl causes a dose-dependent slowing of the EEG.[86] Other synthetic narcotics similar to fentanyl cause similar alterations in the EEG.[87] Narcotic-induced EEG changes lag behind (in time) serum narcotic concentration and may be due to the large blood-brain partition coefficient for fentanyl.

Nitrous oxide produces fast EEG activity (>20 Hz) in concentrations that produce unconsciousness in unpremedicated humans[88] with activity predominantly in the frontal areas and a peak frequency of 34 Hz. Amplitude and quantity of increased activity increases with concentration of nitrous oxide and returns to control over 1 hour following discontinuation of nitrous oxide.

Halothane causes a progressive slowing of EEG frequency as concentration is increased[89] and does not appear to enhance epileptogenic activity.[90] Enflurane causes a dose-dependent loss of fast wave activity[91] with periods of burst suppression occurring with high concentrations. Enflurane may cause generalized seizures with characteristic tonic clonic activity and high-voltage EEG activity in humans,[92] even in concentrations less than that necessary for satisfactory anesthesia.

Isoflurane initially produces a low-amplitude EEG with a frequency of 15 to 35 Hz. With loss of consciousness, 12- to 14-Hz activity is superimposed on 2- to 5-Hz high-amplitude waves.[93] Anesthetic doses of isoflurane produce increasing periods of burst suppression with complete electrocortical silence appearing at end-inspired concentration of 2.5%.[94] The amount of isoelectricity during stable isoflurane anesthesia may be increased by pancuronium[95] and may be opposed by coadministration of nitrous oxide.[96] Although isoflurane decreases EEG frequency and increases amplitude, it does not interfere with the diagnosis of intraoperative ischemia by EEG.[97] Desflurane produces EEG patterns comparable to isoflurane in the equianesthetic doses.[98]

Somatosensory Evoked Potentials

Early components of the SSEP (<40 msec for upper extremity nerve stimulation; <80 msec for lower extremity nerve stimulation) are readily generated for intraoperative monitoring and information about anesthetic effects on those waves will be emphasized. Intravenous agents generally have only moderate effects on early parts of the waveforms and allow generation of waveforms adequate for rapid evaluation. A surprising drug effect on SSEP waveform is increase of amplitude (200 to 600%) caused by etomidate.[99] Waveform augmentation appears to be a cortical effect[99] and has been used clinically to augment abnormally small waves, thus allowing monitoring that would have otherwise not been possible.[100] Volatile anesthetic gases and nitrous oxide are all depressant on SSEP waveform apparently in a dose-

TABLE 12–4
Anesthetic Effects of Somatosensory Evoked Potentials

Drug	Amplitude	Latency
Thiopental	Small or no change	Increase
Etomidate	Increase	Increase
Fentanyl	Modest or no decrease	Modest or no increase
Diazepam	Decrease	Increase
Midazolam	Decrease	Increase
Ketamine	Increase	Increase
Propofol	Decrease	Increase
Nitrous oxide	Decrease	No change
Halothane	Decrease	Increase
Enflurane	Decrease	Increase
Isoflurane	Decrease	Increase

dependent manner.[101–103] With halothane, enflurane, and isoflurane the amplitude is less and latency greater with coadministration of nitrous oxide (60%) (Table 12–4).

Brain Stem Auditory Evoked Responses

BAERs are particularly resistant to anesthetic agents, both intravenous and inhalational. Table 12–5 summarizes the effects of frequently used drugs on the BAERs when used individually. Even propofol in doses used for induction of anesthesia causes disappearance of the 40-Hz auditory steady-state responses.[104]

Motor Evoked Potentials

Table 12–6 summarizes the effects of frequently used anesthetics on MEPs when administered individually. Etomidate is less depressant than thiopental and should be used for anesthesia induction if MEPs are to be measured.[105] Fentanyl and ketamine have only moderate effects and should be compatible with stable monitoring.[105] Glassman and co-workers[105] found that etomidate allowed M-MEP monitoring, whereas thiopental resulted in loss of potentials for 45 minutes. Propofol allows monitoring of MEPs, although it increases onset latency and decreases amplitude.[106] Isoflurane causes a rapid (within 2 minutes) and profound decrease in the amplitude of the compound muscle action potential. Although small compared to preanesthetic amplitudes, the amplitude of the waves is much larger than scalp recorded SSEP waves and might be monitored using conventional averaging technique.

TABLE 12–5
Anesthetic Effects on Brain Stem Auditory Evoked Response

Drug	Latency
Thiopental	Increase
Fentanyl	No change
Propofol	Increase
Ketamine	Increase
Nitrous oxide	Increase
Halothane	Increase
Enflurane	Increase

TABLE 12–6
Anesthetic Effects on Motor Evoked Potentials

Drug	Amplitude	Latency
Etomidate	No change	Increase
Fentanyl	No change?	No change?
Propofol	Decrease	Increase
Diazepam	Decrease	Increase
Ketamine	Decrease	Increase
Nitrous oxide	Decrease	Increase
Halothane	Decrease	Increase
Isoflurane	Decrease	Increase

Sloan and Erian[107] assessed the impact of neuromuscular blockade by vecuronium on compound muscle action potential response to M-MEP in primates during ketamine infusion. M-MEP amplitude reduction was not significant until train-of-four was greatly reduced.

Zenter et al.[108] compared the effects of halothane, enflurane, and isoflurane on MEP monitored at either extremity compound muscle action potential or from the epidural space. They found a dose-dependent decrease in MEP that was similar with all three anesthetics. In contrast, spinal evoked responses were only slightly affected by the anesthetics.

Ischemia/Hypoxia

Electroencephalogram

The EEG is affected by oxygen deprivation to the brain (hypoxia or ischemia) or the inability of the brain to use oxygen. In animals, sudden inhalation of 100% nitrogen changes EEG low-amplitude fast activity to high-amplitude slow activity and is associated with unconsciousness and lack of response to stimulation and complete flattening of the EEG within 40 seconds.[109] Cerebral utilization of oxygen and glucose diminish drastically when electrocortical silence occurs.[110]

Ernsting[111] reviewed the EEG changes of brief, profound hypoxia with a decrease in Pa_{O_2} from 65 to 15 mm Hg over 1 to 2 seconds. With the onset of hypoxia, there is the appearance of activity in the alpha band when the waves are present prior to onset of hypoxia. As the intensity of oxygen lack is increased, electrical activity with a lower frequency occurs until finally the EEG is dominated by delta rhythm. In human volunteers, isocapnic hypoxia (O_2 saturation about 50%) decreases posterior alpha activity and causes the appearance of irregular slow waves over posterior and anterior head regions with amplitude of 50 μV.[112]

Zhongyuan et al.[113] assessed acute and chronic hypoxia (equivalent to about 8% inspired oxygen) in human volunteers. Acute hypoxia produces the abrupt onset of slow waves (3 to 7 Hz) with amplitude of greater than 50 μV most obvious in frontal leads (Fig. 12–6). Less severe acute hypoxia increases alpha frequency and

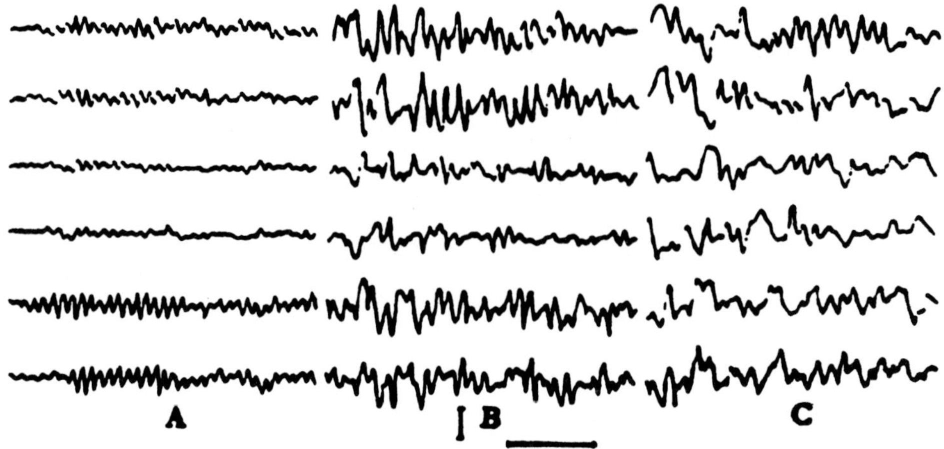

FIGURE **12–6.** The effect of acute hypoxia (Pa_{O_2} ~ 55 mm Hg) on the EEG in unanesthetized humans is shown. *A*, Normoxia. *B* and *C*, During hypoxia in two subjects. (From Zhongyuan S, Deming Z, Zhengzhong G: The influence of acute and chronic hypoxia on the electroencephalogram of human body. Ann Physiol Anthrop 6:111, 1987, with permission.)

decreases alpha amplitude. Some subjects also had onset of theta waves (4 to 7 Hz). During acute hypoxia, EEG changes correlated with mental symptoms and the EEG rapidly returns to normal with reoxygenation.

Somatosensory Evoked Potentials

Branston et al.[114] assessed the effects of ischemia on early components of SSEPs in brain stem, thalamus, and cerebral cortex and found a cephalic to caudal decrease in CBF required to maintain normal electrical activity. Initial changes in cortical SSEP waves occurred at mean arterial blood pressure (MABP) of 30 to 40 mm Hg, but thalamic and medial lemniscus flows are changed only at a lower MABP (<30 mm Hg). At MABP of 20 to 30 mm Hg, SSEP amplitudes in cortex, thalamus, and medial lemniscus were 9, 73, and 91% of control. In terms of blood flow, the threshold for cortical SSEP change was 15 to 20 ml/min/100 gm, for thalamus 10 to 15 ml/min/100 gm, and for medial lemniscus the threshold is 10 ml/min/100 gm.

Graf et al.[115] studied the effect of middle cerebral artery (MCA) occlusion on somatosensory response and found that ischemia is much more severe in the white matter pathways than in the somatosensory cortex and concluded that SSEP loss in such circumstances is due to white matter ischemia. Postischemia recovery of SSEP amplitude correlates with residual flow during ischemia both in the ipsilateral MCA territory and in white matter during ischemia.[116] Animals that developed ischemic lesions of the cortex have more rapid loss and slower recovery of scalp SSEPs than animals who did not subsequently develop lesions after reperfusion.[117]

Friedman et al.[118] found during intracranial aneurysm ablation that prolongation of central conduction time (from spinal cord to scalp), decreased amplitude of scalp recorded waves or disappearance of the SSEP wave was predictive of postoperative sensory or motor deficits of carotid but not basilar artery lesions. They felt that failure of SSEPs to correlate with outcome in basilar aneurysm surgery was because the vascular distribution at risk (posterior cerebral arteries and basilar perforating vessels) does not reliably include either the BAER or SSEP pathways.

Brain Stem Auditory Evoked Response

In a study by Sohmer et al.,[119] EEG became isoelectric at CPP (mean arterial pressure minus intracranial pressure) of 24 mm Hg, whereas BAER became isoelectric at 7 mm Hg. Goitein et al.[120] assessed BAER in 25 children with reduced CPP and found that BAER becomes abnormal when CPP decreases to less than 30 mm Hg.

Sohmer et al.[121] compared the effect of severe hypoxia (Pa_{O_2} 20 to 30 mm Hg) on BAER and SSEP. If MABP was maintained during severe hypoxia, there was no effect on SSEP, but BAER and long-latency auditory EP waves were depressed. However, if MABP was allowed to decrease during hypoxia, all evoked potentials became severely depressed and isoelectric, suggesting that the reason that BAER is altered early during hypoxia is due to sensitivity of the cochlear microphonic to hypoxia rather than failure of brain stem conduction.

Motor Evoked Responses

The proposed utility of MEPs is in those areas in which monitoring of SSEPs has been found to be inadequate, the most notable of which are false-negatives (injury without intraoperative change in SSEP) during spinal surgery.[122]

E-MEP has been assessed in animal studies of spinal cord ischemia using a thoracic aortic cross-clamp model.[123] Aortic cross-clamp produces a characteristic time and spinal level dependent deterioration and loss of MEP. Ischemic cord dysfunction (change in MEP) progressed from distal to proximal cord with changes at the

L4 level occurring after 11 minutes and at the T10 level after 17 minutes. In the same study, reperfusion resulted in MEP return that progressed from proximal to distal. Although spinal cord blood flow was not assessed, this study suggests a significant time lag between events that limit blood flow to the spinal cord and changes in conduction of efferent impulses through the spinal cord. This time lag may be due to the extremely small energy requirement for transmission of impulses via the spinal cord.

Hypothermia

Electroencephalogram

Hypothermia decreases frequency of the EEG, and in patients undergoing hypothermic cardiopulmonary bypass, 76% of patients demonstrate a linear relationship between power in higher frequencies (8 to 10 Hz) and temperature. Approximately 25% of patients demonstrate burst suppression at 26°C.[124] In pigs, EEG becomes flat at 23°C.[125]

Somatosensory Evoked Potentials

Hypothermia increases SSEP latency[126] with latency changes correlated with nasopharyngeal temperature. Latency of the initial waves is prolonged about 1.15 msec/1°C, suggesting that a decrease in temperature of 2° to 3°C will increase latency about 3 msec,[126] an amount of change previously suggested to indicate neural injury. The impact of hypothermia on amplitude is less clear with reports of no change or decreased amplitude with hypothermia.[127] SSEP waves disappear at about 20°C[128] (Fig. 12–7).

Brain Stem Auditory Evoked Responses

An exponential increase in BAER latency occurs as temperature is decreased to 19°C in both primates[129] and

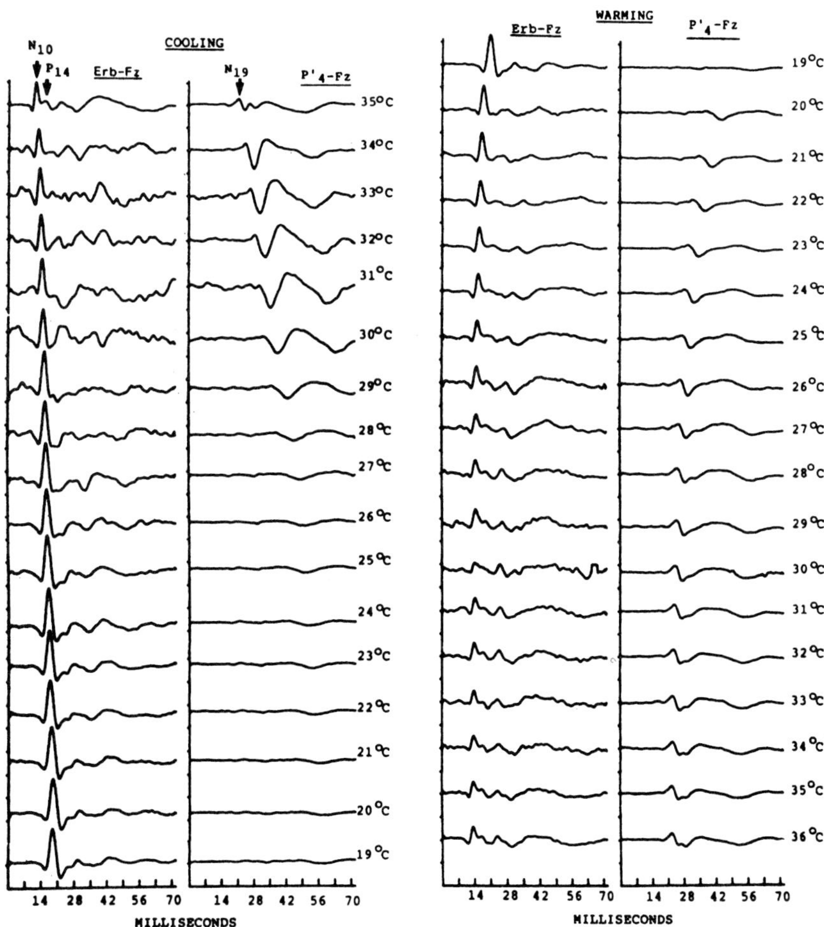

FIGURE 12–7. Short-latency somatosensory evoked potentials (SSEPs) elicited by left median stimulation in a patient during hypothermia and subsequent rewarming. Major SSEP peaks are identified. There is a progressive prolongation of all components with decreasing temperature. Note decrease in the amplitude of N_{19} and increase in the amplitude of N_{10} and P_{14} components during cooling. (From Markand ON, Warren C, Mallik G, et al: Effects of hypothermia on short latency somatosensory evoked potentials in humans. Electroencephalogr Clin Neurophysiol 77: 416, 1990. Copyright 1990, Elsevier Science, with permission.)

rodents.[130] The increase in latency appears greater in the later waves. Waves are easily identifiable at more frequently used levels of hypothermia (29°C) but are delayed by about 33%.

Monitoring in Cardiothoracic and Vascular Procedures

Carotid Endarterectomy

Carotid endarterectomy (CEA) was introduced in 1954, and its frequency peaked in 1985 but declined in 1990, reflecting an uncertainty regarding indications.[131] Recent reports from large studies showed that for specified conditions, surgery is superior to medical therapy alone.[132,133] This patient selection process may increase the importance of neurologic monitoring and intervention. Nevertheless, a recent retrospective analysis of the perioperative records for the 328 patients with 70 to 99% carotid stenosis who received surgery in the North American Symptomatic Carotid Endarterectomy Trial (NASCET) trial[132] demonstrated that cerebral monitoring and use of a shunt are not the standard of practice and do not seem to influence neurologic outcome.[134]

The brain receives 20% of the cardiac output (80% via carotid artery; 20% via basilar artery). Although theoretically protected from consequences of occlusion of a carotid artery by the circle of Willis, only 53% of the population has an intact circle of Willis, with small or absent posterior communication arteries being the most important abnormality.

Neurologic injury associated with CEA can be attributed to ischemia from carotid clamping, perioperative vessel manipulation with release of emboli, or reperfusion hyperemia with subsequent intracerebral hemorrhage. Measurements of CBF have been implemented during CEA, but CBF measurements allow for only noncontinuous assessment of cerebral vascular hemodynamics, and may be difficult to obtain intraoperatively. The threshold for brain infarction (for healthy neural tissue, as opposed to recent infarct) has been experimentally and clinically correlated with a value of 10 ml/100 gm/min, and selective shunting based on CBF measurements has been practiced.[135] The critical CBF (i.e., level below which the majority of patients develop EEG ischemia changes within 3 minutes of carotid occlusion) is 10 ml/100 gm/min, 15 ml/100 gm/min, and 20 ml/100 gm/min for isoflurane, enflurane, and halothane, respectively.[136] Of note, however, are findings of uneventful clinical outcome despite the lack of shunting in patients with EEG changes or CBF values below the supposed ischemic threshold.[137] This finding may indicate that short periods of ischemia may be tolerated without permanent damage. The rare complication of postoperative intracerebral hemorrhage is thought to result from sudden restoration of normal blood flow to brain regions with impaired autoregulation due to vasomotor paralysis from chronic hypoperfusion, resulting in breakthrough bleeding.[138]

Cross filling of anterior and middle cerebral arteries from the contralateral carotid artery through the anterior communicating artery decreases the incidence of EEG changes with cross-clamp from 50% to 21%.[139] Three radiographic findings contralateral to the carotid artery for surgery influence the incidence of cross-clamp ischemia: (1) occlusion of the contralateral internal carotid artery (71% ischemic EEG changes); (2) collateral flow from external carotid artery via ophthalmic artery; and (3) collateral flow from the posterior circulation to the contralateral anterior circulation.[139]

Transcranial Doppler

The utility of TCD in CEA remains unclear.[140] MCA mean velocity was monitored during CEA in 1,420 cases. Reduced levels of MV (relative to preclamp level) were defined as 0 to 15% for severe ischemia, 16 to 40% for mild ischemia, and greater than 41% for no ischemia. In severe ischemia, intraoperative shunting was a significant factor in preventing severe stroke in one study.[141] However, Bornstein et al.[142] used TCD to evaluate MCA peak velocities, before, during, and after CEA under local anesthesia in 50 consecutive patients. A marked decrease in velocities was noted upon clamping as compared to baseline, and an increase in velocity with unclamping. In seven patients who developed focal neurologic deficits, ischemic cerebral events and MCA velocity changes did not correlate, suggesting embolic etiology.

A prospective study[143] of 123 patients with simultaneous monitoring of EEG and TCD detected 75 episodes of embolization in 55 patients. Only one of those patients had a massive embolization following clamp release, and a dense neurologic deficit was present at the end of the operation. In only 2 of 75 patients were EEG changes suggestive of embolization present. TCD measurements were technically successful in 95% of the patients. Therefore, TCD is much more sensitive than EEG for the detection of intracerebral emboli; however, emboli are common but infrequently cause symptoms. In the same study,[143] a reduction of greater than 70% of blood flow velocities was recorded in 16 patients with carotid cross-clamp. Nine of those patients developed a severe (>15%) EEG asymmetry and all but one had intraluminal shunt insertion. Two patients developed moderate (10 to 15%) asymmetry and one of those patients later demonstrated a subcortical infarct. Of five patients who showed no EEG asymmetry, the TCD signal completely disappeared in two, with cross-clamping. These investigators suggest that the EEG remaining nearly normal despite very low MCA velocities probably reflects cerebral cortical perfusion via leptomeningeal anastomoses.

Bass et al.[14] found in a study of 83 patients undergoing CEA that complete intraoperative and postoperative TCD examination was possible in only 60% of patients. Thirteen per cent of patients had incomplete examination because of small or absent transtemporal window. Twenty-three per cent had unsuccessful monitoring due to inability to maintain probe position. In patients with successful monitoring, TCD failed to provide information that altered therapy. All TCD parameters were normal in the one patient who had an operative stroke.

TCD monitoring may demonstrate postoperative hyperemia following carotid surgery. In a series of 250 patients undergoing CEA, four patients with postoperative intracerebral hemorrhage had a 150% increase in MCA flow velocity following cross-clamp release, quite different from the 20% increase seen in patients who did not have intracerebral hemorrhage.[144]

Electroencephalogram

The adequacy of collateral flow to the ipsilateral hemisphere during carotid clamp can be determined by a trial of temporary occlusion with EEG monitoring. Carotid cross-clamping during carotid endarterectomy may produce global hemispheric ischemia in some patients. EEG changes that may occur during carotid cross-clamping include a decrease in amplitude (including slow waves) or an increase in amplitude and decrease in frequency. Unilateral changes are more frequent, but bilateral changes may occur with severely compromised contralateral cerebral blood flow (>90% stenosis). Blume and Sharbrough[145] concluded after reviewing several studies that moderate EEG changes due to cross-clamp can be treated without temporary shunt insertion. However, severe changes with loss of all frequencies except for those below 1-Hz activity probably require placement of a shunt. Even severe changes in EEG following carotid cross-clamp may be self-limited and may resolve before the anticipated salvaging interventions such as temporary shunt placement can be accomplished.[64]

There is little doubt that the EEG reflects instantaneous adequacy of oxygen to the brain. The variability of EEG response and spontaneous resolution of those changes[64] represent time-related return toward normal of cerebral blood flow and cerebral oxygen delivery via collateral channels. General anesthesia, and the lowered cerebral metabolic rate associated with the inhalational and intravenous anesthetics, may be an additional factor in the reversibility of ischemia-induced neuronal dysfunction, as the alterations in brain carbohydrate metabolism or receptor-mediated phenomena could reduce ischemic cellular damage. Furthermore, the length of time that neural tissue can tolerate ischemia without infarction is inversely related to the severity of the reduction of blood flow during the ischemic period.

The effect of isoflurane on the electroencephalogram of patients during CEA does not alter the ability to detect the onset of cerebral ischemia upon temporary occlusion of the internal carotid artery. EEG change usually occurred within 1 minute of occlusion, and involved a marked reduction in frequency and amplitude.[97]

There are reports of EEG changes caused by head and neck manipulations during internal jugular vein catheterizations and intubation.[146,147] Thus, in patients with severely compromised circulation, EEG monitoring should be initiated prior to these risk periods.

Evoked Potentials

Although conventional EEG is still widely used for intraoperative monitoring during CEA, several groups have been gaining experience with SSEP monitoring as an alternative. The cerebral cortex responsible for the scalp recorded upper extremity SSEP waves is perfused by the middle cerebral artery and should be sensitive to decreases in hemispheric flow caused by carotid cross-clamping. Brinkman et al.[148] compared intraoperative SSEP changes during CEA with postoperative neuropsychological performance 7 days after surgery in 14 patients and found that intraoperative loss of early waves in four patients was associated with worsening neuropsychological performance, and two of those patients ultimately had strokes. Patients who had SSEP amplitude decreases of 50% or more performed worse after operation than those with less severe reduction of amplitude.

Results of intraoperative SSEP monitoring in 734 patients undergoing CEA were reported by Horsch et al.[149] In 80% of patients there were no changes in SSEP, reversible changes occurred in 11%, and irreversible changes were found in 0.8% of patients. Monitoring was not possible in 8% of patients due to electrical interference, defective equipment, or initial wave amplitude during 50% nitrous oxide anesthesia that was too small to evaluate. The diagnostic sensitivity of intraoperative SSEP monitoring in predicting neurologic outcome was 60% with a specificity of 100%. Sensitivity indicated the ability to correctly identify a true-positive and specificity indicated the ability to correctly identify a true-negative.

Detection of Perioperative Neurologic Deficits

Esses et al.,[150] reporting on their use of TCD and EEG for monitoring during CEA, revealed one shunted patient who sustained a stroke postoperatively, with changes in both EEG and TCD. Interestingly, the patient's ipsilateral MCA flow velocity had returned to the preoperative value, whereas the EEG changes did not reverse. This indicated that if ischemia is of sufficient duration, restoration of flow will not restore function.

In a study that examined 44 patients undergoing CEA monitored by TCD, EEG, and ^{133}Xe CBF measurements, MCA flow velocity values following a cross-clamp of below 30 cm/sec identified patients with low CBF (<30 ml/100 gm/min), including patients who developed EEG flattening. In patients with flow velocities below 30 cm/sec and a clamp-preclamp flow velocity ratio of less than 0.6, the accuracy of predicting CBF values above or below 20 ml/min/100 gm was 89%. Using a ratio of 0.4, the corresponding accuracy for discriminating EEG flattening was 98%.[151]

EEG and SEP are more sensitive than TCD or stump pressure in demonstrating ischemic changes during CEA. No neurologic deficits were seen immediately after operation when intraoperative EEG or SSEP were unchanged. Complete intraoperative resolution of temporary changes also excluded permanent morbidity. With MCA velocities above 25 cm/sec after clamp application, no deterioration of the neurophysiologic measures occurred. Stump pressure was the weakest predictor of intraoperative ischemia.[152]

Cardiac Surgery

Cardiac surgery is associated with a broad spectrum of neurologic complications. As many as 5% of the approximately 400,000 coronary artery bypass procedures performed annually in the United States result in stroke, and 50 to 80% of patients have neuropsychological deterioration.[153–155] An even higher frequency of these complications has been demonstrated among the 60,000 patients undergoing cardiac valve replacement. In a study of 2,000 patients undergoing coronary artery surgery, 2.8% of patients demonstrated neurologic deficits postoperatively, with an increasing incidence evidenced in patients older than 65 years of age. There was a ninefold greater mortality among patients with neurologic events compared to those without such complications.[156] Neurologic complications following cardiac surgery result in extended hospital stays,[157] longer periods of intubation, and longer intensive care unit (ICU) monitoring, followed by longer term issues such as placement for patients with altered mental status or considerations regarding patients suffering from the sequelae of lowered intellectual function.

The major mechanisms of nervous system injury from cardiac surgery and cardiopulmonary bypass (CPB) are believed to relate to micro- and macroembolic phenomena, and reduced perfusion from reduced flow and decreased arterial blood pressure, possibly in the face of impaired cerebral autoregulation.

Cerebral blood flow normally is regulated by cerebral metabolic rate, Pa_{O_2}, and Pa_{CO_2}, and autoregulated by blood pressure. Cerebral metabolism is depressed by anesthetic effects, and with CPB and profound hypothermia, cerebral blood flow and cerebral oxygen consumption are also reduced greatly. On CPB, CBF is 25 to 35 ml/min/100 gm (~35°C) with $CMRO_2$ of 1.4 to 1.6 ml/min/100 gm. With hypothermia, flow is 15 to 20 ml/min/100 gm and $CMRO_2$ is 0.4 to 0.5 ml/min/100 gm.[158] With normothermia, the ratio of cerebral blood flow to cerebral metabolic rate of oxygen is 20:1, whereas with deep hypothermia the ratio increases to 75:1.[159] Therefore, increased delivery of oxygen relative to demand may contribute to cerebral protection.

Loss of cerebral autoregulation during CPB has been suggested.[160] The method of arterial blood gas and acid-base management during hypothermia significantly influences cerebral hemodynamics and may explain disagreement concerning preservation or loss of autoregulation. The *pH-stat* method attempts to maintain pH at 7.40 by maintaining Pa_{CO_2} at 40 mm Hg after correction for body temperature. With the *α-stat* method, Pa_{CO_2} is maintained at 40 mm Hg, uncorrected for body temperature. With pH-stat management, CBF appears to increase out of proportion to cerebral metabolism, and autoregulation is abolished with CBF becoming pressure dependent.[161,162] In contrast, the α-stat method may produce a lower CBF as a result of a lower CO_2 (actually normocapnia) and potential arteriolar vasoconstriction.

In pediatric patients on CPB, CBF is responsive to changes in Pa_{CO_2} and CBF changes 1.2 ml/100 gm/min for each 1-mm Hg change in Pa_{CO_2}. Deep hypothermia (18° to 22°C) and reduced age (<1 year) decreased the effect of Pa_{CO_2} on CBF.[163]

During stable moderate hypothermic CPB with α-stat management, hypothermia is the most important factor altering $CMRO_2$. During hypothermic CPB using α-stat management, autoregulation is intact.[164] With pH-stat management autoregulation is obtunded. At 28°C, the difference in Pa_{CO_2} between the two management methods is about 16 mm Hg with pH-stat being hypercapnic compared to α-stat. In dogs, CBF decreased to 20% of normothermic at 20°C and $CMRO_2$ decreased to 18% of normothermic value (α-stat). Autoregulation was intact to 40 mm Hg and $CMRO_2$ was maintained to CPP of 30 mm Hg.[165]

Despite the controversial influences on CBF and autoregulation, a significant difference in neurologic outcome based on α-stat versus pH-stat management of CPB has yet to be shown.

Croughwell[166] compared CBF and $CMRO_2$ responses of insulin-dependent diabetic and nondiabetic patients on CPB. In diabetics, CBF was similar at 27° and 37°C degrees; in contrast, CBF increased by 75% with the same increase in temperature in nondiabetic patients. In the diabetic, increase in $CMRO_2$ was maintained by an increase in cerebral oxygen extraction rather than an increase in CBF.

CBF can be measured during cardiac surgery using externally placed gamma detectors and radioactive ^{133}Xe. Although these studies provide valuable information concerning factors influencing CBF during CPB, and the correlation of functional monitoring techniques, such as EEG, with the lower limits of tolerable regional CBF, this information cannot be obtained quickly enough to allow corrective action in individual patients.[158,167]

Transcranial Doppler

TCD has furthered investigation of the effects of profound hypothermic circulatory arrest (PHCA) versus deep hypothermia with continuous low-flow cardiopulmonary bypass (low-flow CPB), which are used in repair of complex congenital heart defects in infants. Presumably, by avoiding cessation of the extracorporeal circulation, but substantially reducing pump flow, continuous cerebral circulation is maintained. The presence or adequacy of cerebral perfusion during low-flow CPB can be monitored by TCD. The effectiveness of low-flow CPB in providing improved cerebral protection, however, remains controversial.[163,168]

In children, low-flow CPB leads to fewer postoperative seizures, a shorter time for return of EEG activity, and a lesser release of brain isoenzyme of creatine kinase compared to total circulatory arrest.[169] Astudillo et al.[170] used TCD to study children who had undergone circulatory arrest. They found that immediately after reinstitution of circulation MCA flow was decreased and diastolic flow was absent. Diastolic flow normalized 54 to 328 minutes following start of perfusion.

Taylor et al.[171] measured cerebral blood flow velocity with TCD in four infants undergoing repair of congenital heart defects and observed an immediate loss of flow in the MCA both during normal pump flow (2.4 L/min/m^2)

and during low-flow CPB (1.2 to 0.6 L/min/m^2). Their determination of CPP during moderate and profound hypothermic CPB (using α-stat acid-base management) suggests that low-flow, hypothermic CPB with low systemic mean arterial pressure provides insufficient CPP to ensure continued cerebral blood flow. Although this finding has been confirmed by other studies,[172–174] it is possible that cerebral perfusion could still be present but undetectable by TCD because of the threshold of resolution for TCD, or alternatively, different clinical settings could produce differing responses to low-flow CPB.

Inadequate perfusion or emboli to the brain may be etiologic factors for postoperative cognitive or motor deficits associated with cardiac surgery. In a study of neuropsychological testing before and 5 to 7 days after coronary artery bypass graft (CABG) surgery, patients with a postoperative decline of 20% on two or more neuropsychological tests averaged twice the number of emboli as those without deficits.[175]

TCD of the carotid artery intraoperatively permits detection and quantification of microemboli. Microemboli are detected most frequently during CPB with the use of bubble oxygenators, and with valve replacement surgery as cardiac ejection is resumed. They are most prevalent intraoperatively and in the first few hours following the removal of the aortic cross-clamp, rather than in the first hour postoperatively.[176]

The incidence of neuropsychological deficit is not significantly greater in those patients who demonstrated angiographically visible carotid artery disease among patients who underwent coronary artery bypass surgery, strongly supporting the conclusion that embolism of small particles is more likely to be important than decreased blood flow as the cause for neurologic damage.[177] Reduced perfusion is not observed during CPB, as compared to a control group with no stenosis, and it is concluded that reduced perfusion was not a significant risk factor for the development of intraoperative stroke in those patients with severe carotid stenosis. This is consistent with clinical observations that the incidence of stroke after CABG in patients with carotid obstruction is not significantly increased.[178]

Large numbers of microemboli occur throughout surgery, but with particularly high numbers (>200 per minute) at the initiation and completion of CPB.[179] Albin et al.[180] found patients undergoing valve replacement entrained more air than CABG patients ($p < .01$), and that the incidence of air increases significantly for valve replacement in the 10-minute interval following the end of CPB ($p < .01$). Furthermore, decreases in MCA flow velocity to below 5 cm/sec occurred in patients for periods ranging from 1 second to 30 minutes.[180]

In patients with left ventricular assist devices (LVADs), such as the intra-aortic balloon pump, TCD permits assessment of the effects of these devices on the cerebral circulation. Subtle changes in the velocity flow profile can be detected and intra-aortic balloon deflation has been associated with a reversal of flow in the intracranial vessels. Although the clinical significance of cessation and reversal of blood flow remains to be determined, TCD may be helpful in devising inflation/deflation timing sequences that may maximize forward flow.[181] Furthermore, emboli and correlative neurologic deficits have been associated with these devices, and preliminary findings suggest that TCD can detect such episodes of embolization and guide physicians to begin intervention that may prevent cerebral infarction.[182]

Electroencephalogram

Deep hypothermia appears to be the major factor limiting the use of EEG in cardiac surgery, as the changes induced by hypothermia and hypoxia can appear to be similar. However, acute ischemic effects can be separated from temperature effects by observing the magnitude of frequency rather than amplitude changes[183,184] or by distinguishing the more gradual and progressive EEG changes due to hypothermia from the more abrupt and occasionally regional differences of inadequate perfusion.[185]

In children undergoing cardiac surgery with deep hypothermia, 16% had abnormal EEG preoperatively, and 17% had abnormal EEG postoperatively. There was no correlation with abnormal EEG and postsurgery ability to advance in school.[186]

Monitoring for burst suppression during barbiturate- or etomidate-induced electrocerebral silence during surgeries requiring deep hypothermia and circulatory arrest is a specific indication for EEG monitoring. Sano et al.[187] found that at the level of burst suppression (in rats) etomidate and thiopental had slight protective effects. The same group, however, showed in another rat ischemia model that when given to burst suppression, thiopental decreased ischemic injury but etomidate and isoflurane worsened brain injury (Cole et al.)[188]

The augmented delta quotient (ADQ) is the ratio of mean amplitude of "augmented" delta frequencies to the mean amplitude of the whole EEG signal. An ADQ of zero indicates no low-frequency component in the EEG and a ratio of 1.0 indicates an EEG composed entirely of low frequencies. Burrows et al.[76] assessed the ADQ to monitor cerebral function during cardiac surgery in 48 patients (2 weeks to 19 years). ADQ for CPB, hypothermia, and general anesthetic could be differentiated from changes caused by cerebral ischemia except in patients less than 18 months during deep hypothermia. Neurologic deficit occurred only if ADQ was abnormal during hypotension for longer than 7 minutes. Those authors found that ADQ was easier to interpret than the compressed spectral array.

In a study by Edmonds et al.[183] quantitative EEG monitoring was evaluated for the intraoperative detection of cerebral dysfunction during myocardial revascularization. They used a 3–standard deviation increase in low-frequency (1.5 to 3.5 Hz) relative power persisting for 5 minutes as the single numeric descriptor of the brain's functional disturbance because of its low variance and insensitivity to fluctuations in body temperature and level of opiate-based anesthesia. Prolonged focal increases in relatively low-frequency power were temperature corrected (at 37°C) to determine a standardized cerebrocortical dysfunction time (CDT_{37}), and proved to be an effective predictor of postoperative disorientation. Interestingly, hypoperfusion, rather than embolization, was implicated as the major cause of the neurologic deficit because of the close relationship between low-frequency power increase and low perfusion pressure. In phase II of that study, the investigators successfully corrected the quantitative EEG abnormality by elevation of MAP to greater than 50 mm Hg and reduced the incidence of postoperative disorientation from 28% to 4%. It is suggested that this form of EEG monitoring may provide the opportunity for timely correction of perfusion abnormalities. Delta CDT_{37} had 68% false-positive but only 8% false-negative results.

While computerized EEG facilitates its use by clinicians during cardiovascular surgery,[189] the limitations of the technique must be clearly recognized. Adams and coworkers suggest that the output of such automated systems be interpreted cautiously.[190] Using the Cadwell Laboratories Cardiovascular Intraoperative Monitoring (CIMON) system (Kennwick, WA), they noted the presence of ischemic patterns and low-frequency (1.5 to 3.5 Hz) power for 5 minutes (termed quantitative EEG cerebral dysfunction) to a similar extent both in patients undergoing automatic defibrillator implantation and in those having abdominal procedures.[190]

Aldrich et al.[191] reported a series of 25 patients with cortical blindness, five of which had undergone CPB (four of five CABG). In four of five patients, vision improved to 20 to 40/100. EEG postoperative abnormalities were present in all patients with computed tomography (CT) scan that showed occipital tip infarct following surgery.

Somatosensory Evoked Potentials

The use of evoked potential monitoring during CPB has certain limitations because of the effect of cooling on latencies and amplitudes measured. Nevertheless, with rewarming, the waveforms should revert toward baseline levels, and in those instances where abnormal waveforms persisted, postoperative neurologic deficits were demonstrated. Hickey et al.[192] used median and ulnar nerve SSEPs to assess peripheral nerve injuries in cardiac patients associated with internal jugular central venous catheter insertion and sternal distraction. Thirteen per cent of patients had transient SSEP changes with CVP insertion that resolved spontaneously within 5 minutes. With sternal distraction, SSEP changed in 70% of patients and 21% of patients had SSEP changes that persisted to the end of the operation and had postoperative neurologic changes.

Jugular Venous Oxygen Saturation

Newer techniques available to monitor the adequacy of cerebral perfusion, particularly during low-flow CPB or PHCA, are monitors of oxygen delivery, such as near infrared spectroscopy and jugular venous oxygen saturation monitoring. Nakajima et al.[193] evaluated jugular bulb catheterization in patients on CPB and found that JBC saturation was maintained during CPB despite a decrease in MABP. They found an inverse relationship between nasopharyngeal temperature and O_2 saturation. Cerebral metabolic monitoring provides meaningful information in assessing cerebral cooling and metabolic suppression, as a gauge of adequate hypothermic, or intermittent perfusion, cerebral protection strategies.[194]

Thoracolumbar Aortic Aneurysm

The incidence of paraplegia or paraparesis following thoracic aneurysm repair is 9%, and 21% with thoracolumbar aneurysm repair.[195] With extensive aortic involvement or dissection, the risk for spinal injury approaches 30 to 40%.[195] Presumably, the more extensive the aneurysm, the longer the segment of aorta that must be removed with associated intercostal or lumbar arteries needing to be reattached, and the longer the aortic occlusion. Thus the need to preserve critical spinal cord blood supply and to limit aortic cross-clamp time becomes apparent. The spinal cord may be highly dependent on collateral flow from the artery of Adamkiewicz, which usually arises from the aorta between the T8 and the L3 nerve roots and may supply up to 50% of the spinal cord.[196] Complications are greater with acute dissection compared to chronic dissection and may relate to development of collateral flow patterns that provide protection when the aorta is clamped.[197]

Many methods of preventing paraplegia following cross-clamping of the descending aorta have been considered and applied, including various surgical techniques, pharmacologic agents and interventions, and monitoring considerations, which aim to preserve and enhance blood flow to the spinal cord, or alert the surgical and anesthetic team to ischemic intolerances. The efficacy of interventions such as hypothermia, ranging from mild to deep hypothermic arrest, and cerebrospinal fluid (CSF) drainage, remain controversial in the literature.[197,198]

Intraoperative spinal cord monitoring techniques require a high sensitivity, and additionally, should be highly specific, as responses to false-positives may influence neurologic and overall morbidity. For example, attempts to avert cord ischemia by shunting or bypass maneuvers, or reimplantation of segmental vessels, requiring placement of additional aortic cross-clamps or prolongation of cross-clamp time may add potential complications.

Somatosensory Evoked Potentials

Maeda et al.[199] studied spinal cord perfusion pressure (SCPP) and SSEP in 19 patients requiring aortic cross-clamp. Ten patients had axillofemoral shunting and nine patients had partial CPB. SSEP changed in five patients, and two of those patients had complete loss of SSEP and developed paraplegia following surgery (SCPP of 32 and 35 mm Hg). In the other three patients, CSF drainage increased SCPP to greater than 40 mm Hg and led to gradual SSEP recovery in two patients. The other patient had reimplantation of intercostal arteries with recovery of SSEP. In the 14 patients without change in SSEP, spinal cord perfusion pressure was greater than 40 mm Hg.

Distal perfusion pressure greater than 60 mm Hg by shunt or bypass preserves SSEP and preserves neurologic function.[200] The incidence of paraplegia was 15% (5 of 33 patients). The incidence of paraplegia with perfusion pressure below 60 mm Hg was 31% when SSEP was lost (5 of 16 patients). Patients with loss of SSEP for more than 30 minutes had a 71% incidence of paraplegia. There were no neurologic deficits if SSEP was lost for less than 30 minutes.

Peripheral somatosensory evoked potentials have limited value in the assessment of spinal cord ischemia during aortic cross-clamping if the extremity from which the evoked potentials are monitored is not perfused. Direct stimulation of spinal cord, bypassing the peripheral nerve, may be expected to avoid the nonspecific effects of vascular insufficiency and peripheral neuropathy on evoked potentials.[201] A potential complication of spinal electrode placement for monitoring purposes is epidural hematoma, particularly in anticoagulated patients; however, this incidence appears to be low.[202]

Stuhmeier et al.[203] used the electrospinogram (ESEP; epidural stimulation at L2, recording at T3) to assess neurologic injury during thoracolumbar aortic aneurysm in 100 consecutive patients. They found that ESEP loss occurring later than 15 minutes after cross-clamp was associated with neurologic deficit in 7% of the patients. If there were no changes in ESEP, no neurologic deficit occurred. In 30% of patients, a neurologic deficit occurred when ESEP was lost within 15 minutes after cross-clamp. A total loss of ESEP for less than 40 minutes had a sensitivity of 100%. There was a specificity of 68% with a positive predictive value of 35% and a negative predictive value of 100%. A recovery after declamping later than 20 minutes had a sensitivity of 93%, a specificity of 86%, a positive predictive value of 52%, and a negative predictive value of 99%. Grabitz et al.[204] studied peridural stimulation of L4–L5 via a second bipolar catheter at T4 and found a correlation of .89 between postoperative motor deficit and the time from declamping to reappearance of the potential.

Motor Evoked Potentials

SEP monitoring is capable of assessing the integrity of only the posterior portion of the spinal cord, as normal somatosensory responses can be seen despite ischemic infarction of the anterior spinal cord resulting in paraplegia.[122,205] MEPs have been proposed as an alternative method to directly monitor the motor tracts of the spinal cord during thoracic aortic occlusion. MEPs are not affected by peripheral nerve ischemia and monitor anterior and lateral column ischemia (motor tracts), in contrast to SEPs, which monitor the posterior and lateral columns. Recent animal studies demonstrate that myogenic motor evoked responses elicited by transcranial stimulation are more sensitive to ischemia than those recorded from the epidural space.[206] The response to balloon occlusion of the infrarenal aorta in rabbits was a 50% reduction in motor evoked potential amplitude from the epidural space over approximately 11 minutes as compared with complete disappearance of the myogenic response within 2 minutes. These responses resulted from spinal cord ischemia, as femoral artery occlusion produced no change in soleus muscle motor evoked responses to transcranial stimulation.

Elmore et al.[207] studied 60 minutes of aortic occlusion in dogs with and without CSF drainage. CSF drainage improved neurologic outcome. MEP was lost in 9 of 20 dogs with neurologic injury and was lost in none of seven animals that were neurologically normal. SSEP was lost in 19 of 20 animals with neurologic injury and was lost in three of seven animals that were neurologically normal. After reperfusion, MEP returned to control in all nine neurologically injured dogs that had lost MEP and were still present at 24 hours. Change in amplitude, latency, or time until loss or return of MEP or SSEP did not predict neurologic injury. With loss of SSEP, sensitivity was 95% and specificity was 67% (probably secondary to peripheral nerve ischemia). Loss of MEP had low sensitivity but 100% specificity and return of MEP did not correlate with functional recovery.

Cerebrospinal fluid drainage with aortofemoral (AF) shunting also improves neurologic outcome in dogs with aortic cross-clamp. CSF drainage did not improve over AF shunting. AF shunting increased spinal cord blood flow. Loss of SSEP had a sensitivity of 92% and a specificity of 68% in predicting neurologic injury, whereas loss of MEP had a sensitivity of 16% and a specificity of 100%.[208]

The authors suggest that the lower sensitivity seen with MEPs may be related to recording over the low thoracic and proximal lumbar spine where potentials are transmitted in the axon of descending corticospinal tracts. Theoretically, these white matter fibers with cell bodies within the cerebral cortex are more resistant to ischemia than the anterior horn cells and interneurons, with cell bodies within ischemic cord, which account histologically for a significant degree of the neurologic deficit after aortic occlusion.[207,208] Intrathecal stimulation and recordings from lower extremity muscles improve the sensitivity of MEPs.[209]

Summary

Unfortunately, there is no simple and completely reliable monitor to detect and prevent neurologic injury. Various modalities of monitoring have been described with emphasis on strengths and limitations of each monitor relative to specific disease entities or operative interventions. A common thread has been that a single monitor rarely provides sufficient information in a wide variety of circumstances. Several examples of complementary monitors, such as EEG and TCD or JBC, which assess different aspects of cerebral physiology, have been provided that improve understanding of the etiology of injury or provide a dynamic picture of physiologic changes leading to injury.

Monitoring plans that provide frequent assessment of various aspects of nervous system function will allow demonstration of cause and effect relative to neurologic injury. Injury, regardless of the type of monitor used, may not be manifested immediately after the insult, frequently producing difficulty in interpretation of the cause-and-effect relationship. Thus, careful consideration of the anticipated abnormalities and an understanding of the limitations of specific monitoring techniques can greatly reduce misinterpretation of data.

References

1. Dong WK, Bledsoe SW, Eng DY, et al: Profound arterial hypotension in dogs: Brain electrical activity and organ integrity. Anesthesiology 58:61, 1983.
2. Dhasmana KM, Saxena PR, Prakash O, VanderZee HT: A study on the influence of ketamine on systemic and regional haemodynamics in conscious rabbits. Arch Pharmacodyn Ther 269: 323, 1984.
3. Schwedler M, Miletich DJ, Albrecht RF: Cerebral blood flow and metabolism following ketamine administration. Can Anaesth Soc J 29:222, 1982.
4. Akeson J, Bjorkman S, Messeter K, et al: Cerebral pharmacodynamics of anaesthetic and subanaesthetic doses of ketamine in the normoventilated pig. Acta Anaesthesiol Scand 37:211, 1993.
5. Kontos HA: Validity of cerebral arterial blood flow calculations from velocity measurements. Stroke 20:1, 1989.
6. Aaslid R, Lindegaard KF, Sorteberg W, Nornes H: Cerebral autoregulation dynamics in humans. Stroke 20:45, 1989.
7. Giller CA: Diameter changes in cerebral arteries during craniotomy. J Cardiovasc Technol 9:301, 1990.
8. Dahl A, Russell D, Nyberg-Hansen R, Rootwelt K: Repeated simultaneous rCBF and TCD measurements. Proceedings of the 6th International Symposium and Tutorials on Cerebral Hemodynamics: Transcranial Doppler, Cerebral Blood Flow and Other Modalities. The Institute of Applied Physiology and Medicine, Seattle, WA, 1992, no. 41.
9. Obrist WD, Jarjour IT, Marks EC, et al: Correlation of transcranial Doppler and cerebral blood flow during xenon inhalation. Proceedings of the 6th International Symposium and Tutorials on Cerebral Hemodynamics: Transcranial Doppler, Cerebral Blood Flow and Other Modalities. The Institute of Applied Physiology and Medicine, Seattle, WA, 1992, no. 42.
10. Hanson S, Grotta JC: Cerebral perfusion rCBF-Xenon, spect. Proceedings of the 6th International Symposium and Tutorials on Cerebral Hemodynamics: Transcranial Doppler, Cerebral Blood Flow and Other Modalities. The Institute of Applied Physiology and Medicine, Seattle, WA, 1992, no. 39.
11. Van der Linden, Wesslen O, Ekroth R, et al: Transcranial Doppler estimated versus thermodilution-estimated cerebral blood flow during cardiac operations. J Thorac Cardiovasc Surg 102: 95, 1991.
12. Nicholls SC, Glickerman DJ, Lam AM: Cerebral embolization: Transcranial Doppler monitoring in the swine model. Proceedings of the 6th International Symposium and Tutorials on Cerebral Hemodynamics: Transcranial Doppler, Cerebral Blood Flow and Other Modalities. The Institute of Applied Physiology and Medicine, Seattle, WA, 1992, no. 77.
13. Spencer MP, Thomas GI, Nicholls SC, Sauvage LR: Detection of middle cerebral artery emboli during carotid endarterectomy using transcranial Doppler ultrasonography. Stroke 21:415, 1990.
14. Bass A, Krupski WC, Schneider PA, et al: Intraoperative transcranial Doppler: Limitations of the method. J Vasc Surg 10:549, 1989.
15. Halsey JH: Effect of emitted power on waveform intensity in transcranial Doppler. Stroke 21:1573, 1990.
16. Brouwers P, Vriens EM, Musbach M, et al: Transcranial pulsed Doppler measurements of blood flow velocity in the middle cerebral artery: Reference values at rest and during hyperventilation in healthy children and adolescents in relation to age and sex. Ultrasound Med Biol 16:1, 1990.
17. Grolimund P, Seiler RW: Age dependence of the flow velocity in the basal cerebral arteries—a transcranial Doppler ultrasound study. Ultrasound Med Biol 14:191, 1986.
18. Jorgensen LG, Perko M, Perko G, Secher NH: Middle cerebral artery velocity during head-up tilt induced hypovolemic shock in humans. Clin Physiol 13:323, 1993.
19. Laumer R, Steinmeier R, Gonner F, et al: Cerebral hemodynamics in subarachnoid hemorrhage evaluated by transcranial Doppler sonography. Part 1. Reliability of flow velocities in clinical management. Neurosurgery 33:1, 1993.
20. Venketasubramanian N, Sacco RL, DiTullio M, et al: Vascular distribution of paradoxical emboli by transcranial Doppler. Neurology 43:1533, 1993.
21. Rommer B, Lunggren B, Brandt L, Saveland H: Transcranial Doppler sonography within 12 hours after subarachnoid hemorrhage. J Neurosurg 70:732, 1989.
22. Dong M, Kofke WA, Acuff J, et al: Transcranial Doppler evaluation of anesthetic induction of neurosurgical patients. J Neurosurg Anesth 1:153, 1989.
23. Giller CA: Transcranial Doppler monitoring of cerebral blood velocity during craniotomy. Neurosurgery 25:769, 1989.
24. Werner C, et al: Increase in blood flow volume in MCA following low-dose ketamine. Anaesthesiol Intensivmed Notfallmed Schmerzther 24:231, 1989.
25. Kochs E, Hoffman WE, Cunnigham F, et al: EEG median frequency, $CMRO_2$, CBF and cerebral blood flow velocity during propofol anesthesia in dogs. J Neurosurg Anesth 3:235, 1991.
26. Eng C, Lam A, Mayberg T, et al: The influence of propofol with and without N_2O on cerebral blood flow volume on CO_2 reactivity in man. Anesth Analg 74:S87, 1992.
27. Cheng MA, Hoffman WE, Baughman VL: Midazolam sedation produces transient decreases in MCA velocity. Proceedings of the 6th International Symposium and Tutorials on Cerebral Hemodynamics: Transcranial Doppler, Cerebral Blood Flow and Other Modalities. The Institute of Applied Physiology and Medicine, Seattle, WA, 1992, no. 17.
28. Werner C, Hoffman WE, Miletich DJ, et al: Sufentanil decreases cerebral blood flow and cerebral blood flow velocity in dogs. J Neurosurg Anesth 2:219, 1990.
29. Werner C, Hoffman WE, Braugham VL, et al: Effects of sufentanil on cerebral blood flow, cerebral blood flow velocity, and metabolism in dogs. Anesth Analg 72:177, 1991.
30. Slee TA, Lam AM, Winn HR, Laohaprasit V: The cerebral hemodynamic and metabolic response to alfentanil in humans. Anesthesiology 75:A171, 1991.
31. Werner C, Hoffman WE, Kochs E, et al: Cerebral blood flow in correlation to cerebral blood flow velocity during isoflurane anesthesia. J Neurosurg Anesth 3:236, 1991.
32. Lam AM, Slee TA, Cooper JO, Bachenberg KL: Nitrous oxide is a more potent cerebrovasodilator than isoflurane in humans. J Neurosurg Anesth 3:244, 1991.
33. Leon JE, Bissonnette B: Cerebrovascular responses to carbon dioxide in children anesthetized with halothane and isoflurane. Can J Anaesth 38:817, 1991.
34. Leon J, Bissonnette B: Does isoflurane affect the cerebrovascular response to carbon dioxide in anesthetized children? Proceedings of the 5th International Symposium and Tutorials on Intracranial Hemodynamics: Transcranial Doppler, Cerebral Blood Flow and Other Modalities. The Institute of Applied Physiology and Medicine, Seattle, WA, 1991, no. 79B.
35. Leon J, Bissonnette B: Does nitrous oxide affect cerebral blood flow velocity under neuroleptanesthesia in children? Proceedings of the 5th International Symposium and Tutorials on Intracranial Hemodynamics: Transcranial Doppler, Cerebral Blood Flow and Other Modalities. The Institute of Applied Physiology and Medicine, Seattle, WA, 1991, no. 79C.
36. Leon J, Bissonnette B: Isoflurane, the most inert volatile agent on cerebrovascular circulation in anesthetized infants and children? Proceedings of the 5th International Symposium and Tutorials on Intracranial Hemodynamics: Transcranial Doppler, Cerebral Blood Flow and Other Modalities. The Institute of Applied and Medicine, Seattle, WA, 1991, no. 79D.
37. Bolognese P, Miller JI, Heger IM, Milhorat TH: Laser-Doppler flowmetry in neurosurgery. J Neurosurg Anesth 5:151, 1993.
38. Dirnagl U, Kaplan B, Jacewicz M, Pulsinelli W: Continuous measurement of cerebral cortical blood flow by laser-Doppler flowmetry in a rat stroke model. J Cereb Blood Flow Metab 9: 589, 1989.
39. Haberl R, Heizer ML, Marmarou A, et al: Laser Doppler assessment of the brain microcirculation: Effect of systemic alterations. Am J Physiol 256:H1248, 1989.

40. Haberl R, Heizer MI, Ellis EF: Laser Doppler assessment of the brain microcirculation: Effect of local alterations. Am J Physiol 256:H1255, 1989.
41. Werner C: Laser Doppler flowmetry: A valid clinical tool? J Neurosurg Anesth 5:139, 1993.
42. Levy WJ, Levin S, Chance B: Near-infrared measurement of cerebral oxygenation. Anesthesiology 83:738, 1995.
43. Hampson NB, Camporesi EM, Stolp BW, et al: Cerebral oxygen availability by NIR spectroscopy during transient hyoxia in humans. J Appl Physiol 69:907, 1990.
44. Pollard V, Prough DS, DeMelo AE, et al: Validation in volunteers of a near-infrared spectroscope for monitoring brain oxygenation in vivo. Anesth Analg 82:269, 1996.
45. Pollard V, Prough DS, DeMelo AE, et al: The influence of carbon dioxide and body position on near-infrared spectroscopic assessment of cerebral hemoglobin oxygen saturation. Anesth Analg 82:278, 1996.
46. Owen-Reece H, Elwell CE, Harkness W, et al: Use of near infrared spectroscopy to estimate cerebral blood flow in conscious and anaesthetized adult subjects. Br J Anaesth 76:43, 1996.
47. Ferrari M, Wilson DA, Hanley F, et al: Noninvasive determination of hemoglobin saturation in dogs by derivative near infrared spectroscopy. Am J Physiol 256:H1493, 1989.
48. Ausman JI, McCormick PW, Stewart M, et al: Cerebral oxygen metabolism during hypothermic circulatory arrest in humans. J Neurosurg 79:810, 1993.
49. Nollert G, Mohnle P, Tassani-Prell P, Reichart B: Determinants of cerebral oxygenation during cardiac surgery. Circulation 92(Suppl):II-327, 1995.
50. Greeley WJ, Bracey VA, Ungerleider RM, et al: Recovery of cerebral metabolism and mitochondrial oxidation state is delayed after hypothermic circulatory arrest. Circulation 84(Suppl III): III-400, 1992.
51. Kurth CD, Steven JM, Nicolson SC: Cerebral oxygenation during pediatric cardiac surgery using deep hypothermic circulatory arrest. Anesthesiology 82:74, 1993.
52. Samra SK, Dorje P, Zelenock GB, Stanley JC: Cerebral oximetry in patients undergoing carotid endarterectomy under regional anesthesia. Stroke 27:49, 1996.
53. Kirkpatrick PJ, Smielewski P, Whitfield PC, et al: An observational study of near-infrared spectroscopy during carotid endarterectomy. J Neurosurg 82:56, 1995.
54. Mason PF, Dyson EH, Sellars V, Beard JD: The assessment of cerebral oxygenation during carotid endarterectomy utilising near infrared spectroscopy. Eur J Vasc Surg 8:590, 1994.
55. McPherson RW, Koehler RC, Traystman RJ: Hypoxia, α_2-adrenergic, and nitric oxide-dependent interactions on canine cerebral blood flow. Am J Physiol 266:H476, 1994.
56. Sutton LN, McLaughlin AC, Dante S, et al: Cerebral venous oxygen content as a measure of brain energy metabolism with increased intracranial pressure and hyperventilation. J Neurosurg 73:927, 1990.
57. Croughwell ND, Frasco P, Blumenthal JA, et al: Warming during cardiopulmonary bypass is associated with jugular bulb desaturation. Ann Thorac Surg 79:745, 1992.
58. Cook DJ, Oliver WC Jr, Orszulak TA, et al: A prospective randomized comparison of cerebral venous oxygen saturation during normothermic and hypothermia cardiopulmonary bypass. J Thorac Cardiovasc Surg 107:1020, 1994.
59. Trubiano P, Heyer EJ, Adams DC, et al: Jugular venous bulb oxyhemoglobin saturation during cardiac surgery; accuracy and reliability using a continuous monitor. Anesth Analg 82:964, 1996.
60. Goetting MG, Preston G: Jugular bulb catheterization: Experience with 123 patients. Crit Care Med 18:1220, 1990.
61. Goetting MG, Preston G: Jugular bulb catheterization does not increase intracranial pressure. Intensive Care Med 17:191, 1991.
62. Taylor GA, Walker LK: Intracranial venous system in newborns treated with extracorporeal membrane oxygenation: Doppler US evaluation after ligation of the right jugular vein. Radiology 183: 453, 1992.
63. Cedwich C, Schramm J, Fahbusch R: Are flash-evoked visual potentials useful for intraoperative monitoring of visual pathway function? Neurosurgery 21:709, 1987.
64. Rampil IJ, Correll JW, Rosenbaum SH, et al: Computerized electroencephalogram monitoring and carotid artery shunting. Neurosurgery 13:276, 1983.
65. Yli-Hankala-A, Jantti V: EEG burst suppression pattern correlates with the instantaneous heart rate under isoflurane anaesthesia. Acta Anaesthesiol Scand 34:665, 1990.
66. Rampil IJ, Laster MJ: No correlation between quantitative electroencephalographic measurements and movement response to noxious stimuli during isoflurane anesthesia in rats. Anesthesiology 77:920, 1992.
67. Rung GW, Wickey GS, Myers JL, et al: Thiopental as an adjunct to hypothermia for EEG suppression in infants prior to circulatory arrest. J Cardiothorac Vasc Anesth 5:337, 1991.
68. Metz S, Slogoff S: Thiopental sodium by single bolus dose compared to infusion for cerebral protection during cardiopulmonary bypass. J Clin Anesth 2:226, 1990.
69. Modica PA, Tempelhoff R: Intracranial pressure during induction of anaesthesia and tracheal intubation with etomidate-induced EEG burst suppression. Can J Anaesth 39:236, 1992.
70. Levy WJ, Shapiro HM, Maruchak G, et al: Automated EEG processing for intraoperative monitoring: A comparison of techniques. Anesthesiology 53:223, 1980.
71. Russ W, Kling D, Sauerwein G, Hempelmann G: Spectral analysis of the EEG during hypothermic cardiopulmonary bypass. Acta Anaesthesiol Scand 32:111, 1987.
72. Hanowell LH, Soriano S, Bennett HL: EEG power changes are more sensitive than spectral edge frequency variation for detection of cerebral ischemia during carotid artery surgery: A prospective assessment of processed EEG monitoring. J Cardiothorac Vasc Anesth 6:292, 1992.
73. Rampil IJ, Matteo RS: Changes in EEG spectral edge frequency correlate with the hemodynamic response to laryngoscopy and intubation. Anesthesiology 67:139, 1987.
74. Ghouri AF, Monk TG, White PF: Electroencephalogram spectral edge frequency, lower esophageal contractility, and autonomic responsiveness during general anesthesia. J Clin Monit 9:176, 1993.
75. Long CW, Shah NK, Loughlin C, et al: A comparison of EEG determinants of near-awakening from isoflurane and fentanyl anesthesia. Anesth Analg 69:169, 1989.
76. Burrows FA, Volgyesi GA, James PD: Clinical evaluation of the augmented delta quotient monitor for intraoperative electroencephalographic monitoring of children during surgery and cardiopulmonary bypass for repair of congenital cardiac defects. Br J Anaesth 63:565, 1989.
77. Lubricky JP, Spadaro JA, Yuan HA, et al: Variability of somatosensory cortical evoked potential monitoring during spinal surgery. Spine 14:790, 1989.
78. York DH, Chabot RJ, Gaines RW: Response variability of somatosensory evoked potentials during scoliosis surgery. Spine 12:864, 1987.
79. McPherson RW, Traystman RJ: The relationship of changes in somatosensory evoked potential and cerebral oxygen consumption during hypoxic hypoxia. Stroke 17:30, 1986.
80. Sohmer H, Freeman S, Malachi S: Multi-modality evoked potentials in hypoxemia. Electroencephalogr Clin Neurophysiol 64: 328, 1986.
81. Katayama Y, Tsubokawa T, Maejima S, et al: Corticospinal direct response in humans: Identification of the motor cortex during intracranial surgery under general anaethesia. J Neurol Neurosurg Psychiatry 51:50, 1988.
82. Cracco RQ: Evaluation of conduction in central motor pathways: Techniques, pathophysiology, and clinical interpretation. Neurosurgery 20:199, 1987.
83. Kiersey DK, Bickford RG, Faulconer A: Electroencephalographic patterns produced by thiopental sodium during surgical operations: Description and classification. Br J Anaesth 22:141, 1950.
84. Waugier A, van-den-Broech WA, Verheyen JL, et al: Electroencephalographic study of the short-acting hypnotics etomidate and methohexital in dogs. Eur J Pharmacol 47:367, 1978.
85. Schwilden H, Schuttler J, Stoeckel H: Quantitation of the EEG and parmacodynamic modelling of hypnotic drugs: Etomidate as an example. Eur J Anaesthesiol 2:121, 1985.
86. Sebel PS, Bovill JG, Wauquier A, Rog P: Effects of high-dose fentanyl on the electroencephalogram. Anesthesiology 55:203, 1981.
87. Smith NT, Dec-Silber H, Sanford TJ, et al: EEGs during high dose fentanyl, sufentanil or morphine-oxygen anesthesia. Anesth Analg 63:386, 1984.

88. Yamamura T, Fukuda M, Takeya H, et al: Fast oscillatory EEG activity induced by analgesic concentrations of nitrous oxide in man. Anesth Analg 60:283, 1981.
89. Gain EA, Paletz SG: An attempt to correlate the clinical signs of flurothane anaesthesia with the electroencephalographic levels. Can Anaesth Soc J 4:289, 1957.
90. Mecarelli O, DeFeo MR, Romanini L, et al: EEG and clinical features in epileptic children during halothane anaesthesia. Electroencephalogr Clin Neurophysiol 52:486, 1981.
91. Persson A, Peterson E, Wahlin A: EEG changes during general anaesthesia with enflurane (Ethrane) in comparison with ether. Acta Anaesthesiol Scand 22:339, 1978.
92. Niejadlik K, Galindo A: Electroencephalographic seizure activity during enflurane anesthesia. Anesth Analg 54:722, 1975.
93. Clark DL, Hosick EC, Adam N, et al: Neural effects of isoflurane (Forane) in man. Anesthesiology 39:261, 1973.
94. Eger EI II, Stevens WC, Cromwell TH: The electroencephalogram in man anesthetized with Forane. Anesthesiology 35:504, 1971.
95. Schwartz AE, Navedo AT, Berman MF: Pancuronium increases the duration of electroencephalogram burst suppression in dogs anethetized with isoflurane. Anesthesiology 77:686, 1992.
96. Yli-Hankala A, Lindgren L, Porkkala T, Jantti V: Nitrous oxide-mediated activation of the EEG during isoflurane. Br J Anaesth 70:54, 1993.
97. Campkin TV, Honigsberger L, Smith IS: Isoflurane: Effect on the encephalogram during carotid endarterectomy. Anaesthesia 40:188, 1985.
98. Rampil IJ, Lockhart SH, Eger EI II, et al: The electroencephalographic effects of desflurane in humans. Anesthesiology 74: 434, 1991.
99. McPherson RW, Sell B, Traystman RJ: Effects of thiopental, fentanyl, and etomidate on upper extremity somatosensory evoked potentials in humans. Anesthesiology 65:584, 1986.
100. Sloan TB, Ronai AK, Toleikis JR, Koht A: Improvement of intraoperative somatosensory evoked potentials by etomidate. Anesth Analg 67:582, 1988.
101. Pathak KS, Ammadio M, Kalamchi A, et al: Effects of halothane, enflurane, and isoflurane on somatosensory evoked potentials during nitrous oxide anesthesia. Anesthesiology 66:753, 1987.
102. Peterson DO, Drummond JC, Todd MM: Effects of halothane, enflurane, isoflurane, and nitrous oxide on somatosensory evoked potentials in humans. Anesthesiology 65:35, 1986.
103. Wolfe DE, Drummond JC: Differential effects of isoflurane/nitrous oxide on posterior tibial somatosensory evoked responses of cortical and subcortical origin. Anesth Analg 67:852, 1988.
104. Plourde G: The responses of propofol on the 40-Hz auditory steady-state response and on the electroencephalogram in humans. Anesth Analg 82:1012, 1996.
105. Glassman SD, Shields CB, Linden RD, et al: Anesthetic effects on motor evoked potentials in dogs. Spine 18:1083, 1993.
106. Kellner BP, Haghighi SS, Oro JJ, Eggers GW Jr: The effects of propofol anesthesia on transcortical electric evoked potentials in the rat. Neurosurgery 30:557, 1992.
107. Sloan TB, Erian R: Effect of vecuronium-induced neuromuscular blockade on cortical motor evoked potentials. Anesthesiology 78:966, 1993.
108. Zenter J, Albrecht T, Heuser D: Influence of halothane, enflurane, and isoflurane on motor evoked potentials. Neurosurgery 31:298, 1992.
109. Herin RA, Hall P, Fitch JW: Nitrogen inhalation as a method of euthanasia in dogs. Am J Vet Res 39:989, 1978.
110. Cartheuser CF: Progressive hypoxia until brain electrical silence: A useful model for studying protective interventions. Can J Physiol Pharmacol 66:1398, 1988.
111. Ernsting J: The effects of hypoxia upon human performance and the electroencephalogram. Int Anesth Clin 4:245, 1966.
112. Rebuck AS, Davis C, Longmire D, et al: Arterial oxygenation and carbon dioxide tensions in the production of hypoxic electroencephalographic changes in man. Clin Sci Mol Med 50:301, 1976.
113. Zhongyuan S, Deming Z, Zhengzhong G: The influence of acute and chronic hypoxia on the electroencephalogram of human body. Ann Physiol Anthrop 6:111, 1987.
114. Branston NM, Ladds A, Symon L, Wang A: Comparison of the effects of ischaemia on early components of the somatosensory evoked potential in brainstem, thalamus, and cerebral cortex. J Cereb Blood Flow Metab 4:68, 1984.
115. Graf R, Kataoka K, Wakayama A, et al: Functional impairment due to white matter ischemia after middle cerebral artery occlusion in cats. Stroke 21:923, 1990.
116. Matsumiya N, Koehler RC, Traystman RJ: Consistency of cerebral blood flow and evoked potential alterations with reversible focal ischemia in cats. Stroke 21:908, 1990.
117. Dowman R, Boisvert DP, Gelb AW, et al: Changes in the somatosensory evoked potential during and immediately following temporary middle cerebral artery occlusion predict somatosensory cortex ischemic lesions in monkeys. J Clin Neurophysiol 7:269, 1990.
118. Friedman WA, Kaplan BL, Day AL, et al: Evoked potential monitoring during aneurysm operation: Observations after fifty cases. Neurosurgery 20:678, 1987.
119. Sohmer H, Gafni M, Havatselet G: Persistence of auditory nerve response and absence of brain-stem response in severe cerebral ischaemia. Electroencephalogr Clin Neurophysiol 58:65, 1984.
120. Goitein KJ, Fainmesser P, Sohmer H: Cerebral perfusion pressure and auditory brain-stem responses in childhood CNS diseases. Am J Dis Child 137:777, 1983.
121. Sohmer H, Freeman S, Malachi S: Multi-modality evoked potentials in hypoxemia. Electroencephalogr Clin Neurophysiol 64: 328, 1986.
122. Lesser RP, Raudzens P, Luders H, et al: Postoperative neurological deficits may occur despite unchanged intraoperative somatosensory evoked potentials. Ann Neurol 19:22, 1986.
123. Laschinger JC, Owen J, Rosenbloom M, et al: Direct noninvasive monitoring of spinal cord motor function during thoracic aortic occlusion: Use of motor evoked potentials. J Vasc Surg 7:161, 1988.
124. Levy WJ: Quantitative analysis of EEG changes during hypothermia. Anesthesiology 60:291, 1984.
125. Reland T, Sulg IA, Bjaertnes L, Jolin A: Neuromonitoring in hypothermia and in hypothermic hypoxia. Arctic Med Res 50: 32, 1991.
126. Van-Rheineck-Leyssius AT, Kalkman CJ, Bovil JG: Influence of moderate hypothermia on posterior tibial nerve. Anesth Analg 65:475, 1986.
127. Stejskal L, Travnicek V, Sourek K, Kredba J: Somatosensory evoked potentials in deep hypothermia. Appl Neurophysiol 43: 1, 1980.
128. Markand ON, Warren C, Mallik G, et al: Effects of hypothermia on short latency somatosensory evoked potentials in humans. Electroencephalogr Clin Neurophysiol 77:416, 1990.
129. Doyle WJ, Fria TJ: The effects of hypothermia on the latencies of the auditory brain-stem response (ABR) in the rhesus monkey. Electroencephalogr Clin Neurophysiol 60:258, 1985.
130. Schorn V, Lennon V, Bickford R: Temperature effects on the brainstem evoked responses (BAERS) of the rat. Proc San Diego Biomed Symp 16:313, 1977.
131. Barnett HJM, Haines SJ: Carotid endarterectomy for asymptomatic carotid stenosis. N Engl J Med 328:276, 1993.
132. North American Symptomatic Carotid Endarterectomy Trial Collaborators: Beneficial effect of carotid endarterectomy in symptomatic patients with high-grade carotid stenosis. N Engl J Med 325:445, 1991.
133. European Carotid Surgery Trialists Collaborative Group: MRC European Carotid Surgery Trial: Interim results for symptomatic patients with severe (70–99%) or with mild (0–29%) carotid stenosis. Lancet 337:1235, 1991.
134. Craen RA, Gelb AW, Eliasziw M, et al: Anesthesia, monitoring and neurologic outcome in carotid endarterectomy: NASCET results. J Neurosurg Anesth 5:303, 1993.
135. Sundt TM: The ischemic tolerance of neural tissue and the need for monitoring and selective shunting during CEA. Stroke 14: 93, 1983.
136. Michenfelder JD, Sundt TM, Fode N, Sharbrough FW: Isoflurane when compared to enflurane and halothane decreases the frequency of cerebral ischemia during carotid endarterectomy. Anesthesiology 67:336, 1987.
137. Ferguson GG: Intraoperative monitoring and internal shunts: Are they necessary in carotid endarterectomy? Stroke 13:287, 1982.

138. Schroeder TV: Cerebral blood flow in carotid surgery. Proceedings of the 5th International Symposium and Tutorials on Intracranial Hemodynamics: Transcranial Doppler, Cerebral Blood Flow and Other Modalities. The Institute of Applied Physiology and Medicine, Seattle, WA, 1991, no. 82.
139. Lopez-Bresnahan MV, Kearse LA, Yanez P, Young TI: Anterior communicating artery collateral flow protection against ischemic change during carotid endarterectomy. J Neurosurg 79:379, 1993.
140. Wilke HJ, Ellis JE, McKinsey JF: Carotid endarterectomy: Perioperative and anesthetic considerations. J Cardiothorac Vasc Anesth 10:928, 1996.
141. Halsey JH Jr: Transcranial Doppler monitoring in carotid endarterectomy: The risks and benefits of shunting. Progress report of the international study group. Proceedings of the 6th International Symposium and Tutorials on Cerebral Hemodynamics: Transcranial Doppler, Cerebral Blood Flow and Other Modalities. The Institute of Applied Physiology and Medicine, Seattle, WA, 1992, no. 64.
142. Bornstein N, Rossi GB, Treves TA, et al: Is TCD effective in avoiding the hazards of carotid surgery. Proceedings of the 5th International Symposium and Tutorials on Cerebral Hemodynamics: Transcranial Doppler, Cerebral Blood Flow and Other Modalities. The Institute of Applied Physiology and Medicine, Seattle, WA, 1991, no. 22.
143. Jansen C, Vriens EM, Elkelboom BC, et al: Carotid endarterectomy with transcranial Doppler and electroencephalographic monitoring. Stroke 24:665, 1993.
144. Ackerstaff RGA, Jansen C, Woll FL, et al: The significance of intra-operative TCD monitoring to predict intracerebral haemorrhage after carotid endarterectomy. Proceedings of the 7th International Symposium and Tutorials on Cerebral Hemodynamics: Transcranial Doppler, Cerebral Blood Flow and Other Modalities. The Institute of Applied Physiology and Medicine, Seattle, WA, 1993, no. 12.
145. Blume WT, Sharbrough FW: EEG monitoring during carotid endarterectomy and open heart surgery. In Niedermeyer E, Lopes da Silva F (eds): Electroencephalography: Basic Principles, Clinical Application and Related Fields, 2nd ed. Baltimore, Urban & Schwarzenberg, 1987.
146. Kim BY, Ngeow JY, Kitabata LM, Swift CA: EEG changes with lateral rotation of the head. Anesthesiology 12:36, 1985.
147. Sablocki AD, Albin MS: The EEG should be monitored during CPB. J Cardiothorac Anesth 3:119, 1989.
148. Brinkman SD, Braun P, Ganji S, et al: Neuropsychological performance one week after carotid endarterectomy reflects intraoperative ischemia. Stroke 15:497, 1984.
149. Horsch S, De Vleeschauwer P, Ktenidis K: Intraoperative assessment of cerebral ischemia during carotid surgery. J Cardiovasc Surg 31:599, 1990.
150. Esses GE, Babikian VL, Cantelmo NL, et al: Intraoperative use of transcranial Doppler and electroencephalography during carotid endarterectomy. Proceedings of the 6th International Symposium and Tutorials on Cerebral Hemodynamics: Transcranial Doppler, Cerebral Blood Flow and Other Modalities. The Institute of Applied Physiology and Medicine, Seattle, WA, 1992, no. 22.
151. Jorgensen LG, Schroeder TV: Transcranial Doppler identification of cerebral ischemia during carotid endarterectomy. Proceedings of the 6th International Symposium and Tutorials on Cerebral Hemodynamics: Transcranial Doppler, Cerebral Blood Flow and Other Modalities. The Institute of Applied Physiology and Medicine, Seattle, WA, 1992, no. 63.
152. Gaab MR, Ubenauf A, Lorenz M, et al: Complex intraoperative monitoring during carotid operations—comparison of EEG, SEP, TCD and stump pressures. Proceedings of the 5th International Symposium and Tutorials on Intracranial Hemodynamics: Transcranial Doppler, Cerebral Blood Flow and Other Modalities. The Institute of Applied and Medicine, Seattle, WA, 1991, no. 87.
153. Breuer AC, Furlan AJ, Hanson MR, et al: Central nervous system complications of coronary artery bypass graft surgery: Prospective analysis of 421 patients. Stroke 14:682, 1983.
154. Shaw PJ, Bates D, Cartlidge NEF, et al: Early neurological complications of coronary artery bypass surgery. Br Med J 291:1384, 1985.
155. Shaw PJ, Bates D, Cartlidge NEF, et al: Neurologic and neuropsychological morbidity following major surgery: Comparison of coronary artery bypass and peripheral vascular surgery. Stroke 18:700, 1987.
156. Tuman KJ, McCarthy RJ, Najafe H, Ivankovich AD: Differential effects of advanced age on neurologic and cardiac risks of coronary artery operations. J Thorac Cardiovasc Surg 104:1510, 1992.
157. Weintraub WS, Jones EL, Craver J, et al: Determinants of prolonged length of hospital stay after coronary bypass surgery. Circulation 80:276, 1989.
158. Schell RM, Kern FH, Greeley WJ, et al: Cerebral blood flow and metabolism during cardiopulmonary bypass. Anesth Analg 76:849, 1993.
159. Greeley WJ, Keern FH, Ungerleider RM, et al: The effect of hypothermic cardiopulmonary bypass and total circulatory arrest on cerebral metabolism in neonates, infants, and children. J Thorac Cardiovasc Surg 101:783, 1991.
160. Greeley WJ, Ungerleider RM, Smith LR, Reves JG: The effects of deep hypothermic cardiopulmonary bypass and total circulatory arrest on cerebral blood flow in infants and children. J Thorac Cardiovasc Surg 97:737, 1989.
161. Lundar T, Lindegaard KF, Froysaker T, et al: Dissociation between cerebral autoregulation and carbon dioxide reactivity during non-pulsatile CPB. Ann Thorac Surg 40:582, 1985.
162. Murkin JM, Farrar JK, Tweed WA, et al: Cerebral autoregulation and flow/metabolism coupling during cardiopulmonary bypass: The influence of $PaCO_2$. Anesth Analg 66:825, 1987.
163. Kern FH, Ungerleider RM, Quill TJ, et al: Cerebral blood flow response to changes in arterial carbon dioxide tension during hypothermic cardiopulmonary bypass in children. J Thorac Cardiovasc Surg 101:618, 1991.
164. Rogers AT, Stump DA, Gravlee GP, et al: Response of cerebral blood flow to phenylephrine infusion during hypothermic cardiopulmonary bypass: Influence of $PaCO_2$ management. Anesthesiology 69:547, 1988.
165. Tanaka J, Shiki K, Asou T, et al: Cerebral autoregulation during deep hypothermic nonpulsatile cardiopulmonary bypass with selective cerebral perfusion in dogs. J Thorac Cardiovasc Surg 95: 124, 1988.
166. Croughwell N, Lyth M, Quill TJ, et al: Diabetic patients have abnormal cerebral autoregulation during cardiopulmonary bypass. Circulation 82(Suppl 5):IV-407, 1990.
167. Prough DS, Rogers AT: What are the normal levels of cerebral blood flow and cerebral oxygen consumption during cardiopulmonary bypass in humans. Anesth Analg 76:690, 1993.
168. Burrows FA, Bissonnette B: Monitoring the adequacy of cerebral perfusion during cardiopulmonary bypass in children using transcranial Doppler technology. J Neurosurg Anesth 5:209, 1993.
169. Newburger JW, Jonas RA, Wernovsky G, et al: A comparison of the perioperative neurologic effects on hypothermic circulatory arrest versus low-flow cardiopulmonary bypass in infant heart surgery. N Engl J Med 329:1119, 1993.
170. Astudillo R, van der Linden J, Ekroth R, et al: Absent diastolic cerebral blood flow velocity after circulatory arrest but not after low flow in infants. Ann Thorac Surg 56:515, 1993.
171. Taylor RH, Burrows FA, Bissonnette B: No flow during low-flow cardiopulmonary bypass. Proceedings of the 5th International Symposium and Tutorials on Intracranial Hemodynamics: Transcranial Doppler, Cerebral Blood Flow and Other Modalities. The Institute of Applied Physiology and Medicine, Seattle, WA, 1991, no. 53.
172. Taylor RH, Burrows FA, Bissonette B: No flow during low-flow cardiopulmonary bypass. J Thorac Cardiovasc Surg 101:362, 1991.
173. Taylor RH, Burrows FA, Bissonette B: Cerebral pressure-flow velocity relationship during hypothermic cardiopulmonary bypass in neonates and infants. Anesth Analg 74:636, 1992.
174. Burrows FA, Bissonette B: Cerebral blood flow velocity patterns during cardiac surgery utilizing profound hypothermia with low-flow cardiopulmonary bypass or circulatory arrest in neonates and infants. Can J Anaesth 40:298, 1993.
175. Stump DA, Tegeler CH, Rogers AT, et al: Neuropsychological deficits are associated with the number of emboli detected during cardiac surgery. Proceedings of the 7th International Symposium

and Tutorials on Cerebral Hemodynamics: Transcranial Doppler, Cerebral Blood Flow and Other Modalities. The Institute of Applied Physiology and Medicine, Seattle, WA, 1993, no. 45.
176. Eicke M, Stump DA, Tegeler CH, Stein CS: Carotid artery microemboli detection following cardiopulmonary bypass. Proceedings of the 5th International Symposium and Tutorials on Intracranial Hemodynamics: Transcranial Doppler, Cerebral Blood Flow and Other Modalities. The Institute of Applied Physiology and Medicine, Seattle, WA, 1991, no. 61.
177. Harrison MJG, Schneidau A, Ho R, et al: Cerebrovascular disease and functional outcome after coronary artery bypass surgery. Stroke 20:235, 1989.
178. von Reutern GM, Hetzel A, Birnbaum D, Schlosser V: Transcranial Doppler ultrasonography during cardiopulmonary bypass in patients with severe carotid stenosis or occlusion. Stroke 19: 674, 1988.
179. Boyajian RA, Baker LA, Tyner JJ, et al: Cerebral blood flow physiology during cardiopulmonary bypass procedures. Proceedings of the 6th International Symposium and Tutorials on Cerebral Hemodynamics: Transcranial Doppler, Cerebral Blood Flow and Other Modalities. The Institute of Applied Physiology and Medicine, Seattle, WA, 1992, no. 67.
180. Albin MS, Hantler C, Mitzel H, et al: Transcranial Doppler (TCD) utilization during open heart surgery: Flow changes and incidence of air microemboli. Proceedings of the 6th International Symposium and Tutorials on Cerebral Hemodynamics: Transcranial Doppler, Cerebral Blood Flow and Other Modalities. The Institute of Applied Physiology and Medicine, Seattle, WA, 1992, no. 81.
181. Brass LM: Reversed intracranial blood flow in patients with an intra-aortic balloon pump. Stroke 21:484, 1990.
182. Knepper LE, Eidelman BH, Thompson J, Kormos RL: Transcranial Doppler monitoring of patients with left ventricular assist devices. Proceedings of the 7th International Symposium and Tutorials on Cerebral Hemodynamics: Transcranial Doppler, Cerebral Blood Flow and Other Modalities. The Institute of Applied Physiology and Medicine, Seattle, WA, 1993, no. 46.
183. Edmonds HL Jr, Griffiths LK, van der Laken J, et al: Quantitative electroencephalographic monitoring during myocardial revascularization predicts postoperative disorientation and improves outcome. J Thorac Cardiovasc Surg 103:555, 1992.
184. Murray A, Glaria AP, Pearson DT: Monitoring of EEG frequency and amplitude during cardiac surgery. Anaesthesia 41:173, 1986.
185. Salerno TA, Lince DP, White DA, et al: Monitoring of electroencephalogram during open heart surgery. A prospective analysis of 118 cases. J Thorac Cardiovasc Surg 76:97, 1978.
186. Iwamoto I, Baba H, Koga Y, et al: The relation between EEG and mental development following cardiac surgery performed under simple deep hypothermia in children. Jpn J Surg 20:158, 1990.
187. Sano T, Patel PM, Drummond JC, Cole DJ: A comparison of the cerebral protective effects of etomidate, thiopental, and isoflurane in a model of forebrain ischemia in the rat. Anesth Analg 76:990, 1993.
188. Cole D, Drummond J, Patel P: The effect of thiopental isoflurane, and etomidate on focal cerebral ischemic injury in rats. J Neurosurg Anesth 5:285, 1993.
189. Edmunds LH Jr, Griffiths LK, Van der Laken J, et al: Quantitative electroencephalographic monitoring during myocardial revascularization predicts postoperative disorientation and improves outcome. J Thorac Cardiovasc Surg 103:555, 1992.
190. Adams DC, Heyer EJ, Emerson RG, et al: The reliability of quantitative electroencephalography as an indicator of cerebral ischemia. Anesth Analg 81:80, 1995.
191. Aldrich MS, Alessi AG, Beck RW, Gilman S: Cortical blindness: Etiology, diagnosis, and prognosis. Ann Neurol 21:149, 1987.
192. Hickey C, Guino LD, Aglio LS, et al: Intraoperative somatosensory evoked potential monitoring predicts peripheral nerve injury during cardiac surgery. Anesthesiology 78:29, 1993.
193. Nakajima T, Kuro M, Hayashi Y, et al: Clinical evaluation of cerebral oxygen balance during cardiopulmonary bypass: Online continuous monitoring of jugular venous oxyhemoglobin saturation. Anesth Analg 74:630, 1992.
194. Kern FH, Schell RM, Greeley WJ: Cerebral monitoring during cardiopulmonary bypass in children. J Neurosurg Anesth 5:213, 1993.
195. Crawford ES, Crawford JL, Safi HJ, et al: Thoracoabdominal aortic aneurysms: Preoperative and intraoperative factors determining immediate and long-term results of operations in 605 patients. J Vasc Surg 3:389, 1985.
196. Wadouh F, Lindemann EM, Ardnt CF, et al: The arteria radicularis magna anterior as a decisive factor influencing spinal cord damage during aortic occlusion. J Thorac Cardiovasc Surg 99:1, 1984.
197. Shenaq SA, Svensson LG: Con: Cerebrospinal fluid drainage does not afford spinal cord protection during resection of thoracic aneurysms. J Cardiothorac Vasc Anesth 6:369, 1992.
198. Nugent M: Pro: Cerebrospinal fluid drainage prevents paraplegia. J Cardiothorac Vasc Anesth 6:366, 1992.
199. Maeda S, Miyamoto T, Murata H, Yamashita K: Prevention of spinal cord ischemia by monitoring spinal cord perfusion pressure and somatosensory evoked potentials. J Cardiovasc Surg 30:565, 1989.
200. Cunningham JN, Laschinger JC, Spencer FC: Monitoring of somatosensory evoked potentials during surgical procedures on the thoracoabdominal aorta. IV. Clinical observations and results. J Thorac Cardiovasc Surg 94:275, 1987.
201. Drenger B, Parker SD, McPherson RW, et al: Spinal cord stimulation evoked potentials during thoracoabdominal aortic aneurysm surgery. Anesthesiology 76:689, 1992.
202. North RB, Drenger B, Beattie C, et al: Monitoring of spinal cord stimulation evoked potentials during thoracoabdominal aneurysm surgery. Neurosurgery 28:325, 1991.
203. Stuhmeier KD, Grabitz K, Mainzer B, et al: Use of the electrospinogram for predicting harmful spinal cord ischemia during repair of thoracic or thoracoabdominal aortic aneurysms. Anesthesiology 79:1170, 1993.
204. Grabitz K, Freye E, Stuhmeier K, Sandmann W: Spinal evoked potential in patients undergoing thoracoabdominal aortic reconstruction: A prognostic indicator of postoperative motor deficit. J Clin Monit 9:186, 1993.
205. Zornow MH, Grafe MR, Tybor C, et al: Preservation of evoked potentials in a case of anterior spinal artery syndrome. Electroencephalogr Clin Neurophysiol 77:137, 1990.
206. DeHaan P, Kalkman CJ, Ubags LH, et al: A comparison of the sensitivity of epidural and myogenic transcranial motor evoked responses in the detection of acute spinal cord ischemia in the rabbit. Anesth Analg 83:1022, 1996.
207. Elmore JE, Gloviczki P, Harper CM, et al: Failure of motor evoked potentials to predict neurologic outcome in experimental thoracic aortic occlusion. J Vasc Surg 14:131, 1991.
208. Elmore JR, Gloviczki P, Harper CM Jr, et al: Spinal cord injury in experimental thoracic aortic occlusion: Investigation of combined methods of protection. J Vasc Surg 15:789, 1992.
209. Svensson LG, Paterl V, Robinson MF, et al: Influence of preservation or perfusion of intraoperatively identified spinal cord blood supply on spinal motor evoked potentials and paraplegia after aortic surgery. J Vasc Surg 13:355, 1992.

SECTION III

CARDIAC ANESTHESIA

CHAPTER 13

Invasive Cardiology: Diagnosis and Therapeutics

Alan N. Tenaglia, M.D.
Joseph A. Proli, M.D.

The history of cardiac catheterization can be traced to the now well-known story of Forssmann, who placed a catheter in his own right heart under fluoroscopic guidance in 1929.[1] Following this, right heart catheterization was used by Klein to measure cardiac output in 1930[2] and by Cournand and Richards to perform hemodynamic measurements in the 1940s.[3,4] Left heart catheterization was first performed in 1950 by Zimmerman,[5] with coronary arteriography first performed by Sones in 1959.[6] The initial coronary angioplasty was performed in 1977 by Gruntzig.[7] Newer therapeutic modalities have been developed over the last several years.

In adults, diagnostic catheterization is used most often to diagnose coronary artery disease. Other common indications include assessment of congestive heart failure, valvular abnormalities, and congenital heart disease. Related therapeutic techniques include percutaneous transluminal angioplasty (PTCA), atherectomy, laser angioplasty, intracoronary stenting, balloon valvuloplasty, and balloon pericardiotomy. Table 13–1 lists various indications and the specific procedures performed.

Cardiac catheterization should only be performed by physicians who are well versed in the techniques involved and at facilities that have adequate equipment and staffing to safely perform procedures. Routine diagnostic catheterization in low-risk patients may be performed on an outpatient basis, but high-risk patients or patients undergoing interventions should only be treated as inpatients in a hospital with on-site cardiothoracic surgical back-up.

Diagnostic Catheterization

General Procedural Aspects

The cardiac catheterization laboratory has several components, including a patient support table, ability to simultaneously monitor several intracardiac pressures, a multichannel electrocardiograph (ECG), and an imaging system. The imaging system has two major functions, fluoroscopy and cineangiography. Fluoroscopy allows visualization of intrathoracic structures by gamma radiation, and cineangiography allows permanent recording of anatomic features using contrast dye and photographic film. Newer systems include the digital recording and storage of images, which may replace cineangiography in the future.

An important aspect of cardiac catheterization is radiation safety. Cardiac catheterization exposes patients to the highest level of radiation of any commonly used radiology study. During a typical cardiac catheterization, the patient receives a total radiation dose of approximately 50 rad which is the equivalent of approximately 250 chest x-rays. Women of child-bearing age should have their pelvis shielded to protect germ cells, which are highly sensitive to gamma radiation. Pregnant patients in general should not undergo catheterization unless absolutely necessary, and in those cases the fetus should be shielded with lead. The cardiac catheterization laboratory is usually completely lined with 1 mm of lead shielding and any windows or doors also contain lead shielding. Operators and other personnel should wear lead aprons. Protective lead eye wear should also be worn to reduce the risk of cataract formation. Radiation exposure to the operator is monitored by mandatory use of film badges, which are reviewed monthly.

Patient preparation includes establishing rapport, a directed history and physical, limited laboratory evaluation, patient education including discussion of risks and benefits, obtaining informed consent, and premedication. The history is important in determining patients at increased risk during cardiac catheterization. Specifically, the history should include medication allergies, especially allergies to contrast, symptoms of heart failure, history of severe peripheral vascular disease, and a history of significant noncardiac disease, all of which increase morbidity and mortality. Young women should be questioned about possible pregnancy. Physical examination is directed towards the heart, lungs, and peripheral vascular system, and adds additional information concerning left ventricular dysfunction, valvular disease, and peripheral vascular disease. Laboratory data should

TABLE 13–1
Indications for Diagnostic and Therapeutic Cardiac Catheterization

Indication	Procedure
Diagnosis	
Chest pain	Left, coronaries
Heart failure	Left, right, coronaries, ± biopsy
Valvular disease	Left, right, ± coronaries
Congenital	Left, right, ± coronaries
Posttransplant	Left, right, coronaries, biopsy
Therapeutics	
Coronary artery disease	PTCA, stent, atherectomy, laser
Valvular stenosis	Valvuloplasty
Pericardial effusion	Balloon pericardiotomy

Left, left heart catheterization including pressure measurements and left ventriculography; right, right heart catheterization including pressure measurements, oxygen saturations, and cardiac output determination; coronaries, coronary arteriography; PTCA, percutaneous transluminal coronary angioplasty.

include a recent electrocardiogram, complete blood count, platelet count, prothrombin time (PT), partial thromboplastin time (PTT), electrolytes, blood urea nitrogen (BUN), creatinine, and a chest x-ray if warranted by the history or physical exam. Significant anemia, bleeding disorders, electrolyte abnormality, or renal insufficiency also increase the risk of cardiac catheterization.

Patients should be informed about the procedures in layperson's terms and all questions answered to the patient's satisfaction. The risks and complications in cardiac catheterization need to be discussed. These include death, myocardial infarction, cerebrovascular accident, arrhythmias, bleeding, perforation, embolus, thrombosis, vascular complications such as pseudoaneurysm and arteriovenous fistula, infection, allergic reaction, renal failure, heart failure, and hemodynamic instability.[8] Major complications occur in less than 1 in 100 cases of diagnostic catheterization.[9,10] Once the procedure has been explained, questions answered, and risks and benefits discussed, the patient must sign consent to undergo cardiac catheterization.

Patients routinely receive a benzodiazepine in combination with an antihistamine as premedication. A common combination is Valium (5 to 10 mg PO) and diphenhydramine (25 to 50 mg IV) just prior to the procedure. Patients with a history of contrast or iodine allergy should receive corticosteroids prior to cardiac catheterization. An accepted regimen is prednisone 50 mg PO q8h times three doses, last dose on call to the cardiac catheterization laboratory.[11] In addition, nonionic contrast media should be used in these patients.

Once the patient has been premedicated and placed on the cardiac catheterization table, the site of vascular entry is prepped and draped in a sterile manner. In most laboratories the femoral artery and vein are used, although right heart catheterization may also be performed via the jugular or subclavian vein and left heart catheterization via the brachial artery. Strict bodily fluid precautions are observed at all times to protect the operators. This should include protective eye wear. Local anesthesia, usually 1% lidocaine without epinephrine, is given subcutaneously and then into the fascia surrounding the common femoral artery and vein. The artery and vein are accessed in a similar manner, using a hollow core needle. A wire is placed through the needle and a vascular sheath is placed over the wire after the needle has been removed. Sheath size varies from 5 to 10 F, depending upon the particular procedure.

During routine left heart catheterization, low-dose heparin (i.e., 2,000 to 3,000 U) is often given after the sheaths are in place. After the procedure, the femoral sheaths are removed and pressure is applied to the site of entry, either by hand or by using a C clamp. Protamine is usually not needed to reverse the effects of heparin before sheath removal.

Right Heart Catheterization

Right heart catheterization is indicated in patients with unexplained dyspnea, valvular heart disease, or suspected intracardiac shunting. It can be performed in an intensive care unit (ICU) without the use of fluoroscopy or at the time of left heart catheterization. Right heart catheterization usually is performed with balloon-tipped flow-directed catheters that have the ability to record pressure and sample blood at distal and proximal ports. There is also a thermistor that allows calculation of cardiac output by the thermodilution method.[12] This is based upon the rate of change of temperature at the thermistor in response to a bolus of saline injected proximally.

Right heart catheterization provides pressure measurements and oxygen content in the inferior and superior vena cava, right atrium, right ventricle, pulmonary artery, and the pulmonary capillary wedge position (which provides indirect measurement of the left atrium). Cardiac output can be determined by the thermodilution method mentioned above or by using oxygen content and the Fick principle:

$$\text{Cardiac output (L/min)} = \frac{O_2 \text{ consumption (ml/min)}}{D(a - v)O_2\ (\text{vol\%}) \times 10}$$

where oxygen consumption is usually assumed based upon patient age and body weight and the arterial-venous oxygen difference is based upon samples of systemic and pulmonary artery blood. In general, the Fick method is more accurate in patients with low cardiac output and the thermodilution method is more accurate in patients with high cardiac output.

Left-to-right and right-to-left shunts may be calculated from changes in oxygen content in the various chambers as follows:

$$\text{Left-to-right shunt} = \frac{O_2 \text{ consumption}}{(S_{AO_2} - P_{AO_2}) \times 10} - \frac{O_2 \text{ consumption}}{(P_{VO_2} - M_{VO_2}) \times 10}$$

TABLE 13–2
Normal Values for Right Heart Catheterization

Chamber	Pressure (mm Hg)	Minimal Change in O_2 Saturation*
Right atrium		
a wave	3–7	11%
v wave	2–7	
Mean	1–7	
Right ventricle		
Systole	17–30	7%
Diastole	1–7	
Pulmonary artery		
Systole	17–30	5%
Diastole	5–13	
Mean	9–19	
Pulmonary wedge		
Mean	5–13	

*This value is minimum increase in oxygen saturation in chamber compared with chamber proximal (mixed venous for right atrium) to detect left-to-right shunt. For example, to detect a ventricular septal defect, the oxygen saturation of blood in the right ventricle needs to be at least 7% greater than the oxygen saturation of blood obtained in the right atrium.

and

$$\text{Right-to-left shunt} = \frac{O_2 \text{ consumption}}{(\text{SA}O_2 - \text{MV}O_2) \times 10} - \frac{O_2 \text{ consumption}}{(\text{PV}O_2 - \text{MV}O_2) \times 10}$$

where $\text{SA}O_2$ = systemic artery oxygen content, $\text{PA}O_2$ = pulmonary artery oxygen content, $\text{PV}O_2$ = pulmonary vein oxygen content, and $\text{MV}O_2$ = mixed venous oxygen content. Table 13–2 lists normal values for right heart catheterization.

Left Heart Catheterization

The purpose of left heart catheterization is to assess the coronary arteries, the left ventricle, and the aortic and mitral valves.

Diagnostic coronary catheters are available with preshaped curves that allow easier access to the left and right coronary arteries. The catheter is advanced over a J-tipped wire through the arterial sheath, retrograde up the aorta and around the aortic arch to the aortic root. The wire is removed, the catheter is flushed and subsequently attached to a pressure manifold. The catheter tip is then gently advanced into the ostium of either the left main coronary artery or right coronary artery for selective coronary angiography using hand injection of dye. A variety of views are obtained by moving the cinecamera in cranial or caudal and left anterior oblique (LAO) or right anterior oblique (RAO) positions. Multiple images are recorded in different views for both the left coronary system and right coronary system. Stenosis severity is usually expressed as percentage diameter stenosis of the diseased segment in relation to an adjacent normal reference segment. Visual assessment is subject to marked variability,[13,14] and this has led to the use of more quantitative methods[15,16] using computer-generated edge detection algorithms, densitometry or, at a minimum, measurements using calipers. These quantitative techniques are still limited by the need for a reference segment, which itself may be inapparently diseased. Normal coronary anatomy is outlined in Figure 13–1.[17]

In addition to coronary arteriography, as part of left heart catheterization a pigtail catheter with multiple sideholes is placed across the aortic valve into the left ventricle. Measurements of aortic and ventricular pressures are made and contrast injected using a power injector. Both LAO and RAO views are obtained. This allows assessment of overall and segmental ventricular function as well as assessment of any mitral regurgitation. Ascending aortography is also sometimes performed to assess the aorta and to document any aortic insufficiency.

Valvular regurgitation is graded on a 4-point scale as noted in Table 13–3. Stenotic valves may be assessed by the Gorlin formula,[18] which is based upon the concept that the pressure gradient between two chambers is related to the flow across the valve and inversely to the size of the valve orifice. Therefore, the valve area may be estimated by the ratio of flow over pressure gradient:

$$A = \frac{\text{CO/(DFP or SEP)(HR)}}{44.3C\Delta P}$$

where A = valve area (cm^2), CO = cardiac output (cm^3/min), DFP = diastolic filling period (sec/beat), SEP = systolic filling period (sec/beat), HR = heart rate (bpm), C = constant (1 for aortic valve, 0.85 for mitral valve), and P = pressure gradient (mm Hg). For mitral regurgitation, the pressure difference between the left atrium and the left ventricle is used and for aortic stenosis the gradient between the left ventricle and aorta is used.

New Imaging Modalities

As discussed above, contrast arteriography is limited, since it provides only a two-dimensional (2D) silhouette of the vessel. There is variability in interpretation and it is also limited in its ability to detect minimal disease, plaque morphology, and topography. Two new imaging techniques—intracoronary ultrasound and angioscopy—have been developed to overcome some of these limitations.

For intracoronary ultrasound imaging a miniature transducer is advanced over a guidewire down the coronary artery. The transducer is then mechanically rotated to provide a 2D cross-sectional image of the arterial wall and lumen. Intracoronary ultrasound has been used as a research tool, for example, to assess the mechanisms of PTCA and other interventional procedures.[19] Its clinical utility is yet to be determined, but it may be particularly valuable in improving results of intravascular stent implantation.[20,21]

During angioscopy, a catheter carrying fiberoptic cables is advanced over a guidewire down the coronary artery. Images of the surface of the artery are then obtained. Angioscopy is especially useful for documenting the presence of thrombus, which is often difficult to assess by angiography.[22]

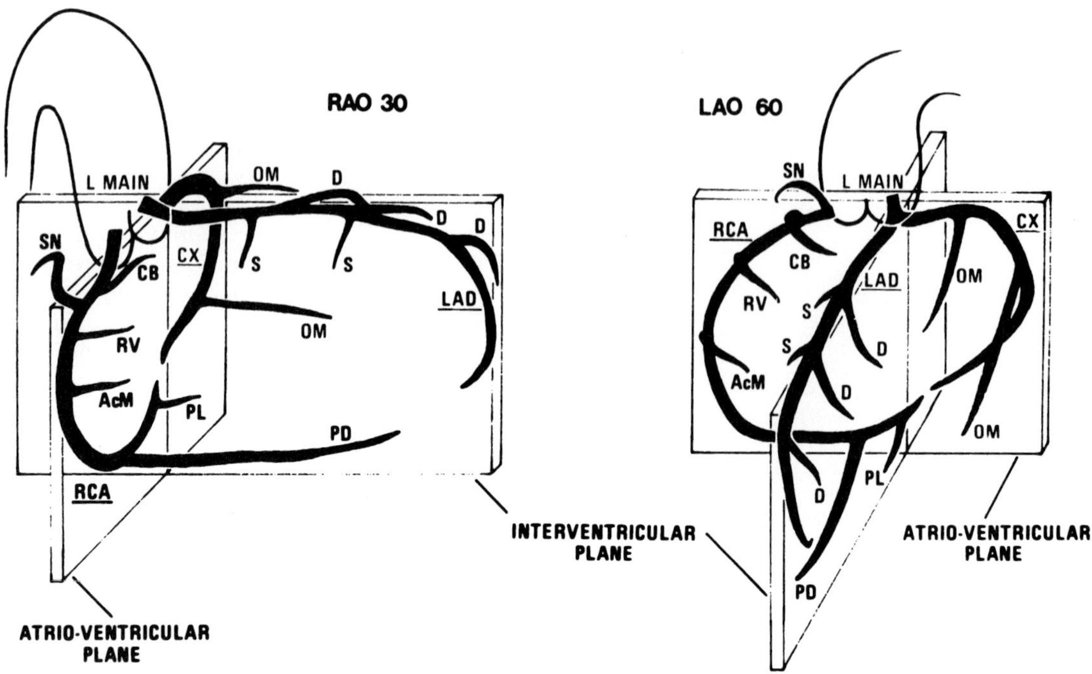

FIGURE 13–1. Representation of coronary anatomy relative to the interventricular and atrioventricular valve planes. Coronary branches are as indicated: L Main, left main; LAD, left anterior descending; D, diagonal; S, septal; CX, circumflex; OM, obtuse marginal; RCA, right coronary; CB, conus branch; S, sinus node; ACM, acute marginal; PD, posterior descending; PL, posterolateral. (From Grossman W: Cardiac Catheterization and Angiography, 3rd ed. Philadelphia, Lea & Febiger, 1986, with permission.)

TABLE 13–3
Grading of Valvular Regurgitation

Grade	Description
1	Contrast enters proximal chamber but clears with each beat
2	Contrast enters proximal chamber, does not clear with each beat, proximal chamber not as dense as injected chamber
3	Proximal chamber as dense as injected chamber
4	Proximal chamber denser than injected chamber

Interventional Cardiac Techniques

In addition to diagnostic catheterization, a number of percutaneous catheter-based therapeutic procedures have been developed.

Percutaneous Transluminal Coronary Angioplasty

The first PTCA was performed in 1977, and since then the procedure has become an accepted therapy for coronary artery disease.[23] PTCA continues to be the mainstay of interventional cardiology, despite the development of several other techniques, including atherectomy, excimer laser angioplasty, and intracoronary stenting.

All patients should receive aspirin (or ticlopidine in aspirin-allergic patients) and large doses of heparin. The activated coagulation time (ACT) is commonly used to monitor adequacy of anticoagulation. During PTCA, the ACT is kept above 300 seconds. A guiding catheter is placed into the coronary ostium. Guiding catheters are larger and stiffer than diagnostic catheters. This may predispose to vascular trauma of the coronary artery and so extra care must be exercised. Next, a small guidewire (0.010 to 0.018 inch) is advanced into the coronary artery past the stenosis. Careful manipulation of the intracoronary guidewire is of critical importance throughout the procedure. Following this, a balloon catheter is advanced over the wire and positioned across the area of stenosis. Contrast is used to inflate the balloon using an inflation device. The balloon is usually inflated with a pressure of several atmospheres and remains inflated for 1 or more minutes. Inflation duration is limited by the development of ischemia as manifested by severe chest pain, marked ECG abnormalities, or hemodynamic or electrical instability. Perfusion catheters are available and have sideholes both proximal and distal to the balloon to maintain blood flow during balloon inflation, which allows for prolonged inflation times.[24] This may be particularly advantageous in sealing off dissections that may develop, as discussed below.

After uncomplicated PTCA, the femoral sheaths are left in place 4 to 6 hours, until the heparin wears off, and are then removed. The patient may then be discharged the next day. In cases with suboptimal results (e.g., procedures complicated by dissection or thrombus), heparin may be continued for 24 hours while the sheaths remain in place and the patient is carefully mon-

TABLE 13–4
Lesion Classification*

Type A (minimally complex)
Discrete (<10 mm)
Readily accessible
Smooth contour
Less than totally occlusive
No major side branch involvement
Concentric
Nonangulated segment (<45 degrees)
Little or no calcification
Not ostial in location
Absence of thrombus
Type B (moderately complex)
Tubular (length 10–20 mm)
Moderate tortuosity of proximal segment
Irregular contour
Moderate or heavy calcification
Bifurcation requiring double guidewires
Eccentric
Moderately angulated (>45 degrees, <90 degrees)
Ostial in location
Total occlusions <3 mo old
Some thrombus present
Type C lesions (severely complex)
Diffuse (length >2 cm)
Extremely angulated segments (>90 degrees)
Inability to protect major side branches
Excessive tortuosity
Total occlusion >3 mo old
Degenerated vein grafts

*Modified from Ryan TJ, Bauman WB, Kennedy JW, et al: Guidelines for percutaneous transluminal coronary angioplasty. J Am Coll Cardiol 22:2033, 1993. Copyright 1993, American College of Cardiology, with permission.

itored. A postprocedure ECG should be obtained in all patients. Routine post-PTCA laboratory data may include cardiac enzymes, electrolytes and renal function tests, and blood count. Patients should be well hydrated following the procedure to avoid the dehydration that sometimes develops due to the diuretic action of contrast dye as well as to limit nephrotoxicity.

In general, acute success rates for PTCA are greater than 90%.[25] Success is most affected by characteristics of the lesions with simple, discrete, nonulcerated, concentric lesions having the highest success rate and more complex lesions having lower success rates (Table 13–4).[26] Acute complications are mainly due to abrupt closure of the vessel, which occurs in 4 to 8% of patients.[27,28] The mechanism of abrupt closure is dissection, thrombus formation, or spasm. Depending upon the etiology, treatment may include prolonged balloon inflation, atherectomy, intracoronary stenting, intracoronary thrombolytics, or intracoronary nitroglycerin. Abrupt closure leads to the major acute clinical complications of PTCA, which include death (1%), myocardial infarction (4%), and emergency bypass operation (3%).[25]

The long-term success of PTCA is limited by the problem of restenosis, which occurs in up to 50% of patients. This is due to a combination of intimal hyperplasia, recoil, and thrombus formation.

Newer interventional devices have been developed to address some of the limitations of PTCA, which include inability to treat certain lesions, abrupt closure, and restenosis.

Intracoronary Stenting

The introduction of stenting has greatly changed interventional cardiology over the last few years. This procedure involves the use of mesh-like cylindric scaffolding devices that can be placed across a stenosis and expanded via balloon into a permanent position within the coronary artery. The stent is left in place and becomes endothelialized in several weeks. The initial experience with stenting was marked by high subacute thrombosis rates.[29,30] However, recent advances, based in part on intracoronary ultrasound assessment demonstrating inadequate stent expansion in the majority of cases, have led to modifications of the stenting procedure.[31] Currently, patients are routinely treated with high-pressure inflations following stenting and with ticlopidine for 2 to 4 weeks, resulting in abrupt closure rates no different than seen with balloon PTCA. Restenosis rates are significantly lower than with routine balloon angioplasty.[29,30]

Rotational Atherectomy

This device utilizes a diamond-tipped burr that rotates over a guidewire and is advanced through atherosclerotic plaque.[32] The plaque is pulverized into small-sized particles that are then cleared by the body. It is especially useful in the treatment of calcified plaque.

Directional Coronary Atherectomy

This device was approved for clinical use in 1990. It is a percutaneous system for cutting and removing atheromatous material. The device is composed of a metal housing, which has an opening on one side and a balloon on the opposite side, and a circular cutter, which can be moved within the housing to cut plaque.

In a large, randomized trial comparing atherectomy to PTCA, clinical outcomes were somewhat worse with atherectomy, although there was a trend towards less restenosis.[33]

Transluminal Extraction Atherectomy

This device consists of a cone-shaped cutting blade that again is advanced over a wire and through the plaque. The rotating blade cuts plaque, which is then suctioned out through the catheter and collected. This device is most useful for thrombus-containing plaques and for old, degenerated vein grafts.

Excimer Laser

This device consists of a catheter with multiple fiberoptic cables that carry xenon chloride excimer laser energy to the lesion.[34] It is also advanced over a wire and acts by ablating tissue. It is most useful for long or totally occluded lesions. It is somewhat limited by the need for a large capital outlay to purchase the laser machine.

Balloon Valvuloplasty

Nonsurgical methods are now available for treating stenotic heart valves.[35] In this procedure, the stenotic valve is crossed with a guidewire and a balloon is positioned across the valve and inflated. The procedure is very successful in pulmonic stenosis in children and for the treatment of many patients with mitral stenosis. Its use in aortic stenosis is limited by high complication rates and high recurrence rates. Complications include valvular regurgitation, septal defects, perforation of the ventricle, and peripheral vascular complications.

Balloon Pericardiotomy

This procedure may be used in treating patients with pericardial effusions who otherwise would be treated surgically, usually with subxiphoid pericardiectomy. The pericardium is entered with a needle, a wire is placed, and a balloon tracked over the wire and positioned across the pericardium.[36] The balloon is inflated to create an opening in the pericardium, allowing fluid to drain into the pleural space. Initial results have been very promising.

Complications

Vascular

Vascular complications include dissection of the common femoral or iliac arteries, arteriovenous fistula, pseudoaneurysm formation at the entry site, and cholesterol embolization from the aorta.[37] Subintimal dissection occurs most commonly secondary to difficulties encountered in advancing guidewires or catheters through diseased or tortuous vessels. Usually these are self-limited and heal satisfactorily. However, if distal flow or significant side branches are affected, surgical repair may be necessary. An arteriovenous fistula is characterized by continuous bruit over the site of entry and swollen tender extremity secondary to increased venous flow. A pseudoaneurysm may be defined as a hematoma in direct communication with arterial blood through a disrupted vessel wall. Arteriovenous fistulae and pseudoaneurysms usually require surgical repair, although small to moderate pseudoaneurysms may resolve with prolonged compression of the artery. The incidence of dissection, arteriovenous fistula, and pseudoaneurysm formation in each is about 0.3 to 0.5%. Cholesterol atheroembolus occurs secondary to trauma of the aorta from interventional hardware. Macroemboli can lead to distal arterial occlusion or infarction of the abdominal viscera or kidneys. Showers of microemboli can cause grammarian obstruction and livido reticularis.

Bleeding

Significant bleeding requiring transfusion is very uncommon during routine catheterization (~0.4%). However, the risk increases with interventional techniques. Intracranial bleeding is the most feared bleeding complication, and is heralded by progressive headache or mental status change. Diagnosis is made by head computed tomography (CT), and therapy involves reversal of anticoagulation including the use of fresh frozen plasma and protamine. Retroperitoneal bleeding also occurs and may be due to needle puncture of the posterior arterial wall during sheath placement. Abdominal CT scan is the diagnostic modality of choice and treatment is generally supportive, including discontinuation of anticoagulation and transfusion as necessary. Groin hematoma is the most common bleeding complication and can generally be treated with prolonged external pressure; a C-clamp device is helpful in this situation.

Hemodynamic Abnormalities

Hypotension during cardiac catheterization or intervention may have one of several etiologies including hypovolemia secondary to patients being NPO, the osmotic diuretic effect of contrast, or occult bleeding; left ventricular dysfunction from dye-induced myocardial toxicity or coronary ischemia; or vasovagal episodes with arterial dilation and bradycardia. Unexplained hypotension warrants the use of invasive hemodynamic monitoring using a pulmonary artery catheter to measure the pulmonary capillary wedge pressure, cardiac output, and systemic vascular resistance. Hypovolemia is usually treated without difficulty by infusion of normal saline, whereas vasovagal episodes respond to atropine 0.5 mg IV.

Arrhythmia

Bradyarrhythmias usually respond to atropine; however, they may require the use of an external pacemaker or temporary transvenous pacing. Hemodynamically significant ventricular tachycardia or fibrillation is treated with electrical countershock beginning at 200 J. Supraventricular tachycardia responds well to adenosine (6 mg IV push).

References

1. Forssmann W: Die sondierung des rechten herzens. Klin Wochenschr 8:2085, 1929.
2. Klein O: Zur bestimmung des zerkulatorischen minutens volumen nach dem fickschen prinzip. Munch Med Wochenschr 77:1311, 1930.
3. Cournand AF, Ranges HS: Catheterization of the right auricle in man. Proc Soc Exp Biol Med 46:462, 1941.
4. Richards DW: Cardiac output by the catherization technique in various clinical conditions. Fed Proc 4:215, 1945.
5. Zimmerman HA, Scott RW, Becker ND: Catheterization of the left side of the heart in man. Circulation 1:357, 1950.

6. Sones FM Jr, Shirey EK, Prondfit WL, Westcott RN: Cinecoronary arteriography. Circulation 20:773, 1959.
7. Guntzig A, Senning A, Siegenthaler W: Non-operative dilatation of coronary artery stenoses. N Engl J Med 301:61, 1979.
8. Krone J, Morton MJ: Complications of Cardiac Catheterization and Angiography: Prevention and Management. Mount Kisco, NY, Futura, 1989.
9. Braunwald E, Swan HJC: Cooperative study on cardiac catheterization. Circulation 111:1, 1968.
10. Kennedy JW, et al: Complications associated with cardiac catheterization and angiography. Cathet Cardiovasc Diagn 8:5, 1982.
11. Lasser EC, Berry CC, Talner LB, et al: Pretreatment with corticosteroids to alleviate reactions to intravenous contrast material. N Engl J Med 317:845, 1987.
12. Weisel RD, Berger RL, Hechtman HB: Measurement of cardiac output by thermodilution. N Engl J Med 292:682, 1975.
13. Detre KM, Wright E, Murphy ML, Takato T: Observer agreement in evaluating coronary angiograms. Circulation 52:979, 1975.
14. Zir LM, Miller SW, Dinswore RE, et al: Interobserver variability in coronary angiography. Circulation 53:627, 1976.
15. Spears JR, Sandor T, Als A, et al: Computerized image analysis for quantitative measurement of vessel diameter for cineangiograms. Circulation 68:453, 1993.
16. Mancini GBJ, Simon SB, McGillem MJ, et al: Automated quantitative coronary arteriography: Morphologic and physiologic validation in vivo of a rapid digital angiographic method. Circulation 75:452, 1987.
17. Grossman W: Cardiac Catheterization and Angiography, 3rd ed. Philadelphia, Lea & Febiger, 1986.
18. Gorlin R, Gorlin G: Hydraulic formula for calculation of area of stenotic mitral valve, other cardiac valves, and central circulatory shunts. Am Heart J 41:1, 1951.
19. Tenaglia AN, Buller CE, Kisslo KB, et al: Mechanisms of balloon angioplasty and directional coronary atherectomy as assessed by intracoronary ultrasound. J Am Coll Cardiol 20:685, 1992.
20. Tenaglia AN, Kisslo K, Kelly S, et al: Ultrasound guidewire directed stent deployment. Am Heart J 125:1213, 1993.
21. Nakamura S, Colombo A, Gaglione A, et al: Intracoronary ultrasound observations during stent implantation. Circulation 89: 2026, 1994.
22. Sherman CT, Litvack F, Grundfest W, et al: Coronary angioscopy in patients with unstable angina pectoris. N Engl J Med 315:913, 1986.
23. Landau C, Lange RA, Hillis LD: Percutaneous transluminal coronary angioplasty. N Engl J Med 330:981, 1994.
24. Tenaglia AN, Quigley PJ, Kereiakes DJ, et al: Coronary angioplasty performed with gradual and prolonged inflation using a perfusion balloon catheter: Procedural success and restenosis rate. Am Heart J 124:585, 1992.
25. Detre K, Houlbkov PHR, Kelsey S, et al: Percutaneous transluminal coronary angioplasty in 1985–1986 and 1977–1981. N Engl J Med 318:266, 1988.
26. Ryan TJ, Bauman WB, Kennedy JW, et al: Guidelines for percutaneous transluminal coronary angioplasty. J Am Coll Cardiol 22:2033, 1993.
27. Tenaglia AN, Fortin DF, Caiff RM, et al: Predicting the risk of abrupt vessel closure after angioplasty in an individual patient. J Am Coll Cardiol 24:1004, 1994.
28. Lincoff AM, Popma JJ, Ellis SG, et al: Abrupt vessel closure complicating coronary angioplasty: Clinical, angiographic, and therapeutic profile. J Am Coll Cardiol 19:826, 1992.
29. Serruys PW, DeJaegere P, Kiemeneij F, et al: A comparison of balloon-expandable-stent implantation with balloon angioplasty in patients with coronary artery disease. N Engl J Med 331:489, 1994.
30. Fischman DL, Leon MB, Baim DS, et al: A randomized comparison of coronary-stent placement and balloon angioplasty in the treatment of coronary artery disease. N Engl J Med 331:496, 1994.
31. Colombo A, Hall P, Nakamura S, et al: Intracoronary stenting without anticoagulation achieved with intracoronary ultrasound guidance. Circulation 91:1676, 1995.
32. Safian RD, Niazi KA, Strzelecki M, et al: Detailed angiographic analysis of high-speed mechanical rotational atherectomy in human coronary arteries. Circulation 88:961, 1993.
33. Topol EJ, Leya F, Pinkerton CA, et al: A comparison of directional atherectomy with coronary angioplasty in patients with coronary artery disease. N Engl J Med 329:221, 1993.
34. Bittl JA, Sanborn TA: Excimer laser-facilitated coronary angioplasty relative risk analysis of acute and follow-up results in 200 patients. Circulation 86:71, 1992.
35. Bashore TM, Davidson CJ: Percutaneous Balloon Valvuloplasty and Related Techniques. Baltimore, Williams & Wilkins, 1991.
36. Ziskind AA, Pearce AC, Lemmon CC, et al: Percutaneous balloon pericardiotomy for the treatment of cardiac tamponade and large pericardial effusions: Description of technique and report of the first 50 cases. J Am Coll Cardiol 21:1, 1993.
37. Muller DWM, Shamir KJ, Ellis SG, Topol EJ: Peripheral vascular complications after conventional and complex percutaneous coronary interventional procedures. Am J Cardiol 69:63, 1992.

CHAPTER 14

Coronary Artery Disease

Jacques YaDeau, M.D., PhD
Stephen J. Thomas, M.D.
Jan Kramer, M.D.

Anesthetic care of the patient undergoing coronary artery bypass grafting (CABG) is, for the most part, no different than for any other operative procedure. Patients undergoing CABG have concurrent diseases and medications that may interact with anesthetics, airways that must be properly managed, and central and autonomic nervous systems that must be adequately anesthetized. The critical differences are that the heart is directly affected by the surgical procedure and, for most patients, extracorporeal circulation is required. It is important to understand that these last two items are *in addition* to the usual anesthetic concerns, not in place of them. This chapter provides an overview of the perioperative care of the CABG patient requiring either cardiopulmonary bypass or minimally invasive coronary surgery.

Anesthesia and Myocardial Ischemia

The goals of the anesthetic for CABG include the "usual suspects" (an unmoving patient with analgesia, anesthesia, and amnesia) plus prevention of myocardial ischemia. The primary objective is to control myocardial oxygen demand (MVO_2) and improve supply so that myocardial oxygen balance is improved, thereby reducing the likelihood that myocardial ischemia will develop.

Determinants of oxygen demand include wall tension, contractility, and heart rate. Wall tension may be approximated by the law of Laplace and is directly proportional to both the pressure in, and the size of, the ventricular cavity. Thus, a small ventricle will have less wall tension and, therefore, less oxygen demand than a large ventricle, all other things being equal. Contractility is the intrinsic vigor of myofibrillar shortening. Heart rate actually plays little part in increasing oxygen demand *per beat*, but does increase oxygen demand *per minute*. The main reason that increased heart rate is proischemic is that it decreases the length of diastole, during which the majority of left ventricular (LV) perfusion is occurring.

Determinants of myocardial oxygen supply are related to the amount of coronary blood flow, determined by both coronary perfusion pressure and resistance to flow in the coronary circulation, and the oxygen-carrying capacity of the blood. The coronary perfusion pressure is often represented by the difference between the systemic diastolic pressure and the left ventricular end-diastolic pressure (LVEDP). While the LVEDP is not an exact description of the true "downstream" pressure, it is a reasonable estimate. The coronary vascular resistance is determined by the degree of vasoconstriction of the coronary arterioles. The concentration of hemoglobin in the blood and the oxygen saturation determine the oxygen-carrying capacity.

Commonly used anesthetic or vasoactive drugs alter most of these determinants. Decreased blood pressure reduces oxygen demand and has potential for significantly decreasing supply. The size of the left ventricle may be decreased by decreasing afterload or by venodilation and preload reduction with nitroglycerin. The heart rate may be controlled with either anesthetics, β-blockers, or calcium entry blockers. Coronary vascular resistance may be decreased by both calcium entry blockers and nitroglycerin. The ideal recipe for preventing or treating myocardial ischemia is to make the heart *slow*, *small*, and *well perfused*. At the same time systemic blood flow must be adequate to meet physiologic needs. A *slow* heart rate allows maximal diastolic time for left ventricular perfusion. A *small* heart has minimal wall tension, which diminishes oxygen demand, and a *well-perfused* heart (normal to high AoDP-LVEDP gradient) has adequate coronary blood flow.

The effects of anesthetics on the coronary circulation have been the subject of some debate. While narcotics, benzodiazepines, and other adjunctive agents may cause coronary vasodilation, this is most likely secondary to the suppression of sympathetic tone induced by these drugs. Inhaled anesthetics, on the other hand, have direct effects on the coronary vasculature. Isoflurane and possibly sevoflurane are the most potent dilators, followed by enflurane and halothane. Isoflurane was suspected of causing ischemia-inducing "coronary steal," at least in the laboratory,[1] but clinical experience demonstrates that it does not cause ischemia in doses under 1 minimal alveolar concentration (MAC). Systemic vasodilation caused by volatile agents may also help lessen myocardial oxygen demand by decreasing wall tension.

Volatile anesthetics are potent myocardial depressants; contractility is decreased in the presence of these drugs. Whether this is a desirable attribute or an unwanted side effect is often a matter of philosophy. Some feel that "optimizing" of cardiac function prior to cardiopulmonary bypass (CPB) is ideal; others opine that cardiac function should be minimized while maintaining adequate systemic blood flow and pressure. Decreased contractility decreases myocardial oxygen demand. The characteristic myocardial depression of volatile anesthetics, therefore, may be desirable for those hearts with good ventricular function (after all, the mainstays of their medical therapy are myocardial depressants). Conversely, myocardial depression may be deleterious to patients with severely impaired contractility and contribute to ventricular dilation and increased myocardial oxygen demand, as well as inadequate systemic flow.

Attempts have been made to quantify these hemodynamic goals in order to provide more complete and accurate perioperative monitoring. Though they emphasize the need for a slow heart rate and adequate coronary perfusion pressure, no index of myocardial oxygen balance is sufficiently sensitive and specific to be used routinely. The rate pressure product (systolic blood pressure times heart rate) correlates with MVO_2 during exercise, but an elevated rate-pressure product does not predict intraoperative ischemia.[2] A rate-pressure ratio (heart rate divided by mean arterial pressure) greater than unity predicts ischemia in dogs,[3] but its inverse, the pressure rate quotient, does not predict myocardial ischemia in patients undergoing CABG.[4]

Significance of Perioperative Ischemia

Perioperative electrocardiographic (ECG) evidence of ischemia has been estimated to occur in 40 to 60% of CABG patients.[5,6] Some of these episodes are associated with hemodynamic abnormalities (tachycardia, hypertension, or hypotension). However, of crucial importance, more than half of these episodes were unaccompanied by hemodynamic changes. The lack of a strong correlation between ischemia and notable alterations in heart rate or blood pressure suggests that ischemia is often caused by decreased myocardial oxygen supply (e.g., increased coronary artery tone or thrombotic coronary occlusion) rather than by increased oxygen demand.[7] Whatever the cause, perioperative ischemia has been associated with poor outcomes in the form of increased incidence of postoperative myocardial infarction. It has been suggested that ischemia shortly after revascularization or in the early postoperative period is a risk factor for adverse cardiac outcome.[8-10]

Preoperative Evaluation

The preoperative visit with the prospective CABG patient is no different than a visit to any other patient. Severity of cardiac disease should be assessed from the history; physical exam; and review of echocardiograph, radionuclide, and angiographic studies. In addition, a review of concurrent disease(s), medications, past anesthetic and surgical history, and family history of anesthetic problems is mandatory. Patients and their families are usually apprehensive about an upcoming CABG. Some of this fear may be alleviated by an explanation of what can be expected both before and after the operation. A frank and detailed discussion of the perioperative plan plays a greater role than premedication in allaying anxiety. In particular, explanation of what to expect on emergence in the intensive care unit (ICU) (tracheal tube, arterial catheter, pulmonary artery or central venous catheter, provisions for pain relief) can obviate the distress that may otherwise arise. One can also use this time to clarify the role of the anesthesiologist in the patient's care. Sedatives administered the evening before and the day of surgery are often helpful adjuncts and may help prevent perioperative ischemia.

Risk

Patients and families often inquire about expected outcome, and a general discussion may be helpful if the patient so desires. It is difficult to assign numeric risk for an individual patient because the exact definition of what constitutes a "risk factor" is unclear. In any operation requiring general anesthesia, there is an anesthetic-related mortality caused by such factors as failure to ventilate, drug overdose, and an idiosyncratic or allergic response to medications. This strictly anesthesia-related risk (estimates of which range from 1 in 10,000 cases[11] to 1 in 200,000 cases[12]) is markedly overshadowed by the 1.1% in-hospital mortality observed in a 1987 study of patients under 65 with normal LV function who underwent their first CABG.[13]

Multiple studies have attempted to define the risk factors for morbidity and mortality following CABG, often with conflicting results. The discrepancies may be due to sample size, patient population, or geographic and secular differences in anesthetic practice, surgical practice, or co-assortment of disease. Generally agreed upon risk factors for morbidity and mortality include age, reoperations, emergency surgery, cross-clamp time, female sex, small body size, decreased left ventricular ejection fraction, dialysis dependence, diabetes mellitus, hypertension, and chronic obstructive pulmonary disease (COPD). The contribution of each of these to overall outcome is unclear.

However, quantitative estimation of risk may serve several useful functions. It can facilitate comparison of outcomes between different institutions by adjusting for differences in patient populations. Risk stratification may allow for more accurate cost projections. Finally, assessment of risk could identify high-risk patients in advance, thereby allowing the anesthesiologist (and the patient, if necessary) to make suitable preparations.

Paiement[14] prospectively attempted to predict outcome for heart surgery (including valvular surgery) by assessing the presence of eight proposed risk factors. They consisted of an ejection fraction less than 0.3, unstable angina or recent myocardial infarction (MI), heart failure, age over 65 years, severe obesity, emergency surgery, reoperation, and other significant and uncontrolled systemic disturbances (such as pulmonary hypertension, chronic lung disease, chronic renal failure, poor hepatic function, cerebrovascular insufficiency, severe arterial hypertension, and severe arrhythmias). One half of the patients had no risk factors and had a 0.4% mortality. Thirty-two percent of the patients had one risk factor and experienced a 3.1% mortality, while 18% of the patients had more than one risk factor and suffered a 12.2% mortality rate.

Higgins, using a retrospective multivariate analysis, developed a severity scoring system to predict mortality and morbidity (defined as MI, use of an intra-aortic balloon pump [IABP], prolonged ventilation, central nervous system complications, acute renal failure, or infection) in patients undergoing CABG.[15] The most significant risk factors were emergency surgery and renal dysfunction. Interestingly, neither history of MI or congestive heart failure nor provider of surgical or anesthetic care predict increased risk. However, left ventricular dysfunction, valve dysfunction, emergency surgery, and reoperation were found to be significant predictors. To validate the accuracy of the severity score, predicted and observed morbidity and mortality were compared in CABG patients over the next 2 years. The model predicted mortality well, but observed morbidity was lower than predicted. The discrepancy was attributed to changes in clinical practice such as routine administration of low-dose dopamine to patients with chronic renal failure, and improved transport of emergent cases to the operating room (OR). This points out a difficulty in using risk estimates based on clinical practice patterns that do not include new routines and protocols.

The presence of left main coronary artery stenosis may pose increased risk. Whether this is due to the stenosis itself (and associated ischemia) or, conversely, to the presence of secondary factors such as arrhythmia, unstable angina, or recent MI, is unclear. It does appear that neither "steal-prone" anatomy nor left main disease predicted increased risk for intraoperative or postoperative ischemic episodes. Despite this, it seems prudent to approach patients with left main coronary artery disease with a heightened level of vigilance.

The contribution of anesthetics or anesthesiologists to the risk of morbidity and mortality of CABG has been examined. In a study aimed at comparing outcomes among different anesthetic agents, only chronic hypertension, poor quality of anastomosis or graft (rated by the surgical staff), prolonged aortic cross-clamp time, and new perioperative myocardial ischemia were predictive of postoperative MI.[16] A similar study of anesthetic choice and outcome[17] found that mortality could be predicted by aortic cross-clamp time, recent MI, preoperative congestive heart failure, inability to use a mammary graft, preoperative dysrhythmias, left main coronary artery disease, high New York Heart Association (NYHA) functional class, and unstable angina. Neither study found that the type of anesthetic made a difference. However, Slogoff's study identified an individual anesthesiologist (the infamous #7) as a risk factor, who had a higher incidence of hemodynamic abnormalities and perioperative ischemia than all others. Hemodynamic control does play an important role in perioperative management of the CABG patient.

Included in the preoperative evaluation should be an assessment of left ventricular function. Left ventricular ejection fraction can be obtained from radionuclide cineangiography or cardiac catheterization. Decreased ejection fraction may pose an independent risk for poor outcome, and evaluation of left ventricular performance is useful for planning an anesthetic. Patients with markedly decreased ejection fraction may benefit from more extensive monitoring and a nondepressant or minimally depressant anesthetic regimen. Consideration can be given to the administration of inotropes prior to the first attempt to separate from CPB.

Cardiovascular medications taken chronically should be continued up to the morning of surgery. Some of these medications, especially β-blockers, may prevent or lessen the degree of perioperative myocardial ischemia. Conversely, calcium entry blockers do not seem to be protective. Presumably, the difference is due to the greater ability of β-blockers to prevent tachycardia. Other common preoperative medications that should be continued include antihypertensives, although angiotensin converting enzyme (ACE) inhibitors may increase the requirement for vasoconstrictors following CPB.

Digoxin is usually continued immediately preoperatively if given for control of heart rate, such as for patients with atrial fibrillation. However, the arrhythmogenic properties of digoxin may be accentuated by the perioperative hypothermia and electrolyte changes. For this reason, if digoxin is being administered to a patient with heart failure for its inotropic properties, consideration should be given to withholding the digoxin on the morning of CABG surgery.

Magnesium is now given frequently following acute MI.[18,19] It appears to reduce the incidence of mortality and heart failure, and may be antiarrhythmogenic. Major side effects include transient hypotension and bradycardia. Although the mechanism of action is unproven, possibilities include coronary and peripheral vasodilation, antiplatelet action, and direct protection of the myocardium from ischemia and reperfusion injury, perhaps by mitigating toxic effects of calcium. Furthermore, magnesium is a cofactor for many enzymes, including sodium (Na), potassium adenosine triphosphatase (K-ATPase), and calcium ATPase (Ca-ATPase), which are involved in maintenance of ionic gradients across cell membranes. Hypermagnesium can cause sedation and prolongation of neuromuscular blockade; but such effects occur at levels of magnesium (2 to 3 mmol/L) that exceed the peak levels reached in treatment of an MI (0.96 to 1.54 mmol/L).[18]

Heparin is commonly administered preoperatively to patients with unstable angina to prevent intracoronary thrombosis. This infusion should be continued at least up to the OR door. The half-life of heparin is on the order of 1 hour, so in most patients the infusion may be stopped prior to induction of anesthesia. However, patients with near-total coronary occlusion symptoms may benefit from continuing the heparin infusion until anticoagulation is achieved prior to CPB. Heparin therapy of several days' duration may induce heparin resistance, an ill-defined entity in which larger than normal doses of heparin may be required to provide sufficient anticoagulation for CPB.

Anesthesia for CABG

Monitoring

Monitoring for CABG includes ECG, pulse oximetry, capnography, and temperature measurement, as in any other type of procedure. Direct arterial pressure monitoring is usually employed because precipitous changes in systemic blood pressure may occur as a result of blood loss, surgical manipulation of the heart, anesthetic administration, and myocardial ischemia. In most but not all institutions, the catheter is inserted prior to induction. The radial artery is the most common site for cannulation due to its easy availability and safety. Other sites include the dorsalis pedis, femoral, and axillary arteries. Arterial tracings vary with the site of measurement. Under normal conditions, aortic systolic pressure is less than or equal to radial systolic pressure, while the peak of the dorsalis pedis arterial pressure wave occurs later than in the radial artery, and is 5 to 20 mm Hg higher.

Immediately after bypass, aortic pressure was higher than radial pressure in 72% of patients, with a mean difference of 20 mm Hg.[20] The pressure gradient returned to normal over a mean time of 20 minutes. The authors recommend direct measurement of aortic pressure whenever treatment of blood pressure is considered following bypass. It was suggested that the aortic-radial artery pressure gradient reflected diversion of blood to a vasodilated forearm vascular bed. However, it appears that the aortic-radial artery mean arterial pressure gradient does not develop during rewarming, but can be observed soon after institution of cardiopulmonary bypass.[21] In this study, common iliac artery pressure was found to accurately reflect the aortic mean pressure. During surgical dissection of the internal mammary artery, the pressure tracing may be dampened or absent in the ipsilateral radial artery.[22] It was suggested that the contralateral (generally the right) radial artery be used if internal mammary grafting is intended.

Whether to monitor central venous pressure alone, or to also monitor pulmonary artery pressure is usually a matter of local custom and often based on severity of the patient's myocardial dysfunction. Neither central venous pressure (CVP) catheters nor pulmonary artery (PA) catheters are particularly useful for the detection of ischemia, as they are both insensitive and nonspecific. Rather, they are best used as indicators of volume status. The pulmonary artery occlusion pressure (PAOP) appears to be better than CVP for the evaluation of cardiac filling only for patients with markedly abnormal left ventricular function.[23] The PA catheter can help evaluate cardiac function further by providing the means to measure stroke volume.

Selected low-risk patients appear to do well with only CVP monitoring during anesthesia for CABG.[24,25] No differences were noted between patients managed initially with a PA catheter compared with those with only a CVP. Some patients initially managed with CVP alone may require insertion of a PA catheter later in the postoperative period for diagnosis and management of hemodynamic derangements. It has been suggested that routine placement of a PA catheter may be unnecessary, and that it increases direct and indirect costs. The choice between a CVP catheter and a PA catheter is further clouded by the unreliability of cardiac output data immediately following CPB. A systematic error is introduced to cardiac output measurement following CPB performed with hypothermia and rewarming. Rapid core cooling within the first 10 minutes after CPB is caused by redistribution of heat to less well-perfused peripheral tissues. The consequent marked baseline drift causes underestimation of cardiac outputs by about 11%.[26]

The risks related to access to the central circulation, such as arterial puncture or pneumothorax, are identical for both PA and CVP catheters. The risk of serious complications specifically related to PA catheterization, such as serious ventricular dysrhythmias, pulmonary artery rupture, and endocardial lesions, has been estimated at 0.1 to 0.5% (ASA Practice Guidelines). The Practice Guidelines state that this risk is acceptable for patients undergoing cardiac surgery, but that deviations from their recommendations "should not necessarily be viewed as inappropriate care." The decision between CVP and PA catheters reflects patient characteristics and institutional practice.

In addition to monitoring volume status and ventricular function, the ever-present possibility of new or worsening ischemia must be considered. ST-segment analyzers are useful aids to following trends, and may prompt recognition of subtle or gradual changes in the ECG.[27] A printout of the ECG for later comparison may be helpful. Changes in ST-segments usually indicate ischemia, but can also be caused by hypothermia, electrolyte imbalance, or baseline drift. OR monitors have a narrower bandwidth than diagnostic ECG machines, which lessens interference caused by muscle movement, electrical noise, or respiratory variation. However, most OR monitors (at least in the monitor mode) appear to overestimate ischemia if compared to standard ECG machines.[28]

Transesophageal echocardiography (TEE) has been touted as a sensitive monitor of myocardial ischemia. Regional wall motion abnormalities that may be detected by TEE may, in fact, be due to ischemia[8,9]; however, they may also be due to abrupt changes in either afterload or preload. TEE is, therefore, a very sensitive monitor for ischemia but not a particularly specific one. Eisenberg noted that, at least in patients undergoing general surgery, TEE offered no advantage over the standard five-lead ECG.[29]

TEE is unique in its ability to evaluate valvular function. It may be used to document pressure gradients across stenotic valves, estimate severity of regurgitant lesions, and provide an overall view of cardiac function as well as investigate regional contractile abnormalities. Cardiac chamber size may also be estimated. This is very useful in those patients with pulmonary hypertension or diastolic dysfunction, where PA catheters may provide misleading information about the volume status. The TEE may also be valuable in patients undergoing CABG by facilitating examination of the descending and part of the ascending aorta in the search for potential sources of emboli.[30]

Electroencephalographic (EEG) monitoring during CPB has been suggested as a means to prevent neurologic problems.[31] Unfortunately, it is difficult to assess EEG abnormalities in the electrically noisy setting of the OR, and a recent study[32] found that the high background variability of the EEG precluded prediction of brain injury by EEG analysis.

Choice of Anesthetic Agents

There has been much debate over the relationship between choice of anesthetic and patient outcome.[33] Studies over the last 20 years have demonstrated that a multitude of different anesthetic regimens involving many combinations of premedications, analgesics, amnestics, neuromuscular blockers, and volatile anesthetics have negligible effect on the development of intraoperative ischemia and morbidity and mortality. This is not to say that all anesthetics are the same. In fact, identifiable differences were found between various combinations of anesthetics. The fact remains, however, that as long as tachycardia and large swings in blood pressure are avoided, it matters little which anesthetic is used.

Slogoff and Keats[16] found no significant difference in the incidence of postoperative MI or pre-CPB ischemia in CABG patients randomly assigned to receive sufentanil (15 to 25 μg/kg at induction, with 5 μg/kg before sternotomy), halothane, enflurane, or isoflurane. Patients receiving volatile anesthetics for maintenance of anesthesia were given 10 μg/kg fentanyl and 0.25 to 0.4 mg/kg diazepam for induction of anesthesia. Pancuronium was given for neuromuscular blockade. The results confirmed "clinical impressions." Patients who received a volatile agent had a higher incidence of hypotension and a lower incidence of hypertension. Patients randomized to receive sufentanil had less postoperative hypertension, but were mechanically ventilated for a longer period postoperatively. The authors suggest that only the 11.7% of the ischemic events that were temporally related to a hemodynamic abnormality (such as tachycardia) could have been a consequence of anesthetic management, and conclude that there is no connection between anesthetic agent and ischemia. Tuman et al.[17] prospectively, but not randomly, compared five anesthetics for CABG surgery: high-dose fentanyl (>50 μg/kg), moderate-dose fentanyl (<50 μg/kg), sufentanil (3 to 8 μg/kg), diazepam/ketamine, or halothane. Sixty percent of the patients given a primarily intravenous technique received supplemental volatile anesthetic. No differences were seen in the incidence of mortality, postoperative MI, or other serious morbid events. The authors of this study emphasize that achieving appropriate intraoperative hemodynamics and aggressively treating arrhythmias and ischemia are more important than the choice of anesthetic agent.

A comparison of four anesthetic drugs (fentanyl, thiopental, enflurane, and propofol) used to maintain anesthesia following premedication and fentanyl induction of premedicated patients demonstrated that hemodynamic stability could be achieved with any of these regimens.[34] Some interesting though not unexpected differences among the groups emerged. For example, 32% of the patients in the fentanyl group required nitroprusside, while none of the patients in the other treatment groups were given nitroprusside. Vasopressor use varied among groups, as well. Patients in the propofol and enflurane groups awakened faster, but this did not result in faster discharge from the ICU.

Thomson et al.[35] studied the cardiovascular effects of inducing anesthesia with 100 μg/kg fentanyl in patients premedicated with either 0.06 mg/kg lorazepam, given orally, or 0.1 mg/kg morphine plus 6 μg/kg scopolamine, given intramuscularly. Atracurium was used for neuromuscular blockade. Similar degrees of sedation and anxiolysis were achieved, but marked differences in intraoperative hemodynamics were noted. The morphine/scopolamine group had a higher mean heart rate with occasional hyperdynamic responses to induction of anesthesia, while patients receiving lorazepam had lower cardiac indices and lower blood pressures, which was attributed to sympatholysis. One patient in the morphine/scopolamine group recalled being intubated. The authors suggest that premedications for high-dose narcotic inductions be chosen on the basis of the desired hemodynamic response.

If hemodynamic perturbations are avoided, the incidence of prebypass ischemia is the same whether pancuronium or vecuronium is used as a relaxant.[36] Patients in this study were premedicated with diazepam, morphine, and scopolamine, and anesthesia was induced with 40 μg/kg fentanyl. Heart rates greater than 90 were treated with propranolol, blood pressures that deviated from preoperative values by more than 20% were treated with enflurane or phenylephrine, and ECGs indicative of ischemia were treated with nitroglycerin. Patients receiving vecuronium had a lower heart rate and cardiac index, and required less propranolol than patients receiving pancuronium. The incidence of postoperative MI was similar in each group. None of the patients with a postoperative MI had prebypass ischemia, but they had significantly longer aortic cross-clamp times than the other patients. The authors conclude that either pancuronium or vecuronium is acceptable, provided tachycardia and extremes of blood pressure are avoided.

Thomson examined the role of both premedication (morphine/scopolamine, or lorazepam, dosed as above) and muscle relaxants (vecuronium or pancuronium, 0.1 mg/kg) on the hemodynamic response to induction with 10 μg/kg sufentanil.[37] Mean arterial pressure decreased in all four groups; the decrease was least in the morphine/scopolamine/pancuronium group. Morphine/scopolamine/pancuronium was associated with a mean heart rate increase of 13.6 following induction, and an increased cardiac index following intubation. Almost half the patients in this group received pharmacologic therapy for this hyperdynamic response. The lorazepam/pancuronium group had an average heart rate increase of 6 bpm; blood pressure and cardiac indices decreased. The morphine/scopolamine/vecuronium group had decreased blood pressures but stable heart rates and cardiac indices. Conversely, the lorazepam/vecuronium group had stable heart rates but diminished blood pressures and cardiac indices. This study suggests that hemodynamic goals be considered when choosing premedication and muscle relaxant. For example, a young, relatively vigorous patient might benefit from the lorazepam/vecuronium combination, while an elderly patient with congestive heart failure could be considered for morphine/scopolamine/pancuronium. The presence of coexisting diseases such as valvular heart disease or cerebrovascular disease will also influence the decision.

Opioids are the traditional mainstay of cardiac anesthesia. Opioids primary virtue, the lack of myocardial depression, is particularly important for patients with decreased ventricular function. Patients with normal myocardial contractility, however, may benefit by use of a myocardial depressant to attenuate increases in MVO_2. The bradycardic response to narcotics is generally beneficial to patients with coronary artery disease. Narcotics such as fentanyl or sufentanil provide stable hemodynamics; appear to decrease stress responses such as increases in antidiuretic hormone (ADH), growth hormone, and catecholamines; but are inconsistent in blunting the sympathetic response that may lead to hypertension. Sympathetic stimulation can be reduced or prevented by supplementation of the narcotic anesthetic with vasodilators, α-agonists such as clonidine, or a volatile anesthetic agent. Drawbacks of narcotic anesthesia include skeletal muscle rigidity, histamine release, lessened ability to titrate the depth of anesthesia, inconsistent provision of amnesia, and increased intravenous fluid requirement. Some side effects, such as histamine release, may be related to the rate of administration of the narcotic. Reports of asystole on induction of anesthesia with high-dose narcotics in patients receiving β-blockers emphasize the necessity of individualized titration of doses. "Full doses" of narcotics can be up to 100 μg/kg of fentanyl or 10 to 15 μg/kg sufentanil. In this current age of fast-tracking and emphasis on shortened length of stay, such high-dose techniques are infrequently employed.

In healthy, unpremedicated patients, fentanyl is unreliable as a sole anesthetic. Unconsciousness appears to be associated with opioid-induced rigidity and apnea.[39] However, when given as a sole medication to unpremedicated volunteers, 15 μg/kg fentanyl produced rigidity, apnea, and unconsciousness lasting an average of 11.5 minutes in only half the subjects. Animal studies of the enflurane-sparing effects of opioids indicate that fentanyl or sufentanil infusions cannot entirely replace enflurane.[39,40] Common anesthetic practice with high-dose narcotic techniques includes premedication with benzodiazepines, individualization of doses, and use of adjuvant anesthetic agents. Intraoperative awareness has been described in a 41-year-old woman after receiving 90 μg/kg fentanyl, despite premedication with morphine and scopolamine.[41] Another case report describes two anesthetics for the same 45-year-old patient; in both cases the patient was premedicated with morphine, and received more than 70 μg/kg fentanyl. The first case was uneventful, and the patient received 10 mg of diazepam. The second anesthetic, for an acutely occluded graft, did not include diazepam, and the patient reported awareness.[42]

CABG patients frequently exhibit hyperdynamic responses to intraoperative stimuli, despite massive doses of narcotics, such as a loading dose of 40 μg/kg sufentanil followed by an infusion of 0.2 μg/kg/min.[43,44] Hypertensive responses occur over a wide range of plasma fentanyl concentrations, indicating that fentanyl alone does not reliably block adrenergic responses to operative stimuli.[45] It is prudent to administer amnestic agents, such as midazolam or diazepam. Droperidol (2.5 to 10 mg) is particularly useful because of its α-antagonist properties. Low-dose potent inhalational agents are often used. Supplemental agents such as enflurane or propofol may allow extubation earlier than if high-dose fentanyl were used as the sole anesthetic.[46] Nitrous oxide (N_2O) can be used as an adjunct to narcotic-based anesthetics but must be discontinued well in advance of institution of CPB. Lower doses of opioids combined with benzodiazepines, volatile anesthetics, or other sedatives are safe, permit earlier extubation, and may help reduce total hospital costs.

Volatile anesthetics have many useful properties as a supplement to narcotic anesthetics, including dose-related and reversible myocardial depression, suppression of sympathetic responses, vasodilation, amnesia, and hypnosis. They are easier to titrate than most intravenous anesthetic agents, a virtue that becomes apparent should the patient's hemodynamic profile suddenly change. However, they generally decrease systolic blood pressure, which can provoke ischemia, and may necessitate the use of vasoconstrictors. They do not provide postoperative analgesia, and may induce dysrhythmias (particularly halothane, when used in conjunction with adrenergic agonists). Concerns have been raised about isoflurane-exacerbated coronary artery steal,[1,47] but these appear to have been overstated.[44] Steal-prone anatomy consists of a total occlusion of a coronary artery, whose subtended myocardium is supplied by collateral flow from a different coronary artery with a significant stenosis. It has been suggested that patients with such anatomy are prone to ischemia if the artery supplying collateral flow were vasodilated. However, several comparisons of anesthetic techniques have shown that patients with steal-prone anatomy do as well with isoflurane-based anesthetics as with anesthetics based on other inhalational agents or opioids.[48–50]

Desflurane has been compared to sufentanil for maintenance of anesthesia.[51] Following thiopental induction, patients were ventilated with 1 to 2 MAC end-tidal desflurane prior to intubation, then 1 MAC after intubation. No opioids were given to patients in the desflurane group prebypass. During CPB, the desflurane patients received sufentanil and midazolam. The sufentanil was discontinued following bypass and the patients ventilated with 1 MAC desflurane. The sufentanil patients received 5 to 10 μg/kg sufentanil for induction, followed by sufentanil infusion of 0.07 μg/kg min. Patients were randomly and prospectively assigned to receive either sufentanil or desflurane. The incidence of adverse cardiac outcomes were similar in both groups, but there were interesting variations in the hemodynamics and therapeutic interventions between the two groups. On induction, the desflurane group required significantly more esmolol for tachycardia, while the sufentanil group received more ephedrine and phenylephrine. More importantly, the desflurane group had a higher incidence of myocardial ischemia on induction: 9% versus 0% by electrocardiographic criteria and 13% versus 0% using echocardiographic criteria. During maintenance of anesthesia, the desflurane group received more interventions with esmolol, phenylephrine, and nitroglycerin, while the sufentanil group had a higher incidence of administration of nitroprusside during and following bypass. The authors conclude that although desflurane is not a desirable induction agent in patients undergoing CABG, it is safe for maintenance of anesthesia. The primary possible advantage of the desflurane technique, that it might allow earlier extubation, was not evaluated.

Desflurane has also been compared to isoflurane for use as the primary anesthetic for CABG surgery.[52] The hemodynamic effects were similar, with the exception that systemic blood pressures before bypass were lower with desflurane. This may have been due to more rapid approach of end-tidal to inspired values because of the low solubility of desflurane.

Sodium thiopental is a commonly used induction agent for volatile-based anesthetics. It is a myocardial depressant and peripheral vasodilator, and in severely compromised patients, consideration may be given to alternative induction agents. Ketamine, while also a direct myocardial depressant, supports blood pressure through release of catecholamines and can be used as either an induction agent or as the primary anesthetic.[17] Attention must be given to avoiding undesirable tachycardia. Etomidate is another option for induction of anesthesia for unstable patients. Unless one is planning a propofol-based anesthetic, a primary virtue of propofol as an induction agent (rapid emergence) is inconsequential in a lengthy CABG operation. Recent trends in cardiac anesthesia include attempting to promote early extubation for patients with uncomplicated courses. Early extubation can be facilitated by avoiding high-dose narcotic techniques, but this requires supplementation of the narcotic anesthetic. Propofol is often chosen, in part because intraoperative use of propofol can be continued into the postoperative period, and allow for early titrated sedation. Benzodiazepines (e.g., 0.2 to 0.3 mg/kg midazolam or 0.5 mg/kg diazepam) can be used for induction of anesthesia. Both provide stable induction hemodynamics but fail to block the hyperdynamic response to intubation.[53,54] However, administration of fentanyl after a benzodiazepine induction may cause significant hypotension, primarily because of vasodilation.[55] The hypotension is associated with decreased plasma catecholamine levels.

Analgesic Alternatives in Cardiac Surgery

The use of high-dose narcotic techniques for cardiac surgery arose from a desire to maintain hemodynamic stability in patients with marginal cardiac reserve and to provide a smooth transition to the prolonged mechanical ventilation that was routine. Later, it became apparent that these techniques also blunted the stress response to surgery, at least during the prebypass period. Despite high-dose opioid anesthesia, significant increases in levels of stress response hormones (cortisol, epinephrine, norepinephrine) occur that persist into the immediate postoperative period.

Cardiac sympathetic nerve activation initiates coronary artery vasoconstriction in patients with coronary artery disease (CAD), disrupting the normal matching of coronary blood flow and myocardial oxygen demand. Increased myocardial work secondary to hypertension, tachycardia, and peripheral vasoconstriction may contribute to myocardial ischemia, tissue hypoxia, and acidosis. Regional anesthesia has been shown to attenuate these responses to bypass, reduce the incidence of postoperative ischemia, reduce postoperative analgesic requirements, and potentially shorten the period of postoperative ventilator support and ICU stay.[56]

Intrathecal and epidural techniques utilizing either opioids or local anesthetics have been evaluated extensively in cardiac surgical patients. They diminish the response to noxious stimuli, reduce inhalation anesthetic requirements and, when administered prior to CPB, significantly reduce postoperative intravenous opioid requirements. However, neuraxial opioids do not consistently alter the stress response to CPB and may actually impede early postoperative extubation due to delayed respiratory depression.[57]

Cardiac sympathetic blockade, achieved with local anesthetics placed in the intrathecal or epidural space, may reduce the incidence of perioperative ischemia and perhaps improve overall outcome. Intrathecal local anesthetics have been used successfully in cardiac surgery and may facilitate early extubation. The anesthetic level necessary to produce sympathetic blockade is associated with significant hemodynamic changes that must be anticipated and treated.[58] Thoracic cardiac sympathetic blockade is associated with a reduction in the serum levels of epinephrine and norepinephrine, and reduced coronary vascular resistance. These effects suggest an improvement in the balance of myocardial oxygen demand and supply.

The benefits of regional anesthesia in cardiac surgery are appealing, but the technique is not altogether without risk. The incidence of undesirable side effects from opioids is similar whether they are given intravenously or neuraxially and include nausea and vomiting, pruritus, urinary retention, and respiratory depression. Early respiratory depression occurs within minutes of opioid injection and is associated with administration of intrathecal or epidural fentanyl or sufentanil. Delayed respiratory depression occurs hours after neuraxial morphine injections as a result of cephalad migration of opioid in cerebrospinal fluid (CSF) and subsequent stimulation of receptors in the ventral medulla. Factors that increase the risk of respiratory depression include large and/or repeated doses of opioids, intrathecal utilization, advanced age, and concomitant use of intravenous sedatives. Consequently, intubation time may be prolonged when neuraxial opioids are given.

In contrast, intrathecal and epidural local anesthetics do not initiate respiratory depression. Instead, the adverse side effects of peridural local anesthetics include hypotension, bradycardia, and potential myocardial depression. Disturbances in myocardial oxygenation may occur in patients with CAD if coronary perfusion pressure significantly decreases following epidural anesthesia.

The dilemma of peridural anesthesia in a soon-to-be anticoagulated patient is yet to be completely resolved. No neurologic complications have been reported in current clinical trials of thoracic epidural anesthesia in cardiac surgical patients as long as certain precautions are taken. These measures include laboratory evidence of normal coagulation parameters and platelet count, catheter insertion the evening before surgery (at least a 60-minute interval between instrumentation and anticoagulation), a surgical delay of 24 hours in the event of traumatic tap, and rigid control of heparin effect and reversal.[59] The risk-to-benefit ratio continues to be examined.

Conduct of the Operation

Important precepts in anesthetizing patients for CABG include preparation and anticipation. Preparation includes knowledge of the patient's cardiovascular status, proposed surgical procedure, and availability of cardioactive support drugs and mechanical devices. Anticipation means knowing the planned course of surgery (we know it does not always go as planned, but there is supposed to be a plan) and the expected anesthetic needs and hemodynamic alteration expected during each phase of the operation.

Prebypass Period

After the patient is placed on the OR table, catheter placement proceeds with the use of local anesthesia and intravenous sedation as needed. Central vascular access, as described previously, can be obtained either before or after induction.

Induction drugs have also been described above. To re-emphasize, for most patients undergoing CABG, myocardial depressants are just fine.

Following anesthetic induction, the initial major stimulus is placement of the tracheal tube. The patient should be sufficiently anesthetized to block deleterious cardiovascular responses. If such a response does occur, it is helpful to keep in mind that it is usually short lived; blood pressure and heart rate return toward normal in 4 to 5 minutes.

Provision of an unobstructed airway is paramount. Patients with difficult airway, full stomachs, hiatal hernia, and the like, present the dilemma of obtaining an airway while at the same time maintaining hemodynamic stability and preventing myocardial ischemia. It is not always possible to do all at once; priorities must be established. However, rapid-sequence inductions, fiberoptic intubations, and awake laryngoscopy can all be performed in CABG patients with concomitant pharmacologic control of hemodynamics.

Initiation of positive-pressure ventilation can be deleterious to a precarious cardiovascular system. Decreased preload can cause hypotension and may require volume infusion. The hemodynamic "sag" that is frequently seen following laryngoscopy can be treated by decreasing the concentration of volatile anesthetic, if any are being used, infusion of volume (which may increase end-systolic volume, with a concomitant decrease in oxygen supply and an increase in myocardial work), or administration of a phenylephrine bolus (which may increase the PAOP and decrease the cardiac output).

The patient must be adequately anesthetized for subsequent stimuli, which occur after chest prepping and draping are completed. Skin incision, sternal split, sternal retraction, reflection of the pericardium, and aortic manipulation are periods of increased surgical stimulation. One study related 99% of intraoperative ischemia to six events: induction, intubation, skin incision, sternal splitting, cannulation, or initiation of cardiopulmonary bypass.[5] Most intraoperative ischemic events occur without hemodynamic changes, but tachycardia, hypotension, and hypertension predispose to ischemia. It is best to anticipate responses to noxious stimuli with additional anesthesia (intravenous or inhalational), vasodilators, or drugs to prevent tachycardia. It is important to remember that sternal splitting and pericardial retraction may also lead to a vagal response and reduced heart rate.

It is common practice to disconnect the patient from the ventilator, allowing the lungs to collapse during median sternotomy. Patients undergoing reoperations, or other patients with scarred pericardiums, are at increased risk for mishaps at this stage of the operation. (Heparin must be available in case the heart is injured and CPB must be instituted immediately using the femoral vessels as cannulation sites.) Sternal retraction follows, and can compromise hemodynamic monitoring by dampening radial artery tracings. It is then necessary to harvest the conduits; saphenous vein and/or internal mammary artery grafts are the most common, although there is interest in complete arterial revascularization using radial arteries as free grafts. Dissection of the internal mammary artery is facilitated by decreasing the tidal volume.

Observation of the chest often provides useful information. It is helpful to visually assess the contractility of the right ventricle. Important information about cardiac rhythm and pulmonary function may also be obtained by visual inspection.

Heparin (300 to 400 U/kg) is often given during placement of aortic pursestring sutures, with determination of the activated clotting time (ACT) 3 to 5 minutes later. The acceptable ACT for initiation of CPB is a matter of local custom, although 480 seconds is oft quoted.[60] If aprotinin is being administered, an ACT of 700 to 800 seconds is appropriate. Arterial cannulation poses several opportunities for mishap, including the potential for blood loss and aortic dissection. If the clamp partially occludes the aorta, a dampened arterial waveform may be noticed. Should this occur, notify the surgeon. Inspect the arterial inflow cannula for bubbles.

Venous cannulation is usually done after aortic cannulation. This order is particularly important in patients with aortic stenosis, hypertrophic cardiomyopathy, or left main CAD. Atrial manipulation can cause hypotension secondary to obstruction to venous return or induce atrial fibrillation. Infusion of fluid from the pump into the aorta, vasoconstriction with phenylephrine, cardioversion, or prompt initiation of CPB are potential sources of relief.

Cardiopulmonary Bypass

Prior to and upon initiation of cardiopulmonary bypass, certain checklists should be reviewed. We use the mnemonic LAMPS to ensure that this review is complete. LAMPS stands for *l*abs, *a*nesthetics/anesthesia machine, *m*onitors, *p*atient/pump, and *s*upport. Laboratory results to be evaluated include the ACT and the hematocrit. Additional anesthetics and muscle relaxants may be needed. Monitors—any additional monitors utilized during CPB (e.g., myocardial temperature, cardioplegia infusion pressure)—should be prepared. The CVP should be working properly and be followed during commencement of bypass to ensure adequate superior vena cava (SVC) drainage. The PA catheter can be withdrawn a few centimeters to prevent advancement caused by surgical manipulation or stiffening of the catheter during hypothermia. The patient's pupils may be evaluated, and the pump cannulae should be inspected for the absence of bubbles in the arterial cannula and of an air lock in the venous cannula. Support indicates the anesthesiologist must be prepared to intervene pharmacologically to manage the patient's cardiovascular system.

Initiation of CPB occurs after release of the venous clamp, with subsequent initiation of arterial flow. The first hemodynamic change is usually a decrease in central venous and pulmonary artery occlusive pressures, reflecting diversion of venous return to the pump. Transition to nonpulsatile flow and dilutional decrease of blood viscosity often leads to decreased mean arterial pressure, which may necessitate higher pump flows or administration of phenylephrine. Once full bypass is achieved, ventilation is discontinued, fluid infusions are stopped except for infusion of drugs, and alarms are adjusted appropriately. The blood flowing through the arterial cannula should be bright red. The CVP should be near zero if venous blood is flowing freely into the venous cannula. The patient should be evaluated for unilateral blanching of the head, which may indicate cannulation of the brachiocephalic artery. Plethora of the head suggests obstruction of the SVC. Distention of the left ventricle may be caused by poor venous drainage, hypervolemia, increased right-to-left shunting, or aortic valvular insufficiency. It can be diagnosed by visible distention of the heart or by noting increases in pulmonary artery pressure. It can be treated by improving venous drainage, placement of a left ventricular vent, or in cases of severe insufficiency, aortic cross-clamping. The same differential diagnosis should be entertained if an elevated PAOP is observed.

Laboratory results to monitor during cardiopulmonary bypass include activated clotting time (ACT), hematocrit, potassium (potassium is contained in the cardioplegic solution), and arterial blood gases. Mixed venous oxygen saturation in the venous return is monitored by many, and pump flows are adjusted accordingly. Because pump primes contain heparin, the ACT is initially prolonged. However, during bypass it may decrease, especially during rewarming, and it is sometimes necessary to give more heparin, particularly if there is a prolonged period of normothermic CPB. Acceptable hematocrits on cardiopulmonary bypass are controversial, but many view a hematocrit in the low to middle 20s as acceptable. Mixed venous oxygen saturation may decrease when warming. If so, it may indicate inadequate tissue perfusion and can be treated by increasing pump flow. It may be necessary to administer vasodilators (e.g., nitroprusside) concomitantly to prevent excessive increases in arterial pressure.

Myocardial protection is usually effected using a cold solution (blood or crystalloid based) to provide local hypothermia, and contains potassium (~30 mEq/L) to cause diastolic arrest. Additional drugs, such as nitroglycerin, mannitol, magnesium, etc., in various combinations are included depending on local custom. There are also some who prefer continuous warm cardioplegia, and cold fibrillatory arrest is used as well.

Cardioplegia can be administered either anterograde (through the aorta into the native coronary arteries) or retrograde (via the coronary sinus). Anterograde administration is performed by infusing cardioplegia into the root of the aorta proximal to an aortic cross-clamp. Retrograde cardioplegia is given via a catheter in the coronary sinus. Measuring the pressure in the cardioplegia line is often helpful in diagnosing misadventures. If elevated, the probe may be misplaced (e.g., in a dissection of the aorta, or at the os of the coronary sinus), or there may be inadequate flow through a tight stenosis to allow runoff of the solution. A very low injection pressure may indicate aortic insufficiency. (Rapid arrest often follows the sequence of progressive hyperkalemia.) The ECG shows, sequentially, ST-segment elevation, widening of the QRS complex, then electrical quiescence. In some cases, ventricular fibrillation occurs prior to complete arrest, often due to maldistribution of cardioplegia solution. Some cardiac surgery teams pack the heart in ice slush to afford topical hypothermia, a practice that may increase the incidence of phrenic nerve paralysis. Failure to arrest the heart can be caused by aortic incompetence, severe coronary artery stenosis, localized aortic dissection, technical errors, or use of the incorrect cardioplegia solution. Nitroglycerin in the cardioplegia solution can cause arterial hypotension. Some teams evaluate myocardial protection by measuring the temperature of the myocardium during cardioplegia. Consideration should be given to performing bypass first to areas that do not cool rapidly, as such areas receive the least protection.

It is not clear what the ideal arterial pressure is for a patient during CPB. Low pressures contribute to a clear operative field, and may facilitate surgery. Additionally, if lower pressure is achieved by decreasing pump output, then components of the blood are less exposed to the denaturing and damaging effects of the oxygenator and pump. It is, however, necessary to maintain sufficient perfusion pressure for organ perfusion. Focal neurologic events occur in about 5 to 8% of patients, while impaired neuropsychiatric performance is much more common. Most, but not all, of these changes are reversible. It is not clear if this is related to decreased perfusion while on cardiopulmonary bypass, or to other factors such as microembolization or the effects of nonpulsatile flow. Hartman et al., in a preliminary study, have shown that high pressure (>70 mm Hg) is associated with better neurologic outcome in patients with atheromatous aortas.[30] Further confirmation of this work is necessary.

Hypotension on CPB should prompt consideration of inadequate venous return, pump difficulties, and peripheral vasodilation. Decreased venous return can be caused by obstruction, hypovolemia, or inadequate pump volume. Pump failure includes pump head occlusion and obstruction in the aortic line. Vasodilation can be caused by pharmacologic agents, temperature changes, or hemodilution.

Hypertension during CPB occurs most commonly while rewarming. Rewarming is a period of peak occurrence of patient awareness, so one should search for other signs of light anesthesia, such as facial diaphoresis. Opioids, amnestic agents, and muscle relaxants are often redosed while rewarming. Other possible etiologies of hypertension include monitor error, excessive flows, and excessive vasoconstriction. Additional anesthetics can be administered as necessary. Hypertension may persist despite such treatment, and consideration should be given to vasodilators such as nitroprusside, nitroglycerin, or sublingual nifedipine. Additionally, vasodilators may promote blood flow to less well-perfused tissues and result in an increased body temperature at the end of rewarming. Sublingual nifedipine has the advantage of potential prophylaxis against coronary artery vasospasm, but is not titratable. Mixed venous saturation is followed to assess adequacy of peripheral perfusion. Decreased mixed venous saturation may indicate the need for increased pump flows. Vasodilators, including volatile anesthetics, can facilitate increased flows.

Urine output is monitored during bypass, though data relating urine output to postoperative renal dysfunction are lacking. Furosemide or low-dose dopamine (1 to 3 mg/kg/min) are administered to patients with preexisting renal dysfunction in order to preserve renal function. Administration of furosemide while on pump may have little effect until rewarming, when a profound diuresis may result. Mannitol contained in pump primes often causes an osmotic diuresis.

Following removal of the aortic cross-clamp, the heart is perfused with warm blood and the cardioplegic solution is washed out. A variety of rhythms from sinus to ventricular fibrillation may result. Defibrillation, if necessary, is performed with paddles applied directly to the heart. Alternative measures to facilitate defibrillation include increasing perfusion pressure (either by increasing flows or with phenylephrine) or administration of a β-blocker. Hyperkalemia, which may ensue from oliguria or recent administration of cardioplegia, can be treated with 10 units regular insulin and 50 gm glucose.

Separation from Bypass

Separation from bypass involves going from a circulation in series (RA → Pump → Ao) to a transitional one (one in parallel RA → Pump → Ao and RA → LA → LV → Ao) and finally to one in series (RA → LA → LV → Ao). The critical part of the process, the length of time spent with two parallel circulations, is usually related to the extent of myocardial dysfunction. Patients with very poor ejection fractions benefit from a slow wean when pacing and vasoactive drugs can be titrated as the heart gradually takes over pumping the entire output. Patients with excellent LV and right ventricular (RV) function can often be separated from bypass rather expeditiously.

A checklist, similar to the one used when commencing bypass and again using the mnemonic LAMPS, is helpful. Labs include arterial blood gases, hematocrit (low 20s), sodium, potassium (usually <5.5, although if rhythm and conduction are normal, a higher level can be tolerated; conversely, patients experiencing difficulty separating seem to do better when the potassium is normal). Some anesthesiologists measure ionized calcium and glucose. The anesthesia machine and associated equipment should be turned on. Depth of anesthesia should be adequate and vaporizers off if concerned about LV function. The lungs should initially be manually inflated to evaluate pulmonary compliance followed by institution of mechanical ventilation. Transducers and monitors should be zeroed and the presence of undamped tracings confirmed. All ECG leads should be reviewed for evidence of conduction abnormalities or ST-segment abnormalities. Temperature should be normal. If a TEE is used, preliminary evaluation of wall motion is possible, although a more complete exam must await ventricular filling. Patient/pump includes a survey of the operative field to assess rhythm, vigor of contraction, bilateral lung excursion, and the presence of "potentially troublesome" bleeding—especially of the variety best corrected while still on bypass. Knowledge of the current pump flow rate and blood pressure will help determine the need for peripheral vasoconstriction (e.g., if a flow of 5.5 L/min only generates a mean blood pressure of 50 mm Hg, it is likely that phenylephrine or calcium will be needed). Support includes electrical (pacing, cardioversion if necessary), pharmacologic (vasoconstrictors, inotropes), and mechanical (IABP or ventricular assist device).

The sequence for separating from bypass is depicted in Figure 14–1 emphasizing a rapid and slow wean based on blood pressure. Figure 14–2 defines various

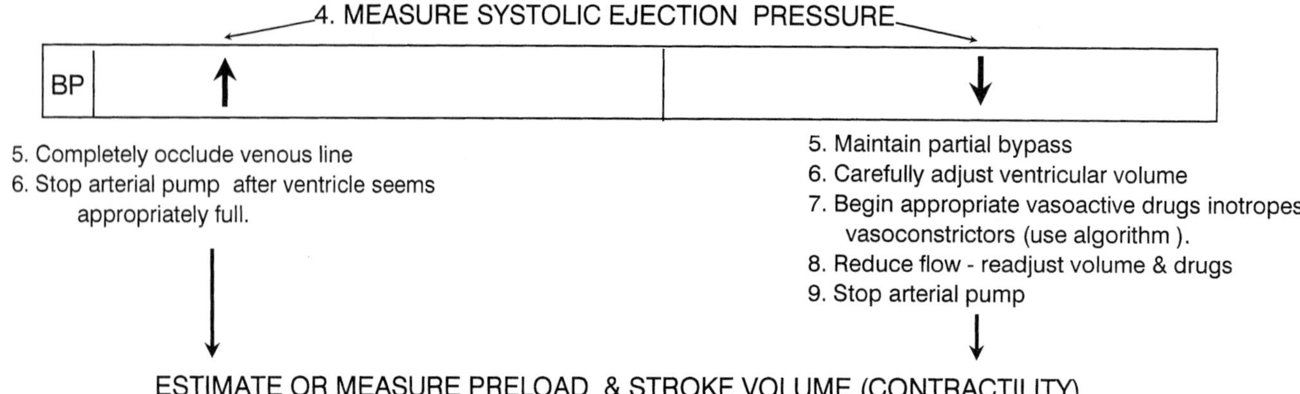

FIGURE **14–1.** General approach to the termination of CPB. (Modified from Amado WJ, Thomas SJ: Cardiac Surgery: Intraoperative management. In Thomas SJ [ed]: Manual of Cardiac Anesthesia, 2nd ed. New York, Churchill Livingstone, 1993, with permission.)

hemodynamic scenarios using blood pressure, ventricular filling pressure (estimated or measured), and stroke volume. A more extensive discussion of pharmacologic manipulations is beyond the scope of this chapter but can be found in Chapter 18 or specific textbooks.[61–63]

Postbypass Period

Once the patient is stable and the technical quality of the grafts thought satisfactory, protamine is administered to bind heparin and restore normal coagulation. When starting the protamine, the perfusionists must be informed so that the cardiotomy suction is turned off to prevent clotting of the pump contents. Some of the adverse effects of protamine appear to be related to the rate and site of administration, so it is advised to give protamine slowly (e.g., over 10 minutes) via a peripheral vein. When given in this fashion, usually no significant hemodynamic changes occur. If adverse effects are noted, the protamine infusion should be slowed or discontinued until the difficulties are rectified. Protamine can cause hypotension from a decrease in the SVR that can be treated with fluid administration, α-adrenergic agonists, and calcium chloride. Myocardial depression and left ventricular failure can also follow protamine administration, requiring inotropic support. In rare instances pulmonary vasoconstriction occurs, manifested by elevation of pulmonary artery, right atrial, and peak airway pressures. Inotropes and calcium chloride usually reverse the problem. In the rare instance, reinstitution of cardiopulmonary bypass may be necessary following rehepar-

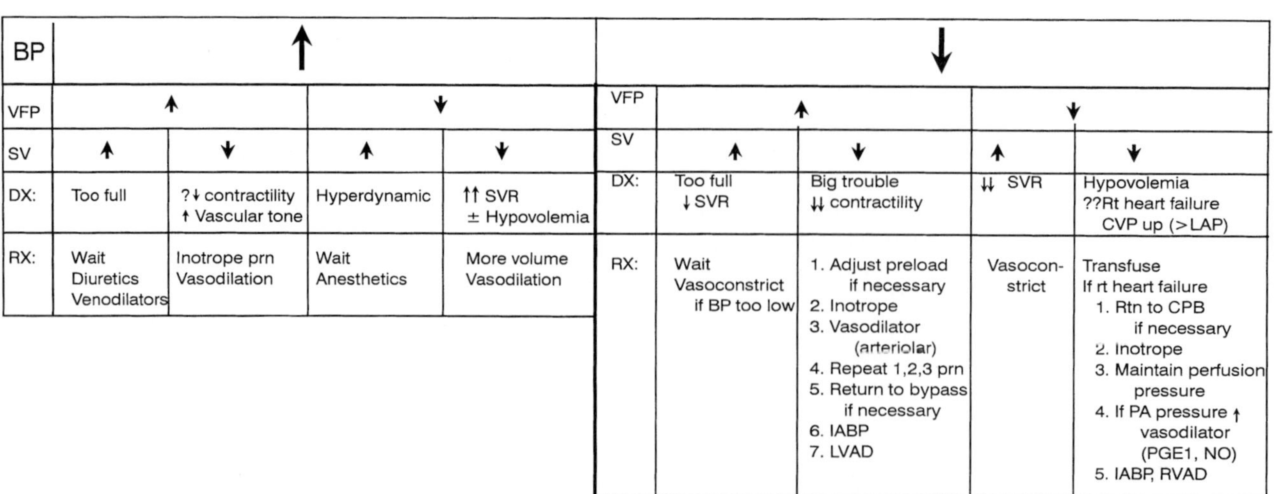

FIGURE **14–2.** Algorithm for the diagnosis and treatment of hemodynamic abnormalities at the termination of CPB. BP, systemic blood pressure; VFP, ventricular fillking pressure; SV, stroke volume; Dx, diagnosis; Rx, treatment; SVR, systemic vascular resistance; CVP, central venous pressure; LAP, left atrial pressure, IABP, intra-aortic balloon pump; LVAD, left ventricular assist device; RVAD, right ventricular assist device. (Modified from Amado WJ, Thomas SJ: Cardiac surgery: Intraoperative management. In Thomas SJ [ed]: Manual of Cardiac Anesthesia. 2nd ed. New York, Churchill Livingstone, 1993, with permission.)

inization. In such cases, protamine has been administered successfully following re-emergence from bypass.

Patients who receive protamine-containing insulin (e.g., NPH) are at increased risk of adverse reactions to protamine. Vasectomized men may also be at increased risk, as they have an increased incidence of protamine-specific antibodies. Anaphylaxis has followed administration of protamine to a vasectomized patient.[64]

Hypokalemia and hypomagnesemia are common following CPB, and may require aggressive repletion. Correction of hypomagnesemia can facilitate correction of hypokalemia. Hypomagnesemia following CPB is more common in patients receiving digitalis or diuretics. A recent double-blind study showed that empiric administration of 2 gm magnesium chloride following CPB diminished the frequency of supraventricular arrhythmias (from 37% to 17%) and increased cardiac indices in the ICU (from 2.5 L/min/m^2 to 2.8 L/min/m^2).[65] Prolonged mechanical ventilation was more common in patients who were hypomagnesemic on postoperative day 1, perhaps because of respiratory muscle weakness.

Surgical events after the patient is weaned from bypass often provoke hemodynamic changes. Decannulation of the heart and aorta can cause blood loss and arrhythmias. Frequently, the surgeons lift the heart to assess distal anastomoses. This is usually tolerated for a brief period, but the surgeons must be informed if excessive hypotension or marked arrhythmias ensue. If the duration of surgical manipulation cannot be limited (e.g., to allow repair of a faulty anastomosis), it may be necessary to reinstitute CPB. Chest closure can cause hypotension related to decreased venous return. The hypotension often resolves in 2 to 5 minutes with administration of fluid. Rarely, chest closure is not tolerated because of a tamponade effect of noncompliant lungs. The sternum can then be left open with or without skin closure until myocardial performance has improved.

If autologous blood was removed prior to heparinization, this can be given as a source of platelets and clotting factors that have not been subjected to CPB. Should postbypass bleeding not be controlled by protamine, autologous blood, and surgical suture, platelets, fresh frozen plasma (FFP), and/or cryoprecipitate may be indicated. Despotis has developed a focused approach to coagulation factor administration based on on-site testing which appears more logical than the shotgun method often employed.[66] Moderate levels of positive end-expiratory pressure (PEEP) are sometimes used in the ICU to attempt to tamponade bleeding.

Most patients improve rapidly following CPB, as the effects of ischemia and residual myocardial stunning dissipate, allowing the anesthesiologist to taper doses of vasoactive drugs, if they were required. Anemia and postbypass hypovolemia are best managed by infusion of autologous blood or cell-saver (red blood cells processed from the pump contents). This has the added advantage of increasing the hematocrit from the low levels caused by hemodilution while on CPB. Cell-saver product contains heparin, and one may wish to administer further protamine in conjunction with large volumes of cell-saver.

The presence of postbypass ischemia requires a search for causes, especially potentially reversible technical ones. Kinking or clotting of the grafts can cause persistent hypotension, signs of ischemia, and arrhythmias, as can spasm of internal mammary artery grafts. Vascular spasm can be managed by administration of nitroglycerin or calcium channel blockers, and by maintenance or elevation of perfusion pressure. Review of the entire ECG or use of the TEE will help identify the ischemic area and hence the involved coronary artery or graft.

Hypoxemia may be noted following CPB. The ventilator settings and pulmonary compliance should be assessed. Atelectasis is a frequent finding, as are other ventilation-perfusion ($\dot{V}/\dot{Q}$) abnormalities, including right-to-left shunting. PEEP is often beneficial, as is manual ventilation with a sharp inspiration and maintenance of plateau pressure at end-inspiration to reinflate atelectatic regions. Care must be taken not to disrupt grafts, especially the mammary artery, with excessively vigorous ventilation. Small tidal volumes are often requested by the surgeons if an internal mammary artery graft is used. Pneumo-, hydro-, or hemothorax should be ruled out by direct inspection if persistent hypoxemia is noted. A markedly diminished cardiac output is another cause of hypoxemia.

Patients can abruptly deteriorate immediately following bypass, and continued vigilance is mandatory. The ST-segment analyzer should be reactivated to facilitate monitoring for ischemia. The blood potassium level should be measured, as aggressive potassium repletion may prevent hypokalemia-associated arrhythmias. Efforts should be made to keep the patient warm, or at least diminish the rate of cooling. These include raising the ambient temperature, warming intravenous fluids, and decreasing fresh gas flows. If a pacemaker is being used, the underlying cardiac rhythm should be evaluated periodically both to assess the recovery from CPB and to determine if the pacemaker will be needed postoperatively. If appropriate, attempts should be made to gradually diminish or discontinue inotropic infusions. A need for increased inotropic support warrants an extensive search for new etiologies. The natural course is for gradual improvement.

A plan should be made for the immediate postoperative period. If the patient is stable hemodynamically, warm, and not bleeding, early extubation 2 to 6 hours following surgery is reasonable. Alternatively, patients requiring pharmacologic or mechanical circulatory support, and those continuing to bleed, require a longer period of mechanical ventilation. Appropriate narcotics and sedatives should be given. Volatile anesthetics effectively reduce hypertension. Their short duration of action is often a virtue, but in the postbypass period, one may wish to give a longer acting agent to facilitate ICU management.

Management of Common Postbypass Problems

Hypertension

Provision of adequate levels of anesthesia, oxygenation, and ventilation are the cornerstones of treatment. Large doses of narcotics or benzodiazepines are best avoided if early extubation is planned. Vasodilators such as nitroglycerin, nitroprusside, hydralazine, nicardipine, and nifedipine or β-blockade with labetalol are also options. Speed of onset and offset and titratability are important factors in the final selection. For example, hydralazine can be used, but its slow onset and long duration of action must be considered. Calcium channel blockers, such as sublingual nifedipine, work well, but titration of drug to effect is relatively difficult given the means of administration and the prolonged action of the drug. Calcium channel blockers have the theoretically appealing, but not conclusively beneficial, property of promoting coronary artery vasodilation. Intravenous verapamil or diltiazem may have undesirable effects on cardiac conduction. Intravenous enalaprilat is an ACE inhibitor and, as with other drugs of its class, consideration should be given to the possibility that it may adversely affect renal function or alter electrolyte balance.

Nicardipine is an effective means of controlling hypertension during CABG. It effectively decreases the blood pressure, both by arterial and venous vasodilation, and also decreases PAP and PAOP. It has theoretical anti-ischemic advantages over nitroprusside, but nitroprusside remains a time-tested treatment. Verapamil infusions have negative inotropic and dromotropic effects, and can lead to elevated PAP and prolonged PQ intervals.[67] On the other hand, if used judiciously, verapamil can be used to treat intraoperative hypertension with associated ischemia.[68]

Labetalol, a combined α_1- and β-adrenergic blocker, is a useful antihypertensive agent. It can be administered in 5- to 20-mg boluses, or by infusion.[69] Mean arterial pressure decreased more with nitroprusside than labetalol, because diastolic blood pressure declined with nitroprusside, but not with labetalol. Nitroprusside caused an increase in heart rate and decreases in CVP and PAOP; labetalol caused a decrease in heart rate and increases in CVP and PAOP. Labetalol may promote beneficial changes in the myocardial oxygen supply/demand ratio. If labetalol is used concomitantly with nitroprusside, generally the total dose of nitroprusside is much lower, lessening the likelihood of cyanide toxicity.[70]

Hypotension

Common causes of hypotension include hypovolemia, anesthetic overdose, cardiac manipulation, arrhythmias, ischemia, and myocardial failure. Assuming normal ventricular compliance, hypovolemia can be assessed by central venous or pulmonary artery pressures. Even in the presence of normal or slightly elevated filling pressures, it is often worth a trial fluid challenge to rule out hypovolemia, as ventricular compliance may be decreased as a result of ischemia or CPB. Direct assessment of ventricular filling, either by inspection if the chest is open, or by TEE, is very useful. A TEE can evaluate volume status directly, rather than extrapolating from pressure to volume. If the chest is open, visual inspection can help assess volume status, and also determines if cardiac manipulation is contributing to hypotension. Initial high filling pressures in a patient without clinical signs of heart failure suggests that the patient depends on elevated venous pressures to maintain normal cardiac output. Acute pulmonary hypertension may be associated with protamine administration, prolonged CPB, hypoxemia, hypercarbia, or acidosis.

Vasoconstrictors are the definitive therapy if hypotension is due to decreased SVR, or may be used initially to provide time to correct an underlying hemodynamic problem. Phenylephrine or norepinephrine are often used. Metaraminol is a useful alternative therapy. Inotropes, such as an epinephrine infusion, are indicated for hypotension with elevated PAOP and decreased stroke volume (e.g., myocardial failure). The resultant increased perfusion pressure and decreased ventricular size are beneficial, but inotropes will tend to increase MVO_2, which may worsen ischemia. Alternatively, infusion of nitroglycerin and phenylephrine can be attempted, in the hopes of relieving ischemia (see "Ischemia," below). If need be, reinstitution of CPB can maintain perfusion pressure while correcting volume status, titrating infusions, or placing an IABP.

Transesophageal echocardiography was used to compare the effects of 2 μg/kg phenylephrine with 0.1 μg/kg norepinephrine in American Society of Anesthesiologists (ASA) I or II patients rendered hypotensive with 1.5% end-tidal isoflurane in 70% N2O.[71] The patients, who were not undergoing CABG, showed similar increases in blood pressure and decreases in heart rate, but phenylephrine caused a transient impairment of myocardial performance (decreased fractional area change and decreased fiber shortening), whereas norepinephrine bolstered myocardial performance. The combined α- and β-adrenergic properties of norepinephrine may make it a superior choice in this setting.

Ischemia

ST-segment elevations or depressions suggest ischemia but may reflect electrolyte disturbances or hypothermia. Patients with intraoperative ischemia may have an increased incidence of postoperative infarcts. There is no evidence that prophylactic nitroglycerin wards off ischemia in patients given fentanyl anesthetics.[72,73] If electrocardiographic signs of ischemia are associated with tachycardia, hypertension, or hypotension, the anesthesiologist should attempt to correct the hemodynamic abnormality. The surgeons should be alerted to progressive severe ischemia, both to search for surgically correctable factors such as a kinked graft or because it may be necessary to rapidly institute CPB.

If ischemia is due to a low output state, it may be necessary to infuse β-agonists or arteriolar dilators, or to use a pacemaker. Nitroglycerin may be used to promote coronary artery dilation and may also decrease preload. If unacceptable hypotension results, a phenylephrine infusion may be instituted.

Seitelberger et al.[74] administered either a nitroglycerin or a nifedipine infusion to patients undergoing elective CABG, in order to examine whether nifedipine diminishes perioperative ischemia. Patients received an etomidate/fentanyl/diazepam/N_2O/pancuronium anesthetic. The nitroglycerin or nifedipine infusion was begun on initiation of CPB. Although hemodynamic parameters were similar for the two groups, nifedipine decreased the incidence of ischemia by three measures: postoperative MI (4% vs. 12%), electrocardiographic transient ischemia (6% vs. 19%), and peak levels of creatine kinase. This difference was attributed to increased myocardial blood flow caused by nifedipine.

A contrasting study[75] demonstrated that intravenous nifedipine was as effective as nitroprusside for the control of hypertension in the recovery room after CABG. The incidence of ischemia, as determined by Holter monitoring, was similar: 5% in the nifedipine group and 4% in the nitroprusside group. Perioperative MIs occurred in 9.5% of the nifedipine group and 10.7% of the nitroprusside group. This study cannot be compared directly with Seitelberger's study, as the infusions were started at different times (initiation of CPB vs. in the recovery room), and for different indications (as anti-ischemic prophylaxis vs. control of hypertension). Intravenous nifedipine is not commercially available in the United States.

Arrhythmias

Sinus tachycardia may be a response to hypovolemia or may indicate the need for further anesthesia (particularly if associated with hypertension or diaphoresis). β-Blockade may be useful once the anesthesiologist is convinced that the patient is adequately anesthetized. Many anesthesiologists emphasize the importance of a slow heart rate before CPB, which allows adequate left ventricular perfusion during diastole and decreases MVO_2. After CPB, the heart is less compliant, and a faster rate may be necessary to maintain the cardiac output. On the other hand, there is evidence that postrevascularization ischemia may be related to tachycardia.[8] This study did not examine whether efforts to reduce tachycardia would be beneficial.

Premature ventricular contractions are usually transient and commonly reflect autonomic imbalance. After considering hypoventilation, cardiac manipulation such as cannulation, inadequate oxygenation, or hypokalemia, the diagnosis of ischemia should be entertained. Therapy for ischemia has been discussed above. Therapy of ventricular irritability includes overdrive pacing or antiarrhythmic drugs.

Postoperative ICU Period

A provocative study by Mangano et al.[10] examined ischemia in patients randomized to either low-dose morphine or intermediate-dose sufentanil infusion (1 μg/kg/hr) in the ICU after CPB. The overall incidence of ischemia and length of ICU stay was the same in both groups, but the area under the ST-time curve was substantially less in the sufentanil group. Given the low incidence of adverse cardiac outcomes, the study was too small to determine whether increasing the dose of opioid in the immediate postoperative period is beneficial.

Supraventricular arrhythmias such as atrial fibrillation occur frequently after CABG. Adverse effects include hemodynamic deterioration, increased risk of stroke, and lengthened hospital stay. A meta-analysis of randomized, controlled trials found that prophylactic β-blockade reduced the odds ratio of developing a supraventricular arrhythmia to 0.28.[76] Neither verapamil nor digoxin significantly reduced the incidence of developing a supraventricular tachycardia, but all three classes of drugs reduced ventricular rate during the arrhythmia. Rates of developing a supraventricular arrhythmia were dependent on the means of detection (continuous Holter monitoring, continuous bedside monitoring, or development of symptoms). Pooled incidence rates were 8.7% for patients on prophylactic β-blockade, with a control group incidence of 34%. A 5-day postoperative course of procainamide decreases the number of episodes of atrial fibrillation.[77] Perhaps because of the small size of the study, procainamide did not significantly decrease the number of patients experiencing atrial fibrillation or the average length of stay. This study needs to be repeated on a larger scale before routine postoperative procainamide can be recommended.

Management of Special Cases

Post-PTCA Emergencies

Percutaneous transluminal coronary angioplasty (PTCA) has become the primary therapy for many patients with atherosclerotic CAD.[78,79] Urgent CABG may be necessary if PTCA was unable to achieve revascularization, or if PTCA was followed by threatened closure of the dilated segment, dissection, hemodynamic instability, or impending infarction. Emergent post-PTCA CABG is usually necessitated by coronary dissection or acute closure. The dissection often occurs outside the area intended for dilation. Cardiologists may treat these emergencies with coronary vasodilators, thrombolytic agents, or reperfusion catheters, which provide a stent for blood flow past the occluded segment.[80] If a reperfusion catheter is placed, it should be withdrawn prior to aortic cross-clamping.

Patients undergoing emergent post-PTCA CABG are more likely to require inotropic agents and IABPs, and have increased morbidity and mortality.[79] If ischemia was present on the preoperative ECG, 57% of patients proceed to Q-wave MI.[81] One study found that patients placed on CPB within 25 minutes of onset of symptoms did better than patients with delayed surgery; no deaths or MIs occurred in the ten patients rushed to CPB, while 14% of the patients in the delayed group had MIs, and 5% died. Although this was a small, nonrandomized study, it supports the intuitively appealing idea that prompt surgery is beneficial.

Thrombolytic therapy is common for an evolving myocardial infarction. Aspirin is also usually given. Patients who have received thrombolytic agents may proceed to emergent CABG following failed PTCA of the infarcted vessel, or may proceed directly to CABG if they have lesions not amenable to PTCA (e.g., left main, complex, or distal disease).[80] Intravenous thrombolytic therapy given within 12 hours of CABG results in a marked increase in postoperative bleeding, use of blood products, and hemodynamic instability. The incidence of such complications can be decreased by postponing the operation, if the patient's condition permits. Intracoronary thrombolytic therapy uses lower total doses of thrombolytic agent, and carries less of a risk for coagulopathy if the patient should proceed to CABG.

CABG for unstable postinfarction angina has been both condemned as too dangerous and advocated as lifesaving. Because of the elevated morbidity and mortality of CABG performed after an MI, some authors view this as a salvage therapy appropriate only after interventional medical therapies fail.[80] Others find the 3.3 to 5.7% mortality encouraging.[82,83] Consideration of markers of increased risk may help delineate patients who would benefit from a post-MI CABG. Multivariate logistical analysis implicated age, urgent or emergent surgery, reoperation, congestive heart failure, and Q-wave MI as risk factors for adverse outcome of post-MI CABGs.[83] Another study found only occurrence of anterior transmural infarction and preoperative use of IABPs as significant risk factors, while a third held that increased mortality was associated with left main disease, female sex, and elevated left ventricular wall motion abnormality scores.[82] Patients undergoing post-MI CABG also have increased morbidity, such as need for prolonged inotropic support, IABPs, and therapy for ventricular arrhythmias.[82] One group recommends waiting until 1 week after MI in elective patients, as this may reduce morbidity and mortality. The improved results may just reflect a survivorship bias. If patients with MI have progressed to cardiogenic shock, the operative mortality is 34%.[84]

Reoperations

Reoperations pose numerous additional anesthetic problems. The patients tend to be older and have had further progression of both coronary artery and coexisting diseases. One must be prepared to rapidly infuse crystalloid or colloid, as bleeding is often increased. The surgeons may transect or lacerate old grafts, or may inadvertently enter cardiac chambers during sternotomy or dissection of the scarred pericardial area. These patients are at increased risk of arrhythmias, and the scarring from the previous surgery leads to difficulty with internal defibrillation. Similarly, epicardial scarring can pose technical difficulties with achieving rapid cannulation if it should become desirable to proceed expeditiously to CPB. Poor myocardial protection may predispose to ischemia during bypass, and prolonged aortic cross-clamp and CPB times should be anticipated. Prolonged CPB times are a marker for poor outcomes, and may result in a post-CPB bleeding diathesis. If insufficient saphenous vein is available, other veins will be used. The source of conduit should be discussed with the surgeons preoperatively, both to facilitate positioning and to avoid inappropriate placement of intravenous and arterial catheters.

Full Stomach

The anesthesiologist cannot postpone an emergent cardiac procedure because of recent ingestion of food. Heavy premedications are contraindicated for patients with full stomachs. A traditional rapid-sequence induction performed on an unstable cardiac patient may cause unacceptable alterations in hemodynamics. Unless the intubation is performed with the patient awake, Sellick's maneuver is indicated. A modified rapid-sequence induction can be performed with 20 to 30 μg/kg fentanyl and 250 μg/kg of pancuronium or vecuronium. Rocuronium (0.9 mg/kg) may now be viewed as the nondepolarizing muscle relaxant of choice for rapid intubation.[85] It will rapidly cause precipitation of thiopental if the two drugs come into contact in the intravenous tubing.[86] Alternatively, in a patient with good left ventricular function, one can induce anesthesia with 1.5 mg/kg succinylcholine, 1.5 mg/kg sodium thiopental, and 1.5 μg/kg sufentanil.

Newer Approaches to Coronary Artery Bypass Surgery

Stimulated by the desire for less patient discomfort and shorter (and less costly) hospital stays, a variety of approaches involving less-invasive surgery, both with and without cardiopulmonary bypass, are being developed. These, in combination with "critical pathways"—defined modes of treatment, clinical end points, and cost analysis—are expanding the spectrum of cardiac surgery. Each of the new procedures has anesthetic implications, most of which are similar to those discussed earlier. However, each also brings a new twist or wrinkle. Whether any of these new techniques will survive rigorous analysis in terms of patient satisfaction, outcome, or cost reduction remains to be seen (see Chapter 13).

CABG Without CPB

CABG without bypass can be performed via a variety of incisions. The minimally invasive direct-vision coronary artery bypass (MIDCAB), used most often for a single left anterior descending artery (LAD) lesion, avoids both a sternotomy and CPB. The most common approach is via a short left paramedian incision, which often requires the removal of one or more costochondral junctions for adequate exposure of both the left internal mammary artery and the LAD. Other approaches include both a ministernotomy, where the sternum is not completely divided, and a complete sternotomy, where it is. Indications include isolated single LAD disease, multivessel disease where angioplasty/stenting is done to vessels on the back of the heart, and patients in whom the risks imposed by CPB might be prohibitive. Calcification of the ascending aorta and renal dysfunction predictably increase the morbidity and mortality of CABG when CPB is used.

The major surgical problems are access and operating on the beating heart. To accomplish this, a variety of ingenious instruments have become available that immobilize the area of the heart where the anastomosis will be placed. The internal mammary artery is dissected from the sternum and anastomosed under direct vision to the LAD. Blood flow through the LAD is interrupted in order to create a bloodless field.

Myocardial ischemia is mandatory while the vessel is occluded and the anastomosis constructed. Hemodynamic deterioration may develop, requiring treatment with vasoactive drugs. Bradycardia was important to minimize cardiac movement when this procedure was initially developed and esmolol and diltiazem were frequently required. These are less critical now, with the newly developed instruments for holding the heart steady. Early extubation is expected. This type of incision is quite painful. Thoracic epidural analgesia or intercostal blocks may be required. In fact, one wag has said "the procedure is minimally invasive, but maximally painful!"

Criticisms of this approach include inadequate length of the mammary artery pedicle, poor visualization of the anastomosis, and the possibility of decreased blood flow to the heart, since the proximal branches of the mammary artery remain intact, potentially creating a "steal" by diverting blood flow to the sternum and chest muscles.[87,88]

Video-Assisted CABG with Cardiopulmonary Bypass

Videoscopic techniques derived from arthroscopic and laparoscopic procedures have been developed for CABG procedures. These techniques involve the creation of anastomoses using instruments placed via several small incisions in the chest wall. CPB is established via percutaneously placed femoral arterial and venous catheters. Cardioplegia is given through the central lumen of a balloon-tipped catheter inflated in the ascending aorta.

These procedures, as one might expect, take longer than similar ones using the standard sternotomy. They also require TEE to aid in placement and positioning of this aortic catheter, which also acts as the aortic cross-clamp. Movement of the catheter has the potential for occluding the innominate artery. These procedures are less invasive; they have been criticized due to the expense of the equipment and the long training period involved.[89]

Transmyocardial Laser

Patients who are not candidates for coronary artery bypass (e.g., lack of suitable conduit, or coronary arteries either obliterated or with poor distal runoff) have been offered this method of neovascularization. Following left anterior thoracotomy, a laser creates small channels completely through the myocardium. These channels form an endothelial lining, presumably bringing blood to areas of myocardium that are unable to be revascularized in any other way.[90]

Anesthetic considerations center on anesthetizing a patient, usually with poor ventricular function, who will not be better immediately after surgery. Anti-ischemia and inotropic regimens may be required. TEE is used to document transmyocardial laser (TML) laser action, which is manifest by bubbles from vaporized hemoglobin.[91]

Currently, the technique is not widely used. Additionally, if it proves to be valuable, it will probably be done in the catheterization lab with a laser catheter.

Radial Artery Conduit

The radial artery has been proposed as an alternative to vein for aortocoronary bypass. It is thought to have a higher long-term patency. This may be simply because it is an artery, already adapted to high-pressure flow, unlike saphenous veins. The radial arterial wall is quite muscular and seems to be prone to spasm both during dissection and after anastomosis to the coronary artery. Infusion of nitroglycerin or diltiazem has been used to prevent spasm. Initial results have demonstrated patency of the radial artery graft that approaches that of the internal mammary artery. Long-term results, however, are available from only a few centers.

References

1. Reiz S, Balfors E, Sorensen MB, et al: Isoflurane—a powerful coronary vasodilator in patients with coronary artery disease. Anesthesiology 59:91, 1983.
2. Urban MK, Gordon MA, Haris SN, et al: Intraoperative hemodynamic changes are not good indicators of myocardial ischemia. Anesth Analg 76:942, 1993.
3. Buffington CW: Hemodynamic determinants of ischemic myocardial dysfunction in the presence of coronary stenosis in dogs. Anesthesiology 63:651, 1985.
4. Harris S, Gordon M, Urban M, et al: The pressure rate quotient is not an indicator of myocardial ischemia in humans: An echocardiographic evaluation. Anesthesiology 87:242, 1993.
5. Slogoff S, Keats A: Does perioperative myocardial ischemia lead to postoperative myocardial infarction? Anesthesiology 62:107, 1985.
6. Hogue CW, Herbst TJ, Pond C, et al: Perioperative myocardial ischemia. Its relation to anatomic pattern of coronary artery stenosis. Anesthesiology 79:514, 1993.
7. Knight A, Hollenberg M, London M, Mangano D: Myocardial ischemia in patients awaiting coronary artery bypass grafting. Am Heart J 117:1189, 1989.
8. Smith R, Leung J, Mangano D: Postoperative myocardial ischemia in patients undergoing coronary artery bypass graft surgery. Anesthesiology 74:464, 1991.
9. Leung J, O'Kelly B, Browner W, et al: Prognostic importance of postbypass regional wall-motion abnormalities in patients undergoing coronary artery bypass graft surgery. Anesthesiology 71:16, 1989.
10. Mangano D, Silicano D, Hollenberg M, et al: Postoperative myocardial ischemia. Therapeutic trials using intensive analgesia following surgery. Anesthesiology 76:342, 1992.
11. Keenan RL, Boyan CP: Cardiac arrest due to anesthesia: A study of incidence and causes. JAMA 253:2372, 1985.

12. Eichhorn JH: Prevention of intraoperative anesthesia accidents and related severe injury through safety monitoring. Anesthesiology 70:572, 1989.
13. Jones EL, Weintraub WS, Craver JM, et al: Coronary bypass surgery: Is the operation different today? J Thorac Cardiovasc Surg 101:108, 1991.
14. Paiement B, Pelletier C, Dyrda I, et al: A simple classification of the risk in cardiac surgery. Can Anaesth Soc J 30:61, 1983.
15. Higgins T, Estafanous F, Loop F, et al: Stratification of morbidity and mortality outcome by preoperative risk factors in coronary artery bypass patients. A clinical severity score. JAMA 267:2344, 1992.
16. Slogoff S, Keats A: Randomized trial of primary anesthetic agents on outcome of coronary artery bypass operations. Anesthesiology 70:179, 1989.
17. Tuman K, McCarthy R, Spiess B, et al: Does choice of anesthetic agent significantly affect outcome after coronary artery surgery? Anesthesiology 70:189, 1989.
18. Horner SM: Efficacy of intravenous magnesium in acute myocardial infarction in reducing arrhythmias and mortality: Meta-analysis of magnesium in acute myocardial infarction. Circulation 86:774, 1992.
19. Yusuf S, Teo K, Woods K: Intravenous magnesium in acute myocardial infarction. An effective, safe, simple, and inexpensive intervention (Editorial). Circulation 87:2043, 1993.
20. Stern D, Gerson J, Allen F, Parker F: Can we trust the direct radial artery pressure immediately following cardiopulmonary bypass? Anesthesiology 62:557, 1985.
21. Rich G, Lubanski R, McLoughlin T: Differences between aortic and radial artery pressure associated with cardiopulmonary bypass. Anesthesiology 77:63, 1992.
22. Kinzer J, Lichtenthal P, Wade L: Loss of radial artery pressure trace during internal mammary artery dissection for coronary artery bypass graft surgery. Anesth Analg 64:1134, 1985.
23. Lieberman R, Orkin F, Jobes D, Schwartz A: Hemodynamic predictors of myocardial ischemia during halothane anesthesia for coronary-artery revascularization. Anesthesiology 59:36, 1983.
24. Tuman K, McCarthy R, Spiess B, et al: Effect of pulmonary artery catheterization on outcome in patients undergoing coronary artery surgery. Anesthesiology 70:199, 1989.
25. Bashein G, Johnson P, Davis K, Ivey T: Elective coronary bypass surgery without pulmonary artery catheter monitoring. Anesthesiology 63:451, 1985.
26. Bazaral M, Petre J, Novoa R: Errors in thermodilution cardiac output measurements caused by rapid pulmonary artery temperature decreases after cardiopulmonary bypass. Anesthesiology 77: 31, 1992.
27. Kotrly K, Kotter G, Mortata D, Kampine J: Intraoperative detection of myocardial ischemia with an ST segment trend monitoring system. Anesth Analg 63:343, 1984.
28. Slogoff S, Keats A, David Y, Igo S: Incidence of perioperative myocardial ischemia detected by different electrocardiographic systems. Anesthesiology 73:1074, 1990.
29. Eisenberg MJ, London MJ, Leung JM, et al: Monitoring for myocardial ischemia during noncardiac surgery: A technology assessment of transesophageal echocardiography and 12-lead electrocardiography. JAMA 268:210, 1992.
30. Hartman GS, Yao FS, Bruefach M III, et al: Severity of aortic atheromatous disease diagnosed by transesophageal echocardiography predicts stroke and other outcomes associated with coronary artery surgery: A prospective study. Anesth Analg 83:701, 1996.
31. Arom KV, Chen DE, Strobl FT: Effect of intraoperative intervention on neurological outcome based on electroencephalographic monitoring during cardiopulmonary bypass. Ann Thorac Surg 48: 476, 1989.
32. Bashein G, Nessly M, Bledsoe S, et al: Electroencephalography during surgery with cardiopulmonary bypass and hypothermia. Anesthesiology 76:878, 1992.
33. Mangano D: Anesthetics, coronary artery disease, and outcome; unresolved controversies. Anesthesiology 70:175, 1989.
34. Mora CT, Dudek C, Torjman MC, White PF: The effects of anesthetic technique on the hemodynamic response and recovery profile in coronary revascularization patients. Anesth Analg 81: 900, 1995.
35. Thomson I, Bergstrom R, Rosenbloom M, Meatherall R: Premedication and high-dose fentanyl anesthesia for myocardial revascularization: A comparison of lorazepam versus morphine-scopolamine. Anesthesiology 68:194, 1988.
36. O'Connor J, Ramsay J, Wynands J, et al: The incidence of myocardial ischemia during anesthesia for coronary artery bypass surgery in patients receiving pancuronium or vecuronium. Anesthesiology 70:230, 1989.
37. Thomson IR, MacAdams CL, Hudson RJ, Rosenbloom M: Drug interactions with sufentanil. Hemodynamic effects of premedication and muscle relaxants. Anesthesiology 76:922, 1992.
38. Streisand J, Bailey P, LeMaire L, et al: Fentanyl-induced rigidity and unconsciousness in human volunteers. Incidence, duration, and plasma concentrations. Anesthesiology 78:629, 1993.
39. Murphy M, Hug C: The anesthetic potency of fentanyl in terms of its reduction of enflurane MAC. Anesthesiology 57:485, 1982.
40. Hall R, Murphy M, Hug C: The enflurane sparing effect of sufentanil in dogs. Anesthesiology 67:518, 1987.
41. Hilgenberg J: Intraoperative awareness during high-dose fentanyl-oxygen anesthesia. Anesthesiology 54:341, 1981.
42. Mummaneni N, Rao T, Montoya A: Awareness and recall with high-dose fentanyl oxygen anesthesia. Anesth Analg 59:948, 1980.
43. Philbin D, Rosow C, Schneider R, et al: Fentanyl and sufentanil anesthesia revisited: how much is enough? Anesthesiology 73:5, 1990.
44. Ramsay J, DeJesus J, Wynands J, et al: Pure opiate vs. opiate volatile anesthesia for coronary bypass surgery. Anesth Analg 68: S233, 1989.
45. Wynands J, Wong P, Townsend G, et al: Narcotic requirements for intravenous anesthesia. Anesth Analg 63:101, 1984.
46. Mora C, Dudek C, Epstein R, et al: Cardiac anesthesia techniques: Fentanyl alone or in combination with enflurane or propofol. Anesth Analg 68:S202, 1989.
47. Becker L: Is isoflurane dangerous for the patient with coronary artery disease? Anesthesiology 66:259, 1987.
48. Pulley D, Kirvassilis G, Kelermenos N, et al: Regional and global myocardial circulatory and metabolic effects of isoflurane and halothane in patients with steal-prone coronary anatomy. Anesthesiology 75:756, 1991.
49. Slogoff S, Keats A, Dear W, et al: Steal-prone coronary anatomy and myocardial ischemia associated with four primary anesthetic agents in humans. Anesth Analg 72:22, 1991.
50. Leung J, Hollenberg M, O'Kelly B, et al: Effects of steal-prone anatomy on intraoperative myocardial ischemia. J Am Coll Cardiol 20:1205, 1992.
51. Helman JD, Leung JM, Bellows WH, et al: The risk of myocardial ischemia in patients receiving desflurane versus sufentanil anesthesia for coronary artery bypass graft surgery. Anesthesiology 77:47, 1992.
52. Thomson I, Bowering J, Hudson R, et al: A comparison of desflurane and isoflurane in patients undergoing coronary artery surgery. Anesthesiology 75:776, 1991.
53. Samuelson P, Reves J, Kouchoukos N, et al: Hemodynamic responses to anesthetic induction with midazolam or diazepam in patients with ischemic heart disease. Anesth Analg 60:802, 1981.
54. Kawar P, Carson I, Clarke R, et al: Haemodynamic changes during induction of anaesthesia with midazolam and diazepam (Valium) in patients undergoing coronary artery bypass surgery. Anaesthesia 40:767, 1985.
55. Tomicheck R, Rosow C, Philbin D, et al: Diazepam-fentanyl interaction—hemodynamic and hormonal effects in coronary artery surgery. Anesth Analg 62:881, 1983.
56. Stenseth R, Bjella L, Berg EM, et al: Thoracic epidural analgesia in aortocoronary bypass surgery. Acta Anaesth Scand 38:826, 1994.
57. Chaney MA: Intrathecal and epidural anesthesia and analgesia for cardiac surgery. Anesth Analg 84:1211, 1997.
58. Blomberg S, Emanuelsson H, Kvist H, et al: Effects of thoracic epidural anesthesia on coronary arteries and arterioles in patients with coronary artery disease. Anesthesiology 73:840, 1990.
59. Sanchez R, Nygard E: Epidural anesthesia in cardiac surgery: Is there an increased risk? J Cardiothorac Vasc Anesth 12:170, 1998.
60. Bull BS, Korpman RA, Huse WM, Briggs BD: Heparin therapy

during extracorporeal circulation. I. Problems inherent in existing heparin protocols. J Thorac Cardiovasc Surg 69:674, 1975.
61. Hemmings HC Jr, Thomas SJ: Termination of cardiopulmonary bypass. In Gravlee GP, Davis RF, Utley JR (eds): Cardiopulmonary Bypass: Principles and Practice. Baltimore, Williams & Wilkins, 1993.
62. Jackson JM, Thomas SJ: Valvular heart disease. In Kaplan JA (ed): Cardiac Anesthesia, 3rd ed. Philadelphia, WB Saunders Co, 1993.
63. Thomas SJ (ed): Manual of Cardiac Anesthesia. New York, Churchill Livingstone, 1984.
64. Adourian U, Shampaine EL, Hirshman CA, et al: High-titer protamine-specific IgG antibody associated with anaphylaxis: Report of a case and quantitative analysis of antibody in vasectomized men [see comments]. Anesthesiology 78:368, 1993.
65. England M, Gordon G, Salem M, Chernow B: Magnesium administration and dysrhythmias after cardiac surgery. A placebo-controlled, double-blind, randomized trial. JAMA 268:2395, 1992.
66. Despotis GJ, Santoro SA, Spitznagel E, et al: Prospective evaluation and clinical utility of on-site monitoring of coagulation in patients undergoing cardiac operation. J Thorac Cardiovasc Surg 107:271, 1994.
67. Wezel H van, Bovill J, Schuller J, et al: Comparison of nitroglycerine, verapamil and nifedipine in the management of arterial pressure during coronary artery surgery. Br J Anaesth 58:267, 1986.
68. Humphrey LS, Blanck TJJ: Intraoperative use of verapamil for nitroglycerin-refractory myocardial ischemia. Anesth Analg 64: 68, 1985.
69. Cruise C, Skrobik Y, Webster R, et al: Intravenous labetalol versus sodium nitroprusside for treatment of hypertension postcoronary bypass surgery. Anesthesiology 71:835, 1989.
70. Friederich JA, Butterworth JF IV: Sodium nitroprusside: Twenty years and counting. Anesth Analg 81:152, 1995.
71. Goertz A, Schnidt M, Seefelder C, et al: The effect of phenylephrine bolus administration on left ventricular function during isoflurane-induced hypotension. Anesth Analg 77:227, 1993.
72. Gallagher JD, Moore RA, Jose AB, et al: Prophylactic nitroglycerin infusions during coronary artery bypass surgery. Anesthesiology 64:785, 1986.
73. Thomson IR, Mutch WA, Culligan JD: Failure of intravenous nitroglycerin to prevent intraoperative myocardial ischemia during fentanyl-pancuronium anesthesia. Anesthesiology 61:385, 1984.
74. Seitelberger R, Zwolfer W, Huber S, et al: Nifedipine reduces the incidence of myocardial infarction and transient ischemia in patients undergoing coronary bypass grafting. Circulation 83:460, 1991.
75. Nathan H, Laganiere S, Dube L, et al: Intravenous nifedipine to treat hypertension after coronary artery revascularization surgery. A comparison with sodium nitroprusside. Anesth Analg 74:809, 1992.
76. Andrews T, Reimold S, Berlin J, Antman E: Prevention of supraventricular arrhythmias after coronary artery bypass surgery. A meta-analysis of randomized control trials. Circulation 84:III-236, 1991.
77. Laub G, Janeira L, Muralidharan S, et al: Prophylactic procainamide for prevention of atrial fibrillation after coronary artery bypass grafting: A prospective, double-blind, randomized, placebo-controlled pilot study. Crit Care Med 21:1474, 1991.
78. King S, Talley JD: Coronary arteriography and percutaneous transluminal coronary angioplasty. Changing patterns of use and results. Circulation 79:I-19, 1989.
79. Talley JD, Jones E, Weintraub W, King S: Coronary artery bypass surgery after failed elective percutaneous transluminal coronary angioplasty: A status report. Circulation 79:I-126, 1989.
80. Barner H, Lea J, Naunheim K, Stoney W: Emergency coronary bypass not associated with preoperative cardiogenic shock in failed angioplasty, after thrombolysis, and for acute myocardial infarction. Circulation 79:I-152, 1989.
81. Golding LAR, Loop FD, Hollman JL, et al: Early results of emergency surgery after coronary angioplasty. Circulation 74:III-26, 1986.
82. Kouchoukos N, Murphy S, Philpott T, et al: Coronary artery bypass grafting for postinfarction agina pectoris. Circulation 79:I-68, 1989.
83. Kennedy J, Ivey T, Misbach G, et al: Coronary artery bypass graft surgery early after acute myocardial infarction. Circulation 70:I-73, 1989.
84. Bolooki H: Emergency cardiac procedures in patients in cardiogenic shock due to complications of coronary artery disease. Circulation 79:I-137, 1989.
85. Magorian T, Flannery KB, Miller RD: Comparison of rocuronium, succinylcholine, and vecuronium for rapid-sequence induction of anesthesia in adult patients. Anesthesiology 79:913, 1993.
86. Chambi D, Omoigui S: Precipitation of thiopental by some muscle relaxants. Anesth Analg 81:1112, 1995.
87. Ancalmo N, Busby JR: Minimally invasive coronary artery bypass surgery: Really minimal? (Editorial). Ann Thorac Surg 64: 928, 1997.
88. Hensley FA Jr: Minimally invasive myocardial revascularization surgery: Here to stay? (Editorial; comment). J Cardiothorac Vasc Anesth 10:445, 1996.
89. Schwartz DS, Ribakove GH, Grossi EA, et al: Single and multivessel port-access coronary artery bypass grafting with cardioplegic arrest: Technique and reproducibility. J Thorac Cardiovasc Surg 114:46, 1997.
90. Horvath KA, Mannting F, Cummings N, et al: Transmyocardial laser revascularization: Operative techniques and clinical results at two years. J Thorac Cardiovasc Surg 111:1047, 1996.
91. Grocott HP, Newman MF, Lowe JE, Clements F: Transmyocardial laser revascularization: An anesthetic perspective. J Cardiothorac Vasc Anesth 11:206, 1997.

C H A P T E R 15

Minimally Invasive Coronary Artery Bypass Grafting

Steven R. Young, M.D.
Robert G. Matheny, M.D.
Steven R. Dryden, M.D.

Minimally invasive coronary artery bypass graft (CABG) surgery is a relatively recent "reinvention" in cardiac surgery. Although many physicians and the lay public view minimally invasive CABG as a "new" procedure, similar approaches have been attempted over the past 30 years and have their roots in reports of Kolesov[1] and Favaloro[2] and others from the late 1960s. These physicians reported early success with thoracotomy and median sternotomy approaches in performing coronary anastomoses without cardiopulmonary bypass.

Classification

Minithoracotomy Without Bypass

As used in this chapter, minimally invasive CABG refers to a coronary bypass operation in which a smaller "minithoracotomy" incision is used, typically in the fourth or fifth intercostal space. In addition, cardiopulmonary bypass is not utilized. Proximal blood flow originates from the internal mammary artery or the inferior epigastric artery, and the distal anastomosis is attached end-to-side past the coronary obstruction. Most commonly, the left internal mammary (internal thoracic) artery is placed to the left anterior descending (LAD) coronary artery and is attached approximately 2 to 3 cm past the first diagonal branch or the right internal mammary is placed to the distal right coronary artery. The terms "minimally invasive direct coronary artery bypass" (MIDCAB), "keyhole," "minimally invasive surgery" (MIS), and "left anterior small thoracotomy" (LAST) surgery are also terms used to describe this surgery.

Alternative Techniques

The Hemopump (Medtronic, Minneapolis, MN) is a catheter-mounted axial-flow pump introduced in a retrograde manner across the aortic valve into the left ventricular cavity. It decompresses the left ventricle while helping to maintain perfusion. Controlled trials are currently underway, and as a device, it could be a useful adjunct in the future.

"Port-Access CABG"[3] (Heartport, Redwood City, CA) is a more complex new technique utilizing femorofemoral cardiopulmonary bypass via the femoral approach. Briefly, this technique uses a coronary sinus retrograde perfusion catheter; a percutaneous pulmonary artery venting catheter; thoracic endoscopy in some instances; and an aortic balloon catheter, which is introduced into the ascending aorta and used for aortic occlusion, aortic root venting, monitoring of aortic root pressure, and delivery of cold cardioplegic solution. Retrograde femoral arterial cardiopulmonary bypass is used. Sternal incision and complications are avoided. Patients' average length of stay in one series was more than a week.[4] Although the technique provides another feasible approach to cardiopulmonary bypass, many clinicians question whether the "Port-Access" technique, as currently developed and utilized, with its higher level of complexity and cost and longer operative time, is as advantageous as other approaches that appear to be simpler and less invasive.[5,6]

Patient Preference

In addition to physician interest, patient preference for a smaller incision, fewer transfusions, shorter length of stay, quicker return to work, decreased morbidity, and the potential for diminished costs have increased interest in less invasive procedures such as angioplasty and minimally invasive CABG. In addition, interest in the procedure has also increased because of efforts to reduce serious complications associated with traditional CABG, including respiratory insufficiency, stroke and other cerebral dysfunction, sternal wound problems, coagulopathy and anemia with resultant transfusion requirement, phrenic and other nerve injury, and microembolization.

New endoscopic and microsurgical techniques, new developments in other surgical instrumentation as discussed in the section to follow, and important improvements in anesthesia and pharmacology have enabled minimally invasive CABG to take a more prominent place in the treatment of coronary artery disease (CAD). Finally, improvements in invasive cardiology, including improved angioplasty techniques, balloon and stent materials, atherectomy, laser, and ultrasound techniques, have presented additional options for revascularization.

Indications

Similar to the early days of percutaneous coronary angioplasty, minimally invasive CABG was initially used only for patients with single-vessel disease. However, as experience increased, physicians have been able to provide therapeutic alternatives for coronary revascularization to a wider variety of patients with multivessel disease.[7,8] Like angioplasty, minimally invasive CABG has enabled patients to avoid a sternum-splitting incision and cardiopulmonary bypass. Additionally, patients with many prohibitive comorbidities (renal dysfunction, aortic calcification, diffuse peripheral vascular disease, Jehovah's Witness faith, hematologic disorders, etc.), for whom revascularization might otherwise not be considered, are now able to undergo surgical revascularization. Invasive cardiology colleagues have been working toward similar goals with their improvements in angioplasty and stents.

Over the last decades, improvements in cardiopulmonary bypass, utilization of cardioplegia, and advances in anesthesia and pharmacology, with the resultant motionless, bloodless surgical field in hemodynamically stable patients, have enabled surgeons to accomplish anastomoses and technical repairs of increasing complexity. These salutary effects of cardiopulmonary bypass, which enable a still and bloodless surgical field, are also requisites for an adequate anastomosis even with "off-pump" surgery. Presently, patients with vessels that can be stabilized on the anterior surface of the heart are ideal candidates for minimally invasive CABG. Posterior descending vessels are also approachable via a subxiphoid incision, often using the inferior epigastric artery for the conduit.

Patient selection is of paramount importance in minimally invasive CABG. Those patients with small, diffusely calcified, diseased coronaries are not ideal candidates for this approach, although some appropriately selected patients with lesions appearing complex and difficult on angiography (type B-2 and C lesions), where long-term results are less favorable, can benefit from the minimally invasive approach. Morbid obesity and an intramyocardial location of the LAD are relative contraindications that may preclude this technique. In some patients, double- or triple-vessel disease may be revascularized by approaching the diagonal, right, and posterior descending vessels as well. Early indications from our hospital are that, in properly selected patients, anastomotic patency with minimally invasive CABG is similar to patency of conduits in patients with traditional CABG utilizing cardiopulmonary bypass (St. Vincent Hospital/Indiana Heart Institute data).

Finally, although there have been improvements in cardiopulmonary bypass in recent decades, ameliorating the side effects of cardiopulmonary bypass has been a primary goal of cardiac anesthesiologists, surgeons, and perfusionists. Indeed, utilization of and improvements in anesthetic techniques, cardioplegia, cardiopulmonary bypass gas and temperature management, serine protease inhibition, and newer generations of membrane oxygenators have decreased bypass-associated morbidity and mortality. Nevertheless, problems persist. When bypass can be avoided altogether, the improvement in patient homeostasis postoperatively can be dramatic. Those patients who are more likely to suffer from the ill effects of cardiopulmonary bypass are more likely to benefit from minimally invasive CABG.

Reoperative CABG

A growing number of patients with failed percutaneous transluminal coronary angioplasty (PTCA)/stenting procedures or patients who have had previous surgical interventions on the LAD and its branches are excellent potential candidates. Obviously, the left arterior mammary artery (LIMA) (or other arterial conduit that will be used) must be available and usable for the reoperative patient to benefit from this approach. In performing a minimally invasive CABG as a reoperation, the previously placed bypass grafts and associated scar tissue around and within the pericardium are left undisturbed, while target vessels are approached laterally so that distal embolization is avoided. The lack of sternotomy and the necessity of dissecting the heart in scar tissue have made the minimally invasive approach particularly advantageous for these "redo" patients. Interestingly, in some cases, the technical aspects of the redo minimally invasive CABG can result in an easier approach than for a primary minimally invasive procedure. In many patients, but especially those scheduled for a "redo," evaluation of the size and quality of the internal mammary artery can be important. Doppler ultrasound, but more particularly angiography, can be particularly helpful in this evaluation. In the future, the bi-spectral index monitor (BIS, Aspect Medical) could prove to be helpful in assessing anesthetic depth.

Surgical Aspects

Although the vast majority of patients undergoing minimally invasive CABG will have the LAD or diagonal coronary artery bypassed, positioning and other operative considerations are quite similar for other vessels. Patients are placed in a supine position without elevating either side of the chest. The arms are padded and tucked at the patient's side in a standard fashion. The patient is then prepped and draped fully, as if standard coronary bypass grafting were to be performed. At this point in the operation, it is not known if the LAD is intramyocardial or if other anatomic considerations will preclude the use of minimally invasive CABG and require full sternotomy with cardiopulmonary bypass. Therefore, the chest, femoral area, and legs are prepped and draped as if traditional CABG may become necessary.

Typically, an 8-cm incision is made, beginning 2 cm lateral to the sternum and carried into the inframammary crease. The fourth intercostal space is generally selected in a patient with a normal body habitus (Fig. 15–1). The inferior aspect of the pectoralis muscle and the fourth intercostal space muscles are divided, and the pleural space is entered. Single-lumen endotracheal intubation appears to be satisfactory and is discussed later. If the lung should interfere with the operative field, it can be tucked away with a warm lap sponge. New retracting devices, both for exposure of the mammary artery and for stabilization of the target coronary artery, assist the surgeon so that the anastomosis can be more easily accomplished. The mamamary artery is dissected free in the space created by the retractor device, which is placed with the superior blade on the fourth rib and the inferior blade on the fifth rib, thus making a window that exposes the entire length of the LIMA. Vascular clips are used on the perforating branches.

The pericardium is then elevated, incised, and retracted laterally. The LAD or other target vessel is exposed. In our institution, to dissect the LAD free, a stabilizing retractor (CardioThoracic Systems, Cupertino, CA) is then utilized (Fig. 15–2). The motion of the heart in the area of the anastomosis can be reduced by 90 to 95% with the placement of the retractor's stabilizing foot. With a tourniquet or snare around the proximal vessel or an intraluminal occluding device, a still bloodless field is then obtained allowing for a safe and technically accurate anastomosis to be created. The authors do not routinely use preconditioning (discussed in detail later) except occasionally for a very large patent LAD. Preconditioning is used more often for the right coronary artery, because of a seemingly higher incidence of rhythm disturbances.

Heparin and lidocaine are given prior to occlusion of the coronary artery. In over 200 patients, we have not seen an episode of ventricular fibrillation, except in a patient brought emergently from the cardiac catheterization lab. Also, although occasional intraoperative ECG

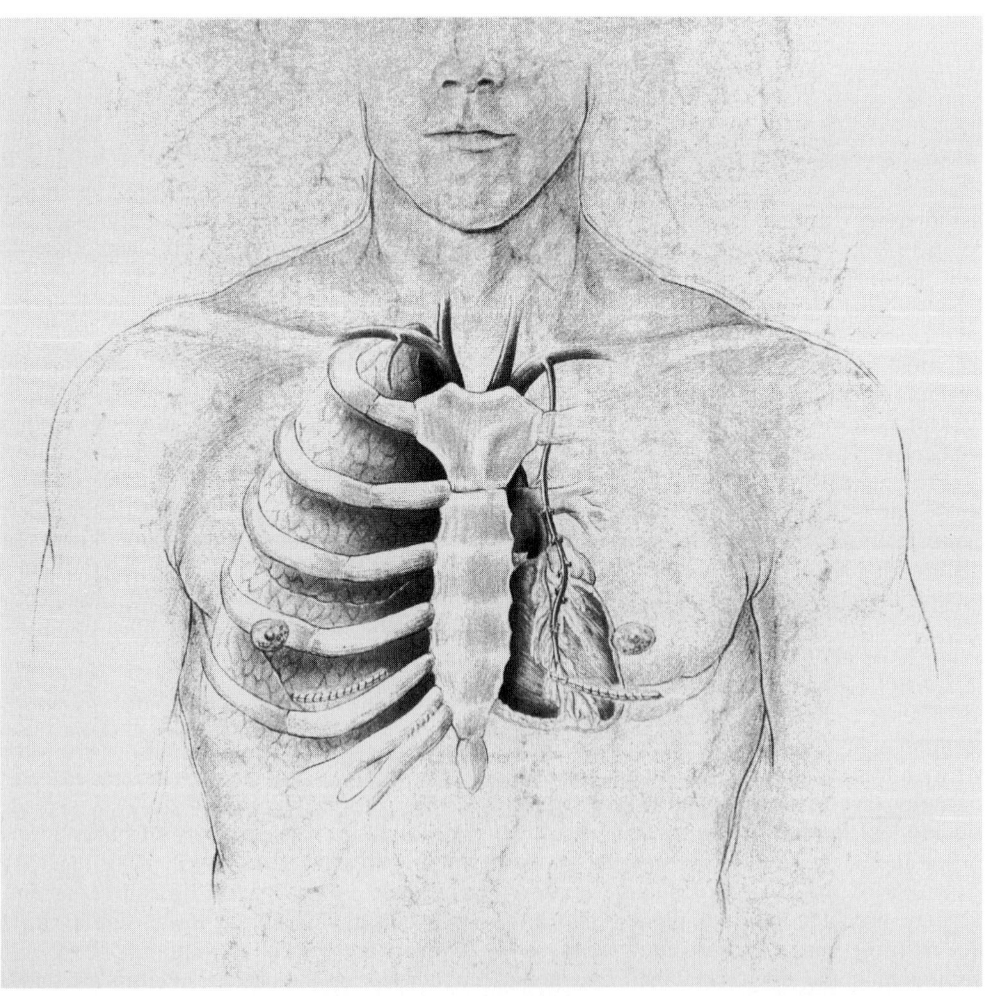

FIGURE **15–1.** Anatomic considerations are seen as the left internal mammary (internal thoracic) artery is anastomosed to the left anterior descending artery in a view that reveals underlying osseus and cardiopulmonary structures involved in a minimally invasive CABG.

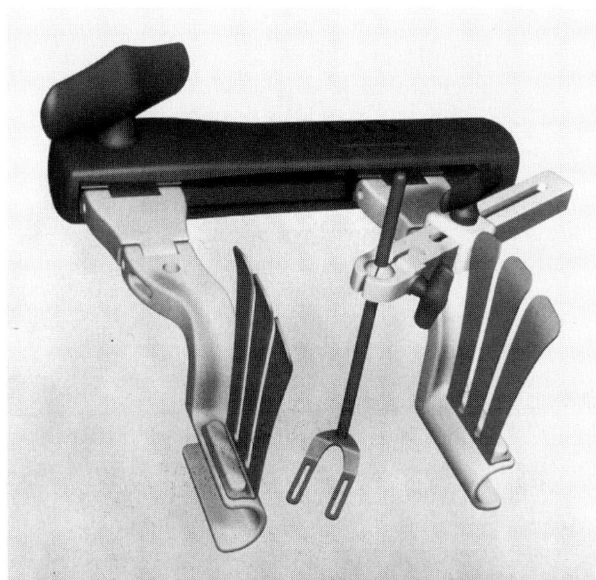

FIGURE **15–2.** Rib and muscle retraction is accomplished with the six malleable retractor arms while the fork-shaped foot device produces cardiac and target coronary artery stabilization. (Courtesy of CardioThoracic Systems, Cupertino, CA.)

changes are seen, worrisome electrocardiographic (ECG) changes or postoperative enzyme increases indicative of perioperative myocardial infarction have been seen in less than 1% of our elective series, even following 20 minutes of occlusion (St. Vincent Hospital/Indiana Heart Institute data).

The anastomosis is performed in a standard fashion with 7-0 or 8-0 Proline suture with the ribs and musculature retracted and the heart and target coronary artery stabilized (Fig. 15–3). After the anastomosis is complete, the flow through the mammary artery is allowed to return prior to removing the snare/occluding device. The integrity of the anastomosis is inspected, and patency and flow are assessed in a number of different ways (discussed later). The pedicle is then secured to the epicardium. In patients with chronic obstructive pulmonary disease (COPD), the pedicle is also secured to the mediastinum so that it will not be distracted medially by the expanding lung. ECG changes seen during LAD occlusion have been seen to revert to normal after opening the mammary-coronary anastomosis. A single chest tube is placed, and in some patients, postoperative analgesia is aided by intraoperative intercostal blocks with bupivacaine or ropivacaine. Patients are observed in the intensive care unit (ICU) (or other setting with a higher level of nursing/monitoring care) for several hours, where attention is paid to pain control, hemodynamics, and evidence of graft patency and ischemia. If the patient is stable, transfer can be accomplished, or the patient can remain in the same room or patient care area but at a reduced level of nursing care staffing or "acuity." In patients who are stable and who have bowel sounds, liquids can be taken later on the day of surgery. Patients without significant comorbid conditions are generally discharged in the following 24 to 48 hours.

Anesthetic Choice

Many minimally invasive CABG patients have single-vessel disease with normal or nearly normal ventricular function. At the other extreme are patients with multi-vessel disease or significant comorbidities who risk suffering severe complications with conventional CABG surgery. Many of these individuals are candidates for an integrated approach in the treatment of coronary artery disease utilizing minimally invasive CABG followed by angioplasty and/or stent placement. Medications in both groups likely include β-blockers, calcium channel block-

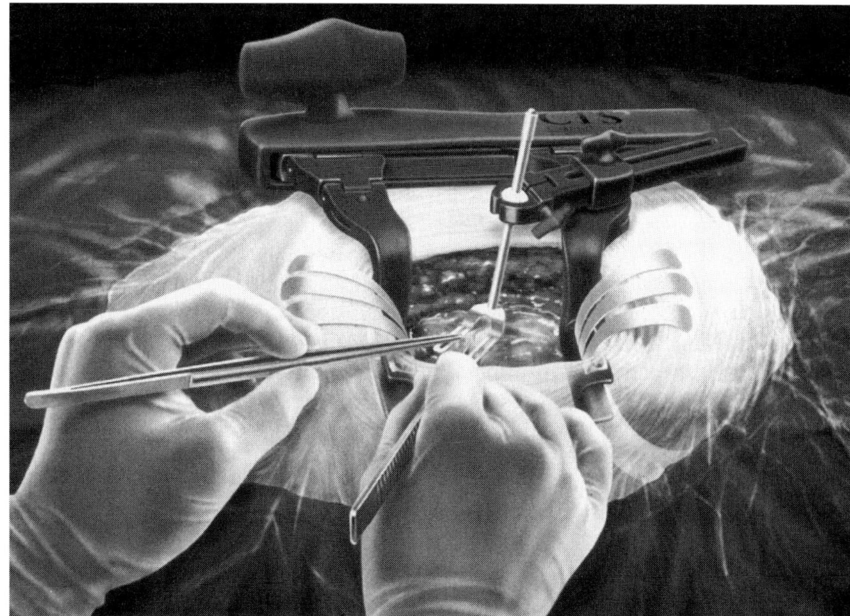

FIGURE **15–3.** During the minimally invasive CABG, adequate visualization, retraction, and coronary stabilization permit the operation to proceed smoothly.

ers, angiotensin converting enzyme (ACE) inhibitors, and nitrates. Current anesthetic strategies focus on goals of hemodynamic stability, optimized surgical conditions, and prevention and treatment of ischemia. Also, techniques aim to improve patient safety, decrease costs and morbidity, shorten intubation time, and diminish ICU and hospital length of stay.

Preoperative Considerations

On the day of surgery, most patients arrive at the hospital 1 to 2 hours preoperatively. Therefore, comprehensive preoperative patient preparation, evaluation, and treatment of comorbidities must be accomplished before the day of surgery. Discussion of risks and plans for anesthesia, monitoring, proposed surgery, postoperative pain control, and consents for procedures (e.g., epidural), where appropriate, are important elements of the preoperative patient interview. An anesthetic plan, with attention to issues raised in this chapter, is formulated and discussed with the surgeon, patient, and appropriate team members.

Traditional preoperative "NPO after midnight" orders and other measures including H_2 receptor blockade and cricoid pressure are important to consider in patients with high risk status, diabetic gastroparesis, morbid obesity, an "anatomically difficult" upper airway, preoperative emergency status, gastrointestinal obstruction or abdominal distention, or gastroesophageal reflux (hiatal hernia).[9] On the other hand, patients who are able to take clear fluids preoperatively are likely to enter the operative period less stressed, less hypoglycemic, and better hydrated. Indeed, current knowledge supports liberalization of NPO guidelines so that clear liquids may be ingested until 2 hours before surgery[9,10] except in patients such as those listed above.

Cardiac medications are continued preoperatively. Heparin may be continued through intraoperative heparinization, although many physicians (ourselves included) choose to discontinue heparin approximately 1 hour before starting invasive monitoring lines. In our institution, intramuscular (IM) or intravenous (IV) premedication with morphine sulfate (0.1 mg/kg) and midazolam (0.025 to 0.05 mg/kg) or other short-acting drugs provides mild anxiolysis, amnesia, and analgesia for monitoring line insertion. Scopolamine and other long-acting drugs must be avoided if early extubation is a goal. Once the patient has been premedicated, 2 to 4 L/min nasal cannula oxygen is applied to keep Spo_2 greater than 91%. Where appropriate, intravenous infusions (such as nitroglycerin or inotropes) and electrocardiographic and hemodynamic monitors may be utilized during preoperative patient transport, although, in our experience, this is usually unnecessary for most patients.

Intraoperative Considerations

In the operating room or induction area, after placing nasal cannula oxygen, ECG leads, external defibrillator pads (with pacing capability), and pulse oximeter, at least one large-bore peripheral intravenous and a radial arterial catheter are started. The V_5 ECG lead usually is placed somewhat closer to a V_6 position, considering the usual planned surgical site. Methods contributing to temperature homeostasis, such as a warm circulating water mattress, forced air warming blanket, airway warming or heat/moisture exchanger, warm operating room, and other techniques continue, although keeping the minimally invasive CABG patient warm is frequently a challenge. A noninvasive blood pressure cuff is placed (usually on the contralateral arm from the arterial catheter), and anesthetic induction commences. In our institution, in an effort to reduce costs, the cardiopulmonary bypass circuit is assembled, but without a fluid prime. Some other institutions do not preassemble any portion of the pump circuit, whereas others use a full set-up.

After induction, appropriate monitors (see later discussion)—including Swan-Ganz right heart catheter, central venous pressure (CVP), and/or transesophageal echocardiography (TEE)—are placed. Many physicians perform right heart catheterization or CVP placement before induction. However, despite alterations in hemodynamics during induction, there are not compelling data from the literature that support the need to place the catheter before the patient is anesthetized. For most patients, expedient placement can be accomplished with a greater degree of patient comfort and asepsis after anesthetic induction. Also, after anesthesia begins, TEE (if desired) is positioned and an initial examination performed (the authors and others[11–13] do not routinely use TEE during minimally invasive CABG). A urinary catheter is anchored, and temperature monitoring probe(s) are placed. If TEE is not used, many anesthesiologists place a gastric tube to decompress the stomach. The multilead electrocardiogram with ST-segment analysis, invasive, and noninvasive pressures are monitored continuously.

Anesthetic induction can be accomplished with a variety of agents including thiopental (2 to 4 mg/kg), propofol (1.0 to 1.5 mg/kg), or etomidate (0.2 to 0.3 mg/kg). In addition, low-dose sufentanil (0.5 to 1.0 μg/kg), remifentanil (0.5 to 1.0 μg/kg/min infusion) or other short-acting opioids can be effective adjuvants. In general, use of short- to intermediate-acting neuromuscular blockers and methods to assess neuromuscular block are important aspects of our anesthetic technique.

A variety of intravenous anesthetic regimens have been described to accomplish the goal of stable hemodynamics and early awakening and extubation following various types of cardiothoracic surgery. Young and Stogsdill in our institution (unpublished data) find that low-dose sufentanil (1.0 μg/kg/hr) plus propofol (4 to 6 mg/kg/hr) compared to low-dose sufentanil plus midazolam (40 μg/kg/hr) achieves significantly more rapid extubation in patients for traditional CABG or valve replacement. With alfentanil (30 μg/kg/hr) and propofol (3 to 6 mg/kg/hr) infusions, more rapid extubation is accomplished when compared to fentanyl-midazolam infusion, with approximately 16% of patients experiencing breakthrough hypertension requiring additional 1-mg alfentanil boluses.[14] Relatively stable cardiac function and hemodynamics are observed in patients administered propofol and alfentanil[15,16] or in patients with ejection fraction less than 50% receiving propofol.[17] Importantly, for maintenance of anesthesia, no major effect on cardiac function is seen using propofol as a supplement to low-dose narcotic anesthesia.[18] The newer rapidly metabolized opioid remifentanil appears promising for use in some patients. However, different postoperative pain strategies will likely be needed with such rapid disappearance of narcotic effect. Most anesthesiologists would agree that a "high-dose" regimen of fentanyl or sufentanil is not well suited for shorter duration minimally invasive CABG procedures due to longer duration of opioid action.

Inhalation anesthetics offer many benefits as maintenance agents for cardiothoracic surgery, including rapid titration, bronchodilation, rapid elimination, and the capability of monitoring end-tidal concentrations. In addition, volatile anesthetics help to protect against ischemia by lessening myocardial oxygen demand. However, inhalation anesthetics (and propofol and narcotics when rapidly administered) can decrease blood pressure and, therefore, coronary perfusion pressure. In the 1980s, in a study that did *not* utilize usual anesthetic adjuvant drugs, isoflurane was reported to induce "coronary steal" (redistribution of blood away from underperfused areas).[19] However, subsequent reports show that isoflurane is, in fact, not detrimental to patients undergoing CABG.[20-22] The use of isoflurane in patients with coronary disease, assuming reasonable attention to hemodynamics, appears to be safe and provides for early extubation.[23] With rapid elimination and "wake up," the newer agents sevoflurane and desflurane may be valuable anesthetics or adjuvants when performing anesthesia for minimally invasive CABG.

Before manipulation of the target coronary artery, heparin (70 to 100 U/kg) and lidocaine 0.5 to 1.5 mg/kg are administered IV. Shortly before the target artery is to be occluded or manipulated, some centers utilize ischemic preconditioning techniques[24,25] (see below). With surgical manipulation, increasing ischemia requiring evaluation and treatment can be observed: ST-segment changes and arrhythmias; segmental wall motion abnormalities or worsened mitral regurgitation on TEE; increases in pulmonary artery diastolic or wedge pressures; and/or unintended substantial changes in cardiac output, blood pressure, heart rate, and/or mixed venous oxygen saturation. At the conclusion of the anastomosis, protamine sulfate (0.75 to 1.0 mg/kg) is typically administered to reverse the smaller dose of heparin given for the minimally invasive CABG. However, for some surgeons, protamine is not administered if the surgical field is "dry."

During the minimally invasive CABG, anesthesiologists are faced with a significant challenge in the quest to avoid intraoperative patient awareness. Medications are given that decrease heart rate, cardiac output, and blood pressure and make assessment of anesthetic depth more problematic. In addition, ventricular dysfunction from surgical manipulation of the heart and ischemia secondary to acute coronary occlusion ensure that maintenance of hemodynamic stability while administering any substantive amount of anesthesia can frequently be difficult.

Postoperative Considerations

After successful surgery and appropriate anesthesia, when there is no evidence of residual hemodynamic, arterial conduit, airway, or bleeding problems, early extubation (defined as extubation in the operating room or in the early postoperative period in the ICU) is possible for the vast majority of patients. Indeed, without cardiopulmonary bypass and the associated problems of respiratory and cerebral dysfunction, coagulopathy, anemia, phrenic injury, inflammatory cascade activation,[26] protein denaturation, and microembolization, early extubation is an achievable goal even in many patients with significant comorbid conditions. Despite some earlier debate in the anesthetic literature concerning the effectiveness of early extubation, it is clear that patients who are extubated earlier are more likely to have shorter ICU and hospital length of stays.[27] During the recovery phase, a number of physicians continue to administer both calcium channel blockers and nitroglycerin (NTG). However, Matheny[8] and Schaff[11] use only NTG. Finally, postoperative pain control is important in diminishing pulmonary dysfunction, tachycardia, and hypertension, all of which increase postsurgical mortality and ICU readmissions.[28,29] In addition, higher levels of catecholamines observed with stress and postoperative pain facilitate platelet aggregation, which contributes to coronary thrombosis.[29,30]

Ischemia Prophylaxis and Treatment

Calcium channel blockers, β-blockers, and nitrates assist in the reduction of cardiac morbidity and mortality from ischemia. Diltiazem helps prevent ischemia during noncardiac surgery in patients at risk for ischemia.[31] In addition to its negative chronotropic effects, diltiazem favorably redistributes blood flow to ischemic and endocardial areas, inhibits platelet aggregation (mediated by metabolites), and decreases myocardial energy demands.[32,33] After a 2- to 5-mg loading dose administered over 10 to 15 minutes, diltiazem is frequently administered as an infusion of 50 mg per 250 ml saline or D_5W at 2.0 to 4.0 mg/hr.[34] Atrioventricular block, congestive heart failure, and hypotension are relative contraindications. Long-term use of atenolol[35] and other β-blockers[36] decreases mortality and cardiovascular morbidity after peripheral vascular surgery. β-Blockers such as atenolol and the shorter duration esmolol increase diastolic filling time and reduce myocardial oxygen demand, apparently by decreasing heart rate. NTG[37] is an important adjuvant in the treatment of myocardial ischemia and is administered as an infusion of 50 mg per 500 ml saline or D_5W at 0.2 to 2.0 μg/kg/min (see "Preconditioning," p 385).

Heart Rate Control

Esmolol, adenosine, anticholinesterase drugs, and bolus doses of synthetic short-acting opioids can be used to induce a slower heart rate during surgical manipulation. Esmolol, a rapidly acting selective β_1-receptor antagonist, is particularly useful in controlling heart rate during surgical distal coronary anastomosis on the beating heart. Increments of 10 to 20 mg can be given as a bolus, while an infusion of 2.5 gm per 250 ml saline or D_5W at 0.05 to 0.2 mg/kg/min is effective for inducing bradycardia.[34] Obviously, great care must be used with any β-blocker in a patient with severe bronchospastic disease, moderate to severe congestive heart failure, or severe ventricular dysfunction. After hundreds of minimally invasive CABG procedures, at the present time in patients with left ventricular dysfunction, the authors are less aggressive in using esmolol than earlier in our experience because of depression of cardiac output and blood pressure. Practically speaking, reversal of esmolol-induced bradycardia usually occurs 10 to 20 minutes after discontinuing the esmolol infusion. Adenosine, an endogenous nucleotide, can assist the surgeon by producing transient (10- to 20-second) atrioventricular block and asystole (and hypotension) when administered as one or two rapid 6-mg IV bolus injections. The anticholinesterase drugs edrophonium (5-mg IV boluses) and neostigmine (0.5-mg IV boluses) can also slow heart rate without diminishing contractility and cardiac output. Of course, the use of anticholinesterase agents can reverse residual neuromuscular blockade, necessitating potential use of a succinylcholine infusion, with some potential for "confusion" at the neuromuscular junction. Finally, a small dose of short-acting opioid can be very effective in producing moderate slowing of the heart rate. Availability of external or internal pacing is important as a back-up with any of these techniques that can produce asystole or *profound* bradycardia.

Hypotension can be reversed without increasing myocardial contractility using a phenylephrine infusion (8 to 10 mg per 250 ml saline or D_5W) to keep systolic blood pressure close to preoperative levels. A bolus of 0.1 to 0.5 mg of phenylephrine or 5 to 25 mg of ephedrine can quickly reverse hemodynamic misfortune. Finally, increasing cardiac output and contractility can be accomplished with infusions of appropriate inotropic drugs such as dobutamine, dopamine, epinephrine, norepinephrine, calcium, and milrinone.

Thermoregulation

As an attainable goal, early extubation is difficult to accomplish if the patient is hypothermic. In fact, hypothermia is cited as the primary contributing factor resulting in delayed extubation[38] and has been implicated in increased blood loss[39] and wound infection[40] in noncardiac surgery. Frank et al.[41] show that maintenance of normothermia is associated with a reduction in perioperative morbid cardiac events from 6.3% in hypothermic (35.4°C) patients to 1.4% in normothermic (36.7°C) patients. In 100 peripheral vascular patients, a sublingual temperature of less than 35°C was found to be the only predictor of postoperative ischemia.[42] In another study in which routine warming measures were used for both groups of patients, forced air warming produced a higher postoperative temperature (36.8° vs. 35.4°C), a significant cost savings, and decreased emergence time (13.9 vs. 9.8 minutes).[43]

Choice of Monitors

Detection of ischemia can be accomplished by utilizing a number of different monitors, each of which has its own advantages and limitations.[45] A complete review is beyond the scope of this chapter and is found elsewhere in this text.

Electrocardiogram

The ECG is easily applied and interpreted and is effective in detecting ischemia,[45–48] especially when observing multiple leads that include the lateral precordial V_5 lead. After CABG, ECG abnormalities predict myocardial injury and increased length of stay.[49] However, as with other monitors, not all ischemia is detected by the ECG.[50]

Pulmonary Artery Catheterization

Connors et al.[51] conclude that a pulmonary artery catheter (PAC) provides measures of cardiovascular performance not otherwise readily clinically available. In our institution, a PAC is utilized in almost all patients and is felt to be valuable in prompting changes in therapy,[52] looking for increases in mean and pulmonary artery diastolic pressure and pulmonary capillary wedge pressures as early indicators of decreased ventricular compliance associated with myocardial ischemia. Although the PAC does not detect all episodes of ischemia, it has additional benefits of being useful for medication administration, can remain in place after the patient is awake and extubated, and is useful in following cardiac index and mixed venous oxygen saturation ($S\bar{v}O_2$) (if an $S\bar{v}O_2$ catheter is used). These authors see little benefit in the substitution of a CVP catheter for a PAC, when looking at a cost-value analysis of the two catheters and when considering that most of the short-term morbidity with either catheter is primarily related to accessing the central circulation. As with other monitoring techniques, knowledge and experience in the use of the PAC are essential if patient benefit is to accrue from its use.[53,54] Tuman and Roizen's discussion summarizes problems in current PAC studies and provides insight into future issues.[54]

Transesophageal Echocardiography

TEE is quite sensitive in detecting ischemia and is used widely for many patients undergoing coronary surgery.[50,55] New segmental wall motion abnormalities thought to be induced by ischemia were seen with TEE in 24 of 50 patients undergoing coronary or major vascular surgery while ischemic changes detected by ECG were seen in only six patients.[56] For the most part, diagnostic capability with TEE is excellent.[51] However, as with other monitors, pitfalls are present including inconsistent interpretation,[57] the need for a higher level of user expertise, questions concerning postinsertion laryngeal dysfunction,[58,59] and lack of usefulness for continuing monitoring in the awake, extubated patient.

One-Lung Ventilation

Initial experiences with minimally invasive CABG procedures resulted in surgical requests for double-lumen endotracheal tube use. Although helpful when using a thoracoscopic approach, further experience from the St. Vincent Hospital/Indiana Heart Institute and other institutions[11,38] has found double-lumen endotracheal anesthesia to be unnecessary when performing a standard anterior minithoracotomy approach for minimally invasive CABG. Instead, a modest reduction in tidal volume and the use of a standard endotracheal tube (ETT) appears to be adequate for surgical needs. Certainly, the use of a standard ETT simplifies airway considerations, especially in the patient with a difficult airway, and ensures a more rapid and less traumatic transition to postoperative mechanical ventilation if the need arises. Importantly, if one-lung ventilation and a PAC are used for the same patient, more reliable data can be obtained if the catheter is positioned in the main pulmonary artery or the pulmonary artery on the side of the lung that is to remain expanded.

When properly utilized, one-lung ventilation (OLV) can lead to diminished excursion of the lung on the operated side. However, double-lumen ETT-OLV problems complicate anesthetic and postoperative care. Obvious difficulties include initial intubation (particularly in a patient with a difficult airway), proper placement, suctioning through a smaller diameter lumen, and the necessity of switching to a standard ETT if postoperative ventilation is necessary.[60] In addition, hypoxemia during OLV remains problematic. Propofol-opioid anesthesia does not inhibit hypoxic pulmonary vasoconstriction,[61] which is crucial in maintaining optimal oxygenation and in preventing ventilation-perfusion mismatch during OLV. Propofol is associated with lower shunt fractions than enflurane during OLV.[62] Also, under OLV, intravenous anesthesia is thought to avoid the hypoxemia associated with the use of inhaled agents. However, in patients undergoing thoracoscopic and esophageal surgery, arterial oxygenation during OLV with 1 minimum alveolar concentration (MAC) of isoflurane is not significantly different than during propofol-alfentanil anesthesia.[63]

Utilization of an ETT with bronchial blocker (Univent, Fuji Systems, Tokyo) presents an effective alternative to the use of a double-lumen ETT. Placement is accomplished with a tube rotation technique and requires use of the fiberoptic bronchoscope to assist with final placement.[60] The same tube with the blocker retracted can be used for postoperative ventilation. Careful discussion with other providers will help prevent improper use and avoid complications, such as improper cuff inflation resulting in blockage of the central lumen of the Univent tube.[64] Benumof provides a thorough discussion of techniques of one-lung anesthesia.[60]

Preconditioning

Preconditioning is defined as a rapid adaptive response to a brief ischemic insult. This adaptive response slows the rate of cell death during a subsequent prolonged period of ischemia.[65] Observations in the 1980s showed that brief repetitive coronary occlusions are not associated with further diminishing levels of adenosine triphosphate (ATP).[66,67] Thus, ongoing degradation of high-energy phosphates appears to slow after a brief ischemic episode. After a brief period of preconditioning, dogs were subjected to 40 minutes of coronary occlusion. With subsequent reperfusion of the same coronary artery, the preconditioned dogs experienced only one quarter the area of infarcted myocardium compared to control animals.[68] Some investigations revealed that preconditioned hearts show less decrease in left ventricular function after ischemia[69] and fewer arrhythmias secondary to preconditioning,[70] although these effects are apparently not as consistent as reduction in infarct size.[24]

Certainly, beneficial effects of preconditioning have not been a consistent finding in all studies. However, the validity of preconditioning under certain circumstances is supported by a number of studies in man.

1. Intermittent angina prior to myocardial infarction can produce cardioprotection,[71] preservation of contractile function,[72] and smaller infarct size.[73]
2. Biochemical assays obtained from acutely preconditioned patients undergoing CABG with cardiopulmonary bypass demonstrate higher ATP tissue levels compared to assays from nonpreconditioned control patients.[74] In addition, human atrial muscle subject to normothermic ischemia appears to have improved viability (as measured by creatine kinase activity) and improved contractile function when compared to controls without preconditioning.[75]
3. Acute tolerance to angina ("walk-through" angina) is commonly seen in man.[24]
4. ST-segment changes and lactate release are reduced following subsequent balloon inflation during coronary angioplasty.[76] Is an improvement in coronary blood flow or preconditioning responsible for this positive finding?

Although the exact mechanism that produces the beneficial effects of preconditioning in certain individuals under select circumstances is not precisely known, the molecule adenosine, the adenosine myocardial A_1 receptor, and an increase in potassium conductance via the ATP-sensitive K^+ channel are thought to be intimately involved in the development of preconditioning.[77] Excellent reviews discuss proposed mechanisms and other aspects of preconditioning in more detail.[24,78–84]

Prior to performing the distal anastomosis during minimally invasive CABG, some physicians precondition utilizing brief 2-, 3-, and 5-minute coronary occlusions followed by a similar time for reperfusion in the target vessel.[25] It remains to be seen whether preconditioning will protect or lessen postischemic dysfunction in this group of cardiac patients.

Postoperative Pain Control

Surgeons recognize that anesthesiologists can make a significant contribution to the success of a patient's minimally invasive CABG through their expertise in management of postoperative pain.[11] Patients undergoing minimally invasive CABG are not pain free. Important issues in patients undergoing minithoracotomy for minimally invasive CABG include if and when to administer epidural or intrathecal opioids, and the use of other adjuvant drugs and techniques.

Given the current state of knowledge in 1997, especially the difficulty in assessing neurologic function while the patient is anesthetized, these authors generally agree with Ralley[85] and others,[86] who question whether preoperative neuraxial opioids–local anesthetics should be used when the potential for full (300 to 400 U/kg) heparinization exists, as it does if a minimally invasive CABG must be converted to a traditional CABG. Although some physicians advocate the use of preoperative neuraxial techniques for patients undergoing cardiac surgery, to date, studies have not showed improved outcomes in cardiac surgery from preoperative neuraxial techniques. Therefore, many physicians, including those at our institution, believe that *preoperative* use of neuraxial techniques for minimally invasive CABG or traditional CABG does not merit the increased neurologic risk of undetected epidural hematoma.[86]

If an epidural technique is selected for the patient undergoing minimally invasive CABG, some individuals before the incision or early in the case begin a continuous epidural infusion with bupivacaine (1.0 mg/ml) with fentanyl (20 μg/ml) at a rate of 4 to 6 ml/hr in younger patients and 2 to 3 ml/hr in the elderly or debilitated. This same epidural infusion can then be continued postoperatively until other modalities of pain control are effective. A complete discussion of epidural indications, techniques, and associated anticoagulation issues is beyond the scope of this chapter.

Postoperative pain control can include pre-, intra-, or postoperative intercostal blockade with 0.5% bupivacaine or ropivacaine.[87–89] In our institution, posterior intercostal nerve blockade is frequently performed by the surgeon via the thoracic cavity under direct vision at the conclusion of the minimally invasive CABG. Performed in this manner, the upper thoracic dermatome intercostal blockade is easily administered, carries a very low risk, and is quite advantageous for postoperative pain relief.

Other important techniques include IV opioid patient-controlled analgesia (PCA), intrapleural local anesthesia, and postoperative neuraxial epidural[90–92] or intrathecal[92,93] analgesia. Many anesthesiologists most commonly administer neuraxial opioids by the epidural route. However, Gwirtz et al. have studied over 4,000 patients who received excellent postoperative pain relief with a single intrathecal opioid injection, a technique that is less invasive, simpler, and less costly than continuous epidural approaches.[93]

In patients without significant renal dysfunction or bleeding, beginning with the conclusion of surgery and continuing postoperatively, IV doses of 15 to 30 mg ketorolac (Toradol)[94] or other nonsteroidal anti-inflammatory drugs can be helpful in pain management. Additionally, intrapleural local anesthetics, application of transcutaneous electrical nerve stimulation (TENS) units, and cryoanalgesia are other less frequently used but helpful adjuncts for postoperative pain. Other issues in postoperative control of thoracic pain are discussed elsewhere in this text and covered thoroughly elsewhere.[91]

Graft Evaluation

Evaluation of mammary artery patency and flow is of vital importance. For graft assessment during or after minimally invasive CABG, many different techniques are in use or under development, including postprocedure angiography, thermal imaging systems,[13] various Doppler techniques including transthoracic Doppler echo and flowmeters (e.g., Transonic Systems, Inc, Ithaca, NY), or continuous wave Doppler echo.[95] With continuous wave Doppler echo, observation of systolic and diastolic flow on the operated side compared to only systolic flow on the nonoperated side appears to be a useful noninvasive indicator of graft flow (Fig. 15–4).

The presence of abnormalities in pulmonary artery catheterization data (increased pulmonary capillary wedge pressure, pulmonary hypertension, and low car-

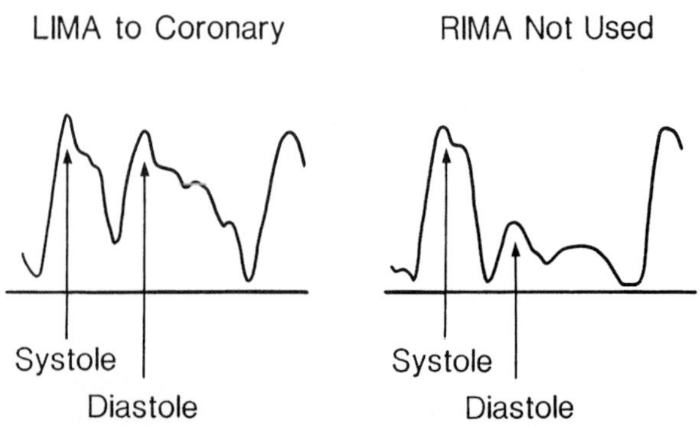

FIGURE **15–4.** Continuous wave Doppler tracings showing diastolic flow to the coronary bed with a successful anastomosis.

diac index),[52] electrocardiogram (ST changes and serious arrhythmias),[46] transesophageal echo (segmental wall motion abnormalities, new or worsened mitral insufficiency),[51,56] and later postoperative biochemical markers (creatine kinase-MB and troponin-T) can assist in the assessment of anastomosis difficulties. If questions remain, angiography should be undertaken.[11] The above measures should assist the surgeon and anesthesiologist in determining the success of the minimally invasive CABG.

Innovations/Questions

Recent surgical[95–100] and anesthetic[101] innovations have improved our abilities to offer patients a wider range of therapeutic choices. The importance of completeness of myocardial revascularization is well understood[102]; for that reason more traditional approaches to CABG are continuing to evolve. Current trends in the 1990s favor streamlined, tailored patient management and have been accelerated by improvements in surgical, anesthetic, and perfusion techniques. Improvements in both traditional[103] and minimally invasive CABG (St. Vincent Hospital/Indiana Heart Institute data) have decreased ICU length of stay and in-hospital length of stay and cost, and have reduced morbidity and mortality.

In the treatment of coronary artery disease, patency of the LIMA-LAD bypass is certainly one of the most critical elements of modern coronary revascularization. Compromise of the integrity of that conduit is not acceptable. Will positive results utilizing minimally invasive CABG continue to live up to early expectations? Will minimally invasive CABG be less costly and confer greater long-term benefit when compared to angioplasty plus stents or other new techniques?[8] Will minimally invasive CABG arterial patency be as successful as traditional CABG? Continued study and advances will expand horizons in the successful treatment of patients with coronary artery disease while achieving lowered morbidity, mortality, and cost.

References

1. Kolesov VI: Mammary artery-coronary artery anastomosis as a method of treatment for angina pectoris. J Thorac Cardiovasc Surg 54:535, 1967.
2. Favaloro RG: Saphenous vein autograft replacement of severe coronary artery occlusion. Ann Thorac Surg 5:334, 1968.
3. Siegel LC, Stevens JH, St Goar FG, et al: Intraoperative monitoring of patients undergoing port-access coronary artery bypass grafting. Anesthesiology 85(Suppl):A160, 1996.
4. Reichenspurner H, Gulielmos V, Daniel WG, Schuler S: Minimally invasive coronary bypass surgery. N Engl J Med 336:67, 1997.
5. Lytle BW: Minimally invasive cardiac surgery. J Thorac Cardiovasc Surg 111:554, 1996.
6. Westaby S, Benetti FJ: Less invasive coronary surgery: Consensus from the Oxford meeting. Ann Thorac Surg 62:924, 1996.
7. Subramanian VA, Sani G, Benetti FJ, Calafiore AM: Minimally invasive coronary bypass surgery: A multi-center report of preliminary clinical experience. Circulation 92:645, 1995.
8. Fry ETA, Hermiller JB, Lips D, et al: Comparison of stents, bypass surgery (CABG), and minimally invasive bypass for isolated LAD revascularization: Patient section, outcomes, and costs. Circulation 94(Suppl I):I-324, 1994.
9. Stoelting RK: "NPO" and aspiration pneumonitis—changing perspectives. Lecture 432. American Society of Anesthesiologists 1995 Annual Refresher Course Lectures. Park Ridge, IL.
10. Strunin L: How long should patients fast before surgery? Time for new guidelines. Br J Anaesth 70:1, 1993.
11. Schaff HV: New surgical techniques: Implications for the cardiac anesthesiologist: Mini-thoracotomy for coronary revascularization without cardiopulmonary bypass. J Cardiothorac Vasc Anesth 11(Suppl 1):6, 1997.
12. Greenspun HG, Adourian UA, Fonger JD, Fan JS: Minimally invasive direct coronary artery bypass (MIDCAB): Surgical techniques and anesthetic considerations. J Cardiothorac Vasc Anesth 10:507, 1996.
13. Gayes JM, Emery RW, Nissen MD: Anesthetic considerations for patients undergoing minimally invasive coronary artery bypass surgery: Mini-sternotomy and mini-thorocotomy approaches. J Cardiothorac Vasc Anesth 10:531, 1996.
14. Collard E, Delire V, Mayne A, et al: Propofol-alfentanil versus fentanyl-midazolam in coronary artery surgery. J Cardiothorac Vasc Anesth 10:869, 1996.
15. Manara AR, Monk CR, Bolsin SN, et al: Total IV anesthesia with propofol and alfentanil for coronary artery bypass grafting. Br J Anaesth 66:716, 1991.
16. Roekaerts PM, Gerrits HJ, Timmerman BE, deLang S: Continuous infusions of alfentanil and propofol for coronary artery surgery. J Cardiothorac Vasc Anesth 9:362, 1995.
17. Hall RI, Murphy JT, Landymore R, et al: Myocardial and hemodynamic changes during propofol anesthesia for cardiac surgery in patients with reduced ventricular function. Anesth Analg 77:680, 1993.
18. Vermeyen KM, DeHert SG, Erpels FA, et al: Myocardial metabolism during anesthesia with propofol-low dose fentanyl for coronary artery bypass surgery. Br J Anaesth 66:504, 1991.
19. Reiz S, Balfors E, Sorensen MD, et al: Isoflurane: A powerful coronary vasodilator in patients with ischemic heart disease. Anesthesiology 59:91, 1993.
20. Slogoff S, Keats AS: Randomized trial of primary anesthetic agents on outcome of coronary artery bypass operations. Anesthesiology 70:179, 1989.
21. Tuman KJ, McCarthy RJ, Spiess BD, et al: Does choice of anesthetic agents significantly affect outcome after coronary artery surgery? Anesthesiology 70:189, 1989.
22. Slogoff S, Keats AS, Dear WE, et al: Steal-prone coronary anatomy in myocardial ischemia associated with four primary anesthetic agents in humans. Anesth Analg 72:22, 1991.
23. Leung JM, Goeher P, O'Kelly BF, et al: Isoflurane anesthesia in myocardial ischemia: Comparative risks versus sufentanil anesthesia in patients undergoing coronary artery bypass surgery. Anesthesiology 74:834, 1991.
24. Kloner RA, Yellon D: Does ischemic preconditioning occur in patients? J Am Coll Cardiol 24:1133, 1994.
25. Jacobsohn E, Ferdinand F, Albertucci M, et al: Minimally invasive CABG: Anesthetic technique and outcome. Anesth Analg 84(Suppl):S91, 1997.
26. Butler J, Rocker G, Westaby S: Inflammatory response to cardiopulmonary bypass. Ann Thorac Surg 55:552, 1993.
27. Smith LR, Milano CA, Molter BS, et al: Preoperative determinants of postoperative costs associated with coronary artery bypass graft surgery. Circulation 90:124, 1994.
28. Rose DK, Cohen MM, DeBoer DP: Cardiovascular events in the post-anesthesia care unit. Anesthesiology 84:772, 1996.
29. Nabel EG, Selwyn AP, Ganz P: Paradoxical narrowing of atherosclerotic coronary arteries induced by increases in heart rate. Circulation 81:850, 1990.
30. Kumpuris AG, Luchi RJ, Waddel CC, Miller RR: Production of circulating platelet aggregates by exercise in coronary patients. Circulation 61:62, 1980.
31. Godet G, Coriat P, Baron JF, et al: Prevention of intraoperative myocardial ischemia during noncardiac surgery with intravenous diltiazem: A randomized trial versus placebo. Anesthesiology 6:241, 1987.
32. Rossen JD, Simonetti I, Marcus ML, et al: The effects of diltiazem on coronary flow reserve in humans. Circulation 80:1240, 1984.

33. Vrolix MC, Sironis D, Piessens JH, et al: Coronary hemodynamics and coronary flow reserve after intracoronary diltiazem in humans. Am J Cardiol 68:1633, 1991.
34. Physicians' Desk Reference. Medical Economics Data, Montvale, NJ, 1997.
35. Mangano DT, Layug EL, Wallace A, et al: Effect of atenolol on mortality and cardiovascular morbidity after noncardiac surgery. N Engl J Med 335:1713, 1996.
36. Pasternack PF, Grossi EA, Baumann FG: Beta blockade to decrease silent myocardial ischemia during peripheral vascular surgery. Am J Surg 158:113, 1989.
37. Coriat P, Daloz M, Bousseau D, et al: Prevention of intraoperative myocardial ischemia. Anesthesiology 61:193, 1984.
38. Juneja R, Mehta Y, Mishra Y, Trehan N: Minimally invasive coronary artery surgery: Anesthetic considerations. J Cardiothorac Vasc Anesth 11:123, 1997.
39. Schmied H, Kurz A, Sessler DI, et al: Mild hypothermia increases blood loss and transfusion requirements during total hip arthroplasty. Lancet 347:289, 1996.
40. Kurz A, Sessler DI, Lenhardt R: Perioperative normothermia to reduce the incidence of surgical wound infection. N Engl J Med 334:1209, 1996.
41. Frank SM, Fleisher LA, Breslow MJ, et al: Perioperative maintenance of normothermia reduces the incidence of morbid cardiac events: A randomized clinical trial. JAMA 277:1127, 1997.
42. Frank SM, Beattie C, Christopherson R, et al: Unintentional hypothermia as associated with postoperative myocardial ischemia. Anesthesiology 78:468, 1993.
43. Metzger SE, Lam J, Harris A, et al: Intraoperative forced-air warming decreases emergence time and operating room costs. Anesth Analg 84(Suppl):S44, 1997.
44. Cheney FW: Should normothermia be maintained during major surgery? JAMA 277:1165, 1997.
45. Barash PG: Monitoring myocardial ischemia: A sequential clinical approach. Lecture 222. American Society of Anesthesiologists 1996 Annual Refresher Course Lectures, Park Ridge, IL.
46. Eisenberg MJ, et al: Monitoring for myocardial ischemia during noncardiac surgery. A technology assessment of transesophageal echocardiography and a twelve-lead electrocardiography. The Study of Perioperative Ischemia Research Group. JAMA 268: 210, 1992.
47. Tuman KJ, McCarthy RJ, Spiess BD, et al: Effect of pulmonary artery catheter on outcome in patients undergoing coronary artery bypass. Anesthesiology 70:199, 1989.
48. Lowenstein E: Review of recent information on myocardial ischemia. Lecture 234. American Society of Anesthesiologists 1996 Annual Refresher Course Lectures, Park Ridge, IL.
49. Jain U, Laflamme C, Ghoshol S, et al: The effect of cardiac injury during coronary artery bypass graft during CABG on LOS. Anesth Analg 84(Suppl):S162, 1997.
50. Cahalan MK: Current role of transesophageal echocardiography. Lecture 172. American Society of Anesthesiologists 1996 Annual Refresher Course Lectures, Park Ridge, IL.
51. Connors AF, McCaffre DR, Gray BA: Evaluation of right-heart catheterization in the critically ill patient without acute MI. N Engl J Med 308:263, 1983.
52. Mimoz O: Pulmonary artery catheterization in crtically ill patients: A prospective analysis of outcome changes and catheter-prompted changes in therapy. Crit Care Med 22:573, 1994.
53. ASA Task Force on pulmonary artery catheterization: Practice guidelines for pulmonary artery catheterization. Anesthesiology 78:380, 1993.
54. Tuman KJ, Roizen MF: Outcome assessment and PA catheterization. Why does the debate continue? Anesth Analg 84:1, 1997.
55. Savage RM, et al: Intraoperative echocardiography is indicated in high-risk coronary artery surgery. Anesth Analg 82(Suppl): SCA25, 1996.
56. Smith JS, et al: Intraoperative detection of myocardial ischemia in high-risk patients: Electrocardiography versus two-dimensional transesophageal echocardiography. Circulation 72:1015, 1985.
57. Rouine-Rapp K, et al: Comparison of segmental wall motion analysis by anesthesiologists and an echocardiographer. Anesth Analg 76(Suppl):361, 1993.
58. Urbanowicz JH, Kernoff RS, Oppenheim G, et al: Transesophageal echocardiography and its potential for esophageal damage. Anesthesiology 72:40, 1990.
59. Kawahito S, Kitahata H, Kimura H, Oshita S: Recurrent laryngeal nerve palsy after cardiovascular surgery—relationship to the placement of transesophageal echo probe. Anesthesiology 85(Suppl):S159, 1996.
60. Benumof JL: Anesthesia for Thoracic Surgery, 2nd ed. Philadelphia, WB Saunders Co, 1995.
61. VanKeer L, VanAken H, Vandermeersch E, et al: Propofol does not inhibit hypoxic pulmonary vasoconstriction in humans. J Clin Anesth 1:284, 1989.
62. Spies C, Zaune U, Pauli MHF, et al: Comparison of enflurane and propofol during thoracic surgery. Anesthetist 40:14, 1991.
63. Reid CW, Slinger PD, Len IS, Orlanis S: A comparison of the effects of propofol-alfentanil versus isoflurane anesthesia on arterial oxygenation during one-long ventilation. J Cardiothorac Vasc Anesth 10:860, 1996.
64. Dougherty P, Hannallah M: A potentially serious complication that resulted from the use of the Univent tube. Anesthesiology 77:835, 1992.
65. Murry CE, Jennings RB, Reimer KA: Preconditioning with ischemia: A delay of lethal cell injury in ischemic myocardium. Circulation 74:1124, 1986.
66. Lange R, Ingwall J, Hale SL, et al: Effects of recurrent ischemia on myocardial high energy phosphate content in canine hearts. Basic Res Cardiol 79:469, 1984.
67. Reimer KA, Murry CE, Yamasawa I, et al: Four brief periods of ischemia cause no cumulative ATP loss or necrosis. Am J Physiol 251:H1306, 1986.
68. Murry CE, Jennings RB, Reimer KA: Preconditioning with ischemia: A delay of lethal cell injury in ischemic myocardia. Circulation 75:1124, 1986.
69. Cohen MV, Liu GS, Downey JM: Preconditioning causes improved wall motion as well as smaller infarcts after transient coronary occlusion in rabbits. Circulation 84:341, 1991.
70. Murry CE, Jennings RB, Reimer KA: In Przyklenk K, Kloner RA, Yellon DM (eds): What is Ischemic Preconditioning: A Concept of Endogenous Cardioprotection. Norwell, MA, Kluwer Academic, 1995.
71. Yoshika WA, Noa T, Inoue S, Abe S, et al: Acute myocardial infarction without warning: Clinical characteristics and significance of preinfarction angina. Cardiology 82:42, 1993.
72. Nakagawa Y, Ito H, Kitakaze M, et al: Effect of angina pectoris on myocardial protection in patients with reperfused anterior wall myocardial infarction: Retrospective clinical evidence of preconditioning. J Am Coll Cardiol 25:1076, 1995.
73. Ottani F, Galvani M, Ferrini D, et al: Prodromal angina limits infarct size: A role for ischemic preconditioning. Circulation 91: 291, 1995.
74. Yellon DM, Alkhulaifi AM, Pugsley WB: Preconditioning the human myocardium. Lancet 342:276, 1933.
75. Cleveland JC, Meldrum DR, Rowland RT, et al: Preconditioning and hypothermic cardioplegia protect human heart equally against ischemia. Ann Thorac Surg 63:147, 1997.
76. Deutsch E, Berger M, Kussmaul WG, et al: Adaptation to ischemia during percutaneous transluminal coronary angioplasty: Clinical, hemodynamic and metabolic features. Circulation 82: 2004, 1990.
77. Tomai F, Crea F, Gaspardone A, et al: Ischemic preconditioning during coronary angioplasty prevented by glibenclamide, a selective ATP-sensitive large K^+ channel blocker. Circulation 90: 700, 1994.
78. Downey JM, Liu GS, Thornton JD: Adenosine and the anti-infarct effects of preconditioning. Cardiovasc Res 27:3, 1993.
79. Vegh A, Szekeres L, Parratt JR: Protective effects of preconditioning of the ischemic myocardium involves cyclooxygenase products. Cardioavasc Res 24:1020, 1990.
80. Li Y, Whittaker P, Klonar RA: The transient nature of the effect of ischemic preconditioning on myocardial infarct size and ventricular arrhythmias. Am Heart J 123:346, 1992.
81. Martin HB, Walter CL: Preconditioning: An endogenous defense against the insult of myocardial ischemia. Anesth Analg 83:639, 1996.
82. Lasley RD, Mentzer RM: Preconditioning and its potential for myocardial protection during cardiac surgery. J Card Surg 10: 349, 1995.

83. Vroom MB, van Wezel HB: Myocardial stunning, hibernation, and ischemic preconditioning. J Cardiothorac Vasc Anesth 10: 789, 1996.
84. Yao Z, Gross GJ: A comparison of adenosine-induced cardioprotection and ischemic preconditioning in dogs. Efficacy, time course, in role of K-ATP channels. Circulation 89:1229, 1994.
85. Raley FE: Neuroaxial anesthesia should not be used in patients undergoing heparinization for surgery. J Cardiothorac Vasc Anesth 10:957, 1996.
86. Vandermeulen ET, van Aken H, Vermylen S: Anticoagulants and spinal-epidural anesthesia. Anesth Analg 79:1165, 1994.
87. Molier R, Covino BG: Cardiac electrophysiologic properties of bupivacaine and lidocaine compared with those of ropivacaine, a new amide anesthetic. Anesthesiology 72:322, 1990.
88. Scott DB, et al: Acute toxicity of ropivacaine compared with bupivacaine. Anesth Analg 69:563, 1989.
89. Johnson MD, Mickles J, Arthur GR, et al: Bupivacaine with and without epinephrine for intercostal nerve block. J Cardiothorac Vasc Anesth 4:102, 1990.
90. Bloomberg S, Emanuelsson H, Kvist H, et al: The effects of thoracic epidural anesthesia on coronary arteries and in arterioles in patients with coronary disease. Anesthesiology 73:840, 1990.
91. Benumof JL: Anesthesia for Thoracic Surgery, 2nd ed. Philadelphia, WB Saunders Co, 1995.
92. Ferrante FM, VadeBoncouer TR: Epidural and subarachnoid analgesia for thoracic surgery. In Gravlee GP, Rauck RL (eds): Pain Management In Cardiothoracic Surgery. Philadelphia, JB Lippincott Co, 1993.
93. Gwirtz KH, Young JV, Walker SG, et al: Intrathecal opioid analgesia for acute postoperative pain: Experience with 4,135 surgical patients at Indiana University Hospitals (Abstract). Anesthesiology 83(Suppl):A730, 1995.
94. Varrassi G, Panella L, Piroli A, et al: The effects of perioperative ketorolac infusion on postoperative pain and endocrine-metabolic response. Anesth Analg 78:514, 1994.
95. Calafiore AM, Giammarco GD, Teodori G, et al: Left anterior descending coronary artery grafting via left anterior small thoracotomy without cardiopulmonary bypass. Ann Thorac Surg 61: 1658, 1996.
96. Calafiore AM, Angelini GD, Bergsland J, Salenro T: Minimally invasive coronary artery bypass grafting. Ann Thorac Surg 62: 1545, 1996.
97. Arom KV, Emery RW, Nicoloff DM: Mini-sternotomy for coronary artery bypass grafting. Ann Thorac Surg 61:1271, 1996.
98. Boonstra TW, Grandjean JG, Mariani MA: Improved method for direct coronary grafting without CPB via anterolateral small thoracotomy. Ann Thorac Surg 63:567, 1997.
99. Landreneau RJ, Mack MJ, Magovern JA, et al: "Keyhole" coronary artery bypass surgery. Ann Surg 224:453, 1996.
100. Robinson MC, Gross DR, Zeman W, Stede-Larsen E: Minimally invasive coronary artery bypass grafting: A new method using an anterior mediastinotomy. J Card Surg 10:529, 1995.
101. Hensley FA: Minimally invasive myocardial revascularization surgery: Here to stay? J Cardiothorac Vasc Anesth 10:445, 1996.
102. Jones EL, Weintraub WS: The importance of completeness of revascularization during long-term follow-up after coronary artery operations. J Thorac Cardiovasc Surg 112:227, 1996.
103. O'Connor CJ, McCarthy RJ, McCarthy WE, et al: Coronary artery bypass surgery in the 1990's: Has outcome changed? Anesthesiology 85(Suppl):A164, 1996.

CHAPTER 16

Valvular Heart Disease

William Zimmerman, M.D.
Joseph P. Mathew, M.D.
Paul Barash, M.D.

Patients with valvular heart disease represent a population in whom appropriate anesthetic care demands a thorough understanding of the pathophysiology of the valvular lesion as well as the interaction with anesthetic agents. This chapter is organized by valvular lesion, and for each lesion there is a discussion of etiology, symptoms, pathophysiology, laboratory data, medical management, and hemodynamic goals. The preoperative hemodynamic considerations for each lesion are specific and are presented both in the text and in table form. The mnemonic PARCOR ("par for the heart") is listed for each valvular lesion and will assist in the understanding of the preoperative preparation and anesthetic concerns of these patients (Table 16–1). In addition, pressure-volume loops and echocardiograms are displayed. Since the premedication, anesthetic techniques, and monitoring strategies are similar in all the lesions, these areas will be discussed at the end of the chapter. Antibiotic prophylaxis and anticoagulation in patients with valvular heart disease will also be presented.

Preoperative Assessment

Aortic Stenosis

Isolated aortic stenosis is the most common valvular lesion.[1] Causes of aortic stenosis in a surgical population are congenital bicuspid aortic valve (38%), degenerative calcification (33%), postinflammatory fibrocalcific disease resulting primarily as a consequence of rheumatic fever (24%), congenitally unicommissural aortic valve (2%), hypoplastic (1%), and indeterminate (2%).[2] Obstruction to left ventricular outflow can also occur above (supravalvular aortic stenosis) or below the valve (hypertrophic obstructive cardiomyopathy). Present in 1 to 2% of the population, bicuspid aortic valves usually become stenotic over time from repeated trauma and fibrosis. Likewise, degenerative calcification is the result of a lifetime of "wear and tear." The latency period is 48 ± 6 years for bicuspid aortic stenosis, 66 ± 12 years for degenerative aortic stenosis, and 39 ± 18 years for rheumatic aortic stenosis.[3]

Symptoms usually are not present unless aortic stenosis is severe (i.e., adult valve area <0.75 cm^2 or 0.5 cm^2/m^2 of body surface area in children). During the latency period, patients are at a small risk of sudden death (<2% per year)[4] and infective endocarditis (<1% per year).[5] However, once symptoms occur, morbidity is high. Mean survival is 45 ± 13 months after the onset of anginal symptoms, 27 ± 15 months after syncope, and 11 ± 10 months after left ventricular failure.[3] The incidence of sudden death can exceed 10% per year in symptomatic patients.[4] Longevity is greatly improved by valve replacement with survival of 75% at 5 years, 61% at 10 years, and 49% at 15 years in a representative series.[6] Congestive heart failure as a result of diastolic and/or systolic dysfunction, angina pectoris as a result of the increased oxygen demand of a hypertrophied myocardium, and syncope as a result of hypotension from decreased cardiac output or transient arrhythmias are the classic triad of symptoms. Sudden death is likely the result of arrhythmias.

On physical examination, a characteristic loud, harsh, midsystolic crescendo-decrescendo murmur is heard best over the first or second right intercostal space.[7] The murmur's duration increases with increased stenosis except in a low-cardiac-output state. Palpation reveals an arterial pulse that has a slow rate of rise, anacrotism, and a low, delayed peak (parvus et tardus pulse). The electrocardiogram (ECG) is consistent with left ventricular hypertrophy (LVH) in 70 to 80% of patients with significant stenosis. Left atrial hypertrophy, seen as a negative P-terminal force in V_1 is evident in 80% of patients' ECGs. The rhythm is usually sinus until late in the course of the disease. The chest roentgenogram exam can be completely normal; however, subtle abnormalities are often present. There may be rounding of the left ventricular apex, atrial enlargement, a moderately enlarged cardiac silhouette, pulmonary edema, poststenotic dilation of the aorta, and calcification of the aortic valve.

TABLE 16–1
Definition of the Mnemonic PARCOR

P	Preload
A	Afterload
R	Heart rate
C	Contractility
O	Oxygen balance (myocardial)
R	Rhythm

An echocardiographic exam provides information about the type of valve pathology, valve area, pressure gradient, extent of left ventricular hypertrophy, and ventricular function (Fig. 16–1). Valve area and the pressure gradient across the aortic valve are commonly used to classify the degree of stenosis. Using the valve area method, hemodynamically significant or "moderate" aortic stenosis occurs when the normal valve area of 2.6 to 3.5 cm^2 is reduced by approximately 30% to 1.0 cm^2. Stenosis is classified as "severe" when the valve area is less than 0.75 cm^2 and "critical" when the valve area is less than 0.4 cm^2. The second method of classification employs echocardiographically measured transvalvular velocities to determine systolic pressure gradients. A left ventricular–aortic gradient less than 25 mm Hg is "mild" stenosis, between 25 and 50 mm Hg is "moderate" stenosis, and above 50 mm Hg is "severe" stenosis. Unlike valve area, which is a "fixed" value, the pressure gradient is dependent on flow velocities across the valve (i.e., cardiac output). Therefore, if contractile function is below normal, as with a failing ventricle, the pressure gradient classification will underestimate the degree of stenosis.

Cardiac catheterization is associated with a mortality rate of 0.19% in patients with aortic valve disease.[8] Catheterization provides information on pressure gradients, left ventricular end-diastolic pressures, ejection fraction, and associated coronary artery disease. Valve area is computed from the measured pressure gradient using the Gorlin formula.[9] The following patients should have coronary angiography prior to valve replacement: patients with coronary risk factors,[10] patients without angina but older than 50 years,[11] and asymptomatic patients between the ages of 35 and 50 without risk factors if they are catheterized for other reasons.[12]

Patients with aortic stenosis must be closely monitored for progression of valvular stenosis and deterioration of left ventricular function so that surgery can be performed at the optimal time. Patients with severe stenosis and angina, syncope, or congestive heart failure are referred for surgery. Asymptomatic patients with severe stenosis and evidence of significant left ventricular dysfunction are also referred for surgery.[13] Patients with severe stenosis but without symptoms or evidence of significant left ventricular failure are still at risk for sudden death and some physicians recommend surgery. The operative mortality of aortic valve replacement for isolated aortic stenosis is less than 5% at major centers.[14,15] Factors that increase operative mortality are emergency operation, patient age older than 70 years, and previous cardiac operation.[16,17] After valve replacement, improvement in dysfunctional ventricles will normalize ejection fraction in 60% of patients.[18]

The heart compensates for aortic stenosis through concentric hypertrophy of the left ventricle, which maintains wall tension and thus preserves the efficiency of the heart (Fig. 16–2). However, hypertrophy also produces diastolic dysfunction and left ventricular filling becomes dependent on atrial contraction. Patients also become susceptible to angina from increased demand for oxygen by the hypertrophied myocardiogram and reduced coronary perfusion pressure as a result of elevated end-diastolic pressures. Only 60% of aortic stenosis patients with chest pain have significant coronary artery disease.[19] In chronic aortic stenosis, the intrinsic contractility of the myocytes diminishes and the left ventricle fails.

The hemodynamic goals for the patient with aortic stenosis are summarized in Table 16–2. The left ventricle must have adequate filling volumes and pressures to function optimally, and since the hypertrophied left ventricle has reduced compliance, adequate filling pressures are usually higher than normal. Furthermore, since the stenotic aortic valve limits increases in cardiac output in response to decreases in systemic vascular resistance (SVR), maintenance of a normal or increased SVR is essential to maintain systemic blood pressure and cardiac perfusion pressure. High heart rates reduce coronary

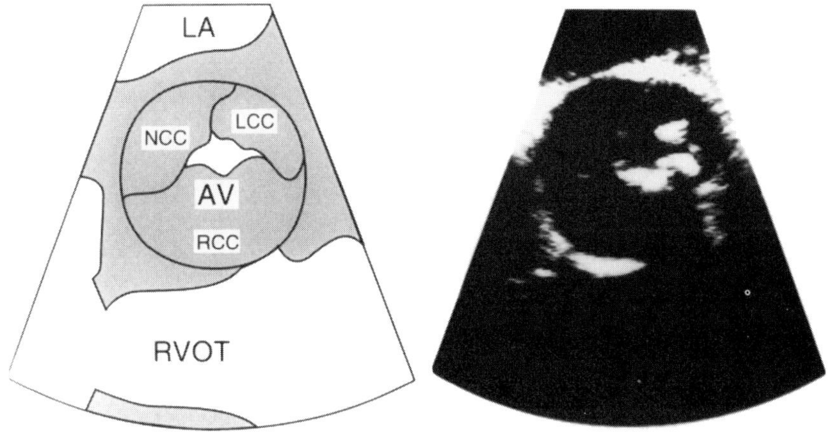

FIGURE **16–1.** Transverse plane echocardiographic image of aortic stenosis. LA, left atrium; AV, aortic valve; RVOT, right ventricular outflow tract; NCC, noncoronary cusp; RCC, right coronary cusp; LCC, left coronary cusp. (From Rafferty TD: Basics of Transesophageal Echocardiography. New York, Churchill Livingstone, 1995, p 167, with permission.)

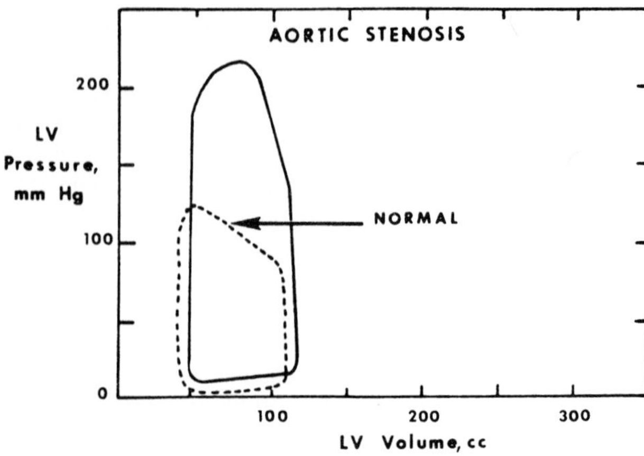

FIGURE **16–2.** Pressure-volume loop for aortic stenosis. LV, left ventricular. (From Jackson JM, Thomas SJ, Lowenstein E: Anesthetic management of patients with valvular heart disease. Semin Anesth 1: 239, 1982, with permission.)

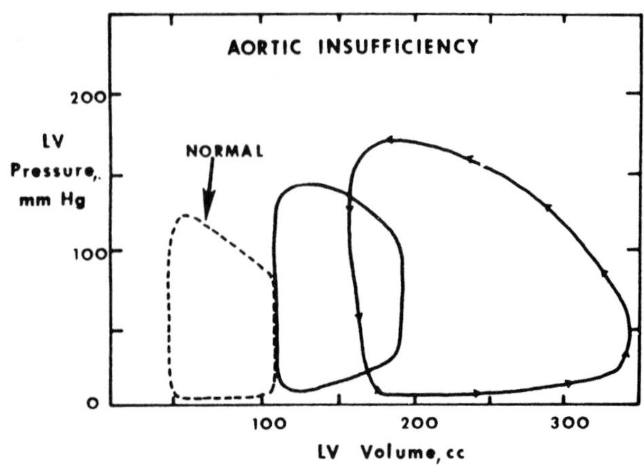

FIGURE **16–3.** Pressure-volume loop for acute and chronic aortic regurgitation. LV, left ventricular. (From Jackson JM, Thomas SJ, Lowenstein E: Anesthetic management of patients with valvular heart disease: Semin Anesth 1:239, 1982, with permission.)

flow and can lead to ischemia. Maintenance of sinus rhythm is important not only for stability of heart rate, but also for preservation of the left atrial contribution to left ventricular filling.

Aortic Regurgitation

Approximately 10% of patients with valvular heart disease have aortic insufficiency. A review of 225 patients who received aortic valve replacement during 1965, 1970, 1975, and 1980 showed the overall causes of insufficiency to be postinflammatory disease (46%), aortic root dilation (21%), incomplete closure of a congenitally bicuspid aortic valve (20%), infective endocarditis (9%), ventricular septal defects (2%), quadricuspid aortic valves (1%), and indeterminate (1%). Except for postinflammatory and indeterminate types, aortic insufficiency was much more common in males. The incidence of postinflammatory disease decreased with time and for patients presenting in 1980, aortic root dilation (37%) was more prevalent than postinflammatory disease (29%).[20] Acute aortic insufficiency is usually produced by infective endocarditis, but a traumatic tear of the cusp supporting structures can also result in acute aortic regurgitation.

Aortic regurgitation volume overloads the left ventricle with diastolic flow through the incompetent aortic valve in addition to filling from the left atrium (Fig. 16–3). In chronic aortic regurgitation, eccentric hypertrophy of the left ventricle maintains nearly normal left ventricle end-diastolic pressure (LVEDP) and wall stress until the left ventricle decompensates. Eccentric hypertrophy increases both the ventricular radius and the wall thickness, and can increase the weight of the heart to as much as 1,000 gm. The increase in radius enables the left ventricle to accept greatly increased diastolic filling (left ventricular end-diastolic volume can be three to four times normal) while maintaining LVEDP near normal limits. The markedly enlarged hearts found in patients with chronic aortic regurgitation are appropriately named "cor bovinum" (cow heart). When contractility is measured in asymptomatic patients with moderate to severe aortic regurgitation using the slope of left ventricular end-systolic pressure-volume relationship, the contractility was significantly lower in patients with aortic regurgitation than in normal patients.[21] In acute aortic regurgitation, the compensatory mechanism of eccentric hypertrophy cannot be utilized. Consequently LVEDP is high, and the left ventricle operates on the steepest portion of the Frank-Starling curve. Often the left ventricular diastolic pressure exceeds the left atrial pressure prior to the end of diastole, which causes the mitral valve to close before the end of diastole.

Patients with acute aortic regurgitation develop sudden cardiovascular collapse. In patients with chronic aortic regurgitation there is an asymptomatic period of approximately 10 years. The first symptoms to develop are exertional dyspnea, palpitations, and an uncomfortable awareness of the heart beats. With disease progression,

TABLE **16–2**
Management of Aortic Stenosis

Preload	Increase to distend the stiff ventricle
Afterload	Decrease is hazardous
Rate	Slow (increase in rate can produce ischemia)
Contractility	Decreased
Oxygen balance	Increased demand as a result of increase in LV mass
Rhythm	Sinus

LV, left ventricular.

the patient develops orthopnea and paroxysmal nocturnal dyspnea. Nocturnal angina with diaphoresis may also occur, the result of low blood pressure during slower heart rates. Abdominal pain from splanchnic ischemia may also be present.

On physical exam, the systolic arterial pressure is increased and the diastolic pressure is decreased, producing a widened pulse pressure; however, as the heart fails, increases in systemic vascular resistance raises the diastolic pressure, which decreases with pulse pressure. The arterial pressure rises abruptly, producing the "water-hammer" pulse, and falls rapidly during late systole. This characteristic pulse can be visualized in the rhythmic movement of the large arteries, head, uvula, and larynx. With auscultation, a diastolic, high-pitched, decrescendo murmur is heard in the left parasternal second or third intercostal space with the patient sitting and leaning forward. Often a low-pitched, middiastolic rumble is heard at the apex, the Austin Flint murmur, which is probably the result of the regurgitant jet producing anterior mitral leaflet shuddering.

Patients with chronic aortic regurgitation are usually in sinus rhythm. Left ventricular volume overload produces a left axis and Q waves in leads I, aVL, V_3, and V_4. With time the Q waves diminish and a pattern of left ventricular hypertrophy prevails. The presence of ST-segment depression and T-wave inversions may predict impaired survival.[22] Conduction defects, such as bundle branch blocks, occur late in the disease course and are associated with left ventricular dysfunction. Dilation and elongation of the ascending aorta and an increased cardiothoracic ratio are usually seen on chest x-ray. Patients with acute aortic regurgitation have nonspecific ST and T-wave changes, but usually do not have evidence of left ventricular hypertrophy.

The presence, severity, and cause of aortic regurgitation can be determined with both transesophageal and transthoracic echocardiography (Fig. 16–4). Regurgitation is usually described as the ratio of the width of the regurgitant jet to the width of the left ventricular outflow tract.[23] Based on this ratio, aortic regurgitation is classified as: Grade I = less than or equal to 0.24, Grade II = ratio 0.25 to 0.46, Grade III = ratio 0.47 to 0.64, Grade IV = greater than or equal to 0.65. Aortography provides the best method of demonstrating the dynamics and estimating the severity of aortic regurgitation. Invasive evaluation is indicated when patients are symptomatic, the cardiothoracic ratio exceeds 0.55, ECG repolarization disturbances are present, left ventricular transverse diameter shortening (as measured by echocardiography) is below 30%, or the left ventricular end-diastolic diameter exceeds 70 mm.[24]

Once aortic regurgitation is symptomatic, patients treated medically have a 75% 5-year survival and a 50% 10-year survival.[25] Asymptomatic patients can have a latency period as long as 30 years; however, rare sudden death has occurred. Surgery can improve longevity and in one series, patients with a normal ejection fraction had a 96% 5-year survival. Patients with subnormal ejection fractions had a 63% 5-year survival, and patients with a subnormal ejection fraction and poor exercise tolerance had a 52% 5-year survival.[26]

Patients with acute aortic regurgitation require prompt surgery, since early death from left ventricular failure is frequent. Patients with chronic aortic regurgitation can be managed with afterload reduction; however, those with severe aortic regurgitation, progressive left ventricular enlargement, and LVH by ECG are referred for surgery. The average operative mortality for aortic valve replacement is 6% and the average 5-year survival is 77%.[27]

The preoperative hemodynamic findings are summarized in Table 16–3. Patients with aortic regurgitation often have ventricular dysfunction and consequently are dependent on adequate preload to maximize contractility and cardiac output. LVEDP should be maintained in the normal range (8 to 12 mm Hg) and blood loss must be quickly replaced to maintain stable hemodynamics. If elevated, afterload should be normalized in order to maximize forward cardiac output by increasing stroke volume and decreasing the regurgitant fraction. However, coronary perfusion pressure must be maintained; and although a low diastolic pressure decreases the regurgitant fraction, it also decreases coronary perfusion. Patients generally benefit from a heart rate of 80 bpm. Even though an elevated heart rate reduces the regurgitant volume and stroke volume such that the regurgitant fraction remains unchanged, tachycardia decreases left ventricular end-diastolic pressure. This reduces wall tension and increases coronary perfusion pressure with a

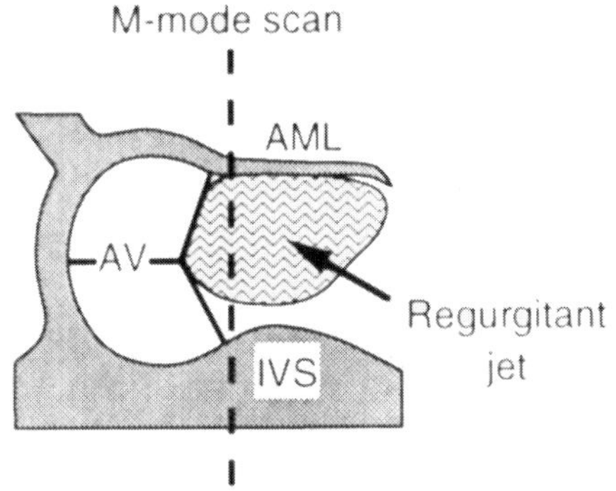

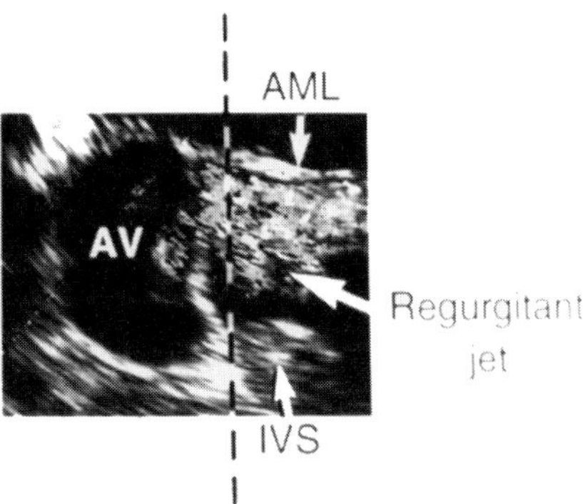

FIGURE **16–4.** Color M-mode examination of aortic regurgitation presented in black and white. AV, aortic valve; AML, anterior mitral leaflet; IVS, interventricular septum. (From Rafferty TD: Basics of Transesophageal Echocardiography. New York, Churchill Livingstone, 1995, p 32, with permission.)

TABLE 16–3
Management of Aortic Regurgitation

Preload	Maintain preload
Afterload	Vasodilator beneficial
Rate	Prevent slow rate (≥80 bpm)
Contractility	Decreased in chronic
Oxygen balance	Increased demand as a result of increase in LV mass
Rhythm	Sinus

bpm, beats per minute; LV, left ventricular.

minimal increase in oxygen demand from the tachycardia. An elevated heart rate is especially important in patients with acute aortic regurgitation. Since patients with acute aortic regurgitation do not have the benefit of eccentric hypertrophy, an increase in the length of diastole (bradycardia) will allow the LVEDP to rise excessively and distend the left ventricle. It may be unwise, however, to induce tachycardia in an otherwise stable patient. Contractility is often compromised in both acute and chronic aortic regurgitation. Sinus rhythm should be maintained if possible, and bradycardia and junctional rhythms should be appropriately treated. In both chronic and acute aortic regurgitation, an intra-aortic balloon pump (IABP) is contraindicated, since diastolic augmentation increases aortic regurgitation.

Mitral Stenosis

Mitral stenosis is the result of postinflammatory disease in 99% of cases. The remaining 1% of cases are congenital in origin.[28] Rheumatic fever is the presumed cause of most postinflammatory disease even though only 50% of these patients have a clear history of rheumatic fever. Women are more predisposed to mitral stenosis with 73% of postinflammatory mitral stenosis being found in females.[28]

After the initial attack of rheumatic fever, patients are usually asymptomatic for 20 to 25 years. Patients with mild disability (New York Heart Association [NYHA] Class II) progress to severe disability (NYHA Class III or IV) in approximately 5 years.[29] The 10- and 20-year survival rates are 69% and 49% in Class II patients, 33% and 0% in Class III, and 0% in Class IV.[30] With surgery a 95% 5-year survival and an 85% 7-year survival can be achieved.[31]

Mitral stenosis causes a pressure gradient across the mitral valve that increases left atrial pressure with subsequent pulmonary congestion. Patients with mitral stenosis are asymptomatic until the mitral valve area has decreased from a normal 4 to 6 cm^2 to 2 cm^2. With this degree of narrowing, heavy exercise produces dyspnea that resolves quickly upon rest. With a valve area of 1.5 cm^2, moderate exertion will produce dyspnea, and with a valve area of 1.2 cm^2, most patients are symptomatic with activities of daily living. As the valve area falls below 1.0 cm^2, the patient may have pulmonary edema at rest. Emotional stress, pregnancy, fever, paroxysmal atrial fibrillation are factors other than activity that can precipitate symptoms of congestive failure by increasing flow across the mitral valve and thus increasing the pressure gradient.

Mitral stenosis reduces left ventricular preload and consequently left ventricular stroke volume (Fig. 16–5). In 40% of patients, anterior or posterior wall motion abnormalities have been described and 16% had ejection fractions below 50%.[32] The contractile dysfunction may be the result of rigid calcification of the mitral valve apparatus or fibrosis of the papillary muscles that is presumed to be the result of smoldering rheumatic fever. Paroxysmal atrial fibrillation is usually seen with mild mitral stenosis, whereas chronic atrial fibrillation is associated with significant mitral stenosis. An acute elevation in left atrial pressure can produce hemoptysis from rupture of small bronchial veins. Left atrial enlargement, enlarged tracheobronchial lymph nodes, and a dilated pulmonary artery may produce hoarseness through compression of the recurrent laryngeal nerve (Ortner's syndrome). Approximately 10% of patients with mitral stenosis experience anginal type chest pain not attributable to coronary artery disease.[33] With disease progression, an elevated pulmonary vascular resistance (PVR) can produce right ventricular failure.

Mitral stenosis patients who have developed elevated pulmonary vascular resistance have a typical appearance called "mitral facies." The pink-purple patches on the cheeks are cyanotic skin changes from low cardiac output. As cardiac output falls, systemic vascular resistance rises to maintain normal blood pressure; however, the palpable pulse becomes weak. The classic murmur of

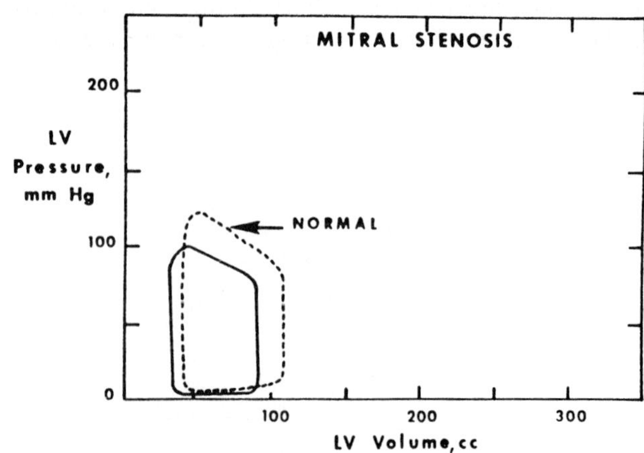

FIGURE 16–5. Pressure-volume loop for mitral stenosis. LV, left ventricular. (From Jackson JM, Thomas SJ, Lowenstein E: Anesthetic management of patients with valvular heart disease: Semin Anesth 1: 239, 1982, with permission.)

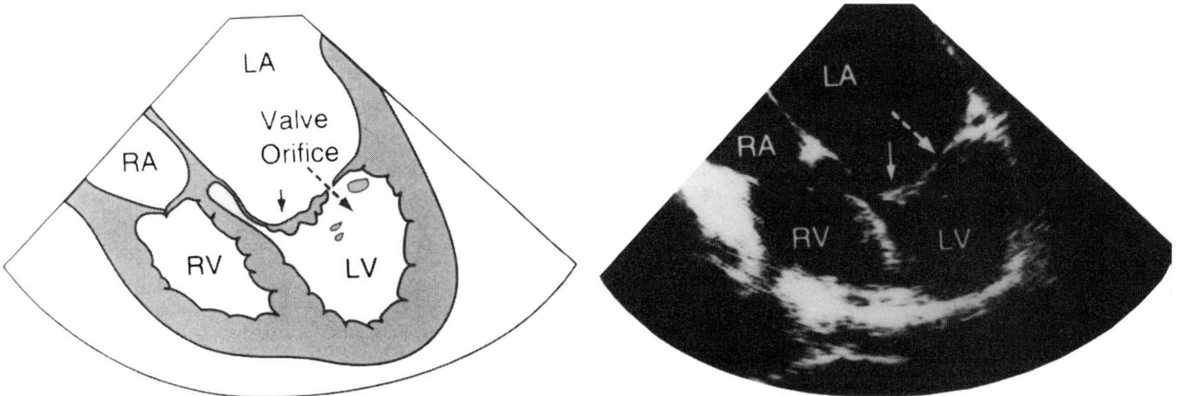

FIGURE **16–6.** Transverse plane echocardiographic image of mitral stenosis. LA, left atrium, LV, left ventricle; RA, right atrium, RV, right ventricle. (From Rafferty TD: Basics of Transesophageal Echocardiography. New York, Churchill Livingstone, 1995, p 147, with permission.)

mitral stenosis is low-pitched, rumbling, and localized to the apical area. It is heard best with the patient in the left lateral recumbent position using the bell of the stethoscope. With disease progression, the murmur is heard throughout diastole and atrial contraction produces presystolic accentuation of the murmur. The murmur intensity increases with maneuvers that increase left atrial pressure (i.e., exercise, squatting, expiration). The P-mitrale pattern on ECG consisting of a wide, notched P wave (>0.12 second) in leads I and II and a flat, biphasic or inverted P wave in lead III is found in 90% of patients with significant mitral stenosis. The underlying rhythm is frequently atrial fibrillation. ECG evidence of right ventricular hypertrophy may be seen. Left atrial enlargement and pulmonary venous congestion are evident on chest x-ray. If mitral stenosis and the resultant left atrial enlargement are not severe, atrial fibrillation should be cardioverted to sinus rhythm after 4 weeks of anticoagulation.

An echocardiographic exam can aid in the diagnosis of mitral stenosis and provide an estimate of valve area (Fig. 16–6). Estimating the valve area uses the pressure half-time—the time required for the blood flow velocity across the mitral valve to decrease to 50% of the peak velocity. Normal pressure half-times are 20 to 60 msec, but in mitral stenosis, they range from 100 to 400 msec. The valve area is then computed by dividing 220 by the pressure half-time. Although echocardiographically derived pressure gradients correlate closely with those obtained at catheterization, this measurement varies too much with cardiac output to be a reliable estimate of valve area. Other echocardiographic findings associated with mitral stenosis include an enlarged left atrium (>4.0 cm), spontaneous echo contrast ("smoke") in the left atrium, and thrombi in the left atrial appendage.

Surgical recommendations for NYHA Class II patients must be individualized and must consider the patient's activity level. In general, Class II patients with valve areas greater than 1.0 cm^2/m^2 body surface area (BSA) are deferred; whereas, Class II patients with valve areas less than 1.0 cm^2/m^2 BSA receive surgical correction. Pregnant patients should receive surgical correction only if they have significant pulmonary congestion despite maximal medical therapy. Open mitral commissurotomy is preferred in the United States, and mortality ranges from 1 to 3%. The commissurotomy is palliative and in time symptoms will recur. At 10 years, 56% of patients who have undergone commissurotomy had functional limitations but only 50% of these patients had evidence of restenosis.[34] Often, repair is not possible during a second operation, and mitral valve replacement is required.

The preoperative hemodynamic considerations for mitral stenosis are summarized in Table 16–4. Since mitral stenosis produces a pressure gradient across the mitral valve, and consequently inhibits left ventricular filling while raising left atrial pressure, the patient can be in pulmonary edema with low left ventricular end-diastolic pressures. Patients with mitral stenosis are frequently hypovolemic as a result of diuretic use. A normal systemic vascular resistance should be maintained, since decreases in SVR produce tachycardia and increases in SVR produce left ventricular dysfunction. Heart rates in the range of 80 bpm usually maximize cardiac output. Tachycardia decreases diastolic time and thus flow

TABLE **16–4**
Management of Mitral Stenosis

Preload	Maintain preload (presents hypovolemic)
Afterload	Increase is poorly tolerated
Rate	About 80 bpm, tachycardia and bradycardia decrease CO
Contractility	Normal
Oxygen balance	Normal
Rhythm	Atrial fibrillation (ventricular response <80 bpm)

CO, cardiac output; bpm, beats per minute.

across the mitral and aortic valve (cardiac output). Approximately a third of mitral stenosis patients will come to surgery in atrial fibrillation. The ventricular response rate in these patients must also be maintained at less than 80 bpm. The PVR should be kept as low as possible to prevent right ventricular failure. Hypoxia, hypercarbia, hypothermia, acidosis, and catecholamine release all increase PVR.

Mitral Regurgitation

Mitral regurgitation can result from disruption of the mitral annulus, mitral leaflets, chordae tendinae, or papillary muscles. An analysis of 97 surgical patients revealed the etiology of mitral regurgitation to be myxomatous degeneration in 62%, ischemia in 30%, infective endocarditis in 5%, and rheumatic fever in 3%.[35] Ischemia can produce regurgitation as a result of papillary muscle dysfunction or left ventricular dilatation. The posterior papillary muscle is supplied by the posterior descending artery and is more vulnerable to ischemia than the anterior papillary muscle, which is supplied by a diagonal and/or a marginal artery. Dilation of the mitral annulus in cardiomyopathy will also produce mitral regurgitation.

Patients with mild mitral regurgitation may be asymptomatic their entire lives. Acute mitral regurgitation (e.g., papillary muscle rupture) produces a sudden volume overload and raises left ventricular end-diastolic and left atrial pressures. The systolic flow into the left atrium markedly elevates left atrial pressure, produces a prominent v wave, and may produce pulmonary edema. With chronic mitral regurgitation, the elevated LVEDP produces eccentric hypertrophy. The left atrium also enlarges, which allows the left atrium to accept the regurgitant volumes with minimal increases in pressure (Fig. 16–7). Eventually volume overload produces contractile dysfunction and the heart begins to decompensate. Surgery can produce a dramatic reduction in left ventricular mass and clinical symptoms. However, when the ventricular dimension at end-systole exceeds 2.6 cm/m^2, fractional shortening is less than 31%, or end-systolic wall stress exceeds 195 mm Hg, the patients remain symptomatic postoperatively and left ventricular mass remains unchanged.[36] A comparison of valve replacement versus medical management showed a 5-year survival of 75% versus 55% and a 10-year survival of 62% versus 22%.[37] In a study comparing valve replacement with repair, patients undergoing repair had improved mortality. The 5-year survival for repair was 91% versus 61% for valve replacement and the 10-year survival was 81% versus 39%.[38]

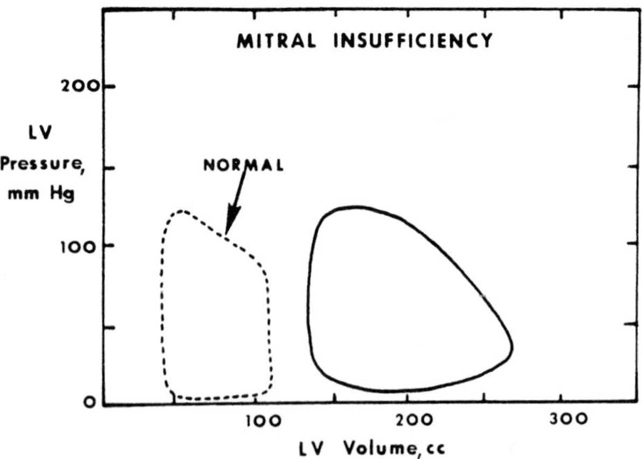

FIGURE **16–7.** Pressure-loop for mitral regurgitation. LV, left ventricular. (From Jackson JM, Thomas SJ, Lowenstein E: Anesthetic management of patients with valvular heart disease: Semin Anesth 1: 239, 1982, with permission.)

Patients usually become symptomatic with a sudden hemodynamic change such as the onset of atrial fibrillation or the rupture of chordae tendinae. Patients who develop symptoms complain of fatigue, progressive dyspnea, and orthopnea. Symptoms of right-sided failure such as painful hepatic congestion, ankle edema, distended neck veins, ascites, and tricuspid regurgitation may be present in patients with associated pulmonary vascular disease. Palpation reveals an apical impulse that is displaced laterally and caudally to the sixth intercostal space. The arterial pulse has a brisk upstroke but the amplitude is small. With auscultation a holosystolic blowing high-pitched murmur is heard loudest at the apex and can radiate to the axilla.

Patients with acute mitral regurgitation usually have sinus tachycardia. Patients with chronic mitral regurgitation have an enlarged left atrium that is seen as the P-mitrale pattern. Approximately two thirds of patients with chronic mitral regurgitation are in atrial fibrillation and 50% of ECGs show LVH. On the chest x-ray, patients with severe acute mitral regurgitation will have a normal cardiac silhouette with signs of pulmonary edema. Patients with chronic mitral regurgitation have an enlarged left atrium and ventricle.

Echocardiography can assess the severity of mitral regurgitation and determine the etiology in most cases (Fig. 16–8). Several criteria have been established to grade mitral regurgitation. One criterion, using color flow Doppler, compares the area of the regurgitant jet to the area of the left atrium. If the area of the regurgitant jet is less than 20% of the left atrial area, the regurgitation is graded as mild; between 20 and 40% the regurgitation is graded moderate; and when greater than 40%, the regurgitation is graded as severe.[39] The pulsed wave Doppler tracing of the pulmonary veins also provides an assessment of the degree of mitral regurgitation (Fig. 16–9). Normally, peak systolic flow is greater than diastolic flow. If peak diastolic flow is greater than systolic flow, either the left atrial pressures are elevated or mild to moderate mitral regurgitation is present. When systolic flow is negative (reversed), severe mitral regurgitation is present. Cardiac catheterization is considered the "gold standard," but with the advent of echocardiography, this test is not necessary for all patients. All patients with risk factors for coronary artery disease will benefit from catheterization to assess the need for bypass surgery.

Once patients become symptomatic, surgery is considered. The timing of surgery weighs the risk of damage to the left ventricle from disease progression versus the

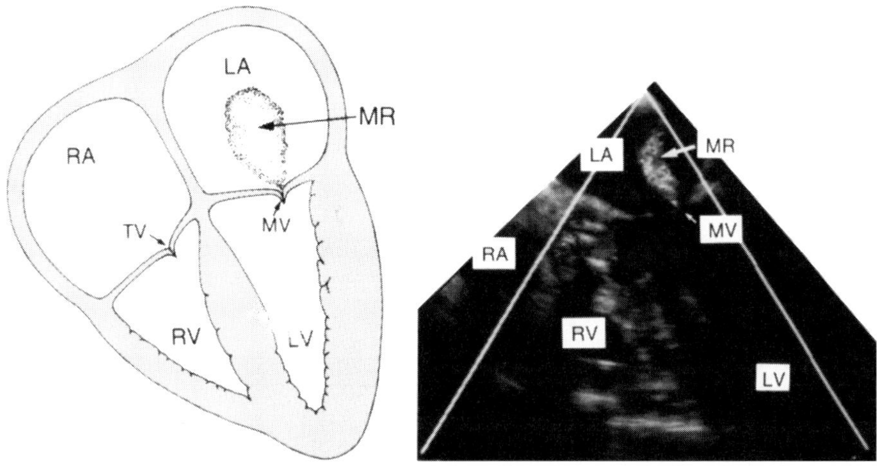

FIGURE **16–8.** Black-and-white print of mitral regurgitation defined by color flow Doppler examination. LA, left atrium, MV, mitral valve, MR, mitral regurgitation; LV, left ventricle; RA, right atrium, TV, tricuspid valve; RV, right ventricle. (From Rafferty TD: Basics of Transesophageal Echocardiography. New York, Churchill Livingstone, 1995, p 33, with permission.)

risks of the surgery itself. Valve repair as opposed to replacement should be performed when possible. The improved survival with valve repair is due to the excellent durability of a repair, a lower rate of infectious endocarditis, a lower incidence of postoperative thromboembolism, and better postoperative left ventricular function. Preservation of the chordae tendinae structures helps maintain the shape of the left ventricle and appears to be responsible for the improvement in left ventricular function. Likewise, with mitral valve replacement, preservation of the valve apparatus results in a reduction of wall stress.[40] Valve repair is not possible when there is extensive calcification of the leaflets, marked alterations of the subvalvular apparatus, or bacterial endocarditis. One study showed mortality was 8.3% for mitral valve replacement and 2.3% for mitral valve repair, and 17% of the replacement group required an intra-aortic balloon pump versus 2% in the repair group.[41]

The preoperative hemodynamic considerations are summarized in Table 16–5. Mitral regurgitation volume overloads the left ventricle and most patients have an increased left ventricular preload. Increases in preload will augment pump function by the Frank-Starling mechanism. However, the left ventricular end-systolic diameter will also increase with increased preload. Since increases in end-systolic diameter can produce annular dilatation and a worsening of mitral regurgitation, an increased left ventricular preload is not always beneficial for the patient, and fluid management must be individualized. Patients may be hypovolemic if diuretic therapy has been instituted. Increases in afterload increase the regurgitant fraction, whereas decreases in afterload decrease the regurgitant fraction. Consequently, patients will benefit from afterload reduction as long as adequate perfusion pressure is maintained. Bradycardia will decrease forward cardiac output and increase the regurgi-

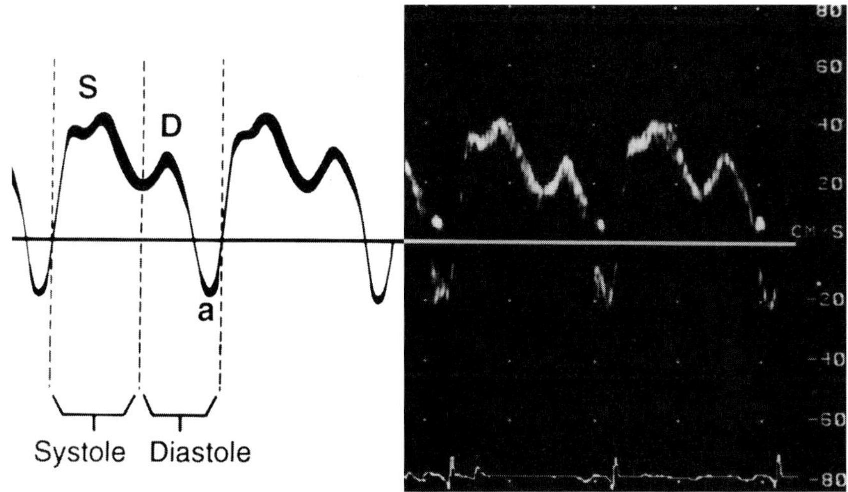

FIGURE **16–9.** Pulsed-wave Doppler tracing representing normal pulmonary vein flow. The timing of the S (systolic), D (diastolic), and *a* (atrial contraction) waveforms are also presented. (From Rafferty TD: Basics of Transesophageal Echocardiography. New York, Churchill Livingstone, 1995, p 85, with permission.)

TABLE 16–5
Management of Mitral Regurgitation

Preload	Decrease
Afterload	Vasodilator beneficial
Rate	Prevent slow rate (<80 bpm)
Contractility	Decreased from rheumatic or coronary artery disease
Oxygen balance	Increased demand as a result of increased mass
Rhythm	Atrial fibrillation

bpm, beats per minute.

tant fraction and left ventricular end-systolic volume. Hemodynamics are usually optimized with a normal to elevated heart rate (>80 bpm). As long as the rate is controlled, atrial fibrillation is well tolerated. Excepting patients with acute mitral regurgitation, contractility is usually reduced as a result of rheumatic or coronary artery disease. Consequently, drugs with a myocardial depressant effect should be used cautiously or not at all.

Tricuspid Regurgitation

Since tricuspid stenosis is extremely rare, this section will focus only on tricuspid regurgitation. In a study of 45 patients at necropsy, the etiology of pure tricuspid regurgitation was "functional" from pulmonary hypertension in 47%, myxomatous disease in 16%, rheumatic in 11%, idiopathic dilated cardiomyopathy in 9%, Ebstein's anomaly in 7%, and miscellaneous in 10%.[42] In the presence of significant pulmonary hypertension, the right ventricle may hypertrophy to compensate for the increased wall stress, but more often the thin-walled right ventricle dilates and fails. Dilation produces tricuspid regurgitation and raises right atrial pressure, which impedes venous return producing edema, ascites, and hepatomegaly. The compliance of the left ventricle also can be decreased by the paradoxical leftward motion of the interventricular septum produced by right ventricular distention.[43]

Symptoms from isolated tricuspid regurgitation in the absence of pulmonary hypertension are minor, and even the complete removal of an infected tricuspid valve is often well tolerated.[44] Patients may be cachectic with evidence of weight loss, cyanosis, and jaundice. There is elevation of the jugular venous pressures with a prominent cv or "s" wave. Auscultation reveals an S_3 that increases with inspiration. The murmur of tricuspid regurgitation is classically high pitched, holosystolic, and loudest over the right sternal border at the level of the fourth intercostal space.

Using two-dimensional and M-mode echocardiography, the etiology of tricuspid regurgitation can often be determined. The diameter of the annulus can also be measured to detect dilation (normal diameter, 2.2 ± 0.3 cm). Tricuspid regurgitation can be demonstrated with injection of agitated saline into the superior vena cava. The microbubbles linger in the right atrium and may actually enter the inferior vena cava and hepatic veins. Using the ratio of the regurgitant jet area divided by the area of the right atrium obtained by color flow Doppler, tricuspid regurgitation is graded as follows: Grade I (mild) ratio less than or equal to 0.2, Grade II (moderate) ratio between 0.2 and 0.34, Grade III (severe) greater than or equal to 0.34 (Fig. 16–10). The presence of a negative waveform (systolic flow reversal) on a pulsed-wave Doppler trace of hepatic venous flow also indicates severe tricuspid regurgitation. Echocardiography can also utilize the velocity of tricuspid regurgitation to mea-

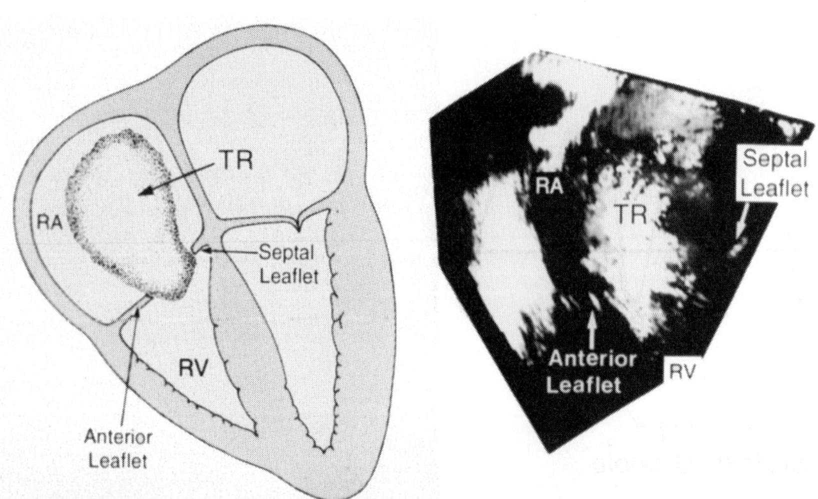

FIGURE 16–10. Black-and-white print of color-flow Doppler–defined tricuspid regurgitation. RA, right atrium; RV, right ventricle; TR, tricuspid regurgitation. (From Rafferty TD: Basics of Transesophageal Echocardiography. New York, Churchill Livingstone, 1995, p 36, with permission.)

TABLE 16–6
Management of Tricuspid Regurgitation

Preload	Increase
Afterload	Vasodilator beneficial
Rate	Rate <80 bpm
Contractility	Decreased with chronic regurgitation
Oxygen balance	Increased demand as a result of increased mass
Rhythm	Atrial fibrillation

bpm, beats per minute.

sure peak systolic pulmonary artery pressure. Trivial tricuspid regurgitation is a common finding in control populations.

The preoperative hemodynamic considerations are listed in Table 16–6. Right ventricular preload should be normal to high, especially if right heart failure is present. Volume assessment with a central venous catheter is difficult, since the right atrium is very compliant and there is a large cv wave on the central venous pressure tracing. Afterload should be decreased to help forward flow. Acidosis, hypercarbia, hypoxia, hypothermia, and nitrous oxide will increase pulmonary vascular resistance and should be avoided. Heart rate should be normal to high and if right heart failure is present, inotropes may be needed to increase contractility. Phosphodiesterase inhibitors such as amrinone and milrinone are particularly effective, since they also decrease PVR. Myocardial oxygen consumption is usually not a problem in pure tricuspid regurgitation. A sinus rhythm is desirable.

Hypertrophic Cardiomyopathy

Patients with hypertrophic cardiomyopathy (HCM) have ventricular hypertrophy without an identifiable cause and usually have microscopic evidence of myocardial fiber disarray. Hypertrophic cardiomyopathy occurs in both a familial pattern (56%) and sporadically (44%).[45] Males are affected more often than females. On a cellular basis, proposed mechanisms for producing myocardial hypertrophy include abnormal calcium kinetics, abnormal sympathetic stimulation, ischemia, and duplication of the gene coding for the myosin heavy chain.

HCM can be classified into the subgroups of nonobstructive, latent obstructive, and resting obstructive. In the nonobstructive form, there is no pressure gradient across the left ventricular outflow tract, but pathologic hypertrophy can cause diastolic dysfunction. In the latent form, a pressure gradient can be produced with provocation such as amyl nitrite inhalation. In the resting obstructive form, a pressure gradient is consistently present. HCM with resting obstruction is also referred to as muscular subaortic stenosis, idiopathic hypertrophic subaortic stenosis (IHSS), and hypertrophic obstructive cardiomyopathy (HOCM). The entire septum is hypertrophied in 72% of patients; the basal two thirds of the septum is hypertrophied in 20% of patients; and only 8% of patients have hypertrophy localized to the basal one third of the septum. It is generally assumed that the pressure gradient is produced by apposition of the anterior mitral leaflet and the hypertrophied septum. Since the hypertrophied septum narrows the left ventricular outflow tract, the velocity of ejected blood is increased and the ejection path is closer to the anterior mitral valve leaflet. The increased velocity in turn creates a Venturi effect, and the anterior mitral valve leaflet is drawn into the outflow tract where contact between the anterior mitral valve leaflet and the hypertrophied septum produces obstruction. Movement of the anterior mitral valve leaflet in this manner is known as systolic anterior motion (SAM). Since the anterior mitral valve leaflet is pulled out of its normal position, mitral regurgitation almost always accompanies hypertrophic obstructive cardiomyopathy. Furthermore, the increased muscle mass and reduced rate of relaxation produces diastolic dysfunction.

Patients with HCM who develop atrial fibrillation should be cardioverted to improve hemodynamics. Amiodarone can suppress both supraventricular and ventricular arrhythmias. An automatic implantible defibrillator (AICD) is another option for arrhythmia control. Medical management is directed toward reducing the left ventricular outflow tract obstruction, improving diastolic relaxation, and preventing arrhythmias. Approximately 10 to 15% of patients with HCM will require surgery, and myomectomy is the most prevalent technique used for correction; however, Cooley has advocated mitral valve replacement to eliminate systolic anterior motion. McIntosh's indications for surgery are: (1) patients who are NYHA Class III or Class IV who have failed medical management and have resting or provocable gradients or (2) patients who survived a sudden death episode and have a resting or provocable gradient greater than 50 mm Hg. A series by Mohr of 115 patients who were operated on for hypertrophic obstructive cardiomyopathy demonstrates the efficacy of surgery. The preoperative pressure gradient was reduced from a mean of 70 mm Hg to 9 mm Hg postoperatively. Preoperative symptoms were relieved in 76% of patients with dyspnea, 83% of patients with angina, and 96% of patients with syncope. The overall operative mortality was 5.2%, but in patients less than 65 years of age the operative mortality was only 1.2%. Patients younger than 65 years of age had a 5-year survival of 93% versus 54% for the older group.[46]

Patients with HCM may be asymptomatic and detected only on family screens for the disease. Symptomatic patients may complain of dyspnea (90%), angina (75%), fatigue, and dizziness. In all patients with hypertrophic cardiomyopathy, sudden death may be the first manifestation of the disease. Patients at high risk for sudden death include those with a young age of diagnosis, family history of HCM and sudden death, syncope (children not adults), and nonsustained ventricular tachycardia detected by 48-hour Holter monitoring (adults not children). Patients with septal hypertrophy localized to the subaortic area have a more favorable prognosis than patients with more extensive septal hypertrophy.[47] HCM usually presents with a murmur at about 20 years of age, NYHA Class II symptoms typically develop by age 30, and NYHA Class III symptoms by age 35. Death occurs approximately at age 40.[48] The yearly sudden death rate is 2.5% for adults and 6% for children.[49]

Patients who are asymptomatic and have a low pressure gradient at the site of obstruction may have a normal physical exam. With increases in the pressure gradient, physical findings develop. A harsh systolic crescendo descrescendo murmur is heard best between the apex and the left sternal border with radiation to the axilla but not to the neck vessels. The murmur will increase with a Valsalva maneuver or changing from a squatting to a standing position.

The most common abnormality on ECG is the pattern of left ventricular hypertrophy and strain. Pathologic Q waves in leads II, III, aVL, or V_4 through V_6 are often present and the basis is presumed to be the left-to-right depolarization of the hypertrophied septum. With 24-hour ambulatory monitoring, high-grade ventricular arrhythmias are found in 66% of patients. The presence of ventricular tachycardia (detected in 25% of patients) increases the incidence of sudden death by 8.6 times.[50]

Echocardiography provides for an excellent evaluation of patients with hypertrophic cardiomyopathy. Asymmetric septal hypertrophy (ASH) can be demonstrated with both two-dimensional and M-mode examination. The normal upper limit of the septum is 12 mm, and a measurement of 14 mm is required to make the diagnosis. A septal measurement of more than 20 mm is strongly suggestive of ASH. In ASH, the septum is hypertrophied disproportionately to the rest of the left ventricle, and to make the diagnosis, the ratio of the thickness of the septum to the posterobasal region should be greater than 1.3 to 1.5. When there is left ventricular outflow obstruction, an examination of the mitral valve will demonstrate systolic anterior motion of the anterior mitral valve leaflet. Doppler interrogation will demonstrate high peak velocity at the site of SAM, and the pressure gradient can be calculated using the modified Bernoulli equation.

The preoperative hemodynamic considerations are summarized in Table 16–7. Since the obstruction will increase as left ventricular chamber size decreases, the left ventricle must be adequately filled. To achieve adequate filling, a high left ventricular filling pressure will be required, since these patients frequently have concomitant diastolic dysfunction. A decrease in afterload will increase the degree of obstruction. Tachycardia lowers preload and thus increases obstruction; these patients will do best with a slow heart rate. Increases in contractility also increase the degree of obstruction. Oxygen consumption is increased by the increase in muscle mass and the high left ventricular end-diastolic pressures decrease supply by decreasing perfusion pressure. Maintaining patients in sinus rhythm is important.

Mitral Valve Prolapse

The etiology of mitral prolapse in the majority of patients is idiopathic myxomatous degeneration. Mitral valve prolapse is also seen in many other disease states, especially in the connective tissue disorders such as Marfan's syndrome. The incidence of mitral valve prolapse is presumed to be 5 to 10% of the population with a predominance in women; however, using two-dimensional echocardiography, only 2 of 100 women were shown to have mitral valve prolapse.[51] Approximately 15% of patients develop progressive mitral regurgitation over a 10- to 15-year period. Patients with mitral valve prolapse are at greater risk for acute hemiplegia and transient ischemic attacks, and the basis is presumed to be embolic. If symptoms of embolization occur, the patient should be anticoagulated. Sudden death as a result of an arrhythmia has also occurred.

Most patients with mitral valve prolapse are asymptomatic. Symptomatic patients complain of palpitations, lightheadedness, chest pain, and fatigability. Auscultation reveals a mid or late systolic click. If mitral regurgitation is present, the murmur of mitral regurgitation may be heard and as with the systolic click, its onset and duration are usually delayed with maneuvers that increase preload. On ECG, biphasic or inverted T waves in leads II, III, and aVF can be seen in some patients. Supraventricular and ventricular arrythmias are seen, especially in those patients with significant mitral regurgitation. On two-dimensional echocardiography, one or both of the mitral valve leaflets are displaced into the left atrium during ventricular systole. The mitral annulus is the reference plane above which the leaflets must prolapse, and prolapse of both leaflets occurs in 75 to 90% of cases. The preoperative hemodynamic considerations are listed in Table 16–8.

TABLE 16–7
Management of Hypertrophic Cardiomyopathy

Preload	Normal to high
Afterload	High
Rate	Rate <80 bpm
Contractility	Decreased
Oxygen balance	Increased demand as a result of increased LV mass
Rhythm	Atrial fibrillation, supraventricular or ventricular tachycardia

bpm, beats per minute; LV, left ventricular.

TABLE 16–8
Management of Mitral Valve Prolapse

Preload	Normovolemia
Afterload	Vasodilator beneficial only when regurgitation is present
Rate	Slow (<80 bpm)
Contractility	Normal
Oxygen balance	Normal
Rhythm	Atrial fibrillation or supraventricular tachycardia

bpm, beats per minute.

Intraoperative Anesthetic Management

Premedication

The primary goals of premedication are to reduce stress and anxiety in the patient being prepared for surgery. Typically, morphine and scopolamine are given in combination at least 90 minutes prior to the start of surgery. Morphine is administered in doses of 0.05 to 0.1 mg/kg intramuscularly (IM) to patients with diminished cardiac reserve, while 0.1 to 0.2 mg/kg is given to the more robust patient. Scopolamine (0.2 to 0.4 mg IM) supplies amnesia and enhances the central nervous system effects of morphine. In the elderly, a smaller dose of scopolamine (0.1 to 0.2 mg) is administered, since severe mental confusion resembling an acute organic brain syndrome might be observed on the basis of scopolamine's autonomic effects. Midazolam (0.05 to 0.1 mg/kg IM) or diazepam (5 to 10 mg orally [PO]) may be used instead of scopolamine. Premedication with respiratory depressants can result in hypoxemia. Therefore, supplemental oxygen should be provided from the time of premedication to induction of anesthesia.

In addition to sedatives, any drugs required for daily maintenance are administered at the time of premedication. Antianginal and antihypertensive therapy should not be withdrawn prior to surgery. Abrupt cessation of β-blocker therapy can result in a hypersympathetic state.[52] Calcium channel blockers are commonly continued in the perioperative period while the potential for side effects is accounted for in the anesthetic management plan. Case reports of low systemic vascular resistance in patients chronically treated with angiotensin converting enzyme (ACE) inhibitors have been presented. However, studies in patients undergoing valvular surgery have not demonstrated significant deleterious hemodynamic events.[53] Any additional maintenance drugs such as insulin, steroids, etc., are administered as indicated. Finally, antibiotics are given according to the protocol established by the American Heart Association (see below).

Monitors

In addition to the monitors outlined in the Standards for Basic Anesthetic Monitoring defined by the American Society of Anesthesiologists, all patients should have a five-electrode ECG placed to have the capability of monitoring all limb leads and the precordial lead V_5. The axis of limb lead II parallels the electrical axis of the heart, thus facilitating the recognition of the P wave and the diagnosis of arrhythmias. Sensitivity for detecting ECG myocardial ischemia using the standard clinical combination of leads II and V_5 is 80% (adding V_4 increases sensitivity to 96%). A Foley catheter for measuring urine flow and bladder temperature should be placed. Additional temperature monitoring sites (pulmonary artery or esophageal) are used to assess and ensure adequate and uniform cooling and warming during bypass. Since blood pressure can change rapidly, a pre-induction arterial catheter is essential.

Since its development more than two decades ago, the pulmonary artery catheter (PAC) has become an important tool in assessing the hemodynamic function of the patient undergoing cardiac surgery. PAC monitoring may be particularly useful in patients with valvular heart disease. The increase in left atrial pressure in many valvular lesions may lead to increases in pulmonary vascular pressure, redistribution of pulmonary blood volume, and pulmonary edema. Variation does exist in the utilization of PACs in patients undergoing cardiac surgery. Attempts to determine if PAC use affects outcome in this patient population have been limited to uncontrolled, observational studies. Guidelines have been developed by the American Society of Anesthesiologists for the use of a PAC.[54]

Modification of the standard PAC has resulted in the ability to pace the myocardium from the PAC and to measure mixed venous oxygen saturations, continuous cardiac outputs, and right ventricular ejection fractions. The benefits of these newer PACs must be balanced against the increased cost as well as the complications of PAC monitoring. These complications include arterial puncture, pneumothorax, air embolism, nerve injury, arrhythmias (especially the development of complete heart block in patients with pre-existent left bundle branch block), intracardiac knotting, thrombosis, infection, pulmonary infarction, and pulmonary artery rupture. Advanced age, hypothermia, pulmonary hypertension, female gender, and deviations from standard insertion techniques have been associated with a greater risk of perforation.

Although not universally available, transesophageal echocardiography (TEE) is strongly recommended. TEE provides intraoperative confirmation of the diagnosis as well as an assessment of the adequacy of valve repair or replacement prior to departing the operating room. TEE is also used for ischemia detection, assessing ventricular preload and contractility, and detection of atherosclerotic plaque in the ascending aorta. While the aortic arch and descending aorta are clearly imaged with TEE, epiaortic scanning is in fact better than TEE at assessing the ascending aorta. Wareing et al.[55] suggested that modification of cannulation and clamping techniques based on intraoperative epiaortic scanning may decrease the frequency of postoperative stroke.

Induction

The perfect anesthetic for valvular surgery is one that does not alter SVR, heart rate, or contractility. Unfortunately, such an agent currently does not exist. Thiopental and ketamine may cause significant hemodynamic alterations. Etomidate, on the other hand, is an intravenous agent that appears to preserve hemodynamic function during induction of anesthesia. As an alternative, narcotic analgesics have been used for induction and maintenance of anesthesia. In a classic study, Lowenstein et al.[56] reported on the benefits of morphine anesthesia (0.5 to 3.0 mg/kg) in a group of patients undergoing valvular heart surgery. Histamine release and the associated decreases in SVR with the use of high doses of morphine requires that H_1- and H_2-receptor antagonists be administered as part of the premedication. Hypovolemia must also be corrected prior to the induction of anesthesia. Barash et al.[57] have shown that fentanyl, a synthetic narcotic (100 times as potent as morphine), can prevent the decrease in left ventricular ejection fraction commonly seen as a response to laryngoscopy. Due to the stabilizing effects on the circulation, high doses of fentanyl are now widely used in cardiac anesthesia. Sufentanil, ten times more potent than fentanyl, was initially advocated as a more "complete" anesthetic. Most studies, however, have served to emphasize the similarities, rather than the differences, between fentanyl and sufentanil. Like fentanyl, sufentanil demonstrates a "ceiling effect" such that breakthrough hypertension is common, especially in patients with normal left ventricular function.

Maintenance

Following induction of anesthesia, additional intravenous agents (narcotics, benzodiazepines) or inhalational anesthetics are necessary. Propofol, an intravenous agent with sedative and hypnotic properties but lacking analgesic effects, has gained popularity in recent years because of its shorter duration of action. Like thiopental, propofol produces ventilatory depression, peripheral vasodilation, and decreases in cardiac output. The high clearance rate for propofol indicates that it be administered as a continuous infusion. The use of propofol intraoperatively as well as for sedation in the intensive care unit may enable early extubation of the cardiac surgical patient.

Since all of the inhalational anesthetic agents are myocardial depressants, they are added to the anesthetic regimen primarily in patients with preserved left ventricular function. Isoflurane differs from enflurane and halothane in that it is a more potent vasodilator. The vasodilating properties may be particularly useful in unloading the diseased left ventricle or the ventricle subject to valvular regurgitation. Controversy exists as to whether isoflurane causes coronary steal. It is likely that the beneficial effects of isoflurane in decreasing myocardial oxygen demand are of greater importance than its effects on coronary tone. In a large trial of four different anesthetic regimens for patients undergoing coronary artery bypass grafting (CABG) surgery, Slogoff and Keats[58] demonstrated no difference in the frequency of myocardial ischemia between isoflurane, enflurane, halothane, and sufentanil even in patients with steal-prone coronary anatomy. Initial studies on the use of nitrous oxide raised concerns over the occurrence of myocardial ischemia when added to a narcotic or inhalational anesthetic. More recent studies, however, indicate that if hemodynamics are controlled, then nitrous oxide does not worsen myocardial ischemia.[59]

Administration of muscle relaxants may also be associated with significant cardiovascular effects. In particular, effects on heart rate may be deleterious to patients with a stenotic lesion. Pancuronium is associated with increases in heart rate. In contrast, vecuronium has no sympathomimetic effects but has been implicated in the generation of bradyarrhythmias when given the high doses of sufentanil.[60] Atracurium offers a unique pathway of degradation (Hoffman elimination) that makes it a useful drug in patients with renal failure. The histamine release and hypotension associated with atracurium have limited its widespread use during cardiac surgery. Doxacurium, pipecuronium, mivacurium, and rocuronium are newer muscle relaxants with varying durations of action that seem also to have no adverse hemodynamic side effects. The benefits of minimal side effects must be balanced against the increased cost of the newer agents.

Antibiotic Prophylaxis

All patients who present for valvular surgery must receive antibiotic prophylaxis, since the frequency of post-surgical endocarditis is 2 to 10% and mortality in these patients can be as high as 59%.[61,62] For cardiac surgery, first-generation cephalosporms are most often used. Guidelines for prevention of bacterial endocarditis in patients undergoing noncardiac surgery or who are not candidates for the standard regimen have been developed by the American Heart Association.[63] In patients with mitral valve prolapse the risk of endocarditis is lower and these patients may not need prophylaxis if mitral regurgitation is absent. Long-term prophylaxis to prevent disease progression may be considered in patients with rheumatic fever; however, such prophylaxis may lead to the development of resistant organisms. Patients who develop valvular regurgitation from endocarditis should receive several days of antibiotics prior to valve replacement, provided they are hemodynamically stable. Tricuspid valvulotomy without prosthetic replacement may be performed in intravenous drug users with intractable endocarditis in order to prevent further infections.

Anticoagulation

Patients with the lesions described in this chapter may require anticoagulation both before and after cardiac as well as noncardiac surgery. The risk of thromboembolism is greatest in patients with mitral stenosis (1 to 5% per year). Without anticoagulation, 13% of mitral stenosis patients experienced systemic embolization with 75% of these emboli settling in the cerebral circulation.[64] Patients who experienced emboli were more likely to have low cardiac output, advanced age, increased left atrial appendage size, and atrial fibrillation (80%). Patients with aortic disease experience thromboembolism at a rate less than 1%. Mitral valve prolapse patients with other predisposing factors are also at risk.

Patients who receive bioprosthetic valves usually are not anticoagulated. If long-term anticoagulation is required, warfarin alone or in combination with aspirin or dipyridamole is used. Anticoagulation predisposes patients to hemorrhage and an international normalized ratio (INR) of 2.3 to 2.4 seems to offer the best risk-benefit ratio.[65] For outpatient surgery, it has been shown that patients with prosthetic valves can safely discontinue warfarin (Coumadin) 6 days prior to noncardiac surgery.[66] However, surgical patients on anticoagulation therapy with Coumadin are usually admitted 3 days prior to surgery. The Coumadin is discontinued and intravenous heparin therapy is initiated. The heparin, in turn, can be discontinued 4 to 6 hours prior to surgery. In the case of emergency surgery, fresh frozen plasma and platelets may be administered in an attempt to normalize coagulation immediately.

References

1. Roberts WC: Valvular, subvalvular, and supravalvular aortic stenosis. Morphologic features. Cardiovasc Clin 5:97, 1973.
2. Passik CS, Ackermann DM, Pluth JR, et al: Temporal changes in the causes of aortic stenosis: A surgical pathologic study of 646 cases. Mayo Clin Proc 62:119, 1987.
3. Horstkotte D, Loogen F: The natural history of aortic valve stenosis. Eur Heart J 9(Suppl E):57, 1988.
4. McAnulty JH: Timing of surgical therapy for aortic valve stenosis. Goals of therapy. Herz 9:341, 1984.
5. Gersony WM, Hayes CJ, Driscoll DJ, et al: Bacterial endocarditis in patients with aortic stenosis, pulmonary stenosis, or ventricular septal defect. Circulation 87(Suppl 1):I-121, 1993.
6. Olesen KH, Rygg IH, Wennevold A, Nyboe J: Aortic valve replacement with the Lillehei-Kaster prosthesis in 262 patients: An assessment after 9 to 17 years. Eur Heart J 12:680, 1991.
7. Perloff JK: Clinical recognition of aortic stenosis: The physical signs and differential diagnosis of the various forms of obstruction to left ventricular outflow. Prog Cardiovasc Dis 10:323, 1968.
8. Pepine CJ, Allen HD, Bashore TM, et al: ACC/AHA guidelines for cardiac catheterization and cardiac catheterization laboratories. J Am Coll Cardiol 18:1149, 1991.
9. Gorlin R, Gorlin SG: Hydraulic formula for calculation of the stenotic mitral valve, other cardiac valves, and central circulatory shunts. Am Heart J 41:1, 1951.
10. Ramsdale DR, Faragher EB, Bennett DH, et al: Preoperative prediction of significant coronary artery disease in patients with valvular heart disease. Br Med J 284:223, 1982.
11. Mullany CJ, Elveback LR, Frye RL, et al: Coronary artery disease and its management: Influence on survival in patients undergoing aortic valve replacement. J Am Coll Cardiol 10:66, 1987.
12. Chatterjee K, Parmley WW: Cardiology: An Illustrated Text. New York, Gower Medical Publishing, 1991, 9.112.
13. Lund O: Preoperative risk evaluation and stratification of long-term survival after valve replacement for aortic stenosis. Circulation 82:124, 1990.
14. Frater RW, Salomon NW, Rainer WG, et al: The Carpentier-Edwards pericardial aortic valve: Intermediate results. Ann Thorac Surg 53:764, 1992.
15. Cohn LH, Allred EN, DiSesa VJ, et al: Early and late risk of aortic valve replacement. A 12 year concomitant comparison of the porcine bioprosthetic and tilting disc prosthetic aortic valves. J Thorac Cardiovasc Surg 88:695, 1984.
16. Magovern JA, Pennock JL, Campbell DB, et al: Aortic valve replacement and combined aortic valve replacement and coronary artery bypass grafting: Predicting high risk groups. J Am Coll Cardiol 9:38, 1987.
17. Galloway AC, Colvin SB, Grossi EA, et al: Ten-year experience with aortic valve replacement in 482 patients 70 years of age or older: Operative risk and long-term results. Ann Thorac Surg 49:84, 1990.
18. Rediker DE, Boucher CA, Block PC, et al: Degree of reversibility of left ventricular systolic dysfunction after aortic valve replacement for isolated aortic stenosis. Am J Cardiol 60:112, 1987.
19. Hakki AH, Kimbiris D, Iskandrian AS, et al: Angina pectoris and coronary artery disease in patients with severe aortic valvular disease. Am Heart J 100:441, 1980.
20. Olson LJ, Subramanian R, Edwards WD: Surgical pathology of pure aortic insufficiency: A study of 225 cases. Mayo Clin Proc 59:835, 1984.
21. Shen WF, Roubin GS, Choong CY, et al: Evaluation of the relationship between myocardial contractile state and left ventricular function in patients with aortic regurgitation. Circulation 71:31, 1985.
22. Spagnuolo M, Kloth H, Taranta A, et al: Natural history of rheumatic aortic regurgitation. Circulation 44:368, 1971.
23. Perry GJ, Helmcke F, Nanda NC, et al: Evaluation of aortic insufficiency by Doppler color flow mapping. J Am Coll Cardiol 4: 952, 1987.
24. Chaterjee K, et al: Cardiology: An Illustrated Text. Philadelphia, JB Lippincott Co, 1991, p 9.21.
25. Rapaport E:P Natural history of aortic and mitral valve disease. Am J Cardiol 35:221, 1975.
26. Bonow RO, Picone AL, Mcintosh CL, et al: Survival and functional results after valve replacement for aortic regurgitation from 1976 to 1983: Impact of preoperative left ventricular function. Circulation 72:1244, 1985.
27. Copeland JG, Griepp RB, Stinson EB, et al: Long term follow up after isolated aortic valve replacement. J Thorac Cardiovasc Surg 74:875, 1977.
28. Olson LJ, Subramanian R, Ackermann DM, et al: Surgical pathology of the mitral valve: A study of 712 cases spanning 21 years. Mayo Clin Proc 62:22, 1987.
29. Braunwald E: Heart Disease, A Textbook of Cardiovascular Medicine, 4th ed. Philadelphia, WB Saunders Co, 1992, p 1015.
30. Olesen KH: The natural history of 271 patients with mitral stenosis under medical treatment. Br Heart J 24:349, 1962.
31. Enriquez-Sarano M, Louvard Y, Darmon D, et al: Should closed-heart mitral commissurotomies still be performed? Arch Mal Coeur Vaiss 77:782, 1984.
32. Colle JP, Rahal S, Ohayon J, et al: Global left ventricular function and regional wall in pure mitral stenosis. Clin Cardiol 7:573, 1984.
33. Reichek N, Shelburne JC, Perloff JK: Clinical aspects of rheumatic valvular disease. Prog Cardiovasc Dis 15:491, 1973.
34. Heger JJ, Wann LS, Weyman AE, et al: Long-term changes in mitral valve area after successful mitral commissurotomy. Circulation 59:443, 1979.
35. Waller BF, Morrow AG, Maron BJ, et al: Etiology of clinically isolated, severe, chronic, pure mitral regurgitation: Analysis of 97 patients over 30 years of age having mitral valve replacement. Am Heart J 104:276, 1982.
36. Zile MR, Gaasch WH, Carroll JD, Levine HJ: Chronic mitral regurgitation: Predictive valve of preoperative echocardiographic indexes of left ventricular function and wall stress. J Am Coll Cardiol 3:235, 1984.
37. Hammermeister KER, Fisher L, Kennedy JW, et al: Prediction of late survival in patients with mitral valve disease from clinical,

hemodynamic, and quantitative angiographic variables. Circulation 57:341, 1978.
38. Yacoub M, Halim M, Radley-Smith R, et al: Surgical treatment of mitral regurgitation caused by floppy valves: Repair versus replacement. Circulation 64(Suppl 2):11-210, 1981.
39. Helmcke F, Nanda NC, Hsiung MC, et al: Color Doppler assessment of mitral regurgitation with orthogonal planes. Circulation 75:175, 1987.
40. Rozich JD, Carabello BA, Usher BW, et al: Mitral valve replacement with and without chordal preservation in patients with chronic mitral regurgitation: Mechanism for differences in postoperative ejection performance. Circulation 86:1718, 1992.
41. Kawachi Y, Oe M, Asou T, et al: Comparative study between valve repair and replacement for pure mitral regurgitation—early and late postoperative results. Jpn Circ J 55:443, 1991.
42. Waller BF: Etiology of pure tricuspid regurgitation. Cardiovasc Clin 17:53, 1987.
43. Kerber RE, Dippel WF, Abboud FM: Abnormal motion of the interventricular septum in right ventricular volume overload. Circulation 48:86, 1973.
44. Arbulu A, Holmes RJ, Asfaw I: Tricuspid valvulotomy without replacement: Twenty years' experience. J. Thorac Cardiovasc Surg 102:917, 1991.
45. Maron BJ, Nichols PF, Pickle LW, et al: Patterns of inheritance in hypertrophic cardiomyopathy: Assessment by M-mode and two-dimensional echocardiography. Am J Cardiol 53:1087, 1984.
46. Mohr R, Schaff HV, Danielson GK, et al: The outcome of surgical treatment of hypertrophic obstructive cardiomyopathy. Experience over 15 years. J Thorac Cardiovasc Surg 97:666, 1989.
47. Wigle ED, Sasson Z, Henderson M, et al: Hypertrophic cardiomyopathy: The importance of the site and extent of hypertrophy. A review. Prog Cardiovasc Dis 28:1, 1985.
48. Adelman AG, Wigle ED, Ranganathan N, et al: The clinical course in muscular subaortic stenosis: A retrospective and prospective study of 60 hemodynamically proved cases. Ann Intern Med 77:515, 1972.
49. McKenna WJ: The natural history of hypertrophic cardiomyopathy. Cardiovasc Clin 19:135, 1988.
50. Maron BJ, Savage DD, Wolfson JK, et al: Prognostic significance of 24 hour ambulatory electrocardiographic monitoring in patients with hypertrophic cardiomyopathy: A prospective study. Am J Cardiol 48:252, 1981.
51. Wann LS, Grove JR, Hess TR, et al: Prevalence of mitral prolapse by two-dimensional echocardiography in healthy young women. Br Heart J 49:334, 1983.
52. Boudoulas H, Lewis RP, Kates RE, Dalamangas G: Hypersensitivity to adrenergic stimulation after propranolol withdrawal in normal subjects. Ann Intern Med 86:433, 1977.
53. Colson P, Ribstein J, Mimran M, et al: Effect of angiotensin converting enzyme inhibition on blood pressure and renal function during open heart surgery. Anesthesiology 72:23, 1990.
54. Practice guidelines for pulmonary artery catheterization: A report by the American Society of Anesthesiologists task force on pulmonary artery catheterization. Anesthesiology 78:380, 1993.
55. Wareing TH, Davila-Roman VG, Barzilai B, et al: Management of the severely atherosclerotic ascending aorta during cardiac operations: A strategy for detection and treatment. J Thorac Cardiovasc Surg 103:453, 1992.
56. Lowenstein E, Hallowell P, Levine FH, et al: Cardiovascular responses to large doses of intravenous morphine in man. N Engl J Med 281:1389, 1969.
57. Barash PG, Tarabadkar S, Giles R, et al: Preservation of global left ventricular function during intubation in patients with ischemic heart disease. Anesthesiology 55:A6, 1981.
58. Slogoff S, Keats AS: Randomized trial of primary anesthetic agents on outcome of coronary artery bypass operations. Anesthesiology 70:179, 1989.
59. Nathan HJ: Control of hemodynamics prevents worsening of myocardial ischemia when nitrous oxide is administered to isoflurane anesthetized dogs. Anesthesiology 71:686, 1989.
60. Starr NJ, Sethna DH, Estafanous FG: Bradycardia and asystole following the rapid administration of sufentanil and vercuronium. Anesthesiology 64:521, 1986.
61. Walter WR, Danielson GK, Giuliani ER, Geraci JE: Prosthetic valve endocarditis. Mayo Clin Proc 57:155, 1982.
62. Geraci JE, Dale AJD, McGoon DC: Bacterial endocarditis and endarteritis following cardiac operations. Wis Med J 62:302, 1963.
63. Dajani AS, Taubert KA, Wilson W, et al: Prevention of bacterial endocarditis. Recommendations by the American Heart Association. Circulation 96:358, 1997.
64. Wood P: An appreciation of mitral stenosis. Part I. Clinical features. Br Med J 1:1051, 1954.
65. Kearon C, Hirsh J: Management of anticoagulation before and after elective surgery. N Engl J Med 336:1506, 1997.
66. Tinker JH, Tarhan S: Discontinuing anticoagulant therapy in surgical patients with cardiac valve prosthesis: Observations in 180 patients. JAMA 239:738 1978.

CHAPTER 17

Cardiopulmonary Bypass: Technology, Pathophysiology, and Pharmacology

John Thompson, M.D.
Richard F. Davis, M.D.

The first clinically successful use of cardiopulmonary bypass (CPB) was in May of 1953, when Dr. John Gibbon successfully used the technique to support the circulation of a 5-year-old girl while he repaired her atrial septal defect. In the 46 years since, the technology involved with CPB has become increasingly specialized and complex. This technological evolution has made a dramatic impact on the treatment and surgical correction of patients with congenital, ischemic, and/or valvular heart disease. In addition, the advances of CPB technology have been utilized in the development of other complex medical devices including artificial hearts, extracorporeal membrane oxygenation (ECMO), and ventricular assist devices (VAD).

The field of cardiac anesthesia has also increased in sophistication and complexity. New methods and techniques have become available to better anesthetize, monitor, and pharmacologically support patients undergoing bypass surgery. The progressive development of CPB technology requires a continual learning process by the cardiac anesthesiologist to stay abreast of current issues, and apply new technology appropriately. Topics of CPB management which constitute a core knowledge base include the following:

1. CPB technology/components
2. Coagulation management
3. Pathophysiology of CPB
4. Overview of bypass sequence of events
5. Pharmacologic considerations of bypass

By-pass Systems and Components

The development of cardiopulmonary bypass is one of the most significant medical advances of the last century. The original concept still holds true today: the patient's blood temporarily bypasses the cardiopulmonary circulation while the cardiopulmonary bypass apparatus performs the dynamic functions of the normal heart and lung. The end result is that the cardiac surgeon operates on a blood-free, nonbeating heart.

This interruption of cardiopulmonary blood flow depends upon three essential functions performed by the CPB apparatus:

1. Oxygenation of venous blood
2. Elimination of carbon dioxide
3. Maintenance of system perfusion

Modern bypass machines effectively perform the primary pulmonary functions of oxygenating and removing CO_2 from the blood; however, technical considerations have limited reproducing the heart's pulsatile flow dynamics. In addition, the CPB apparatus also regulates blood temperature and filters particulate matter prior to the blood reaching the body, much like the native lung. The CPB apparatus itself is composed of a number of individual mechanical parts. Each part has been developed and refined to replace the normal physiologic function of the heart and lung.

The essential components of CPB have remained unchanged over the years, despite refinements and different component designs. Figure 17–1, is a simple overview of the standard CPB setup. The path of blood flow is as follows: desaturated venous blood drains by gravity into a venous reservoir, which is either a separate component or more typically an integral part of both the bubble and membrane type oxygenators. The oxygenated blood then passes through a heat exchanger, several filtering devices, and finally is actively pumped back into the systemic circulation.[1] The order of the above components may vary with different CPB configurations. Additional components may include alarm systems to warn of low blood levels in the oxygenator/reservoir, in-line pressure monitors and blood gas analyzers, and vaporizers to allow the introduction of volatile anesthetic agents during bypass. Bypass machines at first appear overwhelmingly complex and sophisticated. Thus, in order to fully grasp the concepts and physiology of bypass, it is best to simplify the technology and analyze each component individually.

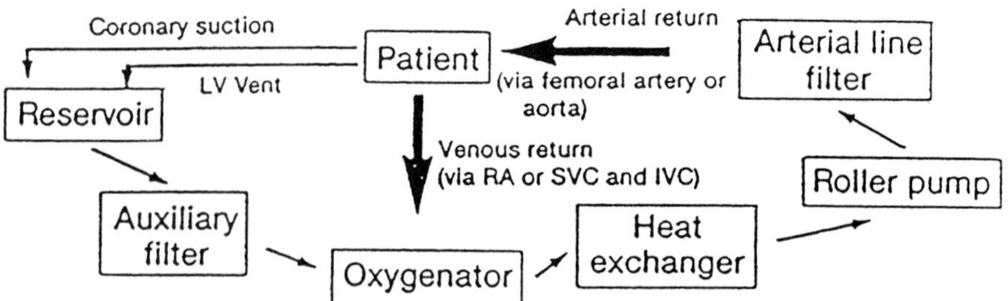

FIGURE **17–1.** The basic circuit for cardiopulmonary bypass. See text for details. (From Tinker JH: Cardiopulmonary bypass: Technical aspects. In Thomas SJ (ed): Manual of Cardiac Anesthesia. New York, Churchill Livingstone, 1984, p 375, with permission.)

Cannula, Tubing and Reservoir

Venous Access

Venous cannulation allows the drainage of blood from the right side of the circulation by either a large, single, two-stage catheter (draining both inferior vena cava and right atrium) or from two separate catheters draining both the superior and inferior venae cavae individually (Fig. 17–2). The single cannula is faster to place, uses one atrial incision, and is technically easier to perform, yet it does not isolate blood flow to the right atrium and is inappropriate when surgery requires access to the right atrium. The double-catheter technique is slower to perform, and more technically difficult in that it requires two atrial incisions. Advantages include optimal caval drainage, access to right atrium, and potentially complete right heart isolation from blood flow, especially when caval tourniquets are utilized. Examples of commonly used venous cannulas are shown in Figure 17–3.

Venous drainage is a passive, gravity-dependent process (siphon) that does not require mechanical assistance. The ability to achieve proper venous drainage is dependent upon several factors, including:

1. Maintaining a height differential between the patient and the reservoir (with the patient being higher)
2. The presence of adequate intravascular volume status
3. Proper placement and/or functioning of the catheters

In addition, the lines must be continuously fluid filled or a vapor lock may potentially develop and disrupt further drainage. When venous drainage exceeds inflow to

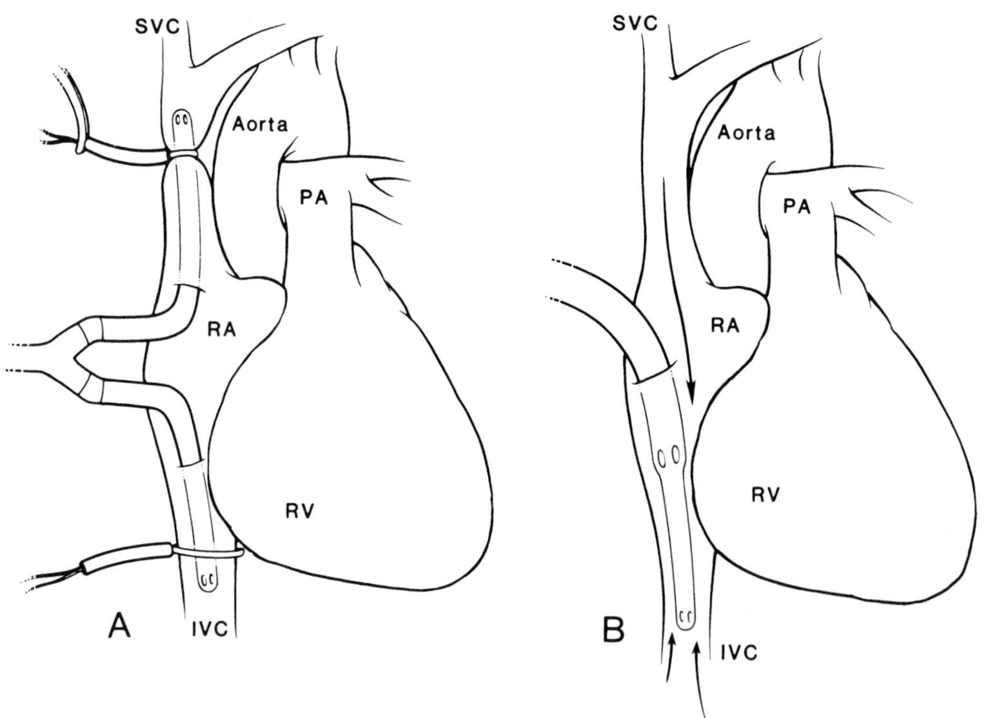

FIGURE **17–2.** Methods of venous cannulation. *A*, Separate cannulation of the superior vena cava (SVC) and inferior vena cava (IVC). Note that there are loops placed around the cavae and venous cannulas and passed through tubing to act as tourniquets or snares. The tourniquet on the SVC has been tightened to divert all of the SVC flow into the SVC cannula and prevent communication with the right atrium (RA). *B*, Single cannulation of right atrium with a "two-stage" cannula. This is typically inserted through the right atrial appendage. Note that the narrower tip of the cannula is in the IVC, where it drains this vein. The wider portion, with additional holes, resides in the right atrium, where blood is received from the coronary sinus and SVC. The SVC must drain via the right atrium. RV, right ventricle; PA, pulmonary artery. (From Hessel EA II: Cardiopulmonary bypass circuitry and cannulation techniques. In Gravlee GP, Davis RF, Utley JR [eds]: Cardiopulmonary Bypass: Principles and Practice. Baltimore, Williams & Wilkins, 1993, p 60, with permission.)

the vena cava, the thin-walled veins or atrium may collapse around the catheter ports, which leads to "chattering" of the venous lines and a decrease in venous return to the machine. Partial clamping of the venous lines will decrease the rate of drainage and allow time to fill the cavae in order to restore normal drainage.

The venous blood drains into a reservoir that has two functions: (1) store the drained deoxygenated blood, and (2) act as an emergency source of blood for the circuit if arterial outflow exceeds venous drainage. All modern CPB machines have an alarm system to alert the perfusionist to a predetermined low-volume threshold to the amount of blood remaining in the reservoir. When the low-volume alarm sounds, the surgeon and the perfusionist must perform an immediate inspection of the circuit and quickly address potential causes of inadequate venous drainage. The most common causes of low reservoir volumes are decreased venous return, or an inadvertent increase in arterial flow. Common flow rates of 2.0 L/min and a reservoir volume of 500 ml only give 15 seconds before the reservoir runs dry. Once the reservoir is drained, air is pumped into the arterial line resulting in a massive air embolus, which is catastrophic and may be lethal. Crystalloid and/or colloid can be quickly added to the reservoir volume by the perfusionist, and arterial flows can be decreased until the surgeons can reposition the venous cannula and restore the adequacy of venous drainage.

Femoral veins are occasionally used as alternative sites to the right atrium/venae cavae but complete bypass is not attainable, because of their smaller relative size and flow limitations. Partial bypass can act as a temporary support, bridging a gap of hemodynamic instability, and allow time until full bypass can be achieved. Femoral access is often done prophylactically for redo open heart cases because of the increased risk of nicking the atrium on dissection, which can lead to uncontrollable hemorrhage and the patient being placed emergently on bypass.

Complications associated with venous cannulation include atrial arrhythmias, atrial/caval lacerations, air embolization, and malposition of catheters. Venous cannulas have been placed through patent atrial defects as well as the azygous, hepatic, and innominate (extracaval) veins. In addition, because of the catheter's large size, caval obstruction occurs and prebypass venous return is frequently impaired. Superior vena cava (SVC) obstruction results in venous facial/neck engorgement (i.e., conjunctival edema) and increased SVC pressures. One method to detect SVC obstruction is to monitor the pressure from the side port of the pulmonary artery catheter (PAC) introducer and monitor for rising pressures as the SVC cannula is inserted. Inferior vena cava (IVC) obstruction is much more difficult to detect, with decreased venous return usually being the earliest warning sign.

Arterial Access

Arterial cannulation allows the return of oxygenated blood to the systemic circulation. The ascending aorta is the most common site of access, primarily because this part of the aorta is large enough to allow the placement of large arterial cannulas. These relatively large catheters allow higher blood flows with less of a pressure differential during blood passage through the catheter. The major causes of morbidity include embolization, aortic dissection, and malposition of the cannula.

Embolization of atheroma and/or other thrombotic material can occur with both arterial cannulation, clamping, and/or manipulation of the aorta. Transcranial Doppler has clearly shown that any manipulation of the ascending aorta results frequent in cerebral embolization.[2,3] These results are further verified by the 5 to 17% incidence of embolic retinal infarctions observed following CPB.[4-6] Steps to reduce the incidence of embolic morbidity include echocardiographic observation of the aorta, and identification of high-risk areas prior to cannulation or manipulation. If the aorta appears completely calcified, then alternative sites such as femoral arteries should be utilized.

Aortic dissection can occur at any time prior to, during, or after CPB, with a frequency rate of 0.02 to 0.35%.[7-9] Dissection is defined as a disruption of the intimal layer, with at least some diversion of blood flow through the extraluminal passage and into the vessel wall. The false passage can become obstructive to major arterial branches, resulting in potential organ/tissue ischemia. Dissection may occur at the arterial cannulation site, the vein graft anastomotic sites, or any segment subjected to complete or partial cross-clamping. The greatest contributing factor to arterial dissection appears to be the presence of arterial hypertension. Because of

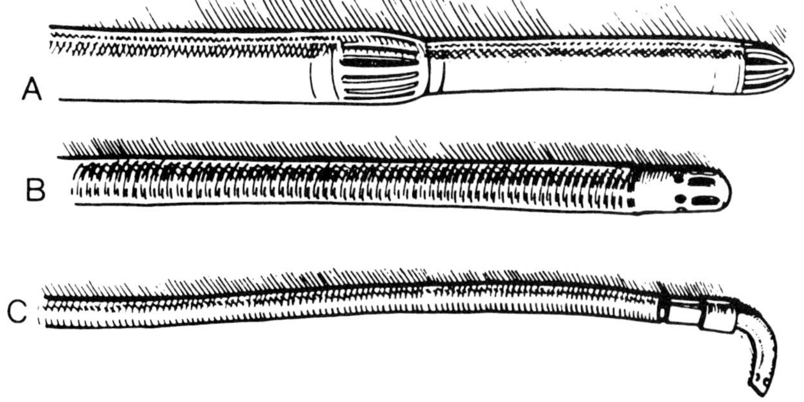

FIGURE **17–3.** Venous cannulae. *A*, Two-stage cannula. *B*, Wire-reinforced plastic cannula for atrial or caval cannulation. *C*, Cannula with right-angled tip usually constructed of metal because the thin wall optimizes the ratio of internal to external diameters. This type of venous cannula is often used for pediatric cases. May be inserted directly into the vena cava near its junction with the right atrium. (From Hensley FA Jr, Martin DE [eds]: The Practice of Cardiac Anesthesia. Boston, Little, Brown & Co, 1990, with permission.)

this, it is common for the surgeon to request transient hypotension with the placement of the arterial cannula. Many methods are effective, including reverse Trendelenburg position, boluses of vasodilating drugs (i.e., nitroprusside, nitroglycerin, or sodium pentothal), or increases in potent inhaled agents. Full anticoagulation is required prior to arterial cannula placement. Recognition of an aortic dissection can occur immediately with cannula placement or be delayed until well into the CPB period. Once dissection has been recognized, the mean arterial pressure (MAP) should be quickly reduced to prevent further propagation. Other risk factors for dissection include the presence of local atheroma plaques and cystic medial necrosis.[8–10]

Once cannulation has been achieved, arterial blood is allowed to back-flow to flush out any air/bubbles and the cannula is attached to the arterial tubing from the machine. Prior to commencing flow, a careful visual inspection is performed by the surgeon to identify and remove any remaining air bubbles. At this time the MAP can rise to preinsertion levels.

Malpositioned aortic cannulas can completely or partially obstruct proximal aortic arch vessels, resulting in reduced perfusion to the right side of the arm and/or face. In addition, the cannula may be positioned to preferentially flow into any one of the great vessels, resulting in focal hyperperfusion and vascular damage due to the high pressures. The anesthesiologist should have heightened awareness at this stage to look for facial color asymmetry, differences in pulse pressures, or differences in blood pressure (BP) measurements in both arms. In one study,[11] electroencephalogram (EEG) monitoring detected perfusion asymmetry in 3.5% of patients (3 of 84).

Alternate sites for arterial cannulation include the femoral arteries. The major drawback of this site is the higher incidence of arterial dissection (0.5 to 0.9%)[12] compared to aortic arch placement. Additional complications include arterial thrombosis, limb ischemia, and arterial site stenosis.[11]

Oxygenators

The development of a practical way to oxygenate venous blood was a major challenge to the early pioneers of CPB technology. Numerous models/techniques were developed in the 1950s, but it was not until 1955 when the Gibbon-type pump oxygenator[13,14] and the DeWall and Lillehei bubble oxygenator[15] were developed that the prototype of modern oxygenators was established. The price of the original oxygenator was prohibitive, but continuous technological advances have produced disposable and relatively inexpensive components, which have led to a dramatic increase in the numbers of cardiac operations over the years.

The term "oxygenator" is a bit of a misnomer because these devices also transport and/or exchange carbon dioxide, potent inhaled agents, and any other gas present in the system into and out of the circulation. There are essentially two types of oxygenators currently in use today, bubble and membrane, and each will be discussed below.

Bubble Oxygenator

The bubble oxygenator was the first type of oxygenator made available for CPB, and its concept is simply to bubble oxygen (O_2) through deoxygenated venous blood. This direct contact between the blood and gas facilitates the transfer of oxygen and carbon dioxide (CO_2) between the two phases. Oxygen flows through a screen mesh, the diameter of which produces a certain bubble size. The number of bubbles depends on the flow of oxygen; 100% oxygen is used because nitrogen is much less soluble in solution and could potentially form gas emboli and escape into the arterial circulation. The exchanging of gases in bubble oxygenators is slightly problematic in the fact that CO_2 is 25 times more soluble and thus more easily diffusible than O_2. The transport of oxygen is optimized by increasing the available surface area of the gas-blood interface, which is accomplished by reducing the size of the gas bubbles. Smaller bubbles enhance the exchange of oxygen. On the other hand, the removal of CO_2 is proportional to total gas flow and is enhanced by larger bubble size. In actuality, the bubble sizes are a compromise between these two extremes.

Once oxygenation has been completed, the blood then enters a defoaming chamber, where it passes through a polyurethane mesh coated with a silicone-based antifoam material. The defoaming process must be rapid enough to maintain blood flow rates, but thorough enough to prevent any bubbles from escaping into the systemic circulation. Final defoaming occurs in the arterial reservoir, where the bubbles are allowed to float to the top of the reservoir and vent to the atmosphere. In addition, the arterial outflow tract is at the bottom of the reservoir, allowing additional time for the air and blood phases to separate. Figure 17–4 is a schematic drawing of a typical bubble oxygenator.

The bubble oxygenator is a simple, efficient, and relatively inexpensive type of oxygenator that does not require a large priming volume, and the pressure drop across the bubble oxygenator is low enough to allow them to be placed upstream of the CPB pump. One limitation of the bubble oxygenator is that oxygenation and carbon dioxide removal cannot be changed independently of one another. Another limitation is the direct trauma to blood components resulting in hemolysis, platelet dysfunction/destruction, and disruption of clotting mechanisms. This impact appears to be time dependent, with increased hematologic trauma with longer bypass times. There is no clinical difference between bubble oxygenator and membrane oxygenator–managed patients, as long as bypass is limited to less than 2 hours.[16]

Membrane Oxygenator

The driving force behind the development of the membrane oxygenator was to more accurately replicate the normal human lung. This is accomplished by separating the gas and the blood phases with a thin permeable membrane. The first membrane oxygenator was introduced into clinical practice in 1956. The prototype was awkward to use, and required large priming volumes.

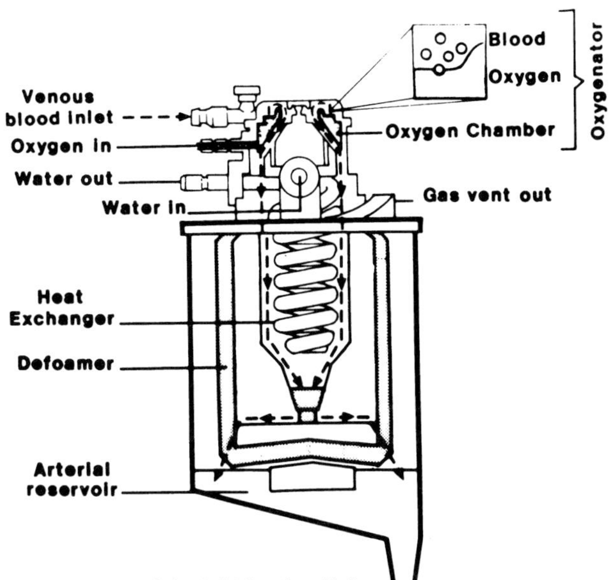

FIGURE 17–4. Schematic of a typical bubble oxygenator showing the mixing chamber, heat exchanger, defoamer, and arterial reservoir. (From High KM, Williams DR, Kurusz M: Cardiopulmonary bypass circuits and design. In Hensley FA, Martin DE [eds]: The Practice of Cardiac Anesthesia. Boston, Little, Brown & Co, 1990, with permission.)

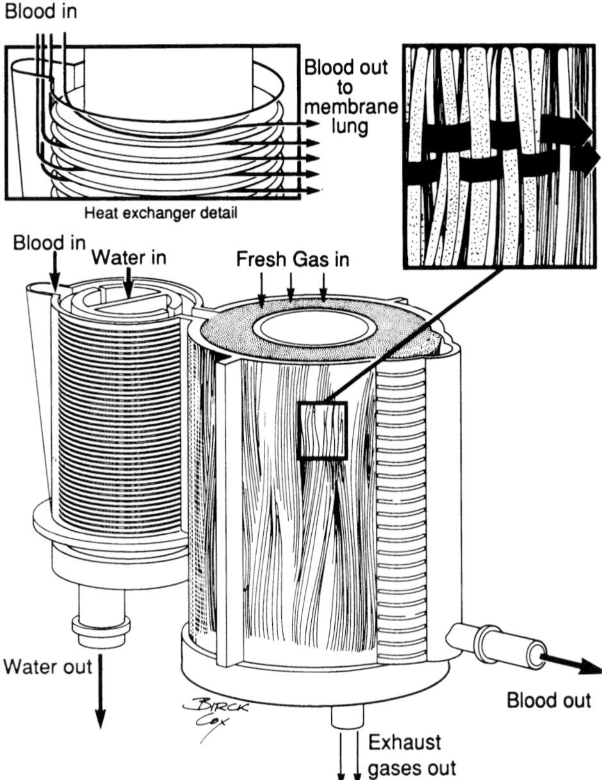

FIGURE 17–5. Schematic diagram of a typical membrane lung. In this case, the heat exchanger (shown in detail in the upper left of the figure) incorporates fins that act as channels through which the blood flows. The blood first passes through the heat exchanger and then through the gas exchange portion of the membrane lung. Both the heat exchanger and gas exchanger portions contain manifolding that distributes blood flow evenly to minimize shunting with the device. (From High KM, Snider MT, Bashein G: Principles of oxygenator function: Gas exchange, heat transfer, and blood-artificial surface interaction. In Gravlee GP, Davis RF, Utley JR [eds]: Cardiopulmonary Bypass: Principles and Practice. Baltimore, Williams & Wilkins, 1993, p 40, with permission.)

However, it led to the development of the modern compact membrane oxygenator, which has a large surface area, ranging from 2 to 4 m^2. Figure 17–5 is a schematic diagram of a typical membrane oxygenator.

There are generally two types of membranes used in membrane oxygenators: microporous and solid membranes. The solid membranes are not commonly used during CPB for cardiac surgery. Instead, they are used in oxygenators designed for ECMO where cardiopulmonary support is required for extended periods of time. The microporous membranes are more commonly used in CPB cases and are made of a thin layer of polypropylene, silicon, Teflon, or other similar gas-permeable material arranged in sheets or fibers. These sheets/fibers contain a vast number of micropores, and these micropores initially allow physical contact between the blood and gas phases when CPB is initiated. The pores themselves are quickly covered by a thin protein layer that effectively separates the blood and gas phases. Because there is no prolonged direct contact between the gas and blood, red blood cells (RBC) and other cellular elements appear to suffer less trauma with membrane oxygenators compared with bubble oxygenators. Another advantage of the membrane oxygenators is the ability to alter FIO_2 and CO_2 independently, which again is not possible in the bubble oxygenator.

One disadvantage is that the membrane oxygenator must be positioned after the pump source because of the higher blood flow resistance through the oxygenator. In addition, there are still significant limitations in duplicating normal lung function, including effectively reproducing the surface area of the normal human lung and decreasing the diffusion distance that gas molecules must travel to effectively be exchanged. In order to compensate for these shortcomings, membrane oxygenators allow for a longer time period in which the blood and the gas phases are exposed to one another. Theoretically, this will result in more complete oxygen saturation and unloading of CO_2. In addition, the gas-permeable sheets have purposeful irregularities on their surface to induce blood mixing and potentially allow deoxygenated blood to swirl closer to the membrane for gas exchange. An added benefit is that 100% O_2 can be used without the threat of oxygen toxicity.

Pumps

There are essentially two types of arterial pumps to provide nonpulsatile systemic perfusion: the nonocclusive roller pump (RP) and the centrifugal blood pump (CP) as seen in Figure 17–6.

The most commonly used pump is the nonocclusive roller type, which uses volume displacement to create forward blood flow. The roller pump commonly has two to three heads, and at least one is in contact with the

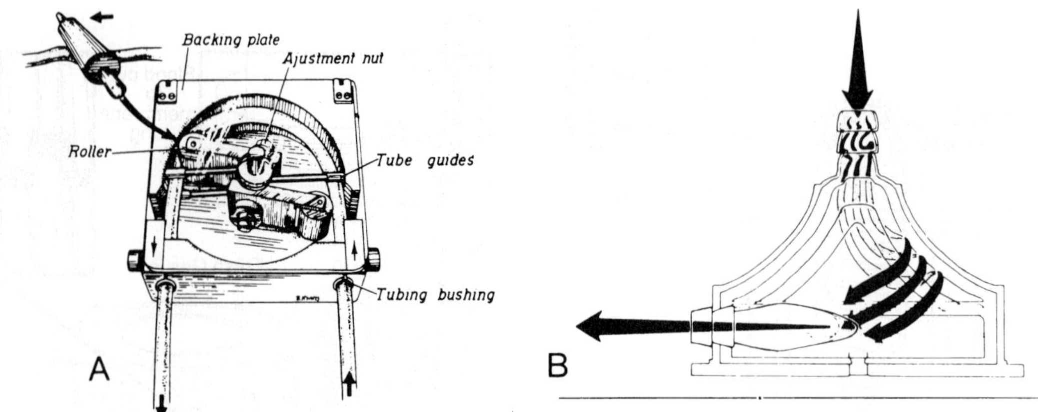

FIGURE **17–6.** Arterial pumps. *A*, Roller pump. *B*, Centrifugal pump. See text for details of their function. (*A* is from Reed CC, Stafford TB: Cardiopulmonary Bypass, 2nd ed. Houston, Texas Medical Press, Inc, 1985; *B* is from Lake CL [ed]: Pediatric Cardiac Anesthesia. Norwalk, CT, Appleton & Lange, 1988, with permission.)

tubing at all times. This contact ensures forward blood displacement, resulting in a generation of blood flow. Electric motors drive the pumps, and are load independent, meaning that the pumps will continue to push the same volume of fluid forward, regardless of the resistance in the line itself. This can lead to large pressure rises in the arterial tubing and potential rupture of tubing interconnections. Modern machines have pressure monitors that alarm and/or reduce flow to decrease the pressure generation and allow time for the surgeon to inspect and correct arterial line kinks. Another drawback of roller pumps is their potential for pumping large volumes of air if the reservoir/oxygenator is allowed to empty. One benefit of the RP is that in the case of power failure a set of hand cranks provide continuous blood flow.

Centrifugal pumps operate by generating a vortex in the pump that in turn creates a centrifugal force, driving the blood through the tubing.[17,18] One benefit of this pump versus the roller type is that there appears to be less insult to the red blood cells and other blood components.[17] The CP also differs in the fact that increases in in-line resistance result in decreased flow rates; thus the CP autoregulates and prevents line rupture. An additional benefit is that if a large quantity of air is introduced into the pump, a disruption between blood layers occurs, diminishing the centrifugal forces, and pumping will decrease or stop. There is also a reduced risk of microbubble air embolization, because smaller bubbles will tend to gravitate to the center of the vortex and avoid being pushed into the systemic arterial line. Disadvantages include the inability to generate pulsatile flow and the potential discrepancy between pump speed and actual flow generated.

Heat Exchangers

The purpose of the heat exchanger (HE) is to rapidly achieve mild, moderate, or profound degrees of hypothermia and to quickly reverse the process in order to prepare the patient for bypass separation. The cooling and warming of the patient's blood occurs via a countercurrent mechanism, which is the most efficient technique for heat exchange. Water of a predetermined temperature flows through a metal coil in an opposite direction of blood flow. The temperature difference between the coil and the blood during rewarming should never exceed 10°C. Avoidance of a gradient prevents the formation of gas microemboli, which can form as gases become less soluble in the blood during rewarming. This phenomenon is the reason that HEs are located before the oxygenator in CPB circuits, in order to filter out air emboli prior to reaching the arterial circulation.

Filters

Standard CPB machines are equipped with both venous and arterial micropore filters. The venous filters primarily remove particulate matter from the cardiotomy suction devices. Arterial filters function to remove air emboli from the arterial tubing prior to the blood entering the body. A typical arterial filter is seen in Figure 17–7. The arterial filter is vented to the atmosphere to prevent gas accumulation that may impede blood flow through the filter. Decreased flow through the filter will increase the in-line pressure and eventually force air through the filter and into the circulation. An extensive review of bypass filters was recently published by Joffe and Silvay.[19]

Anticoagulation

Appropriate systemic anticoagulation is an absolute prerequisite to the initiation of bypass. Bypass circuits are thrombogenic when exposed to blood; thus, temporary, reversible inhibition of coagulation is necessary to allow the patient to undergo bypass surgery. This requires the cardiac anesthesiologist to have a thorough knowledge of both normal and pathologic hemostasis and the implications of heparin and protamine pharmacology in relation to the bypass patient.

Heparin

The anticoagulant properties of heparin were first noted in 1916 and introduced into clinical practice in 1937.[20] It is currently the only anticoagulant drug utilized for CPB in the United States. Heparin continues to be used because of its rapid onset time, easy reversibility, and moderate therapeutic window with relatively few side effects. The only relative contraindication for heparin use during bypass is heparin-induced thrombocytopenia (HIT), the management of which is discussed below. Heparin is a polyanionic mucopolysaccharide extracted from other porcine intestine or bovine lung. The molecule itself is heterogeneous in size, varying with the length of the carbohydrate side chain. The half-life of heparin is 90 to 100 minutes in a normothermic patient, with decreasing temperature prolonging the half-life. It is highly protein bound, and undergoes hepatic metabolism with the metabolite being excreted in the urine. In addition, heparin can also be taken up by endothelial cells[21] where it is neither metabolized nor neutralized by protamine. This intracellular store of heparin in released back into the circulation as the concentration gradient reverses itself. This may explain the phenomenon of heparin "rebound," where a heparin effect is observed 1 to 8 hours after neutralization with protamine was initially successful.

Heparin exerts its pharmacologic effect primarily through its interaction with antithrombin III (AT-III). AT-III is a naturally occurring anticoagulant that inactivates several serine proteases of the coagulation system, including thrombin (factor Ii), and factors IV, IX, and aX. Heparin binds to AT-III and accelerates the formation of inactive complexes 2,000-fold,[22] resulting in a dose-dependent level of anticoagulation.

The use of heparin during cardiopulmonary bypass has been well established. Heparin is given as a single-bolus loading dose in the range of 300 to 400 U/kg, anytime prior to cannula placement. The drug must be injected into a known central access or directly by the surgeon into the right atrium. Heparin doses should always be described in unit values and not by weight because of the variance in biologic activity. A transient episode of hypotension may be seen because the negatively charged heparin chelates a substantial fraction of ionized calcium. An activated coagulation time (ACT) measurement can be obtained 2 minutes after administration of heparin.

Heparin resistance occurs in a variety of clinical settings, where the conventional dose of heparin has minimal anticoagulant effects. Some of the factors associated with heparin resistance are listed in Table 17–1. The mechanism of heparin resistance is still not fully known, however, decreased levels of AT-III is the most likely cause. Intravenous (IV) or subcutaneous (SC) doses of heparin decrease serum AT-III levels 17 to 33%.[23–25] One prominent cause of decreased AT-III levels in CPB patients is the hemodilution that occurs with the onset of bypass. The mixing of prime solution with the patient's blood reduces AT-III levels 50% of normal.[26] Treatment consists of increased heparin doses, up to 800 U/kg, and the administration of fresh frozen plasma (FFP) to increase AT-III levels (usually 2 U in adults).

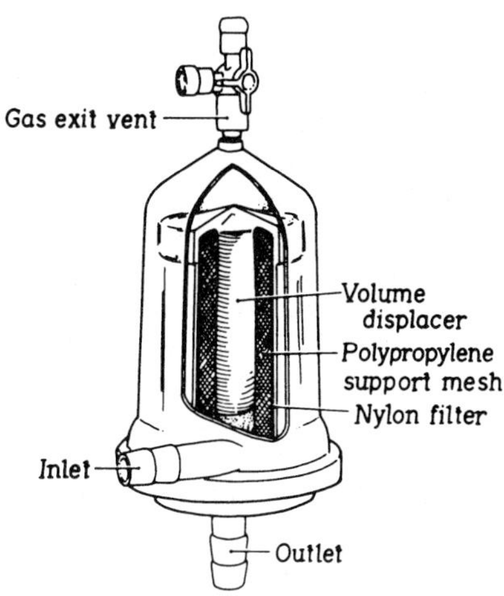

FIGURE **17–7.** An arterial line microfilter and bubble trap (Bentley AF-10). Blood enters tangentially at the bottom and swirls upward, encouraging bubbles to flow to the top, where they escape through a continuous purge line to the cardiotomy reservoir. Blood passes through a microfilter (25 μm) and out the bottom. (From Reed CC, Stafford TB: Cardiopulmonary Bypass, 2nd ed. Houston, Texas Medical Press, Inc, 1985, with permission.)

HIT is a complication of heparin therapy that results in thrombocytopenia, tachyphylaxis, and arterial thrombosis. It commonly occurs 7 to 10 days after starting heparin therapy and is caused by the formation of IgG antibodies that bind and activate platelets, fix complement, and generate platelet aggregation. The major cause of morbidity and mortality is a result of arterial thrombus formation in critical organ beds or distal extremities. The incidence of thrombotic complications is 20% with a resultant 35% mortality rate.[27] The diagnosis is confirmed by a heparin antibody assay (HAT test), where heparin administration results in platelet aggregation. Treatment is simply to stop heparin administration, which also includes the removal of heparin from transducer flush solutions.

The administration of heparin to previously sensitized patients results in a rapid and, at times, severe thrombocytopenia with concomitant formation of platelet aggregates/emboli. A real dilemma exists when a patient with the diagnosis of HIT requires emergent open heart surgery. Therapeutic options include delaying the case (often up to 12 months) until the heparin-induced antibodies are no longer present, plasmapharesis, or Iloprost administration. Iloprost, a prostacyclin analog that can

TABLE **17–1**
Causes of Heparin Resistance

Ongoing active coagulation
AT-III deficiency—congenital or secondary
Prior heparin treatment
Drug interactions (oral contraceptives)
Other medical diseases—hypereosinophilia
Drug error
Advanced age
Intravenous nitroglycerin

produce reversible platelet inhibition by preventing platelet aggregation and adherence to vessel or circuit walls, is considered the drug management of choice for patients with HIT requiring urgent cardiac surgery.[28] The drug is delivered by infusion, started before heparinization and continued through heparin neutralization by protamine. The drug has a rapid half-life (15 to 30 minutes) and platelet function returns rapidly after the infusion is discontinued. This allows the platelets to participate in hemostasis at the end of surgery.

Inadequate anticoagulation during bypass is uniformly lethal to the patient. The presence of clots in the bypass machine is a medical crisis, as the accumulating thrombi prevent forward blood flow through the machine resulting in inadequate systemic perfusion. Thrombi will also clog the filters and eventually rupture the tubing if flows are not decreased. Finally, thrombi can form distal to the filters and embolize systemically. The presence of thrombus within the circuit is essentially untreatable. The only option available is to stop CPB and go to complete circulatory arrest. External cooling of the patient should begin immediately (i.e., ice bags, iced solutions) and open cardiac massage is initiated. A repeat full heparin dose is given from another stock source and another pump oxygenator is quickly primed to serve as a replacement. Once the patient is back on bypass, additional steps may be taken to reduce the ischemic neurologic injury including the administration of steroids, barbiturates, and/or oxygen free radical scavengers. Unfortunately, these steps can only lessen the degree of hypoxic insult, not prevent it.

Tests of Coagulation

ACT is the most commonly used measurement of adequacy of anticoagulation and is a modification of the accelerated Lee-White whole blood clotting time that was first described by Hattersley in 1966.[29] The addition of diatomaceous earth accelerates the generation of factor XIIa,[29] allowing 2 to 3 ml of blood in the tube to clot faster than the WBCT.

Once the heparin has been given, an ACT is measured 2 minutes later. Although institutions differ, an acceptable ACT for bypass is usually greater than 400 seconds. Bull et al.[30] recommended an ACT greater than 480 seconds or longer for CPB. Young et al.,[31] combining a primate study and data from human children, found no fibrin monomers present if the ACT was at least 400 seconds. The tendency is to err on the side of overanticoagulation, as the reverse is lethal. The adequacy of anticoagulation must be established prior to the placement of the arterial and venous lines.

The thromboelastograph (TEG) is an alternative method of measuring coagulation status, where the physical properties of whole blood are plotted and amplified on tracing paper and examined for several parameters. Its applicability in the operating room remains limited and a majority of centers continue to utilize the ACT exclusively.

Alternate Methods of Anticoagulation

The only contraindication to heparin administration is the presence of HIT. Currently, in the United States no alternative drug has been approved for CPB anticoagulation, although some recent research appears encouraging.

Ancrod is an extract of Malayan pit viper venom, which cleaves fibrinogen, leading to fibrinogen levels well below 40 mg/dl. This process can take up to 24 hours, and to reverse the venom's effect requires the transfusion of FFP or cryoprecipitate. Because of the increased use of perioperative blood products, ancrod is not considered a reasonable alternative to heparin and is not available in the United States for clinical use.

Another group of alternative anticoagulant drugs include leech-derived anticoagulant factors, hirudin and dermatan sulfate. Both factors are direct thrombin inhibitors and function independently of AT-III. Walenga et al.[32] successfully used hirudin for full anticoagulation in a dog CPB model. However, the perioperative bleeding was the same when compared to a heparin control group. In addition, the fibrin levels were 20-fold higher in the hirudin-treated group. At this time, hirudin provides no real benefit over heparin and is not likely to gain clinical acceptance. A recent study by Brister and Buchanan[33] compared dermatan sulfate and heparin in a pig model and found that the dermatan sulfate is an effective alternative to heparin during CPB. This study and several others[34–36] have found significantly less bleeding compared with heparin. Further research needs to be done, as dermatan sulfate may prove to be a viable alternative to heparin therapy.

An alternative to systemic heparinization is the development of bypass components that have reduced or completely lack thrombogenic activity. Heparin-bonded circuits are now being examined in clinical trials with favorable initial results. The heparin-bonded surface, interacting with the patient's own AT-III, is effective in preventing thrombus formation. In addition, these circuits also reduce platelet and coagulation activation.[37–39] Because of the presence of bound heparin, a smaller amount of systemic heparin is required to initiate bypass. Potential benefits include less bleeding complications and a smaller dose of protamine will be needed, which in turn may lessen the severity of adverse protamine reactions.[39]

Organ System Pathophysiology

The onset of CPB is associated with a profound impact on virtually every organ system in the body. Yet, despite the systemic insult, CPB is associated with a relatively low incidence of morbidity and mortality. The reason for this low incidence is certainly due to significant improvements in bypass machine designs and an increase in our basic understanding of the pathophysiology associated with bypass. What is not understood is the patient variability in response to the bypass insult. Postbypass organ system dysfunction is a spectrum ranging from mild organ dysfunction to severe multisystem organ failure with a high mortality. The etiology of post-bypass organ dysfunction is dependent on the following four variables:

1. The exposure to the blood to foreign material
2. Changes in blood flow patterns
3. The patient's neurohumoral response
4. Degree of hypothermia

The majority of the pathologic conditions resolve after restoration of normal physiologic conditions; however, some patients develop end-organ injury, which can result in significant morbidity and mortality. The length of bypass is associated with the development of impaired organ dysfunction. The risk to the patient is also complicated by the fact that older, less healthy patients are undergoing open heart procedures and that more of these patients are having redo surgeries or emergency operations after failed catheterization laboratory interventions.

Hemodilution

Hemodilution occurs at the onset of bypass as the patient's blood and the priming volume in the bypass machine mix. Historically, the first CPB cases utilized whole blood to prime the apparatus so hemodilution was not really observed. The 1960s saw the introduction of blood-free priming solutions to reduce blood product use and decrease the risk of infectious disease transmission. Crystalloid and/or colloid solutions became increasingly popular and are utilized almost exclusively in today's bypass cases. Prior to the acceptance of blood-free priming solutions, however, there was considerable concern that the hemodilution effect could potentially lead to a reduced oxygen-carrying capacity and subsequent tissue ischemia. Fortunately, hypothermia became increasingly utilized, which decreased tissue metabolic activity and correspondingly reduced tissue oxygen demand. Thus the use of blood-free solutions became increasingly safe as hypothermia was used on a more frequent basis.

The composition of the modern day priming solutions is variable and center dependent. Common prime solutions utilize a balanced salt solution (i.e., normosol, lactated Ringer's) that is combined with varying amounts of colloid (hydroxyethyl starch, albumin), mannitol, heparin, calcium, magnesium, bicarbonate and steroids.[40] Colloid solutions are commonly added to increase the plasma oncotic pressure. However, a study by Marelli et al.[41] showed the addition of albumin provided no clinical benefit.

The mixing of the adult patient's blood with the typical 1.5 to 2.0 L of prime volume results in a dilutional anemia (hematocrit [Hct] of 20 to 25), and a reduction in the colloid osmotic pressure (COP). Webber and Garnett[42] found a 44% reduction in COP during CPB, while other studies showed similar reductions in COP, ranging from 37 to 60%.[43,44] Albumin is the prime determinant of COP, and appears to decrease during bypass. Webber and Garnett found albumin reduced 32% at the conclusion of bypass. The decrease in COP leads to an increased accumulation of extracellular fluid in numerous organ beds including the heart, musculoskeletal, liver, gastrointestinal, and lungs.[45]

The potential benefits of hemodilution include a reduction in the use of scarce blood products, decreased risk of transfusion-related complications, and reduced transmission of blood-borne disease.[46] In addition, rheologic studies have shown that decreased viscosity of the blood allows improved perfusion in the microcirculation, thus enhancing tissue blood flow and potentially increasing delivery of oxygen and other nutrients. This is particularly important in hypothermic conditions where blood viscosity increases with cooler temperature. If the hypothermic bypass patient had a normal hematocrit, blood may tend to sludge in the microcirculation and impede oxygen delivery to the tissues.

Cardiovascular

The onset of bypass commonly results in a dramatic decrease in the patient's MAP. The mechanism is probably secondary to the reduction in blood viscosity that occurs with the mixing of blood and nonblood priming solutions.[47] In two separate studies by Gordon et al.[47,48] the MAP was found to reasonably correlate with changes in blood viscosity. They examined 20 CPB patients, whose MAP, on initiation of bypass decreased by 56% (±16%) and corresponded with a 40% (±12%) decrease in blood viscosity. Interestingly, five patients had blood added to the prime so that hematocrit and blood viscosity remained constant, and these patients did not have decreases in their MAP.[48] The MAP gradually returns toward normal bypass values as hypothermia increases blood viscosity (Fig. 17–8) and elevated endogenous vasoactive molecules result in vasoconstriction. Other

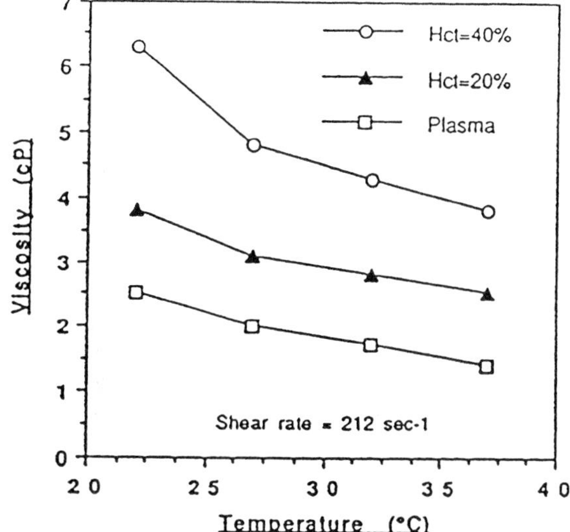

FIGURE **17–8.** Blood viscosity as a function of temperature and hematocrit. Viscosity increases with increasing hematocrit and decreasing temperature. (Data from Rand PW, Lacombe E, Hunt HE, Austin WH: Viscosity of normal human blood under normothermic and hypothermic conditions. J Appl Physiol 19:117, 1964)

causes of hypotension with the commencement of bypass include:

1. Vasodilation secondary to anesthetic agents, vasoactive drugs, or metabolic factors
2. Inappropriately low perfusion flow rates due to either mechanical problems within the circuit or the perfusionist miscalculating the actual flow rate for the patient
3. Cannula malposition into the carotid or subclavian vessels
4. Aortic dissection

Lastly, it must be emphasized to check the accuracy of the measurement itself by flushing and zeroing the transducers prior to initiating any unnecessary interventions. Hypertension is not commonly seen and is discussed in a later section.

Hemodilution itself causes an increase in myocardial interstitial fluid, which could potentially alter contractility and reduce cardiac function. Utley et al.[49] found that in a canine model, 2 hours of bypass resulted in the development of myocardial edema. The addition of albumin to the prime solution did not reduce the degree or incidence of edema formation. The impact of myocardial edema is not known, especially as regards postbypass contractility. Several studies have found no relationship between low COP and any cardiac function parameters.[50–52]

The other major alteration of the cardiovascular system is the loss of pulsatile blood flow during bypass. This topic has been intensely researched and hotly debated, and yet still remains a controversial topic in CPB management. Nonpulsatile blood flow (NPBF) remains the standard of care in a vast majority of bypass cases. However, a few centers continue to research the benefits of pulsatile blood flow. NPBP is technically easier to reproduce and is generated by roller pumps that produce a sine waveform pattern of blood flow. This blood flow pattern is sequentially dampened as the blood passes through successive lengths of tubing and cannulas, resulting in a nonpulsatile mean pressure. In order to make the waveform pulsatile, additional components need to be added to the circuit that add significantly to the complexity and to the cost of the bypass machine.

The comparison between pulsatile and nonpulsatile blood flow remains controversial despite a large volume of research in this area. While a number of studies report benefits of pulsatile blood flow, an equal number fail to show a difference in outcome between the two techniques. The proposed benefit of PBF is that additional hydraulic energy is required to generate the pulse waveform and that this extra energy is translated into improved capillary perfusion, enhanced lymphatic drainage, and increased RBC transit through the tissues.[53] Theoretically, it would seem that the body would prefer the more normal physiology of a pulsatile waveform, yet until a study can show conclusive evidence of superiority this hypothesis remains unproven.

Baroreceptor activity appears to remain intact during pulsatile blood flow (PBF),[54] resulting in less hemodynamic variability in the immediate postbypass period. Canivert et al.[55] demonstrated that the renin-angiotensin axis is attenuated during PBF, resulting in a lower systemic vascular resistance. Other studies, however, fail to demonstrate a decrease in systemic vascular resistance (SVR).[56–60] The comparison of PBF versus NPBF on critical organ beds such as the kidney and the central nervous system (CNS) has also been extensively examined. Several studies[56,61,62] have suggested improved renal blood flow or urine output with PBF. In contrast, a recent study by Badner et al.[63] found no difference in renal function between NPBF- and PBF-managed patients. In patients with pre-existing renal disease, however, PBF may be superior. Olinger et al.[64] found that pulsatile blood flow better preserved renal function in patients with serum creatinine greater than 1.7 mg/dl. A number of studies[65–67] have shown better cerebral perfusion or improved neurologic outcome in both animal and human models treated with PBF. Yet, recent human studies by Henze et al.[68] and Shaw et al.[69] found no difference in neurologic outcome in patients managed with pulsatile versus nonpulsatile blood flow. PBF impact on hormonal levels is interesting in that cortisol levels are not influenced by the presence of pulsation,[70–72] and pancreatic β cell function appears to be better maintained under pulsatile blood flow.[73]

These data suggest that PBF may improve tissue perfusion in certain critical organ beds and better preserve endocrine and autonomic integrity in comparison to NPBF. Yet, despite this evidence NPBF continues to be used almost exclusively for several reasons. First, NPBF is technically easier to generate, requiring less components than PBF; this makes NPBF less costly. Second, the NPBF outcome studies are comparable to PBF and despite volumes of research no true advantage has been clearly identified. And lastly, there are a number of technical difficulties in generating a true pulsatile waveform pattern. The analysis of the pulse waveform is complex, and at this time the technology does not exist to precisely reproduce an arterial pulse. In addition, there is no standard or universally accepted definition of effective pulsatile blood flow currently available, making comparisons between different pulse-generating machines/models virtually impossible. Thus, the creation of an "ideal" pulsatile waveform for individual patients with variable cardiovascular pathophysiologic abnormalities is at this time impossible. For all these reasons, NPBF will continue to be almost exclusively utilized for cardiopulmonary bypass. This topic is further reviewed by Philbin.[74]

Hematologic

Red Blood Cells

A number of factors influence RBC survival during CPB exposure. During CPB, red blood cells become stiffer and lose their distensibility, which may in turn interfere with profusion on the microcirculatory level. Stiffer red blood cells also have shorter lifespans. Red blood cells are directly traumatized by CPB, either by direct exposure to air/artificial surfaces and/or by exposure to unnatural shear stresses. Thus hemolysis is encouraged by higher pump flow rates and the use of bubble oxygenators.[75,76] The greatest cause of RBC damage and hemolysis is the intraoperative suction devices, in particular cardiotomy suction. Accordingly, because of all the potential trauma to the RBC, free hemoglobin levels increase four-fold within 10 minutes of CPB initiation.[77]

An unusual cause of hemolysis during bypass is a result of cold agglutination. This autoimmune disease produces antibodies that cause agglutination of red cells below a specific temperature. Upon rewarming, the red cells are hemolyzed, producing dramatic rises in free hemoglobin levels. In addition, once the process has been initiated, microvascular thrombi can form, leading to critical organ ischemia or infarction. Patients with this diagnosis must have their critical temperature threshold where red cells start to agglutinate identified. There are five types of cold agglutinins, each with a different critical temperature. Bypass management in these patients is problematic, as the temperature must remain above the critical threshold. The benefit of hypothermia, particularly with regard to neurologic and myocardial protection, may be reduced or negated.

Alternative techniques include the use of warm cardioplegia or the use of standard hypothermic management; potential complications are handled afterward. A study by Berreklouw et al.[78] proposed the use of warm cardioplegia to wash all the blood and serum out of the coronary circulation and then infuse the cold cardioplegia solution to protect the myocardium. It is imperative to limit the collateral blood flow during this portion of the surgery. This group also recommended the use of steroids to attenuate the agglutination process.[78] Plasmapharesis has also been used to decrease the cold agglutinin antibody levels. An algorithm to manage patients with cold agglutinins is listed in Figure 17–9.

White Cells

The other cellular elements affected by CPB are white cells. In the first few minutes following the initiation of bypass, the neutrophil count drops rapidly as they become sequestered primarily in the pulmonary circulation and form aggregates in a number of organ systems.[79]

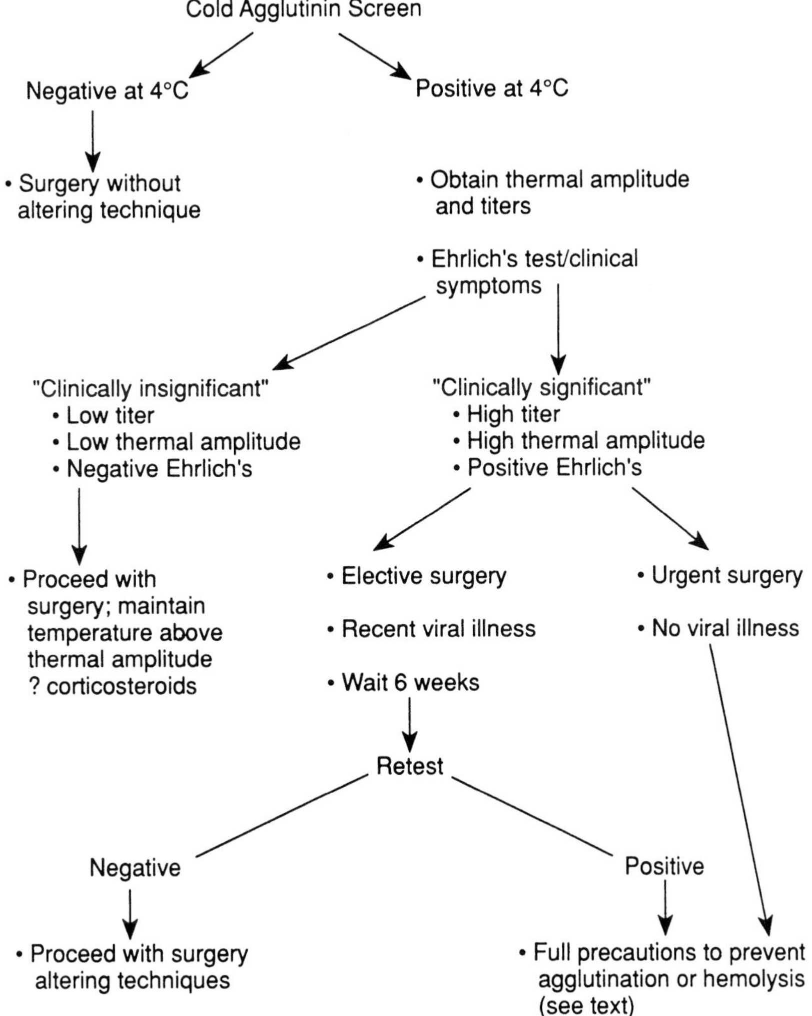

FIGURE 17–9. Algorithm for cold agglutinins in CPB. (From Hockmuth DR, Mills NL: Management of unusual problems encountered initiating and maintaining cardiopulmonary bypass. In Gravlee GP, Davis RF, Utley JR [eds]: Cardiopulmonary Bypass: Principles and Practice. Baltimore, Williams & Wilkins, 1993, p 746, with permission.)

Circulating neutrophils rebound during the rewarming phase of the bypass operation.

The importance of complement activation during bypass was first noted by Parker et al.[80] in 1972. CPB activates complement via the alternate pathway,[80] a result of contact with nonendothelial surfaces. Elevated levels of C5a and C3a have been noted on bypass,[79] and C5a binds rapidly to circulating neutrophils, activating them and causing their sequestration in the lungs and other vascular organs. The activated neutrophils release numerous intracellular contents including oxygen free radicals, superoxides and lysosomal enzymes. The end result is widespread endothelial damage, activation of the coagulation cascade, increase in vascular permeability, and the accumulation of interstitial fluid. Figure 17–10 demonstrates the proposed mechanism of lung injury occurring during bypass. These reactions are usually self-limited; however, the degree of activation is linked to the duration of bypass. Thus, longer bypass times often result in significantly more morbidity as a result.

Renal

Renal blood flow and urine output are often decreased during CPB secondary to decreased flow rates and MAP during bypass. The potential for renal impairment increases with duration of bypass.[81] The loss of pulsatility may also reduce renal blood flow. During low perfusion states, renal blood flow is redistributed from the cortex to the more peripheral medulla. Interestingly, several studies have shown that urine output during bypass has no correlation with postbypass renal function.[82,83] One potential reason for this observation is that the priming solutions often contain mannitol, and the osmotic diuresis may give a false sense of security to the anesthe-

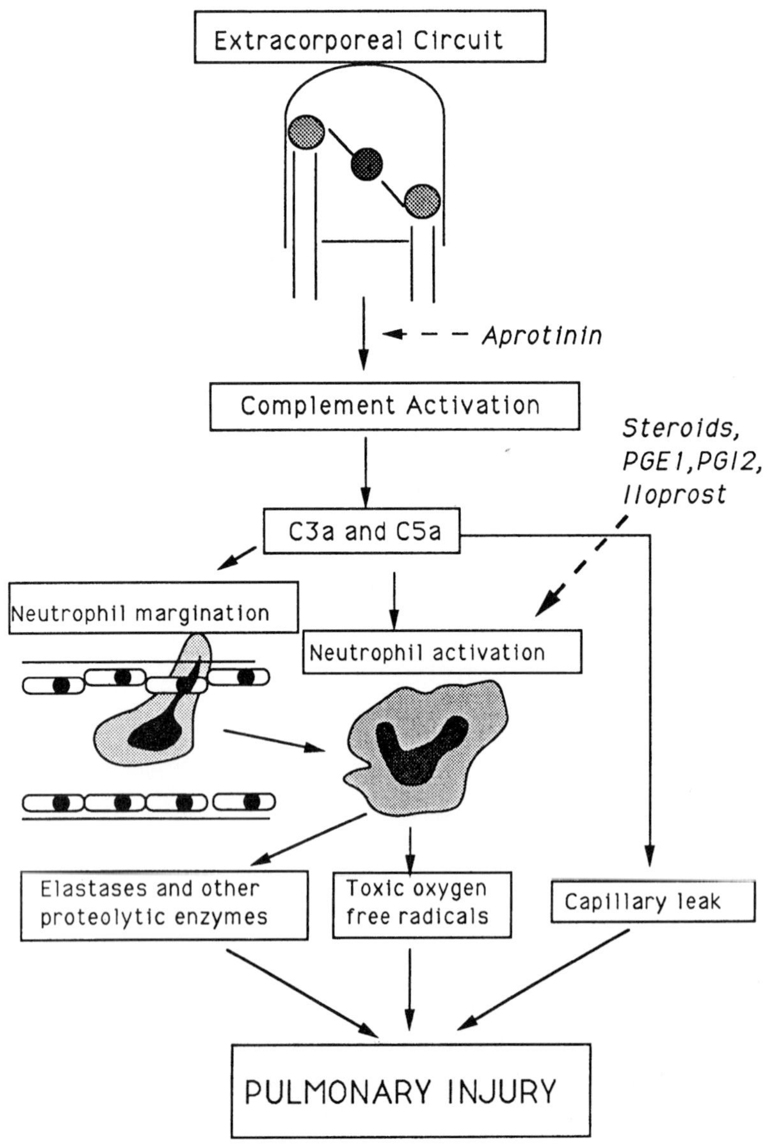

FIGURE **17–10.** A conceptual diagram of the cascade of pathophysiologic events initiated by CPB and leading to pulmonary injury. *Dashed arrows* indicate inhibitory actions. (From Sladen RN, Berkowitz DE: Cardiopulmonary bypass and the lung. In Gravlee GP, Davis RF, Utley JR [eds]: Cardiopulmonary Bypass: Principles and Practice. Baltimore, Williams & Wilkins, 1993, p 473, with permission.)

siologist. Most anesthesiologists prefer the patient to maintain a urine output during bypass of 1 ml/kg/hr. A urine output less than 0.5 ml/kg/hr should be evaluated and is often treated with volume and/or pharmacologic intervention.

The incidence of acute renal failure (ARF) in CPB patients varies from 1.5%[84] to 5.3%.[83,85] Risk factors for the development of ARF include preoperative left ventricular (LV) dysfunction, pre-existing renal insufficiency, and length of bypass exposure. Two studies by Hilberman et al.[82,83] found postbypass ventricular dysfunction and a low cardiac output state to be a major cause of postoperative renal dysfunction/failure. Other causes of perioperative renal dysfunction include cellular or humoral elements released during bypass; endocrine response to stress; and the administration of nephrotoxic drugs before, during, and after the surgery itself. The onset of bypass stimulates the renin-angiotensin axis and can dramatically increase renal vascular resistance.[86] Pharmacologic agents that can contribute to perioperative renal dysfunction include angiographic dyes, antibiotics, and nonsteroidal anti-inflammatory drugs that can inhibit renal artery vasodilating prostaglandins. Angiotensin-converting enzyme inhibitors can lead to renal failure in patients with renal artery stenosis.[87] If iatrogenic renal dysfunction is recognized preoperatively, it may be prudent to delay surgery several days until the insult has resolved. One often overlooked cause of intraoperative renal dysfunction is hemoglobinuria resulting in acute tubular necrosis (ATN).

The development of ARF in the postoperative period can have significant impact on the patient's mortality. In adults, with renal failure requiring dialysis, mortality is 25 to 100%.[84] Additional steps to reduce the severity of ARF include infusions of renal dose dopamine (2 to 5 μg/kg/min), and boluses of mannitol and furosemide. Forced diuresis in the face of oliguria may prevent the development of acute renal failure.[88] The institution of early hemodialysis in postbypass patients with ARF may be beneficial to return of normal renal function and long-term outcome.

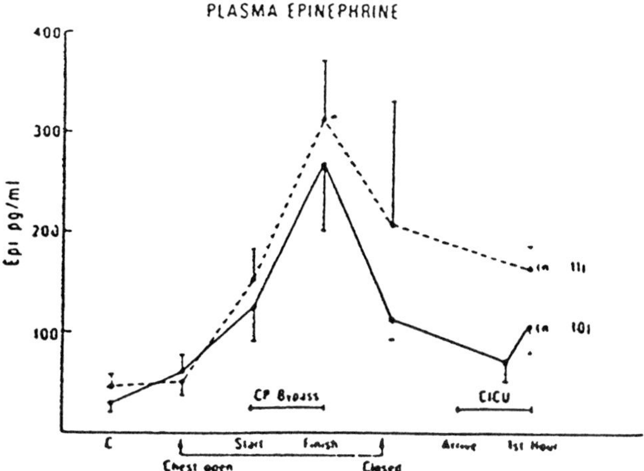

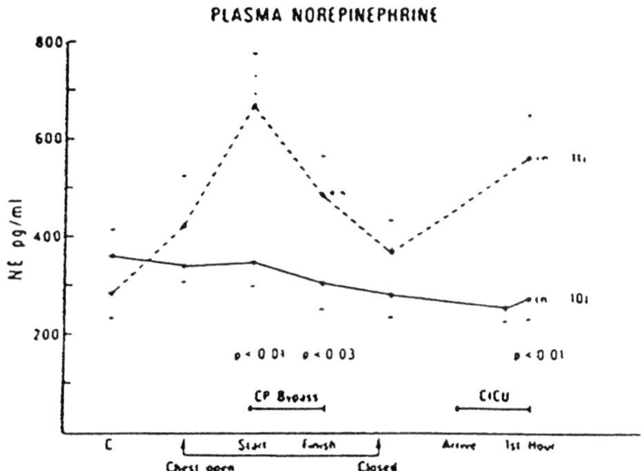

FIGURE 17–11. *Top*, Changes in plasma epinephrine during and after CABG surgery in patients with (*dashed line*) and without (*solid line*) postoperative hypertension. *Bottom*, Changes in plasma norepinephrine during and after CABG surgery in patients with (*dashed line*) and without (*solid line*) postoperative hypertension. (From Wallach R, Karp RB, Reves JG, et al: Pathogenesis of paroxysmal hypertension developing during and after coronary bypass surgery: A study of hemodynamic and humoral factors. Am J Cardiol 46:562, with permission.)

Neuroendocrine

Cardiopulmonary bypass and aortic cross-clamping produces a marked stress response that is manifested by increased levels of "stress" hormones and catecholamines. A number of factors exacerbate catecholamine release during bypass including hypothermia, nonpulsatile blood flow, and sympathetic reflexes initiated by the nonperfused heart and lungs. Replogle et al.[90] found a 200% increase in norepinephrine and a 1,500% increase in epinephrine plasma levels during CPB. Known hypertensive patients who undergo bypass have higher and more prolonged increases in norepinephrine during CPB. In addition, patients who were hypertensive into the postoperative period also had higher levels of catecholamines (Fig. 17–11). The higher epinephrine levels suggest the adrenal medulla stimulation is the primary cause rather than nonspecific sympathetic discharge. Elevated catecholamines may be partly due to the fact that the lungs are the primary organs responsible for norepinephrine metabolism,[91] and during bypass they are obviously excluded from the circulation. Elevated catecholamine levels may alter regional and whole-organ blood flow patterns, potentially to the detriment of the patient. Another danger is that upon reperfusion of the heart high-dose catecholamines may inappropriately increase oxygen consumption and lead to a higher risk of reperfusion injury. High-dose narcotics have been shown to attenuate the stress response,[92,93] although no outcome studies have shown any benefit in controlling the stress response in bypass patients.

Circulating "stress" hormones including glucagon, growth hormone, and cortisol are found in elevated levels during bypass. Cortisol levels continue to increase during the bypass period, but do not peak until the first postoperative day.[94] Hyperglycemia is a common occurrence during CPB and is due to several factors (Fig. 17–12), including a decrease in insulin release during hy-

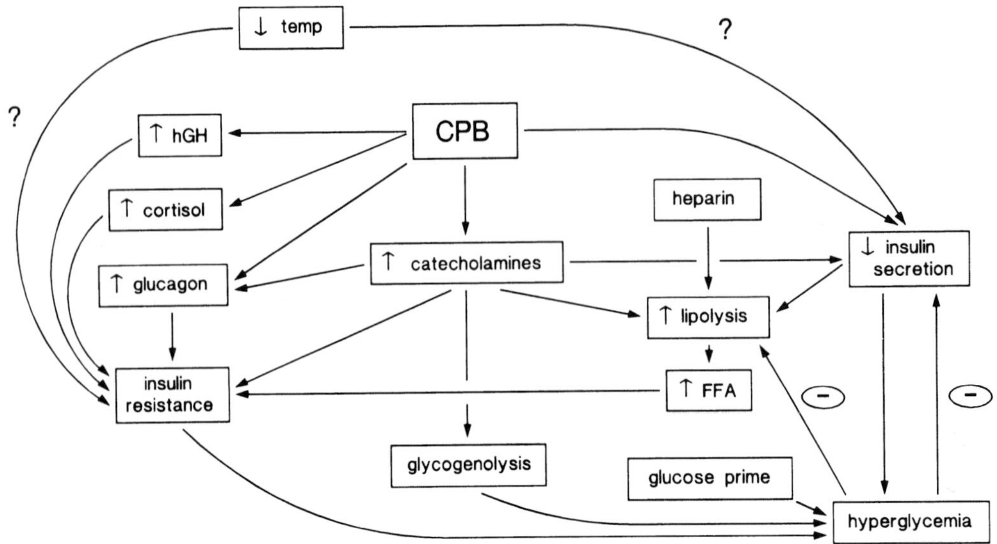

FIGURE 17–12. Schematic representation of metabolic alterations during CPB. A complex system of factors contributes to development of hyperglycemia early after initiation of CPB. Hyperglycemia, in turn, provokes hyperinsulinemia later in the course of CPB and also acts to directly and indirectly restrain lipolysis. This diagram represents a core metabolic response to CPB rather than an exhaustive listing of all interactive factors playing a role in the metabolic and endocrine response to CPB. hGH, human growth hormone. (From Shangraw RE: Metabolic and splanchnic visceral effects of cardiopulmonary bypass. In Gravlee GP, Davis RF, Utley JR [eds]: Cardiopulmonary Bypass: Principles and Practice. Baltimore, Williams & Wilkins, 1993, p 514, with permission.)

pothermic bypass, binding of insulin to the bypass circuit, and increased glycogenolysis.[95] Most anesthesiologists keep serum glucose levels below 220 mg/dl, as osmotic diuresis threshold is close to 250 mg/dl. Blood glucose concentration is frequently controlled with an insulin infusion.

Pulmonary

The lungs appear to be particularly sensitive to the effects of CPB, which in turn can lead to significant morbidity in postbypass patients.[96] CPB can lead to numerous derangements in pulmonary physiology including the development of atelectasis, the worsening of ventilation-perfusion relationships, and increases in both dead space and shunt fractions. Patients can also develop acute lung injury following bypass that is indistinguishable from adult respiratory distress syndrome (ARDS).

The development of atelectasis is a common phenomenon, occurring in up to 70% of postbypass patients.[97] Risk factors for developing atelectasis are listed in Table 17–2. Techniques to prevent atelectasis are discussed in a later section. Dead space ventilation is increased secondary to microemboli filtered by the lungs, and neutrophil sequestration with the release of cytokines and other vasoactive substances that lead to localized vasoconstriction. During CPB, interstitial lung water increases, and as a result some fluid invariably crosses into the alveoli, and pulmonary edema of various degrees can develop. Fluid-filled alveoli increases the shunt fraction, resulting in arterial hypoxemia. The hypoxemia may be further worsened by volatile anesthetics and vasodilators (particularly the nitrovasodilators), as the agents blunt or eliminate the patient's own hypoxic pulmonary vasoconstriction. The increased lung water in most patients resolves in the first 24 hours postoperatively, but a small fraction of patients go on to develop a clinical picture of severe lung injury.

Postbypass or "pump" lung results in a profound disruption of normal pulmonary function and has been associated with preoperative pulmonary dysfunction, length of bypass, and postoperative hemodynamic instability. The cause of pump lung has been attributed to many causes including the loss of surfactant,[98,99] development of interstitial and alveolar fluid accumulation,[100] activation of complement, and the sequestration of white blood cells in the alveoli.[101] Neutrophil activation by complement appears to be the prominent cause of dam-

TABLE 17–2
Etiology of Pulmonary Atelectasis*

Preoperative factors
Smoking, chronic bronchitis (mucus cell hyperplasia, surfactant depletion)
Obesity (decreased FRC)
Cardiogenic pulmonary edema
Intraoperative factors
Passive ventilation of paralyzed diaphragm
Monotonous ventilatory pattern
CPB factors
Surfactant inhibition—plasma, lung distention, lung ischemia
Increased extravascular lung water (complement activation)
Heart rests on immobile left blower lobe
Blind bronchial suctioning—preferential right bronchial drainage, mucosal damage
Open pleural cavity—blood, fluid

*From Sladen RN, Berkowitz DE: Cardiopulmonary bypass and the lung. In Gravlee GP, Davis RF, Utley JR (eds): Cardiopulmonary Bypass: Principles and Practice. Baltimore, Williams & Wilkins, 1993, 469, with permission.

age to the lung parenchyma via the mechanisms discussed in the previous section. Clinically, the patient is hypoxemic with shunt fractions in excess of 30%, chest x-ray reveals bilateral pulmonary infiltrates, lung compliance is decreased, and the pulmonary artery wedge pressure is normal.

Treatment for this condition is fairly nonspecific and depends on the severity of the injury. Mild to moderate injury is often treated conservatively with delayed extubation and gentle diuresis. More severe cases with refractory hypoxia may require increased levels of positive end-expiratory pressure (PEEP) and high inspired oxygen concentrations. Inverse ratio ventilation may be considered. Unfortunately, time is the only real treatment for severe cases and all precautions should be employed to avoid nosocomial infections and iatrogenic complications.

Protamine administration can have significant impact on the pulmonary circulation and will be discussed in a later section.

Neurologic

The impact of bypass on neurologic function is revealed in various other sections. A recent study by Mangano[102] reported a 6% rate of serious neurologic sequelae following cardiopulmonary bypass.

Perioperative Management/ Sequence of Bypass Events

The management of CPB patients can be extremely challenging; thus, it is essential or even mandatory for the anesthesiologist to have a thorough knowledge of each phase of the operation in order to smoothly handle each transition period and anticipate potential complications before they arise. In addition, because of the complexity of the bypass process, surgeons, perfusionists, and anesthesiologists work together as a team and jointly manage the patient on bypass. Clear communication between all the team members and a thorough knowledge of each other's responsibilities helps to ensure the safe conduct of the patient through surgery.

The learning curve for cardiopulmonary bypass is extremely steep and, at first, overwhelming. For the novice anesthesia resident the combination of new technology, illness of the patients, and the number of events makes the bypass process appear formidable. The technology of the bypass process is complex, starting from induction to delivery to the intensive care unit (ICU).

Preoperative Assessment

The purpose of the preoperative visit with respect to CPB is (1) to assess the functional capacity and reserve of the patient's cardiovascular system and (2) to evaluate the functional capacity of other organ systems (i.e., pulmonary, renal, hepatic, and endocrine) and assess their impact on the anesthetic plan.

The major focus of the preoperative visit is to evaluate the patient's functional cardiovascular state and reserve. By integrating the patient history with significant findings on physical examination, and reviewing the pertinent labwork, the cardiac anesthesiologist should be able to assess the patient's LV performance and quantify the degree of cardiovascular dysfunction. Table 17–3 is a review of pertinent findings suggestive of LV dysfunction. The degree of difficulty associated with discontinuation of CPB can thus be assessed.

Patients with CAD frequently have other associated illnesses including hypertension, diabetes mellitus, peripheral vascular disease, chronic obstructive pulmonary disease (COPD), and renal insufficiency. These associated illnesses may have significant impact on the patient's management during CPB. Hypertension, in particular, is commonly associated with coronary artery disease, and if not well controlled preoperatively can lead to exaggerated hemodynamic instability during the case. For this reason, most anesthesiologists prefer to continue the patient's chronic antihypertensive medications up to and including the morning of surgery. Thus β-blockers, calcium channel blockers, and nitrates are all given up to the time of surgery. One class of antihypertensive drugs, the angiotensin-converting enzyme inhibitors (ACEIs), remains controversial. ACEIs are commonly used as first-line therapy for hypertension associated with left ventricular dysfunction and mitral valve insufficiency. A number of reports[103–105] found long-term ACEI use linked to profound intraoperative hypotension, particularly during major invasive surgery

TABLE 17–3
Preoperative Findings Suggestive of Ventricular Dysfunction*

History
- History of MI, intermittent or chronic CHF
- Symptoms of CHF: fatigue, DOE, orthopnea, PND, ankle swelling

Physical examination
- Hypotension/tachycardia (severe CHF).
- Prominent neck veins, laterally displaced apical impulse, S_3, S_4, rales, pitting edema, pulsatile liver, ascites (tricuspid regurgitation)

Electrocardiogram
- Ischemia/infarction, rhythm, or conduction abnormalities

Chest x-ray
- Cardiomegaly, pulmonary vascular congestion/pulmonary edema, pleural effusion, Kerley B lines

Cardiac Testing
- Cath data—LVEDP >18, EF <0.4, CI <2.0 L/min/m^2
- Echocardiography—low EF, multiple regional wall motion abnormalities
- Ventriculography—low EF, multiple areas of hypokinesis, akinesis, or dyskinesis

*From Wray DL, Hughes CW, Fine RH, Thomas SJ: Anesthesia for cardiac surgery. In Barash PG, Cullen BF, Stoelting RK (eds): Clinical Anesthesia. Philadelphia, JB Lippincott Co, 1989, p 1035, with permission.
MI, myocardial infarction; CHF, congestive heart failure; DOE, dyspnea on exertion; PND, paroxysmal nocturnal dyspnea; LVEDP, left ventricular end-diastolic pressure; EF, ejection fraction; CI, cardiac index.

and induction of anesthesia. Thaker et al.[106] treated a group of chronic ACEI users with refractory intraoperative hypotension with IV angiotensin II and were able to restore normal blood pressure. Recently, Licker et al.[107] found long-term ACEI use does not alter the hemodynamic stability of patients undergoing CPB who have preserved LV function. Interestingly, the patients on chronic ACEIs require less anesthetic during the case to maintain a stable blood pressure. One proposed mechanism is that ACEIs prevent the breakdown of endogenous bradykinin leading to a heightened vasodilation state.

Diabetes makes regulation of serum glucose difficult, while hyperglycemia may have an adverse effect on neurologic outcome. Pulmonary disease may not be problematic during bypass, but may preclude early extubation of the patient postoperatively. Patients with known chronic renal dysfunction are at higher risk for postoperative renal failure requiring dialysis. It is important to identify these illnesses and inform the patient that these additional risk factors may impact their outcome.

Anesthesia During CPB

Despite hypothermia, adequate anesthesia must be maintained during CPB. Neuromuscular blockade should be maintained to prevent shivering during induction of hypothermia or inadvertent inspiration, which might result in air entry into open cardiac chambers. Morphine was the first narcotic to be used during bypass procedures[108]; however, because of histamine release and hemodynamic instability, alternate opioids have been utilized. Fentanyl and sufentanil have little hemodynamic impact and have essentially replaced morphine. Benzodiazapines are commonly used dosed intermittently throughout the case to ensure amnesia. Dilution by the primary solution and sequestration of narcotics on oxygenator membrane may necessitate administration of additional doses just before or on initiation of CPB.[109]

The use of volatile agents during bypass is somewhat controversial. The use of volatile agents may reduce the dose of benzodiazapines, which may be important when the patient is being fast-tracked for early extubation. Volatile agents can also be used to treat episodes of hypertension, particularly in the prebypass and bypass phases. An anesthetic vaporizer is often attached to the extracorporeal circuit to add the inhaled agent directly to the patient's blood. Hypertension during bypass can only be treated by direct vasodilators and not with negative inotropes because the heart is replaced by the bypass pump. The only limitation of the inhaled agents is their cardiac depressant effects, which may interfere with discontinuation of CPB if the patient's cardiac function is inadequate. An important point to remember is that if volatile agents are used towards the end of the case they will be gone by the time of arrival in the ICU, which may produce unwanted hypertension in the immediate postbypass period. Appropriate scavenging of volatile agents from the outlet of the extracorporeal circuit must be performed.[110,111]

The placement of the venous and arterial cannulas requires the patient to be fully heparinized to prevent thrombus formation. As discussed previously, a full anticoagulating dose of heparin is 300 to 400 U/kg and an ACT can be measured 1 to 2 minutes after the heparin dose is given.[112] Adequate anticoagulation is an ACT of at least 400 seconds, but because the CPB prime contains additional heparin (5,000 to 10,000), CPB can be started when the ACT reaches 300 seconds. The arterial cannula is usually placed first because it is technically more difficult to do and after placement the perfusionist can give additional volume via the arterial cannula to support the patient's blood pressure. Once the arterial cannula is placed, it is then connected to the arterial tubing from the bypass machine and a careful search is done for any air bubbles left in the tubing. Even a small amount of air may lead to cerebral air embolus with dire neurologic consequences. Because of this, the surgeon may have to perform several reconnections until the line is free of air. The patient is placed in Trendelenburg position and the perfusionist gives a small fluid bolus through the arterial line to check for proper flow dynamics and to confirm placement of the cannula in the aortic lumen. High in-line pressures may indicate improper positioning of the arterial cannula or may be an initial warning of an aortic dissection. The anesthesiologist should palpate both carotids to confirm the cannula is not obstructing right-sided carotid blood flow.

Once the surgeon, perfusionist, and anesthesiologist are satisfied with the functioning and placement of the arterial line, the venous cannula is then placed. Placement of the venous cannula may be associated with episodes of hypotension that usually occur secondary to impaired venous return or an atrial arrhythmia. Frequent premature atrial contractions or atrial fibrillation can produce significant hypotension as the atrial kick is lost. It is important to correlate the hypotension with visual inspection of the surgical field, with particular attention being paid to manual heart manipulations and unexpected blood loss. Usually these situations resolve quickly without intervention, but occasionally IV medications, cardioversion, or the rapid placement of the patient on bypass may be necessary. Large unexpected blood loss is often secondary to an unplanned nicking of the atria and/or vena cava. If the bleeding is not controlled quickly, heparin is given, the femoral artery is cannulated, and "sucker bypass" commences with the cardiotomy suction functioning as the venous cannula.

Final preparations include calibrating all monitoring transducers, emptying the bladder to accurately track urine output while on bypass, and inspecting the patient's eyes for conjunctival edema and pupil size discrepancies. Table 17–4 lists the steps to complete before initiating CPB.

Initiation of Bypass Phase

Bypass begins when the surgeon unclamps the venous lines, and blood begins to enter the extracorporeal circuit. As the heart and lungs begin to receive less volume, the perfusionist gradually increases the bypass flow rates

TABLE 17–4
Checklist Prior to Initiating Cardiopulmonary Bypass*†

Laboratory values
ACT or measure of adequate heparinization
Hematocrit

Anesthesia/machine
Adequate anesthesia and muscle relaxants given
Nitrous oxide off (if used)

Monitor
Arterial pressure—initial hypotension and then return
CVP—indication of inadequate venous drainage
PCWP—LV distention—inadequate drainage, Al—pull back pulmonary artery catheter 1–2 cm

Patient/field
Cannulas in place: no air locks, clamps, or kinks; no bubbles in arterial cannula
Facial appearance
Suffusion (inadequate SVC drainage)
Unilateral blanching (innominate artery cannulation)
Heart
Signs of distention (especially in Al, ischemia)

Support
Usually not required

*From Wray DL, Hughes CW, Fine RH, Thomas SJ: Anesthesia for cardiac surgery. In Barash PG, Cullen BF, Stoelting RK (eds): Clinical Anesthesia. Philadelphia, JB Lippincott Co, 1989, p 1041, with permission.
†The major categories for this table and Table 17–7 are organized using the mnemonic LAMPS.
ACT, activated clotting time; CVP, central venous pressure; PCWP, pulmonary capillary wedge pressure; LV, left ventricle; SVC, superior vena cava; Al, aortic insufficiency.

TABLE 17–5
Initiation of Bypass: On-Bypass Checklist*

1. Assess arterial inflow
   a. Is arterial perfusate oxygenated?
   b. Is direction of arterial inflow appropriate?
   c. Evidence of arterial dissection?
      Patient's arterial pressure persistently low
      Inflow line pressure high
      Pump/oxygenator reservoir level falling
   d. Evidence of arterial cannula malposition?
      Patient's arterial pressure persistently high or low
      Inflow line pressure high
      Unilateral facial swelling, discoloration
2. Assess venous outflow
   a. Is blood draining to the pump/oxygenator's venous reservoir?
   b. Evidence of SVC obstruction?
      Facial venous engorgement or congestion
      CVP elevated
3. Is bypass complete?
   a. High CVP/low PA pressure
      Impaired venous drainage
   b. Low CVP/high PA pressure
      Large bronchial venous blood flow
      Aortic insufficiency
   c. Arterial and PA pressure nonpulsatile?
   d. Desired pump flow established?
4. Discontinue drug and fluid administration
5. Discontinue ventilation

*From Hindman BJ, Lillehaug SL, Tinker JH: Cardiopulmonary bypass and the anesthesiologist In Kaplan JA (ed): Cardiac Anesthesia, 3rd ed. Philadelphia, WB Saunders Co, 1993, p 922, with permission.
SVC, superior vena cava; CVP, central venous pressure; PA, pulmonary artery.

until all systemic perfusion is machine generated. During the first few minutes of the initial bypass period, the anesthesiologist must be particularly vigilant in identifying potential problems and communicating them to the team in order to minimize their impact on the patient.

Fortunately, the onset of bypass in the vast majority of patients is accomplished without difficulty. If the transition to bypass occurs smoothly, the anesthesiologist in conjunction with the perfusionist, adjusts the doses of vasoactive drugs, narcotics, or inhaled agents and corrects metabolic derangements. The anesthesiologist at this point, frequently gives an additional dose of muscle relaxant to prevent subclinical shivering and increase in oxygen consumption associated with hypothermia. The TEE is turned off, all IV fluids are adjusted to maintain venous patency, and the pulmonary artery catheter is withdrawn to prevent accidental perforation of the pulmonary artery as the catheter cools.

Once the machine is at "full flow," all the venous blood is bypassing the cardiopulmonary circulation. Ventilation at this point is discontinued; however, there is no consensus on how to best manage the lungs on bypass. Three methods have been employed: (1) disconnection of the airway from the anesthesia circuit allowing passive lung deflation, (2) maintaining low flow rates and/or low levels of CPAP, and (3) continuing ventilation with reduced tidal volumes. Early studies found a combination of reduced lung compliance and increased shunt fraction with continued ventilation to be most effective[113–115]; thus, most centers do not maintain ventilation, but rather maintain CPAP or allow passive deflation. A study by Boldt et al.[116] found no difference in outcome in patients ventilated with 5 cm H_2O CPAP, 15 cm H_2O CPAP, passive deflation, and continued ventilation on 100% oxygen, although there appeared to be less lung water in patients receiving 5 cm H_2O. Until a definitive study shows a benefit, most anesthesiologists will continue with passive deflation as their treatment of choice.

Despite the majority of patients having a smooth transition to bypass, there are still a number of potential problems that can and do occur. Occasionally, the surgeon needs to correct a minor problem and asks for the bypass flow rates to be reduced or even temporarily halted. The reduced flow rates require the patient to become more dependent upon his or her own native circulation again to maintain systemic perfusion pressures. Because of the initial volume removed on commencing bypass, the patient may become significantly hypotensive, requiring a large volume of fluid and inotropic support to maintain the blood pressure. Fortunately, the majority of these episodes are brief and the perfusionist is able to quickly resume normal bypass flow rates and pressures. There are, however, some complications that may result in serious morbidity and/or mortality to the patient if they are unrecognized and left untreated.

The items listed in Table 17–5 must be memorized by the anesthesiologist and continuously reassessed as the bypass machine takes over cardiopulmonary functions of the patient. Initial attention should be focused on the adequacy of venous drainage and the appearance of "red" oxygenated blood in the arterial line. The blood should be noticeably different in each of the two lines. Adequate arterial saturation is often confirmed by a continuous in-line oximetric monitor. Any abnormality in venous drainage or arterial oxygenation/pressures/flows must be immediately assessed and corrected. Inadequate venous drainage is commonly due to catheter malposition, while any asymmetric swelling or discoloration of the face or eye exam requires the surgeon to check the arterial cannula position. The scenario of elevated inflow line pressures and dampened distal arterial pressures often herald an aortic dissection. In the case of an aortic dissection, the femoral arteries are utilized for partial bypass, and the dissection is surgically corrected and an alternate site on the aortic arch is found. Inadequate arterial oxygenation is due to either an erroneous oxygen supply or a malfunctioning oxygenator. Defective oxygenators are most commonly a result of a manufacturer's defect or damage to the unit itself. In a large retrospective study of CPB accidents, Kurusz et al.[117] reported that oxygenator failure was the third leading cause of accidents after protamine reactions and hypoperfusion. There have been a number of case reports[118,119] reporting oxygenator failure as a result of spilling isoflurane onto the oxygenator resulting in cracks in the outer shell of the units or the connection tubing. These reports have led to the practice of placing bypass vaporizers in areas away from the oxygenators.

Hemodynamically, the onset of bypass commonly produces hypotension for the reasons discussed previously. Hypertension can be due to inadequate analgesia/anesthesia, excessive vasoconstriction from elevated catecholamine levels, right innominate artery receiving preferential flow in a patient with a right radical arterial catheter, and nonzeroed transducers. Elevated pulmonary artery pressures are most commonly caused by an "overwedged" or a kinked catheter. Overwedged catheters should be withdrawn until the pulmonary artery (PA) pressure goes to zero. Another cause of elevated PA pressures is left ventricular distention, a result of excessive pulmonary blood flow from inadequate venous drainage, or from aortic valve insufficiency prior to the placement of the aortic cross-clamp. A high CVP can result from inadequate venous drainage or from the catheter becoming ensnared in a suture securing the venous cannula.

There are a number of complications that are considered catastrophic to the patient if they occur. The presence of air bubbles in the arterial cannula or tubing is a medical emergency and may herald a massive gas embolus that may have catastrophic implications for the patient, including stroke, coronary artery occlusion, and death. The major mechanisms of gas embolism were reported by Kurusz and Wheeldon,[120] who observed 284 incidents of air embolism during open heart cases. Their results are listed in Figure 17–13. The most common cause of air embolus is inattention to venous reservoir levels and the failure by the perfusionist to act quickly enough to prevent air from being pumped into the arterial circulation. If an air embolus is suspected, a therapeutic protocol for massive gas emboli protocol is initiated (Table 17–6). Another rarer cause of gas embolus

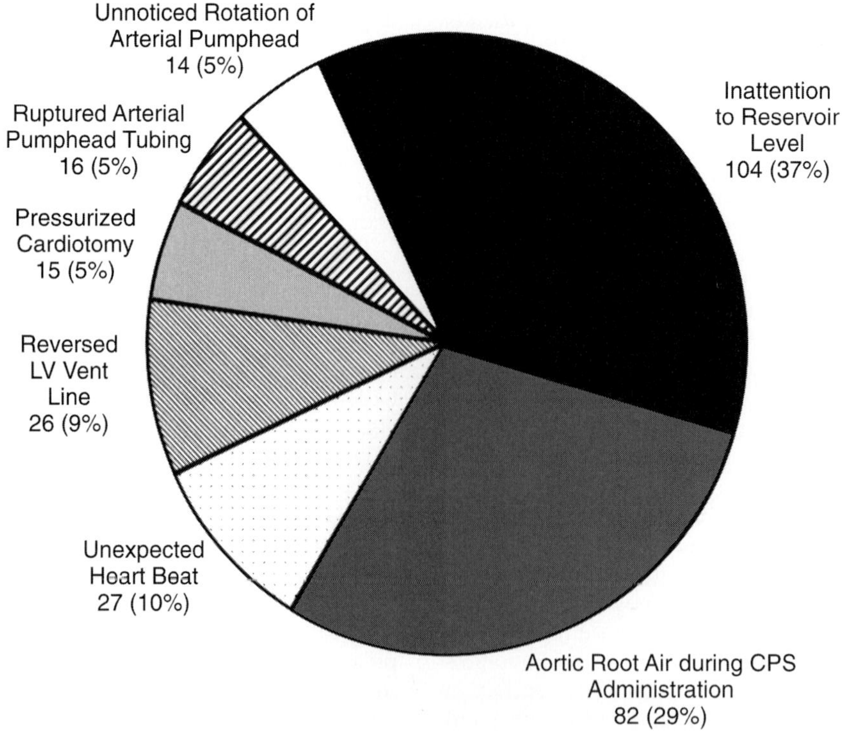

FIGURE **17–13.** Major mechanisms of gas embolism. These were reported by survey respondents who observed 284 incidents of air embolism during clinical cases. CPS, cardioplegic solution; LV, left ventricular. (From Kurusz M, Wheeldon DR: Risk containment during cardiopulmonary bypass. Semin Thorac Cardiovasc Surg 2:400, 1990, with permission.)

TABLE 17–6
Massive Gas Embolism Emergency Protocol*†

1. Stop CPB immediately.
2. Steep Trendelenburg position
3. Remove aortic cannula—vent air from aortic cannulation site.
4. De-air arterial cannula and pump line.
5. Institute hypothermic retrograde SVC perfusion by connecting arterial pump line to the superior vena caval cannula with caval tape tightened. Blood at 20°–24°C is injected into SVC at 1–2 L/min or more, and air plus blood is drained from aortic root cannulation site to the pump.
6. Carotid compression is performed intermittently during retrograde SVC perfusion to allow retrograde purging of air from the *vertebral* arteries.
7. Maintain retrograde SVC perfusion for at least 1–2 min. Continue for an additional 1–2 min if air continues to exit from aorta.
8. In extensive systemic air injection accidents in which emboli to splanchnic, renal, or femoral circulation are suspected, retrograde IVC perfusion may be performed after head de-airing procedures are completed. This is performed while the *carotid arteries are clamped* and the patient is in *head-up position* to facilitate removal of air through the aortic root vent but prevent re-embolization of the brain.
9. When no additional air can be expelled, resume anterograde CPB, maintaining hypothermia at 20°C for at least 40–45 min. Lowering patient temperature is important because increased gas solubility helps to resorb bubbles and because decreased metabolic demands may limit ischemic damage prior to bubble resorption.
10. Induce hypertension with vasoconstrictor drugs. Hydrostatic pressure shrinks bubbles; also, bubbles occluding arterial bifurcations are pushed into one vessel, opening the other branch.
11. Express coronary air by massage and needle venting.
12. Steroids may be administered, although this is controversial; usual dosage of methylprednisolone is 30 mg/kg.
13. Barbiturate coma should be considered if the myocardium will be able to tolerate the significant negative inotropy. Thiopental 10 mg/kg loading dose plus 1–3 mg/kg/hr infusion may be used empirically. If EEG monitoring is available, titration of barbiturate to an EEG burst/suppression (1 burst/min) pattern is preferable.
14. Patient is weaned from CPB.
15. Continue ventilating patient with 100% O_2 for at least 6 hr to maximize blood-alveolar gradient for elimination of N_2.
16. Hyperbaric chamber (if locally available) can accelerate resorption of residual bubbles. However, the risk of moving a critically ill patient must be weighed against the potential benefits.

*Modified from Mills NL, Oschsner JL: Massive air embolism during cardiopulmonary bypass: Causes, prevention, and management. J Thorac Cardiovasc Surg 80:712, 1980, with permission.
†This protocol should be reviewed together by all members of the cardiac team every 3 months.
SVC, superior vena cava; CPB, cardiopulmonary bypass; IVC, inferior vena cava; EEG, electroencephalogram.

is the accidental reversal of the arterial and venous cannulas, which results in blood being removed from the arterial side and inadvertently pumped back into the venous circulation. The diagnosis is suspected with arterial hypotension and critically high venous pressures. Once recognized, CPB is terminated, the patient is placed in steep Trendelenburg position, and the venous and arterial tubes are switched. It is important to not resume flow through the arterial cannula until all the air has been removed from the arterial tubing and the reservoir has adequate volume to resume bypass.

It is important for the anesthesiologist to realize that though these disasters rarely occur, it is critical to be as attentive as possible and to have mentally prepared a crisis algorithm in order to deal with the most common emergencies that may arise. Bad things happen during CPB, but the situation must be identified quickly and corrected as soon as possible in order for the patient to survive the crisis.

Maintenance of Bypass

The primary goal of this period is to obtain desired levels of hypothermia, maintain adequate systemic perfusion, ensure appropriate tissue oxygenation, and manage arterial blood gases. Despite the millions of successful bypass cases that are done each year, significant controversy and unanswered questions still remain in the "ideal" management of these patients. Table 17–7 summarizes steps to maintain a patient on bypass.

Hypothermia

Most centers perform cardiac surgery with some degree of hypothermia, ranging from mild (30°C) to profound (<20°C). Hypothermia decreases cellular metabolism which in turn reduces systemic oxygen/consumption ($\dot{V}O_2$). The $\dot{V}O_2$ is reduced 5 to 7% per degree centigrade,[121] thus a drop of 10°C with bypass will half metabolic activity and accordingly reduce cellular demands. This relationship is critical to protecting certain organ beds (i.e., brain, kidney) from ischemic injury. The use of hypothermia during CPB allows lower pump flow rates, better organ protection, less blood trauma, and improved myocardial protection.[122] A study by Hickey and Hoar[123] showed that a reduction in pump flow rates from 2.1 to 1.2 L/min/m^2 at 25°C centigrade did not affect $\dot{V}O_2$ or reduce tissue perfusion. Lower flow rates de-

TABLE 17–7
Checklist During Cardiopulmonary Bypass*

Laboratory values
- ACT or measure of adequate heparinization
- ABGs (uncorrected)—acidosis
- Hematocrit, potassium, calcium levels

Anesthesia/machine
- Discontinue ventilation

Monitor
- Arterial pressure
  - Hypotension
    - Venous cannula—kink, malposition, clamp, air lock
    - Inadequate venous return (bleeding, hypovolemia, IVC obstruction, table too low)
    - Pump—poor occlusion, low flows
    - Arterial cannula—misdirected, kinked, partially clamped, dissection
    - Vasodilation—anesthetics, hemodilution, idiopathic
    - Transducer or monitor malfunction, stopcocks the wrong way
  - Hypertension
    - Pump—↑ flow
    - Arterial cannula—misdirected
    - Vasoconstriction—light anesthesia, response to temperature changes
    - Transducer or monitor malfunction
- Venous pressure—above level of atrium—obstruction to return
  - LV filling pressure—LA, PCW (if available)—any elevation?
- ECG—electrical quiescence (if cardioplegia used)
- EEG
- Adequacy of perfusion??
  - Flow and pressure??
  - Acidosis
  - Mixed venous oxygen saturation
- Urine output
- Temperature

Patient/field
- Conduct of the operation
- Heart—distention, fibrillation
- Cyanosis, venous engorgement, skin temperature
- Movement
- Breathing, diaphragmatic movement (hypercarbia, light anesthesia)

Support
- Vasodilators, anesthetics, or constrictors to control blood pressure when flow is appropriate

*From Wray DL, Hughes CW, Fine RH, Thomas SJ: Anesthesia for cardiac surgery. In Barash PG, Cullen BF, Stoelting RK (eds): Clinical Anesthesia. Philadelphia, JB Lippincott Co, 1989, p 1042, with permission.
ACT, activated clotting time; ABG, arterial blood gas; IVC, inferior vena cava; LV, left ventricle; LA, left atrium; PCW, pulmonary capillary wedge, ECG, electrocardiogram; EEG, electroencephalogram.

crease the volume of collateral blood return and in turn reduce the inappropriate warming of the myocardium.

Temperature monitoring is an important aspect of bypass management. Systemic cooling from the bypass machine is very efficient, but it is not uniform. Tissues with lower blood flows (i.e., fat, skin, muscle) will cool (and warm) less quickly than tissues with higher blood flows. Core temperature measurements should reflect the temperature in the proximal aorta, and this in turn should be equal to the myocardial temperature.[124] Esophageal probes are frequently used to approximate core temperatures.[125] Esophageal temperature measurements may be affected by direct surface cooling of the heart itself, and may give a falsely low value. It is usually beneficial to measure a distal temperature site to establish a gradient between well-perfused tissues and poorly perfused ones. Large temperature gradients between two sites is considered incomplete rewarming and may result in a 1° to 3°C temperature decrease in the period following surgery as the patient re-establishes temperature homeostasis.[126,127]

During hypothermic circulatory arrest it is critical to know the temperature of the brain in order to maximally protect it with profound levels of hypothermia. The most commonly used site to monitor brain temperature is the nasopharynx. Tympanic membrane temperatures have also been used to approximate brain temperature during bypass.[128]

Despite the benefits of hypothermia, there are some centers that perform bypass surgery with warm cardioplegia and normothermic or slightly hypothermic bypass.[129] One study found significantly lower enzymatic infarction rates and more frequent spontaneous defibrillation episodes in patients who underwent normothermic bypass.[130] This same study found no significant difference in 30-day mortality or nonfatal Q-wave infarction rates. A recent trial was halted prematurely because of a threefold increase in stroke rate of the normothermic group.[131] The increased stroke rate raises serious concerns about the safety of warm bypass. Hypothermia also has several potential disadvantages including shifting of the oxyhemoglobin curve to the left preventing oxygen unloading in the periphery and decreased red cell deformability resulting in microcirculatory stasis. Both of these conditions may result in impaired tissue perfusion and potential cellular ischemia.

Blood-Gas Management

Acid-base management during hypothermic CPB is controversial. The two techniques currently employed are α-stat and pH-stat management.

α-Stat management maintains intracellular pH to keep the ionization state of histidine imidazole constant. The solubility of carbon dioxide increases with lower temperatures, resulting in more CO_2 dissolved in the blood. The decrease in the partial pressure of CO_2 results in "respiratory alkalosis." For example, if P_{CO_2} is 40 mm Hg at 30°C the P_{CO_2} will decrease to 19 mm Hg at 20°C, assuming a constant total CO_2 content. Supporters of α-stat suggest that the respiratory alkalosis is physiologically appropriate because the intracellular protein charge state is preserved during hypothermia. The use of pH-stat regulation maintains pH and P_{CO_2} at normal values, regardless of the blood temperature. This is similar to what hibernating animals do to survive the winter. In order to maintain a normal P_{CO_2} as the patient cools, CO_2 must be added to the ventilating gas mixture. This produces a relative hypercarbia resulting in a temperature-corrected "respiratory acidosis." The supporters of pH-state management argue that this adaptation exists in nature and is universally seen in hibernating animals. Unfortunately, the comparison between animals and humans may be irrelevant because humans never purposefully become hypothermic.

The pertinent question in comparing α- and pH-stat management is which technique has the better outcome. To date no study has shown a difference in overall outcomes. One particular focus between the two techniques is the effect on neurologic outcome. During hypothermic bypass, the cerebral vasculature maintains its responsiveness to P_{CO_2} and modulates cerebral blood flow accordingly.[132] Patients managed by pH-stat tend to have higher cerebral blood flows because of the overall increase in CO_2 content and the loss of cerebral autoregulation.[133-137] The increased cerebral blood flow may potentially direct more microemboli into the cerebral circulation, resulting in higher neurologic morbidity. α-Stat management of patients, in contrast, preserves cerebral autoregulation[134,138,139] and does not appear to have excessive blood flow. In theory, α-stat would have better neurologic outcomes; however, a study by Bashein et al.[140] found no differences in neurologic outcomes in patients randomized between the two management styles. Additional studies suggest that the difference in blood flow between pH- and α-stat is not particularly significant.[141] No difference in several renal parameters between the two management styles were noted by Badner and co-workers.[142]

Blood Pressure and Flow Rate Management

Considerable controversy exists in what the optimal MAP should be once the aorta is cross-clamped. Most centers maintain flow rates in the 50- to 60-ml/kg range, which in turn generates mean arterial pressures between 40 and 60 mm Hg. There are two main issues concerning the appropriate MAP level. The first is myocardial protection and the second is maintaining adequate perfusion to critical organ beds, particularly the CNS and the kidneys.

From a myocardial protection viewpoint, there is evidence in support of both higher and lower perfusion pressures. The supporters of maintaining lower blood pressure believe that lower flows cause less collateral rewarming of the heart and less hematologic trauma.[143] Others feel that higher mean arterial pressures provide superior myocardial protection, allowing at least some oxygenated blood to reach areas not protected by the cold cardioplegia.[144] No study to date has shown any difference in myocardial preservation in comparing the two techniques. Thus, at this time, hemodynamic parameters to protect the myocardium remain institutionally and personally biased.

The preservation of CNS function is of obvious importance during bypass surgery. Cerebral perfusion pressure (CPP) is defined as MAP-CVP or ICP, whichever is higher, and should be maintained above 50 mm Hg. The major factors regulating cerebral blood flow under bypass are Pa_{CO_2} and the degree of cerebral $\dot{V}_{O_2}$. Central $\dot{V}_{O_2}$ is dependent upon anesthetic depth and the temperature of the brain tissue itself. Autoregulation of cerebral blood flow appears to be maintained under α-stat management during bypass. Stockard et al.[145] linked hypotension during bypass with postoperative neurologic dysfunction and recommended that an MAP of at least 50 mm Hg should be maintained during bypass. Several subsequent studies[140,146] have not found an association between neurologic impairment and MAP during CPB. A study by Govier et al.[147] found that during α-stat management, CBF was independent of MAP between 30 and 100 mm Hg at 27°C. Feddersen et al.[148] found that CBF was reduced at an MAP of 30 mm Hg during hypothermic CPB; however, increased oxygen extraction by the brain helped maintain normal cerebral oxygen consumption. These studies suggest that a patient who is free of cerebral vascular disease will tolerate a lower limit MAP of 30 mm Hg without adverse sequelae. In practice, the authors tolerate an MAP of 40 mm Hg, in order to provide some level of protection for the patient. It must be emphasized that this level of MAP only applies to hypothermic patients. As the patient rewarms, the CBF once again becomes autoregulated over normal values of 50 to 150 mm Hg and the MAP must increase accordingly to ensure adequate CBF.

The dilemma for the majority of CPB patients is that the minimal MAP has not been established in patients with severe peripheral vascular disease, diabetes, or other significant illnesses. The presence of vascular disease, particularly carotid artery disease, usually results in the perfusionist maintaining an MAP of at least 60 mm Hg during bypass and pharmacologically preventing it from decreasing below this pre-established threshold. However, there are no data supporting this practice. What is known is that embolic events, not inadequate cerebral perfusion, appear to be the primary cause of neurologic insult.[149] At this time, there are inadequate data to assess the impact of insufficient flow and/or pressure on neurologic outcome.

Adequate renal perfusion pressure is even harder to determine because of the impact of diuretics (mannitol) used in the priming solution. Preoperative renal dysfunction appears to be the most accurate predictor of postoperative renal dysfunction, although length of bypass and postoperative hemodynamic instability also appear to be predictive of renal dysfunction. Slogoff et al.[146] found no correlation between postoperative renal dysfunction and episodes of low flow or pressure during bypass. Renal function appeared to be maintained with pump flows at 1.6 L/min or more.

Rewarming/Awareness

The perfusionist begins to rewarm the patient when the surgeon begins the last phase of the procedure. The rewarming should be gradual, commonly done over a 30-minute period. One concern is that as the patient warms, gases become less soluble in solution and the potential for the formation of gas bubbles exists. For this reason a gradient of only 10°C is maintained between the blood and the heating coils. Hypothermia itself has anesthetic/amnestic effects so the risk of recall is greatest as rewarming progresses. Many anesthesiologists ensure amnesia of the patient by administering additional doses of benzodiazapines. Inhaled agents are often avoided at this step because of their negative inotropic properties.

During the rewarming process, the anesthesiologist prepares for the patient to separate from bypass. It is at this point that all drugs and drug infusions should be prepared and ready for use. During this time the heart may resume a normal sinus rhythm or may need electrical pacing. A small amount of blood may begin to be ejected from the beating ventricle. Visual inspection of the heart is critical in the decision to start inotropic therapy prior to separation from bypass. When the patient is fully warmed the surgeon often asks for an assessment of the patient. It is at this point that a mutual discussion between team members is beneficial and contributes to overall success of the operation.

Termination of Bypass

The period just prior to the discontinuation of bypass can be stressful, as multiple tasks must be done in rapid succession. The importance of being fully prepared to separate the patient from bypass cannot be overstated. Table 17–8 offers a summary of the essential steps that must be completed prior to separation. At this point, the patient should be fully warmed, the lungs should be completely reinflated and ventilation resumed, all transducers should re-zeroed, and all abnormal lab values (Hct, K^+, Mg^{2+}, Ca^{2+}, and pH) should be corrected. The heart rhythm should ideally be sinus with a rate between 80 and 100. Not uncommonly, however, the heart rhythm needs pharmacologic support and/or electrical pacing. If the AV node is intact atrial pacing alone is sufficient; however, with any evidence of heart block, AV sequential pacing is the preferred method. For a full discussion of pacemakers the reader should consult Chapter 32 to learn to identify atrial and ventricular capture.

TABLE 17–8
Preparation for Separation-from-Bypass Checklist*

1. Air clearance maneuvers completed
2. Rewarming completed
   a. Nasopharyngeal temperature 37°–39°C
   b. Rectal/bladder temperature ≥35°C
3. Address issue of adequacy of anesthesia and muscle relaxation
4. Obtain stable cardiac rate and rhythm
   a. Pacing if necessary
5. Pump flow and systemic arterial pressure
   a. Pump flow to maintain mixed venous saturation ≥70%
   b. Systemic pressure restored to normothermic levels
6. Metabolic parameters
   a. Arterial pH, P_{O_2}, P_{CO_2} within normal limits
   b. Hct: 20–25%
   c. K^+: 4.0–5.0 mEq/L
   d. *Possibly* ionized calcium
7. Are all monitoring/access lines functional?
   a. Transducers rezeroed
   b. TEE (if used) out of freeze mode
8. Respiratory management
   a. Atelectasis cleared/lungs reexpanded
   b. Evidence of pneumothorax?
   c. Residual fluid in thoracic cavities drained
   d. Ventilation reinstituted without nitrous oxide
9. Intravenous fluids restarted
10. Inotropes/vasopressors/vasodilators prepared

*From Hindman BJ, Lillehaug SL, Tinker JH: Cardiopulmonary bypass and the anesthesiologist. In Kaplan JA (ed): Cardiac Anesthesia, 3rd ed. Philadelphia, WB Saunders Co, 1993, p 943, with permission.
TEE, transesophageal echocardiography.

Separation from bypass begins with the surgeon gradually occluding venous drainage and the perfusionist slowly decreasing the bypass flow, often in 0.5-L/min increments. This gradual shifting of blood back into the cardiopulmonary circuit allows the atria and ventricles to slowly accommodate to the increase in preload and is the most common technique to prepare the heart for bypass separation. During this time it is imperative for the surgeon and anesthesiologist to clearly communicate with each other and continue to assess the preload and contractility of the heart by direct visual inspection and hemodynamic data. Adequate preload, as determined by the wedge or CVP, is critical to the patient successfully terminating bypass. The perfusionist continues arterial flow until the desired preload is achieved and if contractility is deemed acceptable then the surgeon clamps the venous line, the perfusionist stops arterial flow, and the patient is separated from bypass. This gradual stepwise method is in contrast to more abrupt discontinuation of CPB by simply clamping the venous line and quickly reducing pump flow to zero. This technique is challenging to the patient but is generally well tolerated in patients with good LV function.

The initial few minutes off bypass can be very labile hemodynamically, as sudden changes can occur in preload, contractility, and afterload. This hemodynamic instability can lead to rapid extremes in blood pressure. However, prior to initiating pharmacologic therapy, the accuracy of the arterial pressure must be established. Large discrepancies may exist between the distal radial and proximal arterial pressure measurements. It has been shown in several studies[150,151] that a discrepancy of 10 to 30 mm Hg is found between central aortic pressures and distal radial artery pressures. The difference is thought to be due to arterio-venous shunting in the forearm.[150–152] Transducing the central aortic pressure may be helpful until the chest is closed, but if a difference is still noted, then a femoral arterial catheter should be placed. The difference resolves relatively quickly, often within the first hour in the ICU as the patient becomes normothermic.

Once a true measure of arterial pressure has been identified, the patient's hemodynamic profile separates them into one of several groups. Some patients come off bypass and require no additional support other than a little fine tuning of volume, inotropes, and vasodilators. Others experience transient decreases in their blood and filling pressures and only require volume infusion and/or small boluses of inotropic drugs to restore normal BP. Ephedrine, low-dose epinephrine, and calcium salts are examples of drugs with moderate positive inotropic effects. Calcium chloride is given in 5- to 10-mg/kg boluses to increase the inotropic state of the heart and cause some peripheral vasoconstriction. However, recent studies have questioned routine use of calcium. Calcium administration has been reported to blunt dobutamine-

TABLE **17–9**
Etiology of Right or Left Ventricular Dysfunction After Cardiopulmonary Bypass*

Ischemia
- Adequate myocardial protection
- Coronary spasm
- Technical difficulties
- Emboli (air, thrombus, calcium)
- Inoperative infarction
- Reperfusion injury

Uncorrected structural defects
- Nongraftable vessels
- Kinked or clotted grafts
- Residual valve gradient
- Hypertrophic cardiomyopathy
- Shunts

Excess cardioplegia

Pre-existing dysfunction
- Cardiomyopathy

*From Wray DL, Hughes CW, Fine RH, Thomas SJ: Anesthesia for cardiac surgery. In Barash PG, Cullen BF, Stoelting RK (eds): Clinical Anesthesia. Philadelphia, JB Lippincott Co, 1989, p 1043, with permission.

induced increases in cardiac output by 30%.[153] Calcium has also been linked by postbypass pancreatitis[154] and the potentiation of cellular ischemic reperfusion injury, particularly in the brain and the myocardium.[155] Ionized hypocalcemia should be replaced appropriately, but the use of empiric calcium to treat hypotension remains controversial. To date there is no study suggesting a worse outcome in patients receiving calcium immediately following bypass.

The most challenging postbypass patients are those that separate from bypass and remain hypotensive despite volume and inotrope boluses. The scenario of high filling pressures, low cardiac output, and a distended left ventricle is classic for acute LV failure. This patient should be placed back on bypass and an etiology of the ventricular failure should be sought. Some of the more common causes include pre-existing LV dysfunction; air emboli in the venous grafts; kinked, clotted, or inadequate coronary grafts; excessive cardioplegia; and focal/global areas of ischemia or infarction. A systematic approach to detect the etiology of the LV failure is listed in Table 17–9. Therapeutic maneuvers include repairing the structural defects, removing air from the grafts, and allowing sufficient time to wash-out the residual cardioplegia. Frequently, these steps are therapeutic and the following trial of separation goes smoothly. Unfortunately, these steps are not always effective in restoring more normal LV function and more potent or additional inotropes are required prior to another attempt at bypass separation. The selection of a particular inotrope is heavily influenced by both personal and institutional bias. The rationale for the usage of a specific inotropic agent is beyond the scope of this chapter, yet, by integrating cardiac physiology and pharmacology with the patient's hymodynamic data, an appropriate drug will be selected. If the inotropic therapy is not effective in allowing separation from bypass, then mechanical support is justified in the form of intra-aortic balloon pump (IABP) or VAD. Figure 17–14 details an algorithm to diagnose and treat hemodynamic abnormalities following CPB.

The IABP is the most common mechanical support device with approximately 3% of all cardiac patients utilizing an IABP during their hospital course.[156] Indications for the use of IABP are listed in Table 17–10 and include failure to separate from bypass, cardiogenic shock, acute mitral insufficiency, and prophylactic perioperative placement in selected high-risk patients. Approximately two thirds of the IABPs are placed in the operating room. The IABP is usually placed in the femoral artery and the balloon is advanced so the tip is just distal to the left subclavian artery. In addition, the bal-

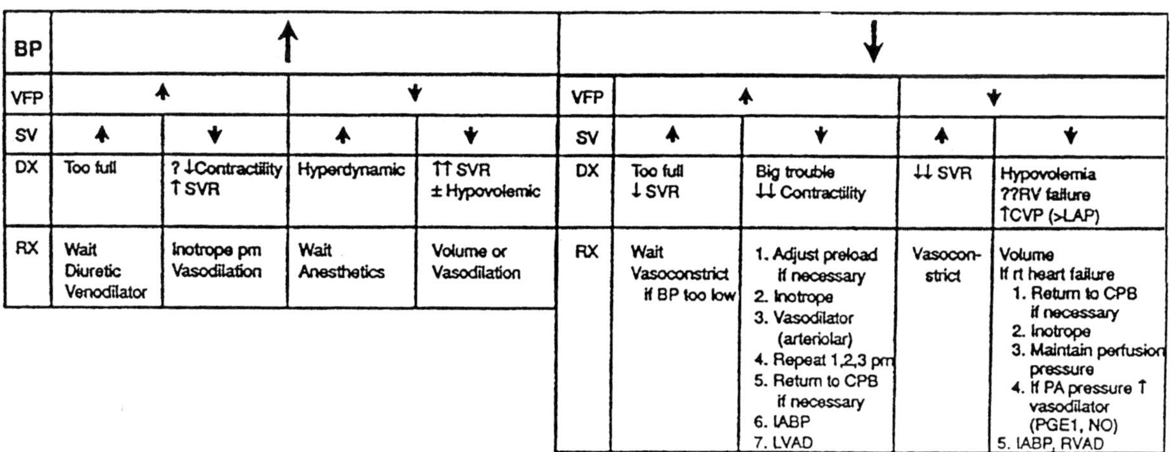

FIGURE **17–14.** Algorithm for the diagnosis and treatment of hemodynamic abnormalities at the termination of CPB. BP, systemic blood pressure, VFP, ventricular filling pressure; SV, stroke volume; Dx, diagnosis; Rx, treatment; SVR, systemic vascular resistance; CVP, central venous pressure; LAP, left atrial pressure; IABP, intra-aortic balloon pump; LVAD, left ventricular assist device; RVAD, right ventricular assist device; PA, pulmonary artery; PGE_1, prostaglandin E_1; NO, nitric oxide; RV, right ventricle. (Modified from Amado WJ, Thomas SJ: Cardiac surgery: Intraoperative management. In Thomas SJ [ed]: Manual of Cardiac Anesthesia, 2nd ed. New York, Churchill Livingstone, 1993, with permission.)

TABLE 17–10
Intra-aortic Balloon Pump Indications and Contraindications*

Indications
Complications of myocardial infarction
Hemodynamic—cardiogenic shock
Mechanical—mitral regurgitation, ventricular septal defect
Intractable dysrhythmias
Extension—postinfarction angina
?? Limitation of infarct size
Acute cardiac instability
Unstable angina—preinfarction angina
PTCA misadventure
Pretransplantation
Cardiac contusion
?? Septic shock
Open heart surgery
Separation from cardiopulmonary bypass
Right or left ventricular failure
Increasing inotropic requirement
Progressive hemodynamic deterioration
Contraindications
Irreversible brain damage
Severe aortic insufficiency
Inability to insert
Irreversible cardiac disease (if not a candidate for transplant)

*From Wray DL, Hughes CW, Fine RH, Thomas SJ: Anesthesia for cardiac surgery. In Barash PG, Cullen BF, Stoelting RK (eds): Clinical Anesthesia. Philadelphia, JB Lippincott Co, 1989, p 1045, with permission.
PTCA, percutaneous transluminal coronary angioplasty.

loon should not occlude the renal arteries and placement should be confirmed radiographically. The balloon works by inflating during diastole, augmenting coronary perfusion pressure, and deflating immediately before systole to reduce LV afterload. The reduction in afterload translates into improved forward blood flow to the peripheral tissues. Timing of the balloon inflation/deflation is critical to maximizing the mechanical support. Tachycardia and atrial/ventricular arrhythmias reduce the effectiveness of the IABP by preventing proper timing of the balloon and the cardiac cycle. Contraindications of IABP use include aortic insufficiency and the inability to insert secondary to severe atherosclerotic disease (Table 17–11). IABPs have been placed in the aortic arch as an alternate site. Complications with IABP use include severe lower extremity ischemia (5%), infection (1%), and direct trauma to the vessel.[157] Balloon rupture is a rare occurrence.

The next level of mechanical support are VADs, which are only utilized in cases of severe cardiac dysfunction. VADs can be used to support the right, left, or both ventricles and actually generate a pulsatile waveform, effectively replacing the failing ventricle. The VADs are used to achieve a cardiac index of 2.2 L/min or greater in order to improve overall organ perfusion. There are a number of different models available including the Biomedicus centrifugal pump[158] and the pneumatically powered Heartmate,[159] which is being utilized for longer term support. VADs are often used as a bridge to cardiac transplantation, but with such a shortage of available organs, these pump devices may become standard treatment in refractory heart failure. McCarthy and Sabik[159] provide an extensive review of this topic.

Postbypass Management

The successful termination of bypass is only the initial phase of hemodynamic recovery, as the patient now becomes solely dependent upon his own native circulation. The postbypass phase requires absolute concentration from the anesthesiologist as the patient's vessels are decannulated, the heparin is antagonized, and the surgeons perform final hemostasis to prepare for closing of the chest.

The venous cannulas are removed first and the volume remaining in these tubings is flushed through into the venous reservoir. If the patient is hemodynamically stable, the surgeon requests administration of protamine. At this point, the arterial cannula is still in place and the perfusionist can continue to give volume transfusions until the venous reservoir is essentially empty. Removal of the arterial cannula varies between institutions. Some surgeons decannulate prior to protamine, while others wait until about half the protamine has been given. The risk of leaving the cannula in place longer is the potential of thrombus formation of the cannula and subsequent embolization. Once the protamine has been started, the cardiotomy suction devices should no longer be used.

Protamine Administration

The reversal of heparin anticoagulation is accomplished with protamine, which is currently the only drug available to neutralize heparin. Protamine is a protein molecule derived from salmon sperm and is highly cationic.

TABLE 17–11
Classification of Protamine Reactions*

Type	Horrow	Moorman, Zapol, Lowenstein
I	Hypotension due to rapid administration	Pharmacologic histamine release
IIa.	Anaphylactic reactions	True anaphylaxis (IgE-mediated)
IIb.	Immediate anaphylactoid reactions	
IIc.	Delayed anaphylactoid reactions	Anaphylactoid reactions
III.	Catastrophic pulmonary vasoconstriction	Pulmonary vasoconstriction (? IgG/complement-mediated) Noncardiogenic pulmonary edema

*From Moorman RM, Zapol WM, Lowenstein E: Neutralization of heparin anticoagulation. In Gravlee GP, Davis RF, Utley JR (eds): Cardiopulmonary Bypass: Principles and Practice. Baltimore, Williams & Wilkins, 1993. Copyright 1993, Excerpta Medica Inc, p 390, with permission.

The positive charge is secondary to the high percentage of the amino acid arginine. The positively charged molecule forms a stable complex with the negatively charged heparin molecule, effectively neutralizing heparin's anticoagulant activity. The dosing for heparin reversal is a bit empiric, but ranges from 1 to 1.3 ml of protamine (10 mg/ml) for every 1,000 U of heparin administered. Roughly 10 mg of protamine will reverse 1000 U of heparin.

Protamine is administered by syringe or in a small volume of fluid, which is infused no faster than 50 mg/min. This corresponds to an infusion time of 5 to 10 minutes. Some anesthesiologists give the protamine in a peripheral vein to dilute the drug concentration and potentially reduce the hypotension and/or pulmonary complications commonly seen with protamine dosing. Rapid administration of protamine increases white blood cell sequestration in the pulmonary circulation.[160] This phenomenon may partly explain the cardiopulmonary side effects seen with this drug. Approximately 5 minutes after the protamine has been given an ACT is checked. An adequate reversal will return the ACT to within 10% of the baseline value.

The administration of protamine results in a number of adverse reactions as noted below and listed in Table 17–11.

1. Protamine, in large doses, may actually have anticoagulant properties. The protamine-heparin complex impairs platelet function and may inhibit thrombin activity; however, these effects are only seen in doses two to four times the normal reversal dose. This should not prevent the use of an additional small dose of protamine to adequately reverse heparin and normalize the ACT.
2. Protamine administration commonly causes hypotension secondary to a decrease in preload and peripheral vasodilation. The hemodynamic effects are most likely histamine related. Hypotension is worsened by rapid administration of the drug and frequently observed in patients who are relatively hypovolemic. Volume infusions and small doses of phenylephrine will often be adequate for the brief episode of hypotension.
3. Protamine allergic reactions are mediated by IgE or IgG antibodies that cause a wide range of clinical responses from mild skin reactions to complete cardiovascular collapse. Diabetic patients who use protamine-containing preparations may develop an immunologic response and may be at increased risk for an adverse reaction.[161] Cross reactivity can potentially exist in patients with a fish allergy[162] or prior vasectomy.[163] Treatment of idiosyncratic protamine reactions are listed in Table 17–12.
4. Protamine can also cause anaphylactoid reactions. These reactions do not involve antibodies. The heparin-protamine complex activates the classic complement pathway. Cellular contents and complement fragments cause the release of a number of vasoactive molecules that produce a clinical picture of an anaphylactic reaction.
5. Catastrophic pulmonary vasoconstriction is a life-threatening medical emergency and occurs in about 1.5% of adult cardiac patients.[164] It can occur after doses as small as 0.14 mg/kg.[165] The syndrome is probably mediated by thromboxane,[160] resulting in pulmonary hypertension, bronchoconstriction, systemic hypotension, and pulmonary edema. The marked elevation in PA pressures leads to RV failure, a rise in right sided pressures, and eventually to biventricular failure. Treatment involves maneuvers to decrease PA pressures with IV infusions of nitrates and/or prostaglandins. Prostaglandins are often infused into the right atrium. Additional steps include

TABLE 17–12
Therapy for Idiosyncratic Protamine Reactions*

Initial Therapy

1. Stop administration of protamine
2. Maintain airway with 100% oxygen
3. Discontinue all anesthetic agents
4. Start intravascular volume expansion (2–4 L of crystalloid with hypotension)
5. Give epinephrine (4–8 μg IV bolus with hypotension, titrate as needed; 0.1–1.0 mg IV with cardiovascular collapse)
6. Reinstitute cardiopulmonary bypass for severe reactions to allow time for drug therapy to take effect

Secondary Treatment

1. Antihistamines (0.5–1 mg/kg diphenhydramine, 300 mg cimetidine, 20 mg famotidine, or 50 mg ranitidine)
2. Catecholamine infusions (starting doses: epinephrine 2–4 μg/min, norepiephrine 2–4 μg/min, *or* isoproterenol 0.5–1.0 μg/min as a drip, titrated to desired effects)
3. Aminophylline (5–6 mg/kg over 20 min with persistent bronchospasm) followed by infusion
4. Corticosteroids (0.25–1,00 gm hydrocortisone; alternatively, 1–2 gm methylprednisolone)†
5. Sodium bicarbonate (0.5–1.0 mEg/kg with persistent hypotension or acidosis)
6. Airway evaluation (prior to extubation)

Specific Treatment for Catastrophic Pulmonary Vasoconstriction

Therapy as above; once diagnosed, treatment of pulmonary hypertension, right heart failure, and bronchoconstriction should include immediate hyperventilation and one or –of the following treatments: nitroglycerin; isoproterenol; aminophylline; prostaglandin E_1; amrinone

*Modified from Levy JH: Anaphylactic Reactions in Anesthesia and Intensive Care. Boston, Butterworth's, 1986, p 104, with permission.
†Methylprednisolone may be the drug of choice if the reaction is suspected to be mediated by complement.

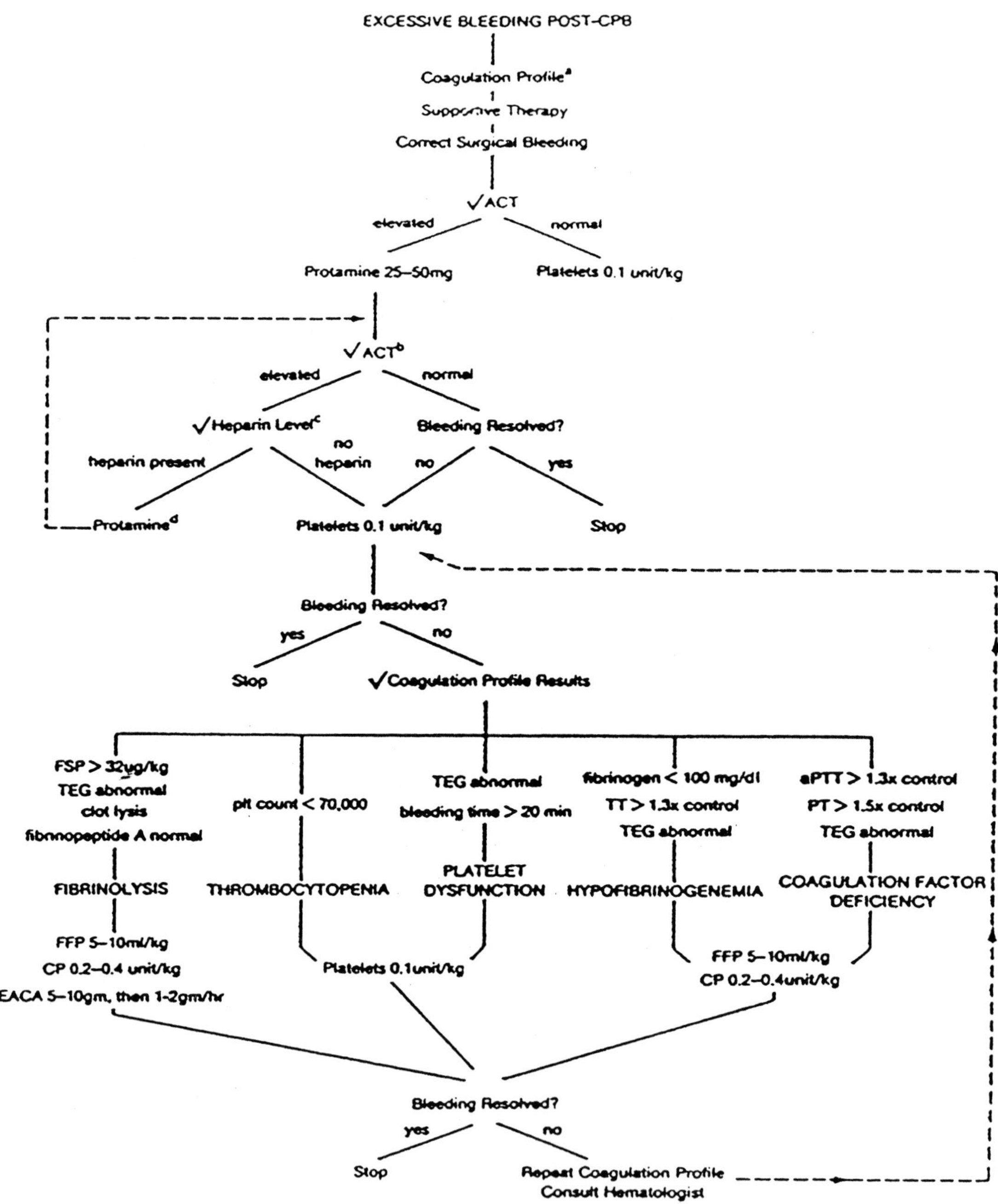

FIGURE **17–15.** An algorithm for the treatment of patients bleeding excessively after CPB. *a*, Commonly includes platelet count, PT, aPTT, TT, fibrinogen level, FSPs. Template bleeding time or TEG is desirable if available and feasible. *b*, Heparin level may be checked at this step. *c*, Most commonly by in vitro whole blood protamine titration (manual or automated); alternatively, by protamine corrected TT. *d*, Protamine dose determined by measured heparin level. Disseminated intravascular coagulation (DIC) is a rare cause of post-CPB hemorrhage and therefore is not included in the outline of coagulation profile results and treatment of post-CPB hemostatic abnormalities shown in the lower portion of the figure. It would be suspected on the occurrence of hypofibrinogenemia, thrombocytopenia, and elevated fibrinopeptides in association with increased FSPs, clot lysis, or a TEG characteristic of fibrinolysis. The treatment of DIC includes identification and arrest of the inciting cause and coagulant replacement with FFP, CP, and platelets. EACA should not be administered to the patient with DIC and secondary fibrinolysis because of the risk of intravascular thrombosis. ACT, activated coagulation time; aPTT, activated partial thromboplastin time; CP, cryoprecipitate; EACA, epsilon-aminocaproic acid; FFP, fresh frozen plasma; FSP, fibrin(ogen) split products; plt count, platelet count; PT, prothrombin time; TEG, thromboelastogram; TT, thrombin time. (From Campbell FW, Jobes DR, Ellison N: Coagulation management during and after cardiopulmonary bypass. In Hensley FA, Martin DE [eds]: The Practice of Cardiac Anesthesia. Boston, Little, Brown & Co, 1990, p 570, with permission.)

rapid volume expansion and bronchodilator therapy. In severe cases, the patient is placed back on bypass to stabilize the hemodynamics. The reinstitution of bypass requires full reheparinization.

Alternatives to protamine reversal of heparin include allowing the drug to be naturally metabolized, but this practice increases blood loss and use of blood products. A study by D'Ambra[166] found recombinant platelet factor 4 was effective in reversing heparin effects and no serious side effects were reported. The development of a specific heparinase may show future promise.

Postoperative Bleeding

The presence of persistent blood loss following adequate heparin reversal is a common postbypass problem. The initial management of a postbypass bleeding patient begins with rechecking the ACT; if it is still elevated, an additional 50 mg of intravenous protamine is given. If the additional dose of protamine has not corrected the ACT or if clinical bleeding persists, then a complete coagulation panel should be sent to evaluate the etiology of the coagulopathy. Coagulation tests can be difficult to interpret in postbypass patients. Prothrombin and partial thromboplastin times are frequently elevated in patients undergoing CPB in the postoperative period and have limited clinical use.[167] Platelet counts give no measure of qualitative function, particularly in patients with recent aspirin ingestion.[168] Despite these limitations, Figure 17–15 presents an algorithm for the therapeutic approach to the bleeding postoperative cardiac patient.

Defects in platelet function are a common cause of bleeding complications. Bypass itself causes a transient decrease in platelet function.[169–171] This is thought to be due to the platelets being partially activated or destroyed by contact with the bypass machine surfaces. Another contributing factor is recent aspirin ingestion, which has been shown to increase blood loss following bypass.[172] Fortunately, normal platelet function usually returns within a few hours following bypass as endogenous sources supply new unaffected platelets.[171] Pharmacologic techniques to improve platelet function following bypass include desmopressin (DDAVP) administration, which causes a release of von Willebrand factor (VWF) and factor VIII from endothelial stores. DDAVP, in a dose of 0.3 μg/kg, raises factor VIII coagulant activity 2- to 20-fold[173] and concomitant elevations in VWF enhances platelet aggregation. DDAVP has only been shown to be effective in certain limited clinical situations: uremia,[174] cirrhosis,[173] and in patients who recently took aspirin.[175] A number of studies[176–179] failed to show any benefit from DDAVP in cardiac surgery patients. Preoperative techniques to reduce platelet dysfunction include platelet-rich plasmapheresis. A recent review article by Boldt[180] discusses plasmapheresis and its clinical applicability in great detail. Prophylactic platelet transfusion following CPB has not been shown to be beneficial.[181]

Deficiency of coagulation factor is not a common cause of postbypass coagulopathies. Hemodilution at the onset of bypass is associated with a 30 to 36% reduction in levels of factors II, V, VII, X, and XI for up to 48 hours following bypass.[169,171] Factor V levels were decreased 80% in a study by Mammen et al.[169] This reduction in and of itself is not enough to cause bleeding, as about only 30% of normal coagulation factors are required for normal hemostasis. Prophylactic administration of FFP has not been shown to be effective in reducing postbypass bleeding.[182] FFP should only be given to patients with laboratory-documented coagulopathies.

Pharmacologic prevention of postbypass bleeding has received substantial attention. Aminocaproic acid and aprotinin are both inhibitors of fibrinolysis. Aminocaproic acid, a synthetic antifibrinolytic, reduces blood loss by 30% compared with controls.[179,183,184] A standard dose is 15 gm total, 5 gm before skin incision, and 10 gm while on bypass. These drugs may potentially cause graft occlusion; however, a number of studies refute this possibility.[179,183–185] Aminocaproic acid should be adjusted when renal insufficiency is present.

Aprotinin is a naturally occurring antifibrinolytic obtained from bovine lung. The drug inhibits plasmin and plasminogen and kallikrein.[186] Early studies showed no benefit with aprotinin use, but subsequent studies using higher doses demonstrated reduced blood loss.[187–194] At least some of the benefit is derived from preserving platelet function.[190]

References

1. Taylor RM: Cardiopulmonary Bypass: Principles and Management. Baltimore, Williams & Wilkins, 1986.
2. Pugsley W, et al: Microemboli and cerebral impairment during cardiac surgery. Vasc Surg 24:34, 1990.
3. van der Linden J, Casimir-Ahn H: When do cerebral emboli appear during open heart operations? A transcranial Doppler study. Ann Thorac Surg 51:237, 1991.
4. Gutman FA, Zeggarra H: Ocular complications in cardiac surgery. Surg Clin North Am 51:1095, 1971.
5. Taugher PJ: Visual loss after cardiopulmonary bypass. Am J Ophthalmol 81:280, 1976.
6. Williams IM: Retinal vascular occlusions in open heart surgery. Br J Ophthalmol 59:81, 1975.
7. Serry C, et al: Superiority of aortic over femoral cannulation for cardiopulmonary bypass, with specific attention to lower extremity neuropathy. J Cardiovasc Surg 19:277, 1978.
8. Taylor PC, et al: Cannulation of the ascending aorta for cardiopulmonary bypass. Experience with 9,000 cases. J Thorac Cardiovasc Surg 71:255, 1976.
9. Murphy DA, et al: Recognition and management of ascending aortic dissection complicating cardiac surgical operations. J Thorac Cardiovasc Surg 85:247, 1983.
10. Reinke RT, et al: Aortoiliac dissection due to aortic cannulation. Ann Thorac Surg 18:295, 1974.
11. Salerno TA, et al: Arch versus femoral artery perfusion during cardiopulmonary bypass. J Thorac Cardiovasc Surg 76:681, 1978.
12. Carey JS, Skow JR, Scott C: Retrograde aortic dissection during cardiopulmonary bypass: "Nonoperative management." Ann Thorac Surg, 24:44, 1977.
13. Jones RE, et al: Apparatus of the Gibbon type for mechanical bypass of the heart and lungs. Mayo Clin Proc 30:105, 1955.
14. Donald DE, et al: Experiences with a heart lung bypass (Gibbon type) in the experimental laboratory. Mayo Clinic Proc 30:113, 1955.
15. Lillihei CW, et al: Direct vision intracardiac surgery in man using a simple, disposable artificial oxygenator. Dis Chest 29:1, 1956.
16. Cosgrove DM, Loop FD: Clinical use of travenol TMO membrane oxygenator. In Ionescu MI (ed): Techniques in Extracorporeal Circulation. London, Butterworths', 1981, p 85.

17. Lynch MF, Peterson D, Baker V: Centrifugal blood pumping for open heart surgery. Minn Med 61:536,1978.
18. Diehl JT, et al: Arterial bypass of the descending thoracic aorta with the Bio-Medicus centrifugal pump. Ann Thorac Surg 44: 422, 1987.
19. Joffe D, Silvay G: The use of microfiltration in cardiopulmonary bypass. J Cardiothorac Vasc Anesth 8:685, 1994.
20. McLean J: The discovery of heparin. Circulation 19:75, 1959.
21. Glimelius B, Busch C: Binding of heparin on the surface of cultured human endothelial cells. Thromb Res 12:773, 1978.
22. Jordan RE, et al: The kinetics of hemostatic enzyme-antithrombin interactions in the presence of low molecular weight heparin. J Biol Chem 225:10,081, 1980.
23. Conard J, et al: Antithrombin III in patients treated with subcutaneous or intravenous heparin. Thromb Res 22:507, 1981.
24. Andersson G, et al: Antithrombin III in patients with acute deep vein thrombosis during heparin treatment (subcutaneous and intravenous) and during and after treatment with oral coumarins. Thromb Res 34:333, 1984.
25. Holm HA, et al: Changes in plasma antithrombin (heparin cofactor activity) during intravenous heparin therapy: Observations in 198 patients with deep venous thrombosis. Scand J Haematol 35:564, 1985.
26. Kesteven PJ, et al: Protamine sulfate and rebound following open heart surgery. J Cardiovasc Surg 27:600, 1986.
27. Godal HC: Heparin induced thrombocytopenia. In Lane DA, Lindahl U (ed): Heparin. Chemical and Biological Properties, Clinical Applications. Boca Raton, FL, CRC Press, 1989, p 533.
28. Kappa JR, et al: Efficacy of Iloprost (ZK 36374) versus aspirin in preventing heparin-induced platelet activation during cardiac operations. J Thorac Cardiovasc Surg 94:405, 1987.
29. Hattersley PG: Activated coagulation time of whole blood. JAMA 196:150, 1966.
30. Bull BS, et al: Heparin therapy during extracororeal circulation. J Thorac Cardiovasc Surg 69:674, 1975.
31. Young JA, Kisker T, Doty DB: Adequate anticoagulation during cardiopulmonary bypass determined by activated clotting time and the appearance of fibrin monomer. Ann Thorac Surg 26:231, 1978.
32. Walenga JM, et al: Potential use of recombinant hirudin as an anticoagulant in a cardiopulmonary bypass model. Ann Thorac Surg 51:271, 1991.
33. Brister SJ, Buchanan MR: Heparin-less cardiopulmonary bypass revisited: A newer strategy to avoid heparin-related bleeding using dermatan sulfate. J Cardiothorac Vasc Anesth 9:317, 1995.
34. Brister SJ, et al: Is heparin the ideal anticoagulant for cardiopulmonary bypass? Dermatan sulfate may be an alternate choice. Thromb Haemost 71:468, 1994.
35. Astrup T, Brakman P, Nissen J: The estimation of fibrinogen—a revision. Scand J Clin Lab Invest 17:57, 1965.
36. Prandoni P, et al: Dermatan sulfate: A safe approach to prevention of postoperative deep vein thrombosis. Br J Surg 79:505, 1992.
37. Borowiec J, et al: Heparin-coated circuits reduce activation of granulocytes during cardiopulmonary bypass. A clinical study. J Thorac Cardiovasc Surg 104:642, 1992.
38. Tong SD, Rolfs MR, Hsu LC: Evaluation of Duroflo II heparin immobilized cardiopulmonary circuits. ASAIO Trans 36:M654, 1990.
39. Von Segesse LK, Weiss BM, Garcia E, et al: Reduction and elimination of systemic heparinization during cardiopulmonary bypass. J Thorac Cardiovasc Surg 103:790, 1992.
40. Tobias MA: Choice of priming fluids. In Taylor KM (ed): Cardiopulmonary Bypass—Principles and Management. Baltimore, Williams & Wilkins, 1986, p 221.
41. Marelli D, et al: Does the addition of albumin to the prime solution in cardiopulmonary bypass affect clinical outcome? J Thorac Cardiovasc Surg 98:751, 1989.
42. Webber CE, Garnett ES: The relationship between colloid osmotic pressure and plasma proteins during and after cardiopulmonary bypass. J Thorac Cardiovasc Surg 65:234, 1973.
43. Sanchez DeLeon R, Patterson JL, Sykes MK: Changes in colloid osmotic pressure and plasma albumin concentration associated with extracorporeal circulation. Br J Anesth 54:465, 1982.
44. English TA, Digerness S, Kirklin JW: Changes in colloid osmotic pressure during and shortly after open intra-cardiac operation. J Cardiovasc Thorac Surg 61:338, 1971.
45. Hall TS: The pathophysiology of cardiopulmonary bypass: The risks and benefits of hemodilution. Chest 107:1125, 1995.
46. Kolins J, Kolins MB: Informed consent, risk, and blood transfusion. J Thorac Cardiovasc Surg 100:88, 1990.
47. Gordon RJ, et al: Changes in arterial pressure, viscosity, and resistance during cardiopulmonary bypass. J Thorac Cardiovasc Surg 69:552, 1975.
48. Gordon RJ, Ravin M, Daicoff R, et al: Effects of hemodilution on hypotension during cardiopulmonary bypass. Anesth Analg 54:482, 1975.
49. Utley JR, et al: Effect of albumin and mannitol on organ blood flow oxygen delivery, water content and renal function during hypothermia, hemodilution, and cardiopulmonary bypass. Ann Thorac Surg 33:250, 1982.
50. Ohqvist G, et al: Pulmonary oxygenation central hemodynamics glomerular filtration following cardiopulmonary bypass with colloid or non-colloid priming solution. Scand J Thorac Cardiovasc Surg 15:257, 1981.
51. Hallowell P, et al: The effects of hemodilution with albumin or Ringers lactate on water balance and blood use in open heart surgery. Ann Thorac Surg 25:22, 1978.
52. Marelli D, et al: Does the addition of albumin to the prime solution in cardiopulmonary bypass affect the clinical outcome. J Thorac Cardiovasc Surg 98:751, 1989.
53. Mavroudis C: To pulse or not to pulse. Ann Thorac Surg 25: 259, 1978.
54. Angell James JE, de Burgh Daly M: Effects of graded pulsatile pressures on the reflex vasomotor responses elicited by changes of mean pressure in the perfused carotid sinus-aortic arch regions of the dog. J Physiol (Lond) 214:51, 1971.
55. Canivert JL, et al: Plasma renin activity and urine beta-2 microglobulin during and after cardiopulmonary bypass: Pulsatile vs nonpulsatile perfusion. Eur Heart J II:1079, 1990.
56. Boucher JK, Rudy LW, Edmunds LH: Organ blood flow during pulsatile cardiopulmonary bypass. J Appl Physiol 36:86, 1974.
57. Singh RKK, Barratt-Boyes BG, Harris EA: Does pulsatile flow improve perfusion during hypothermic cardiopulmonary bypass? J Thorac Cardiovasc Surg 79:827, 1980.
58. Salerno TA, Henderson M, et al: Hypertension after coronary operation. Can it be prevented by pulsatile perfusion? J Thorac Cardiovasc Surg 81:396, 1981.
59. Watkins WD, Peterson MB, et al: Thromboxane and prostacyclin changes during cardiopulmonary bypass with and without pulsatile flow. J Thorac Cardiovasc Surg 84:250, 1982.
60. Nagaoka H, Innami R, Arai H: Effects of pulsatile cardiopulmonary bypass on the renin-angiotensin-aldosterone system following open heart surgery. Jpn J Surg 18:390, 1988.
61. Philbin DM, Levine PH, Emerson CW, et al: Plasma vasopressin levels and urinary flow during cardiopulmonary bypass in patients with valvular heart disease. J Thorac Cardiovasc Surg 78: 779, 1979.
62. Mori A, Watanabe K, Onoe M, et al: Regional blood flow in the liver, pancreas, and kidney during pulsatile and non-pulsatile perfusion under profound hypothermia. Jpn Circ J 52:219, 1988.
63. Badner NH, Murkin JM, Lok P: Renal function is not influenced by differences in pH management and pulsatile/nonpulsatile perfusion during cardiopulmonary bypass (Abstract). Anesthesiology 75:A65, 1991.
64. Olinger GN, Hutchinson LD, Bonchek LI: Pulsatile cardiopulmonary bypass for patients with renal insufficiency. Thorax 38: 543, 1983.
65. Dernevik L, Arvidsson S, William-Olsson G: Cerebral perfusion in dogs during pulsatile and nonpulsatile extracorporeal circulation. J Cardiovasc Surg 26:32, 1985.
66. Anderson K, Waaben J, Husum B, et al: Nonpulsatile cardiopulmonary bypass disrupts the flow-metabolism couple in the brain. J Thorac Cardiovasc Surg 90:570, 1985.
67. Tranmer BI, Gross CE, Kindt GW, Adey GR: Pulsatile versus nonpulsatile blood flow in the treatment of acute cerebral ischemia. Neurosurgery 19:724, 1986.
68. Henze T, Stephan H, Sonntag H: Cerebral dysfunction following extracorporeal circulation for aortocoronary bypass surgery: No difference in neuropsychological outcome after pulsatile versus nonpulsatile flow. Thorac Cardiovasc Surg 38:65, 1990.
69. Shaw PJ, Bates D, Cartlidge, NEF, et al: An analysis of factors

predisposing to neurological injury in patients undergoing coronary bypass operations. Q J Med 72:633, 1989.
70. Azariades M, et al: A qualitative analysis of pulsatile perfusion: Effects on cortisol response to cardiopulmonary bypass surgery. Thorac Cardiovasc Surg 34:163, 1986.
71. Kono K, Philbin DM, Coggin CH, et al: Adrenocortical hormone levels during cardiopulmonary bypass with and without pulsatile flow. J Thorac Cardiovasc Surg 85:129, 1983.
72. Pollock EMM, Pollock JCS, Jamieson MPG, et al: Adrenocortical hormone concentrations in children during cardiopulmonary bypass with and without pulsatile flow. Br J Anaesth 60: 536, 1988.
73. Nagaoka H, et al: Preservation of pancreatic beta cell function with pulsatile cardiopulmonary bypass. Ann Thorac Surg 48: 798, 1989.
74. Philbin DM: Pulsatile blood flow. In Gravlee G, Davis R, Utley J (eds): Cardiopulmonary Bypass: Principles and Practice. Baltimore, Williams & Wilkins, 1993.
75. Alton L, Turina M, Gattiker R: Membrane and bubble oxygenator: A clinical comparison in patients undergoing aortocoronary bypass procedures. Herz 4:56, 1979.
76. Clark RE, Beauchamp RA, Magrath RA, et al: Comparison of bubble and membrane oxygenators in short and long perfusions. J Thorac Cardiovasc Surg 78:655, 1979.
77. Han P, et al: The use of B-thromboglobulin release to assess platelet damage during cardiopulmonary bypass. Presented at the Combined Meeting of the Royal Australasian College of Physicians, Feb. 24–29, 1980, Sydney, Australia.
78. Berreklouw E, et al: Myocardial protection with cold cardioplegia in a patient with cold autoagglutins and hemolysis. Ann Thorac Surg 133:521, 1982.
79. Hammerschmidt DE, Stroncek DF, Bowers TK, et al: Complement activation and neutropenia occurring during cardiopulmonary bypass. J Thorac Cardiovasc Surg 81:372, 1981.
80. Parker DJ, et al: Changes in serum complement and immunoglobulins following cardiopulmonary bypass. Surgery 71:824, 1972.
81. Moghissi K, et al: Acute renal failure and open heart surgery. Br Med J 32:228, 1972.
82. Hilberman M, Derby GC, Spencer RJ: Sequential pathophysiological changes characterizing the progression from renal dysfunction to acute renal failure following cardiac operations. J Thorac Cardiovasc Surg 79:838, 1980.
83. Hilberman M, Myers BD, Carrie BJ: Acute renal failure following cardiac surgery. J Thorac Cardiovasc Surg 77:880, 1979.
84. Gailiunas P, Chawla R, Lazarus JM, et al: Acute renal failure following cardiac operations. J Thorac Cardiovasc Surg 79:241, 1980.
85. Rigden SPA, et al: Acute renal failure complicating cardiopulmonary bypass surgery. Arch Dis Child 57:425, 1982.
86. Tan CK, et al: Levels of circulating norepinephrine and epinephrine before, during and after cardiopulmonary bypass in man. J Thorac Cardiovasc Surg 71:928, 1976.
87. Blythe WB: Renal autoregulation, drugs and acute renal failure. N C Med J 46:413, 1985.
88. Wilkes BM, Mailloux LU: Acute renal failure. Pathogenesis and prevention. Am J Med 80:1129, 1986.
89. Moore RA, Laub GW: Hemofiltration, dialysis, and blood salvage techniques during cardiopulmonary bypass. In Gravlee G, Davis R, Utley JR (eds): CPB: Principles and Practice. Baltimore, Williams & Wilkins, 1993.
90. Replogle R, et al: Catecholamine and serotonin response to cardiopulmonary bypass. J Thorac Cardiovasc Surg 44:638, 1962.
91. Hindman BJ, Lillehaug SL, Tinker JH: Cardiopulmonary bypass and the anesthesiologist. In Kaplan JA (ed): Cardiac Anesthesia, 3rd ed. Philadelphia, WB Saunders Co, 1993, p 919.
92. Stanley TH, Berman L, Green O, Robertson D: Plasma catecholamine and cortisol responses to fentanyl-oxygen anesthesia for coronary operations. Anesthesiology 53:250, 1980.
93. Samuelson PN, Reves JG, Kirklin JK, et al: Comparison of sufentanil and enflurane-nitrous oxide anesthesia for myocardial revascularization. Anesth Analg 65:217, 1986.
94. Scott WJ, Rode R, Castlemain B, et al: Efficacy, complications, and cost of a comprehensive blood conservation program for cardiac operations. J Thorac Cardiovasc Surg 103:1001, 1992.
95. Shangraw RE: Metabolic and splanchnic visceral effects of cardiopulmonary bypass. In Gravlee G, Davis R, Utley JR (eds): Cardiopulmonary Bypass: Principles and Practice. Baltimore, Williams & Wilkins, 1993.
96. Pennock J, et al: The management of the lungs during cardiopulmonary bypass. Surg Gynecol Obstet 145:917, 1977.
97. Sladen RN, Berkowitz DE: Cardiopulmonary bypass and the lung. In Gravlee G, Davis R, Utley JR (eds): Cardiopulmonary Bypass: Principles and Practice. Baltimore, Williams & Wilkins, 1993.
98. Ellison JT, Duke JF, Ellison RG: Pulmonary compliance following open heart surgery and its relationship to ventilation and gas exchange. Circulation 35(Suppl I):I-217, 1967.
99. Mandelbaum J, Giammona ST: Extracorporeal circulation, pulmonary compliance, and pulmonary surfactant. J Thorac Cardiovasc Surg 48:881, 1964.
100. Breckenridge IM, Diggerness SB, Kirklin JW: Increased extracellular fluid after open intracardiac operation. Surg Gynecol Obstet 131:53, 1970.
101. Ratliff NB, Young WG, Hackel DB: Pulmonary injury secondary to extracorporeal circulation. J Thorac Cardiovasc Surg 65:425, 1973.
102. Roach GW, Kanchuger M, Mangano CM, et al: Adverse cerebral outcomes after coronary bypass surgery. N Engl J Med 335:114, 1996.
103. Kataja JH, Kaukinen S, Viinamaki OV, et al: Hemodynamic and hormonal changes in patients pretreated with captopril for surgery of the abdominal aorta. J Cardiothorac Anesth 3:425, 1989.
104. Colson P, Saussine M, et al: Hemodynamic effects of anesthesia in patients chronically treated with angiotensin-converting enzyme inhibitors. Anesth Analg 74:805, 1992.
105. Coriat P, Richer C, Douraki T, et al: Influence of chronic angiotensin-converting enzyme inhibition on anesthesia induction. Anesthesiology 81:299, 1994.
106. Thaker U, Geary V, Chalmers P, Sheikh F: Low systemic vascular resistance during cardiac surgery: Case reports, brief review, and management with angiotensin II. J Cardiothorac Anesth 4:360, 1990.
107. Licker M, Niedhart P, Lustenberger S, et al: Long-term angiotensin-converting enzyme inhibitor treatment attenuates adrenergic responsiveness without altering hemodynamic control in patients undergoing cardiac surgery. Anesthesiology 84:789, 1996.
108. Lowenstein E, Hallowell P, Levine FH, et al: Cardiovascular response to large doses of intravenous morphine in man. N Engl J Med 281:1389, 1969.
109. Rosen DA, Rosen KR, Silvasi DL: In vitro variability in fentanyl absorption by different membrane oxygenators. J Cardiothorac Vasc Anesth 4:332, 1990.
110. Muravchick S: Scavenging enflurane from extracorporeal pump oxygenators. Anesthesiology 47:468, 1977.
111. Miller JD: A device for removal of waste anesthetic gases from the extracorporeal oxygenator. Anesthesiology 44:181, 1976.
112. Gravlee GP, Angert KC, Tucker WY, et al: Early anticoagulation peak and rapid distribution after intravenous heparin. Anesthesiology 68:126, 1988.
113. Mandelbaum J, Giammona ST: Extracorporeal circulation, pulmonary compliance, and pulmonary surfactant. J Thorac Cardiovasc Surg 48:881, 1964.
114. Stanley TH, Liu WS, Isern-Amaral J: The influence of IPPB, CPAP, and IPPB and CPAP during cardiopulmonary bypass on post-bypass and postoperative pulmonary function. Ann Thorac Surg 22:182, 1976.
115. Svennevig JL, Lindberg H, Geiran O, et al: Should the lungs be ventilated during cardiopulmonary bypass? Clinical, hemodynamic, and metabolic changes in patients undergoing elective coronary artery surgery. Ann Thorac Surg 37:295, 1984.
116. Boldt J, King D, Scheld HH, Hempelmann J: Lung management during cardiopulmonary bypass: Influence on extra-vascular lung water. J Cardiothorac Vasc Anesth 4:73, 1990.
117. Kurusz M, et al: Perfusion accident survey. Proc Am Acad Cardiovasc Perfusion 7:57, 1986.
118. Walls JT, Curtis JJ, McClatchey BJ, et al: Adverse effects of anesthetic agents on polycarbonate oxygenators (Letter to the Editor). J Thorac Cardiovasc Surg 96:667, 1988.
119. Cooper S, Levin R: Near catastrophic oxygenator failure (Letter to the Editor). Anesthesiology 66:101, 1987.

120. Kurusz M, Wheeldon DR: Risk containment during cardiopulmonary bypass. Semin Thorac Cardiovasc Surg 2:400, 1990.
121. Michenfelder JD, Theye RA: Hypothermia: Effect on canine brain and whole body metabolism. Anesthesiology 29:1107, 1968.
122. Cameron DE, Gardner TJ: Principles of clinical hypothermia. Card Surg State Art Rev 2:13, 1988.
123. Hickey RF, Hoar PF: Whole body oxygen consumption during low-flow hypothermic cardiopulmonary bypass. J Thorac Cardiovasc Surg 86:903, 1983.
124. Stupfel M, Severinghaus JW: Internal body temperature gradients during anesthesia and hypothermia and effect of vagotomy. J Appl Physiol 9:380, 1956.
125. Benzinger M: Tympanic thermometry in surgery and anesthesia. JAMA 209:1207, 1969.
126. Sladen RN: Temperature and ventilation after hypothermic cardiopulmonary bypass. Anesth Analg 64:816, 1985.
127. Zwischenberger JB, Mirsh MM, Dechert RE, et al: Suppression of shivering decreases oxygen consumption and improves hemodynamic stability during postoperative rewarming. Ann Thorac Surg 43:428, 1987.
128. Davis FM, Barnes PK, Bailey JS: Aural thermometry during profound hypothermia. Anaesth Intensive Care 9:124, 1981.
129. Lichtenstein SV, Ashe KA, El Dalati H, et al: Warm heart surgery. J Thorac Cardiovasc Surg 101:269, 1991.
130. The Warm Heart Investigators: Randomized trial of normothermic versus hypothermic coronary bypass surgery. Lancet 343:559, 1994.
131. Martin TD, Craver JM, Gott JP, et al: Prospective, randomized trial of retrograde warm blood cardioplegia: Myocardial benefit and neurological threat. Ann Thorac Surg 57:298, 1994.
132. Prough DS, Stump DA, Roy RC, et al: Response of cerebral blood flow to changes in carbon dioxide tension during hypothermic cardiopulmonary bypass. Anesthesiology 64:576, 1986.
133. Murkin JM, Farra JK, Tweed A, et al: Cerebral autoregulation and flow/metabolism coupling during cardiopulmonary bypass: The influence of $PaCO_2$. Anesth Analg 66:825, 1987.
134. Rogers AT, Stump DA, Gravlee GP, et al: Response of cerebral blood flow to phenylephrine infusion during hypothermic cardiopulmonary bypass: Influence of $PaCO_2$ management. Anesthesiology 69:547, 1988.
135. Lundar T, Lindegaard KF, Froysaker T, et al: Cerebral perfusion during nonpulsatile cardiopulmonary bypass. Ann Thorac Surg 40:144, 1985.
136. Lundar T, Lindegaard KF, Froysaker T, et al: Dissociation between cerebral autoregulation and carbon dioxide reactivity during nonpulsatile cardiopulmonary bypass. Ann Thorac Surg 40: 582, 1985.
137. Lundar T, Lindegaard KF, Froysaker T, et al: Cerebral carbon dioxide reactivity during nonpulsatile cardiopulmonary bypass. Ann Thorac Surg 41:525, 1986.
138. Brusino FG, Reves JG, Smith LR, et al: The effect of age on cerebral blow flow during hypothermic cardiopulmonary bypass. J Thorac Cardiovasc Surg 97:541, 1989.
139. Johnsson P, Messeter K, Ryding E, et al: Cerebral blood flow and autoregulation during hypothermic cardiopulmonary bypass. Ann Thorac Surg 43:386, 1987.
140. Bashein G, Townes BD, Nessly ML, et al: A randomized study of carbon dioxide management during hypothermic cardiopulmonary bypass. Anesthesiology 72:7, 1990.
141. Hindman BJ, Funatsu N, Harrington J, et al: Differences in cerebral blood flow between alpha-stat and pH-stat management are eliminated during periods of decreased systemic flow and pressure. Anesthesiology 75:A65, 1991.
142. Badner NH, Murkin JM, Lok P: Renal function is not influenced by differences in pH management and pulsatile/nonpulsatile perfusion during cardiopulmonary bypass (Abstract). Anesthesiology 75:A65, 1991.
143. Kolkka R, Hilberman M: Neurological dysfunction following cardiac operation with low-flow, low-pressure cardiopulmonary bypass. J Thorac Cardiovasc Surg 79:432, 1980.
144. Akins CW: Noncardioplegic myocardial preservation for coronary revascularization. J Thorac Cardiovasc Surg 88:174, 1984.
145. Stockard JJ, Bickford RG, Schauble JF: Pressure-dependent cerebral ischemia during cardiopulmonary bypass. Neurology 23: 521, 1973.
146. Slogoff S, Reul GJ, Keats AS, et al: Role of perfusion pressure and flow in major organ dysfunction after cardiopulmonary bypass. Ann Thorac Surg 50:911, 1990.
147. Govier AV, Reves JG, McKay RD, et al: Relationship of cerebral blood flow and perfusion pressure during cardiopulmonary bypass. Anesthesiology 59:A-70, 1983.
148. Feddersen K, Aren C, Nilsson NJ, Radegran K: Cerebral blood flow and metabolism during cardiopulmonary bypass with special reference to effects of hypotension induced by prostacyclin. Ann Thorac Surg 41:395, 1986.
149. Slogoff S, Girgis KV, Keats AS: Etiologic factors in neuropsychiatric complications associated with cardiopulmonary bypass. Anesth Analg 61:903, 1982.
150. Stern DH, Gerson JI, Allen FB, Parker FB: Can we trust the direct radial artery pressure immediately following cardiopulmonary bypass? Anesthesiology 62:557, 1985.
151. Mohr R, Lavee J, Goor DA: Inaccuracy of radial arterial pressure measurement after cardiac operations. J Thorac Cardiovasc Surg 94:286, 1987.
152. Pauca AL, Meredith JW: Possibility of A-V shunting upon cardiopulmonary bypass discontinuation. Anesthesiology 67:91, 1987.
153. Butterworth JF, Zaloga GP, Prielipp RC, et al: Calcium inhibits the cardiac stimulating properties of dobutamine but not of amrinone. Chest 101:174, 1992.
154. Fernandez-Del Castillo C, Harringer W, Warshaw, et al: Risk factors for pancreatic cellular injury after cardiopulmonary bypass. N Engl J Med 325:382, 1991.
155. Cheung JY, Bonventre JV, Malis CD, et al: Calcium and ischemic injury. N Engl J Med 314:1670, 1986.
156. Golding LAR: Postcardiotomy mechanical support. Semin Thorac Cardiovasc Surg 3:29, 1991.
157. Sanfelippo PM, Baker NH, Ewe HG, et al: Experience with intraaortic balloon counterpulsation. Ann Thorac Surg 41:36, 1986.
158. Lee WA, Gillinov AM, Cameron DE, et al: Centrifugal ventricular assist device for support of the failing heart after cardiac surgery. Crit Care Med 21:1186, 1993.
159. McCarthy PM, Sabik JF: Implantable circulatory support devices as a bridge to heart transplantation. Semin Thorac Cardiovasc Surg 6:174, 1994.
160. Morel DR, Zapol WM, Thomas SJ, et al: C5a and thromboxane generation associated with pulmonary vaso- and bronchoconstriction during protamine reversal of heparin. Anesthesiology 66:597, 1987.
161. Sharath MD, Metzger WJ, Richerson HB, et al: Protamine-induced fatal anaphylaxis, prevalence of antiprotamine immunoglobin E anti-body. J Thorac Cardiovasc Surg 90:86, 1985.
162. Knape JTA, Schuller JL, De Haan P, et al: An anaphylactic reaction to protamine in a patient allergic to fish. Anesthesiology 55:324, 1981.
163. Caplan SN, Berman EM: Protamine sulfate and fish allergy (Letter). N Engl J Med 295:172, 1976.
164. Lowenstein E, Zapol WM: Protamine reactions, explosive mediator release and pulmonary vasoconstriction (Editorial). Anesthesiology 73:373, 1990.
165. Lowenstein E: Lessons from studying an infrequent event: Adverse hemodynamic responses associated with protamine reversal of heparin anticoagulation. J Cardiothorac Anesth 3:99, 1989.
166. D'Ambra M: Restoration of the normal coagulation process: Advances in therapies to antagonize heparin. J Cardiovasc Pharm 27(Suppl 1):S58, 1996.
167. Milam JD, Austin SF, Martin RF, et al: Alterations of coagulation and selected clinical chemistry parameters in patients undergoing open heart surgery without transfusions. Am Soc Clin Pathol 76:155, 1981.
168. Ansell J, Tiarks C, McCue J, et al: Amrinone-induced thrombocytopenia. Arch Intern Med 144:949, 1984.
169. Mammen EF, Koets MH, Washington BC, et al: Hemostasis changes during cardiopulmonary bypass surgery. Semin Thromb Hemost 11:281, 1985.
170. Bick RL: Hemostasis defects associated with cardiac surgery, prosthetic devices, and other extracorporeal devices. Semin Thromb Hemost 11:249, 1985.
171. Harker LA, Malpass TW, Branson HE, et al: Mechanism of abnormal bleeding in patients undergoing cardiopulmonary bypass:

Acquired transient platelet dysfunction associated with selective alpha-granule release. Blood 56:824, 1980.

172. Ferraris VA, Ferraris SP, Lough FC, Berry WR: Preoperative aspirin ingestion increases operative blood loss after coronary artery bypass grafting. Ann Thorac Surg 45:71, 1988.
173. Mannucci PM: Desmopressin: A nontransfusional form of treatment for congenital and acquired bleeding disorders. Blood 72: 1449, 1988.
174. Mannucci PM, Remuzzi G, Pusineri F, et al: Deamino-8-D-arginine vasopressin shortens the bleeding time in uremia. N Engl J Med 308:8, 1983.
175. Kobrinsky NL, Gerrard JM, Watson CM, et al: Shortening of bleeding time by 1-desamino-8-D-arginine vasopressin in various bleeding disorders. Lancet 1:1145, 1984.
176. Seear MD, Wadsworth LD, Rogers PC, et al: The effect of desmopressin acetate (DDAVP) on postoperative blood loss after cardiac operations in children. J Thorac Cardiovasc Surg 98:217, 1989.
177. Andersson TLG, Solem JO, Tengborn L, Vinge E: Effects of desmopressin acetate on platelet aggregation, von Willebrand factor, and blood loss after cardiac surgery with extracorporeal circulation. Circulation 81:872, 1990.
178. Hackman T, Gascoyne RD, Naiman SC, et al: A trial of desmopressin (1-desamino-8-D-arginine vasopressin) to reduce blood loss in uncomplicated cardiac surgery. N Engl J Med 321: 1437, 1989.
179. Horrow JC, Van Riper DF, Strong MD, et al: The hemostatic effects of tranexamic acid and desmopressin during cardiac surgery. Circulation 84:2063, 1991.
180. Boldt J: Acute platelet-rich plasmapheresis for cardiac surgery. J Cardiothorac Vasc Anesth 9:79, 1995.
181. Consensus Conference: Platelet transfusion therapy. JAMA 257: 1777, 1987.
182. Roy RC, Stafford MA, Hudspeth AS, Meredith JW: Failure of fresh frozen plasma to reduce blood loss and blood replacement after cardiopulmonary bypass. Anesth Analg 67:S190, 1987.
183. DelRossi AJ, Cernaianu AC, Botros S, et al: Prophylactic treatment of post-perfusion bleeding using EACA. Chest 96:27, 1989.
184. Horrow JC, Hlavacek J, Strong MD, et al: Prophylactic tranexamic acid decreases bleeding after cardiac operations. J Thorac Cardiovasc Surg 99:70, 1990.
185. Sharifi R, Lee M, Ray P, et al: Safety and efficacy of intravesical aminocaproic acid for bleeding after transurethral resection of prostate. Urology 27:214, 1986.
186. Royston D: The serine antiprotease aprotinin (trasylol): A novel approach to reducing postoperative bleeding. Blood Coag Fibrin 1:55, 1990.
187. Verstraete M: Clinical application of inhibitors of fibrinolysis. Drugs 29:236, 1985.
188. Havel M, Teufelsbauer H, Knobl P, et al: Effect of intraoperative aprotinin administration on postoperative bleeding in patients undergoing cardiopulmonary bypass operation. J Thorac Cardiovasc Surg 101:968, 1991.
189. Blauhut B, Gross C, Necek S, et al: Effects of high-dose aprotinin on blood loss, platelet function, fibrinolysis, complement, and renal function after cardiopulmonary bypass. J Thorac Cardiovasc Surg 101:958, 1991.
190. van Oeveren W, Harder MP, Roozendaal KJ, et al: Aprotinin protects platelets against the initial effect of cardiopulmonary bypass. J Thorac Cardiovasc Surg 99:788, 1990.
191. Edmunds LH, Niewiarowski S, Colman RW: Aprotinin (Letter). J Thorac Cardiovasc Surg 101:1103, 1991.
192. Alajmo F, Calamai G, Perna AM, et al: High-dose aprotinin: Hemostatic effects in open heart operations. Ann Thorac Surg 48:536, 1989.
193. Dietrich W, Spannagl M, Jochum M, et al: Influence of high-dose aprotinin treatment on blood loss and coagulation patterns in patients undergoing myocardial revascularization. Anesthesiology 73:1119, 1990.
194. Harder MP, Eijsman L, Roozendaal KJ, et al: Aprotinin reduces intraoperative and postoperative blood loss in membrane oxygenator cardiopulmonary bypass. Ann Thorac Surg 51:936, 1991.

CHAPTER 18

Low Cardiac Output States: Drugs, Intra-Aortic Balloon, and Ventricular Assist Devices

Mark Stafford Smith, M.D., C.M., F.R.C.P.C.
David D. Kaemmer, A.S., B.S., C.C.P.
Robert N. Sladen, M.B., M.R.C.P.(UK), F.R.C.P.C.

Patients undergoing cardiac, thoracic, and vascular surgery are at high risk for perioperative cardiac morbidity, including conditions complicated by low cardiac output syndrome. Therefore, a familiarity with the diagnosis and therapeutic approaches to low-perfusion states is essential for the anesthesiologist caring for these patients. All three types of surgery frequently involve major perioperative blood loss and fluid shifts that may result in low-output states. Clearly, cardiac surgical patients are also vulnerable to low-perfusion states due to the additive effects of pre-existing cardiac disease, the cardiac surgery, and the myocardial stunning associated with cardiopulmonary bypass and aortic cross-clamping. However, thoracic and vascular surgical patients are also at high risk for postoperative cardiac events due to the prevalence of coexisting coronary atherosclerosis and other cardiac conditions in these patients, and the major hemodynamic stresses commonly associated with thoracic and vascular surgical procedures (e.g., aortic cross-clamping). This chapter summarizes the pathophysiology of low cardiac output syndrome, provides a brief description of the physiology of the failing heart and the systemic humoral responses to the low-output state, and gives a logical systematic approach to the hemodynamic management of low cardiac output syndrome.

The Low-Output Syndrome

Definition

The low cardiac output syndrome is a state in which perfusion is inadequate to meet the metabolic demands of a patient, as a result of impaired pumping function of the heart. While the diagnosis of low cardiac output syndrome requires evidence of the manifestations of inadequate perfusion, a low-output state is generally defined as being present when a cardiac index (CI) of less than 2.2 L/min/m^2 exists. Of note, a low cardiac output state is not synonymous with low-output syndrome; clearly a CI of 2.2 L/min/m^2 may exceed the metabolic requirements of a hypothermic anesthetized patient, while a febrile septic patient is likely to be hypermetabolic and require a much greater CI than 2.2 L/min/m^2.

The low cardiac output syndrome is best defined by the clinical manifestations of systemic hypoperfusion (i.e., shock), which result from oxygen delivery that is inadequate to meet tissue demands. Signs and symptoms include tachycardia, hypotension, oliguria, dry mucous membranes, confusion, tachypnea, and cold clammy mottled extremities. If the origin of hypoperfusion is pump failure (i.e., cardiogenic shock) then these symptoms are also associated with the manifestations of acute pulmonary edema. Hemodynamic assessment of these patients reveals a low CI and reduced stroke index, with increased systemic vascular resistance (SVR). Laboratory investigations demonstrate progressive metabolic (lactate) acidosis and disseminated intravascular coagulation (DIC). The natural history of shock, if inadequate oxygen delivery continues, is for compensatory physiologic responses to be overwhelmed as the condition finally becomes irreversible, and death ensues.

Using Ohm's law of the circulation—that is, pressure difference (voltage) = (current) × resistance—the relationship of blood pressure (BP), cardiac output (CO) and SVR can be expressed as:

$$BP = CO \times SVR$$

Implicit in this hemodynamic relationship is the fact that a sustained blood pressure does not necessarily reflect a sustained cardiac output, since increases in SVR can maintain blood pressure in the face of profound reductions in cardiac output. Conversely, tissue perfusion pressure may be inadequate in the face of normal or even high cardiac output with severe drops in SVR.

Finally, this interrelationship provides a basis for the classification of shock states (Fig. 18–1). In this chapter, the low-cardiac-output syndrome will imply the presence of hypovolemic (including hemorrhagic) or cardiogenic shock.

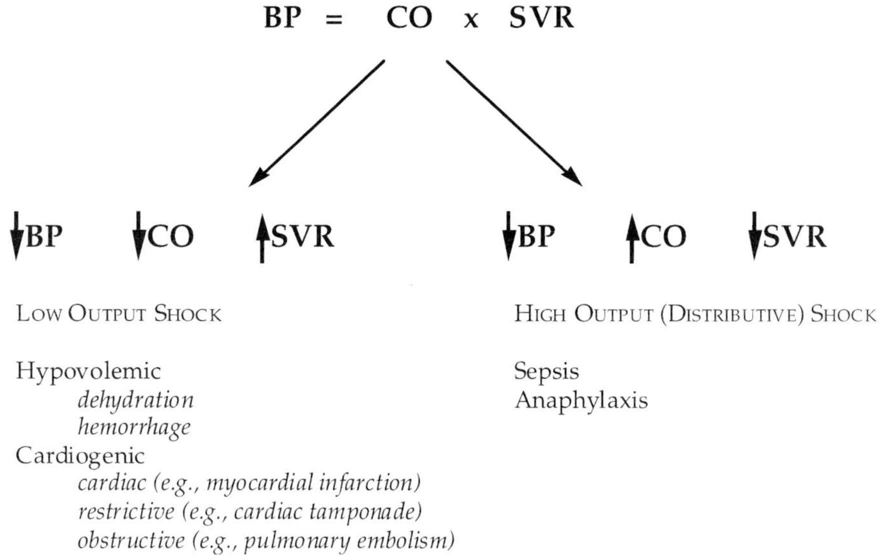

FIGURE **18–1.** Classification of shock states.

Pathophysiology of Shock

Inadequate oxygen delivery to meet the metabolic demands of tissues is the basic underlying problem that leads to the shock state. In the absence of oxygen, anaerobic glycolysis replaces the more efficient aerobic glycolysis as the generator of adenosine triphosphate (ATP). The spiral of decreased cardiac output, hypoperfusion, and shock is further exacerbated by the accumulation of lactic acid from anaerobic glycolysis, and the generation of other vasodilator and cardiodepressant factors. Supply/demand mismatch may be the result of reduced oxygen delivery, as in low cardiac output states, or by excessive metabolic demands, as in sepsis. While supply and demand alterations may coexist in the shock state, the emphasis of this chapter will be to examine issues relating to the problems of oxygen delivery.

Tissue Oxygen Delivery and Consumption

Since oxygen cannot be stored in the body, organisms have evolved elaborate methods for delivering oxygen from the environment to the tissues where it is used in oxidative metabolism.

ARTERIAL OXYGEN CONTENT (Cao_2)

Hemoglobin (Hb) is the most important blood element for carrying oxygen molecules from the lungs to the tissues; each gram of hemoglobin has the potential to carry 1.34 ml of gaseous oxygen; therefore, the oxygen content of hemoglobin in blood is simply calculated as the product of hemoglobin concentration, the saturation of hemoglobin by oxygen (Sao_2), and 1.34 ml/gm Hb. In addition, a small amount of oxygen is dissolved in the blood; the dissolved oxygen content is determined by arterial oxygen tension (Pao_2) and the blood solubility coefficient for oxygen (0.0031 ml/dl). The total arterial oxygen content may therefore be expressed as:

$$Cao_2 = (Hb \times 1.34 \times Sao_2) + (Pao_2 \times 0.0031)$$

For example, in a healthy individual with a hemoglobin concentration of 15 gm/dl breathing room air at sea level, Pao_2 would be 95 mm Hg and hemoglobin would be 100% saturated. Therefore, Cao_2 is $(15 \times 1.34 \times 100\%) + (95 \times 0.0031) = 20.4$ ml O_2 per deciliter of blood. Notably, only 0.3 ml of oxygen per deciliter of blood is transported dissolved in plasma. The important role of hemoglobin in oxygen transport is highlighted by the fact that in order to provide a resting $\dot{V}o_2$ of 248 ml/min solely through dissolved oxygen, a cardiac output of over 80 L/min would be required!

OXYGEN DELIVERY ($\dot{D}o_2$)

The amount of oxygen delivered to the tissues ($\dot{D}o_2$) relies not only on the amount of oxygen carried by arterial blood (Cao_2) but the volume of blood delivered to the tissues over time (i.e., CO):

$$\dot{D}o_2 = Cao_2 \times CO$$

Where $\dot{D}o_2$ = oxygen delivery in milliliters per minute, Cao_2 = arterial blood oxygen content in milliliters O_2 per liter of blood, and CO equals cardiac output in liters per minute. For example, an individual with a normal Cao_2 (200 ml O_2 per liter of blood) with a resting cardiac output of 5 L/min, will have a resting $\dot{D}o_2$ of $200 \times 5 = 1{,}000$ ml/min. The oxygen content of mixed venous blood ($C\bar{v}o_2$) is normally 150 ml O_2 per liter of blood, and reflects unused oxygen returned from the tissues. In the above example, oxygen return would be $150 \times 5 = 750$ ml/min.

Therefore, in an individual at rest, only 250 ml of a possible 1,000 ml of delivered arterial oxygen is actually extracted by the tissues; the remaining 750 ml represents an important reserve mechanism. Interestingly, unlike most tissues at rest, the myocardium extracts about 50% of arterial oxygen content, leaving very little opportunity for further oxygen extraction and requiring the heart to rely mainly on increases in coronary perfusion to increase oxygen supply.

With knowledge of oxygen delivery and oxygen return, we can estimate tissue oxygen consumption ($\dot{V}O_2$) using the Fick equation:

$$\dot{V}O_2 = \text{oxygen delivery } (\dot{D}O_2) - \text{oxygen return}$$

In the above example, therefore, resting $\dot{V}O_2$ is 1,000 − 750 = 250 ml/min. When $\dot{V}O_2$ is increased (e.g., during exercise), more oxygen is made available through increases in cardiac output, tissue oxygen extraction (i.e., reduced oxygen return), or both. However, the myocardium must rely heavily on augmented oxygen delivery ($\dot{D}O_2$) to achieve increased $\dot{V}O_2$, since tissue oxygen extraction for the heart is close to maximum at rest. When the oxygen delivery reserve is exhausted, then tissue oxygen consumption is exceeded by oxygen demand, and anaerobic metabolism occurs with the production of lactic acid.

Lactic Acidosis

Intracellular metabolism of glucose to produce high-energy phosphates (ATP) may occur through two mechanisms: aerobic and anaerobic glycolysis. Anaerobic glycolysis involves ten successive cytoplasmic chemical reactions with the production of 2 M of ATP and 2 M of pyruvic acid for each mole of glucose. When oxygen is available, a further set of reactions occurs in the mitochondria, which involve the activation of pyruvic acid by coenzyme A (acetylcoenzyme A) and entry of the acetyl moiety into the citric acid (Krebs) cycle. The Krebs cycle permits generation of a further 36 M of ATP for each mole of glucose, and results in the waste products of water and carbon dioxide.

In the presence of inadequate tissue oxygen supply, aerobic glycolysis (Krebs cycle) ceases and pyruvate, generated by anaerobic glycolysis, accumulates. By mass action (in the presence of hydrogen ions) pyruvate is converted to lactic acid. While ATP remains essential for cellular integrity, in the presence of decreased oxygen supply ATP production is limited. In addition, local increases in lactic acid cause vasodilation, depressed myocardial function, and decreased vascular sensitivity to catecholamines.[1]

Microcirculatory Changes in Shock

The microcirculation is the pathway through which oxygen is delivered to the tissues. The microcirculation consists of arterioles, meta-arterioles, the capillary bed, and venules. In order for oxygen and nutrient delivery and metabolite removal from tissues to occur, not only is normal global hemodynamic function necessary but microcirculatory integrity is also essential. In fact, one way of describing shock is that state in which inadequate perfusion of the microcirculation exists.

Muscular arterioles regulate capillary flow, and give rise to the smaller, and largely muscle free capillary network. Small muscular precapillary sphincters also serve to direct blood at a capillary level. Meta-arterioles are direct connections between arterioles and venules that bypass capillary beds altogether ("peripheral shunting"). Muscular tone in larger arterioles is highly sensitive to α_1-adrenergic receptor agonist stimulation, which elicits intense vasoconstriction, reducing total blood flow to the affected vascular bed. In contrast, smaller arterioles are influenced more by local factors such as vasodilator prostaglandins and endothelial relaxant factor.[2] Capillary blood flow is therefore dynamically regulated, responding to local and systemic signals, at the level of capillary bed and between capillaries within each bed.

The early endocrine response to low cardiac output is mediated predominantly by the sympathetic adrenal system, and is characterized by intense arteriolar and venular constriction (except in the cerebral and coronary circulation, where blood is preferentially directed). However, substances such as endothelin may be involved in the delayed portion of this effect. Endothelial changes begin to occur as a result of hypoperfusion and the accumulation of lactic acid and other vasodilator substances. This results in decreased catecholamine responsiveness of arterioles.[3] After a critical period, influenced both by host and external modifiers, small precapillary arterioles begin to lose their vascular tone. In the face of persistent venular constriction, as well as obstruction with cellular debris, microcirculatory drainage becomes impaired. The resultant increases in capillary hydrostatic pressure exacerbate leakage of intravascular fluid into the interstitial space. The resulting edema further distances cells from their source of nutrients and oxygen, increasing cell dependence on anaerobic metabolism and aggravating the metabolic acidosis. Stasis of blood within capillary beds also triggers intravascular coagulation. As edema accumulates, global hemodynamic abnormalities increase because of reduced venous return and inadequate preload.

Disseminated Intravascular Coagulation

DIC is a hallmark of shock, and is a consequence of blood stasis within tissues, hypoxia, and acidosis. Endothelial injury resulting from cellular hypoxia not only acts as a stimulus for contact activation of factor XII (Hageman factor) and the intrinsic pathway of coagulation but also activates fibrinolysis by plasmin, and the kinin system. The extrinsic pathway of coagulation is also activated through procoagulants, which are activated by the release of thromboplastins from injured tissues, platelets, and leukocytes. Active fibrinolysis causes the liberation of large amounts of fibrin degradation products, which in turn inhibit fibrin polymerization. DIC is especially likely to occur in situations where shock is associated with hemorrhage and hematoma, where the triggers of hemostasis and fibrinolysis can trigger further consumption of platelets and coagulation factors.[4]

Microthrombosis from DIC leads to end-organ ischemia and infarction and may hasten the onset of multi–organ system failure. However, the role of DIC as a cause of multi–organ system failure or simply as a marker of severe tissue perfusion abnormalities is still disputed. Certainly the consumption of hemostatic factors by DIC can significantly influence the severity of bleeding from surgical wounds and trauma.

Laboratory findings of DIC typically include prolongation of all coagulation tests, and a rapidly falling platelet count (in fact, a normal stable platelet count would make the diagnosis of DIC unlikely). While fibrinogen levels are preserved until later in the course of DIC, the liver's significant reserve for fibrinogen production is ultimately exhausted and fibrinogen levels also decrease. Coexisting fibrinolysis is reflected by increasing levels of fibrin degradation products, in particular the D-dimer. While replacement of blood products and treatment with low-dose heparin infusion with or without antifibrinolytic agents (e.g. ε-aminocaproic acid) will address the immediate problems caused by DIC, only treatment of the underlying low output state, to correct acidosis and hypoxemia by improving tissue perfusion, will address the cause of DIC.

Irreversible Shock

The steady depletion of high-energy phosphate sources seen during shock not only impairs the active transport mechanisms of cell membranes but also compromises the integrity of the cell membrane itself. The resultant leaky cell is unable to maintain the integrity of its contents and leaches potassium out into the extracellular space while allowing sodium and excess water to cause cellular edema. These effects combine to impair cell function and further exacerbate the effects of hypoxia and acidosis. Ultimately, irreparable injury occurs to mitochondria and the cellular oxidative mechanisms, and $\dot{V}O_2$ declines. At this point, even restoration of global circulatory parameters is unable to elicit an appropriate response in regulatory vessels of the microcirculation. Despite improved global perfusion, blood glucose, pyruvate, and lactate continue to accumulate. Shock-damaged mitochondria are unable to generate sufficient high-energy phosphate material, even though oxygen and substrate are now available[5] (fuel is of little use in an irreparably damaged engine). When the microcirculation is irrevocably impaired, irreversible shock has occurred and death is inevitable.

Some experimental evidence suggests that an appropriate response following a period of shock includes increases of oxygen transport variables ($\dot{D}O_2$, $\dot{V}O_2$, cardiac output, etc.) to levels above those prior to the episode, if survival is likely to occur.[6,7] In general, the greater the hypoxic insult, the greater the subsequent increase in oxygen delivery must be if survival is to occur.

Inflammatory Responses to Low Output Shock

Hematologic Responses

GRANULOCYTES

Chemotactic agents are elaborated during the shock state by injured tissues, which attract granulocytes to the area. When granulocytes arrive at the site of cellular injury they undergo leukostasis; a process in which release of lysozyme and myeloperoxidase, as well as free oxygen radicals causes proteolytic injury to normal tissues. Histamine may also be released from basophils through a non–IgE-mediated mechanism.[8] Histamine compounds the disturbances of microvascular regulation, vascular permeability, and extracellular edema by its effects on the microcirculation. The accumulation of granulocytes during leukostasis can also exacerbate tissue perfusion problems from shock by direct obstruction of the microcirculation.[9] This is highlighted by the improved capillary perfusion noted during hemorrhagic shock in neutropenic animals. Gastrointestinal ulceration and transmural necrosis associated with shock has also been attributed to impaired microcirculatory flow,[10] which in a rat model can be significantly improved by neutrophil depletion.[11]

MONOCYTES

Monocytes and macrophages are important scavenger cells that ingest cellular debris and microorganisms that gain access to the bloodstream. Monocytes release various substances that contribute to the pathophysiology of shock, including interleukin-1 and -2, tissue thromboplastin, plasminogen activators, and proteolytic enzymes.

PLATELETS

Endothelial disruption causes platelet activation and release of a variety of vasoactive agents that aggravate the microcirculatory disturbances associated with shock.

Local and Microcirculatory Mediators

EICOSANOIDS

Eicosanoids are important endogenous mediators in shock that are generated from arachidonic acid. Phospholipases release arachidonic acid from cellular membranes in response to primary insults (e.g., tissue injury, ischemia, or hypotension) as well as the presence of substances released during the initial circulatory response to shock (e.g., norepinephrine, angiotensin II, arginine vasopressin, bradykinin, thrombin, adenosine diphosphate [ADP]). Cyclo-oxygenase (prostaglandin synthetase) acts on the arachidonic acid to yield unstable endoperoxides, the precursors to the prostaglandins. Circulating endoperoxides that enter platelets are transformed into thromboxane (TXA_2), a vasoconstrictor that also promotes platelet aggregation. In contrast, endoperoxides that enter capillary endothelial cells are transformed into prostacyclin (PGI_2), which is a vasodilator and also inhibits platelet aggregation, thus maintaining capillary perfusion. The contrasting effects of TXA_2 and PGI_2 normally maintain a balance; however, the overwhelming platelet activation and thromboxane release during shock, especially with hemorrhage, cause severe vasoconstriction and formation of microthrombi, which exacerbates tissue ischemia.[12] Arachidonic acid is also converted in granulocytes to the peptide leukotrienes. The enzyme lipoxygenase is responsible for generating the small peptides that have an array of harmful effects, especially on the lung, and contributes to the pathophysiology of shock. Leukotrienes can cause local vasoconstriction, thrombosis, increased capillary permeability, and the release of several harmful substances (e.g., myocardial depressant factors, lysosomal hydrolases, and proteolytic agents). Further membrane damage and cellular dysfunction result, leading to increased cellular edema, which further limits the utilization of metabolic substrates through impairment of the microcirculation. This cycle of microcirculatory hypoperfusion and cellular injury provokes further leukotriene release. Specific agents designed to interrupt the cascade of endogenous mediators in shock have shown enhanced survival in animals[13–15] that have been subjected to experimental hemorrhagic shock. While these agents offer some hope for treatment of shock in the future, their benefit in human studies has yet to be explored. In contrast, nonspecific inhibitors of eicosanoid production such as nonsteroidal anti-inflammatory drugs (NSAIDs) may not be useful as therapy for shock, since they suppress protective arachidonic acid responses as well as those that promote shock. One such effect is exerted by the vasodilator prostaglandins (e.g., PGI_2), which enhance renal perfusion; it is well recognized that patients receiving NSAIDs are more susceptible to acute renal failure during a hemodynamic insult.[16]

PLATELET ACTIVATING FACTORS

Another family of substances that play a role in the pathophysiology of shock are the platelet activating factors (PAFs). While these substances are derived from the arachidonic acid, they are not eicosanoids. These acetylated phosphoglycerides are generated from cell membrane lipids in response to tissue injury. While these substances are named because of their proaggregatory platelet effects,[17] they also mediate a multiplicity of actions in the inflammatory response to shock. In a hemorrhagic shock model in rats, a specific antagonist to PAFs improved survival and decreased the level of harmful mediators.[18] Interestingly, the benzodiazepine antagonist flumazenil also antagonizes some of the PAF-mediated adverse effects such as coronary vasoconstriction, cardiac depression, and platelet aggregation.[19]

COMPLEMENT ACTIVATION

The organized functioning of the complement system represents a homeostatic mechanism against antimicrobial invasion.[20] The normal functions of the complement system include local effects, including chemotaxis, opsonization, and liberation of anaphylatoxins (which cause membrane disruption and vascular permeability). However, the sustained activation of the complement system observed during shock sets up a harmful systemic inflammatory response leading to tissue damage and organ dysfunction.

CONTACT ACTIVATION SYSTEM (INTRINSIC PATHWAY OF COAGULATION)

When blood is exposed to negatively charged surfaces such as damaged endothelium, the resulting cascade of events involves activation of both coagulation and fibrinolysis.[21] Not only is the intrinsic pathway of coagulation activated, resulting in generation of thrombin, but activation of the complement protein C1 triggers the complement cascade and converts prekallikrein to kallikrein, leading to generation of plasmin. Kallikrein also causes the release of bradykinin from high-molecular-weight kininogen (HMWK). Kinins have a broad range of effects including vasodilation, increased vascular permeability, enhanced prostaglandin activity, induction of pain, and modulation of the renin-angiotensin system.[22] The release of kallikrein is also associated with an amplification of subsequent contact activation such that a cascade of mediator activation and release, and tissue and vascular damage, occurs.

FREE OXYGEN RADICALS

A dangerous cycle of inflammation, increased capillary permeability, and tissue injury is created when free oxygen radicals are liberated and cause peroxidation of lipid membranes. One substrate for the generation of free oxygen radicals is the proteolysis of xanthine dehydrogenase; this enzyme, which is particularly abundant in the lung, intestine, liver, and heart, is converted in the presence of ischemia and calcium to xanthine oxidase. With reperfusion, xanthine oxidase catalyzes release of superoxide and hydrogen peroxide from oxygen. These substances are converted into hydroxyl ions in the presence of iron, which cause tissue injury. Therapeutic strategies involving iron chelation (desferroxamine), and superoxide dismutase, have been shown to diminish injuries associated with free oxygen radicals.[23] Similarly, allopurinol (a xanthine oxidase inhibitor) and vitamin E (an antioxidant) have been shown to increase survival if given prior to experimental hemorrhagic shock in dogs.[24]

ENDOTOXIN

During a low-output state, mesenteric ischemia may lead to loss of mucosal integrity of the gut and depressed activity of the reticuloendothelial system in the liver. This combination sets up the portal circulation as a passage of entry for bacteria and endotoxin, resulting in so-called secondary septic shock. Rush et al. demonstrated that blunt trauma victims are more likely to have positive blood cultures if the injury is associated with hypotension.[25] Endotoxin activates cell membrane enzymes to release arachidonic acid, for subsequent conversion into several proinflammatory mediators including prostaglandins, leukotrienes, thromboxanes, and platelet activating factors. Endotoxin also activates the alternate complement pathway, while bacteria activate the classical complement pathway. Hence, during hemorrhagic shock, the effects of circulating endotoxin may be an added secondary cause of hypotension (due to decreased SVR and myocardial dysfunction) and microcirculatory dysfunction (reduced oxygen consumption and arteriovenous [AV] shunting), and organ damage (low-pressure pulmonary edema, acute renal failure, hepatic dysfunction). Several pieces of evidence indicate that gut sterilization prior to episodes of hypotension and hemorrhagic shock are associated with improved survival.[26,27] Similarly, the existence of an endogenous antibody to endotoxin is associated with lower postoperative infection rates.[28] It has been proposed that the development of a monoclonal endotoxin antibody and the administration of antibiotics could reduce the morbidity and mortality resulting from endotoxemia following mesenteric ischemia.

MYOCARDIAL DEPRESSANT FACTORS

Mesenteric ischemia during a low-output state may lead to disruption of pancreatic acinar cells, liberating harmful proteolytic enzymes into the circulation.[29,30] Animal studies have demonstrated that the release of these digestive enzymes into the circulation during shock states is associated with myocardial dysfunction, mesenteric vasoconstriction (which aggravates the pancreatic ischemia), and depression of reticuloendothelial cell activity.[31]

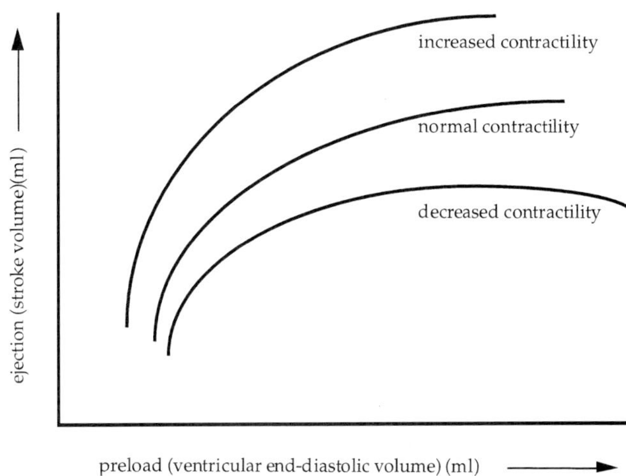

FIGURE **18–2.** The Frank-Starling relationship.

Cardiac Function and Failure

A commonly made assumption is that a normal cardiac output and normal arterial oxygen content are associated with normal tissue oxygen delivery. However, the cascade of events that may occur during a shock state may lead to abnormal distribution of peripheral blood flow with inadequate oxygen supply to the tissues despite a normal cardiac output and arterial oxygen content. Hence, distributive regional blood flow abnormalities that occur in shock are not necessarily reflected in the calculation of $\dot{D}O_2$. However, there is no question that in the presence of a low-cardiac-output state, tissue ischemia resulting from regional blood flow abnormalities can only be aggravated. Therefore, an essential part of therapy for the shock state is to re-establish normal (or supernormal) cardiac output.

Cardiac output represents the product of cardiac ejection (stroke volume [SV]) and the frequency of ejection (heart rate [HR]). In clinical practice, important determinants of cardiac function amenable to therapy include heart rate (and rhythm), preload, afterload, and contractility. While contractility and heart rate are properties intrinsic to the myocardium, preload and afterload are dependent on myocardial and peripheral vascular function. Therapeutic interventions in the shock state generally impact on one or many of these variables.

Preload

The association of increased diastolic ventricular distention (preload) with a corresponding increase in the ventricular ejection has been termed the Frank-Starling hypothesis.[32,33] A graphic relationship between preload and cardiac ejection is typically represented by a left ventricular (LV) function curve (Fig. 18–2). Shifts of the ventricular curve to the left or right are seen with alterations in ventricular compliance, contractility, and afterload, and result in changes in cardiac output in response to a given preload (Fig. 18–3). Myocardial dysfunction from any cause results in a rightward and downward shift in the ventricular function curve, so that cardiac output is decreased for any given preload. The ventricular function curve becomes flattened in the failing heart, such that increases in preload lead only to pulmonary congestion and edema without any significant increase in cardiac output.

Clinical variables commonly used as indicators of preload include jugular venous pulsations, and invasive hemodynamic variables such as central venous pressure (CVP), left atrial pressure (LAP), and pulmonary artery occlusion pressure (PAOP). These variables are useful as indicators of preload most reliably when the ventricles are compliant, and expand normally with added volume. When ventricular compliance is increased (e.g., mitral regurgitation) or decreased (e.g., ventricular hypertrophy), changes in ventricular pressure do not closely reflect changes in ventricular volume. In these settings, imaging of the ventricular volume (e.g., transesophageal echocardiography) may be a more sensitive indicator of ventricular preload.

During hypovolemic states, maintenance of ventricular preload at normal levels occurs at the expense of

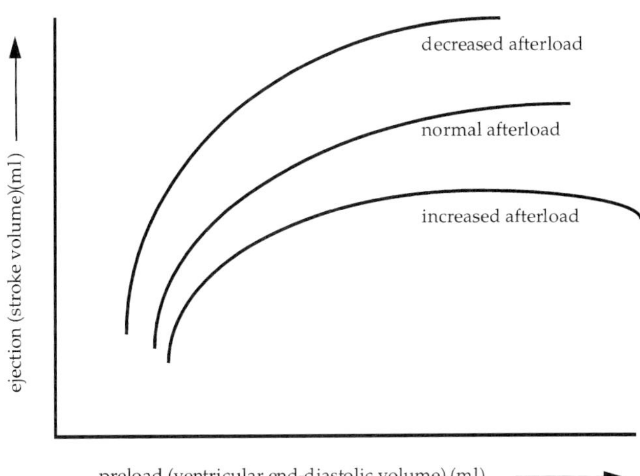

FIGURE **18–3.** Alterations in afterload change the Frank-Starling relationship.

systemic vasoconstriction. Part of this compensation includes diversion of cardiac output preferentially to vital organs such as the brain and the heart. This explains why hypovolemic patients are at significant risk when vasomotor tone is abolished by sedation or anesthesia.

Afterload

An important determinant of the pressure work of ventricular ejection is the impedance to ventricular outflow, or afterload. Changes in afterload can be described in terms of altered ventricular systolic "wall stress" required to successfully eject blood. Laplace's law, which describes the surface tension on a sphere, can be used to relate the variables that influence wall stress and afterload.

$$\text{Wall tension} = Pr/2t$$

Where P = pressure generated in the myocardium during isovolumic contraction, r = intracavitary radius and t = ventricular wall thickness.

The response to an acute increase in afterload is reduced ventricular ejection, which results in accumulation of fluid (preload). Subsequent ventricular ejection is increased (as predicted by the Frank-Starling relationship), and cardiac output is maintained. An interesting observation associated with the phenomenon is augmented ventricular performance, which tends to occur after several beats, possibly reflecting recovery from subendocardial ischemia (the Anrep effect).[34] Clearly, progressive increases in afterload will result in increases in preload with maintenance of cardiac output, until the effect of added preload is to actually reduce ventricular ejection (also predicted by the Frank-Starling relationship). Long-term increases in myocardial afterload (e.g., with aortic stenosis) also stimulate concentric left ventricular hypertrophy. Ventricular hypertrophy is an effective response to chronic increases in afterload; the Laplace relationship predicts that increased ventricular wall thickness and (resulting) decreased intracavitory radius should decrease the overall "wall stress."

Settings in which ventricular function is already operating close to the limit of preload reserve include the ischemic or scarred left ventricle, and interestingly the normal right ventricle. With these conditions ventricular failure can be precipitated by very small acute increases in afterload. The importance of reducing afterload using vasodilator therapy, when possible, is highlighted by the fact that ventricles at the limit of preload reserve are less likely to respond to inotropic stimulation.

Measures of changing systolic wall tension may be derived by calculating the area beneath a ventricular pressure tracing (systolic pressure-time index [SPTI]), and also may be approximated by examining a peripheral arterial tracing. In the absence of fixed obstruction to ventricular ejection (e.g., aortic stenosis), the most important determinant of (left or right) ventricular afterload is peripheral resistance (R), whose relationship to blood pressure and cardiac output may be described using a modification of Ohm's law.

$$\text{BP} = \text{CO} \times \text{R}$$

$$\text{R} = \text{BP/CO}$$

Using these simple formulas, indexes of systemic and pulmonary vascular resistances (SVR, PVR) can be derived;

$$\text{SVR} = (\text{MAP} - \text{CVP/CO}) \times 80 \text{ dyne} \cdot \text{sec} \cdot \text{cm}^{-5}$$

$$\text{PVR} = (\text{MPAP} - \text{PAOP/CO}) \times 80 \text{ dyne} \cdot \text{sec} \cdot \text{cm}^{-5}$$

Where MAP = mean arterial pressure, CVP = central venous pressure, MPAP = mean pulmonary artery pressure, PAOP = pulmonary artery occlusion pressure, and CO = cardiac output. The conversion factor of 80 changes Wood's units to SI units. Normal SVR ranges from 800 to 1500 dyne$\cdot$sec$\cdot$cm^{-5}, whereas normal PVR is 50 to 150 dyne$\cdot$sec$\cdot$cm^{-5}.

Several factors contribute to errors in the estimating of vascular resistance using values derived from a pulmonary artery catheter with thermodilution cardiac output; there is an inherent variability of 10 to 15% (or greater with PAOP measures) in the bedside values obtained, and even small differences between the recorded and true values are multiplied by the conversion factor (80). Other inherent limitations of these derived estimates of vascular resistance relate to the assumptions made in their calculation; for example, CVP acts only as an indirect measure of precapillary arteriole pressure in the calculation of a systemic arterial pressure gradient. Although Ohm's law of the circulation is relatively linear for SVR versus changes in arterial blood pressure and cardiac output, this is not true for the pulmonary circulation. Despite its limitations for calculating vascular resistance, the pulmonary artery catheter provides a useful tool for identifying trends, especially in response to therapeutic interventions. Vascular resistance can be made more meaningful by indexing values to body size, using the cardiac index and the vascular resistance index for calculation.

While vascular resistance is inversely related with arterial radius (to the fourth power), other variables that influence blood viscosity (e.g., blood temperature, hematocrit) also are important determinants of vascular resistance. Finally, fixed ventricular outflow track obstruction (e.g., aortic stenosis) is clearly not a variable amenable to vasodilator therapy or other nonsurgical interventions to alter systemic vascular tone.

Contractility

The intrinsic myocardial force of contraction developed at a given resting myocardial fiber length is an indicator of contractility. Contractility is usually expressed as the velocity of fiber shortening (dl/dt), or by a measured change in ventricular pressure per unit time during contraction (dP/dt). A way of defining the contractile state is to express the extrapolated velocity of myocardial fiber shortening at zero afterload (i.e., when the velocity would be maximal, Vmax).

While cardiac output at a given contractile state is sensitive to variables such as preload and afterload, these variables do not change the intrinsic contractile state (Vmax). Therefore, under the same loading conditions (i.e., preload and afterload), a decrease in cardiac output must reflect a decrease in the contractile state (negative inotropic effect), and vice versa (positive inotropic effect). While clinical measurements of the contractile state are not usually practical, changes in the contractile state can be inferred through sequential construction of ventricular function curves.

Heart Rate

When stroke volume is fixed, heart rate determines cardiac output. Heart rate is also the most important clinical determinant of myocardial oxygen balance. Increases in heart rate not only increase myocardial oxygen consumption but reduce the duration of diastole, thus reducing total diastolic coronary perfusion time, which is the most important period of oxygen delivery to the left ventricle. A second effect associated with tachycardia, more evident in the depressed heart, is a further increase in contractile force with increased heart rate, known as the staircase or *Treppe* phenomenon or Bowditch effect.[35,36] In contrast, decreases in heart rate, even with enhanced stroke volume and coronary perfusion time, may result in insufficient cardiac output to meet oxygen delivery demands. Increased heart rate is an important compensatory response to reductions in stroke volume resulting from hypovolemia or myocardial ischemia, while unwanted bradycardia (e.g., sinus node disease or negative chronotropic agent administration) may exacerbate low-cardiac-output states. However, the importance of tachycardia as a compensatory mechanism is contrasted with its untoward effect on myocardial oxygen balance, especially when compared to other methods of augmenting cardiac output (e.g., preload augmentation, afterload reduction, positive inotropic agents).

Systemic Responses in Low-Output Shock

Compensatory Peripheral Circulatory Responses

The neurohumoral reaction to shock is immediate and prolonged. Mediators of these reflex responses to hypoperfusion include the peripheral vasculature and the kidney. The result of these effects is to activate homeostatic mechanisms to restore intravascular volume and blood pressure.

Sympathoadrenal Responses

The endogenous catecholamines (epinephrine and norepinephrine) mediate the most significant hemodynamic response to shock. Activation of the sympathetic nervous system causes release of epinephrine directly into the circulation from the adrenal medulla, and norepinephrine from the paravertebral sympathetic chain and large prevertebral ganglia. Baseline plasma epinephrine levels are low, but increase rapidly in response to stress. In contrast, basal plasma norepinephrine levels are greater, but increase less during periods of stress due to neuronal reuptake of the majority (85 to 90%) of released hormone. While epinephrine levels decline rapidly after cessation of the stress, norepinephrine levels may be sustained for several days, and are possibly responsible for catabolic effects subsequent to shock.

Catecholamine levels are increased during shock[37] presumably due to the potent combined stimuli of pain, anxiety, reduced pulse pressure, and hypovolemia. At systolic blood pressures less than 70 mm Hg, tonic baroreceptor inhibition of sympathetic nervous system activity is insignificant, and carotid and aortic chemoreceptors further augment sympathetic tone in response to hypoxemia, acidosis, and anemia.

Autonomic responses to low cardiac output and hypotension may differ in hypovolemic and cardiogenic shock states, due to the activation of central cardiopulmonary low-pressure baroreceptors with cardiogenic shock (which cause the release of atrial natriuretic peptide). Gorfinkel et al. demonstrated that in cardiogenic shock, renal blood flow was relatively maintained (75% of normal), while hypovolemic shock was associated with a renal blood flow that was reduced to one tenth of normal values.[38]

The primary physiologic effect of catecholamine release occurs in the circulatory system. Adrenergic receptor subtypes mediate different effects in different tissues; increased myocardial contractility and heart rate are predominantly influenced by β_1-adrenergic receptor activation, whereas peripheral vasoconstriction is mediated mainly by the α_1-adrenergic receptor, which alters relative blood flow to redistribute blood volume to the heart and brain. In addition, blood reservoirs in the large veins (pulmonary circulation, liver, spleen, splanchnic beds, and subcutaneous tissues) are mobilized to supplement the circulating volume. Redistribution of blood volume is also associated with alterations in blood flow to specific organs. For example, splanchnic and hepatic blood flow is significantly decreased, while skin and adipose tissue are almost unperfused, while muscle blood flow is also profoundly affected.

The kidneys, which normally receive 25% of cardiac output, are richly innervated with sympathetic nerve fibers, which profoundly influence their perfusion during shock. Extreme vasoconstriction, especially of renal cortical vessels, can make the kidneys prone to ischemic damage.[39] Relative blood flow within the kidney is thought to be preferentially diverted to nephrons in the juxtamedullary zone, which are responsible for the greatest ability to concentrate urine. This adjustment would allow the kidney to improve its salt water absorption and reduce obligate fluid loss through the urine. Sympathetic stimulation also causes the release of renin, which augments the generation of angiotensin to produce further renal vasoconstriction.

Many of the early symptoms and signs of low-output shock such as tachycardia, oliguria, and cool clammy skin are the result of redistribution of blood volume. While these homeostatic changes may compensate for hypovolemia, prolonged persistent distributive changes may result in ischemic organ damage. Relative renal ischemia may cause renal dysfunction or renal failure, while splanchnic hypoperfusion may result in stress ulceration of the stomach, and enhanced release of bacteria and endotoxin into the circulation, further exacerbating shock. Similarly, pancreatic ischemia and injury causes the release of myocardial depressant factors.

Another important β-adrenergic receptor–mediated metabolic response to shock is the release of glucose stores from the liver (glycogenolysis) and free fatty acids (lipolysis) to provide energy substrates. Epinephrine also suppresses the actions of insulin and lipoprotein lipase, causing hyperglycemia and elevated circulating free fatty acids (the so-called diabetes of injury).

Renin-Angiotensin-Aldosterone System

The rapid response of the autonomic nervous system to shock is accompanied by slower homeostatic mechanisms, which are initiated during the several hours after onset of shock and subsequently sustained for days to weeks. One of these responses results from the renin-angiotensin-aldosterone system.[40,41] Several stimuli associated with shock cause release of renin from the juxtaglomerular apparatus (JGA) in the kidney, including β-adrenergic sympathetic stimulation, in addition to reduced stretch of efferent arterioles, hypoperfusion, and decreased plasma sodium. Once released, renin initiates a process in which angiotensin II is generated from angiotensinogen involving a two step process with angiotensin converting enzyme (ACE).

Angiotensin II is a potent vasoconstrictor; locally in the kidney it causes efferent arteriole vasoconstriction (to maintain glomerular filtration while renal blood flow is diminished), systemically angiotensin II also promotes the release of aldosterone from the adrenal gland. Angiotensin II–related renal vasoconstriction is profound and may exacerbate renal cortical ischemia well beyond a period of hemodynamic insult (e.g., following cardiac surgery[42]). While angiotensin II has a much smaller vasoconstricting effect on systemic vessels, reduced production of angiotensin II through the use of ACE inhibitors profoundly decreases SVR.

Circulating aldosterone initiates changes in renal tubular cells that cause increased production of proteins required to increase sodium and water retention at the distal convoluted tubule, in exchange for potassium. The resulting effects include a sustained intravascular volume expansion and hypochloremic metabolic alkalosis.

Antidiuretic Hormone

Antidiuretic hormone (arginine vasopressin [AVP]) is synthesized in the hypothalamus and stored in the posterior pituitary gland. This hormone acts on vasopressin$_1$ (V_1) receptors in the collecting ducts of the kidney to enhance water reabsorption. The resulting effect is a more concentrated urine, a decreased plasma osmolarity and extensive fluid retention. The other name for antidiuretic hormone, arginine vasopressin, refers to the properties of this hormone at high concentrations to cause vasoconstriction. Release of antidiuretic hormone is stimulated by at least four mechanisms[43]: the homeostatic effects of antidiuretic hormone are mediated through osmoreceptors in the hypothalamus, by stretch receptors in the left atrium and pulmonary veins (which respond to decreased central blood volume), and aortic and carotid barorecepters that respond to decreased systemic arterial blood pressure. In addition to homeostatic mechanisms, other factors may cause inappropriate triggering of the release of antidiuretic hormone to produce a condition known as syndrome of inappropriate antidiuretic hormone secretion (SIADH). Triggers for SIADH include stress, pain, anxiety, and various pulmonary pathology including pneumonia. In settings where hypovolemia exists with normal serum osmolarity, ADH secretion will result in water retention, edema, and hyponatremia. In low-cardiac-output states, extreme baroreceptor stimulation may increase antidiuretic hormone levels sufficiently to contribute to the overall vasopressor response. Interestingly, angiotensin II can also cause antidiuretic hormone release, increasing the overall fluid retention.

Hypothalamic-Endocrine Responses

Cortisol

Shock causes the release of the adrenocorticotropic hormone (ACTH) from the anterior pituitary gland through several different mechanisms. ACTH in turn causes release of glucocorticoids and aldosterone from the adrenal cortex. Cortisol, the primary glucocorticoid, is important in the systemic response to shock.[44] While increases in cortisol production in response to shock take several hours, the effect persists for days. Cortisol has significant effects on many different systems. While it increases responsiveness to catecholamine-mediated myocardial and vascular effects, it also stimulates generation of metabolic substrates through activation of proteolysis and gluconeogenesis. Cortisol also inhibits the actions of insulin, resulting in hyperglycemia. Protein catabolism is an important cause of loss of lean body mass and impaired wound healing in patients following surgery and trauma.

The role of cortisol in modifying the inflammatory effects related to shock are thought to be associated with its ability to inhibit the enzyme phospholipase A_2 (the enzyme that causes release of arachidonic acid from lipid membranes). Arachidonic acid is the substrate for generation of prostaglandins, thromboxanes, leukotrienes, and platelet activating factors, all important mediators in the microcirculatory response to shock.

USE OF STEROIDS IN THE TREATMENT OF LOW-OUTPUT SHOCK

While steroid therapy for shock would make intuitive sense, studies in animals have produced conflicting data in this setting.[45,46] In the treatment of critically ill patients with septic shock, large trials have demonstrated that high-dose methylprednisolone treatments increased mortality in patients with pre-existing renal disease, and increased mortality from septic complications.[47]

Endogenous Opioid Peptides

Endogenous opioids are simultaneously released with steroid hormones due to their generation from the same precursor, pro-opiomelanocortin. The role of endogenous opioids such as β-endorphins in modulating behavior, pain perception, ventilation, vasomotor tone, heart rate, temperature, immunity, and other effects is established.[48] While the majority of endogenous opioid peptides are released from different regions of the brain, there is evidence that enkephalins are also co-released with catecholamines from the adrenal medulla.[49]

USE OF OPIOID ANTAGONISTS IN THE TREATMENT OF LOW-OUTPUT SHOCK

Accumulating evidence suggests that endogenous opioids act at the mu and delta opioid receptors, to have their effects during a shock state.[50] Faden and Holaday demonstrated an improved arterial pressure in rats treated with naloxone (an opioid receptor antagonist) subjected to hemorrhagic shock.[51] Similar naloxone-treated primate models of hemorrhagic and endotoxic shock have demonstrated improved hemodynamics and survival.[52] It has been proposed that naloxone has its effect by inhibiting the endorphin-mediated attenuation of catecholamine effects. In a rat model of hemorrhagic shock, naloxone treatment was associated with reversal of microcirculatory effects from shock.[53] However, naloxone administration may be associated with complications, including acute catecholamine release in patients where reversal of significant narcotic analgesia occurs, causing pain, but also hypertension, arrhythmias, myocardial ischemia, and even pulmonary edema. The role of subtype-selective opioid antagonists with the ability to preserve analgesia, while reversing some of the effects of endogenous opioid agents, may hold promise.[54]

Thyroid Hormones

While thyroid function abnormalities are common in critically ill patients[55] and the endogenous thyroid hormones thyroxin (T_4) and triiodothyronine (T_3) are known to enhance the stress response, the role of the thyroid gland in shock is not entirely clear. General effects of thyroid hormone administration include increased metabolism with elevated oxygen consumption, heat production, and CO_2 production. While the effects of thyroid hormones on cardiac function include their ability to potentiate the actions of catecholamines, glucagon, and cortisol, there is some evidence to suggest that they also have direct intrinsic inotropic and chronotropic effects on the heart. Generally systolic blood pressure increases whereas diastolic pressure is decreased.

Animal studies of shock have demonstrated that survivors have higher brain levels of thyrotropin-releasing hormone (TRH) than nonsurvivors.[56] Primate studies have also demonstrated that TRH administration is associated with improved survival with hemorrhagic (but not endotoxic) shock.[57] TRH administration causes increases in heart rate, body temperature, minute ventilation, and glucose release, which may account for these observations. However, human studies of TRH have not been performed to evaluate its role as a possible therapeutic agent in shock.

Principles of Hemodynamic Management

Whatever the cause of a low-cardiac-output state, effective hemodynamic management is required and must be based upon accurate clinical and hemodynamic data, following a logical intervention sequence (Fig. 18–4).

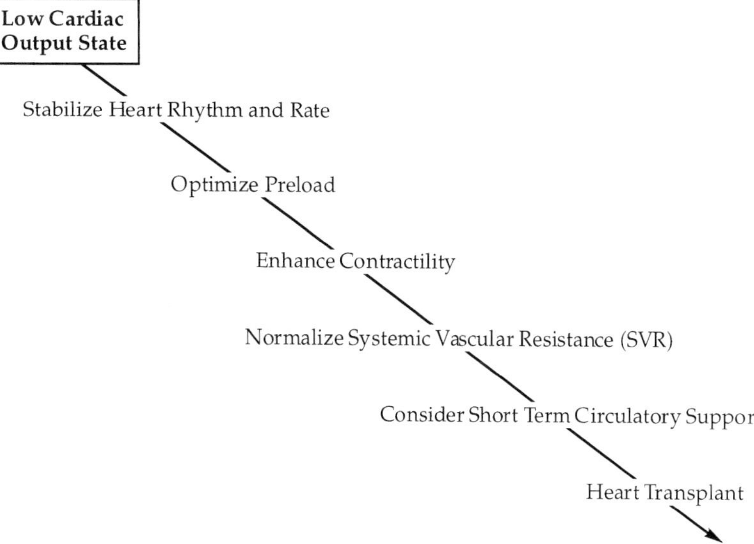

FIGURE **18–4.** A logical approach to the clinical management of a low-cardiac-output state.

Stabilize Heart Rhythm and Rate

Abnormalities of heart rhythm and rate commonly reflect cardiovascular responses to other physiologic disturbances (e.g., hypovolemia, myocardial ischemia, metabolic derangements), and may require correction of the underlying cause for resolution to occur. Tachycardias and other tachyarrhythmias often respond incrementally to such disturbances, and, therefore, may be useful as markers of the effectiveness of corrective therapy. In contrast, bradycardias and bradyarrhythmias are more often related to disorders of the cardiac conduction system or drug effects. In general, until stability of heart rate and rhythm is achieved, hemodynamic assessment of other determinants of cardiac performance and response to therapy is difficult.

Sinus Tachycardia

A normal physiologic response to *low stroke volume* is increased heart rate, whether it is related to reduced ventricular filling (e.g., hypovolemia) or cardiac failure. Other causes of sinus tachycardia (>100 bpm) include pain, acute myocardial ischemia, hypoxemia, and hypercarbia. Clearly, treatment of the underlying cause(s) of sinus tachycardia is more appropriate than interventions that specifically slow the heart (e.g., β-blockers), without regard to the underlying etiology. In fact, for conditions where tachycardia is an appropriate response to low stroke volume, β-blocker therapy may result in acute hemodynamic decompensation.

Interventions that improve stroke volume in a low-output state will generally result in an immediate slowing of heart rate. An example—a hypovolemic patient has a cardiac output of 4.0 L/min before and after intravenous fluids, however, the heart rate has decreased from 120 bpm to 90 bpm during this time. While the cardiac output remains unchanged in this example, cardiac performance is considerably improved (stroke volume has increased from 42 ml/beat to 56 ml/beat). Heart rates above 160 bpm are generally due to supraventricular tachyarrhythmias.

Supraventricular Tachyarrhythmias

The three types of supraventricular tachyarrhythmias are atrial tachycardia, atrial flutter, and atrial fibrillation. In general the etiology of supraventricular tachyarrhythmias is multifactorial. One of the most important contributing factors is elevated circulating levels of catecholamines (endogenous or for inotropic support); while epinephrine and norepinephrine levels are high in all low-cardiac-output states, other factors contributing to catecholamine release include pain, acidosis, hypoxemia, and hypercarbia. Reductions in arrhythmia threshold from metabolic derangements (e.g., hypokalemia, hypomagnesemia, hypercalcemia) may further increase the likelihood of supraventricular tachyarrhythmias. Therapeutic interventions (Tables 18–1 and 18–2) may result in temporary improvements; however, treatment of underlying contributing factors is also essential for long-term hemodynamic stability.

Atrial fibrillation is often a chronic condition, unlikely to be successfully converted to sinus rhythm. Patients with atrial fibrillation are particularly vulnerable to low-cardiac-output states, due to the frequent association of

TABLE 18–1
Treatment of Supraventricular Tachyarrhythmias: Therapeutic Modalities

Modality	Administration	Caveats
DC cardioversion	Use synchronous mode; 50–360 J	Usually reserved for unstable or refractory arrhythmias. Sedation generally necessary in conscious patient.
Adenosine	6–12 mg rapid IV push	Brief period of profound bradycardia common. Heart transplant recipients sensitive to low doses.
Verapamil	2.5 mg q1–2min IV, total 10 mg May be repeated q2–4h	Negative inotropic and vasodilator actions cause acute hypotension. Administration to a patient with VT may be a lethal error.
Diltiazem	0.25–0.35 mg/kg IV over 2 min Infusion 5–15 mg/hr	Infusion not recommended for >24 hr.
Esmolol	"Test doses" 5–10 mg IV q1/2–1min until effect seen Infusion: Load 0.5 mg/kg over 2 min Maintenance 100–300 μg/kg/min	"Test dose" is essential to assess whether effect is beneficial (i.e., conversion or slowing) or adverse (hypotension, decreased CO, bradyarrhythmias).
Procainamide	Infusion: Load 20–30 mg/min IV (max 17 mg/kg) Maintenance 1–4 mg/min Therapeutic range 4–8 μg/ml	Rapid loading may cause hypotension. Metabolite (NAPA) accumulation may precipitate seizures, especially with renal dysfunction: keep levels 10–20 μg/ml.
Digoxin	Load 0.5 mg IV, then 0.25 mg q4h × 2 (total 1.0 mg) Maintenance 0.25–0.125 mg qod, versus renal function Therapeutic range 1–3 ng/ml	Complete onset of action takes 1–2 hr; do not repeat loading doses <q1h even with rapid AF. With AF, dosage guided by ventricular rate, not drug level—but catecholamines make rate difficult to control.
Phenylephrine	IV 50–100 μg prn	Treats acute hypotension caused by PSVT (important with myocardial ischemia); vagal reflex may slow or rarely convert PSVT. Useful with verapamil (see above).

AF, atrial fibrillation; PSVT, paroxysmal supraventricular tachycardia; DC, direct current; IV, intravenous; NAPA, *N*-acetyl procainamide; q1/2–1min, every 30–60 sec; qd, daily; q1hr, hourly; q4hr, 4-hourly; VT, ventricular tachycardia.

TABLE 18–2
Treatment of Supraventricular Tachyarrhythmias: Therapeutic Options

Arrhythmia	Treatment Options	Caveats
Paroxysmal supraventricular tachycardia (PSVT)	DC cardioversion Adenosine Verapamil Digoxin Esmolol Diltiazem	PSVT *must* be differentiated from ST. Negative inotropic effects of verapamil, esmolol may be balanced by improved ventricular filling and SV.
Atrial flutter	DC cardioversion Diltiazem Esmolol Verapamil Digoxin Procainamide	Digoxin slows ventricular response; procainamide more likely to convert. Verapamil slows but seldom converts.
Atrial fibrillation (acute)	Same as atrial flutter	Vagotonic effect of digoxin may promote spontaneous, early conversion. Digoxin essential to slow ventricular response, procainamide more likely to convert.
Multifocal atrial tachycardia (MAT)	Verapamil	Usually refractory to therapy: correct milieu, hypoxemia, RV strain (decrease work of breathing).

AF, atrial fibrillation; RV, right ventricle; ST, sinus tachycardia; SV, stroke volume; DC, direct current.

this disorder with other heart diseases (e.g., rheumatic valve disease), and the absence of an "atrial kick" with atrial fibrillation. Increased ventricular rate in response to elevated catecholamines levels with atrial fibrillation is irregular and unpredictable, frequently compromising ventricular filling (e.g., mitral stenosis) and precipitating a low-cardiac-output state. Pharmacologic interventions aimed at slowing ventricular rate with atrial fibrillation may improve cardiac output, but may also precipitate other arrhythmias (e.g., digoxin toxicity).

A supraventricular tachycardia commonly associated with severe obstructive lung disease is multifocal atrial tachycardia (MAT). This disorder involves chaotic atrial excitation from many atrial locations, and is often difficult to distinguish from atrial fibrillation. MAT rarely responds to digoxin, but drugs that are usually effective such as verapamil and β-blockers may be contraindicated due to associated negative inotropic effects and the risk of aggravating reactive airway disease.

Sinus Bradycardia and Conduction Problems

Although the definition of sinus bradycardia involves rates below 60 bpm, when a low-cardiac-output state exists, much higher heart rates may reflect an *inappropriately low* chronotropic response (e.g., a heart rate of 70 bpm with severe hypovolemia). Disorders of the cardiac conduction system or drug toxicity should be suspected when an inadequate heart rate response to shock is observed. The commonest cause of abnormal heart rate responses is sinus node fibrosis, a disease of aging that is responsible for sick sinus syndrome. Sick sinus syndrome is a condition characterized by episodes of inappropriately slow (or rapid) heart rate, often associated with symptoms including palpitations and syncope. Patients with sick sinus syndrome frequently have exaggerated effects from drugs with chronotropic properties; use of inotropic agents may precipitate episodes of supraventricular tachycardia, while β-blocker therapy may result in profound bradycardia.

The normal myocardial response to hypothermia includes a slowing of the heart rate. The commonest setting for hypothermia-related sinus bradycardia is the operating room, particularly if a patient has received large amounts of unwarmed intravenous fluid (e.g., blood products). Inferior myocardial ischemia or infarction may also precipitate bradycardia or bradyarrhythmias. Digoxin toxicity frequently results in arrhythmias with slowed conduction, which are aggravated by the presence of hyperkalemia and metabolic acidosis. Common abnormal rhythms associated with digoxin toxicity include wandering atrial pacemaker, junctional rhythm, second-degree heart block (Mobitz type I, Wenckebach phenomenon) and complete heart block. Digoxin toxicity may also induce tachyarrhythmias, such as atrial tachycardia with block.

Standard therapy of bradyarrhythmias involves intravenous doses of anticholinergic (e.g., atropine), transcutaneous pacing (TCP), or β-adrenergic agonist (e.g., dopamine or epinephrine) drugs (Table 18–3). Refractory bradycardias may respond to "pharmacologic pacing" with a continuous dopamine or epinephrine infusion, providing a useful bridge to more definitive bradycardia therapy (e.g., a temporary pacemaker). Previously, the β-adrenergic agonist isoproterenol was favored for pharmacologic pacing; however, this drug is more prone to inducing myocardial ischemia than other adrenergic agents with balanced α- and β-adrenergic properties, due to its unopposed β_2-mediated peripheral arterial vasodilatory properties (i.e., tachycardia and hypotension). Electrical pacing is the safest treatment for bradyarrhythmias; unlike pharmacologic therapy, predictable rate control is combined with avoidance of the risk of tachyarrhythmias. Electrical pacing also allows for more aggressive control of some tachyarrhythmias by providing protection from the adverse consequences of drug-related "overshoot" bradyarrhythmias. Temporary transvenous pacemaker wires may be inserted directly into central venous lines, or may be incorporated into pulmonary artery catheters. The recent introduction of transesophageal pacing shows promise as a less invasive al-

TABLE 18–3
Treatment of Bradyarrhythmias

Modality	Administration	Caveats
Transcutaneous pacing (TCP)	Set at 80 bpm 0–200 mA until capture (average 50–100 mA)	Ensure correct placement of electrodes; >50 mA generally requires analgesia/sedation.
Atropine*	0.5–1.0 mg IV q3–5min max 0.03–0.04 mg/kg	Doses <0.5 mg may cause paradoxical bradycardia.
Dopamine	5–20 μg/kg/min	Monitor for myocardial ischemia.
Epinephrine	2–10 μg/min	Monitor for myocardial ischemia.
Isoproterenol	2–10 μg/min	Monitor for myocardial ischemia.

*In general, if intravenous atropine is ineffective, transcutaneous pacing (TCP) should be used to establish a normal heart rate. If TCP is unavailable, "pharmacological pacing" by intravenous infusion of dopamine or epinephrine (or isoproterenol) should be started while more permanent electrical pacing is arranged.
mA, milliamperes; IV, intravenous; q3–5min, every 3–5 min.

ternative temporary pacing technique. Transcutaneous pacing is also effective; however, the associated contraction of major skeletal muscle groups makes this technique unpleasant for the awake patient.[58]

Ventricular Arrhythmias

Factors that cause ventricular ectopy, tachycardia, and fibrillation are similar to those that cause supraventricular tachycardias. Onset of ventricular irritability should always raise suspicion of myocardial ischemia. Even hemodynamically stable ventricular arrhythmias should be carefully and promptly assessed, because of the potential for progression to other malignant arrhythmias (e.g., ventricular fibrillation). The treatment approach to ventricular arrhythmias is summarized in Table 18–4.

Optimize Preload

Identify Optimal Preload

"Optimal" preload is a description of the preload conditions under which the most effective cardiac function (i.e., cardiac output) is achieved with specific afterload and contractility conditions for a single individual (see Figs. 18–3 and 18–4). In contrast, "sufficient" preload (e.g., with hypovolemic shock) reflects filling pressures compatible with adequate vital organ perfusion, evidenced clinically by resolution of signs of a low-output state (e.g., oliguria, confusion, sinus tachycardia). "Optimal" and "sufficient" preload are clearly different from "normal" preload, which is usually present with a central venous pressure of 4 to 12 mm Hg. In cardiogenic shock, the goal of therapy is to provide "sufficient" preload for adequate vital organ perfusion, but

TABLE 18–4
Treatment of Ventricular Tachycardia*

Modality	Administration	Remarks
DC cardioversion	Use synchronous mode for VT, asynchronous for VF; 100–360 J	Use only if pharmacologic therapy fails for stable VT. First-line, emergency treatment for unstable VT or VF.
Lidocaine	IV loading dose 1.0–1.5 mg/kg over 30–60 sec, consider repeat 0.5–0.75 mg/kg in 5 min (max 3 mg/kg) Maintenance infusion 1–4 mg/min Therapeutic level 2–6 μg/ml	First-line therapy for ventricular ectopy; rapid bolus may cause hypotension.
Procainamide	Infusion: Load 20–30 mg/min IV (max 17 mg/kg) Maintenance 1–4 mg/min Therapeutic range 4–8 μg/ml	See Tables 18–1 and 18–2. May provide control of arrhythmias refractory to lidocaine.
Bretylium tosylate	IV loading dose 5–10 mg/kg over 8–10 min (max 30 mg/kg in 24 hours) Maintenance 1–2 mg/min	Indicated for VT or VF unresponsive to cardioversion, lidocaine. May cause transient hypertension followed by quite marked hypotension (catecholamine depletion).
Magnesium sulfate	1–2 gm IV for VF or unstable VT 0.5 gm IV over 10–20 min for stable VT or ventricular ectopy	Use early in resistant arrhythmias.
Epinephrine	1 mg IV q5min	Use with CPR to improve cerebral and myocardial perfusion.

*Stable ventricular tachycardia should be sequentially treated with intravenous lidocaine, procainamide, bretylium, and magnesium until a satisfactory response is achieved. If this is unsuccessful, or if the patient is unstable, DC cardioversion should be used. Conscious patients should be given analgesia/sedation prior to DC cardioversion if possible. Ventricular arrhythmias may remain refractory to cardioversion or pharmacologic therapy until abnormal pH, blood gases, potassium and magnesium are corrected.
DC, direct current; J, joules; IV, intravenous; VF, ventricular fibrillation; VT, ventricular tachycardia; CPR, cardiopulmonary resuscitation.

avoid excessive pulmonary congestion (i.e., requiring supplemental oxygen, or ventilation), which may be the consequence of "optimal" preload.

Restore Deficient Preload

In the presence of a low-cardiac-output state attributed to hypovolemia, initial therapy should be directed toward re-establishing adequate filling pressures. A series of fluid challenges, followed by careful clinical evaluation of response, to guide further management, is recommended. An improvement is indicated by resolution of the signs of a low-output state (i.e., improved urine output, reduced sinus tachycardia, resolution of confusion). Fluid challenges should be continued until either hemodynamic stability is achieved, no further improvement in cardiac output occurs (i.e., the "flat part" of the Frank-Starling curve), or evidence of excessive pulmonary congestion from increased preload is present. In situations where manipulation of preload alone is insufficient to achieve hemodynamic stability, inotropic support should be instituted to increase contractility and improve stroke volume for a given preload.

FLUID SELECTION

Choice of fluid type used to restore preload in a particular situation should be individualized, based upon a knowledge of the patient, and quality of the fluid deficit. While the risks of blood product administration are well known, clearly hypovolemia following major aortic surgery with a large estimated blood loss is likely to require transfusion. In contrast, a low-output state following an anaphylactic reaction is likely due to vasodilation and fluid sequestration (third-space losses) and should not require transfusion. When transfusion is required, selective blood component therapy guided by hematocrit and coagulation monitoring reduces transfusion risk and expense. Hematocrit is a useful tool in guiding fluid management decisions; however, in the setting of acute blood loss, especially when combined with ongoing third-space losses, a normal hematocrit is not a good index of total red cell volume.

Estimates of ideal hematocrit and the "transfusion trigger point" have decreased in recent years, as the risks of transfusion have been highlighted and tolerance of lower hematocrits without excess morbidity demonstrated. This trend in practice should be contrasted, however, with the management goals of low-cardiac-output syndrome, where augmenting oxygen-carrying capacity through increased hematocrit may be one of the few tools available to increase tissue perfusion without further increasing demands on cardiac performance.

The controversy over the choice of crystalloid or colloid solutions for fluid challenges where transfusion is unnecessary remains unresolved. Potential advantages of crystalloid (e.g., Ringer's lactate, 0.9% saline) include freedom from adverse reactions and minimal cost. Advocates of colloid (e.g., 5% albumin, 6% hetastarch, 10% pentastarch) point out the rapid expansion of intravascular volume with these solutions, which draw fluids from the extracellular space because of their osmotic effect.[59] Human protein derivatives are heat treated to prevent disease transmission. However, colloids do nothing to rehydrate the extracellular volume and have been condemned by some for their potential to aggravate interstitial (pulmonary) edema in the setting of capillary leak syndrome. Large volumes of plasma expanders may accelerate the onset of dilutional coagulopathy, and 6% hetastarch coats platelets and impairs platelet aggregation. The disadvantage of crystalloids in the setting of hemorrhagic shock include the very large volumes required versus plasma expanders (4:1) to replace blood loss.[60] Large crystalloid transfusions may produce electrolyte disturbances due to electrolyte differences between these solutions and extracellular fluid (e.g., hyperchloremic metabolic acidosis with 0.9% normal saline).

Use of hypertonic crystalloid solutions (e.g., 3 to 7.5% saline) has been shown to result in improved hemodynamic response to hemorrhagic shock, with less increase in total body water, extravascular lung water, and intracranial pressure[61,62] versus standard crystalloid solution use. However, the same hypertonic solutions used in a model of uncontrolled hemorrhage led to increased bleeding and mortality.[63]

Decrease Excessive Preload

When severe myocardial depression causes a flattening of the Frank-Starling curve (see Figs. 18–2 and 18–3), fluid administration to improve perfusion may result in excessive preload. In addition to respiratory complications and hypoxemia from pulmonary vascular congestion, excessive preload will aggravate cardiac dysfunction by increasing cardiac chamber sizes (and systolic "wall stress"), and raising myocardial oxygen consumption. Elevated left ventricular diastolic pressures will also compress subendocardial vessels, reducing perfusion and aggravating any existing myocardial ischemia. In this setting, supplemental oxygen and the use of pharmacological agents to reduce preload is a priority if acute cardiac failure is to be avoided.

DIURETIC THERAPY

In low-cardiac-output states, humoral responses to low perfusion (see "Cardiac Function and Failure," above) mediate intense renal venoconstriction and diminished renal blood flow, reducing the effectiveness of standard diuretic agents as a preload-reducing strategy. Loop diuretics (e.g., furosemide, ethacrynic acid) and dopamine may be effective in establishing a diuresis.

In animal studies, furosemide administration increases renal cortical blood flow and, when co-administered with dopamine *prior* to an episode of renal ischemia, is protective against renal injury.[64] Rapid intravenous administration of loop diuretics is associated with venodilation in addition to renal effects, and may precipitate hypotension. Lucas et al. were able to increase urine output and renal clearance of sodium, but had no effect on increasing glomerular filtration rate, in critically ill patients with oliguric acute renal failure receiving intravenous furosemide.[65] In addition, several patients developed significant hypotension in the several hours following treatment.[65] The response to loop diuretics is unpredictable in the setting of excessive preload and a low-cardiac-output state, and may precipitate acute hypotension, requiring further fluid therapy. The use of a continuous intravenous furosemide infusion (2.5 to 15 mg/hr) may be better tolerated, while allowing titration to effect, and is more likely to be effective in patients with reduced glomerular filtration rate.[66–68]

"Low-dose" intravenous dopamine infusion (0.5 to 2.0 μg/kg/min) is relatively selective for dopaminergic (DA_1) receptors in the renal and mesenteric vasculature and on renal tubular cells. Receptor activation by dopamine causes vasodilation, increased renal blood flow and glomerular filtration rate, and saliuresis.[69,70] Animal evidence also suggests that dopamine may sustain renal blood flow in the face of norepinephrine-mediated vasoconstriction.[71] This evidence has led many clinicians to routinely institute "renal dose" dopamine infusions in patients at risk for renal dysfunction due to low-cardiac-output states. While this practice is still widely used, it has come into question with recent evidence that dopamine at these doses (in combination with mannitol) may be associated with renal tubular injury in postcardiac surgical patients, where mannitol alone demonstrates a renal protective effect.[72] Even at low doses, intravenous dopamine may have significant β-adrenergic receptor chronotropic effects that may limit its use. The osmotic load associated with mannitol administration makes this drug unsuitable for use in the setting of excessive preload.

Fenoldopam, a relatively pure DA_1 receptor agonist drug (with minor α_2-adrenergic effects at higher doses) has recently become available in North America. While Food and Drug Administration (FDA) approval is currently limited to its use as an antihypertensive agent, the potential of fenoldopam as a replacement for "renal dose" dopamine infusion has yet to be fully explored. In the setting of hypertensive crisis, Shusterman et al. demonstrated that fenoldopam effectively controlled blood pressure, while improving creatinine clearance, urine flow, and sodium excretion in patients with impaired renal function.[73] Similar patients receiving nitroprusside to control blood pressure had no changes in renal function.

VENODILATOR THERAPY

The ability of nitroglycerin (NTG) to reduce excessive preload derives from its potent venodilating properties. Filling pressures rapidly decline in response to low-dose NTG infusion (0.5–1.5 μg/kg/min); however, higher infusion rates also dilate arterioles and may cause significant hypotension. In addition to reduced filling pressures, NTG-mediated beneficial effects on myocardial oxygen balance include direct coronary artery vasodilation, preferential dilation of epicardial (conductance) arterioles, and relative preservation of aortic diastolic pressures (at low NTG doses). The overall effect of NTG is to reduce heart size, improve the transmyocardial filling gradient, and increase blood flow to areas of myocardial ischemia. Excessive reductions in preload may occur with higher doses of NTG, resulting in decreased stroke volume and cardiac output.[74]

Systemic hypotension and reflex tachycardia may complicate the use of higher doses of NTG. In some situations, intravenous phenylephrine infusion will increase blood pressure and reflexly slow heart rate while preserving the beneficial effects of NTG. The adverse effects of increased afterload from phenylephrine exceed the benefit of NTG with PAOP greater than 15 mm Hg.

Therapeutic Options in Refractory Patients

In some patients, a low-cardiac-output state remains after heart rate and rhythm are stabilized and "optimal" preload established. Other therapeutic options include inotropic support or afterload reduction to achieve a greater stroke volume for a given filling pressure (see Figs. 18–2 and 18–3). Both of these therapeutic options have limitations and may precipitate myocardial ischemia; inotropic support requires greater myocardial oxygen consumption, while afterload reduction may reduce transmyocardial filling gradients. However, the risk of myocardial ischemia must be weighed against the adverse consequences of prolonged hypoperfusion. Therapeutic inotropic and afterload-reducing options will now be reviewed.

Enhance Contractility

Myocardial responsiveness to endogenous catecholamines (or exogenous inotropes) diminishes in the presence of acid-base and electrolyte abnormalities. Correction of metabolic acidosis and other electrolyte disorders, which often accompany low-cardiac-output states, is an important first step towards improving cardiac function. Subsequent selection of an inotrope must be based on a thorough understanding of the mechanism of action of each agent, and the interaction of the different agents with the myocyte, the peripheral vasculature, and other peripheral tissues.

Normalize pH and Electrolyte Milieu

Metabolic acidosis, hyperkalemia, and hypocalcemia are the commonest acid-base and electrolyte disorders seen in low-output states. Severe metabolic acidosis ($pH < 7.25$) depresses myocardial response to catecholamines, and with extended periods of shock, the Frank-Starling curve shifts down and to the right. Therapies should be aimed at raising serum pH above 7.25; mechanical hyperventilation (by lowering arterial P_{CO_2}) and intravenous sodium bicarbonate (50 mEq; 50 ml 8% sodium bicarbonate) administration, guided by arterial blood-gas results, are both effective treatments for acidosis. Sodium bicarbonate results in an initial paradoxical intracellular acidosis (associated with the liberation of CO_2) and decreased myocardial contractility, which subsequently leads to improved contractility when CO_2 is cleared.[75] This may explain the clinical experience that

TABLE 18–5
Dosage and Actions of Inotropic and Vasopressor Agents

Drug	Dosage	Predominant Action	Clinical Effects
Adrenergic agents: catecholamines			
Dopamine	1–2 μg/kg/min	Dopaminergic	Saliuresis, inotropy, chronotropy, vasoconstriction
	3–10 μg/kg/min	β_1-adrenergic	
	>10 μg/kg/min	α_1-adrenergic	
Epinephrine	0.02–0.2 μg/kg/min	$\beta_{1,2}$-adrenergic	Inotropy, chronotropy, vasoconstriction
		α_1-adrenergic	
Dobutamine	5–25 μg/kg/min	$\beta_{1,2}$-adrenergic	Inotropy, chronotropy, vasodilation
Norepinephrine	0.01–0.1 μg/kg/min	α_1-adrenergic	Vasoconstriction, inotropy
		β_1-adrenergic	
Adrenergic agents: noncatecholamines			
Phenylephrine	20–80 μg/kg/min	α_1-adrenergic	Vasoconstriction
Nonadrenergic agents: phosphodiesterase inhibitors			
Amrinone	1.5–3 mg/kg (*l*)	PDE-III inhibition	Inotropy, chronotropy, vasodilation
	5–20 μg/kg/min (*m*)		
Milrinone	50 μg/kg (*l*)	PDE-III inhibition	Inotropy, chronotropy, vasodilation
	0.375–0.75 mg/kg/min (*m*)		

(*l*), loading dose; (*m*), maintenance dose; PDE-III, phosphodiesterase III.

hyperventilation and sodium bicarbonate infusion are better tolerated than bolus doses.

Hyperkalemia may result from tissue ischemia, exogenous potassium administration, or renal impairment of potassium clearance. Elevated serum potassium levels exert a negative inotropic effect, while severe hyperkalemia (>6.0 mEq/L) may affect or depress myocardial conduction, the most extreme form being asystolic cardiac arrest. Standard acute therapy of hyperkalemia includes hyperventilation, intravenous calcium supplementation, sodium bicarbonate administration, and balanced doses of short-acting insulin and glucose.

Depressed serum ionized calcium (i.e., <1.0 mM/L) has a significant negative inotropic effect. The commonest setting for this to manifest is during rapid transfusion of citrated blood for resuscitation of hemorrhagic shock, especially in the context of hepatic ischemia (e.g., with aortic cross-clamping). Citrate is normally rapidly metabolized by the liver; however, rapid citrate administration and/or decreased hepatic function may increase serum citrate levels. Citrate binds with free ionized calcium, making it unavailable for other metabolic functions (e.g., coagulation, normal myocardial contraction). If decreased cardiac output is related to hypocalcemia, a rapid response to intravenous 10% calcium chloride administration (5 to 20 mg/kg) would be expected.

Select Appropriate Inotropic Agent

Inotropic support is an important step in re-establishing normal systemic perfusion. Intelligent inotropic agent selection should include consideration of the other myocardial and systemic effects of a drug choice in the context of coexisting conditions in an individual patient. Clearly, an inotropic agent with peripheral vasodilating properties (e.g., milrinone) is not a suitable choice for a patient with hypotension from septic shock. Conversely, the renal artery vasodilating properties of dopamine make this a very appropriate inotrope selection for patients with coexisting renal dysfunction. Some currently available agents, their mechanisms of action, and systemic effects are presented in (Tables 18–5 and 18–6).

MECHANISMS OF CARDIAC INOTROPY

The inotropic state of cardiac muscle depends on the number of cross-bridges formed between the contractile proteins actin and myosin, within myocytes. A third protein, tropomyosin, inhibits the linkage between these proteins. When calcium associates with troponin, the resulting complex alters tropomyosin and permits actin and myosin to interact. The more calcium available, the greater the force of contraction. When calcium dissociates from troponin-C, the process is reversed and relaxation occurs.

Myocyte depolarization is caused by sodium influx through "fast" sodium channels, and subsequently through "slow" calcium channels. Raised intracellular calcium causes release of more calcium from sarcoplasmic reticulum stores.[76] Cyclic adenosine monophosphate (cAMP) is an important regulator of cellular calcium levels.[77] Myocyte cAMP levels are controlled by mechanisms that alter its generation and degradation; activation of several different G-protein–coupled receptors within the cell membrane increases (e.g., β-adrenergic recep-

TABLE 18–6
Activity of Different Inotropic Agents (Receptor Activation or Enzyme Inhibition)

Drug	β_1-AR	β_2-AR	α_1-AR	DA_1	PDE-III
Dopamine	++	++	++	+++	
Epinephrine	++++	++++	++++		
Dobutamine	+++	++	+		
Norepinephrine	++++		++++		
Isoproterenol	++++	++++			
Dopexamine	+/−	++++		++	
Amrinone					−−−
Milrinone					−−−

PDE-III, phosphodiesterase III; AR, adrenergic receptor; DA_1, $dopamine_1$ receptors, + to +++, degrees of adrenergic receptor activation; − to −−−, degrees of enzyme inhibition.

tors) or decreases (e.g., α_2-adrenergic receptors) cAMP formation, while the ubiquitous cytoplasmic enzyme phosphodiesterase III (PDE-III) is responsible for cAMP degradation. *Most inotropic agents currently in use act by influencing the generation (e.g., catecholamines) or degradation (e.g., PDE-III inhibitors) of cAMP.* Inositol triphosphate (IP_3) and diacylglycerol (DAG) are also intracellular mediators of calcium metabolism that are generated by activation of G-protein–coupled receptors (e.g., α_1-adrenergic receptors); however, the inotropic effect of agents influencing IP_3 and DAG levels is modest.[78]

SYMPATHOMIMETIC AMINES (CATECHOLAMINES)

The structural basis for all sympathomimetic amines is a benzene ring with an ethylamine side chain (B-phenylethylamine). Hydroxyl substitutions at the 3 and 4 positions of the benzene ring (catecholamines), or the α and β carbons of the ethylamine side chain differentiate the commonly used inotropic agents.

All sympathomimetic amines cause activation of adrenergic receptors. The differing pattern of activation of the four "classic" adrenergic receptors (α_1, α_2, β_1, and β_2) give each agent a unique combination of adrenergic receptor-mediated effects (Table 18–6). Inotropy is predominantly mediated through β_1-adrenergic receptors, which also mediate chronotropic, dromotropic, and bathmotropic cardiac effects. While increased heart rate and improved conduction may or may not be desirable in a particular setting, clearly generally increasing myocardial excitability brings an unwanted potential for arrhythmia generation. Peripheral effects of sympathomimetic amines result in vasodilation (β_2-adrenergic receptor–mediated, i.e., isoproterenol, dobutamine) or vasoconstriction (α_1-adrenergic receptor–mediated, i.e., norepinephrine, high-dose dopamine).

Dopamine Hydrochloride. Dopamine is a metabolic precursor of the endogenous catecholamines (epinephrine, norepinephrine), that acts directly on dopaminergic, α, and β receptors, and also has about 50% of its activity indirectly through the release of endogenous stores of norepinephrine from nerve terminals.[79] Therefore, in conditions where norepinephrine stores are depleted (e.g., severe myocardial dysfunction), dopamine may have less inotropic activity.

Low ("renal") dose dopamine (0.5 to 2.0 μg/kg/min) is used to selectively activate dopaminergic receptors, causing saliuresis, increased glomerular filtration, and mesenteric and renal artery vasodilation (see above). Dopamine infusion rates between 3 and 10 μg/kg/min cause predominantly β_1-mediated inotropic effects, with some dopaminergic-receptor-mediated effects persisting. The modestly increased myocardial contractility, balanced with preservation of DA_1-mediated effects, offered by dopamine has made this agent a popular first-line inotropic agent. Increased diaphragmatic blood flow and strength have been attributed to dopamine infusion in patients with chronic obstructive lung disease.[80] However, beyond 10 μg/kg/min the α_1-mediated vasoconstricting effects of dopamine become significant, and it offers little benefit compared to the more potent inotropic agents.

Epinephrine. Commonly, when a 7 to 10 μg/kg/min dopamine infusion is failing to provide sufficient inotropic effect, a more potent inotrope such as epinephrine will be added. Epinephrine is direct acting, and has very potent β_1, β_2,and α_1 effects. At low doses (up to 0.02 μg/kg/min) β-mediated effects predominate; however, α_1 activity is significant above doses of 0.01 μg/kg/min.[81] The overall result of epinephrine infusion on systemic vascular resistance is dose dependent; at low doses β_2-mediated vasodilation predominates, while at doses above 0.02 μg/kg/min α_1-mediated vasoconstriction causes blood pressure to rise. Unfortunately, epinephrine infusion usually depresses renal blood flow significantly, despite increased cardiac output and blood pressure. As peripheral vasoconstriction becomes significant, limb ischemia and metabolic acidosis may accompany oliguria. Stimulation of glycogenolysis in the liver may cause hyperglycemia.

Dobutamine. Dobutamine is a direct acting synthetic derivative of isoproterenol. It is composed of a racemic mixture (50:50) of two isoforms with differing activities: the (−)-isomer is an α_1- and β-agonist, while the (+)-isoform is a potent β-agonist, and an α_1-antagonist. The conflicting α_1 effects essentially neutralize each other, leaving the potent β-agonist effect.[82] Dobutamine enhances contractility and causes peripheral vasodilation (and afterload reduction) but has relatively little effect on heart rate. The inotropic and vasodilating properties of this drug make it ideal for patients with right heart failure and pulmonary hypertension. Unlike dopamine, it does not activate DA_1 receptors or cause release of norepinephrine.

Norepinephrine. Norepinephrine is similar to epinephrine in structure but has a significantly different profile of adrenergic receptor activation. Norepinephrine has very potent β_1 activity, almost no β_2 activity, and extremely potent α activity. Generally blood pressure increases in response to norepinephrine do not result from increased cardiac output. Cardiac output may actually decrease due to the predominance of α-mediated vasoconstriction. Prolonged use of this drug at high doses may precipitate acute renal failure and other organ ischemia. Norepinephrine may be useful in the setting of profound peripheral vasodilation (e.g., sepsis) or combined with another vasodilating inotrope (e.g., milrinone).

Isoproterenol. Isoproterenol is a direct-acting synthetic catecholamine with very potent β- and no α-adrenergic activity. Despite its potent inotropic effects, the early appearance of tachycardia, and tachyarrhythmias it is rarely used as an inotropic agent. It has potent bronchodilating effects, and may be useful for temporary "pharmacological pacing" in some circumstances. β_2-mediated peripheral vasodilation and decreased diastolic myocardial perfusion may precipitate myocardial ischemia in some patients.

Dopexamine Hydrochloride. Dopexamine is a synthetic catecholamine with potent β_2 activity, minor DA_1 activity, and weak β_1 activity.[83] Dopexamine also has some of its effects by inhibiting reuptake of circulating norepinephrine. Increased cardiac output with dopexamine is the result of a combination of mild inotropic effect with significant β_2 and DA_1-mediated vasodilation. It causes greater reduction in afterload than dobutamine, and less tachyphylaxis. The future role of this agent in the inotropic armamentarium has yet to be clarified.

PHOSPHODIESTERASE INHIBITORS

Cyclic AMP is the most important intracellular second messenger responsible for calcium regulation and inotropy in myocytes. Selective inhibition of the enzyme responsible for the breakdown of cAMP (PDE-III) represents a different, and often complementary, approach to the actions of inotropic agents that elevate cytoplasmic cAMP levels by activating adrenergic receptors. In contrast, previously available nonselective phosphodiesterase inhibitors (e.g., theophylline) have-side effect profiles that make them unsuitable as inotropic agents.

Amrinone. Amrinone, a bipyridine derivative, has potent vasodilator effects in addition to its inotropic actions. The result is a major reduction in left and right ventricular afterload, due to significant decreases in SVR and pulmonary vascular resistance (PVR).[84] The chronotropic effect of amrinone is relatively less than the inotropic effect, making this agent ideal in the setting of myocardial ischemia. However, hypotension from the peripheral vasodilating effects of PDE-III inhibitors means that some patients require simultaneous infusion of a vasoconstricting agent (e.g., norepinephrine) to maintain adequate myocardial perfusion pressure. Amrinone is particularly beneficial as an inotrope in patients with pulmonary hypertension and right ventricular dysfunction. Also, PDE-III inhibitors are useful in patients who have developed tachyphylaxis due to desensitization, and down-regulation of adrenergic receptors. Unlike sympathomimetic amines, PDE-III inhibitors require an initial loading dose prior to initiation of an infusion. Graded administration of the loading dose is important due to the potential for acute hypotension. In contrast, gradual withdrawal of PDE-III inhibitors is achieved simply by discontinuing the drug infusion, due to the relatively long elimination half-life of these agents.

Milrinone. Milrinone is a bipyridine derivative with similar properties to those of amrinone, but is a considerably more potent PDE-III inhibitor compared to amrinone. It has a better side-effect profile than amrinone,[85] and is commonly infused for long periods in patients with low-cardiac-output states awaiting cardiac transplantation.

CARDIAC GLYCOSIDES

The digitalis glycosides increase intracellular calcium levels to exert their modest inotropic effect. Inhibition of the sodium-potassium ATPase by these drugs results in accumulation of intracellular sodium, which increases the activity of the myocyte sodium-calcium exchange mechanisms, increasing amounts of intracellular calcium. While the inotropic effect of digoxin is modest compared to the other agents discussed, it is the only inotrope with negative chronotropic, dromotropic, and bathmotropic properties. However, this potential benefit of cardiac glycosides must be weighed against the significant potential for drug toxicity with these agents.

ENHANCEMENT OF ADENYLYL CYCLASE AND OTHER NONADRENERGIC MECHANISMS

The recurrent situation where a patient develops tachyphylaxis to previously effective inotropic support stimulates the search for alternate inotropic strategies aimed at mechanisms other than β-adrenergic receptor stimulation and PDE-III inhibition. Cyclic AMP remains the most important intracellular mediator of inotropy in myocytes. Adenylyl cyclase is the enzyme responsible for generation of cAMP from ATP. Adenylyl cyclase activity from β-receptor activation is mediated through a stimulatory "G_s" protein. In addition to β receptors, several other cell surface receptors (e.g., H_2 histamine, vasoactive intestinal peptide, 5-HT_4 serotonin, and prostaglandin E_1 receptors) also interact with the G_s protein, and their agonists have measurable inotropic effects.[78] Stimulation of an inhibitory "G_i" protein causes depression of adenylyl cyclase activity. Inhibition of cell surface receptors (e.g., A_1 adenosine, M_2 muscarinic, and somatostatin receptors) that increase G_i protein activity has also demonstrated inotropic potential.[78] Three cell surface receptors (α_1-adrenergic, endothelin, and angiotensin II receptors) have been identified which also have an inotropic effect through increasing generation of myocyte IP_3 and DAG (other cellular mediators of calcium regulation, see above).[78] The inotropic potential of pharmacologic agents acting at some of these receptors has been clinically tested (e.g., H_2 histamine receptors[86]), but the full potential of the majority continues to be explored.

Historically, many different agents with inotropic potential have been investigated but have not been clinically successful, either because of disappointing inotropic effects or unacceptable side-effect profile; some examples include glucagon,[87] H_2 histamine agonists,[86] forskolin,[88] dibutyryl-cAMP,[89] and thyroid hormone.[90]

Normalize Systemic Vascular Resistance

When evidence of inadequate tissue perfusion due to pump failure persists in the presence of controlled heart rate and rhythm, optimal preload, and maximum inotropic support, improved cardiac output may still be achieved by reducing impedance to ventricular ejection through vasodilator therapy (exchanging pressure work for volume work). Alternately, if inadequate tissue perfusion in this setting is due to hypotension from excessive vasodilation rather than pump failure (e.g., septic shock), vasoconstrictor therapy may be indicated. A review of pharmacologic agents useful in manipulating vascular tone is presented below.

Reduce Excessive Afterload (Vasodilator Therapy)

Vasodilator drugs are generally classified by mechanism of action, but it is clinically important to appreciate the different selectivity of each agent for venodilation (i.e., preload reduction), arterial dilation (i.e., afterload reduction), or both.

NITRIC OXIDE–MEDIATED VASODILATORS

The physiology and pharmacology of the vascular endothelium have become more completely understood in recent years. The important role of nitric oxide (NO) (previously known as endothelium-derived relaxant factor) as a mediator of vascular tone has become evident. The normal physiology of NO production starts with activation of G-protein–coupled receptors (e.g., acetylcholine, adenosine) on endothelial cells, resulting in generation of IP_3. IP_3-mediated calcium release within endothelial cells increases the activity of nitric oxide synthase, a cellular enzyme that generates nitric oxide from the amino acid L-arginine. Nitric oxide is a freely diffusable but unstable gas, which exists only long enough to pass beyond endothelial cells to local vascular smooth muscle cells, where it increases guanylyl cyclase–mediated generation of cyclic guanosine monophosphate (cGMP). Cyclic GMP is a potent second messenger that decreases intracellular calcium levels in smooth muscle, causing relaxation (and vasodilation). Several of the most potent clinically available vasodilators have their effects through NO-mediated smooth muscle relaxation.

Sodium Nitroprusside. Sodium nitroprusside (SNP) consists of a nitroso (—NO) group loosely bound to a ferrous ion (Fe^{2+}) and five cyanide molecules. Dissociation of sodium nitroprusside in the blood results in release of NO, which mediates vascular smooth muscle relaxation. Sodium nitroprusside is a balanced arterial and venodilator that is very useful for afterload reduction due to its potent and titratable effects (Table 18–7). In settings where a low-perfusion state is associated with increased SVR (i.e., >1500 dyne·sec·cm^{-5}), initiation of a low-dose infusion (e.g., 0.2 μg/kg/min) may improve cardiac output. A gradual decline in afterload (mean arterial pressure) is to be expected, and simultaneous preload reduction may require supplemental intravenous fluids. Improved hemodynamic parameters in response to SNP warrant further incremental infusion rate increases with supplemental preload as necessary; infusion rates above 2.0 μg/kg/min for afterload reduction are usually complicated by hypotension. If the starting infusion dose is too high or the patient is hypovolemic, abrupt onset of hypotension will result. Reflex tachycardia and myocardial ischemia may also result from arterial vasodilation, due to the associated decrease in diastolic coronary perfusion pressure, and dilation of coronary conduction and impedance arteries with the potential for shunt away from ischemic areas (i.e., coronary steal).

Toxicity (cyanide and thiocyanate poisoning) may occur with extremely high SNP infusion rates (15 to 40 μg/kg/min) but is very rare within the normal clinical dose range (<8 μg/kg/min).

Nitroglycerin. Nitroglycerin has its effects through NO-mediated relaxation of vascular smooth muscle. Nitroglycerin is a potent venodilator relative to its effects on arterial tone. The benefits of NTG on myocardial oxygen consumption and its effectiveness in reducing preload are discussed above. NTG is not a useful agent to achieve afterload reduction in patients with a low-cardiac-output state.

Hydralazine. Hydralazine is an NO-mediated vasodilator, which has its major effects on systemic arterial vascular tone. These properties make it an ideal drug for selective afterload reduction in patients with low-cardiac-output. Indeed, greater reductions in SVR and increases in cardiac output can be achieved without the requirement of supplemental preload, using hydralazine compared with SNP.[91] Reflex tachycardia does not complicate its use for afterload reduction (unlike for treatment of hypertension), since afterload reduction is complemented by increased stroke volume. Effective dosing is low compared to doses used for control of hypertension (i.e., 2.5 to 7.5 mg IV every 4 hours). Dosing is complicated by genetic

TABLE 18–7
Dosage and Actions of Vasodilator Agents

Drug	Dosage	Predominant Action	Clinical Effects
Nitric oxide-mediated vasodilators			
Sodium nitroprusside	0.25–5 μg/kg/min	Balanced arterial and venous dilation	Potent, rapid acting. Decreases preload and afterload. May induce myocardial ischemia.
Nitroglycerin	0.25–5 μg/kg/min	Predominantly venous dilation	Decreases preload. Enhances myocardial oxygen balance.
Hydralazine	2.5–7.5 mg q4h	Predominantly arterial dilation	Decreases afterload. Worsens myocardial oxygen balance.
Inhaled nitric oxide	0–40 ppm	Pulmonary artery dilation	Effective for "reversible" pulmonary artery vasoconstriction.
Calcium channel blockers			
Nifedipine	10–20 mg sublingual q8h	Predominantly arterial dilation	Decreases afterload. May cause coronary steal.
Nicardipine	3 mg/hr	Predominantly arterial dilation	Decreases afterload. May cause coronary steal.

q4h, ever 4 hours; q8h, every 8 hours; ppm = parts per million of inhaled gas.

variations in drug metabolism (i.e., fast and slow acetylators). Drug effect is 20 minutes after injection, and careful titration of subsequent doses to hemodynamic response is required. Intravenous dosing requirements decrease to every 6 to 8 hours during the 24 to 48 hours after initiation of therapy due to drug accumulation. If transfer to oral therapy is contemplated, a five- to tenfold increase in equivalent oral versus IV dosage is necessary, to take into account the first-pass clearance by the liver.

The slow onset and unpredictable action of hydralazine make this drug unsuitable for early treatment of the low-cardiac-output state, but if a patient has demonstrated dependence on the afterload-reducing effects of SNP for 12 to 24 hours, transfer to hydralazine therapy for afterload may be considered. Hydralazine may be associated with an immune-mediated lupus-like syndrome. It may also worsen myocardial ischemia in patients at risk, because it reduces coronary diastolic perfusion pressure. The predictable actions, better survival benefits,[92] and minimal side effects of ACE inhibitors have made them, rather than hydralazine, the most popular oral drug therapy for chronic afterload reduction.

Inhaled Nitric Oxide. Understanding of the vascular endothelial response to nitric oxide initially prompted experimentation in animal models with inhaled nitric oxide in the setting of pulmonary hypertension. Promising early results have rapidly led to widespread availability and routine use of inhaled nitric oxide (<40 parts per million) for ventilated patients with various low-cardiac-output states involving pulmonary hypertension and right ventricular failure.[93] Benefits are indicated by reduction in pulmonary arterial pressures and evidence of improved right ventricular function with initiation of inhaled NO, and may be titrated to effect. Some individuals demonstrate no response to inhaled NO, presumably due to the "fixed" nature of their pulmonary vascular disorders. The "effervescence" of NO ensures minimal extrapulmonary effects from inhaled NO.

CALCIUM CHANNEL BLOCKERS

Nifedipine. Nifedipine has predominantly vasodilator effects on the coronary, pulmonary, and systemic arterial vessels; also minimal negative inotropic or dromotropic effects. It therefore has suitable properties for afterload reduction with low-cardiac-output states, and has been used for this purpose.[94] However, unpredictable degrees of hypotension, reflex tachycardia, and myocardial ischemia, and reports of hypotensive insult to other organs (e.g., the kidney[95]) have discouraged the use of nifedipine for afterload reduction with low-cardiac-output.

Nicardipine. Nicardipine is a recently introduced calcium channel antagonist. Although nicardipine and nifedipine have very similar actions, nicardipine is water soluble and, therefore (unlike nifedipine), may be given by intravenous infusion.[96] Its slow onset and offset make it unlikely that this drug will replace SNP in the acute management of afterload reduction. Some evidence endorses its use as an oral agent for the management of chronic congestive heart failure.[97,98]

α-ADRENERGIC ANTAGONISTS

Phentolamine. Phentolamine is a nonselective α-adrenergic antagonist. It is no longer used for afterload reduction because it blocks presynaptic α_2-adrenergic receptors, which normally inhibit endogenous norepinephrine release, making patients vulnerable to undesirable reflex tachycardias.

Prazosin. Prazosin is a selective α_1-adrenergic receptor antagonist, which does not have the problems with α_2-receptor inhibition associated with phentolamine. It has balanced venous and arterial vasodilating properties, similar to those of SNP.[99] Difficulty titrating effect in the absence of an intravenous formulation (in the United States), tachyphylaxis, and hypotension have limited the use of prazosin for afterload reduction.

ANGIOTENSIN CONVERTING ENZYME INHIBITORS

Captopril and Enalapril. Captopril, enalapril, and several other ACE inhibitors are currently available. They all have very similar properties, which include balanced venous and arterial vasodilating properties. Their use, and survival benefit, as therapeutic agents for chronic congestive heart failure is well documented.[93] They have also been used successfully (e.g., captopril 25 mg IV every 6 hours) for afterload reduction in low-output states.[100,101] Several other potential benefits of ACE inhibitors include reduced norepinephrine response to exercise, prevention of myocardial depressant factor formation, reduced ventricular arrhythmias, and improved free radical scavenging.[102–105] Potential complications with ACE inhibitors include renal dysfunction, with decreased glomerular filtration rate, and potassium excretion[106] resulting from hypotension, especially associated with hypovolemia.

INODILATOR THERAPY

Inotropic agents that also possess vasodilating properties ("inodilators") are particularly attractive for the therapy of refractory low-cardiac-output states, since they reduce impedance to ventricular ejection in addition to increasing the force of contraction.[107] Inodilating agents include isoproterenol, dopamine in the low-dose range (up to 5 μg/kg/min), dobutamine, milrinone, and amrinone. The potential advantages and disadvantages of each agent were discussed above.

Restore Inadequate SVR (Vasopressor Therapy)

In rare situations, normal vasoconstrictor responses to hypovolemia or low-cardiac-output states may be ineffectual. Examples of such circumstances include persistent effects of drugs (e.g., ACE inhibitors, calcium channel blockers, other long-acting vasodilators), endotoxemia or sepsis, autonomic neuropathy (e.g., diabetes), or arteriovenous shunts (e.g., liver failure). Reestablishing a normal SVR in these situations is often critical, since myocardial and other organ ischemia may be further aggravating an original cause for the low cardiac state. If insufficient vascular tone is suspected (SVR <1000 dyne·sec·cm^{-5}) despite ongoing management of heart rate, preload, and inotropy, then cautious infusion of a vasoconstricting agent is warranted, and should be titrated to obtain the optimum balance between blood pressure and flow. Raising SVR excessively may precipitate further organ ischemia and worsen ventricular function; the goal of therapy should be to maintain mean arterial blood pressure above 60 mm Hg.

Phenylephrine. Phenylephrine is a noncatecholamine α_1-adrenergic receptor agonist. It provides balanced arterial and venoconstriction, commonly associated with a reflex bradycardia. Phenylephrine effects are generally predictable and rapid, and the response to bolus doses (e.g., 50 to 100 μg IV) resolves within several minutes. Phenylephrine is ideal for titrating vascular tone. If hypotension persists a phenylephrine infusion may be used (Table 18–5).

Norepinephrine. Norepinephrine is a potent α_1-adrenergic vasoconstrictor that also possesses significant β-adrenergic receptor activity. It can also provide increased inotropy to compensate for the anticipated increases in afterload, thus reducing the potential for ventricular distention. Although norepinephrine infusion is suitable for hypovolemic or septic shock, the increased myocardial oxygen demands and potential for ventricular rhythm disturbances make this drug a poor choice in circumstances where pump failure is prominent.

Nitro^G-L-Arginine Methyl Ester. Nitro^G-L-arginine methyl ester (L-NAME) is a specific inhibitor of nitric oxide synthase (NOS), the enzyme responsible for the generation of NO in vascular endothelial cells, and at several other locations throughout the body. Experimental use of this drug in settings where massive systemic production of NO by white cells is thought to be the underlying mechanism of vasodilation (i.e., septic shock[108,109]) have shown it to be a potent vasoconstrictor in patients refractory to other vasoconstrictors.[110] However, animal studies suggest that NOS inhibitors decrease renal and cerebral blood flow in septic shock,[111] and in critically ill patients administration of a NOS inhibitor, nitro^G-monomethyl-L-arginine (L-NMMA), was associated with decreased cardiac output. The role of L-NAME–mediated vasoconstriction in critically ill and healthy patients has yet to be fully defined.[108]

Short-Term Mechanical Circulatory Support Techniques

When interventions to optimize cardiac filling and cardiovascular function fail to correct a low-cardiac-output state, the prognosis is generally poor. However, if myocardial function is temporarily reduced (e.g., following cardiopulmonary bypass or myocardial infarction), improved pumping efficiency can be expected as the result of surgery (e.g., closure of an ischemia-induced ventricular septal defect), or a "bridge" to heart transplantation is required, the institution of methods to augment tissue perfusion and assist the heart may be warranted. This section will outline some of the most promising and widely used modalities of short-term cardiac assist techniques currently available.

Intra-Aortic Balloon Pump (IABP)

The Intra-aortic balloon pump (IABP) has been a part of clinical practice since 1968.[113] It is now estimated that over 150,000 intra-aortic balloon catheters are inserted annually. This therapy is accepted as the modality of choice for circulatory support with left ventricular dysfunction or cardiogenic shock inadequately treated by standard therapies, to minimize extension of myocardial infarction, and to treat refractory myocardial ischemia. The IABP utilizes the process of counterpulsation, in which an intra-aortic balloon inflates and deflates during cardiac diastole (aortic valve closure), to displace blood to peripheral vessels (Fig. 18–5). The net effect is to increase cardiac output and coronary and cerebral perfusion, and to decrease ventricular workload. The maximal benefits of counterpulsation are achieved in patients with moderate left ventricular failure due to acute reversible ischemia. Goldberger et al. found survival in a group of 50 patients highly dependent upon the indication for requiring IABP intervention.[114] When IABP was employed for post–myocardial infarction angina, acute ventricular septal defect, unstable angina, or elective perioperative support, the survival rates ranged from 57.6 to 80%. Minimal benefits of IABP are realized in the patient with severe cardiac dysfunction as in cardiogenic shock or severe left ventricular failure. Survival rates for these patients ranged from 20 to 23%.

The Intra-Aortic Balloon Catheter, Insertion, and Hemodynamic Effects. The intra-aortic balloon consists of a long (70-cm) dual-lumen radiopaque catheter with an oblong-shaped balloon on the distal end (Fig. 18–6). The most common adult sizes of IAB catheters range from 30 to 40 ml. The balloon is usually inserted through the femoral artery, either transcutaneously or following surgical vessel exposure. The balloon is positioned in the descending aorta and rapidly inflated and deflated by a pneumatic drive that shuttles helium through an electronically controlled solenoid valve between the IABP console (Fig. 18–7) and the balloon. This inflation-deflation sequence is synchronized with the cardiac cycle, by sensing the "R" wave of the electrocardiogram (ECG) or systolic ejection from an arterial waveform. The ratio of balloon-assisted beats to nonassisted beats may also be controlled (e.g., 1:2 ratio [Figs. 18–8 and 18–9]). Optimal benefit occurs when the balloon is inflated during diastole, simultaneous with aortic valve closure, and remains inflated until immediately prior to initiation of systole (Fig. 18–8). Ventricular myocardial perfusion occurs predominantly during diastole as the relaxation of the myocardium decreases resistance to blood flow though subendocardial capillaries. Diastolic coronary artery blood pressure and the duration of diastole therefore are important factors in subendocardial blood flow. Inflation of the balloon in the aorta displaces blood toward the head vessels and the coronary arteries, thereby augmenting cerebral and coronary perfusion, and

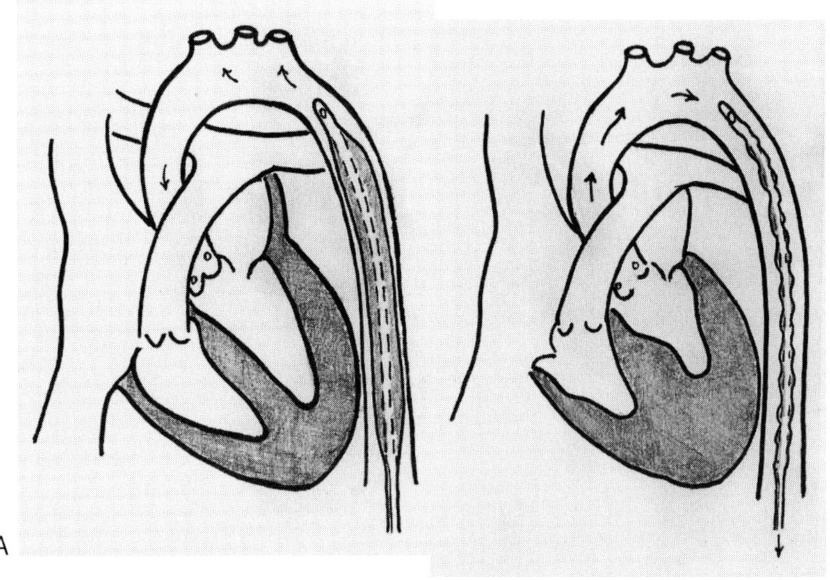

FIGURE **18–5.** Intra-aortic balloon counterpulsation increases cardiac output and coronary and cerebral perfusion, and decreases ventricular workload by inflating (*A*) and deflating (*B*) during cardiac diastole (aortic valve closure) to displace blood to peripheral vessels.

thus is beneficial during periods of myocardial ischemia (Fig. 18–5*A*). This diastolic augmentation may increase diastolic intra-aortic pressure by more than 70%.[115] Just prior to the onset of systole, the balloon is rapidly deflated creating a "sink" in the aorta (Fig. 18–5*B*). The corresponding decrease of 10 to 15%[115] in blood pressure effectively decreases impedance to left ventricular ejection, thereby reducing ventricular afterload, with the result being a decrease in myocardial oxygen consumption. Use of an IABP in a patient with a low-output state usually has numerous early hemodynamic benefits; effective counterpulsation generally results in decreases in heart rate, left ventricular end-diastolic and pulmonary capillary wedge pressures, and increased cardiac output. Other advantages of IABP are reducing peripheral edema, improving urine output, warming of the extremities, and raising the level of consciousness.

Intra-Aortic Balloon Catheter Management. Proper location of the IAB is crucial to optimize function and reduce potential risk of complications. The tip of the balloon should be positioned 1 to 2 cm distal to the left subclavian artery ostium. This offers the safest maximal increase in perfusion pressure during diastole (balloon inflation) and afterload reduction just prior to ventricular systole (balloon deflation). When the IAB catheter is correctly placed, the radiopaque tip can be seen on chest x-ray or fluoroscopy at the second or third intercostal space. It is recommended that the left radial artery pressure be monitored to identify cephalad balloon migra-

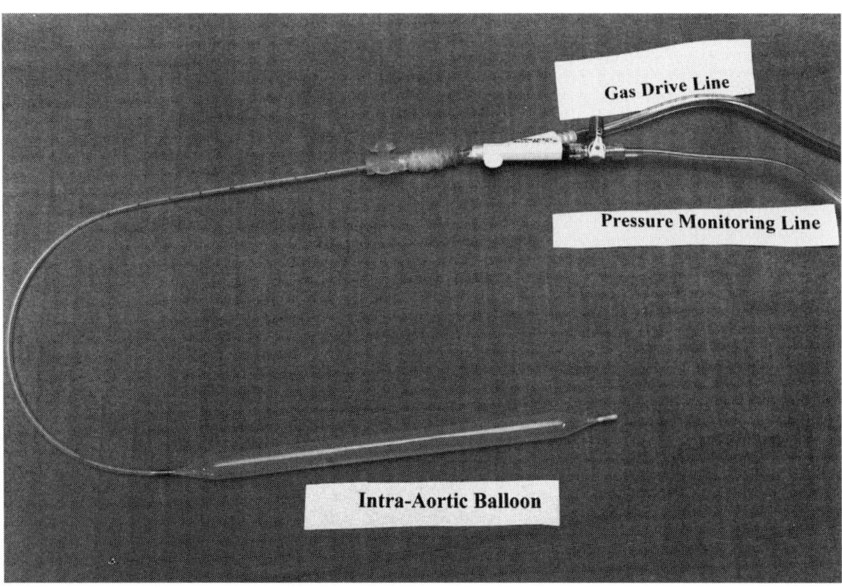

FIGURE **18–6.** A Datascope intra-aortic balloon.

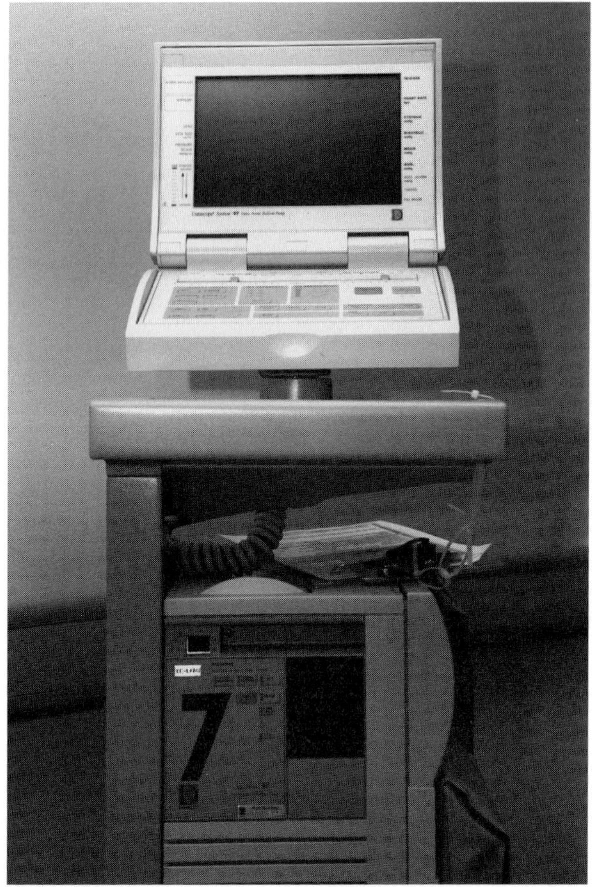

FIGURE **18–7.** A Datascope intra-aortic balloon console.

tion, since this may obstruct or damage the left subclavian artery. Conversely, if the IAB catheter is positioned too distally in the aorta, it will inflate in the narrower abdominal aorta, posing a risk to the balloon, the aorta, and branch vessels, while providing poor hemodynamic support. Confirmation of the IAB catheter tip location by x-ray or transesophageal echocardiography should therefore be obtained as soon as practical following insertion.

An ECG signal and/or arterial pressure waveform are required to trigger the IABP. Trigger options include the R wave of the ECG, an arterial pulse pressure (minimum 15 mm Hg), or ventricular pacemaker spikes. An "internal" setting also allows IABP inflation independent of cardiac activity; the "internal" mode has limited application, although it may be used as a means of generating pulsatile flow during cariopulmonary bypass (CPB). "Internal" mode should not be used if a patient is generating any cardiac output, as asynchronous balloon inflation will obstruct blood flow and also does not generate blood flow during ventricular fibrillation or asystole, despite creating a pressure spike on the arterial monitor.

In order to effectively assist the failing or vulnerable heart, it is important that the IABP be properly synchronized to the timing trigger. Timing the balloon refers to the proper synchronizing of counterpulsation and cardiac ejection; to gain optimal balloon efficiency requires minor shifts in the moment of balloon inflation and deflation with empiric examination of the results upon the arterial pressure waveform. The balloon should be inflated to cause a pressure spike (*diastolic augmentation*) at the dicrotic notch on the arterial waveform (i.e., aortic valve closure). If inflation is initiated too early, the balloon will obstruct blood flow in the aorta (Fig. 18–9*A*). If balloon inflation is initiated too late, the effectiveness of the balloon in reducing ventricular afterload and augmenting coronary perfusion will be compromised (Fig. 18–9*B*). In contrast, balloon deflation should occur just prior to the upsweep of the arterial waveform (aortic valve opening and ventricular ejection). This causes the aortic pressure to be at its lowest level at the onset of ventricular ejection (*systolic unloading*), thus minimizing ventricular workload. If deflation occurs too early, the aorta is not maximally unloaded at the onset of ventricular contraction (Fig. 18–9*C*). If deflation occurs too late, the balloon remains inflated during ventricular ejection, causing impedance to blood flow (Fig. 18–9*D*).

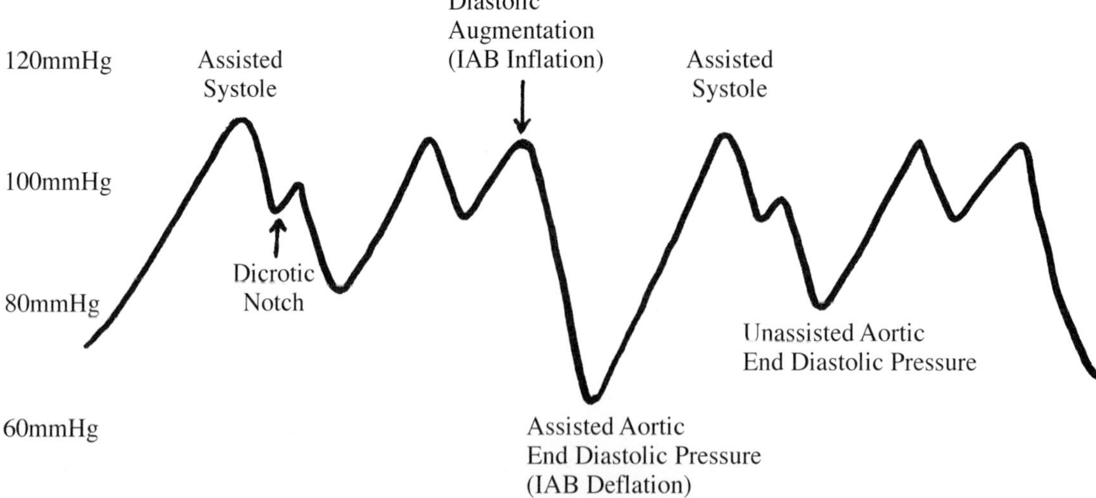

FIGURE **18–8.** Proper timing of intra-aortic balloon inflation and deflation (1:2 ratio).

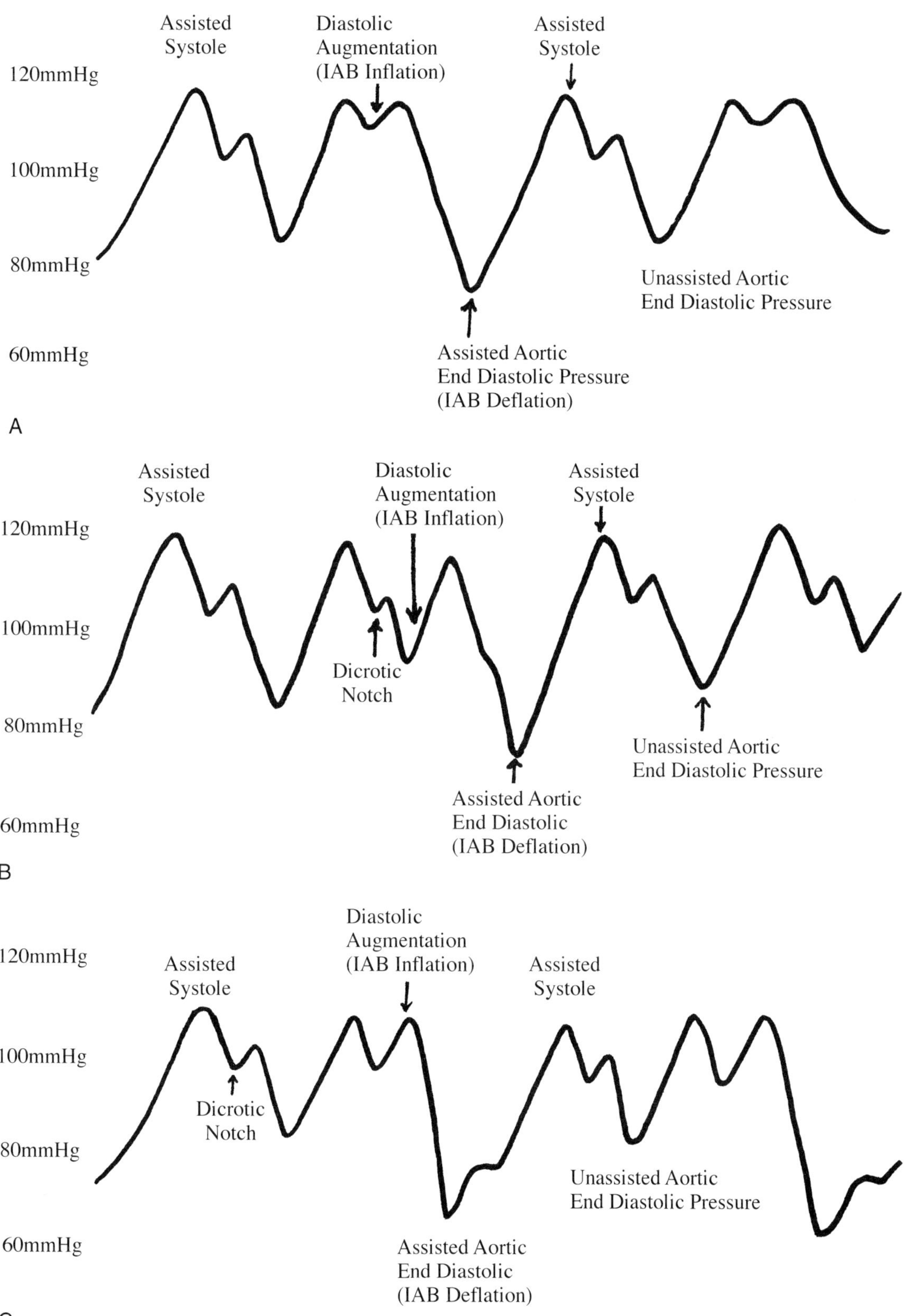

FIGURE **18–9.** Improper timing (1:2 ratio) of intra-aortic balloon inflation (premature [*A*], delayed [*B*], and deflation) (premature [*C*], delayed [*D*]) results in suboptimal increases of cardiac output and decreased ventricular workload. *Illustration continued on following page*

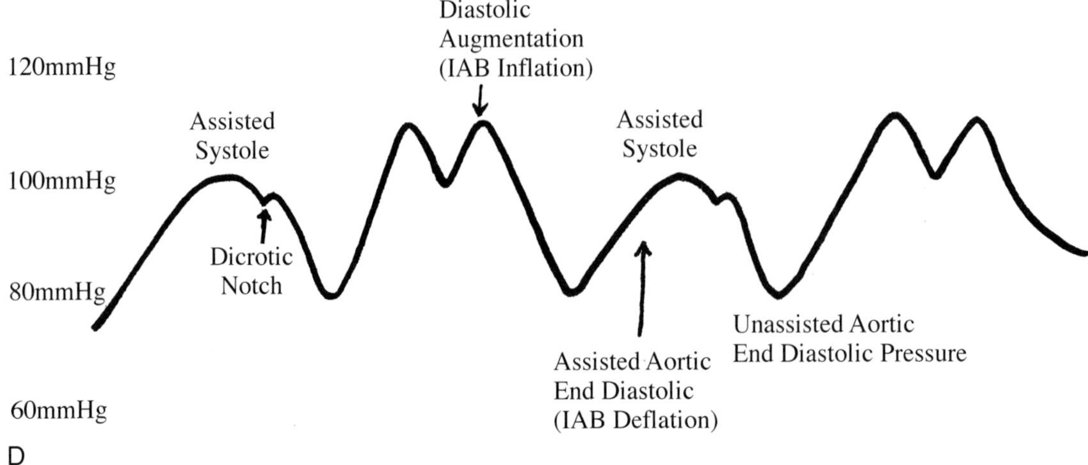

FIGURE **18–9.** *Continued.*

This increases afterload and decreases cardiac output (most of the ventricular volume is ejected during the early phase of ventricular contraction).

The primary means of determining whether a patient is ready to wean from the IAB support is by assessment of the cardiac output. Other clinical signs of improvement include normalized systemic blood pressure with minimal vasopressor and inotropic requirements, CVP and PAOP within normal range, improved urine output, and increased level of consciousness. When the cardiac index is within acceptable range, the amount of inotropic support should be gradually reduced and the patient's hemodynamic status evaluated. Weaning the IAB may be accomplished by ratio or augmentation reduction. Ratio reduction weaning involves incrementally decreasing the ratio of balloon-assisted beats to nonassisted beats (e.g., from 1:1 to 1:2 to 1:4 to 1:8). Ventricular performance can be evaluated by comparing the IAB pulsation to the patient's native arterial waveform. When the ratio has been decreased to 1:8 the IAB catheter is generally removed. Augmentation reduction is a more subtle method than ratio reduction for weaning ventricular assistance; balloon inflation volume is decreased by increments (e.g., 20%), and catheter removal is considered when 20% balloon capacity is tolerated.[116]

Intra-Aortic Balloon Catheter Risks and Complications. Although the benefits of IABP counterpulsation are well documented, the risks presented by this invasive modality are not to be lightly regarded. The overall incidence of serious IABP-related complications ranges from 5 to 10%.[117] Limb ischemia is the commonest complication of percutaneous IAB insertion due to obstruction of blood flow to the iliac and distal femoral artery. The incidence of clinical leg ischemia may approach 30%; generally presenting as the loss of distal pulses and cooling of the extremity. Prompt removal of the catheter is usually adequate treatment; however, approximately 10% of patients have more serious ischemic complications that require additional therapy (e.g., embolectomy, thrombolytic therapy) following IAB catheter removal. Proper preparation of the groin and constant vigilance and care of the site are essential to minimize the risk of infection and bleeding. Heparin anticoagulation must be established prior to IAB insertion. Systemic heparin anticoagulation should be routinely monitored and maintained throughout the duration of IAB pumping to prevent thrombi from forming around the balloon catheter and reduce platelet consumption. Failure to adequately anticoagulate the patient can result in thromboembolic complications, and can even permit adhesions to form between the balloon and the aortic wall, requiring surgical removal of the catheter. The balloon catheter should be removed promptly (within 20 minutes from termination of counterpulsation) to avoid clot.

The IAB is traumatic to blood components; after 24 to 48 hours there is usually evidence of hemolysis and platelet destruction. Blood component replacement therapy may be necessary to avoid anemia and prevent bleeding. Acute aortic dissection is a devastating though rare complication; patients with peripheral vascular disease are at particular risk. Proper balloon size selection is important to optimize function and reduce risk factors associated with IAB pumping. A balloon that is relatively too large may endanger the balloon integrity due to abrasion against atherosclerotic plaque. Furthermore, a balloon that is too long may extend below the renal artery ostia, where there is a greater propensity for calcific atherosclerotic lesions. Elderly and female patients have an increased risk of balloon rupture during IAB pumping. Presumably, increased aortic atherosclerotic plaque is responsible for this in the elderly, while females generally have smaller caliber and shorter aortas. Balloon choice should be based on patient stature (aortic length).[117] In the event of balloon rupture, sensors in the IABP console detect gas leaks and alert the operator; if this occurs pumping should be stopped and the catheter removed. Since the blood pressure in the aorta exceeds intra-balloon pressure during deflation, blood will enter the balloon following rupture and be visible in the balloon gas line. The sequelae of most balloon ruptures are benign due to the functional design and safety mechanisms of the pump.

There are some relative and a few absolute contraindications to IABP therapy. Absolute contraindications in-

TABLE 18–8
Relative and Absolute Contraindications to the Insertion of an Intra-aortic Balloon Pump

Absolute Contraindications to IABP	Relative Contraindications to IABP
Severe aortic insufficiency	Aortic aneurysm
Dissecting aortic aneurysm	Sepsis
Malignant arrhythmias	Severe vascular disease
Asystole	Mild aortic insufficiency
Ventricular fibrillation	
Pulseless electrical activity	

clude those in which IABP therapy will cause further harm to the patient, while the presence of relative contraindications may still warrant a trial of this therapy (Table 18–8).

Ventricular Assist Devices

Rarely, ventricular failure which is refractory to pharmacologic and IABP intervention may be considered reversible (e.g., post cardiac surgery). In these circumstances, the more invasive and supportive ventricular assist devices are currently available. Establishment of most ventricular assist devices requires surgery to insert the cannulas within the great vessels of the chest. Separate left or right ventricular, or even bi-ventricular assistance may be instituted. Several different types of ventricular assist devices have been developed. The two most frequently used will be reviewed below.

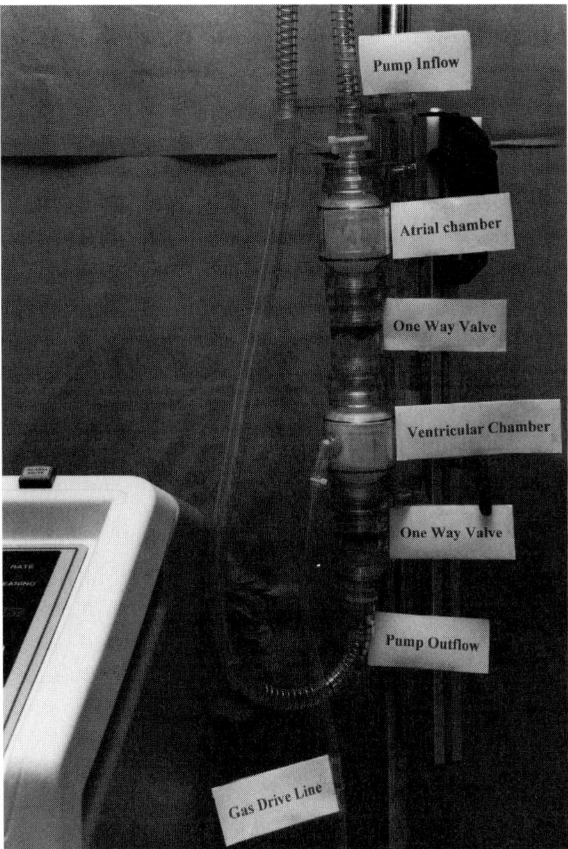

FIGURE **18–10.** The ABIOMED BVS 5000 ventricular assist device.

ABIOMED BVS 5000 SYSTEM

The ABIOMED BVS 5000 consists of two pneumatically driven blood pumps, each capable of pumping 5 L/min, which may be used individually (single ventricular assist), or in combination (biventricular assist). The ABIOMED pump is the only ventricular assist device that is approved by the FDA. This system assists the failing heart by means of allowing blood to bypass the ailing ventricle(s). Circulatory support is provided while unloading the ventricle thus reducing wall tension, improving myocardial perfusion, restoring ATP stores, and therefore allowing the heart muscle the opportunity to recover. Blood flow from the ABIOMED BVS 5000 pump is pulsatile. Proposed advantages of pulsatile flow verses nonpulsatile flow include better myocardial, cerebral, and renal perfusion; improved capillary perfusion; increased oxygen consumption; reduced anaerobic metabolism; and decreased peripheral vascular resistance.

The BVS 5000 system consists of the drive console, two 6 foot lengths of 3/8-inch-diameter tubing, inflow and outflow cannulae, and a blood pump. The housing of the blood pump is made of clear polyethylene, roughly cylindric in shape, approximately 40 cm long and 7.6 cm in diameter and mounted vertically on a pole (Fig. 18–10). Inside the blood pump, two polyurethane bladder-like chambers (atrial and ventricular) are separated by an Angioflex trileaflet valve. These bladders act as the filling and pumping chambers for blood. Blood is ejected from the native atrium and, aided by gravity, fills the pump's "atrial" chamber. This atrial chamber acts as a reservoir, allowing continuous pump filling even during pump systole. This device is a preload-dependent pump sensitive to the patient's own cardiac cycle because the console is able to sense the full ventricular bladder and initiate pump systole. Pump output is regulated by adjusting the height relative to the patient. As the pump position is lowered, there will be faster chamber filling due to gravity, and the pump's ejection rate will increase. Pump output is rate related, as ejection is constant. The console shuttles air into the pump housing, external to the ventricular pumping chamber, displacing/ejecting blood out of the chamber through a second Angioflex trileaflet outflow valve and into the patient. The Angioflex one-way valves insure unidirectional (forward) flow.

The pump inflow cannulation site for left ventricular assist is either posterior to the inter-atrial groove, or through the left atrial appendage. Blood is usually returned from the pump via an end-to-side anastomosis into the ascending aorta. This configuration effectively unloads, and therefore rests, the left ventricle. In contrast, right ventricular assist cannulation sites for the pump inflow are the right atrial appendage, or the mid–free right atrial wall. Blood is returned via an end-to-side anastomosis of the main pulmonary artery. Cannulae exit and enter the chest via subcostal stab wounds, allowing the chest to be closed. Chest closure minimizes the risk of infection and reduces bleeding. Cannulae are connected to the ³⁄₈-inch tubing of the pump circuit.

Systemic heparin anticoagulation is necessary to prevent thromboembolic complications. An activated clotting time (ACT) test of 180 to 200 seconds is necessary when providing pump flow rates greater than 3 L/min, while an ACT of 300 seconds is required for flow rates below 3 L/min. Weaning may be accomplished by reducing pump flow in 0.5-L/min increments until the patient demonstrates hemodynamic stability with pump flows below 2 L/min. Transesophageal or transthoracic echocardiography is ideal for assessment of cardiac performance prior to and during weaning attempts.

Bleeding is the primary complication of this modality, followed by infection. Extreme care must be given to creating and maintaining an air-free circuit. Introduction of air to the circuit may have catastrophic consequences. Contraindications for this mode of circulatory support include uncontrolled hemorrhage, massive air emboli, central nervous system damage, massive transfusion reaction, interstitial pulmonary hemorrhage with inability to maintain adequate ventilation, etc.

Centrifugal Pump Circulatory Assist (Ventricular Assist Device)

One of the most widely used modes of short-term circulatory support is the centrifugal pump circulatory assist system. Like the BVS 5000 system, the centrifugal pump system may be adapted to provide left, right, or biventricular assistance. Its popularity may be attributed to the simplicity of implementation and operation, the availability of components, and the modest cost of the disposable equipment required. Despite the widespread use of the centrifugal pump as a ventricular support device, it has currently not been approved by the FDA for this application.

The centrifugal pump operates on the "constrained vortex" principal and therefore is preload and afterload dependent. It is a nonocclusive, nonpulsatile blood pump in which output is regulated by adjusting pump speed in revolutions per minute (RPM). Different manufacturers (e.g., BioMedicus [Medtronic], Delphin [Sarns 3M], Capiox [Terumo]) maintain slightly varying design characteristics, but the principles of operation and performance remain essentially the same. The pump housing is basically conical in shape and made of clear polyethylene. Inside, sequentially smaller vaneless cones are made to spin by a magnetic linkage to the pump's drive console. These spinning cones produce a centrifugal force on the blood. Negative pressure at the inlet pulls blood into the pump, while the outward force of the swirling blood on the pump wall creates positive pressure. This positive pressure on the pump's lateral wall will translate into flow when a pressure gradient is created between the internal pump and the outlet, the point at which blood exits. Adequate preload must be present in order for the pump to provide optimal flow. Insufficient preload volume or malposition of the inflow cannula are the most likely causes of the pump's inability to flow when utilized as a ventricular assist device. When this condition exists, increasing the RPM fails to increase the pump's output or flow. Inadequate preload is indicated by a rhythmic jumping of the inflow line known as "chatter." Although a constant internal pressure (per RPM) is generated, pump output is inversely proportional and dependent upon the afterload. If the outflow cannula is obstructed or net afterload is increased, the pump output will decrease.

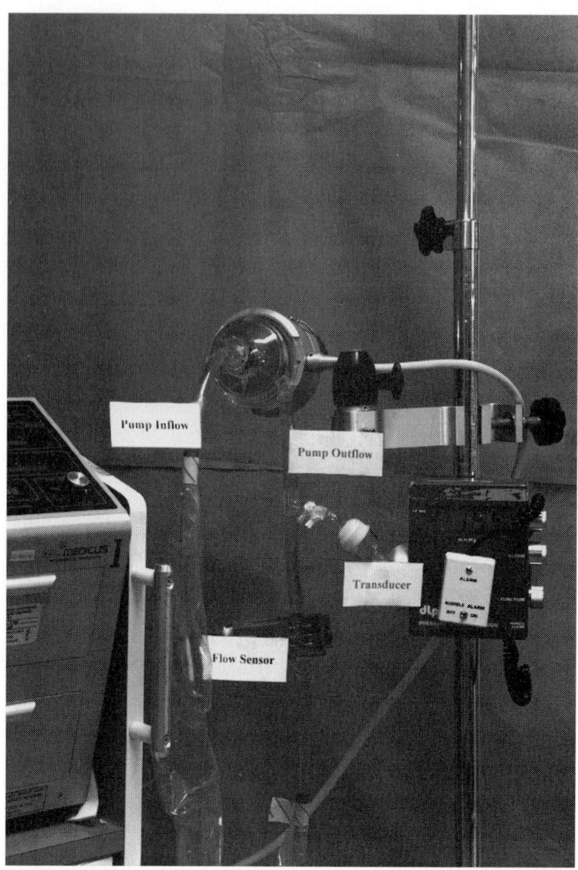

FIGURE **18–11.** The BioMedicus (Medtronic) centrifugal pump ventricular bypass system.

The centrifugal pump ventricular bypass system (Fig. 18–11) consists of an atrial "inflow" cannula leading to the disposable centrifugal pump via a 6-foot length of ³⁄₈-inch tubing. A second 6-foot length of ³⁄₈-inch tubing exits the centrifugal pump to return blood to the patient via the "arterial" cannula. Pre- and postpump pressure monitoring is recommended for troubleshooting flow problems. Cannulation sites and techniques, contraindications, and potential complications for the centrifugal pump ventricular bypass system are similar to those of the ABIOMED BVS 5000 system. Possible advantages of the centrifugal pump system over the BVS 5000 system include reduced cost, less risk of massive air embolus, and a low rate of hemolysis.

SUMMARY

In order to deliver effective treatment to the patient in which a low-cardiac-output state is suspected, an initial assessment should be made; the background to this examination should be a thorough familiarity, not only with the cardiovascular evidence for, and responses to the various hypoperfusion states, but also the systemic humoral response and physiologic consequences of low-cardiac-output syndrome. If a shock state is confirmed, then patient evaluation should be followed by the timely institution of a logical sequence of interventions aimed at optimizing hemodynamic status, and correcting factors that will stabilize oxygen delivery to the microcirculation. While future developments will inevitably change the tools employed to achieve these goals, an attempt has been made to present the basic principles, which will continue to apply.

References

1. Chaudry I, Baue A: Overview of hemorrhagic shock. In Cowley R, Trump B (eds): Pathophysiology of Shock, Anoxia and Ischemia. Baltimore, Williams & Wilkins, 1982, p 203.
2. Garrison R, Cryer H: Role of the microcirculation of skeletal muscle during shock. Pro Clin Biol Res 299:43, 1989.
3. Cryer H, Kaebnick H,, Harris P, Flint L: Effects of tissue acidosis on skeletal muscle microcirculatory responses to hemorrhagic shock in unanesthetized rats. J Surg Res 39:59, 1985.
4. Fine N, Applebaum J, Elquezabal A, Castleman L: Multiple coagulation defects in association with dissecting aneurysms. Arch Intern Med 119:522, 1967.
5. Chaudry I, Ohkawa M, Clemens M, Baue A: Alterations in electron transport and cellular metabolism with shock and trauma. Prog Clin Biol Res 111:67, 1983.
6. Shoemaker W: Pathophysiology, monitoring, and therapy of shock states. Crit Care Clin 2:307, 1987.
7. Kariman K, Jobis F, Saltzman H: Cytochrome a,a3 reoxidation. Early indicator of metabolic recovery from hemorrhagic shock in rats. J Clin Invest 72:180, 1983.
8. Runciman W, Skowronski G: Pathophysiology of haemorrhagic shock. Anaesth Intensive Care 12:193, 1984.
9. Barroso A, Schmid-Schonbein G, Zweifach B, Engler RL: Granulocytes and no-reflow phenomenon in irreversible hemorrhagic shock. Circ Res 63:437, 1988.
10. Ricour C: Stress induced disturbances of the gastrointestinal tract in children. Intensive Care Med 15:S32, 1989.
11. Smith S, Holm R, Perry M, et al: Role of neutrophils in hemorrhagic shock induced gastric mucosal injury in the rat. Gastroenterology 93:466, 1987.
12. Alemayehu A, Sawmiller D, Chou B, Chou C: Intestinal prostacyclin and thromboxane production in irreversible hemorrhagic shock. Circ Shock 23:119, 1987.
13. Bitterman H, Yanagisawa A, Lefer A: Beneficial actions of thromboxane receptor antagonism in hemorrhagic shock. Circ Shock 20:1, 1986.
14. Bitterman H, Smith B, Lefer A: Beneficial actions of antagonism of peptide leukotrienes in hemorrhagic shock. Circ Shock 24: 156, 1988.
15. Bitterman H, Lefer D, Lefer A: A novel mechanism of action of a prostacyclin enhancing agent in hemorrhagic shock. Arch Pharmacol 337:679, 1988.
16. Dunn M: The role of arachidonic acid metabolites in renal homeostasis. Non-steroidal anti-inflammatory drugs renal function and biochemical histological and clinical effects and drug interactions. Drugs 33(Suppl 1):56, 1987.
17. Benveniste J, Henson P, Cochrane C: Leukocyte-dependent histamine release from rabbit platelets. The role of IgE basophils, and a platelet activating factor. J Exp Med 136:1356, 1972.
18. Stahl G, Bitterman H, Terashita Z, Lefer A: Salutary consequences of blockade of platelet activating factor in hemorrhagic shock. Eur J Pharmacol 149:233, 1988.
19. Bitterman H, Lefer D: Beneficial actions of RO 15-1788, a benzodiazepine receptor antagonist in hemorrhagic shock. Methods Find Exp Clin Pharmacol 9:341, 1987.
20. Damerau B: Biological activities of complement-derived peptides. Rev Physiol Biochem Pharmacol 108:151, 1987.
21. Colman R, Schmaier A: The contact activation system: Biochemistry and interactions of these surface mediated defense reactions. CRC Crit Rev Oncol Hematol 5:57, 1986.
22. Nasjletti A, Malik K: Renal kinin-prostaglandin relationship: Implications of function. Kidney Int 19:860, 1981.
23. Smith S, Grisham M, Manci E, et al: Gastric mucosal injury in the rat. Role of iron and xanthine oxidase. Gastroenterology 92: 950, 1987.
24. Darzi A, Feeley M, Coughlan G, et al: Prevention of oxygen free radical generation may protect against the development of irreversible haemorrhagic shock. Br J Surg 75:1251, 1988.
25. Rush B, Sori A, Murphy T, et al: Endotoxemia and bacteremia during hemorrhagic shock: The link between trauma and sepsis? Ann Surg 207:549, 1988.
26. Rush B, Redan J, Flanagan J, et al: Does the bacteremia observed in hemorrhagic shock have clinical significance. A study in germ-free animals. Ann Surg 210:342, 1989.
27. Livingston D, Shumate C, Polk H, Malangoni M: More is better. Antibiotic management after hemorrhagic shock. Ann Surg 208: 451, 1988.
28. Gould F, Harvey J, Dytrych J: Antibody to endotoxic is associated with decreased frequency of postoperative infection. Am J Obstet Gynecol 160:317, 1989.
29. Brand E, Cowgill R, Lefer A: Further characterization of a myocardial depressant factor present in hemorrhagic shock. J Trauma 9:216, 1969.
30. Lefer A, Spath J: Pancreatic hypoperfusion and the production of a myocardial depressant factor present in hemorrhagic shock. Ann Surg 179:868, 1974.
31. Reilly J, Cunnion R, Burch-Whitman C, et al: A circulating myocardial depressant substance is associated with cardiac dysfunction and peripheral hypoperfusion (lactic acidemia) in patients with spectic shock. Chest 95:1072, 1989.
32. Frank O: Zur Dynamik des Herzmuskels. Z Biol 32:370, 1895.
33. Patterson S, Starling E: On the mechanical factors which determine the output of the ventricles. J Physiol 48:357, 1914.
34. Berne R, Levy M: Regulation of the heartbeat. In Berne R, Levy MN (eds): Physiology, 2nd ed. St. Louis, CV Mosby Co, 1988, p 463.
35. Sands S, Winegard S: Treppe and total calcium content of the frog ventricle. Am J Physiol 218:908, 1970.
36. Bodenheimer M, Banka V, Helfant RH: Effect of heart rate on zonal tension and ischemia following coronary occlusion: Optimal rate for Treppe versus ischemia. Cardiovasc Res 10:336, 1976.
37. Woolf P: Endocrinology of shock. Ann Emerg Med 15:1401, 1986.
38. Gorfinkel H, Szidon J, Hirsch L, et al: Renal performance in experimental cardiogenic shock. Am J Physiol 222:1260, 1972.
39. Nelimarka O, Halkola L, Niinikoski J: Distribution of renal cortical and medullary tissue oxygenation in hemorrhagic shock. Acta Chir Scand 148:213, 1982.
40. Schrier R: Effects of the adrenergic nervous system and catecholamines on systemic and renal hemodynamics, sodium and water excretion and renin secretion. Kidney Int 6:291, 1974.
41. Levens N, Peach M, Carey R: Role of the intrarenal renin-angiotension system in the control of renal function. Circ Res 48:157, 1981.
42. Moran S, Myers B: Pathophysiology of protracted acute renal failure in man. J Clin Invest 76:1440, 1985.
43. Khambatta H, Baratz R: IPPB, plasma ADH, and urine flow in conscious man. J of Appl Physiol 33:362, 1972.
44. Genuth G: The adrenal gland. I. Berne R, Levy MN (eds): Physiology, 2nd ed. St. Louis, CV Mosby Co, 1988, p 962.
45. Hall E, Yonkers P, McCall J: Attenuation of hemorrhagic shock by the non-glucocorticoid 21-aminosteroid U74006F. Eur J Pharmacol 147:299, 1988.
46. Engelbrecht F, Mattheyse F, Mouton W: Experimental evaluation of the prophylactic and therapeutic effects of hydrocortisone in hemorrhagic shock. S Afr Med J 67:637, 1985.
47. Bone R, Fisher C, Clemmer T, et al: A controlled clinical trial of high-dose methylprednisolone in the treatment of severe sepsis and septic shock. N Engl J Med 317:653, 1987.
48. Cheung A, Chernow B: The stress response to critical illness. Probl Anesth 3:165, 1989.

49. Sakimoto S, Stone L, Woolf P, Liang-Chang-Seng: Opiate receptor antagonism in right-sided congestive heart failure: Naloxone exerts salutary effects through its action on the central nervous system. Circ Res 65:103, 1989.
50. Curtis M, Lefer A: Effectiveness of ethylketocyclazocine in hemorrhagic shock. Adv Shock Res 10:101, 1983.
51. Faden A, Holaday J: Opiate antagonists: A role in the treatment of hypovolemic shock. Science 205:317, 1979.
52. Gurll N, Reynolds D, Holaday J: Evidence for a role of endorphins in the cardiovascular physiology of primate shock. Crit Care Med 16:521, 1988.
53. Zhao K, Zhu Z, Woo G, Haun X: Effect of naloxone on microcirculatory behavior during irreversible hemorrhagic shock. Microvasc Res 34:84, 1987.
54. Muldoon S, McKenzie J, Collins F: Pressor effect of nalbuphine in hemorrhagic shock is dependent on the sympathoadrenal system. Circ Shock 26:89, 1988.
55. Wartofsky L, Burman K: Alterations in thyroid function in patients with systemic illness: The "euthyroid sick syndrome." Endocrinol Rev 3:164, 1982.
56. Mizobe T, Okuda C: Changes in brain thyrotropin-releasing hormone in reversible and irreversible hemorrhagic shock in the rat. Circ Shock 26:245, 1988.
57. Gurll N, Holaday J, Reynolds D, Ganes E: Thyrotropin releasing hormone: Effects in monkeys and dogs subjected to experimental circulatory shock. Crit Care Med 15:574, 1987.
58. Zoll P, Zoll R, Falk R, et al: External noninvasive temporary cardiac pacing: Clinical trials. Circulation 71:937, 1985.
59. Hankeln K, Radel C, Beez M, et al: Comparison of hydroxyethyl starch and lactated Ringer's solution on hemodynamics and oxygen transport of critically ill patients in prospective crossover studies. Crit Care Med 17:133, 1989.
60. Hein L-G, Albrecht M, Dworschak M, et al: Long-term observation following traumatic-hemorrhagic shock in the dog: A comparison of crystalloid vs. colloidal fluids. Circ Shock 26: 353, 1988.
61. Nakayama S, Sibley L, Gunther R, et al: Small-volume resuscitation with hypertonic saline (2,400 mOsm/liter) during hemorrhagic shock. Circ Shock 13:149, 1984.
62. Chudnofsky C, Dronen S, Syverud S, et al: Intravenous fluid therapy in the prehospital management of hemorrhagic shock: Improved outcome with hypertonic saline/6% dextran 70 in a swine model. Am J Emerg Med 7:357, 1989.
63. Gross D, Landau E, Klin B, Krausz M: Treatment of uncontrolled hemorrhagic shock with hypertonic saline solution. Surg Gynecol Obstet 170:106, 1990.
64. Lindner A, Cutler R, Goodman W: Synergism of dopamine plus furosemide in preventing acute renal failure in the dog. Kidney Int 16:158, 1979.
65. Lucas C, Zito J, Carter K, et al: Questionable value of furosemide in preventing renal failure. Surgery 82:314, 1977.
66. Lawson D, Gray J, Henry D, Tilstone W: Continuous infusion of furosemide in refractory oedema. Br Med J 2:476, 1978.
67. Copeland J, Campbell D, Plachtka J, et al: Diuresis with continuous infusion of furosemide after cardiac surgery. Am J Surg 164:796, 1983.
68. Krasna M, Scott G, Sholz P, et al: Postoperative enhancement of urinary output in patients with acute renal failure using continuous furosemide therapy. Chest 89:294, 1986.
69. Schwartz L, Bissell M, Murphy M, Gewertz B: Renal effects of dopamine in vascular surgical patients. J Vasc Surg 8:367, 1988.
70. Murphy M: The therapeutic role of drugs acting on cardiovascular dopamine receptors. J Cardiothoracic Anesth 4:23, 1990.
71. Schaer G, Fink M, Parrillo J: Norepinephrine alone versus norepinephrine plus low-dose dopamine: Enhanced renal blood flow with combination pressor therapy. Crit Care Med 13:492, 1985.
72. Carcoana O, Garwood S, Mathew J, et al: Renal protection with dopamine and/or mannitol: Does it make a difference? Anesth Analg 84:SCA11, 1997.
73. Shusterman N, Elliott W, White W: Fenoldopam, but not nitroprusside, improves renal function in severely hypertensive patients with impaired renal function. Am J Med 95:161, 1993.
74. Stratton M: Use of nitrates in patients with acute myocardial infarction. Clin Pharm 3:32, 1984.
75. Ayus J, Krothapalli R: Effect of bicarbonate administration on cardiac function. Am J Med 87:5, 1989.
76. Fabioto A: Calcium-induced release of calcium from the cardiac sarcoplasmic reticulum. Am J Physiol 245:C1, 1983.
77. Colucci W, Wright R, Braunwald E: New positive inotropic agents in the treatment of congestive heart failure: Mechanisms of action of recent clinical developments (first of two parts). N Engl J Med 314:290, 1986.
78. Brodde O-E, Broede A, Daul A, et al: Receptors in the nonfailing human heart. Basic Res Cardiol 87(Suppl):1, 1992.
79. Goldberg L: The dopamine vascular receptor: New areas for biochemical pharmacologists. Biochem Pharmacol 24:651, 1975.
80. Aubier M, Murciano D, Menu Y, Boczkowski J: Dopamine effects on diaphragmatic strength during acute respiratory failure in chronic obstructive pulmonary disease. Ann Intern Med 110: 17, 1989.
81. Freyschuss U, Hjemdahl P, Juhlin-Dannfelt A, Linde B: Cardiovascular and metabolic responses to low dose adrenaline infusion: An invasive study in humans. Clin Sci 70:199, 1986.
82. Majerus T, Dasta J, Bauman J, et al: Dobutamine; ten years later. Pharmacotherapy 9:245, 1989.
83. Smith G, O'Connor S: A symposium: Focus of heart failure—current experiences in basic research and clinical studies on dopexamine hydrochloride (Dopacard): An introduction to the pharmacologic properties of Dopacard (dopexamine hydrochloride). Am J Cardiol 62:9C, 1988.
84. Baim D: Effects of amrinone on myocardial energetics in severe congestive heart failure. Am J Cardiol 56:16B, 1985.
85. Copp M, Hill A, Feneck R: Overview of the effects of intravenous milrinone in acute heart failure following surgery. Eur J Anaesth 9(Suppl 5):35, 1992.
86. Baumann G, Felix B, Riess G, et al: Effective stimulation of cardiac contractility and myocardial metabolism by impromidine and dimaprit—two new H2-agonist compounds—in the surviving catecholamine-insensitive myocardium after coronary occlusion. J Cardiovasc Pharmacol 4:543, 1982.
87. Lvoff R, Wilcken D: Glucagon in heart failure and in cardiogenic shock: Experience in 50 patients. Circulation 45:534, 1972.
88. Linderer T, Biamino G, Gruggeman T, et al: Hemodynamic effects of forskolin, a new drug with combined inotropic and vasodilating properties. J Am Coll Cardiol 3:562, 1984.
89. Matsue S, Murakami E, Takekoshi N, et al: Hemodynamic effects of dibutyryl clinic AMP in congestive heart failure. Am J Cardiol 51:1364, 1983.
90. Bennett-Guerrero E, Jimenez JL, White WD, et al: Cardiovascular effects of intravenous triiodothyronine in patients undergoing coronary artery bypass graft surgery. A randomized, double-blind, placebo-controlled trial. Duke T3 study group [see comments]. JAMA 275:687, 1996.
91. Sladen R, Rosenthal M: Specific afterload reduction with parenteral hydralazine following cardiac surgery. J Thorac Cardiovasc Surg 78:195, 1979.
92. Cohn JN, Johnson G, Ziesche S, et al: A comparison of enalapril with hydralazine-isosorbide dinitrate in the treatment of chronic congestive heart failure [see comments]. N Engl J Med 325:303, 1991.
93. Troncy E, Francoeur M, Blaise G: Inhaled nitric oxide: Clinical applications, indications, and toxicology. Can J Anaesth 44:973, 1997.
94. Reicher-Reiss H: Calcium antagonists in heart failure. Eur Heart J 9(Suppl H):101, 1988.
95. Eicher J, Morelon P, Chalopin J, et al: Acute renal failure during nifedipine therapy in a patient with congestive heart failure. Crit Care Med 16:1163, 1988.
96. Turlapaty P, Vary R, Kaplan J: Nicardipine, a new intravenous calcium antagonist: A review of pharmacology, pharmacokinetics, and perioperative applications. J Cardiothorac Anesth 3:344, 1989.
97. Natsume T: Therapeutic advances in the treatment of left ventricular hypertrophy. Eur Heart J 14(Suppl D):33, 1993.
98. Sy J, Vitarelli A, Gheorghiade M: Nicardipine in heart failure: Distinguishing its acute beneficial from its chronic effects. Minerva Cardioangiol 41:535, 1993.
99. Miller R, Awan N, Maxwell K, et al: Sustained reduction of cardiac impedance and preload in congestive heart failure with

the antihypertensive vasodilator, prazosin, N Engl J Med 297: 303, 1977.
100. Flynn K, Coughlan M, Phelan D, et al: Letters to the Editor: Intravenous captopril in acute heart failure. Lancet 1(8578):173, 1988.
101. Lipkin D, Frenneaux M, Maseri A: Letters to the Editor: Beneficial effect of captopril in cardiogenic shock. Lancet 2:327, 1987.
102. Corbalan R, Jalil J, Chamorro G, et al: Effects of captopril versus milrinone therapy in modulating the adrenergic nervous system response to exercise in congestive heart failure. Am J Cardiol 65:644, 1990.
103. Trachete G, Lefer A: Mechanism of the protective effect of angiotensin-converting enzyme in hemorrhagic shock. Proc Soc Exp Biol Med 162:54, 1979.
104. Cleland J, Dargle H, Hodsman G, et al: Captopril in heart failure. A double blind controlled trail. Br Heart J 52:530, 1984.
105. Lefer A: The pathophysiologic role of myocardial depressant factor as a mediator of circulatory shock. Klin Wochenschr 60: 713, 1982.
106. Dzau V: Renal effects of angiotensin-converting enzyme inhibition in cardiac failure. Am J Kidney Dis 10(Suppl 1):74, 1987.
107. Kaplan J, Guffin A: The inodilators: An expanding role in the perioperative period. J Cardiothoracic Anesth 4:27, 1990.
108. Wolfe TA, Dasta JF: Use of nitric oxide synthase inhibitors as a novel treatment for septic shock. Ann Pharmacother 29:36, 1995.
109. Kilbourn RG, Traber DL, Szabo C: Nitric oxide and shock. Dis Mon 43:277, 1997.
110. Petros A, Bennett D, Vallance P: Effect of nitric oxide synthase inhibitors on hypotension in patients with septic shock [see comments]. Lancet 388:1557, 1991.
111. Offner PJ, Robertson FM, Pruitt BA Jr: Effects of nitric oxide synthase inhibition on regional blood flow in a porcine model of endotoxic shock. J Trauma 39:338, 1995.
112. Petros A, Lamb G, Leone A, et al: Effects of a nitric oxide synthase inhibitor in humans with heptic shock. Cardiovasc Res 28:34, 1994.
113. Bregman D: Mechanical support of the failing heart. Curr Probl Surg 13:1, 1976.
114. Goldberger M, Tabak S, Shah P: Clinical experience with intra-aortic balloon counterpulsation in 112 consecutive patients. Am Heart J 111:497, 1986.
115. Bolooki H: Current status of circulatory support with an intra-aortic balloon pump. Cardiol Clin 3:123, 1985.
116. Quail J: Comprehensive Intra-aortic Balloon Counterpulsation. St. Louis, MO, Mosby Publishing Company, 1993.
117. Goldman B, Hill T, Rosenthal G, et al: Complications associated with use of the intra-aortic balloon pump. Can J Surg 25:153, 1982.

CHAPTER 19

Heart and Lung Transplantation

Carol L. Lake, M.D., M.B.A

The initial heart transplant was performed in South Africa by Dr. Christian Barnard in 1967. At the present time cardiac transplantation is performed in about 3,500 patients annually worldwide with ~2,500 of those performed in the United States (Fig. 19–1). Lung transplantation was first performed in humans in 1963 by Hardy.[1] In 1981, the Stanford group performed the first combined heart-lung transplantation.[2] Despite early difficulties with rejection and the lack of effective immunosuppressive drugs, survival rates steadily increased in the 1980s and have remained stable in recent years. The 1997 United Network for Organ Sharing (UNOS) report indicates 1-year survival rates of 81.5% for heart transplant, 70.4% for lung transplant, and 61.9% for heart-lung transplant.[3] Today heart and lung transplantation are increasingly used to treat end-stage cardiac and pulmonary disease. Use of these procedures is limited only by the availability of donor organs.

Cardiac transplantation is primarily funded by Medicare and private insurance. However, the Healthcare Financing Administration (HCFA) established a process for approval of centers performing transplantation in 1986.[4] In order to obtain HCFA approval and receive Medicare reimbursement, the qualifications and training of the transplant physicians and other aspects of the transplant program, including analysis of results, are carefully assessed. The outcomes following transplantation are better (lower mortality rates) in centers meeting the Medicare criteria.[5] Survival is also better in centers performing more than 50 transplants annually.

Heart Transplantation

Indications

General indications for cardiac transplantation include any form of end-stage cardiac disease in which survival or quality of life cannot be assured by conventional forms of therapy. An indication for transplantation must be accompanied by the absence of contraindications such as concomitant disease limiting survival.[6] Exclusion from consideration for transplantation results from pulmonary hypertension, infection, or malignancy. Transplantation is relatively contraindicated in patients with "physiologic" age greater than 55 to 60 years, obstructive/restrictive lung disease, advanced hepatic disease, renal insufficiency, morbid obesity, peripheral vascular disease, and active peptic ulcer disease. A recently described indication for transplantation is after unsuccessful minimally invasive direct coronary artery bypass.[7] Both the American College of Cardiology Consensus Conference in 1992 and the UNOS Board of Directors Guidelines for Cardiac Transplantation emphasize the need to maximize other state-of-the-art therapy before considering cardiac transplantation.[6,8] The timing of transplantation can be difficult. A balance must be struck between transplantation of less severely ill patients who may survive without transplantation versus moribund patients with severe multiorgan failure.

Patient Selection

Patients with the highest probability of benefit from transplantation and the lowest probability of survival without transplantation are selected through objective assessment of their functional capacity.[6] Functional capacity is usually determined by peak oxygen uptake during maximal exercise with a value of 14 ml/kg/min or less indicating need for transplantation.[9] However, the peak oxygen uptake value must be interpreted in the context of patient age and lifestyle. Aaronson and co-workers used a model with seven noninvasive parameters (peak $\dot{V}O_2$, mean resting heart rate, resting heart rate, ischemic cardiomyopathy, left ventricular ejection fraction, intraventricular conduction defect, and plasma sodium concentration) for prediction of survival and risk stratification of patients undergoing cardiac transplantation.[10]

Donor Management

Following the declaration of brain death in the donor, the transplantation procedure begins with the harvesting

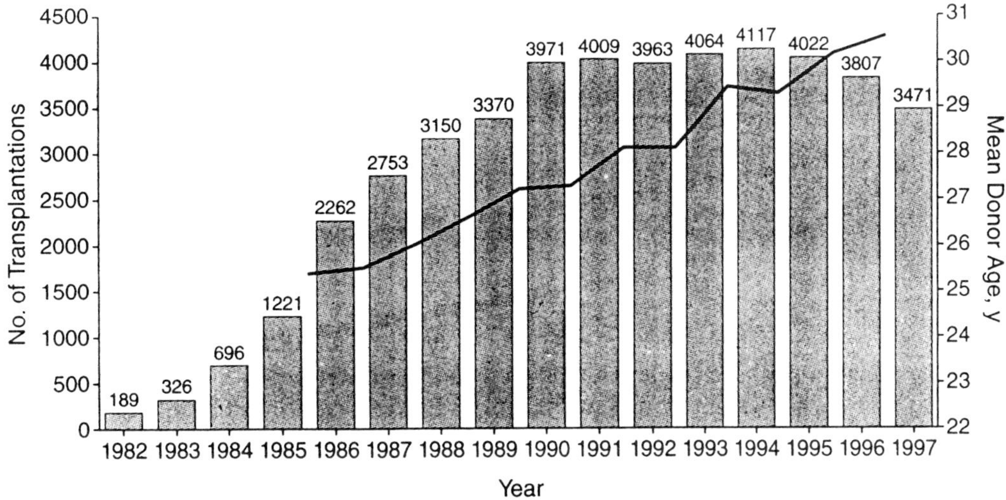

FIGURE **19–1.** Number of heart transplants worldwide in the past two decades. The black line indicates the age of the transplant donors. (From Hosenpud JD, Bennett LE, Keck BM, et al: The Registry of the International Society for Heart and Lung Transplantation. 15th Official Report—1998. J Heart Lung Transplant 17:656, 1998, with permission.)

of the heart. The goal is to keep the donor in good condition during procurement, specifically avoiding hypotension, hypovolemia, hypoxemia, and hypothermia. Donors are usually treated with antibiotics. Cardiovascular management includes maintenance of central venous pressure between 5 and 10 mm Hg, mean arterial pressure between 70 and 90 mm Hg. Peripherally acting vasoconstrictors, rather than positive inotropic drugs, are used to maintain arterial pressure, which is often reduced by brain death. If hypertension is present, it should be vigorously treated with nitroprusside. Fluid administration (lactated Ringer's, albumin, or other crystalloid) is used to maintain the central venous pressure. If the hematocrit is less than 20%, transfusion of the donor should be performed. Respiratory management of the donor includes maintenance of adequate blood gases with volume ventilation, positive end-expiratory pressure (PEEP) if necessary, and a fractional inspired oxygen (FIO_2) level of 1.0.

Donor Heart Procurement

The United Network for Organ Sharing operates the Organ Procurement and Transplantation Network on contract from the federal government. A central registry of waiting cardiac recipients, categorized by blood type and body size, is maintained. Available hearts are offered to the appropriate recipient with the longest time on the waiting list in the local area. If no recipient is available locally, the next appropriate recipient in a 1,000-mile radius is chosen. This distance requirement is essential to avoid greater than 3 hours of ischemic preservation time.

The donor chest and abdomen (if liver and kidneys are to be harvested) are opened through a midline incision. The heart is mobilized and heparin, 30,000 units, administered into the superior vena cava before it is ligated. A catheter is inserted into the ascending aorta for the administration of cardioplegia. The ends of the superior and inferior venae cavae are clamped and the heart is allowed to beat empty for five to six beats prior to administration of cold cardioplegia into the ascending aorta. During infusion of cardioplegia, the left ventricle should be undistended but the aorta should be distended. Topical hypothermia is applied to the pericardial space. Once the cardioplegia is infused, the aorta, superior and inferior venae cavae, followed by the pulmonary veins are transected and the heart is removed.

Recipient Anesthetic Management

Preoperative Evaluation

Patients should be evaluated by the anesthesiologist at the time they are placed on the transplant registry. In addition to the complete cardiovascular studies that will be performed in preparation for the transplant, the anesthesiologist will want to review the patient's airway, prior surgical and anesthetic history, current medications, and disease in other organ systems that may affect the anesthetic plan. Patients with severe heart failure are likely to have hypokalemia secondary to diuretic therapy, hyper- or hypovolemia depending upon diuretic effects, increased adrenergic activity, slow circulation time, respiratory insufficiency, orthopnea, poor nutrition, and down-regulated catecholamine receptors in the heart. Their medications may include angiotensin-converting enzyme inhibitors, nitrates, digoxin, diuretics, or β-adrenergic antagonists such as carvedilol. A more detailed discussion of the pathophysiology and pharmacology of heart failure can be found elsewhere.[11] In most instances, patients for cardiac transplantation will be ambulatory outpatients. However, in other circumstances, the patient may have heart failure requiring inotropic drug infusions, insertion of an intra-aortic counterpulsation balloon, or a ventricular assist device.[12] These therapies are discussed in Chapter 18.

Preoperative Preparation

Premedication, consisting of morphine 1 to 2 mg, fentanyl 1 μg/kg, or midazolam, 1 to 2 mg can be given intravenously in the operating room if the patient's hemodynamic condition permits. Antibiotics and immunosuppressive drugs are administered preoperatively according to the protocol of the transplant center.

Equipment for cardiac transplantation includes a standard anesthesia machine equipped with a sterile anesthetic circuit, humidifier, and sterile equipment for airway instrumentation. Monitoring devices include a hemodynamic monitor with multiple pressure modules, cardiac output, arterial oxygen saturation (Sao_2), transesophageal echocardiography (TEE), and respiratory gas analysis. Intravascular catheters are inserted into two peripheral veins, a radial artery, and a central vein, usually the left internal jugular vein. The right internal jugular vein is not used so that it can be utilized for postoperative ventricular biopsies to monitor rejection. Alternatively, a pulmonary artery catheter may be inserted with its tip placed in the superior vena cava until the transplantation is complete and it can be advanced into the pulmonary circulation.[13] Another alternative is to place the pulmonary artery catheter into the wedge position and then withdraw it when the native heart is removed, repositioning it into the transplanted heart. However, the placement of a pulmonary artery catheter adds to the risk of infection in the immunocompromised patient. All intravascular catheters must be inserted using strict sterile technique (sterile preparation and draping, use of sterile gown and mask during the procedures, and placement of a sterile occlusive dressing on the site). A catheter is placed in the bladder following anesthetic induction. External defibrillator pads should be placed if the patient has had prior cardiac surgery because internal defibrillator paddles may not be applied if adhesions are present.

In addition to the usual drugs prepared for induction and maintenance of anesthesia, cardioactive drugs should be readily available. Syringes of phenylephrine (0.5 mg/ml), calcium chloride (100 mg/ml), lidocaine (20 mg/ml), and epinephrine (4 μg/ml) should be prepared. Infusions of dobutamine, dopamine, epinephrine, nitroprusside, nitroglycerin, amrinone/milrinone, and norepinephrine should be immediately available. An infusion of isoproterenol for administration at 1 to 4 μg/min will be used to maintain heart rate following transplantation.

Anesthetic Management

In most instances the patient will have a full stomach and require rapid sequence induction to limit the aspiration risk. The immunosuppressive drugs cyclosporine and azathioprine are usually given orally preoperatively. Drugs to increase gastric emptying (metoclopramide) or increase gastric pH (ranitidine) can be given preoperatively. The choice of anesthesia depends upon the patient's physical status at the time of induction.[13] Sufentanil 3 to 5 μg/kg, fentanyl 5 to 20 μg/kg, ketamine 0.5 to 1 mg/kg, or etomidate 0.2 to 0.3 mg/kg preceded by intravenous lidocaine can be used for rapid sequence induction of the cardiac transplant patient. If the need for rapid intubation is less acute, a slower induction and longer acting nondepolarizing neuromuscular blocking agents can be used. Either sufentanil or fentanyl, in conjunction with midazolam or low concentrations of volatile agents such as isoflurane, is used for maintenance of anesthesia.

It is important to remember that patients with chronic low cardiac output have prolonged circulation times and apparent reduction in the volume of distribution of drugs. Smaller doses of narcotics may be needed if the cardiac transplant patient has coexisting hepatic or renal impairment affecting drug metabolism.

The prebypass period requires a careful balance between noncardiac organ perfusion and sufficient inotropic support to maintain the native heart until cardiopulmonary bypass is instituted. However, in the choice of inotropes, systemic perfusion outweighs any deleterious effects on the native heart. Transesophageal echocardiography is helpful to detect intracardiac thrombus, ventricular volume and contractility, and aortic atherosclerosis in the recipient in the prebypass period.

As during any other major cardiac operation, arterial blood gases, hematocrit, and serum potassium are measured preoperatively, after tracheal intubation, after sternotomy, after 5 minutes on cardiopulmonary bypass, at 30-minute intervals on bypass, 5 minutes after discontinuation of bypass, and at 30 minutes following bypass before return to the intensive care unit. Hematocrit is also measured after blood transfusions and after any significant blood loss. Hemostasis and anticoagulation are verified using automated activated clotting times at appropriate intervals before, during, and following cardiopulmonary bypass. Other laboratory studies are performed as indicated by patient condition.

Surgery

The surgical technique has changed little over the 30+ years of cardiac transplantation from that described by Lower and Shumway.[14] The recipient's chest is opened through a median sternotomy. Cannulation of the great vessels is performed as for other cardiac procedures with cardiopulmonary bypass. Bicaval cannulation is performed and tapes are placed around the venous cannulas. Cardiectomy is performed, leaving the posterior right atrium attached to the venae cavae and the posterior interatrial septum with the posterior left atrium at the level of the entrance of the four pulmonary veins (Fig. 19–2*A*). The initial anastomosis of the new heart is made to the recipient's left atrial free wall, followed by the right atrium to the free right atrial wall and septum, followed finally by aortic and pulmonary artery anastomoses.

One modification of the technique is bicaval anastomosis, described by Dreyfus and co-workers[15] (Fig. 19–2*B*). With this variation, the anatomic integrity of the right atrium is preserved by using anastomoses at the level of the superior and inferior venae cavae. The advantages of this technique are better preservation of sinoatrial node and tricuspid valve function.

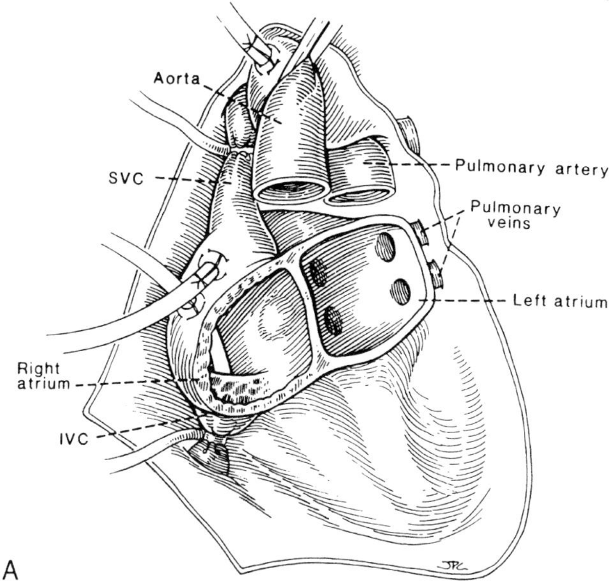

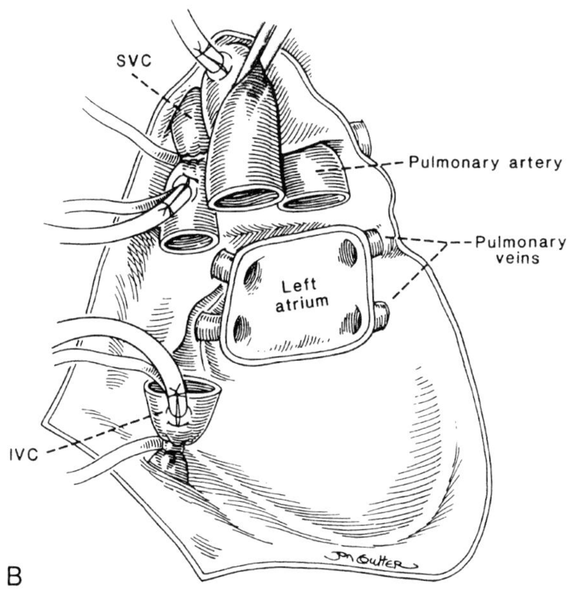

FIGURE **19–2.** *A*, The appearance of the mediastinum after removal of the native heart but before allograft transplantation using the classic orthotopic technique. *B*, The mediastinum prepared for transplantation using the bicaval anastomotic technique. (From Quinlan JJ, Firestone S, Firestone LJ: Anesthesia for Heart, Lung and Heart-Lung Transplantation. In Kaplan JA, Reich DL, Konstadt SN [eds]: Cardiac Anesthesia, 4th ed. Philadelphia, WB Saunders Co, 1999, with permission.)

Reperfusion

As the pulmonary anastomosis is completed, the heart is reperfused and begins to fibrillate, often defibrillating spontaneously. All air must be removed from the heart prior to attempting to wean from bypass. The transplanted heart must undergo a period of warming and perfusion, usually at least 10 minutes to ensure that cardioplegia has been washed out, endothelial function is returning, and myocardial contractility is becoming normal.

Termination of Cardiopulmonary Bypass

Transesophageal echocardiography can evaluate adequacy of de-airing of the heart and its function prior to attempted discontinuation of bypass. Discontinuation of cardiopulmonary bypass may require the administration of isoproterenol, 2 to 6 μg/min, to increase the heart rate to 100 to 120 bpm. The cardiac output of the denervated transplanted heart is rate dependent. However, the denervated heart retains a relatively normal Frank-Starling curve. Central venous pressure should be increased to 5 to 10 mm Hg by transfusion from the oxygenator. An increased central venous pressure appears to be the mechanism by which transplanted hearts compensate for denervation. With the exception of the 1 to 2% of patients who experience donor heart failure secondary to prolonged ischemia, severe pulmonary hypertension, or a marginal heart for transplantation, discontinuation of bypass is usually uncomplicated.[16]

The sinoatrial node of both donor and recipient heart is usually present but no electrical conduction occurs across thc atrial suture line. The donor sinoatrial node determines the heart rate, although two P waves are often seen on electrocardiogram (ECG). Temporary pacemaker wires are placed, although pacing does not produce the same improvement in cardiac output as does isoproterenol.

Protamine is administered following aortic decannulation while transfusion from the oxygenator may be continued through the venous cannula if necessary. Except for the hemodynamic differences presented earlier and administration of immunosuppressive drugs, the postbypass period is similar to that observed following other cardiac operations. Arterial hypertension is a more common problem postoperatively than hypotension. Systolic pressures over 150 mm Hg should be treated acutely with nitroprusside and chronically with calcium channel blockers.

Postoperative Management

Isoproterenol is often administered continuously in the postbypass period regardless of the apparent condition of the heart. The rate of the transplanted heart at rest is 90 to 100 bpm. Arrhythmias are more common in transplanted hearts, particularly in the early postoperative period. Mechanisms for arrhythmogenesis include surgical trauma to the cardiac conduction system, ischemia during preservation, and atrial suture lines. Sinus node dysfunction, manifest by bradycardia, occurs in 50% of patients in the first few weeks after transplantation. Sinus bradycardia significantly reduces cardiac output, necessitating placement of an atrial pacemaker in 7.4% of patients.[17] The surgical technique of anastomosis to the venae cavae, rather than the atrium, minimizes sinus node damage.[18] Sinus node function improves in the first 3 months following transplantation in 55% of the patients who initially have bradycardia and dysrhythmias.[19] Symptomatic bradycardia occurring more than 1 year following transplantation in 5% of patients is thought to be due to disease in the atrioventricular node.[20] Incomplete right bundle branch block occurs in as many as

70% of patients following transplantation. It may be associated with prolonged donor ischemia time or episodes of rejection.[21] Atrial premature beats, atrial fibrillation or flutter are also common after transplantation, occurring in 76% and 18% of patients, respectively.[22] Ventricular premature beats occur in 100% of patients after transplantation. However, they commonly decrease after the early postoperative period and are not associated with rejection. Sustained or complex ventricular arrhythmias or sudden death episodes are usually associated with either rejection or coronary atherosclerosis. Standard antidysrhythmic drugs and cardioversion are used to treat postoperative dysrhythmias. Following transplantation, tachycardia is not useful as a sign of anesthetic lightness because the heart is denervated and unresponsive to neurogenic stimuli.

Myocardial depression should be avoided in the transplanted heart, since measured cardiac outputs at rest are often less than normal. However, theoretically, the contractility and contractile reserve of the transplanted heart should be normal. Alterations in cardiac output occur through the Anrep (ventricular performance increases several beats following initial stretching of myocardial fibers owing to abruptly increased aortic or left ventricular pressure) and Bowditch (treppe or staircase phenomenon in which a progressive increase in contractile force is associated with a sudden increase in heart rate) effects. The Anrep effect results from more rapid activation of the contractile process, while the Bowditch effect results from variation in myofibril calcium sensitivity and alteration of activator calcium. Cardiac output and stroke volume increase in the first 2 to 4 days following transplantation.

Hyperacute rejection, an exaggerated immune response occurring within minutes or hours of transplantation, may be secondary to preformed donor-specific antibodies in the recipient. Without mechanical support until retransplantation can be accomplished, hyperacute rejection is fatal. Other forms of rejection are discussed later in this chapter. Another rare complication presenting early after transplantation is refractory hypoxemia secondary to patency of the foramen ovale in the transplanted heart.[23] Short-term and long-term survival rates are seen in Figures 19–3*A* and 19–4.

Anesthetic Management of the Patient Following Cardiac Transplantation

Preoperative Evaluation

The majority of heart transplant recipients return to New York Heart Association functional Class I following transplantation. Survival at 1 year following transplantation is about 80%. As seen in Figure 19–3*B*, survival decreases with increasing age of the recipient, particularly over age 65 years.[24] Other factors associated with reduced 1-year survival in the most recent UNOS report are older donors, older recipients, longer preservation times, repeat transplantation, and poor preoperative status of the recipient (requiring mechanical ventilation, intra-aortic balloon pump, left ventricular assist device, or intensive care).[3] Although most cardiac transplant patients do not perceive any limitations to activity, only 53% of them are working.[24]

Subsequent surgical procedures may be required for disease acquired as a consequence of immunosuppression such as malignancy, infection, and steroid-induced osteoporosis or unrelated problems. Well-known complications associated with cardiac transplantation include hypertension (resulting from immunosuppressive drugs such as tacrolimus and cyclosporine), hyperlipidemia (associated with steroid therapy), osteoporosis (resulting from steroid therapy), malignancy (associated with prolonged immunosuppression), and gastrointestinal complications (biliary disease, pancreatitis, peptic ulcer disease).

Preoperative evaluation should include review of recent ECGs, chest x-ray, myocardial biopsy results, hemoglobin, blood urea nitrogen (BUN), creatinine, electrolytes, and liver function tests. An echocardiogram to evaluate ventricular function or exercise stress test to check for graft coronary artery disease should be performed if possible. If the patient has a pacemaker, its function should be evaluated preoperatively. Checking for rejection and infection are essential additional components of the preoperative evaluation.

Evaluation for Rejection

Cardiac transplant recipients usually experience two to three episodes of rejection within the first year after transplant. Rejection is most likely in the first 3 to 6 months and decreases after that time.[25] Rejection has no specific clinical signs in its early stages. However, fatigue, relative hypotension (decrease in systolic pressure >20 mm Hg below control), an S_3 gallop, elevated jugular venous pressure, and other symptoms of left ventricular dysfunction may be present. These findings, as well as pericardial effusion, worsening systolic/diastolic function on echocardiography, and atrial/ventricular arrhythmias, should prompt emergent myocardial biopsy. Endomyocardial biopsy remains the "gold standard" for evaluation of rejection, although signal-averaged electrocardiography and serum troponin T levels show promise as noninvasive methods to detect rejection. A percutaneous transvascular approach through the right internal jugular vein with echocardiographic or fluoroscopic guidance is used to obtain a specimen using a bioptome forceps. The procedure is performed on outpatients at weekly intervals for the first 4 weeks postoperatively and then every other week for the second postoperative month, monthly from 2 to 6 months postoperatively, and every 3 months until the end of the first postoperative year. The schedule of myocardial biopsies is individualized after the first year but biopsies continue at least one to two times per year in subsequent years. Light microscopic examination of the myocardium allows grading of rejection using the International Society for Heart and Lung Transplantation (ISHLT) accepted scale of grade 0 to 4 with grade 4 having the most severe evidence of rejection.[26] Characteristics of severe rejection include diffuse aggressive polymorphous infiltrate with edema, hemorrhage, vasculitis, and necrosis.

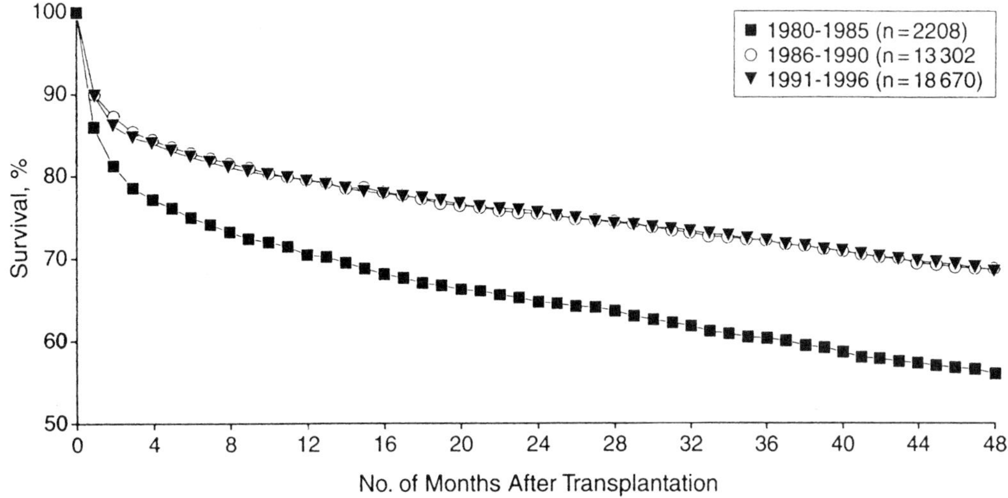

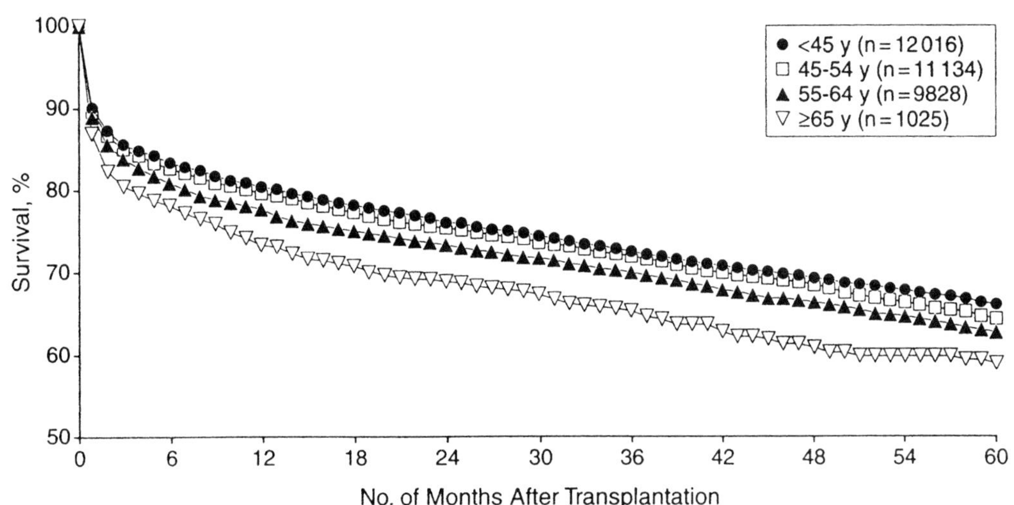

FIGURE **19–3.** *A*, Adult heart transplant actuarial survival by era of transplantation. Survival has improved since 1986. The survival is 8.0 years for patients transplanted between 1991 and 1996 versus only 5.4 years for those transplanted between 1980 and 1986. *B*, Adult heart transplant actuarial survival by patient age at the time of transplantation. Younger patients are significantly more likely to survive than older patients. (From Hosenpud JD, Bennett LE, Keck BM, et al: The Registry of the International Society for Heart and Lung Transplantation. 15th Official Report—1998. J Heart Lung Transplant 17:656, 1998, with permission.)

There are three types of rejection of cardiac allografts: (1) hyperacute, (2) acute vascular, and (3) acute cellular. The most common form is acute cellular rejection, and 50% of these episodes occur in the first 2 to 3 months following transplantation. Episodes of acute cellular rejection occurring early following transplantation are more severe than later episodes. Acute cellular rejection episodes tend to decrease with time. Among the factors associated with increased risk of acute cellular rejection are female gender, young age, non-O blood types, panel reactive antibody (PRA) screen greater than 10%, positive donor-specific crossmatch, human leukocyte antigen (HLA) mismatch, cytomegalovirus (CMV) infection, OKT3 murine monoclonal antibody sensitization, and presence of anti-HLA antibodies.[27]

Acute vascular rejection is diagnosed on myocardial biopsy. Light microscopy and immunofluorescent staining reveal immunoglobulin and complement deposition on vascular endothelium and endothelial swelling. Acute vascular rejection results in a greater incidence of mortality, tenfold increase in allograft coronary artery disease, hemodynamic compromise, and decreased long-term survival.[28] The hyperacute type was discussed earlier.

Immunosuppressive Drugs

Most patients will be on a three-drug regimen consisting of cyclosporine, azathioprine, and corticosteroids. Drug protocols vary by transplantation center. Table 19–1 details the mechanism of action, potential interactions, and toxicity of commonly used immunosuppressive drugs. The most intense immunosuppression is usually administered immediately following surgery and tapered at a

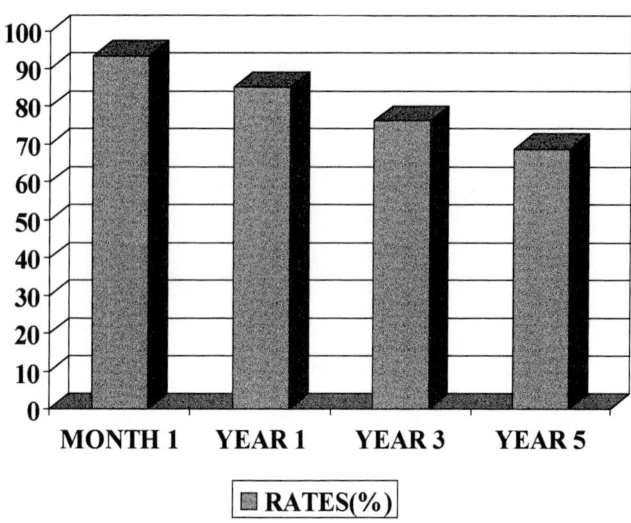

FIGURE **19–4.** Survival following cardiac transplantation decreases over time with a 68.9% surviving for five years. (Data from the United Network for Organ Sharing Annual Report, 1997.)

later time. Early postoperative lympholytic or "induction" therapy includes polyclonal antithymocyte globulin or the monoclonal anti-CD3 OKT3. The advantages of induction therapy are that it allows a delay in the introduction of cyclosporine in patients with marginal renal function and delays the first rejection episode to a time when the patient has recovered more completely from the effects of end-stage cardiac failure.[29] Corticosteroids are commonly reduced to minimal levels as time from transplantation progresses. However, augmented doses of corticosteroid are the mainstay for treating rejection episodes. When rejection is resistant to steroids, daily courses of lympholytic therapy with antithymocyte globulin or OKT3, adjunctive methotrexate, total lymphoid irradiation, and photopheresis have been used.[6] Rejection causing graft failure within the first 6 months after transplantation may necessitate retransplantation.

Several newer immunosuppressive drugs have become part of the antirejection armamentarium. One of these is tacrolimus, which has been found to be effective in rescue therapy for intractable cardiac rejection as a substitute for cyclosporine.[30] However, tacrolimus has no advantage over cyclosporine as a part of the standard regimen.[31] A second drug is mycophenolate mofetil, which has been used as a substitute for azathioprine. One tentative advantage of mycophenolate mofetil may be reduced coronary atherosclerosis.[32] Other antirejection drugs currently under investigation are rapamycin, deoxyspergualin, and leflunomide. All immunosuppressive drugs must be continued throughout the perioperative period.

Perioperative Management

ANATOMY AND PHYSIOLOGY OF THE TRANSPLANTED HEART

Anatomic Connections. Because portions of both native and donor right atria are present, two P waves may be seen on the electrocardiogram. Native sinus node activity is not transmitted across the midatrial suture line.[33] Asynchronous contraction occurs between the native and allograft atria, reducing the usual 15 to 20% atrial contribution to ventricular stroke volume, the "atrial kick." Mitral regurgitation is common because of alterations in

TABLE **19–1**
Immunosuppressive Drugs

Drug	Mechanism of Action	Interactions	Toxicity
Azathioprine	Decreased synthesis/utilization of RNA/DNA precursors	Allopurinol slows its metabolism	Anemia, leukopenia, cholestatic jaundice, hepatitis, pancreatitis
Steroids	Inhibition of release/action of leukokines; interference with antigen-receptor interactions	None	Pituitary-adrenal suppression with cushingoid features, psychoses, glucose intolerance, hypertension, skin fragility, ulcers, osteoporosis, etc
Cyclosporine	Inhibits synthesis of interleukin 1 and other lymphokines; causes lymphocytolysis	Metabolism decreased by metoclopramide, cimetidine, verapamil, diltiazem, alcohol, and other drugs	Hypertension, nephrotoxicity, hepatotoxicity
Tacrolimus	Inhibits production of interleukin 2 and other lymphokines	Similar to cyclosporine	Nephrotoxicity, glucose intolerance, hypertension, neurotoxicity
Mycophenolate mofetil	Inhibition of inosine monophosphate dehydrogenase	Increases level of acyclovir	Irritation of gastrointestinal tract (diarrhea, ulcers, perforation, bleeding)
Muromonab-CD3 Antibody (OKT3)	Inhibits antigen recognition by binding to the CD3 surface antigen of lymphocytes, lymphocyte opsonization	None	Gastrointestinal problems, cytokine release syndrome (fever, chills, hypotension, pulmonary edema)
Antithymocyte globulin	Opsonization of lymphocytes	None	Allergic reactions, serum sickness, fever, chills

left atrial geometry caused by transplantation.[34] Moderate to severe tricuspid regurgitation is often present.[35] Spontaneous echocardiographic contrast has been demonstrated in the left atrium of 55% of patients in one series and was associated with reduced ejection fractions.[36] Otherwise, the anatomic arrangements are normal.

Ventricular Function. Myocardial metabolism is normal. A restrictive hemodynamic pattern is seen with volume administration in the early weeks following transplantation.[37] Donor-recipient size mismatches and graft rejection have been associated with the restrictive filling pattern. It usually resolves within weeks but may be present subclinically for a longer time. Otherwise, systolic ventricular function as determined by ejection fraction and contractile reserve should be normal unless rejection is present.[38] Left ventricular volume increases but left ventricular mass is normal.[39] Diastolic relaxation and compliance may be abnormal, necessitating higher filling pressures to maintain cardiac output, particularly in the early postoperative period. Diastolic function appears to normalize over time.[40] Resting diastolic peak filling rates and time to peak diastolic filling are normal.[38] The Frank-Starling mechanism remains intact. The transplanted heart functions on a steeper, leftward-shifted ventricular pressure-volume curve (Table 19–2).

The overall response of the transplanted heart to exercise is subnormal, probably because of denervation.[41] In response to exercise, cardiac output increases initially by an increase in stroke volume and the Frank-Starling mechanism causing increased stroke volume.[42] Blood pressure increases in response to physical or mental stress.[43] Velocity and extent of fiber shortening, right and left ejection fractions, and peak diastolic filling rate increase during exercise. Only as exercise continues will cardiac output increase by an increase in heart rate caused by increased catecholamines. All responses to stress are abnormally slow in the cardiac transplant recipient because of its denervation, although they ultimately occur.[44] The peak right and left ventricular ejection fractions attained during exercise are significantly lower than those of normal humans. These reduced responses to exercise are still present 2 to 6 years after transplantation and are associated with decreased peripheral oxygen delivery and utilization[45] (see Table 19–2).

TABLE 19–2
Cardiac Function Following Transplantation

Myocardial metabolism normal
Ventricular function slightly reduced
Contractile reserve normal
Frank-Starling mechanism intact
Left ventricular mass/end-diastolic wall thickness are normal
Diastolic relaxation abnormal
Preload dependence for ventricular output
Exercise response
Cardiac output increases owing to increased venous return
Heart rate increases owing to catecholamine increases

Denervation. During transplantation, sympathetic postganglionic, parasympathetic preganglionic, and afferent nerves to the heart are transected. The loss of efferent sympathetic innervation prevents the heart from rapidly changing rate and contractility in response to exercise, hypovolemia, or vasodilatation. Afferent nerve interruption impairs renin-angiotensin-aldosterone regulation, vasoregulatory responses to changes in cardiac filling pressures, and eliminates the afferent signals perceived as angina. Sectioning of the postganglionic sympathetic fibers causes depletion of norepinephrine at the nerve terminal. Catecholamine uptake at the nerve terminals is impaired, resulting in accumulation of circulating catecholamines at the receptors. There is a relative preponderance of β_2-receptors in transplanted hearts, suggesting that nonselective β-agonists rather than selective β_1-agonists should be used to enhance cardiac performance. An increased sensitivity to β-adrenergic agents, particularly norepinephrine, has been described by some authors[46] but is not generally accepted.[47]

Heart rate is determined by the donor sinoatrial node. Loss of vagal effects on both the sinus and atrioventricular (AV) nodes results in an increased resting heart rate of 90 to 100 bpm. Heart rate is unresponsive to drugs or physiologic compensatory mechanisms such as carotid sinus massage. Arrhythmias are particularly prominent during the first 6 months following transplantation and may be exacerbated by episodes of rejection.

Cardiac reinnervation may occur over time, as indicated by a number of physiologic studies.[48,49] The physiologic evidence of reinnervation includes release of cardiac norepinephrine in response to tyramine infusion,[50] physiologic responses to tyramine infusions,[48] and occurrence of angina pectoris.[51] Sympathetic reinnervation may occur before, or in the absence of parasympathetic reinnervation.[52] However, while parasympathetic reinnervation has been demonstrated in animals, only sympathetic reinnervation has been demonstrated in human cardiac transplants.[53]

CORONARY CIRCULATION

Autoregulation. Resting coronary flow is usually increased because of loss of basal adrenergic tone. Coronary autoregulation is intact in the transplanted heart and flow remains dependent upon pH and P_{CO_2}. The coronary circulation remains responsive to adrenoceptor agonists and antagonists (Table 19–3). Coronary vasospasm has been reported in transplanted hearts. In the denervated heart, acetylcholine is a coronary vasoconstrictor.

TABLE 19–3
Changes in Coronary Circulation Following Transplantation

Resting coronary flow increased by absence of α-adrenergic tone
Coronary flow regulated by pH and P_{CO_2} with intact autoregulation
Vasospasm and vasoconstriction in response to acetylcholine possible
Coronary atherosclerosis accelerated and silent ischemia likely

Accelerated Atherosclerosis. One of the main complications limiting survival following cardiac transplantation is the development of diffuse obliterative coronary arteriopathy. This complication affects 10 to 20% at 1 year, 25 to 45 % at 3 years, and 50% of patients within 5 years of transplantation.[54] The arteriopathy is concentric, longitudinal, and diffuse, affecting the epicardial coronary arteries and all of their branches.[6] Collateral formation is uncommon. On angiography, the extent of disease may be somewhat difficult to determine because of the diffuse narrowing of the arteries. Intravascular ultrasound is more sensitive than angiography in the detection of the severe intimal thickening.[55] Other diagnostic techniques include dobutamine stress echocardiography and stress thallium scintigraphy, both of which predict adverse cardiac events and mortality.[56,57] The accelerated atherosclerotic process is not unique to the heart and occurs in all other transplanted organs. However, traditional risk factors for coronary artery disease may exacerbate the problem.

Silent Ischemia. Silent coronary disease secondary to accelerated atherosclerosis is present in 25 to 44% of those surviving beyond 3 years due to disruption of afferent nerve fibers responsible for ischemic pain. Thus, the presenting signs are those resulting from ischemia such as left ventricular dysfunction, ventricular arrhythmias, or even sudden death. Survival following angiographically demonstrated arteriopathy is reported at 63% for any lesion producing greater than 40% vessel occlusion.[58] Interventional coronary procedures have been used to manage the arteriopathy with initial success and safety. However, progression of arteriopathy occurred so that only short-term palliation was evident.[59] Retransplantation has been used successfully to manage coronary arteriopathy with outcomes similar to those of primary transplantation.[60]

Preload-Afterload Dependence. Postural changes in blood pressure are enhanced in the patient with a transplanted heart. Venous return must be maintained to ensure adequate cardiac output.

PRACTICAL ANESTHETIC CONSIDERATIONS

Infection Concerns. Cardiac transplant recipients are always at risk for infection, particularly when high doses of immunosuppressive therapy are needed. All types of infections—viral, bacterial, protozoal, and fungal—may occur. Infections are particularly common within the first month after transplantation because of nosocomial infections. Two to 5 months later, opportunistic infections such as CMV, fungi, and pneumocystic predominate. Some infections result from transplants from donors seropositive for CMV, herpes simplex, or Epstein-Barr viruses into seronegative recipients. Prophylactic therapy with sulfamethoxazole and trimethoprim for *Pneumocystis carinii*, gancyclovir for CMV, acyclovir for herpes simplex, pyrimethamine for toxoplasmosis, and nystatin for *Candida* is effective.[61,62] The lung is the most common site of infection, so that a screening chest x-ray is essential prior to anesthesia. Aseptic precautions in the instrumentation and management of the airway and vascular access sites are mandatory. Antibiotic coverage for the perioperative period is recommended.

Monitoring. The choice of monitoring devices beyond those recommended for all anesthetics is determined by the surgical procedure if the patient's cardiac function is satisfactory. Invasive monitoring should be limited to minimize the risk of infection. The ECG should be monitored for both ischemia and arrhythmias. The presence of two P waves, one from the native atrium and the other from the transplanted atrium is expected.

Anesthetic Techniques. Because patients with transplanted hearts usually have increased systemic vascular resistance and are dependent upon venous return for cardiac output, any technique that may suddenly reduce either venous return or vascular resistance must be carefully monitored and conducted. Regional anesthetics such as spinal or epidural require adequate fluid preloading to avoid hypotension. Incremental dosing through an epidural catheter poses less risk of hypotension in the transplant patient. Joshi and co-workers reported that cardiac transplant patients tolerated pneumoperitoneum for laparoscopic cholescystectomy without adverse effects. Cardiac index and mean arterial pressure returned to control values with pneumoperitoneum while central venous pressure and pulmonary artery wedge pressure increased.[63]

Interactions of Anesthetic Drugs and Immunosuppressive Drugs. Cyclosporine adversely affects renal function so that drugs excreted by the kidney may not be readily cleared. It has also been reported to enhance neuromuscular blockade from atracurium and vecuronium.[64] Potentiation of fentanyl by cyclosporine has also been described in animal studies.[65] Other investigators have not reported clinically significant potentiation in human transplant patients.[66,67] An additional bolus of steroid is usually given in the perioperative period.

Effects of Specific Drugs in Transplanted Hearts. Only drugs that act directly on the heart will be effective. Drugs acting through the autonomic nervous system will generally be ineffective. Drugs with both direct and indirect effects will demonstrate only direct actions. Cardiac α- and β-adrenoceptors are intact without evidence of denervation hypersensitivity. Denervated hearts also respond normally to glucagon, norepinephrine, epinephrine, and propranolol. Phenylephrine, a direct vasoconstrictor, is also effective and should be readily available when anesthetizing cardiac transplant recipients. Acute administration of digoxin has no electrophysiologic effects, but chronic administration depresses atrioventricular conduction. Quinidine slows atrioventricular conduction and sinus rate in transplanted hearts. Drugs with both direct and indirect effects exert only their direct effects in patients with transplanted hearts. The vagotonic effects of neostigmine would not be expected in transplanted hearts. However, Backman and colleagues and Beebe and co-workers reported bradycardia following neostigmine in patients with transplanted hearts.[68,69] Likewise, vagolytic drugs such as atropine would not be expected to be effective in transplanted hearts. However, atropine reversed the neostigmine-induced bradycardia in the patients reported by Backman and Beebe.[68,69] Infusions of isoproterenol should be available to treat bradycardia unresponsive to atropine. Ephedrine may also be used to treat bradycardia or hypotension. Propranolol blocks the effects of isoproterenol and norepinephrine at the sinoatrial node. Pancuronium does not exert its vagolytic effect in a transplanted heart. Whether succinylcholine produces bradycardia in the transplanted heart is unclear. However, atropine may not reverse succinylcholine-induced bradycardia so succinylcholine is usually avoided in patients with cardiac transplants.

Postoperative Concerns. Early extubation is desirable to minimize the risk of pulmonary infection from prolonged mechanical ventilation. The function of other organs compromised by immunosuppressive drugs or chronic heart failure such as the liver or kidneys should be closely monitored by laboratory testing. Because these patients are at risk for silent ischemia, the ECG should be carefully observed using ST-segment trend analysis, if possible. Immunotherapy should be resumed at preoperative doses using alternative routes if necessary because oral intake is precluded by the surgical procedure or ileus. Fluid balance must be carefully monitored, as hypovolemia or hypervolemia are both undesirable. Evidence of infection should be sought and promptly investigated and treated.[70]

Lung Transplantation

Lung transplantation became feasible as a result of the pioneering work of Dr. Joel Cooper in Toronto to reduce the incidence of dehiscence of the bronchial anastomosis and improved antirejection protocols.[71–73] While heart-lung transplantation was initially performed for patients with end-stage pulmonary disease, the recognition that the right heart dysfunction was reversible following lung transplantation has led to the preferential use of single or double-lung transplantation. Single, double, or heart-lung transplantation are increasingly important therapeutic options for many patients with end-stage pulmonary disease.[74]

Indications

The most common etiology of pulmonary failure requiring transplantation is idiopathic pulmonary fibrosis, followed by emphysema. Less common indications are bronchiectasis, sarcoidosis, Eisenmenger's syndrome, bronchiolitis obliterans, primary pulmonary hypertension, eosinophilic granuloma of the lung, lymphangioleiomyomatosis, and α_1-antitrypsin deficiency. Bilateral lung transplantation is often considered for patients with cystic fibrosis, bronchiectasis, emphysema, α_1-antitrypsin deficiency, primary pulmonary hypertension, or Eisenmenger's syndrome.[75] Patients with the latter two indications often require heart-lung transplantation. Single lung transplantation is not usually performed in patients with cystic fibrosis because of the risk of infectious contamination of the transplanted lung by the native lung. Bilateral lung transplantation has been reported to reduce early postoperative mortality in patients with chronic obstructive pulmonary disease as compared to single lung transplantation.[76]

Patient Selection

Criteria for consideration of a patient for lung transplantation include age less than 60 years, absence of major systemic illness or end-organ disease, no prior major thoracic surgery, minimal or no systemic steroid therapy, participation in a pulmonary rehabilitation program, adequate nutritional status, no major psychiatric or substance abuse history, and adequate financial and psychosocial support.[91] Older patients with severe bullous emphysema are usually considered for lung volume reduction surgery rather than lung transplantation.[77] Other chronic diseases or organ damage secondary to pulmonary disease may complicate an otherwise successful lung transplant. Likewise, prior thoracic surgery is likely to distort intrathoracic anatomy with adhesion formation, increasing the risk during surgical dissection. Postoperative complications are also reduced by good nutrition, body weight within 10% of ideal, and increasing activity/strength through an exercise program. Because patients with transplanted organs and their families face significant stresses, mental health and psychosocial support are essential prerequisites.

The evaluation for lung transplantation includes pulmonary consultation, pulmonary function tests, arterial blood gases, chest radiograph, computed tomography of the chest, sputum culture and antibiotic sensitivity analysis, and quantitative ventilation/perfusion scan to evaluate the native lungs. Cardiology consultation with echocardiography, right heart catheterization (and left heart catheterization if greater than 50 years of age or other indications are present), duplex examination of the deep venous system, and duplex examination of carotid arteries and arterial system (if indicated) is performed. Other consultations are requested from thoracic surgery, physical therapy/rehabilitation medicine, social service, nutrition, and mental health professionals.[75] Resting arterial blood-gas values on room air of $Pa{O_2}$ less than 55 mm Hg and $Pa{CO_2}$ greater than 50 mm Hg are associated with less than 50% 2-year survival rates without transplantation.[78] An FEV_1 of 20% of predicted also suggests need for transplantation.

Donor Management

Successful lung transplantation requires functional lungs following procurement and preservation. Criteria for lung donors have been summarized by Gayes and coworkers in Table 19–4. In addition to the activities used to preserve other organs for transplantation, lung preservation requires precise fluid administration to prevent pulmonary edema while treating hypotension and fluid loss. Central venous pressure is maintained at less than 10 mm Hg or pulmonary wedge pressure below 12 mm

TABLE 19–4
Donor Criteria for Lung Transplantation*

Age <55 years
Negative pulmonary history
Absence of pulmonary trauma or only mild parenchymal damage in contralateral lung not targeted for harvesting
Absence of sepsis
No prior thoracic surgery
No organisms or white cells on Gram's stain of tracheobronchial aspirate
Normal endobronchial anatomy on bronchoscopy
ABO blood type match
Lung size to within 2 cm of the transverse and apex-to-base measurements of the planned recipient
Arterial blood gas values:
Pa_{O_2} >100 mm Hg on F_{IO_2} 0.4 or > 350 mm Hg on F_{IO_2} 1.0 without PEEP
Pa_{CO_2} <40 mm Hg at tidal volume of 15 ml/kg and respiratory rate of 10–14 min
Peak inspiratory pressure of <20 cm H_2O at tidal volume of 15 ml/kg

*Modified from Gayes JM, Giron L, Nissen MD, Plut D: Anesthetic considerations for patients undergoing double-lung transplantation. J Thorac Cardiovasc Anesth 4:486, 1990, with permission.

Hg. However, the development of diabetes insipidus (DI), associated with brain death, causes excessive urinary losses. Administration of vasopressin, 5 to 10 IU subcutaneously or intramuscularly every 8 hours or 10 to 40 μg of intranasal desmopressin or 0.3 μg/kg intravenously over 30 minutes accompanied by administration of fluid at 100 ml/hr plus the previous hours' urinary output will control DI. Any electrolyte abnormalities should be corrected. Optimal urine output is 1 ml/kg/hr.

Respiratory management includes maintenance of the Pa_{O_2} about 100 mm Hg on the lowest possible F_{IO_2}. Arterial blood gases should be evaluated every 2 hours. Ventilatory gases should be warmed and humidified to prevent drying of airway secretions and to maintain body temperature. Careful tracheobronchial toilet should be performed, including aseptic suctioning and instillation of small volumes of normal saline every 2 hours.

Matching of donor lungs with the recipient is a critical part of the donor selection process. A single transplanted lung should have an approximately ideal total lung capacity for the recipient. Lungs that are too large for the recipient may interfere with venous return, develop atelectasis, or produce cardiac compression.[75] Recipient height is the most important single indicator of total lung capacity. Another size criteria is a donor/recipient inframammary chest circumference ratio of 0.89.[79]

Donor hypotension results from the loss of vasomotor tone associated with brain death. Mean blood pressure in the donor is maintained at values greater than 70 mm Hg by judicious fluid administration and administration of vasopressors, usually dopamine in doses of 2 to 10 μg/kg/min or phenylephrine 1 to 3 μg/kg/min.

Lung Procurement

The lungs are prepared before harvesting of the heart if both organs are to be removed for transplantation. The lungs should be ventilated with a tidal volume of at least 20 ml/kg and continuous positive airway pressure (CPAP) of 30 cm H_2O should be applied immediately before stapling the trachea. An oxygen-containing mixture is used for lung inflation during ischemia. The pulmonary artery is cannulated with an 18-gauge catheter and flushed with 50 to 60 ml/kg of 4°C modified Euro-Collins "pulmonoplegia" containing prostaglandin E_1 (PGE_1) or prostacyclin at a perfusion pressure of 20 to 30 mm Hg as the aorta is cross-clamped.[80] The lungs and heart are usually removed en bloc if both organs are to be transplanted. When only the lungs are harvested, the surgical technique is similar to pneumonectomy performed for other reasons. As long a piece of main pulmonary artery and bronchus as possible is removed with the lung (Fig. 19–5). Lung ischemia time is measured from the time of removal to reperfusion in the recipient. The lungs are immersed in cold Euro-Collins solution during ischemia, as hypothermia reduces the lung's metabolic rate and delays the depletion of metabolic substrates. Times of 4 to 8 hours or less are essential to limit reperfusion injury.

Recipient Anesthetic Management

Preoperative Evaluation

Evaluation of the lung transplant patient by the anesthesiologist should occur at the time the patient is listed as a transplant candidate. All of the essential information about cardiopulmonary function (spirometry, lung volume measurements, ventilation/perfusion scans, right heart catheterization, exercise capacity, and echocardiography), other medical conditions, prior surgical and anesthetic experiences or complications, medications, and allergies should be reviewed. Adequate right heart function is particularly critical, since the pulmonary artery is cross-clamped during operation, acutely increasing pulmonary vascular resistance. Patients should be counseled about the risks of the proposed anesthetic and surgical care and the perioperative plan including insertion of vascular cannulae, epidural catheter, and other events. Since the actual surgical and anesthetic procedure may occur weeks or months after this initial evaluation, it is essential to review recent developments in the patient's condition such as changes in exercise tolerance, activity, home oxygen requirements, recent in-

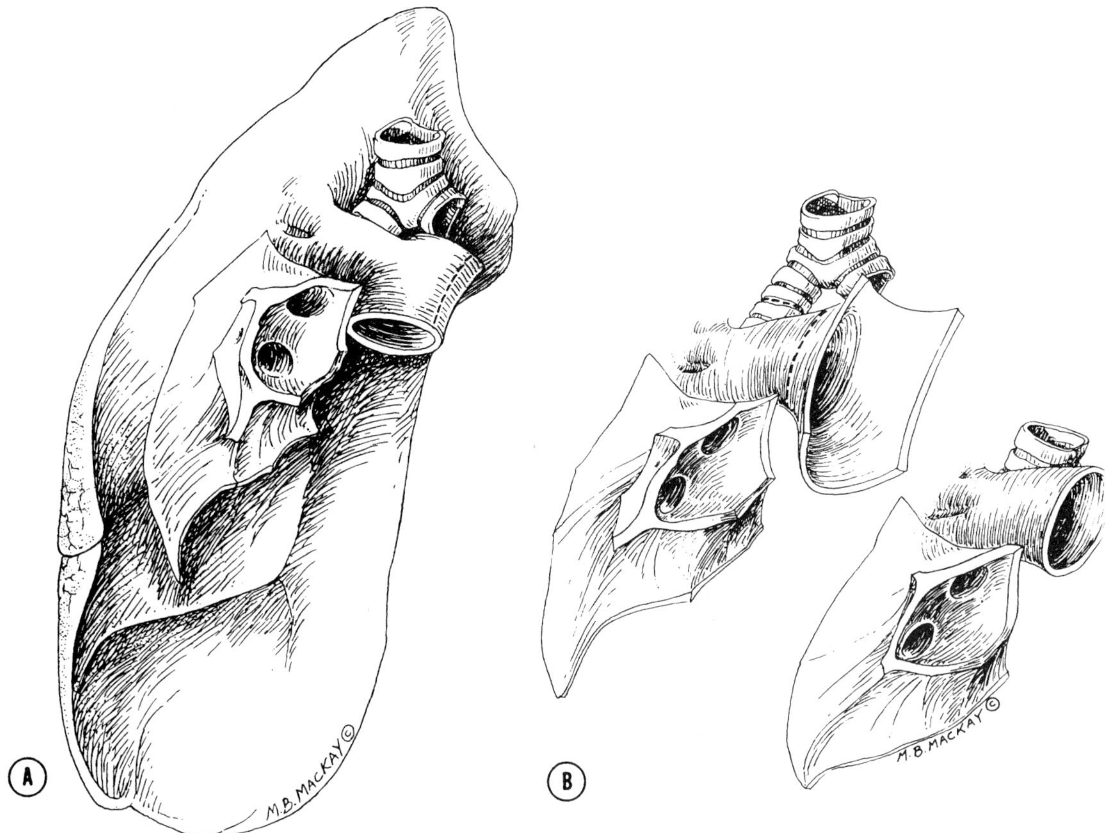

FIGURE **19–5.** *A*, Surgical preparation of a right donor lung. After the heart-lung bloc is removed, the lung is dissected free. The airway is initially divided at the distal trachea and left mainstem bronchus. A cuff of the main pulmonary artery is left attached to the right pumonary artery. A large flap of pericardium is left attached to the lung hiilum. *B*, The donor bronchus has been transected two rings above the origin of the right upper lobe bronchus. If necessary, a portion of the main pulmonary artery is left attached to the right pulmonary artery but often the right pulmonary artery is transected at its origin. (From Cooper JD, Pearson FG, Patterson GA, et al: Technique of successful lung transplantation in humans. J Thorac Cardiovasc Surg 93:173, 1987, with permission.)

fections, and NPO status immediately before the procedure.

Preoperative Preparation

The use of sedative premedication is minimized in these patients to avoid respiratory depression. Careful preoperative counseling is of great benefit in limiting the need for premedication in these highly motivated and cooperative patients. Supplemental oxygen at the same FIO_2 used at home is provided to patients during transport to the operating room and during the preparation phase. The goal is to maintain an SpO_2 of 90 to 95%. If bronchospasm is present or likely in the transplant patient, bronchodilator therapy should be administered before anesthetic induction.

Vascular cannulation includes at least two large-bore intravenous catheters, a radial arterial catheter, and a central venous or pulmonary artery catheter with thermodilution cardiac output capability. Each of these cannulations should be performed using standard technique described elsewhere in this book (see Chapter 9) under strict aseptic technique with sterile gowns, gloves, and equipment. The right internal jugular vein may be used, since it will not be needed for myocardial biopsies as in heart transplant recipients. For single lung transplantation, the tip of the pulmonary artery catheter can be positioned in the contralateral lung.

Postoperative pain relief is essential for lung transplant patients to facilitate early extubation and minimize the need for long-term artificial ventilation. A thoracic epidural catheter is often inserted at the T6–T9 level for this purpose with a test dose of lidocaine 1 to 1.5%, 3 to 5 ml administered to ensure accurate placement. Epidural catheters are not placed if the patient is expected to require cardiopulmonary bypass because of the risk of epidural hematoma associated with systemic anticoagulation. Pain relief for patients requiring bypass is achieved postoperatively when hemostatic function is normal.

Equipment preparation for lung transplantation includes a standard anesthesia machine with a ventilator capable of adjustable flow rates and volume, capnography, transesophageal echocardiography, hemodynamic monitors with multiple pressure modules, pulse oximetry (SpO_2) with multiple probes, ECG with ST-segment monitoring, and cardiac output, temperature probes (nasopharyngeal or urinary bladder), infusion pumps, blood warmer, rapid infusion system, fiberoptic bronchoscopes, range of double lumen/Univent tracheal tubes, and devices for delivery of bronchodilators into the anesthetic circuit. In addition to the standard anesthetic drugs (e.g., induction agent, inhalation anesthetics, neuromuscular blockers), vasoactive infusions (dobutamine, dopamine, epinephrine, isoproterenol, phenylephrine, nitroprusside, PGE_1, amrinone/milrinone) should be readily available.

Anesthesia

If premedication has not been given to the patient, fentanyl 1 to 2 μg/kg or midazolam 0.5 to 1.0 mg may be administered immediately prior to induction while preoxygenation is performed. Induction of anesthesia is performed in a slow and controlled manner using either etomidate 0.2–0.3 mg/kg, thiopental 50-mg increments, or ketamine 1 to 2 mg/kg (for patients with significant reactive airway disease). In some patients induction may need to be accomplished in the sitting position owing to severe dyspnea, orthopnea, or orthodeoxia. Neuromuscular blockade is administered and tracheal intubation is performed. Because all of these patients are considered as full stomachs (oral immunosuppressive drugs given preoperatively as well as the emergent nature of the procedure), rapidly acting neuromuscular blocking drugs are preferable to accomplish a modified rapid sequence induction. Anesthetic maintenance is usually a balanced technique including judicious doses of opioids with isoflurane or other volatile agent. Nitrous oxide is avoided to maximize oxygenation and avoid expansion of bullae. The transesophageal echocardiography transducer is inserted following tracheal intubation and used to monitor right ventricular function and intracardiac air.

The airway is instrumented and a left-sided double-lumen tube placed for bilateral sequential or right single lung transplantation. A tracheal tube with a bronchial blocker (Univent) is often used for left single lung transplantation, although a correctly positioned left endobronchial tube is also usable. Correct positioning of the tracheal tube is confirmed via fiberoptic bronchoscopy. Reevaluation of the tracheal tube position following positioning of the patient for the surgical procedure is essential. Fiberoptic bronchoscopy may also be required at any point during the procedure when single lung ventilation becomes compromised. Common problems associated with tracheal tubes during lung transplantation include: cuff herniation into the tracheal from overinflation or placement too proximal, endobronchial or Univent tube placed too far distally, tube in the wrong bronchus, or tube partially obstructed by secretions.

Ventilation with tidal volumes of 7 to 10 ml/kg, respiratory rates of 10 to 20 breaths per minute, and an FIO_2 that maintains SpO_2 at greater than 96% or SvO_2 greater than 70% usually result in adequate arterial blood gases during recipient pneumonectomy. Hypercarbia and hypoxia are the most common problems during removal of the native lung. Hypercarbia develops because effective ventilation is reduced by the exclusion of one lung and is exacerbated by coexisting obstructive pulmonary disease. Slower respiratory rates may be required to allow adequate expiratory time to prevent gas trapping and "auto-PEEP," which can be quite significant in some patients. Hyperinflation can be so severe as to cause cardiac compression and hemodynamic compromise. A 30-second period of apnea with the breathing circuit open to atmosphere can be life-saving. During one-lung ventilation, a slight increase in respiratory rate, reduction in tidal volume, and tolerance of a slight increase in $PaCO_2$ is preferable to overinflating the ventilated lung.[81] Use of pressure-control, rather than volume-control ventilator mode, may be helpful during intraoperative ventilation of patients with severe obstructive disease.[77] Because most anesthesia machine ventilators are volume-controlled, use of an intensive care unit (ICU) ventilator may produce optimal gas exchange while minimizing barotrauma. With a pressure-control ventilator mode, inspiratory flow occurs until a pressure-control limit is reached. Tidal volume varies slightly from breath to breath depending upon lung and chest wall compliance. Changes in tidal volume alert the anesthesiologist that a change in lung compliance has occurred.

Hypoxemia during bronchial exclusion results in increased shunting through perfused but unventilated alveoli. When desaturation occurs intraoperatively during one-lung ventilation, positive end-expiratory pressure of 5 to 7 cm H_2O applied to the dependent lung may be helpful. Alternatively, CPAP may be applied to the nonventilated lung. Hypoxemia during bronchial exclusion results in increased shunting through perfused but nonventilated alveoli. However, optimal ventilator settings (flow rates and volumes) minimize the need for positive airway pressure during one-lung anesthesia. Reinflation of the nonventilated lung may be required to correct persistent problems with desaturation. Usually, problems with desaturation are temporary and relieved by clamping of the pulmonary artery.

If arterial oxygen saturation cannot be maintained at normoxic levels (SaO_2 less than 90% on $FIO_2 = 1$, SvO_2 <60% on $FIO_2 = 1$), even with optimal ventilation, circulatory support (CI <2 L/m^2/min), and treatment of pulmonary hypertension, cardiopulmonary bypass must be instituted. Cardiopulmonary bypass techniques include femoral-femoral bypass for left lung transplants and aorto–right atrial bypass for right lung transplantation. Usual bypass flow rates are 2.5 L/m^2/min. However, these flow rates may be difficult to maintain during femoral-femoral bypass because of inadequate venous drainage. The need for extracorporeal circulatory support is predicted by severe preoperative pulmonary hypertension and restrictive lung disease, while patients with chronic obstructive pulmonary disease rarely require bypass.[82,83] Use of cardiopulmonary bypass has been reported to worsen endothelial dysfunction in the transplanted lung.[84]

Reperfusion Management

Transplanted lungs are prone to reperfusion injury, the severity of which depends upon the duration of ischemia and effectiveness of preservation techniques. Steroids are often administered immediately prior to reperfusion to complement the immunosuppression with azathioprine and cyclosporine begun preoperatively. Reperfusion injury usually manifests as pulmonary hypertension with worsening of shunting and right ventricular failure. Denervated pulmonary vascular tone is determined by circulating humoral factors. Endothelin is increased immediately following lung transplantation, while endothelial-derived relaxing factor is reduced.[85,86] The condition improves over 4 to 5 hours but may require pharmacologic therapy with PGE_1, phosphodiesterase inhibitors such as amrinone or milrinone, nitroglycerin infusion, dobutamine, or isoproterenol to support the right ventricle and produce pulmonary vasodilation during the intervening period. Inhaled nitric oxide at concentrations of 20 to 60 ppm also produces selective pulmonary vasodilation in patients with severe pulmonary allograft dysfunction.[87] The systemic vasodilation produced by prostaglandin, phosphodiesterase inhibitors, or isoproterenol may necessitate vasopressor support with norepinephrine to maintain arterial pressure. Optimal ventilatory management to maintain Po_2, Pco_2, and ventilatory pressures and volumes is also helpful to control pulmonary hypertension. Once the transplanted lung is in place, distal suctioning should be avoided except under direct bronchoscopic view to prevent disruption of the bronchial anastomosis. Judicious fluid management is essential to avoid fluid accumulation in the newly transplanted lung with its disrupted lymphatic system. Diuretics are also helpful in minimizing the interstitial edema. Immediate improvement in right ventricular failure and pulmonary hypertension occurs.

Surgical Technique

Single lung transplantation is performed via a posterolateral thoracotomy with removal of the native lung and transplantation of the new lung. Bilateral sequential lung transplantation is usually performed through a median sternotomy-bithoracotomy, the so-called clamshell approach (Fig. 19–6). In both single and double lung transplantation, the femoral area is surgically prepared in the event that cardiopulmonary bypass is needed. Careful positioning of the patient is essential to avoid damage to peripheral nerves in the upper extremities.

With double lung transplantation, the right lung is usually transplanted first, followed by the left lung. Alternatively, the lung with the worst function may be removed first so that the newly transplanted lung will support the patient during the sequential lung transplant without a need for cardiopulmonary bypass. For a single lung transplantation, the choice of which side to transplant depends upon the localization of the patient's disease, previous surgery, presence of bullae, necessity for cardiopulmonary bypass, and the orientation of the donor lung.[88] However, the left lung is easier to remove and reimplant because there is a longer length of the recipient bronchus for anastomosis and the left atrium is easily clamped proximal to the pulmonary veins.[73,89] Preservation of the patient's right lung may also theoretically retain more of the lymphatic drainage of the pulmonary parenchyma.[89] The details of the surgical procedure are presented in Figures 19–7 and 19–8. In the recipient, the pulmonary artery is isolated as proximally

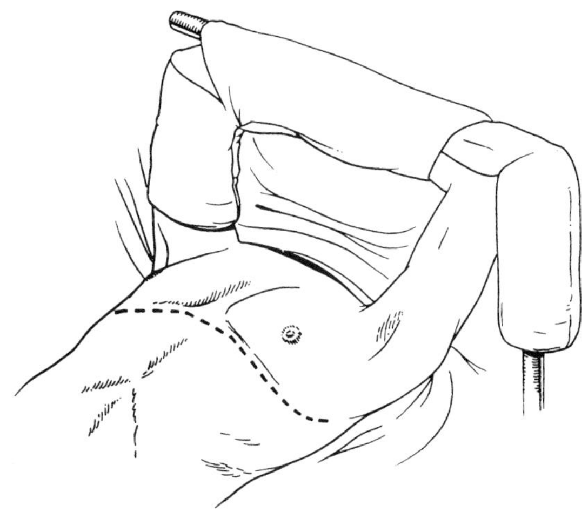

FIGURE **19–6.** The clamshell incision for bilateral sequential lung or heart-lung transplantation. (From Quinlan JJ, Firestone S, Firestone LJ: Anesthesia for heart, lung and heart-lung transplantation. In Kaplan JA, Reich DL, Konstadt SN [eds]: Cardiac Anesthesia, 4th ed. Philadelphia, WB Saunders Co, 1999, with permission.)

as possible. The first branch of the pulmonary artery is divided separately as is its descending branch in order to leave as long a pedicle as possible.[73] The pulmonary veins are located intrapericardially. Temporary occlusion of the pulmonary artery allows observation of patient hemodynamic responses. Pulmonary veins are divided outside the pericardium. The last part of recipient pneumonectomy is bronchial ligation. The bronchus should be divided just proximal to the upper lobe takeoff with extreme care to avoid dissection around the main bronchus.[73]

Considerable retraction of the mediastinum and chest wall is needed during the anastomosis of the pulmonary vessels and bronchi. The bronchial anastomosis is performed first, the pulmonary artery second, and the left atrial anastomosis last. Hemodynamic instability is a frequent consequence of the retraction and dissection. The technique of bronchial anastomosis is particularly critical in order to minimize the likelihood of bronchial dehiscence. The donor bronchus is telescoped inside the recipient bronchus to ensure a well-perfused and strong anastomosis. The earlier technique of bronchial support with an omental flap or pericardial fat pad provides no added benefits. Although bronchial revascularization is anatomically and technically feasible,[90] reestablishment of the bronchial circulation is not usually performed so that circulation to the donor portion of the bronchial anastomosis is dependent upon the native bronchus or omental flap. However, the procedure of telescoping the donor bronchus inside the recipient bronchus has minimized the need for an omental flap in recent years. When anastomosis of the left bronchus is performed, the double-lumen tube may need to be slightly withdrawn, although the anastomotic site is usually sufficiently distal to easily accommodate placement of a left endobronchial tube during bilateral sequential lung transplantation. Deairing of the left atrium and pulmonary circulation is performed via the pulmonary artery immediately prior to

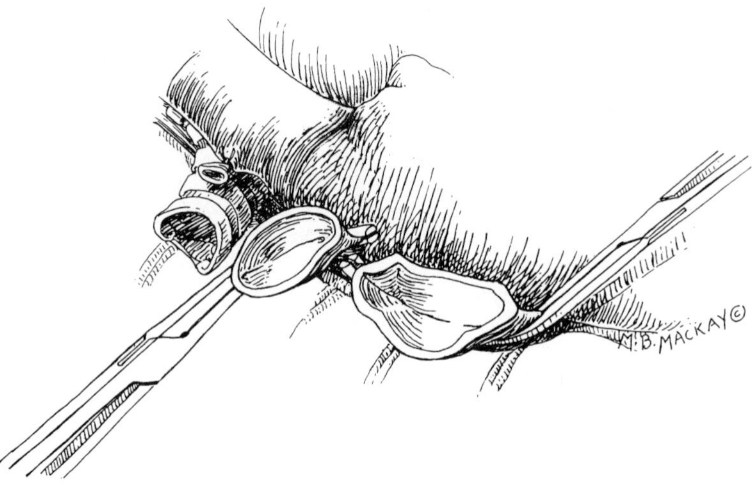

FIGURE **19–7.** The recipient's right hilum is prepared for allograft by clamping the pulmonary artery as proximally as possible, clamping the left atrium intrapericardially, and dividing the recipient bronchus just proximal to the right upper lobe origin. (From Cooper JD, Pearson FG, Patterson GA, et al: Technique of successful lung transplantation in humans. J Thorac Cardiovasc Surg 93:173, 1987, with permission.)

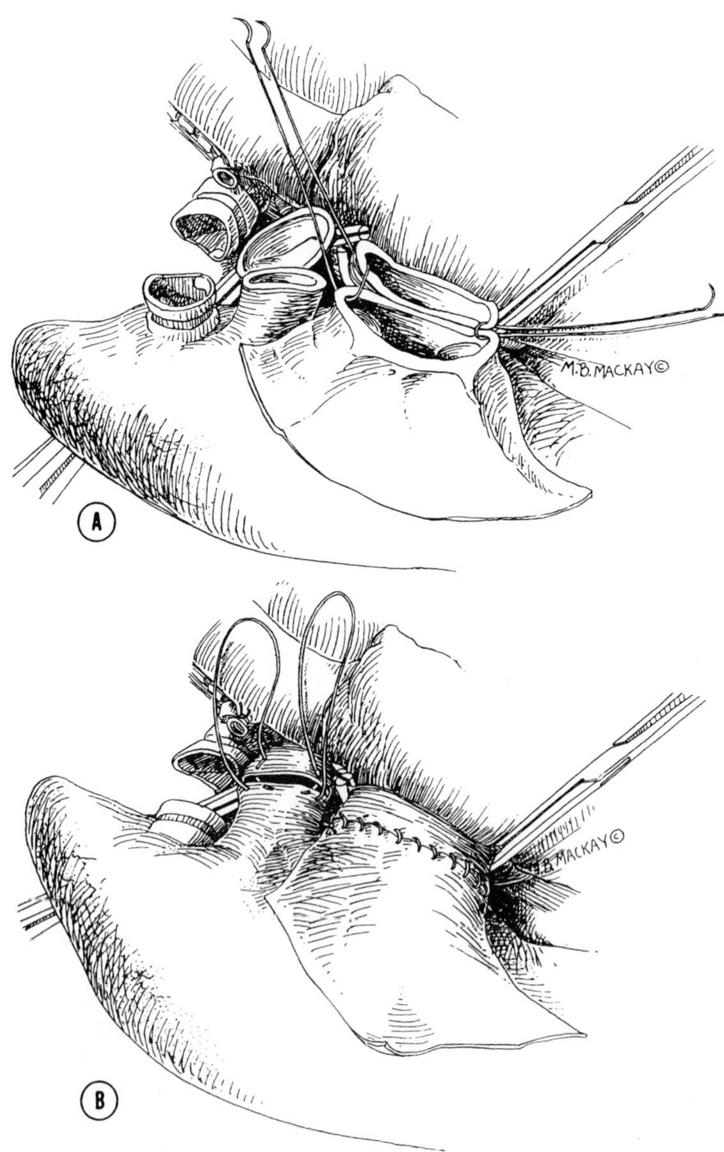

FIGURE **19–8.** Positioning of the donor lung in the recipient's mediastinum and demonstration of the atrial, pulmonary arterial, and bronchial anastomoses. (From Cooper JD, Pearson FG, Patterson GA, et al: Technique of successful lung transplantation in humans. J Thorac Cardiovasc Surg 93:173, 1987, with permission.)

completion of the left atrial anastomosis. The end-tidal carbon dioxide is a valuable indicator of air embolism during unclamping of the atrial anastomosis. Completion of both the pulmonary artery and left atrial anastomoses and unclamping of these vessels restores lung circulation. However, lung reperfusion may exacerbate shunting and hypoxemia until the bronchial anastomosis is completed.

Reperfusion of the transplanted lung following completion of the vascular anastomosis may be associated with hemodynamic and respiratory compromise. Events may include pulmonary hypertension associated with calcium influx into vascular smooth muscle, ventilation/perfusion mismatching, or right heart failure. Treatment of pulmonary hypertension was outlined in the section on anesthetic management.

Immunosuppressive agents are given to coincide with lung reperfusion. These include cyclosporine, azathioprine, corticosteroids, and antilymphocyte globulin. The exact doses and schedule of administration should be verified with transplant specialists.

Postoperative Care

The double-lumen endobronchial tube is replaced with a single-lumen tube prior to leaving the operating room. Bronchoscopy is performed to verify position and perform tracheobronchial toilet. Patients are then transported to the ICU intubated, anesthetized, and manually ventilated. Fluid and hemodynamic management are optimized using inotropic drugs and diuretics to maintain systemic blood pressure, urine output, and oxygen delivery. Steroids for immunosuppression are not usually administered until healing of the bronchus has occurred (~14 days), but azathioprine and cyclosporine are continued in the immediate postoperative period. Broad-spectrum antibiotics are administered to control any pathogens cultured from either donor or recipient.

Early extubation or weaning from mechanical ventilation minimizes the risk of nosocomial infection and barotrauma in the transplanted lung. During mechanical ventilation, gas trapping in the native lung must be avoided by judicious tidal volumes and adequate expiratory times. Independent ventilation of the two lungs may be required following single lung transplantation if severe graft dysfunction is present. Low levels of PEEP are used during ventilation except in the patient with chronic obstructive pulmonary disease receiving a single lung where the compliant native lung might be overinflated. Before extubation, the patient must meet normal respiratory parameters, level of consciousness, adequate upper airway reflexes, recovery of neuromuscular function, and have adequate pain relief before extubation.

Following transplantation, the airway distal to the bronchial anastomosis is denervated, reducing the cough reflex and increasing the risk of silent aspiration. Lung transplant patients must be encouraged to cough, since the subepithelial mechanoreceptors in the bronchi and bronchioles are denervated and unresponsive to stimuli. The ventilatory response to carbon dioxide is also abnormal, possibly owing to vagotomy.[91] Some heart-lung transplant patients will maintain $Pa\text{CO}_2$ of 45 to 50 immediately following surgery, but otherwise, their respiratory function is normal.[98] The transplanted lung is not subject to vagal influences, resulting in bronchodilation and loss of protective bronchoconstriction following small airway irritant receptor stimulation. Nevertheless, bronchoconstriction can occur in transplanted lungs and may signal early rejection.[92] Vagal stimulation to cilia and mucous glands is also absent following transplantation, which may also affect removal of dust or irritant substances from the tracheobronchial tree. The loss of lymphatics in the transplanted lung causes difficulties with removal of pulmonary edema fluid or particulate matter filtered by the lung (such as platelet aggregates in transfused blood). Finally, the bronchial circulation, the principal nutrient circulation to lung tissue, is disrupted in the transplanted lung. Pulmonary reinnervation has not been demonstrated in humans during prolonged follow-up.[93] Despite all of these changes following lung transplantation, respiratory function and gas exchange are usually nearly normal.

Pain relief is provided via thoracic or lumbar epidural once normal coagulation is ensured postoperatively. The epidural catheter may be used to provide pain relief of up to 5 days if necessary. Removal of nasogastric tubes and early oral feeding is also beneficial to minimize bacterial overgrowth in the stomach with the risk of nosocomial infection from silent aspiration. Rapid mobilization of the patient and physical therapy are essential elements for recovery from lung transplantation. Retransplantation of the lung is rarely performed but has been indicated for chronic rejection, early graft failure, or intractable airway problems.[94]

Chest x-rays are performed twice daily while the patient is in the hospital and weekly following discharge. Bronchostenosis at the site of the anastomosis is a well-known complication of lung transplantation.[95] Lung rejection is monitored by serial chest x-rays, changes in clinical condition as determined by pulmonary function testing, alterations in gas exchange, and bronchoscopy. Clinical signs of rejection are nonspecific but may include nonproductive cough, shortness of breath, low-grade fever, or changes in measured pulmonary function. A chest radiograph may demonstrate nonspecific findings of perihilar infiltrates, interstititial edema, or pleural effusions, particularly within the first 6 months following transplantation. Rejection of a lung allograft has two components: (1) a vascular component with endothelial inflammation, and (2) the airway component that may cause bronchiolitis obliterans.[96] Endoscopic transbronchial biopsy is performed once a month for the first 3 months, at 6 months and 1 year following transplantation, and when rejection is suspected. Bronchoalveolar lavage is also performed to establish the diagnosis of rejection.[97] Pulmonary rejection is graded using the scale of the International Society of Heart and Lung Transplantation and is similar to that used to evaluate cardiac rejection. The extent of lymphocytic infiltration, bronchiolar inflammation, and size of the involved airways are determinants of rejection severity. Long-term immunosuppression includes cyclosporine, azathioprine, and prednisone. A variety of immunosuppressive protocols have been used to treat rejection episodes.

Anesthetic Management of the Patient Following Lung Transplantation

As with cardiac transplant patients, the lung transplant patient must be evaluated for the known complications of the procedure, chronic immunosuppression, and infection prior to anesthesia. Most lung transplant patients report dramatic improvements in their quality of life following transplantation. Pulmonary function is usually nearly normal unless bronchiolitis obliterans has developed.

Combined Heart and Lung Transplantation

The etiology of cardiopulmonary failure requiring heart-lung transplantation is usually primary pulmonary hypertension or Eisenmenger's syndrome. Contraindications are similar to those for isolated heart or lung transplantation; namely, life-threatening concurrent illness, peptic ulcer disease, significant psychiatric problems, substance abuse, active infections, and end-stage hepatic or renal disease. The principles of donor management are those described previously for heart and lung transplantation.[98]

Recipients of combined heart-lung transplants require complete preoperative evaluation at the time of their designation as potential recipients. When organs become available, changes in cardiopulmonary parameters are noted, laboratory studies including electrolytes and hemoglobin are measured, and medications such as oxygen and vasodilators are continued up to anesthetic induction. The anesthesia machine, airway equipment, and drugs are prepared as previously described using strict aseptic technique. Intravascular catheters including radial artery and left internal jugular central venous cannulas are inserted using sterile technique. Rapid sequence induction using etomidate, fentanyl or sufentanil, and lidocaine is performed to minimize the risk of aspiration in these seriously compromised patients. Ketamine is usually avoided because of the risk of worsening pulmonary hypertension. The tracheal tube should be inserted to a depth just below the vocal cords and inflated only to occlusion pressure to avoid ischemia of the tracheal mucosa near the anastomotic site.

The surgical procedure is accomplished via median sternotomy. After initiation of cardiopulmonary bypass using bicaval cannulation, the aorta is cross-clamped and the heart removed leaving a cuff of right atrium. The left lung is removed first, followed by the right lung. Careful attention is given to avoid the phrenic and recurrent laryngeal nerves during dissection because of the undesirable postoperative consequences of damage to these nerves. The donor organs are placed in the chest and the tracheal anastomosis is performed first. Following completion of the anastomosis, manual inflation of the lungs at 4 to 6 times per minute is performed at a tidal volume of 400 ml. The right atrial anastomosis is then completed, and ventilation with 40% oxygen and air at 5 cm PEEP is begun. The aortic anastomosis is completed last. After aortic unclamping, isoproterenol infusion is begun to maintain heart rate at 100 bpm. Cardiopulmonary bypass is usually discontinued without difficulty.

In the postbypass period, control of bleeding is often a problem because of the extensive bronchial collateral circulation in the recipient. All of the autologous blood from the extracorporeal circuit is returned to the patient and other blood products are transfused as necessary. Crystalloid infusion is restricted to minimize pulmonary edema.

Early extubation postoperatively is desirable to minimize pulmonary infection. Tracheal suctioning or reintubation must be performed carefully because of the close proximity of the tracheal anastomosis and the risk of its disruption. Immunosuppressive therapy is continued using combinations of methylprednisolone, azathioprine, antithymocyte globulin, cyclosporine, or other drugs. The previously described consequences of denervated heart and lungs and the risk of infection are applicable to these patients as well.

Following transplantation, PaO_2 increases from pretransplant levels and pulmonary function increases progressively so that gas exchange is nearly normal.[99,100] While rejection can affect either transplanted organ, the lung is more commonly rejected. Early cardiac rejection is rare in heart-lung transplant patients. The lung is also more prone to infection. Infection may be difficult to differentiate from rejection, as both cause symptoms of cough, fever, and dyspnea on exertion. Multiple episodes of rejection are associated with the development of obliterative bronchiolitis. Prophylaxis against CMV, *Pneumocystis*, and fungal infections is highly recommended for heart-lung recipients because of the vulnerability of the lung to infection.

Other complications following heart-lung transplantation are similar to those reported for either organ transplanted alone. These include allograft coronary artery disease, lymphoproliferative disease or lymphoma, malignancy, and the sequelae of chronic immunosuppression. Causes of mortality include graft failure, bronchiolitis, infection, transplant coronary disease, and malignancy.

References

1. Hardy JD, Webb WR, Dalton ML, et al: Lung homo-transplantation in man. JAMA 186:1065, 1963.
2. Reitz BA, Hunt SA, Gaudiana V, et al: Clinical heart lung transplantation. Transplant Proc 15:1256, 1983.
3. Lin H-M, Kauffman HM, McBriode MA, et al: Center specific graft and patient survival rates. 1997 United Network for Organ Sharing (UNOS) report. JAMA 280:1153, 1998.
4. Medicare programs: Criteria for Medicare coverage of heart transplants. Federal Register 10935, 1987.
5. Krakuer H, Shakar SS, Kaye MP: The relationship of clinical outcomes to status as a Medicare-approved heart transplant center. Transplantation 59:840, 1995.
6. Hunt SA: Current status of cardiac transplantation. JAMA 280: 1692, 1998.

7. Reardon MJ, Letson GV, Anderson JE, et al: Orthotopic cardiac transplantation after minimally invasive direct coronary artery bypass. J Thorac Cardiovasc Surg 117:390, 1999.
8. Hunt SA: 24th Bethesda Conference: Cardiac Transplantation. J Am Coll Cardiol 22:1, 1993.
9. Mancini DM, Eisen H, Kussmaul W, et al: Value of peak exercise oxygen consumption for optimal timing of cardiac transplantation in ambulatory patients with heart failure. Circulation 83:778, 1991.
10. Aaronson KD, Schwartz JS, Chen TM, et al: Development and prospective validation of a clinical index to predict survival in ambulatory patients referred for cardiac transplant evaluation. Circulation 95:2660, 1997.
11. Lake CL: Chronic treatment of congestive heart failure. In Kaplan JA, Reich DL, Konstadt SN (eds): Cardiac Anesthesia. Philadelphia, WB Saunders Co, 1999, p 131.
12. Hunt SA, Frazier OH: Mechanical circulatory support and cardiac transplantation. Circulation 97:2079, 1998.
13. Hensley FA, Martin DE, Larach DR, et al: Anesthetic management for cardiac transplantation in North America—1986 survey. J Cardiothorac Anesth 1:429, 1987.
14. Lower RR, Shumway NE: Studies of orthotopic homotransplantation of the canine heart. Surg Forum 11:18, 1960.
15. Dreyfus F, Jebara V, Mihaileanu MD, Carpentier A: Total orthotopic heart transplantation: An alternative to the standard technique. Ann Thorac Surg 52:1181, 1991.
16. Calkins MD, Kuzma PJ, Karan SM: Understanding the cardiac transplant patients and anesthetic management for noncardiac surgery. Am J Anesth 25:25, 1998.
17. DiBiase A, Tse TM, Schnittger I, et al: Frequency and mechanism of bradycardia in cardiac transplant recipients and need for pacemakers. Am J Cardiol 67:1385, 1991.
18. Rothman SA, Jeevanandam V, Combs WG, et al: Eliminating bradyarrhythmias after orthotopic heart transplantation. Circulation 94(Suppl II):II278, 1996.
19. Heinz G, Hirschl M, Buxbaum P, et al: Sinus node dysfunction after orthotopic cardiac transplantation: Postoperative incidence and long-term implications. Pacing Clin Electrophysiol 15:731, 1992.
20. Weinfeld MS, Kartashov A, Piana R, Hauptman PJ: Bradycardia: A late complication following cardiac transplantation. Am J Cardiol 78:969, 1996.
21. Villa AE, deMarchena EJ, Myerburg RJ, et al: Comparison of paired orthotopic cardiac transplant donor and recipient electrocardiograms. Am Heart J 127:70, 1994.
22. Scott CD, Dark JH, McComb JM: Arrhythmias after cardiac transplantation. Am J Cardiol 70:1061, 1992.
23. Ouseph R, Stoddard MF, Lederer ED: Patent foramen ovale presenting as refractory hypoxemia after heart transplantation. J Am Soc Echocardiogr 10:973, 1997.
24. Hosenpud JD, Bennett LE, Keck BM, et al: The registry of the International Society for Heart and Lung Transplantation: 15th official report—1998. J Heart Lung Transplant 17:656, 1998.
25. Hunt SA: Complications of heart transplantation. J Heart Transplant 3:70, 1983.
26. Billingham ME, Cary NR, Hammond ME, et al: A working formulation for the standardization of nomenclature in the diagnosis of heart and lung rejection. Heart Rejection Study Group. The International Society for Heart Transplantation. J Heart Transplant 9:587, 1990.
27. Kubo SH, Naftel DC, Mills RM, et al: Risk factors for late recurrent rejection after heart transplantation: A multiinstitutional, multivariable analysis. J Heart Lung Transplant 14:409, 1995.
28. Miller LW, Schlant RC, Kobashigawa J, et al: Task Force #5: Complications. 24th Bethesda Conference: Cardiac Transplantation. J Am Coll Cardiol 22:41, 1993.
29. Starnes VA, Oyer PE, Stinson ED, et al: Prophylactic OKT3 used as induction therapy for heart transplantation. Circulation 80(Suppl 3):79, 1989.
30. Armitage JM, Kormos RL, Griffith BP, et al: A clinical trial of FK506 as primary and rescue immunosuppression in cardiac transplantation. Transplant Proc 23:1149, 1991.
31. Pham SM, Kormos RL, Hattler BG, et al: A prospective trial of tacrolimus (FK506) in clinical heart transplantation: Intermediate-term results. J Thorac Cardiovasc Surg 111:1, 1996.
32. Gregory CR, Prastt RE, Huie P, et al: Effects of treatment with cyclosporine FK 506, rapamycin, mycophenolic acid, or deoxyspergualin on vascular smooth muscle proliferation in vitro and in vivo. Transplant Proc 25:770, 1993.
33. Valantine HA, Appleton CP, Hatle LV, et al: Influence of recipient atrial contraction on left ventricular filling dynamics of the transplanted heart assessed by Doppler echocardiography. Am J cardiol 59:1159, 1987.
34. Stevenson LW, Dadourian BJ, Kobashigawa J, et al: Mitral regurgitation after cardiac transplantation. Am J Cardiol 60:119, 1987.
35. Lewen MK, Brigg RJ, Miller LW, et al: Tricuspid regurgitation by Doppler echocardiography after orthotopic cardiac transplantation. Am J Cardiol 59:1371, 1987.
36. Derumeaux G, Mouton-Schleifer D, Soyer R, et al: High incidence of left atrial thrombus detected by transesophageal echocardiography in heart transplant recipients. Eur Heart J 16:120, 1995.
37. Young JB, Winters WL, Bourge R, Uretsky BF: Task Force #4: Function of the heart transplant recipients. 24th Bethesda Conference: Cardiac Transplantation. J Am Coll Cardiol 22:31, 1993.
38. Verani MS, George Se, Leon CA, et al: Systolic and diastolic ventricular performance at rest and during exercise in heart transplant recipients. J Heart Transplant 7:145, 1988.
39. Stiver EP, Siegel LC: Physiology of the transplanted heart. Int Anesth Clin 33:11, 1995.
40. St. Goar FG, Gibbons R, Schnittger I, et al: Left ventricular diastolic function. Doppler echocardiographic changes soon after cardiac transplantation. Circulation 82:872, 1990.
41. Ehrman J, Keteyian S, Fedel F, et al: Cardiovascular responses of heart transplant recipients to graded exercise testing. J Appl Physiol 73:260, 1992.
42. Pope Se, Stinson EB, Daughters GT, et al: Exercise response of the denervated heart in long-term cardiac transplantation recipients. Am J Cardiol 46:213, 1980.
43. Sehested J, Reinicke G, Ishino K, et al: Blunted humoral responses to mental stress and physical exercise in cardiac transplant recipients. Eur Heart J 16:852, 1995.
44. Pflugfelder PW, Purves PD, McKenzie FN, et al: Cardiac dynamics during supine exercise in cyclosporine-treated orthotopic heart transplant recipients: Assessment by radionuclide angiography. J Am Coll Cardiol 10:336, 1987.
45. Kao AC, Van Trigt P, Shaeffer-McCall G, et al: Allograft diastolic dysfunction and chronotropic incompetence limit cardiac output response to exercise two to six years after heart transplantation. J Heart Lung Transplant 14:11, 1995.
46. Yusuf S, Theodoropoulos S, Mathias CJ, et al: Increased sensitivity of the denervated human transplanted heart to isoadrenaline both before and after beta adrenergic blockade. Circulation 75:696, 1987.
47. Pargger H, Kaufman MA, Schouten R, et al: Hemodynamic responses to electroconvulsive therapy in a patient 5 years after cardiac transplantation. Anesthesiology 83:625, 1995.
48. Burke MN, McGinn AL, Homans DC, et al: Evidence for functional sympathetic reinnervation of left ventricle and coronary arteries after orthotopic cardiac transplantation in humans. Circulation 91:72, 1995.
49. Bernardi L, Bianchini B, Spadacini G, et al: Demonstrable cardiac reinnervation after human heart transplantation by carotid baroreflex modulation of RR interval. Circulation 92:2895, 1995.
50. Wilson RF, Christensen BV, Oliari MT, et al: Evidence for structural sympathetic reinnervation after orthotopic cardiac transplantation in humans. Circulation 83:1210, 1991.
51. Stark RP, McGinn AL, Wilson RF: Chest pain in cardiac transplant recipients: Evidence of sensory reinnervation after cardiac transplantation. N Engl J Med 324:1791, 1991.
52. Mancinci D: Surgically denervated cardiac transplant. Circulation 96:6, 1997.
53. Givertz MM, Hartley LH, Colucci WS: Long-term sequential changes in exercise capacity and chronotropic responsiveness after cardiac transplantation. Circulation 96:232, 1997.
54. Olivari MT, Homans DC, Wilson RF, et al: Coronary artery disease in cardiac transplant patients receiving triple-drug immu-

nosuppressive therapy with cyclosporine and prednisone. Circulation 80(Suppl 3):111, 1989.
55. Mehra MR, Ventura HO, Stapleton DD, et al: Presence of severe intimal thickening by intravascular ultrasonography predicts cardiac events in cardiac allograft vasculopathy. J Heart Lung Transplant 14:632, 1995.
56. Akosah KO, Mohanty PK, Funai TM, et al: Noninvasive detection of transplant coronary artery disease by dobutamine stress echocardiography. J Heart Lung Transplant 13:1024, 1994.
57. Verhoueven PPAM, Lee FA, Ramahi TM, et al: Prognostic value of noninvasive testing one year after orthotopic cardiac transplantation. J Am Coll Cardiol 28:183, 1996.
58. Keogh AM, Valantine HA, Hunt SA, et al: Impact of proximal or midvessel discrete coronary artery stenoses on survival after heart transplantation. J Heart Lung Transplant 11:892, 1992.
59. Halle AA, DiSciascio G, Massein EK, et al: Coronary angioplasty, atherectomy, and bypass surgery in cardiac transplant recipients. J Am Coll Cardiol 26:120, 1995.
60. John R, Chen JM, Weinberg A, et al: Long-term survival after cardiac retransplantation: A twenty-year single-center experience. J Thorac Cardiovasc Surg 117:543, 1999.
61. Olsen SL, Eastburn TE, Renlund DG, et al: Trimethoprim sulfamethoxazole prevents Pneumocystis carinii pneumonia in cardiac transplant recipients. J Heart Transplant 9:20A, 1990.
62. Merigan TC, Renlund DG, Keay S, et al: A controlled trial of ganciclovir to prevent cytomegalovirus disease after heart transplantation. N Engl J Med 326:1182, 1992.
63. Joshi GP, Tillman Hein HA, Ramsay MAE, Foreman ML: Hemodynamic response to anesthesia and pneumoperitoneum in orthotopic cardiac transplant recipients. Anesthesiology 85:929, 1996.
64. Gramstad L, Gjerlow JA, Hysing ES, et al: Interaction of cyclosporine and its solvent, cremaphor, with atracurium and vecuronium. Br J Anaesth 58:1149, 1986.
65. Cirella VN, Pantuck CB, Lee YJ, et al: Effects of cyclosporine on anesthetic action. Anesth Analg 66:703, 1987.
66. Cheng DC, Ong DD: Anesthesia for noncardiac surgery in heart-transplanted patients. Can J Anaesth 40:981, 1993.
67. Melendez JA, Delphin E, Lamb J, et al: Noncardiac surgery in heart transplant recipients in the cyclosporine era. J Cardiothorac Vasc Anesth 5:218, 1991.
68. Backman SB, Ralley FE, Fox GS: Neostigmine produces bradycardia in a heart transplant patient. Anesthesiology 78:777, 1993.
69. Beebe DS, Shumway SJ, Maddock R: Sinus arrest after intravenous neostigmine in two heart transplant recipients. Anesth Analg 78:779, 1994.
70. Shaw IH, Kirk AJB, Conacher JD: Anaesthesia for patients with transplanted hearts and lungs undergoing non-cardiac surgery. Br J Anaesth 67:772, 1991.
71. Cooper JD: The evolution of techniques and indications for lung transplantation. Ann Surg 212:249, 1990.
72. Cooper JD: Technique to reduce air leaks after resection of emphysematous lung. Ann Thorac Surg 57:1038, 1994.
73. Cooper JD, Patterson GA, Turlock EP: Results of single and bilateral lung transplantation in 131 consecutive recipients. Washington University Lung Transplant Group. J Thorac Cardiovasc Surg 107:460, 1994.
74. Trulock EP: Lung transplantation. Am J Respir Crit Care Med 155:789, 1997.
75. Wood DE, Raghu G: Lung transplantation. Part I: Indications and operative management. West J Med 165:355, 1996.
76. Bavaria JE, Kotloff R, Palevsky H, et al: Bilateral versus single lung transplantation for chronic obstructive pulmonary disease. J Thorac Cardiovasc Surg 113:520, 1997.
77. Moore PG: Anesthetic management for lung transplantation and lung volume reduction. In Lake CL, Sperry RJ, Rice LJ (eds): Adv Anesth 14:95, 1996.
78. American Thoracic Society: ATS Guidelines: International guidelines for the selection of lung transplant candidates. Up To date, Inc, 1998, p 1–10.
79. Park SJ, Houck J, Pifarre R, et al: Optimal size matching in single lung transplantation. J Heart Lung Transplant 14:671, 1995.
80. Aoe M, Trachiotis GD, Okabayashi K, et al: Administration of prostaglandin E1 after lung transplantation improves early graft function. Ann Thorac Surg 58:655, 1994.
81. Quinlan JJ, Buffington CW: Deliberate hypoventilation in a patient with air trapping during lung transplantation. Anesthesiology 78:1177, 1993.
82. Hirt SW, Haverich A, Wahlers T, et al: Predictive criteria for the need of extracorporeal circulation in single-lung transplantation. Ann Thorac Surg 54:676, 1992.
83. deHoyos A, Demajo W, Snell G, et al: Preoperative prediction for the use of cardiopulmonary bypass in lung transplantation. J Thorac Cardiovasc Surg 106:787, 1993.
84. Fullerton DA, McIntyre RC, Mitchell MB, et al: Lung transplantation with cardiopulmonary bypass exaggerates pulmonary vasomotor dysfunction in the transplanted lung. J Thorac Cardiovasc Surg 109:212, 1995.
85. Shennib H, Serrick C, Saleh D, et al: Plasma endothelin-1 levels in human lung transplant recipients. J Cardiovasc Pharmacol 26(Suppl 3):S516, 1995.
86. Flavahan NA, Aleskowitch TD, Murray PA: Endothelial and vascular smooth muscle responses are altered after left lung autotransplantation. Am J Physiol 266:H2096, 1984.
87. Date H, Triantafillou AN, Trulock EP, et al: Inhaled nitric oxide reduces human lung allograft dysfunction. J Thorac Cardiovasc Surg 111:913, 1996.
88. Cooper JD, Pearson FG, Patterson GA, et al: Technique of successful lung transplantation in humans. J Thorac Cardiovasc Surg 93:173, 1987.
89. Conacher ID, McNally B, Choudhry AK, McGregor CGA: Anaesthesia for isolated lung transplantation. Br J Anaesth 60:588, 1988.
90. Schmid RA, Boehler A, Speich R, et al: Bronchial anastomotic complications following lung transplantation: Still a major cause of morbidity? Eur Respir J 10:2872, 1997.
91. Gayes JM, Giron L, Nissen MD, Plut DA: Anesthesia and double lung transplantation. Cardiac Surgery: State of the Art Reviews 3:595, 1989.
92. Casella ES, Humphrey LS: Bronchospasm after cardiopulmonary bypass in a heart-lung transplant recipient. Anesthesiology 69:135, 1988.
93. Higenbottam T, Jackson M, Woolman P, et al: The cough response to ultrasonically nebulized distilled water in heart-lung transplantation patients. Am Rev Respir Dis 140:58, 1989.
94. Novick RJ, Kaye MP, Patterson B, et al: Redo lung transplantation: A North American-European experience. J Heart Lung Transplant 12:5, 1993.
95. Keller C, Frost A: Fiberoptic bronchoplasty. Description of a simple adjunct technique for the management of bronchial stenosis following lung transplantation. Chest 102:995, 1992.
96. Yousem SA, Berry GJ, Cagle PT, et al: Revision of the 1990 working formulation for the classification of pulmonary allograft rejection: Lung Rejection Study Group. J Heart Lung Transplant 15:1, 1996.
97. Trulock EP, Ettinger NA, Brund E, et al: The role of transbronchial lung biopsy in the treatment of lung transplant recipients. Chest 102:1049, 1992.
98. Finch EL, Jamieson SW: Anesthesia for combined heart and lung transplantation. Contemp Anesth Pract 10:107, 1987.
99. Theodore J, Jamieson SW, Burke CM, et al: Physiologic aspects of human heart-lung transplantation. Chest 86:349, 1984.
100. Dawkins KD, Jamieson SW, Hunt SA, et al: Long term results, hemodynamics, and complications after combined heart and lung transplantation. Circulation 71:919, 1985.

SECTION IV

VASCULAR ANESTHESIA

CHAPTER 20

Endovascular Surgery

Donald Lea Akers, Jr., M.D.

Endovascular surgery began in the 1960s with the introduction of balloon angioplasty. This device has been both modified and redesigned and is now an integral part of the management of the patient with peripheral vascular disease. Over the last several years there has been an explosion of intravascular devices designed to increase the nonoperative management of peripheral vascular and coronary disease. The ability to treat vascular disease without significant operative intervention and achieve similar long-term results to conventional surgical treatment has been the goal of all these devices. Once introduced to the clinician, these devices have often been presented as a significant advancement in the treatment of the atherosclerotic patient. Unfortunately, the initial wave of enthusiasm is usually replaced with skepticism and cautious reappraisal, as the long-term results of all these devices, with the exception of balloon angioplasty, can only be termed as disappointing. There is still some limited applicability for these devices in peripheral vascular disease, and more importantly there is still a definite need for further investigation and refinement of these techniques, as there is clearly a place for them in the future management of the patient with peripheral vascular disease.

The current armamentarium of the endovascular surgeon consists of several devices, including balloon angioplasty, angioscopy, atherectomy, and laser. In addition some more recently developed modalities will also be discussed, including intravascular stents, intravascular ultrasound, and intravascular graft placement. The indications for use and the long-term results will be reviewed, and several new applications will be presented as well. Special intraoperative and interventional problems encountered with each of these will also be presented. These techniques have some applications in the current treatment of vascular disease and may have potential benefits in the future; however, it must be recognized that careful evaluation and investigation of all techniques are necessary to determine not only short-term results but long-term patency.

Angioplasty

Angioplasty was first introduced as a technique by Dotter in 1964, when he treated an elderly female with gangrene who refused surgical intervention.[1] In 1965 Dotter modified this technique by employing a Fogarty embolectomy catheter to dilate an iliac artery lesion. Since those early interventions, many advances and modifications have occurred resulting in the current technique of guidewire-directed balloon angioplasty utilizing polyethylene balloons. These balloons allow the radial direction of forces, and thus do not permit the force to be directed away from the primary lesions. Angioplasty was initially thought to function by compressing the atherosclerotic plaque, resulting in an increased diameter of the lumen. However, it has now been demonstrated that angioplasty functions by disrupting the plaque at its thinnest portion and dilating the underlying adventitia. After dilatation the vessel will remodel with time. This results in a larger channel for flow.[2] Figure 20–1 shows a vessel following balloon angioplasty, demonstrating the process. This figure demonstrates the disruption that accompanies the dilatation and results in a larger flow channel. The artery then remodels over time, resulting in an increase in both lumen and vessel size. In view of the injury, it is surprising that the vessel does not immediately thrombose following dilation. The vessel patency is maintained, however, by the pressure of the arterial flow. The arterial pressure forces the intimal flaps against the wall in the direction of arterial flow and maintains the vascular lumen. In addition, these flaps probably occur in a longitudinal plane and thus act in a different manner from the transverse intimal flap. It has been suggested that when angioplasty does not remove the pressure gradient across a lesion it often fails because of the propensity of the lesion to close in the face of diminished pressure.

Angioplasty was originally a technique utilized in those situations where the patient was deemed an unsuitable surgical candidate. However, with increasing ex-

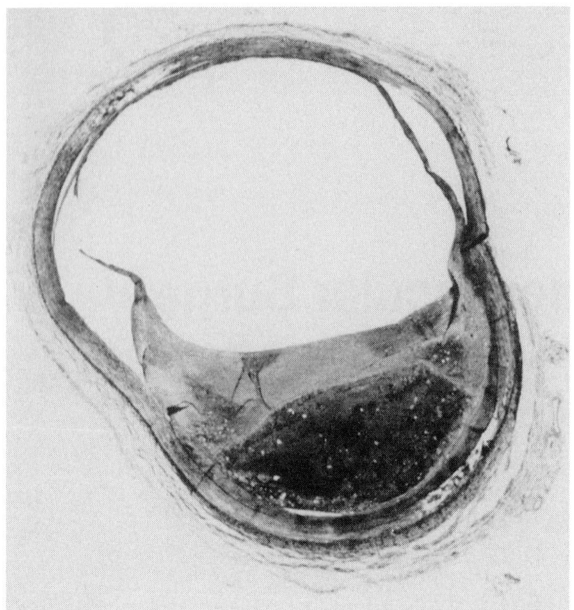

FIGURE **20–1.** Superficial femoral artery following balloon angioplasty. The process of angioplasty has reduced the stenosis by dilating the thinnest portion of the vessel. There has been no change in the configuration of the plaque. Note the small intimal flaps at the edge of the plaque. (From Zarins CK, Glagov S: Histopathology of plaque dilatation and remodeling following balloon angioplasty. In Moore WS, Ahn SS [eds]: Endovascular Surgery. Philadelphia, WB Saunders Co, 1989, with permission.)

perience it has become a separate modality in the treatment of vascular disease. Indeed, it is now felt by some to be overutilized, especially in the patient who presents with minimal symptoms of claudication. This aggressive approach in the management of peripheral vascular disease is reflected in their patient selections. Spence et al. reported their indications for balloon dilatation as 81% for patients with claudication compared to 19% for patients with rest pain.[3] This is in stark contrast to the indications reported by most vascular surgeons. Leather et al. reported limb salvage as the indication in 91% of 1,000 infrainginual reconstructions.[4] Szilagyi et al. reported that 65% of aortoiliac reconstructions were for claudication while 35% were for rest pain and gangrene.[5] It is important that the indications for the procedures be well delineated when comparing studies in patients who undergo interventions. Both surgical revascularization and angioplasty have better results when performed for indications of claudication instead of rest pain. The indications for angioplasty should include (1) intermittent claudication of *sufficient* severity that it adversely affects the patient's lifestyle, (2) pain at rest, (3) ischemic tissue changes including ulceration and gangrene, (4) impaired distal wound healing, and (5) simplification of surgical revascularization.

Contraindications for balloon angioplasty include (1) availability of a safer, simpler, less time-consuming or more effective surgical alternative; (2) distal embolization syndrome ("blue toe syndrome") or deep ulcerations; (3) embolic occlusions; (4) long segments of diffuse disease; (5) long occlusions and (6) acute thrombotic occlusions.[6] Recently, guidelines for evaluating and reporting the results of interventional procedures was adopted by the Society for Interventional Radiology.[7] These standards reflect many of the guidelines established by the Society for Vascular Surgery for the treatment of surgical revascularization. By utilizing these guidelines the results reported in the literature will become more standardized and allow a more open and honest discussion of the results of angioplasty procedures. In addition, patient classification is delineated (Table 20–1). This allows a comparison between interventional procedures and surgical revascularization in comparable patient groups. This is important because, as mentioned previously, much of the angioplasty data reflect intervention on patients with claudication, while surgical re-

TABLE **20–1**
Clinical Categories of Chronic Limb Ischemia

Grade	Category	Clinical Description	Objective Criteria
	0	Asymptomatic, no hemodynamically significant occlusive disease	Normal results of treadmill*/stress test
I	1	Mild claudication	Treadmill exercise completed, postexercise AP is greater than 50 mm Hg but more than 25 mm Hg less than normal
	2	Moderate claudication	Symptoms between those of categories 1 and 3
	3	Severe claudication	Treadmill exercise cannot be completed, postexercise AP is less than 50 mm Hg
II	4	Ischemic rest pain	Resting AP of 40 mm Hg or less, flat or barely pulsatile ankle or metatarsal plethysmographic tracing, toe pressure less than 30 mm Hg
III	5	Minor tissue loss, nonhealing ulcer, focal gangrene with diffuse pedal ischemia	Resting AP of 60 mm Hg or less, ankle or metatarsal plethysmographic tracing flat or barely pulsatile, to pressure less than 40 mm Hg
	6	Major tissue loss, extending above transmetatarsal level, functional foot no longer salvageable	Same as for category 5

*From Rutherford RB, Becker GJ: Standards for evaluating and reporting the results of surgical and percutaneous therapy for peripheral arterial disease. Radiology 181:277, 1991, with permission.
*Five minutes at 2 mph on a 12 degree incline.
AP, ankle pressure.

vascularization is more commonly performed on patients with threatened limb loss. It cannot be overemphasized that misuse or inappropriate use of this modality can have catastrophic consequences. It should be especially noted that the presence of a lesion is not an indication for angioplasty.

Angioplasty can be performed as a separate procedure in the radiology suite or it can be performed in the operating room either alone or in combination with a reconstructive procedure. If both angioplasty and surgical reconstruction are required to treat multilevel disease it is usually optimal to perform the angioplasty several days prior to the operative procedure in order to determine the outcome of the balloon intervention. On occasion, however, it may be necessary to treat both lesions simultaneously, as a lesion may not be recognized as hemodynamically significant until revascularization has been performed. In these situations operative angioplasty may have to be performed. If a lesion is found at the time of arteriogram, the significance can be investigated with the measurement of a pressure gradient across the stenosis. If there is no gradient or the findings are equivocal, then further evaluation of the stenosis can be performed with the intra-arterial administration of a vasodilator.[8] Occasionally, the patient will have significant outflow disease that will cause the angiographic studies to be falsely negative and only after revascularization will the gradient be recognized. Evaluation of inflow lesions at the time of surgery is equivalent to angiographic studies. The determination of the pressure across the stenosis can demonstrate whether or not the stenosis is significant. Again, if the initial pressure findings are somewhat equivocal then a vasodilator can be administered to further determine the significance. If the stenosis is significant then this lesion can be considered for balloon angioplasty.[9]

Documentation of the success of angioplasty requires both physiologic evaluation as well as arteriographic studies. This can be performed with intra-arterial pressure measurements following dilation and postangioplasty vascular laboratory studies. Vascular laboratory studies should include ankle-brachial indices (ABIs) and treadmill testing if the patient is being evaluated for claudication. Figure 20–2 demonstrates a typical lesion treated with angioplasty. This patient presented with less than a block claudication that was significantly inhibiting her lifestyle. Her arteriogram demonstrated a high-grade lesion in her iliac artery. Pressure measurements demonstrated a 40-mm Hg gradient across the lesion. Following the angioplasty, pressures were measured in the artery and there was no residual gradient. The patient had resolution of her symptoms. Repeat vascular laboratory studies demonstrated a good functional result, as the patient could now ambulate for 5 minutes on the treadmill with no recurrence of his symptoms. The patient was seen in follow-up at 3 and 6 months after angioplasty and underwent repeat vascular laboratory testing. These tests again included treadmill testing and indicated that vessel patency following the procedure had been maintained. It is important that postangioplasty evaluations be performed in order to document the long-term durability of the procedure.

The long-term results from angioplasty indicate that in certain situations it has a significant benefit. However, the variability of reporting initial technical success and long-term patency has clouded the data. Some reports do not include initial technical failures in their analysis of long-term patency. Initial failure of angioplasty has been

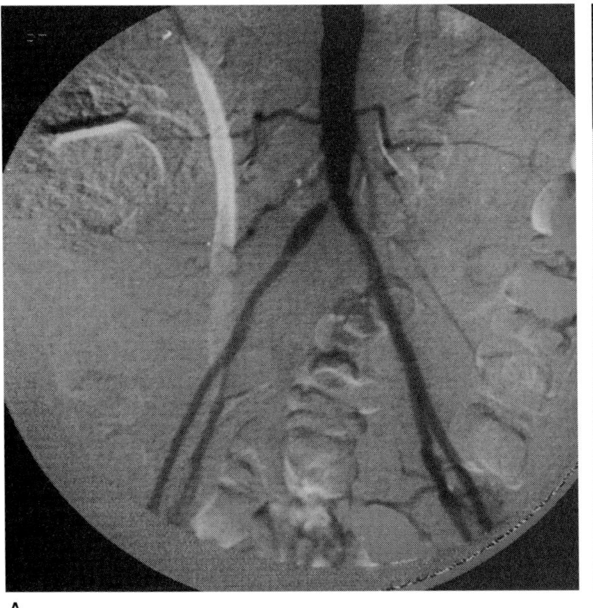

A

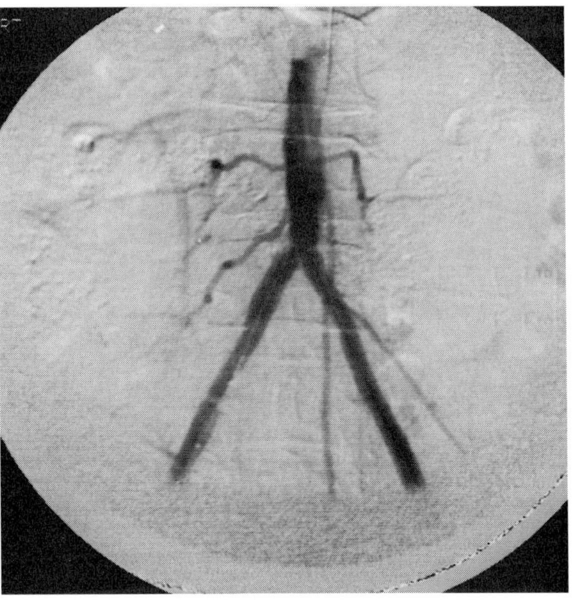

B

FIGURE **20–2.** Arteriogram of a 58-year-old woman who presented with a half block claudication. *A*, The lesion is prior to angioplasty demonstrating a high-grade stenosis of the common iliac artery. *B*, The common iliac artery following balloon angioplasty demonstrating complete resolution of the stenosis. Pressure measurements were obtained both before angioplasty and after dilatation. The pressure gradient present before the angioplasty had completely resolved following the procedure. The stenosis is now resolved.

reported to range from 5% for short segment iliac stenosis to 30% for significant femoral and popliteal disease.[10-12] Other studies only discuss the patients' symptoms and do not have any objective criteria on which to evaluate long-term patency. Tegtmeyer et al. had objective follow-up (i.e. ABIs or measurement of pressure gradients) in only 39% of their patients.[10] This is especially interesting, since the majority of angioplasty procedures are done for claudication, which often improves only with an exercise program. The results of any balloon procedure should be confirmed by vascular laboratory evaluation. Diminishing ABIs or lessening of the flow within the vessel should be considered as an indication of a failing angioplasty and should be aggressively evaluated.

Even with these limitations in the reporting of data there is a definite benefit of angioplasty in certain situations. The best results with angioplasty occur in the larger arteries. Angioplasty of limited iliac lesions has the best initial success and long-term patency reports. Several studies indicate that the initial technical success is 90 to 95% with 1-, 3-, and 5-year patency rates of 90, 80, and 60% respectively.[10,11,13] Long-term durability of the procedure was recently evaluated by Johnston et al. from the University of Toronto.[14] They evaluated 667 patients who had undergone balloon dilation of iliac vessels and had been followed for up to 6 years. The patency of isolated common iliac artery lesions was 68% at 3 years and 60% at 5 years. Angioplasty of external iliac artery lesions had a 57% success rate in men but only a 34% success rate in women. In patients with occluded iliac arteries that could be traversed with a guidewire, the 3-year patency rate following dilation was 48%. The patency rate decreased to 17% in those patients with tandem lesions. Hartnell et al. evaluated the role of balloon angioplasty in the treatment of patients with critical limb ischemia.[15] They found improvement in only 17 of 45 patients at 1 month following angioplasty. These results significantly question the role of balloon angioplasty of the iliac artery in patients with limb-threatening ischemia.

Angioplasty has also been offered as an alternative to surgery in superficial femoral artery disease. It has been argued that angioplasty is less invasive and offers a comparable result to surgery. The initial success rate is usually 80 to 85% and the 1-, 3-, and 5-year patency is 75, 65, and 45%, respectively.[16,17] These results are comparable to arterial reconstruction with synthetic material but significantly inferior to results obtained with autogenous tissue. A more recent study has reported that the 2-year efficacy for claudicants is only 49%, leading the authors to question the benefit of angioplasty in superficial femoral artery lesions.[18] While there may be a role for angioplasty in these lesions, the indications for the procedure are becoming more stringent.

Balloon dilatation has also been attempted for the tibial vessels with some success. Bakal et al. reported a series of 53 patients who had a technical success rate of 72%; however, long-term patency was not reported.[19] Triman et al. reported on 25 patients that underwent balloon angioplasty of the infrageniculate popliteal or the tibioperoneal trunk.[20] Their initial technical success rate was only 59% and their patency at 1, 2, and 3 years was 59, 32, and 20%, respectively. They concluded that there was very little benefit to these patients and have recommended against routine use in this patient population. In patients with infrapopliteal vascular disease surgery is the superior alternative and angioplasty should be used in only extraordinary circumstances, until more information is available.

Angioplasty has also been utilized in several other locations. Isolated stenosis of the abdominal aorta has been treated by balloon dilation with some success.[21] A cumulative patency of 70% at 5 years was reported with only one reported case of an aortic rupture.[22] The number of patients treated by this method continues to be small but the results do appear to be promising. Angioplasty of the mesenteric vessels has also been reported.[23] The major difficulty with the celiac artery and the superior mesenteric artery is that most lesions are orificial and, as has been shown in the renal arteries, balloon angioplasty is usually associated with poor results in this location. Although the numbers are small, the results indicate that this may be a feasible option in patients with other significant comorbid conditions. Balloon angioplasty has also been utilized in the treatment of subclavian artery lesions.[24] Embolism to the vertebral system was initially a major concern. However, the early reports suggest that this may not be a significant factor. The patient numbers reported for this procedure continue to be small and follow-up is limited. Further investigation is needed in order to determine the role of angioplasty in these lesions.

Angioplasty of the carotid artery has also been described.[25-27] The role of angioplasty in this group of patients, however, continues to be very controversial. Angioplasty is offered as an alternative to surgery using the rationale that it has the potential to be less invasive, to be more economical, and to have less morbidity.[28] European investigators have suggested that the results from angioplasty are equivalent to carotid endarterectomy.[29,30] However, reports from the United States seem to question these conclusions.[31] Jordan et al. reported that the cost of carotid angioplasty is significantly higher than surgical therapy. The stroke and death rate of angioplasty was 9.3% versus 3.6% for surgery, a significant increase in morbidity and mortality.[31] The overall complication rate of angioplasty has also been reported to be significantly higher than carotid endarterectomy. In addition, there are few data available on the long-term outcome of carotid angioplasty. However, even with the significant increase in mortality and morbidity in the angioplasty group, there continues to be a significant interest in this modality. The role of angioplasty of the carotid artery will probably await the outcome of a randomized prospective trial of balloon angioplasty versus carotid endarterectomy. Morbidity of balloon angioplasty generally has been stated to range from 5 to 15%, with a mortality of approximately 1 to 2%. It is generally accepted that this rate decreases with the increasing experience of the interventionalist. The incidence of complications associated with angioplasty is reported to range between 4 and 22%.[32] Fortunately, most of these complications are minor and do not require surgical intervention for treatment. The most common complication is that of groin hematoma or a pseudoaneurysm of the entry vessel. Most hematomas are small, but 2 to 8% of cases require surgical treatment.[33] Acute occlusion of the dilated vessel occurs in 1 to 7% of patients.[33] This is usually the result of thrombosis of the vessel but may also be caused by an intimal flap or vasospasm. Technical failure of the procedure can occur as a result of perforation of the vessel or subintimal dissection with the guidewire. Arterial rupture can occur from overinflating the vessel, usually the result of improper selection of the balloon catheter. Obvious distal embolization has been reported to be rare, occurring in less than 1% of cases.[34] However, recent reports suggest that microembolization may be a much more common phenomenon than originally thought.[35] Fortunately, these more serious complications, including embolization, thrombosis, and vessel rupture, occur less frequently. However, a recent report suggests that the complication rate may be as high as 26% with a 13% incidence of significant complications.[36] These complications can necessitate either urgent or emergent surgery, often in an unstable patient or a patient that was deemed as unsuitable for surgical intervention. It must always be recognized that a patient being evaluated for angioplasty must also be evaluated as a potential surgical candidate, as the failed interventional procedure may lead to the operating room. Obviously, angioplasty can be a double-edged sword.

Intravascular Stents

Acute occlusions or failure of percutaneous transluminal balloon angioplasty can occur as a result of intimal flaps, vessel dissection, elastic recoil, or residual vessel irregularities.[37] Gardiner et al. reported that acute occlusions of transluminal angioplasty occur in 1 to 2% of peripheral procedures.[38] Extensive dissection of the iliac system may occur in as many as 4 to 5% of iliac angioplasties.[39] The development and use of intravascular stents in conjunction with angioplasty may assist in the improvement of the long-term patency. Intravascular stents function by mechanically preventing elastic recoil and compressing intimal flaps and dissections against the vessel wall. Eventually the stent becomes incorporated into the vessel wall with a neoendothelium developing over a 4- to 6-week period of time.[36] Intravascular stents are characterized as either balloon-expanding or self-expanding depending on the method of deployment. Figure 20–3 demonstrates the Palmaz stent, a balloon-expandable stent. A Strecker balloon-expandable stent and a Gianturco-Roubin balloon-expandable coil spring stent, two of the more commonly utilized balloon expandable stents, are shown in Figure 20–4. The self-expending stents include the Wallstent and the Gianturco self-expanding "Z" stent shown in Figure 20–5. The descriptions of the actual characteristics of these stents is beyond the scope of this chapter, however, certain attributes are important in the function of these stents. The stents should be easily compressible in order for the delivery system to be as small as possible. The surface area of these stents should be minimal. They should be flexible and have significant durability.

The placement of intravascular stents has been suggested as a mechanism to improve long-term patency of balloon angioplasty. Currently, there are several stents undergoing investigation and being utilized in certain clinical situations. An early study of the Palmaz stent described improvement in a small patient population with a follow-up of only 6 to 12 months. Fourteen of the patients in this series were treated for claudication and only one for threatened limb loss.[40] This paper did not address the question of neointimal hyperplasia or long-term patency with these stents. Another early report indicated that the placement of the stents in the iliac artery position was technically feasible and that early patency results are adequate.[41] The self-expanding Pal-

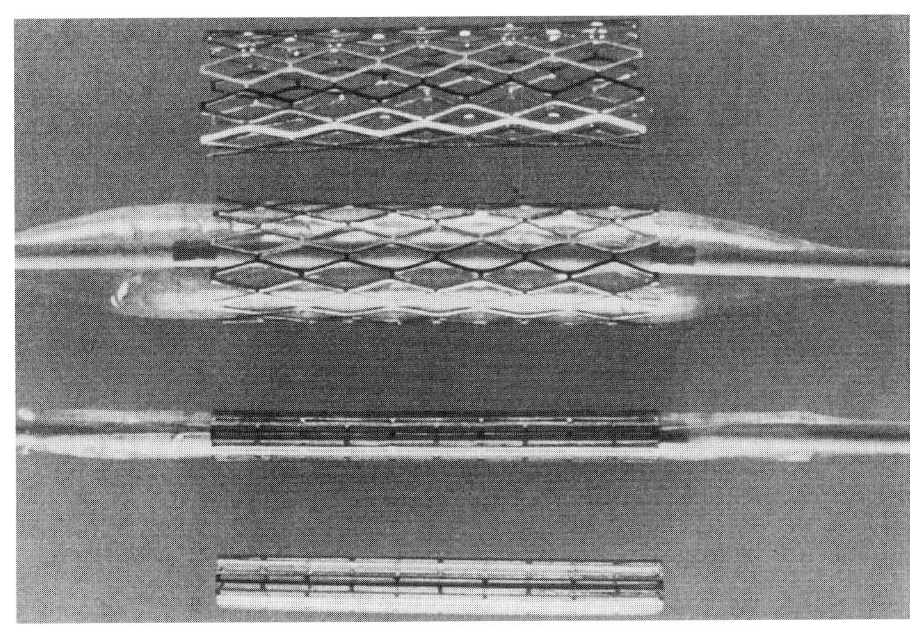

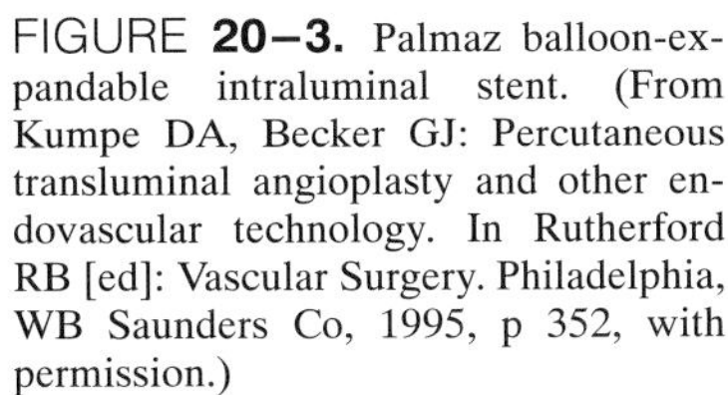

FIGURE **20–3.** Palmaz balloon-expandable intraluminal stent. (From Kumpe DA, Becker GJ: Percutaneous transluminal angioplasty and other endovascular technology. In Rutherford RB [ed]: Vascular Surgery. Philadelphia, WB Saunders Co, 1995, p 352, with permission.)

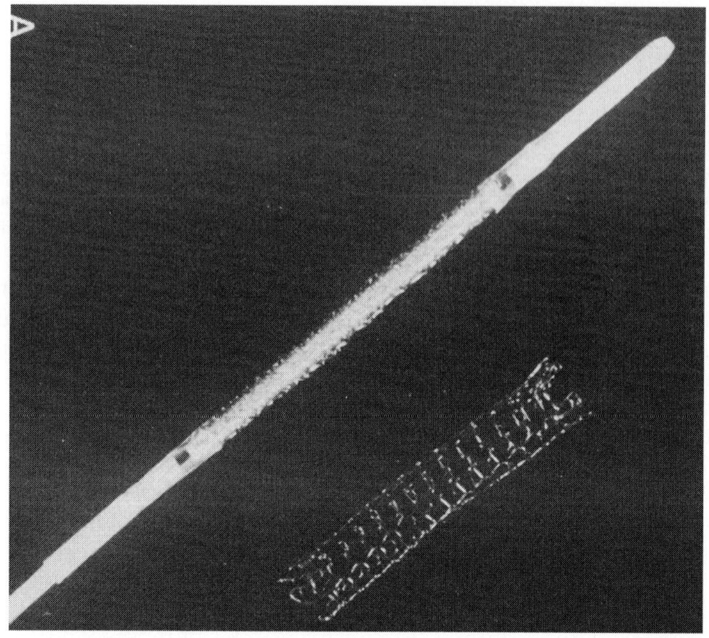

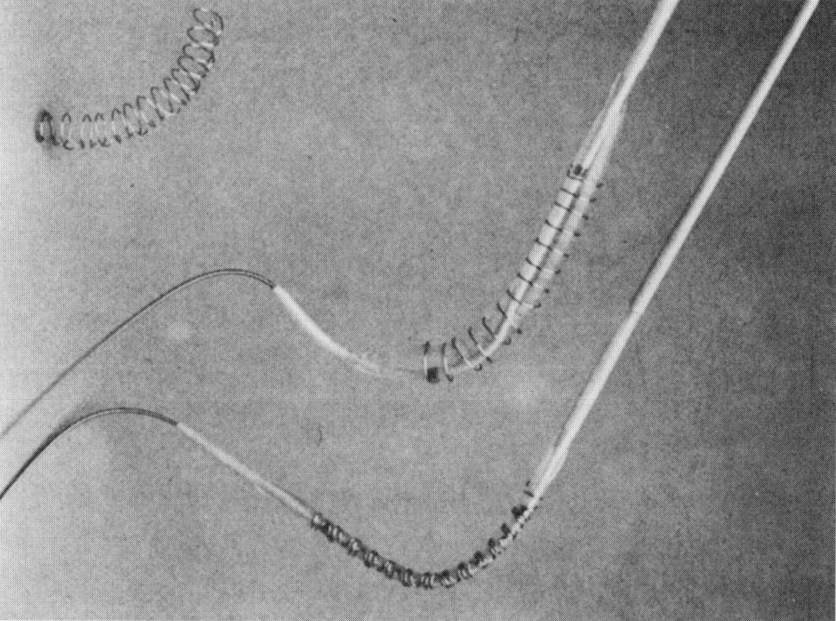

FIGURE **20–4.** Balloon-expandable stents. *A*, Strecker balloon-expandable stent. *B*, Gianturco-Roubin balloon-expandable stent. (From Kumpe DA, Becker GJ: Percutaneous transluminal angioplasty and other endovascular technology. In Rutherford RB [ed]: Vascular Surgery. Philadelphia, WB Saunders Co, 1995, p 352, with permission.)

maz stent has recently obtained Food and Drug Administration (FDA) approval for use in iliac artery angioplasty based on a larger, prospective series.[36] Palmaz reported his experience with the use of the stent in iliac artery angioplasty. He evaluated 587 Palmaz stents placed in 486 patients.[42] These results demonstrated a good clinical outcome in 91% of patients at 1 year, 84% at 2 years, and 69% at 43 months. These results do demonstrate an improvement over standard angioplasty; however, the study has been criticized because the follow-up assessment was based on clinical assessment instead of laboratory evaluation. A second criticism is that the majority of these patients were treated for claudication only. They also reported a complication rate of 10%. This increased complication rate is primarily associated with the larger size of the introducer balloon. Most of the complications occurred at the insertion site.

The initial success with iliac artery stent placement has prompted some authors to suggest that primary stent placement with balloon angioplasty may improve long-term patency. Palmaz recently reported the results of a multicenter study comparing primary stent placement versus angioplasty.[43] The results indicated a statistically improved patency rate in the stented patients. The patency was improved 10 to 15% in this group of patients. However, this group of patients consisted almost entirely of patients with claudication with only 3% of the patients experiencing ischemic rest pain. Still, the results suggest

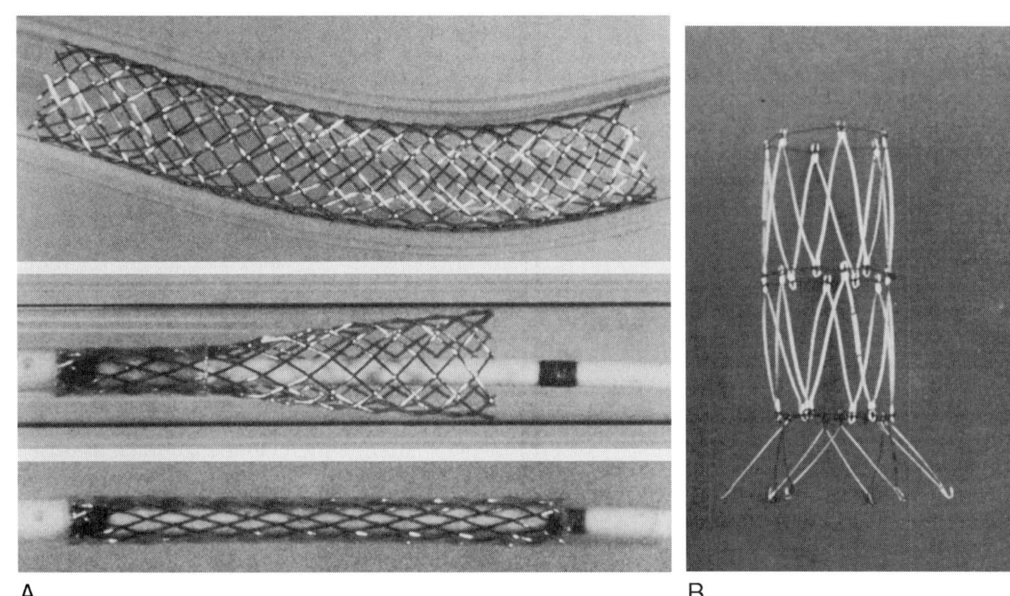
A

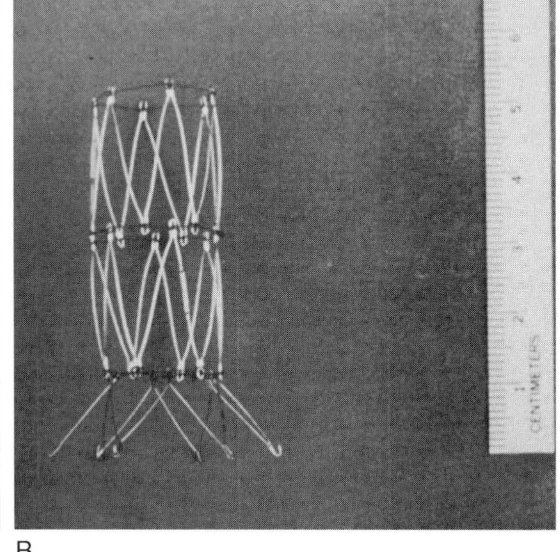
B

FIGURE **20–5.** Self-expanding stents. *A*, Wallstent. *B*, Gianturco self-expanding "Z" stent. (From Kumpe DA, Becker GJ: Percutaneous transluminal angioplasty and other endovascular technology. In Rutherford RB [ed]: Vascular Surgery. Philadelphia, WB Saunders Co, 1995, p 352, with permission.)

that there may be some benefit from primary stenting in patients with iliac occlusive disease. Additional studies suggest that stenting iliac arteries may be beneficial in occluded iliac vessels.[36,44] Martin et al. reported a 93% initial success rate with a similar 6-month patency.[45] Although the results are promising they must be viewed with caution. These results represent mainly clinical follow-up in claudicators. In addition, long-term patency with the placement of stents still awaits longer evaluation. The possibility of development of neointimal hyperplasia with these stents still needs to be fully elucidated.

The Wallstent, a self-expanding stent, has been used extensively in Europe, and a recent study from Germany reported the use of the stent in both iliac arteries and the superficial femoral arteries.[46] Early reports show good results, but severe neointimal hyperplasia occurred in 14% of patients resulting in further treatment.[47] Neointimal hyperplasia has also been an impediment in the development of other stents. Bertrand et al., using the Medivent stent, reported a 67% incidence of restenosis over 2 years.[48] The Nitinol stent, composed of an alloy of nickel and tantalum, functions as a thermal expansion stents. It is extremely pliable at room temperature but reverts to its original configuration at body temperature. The major problem with this stent continues to be the significant neointimal hyperplasia.[49]

The early technical success with intravascular stents in the iliac system has prompted investigation in the femoropopliteal arterial system. Early work with the Palmaz stent in femoropopliteal disease demonstrated 85% patency after 6 months.[36] The acute occlusion rate was 4 to 5%. Another study utilizing the Wallstent reported a 70% 6-month patency in 65 patients with an acute occlusion rate of 7 to 25%.[49] These authors suggest that stents may increase overall patency in the femoropopliteal region. A recent report by Do-dai-Do et al., however, seriously questions this conclusion, as they found no difference in patency at 1 year between the patients that underwent angioplasty versus those that had angioplasty plus stent placement.[50] The final role of stents in the management of femoropopliteal occlusive disease has not been delineated and their use in this disease at this time should be considered investigational.

The placement of stents has also been evaluated in the treatment of both central venous obstruction and dialysis access grafts. They have been demonstrated to have a role in these situations. Rösch et al. placed stents across venous obstructions in patients with malignancies, mediastinal or retroperitoneal fibrosis, and chronic dialysis fistulas.[51] These devices appear to have reasonable short-term results and may be a good alternative in the high-risk surgical patient with venous obstruction. Solomon et al. reported on six patients who underwent stent placement for palliation of superior vena cava syndrome secondary to malignancy.[52] They achieved significant improvement in five patients. In another report, Rösch reported on 22 patients who underwent stent placement for treatment of superior vena cava syndrome.[53] Significant relief was reported in all patients with only one reoccurrence at 9 months. Clearly, the use of these stents can provide significant palliation in this group of patients.

Patients with central stenosis secondary to hemodialysis have also been successfully treated with venous stenting. Shoenfeld et al. reported on 19 lesions treated with venous stent placement.[54] They reported a 68% primary and 93% secondary patency rate; however, this was over a limited time period. Katz et al. reported on 45 patients who underwent angioplasty of the central veins and found that the technique was more effective in patients that had failing grafts as opposed to those with occluded grafts.[55] These stents do appear to have a role in these central lesions. The use of stents in the more distant sites of hemodialysis access, however, have not been as successful. Quinn et al. reported on 20 access grafts managed with self-expandable stents.[56] The primary patency rate of these procedures was only 25%, with a secondary patency rate of 34%. They concluded that these lesions were not very amenable to the placement of stents.

Recent developments in intravascular stenting include a biodegradable stent and stents that have been endothelial seeded.[57,58] Both of these techniques are an attempt to manage the significant problem of neointimal hyperplasia; however, minimal data on their use are currently available. Stents also play a major role in the endoluminal graft treatment of aortic aneurysms, which will be discussed later. Current investigations of intravascular stents include pretreatment with pharmacologic agents that can be delivered directly to the area being treated. This may have a profound benefit when agents are identified that can inhibit neointimal hyperplasia. Intravascular stents may have significant use in the future management of peripheral vascular disease; however, the role of this modality still needs to be clearly defined. In addition, the maximum benefit of this modality will not be achieved until the significant problem of neointimal hyperplasia is resolved.

Angioscopy

Direct visualization of the arterial tree has the potential to offer significant advantages in the treatment of peripheral vascular disease. The development of a small-diameter angioscope that has good resolution has increased the attractiveness of intraoperative angioscopy. The performance of angioscopy requires three essential components: (1) an angioscope, (2) a light source, and (3) an irrigation system. Figure 20–6 demonstrates one currently available system. It should be noted that the size of the angioscope results in it being very fragile, and thus one of the drawbacks of the system is the expense, as these instruments have to be frequently replaced. Angioscopy has been found to be useful in thrombectomies, for inspection of anastomoses, and in the performance of the in situ bypass.[59–61] In addition, many other possible uses for angioscopy are currently being investigated.

Angioscopes are currently available either as disposable or reusable instruments. The disposable angioscopes offer the potential for less expensive equipment. However, the reusable angioscopes have better optics and have some steering capabilities. The only major limitations to the reusable angioscopes is the significant loss of time associated with damage to the instruments and the cost of the system, which can be as much as $50,000. Angioscopes have been reduced in size to such an extent that now almost all vascular procedures are accessible for evaluation. The angioscopes now available can usually be coupled to video display screens currently in use in most operating theaters. Each system, however, requires a light source that is usually recommended by the manufacturer and this can be a significant expense. The lack of an irrigation system, which will be discussed in somewhat more detail later, was initially a major problem with angioscopy, as a significant volume of fluid was administered to the patient during the procedure. Currently, there are several systems available that regulate the administration of fluid during angioscopy.

Angioscopy is most often performed at the time of surgery. The technique involves the isolation of the vessel that has been selected for the introduction of the angioscope. Control of the normal blood flow can be accomplished in one of two ways. In evaluating a more proximal lesion, a balloon occlusion catheter can be introduced that will obstruct the inflow.[62] The irrigation system will then control collateral flow. Distal evaluation can be accomplished with occlusion of the inflow with standard vascular clamps and then distal visualization utilizing the irrigation system to control the collateral

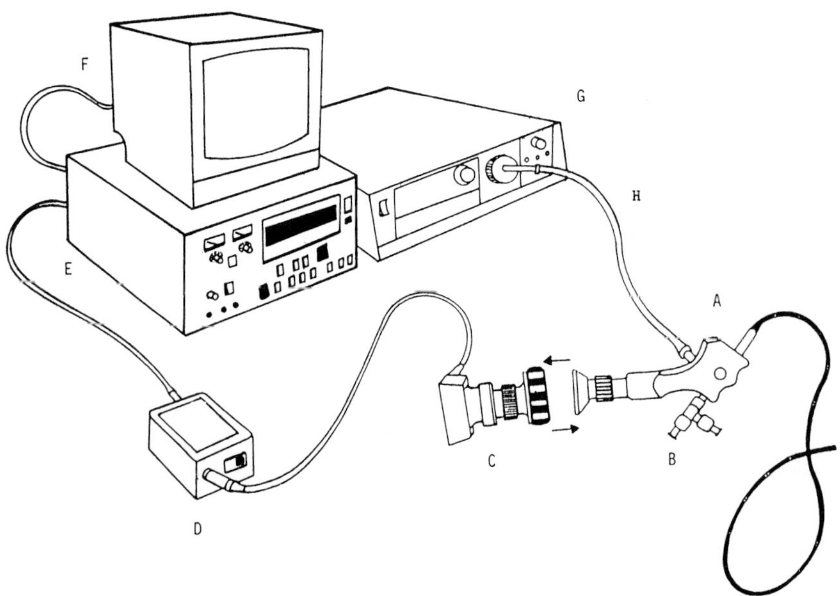

FIGURE **20–6.** Components of an angioscopic system. *A*, angioscope; *B*, irrigation port; *C*, miniature camera; *D*, camera control unit; *E*, videocassette recorder; *F*, monitor; *G*, light source, *H*, light source cable. (From Hernàndez JJ, Quiñones-Baldrich WJ: Angioscopy: Essential, desirable, and optional components. In Moore WS, Ahn SS [eds]: Endovascular Surgery. Philadelphia, WB Saunders Co, 1989, with permission.)

flow provided by side branches. The patient requires continual close monitoring with special attention to the length of ischemia time and the amount of fluid administered.

The use of angioscopy in the performance of a femoral distal in situ bypass has been well described. Miller et al. described their experience with the use of angioscopy and found a significant difference between blind valvulectomy and angioscopically directed valve lysis.[63] A study by Gilbertson et al. states that angioscopy was superior to intraoperative angiography in determining technical problems with the graft.[64] A recent prospective study, however, suggests that angioscopy may not provide any additional benefit in the performance of infrainginual reconstruction. Clair et al. evaluated 59 patients who underwent standard infrainginual revascularization, 32 with an angioscope and 27 without an angioscope.[65] They found no difference in operative morbidity, length of stay, or midterm graft patency. A more novel approach of infrainginual revascularization utilizing the benefits of the angioscope has recently been reported. A cooperative study reported its results utilizing angioscopy to both lyse the valves and occlude the side branches during the performance of the in situ bypass, thus eliminating the need for the long medial leg incision.[66] The major limitation was the length of time required for the procedure and the inability to occlude the smaller branches. Further refinement of this technique suggests that the length of stay of the patients is significantly reduced. The patients who underwent this closed technique had an average length of stay of 4±2 days. While this is currently investigational, if perfected it could offer significant advantages over the current technique. In addition to the lysis of the valves and the inspection of the vein, the angioscope allows the surgeon to visualize the distal anastomosis, evaluating it for technical problems.

Angioscopy also has significant advantages during thrombectomies and embolectomies. Intraoperative arteriograms may miss vessel injuries, such as intimal tears or dissections. Often arteriograms cannot determine the presence of residual thrombus. White et al. found that 67% of graft limbs had pseudointimal flaps and 33% had residual thrombus following blind thromboembolectomy.[67] Angioscopy can determine if the procedure has been adequate and also evaluate for the presence of distal embolization. Angioplasty can give additional information about significant atherosclerotic disease or myointimal hyperplasia, which will result in early failure of any thrombectomy. Techniques are currently being developed that will allow the endovascular treatment of lesions found at the time of angioscopy.[68]

Angioscopy can evaluate any anastomosis. This can determine the technical adequacy of the repair. Its use in situ grafting has already been described. Angioscopy has also been utilized in both aortoiliac and aortofemoral grafting. Other less frequent locations include renal arteries after transaortic renal artery endarterectomy and carotid evaluation following carotid endarterectomy.[69,70] These experiences have been limited and at the current time should be considered investigational. However, as the experience increases there will be more and more utilization of the angioscope.

Complications from angioscopy have been relatively minor. In order to maintain a bloodless field, fluids were originally administered under pressure through the angioscope. This was accomplished by delivering intravenous fluids into the vascular tree with a pressure bag. Early complications with angioscopy were mostly related to the significant volume administered to the patient during the procedure, resulting in a number of patients developing pulmonary edema. Currently, the development of irrigation systems allows delivery of minimal fluids while maintaining a clear vascular field. Van Steigman et al. reported an average of 277 ml for an angioscopic procedure with a range of 100 to 750 ml.[71] A second potential complication results from the passage of the angioscope, which can cause significant vessel injury. There is a direct relationship between the size of the vessel and the potential for injury, with the smaller vessels being more susceptible to injury. Damage to the endothelium can also occur, which results in a reduction of prostacyclin production. This was demonstrated by Hashizume et al.[72] Repeated traumatic passages of the angioscope resulted in a significant reduction in the production of prostacyclin that required 3 to 4 weeks to recover. There have also been reports of remote organ injury resulting both from ischemia time to perform the procedure and from distal embolization. However, with a careful technique the overall incidence of injury continues to be remarkably small.[73]

Angioscopy has the potential to be of great benefit in the evaluation and treatment of peripheral vascular disease. The ability to directly visualize the vascular system allows for the recognition of technical problems before they have the opportunity to induce thrombosis. Angioscopy determines the significance of both proximal and distal disease to better assist in the determination of the best operative therapy. However, repeated passage of the angioscope, may induce endothelial damage, which could possibly initiate either aggressive atherosclerosis or neointimal hyperplasia. The results of early studies concerning the use of angioscopy are mixed in terms of the clinical usefulness. Angioscopy has significant potential, but the true value of this technique will require long-term evaluation.

Atherectomy

Whereas angioplasty simply dilates the vessel, atherectomy devices were designed to remove the atherosclerotic plaque. These devices would then, theoretically, create a less thrombogenic surface and not be associated with the significant intimal damage associated with angioplasty. Several atherectomy catheters were approved for clinical use in both peripheral vascular disease and coronary disease in the late 1980s, and the use of these catheters increased significantly in the early 1990s. The initial enthusiasm associated with these devices has waned recently, as several reports have suggested that the results from atherectomy are no better than what is achieved with angioplasty.

The ability to mechanically remove atherosclerotic plaque without operative intervention is the ultimate goal of all the atherectomy catheters. Currently, directional atherectomy can be performed in either the radiology suite or the operating room. These procedures are employed by either the interventional radiologist, the cardiologist, or the vascular surgeon, depending on the clinical situation. There are four catheters available for clinical use. These are (1) the Simpson Atherocath, (2) the Omnicath, (3) the Auth Rotablator, and (4) the Transluminal Endarterectomy Catheter (TEC). All four catheters remove the atherosclerotic plaque from the vessel wall. The difference between systems is the technique of removal and the handling of the plaque after it is removed.

The only system currently in widespread use in peripheral vascular disease is the Simpson Atherocath which has both a peripheral and coronary capability. It has been utilized in the treatment of both stenotic lesions and occlusions. As with all of the endovascular devices, larger vessels have a better long-term result. The Simpson Atherocath is a side-biting atherectomy catheter that has a side-biting channel. The atherectomy catheter can be introduced either percutaneously or under direct vision in the operating room; however, the procedure requires fluoroscopy. Catheter size ranges from 4 to 11 French.[74] The Simpson Atherocath either has a guidewire attached to the distal end or can be passed over a guidewire. The plaque is traversed and the open port of the Simpson Atherocath is approximated next to the most significant lesion. The catheter position is maintained by inflation of the balloon and the Atherocath is engaged serially, removing small sections of plaque (Fig. 20–7). This results both in the removal of significant plaque and in balloon dilatation of the vessel. Early results have demonstrated the technical ability of this catheter, with initial success rates of 90%.[75] Short-term results have also been promising, with minimal 6-month restenosis. A recent study also presented a 1-year patency of 85%; however, these results are in contrast with another study that reported that at 1 year the outcome is somewhat less promising, as 25% of patients require either surgery or repeat atherectomy.[76,77]

A more recent study by Broegindeweij et al. suggests that the long-term patency rates in peripheral vascular patients treated with atherectomy devices may be worse than with simple balloon angioplasty.[78] They randomized 30 patients to either angioplasty or atherectomy who had either superficial femoral or popliteal artery disease. The patency rate at 9 months was 78% for the angioplasty group and 25% for the atherectomy patients. The major problem with all of these studies is the selection of patients. The majority of patients are having these procedures performed for claudication.[79] The Simpson atherectomy catheter may also have a role in the treatment of vein graft stenosis. Dolmatch et al. have reported a 92% technical success rate in treating 18 infrainguinal vein grafts.[80] They also reported an 88% vein graft patency at 14-month follow-up. These results are definitely an improvement over balloon angioplasty.

The second atherectomy device is the Omnicath (Fig. 20–8). This is also an extirpative catheter currently for investigational use only. The Omnicath is also a side-biting atherectomy catheter; however, it is different from the Simpson Atherocath in several significant ways. The catheter is held in place by a deflector wire system as

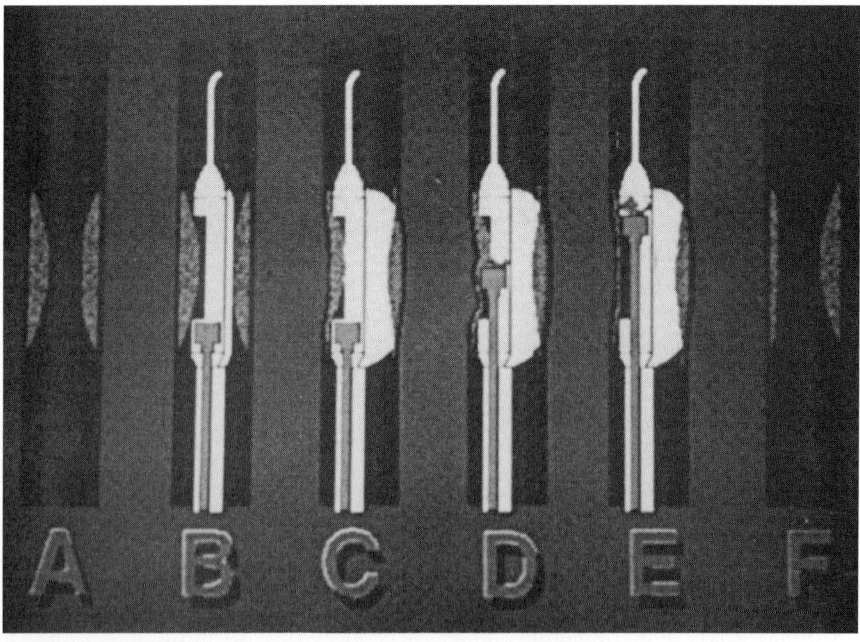

FIGURE **20–7.** The Simpson Atherocath and the atherectomy procedure. *A*, The lesion prior to passage of the catheter. *B*, The catheter passed across the lesion. *C*, The balloon inflated to maintain the catheter's position. *D*, The cutter is advanced. *E*, The specimen is trapped in the housing. *F*, The postatherectomy vessel demonstrating improvement in the diameter of the vascular channel. (From Hinohara T, Robertson GC, Selmon MR, Simpson JB: Transluminal atherectomy: The Simpson atherectomy catheter. In Moore WS, Ahn SS [eds]: Endovascular Surgery. Philadelphia, WB Saunders Co, 1989, with permission.)

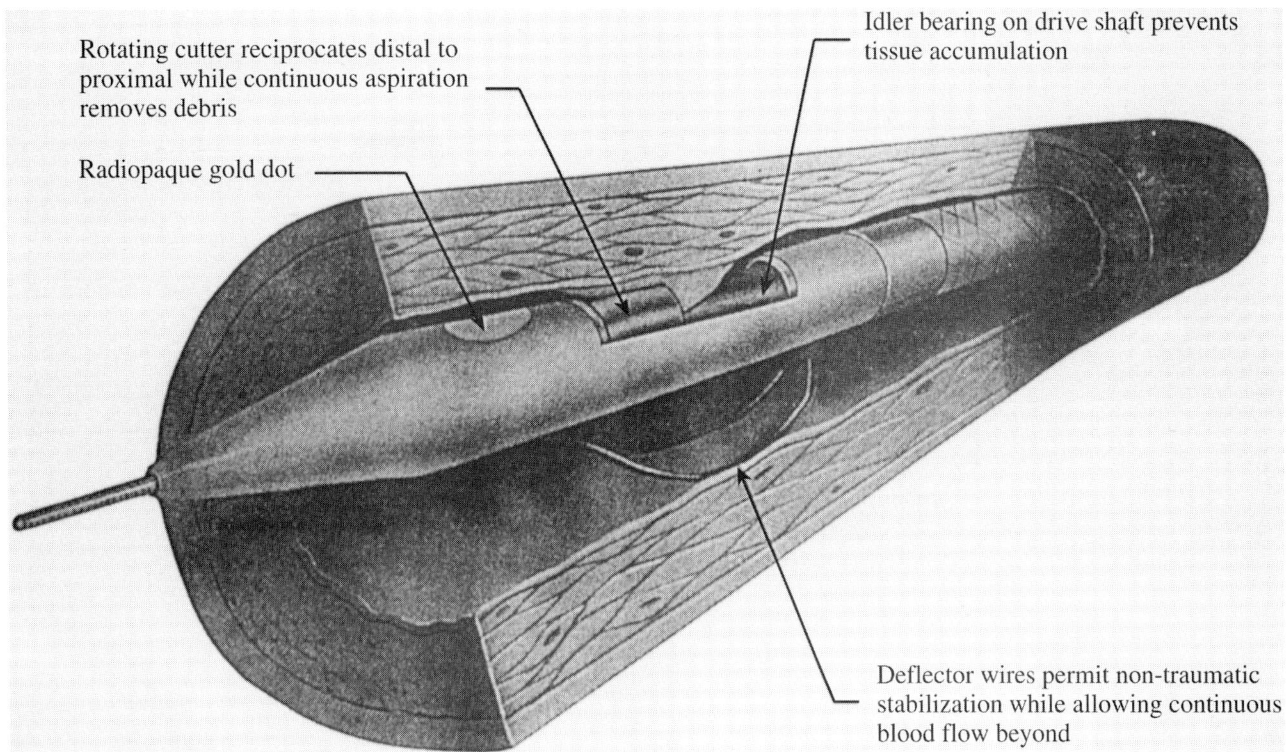

FIGURE **20–8.** The Omnicath atherectomy catheter. Note the deflector wires which allow nontraumatic stabilization of the catheter. (From In Moore WS [ed]: Vascular Surgery: A Comprehensive Review. Philadelphia, WB Saunders Co, 1998, with permission.)

opposed to a balloon, thus reducing the potential for injury to the adjacent vessel. In addition, the blade cuts the plaque from distal to proximal, resulting in the ability to continuously aspirate the debris. The effectiveness of this system is still unclear, as the clinical data are still early; however, animal models suggest that this system is technically feasible with minimal neointimal hyperplasia at 6 weeks.[81]

The Auth Rotablator is also a high-speed rotational atherectomy device. The major difference is a guidewire capability, which appears to reduce the perforation rate. The design is a high-speed rotational burr embedded with multiple diamond chips (Fig. 20–9).[82] This is a high-speed drill that achieves a rotational speed of 100,000 to 200,000 rpm. The basic tenent is that the plaque will be reduced to such small particles that there will be no distal embolization.[83] Unfortunately, this has not been the case, as the major complicating factor with the Rotablator has been the occurrence of distal emboli. A recent report in an animal model, however, suggests that the pattern of distal embolization may not differ much from that which occurs following angioplasty.[84] Clinical trials with the Auth Rotablator have been disappointing, and its use at the present time is limited. An early report from UCLA indicated a 72% initial success rate.[85] In addition, the patency rate at 2 years was only 12%. A multicenter trial had similar poor results with the Auth Rotablater.[86] The initial success rate was 89% and the patency rate was 47% at 6 months, 31% at 12 months, and 18.6% at 24 months. The complication rate was significant and included hemoglobinuria in ten cases (13%), emboli in eight cases (10%), dissection in five cases (6%), perforation in three cases (4%), hematoma in four cases (5%), and infection in one case (1%). They reported nine early thromboses (11%) and two device-related amputations (2.5%). These results suggest that the Auth Rotablator has some significant technical problems that will have to be resolved prior to extending the clinical applications. Even so, the long-term patency rates suggest that this device has a poorer outcome than balloon angioplasty.

The TEC is also a rotational system but functions at a much lower speed (750 rpm). It was first introduced to clinical use in 1989.[87] Larger segments of debris are formed; however, this catheter is connected to a vacuum chamber that is designed to remove the debris as it is being formed. This system is designed in 5- through 9-French sizes, allowing access to all vessels from the iliacs to the infrapopliteal arteries. The major drawback of this device is the inability to treat eccentric lesions. The TEC can be used alone or in conjunction with balloon angioplasty. There are minimal clinical data available but early clinical trials in a small sample population indicate that the system is technically capable of opening both stenoses and short occlusions; however, 6-month patency rates demonstrate a 25% restenosis rate.[87] Reid et al. reported a prospective study comparing the TEC catheter to the Simpson Atherectomy Catheter and the Kensy Atherectomy Catheter. The results were disappointing in regards to all three catheters, but the TEC had the worst results, with a primary patency of 0%.[88] This catheter has been associated with a high restenosis

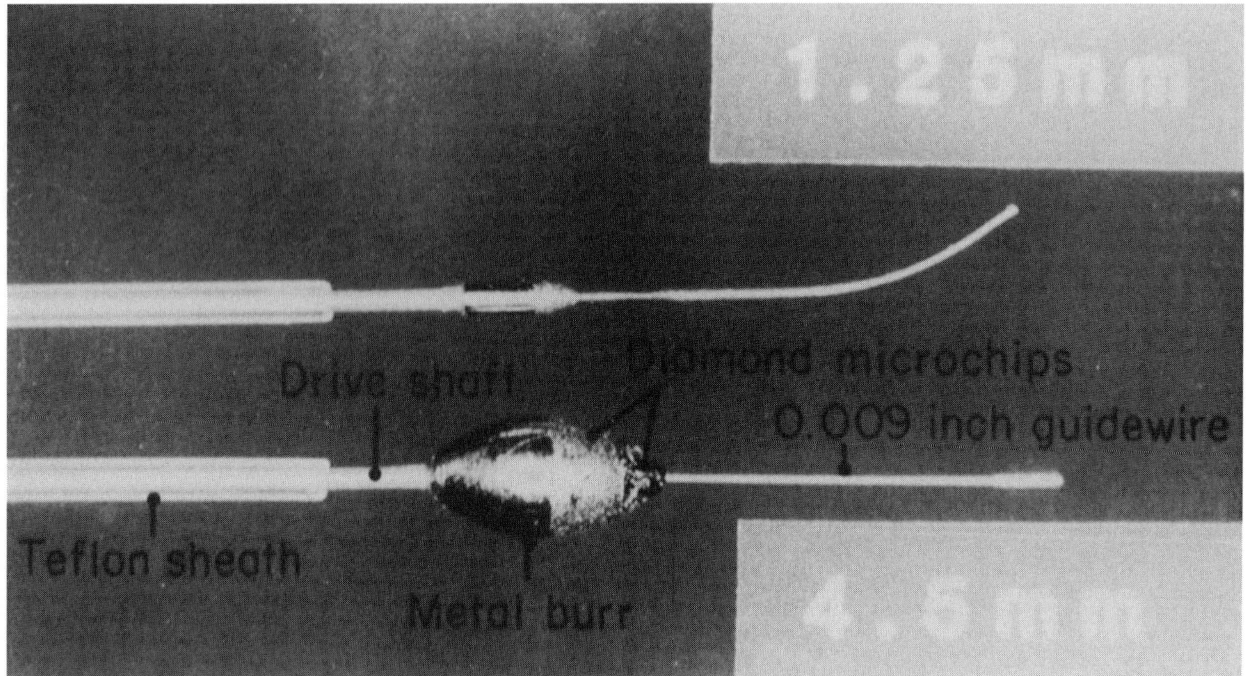

FIGURE **20–9.** The Rotablator. Shown are the 1.25-mm and the 4.5-mm atherectomy catheters. Notice the diamond microchips embedded into the distal portion of the 4.5-mm burr. (From Ahn SS: The Rotablator—high-speed rotary atherectomy: Indications, technique, results, and complications. In Moore WS, Ahn SS [eds]: Endovascular Surgery. Philadelphia, WB Saunders Co, 1989, with permission.)

rate and often requires an adjunctive balloon angioplasty to achieve an adequate result. As with the Rotablator, final determination of the clinical value of the TEC will depend on long-term clinical trials in a much larger patient population.

The ability to mechanically remove atherosclerotic plaque by a minimally invasive technique could potentially offer significant benefit to the vascular patient. However, the currently available atherectomy devices have not been the salvation as initially promised. The long-term results are not much better than with balloon angioplasty. In addition, with the risk of distal embolization, perforation, and subsequent neointimal hyperplasia, they may actually worsen the lesion or convert a stable situation into one that requires surgical intervention. The true use of these instruments in the treatment of vascular surgery demands extended clinical trials with excellent objective long-term patency evaluation. The ability to control neointimal hyperplasia with pharmacologic interventions may eventually lead to an expansion of the role of atherectomy devices in the management of peripheral vascular disease.

Laser

The word laser is actually an acronym for *l*ight *a*mplification by the *s*timulated *e*mission of *r*adiation. Laser surgery was initially presented as a technique to open completely obstructed blood vessels without surgery (i.e., "surgery without scalpels"). This concept was presented to the public, prior to any significant long-term clinical trials, as the ability to treat significant peripheral vascular disease without conventional surgical intervention. The initial studies suggested that the technique was technically feasible and, based on that data, and the significant marketing potential, every facility in the United States rushed to become laser capable. Unfortunately, studies with long-term patency reports suggest that not only does laser not add anything to the current treatment of atherosclerosis but that in some instances it may actually accelerate the process. Indeed, after the initial wave of enthusiasm for laser therapy with its intense marketing campaign, endovascular laser surgery is undergoing careful critical reappraisal.

The majority of lasers now available utilize thermal energy, the primary types being the argon laser, the CO_2 laser, and the yttrium-aluminum-garnet (YAG) crystal laser. These instruments utilize laser energy either directly on the lesion or to heat a metal probe that is directed at the lesion. This energy causes either disintegration of the structure of the plaque or ablation of plaque. The heat generated by the laser can range from 60°C to several hundred degrees centigrade. Initially these catheters were associated with a rather significant perforation rate, and the channel created was limited.[89,90] These systems now have been coupled with balloon angioplasty (laser assisted balloon angioplasty [LABA]) to reduce the energy required to open the vessel and to increase the lumen of the vessel. This should decrease the perforation rate and increase the long-term patency results. As the technique improves, the perforation rate should decrease, but a recent report indicated that perforation still occurred in 33% of their procedures.[91] The long-term patency results with these techniques have also been disappointing.[89,92,93] Most studies fail to show any benefit over balloon angioplasty. Recent reports document less than a 50% patency at 12 months.[94] Even those studies that support the use of laser have significant limitations. A recent multicenter trial reported that the major indication for the procedure is claudication, and the long-term results are no better than balloon angioplasty.[95] An overall review of the literature reveals that the major complication rate of LABA continues to be 10% and only 50 to 60% or less of the technically successful procedures remain open past 1 year.[89,91–96] The majority of the failures require surgery, thus in one aspect the use of laser therapy may have actually increased the need for surgical intervention.

Recent developments in laser technology include the clinical trials of the excited dimer (Excimer) laser and the MCM Smart Laser. The Excimer laser employs short-duration, high-energy pulses of ultraviolet light, which results in tissue ablation with minimal thermal energy. The aim of this laser technology is that the significant problems encountered with the high energy, and thus heat, generated from thermal probes would be eliminated. Two recent clinical studies have not demonstrated a significant advantage.[97,98] In the study by McCarthy et al., there was only a 58% initial technical success rate and only a 47% 9-month patency rate of those arteries that were able to be canalized. The MCM Smart Laser, in simplistic form, is designed to "recognize" atherosclerotic disease through spectroscopy and then utilize an argon probe to destroy the atherosclerotic plaque. This technique has much promise but early results continue to have significant technical complications.[99]

The use of laser surgery to remove atherosclerotic plaque has some very attractive potential benefits. Unfortunately, the initial reports have been somewhat disappointing. The initial marketing campaign with laser surgery has now given way to some very sobering prospective studies that suggest that long-term patency of laser-treated lesions may not be comparable to simple balloon angioplasty. It has been suggested that laser surgery may cause an aggressive atherosclerotic process in the vessel after treatment. Clearly, more significant work with laser surgery must be performed before laser therapy becomes a significant part of the treatment of atherosclerotic peripheral vascular disease.

Intravascular Ultrasound

The ability to visualize the internal aspect of both arteries and veins and to determine the presence and absence of lesions has been the driving force behind the development of intravascular ultrasound (IVS).[100–102] IVS incorporates small ultrasonic transducers on the tips of catheters. This permits a cylindrical phased array in the vessel. In addition, IVS provides information about the nature of the plaque that cannot be determined via angiography or angioscopy. IVS has been demonstrated to be superior to single-plane angiography in evaluating the vascular system.[103] IVS's ability to visualize defects in the lumen and the evaluation of vessel diameter is equivalent to angioscopy. It has also been suggested that intravascular ultrasound can provide information regarding the morphology of the atherosclerotic plaque.[104] This may become important if a relationship can be established between plaque morphology and the potential for that plaque to rupture. IVS also eliminates the need for contrast, thus reducing the risk of acute renal failure. There is also no need for fluid administration as with angioscopy. Several recent studies have presented potential uses for this device. Neville et al. reported on an experimental model where IVS was successful in detecting arterial intimal defects.[105] Cayvelle et al. utilized IVS in monitoring intravascular stent placement.[106] Several authors have reported on the use of IVS in venous disease, specifically in determining the level of vena cava occlusion.[107,108] The major difficulty with IVS at the present time is that the small size of the catheter, and thus the transducer, requires a fairly high-frequency probe. This has resulted in some problems with image distortion.[109] In addition, IVS requires the catheter to be able to cross the lesion, which may not be possible with some highly stenotic lesions. Intravascular ultrasound may have some definite therapeutic advantages over some currently available techniques in the endovascular surgery management of peripheral vascular disease; however, significant investigation is still required.

Intravascular Graft Placement

The use of endoluminal grafts to treat aneurysmal disease, arteriovenous fistula, and peripheral vascular disease has become a potentially significant advance in the management of this patient population. These procedures significantly reduce the morbidity and mortality associated with the standard operative approaches. The development of this technology utilizes several of the modalities of endovascular surgery including intravascular stents, intravascular ultrasound, and balloon angioplasty. Currently, the endovascular graft placement for the treatment of abdominal aortic aneurysms has entered phase II trials and is now utilized in selected patients. In addition, endovascular modalities have been used in the treatment of certain traumatic lesions.

Early experimental studies have determined that abdominal aortic aneurysms could be treated with endoluminal graft placement.[110,111] Figure 20–10 demonstrates the technique. The femoral artery is exposed through a standard operative exploration. The graft is then introduced into the appropriate location in the abdominal aorta through the femoral artery. The graft is then secured in place with balloon inflation of an intravascular stent. A second stent is then placed at the distal end of the graft to prevent reflux around the graft.[112] This technique has been demonstrated successfully in the animal model with the study by Laborde demonstrating graft patency at 6 months.[110]

This technique was first taken from the laboratory to the clinical arena in Brazil. Parodi originally reported a series in which five patients were treated with endoluminal graft placement. Four patients had successful

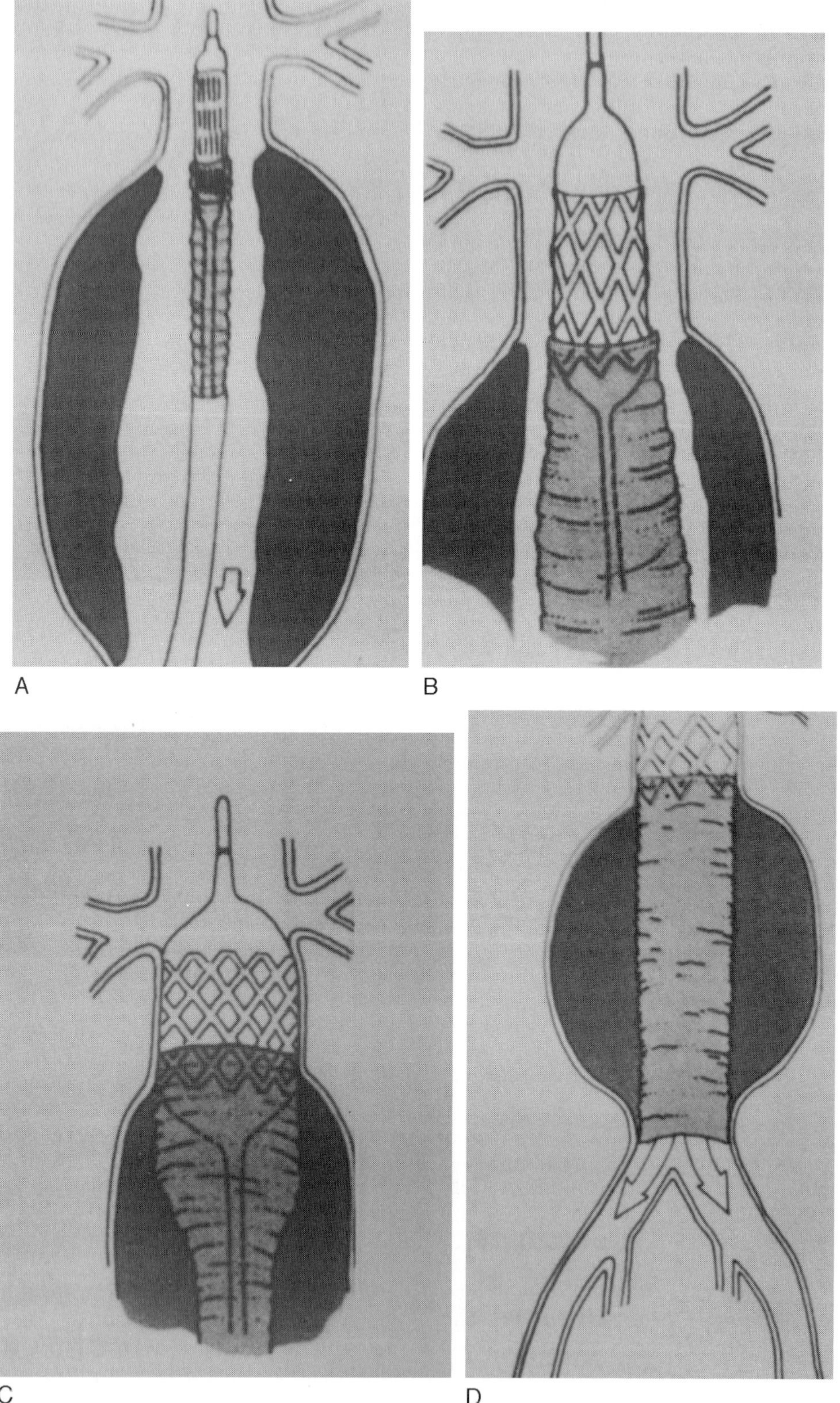

FIGURE **20–10.** Exclusion of an aneurysm by endovascularly placed graft. *A*, The delivery system is placed with the proximal portion of the graft and stent at the infrarenal neck of the aneurysm. *B*, The stent and graft are inflated securing the graft in position. *C*, The inflated graft and stent is noted to be seated below the origin of the renal arteries. *D*, The graft is then pulled to length and the distal end of the graft is secured with a second stent (not shown). (From Parodi JC, Palmaz JC, Barone HD: Transfemoral intraluminal graft implantation for abdominal aortic aneurysms. Ann Vasc Surg 5:491, 1991, with permission.)

placement of the graft, the fifth patient required standard repair secondary to the graft having been placed in the incorrect position. No other significant problems developed demonstrating the technical feasibility of the technique. May et al. reported 25 patients that underwent attempted endoluminal graft placement.[113] Successful graft placement was achieved in 17 patients (67%). The reason for graft placement failure in the remaining eight patients were stent migration (three), access problems (two), balloon malfunction (one), both limbs of a bifurcated graft in one iliac artery (one), and graft thrombosis (one). Several more recent studies continue to document the feasibility of this technique.[114,115] The overall application of this technique at the present time is limited, as it is currently utilized only in prospective trials. The placement of the graft requires several prerequisites for success. The arterial anatomy must be amenable to the placement of the graft. Thus, patients with occlusive disease or significantly tortuous vessels are not candidates. In addition there must be an easily identifiable neck of the aneurysm in order to secure the graft below the renal arteries. All patients with suprarenal extension of their aneurysm are currently excluded from the study. There must also be an identifiable neck at the distal end of the aorta to allow the distal end of the graft to be secured. The significant requirements of the endovascular graft are reflected by the fact that early prospective trials have found that only 10 to 15% of aneurysms are amenable to stent graft treatment.[116,117] The patency of the inferior mesenteric artery must be carefully assessed to make certain that mesenteric ischemia does not develop following deployment of the graft. This is especially important in the bifurcated graft system, as the internal iliac arteries are a major collateral blood supply to the colon. Bifurcated aortic grafts have been developed but their use is still in the early stages. The first U.S. graft was placed in the latter part of 1994 at UCLA (personal communication). The long-term fate of these grafts is still unknown.

The endovascular repair of abdominal aortic aneurysms is still very early in the investigational phase and no long-term results can currently be reported. Some initial technical problems have been recognized including the fact that the early grafts were not secured with stent placement on the distal aorta and several grafts have had to be repaired secondary to reflux around the graft. In addition, the fate of collateral vessels emptying into the aneurysm is unknown. It is believed that these vessels will eventually thrombose but the possibility exists that the vessels may remain patent and additional growth of the aneurysm may occur. This could lead to eventual rupture of the aneurysm as a result of the patent branches of the infrarenal aorta. Indeed, a recent report by Lumsden et al. documents the rupture of two infrarenal abdominal aortic aneurysms following endovascular repair.[118] The durability of the graft itself has also not been completely evaluated. In order to place this graft endovascularly, it must be compressible to minimize the size of the delivery system. This has required the construction of the graft to be made of a thinner material. The result of the long-term stress applied to this material is unknown at the present time. The ability to treat aneurysmal disease in this fashion would eliminate the need for operative intervention, hopefully reducing the morbidity and mortality associated with the disease and the surgical treatment. This technique, however, is still very early in its investigation and further investigation, including long-term follow-up, will be required. Current utilization of this technique should be confined to clinical trials so that the short- and long-term clinical effectiveness of this modality can be determined.

Endovascular graft placement has also been applied to peripheral lesions.[119,120] Marin et al. recently presented their experience with transluminally placed grafts for trauma. They employed seven stented grafts to treat six pseudoaneurysms and one arteriovenous fistula. Figure 20–11 is a schematic demonstrating the mechanism for placing the graft. These grafts were introduced either percutaneously or at a site that was remote from the area of trauma. The average length of stay for these patients was 5.5 days. All seven grafts have remained patent with a mean follow-up of 6.5 months with one graft noted to be patent at 14 months. In cases where the fistula has had time to mature this technique allows treatment without having to explore the often highly vascularized area around the fistula. More recently the same group has described their experience with the treatment of occlusive arterial disease with endoluminal graft placement.[121] They treated 100 arterial lesions in 92 patients with 96 endovascular grafts. This modality employs stented grafts in the treatment of both iliac and superficial femoral disease. The initial technical success was good and the early results are promising. However, long-term data are not yet available and it is unclear what advantage this technique offers over the standard open technique in the treatment of occlusive lesions. The long-term clinical applications of these techniques are not clear.

Endoluminal graft placement is an exciting development in the treatment of vascular disease. It has the potential to revolutionize the current treatment modalities in both aneurysmal disease and some forms of traumatic injury. It must be recognized, however, that this technique is still investigational and requires additional short- and long-term studies to elucidate its role in the treatment of this patient population.

Summary

The concept of managing peripheral vascular disease without surgery is very attractive. Patients with significant peripheral vascular disease are high-risk surgical candidates and often have disease processes that affect multiple organ systems. Any treatment that can significantly reduce the operative risk would obviously benefit this group of patients. Unfortunately many of the new modalities have not achieved their initial promise. Angioplasty has demonstrated significant benefit in the management of the isolated iliac artery stenosis. The benefit of angioplasty in patients with isolated superficial femoral artery stenosis is less clear. Atherectomy and laser-assisted balloon angioplasty have not had the benefit that was hoped for. In fact, in several studies these

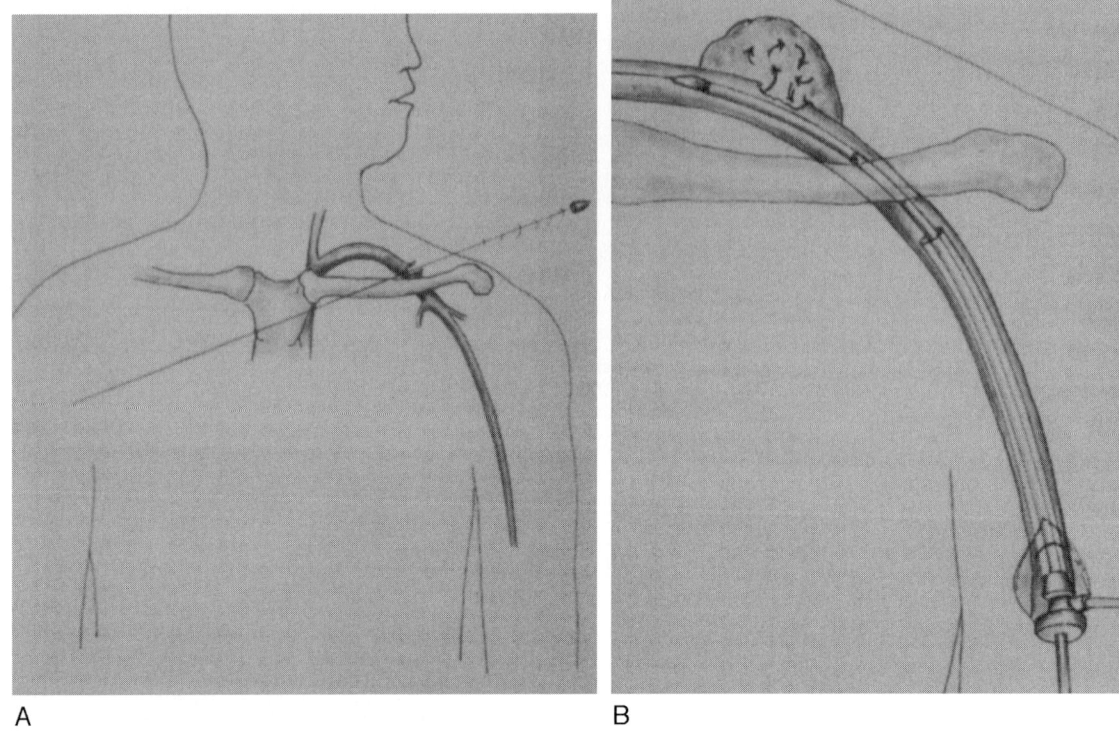

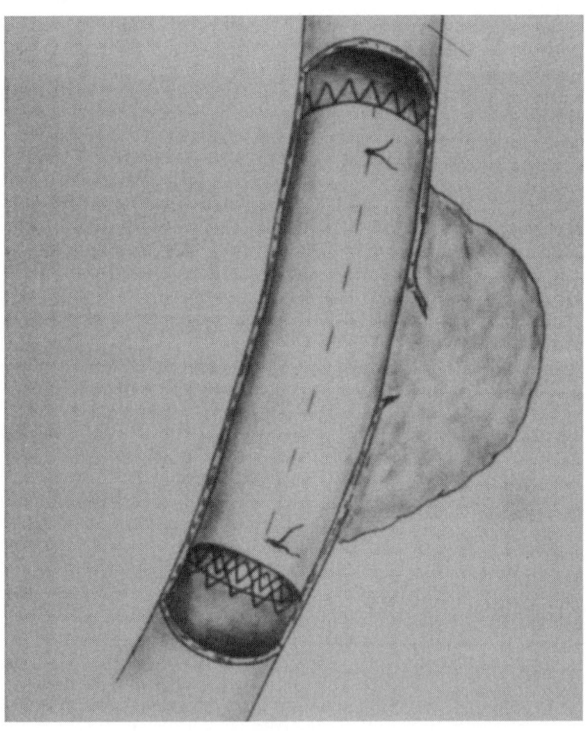

FIGURE **20–11.** Endoluminal placement of a graft for a pseudoaneurysm of the subclavian artery. *A*, A partial injury to the subclavian artery is indicated by the course of the bullet. *B*, The stented graft is introduced from a site remote from the injury. *C*, The stent is deployed, traversing the area of injury, eliminating the injured artery from the circulation. (From Marin ML, Veith FJ, Panetta TF, et al: Transluminally placed endovascular stented graft repair for arterial trauma. J Vasc Surg 20:466, 1994, with permission.)

instruments have actually worsened the disease process, sometimes resulting in urgent surgical intervention. The long-term results from the use of these instruments are now demonstrating that there are some significant deficiencies and/or complications that must be addressed. There is a role for endovascular surgery, but it will take additional prospective clinical trials to determine what that role will be. The outcome must not only consider who has benefitted (i.e., the percentage of patients with claudication who improved and the limb salvage rate) but also the number of patients who experienced a significant worsening of their disease state due to the "noninvasive" intervention. A procedure cannot be deemed as successful if it converts a significant number of stable patients who experience claudication into patients who require operative intervention. The long-term results, including morbidity and mortality of the procedure, must be compared to the results obtained surgically in order to determine if their is clearly a benefit of these procedures over surgery.

References

1. Dotter CT, Judkins MP: Transluminal treatment of arteriosclerotic obstruction: Description of a new technic and a preliminary report of its application. Circulation 30:654, 1974.
2. Zarins CK, Lu C-T, Gerwetz BL, et al: Arterial disruption and remodeling following balloon dilatation. Surgery 92:1086, 1982.
3. Spence R, Freiman D, Gatenby R, et al: Long-term results of transluminal angioplasty of the iliac and femoral arteries. Arch Surg 116:1377, 1981.
4. Leather RP, Shah DM, Chang BB, Kaufman JL: Resurrection of the in situ saphenous vein bypass: 1,000 cases later. Ann Surg 208:435, 1988.
5. Szilagyi DE, Elliott JP Jr, Smith RF, et al: A thirty-year survey of the reconstructive surgical treatment of aortoiliac occlusive disease. J Vasc Surg 3:421, 1986.
6. Deutsch LS: Techniques of percutaneous balloon angioplasty including aortoiliac and femoropopliteal systems: Indications, results, and complications. In Moore WS, Ahn SS (eds): Endovascular Surgery. Philadelphia, WB Saunders Co, 1989, p 163.
7. Rutherford RB, Becker GJ: Standards for evaluating and reporting the results of surgical and percutaneous therapy for peripheral arterial disease. Radiology 181:277, 1996.
8. Flanigan DP, Ryan TJ, Williams LR, et al: Aortofemoral or femoropopliteal revascularization? A prospective evaluation of the papaverine test. J Vasc Surg 1:215, 1984.
9. Pfeiffer RB Jr, String ST: Adjunctive use of the balloon dilatation catheter during vascular reconstructive procedures. J Vasc Surg 3:841, 1986.
10. Tegtmeyer CJ, Hartwell GT, Selby JB, et al: Results and complications of angioplasty in aortoiliac disease. Circulation 83(Suppl 2):153, 1991.
11. Wilson SE, Wolf GL, Cross AP, and the principal investigators of Veterans Administration Cooperative Study No 199: Percutaneous transluminal angioplasty vs. operation for peripheral arteriosclerosis: Report of a prospective randomized trial in a selected group of patients. J Vasc Surg 9:1, 1989.
12. Becker G, Katzen B, Dake M: Noncoronary angioplasty. Radiology 170:921, 1989.
13. Johnston KW, Rae M, Hogg-Hohnston SA, et al: 5-year results of a prospective study of percutaneous transluminal angioplasty. Ann Surg 206:403, 1987.
14. Johnston KW: Iliac arteries: Reanalysis of results of balloon angioplasty. Radiology 186:207, 1993.
15. Hartnell G, Wakeley C, Wyatt M, Horrocks M: Is iliac angioplasty indicated in the treatment of critical limb ischaemia? J Intervent Radiol 7:101, 1992.
16. Hewes R, White R, Murray R, et al: Long-term results of superficial femoral artery angioplasty. AJR 146:1025, 1986.
17. Milford MA, Weaver FA, Lundell CJ, et al: Femoropopliteal percutaneous transluminal angioplasty for limb salvage. J Vasc Surg 8:292, 1988.
18. Stanley B, Teague B, Raptis S, et al: Efficacy of balloon angioplasty of the superficial femoral artery and popliteal artery in the relief of leg ischemia. J Vasc Surg 23:679, 1996.
19. Bakal CW, Sprayregen S, Scheinbaum K, et al: Percutaneous transluminal angioplasty of the infrapopliteal arteries: Results in 53 patients. AJR 154:171, 1990.
20. Treiman GS, Treiman RL, Ichikawa L, et al: Should percutaneous transluminal angioplasty be recommended for treatment of infrageniculate popliteal artery or tibioperoneal trunk Stenosis? J Vasc Surg 22:457, 1995.
21. Odurny A, Colapinto RF, Sniderman KW, Johnston KW: Percutaneous transluminal angioplasty of abdominal aortic stenoses. Cardiovasc Intervent Radiol 3:1, 1989.
22. Berger T, Sorensen R, Konrad J: Aortic rupture: A complication of transluminal angioplasty. AJR 146:373, 1986.
23. Warnock NG, Gaines PA, Beard JD, Cumberland DC: Treatment of intestinal angina by percutaneous transluminal angioplasty of a superior mesenteric artery occlusion. Clin Radiol 45:18, 1992.
24. Becker GJ, Katzen BT, Dake MD: Noncoronary angioplasty: State of the art. Radiology 170:921, 1989.
25. Bockenhemer SAM, Mathias K: Percutaneous transluminal angioplasty in arteriosclerotic internal carotid artery stenosis. Am J Neuroradiol 4:791, 1983.
26. Wiggli U, Gratzl O: Transluminal angioplasty of stenotic carotid arteries: Case reports and protocol. Am J Neuroradiol 4:793, 1983.
27. Kachel R, Basche S, Heerklotz I, et al: Percutaneous transluminal angioplasty (PTA) of supra-aortic arteries, especially the internal carotid artery. Neuroradiology 33:191, 1996.
28. Yadav JS, Roubin GS, Iyer S, et al: Elective stenting of the extracranial carotid arteries. Circulation 95:376, 1997.
29. Kachel R: Results of balloon angioplasty in the carotid arteries. J Endovasc Surg 3:22, 1996.
30. Sivaguru A, Venables GS, Beard JD, et al: European Carotid Angioplasty Trial. J Endovasc Surg 3:16, 1996.
31. Jordan WD Jr, Schroeder PT, Fisher WS, et al: A comparison of angioplasty with stenting vs. endarterectomy for the treatment of carotid artery stenosis. Ann Vasc Surg 11:2, 1997.
32. Mahler F, Triller J, Weidmann P, et al: Complications in percutaneous dilatation of renal arteries. Nephron 44:60, 1986.
33. Gardiner GA, Meyerowitz MF, Stokes KR, et al: Complications of transluminal angioplasty. Radiology 146:57, 1983.
34. Kumpe DA, Becker GJ: Percutaneous transluminal angioplasty and other endovascular technology. In Rutherford RB (ed): Vascular Surgery. Philadelphia, WB Saunders Co, 1995, p 352.
35. Ring EJ, Freiman DB, McLean GK, et al: Percutaneous recanalization of common iliac artery occlusions: An unacceptable complication rate? AJR 139:587, 1982.
36. Weibull H, Bergqvist D, Jonsson D, et al: Complications after percutaneous transluminal angioplasty in the iliac, femoral, and popliteal arteries. J Vasc Surg 5:681, 1987.
37. Katzen BT, Becker GJ: Intravascular stents: Status of development and clinical application. Surg Clin North Am 72:941, 1992.
38. Gardiner GA Jr, Meyerowitz MF, Sokes KR, et al: Complications of angioplasty. Radiology 159:201, 1986.
39. Becker GJ: Intravascular stents: General principles and status of lower-extremity arterial applications. Circulation 83(Suppl 1): 122, 1991.
40. Palmaz JC, Richter GM, Noeldge G, et al: Intraluminal stents in atherosclerotic iliac artery stenosis: Preliminary report of a multicenter study. Radiology 168:727, 1988.
41. Cikrit DF, Becker GJ, Dalsing MC, et al: Early experience with the Palmaz expandable intraluminal stent in iliac artery stenosis. Ann Vasc Surg 5:150, 1991.
42. Palmaz JC, Laborde JC, Rivera FJ, et al: Stenting of the iliac arteries with the Palmaz stent: Experience from a multicenter trial. Cardiovasc Intervent Radiol 15:291, 1992.
43. Palmaz JC, Garcia O, Schatz RA, et al: Placement of balloon expandable stents in iliac arteries: First 171 patients. Radiology 174;969, 1990.
44. Strecker EP, Liermann DD, Barth KH, et al: Expandable tubular tantalum stents for treatment of arterial occlusive disease, with special reference to the iliac arteries. Radiology 173:268, 1989.
45. Martin EC, Katzen BT, Benenati JF, et al: Multicenter trial of the Wallstent in the iliac and femoral arteries. J Vasc Intervent Radiol 6:843, 1995.
46. Joffre F, Rousseau H, Puel J: Arterial stenting. J Intervent Radiol 4:155, 1989.
47. Günther RW, Vorwerk D, Bohndorf K, et al: Iliac and femoral artery stenoses and occlusions: Treatment with intravascular stents. Radiology 172:725, 1989.
48. Bertrand ME, Rickards AF, Serruys PW: Coronary stent implantation for primary and secondary prevention of restenosis after PTCA. Results of a pilot multicenter trial. Eur Heart J 9(Suppl A):55, 1988.
49. Zollikofer CL, Antonucci F, Pfyffer M, et al: Arterial stent placement with use of the Wallstent: Mid-term results of clinical experience. Radiology 179:457, 1991.
50. Do-dai-Do, Triller J, Walpoth BH, et al: A comparison study of self-expandable stents vs balloon angioplasty alone in femoropopliteal artery occlusions. Cardiovasc Intervent Radiol 15:306, 1992.
51. Rösch J, Uchida BT, Hall LD, et al: Expandable wire stents in treatment of venous obstructions (Abstract). Radiology 299:177, 1990.

52. Solomon N, Wholey MH, Jarmolowski CR: Intravascular stents in the management of superior vena cava syndrome. Cathet Cardiovasc Diagn 23:245, 1991.
53. Rösch J, Uchida BT, Hall LD, et al: Gianturco-Rösch expandable Z-stents in the treatment of superior vena cava syndrome. Cardiovasc Intervent Radiol 15:319, 1992.
54. Shoenfeld R, Hermans H, Novick A, et al: Stenting of proximal venous obstructions to maintain hemodialysis access. J Vasc Surg 19:532, 1994.
55. Katz SG, Kohl RD: The percutaneous treatment of angioaccess graft complications. Am J Surg 170:238, 1995.
56. Quinn SF, Schuman ES, Hall GF, et al: Venous stenoses in patients who undergo hemodialysis: Treatment with self-expandable endovascular stents. Radiology 183:499, 1992.
57. Penn IM, Levine SL, Schatz RA: Intravascular stents as an adjunct to endovascular intervention. In Moore WS, Ahn SS (eds): Endovascular Surgery. Philadelphia, WB Saunders Co, 1989, p 258.
58. Dichek DA, Neville RF, Zwiebel JA, et al: Seeding of intravascular stents with genetically engineered endothelial cells. Circulation 80:1347, 1989.
59. White GH, White RA, Kopchok GE, et al: Intraoperative video angioscopy compared with arteriography during peripheral vascular operations. J Vasc Surg 6:488, 1987.
60. Fleisher HL III, Thompson BW, McCowan TC, et al: Angioscopically monitored saphenous vein valvulotomy. J Vasc Surg 4:360, 1986.
61. Vollmar JF, Hutschenreiter S: Vascular endoscopy for thromboendarterectomy. In Moore WS, Ahn SS (eds): Endovascular Surgery. Philadelphia, WB Saunders Co, 1989, p 87.
62. LeMuraglia GM, Brewster DC, Moncure AC, et al: Angioscopic evaluation of unilateral aortic graft limb thrombectomy: Is it helpful? J Vasc Surg 17:1069, 1993.
63. Miller A, Stonebridge PA. Tsoukas AI, et al: Angioscopically directed valvulotomy: A new valvulotome and technique. J Vasc Surg 13:813, 1991.
64. Gilbertson JJ, Walsh DB, Zwolak RM, et al: A blinded comparison of angiography, angioscopy, and duplex scanning in the intraoperative evaluation of in situ saphenous vein bypass grafts. J Vasc Surg 15:121, 1992.
65. Clair DG, Golden MA, Mannick JA, et al: Randomized prospective study of angioscopically assisted in situ saphenous vein grafting. J Vasc Surg 19:992, 1994.
66. Rosenthal D, Herring MB, O'Donovan T, et al: Endovascular in situ femoropopliteal bypass: A multicenter preliminary report. J Vasc Surg 16:453, 1992.
67. Crikit DF, Dalsing MC, Lalka SG, et al: Early results of endovascular-assisted in situ saphenous vein bypass grafting. J Vasc Surg 19:778, 1994.
68. White GH, White RA, Kopchok GE, et al: Endoscopic intravascular surgery removes intraluminal flaps, dissections, and thrombus. J Vasc Surg 11:280, 1990.
69. Mehigan JT, Decampli WM: Angioscopic control of carotid endarterectomy. In Moore WS, Ahn SS (eds): Endovascular Surgery. Philadelphia, WB Saunders Co, 1989, p 95.
70. Vollmar JF, Loeprecht H, Hutschenreiter S: Advances in vascular endoscopy. Thorac Cardiovasc Surg 35:334, 1987.
71. Van Stiegmann G, Pearce WH, Bartle EJ, Rutherford RB: Flexible angioscopy seems faster and more specific than arteriography. Arch Surg 122:279, 1987.
72. Hashizume M, Yang Y, Galt S, et al: Intimal response of saphenous vein to intraluminal trauma by simulated angioscopic insertion. J Vasc Surg 5:862, 1987.
73. Towne JB: Complications of vascular endoscopy. In Moore WS, Ahn SS (eds): Endovascular Surgery. Philadelphia, WB Saunders Co, 1989, p 114.
74. Hinohara T, Robertson GC, Selmon MR, Simpson JB. Transluminal atherectomy: The Simpson atherectomy catheter. In Moore WS, Ahn SS (eds): Endovascular Surgery. Philadelphia, WB Saunders Co, 1989, p 310.
75. Hinohara T, Selmon MR, Robertson GC, et al: Directional atherectomy: New approaches for treatment of obstructive coronary and peripheral vascular disease. Circulation 81(Suppl IV):IV-79, 1990.
76. von Pölnitz A, Nerlich A, Berger H, Höfling B: Percutaneous peripheral atherectomy: Angiographic and clinical follow-up of 60 patients. J Am Coll Cardiol 15:682, 1990.
77. Graor RA, Whitlow PL: Transluminal atherectomy for occlusive peripheral vascular disease. J Am Coll Cardiol 15:1552, 1990.
78. Broegindewij D, Kemper FJM, Tielbeei AV, et al: Recurrence of stenoses following balloon angioplasty and Simpson atherectomy of the femoro-popliteal segment: A randomized comparative 1-year follow-up study using colour flow duplex. Eur J Vasc Surg 6:164, 1992.
79. Dalman RL, Taylor LM, Porter, JM: Current status of endovascular procedures for treatment of lower extremity atherosclerotic occlusive disease. Curr Prob Surg 28:103, 1991.
80. Dolmatch BL, Gray RJ, Horton KM, et al: Treatment of anastomotic bypass graft stenosis with directional atherectomy: Short-term and intermediate results. J Vasc Intervent Radiol 6: 105, 1995.
81. Mazur W, Ali NM, Rodgers GP, et al: Directional atherectomy with the Omnicath: A unique new catheter. Cathet Cardiovasc Diagn 31:79, 1994.
82. Prevosti LG, Cook JA, Unger EF, et al: Particulate debris from rotational atherectomy: Size, distribution, and physiological effect. Circulation 78(Suppl II):83, 1988.
83. Ahn SS, Arca M, Brauel G, et al: Histologic and morphologic effects of rotary atherectomy on human cadaver arteries. Ann Vasc Surg 4:563, 1990.
84. Titus BG, Auth DC, Ritchie JL: Distal embolization during mechanical thrombolysis: Rotational thrombectomy vs balloon angioplasty. Cathet Cardiovasc Diag 19:279, 1990.
85. Ahn SS, Eton D, Yeatman LR, et al: Intraoperative peripheral rotary atherectomy: Early and late clinical results. Ann Vasc Surg 6:272, 1992.
86. The Collaborative Rotablator Atherectomy Group: Peripheral atherectomy with the Rotablator: A multicenter report. J Vasc Surg 19:509, 1994.
87. Wholey MH, Jarmolowski CR, Fein D, et al: Multicenter trial with the transluminal endarterectomy catheter in 200 patients with peripheral vascular occlusive disease. Radiology 173(P): 267, 1989.
88. Reid JD, Hsiang YH, Doyle DL, et al: Atherectomy. Early use of three different methods. Can J Surg 35:242, 1992.
89. Ginsburg R: Laser angioplasty as an adjunct to balloon dilatation. In Moore WS, Ahn SS (eds): Endovascular Surgery. Philadelphia, WB Saunders Co, 1989, p 389.
90. Matsumoto T, Okamura T, Rajyaguru V: Laser arterial disobstructive procedures in 148 lower extremities. J Vasc Surg 10: 169, 1989.
91. Wright JG, Belkin M, Greenfield AJ, et al: Laser angioplasty for limb salvage: Observations on early results. J Vasc Surg 10:29, 1989.
92. Perler BA, Osterman FA, White RI Jr, Williams GM: Percutaneous laser probe femoropopliteal angioplasty: A preliminary experience. J Vasc Surg 10:351, 1989.
93. Pilger E, Lammer J, Bertuch H, et al: Nd:YAG laser with sapphire tip combined with balloon angioplasty in peripheral arterial occlusions long term results. Circulation 83:141, 1991.
94. Sanborn TA, Cumberland DC, Greenfield AJ, et al: Peripheral laser-assisted balloon angioplasty: Initial multicenter experience in 219 peripheral arteries. Arch Surg 124:1099, 1989.
95. Rosenthal D, Pesa FA, Gottsegen WL, et al: Thermal laser-assisted balloon angioplasty of the superficial femoral artery: A multicenter review of 602 cases. J Vasc Surg 14:152, 1991.
96. Miller BV, Sharp WJ, Shamma AR, et al: Surveillance for recurrent stenosis after endovascular procedures. Arch Surg 126: 867, 1991.
97. McCarthy WJ, Vogelzang RL, Nemcek AA Jr, et al: Excimer laser-assisted femoral angioplasty: Early results. J Vasc Surg 13: 607, 1991.
98. Litvack F, Grundfest WS, Adler L, et al: Percutaneous excimer-laser and excimer-laser assisted angioplasty of the lower extremities: Results of initial clinical trial. Radiology 172:331, 1989.
99. Geschwind HJ, Aptecar E, Boussignac G, et al: Results and follow-up after percutaneous pulsed laser-assisted balloon angioplasty guided by spectroscopy. Circulation 83:787, 1991.
100. Nissen SE, Grines CL, Gurley JC, et al: Application of a new phased-array ultrasound imaging catheter in the assessment of vascular dimensions: In vivo comparison to cineangiography. Circulation 81:660, 1990.
101. Isner JM, Rosenfield K, Losordo DW, et al: Percutaneous intra-

vascular US as adjunct to catheter-based interventions: Preliminary experience in patients with peripheral vascular disease. Radiology 175:61, 1990.
102. Pandian NG, Kreis A, Brockway B, et al: Intravascular high frequency two-dimensional ultrasound detection of arterial dissection and intimal flaps. Am J Cardiol 65:1278, 1990.
103. Tabbara M, White R, Cavaye D, Kopchok G: In vivo human comparison of intravascular ultrasonography and angiography. J Vasc Surg 14:496, 1991.
104. Keren G, Douek P, Oblon C, et al: Atherosclerotic saphenous vein grafts treated with different interventional procedures assessed by intravascular ultrasound. Am Heart J 124:198, 1992.
105. Neville RF Jr, Yasuhara H, Watanabe BI, et al: Endovascular management of arterial intimal defects: An experimental comparison by arteriography, angioscopy, and intravascular ultrasonography. J Vasc Surg 13:496, 1991.
106. Cayvelle DM, Tabbara MR, Kopchok GE, et al: Intraluminal ultrasound assessment of vascular stent deployment. Ann Vasc Surg 5:241, 1991.
107. Sarfati PO, Bonnichon P, Pariente D, Chapuis Y: Intraoperative ultrasonography for location of proximal limit of inferior vena caval thrombosis. Ann Vasc Surg 5:459, 1991.
108. Cavaye DM, French WJ, White RA, et al: Intravascular ultrasound imaging of an acute dissecting aortic aneurysm: A case report. J Vasc Surg 13:510, 1991.
109. West AI: Endovascular ultrasound. In Moore WS, Ahn SS (eds): Endovascular Surgery. Philadelphia, WB Saunders Co, 1989, p 518.
110. Mirich D, Wright KC, Wallace S, et al: Percutaneously placed endovascular grafts for aortic aneurysms: Feasibility study. Radiology 170:1033, 1989.
111. Laborde JC, Parodi JC, Clem MF, et al: Intraluminal bypass of abdominal aortic aneurysms: Feasibility. Radiology 184:185, 1992.
112. Parodi JC, Palmaz JC, Barone HD: Transfemoral intraluminal graft implantation for abdominal aortic aneurysms. Ann Vasc Surg 5:491, 1991.
113. May J, White GH, Waugh RC, et al: Results of endoluminal grafting of abdominal aortic aneurysms. J Vasc Surg (submitted).
114. Chuter TAM, Green RM, Ouriel K, DeWeese JA: Infrarenal aortic aneurysm structure: Implications for transfemoral repair. J Vasc Surg 20:44, 1994.
115. Chutter TAM, Green RM, Ouriel K, et al: Transfemoral endovascular aortic graft placement. J Vasc Surg 18:185, 1993.
116. Moore WS, for the EVT Investigators: Transfemoral endovascular repair of abdominal aortic aneurysm: Results of the North American EVT phase 1 trial: J Vasc Surg 23:543, 1996.
117. Armon MP, Yusuf SW, Latief K, et al: Anatomical suitability of abdominal aortic aneurysms for endovascular repair. Br J Surg 84:178, 1997.
118. Lumsden AB, Allen RC, Chaikof EL, et al: Delayed rupture of aortic aneurysms following endovascular stent grafting. Am J Surg 170:174, 1995.
119. Marin ML, Veith FJ, Panetta TF, et al: Percutaneous transfemoral insertion of a stented graft to repair a traumatic femoral arteriovenous fistula. J Vasc Surg 18:1056, 1993.
120. Marin ML, Veith FJ, Panetta TF, et al: Transluminally placed endovascular stented graft repair for arterial trauma. J Vasc Surg 20:466, 1994.
121. Marin ML, Veith FJ, Cynamon J, et al: Initial experience with transluminally placed endovascular grafts for the treatment of complex vascular lesions. Ann Surg 222:449, 1995.

CHAPTER 21

Intrathoracic Aortic Surgery

Katherine Marschall, M.D.

Pathogenesis of Aneurysms

Intrathoracic aortic lesions include "true" aneurysms such as those caused by atherosclerosis, syphilis, and some degenerative diseases; "false" aneurysms such as those caused by acute trauma; and nonaneurysmal but extremely destructive aortic lesions such as acute aortic dissection.

True aneurysms involve all three layers of the aortic wall. There is an initial degeneration of the aortic media that allows the aortic wall to stretch; as it increases in size there is a corresponding increase in wall tension that leads to further dilation and further increases in wall tension, and rupture becomes increasingly likely. With a false aneurysm there is disruption of the intimal and medial layers of the aortic wall, with adventitia or perivascular clot providing the only "cover" to the aorta in that location.

For aneurysms to form there needs to be some basic defect in elastin production or function that leads to elastin overload, followed by collagen overload, followed by dilation of the aorta. In addition to these structural defects, there must also be an excessive force or pressure load on the aorta.

Overview of Aortic Pathology

The diseases associated with intrathoracic aortic pathology include acute or chronic aortic dissection in patients with degenerative disease of the aortic media (cystic medial necrosis, Marfan's syndrome, and other connective tissue diseases associated with loss of elastin or collagen and medial degeneration associated with aging), acute and chronic traumatic injury, syphilis, and atherosclerosis.[1]

Aortic Dissection

Acute aortic dissection is a rare but catastrophic lesion affecting aortic tissue. The pathogenesis of the initial rupture or tear in the intima is not understood, but once this has occurred, there is separation of the intramural layers of the aorta by the force of the stream of blood, the dissection usually occurring at the junction of the middle and outer layers of the media. The dissection progresses distally, involving all or a portion of the circumference of the aorta, and when it reaches branches of the aorta, these may either be sheared off or the dissecting process may extend along them for varying distances. This results in a diminution or complete interruption of blood supply in the area subserved by the branch. The course and extent of dissections are variable. In the most severe and acute form of the disease there will be a rapid dissection and finally a terminal perforation through the adventitia into the pericardium, mediastinum, or pleural or abdominal cavities with death ensuing within a few hours or days. In a more subacute form, the process begins abruptly, but the progression of the dissection is more gradual, over days or weeks, and then terminal adventitial rupture and death ensue. In a chronic dissection there is re-entry of the dissected passage back into the true lumen of the aorta. The false passage may become endothelialized or may be obliterated by fibrous tissue organization.

Acute aortic dissection is not associated with true aneurysm formation and therefore the term "dissecting aortic aneurysm" is inaccurate and should be reserved for chronic aortic dissections that actually develop aneurysmal dilation of the aorta. In the acute phase the condition is best described by the term "acute dissection of the aorta."

What predisposes the aorta to this particular kind of injury? Traditionally it has been taught that there is an abnormality in the aortic media in these patients, particularly cystic medial necrosis or the elastin/collagen abnormalities of the inherited connective tissue disorders such as Marfan's syndrome and Ehlers-Danlos syndrome.[2] These medial defects make the aortic wall weaker and more susceptible to separation of its layers. In the various forms of medial degeneration there may be cystic or noncystic medial necrosis, some loss of smooth muscle cells and elastic tissue in the media, scarring and fibrosis, and hyalin changes. Interestingly, it has been found that older people with "normal" aortas have some of the changes of cystic medial necrosis—fragmentation of elastin fibers, fibrosis, and other cellular abnormalities—suggesting that there is a correlation between the degree of these changes and the age of the patient. This correlation suggests that medial degeneration is a natural process associated with aging and that the differences in the aorta media between those who do and do not have aortic dissection are quantitative rather than qualitative.[3]

Aortic dissections more commonly involve the ascending aorta, less commonly the descending aorta, and they are often present in younger patients. Since the age and anatomic distributions of these lesions are opposite to that typically found with atherosclerosis, it does not appear that these changes are a result of atherosclerosis.

Other conditions associated with dissection include hypertension, especially in older patients. Half of dissections in women under the age of 40 occur during pregnancy, typically during the third trimester or during labor, and in half of these hypertension will be present.[4]

Several hemodynamic events occur inside the aorta with each cardiac cycle and these have their greatest effects on the ascending aorta as demonstrated by the more marked age-related degenerative changes in the ascending aorta. The ascending aorta is also subjected to the most external motion and flexion with each systole. In addition there may be a direct traumatic effect on the ascending aorta as blood is ejected from the heart against the aortic wall. The combination of some medial degeneration, recurring flexion of the aorta, and various tensions applied to the aortic intima by hydrodynamic forces operating within the aorta may lead to an intimal tear and the initiation of a dissection.[5] The tear occurs in the ascending aorta in 60 to 65%, in the aorta arch in 5 to 10%, and in the descending thoracic aorta in 30 to 35% of patients.

Subsequent propagation of the dissecting hematoma is related to hydrodynamic forces in the aorta, and experimental evidence indicates that the most important of these are the amplitude of the pulse wave in the aorta (which directly relates to dP/dt_{max} in the heart) and absolute blood pressure. Laboratory models implicate pulsatile flow as the more important factor in the propagation of a dissection. Wheat and Palmer performed elegant laboratory experiments creating a model aorta which showed that once an intimal tear in this aorta was created, no extension of this dissection would occur if flow through this "aorta" was laminar. However, when pulsatile flow was initiated, dissection extended rapidly. In the laminar flow state, there was no pressure gradient between the torn intima and the adjacent portions of the aorta, and this gradient is the driving force for extending the dissection (Fig. 21–1). Wheat and Palmer deduced that if one could modify the shape of the pressure curve in the aorta—that is, flatten it (reduce dP/dt_{max})—one would minimize this pressure gradient and slow down, or even arrest the dissection process.[5]

Information from the veterinary literature indicated that turkeys who naturally have a high incidence of aortic dissection and death at a young age had a remarkable reduction in early mortality when a small amount of reserpine was added to their feed. From this information and that obtained from their laboratory models, Wheat and Palmer inferred that the reserpine was not changing the blood pressure in the turkey so much as it was flattening the amplitude of the pulsatile wave in the aorta. This reduction in what they called "impulse" or dP/dt_{max} was responsible for the improved survival of the turkeys. They then transferred these data from veterinary and laboratory observation to the medical management of patients with acute aortic dissection.[6]

Some endocrine disorders have been associated with dissection probably through the development of hypertension. Bicuspid aortic valve with or without aortic stenosis and coarctation of the aorta are the most common congenital cardiovascular abnormalities associated with aortic dissection.

Trauma may result in intimal disruption and a dissecting hematoma either from a deceleration injury such as in a motor vehicle accident or from iatrogenic causes including dye injections during arteriography with dye being injected into the aortic wall, placement of the arterial cannula for initiation of extracorporeal circulation, and after some aortic valve or aortic graft operations.

Most patients presenting with aortic dissection complain of sudden onset of intense, unremitting, excruciating pain that may be described as tearing or ripping and is usually located in the back between the scapulae. The pain is often accompanied by a fear of imminent death. Initial pain that subsides and then recurs usually signifies a resumption of the propagation of the dissection. Patients can present in any number of ways depending on the path of the dissection. There may be transient or permanent paralysis or blindness, gastrointestinal symptoms, abdominal pain, nausea and vomiting, melena or hematemesis, dyspnea or hemoptysis, heart failure, anuria or hematuria, and limb pain. Patients are in acute distress and are typically pale or ashen and appear to be in shock even though their blood pressure may be very high. The finding of unequal or absent pulses in the limbs is highly suggestive of acute aortic

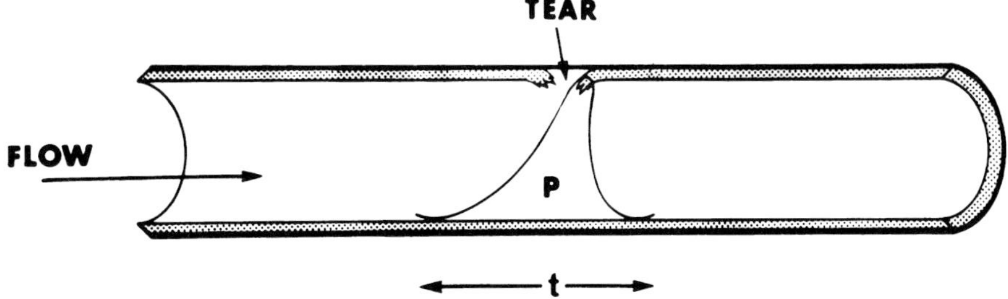

FIGURE **21–1.** A model aorta with an "intimal tear." Under pulsatile conditions, depending upon the sharpness of the pressure curve *P* at any time *t*, a pressure gradient exists between the torn and the intact portions of the aortic wall and this gradient is the driving force for extending a dissection. (From Palmer RF, Wheat MW Jr; Treatment of dissecting aneurysms of the aorta. Ann Thorac Surg 4:38, 1967, with permission.)

dissection. The diastolic murmur of aortic insufficiency is present in about a quarter of patients and this new murmur is also highly suggestive of acute aortic dissection.

Supportive laboratory findings include the electrocardiogram (ECG), since acute myocardial infarction (MI) is in the differential diagnosis. A plain x-ray of the chest may show widening of the mediastinum. Today, a definitive diagnosis of acute aortic dissection can be made most rapidly by transesophageal echocardiography (TEE), which is capable of making the diagnosis in over 95% of patients.[7–10] The echo can usually outline the location of the intimal tear and define which segment(s) of the aorta are involved (Fig. 21–2). The most sensitive and specific noninvasive test to diagnose aortic dissection is magnetic resonance imaging (MRI). MRI is virtually always able to make the diagnosis of aortic dissection, to outline the location of the intimal tear as well as re-entry sites, and to show abnormalities that extend into the branches of the aorta at any location from the aortic valve down to and beyond the aortic bifurcation.[10] The disadvantages of MRI in the acute management of aortic dissection include the length of time for the test, the necessity to transport the patient to and from the scanner, and the difficulties with intensive monitoring of these critically ill patients during the scan. The quality of the data obtained from transesophageal echocardiography and magnetic resonance imaging is excellent and obviates the need for arteriography in most patients.[9,10] The significant risks associated with an aortic

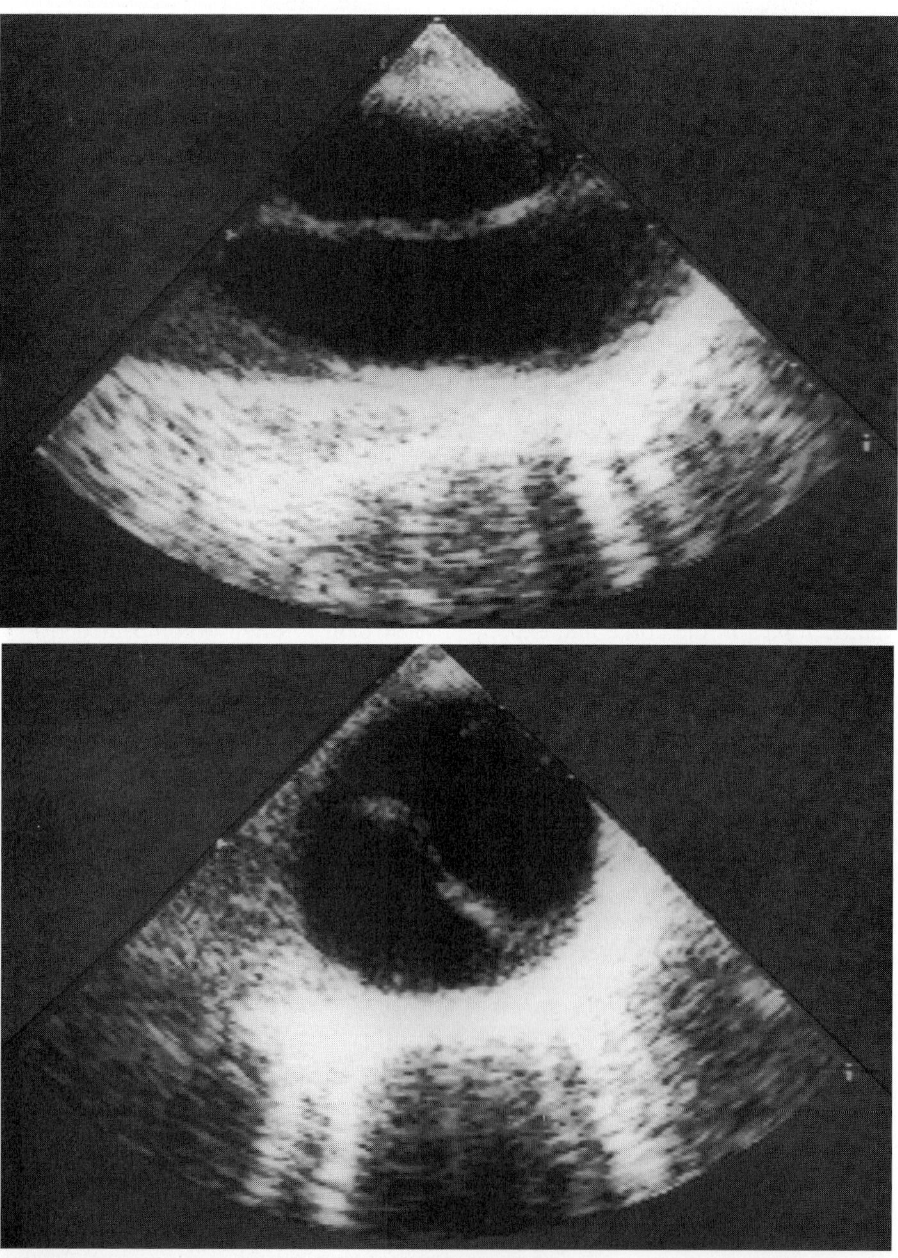

FIGURE **21–2.** Images of acute aortic dissection as seen by transesophageal echocardiography. The raised intimal flap is clearly visible in the aortic arch (*top*) and the descending thoracic aorta (*bottom*).

angiogram are obviated as well, including entry into the false lumen, propagation of the dissection during dye injection, and perforation of the adventitia with the catheter or the dye injection. The findings of the noninvasive tests, namely, transesophageal echocardiography and magnetic resonance imaging, have been shown to correlate very well with the morphologic findings found at surgery or autopsy.[10]

The diagnosis of aortic dissection can be made within a few hours of the time of hospital admission and appropriate therapy planned. The prognosis of untreated dissection is extremely poor—mortality averages 1% per hour for the first 48 hours, and approaches 90% by 1 week.[2] The likelihood of survival beyond a few months is extremely low. Some have suggested likening the mortality of acute aortic dissection to that of an extremely aggressive cancer, and so very aggressive approaches toward controlling this disease are warranted.

Classification Systems

Two classification systems have evolved to describe the location of acute dissections; from these anatomic classifications treatment regimens have evolved. The DeBakey classification divides dissections into types I, II, and III (Fig. 21–3).[11] A type I dissection involves the ascending aorta and can extend for variable distances beyond it, so it may include the arch and descending thoracic aorta as well. A type II dissection involves only the ascending aorta, and a type III dissection begins distal to the left subclavian artery and extends for variable distances beyond that.

The Stanford classification divides dissections into types A and B (Fig. 21–4).[12] Type A dissections involve the ascending aorta and may involve other portions of the aorta as well. Type B dissections involve portions of the aorta other than the ascending aorta.

The earliest efforts at surgical management of aortic dissection were aimed at trying to simulate surgically what happened naturally to survivors of acute dissection, namely, development of a re-entry site and return of the blood flow from the false lumen back into the true lumen.[13] Most patients that appeared with a chronic dissection had evidence of this "double-barreled" aorta. It became clear in a short period of time that surgery to simulate this condition was not helpful, and the search began for ways to recreate normal aortic mural integrity. The intimal tear was oversewn whenever possible so that blood would stop entering the false lumen. Weakened sections of aorta were replaced by tubular grafts. Acute aortic regurgitation was treated by resuspension of the aortic valve or valve replacement if necessary. There have been many refinements in surgical techniques, in the quality of graft materials, in cardiopulmonary bypass, and in alternative ways to perfuse major portions of the body during aortic resection, and all of these have helped improve outcomes in these patients.[14–16]

At the present time, management of the patient with acute dissection requires early recognition of the problem and initiation of medical management once the diagnosis is either suspected or confirmed. Medical management consists of drug therapy aimed at reducing the rate of rise of the aortic pressure pulse. Drugs that reduce left ventricular dP/dt_{max} are effective in this regard. Propranolol has become the drug of choice to use in acute aortic dissection, either alone to reduce "impulse" or in combination with a vasodilator such as nitroprusside to

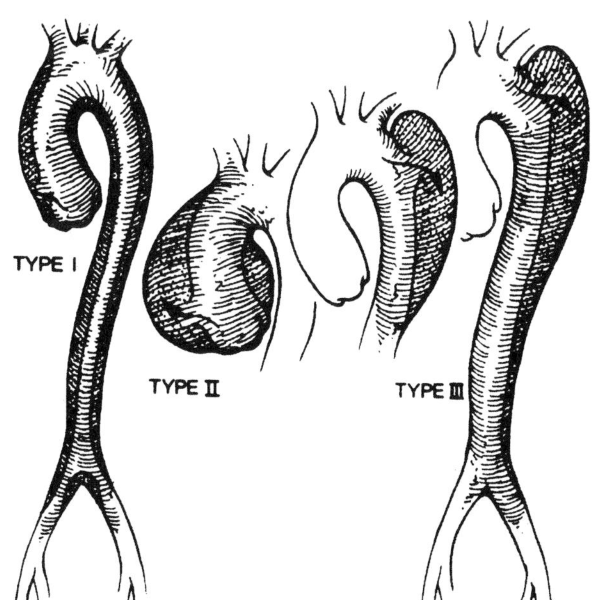

FIGURE **21–3.** DeBakey classification of aortic dissections into three types depending on the site and extent of the dissecting process. *Arrows* indicate the most common sites of the initial intimal tear in each type. (From DeBakey ME, Henly WS, Cooley DA, et al: Surgical management of dissecting aneurysms of the aorta. J Thorac Cardiovasc Surg 49:130, 1965, with permission.)

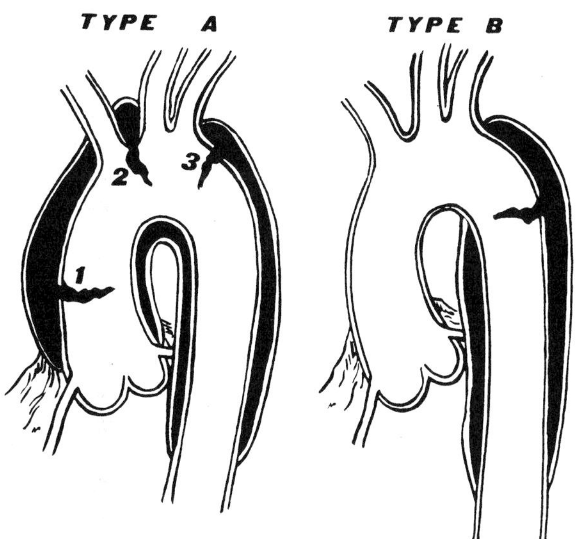

FIGURE **21–4.** Stanford classification of aortic dissections based upon the presence or absence of involvement of the ascending aorta. The primary intimal tear in type A dissections can be in the ascending aorta (1), arch (2), or descending aorta (3). The intimal tear is usually distal to the left subclavian artery in a type B dissection. (From Miller DC, Stinson EB, Oyer PE, et al: Operative treatment of aortic dissections. J Thorac Cardiovasc Surg 78:365, 1979, with permission.)

reduce absolute blood pressure to normal in hypertensive patients. Medical therapy is continued until the patient comes to the operating room for surgical repair and is continued in those patients who will receive only medical management in the acute phase and, indeed, medical therapy is lifelong in all patients whether treated medically or surgically to help prevent recurrent dissection.[3,17]

At the present time, most feel that dissections involving the ascending aorta (type I, II, or A) should be treated surgically and aggressively in the acute phase.[12,16–18] Many feel that dissections limited to the descending aorta (type III or B) should also be treated surgically, though there is controversy about this.[12,16,18–20] There are some who feel that more distal dissections, as long as they are not complicated by loss of flow in major aortic tributaries, will do well with medical therapy alone.[15,21,22]

Survival in the acute phase of aortic dissection appears to be highly correlated with the presence of complications, such as neurologic deficits; pericardial tamponade; hemothorax; hemoperitoneum; or myocardial, mesenteric, or renal infarction (Fig. 21–5).[12,15,18] The presence of aortic insufficiency by itself, however, does not influence early survival. Long-term survival in all patients with aortic dissection is related to complications of coronary artery disease such as myocardial infarction, congestive heart failure, and sudden death, or to recurrent rupture or complications of the dissection itself.[14,23] Often, late death is related to reoperation for some dissection-related problem. Thus long-term evaluation of these patients requires attention to the presence of concomitant coronary artery disease as well as continued surveillance of the entire aorta for evidence of complications related to dissection such as new dissection, aneurysm formation in the area of a previous dissection, or complications of surgical repair. In addition, intensive medical therapy to control the hydrodynamic forces that may initiate or propagate dissection is also necessary.

Traumatic Thoracic Aneurysms

There are two kinds of injuries that can result in a traumatic thoracic aneurysm or aortic rupture: deceleration injuries that occur most commonly to passengers in automobile accidents and acceleration injuries usually involving pedestrians struck by cars. Deceleration and acceleration injuries create very similar damage to the thoracic aorta.[24–26] The site of rupture will be just distal to the ligamentum arteriosum because that is the point at which the aorta is fixed (Fig. 21–6). The aortic arch is held in place by the innominate, carotid, and subclavian vessels and the distal part of the aortic arch is supported by the ligamentum arteriosum. The distal portion of the descending thoracic aorta is attached at the diaphragm. Between the point of the ligamentum arteriosum and the diaphragm only the pleura and intercostal arteries prevent or retard the forward motion of the thoracic aorta in a rapid deceleration. The blood-filled thoracic aorta acts very much like a solid viscus adding weight and force to this forward motion, so typically the rupture occurs just distal to the left subclavian artery. Aortic injury can vary from harmless intimal tears to intimal tears which can create a dissection to complete severance which often results in death at the scene of the accident. Some patients may survive to reach the hospital because they form a false aneurysm of periadventitial clot around the site of injury. Other patients may go on to develop chronic, usually saccular aneurysms and present for surgery at a later time.[27]

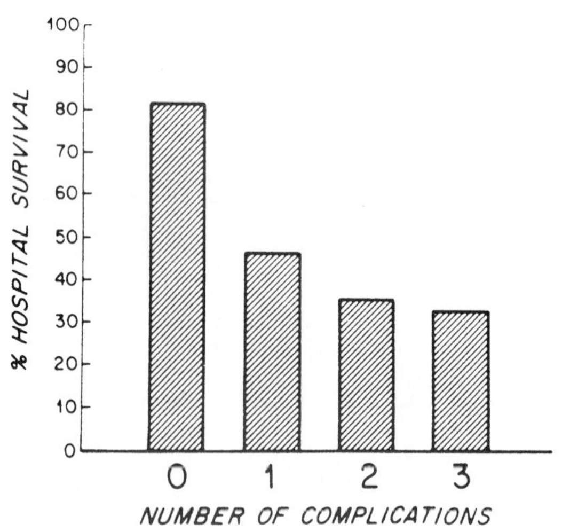

FIGURE **21–5.** Percentage hospital survival as a function of the number of major complications resulting from the aortic dissection. These include neurologic deficit; pulse loss; cardiac tamponade; hemothorax; hemoperitoneum; and myocardial, mesenteric, or renal infarction but do not include aortic insufficiency. (From Doroghazi RM, Slater EE, DeSanctis RW, et al: Long-term survival of patients with treated aortic dissection. J Am Coll Cardiol 3:1026, 1984, with permission.)

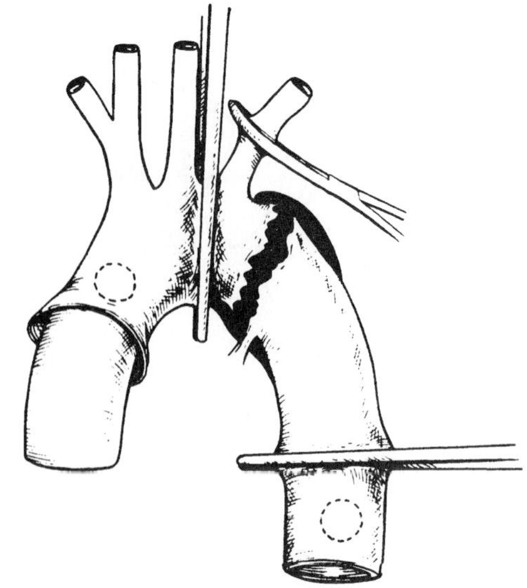

FIGURE **21–6.** Drawing of the usual site of traumatic injury to the descending thoracic aorta near the origin of the left subclavian artery. The sites for clamping to achieve hemostasis in this situation are also noted. (From Turney SZ, Attary S, Ayella R, et al: Traumatic rupture of the aorta. J Thorac Cardiovasc Surg 72:727, 1976, with permission.)

Care of patients with acute traumatic thoracic aneurysms is complicated by the fact that there may already have been significant hemorrhage, either from the aortic injury or from other associated injuries, and hypovolemic shock may be present before these individuals arrive in the operating room. The overall risk of major organ damage is therefore quite high.[25,28] In addition, the presence of other suspected or unsuspected associated injuries makes intraoperative systemic anticoagulation extremely hazardous and, indeed, potentially fatal.

Atherosclerosis

Traditionally, in all aortic aneurysms with evidence of atherosclerosis, this disease entity was assumed to be the primary cause of the aneurysm. However, recent work suggests that in many patients the atherosclerotic changes in aneurysms are secondary.[29] In 1984 the first report of familial clustering of aneurysms was published and a sixfold increase in the risk-odds ratio for an aneurysm was noted among first-degree relatives of an aneurysm proband.[30–32] Aneurysms typically have a 3:1 to 8:1 male predominance. There have been reports of a marked increase in risk in families with an affected mother, suggesting X-linked inheritance.[33] Others suggest autosomal or multifactorial inheritance.[33]

Genes could be responsible for aneurysm formation by affecting elastin in several ways.[34] There could be a genetically altered basic structure of elastin that reduces its strength. There could be accelerated proteolysis resulting in elastin degradation. Or there could be a reduction in the concentrations of protease inhibitors such as α_1-antitrypsin or tissue inhibitor of metalloprotease. The relationship between protease inhibitors and elastase is analogous to that between the coagulation and fibrinolytic systems (i.e., there is a balance between build-up and breakdown of elastin). In the presence of α_1-antitrypsin deficiency, there will be an increase in elastolytic activity. Biochemical analyses of aneurysmal aortic tissue has demonstrated a marked decrease in elastin content and 10% of specimens had measurable decreases in α_1-antitrypsin concentrations.[33]

Smoking is a defined risk factor for development of atherosclerosis as well as for aortic aneurysmal disease. The link to aneurysm formation may be the decrease in α_1-antitrypsin activity and the increase in neutrophil elastase activity noted in patients with emphysema.[34]

Atherosclerosis itself may contribute to development of aortic aneurysms in several ways.[35] Elastin and collagen are synthesized by smooth muscle cells in the aortic wall and a stimulus for their production is the pulsation in the aortic wall. When these oscillations are attenuated in an aortic wall stiffened by atherosclerosis, then production may decrease. In the distal (abdominal) aorta the media is devoid of vasa vasorum and nutrition is largely dependent on diffusion of nutrients from the aortic lumen. Such diffusion may be compromised when the subendothelial region is thickened by atherosclerosis. So these and other effects of atherosclerosis may decrease the reparative capabilities of the aortic wall and result in gradual depletion of elastin and collagen with subsequent aneurysm formation.

The major risks of aortic surgery include hemorrhage, vital organ ischemia, and atheroembolism, so anesthetic considerations must include plans for maintaining cardiovascular stability, preservation of vital organ function, blood conservation, and temperature control. It is very useful to divide the aorta into four regions based on the location of the aneurysm and the aortic cross-clamp, since these will determine the degree of cardiovascular stress; the risk of organ ischemia; and the need for special procedures such as cardiopulmonary bypass, passive or active shunts, moderate or profound hypothermia, and circulatory arrest. The four anatomic regions of the aorta are: (1) the ascending aorta including the aortic root, (2) the aortic arch, (3) the descending thoracic aorta, and (4) the thoracoabdominal aorta.

Surgery on the Ascending Aorta

There are four basic surgical considerations for repair of ascending aortic aneurysms or dissections. There must be: (1) complete removal of the aneurysm; (2) restoration of aortic continuity; (3) correction of aortic valve incompetence, if present; and (4) unimpeded flow of blood into the coronary arteries. The problems of ascending aortic surgery are present in their most complex form when the aortic pathology involves not only the ascending aorta but also the aortic root.[36] The aortic root is that portion of the ascending aorta from the annulus fibrosis to 2 cm superior to the coronary artery ostia (Fig. 21–7). Aneurysms of the aortic root arise from the first few centimeters of the ascending aorta and always involve the aortic valve and that portion of the aorta containing the coronary artery ostia.

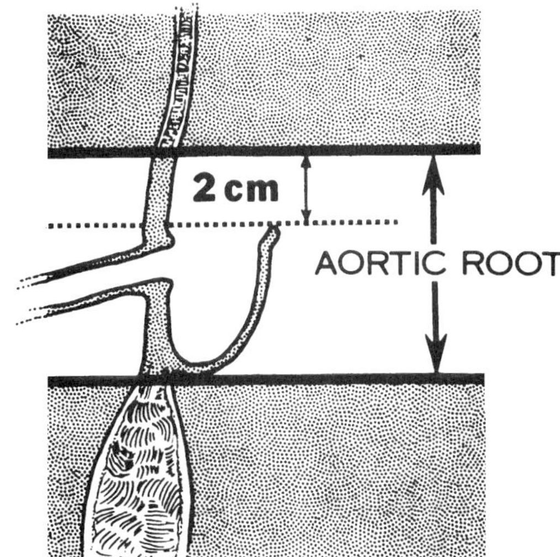

FIGURE **21–7.** The aortic root shown as the first portion of the ascending aorta from the aortic annulus fibrosis to 2 cm superior to the coronary artery ostia. (From Wheat MW Jr, Boruchow IB, Ramsey HW: Surgical treatment of aneurysms of the aortic root. Ann Thorac Surg 12:593, 1971, with permission.)

The most common cause of disease in the aortic root is anuloaortic ectasia, which is dilation of the sinuses of Valsalva with associated moderate or severe aortic valvular incompetence, superior displacement of the coronary ostia, and varying degrees of dilation of the more distal ascending aorta. Acute or chronic dissection of the ascending aorta is another common cause of lesions in the aortic root.[37] Other etiologies include aneurysms of the sinus of Valsalva following previous graft replacement of the ascending aorta or previous aortic valve replacement. Poststenotic dilatation from aortic stenosis and some forms of luetic aortitis may also create a diseased aortic root.

The two surgical methods currently used to repair the aortic root and ascending aorta are: (1) supracoronary artery tube graft replacement of the ascending aorta with aortic valve repair or replacement or (2) replacement of the aortic valve and ascending aorta with a composite graft that consists of a woven Dacron tube graft containing an aortic valve prosthesis.[38–40] The composite graft can be purchased with any kind of aortic valve already in place or one can sew an aortic valve into a tube graft prior to inserting the unit into a patient.

Obviously, insertion of a composite graft requires reimplantation of the coronary arteries. Proponents of composite graft use feel that it is important to have complete resection of ectatic aorta.[38,39,41,42] A conservative or incomplete resection leaves behind a persistent pathologic zone that may be the site of later dissection or aneurysm formation involving the sinus of Valsalva.

Replacement of the ascending aorta requires cardiopulmonary bypass (CPB). Occasionally it may be quite difficult to cannulate the right atrium or the vena cava because of the size of the aneurysm; in such a situation, one can decompress the aneurysm using an initially low bypass flow, and as exposure of the atrium improves, full cannulation and full CPB can be instituted. Alternatively, one can utilize femorofemoral bypass.

The aorta will be cross-clamped just proximal to the innominate artery, opened, and examined. For composite graft insertion, the aortic valve will be removed, the coronary arteries with a rim of aortic tissue left around their origins will be removed from the native aorta, the composite graft will be sewn in, and the coronary arteries will be reimplanted into the aortic graft. Concomitant coronary artery bypass grafting may be necessary in some patients. This procedure can be accomplished by inserting a tube graft of smaller diameter between the aortic graft and the distal coronary artery, or by a venous interposition between the aortic graft and the distal coronary artery. A group from France has suggested using a small Dacron tube that attaches to both coronary arteries as the conduit of choice for providing coronary blood flow.[42]

If a composite graft is not used, then surgery will consist of repair or replacement of the aortic valve followed by placement of a tube graft above the origins of the coronary arteries.[40,43] There is no need for reimplantation or manipulation of the coronaries. For diseases of the ascending aorta that begin superior to the origins of the coronary arteries, a simple tube graft is adequate for aortic replacement (Fig. 21–8). However, since aneurysmal disease in the ascending aorta often causes dilation of the aortic valve ring, it is often necessary to resuspend or repair the aortic valve in addition to inserting the supracoronary tube graft. Aortic valve resuspension has traditionally been done utilizing some form of suturing technique with the sutures passing through the aortic wall. These sutures can make the aortic wall more fragile and bleeding can occur at the suture sites. To obviate these problems, Seguin et al. have recently suggested simply "gluing" the two aortic layers of the aortic root with fibrin "glue" without the use of any sutures.[44] They feel that this technique not only achieves resuspension of the valve but also reinforces the aortic root before replacement of the ascending aorta.

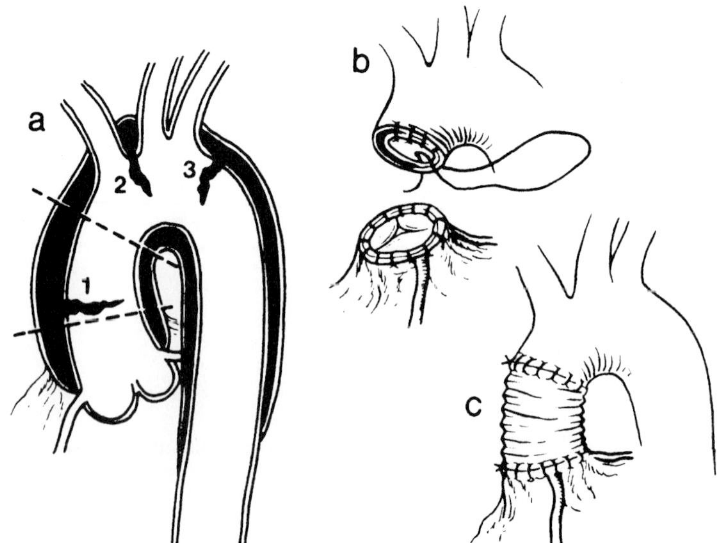

FIGURE **21–8.** Operative technique utilized for repair of type A aortic dissection. The segment of ascending aorta containing the intimal tear is exposed, resected, and replaced with a tubular Dacron graft. The aortic valve is resuspended if necessary and the false lumen oversewn and closed proximally and distally prior to performing the anastomoses. The proximal anastomosis is above the level of the coronary ostia. (From Miller DC, Stinson EB, Oyer PE, et al: Operative treatment of aortic dissections. J Thorac Cardiovasc Surg 78: 365, 1979, with permission.)

Once the aortic conduit is sewn in place, most will take the remaining native ascending aortic tissue, trim it, and cover over the tube graft with this native tissue, the so-called graft-inclusion technique. The principal advantage of this graft-inclusion technique is to reduce the risk of infection by reducing exposure of the graft material to other structures. A significant disadvantage is that bleeding can occur between the aortic graft and this native aortic "cover." If excessive pressure builds up in the space between the graft and the covering tissue, there could be compression of the graft and consequent reduced vital organ blood flow. Cabrol has recommended that a fistula about 1 cm in diameter be created between this graft/aortic wrap space and the right atrium, a technically simple maneuver (Fig. 21–9).[38] Such a fistula has two major advantages: (1) it serves to decompress the graft/aortic wrap space should there be a significant amount of bleeding there, and (2) this blood is recycled through the right atrium into the general circulation and is not lost. Once bleeding stops, the fistula begins to close. In 95% of patients the fistulous tract closes completely.

Dissection of the ascending aorta is a rare but often catastrophic complication of cardiac surgery.[45] The initiating event is typically intimal injury from surgical manipulation of the ascending aorta (e.g., by placement of the partial occluding clamp, the aortic cross-clamp, or the cardioplegia injection cannula or anastomosis of the proximal end of a vein graft). This complication occurs with an incidence of only 0.3% but has very high morbidity and mortality. Critical events associated with this form of dissection include failure to wean from cardiopulmonary bypass, heart failure, cardiac tamponade, and hemorrhage. Of course, any of the other complications of aortic dissection can occur as well.

The dissection is usually apparent immediately, but occasionally it may not be obvious until the postoperative period when the hydrodynamic forces necessary for propagation of a dissection are enhanced by the hyperdynamic and hypertensive state that often follows open heart surgery. The importance of postoperative hemodynamic control cannot be overstated. Intraoperative aortic dissection usually presents as an aortic wall hematoma that can be pulsatile. Unlike the common subadventitial hematomas, dissections bleed briskly when the overlying media and adventitia are incised.

An acute ascending aortic dissection during heart surgery may, if it is a very limited dissection, be treated by closed plication. The dissecting hematoma is contained within a partial occlusion clamp and then plicated with Teflon felt pledgettes. If the dissection is more complex and extensive, then Dacron graft replacement of the ascending aorta may be required. The aortic perfusion cannula is moved elsewhere and a Dacron graft is attached in such a way that it includes all the surgical sites on the aorta involved in the dissection.

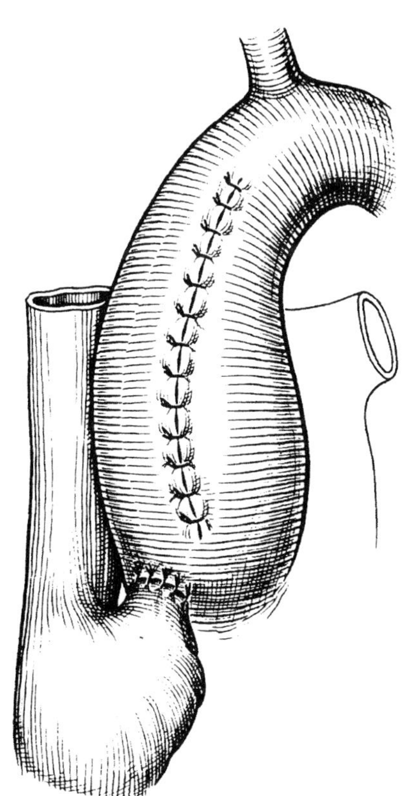

FIGURE **21–9.** The periprosthetic space is drained into the right atrium by creating a 1-cm fistula between that space and the right atrial appendage. (From Cabrol C, Pavie A, Gandjbakhch I, et al: Complete replacement of the ascending aorta with reimplantation of the coronary arteries. J Thorac Cardiovasc Surg 81:309, 1981, with permission.)

Anesthetic Considerations

1. The patient usually will be supine with the surgery performed through a median sternotomy and facilitated by the use of CPB. CPB is usually atrioaortic (arch cannulation) but may be atriofemoral or femorofemoral. Mild hypothermia is usually used.
2. The aorta will usually be clamped proximal to the innominate artery. If the ascending aortic pathology involves or ends very close to the innominate artery, clamping will be required between the innominate artery and the left carotid artery. In this circumstance, total circulatory arrest will be necessary. The arterial catheter for pressure monitoring should be inserted into the left radial artery.
3. Blood pressure should be carefully controlled. In the presence of aortic dissection, dP/dt_{max} must be controlled. β-Adrenergic receptor blocking drugs are excellent for this. Use of inotropic drugs in the presence of aortic dissection is very hazardous because of the significant increase in impulse that they produce.
4. The risk of hemorrhage is moderate. Bleeding may occur from the aortic suture lines, through the graft itself or, if a graft-inclusion technique was used, into the graft/aortic wrap space. This last form of bleeding may not be apparent clinically. The bypass pump and reservoir, a cell-saver system, and two or more large-bore intravenous catheters should be adequate to control hemorrhage. A dilutional coagulopathy or a pro-

longed period of cardiopulmonary bypass will require administration of platelets and fresh frozen plasma.
5. Beware aortic valve dysfunction if the aortic valve has been repaired or resuspended.
6. Beware coronary ischemia if the coronary arteries have been manipulated or reimplanted.
7. Beware low-output syndrome from graft compression if the graft-inclusion technique was used without a Cabrol maneuver.
8. Transesophageal echocardiography may be particularly useful to evaluate the presence and degree of aortic valve incompetence before and after ascending aortic repair and to monitor the extent of and changes in aortic pathology in the presence of acute aortic dissection.

Surgery on the Aortic Arch

Resection and replacement of the aortic arch has been and continues to be one of the most demanding technical and tactical challenges facing a cardiovascular operating team. A historical overview of surgery for aortic arch aneurysms demonstrates the progressive understanding of the complexity of the surgical problems in this area as well as the evolution of techniques to overcome these problems. The earliest efforts at aortic arch surgery consisted of ligating the neck of saccular aneurysms in the arch.[46] Later, others successfully resected saccular aneurysms of the arch by lateral aortorrhaphy. More complex aneurysms required the development of methods to maintain the cerebral circulation and to prevent left ventricular failure during the time that the aortic arch was clamped. Initial efforts involved the use of temporary shunts to bypass blood from the more proximal to the more distal aorta as well as to the head vessels, and later others used temporary shunting along with prosthetic grafts.[47] The first successful replacement of the aortic arch was reported by DeBakey and associates.[48] They replaced the entire arch with a homograph. Surgery was performed using cardiopulmonary bypass and selective perfusion of the brachiocephalic vessels. Since then much has been written investigating cardiopulmonary bypass, selective perfusion of one or both cerebral blood vessels, moderate hypothermia with circulatory arrest, or profound hypothermia with circulatory arrest as ways to solve the problems associated with aortic arch surgery.

The three major challenges of aortic arch replacement are: (1) myocardial preservation and reduction of myocardial stress, (2) preservation of the integrity of the central nervous system, and (3) reduction in the risk of hemorrhage.

The difficulties relating to myocardial stress and myocardial preservation have essentially been eliminated by the use of cardiopulmonary bypass, cold cardioplegia (whether blood or crystalloid), and topical hypothermia to the heart. Preservation of the brain is an ongoing challenge. Everyone utilizes some degree of hypothermia during arch surgery, but the advantages and disadvantages of other brain protection techniques continue to be debated. Thus, a review of the effects of hypothermia on hemodynamics and major organ metabolism and function is in order.[49]

Hypothermia

Hypothermia causes a significant reduction in oxygen consumption that is directly related to the magnitude of the decrease in temperature. At approximately 28°C oxygen consumption decreases 50% and at 18°C oxygen consumption decreases 78%. As blood cools, the oxyhemoglobin dissociation curve shifts leftward. This unfavorable relationship between oxygen supply and tissue demand can be problematic if large internal temperature gradients are present, as, for example, when warm tissue is being perfused by cold blood. However, as the temperature of the blood decreases, there is an increase in the solubility of oxygen in plasma, so the shift in the oxyhemoglobin dissociation curve is counterbalanced by the increased solubility of oxygen in plasma, by increased tissue binding of oxygen, and by decreased tissue oxygen demand. Carbon dioxide production is reduced as a result of the decrease in metabolic rate. Studies suggest that if the arterial P_{CO_2} is maintained close to 40 mm Hg by the addition of carbon dioxide to the inspired gas mixture, this may help to minimize the peripheral vasoconstriction that occurs during cooling, and thereby improve peripheral perfusion and reduce uneven cooling between body compartments[50] (see also Chapter 37).

Metabolic acidosis may develop during hypothermia. Possible causes for this include peripheral hypoperfusion, unequal cooling, a discrepancy between oxygen supply and tissue requirements, and increased production of lactate. There might also be a reduction in the metabolism of lactate and other organic acids. It would seem that rewarming and the restoration of circulation do produce a spontaneous correction in the metabolic acidosis. The blood, liver, and kidneys are among the first organs to return to normal temperature during core rewarming and therefore they should be able to metabolize and dispose of the accumulated acid materials as is their usual function.

Glucose metabolism is altered during hypothermia. Serum glucose concentrations increase as do plasma insulin levels and plasma catecholamine concentrations. Exposure to cold typically induces an adrenal stress response, causing an increase in glucose production, increases in free fatty acid concentrations, and perhaps the dysrhythmias that occur with progressive cooling.

There are a number of hemodynamic effects of hypothermia. Cardiac output progressively decreases as the temperature declines due to some reduction in the stroke volume, but mainly to a decrease in heart rate. As the myocardium cools there is an increase in left ventricular end-diastolic pressure (LVEDP) and a decrease in left ventricular compliance. Some have measured a decrease in contractility, but these changes are not of sufficient magnitude to indicate a severely failing heart.

Several phenomena contribute to alterations in regional perfusion during hypothermia. These include a change in blood viscosity (it increases twofold at 20°C), changes in systemic vascular resistance (SVR), and a redistribution of blood flow. Blood viscosity is altered as a result of hemoconcentration, erythrocyte aggregation, and lower flow rates. Erythrocyte aggregation may cause changes in peripheral perfusion independent of effects on blood viscosity, because it reduces the velocity of erythrocyte flow in small blood vessels and decreases the surface area available for gas exchange by blocking some capillaries. Some have suggested that low-molecular-weight dextran or hemodilution (removal of blood and replacement with a crystalloid infusion) may partially counteract the effects of viscosity and erythrocyte aggregation on regional perfusion.[51,52]

Peripheral vascular resistance increases during hypothermia due to hemoconcentration, changes in blood velocity, and sympathetic stimulation. The distribution of blood flow to organ systems is also altered. Heart blood flow remains relatively unchanged, but brain, kidney, and other major organs have a reduction in flow.

Can the process of profound cooling and rewarming actually injure major organ systems? Histologic studies have shown myofibrillar degeneration in cardiac tissue, but these lesions do not seem to be functionally significant. Most report that there is no significant change in hemodynamic function after varying periods of hypothermia and rewarming.

During rewarming cerebral oxygen consumption increases 15% above precooling levels, even though cerebral blood flow may be somewhat less than it was previously. There is an increase in oxygen extraction from the delivered blood. Measurement of changes in cerebral activity by the electroencephalogram (EEG) is consistent with the decrease in cerebral metabolic function that occurs with cooling. The EEG is a flat line at 20°C. The EEG slowly returns to prehypothermia activity, the delay probably due to alterations in cerebral blood flow and alterations in cellular membrane permeability causing a temporary cerebral edema. There have been alterations visible on histologic sections of brain tissue after profound hypothermia, particularly when the temperature was decreased below 15°C. The etiology of these cellular changes may be related to a temperature gradient between the blood and the cerebral tissue, the greater the blood temperature/brain tissue gradient, the more extensive the brain "damage." Others suggest that the cerebral damage seen by earlier investigators was a result of low cerebral carbon dioxide tensions and consequent cerebral vasoconstriction.[53] They argue that P_{CO_2} levels kept near 40 mm Hg throughout hypothermia may reduce the risk of cerebral injury at any temperature.

Despite the histologic changes in brain tissue that have been seen with hypothermia, it is generally agreed that the tolerance of the brain to circulatory arrest increases when a patient is cooled. Sade et al. have shown that cerebral macrocirculatory obstruction, what is called the "no-reflow" phenomenon, occurs within a half hour of circulatory arrest at normal body temperature but can be delayed for up to 2 hours by systemic hypothermia to 20°C. By 3 hours of circulatory arrest, obstructive lesions are almost universally present. The tolerable limits of the brain to circulatory arrest in adult patients are unclear, but most agree that 1 hour is probably "safe" in most people. Debate continues about whether there is a need for profound hypothermia (15° to 18°C) or whether moderate hypothermia (22° to 24°C) can be equally effective in preventing neurologic injury and more beneficial in terms of rewarming time and total bypass time.

Another approach to maintenance of cerebral integrity during surgery on the aortic arch is cerebral perfusion during circulatory arrest. This perfusion can be accomplished in several ways. Most commonly a perfusion catheter is placed in the innominate artery, the left carotid artery, or both, the catheters being attached to individual pump heads on the bypass machine (Fig. 21–10.[55–57] Suggested flow rates range from 100 to 150 ml/min.

Several Japanese investigators have suggested that "retrograde" cerebral perfusion may be efficacious.[58,59] One method of performing retrograde perfusion is by positioning the patient in steep Trendelenburg position so that the central venous pressure (CVP) is about 15 mm Hg and this pressure differential between the central venous circulation, particularly the superior vena cava, and the open origins of the great vessels provides perfusion of the brain (Fig. 21–11). Others have modified the cardiopulmonary bypass circuitry to allow oxygenated blood to be delivered to the superior vena cava in a continuous low-volume, low-pressure manner during circulatory arrest.[60,61] An effluent of dark (i.e., desatur-

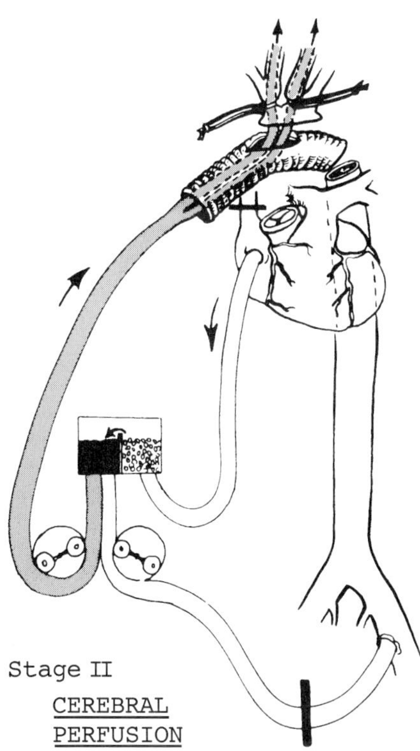

FIGURE **21–10.** Circulation has been arrested and cerebral perfusion via the carotid arteries begun. The superior vena cava is clamped to retain blood in the cerebral vasculature and prevent entrapment of air. (From Cooley DA, Ott DA, Frazier OH, et al: Surgical treatment of aneurysms of the transverse aortic arch: Experience with 25 patients using hypothermic techniques. Ann Thorac Surg 32:260, 1981, with permission.)

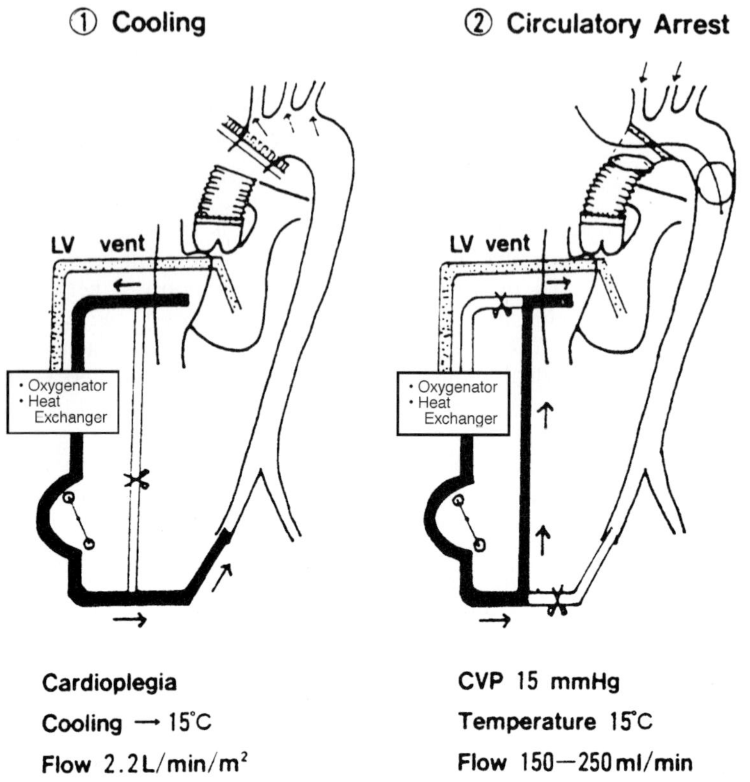

① Cooling

LV vent

• Oxygenator
• Heat Exchanger

Cardioplegia

Cooling → 15°C

Flow 2.2L/min/m²

② Circulatory Arrest

LV vent

• Oxygenator
• Heat Exchanger

CVP 15 mmHg

Temperature 15°C

Flow 150—250ml/min

FIGURE **21–11.** After cooling the body, circulatory arrest is begun. Cerebral perfusion is performed through a venous drainage line in a shunt circuit of the cardiopulmonary bypass circuit. Flow is adjusted to maintain a central venous pressure of 15 mm Hg with the patient in Trendelenburg position. The descending aorta is occluded with a balloon catheter to prevent entrapment of air in the descending aorta. (From Takamoto S, Matsuda T, Harada M, et al: Simple hypothermic retrograde cerebral perfusion during aortic arch surgery. J Cardiovasc Surg 33:560, 1992, with permission.)

ated) blood from the innominate and left carotid arteries during this time suggests that aerobic metabolism of the brain is maintained due to oxygen and substrate availability.

Potential disadvantages of cerebral perfusion during circulatory arrest include cerebral hemorrhage or cerebral edema from "overperfusion" and the technical difficulties of working around perfusion catheters in the surgical field if anterograde perfusion is employed. However, several groups have shown a remarkable reduction in the stroke rate associated with aortic arch repair and circulatory arrest when retrograde cerebral perfusion was utilized.[62–64] In addition to the potential to reduce neurologic injury related to cerebral ischemia during circulatory arrest, retrograde cerebral perfusion may have other benefits including removal of debris and air by the perfusate.

The initial success of retrograde cerebral perfusion in reducing brain injury and the concern about other complications related to aortic clamping in certain types of aneurysms have led to the development of techniques of hypothermic *total-body* retrograde perfusion.[65] This consists of continuous cerebral perfusion through the superior vena cava, intermittent retrograde coronary perfusion through the coronary sinus, and continuous abdominal visceral perfusion through the inferior vena cava. The full consequences of this practice remain to be determined.

Hypothermia effectively reduces the metabolism of the liver and kidney, allowing these organs to be protected for prolonged periods against anoxia. There are minimal histological changes associated with circulatory arrest in these organs.

Surgical Considerations

Surgery on the aortic arch is accomplished during a period of circulatory arrest with moderate or profound systemic hypothermia. The level of hypothermia desired is achieved by a combination of surface cooling prior to institution of cardiopulmonary bypass and then rapid core cooling utilizing the heat exchanger in the bypass circuit. An alternative method is passive temperature drift prior to bypass followed by rapid core cooling on cardiopulmonary bypass. Temperature must be measured from a core location, either rectal, nasopharyngeal, or tympanic membrane, with the latter correlating best with actual brain temperature. When the desired degree of cold has been achieved, the bypass pump is turned off and there is a state of no blood flow, which is the definition of circulatory arrest. This no-flow state allows the surgeon to open the aorta and conduct the arch repair in a virtually bloodless field. The blood in the body can be drained out through the venous drainage system into the pump during the time of circulatory arrest, but it is better to leave the blood in the body, as this cuts down on the likelihood of air entrainment and air embolism when circulation is restored.

Rapid cooling can be associated with several potential problems including vasoconstriction that limits perfusion and further cooling and the existence of temperature gradients between different body regions. Rapid and incomplete cerebral cooling has been implicated in postoperative neurologic deficits after hypothermic arrest. External cooling of the head, for example, by packing the head in ice, during circulatory arrest may help prevent temperature gradients from developing in the brain

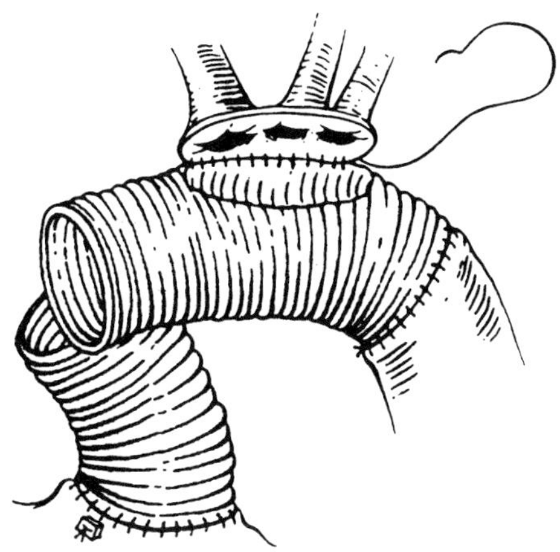

FIGURE **21–12.** Operative procedure for aortic arch replacement. Note that the superior portion of the aortic arch is trimmed to leave a cuff of tissue around the orifices of the three vessels. This aortic cuff is then anastomosed to the arch graft. (From Griepp RB, Stinson EB, Hollingsworth JF, et al: Prosthetic replacement of the aortic arch. J Thorac Cardiovasc Surg 70:1051, 1975, with permission.)

during circulatory arrest. Rapid cooling and rewarming might produce gaseous microemboli that could create neurologic injury. Rewarming should be gradual with the temperature gradient between the blood and the patient not exceeding 10°C (see Chapter 37).

Operative techniques have been modified to expedite arch repairs so that the period of circulatory arrest is as short as possible. A very significant modification was suggested by Bloodwell et al. and involved anastomosis of the three great vessels as a single unit to the prosthetic arch graft.[66] This cuts down substantially on both the number of anastomoses and the time required to effect an arch repair (Figs. 21–12 and 21–13). During the period of circulatory arrest, the distal anastomosis is constructed and the arch vessels are reimplanted into the graft. Many surgeons avoid the use of vascular clamps in the repair of aortic arch aneurysms, and, instead, favor performing what is called "open" aortic repair.[67] This obviates problems of distortion of the aortic lumen by a cross-clamp or further injury to the aorta by a cross-clamp as might occur with acute aortic dissection. In an open repair, the distal anastomosis is constructed from within the aorta. Once these two anastomoses (the distal anastomosis and the great vessel anastomosis) are complete, the aorta is "de-aired" and flow is gradually restarted in the cardiopulmonary bypass circuit. Flow will come retrograde up the aorta from the femoral arterial canula, move air and debris ahead of it, and vent the air and debris out the proximal end of the graft. Great care must be taken to de-air the branches of the aortic arch. Typically the great vessels have had small clamps placed on them during the repair to prevent embolism of atheromatous debris or thrombus into the brain from the aneurysm. Considerable care must be taken then to "milk out" all air, clot, and debris before the clamps are removed and flow is re-established to the brain.

Once the aorta has been cleansed and blood flow resumed, a clamp can be put on the proximal end of the tube graft so that blood flow can occur to all parts of the body except the heart itself and systemic rewarming can begin. Rewarming thus takes place while the proximal portion of the arch anastomosis is constructed (Fig. 21–14). Rewarming should take place gradually. It is recommended that core temperature not increase more than 1°C every 3 minutes. The period of rewarming, especially if profound hypothermia has been used, extends the period on cardiopulmonary bypass and may be associated with the coagulation disturbances that are common with long bypass times. Once the patient is fully rewarmed, the heart can be restarted, myocardial function assessed, and the patient weaned from cardiopulmonary bypass in the usual manner.

Most large series reporting on the use of hypothermic circulatory arrest indicate that global neurologic injuries are quite uncommon.[68–76] Most neurologic injuries are focal and probably related to embolization of air, atherosclerotic material, or thrombotic material from the aneurysm. The techniques of profound and moderate hypothermic circulatory arrest are safe and "protective" in most patients, at least in terms of global brain injury.

Surgery on the aortic arch has a serious potential for hemorrhage. There may be surgical bleeding from a number of surgical sites, the anastomoses, or through the

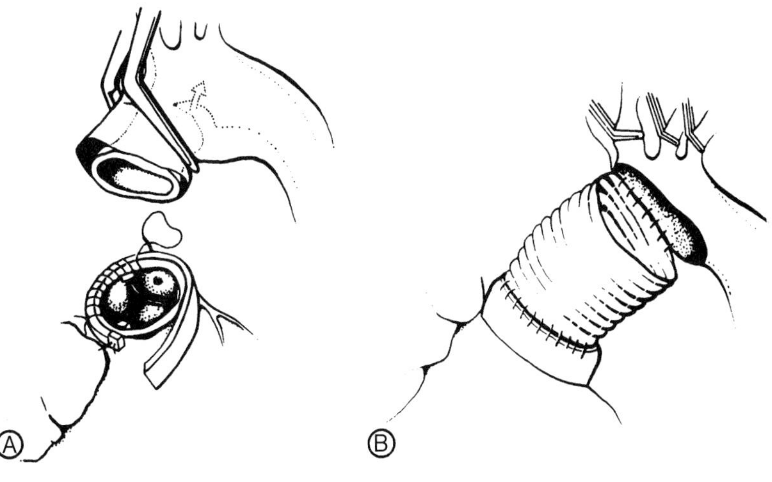

FIGURE **21–13.** Operative procedure for repair of a proximal aortic dissection. *A*, Resuspension of the aortic valve and replacement of the ascending aorta is performed during core cooling. *B*, During circulatory arrest the inside of the arch is inspected and the portion of the arch containing the intimal tear is resected. Note that the arch anastomosis is beveled to allow resection of a substantial portion of the arch and still have only one distal anastomosis to perform. (From Ergin MA, O'Connor J, Guinto R, et al: Experience with profound hypothermia and circulatory arrest in the treatment of aneurysms of the aortic arch. J Thorac Cardiovasc Surg 84:649, 1982, with permission.)

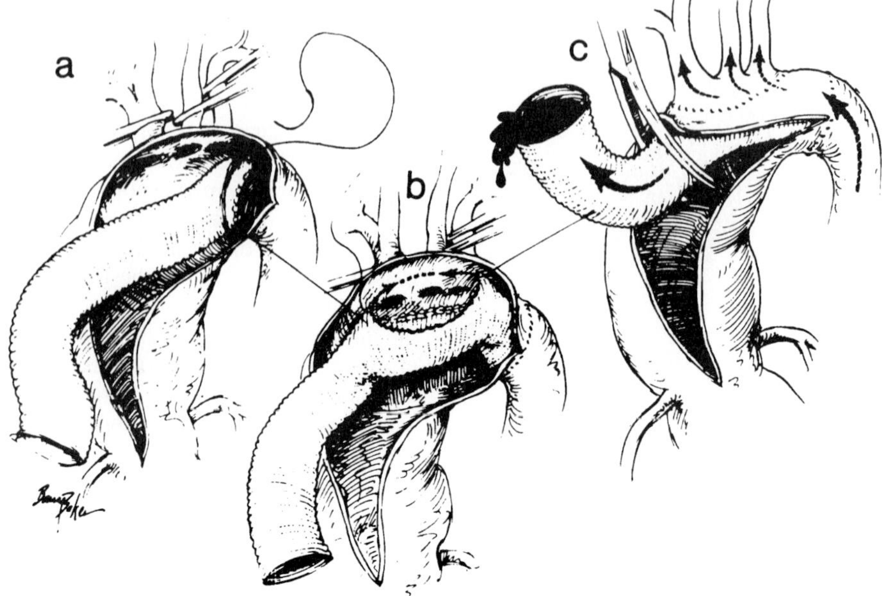

FIGURE **21–14.** Technique for replacement of the ascending aorta and aortic arch. The distal anastomosis is performed after removing all clot and debris. An oval opening is made in the side of the graft and the brachiocephalic vessels are anastomosed. With the head down, the proximal end of the graft is elevated and allowed to fill proximal to the origin of the great vessels which are then unclamped. The graft is then clamped proximally, full perfusion with rewarming is begun, and the proximal anastomosis is completed. (From Crawford ES, Saleh SA: Transverse aortic arch aneurysm. Ann Surg 194:180, 1981, with permission.)

graft itself. Various kinds of cloth grafts have been utilized for aortic surgery and various regimens for "preclotting" the grafts have been proposed. But the longer one remains on bypass the more likely it is that the graft will become unclotted and porous and bleeding will occur directly through it. At present, most surgeons "preclot" the graft with plasma or albumin and "bake" it in the autoclave, which creates a smooth proteinaceous coating that fills the interstices of the graft, making it much less permeable and much more resistant to fibrinolysis.[77] Hypothermia, circulatory arrest, and rewarming require considerable time on cardiopulmonary bypass, so the risk of developing a coagulopathy is significant. The etiology of the coagulation disorder would include the reduction in both platelet number and function associated with bypass. Hypothermia causes a reversible change in platelet activity, with the platelets being much less functional at low temperatures, but returning to near normal function when normal body temperature is restored.[78] Hypothermia also increases fibrinolytic activity and antithrombin activity and decreases plasma concentrations of prothrombin and factor VII, so a multifactorial coagulation disorder may develop. Several methods of dealing with the problem of hemorrhage have evolved, including the development of low-porosity grafts with adequate preclotting. Many suggest empirically administering a generous supply of coagulation materials to the patient at the termination of cardiopulmonary bypass, including platelet and plasma infusions to correct the deficits that are likely to be present and ε-aminocaproic acid (Amicar) or tranexamic acid to impede fibrinolysis. Many surgeons utilize a graft cuddling (surrounding) technique, that is, wrapping the remaining portions of the original aortic wall back around the cloth graft to tamponade bleeding that might occur through and around the graft. Finally, the development of automated transfusion devices, such as the Level One and the Rapid Infuser System (Hemonetics), has reduced the risk of death from hemorrhage. These devices facilitate administration of large volumes of *warmed* fluids and blood products to patients with severe hemorrhage.

Aneurysms of the aortic arch are frequently not localized lesions susceptible to simple graft replacement, but rather are part of more complex and extensive disease of the vascular system. These patients may have concurrent severe disease in the descending thoracic aorta or the thoracoabdominal aorta; extensive replacement of the aorta may be required. Typically a series of staged operations is planned. Staging the operative repair of aortic segments is helpful to avoid stressing a patient beyond the limits of tolerance. Further, such staging allows the surgeon to select the approach most optimal for replacing a specific segment. In that way the reconstruction can be precise and minimally affect adjacent structures. The aortic segment associated with the greatest immediate threat to life is replaced first and subsequent operation is performed when recovery permits.

Anesthetic Considerations

1. The patient will be supine with the surgery performed through a median sternotomy.
2. Atriofemoral or femorofemoral bypass will be utilized to cool the body prior to and warm the body after the period of circulatory arrest.

3. Moderate or profound systemic hypothermia will be used in association with circulatory arrest. Tympanic temperature monitoring to estimate actual brain temperature might supplement the usual method of core temperature monitoring.
4. The patient is kept well hydrated prior to cooling. Hemodilution may partially counteract the hypothermia-induced effects on blood viscosity, erythrocyte aggregation, and regional perfusion.
5. The head should be packed in ice during core cooling and kept cold until the period of circulatory arrest is over. Be careful to protect the nose, eyes, and earlobes from "frostbite."
6. Local belief in efficacy may call for administration of barbiturates, corticosteroids, or other "cerebroprotective" drugs prior to the institution of circulatory arrest.
7. The patient should be slowly rewarmed to reverse the physiologic and metabolic consequences of hypothermia, especially the vasoconstriction, metabolic acidosis, shift of the oxyhemoglobin dissociation curve, alterations in glucose/insulin metabolism, the adrenal stress response, and platelet dysfunction.
8. Blood pressure should be carefully controlled. In the presence of aortic dissection, dP/dt_{max} must be minimized to that amount just permitting adequate tissue perfusion. β-Adrenergic receptor blocking agents are excellent at facilitating this. Use of inotropic drugs in the presence of aortic dissection could be very hazardous because of the increase in dP/dt_{max} produced.
9. The risk of hemorrhage is great and may be due to surgical bleeding, graft porosity, and/or a coagulopathy. The bypass pump and reservoir, a cell-saver system, two or more large-bore intravenous catheters, and an automated transfusion system should be available to facilitate volume resuscitation.
10. An anesthetic technique that allows for complete neurologic assessment within a few hours of surgery is very desirable. Long-acting anesthetics or anesthetic adjuncts with psychotropic properties might be avoided.

Surgery on the Descending Thoracic Aorta

Surgery on the descending thoracic aorta presents two serious clinical problems. First, temporary occlusion (cross-clamping) of the descending thoracic aorta creates major hemodynamic alterations in the areas proximal to and distal to the clamp.[79–81] Such temporary occlusion causes severe proximal hypertension, and distal (beyond the clamp) hypotension. Often, severe left ventricular stress and dysfunction result from the severe proximal hypertension. Ischemia of the abdominal viscera and the spinal cord can result from the distal hypotension. Second, there is a significant risk of hemorrhage from surgical bleeding and/or coagulation disorders.

Hemodynamic Effects of Temporary Thoracic Aortic Occlusion (Cross-Clamping)

The principal hemodynamic effect of temporarily occluding the aorta just distal to the left subclavian artery is severe proximal aortic hypertension. A rise in mean arterial pressure, central venous pressure, mean pulmonary artery pressure, and mean capillary wedge pressure occurs. These increases, according to the work of Kouchoukos et al., average 35, 56, 43, and 90%, respectively.[82] Cardiac index decreases an average of 29%. Heart rate does not change. Their work and the work of others suggest that left ventricular dysfunction—a reduction in cardiac output and marked increase in left ventricular end-diastolic pressure—accompanies the hypertension associated with occluding the proximal descending thoracic aorta.

Work by Stokland et al. (in dogs) and Gelman et al. suggests quite a different mechanism to explain these changes. These investigators found that aortic clamping results in a redistribution of blood volume from the lower to the upper part of the body.[80,83] Superior vena caval blood flow increased by 120%. Although CVP remained constant, left ventricular pressures and dimensions, did change considerably. An increase in LVEDP and volume was attributed to a transfer of blood to the upper part of the body. The larger diastolic volumes activated the Frank-Starling mechanism, promoting an increase in, or at least a maintenance of, left ventricular stroke volume. The increase in afterload balanced the enhanced Frank-Starling mechanism and stroke volume remained essentially unchanged. These authors suggest then that the changes in left ventricular end-diastolic volume (LVEDP) are a function of redistribution of blood volume rather than a sign of heart failure.

The work of Roberts et al.[79,80] in dogs demonstrated that left ventricular systolic and diastolic pressures increased and cardiac output decreased during descending thoracic aortic cross-clamping. Heart rate did not change. Dogs who had some form of shunt inserted had lesser hemodynamic alterations than the control group. However, at 1 hour after release of the cross-clamp there were no significant differences in hemodynamic function between the groups. Left ventricular function curves measured after release of the cross-clamp were similar in all dogs in the study. Biopsy specimens showed preservation of myocardial high-energy phosphate stores and no significant changes in ultrastructure.[79] The authors were unwilling to extrapolate these observations to man because many of the patients who come for descending thoracic aortic surgery have evidence of coronary artery disease or hypertensive heart disease and pre-existing myocardial dysfunction. The effects of aortic cross-clamping in such individuals may differ markedly from the laboratory situation. Cross-clamping of the aorta may cause subendocardial ischemia in the hypertrophied ventricle or create a significant imbalance in myocardial oxygen supply and demand in a ventricle with significant coronary artery disease. In clinical experience it is not uncommon to see overt evidence of myocardial ischemia or alterations in left ventricular systolic or diastolic function both during and after descending thoracic aortic cross-clamping.

Organ systems distal to the thoracic aortic cross-clamp are exposed to the risk of hypoperfusion. Many studies show significant reductions in renal, hepatic, and mesenteric blood flow during the time of clamping, with some improvement after the clamp is removed, though it may be hours after clamp removal before blood flow returns to normal. Ohyama et al. in a primate model demonstrated that, after clamp release, renal blood flow was only 49% of baseline.[81] Roberts' studies in dogs demonstrated that, at 1 hour after clamp release, renal function in all the dogs was 50 to 85% of baseline.[79]

The renin-angiotensin system is active in the alterations in visceral blood flow during and after thoracic aortic clamping. Joob et al. showed that administration of a converting enzyme inhibitor caused a remarkable increase in renal blood flow in the period immediately following aortic unclamping.[84] Blood flow to the organs distal to the thoracic aortic clamp may be pressure dependent. Gelman and associates noted that renal cortical blood flow correlated directly with mean distal aortic blood pressure.[85] Changes in liver blood flow are similar to those of renal blood flow before, during, and after thoracic aortic cross-clamping. Changes in spinal cord blood flow may be very complex as will be described in detail later.

Techniques to Control the Hemodynamic Effects of Thoracic Aortic Cross-Clamping

There has been considerable experimentation in an effort to develop techniques, either pharmacologic or mechanical, that would reduce cardiac stress and preserve kidney, liver, mesenteric, and spinal cord blood flow during the time of thoracic aortic cross-clamping. These include passive or active aortic shunts, partial cardiopulmonary bypass, and infusion of potent vasodilator drugs.

Infusion of sodium nitroprusside is the most widely used technique to control the proximal hypertension associated with descending aortic surgery. Nitroprusside can allow one to control proximal aortic pressure at or close to baseline values. There is a measurable increase in myocardial and cerebral blood flow during nitroprusside infusion, which may indicate a loss of autoregulation of blood flow in these organs, but this does not appear to be a significant problem as long as perfusion pressure is maintained.

Nitroprusside is also active on the vasculature distal to the aortic clamp and distal hypotension could be exacerbated. In fact, there are considerable data showing that nitroprusside infusion is accompanied by derangements in the circulation to organs distal to the level of aortic occlusion.[85–87] Visceral blood flow beyond the occlusion clamp is dependent on perfusion pressure and independent of cardiac output. So vasodilation in this area can be very harmful and represents a critical danger to the kidneys, mesentery, liver, and spinal cord. Thus, I believe that nitroprusside infusion should be used with *extreme caution* during aortic cross-clamping.

Mechanical modalities to control upper and lower body blood flow and pressure during thoracic aortic cross-clamping can be divided into three groups: (1) cardiopulmonary bypass, (2) passive shunts, and (3) active shunts. Femorofemoral cardiopulmonary bypass (pump plus oxygenator) with full heparinization is one option.[88–93] Passive shunts are aortoaortic shunts with one end proximal to the aorta cross-clamp and the other end in the aorta distal to the clamp (Figs. 21–15 and 21–16).[94–96] The proximal end of the shunt can be placed in the ascending aorta, the aortic arch, the left subclavian artery, the left atrium, or the left ventricular apex.[98–104] There is some concern about using the left subclavian artery for the proximal end of the shunt because the internal mammary artery is a branch of the left subclavian and it provides some collateral blood flow to the intercostal arteries and thus to the spinal cord via radicular branches. So there is concern that a shunt in the left subclavian artery might reduce spinal cord blood flow during the time when spinal cord blood flow is of grave concern. Most surgeons use a more proximal aortic location for the proximal end of a passive shunt. If the descending thoracic aneurysm is relatively short, the distal end of the shunt can be located above the diaphragm, but if the aneurysm extends down to or even slightly below the diaphragm, the distal end of the shunt must be located in the femoral or iliac artery. Shunts are made from heparin-bonded tubing so the need for systemic heparinization is obviated. Flow in these shunts is passive—it is not directly controlled by the surgeon. The diameter of the shunt, the pressure differential between the proximal and distal ends of the shunt, and the flow characteristics of the location of the proximal end of the shunt are what determine shunt flow. As Poiseuille's law states, the diameter of the shunt is the most important determinant of shunt flow. It is recommended that shunts

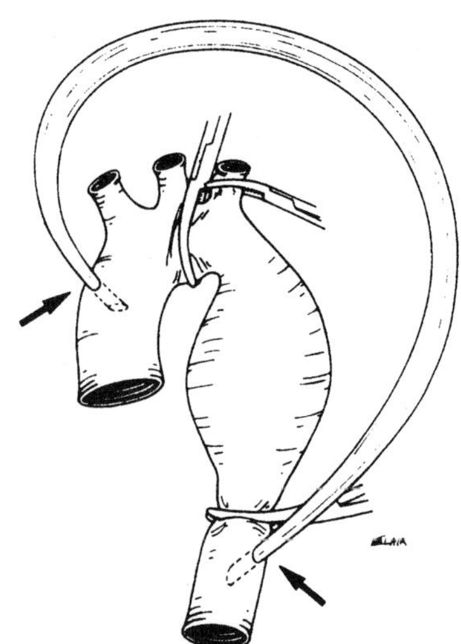

FIGURE **21–15.** *Arrows* indicate typical sites for proximal and distal insertion of a Gott aortoaortic passive shunt. (From Verdant, A, Page A, Cossette R, et al: Surgery of the descending thoracic aorta: Spinal cord protection with the Gott shunt. Ann Thorac Surg 46:147, 1988, with permission.)

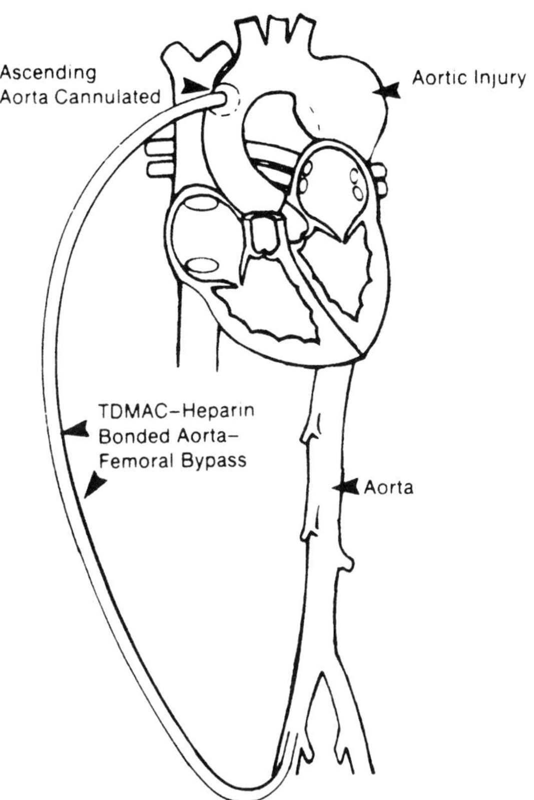

FIGURE **21-16.** Details of insertion of an aortofemoral artery passive shunt. The anatomy did not allow for insertion of the distal end of the shunt above the diaphragm. (From Olivier HF, Maher TD, Liebler GA, et al: Use of the BioMedicus centrifugal pump in traumatic tears of the thoracic aorta. Ann Thorac Surg 38:586, 1984, with permission.)

be at least 9 mm in diameter.[105] The location of the proximal end of the shunt will determine the amount and pulsatility of distal aortic flow. If the shunt is placed in the left ventricle, flow will be more pulsatile than if the shunt is placed in the left atrium or the proximal aorta.[106] However, flow is greater through a passive shunt with its proximal end in the aorta. Whether the advantage of the higher flow from an aortic to aortic shunt is offset by the loss of pulsatility is unclear (Fig. 21-17). It is difficult to translate laboratory evidence of differences in the hemodynamic characteristics of passive aortic shunts to the clinical situation. Wolfe et al. and Pett et al. have demonstrated that aortoaortic and aortofemoral shunts are more effective in decompressing the left ventricle and reducing left ventricular stroke work, wall tension, and myocardial oxygen demand than ventriculoaortic shunts.[99,106]

Flow through passive shunts is estimated clinically—by visual and palpable estimates of flow by the surgeon, by measurement of distal aortic pressure, the adequacy of urine output, and serial measurement of arterial blood gases for evidence of metabolic acidosis. These parameters determine that flow is satisfactory though the actual flow is unknown.

Active shunts are also composed of heparin-bonded tubing, but they differ from passive shunts because in the course of the shunt there is a pump to control shunt flow precisely. The typical circuit is connected from left atrium to femoral artery, the particular advantages of this choice of connections is the technical ease of insertion —the left atrium (LA) is easily accessed in the surgical field in the right lateral decubitus position—and the blood in the left atrium is oxygenated so there is no need

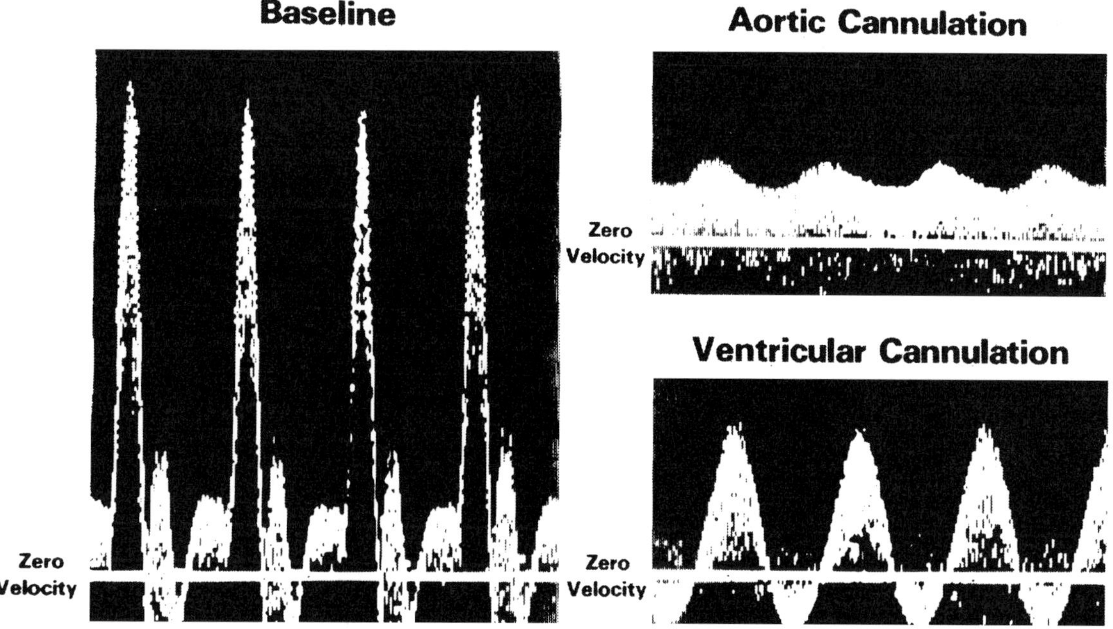

FIGURE **21-17.** Representative femoral artery flow velocities measured in dogs with aortic arch to distal thoracic aorta shunts (aortic cannulation) and left ventricular apex to distal thoracic aorta shunts (ventricular cannulation). Note differences in flow velocities and pulsatility compared to baseline. Aortic cannulation was nonpulsatile but maintained greater mean distal perfusion (From Pett SB, Wernly JA, Akl BF: Observations on flow characteristics of passive external aortic shunts. J Thorac Cardiovasc Surg 93:447, 1987, with permission.)

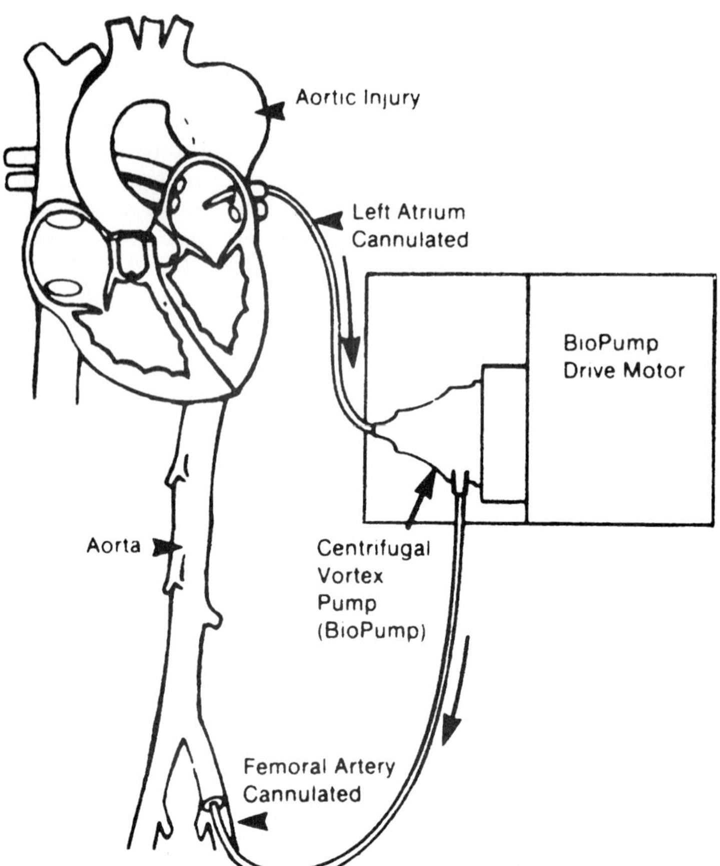

FIGURE **21–18.** Details of insertion of a left atrium–femoral artery active shunt. Note in-line Biopump. (From Olivier HF, Maher TD, Liebler GA, et al: Use of the BioMedicus centrifugal pump in traumatic tears of the thoracic aorta. Ann Thorac Surg 38:586, 1984, with permission.)

for an oxygenator in the circuit (Fig. 21–18). Some pump systems provide pulsatile flow but most use nonpulsatile flow. In the past a standard roller pump was used most often to "drive" the active shunt, but today most use the *Biomedicus* centrifugal pump.[107–114] This kinetic pump propels blood by centrifugal forces generated by a vortex within the pump head. These properties make air embolism less likely, which is important, since there is no reservoir in the circuit. The pump is also inflow responsive and resistance dependent. Forward propulsion of blood will decrease or stop if inflow is restricted or high pressure develops in the outflow line as a result of obstruction. The pump is relatively atraumatic to blood constituents. Flow rates can be adjusted from 0.5 to 4.5 L/min as necessary to maintain LA pressure and proximal aortic pressure at the desired level. The LA pressure is a measure of the degree of decompression of the left ventricle accomplished with the shunt. The proximal aortic pressure indicates the degree of left ventricular afterload reduction that has been accomplished. Typically, flow rates are adjusted to maintain a mean arterial pressure of 60 to 80 mm Hg in the proximal aorta and 60 mm Hg in the distal aorta. Because there is no reservoir in this shunt circuit, devices for blood scavenging and transfusion will be required. Transfusion can be used to maintain the desired left atrial or proximal aortic pressures. The left atriofemoral artery active shunt with the *Biopump* allows amelioration of most of the hemodynamic problems resulting from temporary descending thoracic aortic occlusion. Furthermore, the potential for bleeding problems associated with full systemic heparinization required for a cardiopulmonary bypass circuit is avoided. Compared to passive shunts, the active shunt provides the capability to control shunt flow and thereby control myocardial preload and afterload and to regulate proximal and distal aortic pressures. In addition, the centrifugal pump has proven very safe due to the low risk of air embolism or other pump malfunctions.

Despite considerable research done in the use of partial bypass, passive, and active shunts, there still exists considerable controversy about the value of these adjuncts for descending thoracic aortic surgery in reducing the risk of renal failure, paraplegia, or cardiovascular complications.[114–119] Crawford from his personal experience (which is *very extensive* and highlighted by very short aortic cross-clamp times) was not convinced of a benefit to the use of adjuncts in descending thoracic aneurysm repair surgery.[114,115,117] However, it may not be realistic to translate Crawford's extraordinary experience into that of the ordinary medical center in the United States. Surgery on the descending thoracic aorta may not always be performed by such an experienced surgeon, as descending thoracic aneurysms are uncommon and few U.S. medical centers do large numbers of these operations. Adjuncts may have a place in many hospitals to allow extra time to determine the need for reimplantation of critical intercostal or lumbar arteries and to decide any other special aspects of the surgical repair. Thus, use of particular adjunctive therapies is often a matter of local custom but the left atriofemoral artery active shunt using a centrifugal pump would seem an attractive current option.

The Risk of Spinal Cord Injury During Descending Aortic Surgery

The most dreaded complication of descending thoracic aortic aneurysm repair is paraplegia: this complication creates striking alterations in the patient's subsequent lifestyle. The reasons for the development of pararesis or paraplegia are several. First of all, the blood supply to the spinal cord is complex (Fig. 21–19). Considerable variability exists in which intercostal or lumbar arteries are important in providing spinal cord blood flow and we are without a reliable way to ascertain preoperatively the sources of spinal cord blood flow. Second, the presence and status of collateral spinal cord blood flow may be very important during the time that distal aortic perfusion pressure is low. Older patients may have arteriosclerosis involving the vessels providing collateral spinal cord blood flow that may compound the effects of distal aortic hypotension. Patients with acute aortic dissection who have sudden changes in intercostal or lumbar artery blood flow may be at particular risk, since they have not had time to develop a significant collateral circulation. Conversely, patients with coarctation of the aorta have a very low incidence of paraplegia because they have very extensive collateral circulation. Third, blood flow to the spinal cord may be quite tenuous immediately after descending thoracic aneurysm repair and for several days thereafter. Episodes of hypotension during this time may lead to "late" paraplegia or paraparesis. Clinically, it is impossible to know if spinal cord blood supply is tenuous; therefore, aggressive support of the blood pressure and prevention of hypotension are required for many days after surgery.

Many variables affect spinal cord blood flow that are not under our control. Thus, regardless of the technique chosen to manage the period of thoracic aortic occlusion, and despite our best care and efforts on the patient's behalf, there will be some instances of paraparesis or paraplegia. Patients should be advised preoperatively about this risk, which at the present time is about 10%.

Why is it that the spinal cord is so sensitive in injury during descending thoracic or thoracoabdominal aortic surgery? And why have we made so little progress in reducing the risk of paraplegia? The basic reason that spinal cord injury is a persistent problem is that spinal cord blood flow patterns are unique from individual to individual and no method exists to routinely assess spinal cord blood flow in patients coming for aortic surgery.

In early human embryonic stages of development, radicular arteries perfuse each segment of the spinal cord: cervical, thoracic, lumbar, and sacral. However, in the course of development "desegmentation" of spinal cord blood flow occurs and a number of radicular arteries involute. When one reaches the adult stage, the actual number of radicular arteries supplying the spinal cord in man is less than five in half the population and five to eight in the other half (Fig. 21–20).[120] Each remaining

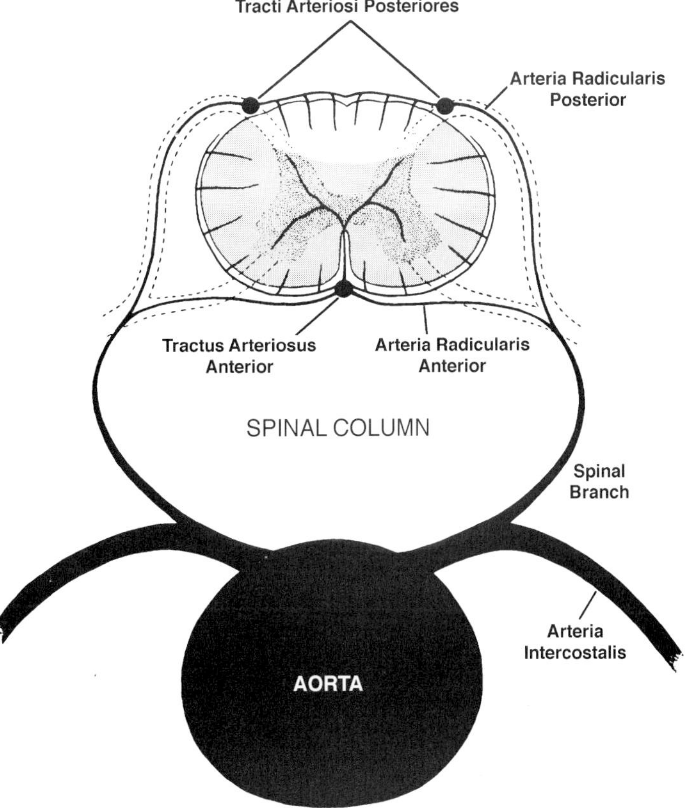

FIGURE **21–19.** Cross section of the spinal cord and its vascular supply. An intercostal artery gives off radicular branches right and left that combine to form the anterior spinal artery (tractus arteriosus anterior). (From Adams HD, Van Geertruyden HH: Neurologic complications of aortic surgery. Ann Surg 144:574, 1956, with permission.)

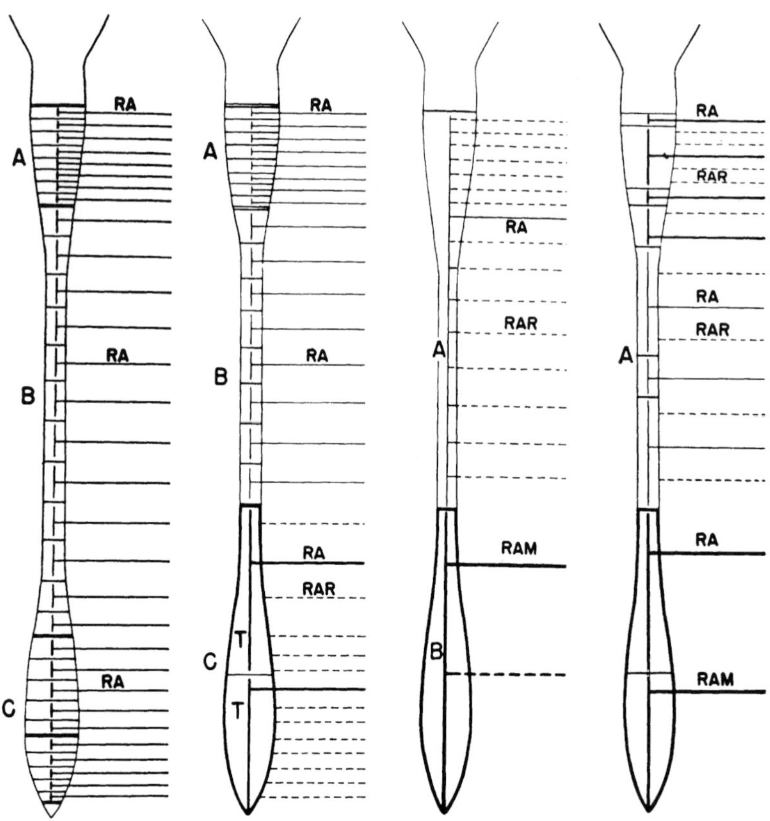

FIGURE **21–20.** Stages in the phylogenetic development of the spinal cord vascular system. From left to right: 1, The initial state in which each segment is supplied by its individual radicular artery. 2, A later stage of development with two radicular arteries remaining after regression of most of the segmental arteries in the lower thoracic and lumbosacral spinal cord. The anterior spinal artery is being formed by fusion of adjacent ascending and descending branches of the purely segmental primitive radicular arteries. 3, A further stage in development demonstrating a typical pattern—complete desegmentation of the vascular supply of the cervical and upper thoracic region. The lower thoracic and lumbosacral spinal cord is supplied by the great radicular artery and a very well-developed anterior spinal artery. 4, Another important pattern showing a larger number of radicular arteries persisting at all levels with a less well-developed anterior spinal artery. A, cervical cord; B, thoracic cord; C, lumbosacral cord; RA, radicular artery; RAM, great radicular artery; T, anterior spinal artery. (From Adams HD, Van Geertruyden HH: Neurologic complications of aortic surgery. Ann Surg 144:574, 1956, with permission.)

radicular artery thus assumes much more importance and supplies more than one segment of the spinal cord.[121] One of these radicular arteries becomes the largest and is responsible for blood flow to most of the thoracolumbar spinal segments. This branch is known as the great radicular artery of Adamkiewicz or the arteria radicularis magna or the great radicular artery. In any individual it is difficult to determine where the artery of Adamkiewicz originates, but pathologic studies help make approximations about this location (Fig. 21–21).[122,123] The artery of Adamkiewicz enters the spinal cord at the level of T5–T8 in man in 15% of people, between T9 and T12 in 60%, around L1 in 14%, L2 in 10%, L3 in about 1.5%, and L4–L5 in 0.2%. Thus, there is considerable variability in the origin of the artery of Adamkiewicz.

As a further complication of the anatomy, the artery of Adamkiewicz enters the spinal cord and sends one larger branch inferiorly and one smaller branch superiorly. The anterior spinal artery in man is a single lon-

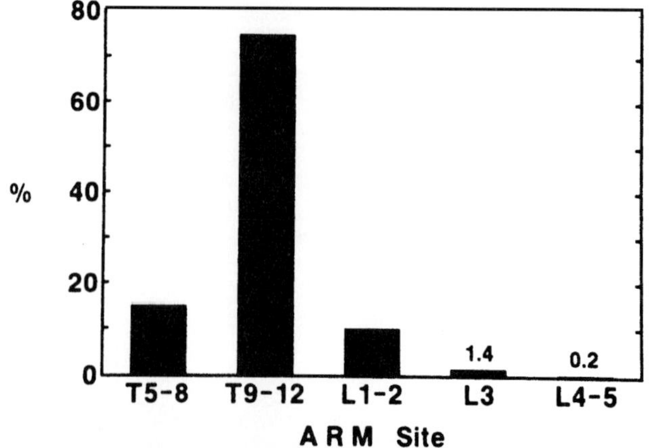

FIGURE **21–21.** Approximate frequency of origin of the great radicular artery (ARM) according to vertebral levels in humans. (From Svensson LG, Patel V, Coselli JS, et al: Preliminary report of localization of spinal cord blood supply by hydrogen during aortic operations. Ann Thorac Surg 49:528, 1990, with permission.)

gitudinal blood vessel from the top to the bottom of the spinal cord, but its diameter may be considerably larger or smaller in certain areas. Interestingly, one of these narrow areas is in the region where the artery of Adamkiewicz enters the anterior spinal artery (Fig. 21–22).[124] So great radicular artery blood flow preferentially goes to the inferior branch, leaving the more superior branch relatively less perfused. There is 50 times more resistance to flow in the superior direction than in the inferior direction.[125] Clinically, the largest blood vessel supplying the spinal cord gives its blood to a relatively small area of the spinal cord. While the thoracolumbar portion of the spinal cord superior to the great radicular artery can be perfused via collateral circulation originating in the vertebral arteries, this area is at risk during descending thoracic aneurysm repair and is a long distance downstream from its source of collateral circulation.

With such variability and complexity of spinal cord blood supply, preoperative knowledge of the origin of the artery of Adamkiewicz and other radicular arteries could facilitate a rational surgical plan to prevent spinal cord injury (Fig. 21–23). However, no method for the safe and accurate localization of these radicular arteries is as yet available. The one available test is highly selective angiography of the aorta.[126] In this procedure, each intercostal and lumbar artery is injected with contrast to determine which supplies a radicular artery. This technically difficult procedure requires an amount of contrast dye that may be nephrotoxic, and also poses the risk of paraplegia. Paraplegic risk from the procedure is thought to result from embolization of aortic plaque, debris, or air. This procedure is considered too dangerous for routine use. Recent work by Svensson et al. describes a method by which critical intercostal and lumbar arteries could be identified intraoperatively.[123] This technique utilizes a specially designed catheter with platinum and

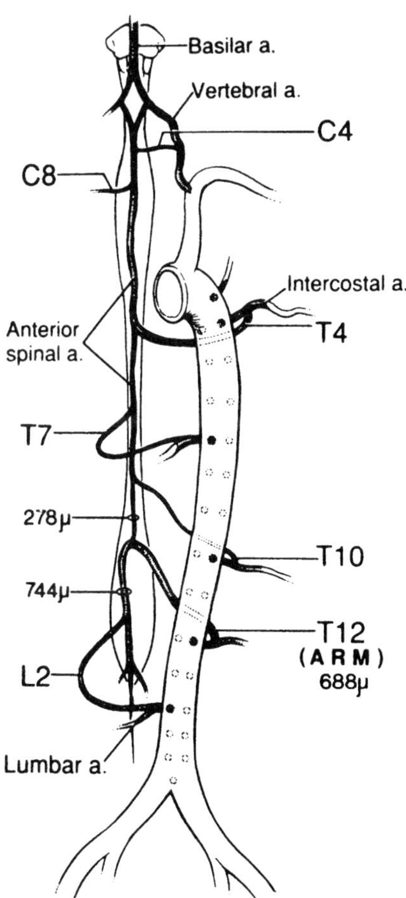

FIGURE **21–22.** Statistical composite of spinal cord blood supply in primates, which simulates that in humans. The sites of the radicular arteries reflect the most common levels of origin and arrangements found on anatomic dissection. Note that the point at which the great radicular artery (ARM) enters the anterior spinal artery is 2.6 times wider below than above this entry point so blood flow will preferentially go caudad. (From Svensson LG, Patel V, Coselli, JS, et al: Preliminary report of localization of spinal cord blood supply by hydrogen during aortic operations. Ann Thorac Surg 49:528, 1990, with permission.)

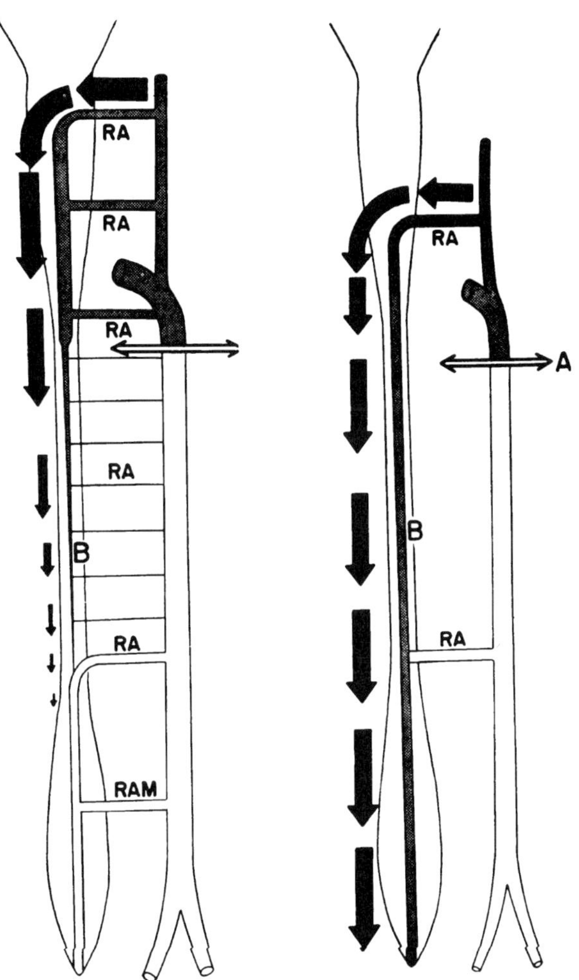

FIGURE **21–23.** The effect of occlusion of the aorta distal to the left subclavian artery at point *A* in an individual (*left*) with many persistent segmental arteries in the thoracic region and a resulting less well-developed anterior spinal artery. There is poor blood supply to the lower spinal cord during aortic occlusion, and ischemic damage may occur. The same occlusion in an individual (*right*) with only two remaining radicular arteries and a very well-developed anterior spinal artery. There is excellent blood supply to the lower spinal cord during occlusion, and ischemic damage is unlikely. RA, radicular artery; B, anterior spinal artery. (From Adams HD, Van Geertruyden HH: Neurologic complications of aortic surgery. Ann Surg 144:574, 1956, with permission.)

stainless steel electrodes inserted intrathecally. It is not passed as far up along the spinal cord as the actual segments of origin of the critical intercostals, but it can make measurements from four or five segments below. Saline solution saturated with hydrogen is injected sequentially into the ostia of each intercostal and/or lumbar artery and the generated current impulses are measured by the platinum electrode. A large hydrogen-induced current impulse (HICI) indicates the location of a radicular artery (Fig. 21–24). Radicular arteries above 180 μm in diameter (a significant size in man) can be located. The procedure takes 6 to 10 minutes to complete. This technique is the first "real-time" method to outline the anatomy of the radicular arteries including the great radicular artery. Such refined information can affect the surgical plan in several ways: (1) it will be known if the origins of the principal spinal cord blood supply are contained within the cross-clamp, (2) the presence of few radicular arteries suggests that collateral flow from the upper anterior spinal artery is good, and (3) specific intercostal and lumbar arteries can be reattached to aid in spinal cord preservation.

During surgery on the descending thoracic aorta, many factors can produce spinal cord injury and neuromuscular dysfunction. The incidence and severity of spinal cord dysfunction is related to both the degree and duration of ischemia. However, safe time limits of tolerance of the spinal cord to ischemia have never been clearly defined in humans. While most surgeons and anesthesiologists work under the assumption that there is a 30-minute grace period before permanent spinal cord injury occurs, some data suggest that a period as short as 18 minutes may be associated with severe injury.[120] Important factors in the creation of spinal cord ischemia include the length of time that the aorta is occluded, the distal aortic perfusion pressure during the time of clamping, the cerebrospinal fluid (CSF) pressure during aortic occlusion, the surgical sacrifice of "critical" intercostal or lumbar arteries during the repair, the presence of perioperative hypotension, and reperfusion phenomena.[127–130]

If the critical spinal cord blood supply has not been mechanically excluded by the surgical clamps and the anterior spinal artery is well developed, then distal aortic blood pressure will be very important in helping to prevent spinal cord ischemia during the time of aortic cross-clamping. With clamp-and-sew techniques, distal aortic pressure is usually very low. The use of passive or active shunts or partial cardiopulmonary bypass is associated with much better maintenance of distal aortic blood flow and blood pressure. Laschinger et al. in elegant studies using somatosensory evoked potentials (SSEP) as a monitor of spinal cord function suggests that a mean distal aortic perfusion pressure of at least 60 mm Hg is necessary to eliminate or ameliorate the risk of spinal cord injury during aortic occlusion (Fig. 21–25).[131]

Spinal cord perfusion pressure is more than simply distal aortic blood pressure. Spinal cord perfusion pressure is defined as the difference between anterior spinal artery pressure (which is approximated by mean distal aortic blood pressure) and CSF pressure. Spinal cord perfusion perssure can be enhanced by increasing distal aortic pressure, lowering CSF pressure, or both.

Many investigators have shown that descending thoracic aortic occlusion increases CSF pressure probably because proximal aortic hypertension increases blood flow to the brain and this major increase in intracranial pressure is compensated for by adjustments in the intracranial volume and pressure of CSF.[132–134] Proximal aortic hypertension may also increase blood flow to the upper portions of the spinal cord making it less compliant and further increasing CSF pressure.

Research directed at reducing CSF pressure during aortic clamping has followed several paths. Simply draining CSF prior to the application of the aortic clamp does measurably reduce CSF pressure, but the clinical

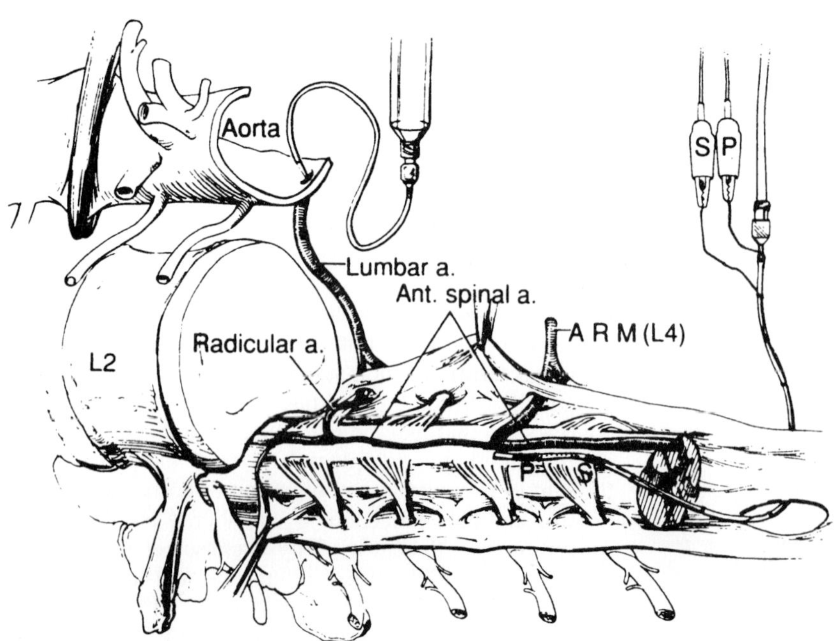

FIGURE **21–24.** Localization of spinal cord blood supply by hydrogen. The proximal aorta is clamped and the more distal portions opened. Saline solution saturated with hydrogen is injected into a lumbar artery giving off a radicular artery that supplies the anterior spinal artery. The more distal platinum electrode (P) detects the hydrogen-induced current impulses. S, stainless steel electrode. (From Svensson LG, Patel V, Coselli JS, et al: Preliminary report of localization of spinal cord blood supply by hydrogen during aortic operations. Ann Thorac Surg 49:528, 1990, with permission.)

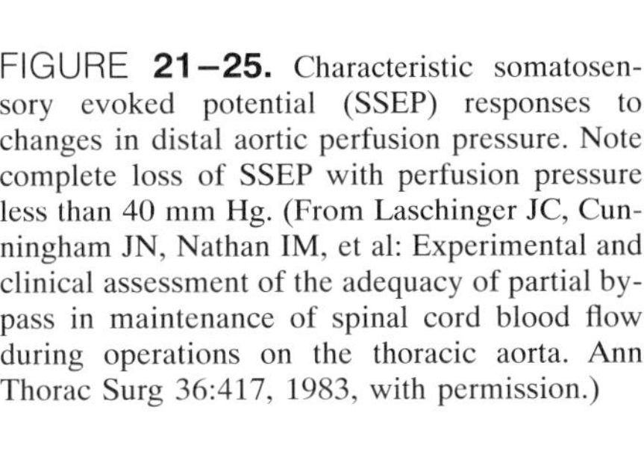

FIGURE **21–25.** Characteristic somatosensory evoked potential (SSEP) responses to changes in distal aortic perfusion pressure. Note complete loss of SSEP with perfusion pressure less than 40 mm Hg. (From Laschinger JC, Cunningham JN, Nathan IM, et al: Experimental and clinical assessment of the adequacy of partial bypass in maintenance of spinal cord blood flow during operations on the thoracic aorta. Ann Thorac Surg 36:417, 1983, with permission.)

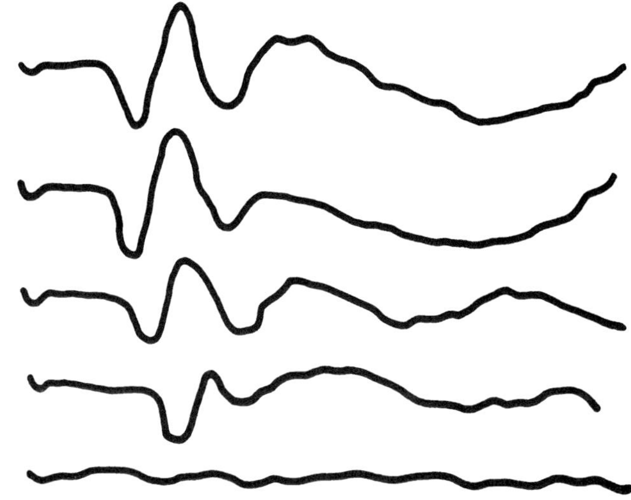

results in terms of eliminating or ameliorating spinal cord injury have varied (Fig. 21–26).[132–137] CSF drainage alone does not appear to be adequate to eliminate the problem of spinal cord ischemia during aortic clamping.[135] Svensson and others have suggested that papaverine be administered intrathecally to produce anterior spinal artery vasodilation and thereby improve spinal cord blood flow.[138–140] Preliminary work demonstrates some beneficial affects from the combination of papaverine and CSF drainage. Papaverine may have some calcium channel-blocking properties and might act as a free radical scavenger or have other biochemical effects that could be useful in addition to its vasodilating properties.

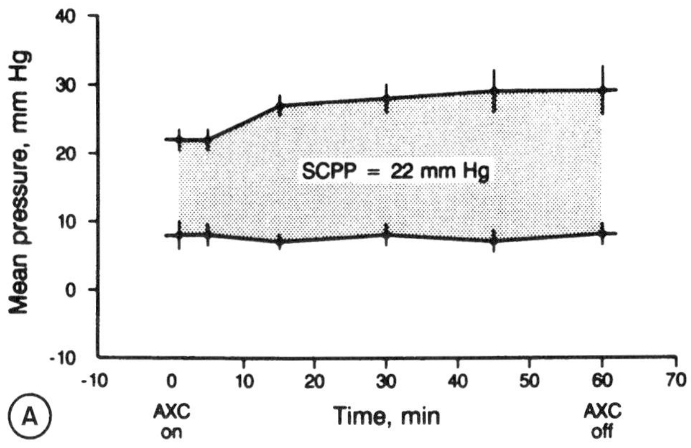

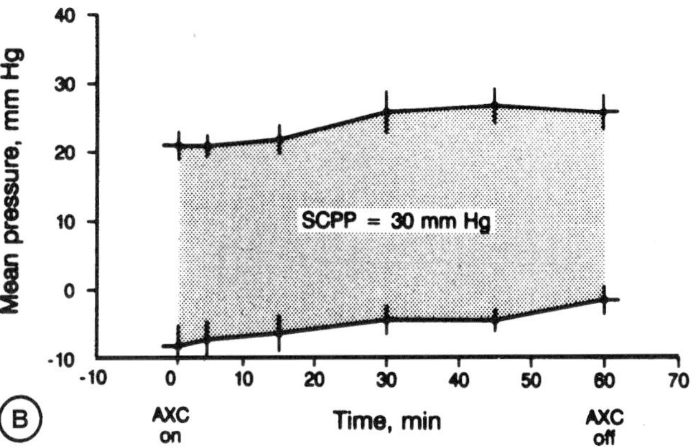

FIGURE **21–26.** Spinal cord perfusion pressure (SCPP) is greater in the spinal fluid drainage group (*B*) than in the control group (*A*). *Upper curves*, Distal aortic blood pressure. *Lower curves*, Cerebrospinal fluid pressure. (From McCullough JL, Hollier LH, Nugent M: Paraplegia after thoracic aortic occlusion: Influence of cerebrospinal fluid drainage. J Vasc Surg 7:153, 1988, with permission.)

Perhaps the most significant research related to spinal cord perfusion pressure and spinal cord ischemia has been the elucidation of the deleterious affects of systemic vasodilators such as sodium nitroprusside. These systemic dilators have been used to control proximal aortic hypertension during aortic clamping; such agents reduce proximal aortic blood pressure but they also reduce distal aortic pressure, which may already be quite low. Nitroprusside administration can reduce distal aortic blood pressure to profoundly low levels (Fig. 21–27). Vasodilators also increase CSF pressure probably via an increase in cerebral blood volume (Fig. 21–28),[85–87,142] so these drugs can affect both sides of the spinal cord perfusion pressure equation in a deleterious manner. Distal aortic pressure is lowered while CSF pressure is increased. There may also be a nitroprusside steal phenomenon in the outflow vessels of the distal aorta. The anterior spinal artery and spinal cord collaterals are relatively high-resistance blood vessels and blood flow may be directed away from these to other lower resistance arteries. Given the many potential or actual adverse effects of systemic vasodilators such as nitroprusside in reducing spinal cord blood flow, their use in controlling proximal aortic hypertension during aortic cross-clamping should be sharply curtailed. It may be much safer to control proximal aortic hypertension with shunting techniques, partial bypass or phlebotomy than to use a systemic vasodilator alone for that purpose.

A number of adjunctive techniques are in use to help preserve spinal cord blood supply and ameliorate or eliminate spinal cord ischemia during thoracic or thoracoabdominal aortic surgery. These adjuncts can be classified into three major categories: first, those that help detect spinal cord ischemia intraoperatively; second,

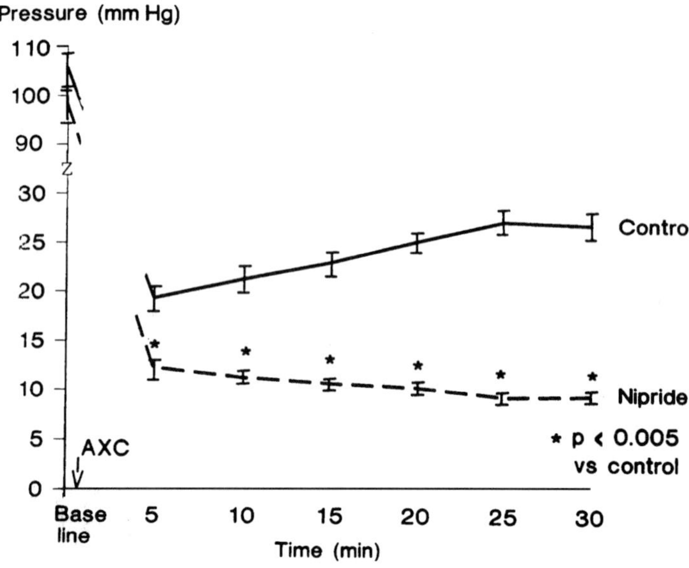

FIGURE **21–27.** Comparison of distal aortic blood pressure between control and nitroprusside-treated animals at baseline and during aortic cross-clamping. (From Marini CP, Grubbs PE, Toporoff B, et al: Effect of sodium nitroprusside on spinal cord perfusion and paraplegia during aortic cross-clamping. Ann Thorac Surg 47:379, 1989, with permission.)

those that help ameliorate the ischemia; and third, those that prevent ischemia.

At the present time the principal modality used to detect intraoperative spinal cord ischemia is evoked potential monitoring, specifically, SSEP monitoring.[143] These evoked potentials are measured by subcutaneous electrodes in the scalp recording stimulation of the posterior and lateral column spinal cord structures after stimulation of peripheral sensory nerves, usually the posterior tibial nerve. The nerves are stimulated every 1 to 2 minutes looking for changes in latency and amplitude of the evoked response. A prolongation in latency or a reduction in amplitude indicates the presence of spinal cord ischemia. Laschinger et al.'s considerable work with SSEP monitoring during descending thoracic aortic surgery has elucidated several characteristic patterns of evoked potential responses.[144–149] A type I SSEP response is a rapid loss of the evoked potential after cross-clamping.[144,146,150] This response would occur with clamp-and-sew techniques without an adjunct for distal aortic perfusion (Fig. 21–29). The type II SSEP response shows maintenance of an adequate evoked potential that occurs when distal aortic pressure is "adequate," that is, a mean pressure of at least 60 mm Hg maintained by use of various shunting or bypass techniques (Fig. 21–30).[144,147,151] A type III SSEP response is the loss of the evoked potential after interruption of critical intercostal arteries.[137,141] This ischemic response would be noted after exclusion of the aneurysmal aortic segment despite adequate distal perfusion pressures and can return following appropriate intercostal artery reimplantation (Fig. 21–31).

There have been reports of failure of SSEP to detect spinal cord ischemia intraoperatively and certainly the SSEP is unable to indicate when ischemia is irreversible.[152] More recent research investigates the utility of motor evoked responses during aortic surgery.[153] Indeed, the spinal cord area of interest is the anterior horn with

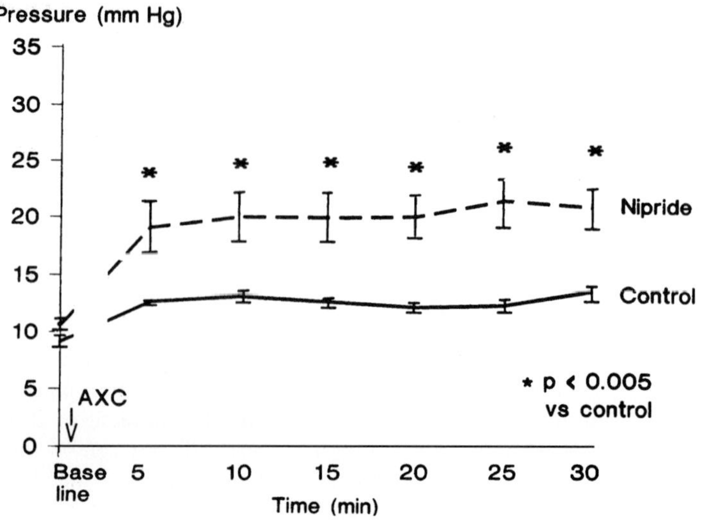

FIGURE **21–28.** Comparison of cerebrospinal fluid pressure between control and nitroprusside-treated animals at baseline and during aortic cross-clamping. (From Marini CP, Grubbs PE, Toporoff B, et al: Effect of sodium nitroprusside on spinal cord perfusion and paraplegia during aortic cross-clamping. Ann Thorac Surg 47:379, 1989, with permission.)

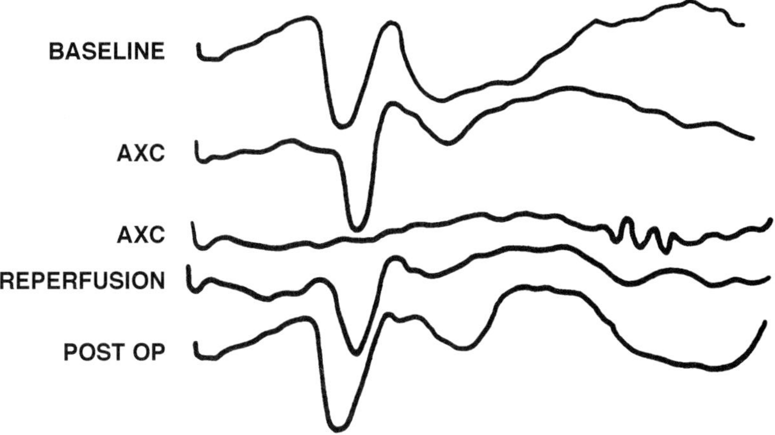

FIGURE 21–29. Type I SSEP response. Note early changes in latency at 4 minutes after aortic clamping (AXC) with progression to cessation of spinal cord conduction at 7 minutes of clamping. Following distal aortic reperfusion, there is slow return of spinal cord conduction with normal conduction seen at 24 hours after surgery. (From Cunningham JN, Laschinger JC, Merkin HA, et al: Measurement of spinal cord ischemia during operations upon the thoracic aorta. Ann Surg 196:285, 1982, with permission.)

its motor neurons that are not evaluated with SSEPs. At the present time there are no other monitors of spinal cord integrity or devices that measure any aspect of spinal cord function in real time for use during aortic surgery, other than potentials.

Adjuncts to ameliorate the effects of spinal cord ischemia include hypothermia, various pharmacologic modalities, oversewing or clamping intercostal arteries during the surgical repair, and reimplantation of "critical" intercostal and lumbar arteries. Hypothermia reduces oxygen consumption of neural tissue about 5% for every degree Celsius reduction in temperature from 37° to 22°C. Considerable technical difficulty occurs when using hypothermia during descending thoracic or thoracoabdominal aortic aneurysm repair.[154] With the use of moderate or profound hypothermia, ventricular fibrillation can occur at 28°C, thereby creating the need for immediate therapy (usually cardiopulmonary bypass).

Can the spinal cord be cooled with minimal effects on core temperature? Hypothermic regional perfusion of the spinal cord is a technique where the area of the aorta contained within the cross-clamps is perfused with iced solutions (Figs. 21–32 and 21–33).[155,156] The only outflow for the iced solution from this segment of the aorta is the intercostal or lumbar arteries (i.e., the sources of the radicular spinal arteries), and so this cold fluid should be transported directly to the spinal cord. Perfusion cooling of the spinal cord can reduce spinal cord temperature to about 20°C with an iced perfusate of 5°C. Systemic temperature may be reduced by only 2°C and spinal cord temperature remains substantially below systemic temperature for quite some time. Recently, Davison et al. demonstrated the feasibility of achieving regional hypothermia of the spinal cord by infusion of iced saline solution at 4°C through an epidural catheter placed at T11–T12.[157] A subarachnoid thermistor catheter was placed at L3–4 and was used to monitor the decline in CSF temperature during the epidural infusion of iced solution as well as to measure CSF pressure and provide for CSF drainage. CSF temperature decreased to about 25°C and core body temperature was not significantly affected by the epidural infusion of iced saline. Coles et al. showed in dogs a remarkable reduction in spinal cord injury with perfusion cooling of the spinal cord with an asanguineous iced Ringer's lactate solution.[155] Histologic specimens of spinal cord tissue showed only minor abnormalities in the animals exposed to hypothermia, whereas those with a normothermic spinal cord during aortic clamping had substantial derangements in spinal cord cellular architecture. Clinical signs of spinal cord injury were also apparent in the normothermic group. Thus regional hypothermia of the spinal cord may become more widely used for spinal cord protection during descending thoracic aneurysm repair.

Thoracic aortic aneurysms may occasionally be so complex as to require circulatory arrest. In this circum-

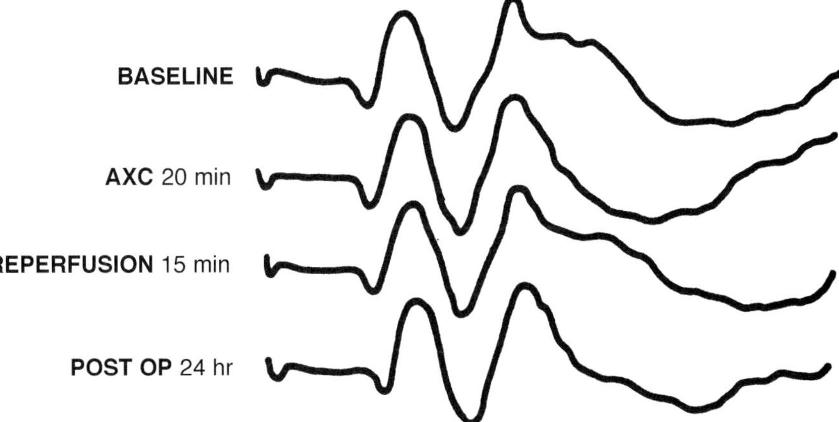

FIGURE 21–30. Type II SSEP response. Note maintenance of baseline latency and amplitude throughout the aortic cross-clamp (AXC) interval. Normal distal aortic perfusion pressure was maintained during this time by use of passive shunts or cardiopulmonary bypass. (From Cunningham JN, Laschinger JC, Merkin HA, et al: Measurement of spinal cord ischemia during operations upon the thoracic aorta. Ann Surg 196:285, 1982, with permission.)

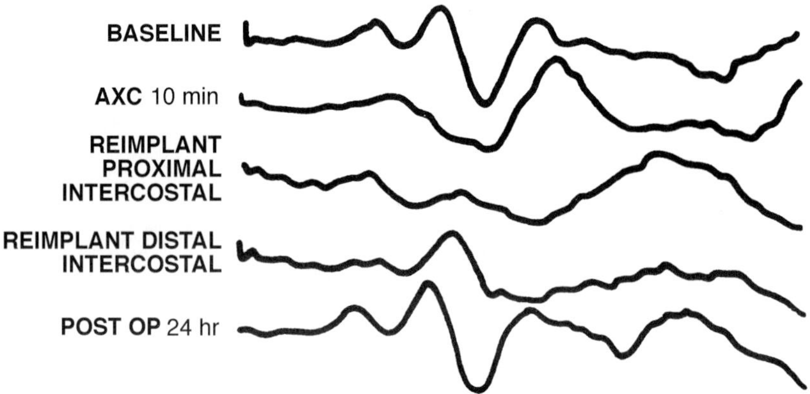

FIGURE **21–31.** Type III SSEP response. Ischemic spinal cord dysfunction is noted following aortic cross-clamping (AXC) despite adequate distal perfusion pressure provided by an extra-anatomic shunt. This response signifies interruption of critical intercostal arteries in the excluded aortic segment, and the abnormal SSEP response is reversed by appropriate intercostal reimplantation and is normal by 24 hours after operation. (From Cunningham JN, Laschinger JC, Merkin HA, et al: Measurement of spinal cord ischemia during operations upon the thoracic aorta. Ann Surg 196:285, 1982, with permission.)

stance cardiopulmonary bypass is necessary to promote the deep cooling necessary prior to circulatory arrest. The indications for this complex surgery include controlling hemorrhage, permitting operation without the need for clamping certain portions of the aorta, or improving surgical exposure. Upon entering the chest, if critical bleeding begins and cannot be controlled or if uncontrolled bleeding occurs because of the application of a clamp or other surgical manipulation, circulatory arrest may be necessary. The aneurysm may be extremely large and the risk of damaging it while opening the chest may be very great. There may be a right-sided aortic arch and technical difficulties exposing some parts of the aorta. To aid in dealing with these very complex situations hypothermic circulatory arrest may be required. Crawford reported on a large series of patients requiring circulatory arrest for descending thoracic aneurysm repair.[90] Even with this technique, the surgery was much more complicated and associated with greater mortality or morbidity. Pulmonary complications (probably due to pulmonary injury from retraction and intrapulmonary hemorrhage) and paraplegia were not uncommon, but the period of circulatory arrest did allow for

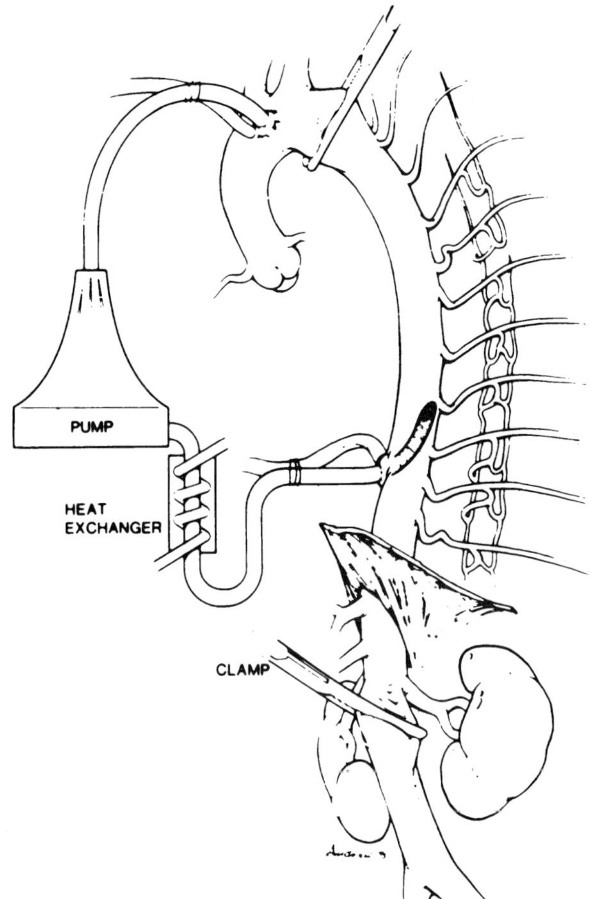

FIGURE **21–32.** A perfusion cooling circuit utilizing a Biomedicus pump and heat exchanger. (From Colon R, Frazier OH, Cooley DA, et al: Hypothermic regional perfusion for protection of the spinal cord during periods of ischemia. Ann Thorac Surg 43:639, 1987, with permission.)

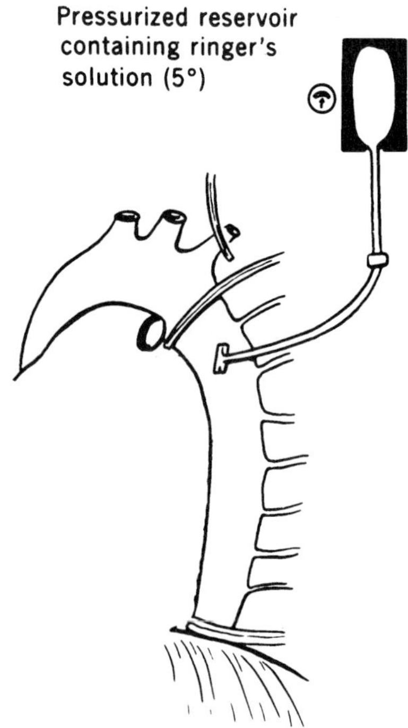

FIGURE **21–33.** Regional cooling of the spinal cord achieved by gravity-controlled infusion of iced Ringer's lactate solution. (From Coles JG, Wilson GJ, Sima AF, et al: Intraoperative management of thoracic aortic aneurysm. J Thorac Cardiovasc Surg 85:292, 1983, with permission.)

technical accomplishments that would have been impossible otherwise.

An enormous body of literature addresses the potential benefits of various drugs to prevent or ameliorate neurologic injury associated with aortic surgery or other insults to the spinal cord. Theories for the beneficial effects of these drugs include the following:

1. Certain drugs may stabilize neuronal membranes and thereby lessen ischemic damage. Such drugs might include corticosteroids, magnesium, and thiopental.
2. Some drugs are thought of as free radical scavengers and may counteract the damaging effects of oxygen free radicals. Papaverine may be in this group.[158]
3. Some drugs may improve collateral spinal cord blood flow. Papaverine might also do this.
4. Some drugs may prevent reperfusion injury resulting from calcium ion fluxes. Calcium channel blockers may do this.[158]

Corticosteroids in high doses—30 mg/kg methylprednisolone—given before and 4 hours after aortic occlusion may lengthen the tolerable period of ischemia of the spinal cord prior to permanent injury.[159] Large studies show that corticosteroids given within 8 hours ameliorate some of the neurologic deficits that occur following acute spinal cord trauma.[160] The operative setting provides the opportunity to administer the steroids *prior to* potential neurologic injury; acute corticosteroid usage has minimal systemic side effects. Significant steroid-induced hyperglycemia can be controlled with insulin administration so that, as with acute brain injury, the spinal cord neural tissue is not exposed to a high-glucose environment.

Naloxone was purported to have beneficial effects in acute spinal cord injury, but large trials have been unable to show that the drug is any more effective than placebo.[160]

There has been a description of a spinal cord "steal" phenomenon that can occur as a result of back-bleeding by intercostal and lumbar arteries while the aorta is open for repair (Fig. 21–34).[161] In this situation, the direction of collateral flow from the mammary anastomotic system to the radicular artery system can be reversed. Spinal cord perfusion is thereby reduced. Thus control of this back-bleeding by either oversewing or occluding the intercostal and lumbar vessels during aortic repair may be important.

Additionally, spinal cord injury may be reduced by reimplantation of those intercostal and lumbar arteries that provide the "critical" blood supply to the spinal cord. However, in the absence of knowledge about the exact anatomy of spinal cord blood supply in an individual patient, the problem has been addressed in two ways: (1) intercostals have been reimplanted "blindly," that is, with the surgeon selecting the largest ones (and so presumably the most important ones) for reimplantation; and (2) intercostals have been reimplanted based on the results of SSEP monitoring,[148] or hydrogen ion wash-out techniques[116] (see above). The SSEP or ion wash-out techniques can help define which intercostals are "critical" or at least can narrow down the area con-

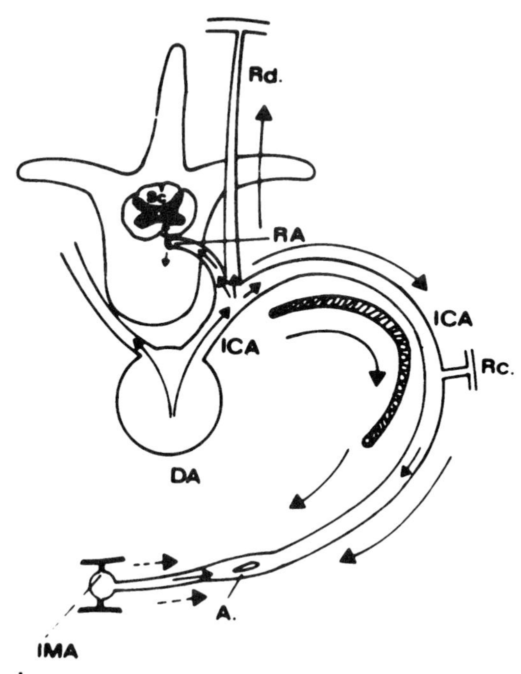

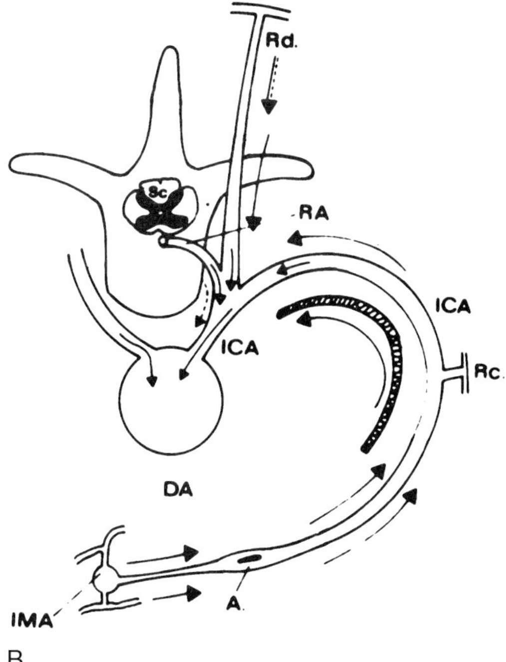

FIGURE **21–34.** Mechanism of a steal phenomenon as a cause of spinal cord injury. Direction of blood flow before (*A*) and after (*B*) cross-clamping of the descending aorta (DA). After cross-clamping blood tends to drain away from the spinal cord rather than toward it. ICA, intercostal artery; RA, radicular artery; Rd, dorsal ramus of the intercostal artery; Rc, cutaneous ramus of the intercostal artery; IMA, internal mammary artery; A, anastomosis of mammary artery; SC, spinal cord. (From Wadouh F, Arndt CF, Oppermann E, et al: The mechanism of spinal cord injury after simple and double aortic cross-clamping. J Thorac Cardiovasc Surg 92:121, 1986, with permission.)

taining the most important spinal feeder vessels so that appropriate islands of aorta containing pairs of these arteries can be attached to the aortic graft.

As with all aortic surgery, a plan for dealing with hemorrhage needs to be in place particularly if cardiopulmonary bypass is not used. Clamp-and-sew techniques and active and passive shunt techniques can (and many think *must*) be supplemented by a cell saver to carry shed blood out of the field wash, and concentrate the blood and return the blood to the patient. The Rapid Infuser System (Hemonetics Corp.) may be the best currently available transfusion device to use in this situation. In addition to recycled blood, the rapid infuser can infuse up to 1,500 ml/min of blood, blood products, colloid, or crystalloid solutions *fully warmed* to 37°C.[162] When attached to two large-bore intravenous catheters (8.5- or 9.0-Fr introducer sheaths), this device allows one to keep up with the sometimes massive hemorrhage that can be seen with aortic surgery. This rate of fluid infusion can be truly life-saving.

Anesthetic Considerations

1. The patient will be in the right lateral decubitus position for the surgery and the aorta will be accessed via a left thoracotomy.
2. One-lung ventilation is often necessary to facilitate exposure of the descending aorta. A left-sided double-lumen endotracheal tube or an endotracheal tube containing a branchial blocker (Univent tube) can be inserted and its position verified by fiberoptic endoscopy both before and after right lateral decubitus positioning. As with all cases involving one-lung ventilation, positive end expiratory pressure (PEEP) valves and a continuous positive airway pressure (CPAP) apparatus should be immediately available should oxygenation become a problem. Use of partial cardiopulmonary bypass will aid in oxygenation.
3. Hemodynamic monitoring often employs two intra-arterial catheters: one to measure proximal aortic pressure and one to measure distal aortic pressure. The only exception to this custom is surgery that will be done with a clamp-and-sew technique without adjuncts.
4. Individuals involved in the operation must function as a team and all understand the particular types and time frames for using the mechanical adjuncts.
5. Proximal aortic hypertension may be best treated by shunting techniques. Active shunts are particularly useful and allow for tight control of left atrial and proximal aortic pressures. Phlebotomy may also be useful to prevent the hemodynamic consequences of cross-clamping and reduce CSF pressure.[163] Nitroprusside or other vasodilator drug infusions should be avoided unless distal aortic perfusion is augmented by bypass or shunt techniques.
6. Distal aortic hypotension may be best treated by the use of shunts or partial bypass. Active shunts and bypass allow for control of flows to achieve the distal aortic pressure desired, usually 60 mm Hg or greater. If SSEP and/or motor evoked potential monitoring is being used, a more objective measure of the adequacy of distal aortic pressure is available.
7. If evoked potential monitoring is to be used and guide therapy, an anesthetic technique that does not interfere with such monitoring must be selected.
8. Local custom may call for administration of drugs for "renal protection" or "spinal cord protection" prior to aortic clamping. Such drugs may include mannitol, furosemide, dopamine, corticosteroids, thiopental, etc.
9. An epidural catheter can be inserted intrathecally after the patient is turned into the right lateral decubitus position if CSF drainage or drainage plus intrathecal papaverine is planned. The catheter should be attached to a sterile system for measurement of CSF pressure and drainage of CSF by gravity. Sterile, preservative-free papaverine—3 ml of 1% solution (30 mg)—can be injected through the catheter.
10. Hemorrhage may be very severe. Two or more large-bore intravenous catheters, a cell-saver system, and an automated transfusion device can be lifesaving, and a rapid infuser system is highly recommended. Both surgical bleeding and/or a coagulopathy may be present. Administration of plasma and platelets is frequently necessary due to dilutional coagulopathy.
11. Hypotension after graft replacement may cause "late" paraparesis or paraplegia.

Surgery on the Thoracoabdominal Aorta

Repair of thoracoabdominal aortic aneurysms is an extremely complex procedure.[164–167] Crawford, who had the largest experience by far with this kind of surgery, classified thoracoabdominal aneurysms into four types: type I involves the proximal descending thoracic aorta down to the upper abdominal aorta, type II involves the proximal descending aorta to below the renal arteries, type III involves the distal descending and abdominal aorta, and type IV involves most of the abdominal aorta (Fig. 21–35).[166]

In a review of 1,509 patients undergoing 1,679 thoracoabdominal aortic repairs, a number of variables were associated with early death.[168] These included older age, higher preoperative serum creatinine concentration, concurrent proximal aortic aneurysms, the presence of significant coronary artery disease or significant chronic lung disease, and longer total aortic occlusion time. Postoperative conditions contributing to death included cardiac complications, stroke, renal failure, and gastrointestinal hemorrhage.

Major morbidity related to renal failure, spinal cord injury, and hemorrhage. Renal failure, defined as a postoperative serum creatinine exceeding 3 mg/dl or the need for dialysis, occurred in 18% of patients. Dialysis was required in 9%. The most important risk factor for development of postoperative renal failure was impaired

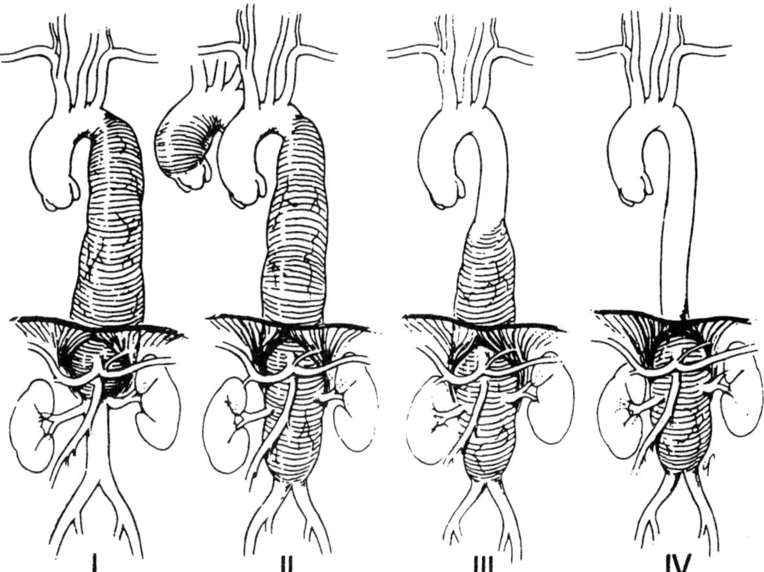

FIGURE **21–35.** Drawing illustrates Crawford classification of thoracoabdominal aortic aneurysms according to the extent of involvement of the thoracoabdominal aorta. (From Crawford ES, Coselli JS: Thoracoabdominal aneurysm surgery. Semin Thorac Cardiovasc Surg 3:300, 1991, with permission.)

preoperative renal function. Iced perfusion of the kidneys, particularly the left kidney, may help to improve the tolerance of the kidneys to ischemia and reduce the risk of renal failure.[169]

The incidence of paraparesis or paraplegia was 16%. Risk factors for spinal cord injury included total aortic cross-clamp time, the amount of aorta repaired, whether or not rupture had taken place prior to surgery, patient age, and a history of renal dysfunction.

The greatest risk of complications occurred in patients with type II aneurysms, that is, from the proximal descending aorta to below the renal arteries. All the important viscera—liver, kidneys, mesentery, spinal cord—are fed by branches of the aorta involved in the aneurysmal segment and it may not be technically feasible to utilize distal aortic perfusion techniques. Because such surgical repairs are complex, aortic occlusion periods tend to be long and the likelihood of visceral ischemia is high.[170–172] In addition, the multiple anastomotic sites increase the risk of severe hemorrhage. A graft-inclusion technique may reduce the risk of hemorrhage somewhat, but serious surgical bleeding and dilutional coagulation disturbances remain common events during these operations.[173]

Despite the complexity of such surgery, the 30-day survival from Crawford's team was 92%. However, in most medical centers this kind of surgery is performed very infrequently and the anticipated results are likely to be less exemplary than those. Patients should understand that, regardless of the anesthetic management or the skill of the anesthesiologist, the use of adjunctive procedures, or the skill of the surgeon, this surgery has great risk of neurologic or renal injury and a moderate risk of gastrointestinal dysfunction. These risks need to be compared to the 75% two-year risk of aneurysmal rupture. Thus, thoracic aortic reconstructive surgery may test the mettle of a medical center: this very aggressive surgery requires considerable preoperative planning, meticulous attention to detail, and superbly coordinated teamwork by all providing perioperative care.

The Future

Perhaps the most exciting event in the field of aortic surgery in the past 5 years has been the development of transluminally placed endovascular stent-graft devices used as alternatives to surgical repair of aortic aneurysms. This technique began as a method of transfemoral repair of abdominal aortic aneurysms but has been extended to treatment of aneurysms of the descending thoracic aorta as well.[174–176] Repair is done in the operating room under general anesthesia. One femoral artery or the lower abdominal aorta is surgically exposed and the device, containing a premeasured graft with proximal and distal self-expanding fixation devices, is inserted through the open arteriotomy under fluoroscopic control. The endovascular stent-graft is custom designed for each patient and is composed of a stainless steel endoskeleton of stent elements and a covering of woven Dacron. Its diameter, length, taper, and curvature are based on measurements obtained from each patient's computed tomography (CT) scan.

The technique of endovascular stent-graft repair of thoracic and/or abdominal aortic aneurysms is still in its infancy. However, it is an exciting field, as it portends the feasibility of repairing aneurysms *without* the serious hemodynamic, hemorrhagic, and homeostatic derangements that plague aneurysm surgery at the present time. Indeed, anesthetic management could become a relatively simple matter. We shall see!

References

1. Bickerstaff LK, Pairolero PC, Hollier LH, et al: Thoracic aortic aneurysms: A population-based study. Surgery 92:1103, 1982.
2. Anagnostopoulos CE, Prabhakar MJS, Kittle CF: Aortic dissections and dissecting aneurysms. Am J Cardiol 30:263, 1972.
3. Wheat MW Jr: Acute dissecting aneurysms of the aorta: Diagnosis and treatment. Am Heart J 99:373, 1979.
4. Pumphrey CW, Fay T, Weir I: Aortic dissection during pregnancy. Br Heart J 55:106, 1986.

5. Palmer RF, Wheat MW Jr: Treatment of dissecting aneurysms of the aorta. Ann Thorac Surg 4:38, 1967.
6. Wheat MW Jr, Palmer RF, Bartley TD, et al: Treatment of dissecting aneurysms of the aorta without surgery. J Thorac Cardiovasc Surg 50:364, 1965.
7. Mathew T, Nanda NC: Two-dimensional and Doppler echocardiographic evaluation of aortic aneurysm and dissection. Am J Cardiol 54:379, 1984.
8. Goldman AP, Kotler MN, Scanlon MH, et al: The complementary role of magnetic resonance imaging, Doppler echocardiography, and computed tomography in the diagnosis of dissecting thoracic aneurysms. Am Heart J 111:970, 1985.
9. Cigarroa JE, Isselbacher EM, DeSanctis RW, et al: Diagnostic imaging in the evaluation of suspected aortic dissection. N Engl J Med 328:35, 1993.
10. Nienaber CA, von Kodolitsch Y, Nicolas V, et al: The diagnosis of thoracic aortic dissection by noninvasive imaging procedures. N Engl J Med 328:1, 1993.
11. DeBakey ME, Henly WS, Cooley DA, et al: Surgical management of dissecting aneurysms of the aorta. J Thorac Cardiovasc Surg 49:130, 1965.
12. Miller DC, Stinson EB, Oyer PE, et al: Operative treatment of aortic dissections. J Thorac Cardiovasc Surg 78:365, 1979.
13. DeBakey ME, Cooley DA, Creech O Jr: Surgical considerations of dissecting aneurysm of the aorta. Ann Surg 142:586, 1955.
14. DeBakey ME, McCollum CH, Crawford ES, et al: Dissection and dissecting aneurysms of the aorta: Twenty-year follow-up of five hundred twenty-seven patients treated surgically. Surgery 92:1118, 1982.
15. Doroghazi RM, Slater EE, DeSanctis RW, et al: Long-term survival of patients with treated aortic dissection. J Am Coll Cardiol 3:1026, 1984.
16. Ergin MA, Galla JD, Lansman S, et al: Acute dissections of the aorta: Current surgical treatment. Surg Clin North Am 65:721, 1985.
17. Kolff J, Bates RJ, Balderman SC, et al: Acute aortic arch dissections: Reevaluation of the indications for medical and surgical therapy. Am J Cardiol 39:727, 1977.
18. Miller DC, Mitchell RS, Oyer PE, et al: Independent determinants of operative mortality for patients with aortic dissections. Circulation 70(Suppl I):I-153, 1984.
19. Reul GJ, Cooley DA, Hallman GL, et al: Dissecting aneurysm of the descending aorta. Arch Surg 110:632, 1975.
20. DeBakey ME, McCollum CH, Graham JM: Surgical treatment of aneurysms of the descending thoracic aorta. J Cardiovasc Surg 19:571, 1978.
21. Jex RK, Schaff HV, Piehler JM, et al: Early and late results following repair of dissections of the descending thoracic aorta. J Vasc Surg 3:226, 1986.
22. Neya K, Omoto R, Kyo S, et al: Outcome of Stanford Type B acute aortic dissection. Circulation 86(Suppl II):II-1, 1992.
23. Haverich A, Miller DC, Scott WC, et al: Acute and chronic aortic dissection—determinants of long-term outcome for operative survivors. Circulation 72(Suppl II):II-22, 1985.
24. Gerbode F, Braimbridge M, Osborn JJ, et al: Traumatic thoracic aneurysms: Treatment by resection and grafting with the use of an extracorporeal bypass. Surgery 42:975, 1957.
25. Turney SZ, Attar S, Ayella R, et al: Traumatic rupture of the aorta. J Thorac Cardiovasc Surg 72:727, 1976.
26. Mattox KL: Contemporary issues in thoracic aortic surgery. Semin Thorac Cardiovasc Surg 3:281, 1991.
27. Finkelmeier BA, Mentzer RM Jr, Kaiser DL, et al: Chronic traumatic thoracic aneurysm. J Thorac Cardiovasc Surg 84:257, 1982.
28. Cowley RA, Turney SZ, Hankins JR, et al: Rupture of thoracic aorta caused by blunt trauma. J Thorac Cardiovasc Surg 100: 652, 1990.
29. Ernst CB: Abdominal aortic aneurysm. N Engl J Med 328:1167, 1993.
30. Norrgard O, Rais O, Anguist K: Familial occurrence of abdominal aortic aneurysms. Surgery 95:650, 1984.
31. Tilson M, Seashore M: Human genetics of the abdominal aortic aneurysm. Surg Gynecol Obstet 158:129, 1984.
32. Tilson M, Seashore M: Fifty families with abdominal aortic aneurysms in two or more first-order relatives. Am J Surg 147: 551, 1984.
33. Reilly JM, Tilson MD: Incidence and etiology of abdominal aortic aneurysms. Surg Clin North Am 69:705, 1989.
34. Cheatle TR, Scurr JH: Abdominal aortic aneurysms: A review of current problems. Br J Surg 76:826, 1989.
35. Dobrin PB: Pathophysiology and pathogenesis of aortic aneurysms. Surg Clin North Am 69:687, 1989.
36. Wheat MW Jr, Boruchow IB, Ramsey HW: Surgical treatment of aneurysms of the aortic root. Ann Thorac Surg 12:593, 1971.
37. Gallotti R, Ross DN: The Marfan syndrome: Surgical technique and follow-up in 50 patients. Ann Thorac Surg 29:428, 1980.
38. Cabrol C, Pavie A, Gandjbakhch I, et al: Complete replacement of the ascending aorta with reimplantation of the coronary arteries. J Thorac Cardiovasc Surg 81:309, 1981.
39. Kouchoukos NT, Karp RB, Blackstone EH, et al: Replacement of the ascending aorta and aortic valve with a composite graft. Ann Surg 192:403, 1980.
40. Cooley DA, DeBakey ME: Surgical considerations of intrathoracic aneurysms of the aorta and great vessels. Ann Surg 135: 660, 1952.
41. Kouchoukos NT, Marshall WG, Wedige-Stecher TA: Eleven-year experience with composite graft replacement of the ascending aorta and aortic valve. J Thorac Cardiovasc Surg 92: 691, 1986.
42. Cabrol C, Pavie A, Mesnildrey P, et al: Long-term results with total replacement of the ascending aorta and reimplantation of the coronary arteries. J Thorac Cardiovasc Surg 91:17, 1986.
43. Kidd JN, Reul GJ, Cooley DA, et al: Surgical treatment of aneurysms of the ascending aorta. Circulation 54(Suppl III):III-118, 1976.
44. Seguin JR, Picard E, Frapier J, et al: Aortic valve repair with fibrin glue for type A acute aortic dissection. Ann Thorac Surg 58:304, 1994.
45. Murphy DA, Craver JM, Jones EL, et al: Recognition and management of ascending aortic dissection complicating cardiac surgical operations. J Thorac Cardiovasc Surg 85:247, 1983.
46. Tuffier TH: Intervention chirurgicale directe pour un aneurysme de la crosse de l'aorte: Ligature du sac. Presse Med 10:267, 1902.
47. Muller WH, Warren DW, Blanton FS: A method for resection of aortic arch aneurysms. Ann Surg 151:225, 1960.
48. DeBakey ME, Beall AC, Cooley DA, et al: Resection and graft replacement of aneurysms involving the transverse arch of the aorta. Surg Clin North Am 46:1057, 1966.
49. Black PR, Van Devanter S, Cohn LH: Effects of hypothermia on systemic and organ system metabolism and function. J Surg Res 20:49, 1976.
50. Callahan PB, Lister J, Paton BC, et al: Effects of varying carbon dioxide tensions on the oxyhemoglobin dissociation curves under hypothermic conditions. Ann Surg 154:903, 1961.
51. Grossman R, Lewis FJ: The effects of cooling and low molecular weight dextran on blood sludging. J Surg Res 4:360, 1964.
52. Suzuki M, Penn I: The effects of therapeutic agents on the microcirculation during general hypothermia. Surgery 60:867, 1966.
53. Belsey RHR, Dowalshashi K, Keen G, et al: Profound hypothermia in cardiac surgery. J Thorac Cardiovasc Surg 56:497, 1968.
54. Sade R, Fisher EG, Castaneda AR: Hypothermic circulatory arrest: Cerebral circulation and metabolism. Eur Surg Res 14:71, 1976.
55. Cooley DA, Ott DA, Frazier OH, et al: Surgical treatment of aneurysms of the transverse aortic arch: Experience with 25 patients using hypothermic techniques. Ann Thorac Surg 32:260, 1981.
56. Frist WH, Baldwin JC, Starnes VA, et al: A reconsideration of cerebral perfusion in aortic arch replacement. Ann Thorac Surg 42:273, 1986.
57. Tabayashi K, Niibori K, Iguchi A, et al: Replacement of the transverse aortic arch for type A acute aortic dissection. Ann Thorac Surg 55:864, 1993.
58. Ueda U, Miki S, Kusuhara K, et al: Surgical treatment of the aneurysm or dissection involving ascending aorta and aortic arch utilizing circulatory arrest and retrograde perfusion. J Jp Assoc Thorac Surg 36:161, 1988.
59. Takamoto S, Matsuda T, Harada M, et al: Simple hypothermic retrograde cerebral perfusion during aortic arch surgery. J Cardiovasc Surg 33:560, 1992.

60. Coselli JS: Retrograde cerebral perfusion via a superior vena caval cannula for aortic arch aneurysm operations. Ann Thorac Surg 57:1668, 1994.
61. Bavaria JE, Woo YJ, Hall RA, et al: Retrograde cerebral and distal aortic perfusion during ascending and thoracoabdominal aortic operations. Ann Thorac Surg 60:345, 1995.
62. Kitamura M, Hashimoto A, Akimoto T, et al: Operation for type A aortic dissection: Introduction of retrograde cerebral perfusion. Ann Thorac Surg 59:1195, 1995.
63. Pagano D, Carey JA, Patel RL, et al: Retrograde cerebral perfusion: Clinical experience in emergency and elective aortic operations. Ann Thorac Surg 59:393, 1995.
64. Coselli JS, Buket S, Djukanovic B: Aortic arch operation: Current treatment and results. Ann Thorac Surg 59:19, 1995.
65. Yasuura K, Okamoto H, Ogawa Y, et al: Resection of aortic aneurysms without aortic clamp technique with the aid of hypothermic total body retrograde perfusion. J Thorac Cardiovasc Surg 107:1237, 1994.
66. Bloodwell RD, Hallman GL, Cooley DA: Total replacement of the aortic arch and the "subclavian steal" phenomenon. Ann Thorac Surg 5:236, 1968.
67. Livesay JJ, Cooley DA, Duncan JM, et al: Open aortic anastomosis: Improved results in the treatment of aneurysms of the aortic arch. Circulation 66(Suppl I):I-222, 1982.
68. Griepp RB, Stinson EB, Hollingsworth JF et al: Prosthetic replacement of the aortic arch. J Thorac Cardiovasc Surg 70:1051, 1975.
69. Ott DA, Frazier OH, Cooley DA: Resection of the aortic arch using deep hypothermia and temporary circulatory arrest. Circulation 58(Suppl I):I-227, 1978.
70. Ergin MA, Griepp RB: Progress in treatment of aneurysms of the aortic arch. World J Surg 4:535, 1980.
71. Galloway AC, Colvin SB, LaMendola CL, et al: Ten-year experience with 165 aneurysms of the ascending aorta and aortic arch. Circulation 80(Suppl I):I-249, 1989.
72. Culliford AT, Ayvaliotis B, Shemin R, et al: Aneurysms of the ascending aorta and transverse arch. J Thorac Cardiovasc Surg 83:701, 1982.
73. Crawford ES, Saleh SA: Transverse aortic arch aneurysm. Ann Surg 194:180, 1981.
74. Ergin MA, O'Connor J, Guinto R, et al: Experience with profound hypthermia and circulatory arrest in the treatment of aneurysms of the aortic arch. J Thorac Cardiovasc Surg 84:649, 1982.
75. Crawford ES, Snyder DM: Treatment of aneurysms of the aortic arch. J Thorac Cardiovasc Surg 85:237, 1983.
76. Sweeny MS, Cooley DA, Reul GJ, et al: Hypothermic circulatory arrest for cardiovascular lesions: Technical considerations and results. Ann Thorac Surg 40:498, 1985.
77. Livesay JJ, Cooley DA, Reul GJ, et al: Resection of aortic arch aneurysms: A comparison of hypothermic techniques in 60 patients. Ann Thorac Surg 36:19, 1983.
78. Valeri CR, Cassidy G, Khuri WS, et al: Hypothermia-induced reversible platelet dysfunction. Ann Surg 205:175, 1987.
79. Roberts AJ, Nora JD, Hughes WA, et al: Cardiac and renal responses to cross-clamping of the descending thoracic aorta. J Thorac Cardiovasc Surg 86:732, 1983.
80. Stokland O, Miller MM, Ilebekk A, et al: Mechanisms of hemodynamic responses to occlusion of the descending thoracic aorta. Am J Physiol 238:H423, 1980.
81. Oyama M, McNamara JJ, Suehiro GE, et al: The effects of thoracic aortic cross-clamping and declamping on visceral organ blood flow. Ann Surg 197:459, 1983.
82. Kouchoukos NT, Lell WA, Karp RB, et al: Hemodynamic effects of aortic clamping and decompression with a temporary shunt for resection of the descending thoracic aorta. Surgery 85:25, 1979.
83. Gelman S, Khazaeli MB, Orr R, et al: Blood volume redistribution during cross-clamping of the descending aorta. Anesth Analg 78:219, 1994.
84. Joob AW, Harman PK, Kaiser DL, et al: The effect of renin-angiotensin system blockade on visceral blood flow during and after thoracic aortic cross-clamping. J Thorac Cardiovasc Surg 91:411, 1986.
85. Gelman S, Reves JG, Fowler K, et al: Regional blood flow during cross-clamping of the thoracic aorta and infusion of sodium nitroprusside. J Thorac Cardiovasc Surg 85:287, 1983.
86. Symbas PN, Pfaender LM, Drucker MH, et al: Cross-clamping of the descending aorta. J Thorac Cardiovasc Surg 85:300, 1983.
87. Marini CP, Grubbs PE, Toporoff B, et al: Effect of sodium nitroprusside on spinal cord perfusion and paraplegia during aortic cross-clamping. Ann Thorac Surg 47:379, 1989.
88. Neville WE, Cox WD, Leininger B, et al: Resection of the descending thoracic aorta with femoral vein to femoral artery oxygenation perfusion. J Thorac Cardiovasc Surg 56:39, 1968.
89. Hug HR, Taber RE: Bypass flow requirements during thoracic aneurysmectomy with particular attention to the prevention of left heart failure. J Thorac Cardiovasc Surg 57:203, 1969.
90. Crawford ES, Coselli JS, Safi HJ: Partial cardiopulmonary bypass, hypothermic circulatory arrest, and posterolateral exposure for thoracic aortic aneurysm operation. J Thorac Cardiovasc Surg 94:824, 1987.
91. Kazui T, Komatsu S, Yokoyama H: Surgical treatment of aneurysms of the thoracic aorta with the aid of partial cardiopulmonary bypass: An analysis of 95 patients. Ann Thorac Surg 43: 622, 1987.
92. Carson DE, Karp RB, Kouchoukos NT: Surgical treatment of aneurysms of the descending thoracic aorta: An analysis of 85 patients. Ann Thorac Surg 35:58, 1983.
93. Culliford AT, Ayvaliotis B, Shemin R, et al: Aneurysms of the descending aorta. J Thorac Cardiovasc Surg 85:98, 1983.
94. Kahn DR, Vathayanon S, Sloan H: Resection of descending thoracic aneurysms without left heart bypass. Arch Surg 97:336, 1968.
95. Gott VL: Heparinized shunts for thoracic vascular operations. Ann Thorac Surg 14:219, 1972.
96. Donahoo JS, Brawley RK, Gott VL: The heparin-coated vascular shunt for thoracic aortic and great vessel procedures: A ten-year experience. Ann Thorac Surg 23:507, 1977.
97. Connors JP, Ferguson TB, Roper CL: The use of the TDMAC-heparin shunt in replacement of the descending thoracic aorta. Ann Surg 181:735, 1975.
98. Lawrence GH, Hessel EA, Sauvage LR, et al: Results of the use of the TDMAC-heparin shunt in the surgery of aneurysms of the descending thoracic aorta. J Thorac Cardiovasc Surg 73:393, 1977.
99. Wolfe WG, Kleinman LH, Wechsler AS, et al: Heparin-coated shunts for lesions of the descending thoracic aorta. Arch Surg 112:1481, 1977.
100. Cukingnan RA, Fee HJ, Carey JS: Repair of lesions of the descending thoracic aorta with the TDMAC-heparin shunt. J Thorac Cardiovasc Surg 75:227, 1978.
101. Hilgenberg AD, Rainer WG, Sadler TR Jr: Aneurysm of the descending thoracic aorta. J Thorac Cardiovasc Surg 81:818, 1981.
102. Verdant A, Page A, Cossette R, et al: Surgery of the descending thoracic aorta: Spinal cord protection with the Gott shunt. Ann Thorac Surg 46:147, 1988.
103. Murray GF, Young WG Jr: Thoracic aneurysmectomy utilizing direct left ventriculofemoral shunt (TDMAC-heparin) bypass. Ann Thorac Surg 21:26, 1976.
104. Frantz PT, Murray GF, Shallal JA, et al: Clinical and experimental evaluation of left ventriculoiliac shunt bypass during repair of lesions of the descending thoracic aorta. Ann Thorac Surg 31:551, 1981.
105. Molina JE, Cogordan J, Einzig S, et al: Adequacy of ascending aorta-descending aorta shunt during cross-clamping of the thoracic aorta for prevention of spinal cord injury. J Thorac Cardiovasc Surg 90:126, 1985.
106. Pett SB, Wernly JA, Akl BF: Observations on flow characteristics of passive external aortic shunts. J Thorac Cardiovasc Surg 93:447, 1987.
107. Connolly JE, Wakabayashi A, German JC, et al: Clinical experience with pulsatile left heart bypass without anticoagulation for thoracic aneurysms. J Thorac Cardiovasc Surg 62:568, 1971.
108. Wakabayashi A, Connolly JE, Stemmer EA, et al: Heparinless left heart bypass for resection of thoracic aortic aneurysms. Am J Surg 130:212, 1975.
109. Wakabayashi A, Connolly JE: Prevention of paraplegia associated with resection of extensive thoracic aneurysms. Arch Surg 111:1186, 1976.

110. Olivier HF, Maher TD, Liebler GA, et al: Use of the BioMedicus centrifugal pump in traumatic tears of the thoracic aorta. Ann Thorac Surg 38:586, 1984.
111. Diehl JT, Payne DD, Rastegar H, et al: Arterial bypass of the descending thoracic aorta with the BioMedicus centrifugal pump. Ann Thorac Surg 44:422, 1987.
112. Hess PJ, Howe HR Jr, Robicsek F, et al: Traumatic tears of the thoracic aorta: Improved results using the Bio-Medicus pump. Ann Thorac Surg 48:6, 1989.
113. Vasilakis A, Rozar GE, Hill RC, et al: Left atrial to femoral arterial bypass using the Biomedicus pump for operations of the thoracic aorta. Am Surg 56:802, 1990.
114. Crawford ES, Fenstermacher JM, Richardson W, et al: Reappraisal of adjuncts to avoid ischemia in the treatment of thoracic aortic aneurysms. Surgery 67:182, 1970.
115. Crawford ES, Rubio PA: Reappraisal of adjuncts to avoid ischemia in the treatment of aneurysms of descending thoracic aorta. J Thorac Cardiovasc Surg 66:693, 1973.
116. Najafi H, Javid H, Hunter J, et al: Descending aortic aneurysmectomy without adjuncts to avoid ischemia. Ann Thorac Surg 30:326, 1980.
117. Crawford ES, Walker HSJ, Saleh SA, et al: Graft replacement of aneurysm in descending thoracic aorta: Results without bypass or shunting. Surgery 89:73, 1981.
118. Livesay JJ, Cooley DA, Ventemiglia RA, et al: Surgical experience in descending thoracic aneurysmectomy with and without adjuncts to avoid ischemia. Ann Thorac Surg 39:37, 1985.
119. Najafi H: Descending aortic aneurysmectomy without adjuncts to avoid ischemia: 1993 update. Ann Thorac Surg 55:1042, 1993.
120. Adams HD, Van Geertruyden HH: Neurologic complications of aortic surgery. Ann Surg 144:574, 1956.
121. Brewer LA III, Fosburg RG, Mulder GA, et al: Spinal cord complications following surgery for coarctation of the aorta. J Thorac Cardiovasc Surg 64:368, 1972.
122. Wadouh F, Lindemann E, Arndt CF, et al: The arteria radicularis magna anterior as a decisive factor influencing spinal cord damage during aortic occlusion. J Thorac Cardiovasc Surg 88:1, 1984.
123. Svensson LG, Patel V, Coselli JS, et al: Preliminary report of localization of spinal cord blood supply by hydrogen during aortic operations. Ann Thorac Surg 49:528, 1990.
124. Svensson LG, Klepp P, Hinder RA: Spinal cord anatomy of the baboon: Comparison with man and implications on spinal cord blood flow during thoracic aortic cross-clamping. S Afr J Surg 24:32, 1986.
125. Svensson LG, Rickards E, Coull A, et al: Relationship of spinal cord blood flow to vascular anatomy during thoracic aortic cross-clamping and shunting. J Thorac Cardiovasc Surg 91:71, 1986.
126. Williams GM, Perler BA, Burdick JF, et al: Angiographic localization of spinal cord blood supply and its relationship to postoperative paraplegia. J Vasc Surg 13:23, 1991.
127. Hollier LH: Protecting the brain and spinal cord. J Vasc Surg 5: 524, 1987.
128. Laschinger JC, Izumoto H, Kouchoukos NT: Evolving concepts in prevention of spinal cord injury during operations on the descending thoracic and thoracoabdominal aorta. Ann Thorac Surg 44:667, 1987.
129. Kouchoukos NT: Spinal cord ischemic injury: Is it preventable? Semin Thorac Cardiovasc Surg 3:323, 1991.
130. Shenaq SA, Svensson LG: Paraplegia following aortic surgery. J Cardiothorac Vasc Anesth 7:81, 1993.
131. Laschinger JC, Cunningham JN, Catinella FP, et al: Detection and prevention of intraoperative spinal cord ischemia after cross-clamping of the thoracic aorta: Use of somatosensory evoked potentials. Surgery 92:1109, 1982.
132. Miyamoto K, Ueno A, Wada T, et al: A new and simple method of preventing spinal cord damage following temporary occlusion of the thoracic aorta by draining the cerebrospinal fluid. J Cardiovasc Surg 1:188, 1960.
133. Blaisdell FW, Cooley DA: The mechanism of paraplegia after temporary thoracic aortic occlusion and its relationship to spinal fluid pressure. Surgery 51:351, 1962.
134. McCullough JL, Hollier LH, Nugent M: Paraplegia after thoracic aortic occlusion: Influence of cerebrospinal fluid drainage. J Vasc Surg 7:153, 1988.
135. Crawford ES, Svensson LG, Hess KR, et al: A prospective randomized study of cerebrospinal fluid drainage to prevent paraplegia after high-risk surgery on the thoracoabdominal aorta. J Vasc Surg 13:36, 1990.
136. Grubbs PE, Marini C, Toporoff B, et al: Somatosensory evoked potentials and spinal cord perfusion pressure are significant predictors of postoperative neurologic dysfunction. Surgery 104: 216, 1988.
137. Woloszyn TT, Marini CP, Coons MS, et al: Cerebrospinal fluid drainage and steroids provide better spinal cord protection during aortic cross-clamping than does either treatment alone. Ann Thorac Surg 49:78, 1990.
138. Svensson LG, Stewart RW, Cosgrove DM III, et al: Intrathecal papaverine for the prevention of paraplegia after operation on the thoracic or thoracoabdominal aorta. J Thorac Cardiovasc Surg 96:823, 1988.
139. Grum DF, Svensson LG, Blum J: Intrathecal papaverine for thoracic aortic aneurysm resection: A preliminary report. Anesthesiology 69:A894, 1988.
140. Svensson LG, Grum DF, Bednarski M, et al: Appraisal of cerebrospinal fluid alterations during aortic surgery with intrathecal papaverine administration and cerebrospinal fluid drainage. J Vasc Surg 11:423, 1990.
141. Ogata M, Marshall BM, Lougheed WM: Observations on the effect of intrathecal papaverine in experimental vasospasm. J Neurosurg 38:20, 1973.
142. Nugent M, Kaye MP, McGoon DC: Effects of nitroprusside on aortic and intraspinal pressures during thoracic aortic cross-clamping. Anesthesiology 61:A68, 1984.
143. Marini CP, Cunningham JN: Evoked potentials: Ten-year experience with a valuable research and clinical tool. Semin Thorac Cardiovasc Surg 3:286, 1991.
144. Cunningham JN, Laschinger JC, Merkin HA, et al: Measurement of spinal cord ischemia during operations upon the thoracic aorta. Ann Surg 196:285, 1982.
145. Laschinger JC, Cunningham JN, Nathan IM, et al: Intraoperative identification of vessels critical to spinal cord blood supply—use of somatosensory evoked potentials. Curr Surg 41:107, 1984.
146. Laschinger JC, Cunningham JN, Cooper MM, et al: Monitoring of somatosensory evoked potentials during surgical procedures on the thoracoabdominal aorta. Part I. J Thorac Cardiovasc Surg 94:260, 1987.
147. Laschinger JC, Cunningham JN, Baumann FG, et al: Monitoring of somatosensory evoked potentials during surgical procedures on the thoracoabdominal aorta. Part II. J Thorac Cardiovasc Surg 94:266, 1987.
148. Laschinger JC, Cunningham JN, Baumann FG, et al: Monitoring of somatosensory evoked potentials during surgical procedures on the thoracoabdominal aorta. Part III. J Thorac Cardiovasc Surg 94:271, 1987.
149. Cunningham JN, Laschinger JC, Spencer FC: Monitoring of somatosensory evoked potentials during surgical procedures on the thoracoabdominal aorta. Part IV. J Thorac Cardiovasc Surg 94: 275, 1987.
150. Coles JG, Wilson GJ, Sima AF, et al: Intraoperative detection of spinal cord ischemia using somatosensory cortical evoked potentials during thoracic aortic occlusion. Ann Thorac Surg 34: 299, 1982.
151. Laschinger JC, Cunningham JN, Nathan IM, et al: Experimental and clinical assessment of the adequacy of partial bypass in maintenance of spinal cord blood flow during operations on the thoracic aorta. Ann Thorac Surg 36:417, 1983.
152. Crawford ES, Mizrahi EM, Hess KR, et al: The impact of distal aortic perfusion and somatosensory evoked potential monitoring on prevention of paraplegia after aortic aneurysm operation. J Thorac Cardiovasc Surg 95:357, 1988.
153. Svensson LG, Patel V, Robinson MF, et al: Influence of preservation or perfusion of intraoperatively identified spinal cord blood supply on spinal motor evoked potentials and paraplegia after aortic surgery. J Vasc Surg 13:355, 1991.
154. Pontius RG, Brockman HL, Hardy EG, et al: The use of hypothermia in the prevention of paraplegia following temporary aortic occlusion: Experimental observations. Surgery 36:33, 1954.

155. Coles JG, Wilson GJ, Sima AF, et al: Intraoperative management of thoracic aortic aneurysm. J Thorac Cardiovasc Surg 85:292, 1983.
156. Colon R, Frazier OH, Cooley DA, et al: Hypothermic regional perfusion for protection of the spinal cord during periods of ischemia. Ann Thorac Surg 43:639, 1987.
157. Davison JK, Cambria RP, Vierra DJ, et al: Epidural cooling for regional spinal cord hypothermia during thoracoabdominal aneurysm repair. J Vasc Surg 20:304, 1994.
158. Svensson LG, Von Ritter CM, Groeneveld HT, et al: Cross-clamping of the thoracic aorta. Ann Surg 204:38, 1986.
159. Laschinger JC, Cunningham JN, Cooper MM, et al: Prevention of ischemic spinal cord injury following aortic cross-clamping: Use of corticosteroids. Ann Thorac Surg 38:500, 1984.
160. Bracken MB, Shepard MJ, Collins WF, et al: A randomized, controlled trial of methylprednisolone or naloxone in the treatment of acute spinal-cord injury. N Engl J Med 322:1405, 1990.
161. Wadouh F, Arndt CF, Oppermann E, et al: The mechanism of spinal cord injury after simple and double aortic cross-clamping. J Thorac Cardiovasc Surg 92:121, 1986.
162. Rothen HU, Lauber R, Mosimann M: An evaluation of the rapid infusion system. Anaesthesia 47:597, 1992.
163. Mutch WAC, Thomson IR, Teskey JM, et al: Phlebotomy reverses the hemodynamic consequences of thoracic aortic cross-clamping: Relationships between central venous pressure and cerebrospinal fluid pressure. Anesthesiology 74:320, 1991.
164. Crawford ES: Thoraco-abdominal and abdominal aortic aneurysms involving renal, superior mesenteric, and celiac arteries. Ann Surg 179:763, 1974.
165. Crawford ES, Snyder DM, Gwen GC, et al: Progress in treatment of thoracoabdominal and abdominal aortic aneurysms involving celiac, superior mesenteric, and renal arteries. Ann Surg 188:404, 1978.
166. Crawford ES, Coselli JS: Thoracoabdominal aneurysm surgery. Semin Thorac Cardiovasc Surg 3:300, 1991.
167. Cox GS, O'Hara PJ, Hertzer NR, et al: Thoracoabdominal aneurysm repair: A representative experience. J Vasc Surg 15:780, 1992.
168. Svensson LG, Crawford ES, Hess KR, et al: Experience with 1509 patients undergoing thoracoabdominal aortic operations. J Vasc Surg 17:357, 1993.
169. Crawford ES, Crawford JL, Safi HJ, et al: Thoracoabdominal aortic aneurysms: Preoperative and intraoperative factors determining immediate and long-term results of operations in 605 patients. J Vasc Surg 3:389, 1986.
170. Kouchoukos NT, Wareing TH, Izumoto H, et al: Elective hypothermic cardiopulmonary bypass and circulatory arrest for spinal cord protection during operations on the thoracoabdominal aorta. J Thorac Cardiovasc Surg 99:659, 1990.
171. Hollier LH, Money SR, Naslund TC, et al: Risk of spinal cord dysfunction in patients undergoing thoracoabdominal aortic replacement. Am J Surg 164:209, 1992.
172. Kelly IP, Attwood SEA, MacGowan S, et al: Thoracoabdominal aortic aneurysm replacement using hypothermic circulatory arrest. Ir J Med Sci 162:88, 1993.
173. Cohen JR, Angus L, Asher A, et al: Disseminated intravascular coagulation as a result of supraceliac clamping: Implications for thoracoabdominal aneurysm repair. Ann Vasc Surg 1:552, 1987.
174. Moore WS, Vescera CL: Repair of abdominal aortic aneurysm by transfemoral endovascular graft placement. Ann Surg 220: 331, 1994.
175. Moore WS: The role of endovascular grafting technique in the treatment of infrarenal abdominal aortic aneurysm. Cardiovasc Surg 3:109, 1995.
176. Dake MD, Miller DC, Semba CP, et al: Transluminal placement of endovascular stent-grafts for the treatment of descending thoracic aortic aneurysms. N Engl J Med 331:1729, 1994.

CHAPTER 22

Anesthesia for Abdominal Aortic Revascularization

John E. Ellis, M.D.
Michael F. Roizen, M.D.
John A. Youngberg, M.D.

Goals of Anesthesia For Aortic Revascularization

The goals of anesthesia for vascular surgery are to minimize patient morbidity and maximize surgical benefit. In the current environment, we must also achieve these goals in the most cost-effective manner. The morbidity from these procedures has decreased rapidly, from a 6-day mortality of greater than 25% for major aortic reconstruction in the mid-1960s to a 1 to 5% mortality today. We believe that advances in preoperative preparation and perioperative anesthetic management are responsible for much of these improvements. The anesthesiologist has had as great an influence in reducing the morbidity and costs of vascular surgery as in any other surgical procedure.

This chapter discusses the pathophysiology of atherosclerotic vascular disease and the general medical problems common in patients presenting for aortic reconstruction, particularly coronary artery disease. We believe the heart should be the major focus of the anesthesiologist's attention insofar as myocardial dysfunction remains the single most important cause of morbidity following vascular surgery[1–11] (Table 22–1). However, preservation of other organ systems (particularly renal and central nervous) is also crucial. This chapter will review current controversies over the selection of anesthetic techniques, monitoring modalities, and organ protection strategies. The specific surgical goals, anatomy, and complications for aortic revascularization will be placed in the context of optimal anesthetic management. The different scenarios that lead to emergency surgery for these conditions and their appropriate management will also be discussed.

Vascular Disease: Epidemiologic, Medical, and Surgical Aspects

Pathophysiology of Aortic Atherosclerosis

Atherosclerosis is a generalized disorder of the arterial tree associated with a number of recognized predisposing risk factors, including advanced age, altered serum lipid and lipoprotein profiles, hypertension, cigarette smoking, obesity and physical inactivity, male gender, diabetes mellitus, and lifestyle. It is a degenerative process characterized by the formation of initial plaques consisting of oxidized lipid accumulations and inflammatory cells, smooth muscle cells, connective tissue fibers, and calcium deposits. Putative etiologies are endothelial damage caused by hemodynamic shear stress, hypercoagulability resulting in thrombosis, and the destructive effects of oxidized low-density lipoproteins. Disruption of the fibrous cap over a lipid deposit can lead to ulceration within the plaque. Vasoactive influences can result in spasm and acute thrombosis.

Morbidity associated with aortic atherosclerosis arises from plaque enlargement and plaque ulceration or embolization, or atrophy of the media due to atherosclerosis disease may weaken the artery wall, producing aneurysmal dilatation. Sheer stress at the aortic bifurcation tends to produce damage (either media destruction and dilation or plaque accumulation) at this point and at bifurcation (trifurcations) of distal vessels.

Natural History of Patients with Aortic Disease

Elderly patients with symptomatic or even asymptomatic peripheral vascular disease have greatly increased mortality rates, particularly from cardiovascular causes (6- to 15-fold increases).[12,13] The prevalence of claudication is approximately 2% among older adults, which represents only about one tenth of patients with asymptomatic lower extremity atherosclerosis. Abdominal aortic aneurysms (AAAs) occur predominantly in white men. Whereas studies showing wide regional variations in surgical rates have been used to suggest physician overuse of technologies, some data suggest the opposite—that all patients who could benefit do no receive such interventions, with potentially adverse results due to lack of interventions.[14]

TABLE 22–1
Perioperative Mortality Associated with Cardiac Events*

Aortic Reconstruction References, Year	Deaths/Total No. of Patients (%)	% Mortality Caused by Cardiac Dysfunction
Szilagyi et al.,[1] 1966	59/401 (14.7)	48
Whittemore et al.,[2] 1980	1/110 (0.9)	100
Crawford et al.,[3] 1981	41/860 (4.8)	54
Benefiel et al.,[4] 1986	3/96 (3.1)	67
Johnston,[5] 1989	32/666 (4.8)	69
Golden et al.,[6] 1990	8/500 (1.6)	75
Krupski et al.,[7] 1993	1/53 (1.9)	100
Lachapelle et al.,[8] 1992	7/146 (4.8)	71
Suggs et al.,[9] 1993	3/247 (1.2)	66
Baron et al.,[10] 1994	20/457 (4.4)	50
L'Italien et al.,[11] 1995	16/321 (5.0)	62

*From Ellis JE, Roizen MF, Mantha S, et al: Anesthesia for vascular surgery. In Barash PG (ed): Clinical Anesthesia, 3rd ed. Philadelphia, Lippincott-Raven, 1996, with permission.

The first abdominal aortic repair was performed by Dubost in 1951. Subsequent advances in vascular surgery have been due to improved radiologic contrast agents and prosthetic graft materials, as well as improved perioperative anesthetic and medical management. The goals of vascular surgery are to provide an enduring restoration of normal perfusion, so as to improve functional status or prevent death from aneurysm rupture. Current challenges remain: to perform revascularization less invasively and with less morbidity.

Clear evidence of the benefit of early elective intervention in aortic aneurysmal disease utilized life table analysis to detail improved outcome. To put this in perspective, electively operating on someone with a 6-cm aneurysm and repairing that aneurysm extends life about 6 years on average (makes the RealAge or physiologic age 6.4 years younger).[1,15] Improvements in organ protection recently reveal that perioperative therapy can make the RealAge 10.1 years younger.[15,16] The rest of this chapter reveals the mechanisms and techniques for doing so. While anesthetic techniques and strategies make a difference to outcome, surgical techniques are being developed to lessen surgical morbidity and even the need for skillful anesthetic practices.

The success of laparoscopic surgery has spurred the development of other minimally invasive procedures. Radiologists and surgeons have reported the placement of endovascular stents to treat patients with thoracic and abdominal aortic aneurysms. A number of recent articles have appeared reporting up to a 95% success rate employing transluminal endovascular graft placement for the treatment of aortic aneurysms.[17–20] Although outcome studies for many of these procedures are lacking, logic would support their investigation if they are associated with less risk and cost than traditional surgery. The practice of anesthesia for aortic revascularization will surely change as the interventional strategies evolve.

Medical Therapy for Atherosclerosis

The goals of medical therapy for atherosclerotic vascular disease are to prevent atherosclerotic progression and cardiovascular morbidity.[21] Lifestyle changes, such as blood pressure control, stress management, exercise, diet modification, antioxidant and antiplatelet use, and cessation of smoking are by far the most effective "medical" therapies.

In fact, aggressive early use of such therapies can probably eliminate over 70% of aortic aneurysmal disease. These lifestyle changes can make a smoking hypertensive person without end-organ damage have a physiologic (RealAge) 20 years younger than without normalization of blood pressure and cessation of smoking.[15]

Antiplatelet therapy is a mainstay of medical therapy for peripheral vascular disease. Chronic aspirin therapy or cyclo-oxygenase type 2 inhibitor (COX-2) therapy may retard the progression of atherosclerosis and prevent morbid cardiovascular events. Therefore, many patients presenting for vascular surgery will be taking aspirin and other agents that have antithrombotic effects such as vitamin E.[22,23] Consideration of the adverse effects of aspirin, including increased bleeding tendency, gastritis, and renal vasoconstriction must be weighed against these benefits. In general, we recommend that patients continue to take aspirin until the day of surgery and individualize the choice. When patients develop acute ischemia, systemic anticoagulation may be instituted. The agents used may range from dextran, to enhance microcirculatory blood flow, to heparin, Coumadin, or thrombolytics. Therefore, when patients present to us for urgent surgery to reverse acute ischemia, we specifically ask them and their surgeons about recent or planned anticoagulation. Not infrequently, we are told that a patient has recently received a bolus dose of heparin or a thrombolytic; in these situations, we will almost always forego regional anesthesia.

Overview of Medical Problems in Peripheral Vascular Disease Patients

Many disorders are associated with vascular disease; however, diabetes, smoking and its sequelae, chronic pulmonary disease, hypertension, and ischemic heart disease are the most common (Table 22–2). Understanding the end-organ effects of these diseases can guide appropriate perioperative therapy.[24] It would be suboptimal to administer anesthesia to patients with uncontrolled medical conditions such as severe hypertension, a recent myocardial infarction, uncontrolled diabetes and hyperglycemia, or untreated pulmonary infections. However, an expanding aneurysm can force one's hand. In such situations, attempts to rapidly control chronically deranged blood pressure (which could precipitate cerebral ischemia) or electrolytes (which could, for example, result in accidental administration of a bolus of potassium) may be more hazardous than leaving the condition untreated or trying to control the abnormality slowly.

TABLE 22–2
Factors Influencing Outcome After Vascular Surgery*

	Factors
Patient factors	Age ≥60 yr: 68% History of cigarette smoking: 88% Co-existing diseases Hypertension: 40–68% Coronary artery disease: 40–60% Dysrhythmia: 36% Diabetes mellitus: 8–44% Congestive heart failure: 5–29% Chronic obstructive pulmonary disease: 25–50% Renal insufficiency: 5–15% Postoperative hypercoagulable state
Surgical factors	Expertise of the surgeon Emergency/semiemergency state Major fluid shifts Clamping and unclampiing of major vessels Intraoperative hypotension Intraoperative hypertension
Institution-specific factors	University/community center Facilities for major preoperative work-ups Expertise in the interpretation of preoperative testing modalities especially for coronary artery disease

*From Ellis JE, Roizen MF, Mantha S, et al: Anesthesia for vascular surgery. In Barash PG (ed): Clinical Anesthesia, 3rd ed. Philadelphia, Lippincott-Raven, 1996, with permission.

Other causes of morbidity following aortic revascularization include pulmonary infections, graft infections, renal insufficiency and failure, hepatic failure, cerebrovascular accidents, and spinal cord ischemia resulting in paraplegia. The incidence of these other causes of morbidity has declined substantially in the past 20 years; in particular, death from renal failure after abdominal aortic reconstruction has declined from 25% to less than 1% at present.[25–27] Much of the elimination of renal failure has resulted from better perioperative fluid management. Still, even in the 1990s, perioperative mortality and the factors limiting patient prognosis after vascular surgery are primarily related to the heart (Table 22–1). We will therefore examine more closely the effects of known or suspected coronary artery disease on patient management before, during, and after vascular surgery.

Coronary Artery Disease in Patients with Peripheral Vascular Disease

Hertzer et al.[28] performed coronary angiography is 1,001 consecutive patients presenting for vascular surgery and identified severe correctable coronary artery disease in 25% of the entire series. The incidence of significant coronary artery disease (stenosis >70%) detected by angiography was 37% in patients without any clinical indications of coronary artery disease and 78% in those with clinical indications. In another study, angiographic triple-vessel or left main coronary artery disease was found in 10.2% of asymptomatic and 14.3% of symptomatic patients awaiting vascular surgery.[29] These patients with severe coronary artery disease are not only at high risk for surgery but also the most likely to benefit from coronary revascularization.

Short-term postoperative morbidity and mortality after vascular surgery is higher than after other types of noncardiac surgery. Cardiac-related death, myocardial infarction (MI), cardiogenic pulmonary edema, unstable angina, and dysrhythmias may occur after vascular surgery. The rates of cardiac-related death range from 0% to 8% and the infarction rate ranges from 0% to 15.3%.[30,31]

Long-term morbidity and mortality following vascular surgery are also greatly influenced by the presence of coronary artery disease. Although the presence of uncorrected coronary artery disease appears to double 5-year mortality after vascular surgery, coronary artery bypass graft (CABG) is associated with improved survival in patients with triple-vessel coronary artery and peripheral vascular disease.[32,33] The prevalence of asymptomatic coronary artery disease and the substantial short-term and long-term cardiac morbidity and mortality in patients undergoing vascular surgery have led investigators and clinicians to propose and undertake extensive preoperative work-ups to detect underlying coronary artery disease.

Controversy persists as to whether preoperative identification of patients most likely to have perioperative cardiovascular events related to myocardial ischemia benefits patients. Invasive interventions may benefit patients with vascular disease but are generally more risky than in other groups of patients.[34] Many believe that more invasive monitoring and preparatory coronary revascularization may be "survival tests" that are accompanied by increased short-term morbidity; others believe that these procedures lead to better long-term survival. Patients who have survived coronary revascularization have fewer cardiac complications after vascular surgery.[32]

Data flow from the Coronary Artery Surgery Study (CASS) study indicates that prior percutaneous transluminal coronary angioplasty (PTCA) or CABG confers 4-year prolongation of life (4 years younger RealAge) after vascular surgery, about the same benefit as perioperative β-blockade.[15,16,35] Do the two provide the same benefit, or is there additional benefit of one added to the other? We as yet do not know the answer to these questions, but the magnitude of a 4-year younger RealAge benefit (equivalent to a 13% reduction in 2-year mortality) is what optimal perioperative management is striving for compared to average perioperative management.[15,16]

Three essential purposes are served by preoperative cardiac risk stratification. The first would be to forego surgery or perform a more conservative surgical procedure in those at high risk. The second goal would be to determine which patients should undergo myocardial revascularization. This goal requires that we identify patients with left main coronary artery disease or triple-vessel coronary artery disease and poor left ventricular function, as these patients are most likely to benefit from coronary revascularization in the long run.[33] Finally, because most myocardial ischemia and infarction occur in the early postoperative period, a third rationale for preoperative segregation of high-risk patients is to target those who might benefit from aggressive therapy in the first 24 to 72 hours after surgery. Risk-reducing interventions may include invasive monitoring, stress-reducing anesthetic techniques, or prolonged intensive care unit (ICU) stay. These attempts to reduce morbidity vary widely in cost and their effectiveness is controversial. The choice of risk-reducing strategies depends upon the surgical procedures, the discretion of the anesthesiologists and surgeons, and institutional protocols (clinical pathways).

The patient's history and bedside examination before aortic revascularization can provide important prognostic information. For example, Pryor et al.[36] found that evaluation of the clinical history, physical examination, electrocardiogram, and chest radiography could predict left main coronary artery disease, triple-vessel disease, and 3-year survival. Although this work was performed in a general population of patients with suspected coronary artery disease and may not be readily extrapolated to patients who need aortic revascularization or remodeling, basic clinical evaluation is obtained with minimal additional cost. Studies have identified known coronary artery disease, congestive heart failure (CHF), advanced age, severely limited exercise tolerance, chronic renal insufficiency, severe uncontrolled hypertension with left ventricular hypertrophy, and the use of digoxin as risk factors for the development of perioperative cardiac morbidity.[30] In most clinical series, congestive heart failure (whether diagnosed by an S_3 gallop or basilar rales on physical examination or history) is associated with the highest risk.[37]

The clinician also tries to identify patients who have previously suffered a myocardial infarction. Previous work has suggested that risk of reinfarction depends primarily on the amount of time passed since infarction, the type of infarct, and functional state.[38] We believe, however, that risk stratification as described below with specialized testing may identify patients who are at relatively low risk despite a recent infarction. In addition, studies using aggressive hemodynamic monitoring and intensive postoperative care suggest that the rate of reinfarction after a recent infarction is currently much lower in some centers.[39,40]

Exercise tolerance may also be a useful prognostic indicator, although claudication, orthopedic problems, and frailty may limit a patient's capabilities. Patients with excellent exercise capacity have greatly reduced risk.[41] We believe that if patients can walk briskly (>4 mph) for two blocks with neither angina nor dyspnea and have no other indicators of coronary artery disease, they are very unlikely to have left main disease, triple-vessel disease, or severe left ventricular dysfunction (ejection fraction >35%).[41,42] Such patients can possibly undergo surgery without specialized noninvasive testing because they are unlikely to be at risk for adverse perioperative outcomes. Others have proposed multifactorial indices. such as Goldman's index,[36] to risk stratify patients. However, many investigators in the 1980s challenged risk stratification based on bedside clinical information, claiming that specialized preoperative tests, such as Holter monitoring or thallium scintigraphy, were more accurate than clinical indicators for predicting perioperative cardiac complications.

Given the costs and risks involved in coronary angiography, it is not practical to subject all vascular patients to this test before surgery. Therefore, many patients undergo noninvasive testing to evaluate cardiovascular risk before vascular surgery.[43] The use of screening tests has remained controversial, with some studies showing great prognostic value[44] and others showing that they are no better than the basic clinical evaluation.

One limitation of specializing testing, including coronary angiography, is the fact that myocardial infarction and cardiac-related mortality need not necessarily be due to severely narrowed coronary arteries. Recent evidence suggests that the rupture of previously nonocclusive lipid-laden, macrophage-rich coronary plaques can cause spasm and initiate unstable angina, acute myocardial infarction, and sudden death.[45] Therefore, testing that attempts to induce ischemia will miss some patients who have nonobstructive plaques that can rupture and cause transmural infarction.

The early experience[46] with dipyridamole-thallium scintigraphy yielded two important observations: an old myocardial infarction ("fixed" defect) was not a risk factor in itself, and an area of redistribution (i.e., myocardium at risk) was associated with an adverse outcome. Dipyridamole-thallium scintigraphy was most helpful in the risk stratification of patients whose risks were intermediate based on clinical evaluation. In these studies, patients who had low clinical risk or a negative dipyridamole-thallium study had a low rate of adverse cardiac events after vascular surgery. Mangano et al.[47] and Baron et al.[10] have challenged the effectiveness of dipyridamole-thallium scintigraphy for the routine preoperative screening of vascular surgery patients. Alternatively, quantifying the degree of redistribution may improve the discriminating ability of thallium scintigraphy; the presence of more than two reversible effects or defects in distribution in the left anterior descending artery increases cardiac risk.[48] Patients with a markedly positive dipyridamole-thallium scan should probably undergo coronary angiography in anticipation of myocardial revascularization.[44] When we (Roizen and Ellis) analyzed the studies in the literature evaluating thallium scintigraphy before vascular surgery, we found that a positive scan increased a patient's chances of having a postoperative cardiac event by a factor of 4.6.[49]

Determination of systolic left ventricular function may provide prognostic information, because of the association of congestive heart failure with morbid postoperative events. Radionuclide ventriculography can define systolic and diastolic function.[50] If ejection fraction does not increase at least 5% with exercise, myocardial ischemia is also presumed. Most investigators attempting to predict operative risk have evaluated only systolic function; however, we are becoming increasingly aware that diastolic dysfunction is also a problem, particularly for hypertensive patients. In the late 1990s, radionuclide ventriculography is being used less frequently for preoperative risk assessment. It has been supplanted by transthoracic echocardiography, which reveals cardiac structure as well as function.

In the past, a pulmonary artery catheter was sometimes placed preoperatively to measure hemodynamics and perform risk stratification, but because catheter placement requires preoperative admission to an ICU, it is rarely used in an era when patients are often admitted on the day of surgery. Pulmonary artery catheterization may still occasionally prove useful for preoperative optimization of unstable patients who require relatively urgent surgery. Low baseline ejection fraction may predict long-term cardiac mortality better than perioperative morbidity and mortality. If patients have congestive heart failure and an ejection fraction less than 35%, they will generally live longer if they receive chronic angiotensin-converting enzyme (ACE) inhibitor treatment. Our (Roizen and Ellis) meta-analysis showed that patients who have an ejection fraction less than 35% by radionuclide ventriculography are 3.7 times more likely to have a postoperative cardiac event.[49]

Raby et al. found that of the 18% of patients who had ischemia detected by Holter electrocardiographic (ECG) monitoring before vascular surgery, approximately one third had cardiac complications, while only 1% of patients without ischemia had complications.[51] Our (Roizen and Ellis) meta-analysis for Holter monitoring of preoperative ischemia suggests that an ischemia Holter recording before surgery increases the risk of a postoperative cardiac event by 2.7-fold.[49] The biggest limitation of ambulatory ECG for preoperative risk stratification is the high percentage (at least one fourth in our practice) of patients with baseline ECG abnormalities that obscure the diagnosis of new myocardial ischemia. These abnormalities include left ventricular hypertrophy with "strain,'' bundle branch block, pacemakers, and the effects of digoxin or minoxidil. Also, nonspecific ST-segment changes may occur perioperatively due to changes in body temperature, serum electrolytes, ventilation, or body position.

Dobutamine (5 to 30 μg/kg/min) stress echocardiography[52] can detect changes in regional wall motion. In one study, sensitivities in detecting one-, two-, and three-, and multivessel disease were 62.5%, 85.7%, and 94.7%, respectively.[53] In our (Roizen and Ellis) meta-analysis, we found that a positive dobutamine stress test increased the risk of a postoperative cardiac event by 6.2-fold.[49]

Clinicians who read the often conflicting studies in the literature may be perplexed about choosing the best test or pathway for their patients. According to Bayes' theorem, as the prior probability of a disease in a population increases, the predictive value of a positive test increases and the predictive value of a negative test decreases. For example, if the results of a dipyridamole-thallium scan for an 80-year-old patient with a history of diabetes and congestive heart failure were negative, the likelihood is good that the screening test is false-negative. Indeed, little is gained by having such a high-risk patient undergo a screening test because the test result is likely to be positive and suspect if negative.

One method that combines evidence from multiple studies to evaluate the effectiveness of therapies or other interventions is meta-analysis.[54] Our (Roizen and Ellis) meta-analysis of preoperative cardiac testing strategies allows the following conclusions.[49] With the exception of dobutamine stress echocardiography, each of the tests demonstrated a bias for better predictive value in earlier studies. This may have been due to pretest referral bias in early studies where patients were not recruited consecutively (sicker patients were chosen for earlier studies). Improvements in perioperative care over time may also explain the phenomenon of decreasing predictive value. All fours tests (dipyridamole-thallium scanning, radionuclide ventriculography, Holter monitoring, and dobutamine stress echocardiography) are "effective'' (the 95% confidence intervals for relative risk are >1.0) in predicting cardiac death or myocardial infarction following vascular surgery. Dobutamine stress echocardiography appears to be the best among these four tests and Holter monitoring the least effective. This conclusion is subject to revision because the 95% confidence intervals for relative risk overlap.

Decision analysis is an explicit analytic tool designated to facilitate complex clinical decisions in which many variables must be considered simultaneously. A decision tree containing a map of all relevant courses of action and their associated outcomes is constructed with the probabilities and utilities (values) of different clinical possibilities (e.g., the likelihood of mortality after preparatory CABG or of myocardial infarction after aortic revascularization). The optimal decision, which is the course of action with the highest overall expected survival rate and lowest cost, is then calculated. Fleisher et al.[55] used decision analysis to examine the effect of perioperative screening with dipyridamole-thallium scans before abdominal aortic surgery on 30-day cardiac-related mortality. The authors found that the decision to perform preoperative testing and coronary revascularization before surgery for abdominal aortic aneurysm was a function of an institution's mortality rates for myocardial revascularization and for vascular surgery performed without preoperative interventions. The authors suggested that in patients with low prior probability of coronary artery disease, aortic revascularization should be performed without cardiac screening. Their analysis demonstrates the importance of local institutional factors (particularly the institution's mortality rates for myocardial revascularization vs. those for vascular surgery) in determining the optimal preoperative strategy. The outcomes of different testing strategies must be compared with their costs. Recently, Bry et al.[56] examined the cost-effectiveness of dipyridamole-thallium scanning for screening before aortic surgical procedures in preventing 30-day postoperative cardiac death or MI. The calculation yielded a cost-effectiveness ratio of $392,253 per life saved and $181,039 per MI averted.

Chapter 2 of this book deals with cost-effectiveness in great detail. Another way of examining the issue is reduction in age or an increase in functional longevity. As stated earlier, optimal perioperative medical management for aortic revascularization can result in making a person's RealAge about 4.1 years younger, of which myocardial functional preservation accounts for about 80% of such benefit.[15,16]

Preoperative Coronary Revascularization

Myocardial revascularization may have long-term benefits in patients with triple-vessel coronary disease or poor left ventricular function.[33] The range of options for preparatory coronary revascularization continues to expand rapidly. These include traditional surgical revascularization (CABG), transmyocardial laser therapy, PTCA, excimer laser, rotoblader, coronary stent placement, and endoscopic CABG. However, mortality rates associated with CABG are 2.4-fold higher in patients with peripheral vascular disease (7.7% vs. 3.2%) compared to those without peripheral vascular disease.[57] Higher complication rates can be anticipated for the newer revascularization techniques when performed in patients with peripheral vascular diseases.[34]

Initial observational studies of PTCA performed before major noncardiac surgery suggest that patients who survive successful PTCA do well. However, complications associated with PTCA are significant (emergency CABG, myocardial infarction, early and late occlusion, and requirements for chronic anticoagulation)[58]; further studies are needed to define the role of PTCA and the newer revascularization modalities in the preoperative preparation of vascular surgery patients. Anticoagulation may be continued after these procedures and may preclude the use of regional anesthesia.

Once the patient has recovered from successful coronary revascularization, aortic revascularization is usually then performed. Elective abdominal aortic aneurysm repair should probably be performed before, simultaneously, or within 2 weeks of CABG because of the increased risk of aneurysm rupture after this period.[59]

Mohr et al. reported a 12% 30-day mortality rate in 25 patients who underwent combined CABG and AAA procedures.[60] All of these patients had severe coronary artery disease with a left ventricular ejection fraction less than 35% and/or unstable angina. Vicaretti et al. reported a 6.7% mortality rate in 15 patients undergoing combined CABG and AAA procedures.[61] There may be less potential benefit combining CABG and surgery for occlusive aortic disease.

Our (Roizen and Ellis) recommendations for preoperative cardiac evaluation are summarized in Table 22–3. We seek to identify and refer for myocardial revascularization patients with three-vessel disease, ejection fraction of less than 35%, or left main disease. Less severe cases of coronary artery disease (two-vessel or single-vessel) can probably benefit from the current state of the art in perioperative care. We refer patients with unstable symptoms directly for coronary angiography rather than noninvasive testing. When patients can walk briskly for two blocks with neither angina nor dyspnea, we recommend that they undergo surgery directly without noninvasive testing because they are unlikely to have adverse perioperative outcomes or to have severe coronary disease. The bedside clinical evaluation (patient history, electrocardiography, and chest radiography) helps us to optimize cardiac risk stratification in these patients. Patients with stable symptoms who cannot walk two blocks briskly are at intermediate risk and may benefit from noninvasive testing. We obtain dobutamine stress echocardiography in these situations. Semiquantitative interpretation of both dipyridamole-thallium scintigraphy and dobutamine stress echocardiography may allow us to refer only high-risk patients for catheterization. Less severe cases of coronary artery disease identified by weakly positive results on these tests may benefit from current state-of-the-art perioperative care, but these patients require careful follow-up after surgery to look for progression of coronary artery disease.

Perioperative Cardiac Monitoring

The goals of perioperative cardiac monitoring are to detect myocardial ischemia and abnormalities of preload, afterload, and ventricular function. Such monitoring may prevent myocardial infarction and allow better perfusion

TABLE **22–3**
Cardiac Risk Stratification Before Vascular Surgery*

Presentation	Interventions	Strength of Recommendation
Unstable angina or current CHF	Coronary angiography (CATH)	Strongly recommended
≥4 risk factors on basic evaluation	CATH	Recommended
Inability to walk two blocks becuse of claudication or cardiac symptoms	Noninvasive test by DTS or DSE	Recommended
2 or 3 risk factors on basic evaluation	Noninvasive test by DTS or DSE	Optional
Strongly positive DTS or DSE results	CATH	Recommended
Weakly positive DTS or DSE results	Surgery under perioperative risk-reducing strategies; follow-up after surgery for progression of CAD,	Optional
	or CATH	Optional
High-risk anatomic subgroups on CATH	Coronary artery bypass graft (CABG) surgery	Strongly recommended
Two-vessel or single-vessel disease on CATH	Percutaneous transluminal coronary angioplasty or CABG as appropriate, *or*	Optional
	Surgery under perioperative risk-reducing strategies	Optional

*From Ellis JE, Roizen MF, Mantha S, et al: Anesthesia for vascular surgery. In Barash PG (ed): Clinical Anesthesia, 3rd ed. Philadelphia, Lippincott-Raven, 1996, with permission.
DTS, dipyridamole-thallium scintigraphy; DSE, dobutamine stress echocardiography; CHF, congestive heart failure.

and preservation of other organs such as the liver, kidney, gut, and spinal cord.

Detection of Perioperative Myocardial Ischemia

ECG monitoring remains the mainstay of perioperative detection of myocardial ischemia. ECG evidence of ST-segment depression is a more common indicator of myocardial ischemia in vascular surgery patients than is ST-segment elevation. ST-segment depression occurs in 20 to 50% of patients undergoing vascular surgery. London et al.[67] showed that in patients with risk factors for significant coronary artery disease, the greatest sensitivity for the detection of myocardial ischemia was achieved by intraoperative use of either lead V_5 (sensitivity 75%) or lead V_4 (sensitivity 61%). Simultaneous viewing of leads V_4 and V_5 had a sensitivity of 90% compared with a sensitivity of 80% for the combination of leads II and V_5. Because clinicians often fail to detect intraoperative ischemic ECG changes when viewing oscilloscopes, automated ST-segment monitors promise to increase the detection of such ECG changes. We have documented that the sensitivity of ST segment monitors for transesophageal echocardiography (TEE)-diagnosed myocardial ischemia is 40% and 75% for ECG-diagnosed ischemia.[63] Although these monitors are not always accurate, we believe they are useful as alarms for busy clinicians.

Perioperative Holter monitoring has shown that the intraoperative period may be the least stressful for patients with coronary artery disease. Patients undergoing aortic revascularization are most likely to manifest myocardial ischemia in the immediate postoperative period with its associated pain, adrenergic stress, hypothermia, hypercoagulability, anemia, shivering, and sleep deprivation. Several studies have reported that postoperative myocardial ischemia begins earlier than has previously been thought, usually on the day of vascular surgery or the next day (Table 22–4).[64–67] At present, our clinical practice is to obtain a 12-lead ECG on the day after surgery in high-risk patients, when the patient has symptoms, and on day 3. We believe that such a strategy will detect most ischemia that is severe and protracted enough to represent a prodrome to infarction.[68] Unfortunately, approximately one fourth of vascular surgery patients will have baseline ECG abnormalities (left bundle branch block, paced rhythm, digoxin effect, left ventricular hypertrophy with strain) that preclude the detection of myocardial ischemia.

Other monitoring devices for detecting myocardial ischemia may be used. Kaplan and Wells[69] concluded that pulmonary capillary wedge pressure (PCWP) could be more sensitive than the ECG in the detection of ischemia. They recommended pulmonary artery catheters to detect papillary muscle dysfunction, mitral regurgitation, and a v-wave on the PCWP tracing; however, subsequent work in patients undergoing vascular surgery has shown that both sensitivity and specificity of PCWP abnormalities for ischemia are relatively low, usually only around 40%.[70,71] Our own group found that 90% of patients developed wall motion abnormalities on TEE when the aorta was cross-clamped above the celiac artery; however, the PCWP remained normal in greater than 80% of these episodes.[72] We therefore do not routinely use PCWP as a monitor for myocardial ischemia but believe the pulmonary artery catheter can provide useful infor-

TABLE **22–4**

Incidence and Prognosis of Postoperative Myocardial Ischemia Detected by Continuous ECG Monitoring*

Reference (year)	No of Patients	Patient Group	Incidence of Postoperative Myocardial Ischemia	Incidence of Complications
Mangano[134] (1990)	474	Veterans; noncardiac surgery; known or suspected coronary artery disease	194/474 (41%)	15/194 (8%) 2 deaths 8 infarctions 1 unstable angina
Ouyang[64] (1989)	24	Vascular surgery; known coronary artery disease	15/24 (62%)	7/15 (47%) 2 infarctions 5 unstable angina
McCann[65] (1989)	50	Lower extremity vascular surgery	19/50 (38%) (overall perioperative ischemia)	4/19 (21%) 2 deaths 2 infarctions
Pasternack[66] (1989)	200	Vascular surgery	57/200 (28%)	11/57 (19%) 2 deaths 9 infarctions
Landesberg[67] (1993)	151	Vascular surgery	88/151 (58%) (overall perioperative ischemia)	8/88 (9%) 6 infarctions 2 unstable angina

*Modified from Ellis JE, Roizen MF, Mantha S, et al: Anesthesia for vascular surgery. In Barash PG (ed): Clinical Anesthesia, 3rd ed. Philadelphia, Lippincott-Raven, 1997, with permission.

mation about a patient's intravascular volume status, myocardial performance, and organ perfusion.

TEE has also been proposed as a monitor for intraoperative myocardial ischemia. In animal studies and in models of coronary angioplasty during balloon inflation, mechanical dysfunction precedes surface ECG changes when myocardial ischemia is produced. Supporting these observation, Smith et al.[73] found that regional wall motion abnormalities were more sensitive than ST-segment change on the ECG in detecting intraoperative ischemia in patients with coronary artery disease undergoing major vascular and coronary surgery. However, Eisenberg et al. concluded that ischemia monitoring with TEE during noncardiac surgery appeared to have little incremental clinical value over preoperative clinical data and Holter monitoring in predicting perioperative ischemic outcome.[74] The benefit of TEE may depend on the skill of the user.

Traditionally, creatine kinase myocardial band (CK-MB) isoenzyme determination has been used to document myocardial damage after vascular surgery. Limitations of this method include false-positive results due to skeletal muscle damage during surgery. The cardiac troponins appear to offer increased sensitivity, primarily because of their prolonged diagnostic window, and may offer enhanced specificity in patients with surgical skeletal muscle damage.[75] In a recent study of 96 vascular surgery patients, all eight patients who received a diagnosis of perioperative infarction (based on new echocardiographic abnormalities in segmental wall motion) had elevations of cardiac troponin I. This study showed that most myocardial infarctions occurred and could be detected on the first postoperative day.[76]

Management of Perioperative Myocardial Ischemia and Infarction in Vascular Patients

In the modern era, rates of myocardial infarction in patients undergoing urgent aortic revascularization can be reduced to less than 10%, but the rates are significantly lower for patients undergoing elective vascular repair. In one series,[77] half of the MIs occurred in patients undergoing urgent or emergent surgery. These patients presumably did not have the luxury of undergoing extensive preoperative evaluation and preparation.

Stable coronary ischemic syndromes presumably occur with increased oxygen demand by the myocardium in a setting of fixed coronary plaques. Unstable syndromes are thought to be the result of active lesions caused by plaque rupture with local thrombus and vasoreactivity that produce intermittent critical decreases in coronary oxygen supply.[44] The period following vascular surgery is characterized by adrenergic stress.[78] The postoperative adrenergic response can predispose to myocardial ischemia in numerous ways, including tachycardia and decreased diastolic time, coronary vasoconstriction, and platelet aggregation.[79] Factors increasing the likelihood of postoperative myocardial ischemia that the anesthesiologist can control include tachycardia, hypertension, hypotension, anemia, hypothermia, shivering, endotracheal suctioning, and less than optimal analgesia. Other factors, such as postoperative hypercoagulability,[80] rapid-eye-movement (REM) sleep rebound, and mild postoperative hypoxemia[81] are more speculative etiologies.

Postoperative myocardial ischemia confers increased risk to vascular surgical patients (Table 22–4). Landesberg et al. found that patients experienced twice as much ischemia after vascular surgery than before or during surgery.[67] Ischemia that lasted longer than 2 hours was associated with a 32-fold increase in the risk of postoperative morbid cardiac events. In this study, postoperative MI was usually preceded by long periods of severe ST-segment depression. Aggressive efforts at prevention or treatment of ischemia during these periods may improve patient outcome. We (Roizen and Ellis) refer patients with documented severe postoperative myocardial ischemia (>2 hours; >2-mm ST-segment depression) emergently to a cardiologist because we consider perioperative PTCA a viable option and because 70% of all adverse cardiac outcomes in a 2-year postoperative follow-up program were preceded by in-hospital postoperative ischemia.[82]

Various strategies have been proposed to reduce cardiac morbidity during and after vascular surgery including the prophylactic use of antianginal drugs, and special anesthetic techniques.[83] We believe it is crucial that patients continue to receive their chronic antianginal and antihypertensive medications before and after surgery. Often, the parenteral route for administration of these medications may be necessary following surgery. Recent reports suggest that chronic administration of the calcium entry blocker nifedipine may increase mortality.[84] We are less likely to use nifedipine as first-line therapy. Prophylactic intravenous (IV) nitroglycerin 0.9 μg/kg/min failed to reduce the incidence of perioperative myocardial ischemia (30% in control group vs. 32% in nitroglycerin group) in patients with known or suspected coronary artery disease undergoing noncardiac surgery.[85] In this study, the preponderance of myocardial ischemia occurred during emergence from anesthesia, which is associated with acute increases in heart rate. β-Adrenergic blocking drugs, through their ability to suppress perioperative tachycardia, appear more efficacious than other anti-ischemic drugs in preventing myocardial ischemia and perhaps infarction after vascular surgery.[66] The β-adrenergic blocking agents, however, may increase vascular resistance, decrease cardiac output, and aggravate bronchospastic conditions and conduction delays.

High-dose sufentanil anesthesia may reduce the stress response and improve overall outcome after abdominal aortic surgery.[4] The postoperative infusion of sufentanil 1 μg/kg/min reduced the severity of myocardial ischemia (ST-segment changes) following CABG, although clinical outcome was not improved.[86] High-dose narcotics may mandate overnight ventilation, which may not be a cost-effective therapy. Another approach using intensive analgesia involves the use of epidural analgesia. Epidural local anesthetics may reduce perioperative myocardial ischemia because preload and afterload are reduced, the postoperative adrenergic and coagulation responses are reduced and, with thoracic administration, the coronary arteries are dilated. Despite these effects on intermediate variables, improvement in cardiac outcomes has not been demonstrated.[87,88] Concerns about respiratory depression, neuroaxis hematomas, and the expense and reimbursement for surveillance have limited the use of peridural narcotics in greater numbers of patients. Although epidural anesthesia may improve outcome in other organ systems,[89] its ability to reduce the rate of myocardial infarction remains speculative.

Given the prominent role of coronary thrombosis in causing coronary syndromes and the hypercoagulable state after aortic reconstruction, future development in the treatment of postoperative myocardial ischemia may include drugs with antiplatelet or anticoagulant effects, such as aspirin, warfarin, heparin, or its analogues or platelet receptor blocking agents. Increased postoperative hemorrhage, however, makes the use of anticoagulant therapy problematic in surgical patients. At present, we do not know how to balance these risks and benefits, or which patients might benefit most from such therapy.

α_2-Adrenergic agonists decrease noradrenergic central nervous system transmission and produce sedation, anxiolysis, and analgesia. Clonidine premedication reduces hypertension, tachycardia, norepinephrine levels, and the incidence of intraoperative myocardial ischemia in patients undergoing vascular reconstruction.[90] However, prophylactic use of the α_2-adrenergic agonists dexmedetomidate in vascular surgery patients may require greater intraoperative pharmacologic intervention to support blood pressure and heart rate.[91] Use of atenolol (50 mg qd) for a week perioperatively in patients with an average age of 70 years who underwent procedures like aortic revascularization prolonged life (made the patient's RealAge younger by 3.7 years).[15,16] Unless contraindicated, already used, or part of a study precluding such use, we (Roizen and Ellis) routinely employ β-blockade with atenolol perioperatively (after gaining surgical consent) in patients undergoing aortic revascularization, even emergent aortic revascularization.

Anemia (hematocrit <28%) may increase the incidence of postoperative myocardial ischemia in high-risk patients undergoing noncardiac surgery.[92] Therefore, we are more likely to transfuse high-risk patients, or those who demonstrate myocardial ischemia, with packed red blood cells to augment the hematocrit to 30%. Hypothermia is also associated with increased adrenergic tone and postoperative myocardial ischemia in vascular surgery patients.[93] We aggressively warm patients and conserve heat during and after such surgery. Suctioning, extubation, and weaning from mechanical ventilation may also produce myocardial ischemia. Therefore, we attempt to extubate patients in the operating room with the same attention to the control of hemodynamics as during induction. If patients require postoperative ventilation, we provide adequate sedation, analgesia, and occasionally even paralysis (which can prevent shivering and its attendant increases in oxygen consumption). We treat tachycardia aggressively, often with β-adrenergic blocking agents, after we have corrected other potential causes such as fever, anemia, and hypovolemia.

Occasionally, in patients with evolving myocardial infarction, using an intra-aortic balloon pump (IABP) to improve coronary blood flow while decreasing workload is indicated. Definitive studies of its effectiveness are lacking, and IABP placement can be difficult and risky in patients with aortic reconstruction.[94] Some patients may be referred to interventional cardiologists immediately after surgery for emergent cardiac catheterization, selective thrombolysis, and PTCA for unstable angina or evolving postoperative myocardial infarction.[95]

Other Medical Problems in Vascular Surgery Patients

Hypertension occurs in the majority of aortic revascularization patients and may produce end-organ damage to the heart and kidneys. The hypertrophied left ventricle is at risk for subendocardial ischemia, even in the absence of obstructive coronary artery disease. Hypertrophied hearts may be more prone to diastolic dysfunction, which can result in "flash" pulmonary edema in the postoperative period. Therefore, antihypertensive medication should be continued in the vast majority of cases through surgery. One often adds β-blockade with atenolol (50 mg qd or bid) to a patient's regimen perioperatively. β-Adrenergic blocking drugs are well tolerated in patients with claudication, despite theoretical concerns about peripheral vasoconstriction and bronchospasm. Calcium channel antagonists are also frequently used, as are ACE inhibitors. The ACE inhibitors may contribute to prerenal azotemia in patients with renal artery stenosis, while diuretics may produce hypokalemia.

One benefit of the modern system of same-day admission is that it allows us to interview many patients in a preanesthesia clinic a week or so before surgery. At that time, if hypertension is poorly controlled, we consult with the patient's internist or cardiologist and adjust or begin the antihypertensive regimen. Lowering blood pressure gradually in this way before surgery allows for restoration of normal intravascular volume and results in a more stable perioperative course.

Diabetic patients have a greatly increased risk for peripheral vascular disease. Aggressive treatment (home glucose monitoring program) to maintain euglycemia has recently been shown to promote wound healing, reduce renal failure, delay amputations and development of CHF, and to forestall retinopathy and the development of proteinuria.[96] Treatment prolongs functional life (makes the diabetic patient's RealAge 6 years younger after just 11 years of tight control). Coronary disease is ubiquitous in diabetic patients requiring vascular surgery.[48] Diabetic patients generally have higher risks of myocardial infarction (5.2% vs. 2.1%) and wound infection (2.6% vs. 0.6%) compared with nondiabetics undergoing abdominal aortic aneurysm.[97] The dramatic increase in the risk of postoperative death (7%) in diabetic patients with autonomic neuropathy suggests that simple tests to identify such patients might be part of the preoperative work-up.[98] Patients with diabetes and severe coronary artery disease may live longer if they undergo CABG rather than PTCA.[99] We (Roizen and Ellis) typically give our diabetic patients one third to one half of their usual insulin dose on the morning of surgery, begin an IV infusion of glucose-containing fluid, and check a "finger-stick" glucometer reading before commencing with an anesthetic. We attempt to maintain intraoperative euglycemia by frequently monitoring and guiding plasma glucose levels. We are especially concerned about glucose management during carotid and thoracic aortic procedures, where hyperglycemia may exacerbate neurologic injury.

Patients with vascular disease may have hypercoagulable states.[100] Hypercoagulable states are more common in younger patients presenting for vascular surgery and in those patients with vascular thrombosis in unusual locations. Hypercoagulable responses to surgery may also predispose patients to vascular graft occlusion after surgery. Postoperative abnormalities include elevated fibrinogen levels, antithrombin III deficiency, impaired fibrinolysis, protein C deficiency, and protein S deficiency.[101] Heparin-induced intravascular thrombosis can occur paradoxically on an immunologic basis (IgG) after several days of exposure to heparin. This problem, which can be fatal, appears to be increasing in incidence, particularly in patients who have had previous vascular surgery and heparin exposure.[102] Patients typically present with thrombocytopenia, a normal prothrombin time, and normal fibrinogen levels. We have seen patients with acute limb ischemia 1 to 2 weeks after cardiac or vascular surgery in whom this disorder was subsequently diagnosed. At present, these patients are usually managed with avoidance of all heparin (including in the flush solution for invasive catheters). Dextran 40 and Coumadin are frequently used in place of heparin; Coumadin may increase the risks of regional anesthesia.

Patients with aortic disease have frequently abused tobacco. Preoperative spirometry may help identify patients likely to have postoperative pulmonary complications. In one study of vascular surgery patients, the incidence of postoperative pulmonary complications (pneumonia, ventilator dependence >48 hours, or the adult respiratory distress syndrome) was 12.9%. Patients with forced expiratory volume in 1 second (FEV_1) less than 2.0 1/sec had a much higher incidence of pulmonary complications (22.5% vs. 5.8% for FEV_1 >2.0 1/sec). Respiratory failure is much more common in patients undergoing repair of aortic aneurysm (~30%) than surgery for lower extremity occlusive disease (8%) or for carotid procedures (5%).[103]

Renal insufficiency or failure exists in many patients who present for arterial reconstruction. Patients with preexisting renal insufficiency have an increased risk of postoperative renal failure, which markedly increases the chance of death.[26,27] If patients receive chronic dialysis treatments, we prefer that they receive dialysis on the day before or the same day as surgery. Some patients will actually be hypovolemic as a result, which can contribute to hypotension upon induction of general or regional anesthesia. Many dialysis patients receive recombinant erythropoition, which normally increases the hematocrit to approximately 30%. Left ventricular hypertrophy and mitral annular calcification are more common in dialysis patients and may predispose to pulmonary edema in the perioperative period; electrocardiography and echocardiography may help the clinician to make these diagnoses. In addition, we usually seek laboratory and electrocardiographic evidence of hyperkalemia and avoid succinylcholine when possible if we suspect hyperkalemia. We are careful when positioning patients to avoid putting pressure on the arm used for hemodialysis; we also do not measure blood pressure in that arm. Vascular access may be difficult in patients who have had multiple arteriovenous fistulae placed for hemodialysis. We also anticipate a more difficult abdominal dissection in some patients who have received peritoneal dialysis.

Aortic Reconstruction

Aneurysmal Disease

Aneurysms pose an ever-present threat to life because of their unpredictable tendency to rupture or to embolize debris. Mortality from rupture may be as high as 85% and even patients who receive emergent surgery have mortality rates one half of that. Therefore, early recognition and aggressive surgical management are warranted, even in the absence of symptoms. Thoracoabdominal aneurysms occur in patients with hypertension or other risk factors for atherosclerotic disease. Abdominal aortic aneurysms are not uncommon in elderly patients. For example, in a study of male patients 65 to 80 years of age undergoing ultrasound scan of the urinary tract, the prevalence of coincidental abdominal aortic aneurysm was nearly 10%.[104]

The size of the aneurysm is the most important predictor of subsequent rupture and mortality. A prospective study followed 300 consecutive patients (mean age, 70 years; 70% men) who presented with abdominal aortic aneurysm (average size, 4.1 cm) and were initially managed nonoperatively. The diameter of the aneurysm increased by a median of 0.3 cm/year. The 6-year cumulative incidence of rupture was 1% among patients with aneurysms smaller than 4.0 cm and 2% for aneurysms 4.0 to 4.9 cm in diameter. By comparison, the 6-year cumulative incidence of rupture was 20% among patients with aneurysms larger than 5.0 cm in diameter.[105] Another study showed that larger aneurysms expand even more rapidly.[106] Patients with aneurysms of the abdominal aorta who do not undergo operation have an 80% 5-year mortality, predominantly secondary to rupture.

Should these patients undergo surgery for asymptomatic aneurysms? This question was addressed by Szilagyi et al.[1] in 1966 when they reported that for aneurysms larger than 6 cm in diameter, surgery approximately doubled a patient's life expectancy. Since then, perioperative mortality has declined from 18 to 25% in the mid-1960s, to 8 to 12% in the early 1970s, to 2 to 4% in the 1990s. Thus outcome after aortic reconstructive surgery has improved dramatically over the past four decades (Table 22–1). Crawford et al.[3] attributed most of the reduction in morbidity in patients who had infrarenal resections before 1971 to improvement in operative techniques and, after 1981, to improvements in anesthesia, monitoring, and supportive care. However, perioperative mortality from supraceliac aneurysms still exceeds 4%. Most morbidity is myocardial in origin, and most myocardial morbidity occurs postoperatively.[30] Mortality in patients undergoing repair of small abdominal aortic aneurysm is less than the mortality for patients having larger aneurysms resected (2.6% vs. 5.5%).[107] Consequently, even patients with abdominal aortic aneurysms less than 6 cm in diameter are considered candidates for aortic reconstructive surgery. This change has resulted from three factors: (1) the lower current morbidity associated with elective repair, (2) the persistently higher mortality (45 to 90%) associated with emergency aortic reconstruction, and (3) the unpredictability of aneurysm enlargement and rupture.

Although patients undergoing surgery for aneurysmal disease have higher perioperative morbidity and mortality (by a factor of 2) and a lower median survival time even in older studies (5.8 vs. 10.7 years) than do patients undergoing aortic reconstruction for occlusive disease, successful surgical repair of an abdominal aortic aneurysm is associated with prolonged life expectancy or reduced RealAge (the Real Age is 6.1 years younger in recent average operative results).[15] Still, life expectancy after successful abdominal aortic aneurysm repair is diminished (62% vs. 85% expected at 5 years). This suggests that in addition to resection of small aneurysms, attention to coronary artery disease, which is the cause of most of the late deaths, is probably required to prolong life in these patients. Strategies, including consideration of perioperative β-blockade or preoperative PTCA or CABG, can prolong functional life or reduce physiologic aging by an additional 4.1 years.[15,16]

Occlusive Disease

The pathologic conditions that give rise to chronic visceral ischemia include atherosclerotic occlusive disease, fibromuscular dysplasia, inflammatory arteriopathies, external compression, and aneurysmal atherosclerotic disease. Chronic ischemia in atherosclerotic arteries or acute occlusive disease occurs more commonly in the elderly, who often are hypertensive, and in persons who have abused tobacco. In most cases, symptomatic disease of the mesenteric artery is due to atherosclerotic narrowing of the origins of the three major visceral vessels: the celiac, superior mesenteric, and inferior mesenteric arteries. The extensive collateral network of the gut is usually sufficient to maintain an adequate intestinal blood supply if only one of these vessels is occluded. However, single-vessel lesions may be important when previous intra-abdominal surgery has interrupted collateral pathways. When there is occlusive disease in the celiac and superior mesenteric arteries, the major mesenteric supply often comes from the inferior mesenteric artery via the marginal artery. If the inferior mesenteric artery (L1–L5) is not revascularized during infrarenal aortic grafting, the risk of bowel ischemia is present, with a reported incidence of colonic infarction after aortic operations of 1 to 2% and that of small bowel infarction of 0.15%, and with a mortality of up to 90% after the occurrence of such infarction that accounts for 10% of deaths postoperatively.[108]

Acute mesenteric occlusion can be of either embolic or thrombotic origin. Embolic occlusions commonly have a cardiac source and may follow a recent myocardial infarction. Thrombotic occlusions may occasionally be due to aortic dissection or trauma but are usually the result of progressing atherosclerosis. Sudden occlusion of the superior mesenteric artery without the previous development of collateral vessels can lead to bowel infarction within a few hours. The diagnosis can be strongly suspected in patients with cardiac disease who suddenly develop severe central abdominal pain, with minimal physical signs. If surgical intervention occurs in the first 4 to 6 hours before gangrene of the bowel develops, revascularization will reduce the otherwise high morbidity and mortality.

Occlusive disease of the abdominal aorta tends to be progressive, with compromise of the distal circulation leading to disabling claudication or limb-threatening ischemia. In the case of aortoiliac occlusive disease, surgical intervention is indicated only for the relief of disabling symptoms. Compared with abdominal aortic aneurysm surgery, the age of patients undergoing aortoiliac reconstruction is approximately 10 years younger, the surgical mortality is lower, and life expectancy after surgery is higher.

In correcting occlusive disease of the aortoiliac segment, the surgeon endeavors to return to near normal the inflow to the limbs at the groin while maintaining flow to the internal iliac and visceral branches. Patients who have critical limb ischemia and stenotic aortoiliac disease also commonly have occlusive lesions of the femoral, popliteal, or tibial vessels. While the prevalence of distal femoral-popliteal occlusive disease in patients undergoing repair of an abdominal aortic aneurysm is only about 11%, the prevalence is almost 50% in patients presenting for occlusive aortoiliac procedures.[109] The long-term patency of the aortobifemoral bypass depends on adequate "run-off"; that is, the status of distal occlusive disease in the femoral segment. The need for subsequent femoral-popliteal bypass can be reduced greatly if the profunda femoris artery is opened by profundoplasty performed concomitantly with the aortobifemoral bypass. This may prolong surgery but is beneficial to the patient. Despite profundoplasty, some patients will still require subsequent distal revascularization.

Pathophysiology of Aortic Occlusion and Reperfusion

Occlusion of the aorta, particularly at the supraceliac level, has consequences for many organ systems, including the cardiovascular system and visceral organs to which blood flow may be impaired. Supraceliac aortic occlusion carries higher risk for patients,[110] particularly when concomitant renal or visceral revascularization is required. Visceral organ ischemia is usually responsible for mortality rates that can approach 25%, although institutions where these procedures are performed routinely have reported substantially lower mortality rates.

Prolonged cross-clamp times are associated with increased risks of visceral ischemia. Complications include renal failure, mesenteric/colonic ischemia, hepatic ischemia with coagulopathy, and spinal cord ischemia.

Arterial hypertension routinely occurs after aortic occlusion. The mechanisms of this response have remained controversial. Beyond increased afterload, etiologies proposed include changes in preload, blood volume distribution, myocardial performance, and activation of the sympathetic nervous system. The pathophysiology of aortic clamping and unclamping have been extensively summarized by Gelman.[111]

The level at which the aorta is occluded affects the degree of hemodynamic response. Blood volume shifts from the lower to the upper half of the body during high aortic cross-clamp due to lower splanchnic venous capacitance. This results in increased left ventricular preload. Our (Roizen) work using TEE has demonstrated a 28% increase in left ventricular end-diastolic area with supraceliac aortic occlusion (Table 22–5).[112,113] Most studies concur that cardiac output decreases with supraceliac occlusion, especially in patients with underlying coronary disease, despite compensatory mechanisms that seek to augment contractility in the setting of elevation of preload and afterload. Although elevated systemic arterial pressure may also be helpful by increasing coronary perfusion, increased preload and afterload associated with high thoracic aortic occlusion also increase myocardial oxygen demand and can produce myocardial ischemia. Renin activity increases with suprarenal or infrarenal aortic occlusion and may contribute to hypertension. Epinephrine and norepinephrine levels consistently increase after aortic occlusion. These changes may help the myocardium increase contractility to adapt to elevated afterload and preload, but our work suggests that these responses are associated with postoperative cardiac and renal dysfunction.[4]

Our (Roizen) work with TEE has shown that myocardial dysfunction is routine in patients undergoing supraceliac aortic occlusion. In these patients, mean arterial pressure rises 54%, PCWP rises 38%, and ejection fraction decreases by 38% (Table 22–5). Additionally, 92% of the patients studied had myocardial ischemia, as evidenced by abnormal wall motion and thickening.[112] Abnormal wall motion generally persists despite aggressive nitrate therapy but usually resolves promptly after aortic unclamping. Nitrates can be used to treat increases in preload, but they will not prevent all wall motion abnormalities. Care must be taken so that decreased blood flow distal to supraceliac aortic occlusion does not promote visceral ischemia. This sets up competing goals because a higher blood pressure may be good for vital organ perfusion, but bad for the heart. In general, we (Roizen and Ellis) tolerate arterial pressures up to 200 mm Hg during supraceliac occlusion, unless other means are used to perfuse the lower part of the body or prolong the tolerable period of visceral ischemia.

Hemodynamic and echocardiographic changes are much more modest in patients undergoing infraceliac or infrarenal aortic occlusion (Table 22–5). The neuroendocrine changes are also less severe in patients undergoing infrarenal aortic occlusion compared with supraceliac occlusion. With infrarenal aortic occlusion, blood volume from the infrasplanchnic vasculature may shift to the compliant splanchnic vasculature, producing relatively small changes in cardiac preload. The hemodynamic responses to cross-clamping and unclamping are further attenuated in patients undergoing aortic occlusion for reconstruction of occlusive disease compared with those having aneurysm repair. Patients with occlusive disease likely have developed collateral circulation, which can continue to perfuse the lower body during aortic cross-clamping.

Unclamping of the thoracic aorta can result in severe hypotension. Reactive hyperthermia after reperfusion may be attenuated by aggressive fluid loading just before reperfusion and gradual release of the aortic clamp. Hypotension may also be due to humoral factors. Tissues distal to aortic occlusion become acidotic; however, treatment with bicarbonate does not reliably prevent hypotension upon reperfusion. Treatment with bicarbonate does result in hypercarbia, and ventilation must be increased proportionally.

Humoral factors that may contribute to organ dysfunction after aortic occlusion include acidosis, the renin-angiotensin system, the sympathetic nervous sys-

TABLE 22–5
Effect of Level of Aortic Occlusion on Changes in Cardiovascular Variables*

	% Change in Variable by Level of Aortic Occlusion		
Cardiovascular Variable	Supraceliac	Suprarenal-infraceliac	Infrarenal
Mean arterial blood pressure	54	5†	2†
Pulmonary capillary wedge pressure	38	10†	0†
End-diastolic area	28	2†	9†
End-systolic area	69	10†	11†
Ejection fraction	−38	−10†	−3†
Abnormal motion of wall (% of patients)	92	33	0
New myocardial infarctions (% of patients)	8	0	0

*From Ellis JE, Roizen MF, Mantha S, et al: Anesthesia for vascular surgery. In Barash PG (ed): Clinical Anesthesia, 3rd ed. Philadelphia, Lippincott-Raven, 1997, as adapted from Roizen MF, Ellis JE, Foss JF, et al: Intraoperative management of the patient requiring supraceliac aortic occlusion. In Veith FJ, Hobson RW, Williams RA, SE W (eds): Vascular Surgery, 2nd ed. New York, McGraw-Hill, 1994, with permission.

†Statistically different ($p<.05$) from group undergoing supraceliac aortic occlusion.

tem, oxygen free radicals, prostaglandins, platelet and neutrophil sequestration, complement activation, and cytokine release. Tissue hypoxia leads to metabolism of adenosine triphosphate (ATP) producing adenosine, hypoxanthine, xanthine oxidase, and oxygen free radicals. Some investigators recommend the use of mannitol before aortic clamping and unclamping because mannitol functions as a hydroxyl free radical scavenger and may prevent tissue injury. Mannitol decreases the production of thromboxane after aortic unclamping, possibly decreasing leukocyte deposition in the lung after aortic surgery.[113] Prostaglandins are increased with aortic occlusion, but studies are hampered by confounding factors, such as prostacyclin release, which can result from mesenteric traction. The response to mesenteric traction can cause profound vasodilation and facial flushing, which can be treated with α-agonists or pretreated with aspirin or nonsteroidal anti-inflammatory drugs (NSAIDs).[114] Nonsteroidals are cyclo-oxygenase inhibitors and therefore reduce the production of prostacyclin. A metabolite of prostacyclin is 6-keto-PGF_1-α which produces vasodilation. Other cyclo-oxygenase inhibitors such as aspirin may produce similar effects. We ask our surgeons to release mesenteric traction while we restore intravascular volume and provide pharmacologic support of afterload; we generally prefer not to use NSAIDs because of their effects on platelet function. C3a and C5a increase during abdominal aortic aneurysm surgery and can produce smooth muscle contraction and pulmonary hypertension, but patients often receive aspirin preoperatively in doses great enough to obtund this reflex. Hypoxic insult to the intestines during aortic occlusion and increased gut permeability can produce endotoxemia during aortic reconstruction. Sludging in tissues distal to aortic occlusion may produce microaggregates, which can exacerbate pulmonary and other tissue injury.

Spinal cord ischemia occurs in 1 to 11% of operations involving repair of the distal descending thoracic aorta. An understanding of the spinal cord blood supply explains this serious complication.[115] The two posterior arteries, which together supply only 25% of the blood to the cord, are formed from the anastomoses of the posterior branch of the vertebral artery and the ascending branch of the bifurcation of the second posterior radicular artery. The anterior spinal artery, which supplies blood to the anterolateral 75% of the cord, is formed throughout by a series of radicular arteries. The midthoracic region, supplied by the anterior spinal artery, usually receives only one afferent vessel, which arises from a left or right intercostal vessel. The afferent arteries to the posterior spinal cord from T2 to T8 have poor collateralization. The blood supply to the thoracolumbar cord (from T8 to the conus terminalis) is derived from the radicular artery, known as the artery of Adamkiewicz. It arises from the left side in 60% of cases. In 75% of cases it joins the anterior spinal artery between T8 and T12, and in 10% of cases it joins between L1 and L2. Although other radicular arteries supply this third section of the cord, much of the blood flow in the anterior spinal artery is dependent on the artery of Adamkiewicz.[116] Because flow in the spinal arteries is dependent on collateralization and is often bidirectional, the blood supply to the spinal cord can be "stolen" and "given" to the rest of the body when "systemic" pressures are lower. Such a situation may arise when a single high aorta-occluding clamp is applied. Spinal cord ischemia is a devastating complication and considerable energy is spent trying to prevent it. To date, the only definitive preventive methods are rapid surgical reconstruction, moderate hypothermia, and maintenance of normal cardiac function.

Infrarenal aortic reconstruction may be associated with a 3% incidence of renal failure, while rates for supraceliac occlusion may be five times as great. With suprarenal occlusion, renal blood flow decreases by greater than 80%. These significant reductions in renal perfusion are not improved by mannitol or dopamine infusion.[117] Even when the aorta is occluded below the renal arteries, renal hypoperfusion may result. In one study, infrarenal aortic cross-clamping decreased renal blood flow by 38%, increased renal vascular resistance by 75%, and redistributed blood flow from the renal cortex. These changes persisted for at least 1 hour after release of the aortic clamp, but early signs of renal tubular damage, such as the appearance of lysozyme in the urine, were never observed.[118] In a study series of patients undergoing thoracoabdominal aneurysm resection, 13% required dialysis; this complication occurred more frequently in patients with preoperative renal dysfunction, a greater extent of aortic replacement, and in those who developed coagulopathy, paraplegia, or paraparesis.[119] We believe that the incidence of renal failure is related to the amount and site of aorta involved and preoperative renal dysfunction.

Patients undergoing thoracoabdominal aneurysm resection have a particularly high incidence of pulmonary complications. Aortic reperfusion may result in pulmonary sequestration of microaggregates and neutrophils that may contribute to postoperative respiratory dysfunction. Pulmonary vascular resistance routinely rises after reperfusion; increased permeability and pulmonary edema are not uncommon. As noted above, mannitol may attenuate these responses.[113]

Surgical Procedures for Aortic Reconstruction

In vascular surgery, understanding the pathophysiology of the disease and anticipating the surgical approach and techniques allow the anesthesiologist to serve the patient most effectively. The surgical goal in these operations is to create an enduring restoration of the normal circulation to the viscera while minimizing the duration of ischemia to viscera, especially to the renal, intestinal, and spinal cord circulations.

Generous exposure of the thoracic and abdominal aorta and its major branches can be obtained with a left thoracoabdominal incision and retroperitoneal dissection. The thoracoabdominal approach is favored for complex thoracoabdominal aortic replacement in the presence of stenotic or aneurysmal disease. The visceral branches are often excised from the parent aorta with a button of aortic wall. If the patient also has mesenteric occlusive disease (approximately one fourth of patients undergoing thoracoabdominal aortic aneurysm surgery), endarterectomy of these branch vessels can be performed before attachment to small openings cut in the graft at appropriate positions. If only mesenteric revascularization is to be performed and aortic replacement is not employed, endarterectomy of any or all the major branches of the aorta may be performed with this exposure.

Elective surgery for asymptomatic mesenteric occlusive disease is generally not justified because the risks of surgery often outweigh the possible gains. Perioperative mortality ranges from 7.5% to 18%. Cardiac disorders, postoperative hemorrhage, and early graft occlusion with bowel infarction are the major causes of perioperative death. Surgery is indicated for symptomatic patients and for a small group of asymptomatic patients with proven major occlusive disease of mesenteric vessels who are to undergo a concomitant intra-abdominal procedure that is likely to interrupt collateral pathways. Such procedures include aortic reconstruction for occlusive or aneurysmal disease and colonic, small bowel, or gastric resections. Surgery may be performed for acute or chronic visceral ischemia. Better long-term results for chronic visceral ischemia may be obtained in elective procedures by performing as complete a revascularization as possible.[120] If single-vessel endarterectomy is performed, it may be carried out for either the celiac axis or the superior mesenteric artery. To overcome the problem of kinking from the infrarenal location, surgeons have used externally supported Gore-Tex grafts. A transabdominal approach is satisfactory for most procedures, including supraceliac grafting. A left thoracoretroperitoneal approach as used for thoracoabdominal aneurysms may be advantageous for transaortic endarterectomy of the celiac axis and the superior mesenteric artery.

Reconstruction of the infrarenal aorta is performed either to replace a segment in the presence of aneurysmal degenerative disease or to increase inflow to and outflow from a vessel with stenosing occlusive disease. Although the natural history of the two diseases is different, the segmental nature of the disease processes, with relatively normal vessels above and below the lesion, provides the basis for reconstruction in each. Recommended preoperative evaluations of the patient's anatomy include palpation alone, ultrasonography, computed tomography, digital subtraction angiography, aortography, and magnetic resonance imaging. Aortography exposes the patient to risks and increases costs but allows determination of the presence of iliac occlusive or aneurysmal disease, renal artery aneurysmal or occlusive disease, and visceral artery lesions in addition to identification of the critical arteries with respect to the aortic lesion.

The most popular surgical exposure for either occlusive or aneurysmal abdominal aortic disease is through a vertical anterior midline abdominal incision, with a transperitoneal approach to the retroperitoneal structures. Another approach is a retroperitoneal one anterior to the kidney. In a randomized, prospective trial that compared the transabdominal with the retroperitoneal approach to the aorta for routine infrarenal aortic reconstruction, there was no difference in pulmonary complications. The retroperitoneal approach was associated with less ileus and small bowel obstruction, shorter stays in the hospital and ICU, and lower hospital costs. It was accompanied, however, by an increase in long-term incisional pain.[121]

After the relevant portions of the aorta and the iliac arteries are exposed, the aneurysmal segment of the aorta is replaced with a graft. Before aortic occlusion, heparin is commonly administered systemically to reduce thromboembolic complications. Distal ischemia complicating aortic surgery is not generally due to thrombosis, but rather to dislodgment of atheroemboli from the diseased aorta. The recognition of the embolic nature of distal ischemic problems prompted Starr et al.[122] to perform aneurysm resections without administration of heparin. Thus, in the absence of major distal occlusive disease, systemic heparinization may be unnecessary in the repair of abdominal aortic aneurysms.

A tube graft (i.e., end-to end anastomoses on both sides) in which the graft is covered with old aorta is often used for aneurysmal resection. When the iliac vessels are not aneurysmal or stenotic, a tube graft may be used as replacement for the diseased aorta, thus making the procedure faster with less blood loss. The standard graft material, in use since the late 1950s, has been Dacron, in either knitted or woven form. Dacron grafts appear to be associated with rare episodes of anaphylactic reactions, which may be related to the stabilizers used in their manufacture.[123] More recently, polytetrafluoroethylene grafts, which are less porous, have become available.

Arterial reconstruction surgery has been developed on the basis of the principle of anatomic correctness. Although this is usually the easiest and best option, situations do occur that require less advantageous revascularization procedures. Such situations include repeat surgery, surgery for graft infection, the presence of contraindications to transabdominal surgery (e.g., sepsis, adhesions, radiation therapy, malignancy), as well as less traumatic alternatives in frail, elderly, high-risk patients. In general, the price paid when alternative techniques such as axillofemoral bypass are used is reduced long-term patency (~50% at 3 years).[124] Temporary axillofemoral bypass may also be performed to decompress the upper half of the body during surgery requiring thoracic aortic occlusion. Another option for reconstruction in the presence of unilateral iliac occlusive disease is femorofemoral bypass, either alone or in combination with axillo-unifemoral or aorto-unifemoral bypass. These procedures have lower long-term patency rates than anatomically correct revascularization. Newer endovascular and laparoscopic techniques have been tried to replace or strengthen existing aneurysmal aortic dilatations or to reconstruct atherosclerotic aortas. These techniques do not have a proven long-term benefit yet, and the quality of perioperative care has increased so that the serious complication rate is less than 10% for most patients who undergo elective infrarenal aortic reconstruction. Emergency procedures for failed endovascular or laparoscopic aortic procedures or subsequent complications may well have a much greater risk.

Several situations may cause the surgeon to change from an infrarenal procedure, which is less risky to the heart and other organs, to a suprarenal procedure. Aneurysms of the abdominal aorta involve the pararenal aorta in up to 20% of cases. Also, significant stenosis of the renal artery may coexist and require repair. Significant stenosis of the celiac trunk or superior mesenteric artery may be repaired at the time of abdominal aortic reconstruction. The patient who has previously undergone aortic surgery, para-aortic lymph node dissection, or radiotherapy will frequently require anastomosis to a higher graft origin. Ruptured aneurysms often must be controlled initially by supraceliac clamping. In these cases, great care must be taken so that material is not dislodged into the renal arteries during manipulation and clamping.

Protecting the Spinal Cord and Visceral Organs

Thoracic aortic occlusion reduces distal blood flow tremendously. In 1 to 11% of operations involving repair of the distal descending thoracic aorta, spinal cord ischemia does occur. The incidence of paraplegia depends on factors such as pre-existing aortic disease, level of aortic cross-clamping, duration of clamping, central spinal fluid pressure, collateral circulation, and prophylactic measures instituted. The reported incidence of spinal cord injury associated with major vascular surgery varies from 24% following acute rupture of the abdominal aorta to 0.19% following repair of nonruptured abdominal aneurysms.[125,126] The incidence of paraplegia is also related to the site of the aneurysm. Crawford et al. reported an incidence of paraplegia of 12%, 26%, 3%, and 3%, respectively, if the aneurysm was thoracic descending, total descending, lower thoracic plus abdominal, or only abdominal.[127] Duration of aortic cross-clamping influences the incidence of paraplegia. Warm ischemic time of the spinal cord has been reported to be approximately 20 to 30 minutes[125,128] (Fig. 22–1).

A number of prophylactic measures have been employed in an attempt to decrease the incidence of spinal cord injury. Drainage of cerebral spinal fluid (CSF) was proposed by McCullough et al. in 1988 as a measure to increase spinal cord perfusion pressure (SCPP).[129] Both Svensson et al. and Grum have reported that combining CSF drainage with the intrathecal administration of papaverine may provide a degree of spinal cord protection.[130–132] Cerebral spinal fluid is withdrawn to maintain CSF pressure between 5 and 15 mm Hg. Svensson recommended an upper limit of 50 ml of CSF drainage in total. Because 3 ml of 1% papaverine injected at room temperature produced hypotension, warming the papaverine to 37°C was recommended.[133] Papaverine is a smooth muscle relaxant, blocks calcium entry into the cell, and is reported to be an indirect oxygen free radical scavenger. Crawford et al. reported that CSF drainage is not effective as a sole therapy.[127] CSF drainage may be offset in part by an increase in venous pressure. Spinal cord perfusion pressure may increase with increased CSF pressure via autoregulation, and CSF pressure may not be uniform intrathecally.

The use of a calcium channel blocker may produce a degree of spinal cord protection in dogs.[135] Ischemic preconditioning of the spinal cord has been reported to offer some degree of protection in both the dog and rabbit models.[136,137] In a dog model, the use of corticosteroids may lessen the risk of spinal cord injury following aortic cross-clamping.[138] If initiated within 8 hours of injury, 30 mg/kg of methylprednisolone followed by 5.4 mg/kg/hr for 24 hours has been reported to improve neurologic outcome after cord injury in humans.[139,140] In the Third National Acute Spinal Cord Injury Trial involving 499 patients, 24 hours of methylprednisolone therapy was indicated when initiated within 3 hours of injury, whereas 48 hours of therapy was indicated when initiated 3 to 8 hours after cord injury. Treatment with tirilazad for 48 hours was as effective as therapy with methylprednisolone.[141]

Glutamate is an excitatory neurotransmitter and cerebral ischemia increases glutamate release. Glutamate activates the *N*-methyl-D-aspartate (NMDA) channel. The

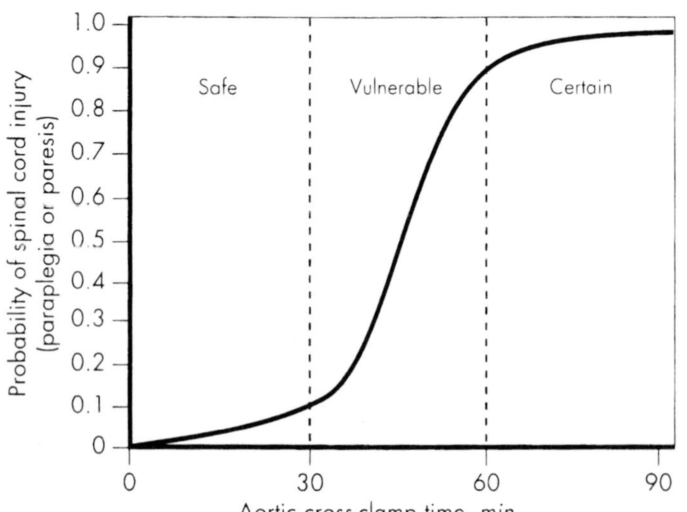

FIGURE 22–1. Risk of paraplegia or paresis in relation to aortic cross-clamp time. Although there is no absolute safe period of aortic cross-clamp time, the risk of paraplegia or paresis increases logarithmically at approximately 30 minutes and cord damage is almost certain at 60 minutes. (From Youngberg JA: Vascular surgery. In Muravchick S (ed): Atlas of Anesthesia, vol 5: Subspecialty Care, New York, Churchill Livingstone, 1998, with permission, as adapted from Svensson and Loop[128].)

NMDA channel allows calcium influx.[142] Magnesium has been reported to have some effect at blocking the NMDA channel.[143] Low magnesium levels can be associated with dysrhythmias, hypertension, coronary artery spasm, apathy, depression, muscle spasms, and stroke.[143] Magnesium has been reported to offer some degree of protection against central nervous system (CNS) injury.[144,145] Rabbits cooled to 3°C and given 5 mmol/kg of magnesium experienced a threefold increase in ischemic time when compared to control animals.[144] Magnesium activates alkaline phosphates and pyrophosphates and affects calcium uptake, adenyl cyclase generation of cyclic adenosine monophosphate (AMP), and membrane sodium-potassium ATP-ase in addition to producing vasodilation and the familiar curariform activity at the neuromuscular junction. Magnesium sulfate can be given intravenously at a rate of 40 mmol (10 gm) in 24 hours followed by 24 mmol/day for 2 to 5 days for slow replacement, or on an emergent basis as 8 mmol (2 gm) in 10 to 20 ml of D_5W over 10 to 20 minutes followed by 20 mmol (5 gm) in 500 ml D_5W over 3 to 12 hours.[146] The excellent review article on this topic by Mark Gomez is recommended.[143]

Iced saline has been administered into the epidural space to provide a degree of cord protection.[147] In a series of 70 patients who received iced saline (4°C) into the epidural space, the volume infused was 1442 ± 718 ml and the CSF temperature was lowered to 24 ± 3°C. CSF pressure increased from 13 ± 8 mm Hg to 31 ± 6 mm Hg during aortic cross-clamping. Mean arterial pressure was maintained 30 to 40 mm Hg above CSF pressure. Neurologic deficit rate was 2.9% compared to an historic control of 23%.[148]

Some investigators have recommended the use of CSF drainage combined with distal aortic perfusion (DAP) in an effort to decrease cord injury. When CSF drainage was combined with DAP in patients undergoing thoracoabdominal aortic aneurysm repair, incidence of neurologic sequelae in type II aneurysm patients was significantly lower than in controls who received neither therapy.[149] Statistical significance was not achieved in type I aneurysms.

Some surgeons place a Gott shunt, a heparinized tube that can decompress the heart and also provide distal perfusion.[150] The Gott shunt can be placed proximally into the ascending aorta (the most common site), the aortic arch, the descending aorta, or the left ventricle, and inserted distally into the descending aorta (most commonly), the femoral artery, or the abdominal aorta. In one study flows to the lower half of the body via the shunt average 1,100 ml/min, and distal pressure during shunting averaged 64.5 mm Hg.[151] Even with a Gott shunt or partial bypass, there is an obligatory time of visceral ischemia when the visceral blood supply arises from a point between the proximal and distal clamps. Placement of a shunt may result in atheroembolism, which can produce rather than prevent ischemic injury and death. Other surgeons may place a temporary ex vivo right axillofemoral bypass graft before positioning for thoracotomy. After the thoracic aortic surgery is completed, the axillofemoral graft is removed. The placement of a shunt or distal perfusion attenuates the hemodynamic response to aortic unclamping, reduces acidosis,[152] and could conceivably ameliorate the hormonal and metabolic changes that accompany aortic occlusion.

Other groups have chosen to use partial bypass, either from the left atrium or ascending aorta, to the iliac or femoral artery to provide distal perfusion and decompress the heart. A heat exchanger may be used to induce hypothermia, which may be neuroprotective. Segmental sequential surgical repair may minimize the duration of ischemia to any given vascular bed.[153] Intercostal artery reattachment in hopes of preserving blood flow to the anterior spinal cord may also be beneficial. After reperfusion, the heat exchanger can be used to warm the patient. Other potential advantages of left atrial–left femoral artery shunt with centrifuge pump support are better operative field exposure, afterload reduction, avoidance of clamp injury, and maintenance of stable distal aortic perfusion without heparin.[154]

Using rapid autotransfusion, some surgeons repair aneurysms of the descending thoracic and thoracoabdominal aorta by using an "open" technique, in which a single cross-clamp is placed proximal to the aneurysm to exsanguinate the lower body.[155] A relatively low incidence of spinal cord injury (8.5%) and renal insufficiency (5.6% dialysis) using this technique may result from the free draining of the intercostal and lumbar arteries during aortic occlusion, which decreases CSF and central venous pressures and increases spinal cord perfusion gradients. A markedly reduced incidence of neurologic deficits has been reported when distal aortic perfusion is combined with drainage of cerebrospinal fluid.[156] SCPP is equated to the distal mean arterial pressure (MAP) minus the CSF pressure such that SCPP = MAP − CSF pressure. Cerebrospinal fluid drainage is used with the aim of improving the pressure gradient, allowing spinal cord blood flow as aortic occlusion lowers distal arterial pressures and increases the central venous pressure. As in almost all other successful series, patients with short aortic occlusion times (<30 minutes) had fewer neurologic deficits.

The development of acute renal failure after aortic reconstruction is associated with a high morbidity and mortality of greater than 30%. This complication is most frequent in patients with ruptured aneurysms who have significant hypotensive episodes and in those for whom suprarenal aortic clamping is required. Approximately one fourth of patients undergoing thoracoabdominal aortic aneurysm repair have occlusive visceral disease, which may also be corrected to reduce the risk of renal failure without increasing the risk of gastrointestinal complications.[114] As in the preservation of other organ function, we believe that maintenance of cardiac function represents the best prophylaxis against renal failure.

In the late 1990s, renal insufficiency remains a predictor of morbidity and mortality after aortic reconstruction procedures, and acute renal failure after surgery continues to have an approximately 50% mortality associated with it, little difference from 30 years ago. But improvements in outcome may soon be reported in the literature.

In a study from Leicester in Great Britain, reporting 13 years of surgical experience with aortic revascularization in 671 patients, 13% developed renal failure after AAA, but 41% of all patients in the series had emergency repair for rupture. In the elective patients, cardiac and renal failure preoperatively were associated with death; in the emergency patients, pulmonary and renal failure were associated with death.[157] In Madison, Wisconsin, renal failure occurred in 10.3% of patients who had renal revascularization, with preoperative elevations in creatinine as the only prognostic finding.[158] At the University of Pittsburgh, preoperative renal insufficiency as well as postoperative renal failure predicted increased length of stay and charges, whereas age, gender, and coronary artery disease did not.[159] The Veterans Administration database confirms this result in 8,702 patients operated upon for aortic revascularization between 1991 and 1994.[160] Acute renal failure increased the odds ratio for death to 9.58, higher than that for pneumonia, pulmonary failure, stroke, or MI by more than a factor of 2. In Montreal, for 112 patients with ruptured AAAs and a median age of 72.4 years, in-hospital mortality was 49% with worse outcome predicted by low systolic blood pressure or cardiac arrest preoperatively; results from Worcester in 105 patients operated on for ruptured aneurysms between 1982 and 1993 were similar.[161,162] In the cases at Worcester, 31 patients developed acute tubular necrosis (ATN) and 19 of the 105 required dialysis. Placement of a peritoneal dialysis catheter at the time of rupture repair did not affect mortality but seemed to make postoperative care easier.

At the Mayo Clinic in a series of aortic operations between 1970 and 1993,[163] 1,643 patients were revascularized. There was a gradual increase in age of patients undergoing surgery from 63.5 years in the first decade to 68 years in the last 13 years. Creatinine increased preoperatively 15% in the first decade and 31% in the last 13 years with levels between 2 and 2.9 mg/dl. These patients had a 9% rate of dialysis postoperatively compared to a 35% rate for patients with a creatinine greater than 3 mg/dl. Thus, in this series, aortic rupture is associated with about the same 50% mortality rate as it was 15 years ago. Dialysis is associated with about a 50% mortality rate as it was 25 years ago, and preoperative elevation of creatinine still predicts postoperative complications, need for dialysis, and mortality. One study does predict improvement in outcome after need for dialysis (from the Mayo Clinic).[164] In comparing renal failure in the ICU between 1977 and 1979 and 1991 and 1992, there was a hospital survival rate of 32% in the first group versus 52% in the second. The 1-year survival rate was 21% versus 30% in the second group. The report included all patients requiring acute dialysis not just dialysis postoperatively. Also, in the last several years, two new pathologic entities have been associated with renal insufficiency perioperatively. The first concerns cholesterol emboli after endovascular surgery. In one study, 2.9% of patients who had endovascular repair had cholesterol emboli and 13% of those patients developing acute tubular necrosis.[165] Rhabdomyolysis appears to occur in about 10% of patients having aortic revascularization but was not found to be a risk factor for renal failure postoperatively.[166] At Baylor, of 234 patients who had thoracoabdominal aneurysm repair,[167] 17.5% developed acute tubular necrosis as diagnosed by a 1 mg/dl or more increase in creatinine for two consecutive days. Of the total group, 15% required dialysis and 49% of patients with acute renal failure died. In 18 of the 21 survivors after dialysis, renal failure resolved. Preoperative creatinine above 2.8% mg/dl made the odds ratio for dialysis 10.3, similar to the odds ratio in the Mayo Clinic series[163] in which a creatinine above 3 mg/dl preoperatively and aortic aneurysm repair led to a 35% dialysis rate. Inability to do an aortic inflow procedure when it was needed resulted in an axillobifemoral bypass, which led to a uniformly bad 2-year prognosis (death or occluded grafts).[168]

At the Cleveland Clinic, 490 males and 92 females had aortic revascularization between 1983 and 1988, with 29 perioperative deaths. Survival rates correlated with age, preoperative creatine level, and the coronary angiographic classification in that study.[169] None of these studies considered the dialysis membrane and the treatment of patients with acute renal failure. In another setting, Hakim and colleagues reported that using a polymethyl methacrylate membrane resulted in a much better outcome than with the cuprophane dialysis membrane. The polymethyl methacrylate membrane had a more limited effect on complement activation. With the cuprophane dialysis membrane 37% of patients recovered from renal dysfunction, while 62% recovered function with the new membrane.[170]

Previous work from our group (Roizen) has shown that intraoperative urinary output is not predictive of postoperative renal function. In 137 patients undergoing aortic reconstruction (38 at the supraceliac level), we found no significant correlation between intraoperative mean urinary output, or lowest hourly urinary output, and changes from preoperative to postoperative levels of creatinine or blood urea nitrogen.[171] Thus, urinary output, which is believed to be an index of perfusion and is therefore monitored routinely during surgery, was not predictive of postoperative renal function in normovolemic patients. When patients who underwent aortic occlusion at the suprarenal level were compared with those who underwent occlusion at the infrarenal level, there was no difference in postoperative renal function. Rather, *preoperative* renal dysfunction was the most powerful predictor of *postoperative* renal dysfunction.

The use of mannitol, furosemide, or dopamine as an isolated therapeutic intervention, however, has not been clearly shown to prevent renal failure. While not associated with a better outcome in a randomized study, mannitol was associated with less elevation of the intermediate variables indicating renal dysfunction and injury.[172] In the study, 28 patients were randomly assigned to an infusion of mannitol 0.3 gm/kg or saline at an equal volume intraoperatively for infrarenal aortic aneurysm repair. One patient in the control group developed renal failure, and there was greater diuresis in the mannitol group, but urinary albumin and N-acetyl glucosaminidase were lower in mannitol-treated patients. Whether the reductions were caused by the increased diuresis or were the result of decreased renal injury remains to be determined. We believe that preoperative renal function and the maintenance of intravascular volume and normal myocardial function are the most important determinants of postoperative renal function. Recent work in patients with diabetes and chronic renal insufficiency undergoing coronary angiography has demonstrated that maintaining intravascular volume is superior to the use of furosemide.[173] These results may be particularly applicable to vascular surgery patients who frequently undergo angiography shortly before surgery.

If prolonged renal ischemia is anticipated, selective profound hypothermia and the direct intra-arterial infusion of mannitol into the renal arteries may decrease the incidence of postoperative renal impairment. Our management, however, is biased by the results of our own studies. Thus, when intraoperative urinary output is less than 0.125 ml/kg/hr, we (Roizen and Ellis) exclude mechanical problems in urine collection and ensure the adequacy of left-sided cardiac filling volumes or pressures. We then continue to monitor but do not usually treat. Urinary output usually returns to acceptable levels within 2 hours. If it does not, or if we are uneasy about low urinary output, 2 to 5 mg of furosemide or mannitol 0.25 mg/kg is administered intravenously to stimulate urine production. Dopamine at 3 to 5 μg/kg/min may be used, but its prophylactic value has not been proven in patients undergoing aortic surgery, and it is not effective in preventing postoperative renal dysfunction in patients undergoing liver transplantation.[174] Thus, virtually all investigators have concluded that maintenance of adequate intravascular volume and preservation of myocardial function largely prevents renal insufficiency.

Distal aortic perfusion had no effects on prediction or prevention of renal dysfunction postoperatively when compared with simple clamping.[175]

Thus, over the most recent half decade, we have learned that as before, poor renal function and old age preoperatively predicts poor renal function postoperatively, that mannitol may improve outcome, that the technique of distal perfusion versus clamp alone does not affect prognosis, and that there is hope in choice of analgesia and choice of dialysis membrane material in improving renal outcome after abdominal aortic aneurysm repair.

Monitoring and Anesthetic Choices for Aortic Reconstruction

Arterial catheters are considered routine monitors in patients undergoing aortic reconstruction. In patients undergoing thoracic aortic clamping with distal perfusion, we will measure distal arterial pressure as well. Pulmonary artery catheters (PACs) are commonly inserted in patients undergoing suprarenal aortic cross-clamp and selectively used in patients undergoing infrarenal clamp. In some relatively healthy patients, the risk of pulmonary artery catheterization probably exceeds the benefit.[176] However, do we place PACs routinely in patients with a history of CHF, diabetes with end-organ damage, cor pulmonale, renal insufficiency, or poor left ventricular function (ejection fraction <35%) on preoperative or intraoperative echocardiography.

If we elect to drain cerebrospinal fluid, we (Roizen and Ellis) use two regular epidural trays and place catheters into the intrathecal space at L3–4 and L4–5. We use two catheters because one often kinks. We allow cerebrospinal fluid to drain passively, typically removing 50 ml before aortic cross-clamp and another 50 ml during aortic occlusion. Catheters with a one-way pressure valve allow drainage only when the cerebrospinal fluid pressure exceeds 5 to 10 mm Hg. Some clinicians have used larger needles made specifically for lumbar cerebrospinal fluid drainage.[153] These are placed the night before surgery in case a "bloody tap" results, so that clotting may be assured. We generally wait until coagulopathy, which is common after thoracoabdominal repair, has resolved to remove cerebrospinal fluid drains, usually on the first or second postoperative day.

Nitrous oxide can be used with opioids or with the inhalational drugs. However, it increases afterload and myocardial work while depressing myocardial inotropic performance and output. In one study of patients undergoing abdominal aortic surgery, nitrous oxide increased the need for nitroglycerin to treat elevated PCWP and myocardial ischemia, although clinical outcome was not affected.[177] Nitrous oxide may decrease renal and splanchnic blood flows[178] and may have long-lasting toxic effects by causing nutritional, neurologic, and immunologic deficits.

In a prospective, controlled study, patients were randomly assigned to receive either an isoflurane- or sufentanil-based anesthetic for aortic reconstruction. Intraoperatively and postoperatively, systemic and pulmonary capillary blood pressures and heart rates were kept within 20% of mean preoperative (baseline) values. Sufentanil anesthesia alone was associated with less major (cardiac and renal) morbidity than isoflurane anesthesia.[4] Sufentanil may have a protective effect because of its superior blockade of the adrenergic stress response.[179] Further study is needed to determine whether all opioids are protective or whether the combination of sufentanil and isoflurane can produce an outcome equivalent to or better than that achieved with sufentanil alone. A disadvantage of the opioids is that they linger into the postoperative period. However, in more than 50% of the patients who received a high-dose, opioid-nitrous oxide anesthetic technique (sufentanil 15 to 20 μg/kg) for suprarenal aortic reconstruction,[4] tracheal extubation was accomplished in the operating room. High-dose opioid anesthetics also produce excellent postoperative analgesia.

Combined general-epidural and general-spinal anesthetics have been used successfully for aortic reconstruction.[180] For patients requiring thoracotomy, the analgesia provided by thoracic epidural infusion of narcotics and/or local anesthetics may be particularly helpful in improving spirometric function. Thoracic epidural local anesthetics can also dilate coronary arteries[181] and help to prevent stress-induced elevations in PCWP. Some clinicians are reluctant to use epidural anesthesia for supraceliac aortic reconstruction because of concerns about concurrent heparinization and the associated incidence of paraplegia. In such patients, the use of peridural narcotics without local anesthetics can preserve sensory and

TABLE 22–6
Anesthetic Technique and Outcome After Major and/or Vascular Surgery*

Series	Technique	Comment
Yeager et al.[89]	General + epidural vs. general	Fewer complications and lower cost in epidural + general
Haku et al.[191]	General + epidural vs. general	No difference
Shah et al.[189]	Regional vs. general	No difference
Baron et al.[193]	General + epidural vs. general	No difference
Rivers et al.[190]	Epidural vs. general	No difference
Bode et al.[192]	Regional vs. general	No difference

*From Youngberg JA: Vascular surgery. In Muravchick S (ed): Atlas of Anesthesia, Vol. 5: Subspecialty Care. New York, Churchill Livingstone, 1998, with permission.

motor function and can allow early assessment of neurologic integrity. Because urinary catheters are typically left in place for at least 36 hours after aortic reconstruction surgery, urinary retention usually is not a major issue. We often use intrathecal or epidural narcotics after supraceliac aortic occlusion. Animal studies have shown that intrathecal naloxone improves neurologic function after thoracic aortic occlusion, but results in humans have been inconclusive.[182] Another disadvantage of epidural local anesthetics is that although patients must receive increased amounts of IV fluids, they are still likely to become hypotensive after reperfusion.[183] Therefore, we are prepared for the possibility of fluid overload toward the end of the procedure. Alternatively, infusions of dopamine or dobutamine may be used to maintain systemic vascular resistance and contractility in the presence of the sympathectomy induced by the use of local anesthetics for regional block.[184]

We believe that prophylaxis of stress and pain by any mechanism (epidural anesthetics, opiate infusion, or α_2-agonists) may result in lower morbidity in those least able to tolerate the myocardial and cardiovascular demands of stress.

The choices of muscle relaxants for use today are many. We choose an agent based primarily on the hemodynamic goals, the patient's renal function, and on whether or not the patient's trachea will be extubated in the operating room.

As anesthesiologists we must address the issue of regional versus general versus a combined technique in patients undergoing abdominal aortic or peripheral vascular procedures. The stress response is associated with increases in serum level of prolactin, growth hormone, adrenocorticotropic hormone (ACTH), ADH, cortisol, aldosterone, renin, epinephrine, and norepinephrine. Preoperative visits and preparation of the patient are important parts in decreasing patient anxiety and level of stress.[185–187] Pflug and Halter reported that the stress response was partly attenuated with a spinal anesthetic at a high thoracic dermatome level in contrast to a "light" general ansthetic.[188]

Early reports such as that by Yeager et al. in 1987 seemed to indicate that a combined regional and general anesthetic might be superior to a general anesthetic alone.[89] More recent studies, however, have failed to demonstrate a significant outcome difference between regional or a regional plus general anesthetic technique and general anesthesia alone[189–193] (Table 22–6). Some investigators have reported better graft patency and fewer reoperations when employing an epidural anesthetic with or without general anesthesia when compared to general anesthesia alone in patients undergoing pe-

TABLE 22–7
Graft Patency and Regional Anesthesia*,†

Series	Technique	Comment
Bengtson et al.[196]	Epidural anesthesia vs. general anesthesia	Greater increase in with general. Epidural may blunt anaphylatoxin activity
Tuman et al.[195]	General anesthesia + epidural analgesia vs. general anesthesia + PCA	Graft failure 1/40 in general + epidural vs. 7/40 in general + PCA
Rosenfeld et al.[194]	Epidural anesthesia/analgesia vs. general anesthesia + PCA	PAI-1 levels higher in general group. Epidural inhibits fibrinolysis 17% graft failure in general vs. 5% in epidural
Christopherson et al.[87]	Epidural anesthesia + fentanyl epidural analgesia vs. general anesthesia + PCA	Regrafting rate 2 in epidural/epidural group vs. 11 in general/PCA group

*From Youngberg JA: Vascular surgery. In Muravchick S (ed): Atlas of Anesthesia, Vol. 5: Subspecialty Care. New York, Churchill Livingstone, 1998, with permission.
†There is emerging data in the literature that the use of epidural anesthesia and/or analgesia may be associated with a higher vascular graft patency rate.
PCA, patient-controlled (IV) anesthesia, PAI-1, plasminogen activator inhibitor 1.

ripheral vascular surgery[87,194–196] (Table 22–7). In contrast, Pierce et al. reported no difference in graft patency or reoperation rates when comparing regional to general anesthesia.[197] The effects of local anesthetics (especially lidocaine) may play a role in the beneficial results with respect to patency rates reported by some authors. Lidocaine inhibits neutrophil hydrogen peroxide and lysosomal enzyme release, decreases whole blood and plasma viscosity, inhibits leukocyte adherence to endothelial cells, increases prostacyclin release, and attenuates procoagulant response to tumor necrosis factor-α.[198] Sharma and Philip reported that general anesthesia is associated with an accelerated coagulability in patients undergoing cesarean section.[199] Carpenter reported a decreased duration of ileus and increased gastrointestinal blood flow with epidural anesthesia.[200] In the canine model of coronary stenosis, thoracic epidural anesthesia was associated with an improved endocardial/epicardial blood flow ratio.[201,202] Similar results are reported with a T1–T6 level thoracic epidural in patients.[181] A lumbar epidural may not achieve the same beneficial results, however, even when a high thoracic level is achieved.[203,204]

A major potential risk of regional anesthesia is the development of an epidural hematoma leading to cord ischemia. In Rao and El-Etr's series, 847 spinals and 3,164 epidurals were performed without evidence of an epidural hematoma.[205] However, the investigators cancelled surgery for 24 hours if blood was encountered during needle or catheter insertion, moderate doses of heparin were used (2,600 ± 400 units every 6 hours), and the catheters were removed when coagulation studies approached normal values. Baron et al. reported the safety of epidural anesthesia in 912 patients and Odoom et al. reported no hematomas in 1,000 patients.[206,207] In contrast other investigators have reported isolated cases of epidural hematomas[208,209] (Table 22–8). Low-molecular-weight heparin (LMWH) with epidural or spinal anesthesia is potentially somewhat more hazardous. Horlocker et al. reported a significant increase in the incidence of epidural hematomas in patients who received LMWH before or after an epidural and/or placement of an epidural catheter.[210] Spinal hematoma was reported in 30 patients undergoing spinal or epidural anesthesia while receiving LMWH perioperatively between May 1993 and November 1997. As of April 1998 a total of 40 cases have been reported. The residual anticoagulant effects of LMWH are only partially reversed by protamine. The plasma half-life of LMWH is approximately two to four times that of standard heparin. Signs of an epidural hematoma can develop well after catheter removal in patients receiving LMWH. Twenty-four hours or more may elapse between catheter removal and the onset of neurologic dysfunction. The median time between initiation of LMWH and neurologic dysfunction was 3 days.[207] As opposed to the usual sign of radicular back pain the initial complaint was new-onset weakness or numbness. Surgical intervention should be sought within 8 hours of the onset of symptoms.[210] Many anesthesiologists avoid the use of spinal or epidural anesthesia/analgesia in patients who are receiving or will receive LMWH perioperatively. LMWH therapy should not be initiated for 12 to 24 hours after catheter placement if one decides to perform a continuous epidural technique.[210] The catheter should be removed when anticoagulant activity is lowest.

Management of Elective Aortic Surgery

For patients undergoing elective surgery, prehydration is begun at maintenance rates as soon as all oral intake is stopped. We believe that maintenance of a normal hydration status reduces variations in blood pressure on induction of anesthesia. After the patient's preoperative condition has been optimized, the range of hemodynamic variables for that patient is determined. Anesthetic management is then adjusted to keep the patient within 20% of this range. Anticholinergic drugs are usually avoided because they produce dry mouth and tachycardia, which increases myocardial oxygen consumption. The patient should be given antihypertensive medication, including β-blockade, and diuretics before being brought to the operating room. Many diabetic patients who re-

TABLE 22–8
Risk of Peridural Hematoma*,†

Series	Complications/Patients	Comments
Rao and El-Etr[205]	0/4011	Heparin dose: 2,600 ± 400 units q6h remove catheter when coagulation studies normal
Ruff and Dougherty[208]	5/342	Traumatic, on aspirin
Odoom and Sih[207]	0/1000	ACT <200 sec, no hemophilia, leukemia, or thrombocytopenia
Baron et al.[206]	0/912	Heparin dose to activated partial thromboplastin time 2.5 × normal
Dickman et al.[209]	2 cases	Thrombolysis therapy or on long-term heparin

*Modified from Youngberg JA: Vascular surgery. In Muravchick S (ed): Anesthesia Atlas, Vol. 5: Subspecialty Care. New York, Churchill Livingstone, 1998, with permission.

†Although the incidence of peridural hematomas following regional anesthesia in patients who are or will be anticoagulated is relatively small, the potential is real and the patient should be observed for signs and symptoms such as back pain and delayed recovery from a local anesthetic injection. If a peridural hematoma is suspected, the patient should be scheduled for an MRI and evaluated for possible exploration and decompression.

ACT, activated coagulation time.

quire insulin are given an insulin infusion throughout surgery. Preoperative considerations and drug therapy for diabetic patients have already been described earlier in this chapter, and β-blockers (atenolol 50 mg)[16] are usually added after consultation with a surgeon.

For the half hour immediately before cross-clamping and aortic occlusion, the patient is kept slightly hypovolemic by examining the ventricular volume by means of echocardiography or by keeping PCWP at 5 to 15 mm Hg. At the time of occlusion we are prepared to give a vasodilating drug. The difference in our management of aortic occlusion at different levels (e.g., supraceliac vs. infrarenal) is that we rigorously and meticulously plan the management and execute the procedure for all occlusions at renal vessels or above.

Without evidence to the contrary, it is assumed that a little hypertension is just as harmful as a little hypotension. For example, in extreme cases, we might permit the systolic blood pressure of a patient whose preoperative range was 110 to 170 mm Hg to decrease to as low as 90 mm Hg, or to increase to as high as 190 mm Hg. If values approach or exceed these limits, we execute our contingency treatment plan. Hypertension may be treated by increasing the amount of anesthetic, infusing nitroprusside, or tilting the patient head-up. Hypotension may be treated by placing the patient in a head-down position, infusing more fluid, or beginning a dilute infusion of phenylephrine at a rate that restores systolic blood pressure to about 100 mm Hg.

Our accepted range for a patient's heart rate is similarly based on preoperative determinations. If a normal range of 60 to 90 bpm is established preoperatively, we initiate treatment once these limits are exceeded intraoperatively. Bradycardia is better tolerated than tachycardia during these operations, because minimizing myocardial oxygen demand is one of our primary concerns. If the intravascular fluid volume is acceptable, we treat tachycardia aggressively, by increasing the level of anesthesia with more opioid or volatile agent, or with an IV infusion of a β-adrenergic receptor blocking drug. Imaging with TEE allows some latitude in the range of acceptable values before intervention must be undertaken. However, PCWPs are not allowed to remain abnormal (i.e., <5 mm Hg or >15 mm Hg) in the face of normal ventricular compliance during this procedure, assuming that these values correlate with the echocardiographic values. Increases in pulmonary artery pressures are treated aggressively with more anesthetic, nitroglycerin, or nitroprusside. For low filling pressures, more fluid is infused, except in the 1- or 2-minute interval immediately before application of the aortic cross-clamp.

Our approach is different when we are concerned about spinal cord perfusion in patients in whom the aorta will be occluded at the thoracic level without distal perfusion. In these instances, we will accept some proximal hypertension while the aorta is occluded in the hope of obtaining higher distal perfusion pressures and preventing distal ischemia.[111] This choice may come at the expense of myocardial well-being.

The application of a cross-clamp to the supraceliac aorta probably produces the greatest hemodynamic stress ever experienced by a patient. In fact, 92% of the patients whom we (Roizen and Ellis) studied had ischemia, as evidenced by abnormal motion and thickening of the left ventricle (Table 22–5).[112] More distal levels of temporary occlusion are less stressful hemodynamically. Stabilizing pulmonary and systemic arterial pressures by administering vasodilating drugs before and during suprarenal cross-clamping may not be sufficient to normalize myocardial performance. We have used phosphodiesterase inhibitors, which increase contractility and reduce afterload, before application of the aortic cross-clamp, but we still see myocardial dysfunction with supraceliac occlusion.

Another technique for maintaining normal volumes during cross-clamping is controlled volume depletion; that is, the removal of a specific amount of blood from the patient just before or during application of the cross-clamp for a short period of time. During the minutes remaining just before the cross-clamp is removed, this amount of blood is replaced. Although we have used this technique, we do not advocate its routine use. A third technique for maintaining normal hemodynamic values is the use of volatile anesthetics, rather than nitroglycerin or nitroprusside, as the vasodilating agent. This technique is usually effective, but close observation is necessary to ensure that myocardial dilation and dysfunction do not occur. This technique is not recommended for routine use.

Administration of exogenous vasoconstrictors is avoided if possible. In patients undergoing carotid endarterectomy, phenylephrine doubles the incidence of wall motion abnormalities observed by echocardiography compared to patients whose blood pressure is maintained simply by light anesthesia and endogenous vasoconstrictors.[211] Phenylephrine causes the heart to dilate in patients with coronary artery disease, whereas norepinephrine raises blood pressure without causing myocardial contractile depression.[212]

To ensure adequate volume at the time of cross-clamp removal, blood lost during occlusion is replaced with crystalloid or colloid, warmed cell-saver blood, or banked blood to keep the hematocrit slightly above 30%, because it will decrease to 30% in the postocclusion period. We believe that this is the minimal acceptable value for patients in this risk group. Guided by filling pressures or echocardiographic estimates of volume, we are careful not to dilate the left ventricle to an abnormal size.

We routinely use autotransfusion devices and prefer to have a second person (usually a technician) to operate them. Because a large part of the vascular tree is excluded from circulation during temporary aortic occlusion, blood loss can be considerable during supraceliac cross-clamping without the onset of hypotension or tachycardia. Therefore, if we find ourselves decreasing the concentration of volatile anesthetic or the infusion rate of vasodilators, or worse, find ourselves giving vasopressors while the aorta is still occluded, we order more blood and seek to correct what is now severe hypovolemia.

Because maintenance of normal intravascular volume status is so important, observation of the surgical field is of key importance. When any blood vessel is dissected, the anesthesiologist and surgeon must communicate closely; blood loss can occur with astonishing rapidity, when the attention of the anesthesiologist may not be directed to the operative field. Blood loss into the pleural or retroperitoneal cavity may not be readily detected. Watching the volumes in the suction bottles supplements the data, as does observation of left ventricular cavity size on echocardiography. In addition, evisceration of bowel, often necessary for optimal exposure of the thoracoabdominal aorta, further depletes intravascular volume.

Thus, immediately before and during removal of the cross-clamp, we stop infusing vasodilators. We allow blood pressure, PCWP, and filling volumes to go as high as possible without the occurrence of myocardial ischemia. The surgeon then opens the aorta gradually to ensure that severe hypotension does not develop and that there is not too much bleeding from the suture line. Pathophysiologic events on removal of the aortic cross-clamp are associated with inadequate preload. We therefore infuse crystalloid, colloid, or blood; often 2 units of cell-saver blood is pressured into venous access sites just before reperfusion. Guided by filling pressures or echocardiographic estimates of volume, or both, we are careful not to dilate the left ventricle.

Moderate hypotension (i.e., a decrease in systolic pressure of 40 to 60 mm Hg) typically accompanies removal of the aortic cross-clamp, regardless of whether the clamp is replaced so that blood flow to only one leg is obstructed. Our observations of the echocardiogram lead us to believe that hypotension is caused mainly by relative volume depletion. If hypotension persists for more than 4 minutes after removal of the clamp and does not return toward normal after blood deficits have been replaced, we search for other causes, including hidden blood loss or myocardial dysfunction. Myocardial dysfunction may be caused by inadequate metabolism of the citrate present in replacement blood; such blood has not gone to the liver, where citrate is metabolized. This problem can be treated by administration of calcium, which is chelated by citrate. If necessary, the surgeon can reclamp or occlude the aorta, preferable below the renal arteries. Thus, volume replacement and maintenance are mainstays of therapy before, during, and immediately after removal of the aortic cross-clamp. At this point in the procedure, pulmonary artery pressures may not be low because reperfusion of ischemic tissues is associated with the release of lactic acid and other unknown mediators that can cause pulmonary vasoconstriction. Mannitol prophylaxis may prevent part of this response, and we frequently give mannitol 0.5 to 1.0 gm/kg immediately before release of the clamp.[213] Removal of the clamp from the second leg usually causes fewer hemodynamic effects, presumably because of collateral blood flow across the pelvis.

During closure, we again ensure adequate organ perfusion as well as hemodynamic and temperature homeostasis, and we reverse the effects of muscle relaxants. Reversal is easier when patients are warm. Hypothermia after aortic reconstruction is associated with other complications, including coagulopathy, low cardiac output states, and significantly higher incidences of organ dysfunction and deaths.[214] Whether hypothermia causes these problems or is a marker for sicker patients who undergo more extensive operations is unclear. We usually use forced-air warming on the upper portion of the body in these patients, although their lateral position and extensive exposure during thoracic procedures sometimes makes maintaining normothermia difficult.

During emergence from anesthesia, we often use infusions of nitroglycerin and/or esmolol to prevent hemodynamic variations outside the patient's normal range. If ventilation is adequate (as is common 6 hours after the initial dose of sufentanil), the trachea is extubated; otherwise, controlled ventilation is maintained until spontaneous ventilation is judged to be adequate. If we elect to use a predominantly inhalational anesthetic technique, we often place an epidural catheter and administer epidural local anesthetics and opioids for postoperative analgesia. When the sufentanil-based technique described above is used, rarely is much additional pain therapy needed for 24 hours. Continuing care into the postoperative period is important for patient outcome.

Anesthesia for Emergency Aortic Surgery

The most common cause of emergency aortic reconstruction is a leaking or ruptured aortic aneurysm or a failed endoscopic or endovascular procedure. Ruptured aneurysms can be atherosclerotic, mycotic, syphilitic, or inflammatory, or may occur in patients with the marfanoid syndrome. In one Swedish study, ruptured abdominal aortic aneurysms were found in 5.6 of 100,000 persons (8.4 of 100,000 men and 3.0 of 100,000 women). The age-specific incidence was highest (113 of 100,000) in men 81 to 90 years of age and (68 of 100,000) in women older than 90 years. These ruptures are ten times more common in male than in female patients of the same age, whereas aortic aneurysms in general have a 4:1 male-to-female preponderance. Retrospective analysis of data from multiple registries in Sweden reported an incidence of 5 per 100,000 of ruptured thoracic aneurysms. Even though 41% of patients were alive upon arrival at an emergency hospital, the overall mortality rate approaches 100%. Therefore, efforts should be made to increase the number of elective operations performed for aortic aneurysms before they rupture.[215,216]

Symptoms of ruptured abdominal aortic aneurysms include pain, faintness or frank collapse, and vomiting. Pain in the back, abdomen, or both is almost always present. Therefore, many surgeons believe that pain in combination with a known abdominal aortic aneurysm or pulsatile abdominal mass indicates dissection or rupture and the immediate need for surgical exploration until proven otherwise. Ruptures most commonly occur in the retroperitoneum. This site permits tamponade of the hemorrhage; however, retroperitoneal hemorrhage and subsequent hematoma can displace the left renal vein, inferior vena cava, and intestine, possibly leading to damage to these structures during the surgical approach.

Venous hemorrhage is often much more difficult to control than arterial hemorrhage.

Approximately 25% of aneurysms rupture into the peritoneal cavity, a site associated with a great degree of exsanguination. Other sites of rupture include adjacent structures after formation of fistulae with the inferior vena cava, iliac veins, or renal veins. Aortoenteric fistulae most commonly rupture into the fixed third position of the duodenum. These fistulae usually occur between the overlaying bowel and a portion of the aorta that has previously undergone resection and grafting for an existing aneurysm. The mortality from these fistulae is high, often exceeding 50%. In rare cases, an abdominal aortic aneurysm may dissect proximally, resulting in hemopericardium. The overall mortality rates vary in published series from 15% to 90%, and the time from the onset of symptoms to control of bleeding appears to be the key to determining outcome. The importance of controlling bleeding gives credence to the inescapable sense of urgency that accompanies such events. Other factors that adversely affect outcome[217] are a history of chronic hypertension, age greater than 80 years, heart disease, renal insufficiency, a hematocrit less than 32.5% at diagnosis, hypotension at diagnosis, surgery lasting longer than 400 minutes, hypotension lasting longer than 110 minutes, a systolic blood pressure less than 100 mm Hg at the end of the operation, and blood loss greater than 11,000 ml.

Management of hemodynamically unstable patients is challenging. Shock frequently accompanies aortic rupture. However, the absence of hypotension does not rule out the possibility of rupture, and shock may occur suddenly. Patients with dissection may have severe hypertension, which must be controlled immediately if rupture is to be prevented. Rapid diagnosis with immediate laparotomy and control of the proximal aorta are of the highest priority. If systolic blood pressure is greater than 90 mm Hg, some clinicians advocate the administration of oxygen by face mask, with tracheal intubation performed only after proximal control of the aorta has been achieved. Because experienced anesthesia personnel can usually intubate the trachea rapidly, and because of the substantial threat of aspiration pneumonitis, we prefer an awake intubation or a rapid sequence tracheal intubation after small doses of etomidate (0.1 mg/kg) and a steroid. We believe that this method causes little morbidity, creates only a slight delay, and prevents a potentially serious complication. However, if the patient has lost consciousness or has marked hypotension unresponsive to rapid volume infusion, the probability of rupture into the free peritoneal cavity is high. In this case, the trachea is immediately intubated in a rapid sequence fashion, usually with the aid of muscle relaxants and perhaps a small dose of etomidate; ventilation with 100% oxygen is also started. Almost simultaneously, laparotomy is begun so that the surgeon can clamp the aorta.

We attempt to replace volume to normalize systemic blood pressure (at this time, often the only guide to volume replacement in the patient with an uncontained rupture). However, when rupture is suspected, rapid control of the proximal portion of the aorta is probably more important than is optimizing the patient's preoperative condition. A difference from elective surgery is that heparin is not administered before aortic cross-clamping.

The patient is resuscitated quickly (before induction of anesthesia, if possible) with type-specific non–cross-matched blood and crystalloid administered via large-bore venous catheters by roller pumps or pressured bags. If type-specific blood is not available, O-negative washed blood cells may be given. We emphasize the importance of large-bore catheters placed in the most easily accessible veins. A 14-gauge catheter placed in each antecubital fossa is more useful for rapid volume expansion than are attempts at placement of a pulmonary artery catheter. We recommend the use, when possible, of fluid warmers that deliver rapid volumes of normothermic fluids.

Once the aorta is controlled with a cross-clamp and blood pressure and perfusion are restored, additional venous access and a radial or brachial arterial line are secured. It is often necessary to have a second anesthesiologist secure vascular access while the first is securing the airway, monitoring blood pressure, and administering volume. Attention may be turned to placing a pulmonary artery catheter once blood pressure is adequate. Even more quickly, an echocardiographic probe can be inserted for rapid assessment of left ventricular volume and contractility. At this point, volume administration is guided by means of PCWP or by the echocardiogram (left ventricular end-diastolic area). High-normal filling pressures are desirable for attenuation of hypotension after removal of the aortic clamp. Some patients will require infusions of dopamine, epinephrine, or norepinephrine to sustain an adequate blood pressure. These patients are often profoundly acidotic; if we administer sodium bicarbonate, we increase ventilation to help eliminate the extra carbon dioxide produced. Continued metabolic acidosis may foretell a poor prognosis. Augmentation of cardiac output with dopexamine increases oxygen delivery perioperatively, with only a limited increase in total body or myocardial oxygen demand, and may improve survival.[218] However, similar studies with dobutamine have yielded opposite conclusions.[219] At the present time, given the high incidence of cardiac-related morbidity, we restrict our use of inotropic support to patients with hypotension or low cardiac output (cardiac index <2 $L/min/m^2$) despite adequate filling pressures. We do not hesitate to administer muscle relaxants and administer large doses of opioids to these patients if they are hemodynamically stable, because they usually require postoperative mechanical ventilation of the lungs and sedation to minimize cardiovascular stress.

Hemodynamically stable patients constitute a second group of patients in whom shock is reversible with volume administration. In such patients, it may be assumed that hemorrhage has been at least partially contained. However, because rapid exsanguination can occur at any time, patients are transported immediately to the operating room for emergency laparotomy, and the same urgency is maintained. Venous access is then ensured. If the blood pressure and heart rate are stable when the patient arrives, sterile preparation of the abdomen is begun. The intravascular volume status may be assessed by observation of the patient for a decrease in systemic blood pressure or an increase in the heart rate when the head is raised 10 to 15 degrees. Administration of a 25-mg bolus of thiopental IV may also aid in the assessment of volume. Normally, induction of anesthesia is delayed until the patient's abdomen is prepared and draped and the surgeon is ready. Thus, in this situation, minimal extra time is spent on inserting and attaching monitors.

Preoxygenation is followed by rapid-sequence induction of anesthesia with small doses of a narcotic and an induction agent, often etomidate, a rapidly acting muscle relaxant, application of cricoid pressure, and tracheal intubation. To blunt the hemodynamic effects of laryngeal visualization and tracheal intubation, one may administer an IV bolus of lidocaine or esmolol, or an additional narcotic or an induction agent. However, hypotension may easily occur following induction, in which case we administer 100% oxygen, elevate the patient's legs, and rapidly administer blood and fluids. If these measures fail to restore adequate blood pressure and perfusion, we infuse phenylephrine or dopamine until the aorta can be occluded.

Because of hypothermia from massive fluid resuscitation and the aortic occlusion above the hepatic artery, replaced blood may not pass through the liver in amounts adequate to allow for the metabolism of citrate. Therefore, if either hypotension due to poor myocardial contractility (which may be easily assessed with echocardiography) or coagulopathy develops, administration of calcium may be therapeutic. It has been suggested that the aggressive fluid resuscitation of trauma patients in the emergency room before transport to the operating room may result in increased mortality, perhaps by causing hypothermia or dilutional coagulopathy, or by raising blood pressure and increasing bleeding.[220] At present, however, we cannot recommend allowing patients to remain hypotensive but believe that attention should be paid to maintaining temperature, adequate hematocrit, and coagulation in addition to simply normalizing intravascular volume.

Some patients may be initially treated with a military antishock trouser (MAST) suit. This temporizing measure allows transport of the patient to the operative room with less hemorrhage and, some believe, with clot formation and temporary sealing of the aortic rent. If possible, pressure in the MAST suit should be removed in stages rather than all at once, and only after the surgeons are scrubbed and ready to begin. Reducing the pressure at once increases blood flow (reactive hyperemia) in all areas simultaneously, thereby causing a large and precipitous decrease in blood pressure and filling volumes of the heart. The cumbersome nature of this device limits its use.

We routinely use autotranfusion in patients with actual or suspected rupture of an aortic aneurysm. This device can be operated by a separate team, allowing the primary anesthesiologist to direct all of his or her attention to the patient's volume status, gas exchange, and depth of anesthesia. Our mnemonic for treatment of such patients is "wovcath," for *w*onder what (if any) anesthetic to give, *o*xygen, *v*ecuronium, *c*oagulation, *a*cid-base change, *t*emperature change, and *h*emodynamic change. The mnemonic lists, in reverse order, the important aspects of patient care that we try to remember when everything about these patients invites disorganization.

After successful surgery for ruptured abdominal aortic aneurysm, the survival rate is about 50% at 1 month and 33% at 3 years, much lower than survival rates after elective operation. Survival is highest if intraoperative urine output is 200 ml or higher and respiratory failure or myocardial infarction does not occur. The decision to repair a ruptured abdominal aortic aneurysm can be made on clinical grounds. However, after surgery (when information on intraoperative and postoperative variables is also available), these prognostic variables assist clinical judgment and guide discussions of prognosis with the family.[216]

The complications that occur during aortic occlusion can usually be linked to the heart, central nervous system, or kidneys. Organ dysfunction can be minimized by maintaining intraoperative values for hemodynamic variables within the normal preoperative range, ensuring that cardiac dilation does not occur at any point, and minimizing episodes of tachycardia. Attention to details of preoperative drug therapy, preoperative hydration, and temperature homeostasis may also promote an improved outcome. Furthermore, vigilance must continue into the postoperative period if morbidity and mortality are to be minimized. As opposed to elective aortic reconstruction, in which preserving myocardial function is the primary goal, in emergency resection the crucial factor for patient survival is first rapid control of blood loss and reversal of hypotension, and then preservation of myocardial function.

Conclusions

Patients undergoing aortic reconstruction are generally elderly individuals who have a physiologic or RealAge that is even older. Vascular disease is a generalized process; thus, patients having surgery for a specific vascular disorder are likely to have atherosclerotic disease elsewhere in the vascular system. Most of the patients have coronary artery disease. The skills of the anesthesiologist can therefore greatly influence outcome in vascular surgery. The considerations for preoperative patient evaluation are the same as for patients with cardiac disease undergoing other noncardiac procedures. Many have a history of smoking, and chronic obstructive pulmonary disease, renal insufficiency, and lipid abnormalities are frequently present. The major morbidity in each of the operations relates to myocardial well-being; therefore, the heart should be the major focus of the anesthesiologist's attention. Attempts to segregate patients who have significant coronary artery disease by use of preoperative testing are controversial. The benefits of coronary revascularization are likely to persist long after vascular surgery in patients with triple-vessel coronary artery disease.

In aortic reconstruction, ensuring intact myocardial function is probably the best way of making certain that spinal cord, visceral, and renal perfusion will be adequate.

In addition, vigilance in ensuring routine prehydration and use of a warming device are probably more important to outcome than is the occasional brilliance. We prefer the diligent, compulsive practitioner to the occasionally brilliant one. Nowhere is such diligence needed more than in the postoperative period, when most morbidity related to the heart occurs. Perhaps it is most important to remember that the best patient results are achieved when intraoperative vigilance is extended to the preoperative and postoperative periods as well.*

References

1. Szilagyi DE, Smith RF, Derusso FJ, et al: Contribution of abdominal aortic aneurysmectomy to prolongation of life. Ann Surg 164:678, 1966.
2. Whittemore AD, Clowes AW, Hechtman HB, et al: Aortic aneurysm repair: Reduced operative mortality associated with maintenance of optimal cardiac performance. Ann Surg 192:414, 1980.
3. Crawford ES, Saleh SA, Babb JW III, et al: Infrarenal abdominal aortic aneurysm: Factors influencing survival after operation performed over a 25-year period. Ann Surg 193:699, 1981.
4. Benefiel DJ, Roizen MF, Lampe GH, et al: Morbidity after aortic surgery with sufentanil versus isoflurane anesthesia. Anesthesiology 65:A516, 1986.
5. Johnston KW: Multicenter prospective study of nonruptured abdominal aortic aneurysm: II. Variables predicting morbidity and mortality. J Vasc Surg 9:437, 1989.
6. Golden MA, Whittemore AD, Donaldson MC, Mannick JA: Selective evaluation and management of coronary artery disease in patients undergoing repair of abdominal aortic aneurysms: A 16-year experience. Ann Surg 212:415, 1990.
7. Krupski WC, Layug EL, Reilly LM, et al: Comparison of cardiac morbidity rates between aortic and infrainguinal operations: Two-year follow-up. Study of Perioperative Ischemia Research. J Vasc Surg 18:609, 1993.
8. Lachapelle K, Graham AM, Symes JF: Does the clinical evaluation of the cardiac status predict outcome in patients with abdominal aortic aneurysms? J Vasc Surg 15:964, 1992.
9. Suggs WD, Smith RB III, Weintraub WS, et al: Selective screening for coronary artery disease in patients undergoing elective repair of abdominal aortic aneurysms. J Vasc Surg 18:349, 1993.
10. Baron JF, Mundler O, Bertrand M, et al: Dipyridamole-thallium scintigraphy and gated radionuclide angiography to assess cardiac risk before abdominal aortic surgery. N Engl J Med 10, 330:663, 1994.
11. L'Italien GJ, Cambria RP, Cutler BS, et al: Comparative early and late cardiac morbidity among patients requiring different vascular surgery procedures. J Vasc Surg 21:935, 1995.
12. Criqui MH, Langer RD, Fronek A, et al: Mortality over a period of ten years in patients with peripheral arterial disease. N Engl J Med 326:381, 1992.
13. Olshansky SJ, Carnes BA, Cassel CK: The aging of the human species. Sci Am 268:46, 1993.
14. Kravitz RL, Laouri M, Kahan JP, et al: Validity of criteria used for detecting underuse of coronary revascularization. JAMA 274:632, 1995.
15. Roizen MF: Real Age: Are You As Young As You Can Be? New York, Harper Collins, 1999.
16. Mangano DT, Layug EL, Wallace A, Tateo I: Effect of atenolol on mortality and cardiovascular morbidity after noncardiac surgery. Multicenter Study of Perioperative Ischemia Research Group. N Engl J Med 335:713, 1996.
17. Inoue K, Iwase T, Sato M, et al: Clinical application of transluminal endovascular graft placement for aortic aneurysms. Ann Thorac Surg 63:522, 1997.
18. Blum U, Voshage G, Lammer J, et al: Endoluminal stent-grafts for infrarenal abdominal aortic aneurysms. N Engl J Med 336: 13, 1997.
19. Yusuf SW, Whitaker SC, Chuter TAM, et al: Early results of endovascular aortic aneurysm surgery with aortouniiliac graft, contralateral iliac occlusion and femorofemoral bypass. J Vasc Surg 25:165, 1997.
20. Dake MD, Miller DC, Semba CP, et al: Transluminal placement of endovascular stent-grafts for the treatment of descending thoracic aortic aneurysms. N Engl J Med 331:1729, 1994.
21. Cooke JP, Ma AO: Medical therapy of peripheral arterial occlusive disease. Surg Clin North Am 75:569, 1995.
22. Hodis HN, Mack WJ, LaBree L, et al: Serial coronary angiographic evidence that antioxidant vitamin intake reduces progression of coronary artery atherosclerosis. JAMA 273:1849, 1995.
23. Roizen MF: Vitamins, minerals and supplements: The right ones in the right doses can make your Real Age younger, while the wrong ones or wrong doses make you older. Real Age: Are You As Young As You Can Be? New York: Harper Collins, 1999.
24. Roizen MF: Anesthetic implications of concurrent diseases. In Miller RD (ed): Anesthesia, 4th ed. New York, Churchill Livingstone; 1994, p 903.
25. Knos GB, Berry AJ, Isaacson IJ, Weitz FI: Intraoperative urinary output and postoperative blood urea nitrogen and creatine levels in patients undergoing aortic reconstructive surgery. J Clin Anesth 1:181, 1989.
26. Kellen M, Aronson S, Roizen MF, et al: Predictive and diagnostic tests for renal failure: A review. Anesth Analg 78:134, 1994.
27. Novis BK, Roizen MF, Aronson S, Thisted RA: Association of preoperative risk factors with postoperative acute renal failure. Anesth Analg 78:143, 1994.
28. Hertzer NR, Beven EG, Young JR, et al: Coronary artery disease in peripheral vascular patients: A classification of 1000 coronary angiograms and results of surgical management. Ann Surg 199: 223, 1984.
29. Kresowik TF, Bower TR, Garner SA, et al: Dipyridamole-thallium imaging in patients being considered for vascular procedures. Arch Surg 128:299, 1993.
30. Mangano DT: Perioperative cardiac morbidity. Anesthesiology 72:153, 1990.
31. Rihal CS, Gersh BJ, Whisnant JP, et al: Influence of coronary heart disease on morbidity and mortality after carotid endarterectomy: A population-based study in Olmsted County, Minnesota 1970–1988. J Am Coll Cardiol 19:1254, 1992.
32. Hertzer NR: Basic data concerning associated coronary disease in peripheral vascular patients. Ann Vasc Surg 1:616, 1987.
33. Rihal CS, Eagle KA, Mickel MC, et al: Surgical therapy for coronary artery disease among patients with combined coronary artery and peripheral vascular disease. Circulation 91:46, 1995.
34. Muller DW, Shamir KJ, Ellis SG, Topol EJ: Peripheral vascular complications after conventional and complex percutaneous coronary interventional procedures. Am J Cardiol 69:63, 1992.
35. Eagle KA, Rihal CS, Foster ED, et al: Long-term survival in patients with coronary artery disease: Importance of peripheral vascular disease. The Coronary Artery Surgery Study (CASS) Investigators. J Am Coll Cardiol 23:1091, 1994.
36. Pryor DB, Shaw L, McCants CB, et al: Value of the history and physical in identifying patients at increased risk for coronary artery disease. Ann Intern Med 118:81, 1993.
37. Goldman L, Caldera DL, Southwick FS, et al: Cardiac risk factors and complications in noncardiac surgery. Medicine 57:357, 1978.
38. Fleisher LA, Barash PG: Preoperative cardiac evaluation for noncardiac surgery: A functional approach. Anesth Analg 74: 586, 1992.
39. Rao TLK, Jacobs KH, El-Etr AA: Reinfarction following anesthesia in patients with myocardial infarction. Anesthesiology 59: 499, 1983.
40. Shah KB, Kleinman BS, Sami H, et al: Reevaluation of perioperative myocardial infarction in patients with prior myocardial infarction undergoing noncardiac operations. Anesth Analg 71: 231, 1990.
41. Detsky AS, Abrams HB, Forbath N, et al: Cardiac assessment

*Much of this material is taken from other works written by the authors, including Chapter 27 in Miller: Anesthesia, 4th ed., Churchill Livingstone, New York, 1994, and Chapter 33 in Barash Clinical Anesthesia, 3rd ed., Lippincott-Raven, 1996, with permission.

for patients undergoing noncardiac surgery: A multifactorial clinical risk index. Arch Intern Med 146:2131, 1986.
42. Bittner V, Weiner DH, Yusuf S, et al: Prediction of mortality and morbidity with a 6-minute walk test in patients with left ventricular dysfunction. JAMA 270:1702, 1993.
43. Fleisher LA, Beattie C: Current practice in the preoperative evaluation of patients undergoing major vascular surgery: A survey of cardiovascular anesthesiologists. J Cardiothorac Vasc Anesth 7:650, 1993.
44. Lette J, Waters D, Lassonde J, et al: Postoperative myocardial infarction and cardiac death: Predictive value of dipyridamole-thallium imaging and five clinical scoring systems based on multifactorial analysis. Ann Surg 211:84, 1990.
45. Fuster V, Badimon L, Badimon JJ, Chesebro JH: The pathogenesis of coronary artery disease and the acute coronary syndromes. N Engl J Med 326:242, 1992.
46. Eagle KA, Singer DE, Brewster DC, et al: Dipyridamole-thallium scanning in patients undergoing vascular surgery: Optimizing preoperative evaluation of cardiac risk. JAMA 257: 2185, 1987.
47. Mangano DT, London MJ, Tubau JF, et al: Dipyridamole thallium-201 scintigraphy as a preoperative screening test: A reexamination of its predictive potential. Study of Perioperative Ischemia Research Group. Circulation 84:493, 1991.
48. Lane SE, Lewis SM, Pippin JJ, et al: Predictive value of quantitative dipyridamole-thallium scintigraphy in assessing cardiovascular risk after vascular surgery in diabetes mellitus. Am J Cardiol 64:1275, 1989.
49. Mantha S, Roizen MF, Barnard J, et al: Relative effectiveness of four preoperative tests for predicting adverse cardiac outcomes after vascular surgery: A meta-analysis. Anesth Analg 79: 422, 1994.
50. Zaret BL, Wackers FJ: Nuclear cardiology. N Engl J Med 329: 775, 1993.
51. Raby KE, Goldman L, Creager MA, et al: Correlation between preoperative ischemia and major cardiac events after peripheral vascular surgery. N Engl J Med 321:1296, 1989.
52. Langan EM III, Youkey JR, Franklin DP, et al: Dobutamine stress echocardiography for cardiac risk assessment before aortic surgery. J Vasc Surg 18:905, 1993.
53. Sahin M, Karakelleoglu S, Alp N, et al: Diagnostic value of dobutamine stress echocardiography in coronary artery disease. Thorac Cardiovasc Surg 42:285, 1994.
54. Oxman AD, Cook DJ, Guyatt GH. Users' guides to the medial literature. VI. How to use an overview. Evidence-based Medicine Working Group. JAMA 272:1367, 1994.
55. Fleisher LA, Skolnick ED, Holroyd KJ, Lehmann HP: Coronary artery revascularization before abdominal aortic aneurysm surgery: A decision analytic approach. Anesth Analg 79:661, 1994.
56. Bry JD, Belkin M, O'Donnell TF Jr, et al: An assessment of the positive predictive value and cost-effectiveness of dipyridamole myocardial scintigraphy in patients undergoing vascular surgery. J Vasc Surg 19:112, 1994.
57. Birkmeyer JD, O'Connor GT, Quinton HB, et al: The effect of peripheral vascular disease on in-hospital mortality rates with coronary artery bypass surgery. Northern New England Cardiovascular Disease Study Group. J Vasc Surg 21:445, 1995.
58. Huber KC, Evans MA, Breshnahan JF, et al: Outcome of noncardiac operations in patients with severe coronary artery disease successfully trated preoperatively with coronary angioplasty. Mayo Clin Proc 67:15, 1992.
59. Blackbourne LH, Tribble CG, Langenburg SE, et al: Optimal timing of abdominal aortic aneurysm repair after coronary artery revascularization. Ann Surg 219:693, 1994.
60. Mohr FW, Falk V, Autschbach R, et al: One-stage surgery of coronary arteries and abdominal aorta in patients with impaired left ventricular function. Circulation 91:379, 1995.
61. Vicaretti M, Fletcher JP, Richardson A, et al: Combined coronary artery bypass grafting and abdominal aortic aneurysm repair. Cardiovasc Surg 2:340, 1994.
62. London MJ, Hollenberg M, Wong MG, et al: Intraoperative myocardial ischemia: Localization by continuous 12-lead electrocardiography. Anesthesiology 69:232, 1988.
63. Ellis JE, Shah MN, Briller JE, et al: A comparison of methods for the detection of myocardial ischemia during noncardiac surgery: Automated ST-segment analysis systems, electrocardiography and transesophageal echocardiography. Anesth Analg 75: 764, 1992.
64. Ouyang P, Gerstenblith G, Furman WR, et al: Frequency and significance of early postoperative silent myocardial ischemia in patients having peripheral vascular surgery. Am J Cardiol 64: 1113, 1989.
65. McCann RL, Clements FM: Silent myocardial ischemia in patients undergoing peripheral vascular surgery: Incidence and association with perioperative cardiac morbidity and mortality. J Vasc Surg 9:583, 1989.
66. Pasternack PF, Grossi EA, Baumann FG, et al: Beta blockade to decrease silent myocardial ischemia during peripheral vascular surgery. Am J Surg 158:113, 1989.
67. Landesberg G, Luria MH, Cotev S, et al: Importance of long-duration postoperative ST-segment depression in cardiac morbidity after vascular surgery. Lancet 341:715, 1993.
68. Charlson ME, MacKenzie CR, Ales K, et al: Surveillance for postoperative myocardial infarction after noncardiac operations. Surg Gynecol Obstet 167:407, 1988.
69. Kaplan JA, Wells PH: Early diagnosis of myocardial ischemia using the pulmonary arterial catheter. Anesth Analg 60:789, 1981.
70. Haggmark S, Hohner PK, Ostman M, et al: Comparison of hemodynamic, electrocardiographic, mechanical, and metabolic indicators of intraoperative myocardial ischemia in vascular surgical patients with coronary artery disease. Anesthesiology 70: 19, 1989.
71. Van Daele ME, Sutherland GR, Mitchell MM, et al: Do changes in pulmonary capillary wedge pressure adequately reflect myocardial ischemia during anesthesia? A correlative preoperative hemodynamic, electrocardiographic and transesophageal echocardiographic study. Circulation 81:865, 1990.
72. Roizen MF, Beaupre PN, Alpert RA, et al: Monitoring with two-dimensional transesophageal echocardiography: Comparison of myocardial function in patients undergoing supraceliac suprarenal-infraceliac or infrarenal aortic occlusion. J Vasc Surg 1:300, 1984.
73. Smith JS, Cahalan MK, Benefiel DJ, et al: Intraoperative detection of myocardial ischemia in high-risk patients: Electrocardiography versus two-dimensional transesophageal echocardiography. Circulation 72:1015, 1985.
74. Eisenberg MJ, London MJ, Leung JM, et al: Monitoring for myocardial ischemia during noncardiac surgery: A technology assessment of transesophageal echocardiography and 12-lead electrocardiography. The Study of Perioperative Ischemia Research Group. JAMA 268:210, 1992.
75. Mangano DT: Beyond CK-MB: Biochemical markers for perioperative myocardial infarction. Anesthesiology 81:1317, 1994.
76. Adams JE III, Sicard GA, Allen BT, et al: Diagnosis of perioperative myocardial infarction with measurement of cardiac troponin I. N Engl J Med 330:670, 1994.
77. Taylor LM Jr, Yeager RA, Moneta GL, et al: The incidence of perioperative myocardial infarction in general vascular surgery. J Vasc Surg 15:52, 1992.
78. Breslow MJ: The role of stress hormones in perioperative myocardial ischemia. Int Anesthesiol Clin 30:81, 1992.
79. Trip MD, Cats VM, van Capelle FJL, Vreeken J: Platelet hyperreactivity and prognosis in survivors of myocardial infarction. N Engl J Med 322:1549, 1992.
80. Rosenfield BA: Perioperative homeostatic changes and coronary ischemic syndromes. Int Anesthesiol Clin 30:131, 1992.
81. Reeder MK, Goldman MD, Loh L, et al: Postoperative hypoxaemia after major abdominal vascular surgery. Br J Anaesth 68: 23, 1992.
82. Mangano DT, Browner WS, Hollenberg M, et al: Long-term cardiac prognosis following noncardiac surgery. JAMA 268:233, 1992.
83. Ellis JE, Busse JR, Foss JF, Roizen MF: Postoperative management of myocardial ischemia. Anesthesiol Clin North Am 9:609, 1991.
84. Furberg CD, Psaty BM, Meyer JV: Nifedipine: Dose-related increase in mortality in patients with coronary heart disease. Circulation 92:1326, 1995.
85. Dodds TM, Stone JG, Coromilas J, et al: Prophylactic nitroglycerin infusion during noncardiac surgery does not reduce perioperative ischemia. Anesth Analg 76:705, 1993.

86. Mangano DT, Siliciano D, Hollenberg M, et al: Postoperative myocardial ischemia: Therapeutic trials using intensive analgesia following surgery. Anesthesiology 76:342, 1992.
87. Christopherson R, Beattie C, Frank SM, et al: Perioperative morbidity in patients randomized to epidural or general anesthesia for lower extremity vascular surgery: Perioperative Ischemia Randomized Anesthesia Trial Study Group. Anesthesiology 79: 422, 1993.
88. Tuman KJ, McCarthy RJ, March RJ, et al: Effects of epidural anesthesia and analgesia on coagulation and outcome after major vascular surgery. Anesth Analg 73:696, 1991.
89. Yeager MP, Glass DD, Neff RK, Brinck-Johnsen T: Epidural anesthesia and analgesia in high-risk surgical patients. Anesthesiology 66:729, 1987.
90. Ellis JE, Drijvers G, Pedlow S, et al: Premedication with oral and transdermal clonidine provides safe and efficacious postoperative sympatholysis. Anesth Analg 79:1133, 1994.
91. Talke P, Li J, Jain U, et al: Effects of perioperative dexmedetomidine infusion in patients undergoing vascular surgery. The Study of Perioperative Ischemia Research Group. Anesthesiology 82:620, 1995.
92. Nelson AH, Fleisher LA, Rosenbaum SH: Relationship between postoperative anemia and cardiac morbidity in high risk vascular patients in the intensive care unit. Crit Care Med 21:860, 1993.
93. Frank SM, Beattie C, Christopherson R, et al: Unintentional hypothermia is associated with postoperative myocardial ischemia. The Perioperative Ischemia Randomized Anesthesia Trial Study Group. Anesthesiology 78:468, 1993.
94. Miller JS, Dodson TF, Salam AA, Smith RB III: Vascular complications following intra-aortic balloon pump insertion. Am Surg 58:232, 1992.
95. Roth S, Shay J, Chua KG: Coronary angioplasty following acute perioperative myocardial infarction. Anesthesiology 71:300, 1989.
96. Reichard P, Nilsson BY, Rosenqvist U: The effect of long-term intensified insulin treatment on the development of microvascular complications of diabetes mellitus. N Engl J Med 329:304, 1993.
97. Treiman GS, Treiman RL, Foran RF, et al: The influence of diabetes mellitus on the risk of abdominal aortic surgery. Am Surg 60:436, 1994.
98. Charlson ME, MacKenzie CR, Gold JP: Preoperative autonomic function abnormalities in patients with diabetes mellitus and patients with hypertension. J Am Coll Surg 179:1, 1994.
99. National Heart, Lung, and Blood Institute: Clinical alert: Bypass over angioplasty for patients with diabetes. September 21, 1995.
100. Donaldson MC, Weinberg DS, Belkin M, et al: Screening for hypercoagulable states in vascular surgical practice: A preliminary study. J Vasc Surg 11:825, 1990.
101. Eason JD, Mills JL, Beckett WC: Hypercoagulable states in arterial thomboembolism. Surg Gynecol Obstet 174:211, 1992.
102. Demasi R, Bode AP, Knupp C, et al: Heparin-induced thrombocytopenia. Am Surg 60:26, 1994.
103. Kispert JF, Kazmers A, Roitman L: Preoperative spirometry predicts perioperative pulmonary complications after major vascular surgery. Am Surg 58:491, 1992.
104. Phillips SM, King D: The role of ultrasound to detect aortic aneurysms in "urological" patients. Eur J Vasc Surg 7:298, 1993.
105. Guirguis EM, Barber GC: The natural history of abdominal aortic aneurysms. Am J Surg 162:481, 1991.
106. Limet R, Sakalihassan N, Albert A: Determination of the expansion rate and incidence of rupture of abdominal aortic aneurysms. J Vasc Surg 14:540, 1991.
107. Hallet JW Jr, Naessens JM, Ballard DJ: Early and late outcome of surgical repair for small abdominal aortic aneurysms: A population-based analysis. J Vasc Surg 18:684, 1993.
108. Zelenock GB, Strodel WE, Knol JA, et al: A prospective study of clinically and endoscopically documented colonic ischemia in 100 patients undergoing aortic reconstructive surgery with aggressive colonic and direct pelvic revascularization, compared with history controls. Surgery 106:771, 1989.
109. Szilagyi DE, Elliott JP Jr, Smith RF, et al: A 30-year survey of the reconstructive surgical treatment of aorto-iliac occlusive disease. J Vasc Surg 3:421, 1986.
110. Nypavar TJ, Shepard AD, Reddy DJ, et al: Supraceliac aortic cross-clamping: Determinants of outcome in elective abdominal aortic reconstruction. J Vasc Surg 17:868, 1993.
111. Gelman S: The pathophysiology of aortic cross-clamping and unclamping. Anesthesiology 82:1026, 1995.
112. Roizen MF, Ellis JE, Foss JF, et al: Intraoperative management of the patient requiring supraceliac aortic occlusion. In Veith FJ, Hobson RW, Williams RA, SE W (eds): Vascular Surgery, 2nd ed. New York, McGraw-Hill, 1994.
113. Paterson IS, Klausner JM, Goldman G, et al: Pulmonary edema after aneurysm surgery is modified by mannitol. Ann Surg 210: 796, 1989.
114. Latson TW, Reinhart DJ, Allison PM, et al: Ketorolac tromethamine may be efficacious in treating hypotension from mesenteric traction. J Cardiothorac Vasc Anesth 6:456, 1992.
115. Piccone W, DeLaria GA, Najafi H: Descending thoracic aneurysms. In Bergan JJ, Yao JST (eds): Aortic Surgery. Philadelphia, WB Saunders, 1989, p 249.
116. Williams GM, Perler BA, Burdick JF, et al: Angiographic localization of spinal cord blood supply and its relationship to postoperative paraplegia. J Vasc Surg 13:23, 1996.
117. Pass LJ, Eberhart RC, Brown JC, et al: The effect of mannitol and dopamine on the renal response to thoracic aortic cross-clamping. J Thorac Cardiovasc Surg 95:608, 1988.
118. Gamulin Z, Forster A, Morel D, et al: Effects of infrarenal cross-clamping on renal hemodynamics in humans. Anesthesiology 61:394, 1984.
119. Svensson LG, Crawford ES, Hess KR, et al: Thoracoabdominal aortic aneurysms associated with celiac, superior mesenteric, and renal artery occlusive disease: Methods and analysis of results in 271 patients. J Vasc Surg 16:378, 1992.
120. Crawford ES, Morris GC Jr, Myhre HO, et al: Celiac axis, superior mesenteric artery, and inferior mesenteric artery occlusion: Surgical considerations. Surgery 82:856, 1977.
121. Sicard GA, Reilly JM, Rubin GB, et al: Transabdominal versus retroperitoneal incision for abdominal aortic surgery: Report of a prospective randomized trial. J Vasc Surg 21:174, 1995.
122. Starr DS, Lawrie GM, Morris GC Jr: Prevention of distal embolism during arterial reconstruction. Am J Surg 138:764, 1979.
123. Roizen MF, Rodgers GM, Valone FH, et al: Anaphylactoid reactions to vascular graft material presenting with vasodilation and subsequent disseminated intravascular coagulation. Anesthesiology 71:331, 1989.
124. Donaldson MC, Louras JC, Bucknam CA: Axillofemoral bypass: A tool with a limited role. J Vasc Surg 3:757, 1986.
125. Elliot J, Szilagyi D, et al: Spinal cord ischemia: Secondary to surgery of the abdominal aorta. In Bernhard V, Towne J (eds): Complication in Vascular Surgery. Orlando, Grune & Stratton, 1985.
126. Katz NM, Blackstone EH, Kirklin JW, Karp RB: Incremental risk factors for spinal cord injury following operation for acute traumatic aortic transection. J Thorac Cardiovasc Surg 81:669, 1981.
127. Crawford ES, Svensson LG, Hess KR, et al: A prospective randomized study of cerebrospinal fluid, drainage to prevent paraplegia after high-risk surgery on the thoracoabdominal aorta. J Vasc Surg 13:36, 1991.
128. Svensson LG, Loop FD: Prevention of spinal cord ischemia in aortic surgery. In Bergen JJ, Yao JST (eds): Arterial Surgery: New Diagnostics and Operative Techniques. New York, Grune & Stratton, 1988, p 273.
129. McCullough JL, Hollier LH, Nugent M: Paraplegia after thoracic aortic occlusion: Influence of cerebrospinal fluid drainage. J Vasc Surg 7:153, 1988.
130. Svensson LG, Von Ritter CM, Groeneveld HT, et al: Cross-clamping of the thoracic aorta. Influence of aortic shunts, laminectomy, papaverine, calcium channel blocker, allopurinol, and superoxide dismutase on spinal cord blood flow and paraplegia in baboons. Ann Surg 204:38, 1986.
131. Svensson LG, Grum DF, Bednarski M, et al: Appraisal of cerebrospinal fluid alterations during aortic surgery with intrathecal papaverine administration and cerebrospinal fluid drainage. J Vasc Surg 11:423, 1990.
132. Grum DF, Svensson LG: Changes in cerebrospinal fluid pressure and spinal cord perfusion pressure prior to cross-clamping of the

thoracic aorta in humans. J Cardiothorac Vasc Anesth 5:331, 1991.

133. Svensson LG, Stewart RW, Cosgrove DM III, et al: Intrathecal papaverine for the prevention of paraplegia after operation on the thoracic or thoracoabdominal aorta. J Thorac Cardiovasc Surg 96:823, 1988.
134. Mangano DT, Browner WS, Hollenberg M, et al: Association of perioperative myocardial ischemia with cardiac morbidity and mortality in men undergoing noncardiac surgery. N Engl J Med 323:1781, 1990.
135. Hill AC, Schechter WP, Mori H, et al: The effect of verapamil on cerebral cortical and spinal cord blood flow during proximal descending thoracic aortic occlusion. J Trauma 28:1214, 1988.
136. Seibel PS, Theodore P, Kron IL, Tribble CG: Regional adenosine attenuates postischemic spinal cord injury. J Vasc Surg 18:153, 1993.
137. Matsuyama K, Chiba Y, Ihaya A, et al: Effect of spinal cord preconditioning on paraplegia during cross-clamping of the thoracic aorta. Ann Thorac Surg 63:1315, 1997.
138. Laschinger JC, Cunningham JN Jr, Cooper MM, et al: Prevention of ischemic spinal cord injury following aortic cross-clamping. Use of corticosteroids. Ann Thorac Surg 38:500, 1984.
139. Bracken MB, Shepard MJ, Collins WF, et al: A randomized, controlled trial of methylprednisolone or naloxone in the treatment of acute spinal cord injury. Results of the Second National Acute Spinal Cord Injury Study. N Eng J Med 322:1405, 1990.
140. Bracken MB, Holford TR: Effect of timing of methylprednisolone or naloxone administration on recovery of segmental and long-tract neurologic function in NASCIS 2. J Neurosurg 79: 500, 1993.
141. Bracken MB, Shepard MJ, Holford TR, et al: Administration of methylprednisolone for 24 or 48 hours or tirilazad mesylate for 48 hours in the treatment of acute spinal cord injury. Results of the Third National Acute Spinal Cord Injury Randomized Controlled Trial. JAMA 277:1597, 1997.
142. Milde LN, Waglinski MR: Pathophysiology of metabolic brain injury. In Cottrell JE, Smith DS (eds): Anesthesia and Neurosurgery. St. Louis, CV Mosby, 1994.
143. Gomez MN: Magnesium and cardiovascular disease. Anesthesiology 89:222, 1998.
144. Vacanti FX, Ames A III: Mild hypothermia and Mg^{++} protect against irreversible damage during CNS ischemia. Stroke 15: 695, 1984.
145. Kass IS, Cottrell JE, Chambers G: Magnesium and cobalt, not nimodipine protect neurons against anoxic damage in the rat hippocampal slice. Anesthesiology 69:710, 1988.
146. Gambling DR, Birmingham CL, Jenkins LC: Magnesium and the anaesthetist. Can J Anaesth 35:644, 1988.
147. Davison JK, Cambria RP, Vierra DJ, et al: Epidural cooling for regional spinal cord hypothermia during thoracoabdominal aneurysm repair. J Vasc Surg 20:304, 1994.
148. Cambria RP, Davison JK, Zannetti S, et al: Clinical experience with epidural cooling for spinal cord protection during thoracic and thoracoabdominal aneurysm repair. J Vasc Surg 25:234, 1997.
149. Safi HJ, Hess KR, Randel M, et al: Cerebrospinal fluid drainage and distal aortic perfusion: Reducing neurologic complications in repair of throacoabdominal aortic aneurysm types I and II. J Vasc Surg 23:223, 1996.
150. Kouchoukos NT, Lell WA, Karp RB, Samuelson PN: Hemodynamic effects of aortic clamping and decompression with a temporary shunt for resection of the descending thoracic aorta. Surgery 85:25, 1979.
151. Verdant A, Cossette R, Page A, et al: Aneurysms of the descending thoracic aorta: Three hundred sixty-six consecutive cases resected without paraplegia. J Vasc Surg 21:385, 1995.
152. Van Norman GA, Pavlin EG, Eddy AC, Pavlin DJ: Hemodynamic and metabolic effects of aortic unclamping following emergency surgery for traumatic thoracic aortic tear in shunted and unshunted patients. J Trauma 31:1007, 1991.
153. Frank SM, Parker SD, Rock P, et al: Moderate hypothermia, with partial bypass and segmental sequential repair for thoracoabdominal aortic aneurysm. J Vasc Surg 19:687, 1994.
154. Walls JT, Boley TM, Curtis JJ, Schmaltz RA: Experience with four surgical techniques to repair traumatic aortic pseudoaneurysm. J Thorac Cardiovasc Surg 106:283, 1993.
155. Scheinin SA, Cooley DA: Graft replacement of the descending thoracic aorta: Results of "open" distal anastomosis. Ann Thorac Surg 58:19, 1994.
156. Safi HJ, Bartoli S, Hess KR, et al: Neurologic deficit in patients at high risk with thoracoabdominal aortic aneurysms: The role of cerebral spinal fluid drainage and distal aortic perfusion. J Vasc Surg 20:434, 1994.
157. Sayers RD, Thompson MM, Nasim A, et al: Surgical management of 671 abdominal aortic aneurysms: A 13 year review from a single centre. Eur J Vasc Endovasc Surg 13:322, 1997.
158. Acher CW, Belzer FO, Grist TM, et al: Late renal function in patients undergoing renal revascularization for control of hypertension and/or renal preservation. Cardiovasc Surg 4:602, 1996.
159. Muluk SC, Painter L, Sile S, et al: Utility of clinical pathway and prospective case management to achieve cost and hospital stay reduction for aortic aneurysm surgery at a tertiary care hospital. J Vasc Surg 25:84, 1997.
160. Kazmers A, Jacobs L, Perkins A: The impact of complications after vascular surgery in Veterans Affairs Medical Centers. J Surg Res 67:62, 1997.
161. Panneton JM, Lassonde J, Laurendeau F: Ruptured abdominal aortic aneurysm: Impact of comorbidity and postoperative complications on outcome. Ann Vasc Surg 9:535, 1994.
162. Hajarizadeh H, Rohrer MJ, Herrmann JB, Cutler BS: Acute peritoneal dialysis following ruptured abdominal aortic aneurysms. Am J Surg 170:223, 1995.
163. Hallet JW Jr, Textor SC, Kos PB, et al: Advanced renovascular hypertension and renal insufficiency: Trends in medical comorbidity and surgical approach from 1970 to 1993. J Vasc Surg 212:750, 1995.
164. McCarthy JT: Prognosis of patients with acute renal failure in the intensive-care unit: A tale of two eras. Mayo Clin Proc 71: 117, 1996.
165. Sharma PV, Babu SC, Shah PM, Nassoura ZE: Changing patterns of atheroembolism. Cardiovasc Surg 4:573, 1996.
166. Bertrand M, Godet G, Fleron MH, et al: Lumbar muscle rhabdomyolysis after abdominal aortic surgery. Anesth Analg 85:11, 1997.
167. Safi HJ, Harlin SA, Miller CC, et al: Predictive factors for acute renal failure in thoracic and thoracoabdominal aortic aneurysm surgery. J Vasc Surg 24:338, 1996.
168. Ligush J Jr, Criado E, Burnham SJ, et al: Management and outcome of chronic atherosclerotic infrarenal aortic occlusion. J Vasc Surg 24:394, 1996.
169. Starr JE, Hertzer NR, Mascha EJ, et al: Influence of gender on cardiac risk and survival in patients with infrarenal aortic aneurysms. J Vasc Surg 23:870, 1996.
170. Hakim RM, Wingard RL, Parker RA: Effect of the dialysis membrane in the treatment of patients with acute renal failure. N Engl J Med 331:1338, 1994.
171. Alpert RA, Roizen MF, Hamilton WK, et al: Intraoperative urinary output does not predict postoperative renal function in patients undergoing abdominal aortic revascularization. Surgery 95:707, 1984.
172. Nicholson ML, Baker DM, Hopkinson BR, Wenham PW: Randomized controlled trial of the effect of mannitol on renal reperfusion injury during aortic aneurysm surgery. Br J Surg 83: 1230, 1996.
173. Solomon R, Werner C, Mann D, et al: Effects of saline, mannitol and furosemide to prevent acute decreases in renal function induced by radiocontrast agents. N Engl J Med 331:1416, 1994.
174. Swygert TH, Roberts LC, Valek TR, et al: Effect of intraoperative low-dose dopamine on renal function in liver transplant recipients. Anesthesiology 75:571, 1991.
175. Bonatti J, Watzka S, Antretter H, et al: Spinal cord protection in descending and thoracoabdominal aortic surgery—the role of distal perfusion. Thorac Cardiovasc Surg 44:136, 1996.
176. Practice guidelines for pulmonary artery catheterization: A report by the American Society of Anesthesiologists Task Force on Pulmonary Artery Catherterization. Anesthesiology 78:380, 1993.
177. Hohner P, Backman C, Diamond G, et al: Anesthesia for abdominal aortic surgery in patients with coronary artery disease, Part

II: Effects of nitrous oxide on systemic and coronary haemodynamics, regional ventricular function and incidence of myocardial ischaemia. Acta Anesthesiol Scand 38:793, 1994.
178. Seyde WC, Ellis JE, Longnecker DE: The addition of nitrous oxide to halothane decreases renal and splanchnic flow and increases cerebral blood flow in rats. Br J Anaesth 58:63, 1986.
179. Gold MS, DeCrosta D, Rizzuto C, et al: The effect of lumbar epidural and general anesthesia on plasma catecholamines and hemodynamics during abdominal aortic aneurysm repair. Anesth Analg 78:225, 1994.
180. Breslow MJ, Jordan DA, Christopherson R, et al: Epidural morphine decreases postoperative hypertension by attenuating sympathetic nervous system hyperactivity. JAMA 261:3577, 1989.
181. Blomberg S, Emanuelsson H, Kvist H, et al: Effects of thoracic epidural anesthesia on coronary arteries and arterioles in patients with coronary artery disease. Anesthesiology 73:840, 1990.
182. Bracken MB, Shepard MJ, Collins WF Jr, et al: Methylprednisolone or naloxone treatment after acute spinal cord injury: 1-year follow-up data. Results of the Second National Acute Spinal Cord Injury Study. J Neurosurg 76:23, 1992.
183. Lunn JK, Dannemiller FJ, Stanley TH: Cardiovascular responses to clamping of the aorta during epidural and general anesthesia. Anesth Analg 58:372, 1979.
184. Raner C, Biber B, Lundberg J, et al: Cardiovascular depression by isoflurane and concomitant thoracic epidural anesthesia is reversed by dopamine. Acta Anaesthesiol Scand 38:136, 1994.
185. Egbert LD, Battit GE, Turndorf H, Beecher HK: The value of the preoperative visit by an anesthetist. A study of doctor-patient rapport. JAMA 185.553, 1963.
186. Egbert LD, Battit GE, Welch CE, Bartlett MK: Reduction of postoperative pain by encouragement and instruction of patients: A study of doctor-patient rapport. N Engl J Med 270:825, 1964.
187. Anderson EA: Preoperative preparation for cardiac surgery facilitates recovery, reduces psychological distress, and reduces the incidence of acute postoperative hypertension. J Consult Clin Psychol 55:513, 1987.
188. Pflug AE, Halter JB: Effect of spinal anesthesia on adrenergic tone and the neuroendocrine responses to surgical stress in humans. Anesthesiology 55:120, 1981.
189. Shah KB, Kleinman BS, Sami H, et al: Reevaluation of perioperative myocardial infarction in patients with prior myocardial infarction undergoing noncardiac operations. Anesth Analg 71:231, 1990.
190. Rivers SP, Scher LA, Sheehan E, Veith FJ: Epidural versus general anesthesia for infrainguinal arterial reconstruction. J Vasc Surg 14:764, 1991.
191. Haku E, Hayashi M, Kato H: Anesthetic management of abdominal aortic surgery: A retrospective review of perioperative complications. J Cardiothorac Anesth 3:587, 1989.
192. Bode RH Jr, Lewis KP, Zarich SW, et al: Cardiac outcome after peripheral vascular surgery. Comparison of general and regional anesthesia. Anesthesiology 84:3, 1996.
193. Baron JF, Bertrand M, Barre E, et al: Combined epidural and general anesthesia versus general anesthesia for abdominal aortic surgery. Anesthesiology 75:611, 1991.
194. Rosenfeld BA, Beattie CH, Christopherson R, et al: The effects of different anesthetic regimens on fibrinolysis and the development of postoperative arterial thrombosis. Anesthesiology 79:435, 1993.
195. Tuman KJ, McCarthy RJ, March RJ, et al: Effects of epidural anesthesia and analgesia on coagulation and outcome after major vascular surgery. Anesth Analg 73:696, 1991.
196. Bengston A, Lannsjo W, Heideman M: Complement and anaphylatoxin responses to cross-clamping of the aorta. Studies during general anesthesia with or without extradural blockade. Br J Anaesth 59:1093, 1987.
197. Pierce ET, Pomposelli FB Jr, Stanley GD, et al: Anesthesia type does not influence early graft patency or limb salvage rates of lower extremity arterial bypass. J Vasc Surg 25:226, 1997.
198. Rosenfeld BA: Benefits of regional anesthesia on thromboembolic complications following surgery. Reg Anesth 21(Suppl 6):9, 1996.
199. Sharma SK, Philip J: The effects of anesthetic techniques on blood coagulability in parturients as measured by thromboelastography. Anesth Analg 85:82, 1997.
200. Carpenter RL: Gastrointestinal benefits of regional anesthesia/analgesia. Reg Anesth 21(Suppl 6):13, 1996.
201. Klassen GA, Bramwell RS, Bromage PR, Zborowska-Sluis DT: Effect of acute sympathectomy by epidural anesthesia on the canine coronary circulation. Anesthesiology 52:8, 1980.
202. Davis RF, DeBoer LWV, Maroko PR: Thoracic epidural anesthesia reduces myocardial infarct size after coronary artery occlusion in dogs. Anesth Analg 65:711, 1986.
203. Baron JF, Coriat P, Mundler O, et al: Left ventricular global and regional function during lumbar epidural anesthesia in patients with and without angina pectoris. Influence of volume loading. Anesthesiology 66:621, 1987.
204. Saada M, Duval AM, Bonnet F, et al: Abmormalities in myocardial segmental wall motion during lumbar epidural anesthesia. Anesthesiology 71:26, 1989.
205. Rao TLK, El-Etr AA: Anticoagulation following placement of epidural and subarachnoid catheters: An evaluation of neurological sequelae. Anesthesiology 55:618, 1981.
206. Baron HC, LaRaja RD, Rossi G, Atkinson D: Continuous epidural analgesia in the heparinized vascular surgical patient: A retrospective review of 912 patients. J Vasc Surg 6:144, 1987.
207. Odoom JA, Sih IL: Epidural analgesia and anticoagulant therapy. Experience with one thousand cases of continuous epidurals. Anaesthesia 38:254, 1983.
208. Ruff RL, Dougherty JH Jr: Complications of lumbar puncture followed by anticoagulation. Stroke 12:879, 1981.
209. Dickman CA, Shedd SA, Spetzler RF, et al: Spinal epidural hematoma associated with epidural anesthesia: Complications of systemic heparinization in patients receiving peripheral vascular thrombolytic therapy. Anesthesiology 72:942, 1990.
210. Horlocker TT, Wedel DJ: Spinal and epidural blockade and perioperative low molecular weight heparin: Smooth sailing on the Titanic. Anesthesiology 86:1153, 1998.
211. Smith JS, Roizen MF, Cahalan MK, et al: Does anesthetic technique make a difference? Augmentation of systolic blood pressure during carotid endarterectomy: Effects of phenylephrine versus light anesthesia and of isoflurane versus halothane on the incidence of myocardial ischemia. Anesthesiology 69:846, 1988.
212. Goertz AW, Lindner KH, Seefelder C, et al: Effect of phenylephrine bolus administration on global left ventricular function in patients with valvular aortic stenosis. Anesthesiology 78:834, 1993.
213. Paterson IS, Klausner JM, Goldman G, et al: Pulmonary edema after aneurysm surgery is modified by mannitol. Ann Surg 210:796, 1989.
214. Bush HL Jr, Hydo LJ, Fischer E, et al: Hypothermia during elective abdominal aortic aneurysm repair: The high price of avoidable morbidity. J Vasc Surg 21:392, 1995.
215. Johansson G, Markstrom U, Swedenborg J: Ruptured thoracic aortic aneurysms: A study of incidence and mortality rates. J Vasc Surg 21:985, 1995.
216. Johnston KW: Ruptured abdominal aortic aneurysm: Six-year follow-up results of a multicenter prospective study. Canadian Society for Vascular Surgery Aneurysm Study Group. J Vasc Surg 19:888, 1994.
217. Wakefield TW, Whitehouse WM Jr, Shu-Chen W, et al: Abdominal aortic aneurysm rupture: Statistical analysis of factors affecting outcome of surgical treatment. Surgery 91:586, 1982.
218. Boyd O, Grounds RM, Bennett ED: The use of dopexamine hydrochloride to increase oxygen delivery perioperatively. Anesth Analg 76:372, 1993.
219. Hayes MA, Timmins AC, Yau EH, et al: Elevation of systemic oxygen delivery in the treatment of critically ill patients. N Engl J Med 330:1717, 1994.
220. Bickell WH, Wall MJ Jr, Pepe PE, et al: Immediate versus delayed fluid resuscitation for hypotensive patients with penetrating torso injuries. N Engl J Med 331:1105, 1994.

CHAPTER 23

Cerebral Vascular Surgery

C. Philip Larson, Jr., M.D.C.M.
John A. Youngberg, M.D.

Cerebrovascular surgical procedures for which anesthesia is required include ligation of intracranial aneurysms, excision of arteriovenous malformations, revascularization procedures, and repair of stenotic or ulcerative lesions of the extracranial cerebral vessels. Although the etiology and presenting symptoms and signs of these cerebrovascular abnormalities are different, they share many of the same general principles of anesthetic management, and can be considered as a group. Important differences in anesthetic management will be noted.

Cerebral Aneurysms

Intracerebral aneurysms are relatively common (about 6% of the population have them), but most are small, innocuous, and remain undetected throughout life. Twenty to 30% of patients will have multiple aneurysms, usually two or three. The most common sites for intracerebal aneurysms are in the anterior circulation at points of bifurcation in the internal carotid artery (30%), anterior cerebral and anterior communicating arteries (40%), middle cerebral artery (20%), and vertebrobasilar system (<10%).[1] The etiology of most aneurysms is not known, but there is evidence to suggest that they may be either congenital or acquired. Two lines of evidence support the concept that they are congenital in origin. First, intracerebral aneurysms occur more commonly in patients with certain genetic connective tissue disorders such as polycystic disease of the kidneys, coarctation of the aorta, fibromuscular hyperplasia, Marfan's syndrome, and Ehlers-Danlos syndrome.[2] Second, it has recently been established that the incidence of intracranial aneurysms is higher in first- or second-generation relatives of a patient with a confirmed intracerebral aneurysm than in the general population.[3] Several patterns of inheritance are possible, with autosomal transmission being the most likely.[3] Evidence favoring the acquired etiology is the fact that intracranial arteries lack the strong layers of tunica media and internal and external elastic lamina that are seen on extracranial arteries of similar size. Upon histologic analysis some aneurysms appear to be comprised only of a layer of intima, fibrous tissue, and adventitia. This layer may be especially thin at the aneurysmal dome, the usual point of rupture. Environmental factors may also play a role in subarachnoid hemorrhage. Untreated hypertension, longstanding history of cigarette smoking, heavy use of alcohol, and postmenopausal status all appear to be associated with a higher incidence of subarachnoid hemorrhage.[4]

In about 1 in 10,000 persons they will enlarge, become thin-walled and, in most cases, become symptomatic by rupturing, causing a subarachnoid hemorrhage.[1] Most patients have warning symptoms and signs before the first major bleed, but these tend to be mild, nonspecific (headache, dizziness, orbital pain, slight motor or sensory disturbance), and are generally disregarded by both patients and physicians. Blood in the subarachnoid space may cause symptoms and signs of meningeal irritation such as stiff neck, and back or leg pain. Seldom do aneurysms produce symptoms by enlarging to the point that they compress adjacent neural tissue or cause large increases in intracranial pressure (ICP). The exception to this are giant aneurysms, which are so labeled when they exceed 2.5 cm in diameter. Giant aneurysms represent about 5% of all aneurysms, occur about twice as often in women as in men, and usually become symptomatic in the fourth or fifth decade of life.[5]

Most patients are between 40 and 60 years of age when their subarachnoid hemorrhage occurs, but it may occur at any age, although it is very rare in children. The consequences of rupture are often devastating. About 10% of patients die before arrival at hospital, and another 40% die within the first month after the hemorrhage; of those who survive, over 30% have major neurologic deficits.[4] The subsequent neurologic dysfunction will vary depending upon the site and extent of the hemorrhage. These patients may complain of severe headache, often accompanied by nausea and vomiting, be confused and disoriented have a motor deficit of one or more extremities, or be comatose. A major complication of an intracerebral hemorrhage is the development of cerebral vasospasm or vasoconstriction of cerebral vessels. The vasospasm may be local or diffuse, and may be mild or severe. If severe, it causes worsening of the ischemic neurologic deficits. It usually occurs about the third day after the bleed, peaks at about 7 days, and is usually resolved by 14 days. The exact mechanism for the vasospasm is not known, but it is believed that the precipitating agent is free oxyhemoglobin, which in turn may cause the release of vasospastic substances such as serotonin, prostaglandin, or potassium from brain cells. There is no definitive treatment for cerebral vasospasm, but measures such as administration of calcium channel blocking drugs to induce cerebral vasodilatation, vigorous hydration to induce hypervolemic hemodilution, and maintenance of a high normal blood pressure are believed by many to lessen the severity of the ischemia by increasing cerebral blood flow (CBF) and improving the rheologic characteristics of blood.

While cerebral aneurysms may be detected by helical computed tomography (CT) or magnetic resonance imaging (MRI) angiography, conventional cerebral angiography will best define the exact size and location of the aneurysm, and identify whether multiple aneurysms are present. Although low, the risks of morbidity or mortality from conventional angiography are greater than from CT or MRI angiography. CT scanning is very useful for diagnosis of acute intracranial or subarachnoid hemorrhage, while MRI is more useful when the hemorrhage is more than several days old.[4]

Surgical treatment has clearly decreased the long-term mortality from a rebleed and is preferred to medical treatment, provided the patient can withstand the operation.[4] If no treatment is offered, about 70% of patients ultimately die from the bleed or related complications (rebleed, vasospasm, or medical complications).[1] Some patients will also develop hydrocephalus following recovery from a subarachnoid hemorrhage presumably from clot occlusion of the ventricular system, and will require a ventriculoperitoneal shunt to relieve the increased ICP. The combined operative mortality and major morbidity from ligation of cerebral aneurysms is less than 10% in institutions where these operations are performed regularly.[1] Timing of the operation is critical. Generally, neurosurgeons will wait 10 to 14 days after a major bleed to ligate an aneurysm. This delay allows the patient's neurologic status to stabilize and for the brain to recover from the edema and vasospasm that may accompany the ischemic episode. However, if the intracranial hemorrhage is very recent and the neurologic injury from the bleed is not severe, many neurosurgeons will elect to operate immediately to avoid the potentially disastrous consequences of a subsequent hemorrhage.

The essential goal of surgery is to isolate the thin-walled aneurysm from arterial pressure, usually by the application of a spring clip at its attachment to the parent artery. Less often, aneurysms are ligated with a surgical tie, wrapped in plastic gauze, or coated with methyl methacrylate or silicone adhesives. In the past, neurosurgeons usually wanted the patient's blood pressure to be markedly decreased just prior to clipping or ligation of an aneurysm to decrease the pressure on the aneurysmal wall and lessen the risk of acute hemorrhage. More recently many neurosurgeons choose instead to surgically collapse the aneurysm by applying a temporary clip on the major feeding vessel(s) to the aneurysm.[6] Under these circumstances, hypertension rather than hypotension is desired to maintain a high collateral perfusion pressure in the head during the period of temporary occlusion of the feeding vessel(s). Once the aneurysm is occluded, then the blood pressure should be returned to a more normal level.

Giant aneurysms are a particularly difficult surgical challenge.[7,8] First, their large size makes direct visualization of the vascular anatomy difficult. Second, vascular branches essential to maintaining flow to normal brain may be an integral part of the giant aneurysm and cannot be included in the clipping without causing permanent neurologic injury. Third, standard aneurysm clips may not occlude a large, turgid aneurysm, or may slip or move once applied. And lastly, giant aneurysms may rupture during dissection or clip application with resultant severe neurologic morbidity or mortality. As a result, a special anesthetic and surgical management has evolved utilizing high-dose thiopental (and more recently propofol) administration, deep hypothermia to 18°C achieved with femorofemoral cardiopulmonary bypass, and temporary circulatory arrest.[7,8] These techniques both decompress the giant aneurysm, making it easier to clip, and offer greater protection to the brain while circulatory arrest is in effect. It is expected that the duration of cardiac arrest may be as long as 45 minutes.

The newest form of treatment of intracranial aneurysms is endovascular occlusion performed by neuroradiologists in the radiology suite. Under radiologic guidance, soft metallic coils are deposited within the lumen of an aneurysm, and electrical current is applied to generate a thrombus within the aneurysm.[4] The long-term success of this treatment remains to be established. As with surgical treatment, patients require general anesthesia because of the long duration of the procedure and the need for absolute immobility while it is being done.

Arteriovenous Malformations

Arteriovenous malformations (AVMs) are aggregations of twisted, dilated, arterial-to-venous communications without any intervening capillary circulation.[9] They are congenital in origin and represent the persistence of embryonic arteriovenous shunts. They may occur anywhere in the brain or spinal cord, but are most commonly found in a cerebral hemisphere (65%), a posterior fossa (20%), or in a deep midline structure (15%).[10] AVMs may also be associated with one or more aneurysms. AVMs occur with equal frequency in men and women. AVMs vary in size from small lesions called cryptic malformations to very large lesions that occupy a major portion of a cerebral hemisphere. On histologic examination the vessel walls are thin and lack a muscular layer. As a consequence, the vessels exhibit loss of normal vasomotor control or responsiveness to changes in carbon dioxide.

The most common presenting clinical picture of AVMs is that of a seizure disorder usually beginning in young adulthood (late teens or early 20s). Other symptoms and signs including headache, motor or sensory deficits, ataxia, cranial nerve dysfunction, visual symptoms or memory loss resulting from the pressure of a mass lesion, an intracerebral hemorrhage from the AVM, or high-flow arteriovenous shunts causing an intracerebral steal. The high-flow shunts may cause a bruit in the head. The diagnosis is generally established by cerebral angiography. However, stereotactic localization using either CT or MRI is necessary to identify the very small AVMs or those deep-seated in the corona radiata, basal ganglia, visual center, cerebellar white matter, or corpus callosum. In adults the stereotactic frame is placed on the patient's head under local anesthesia. The patient is then taken for CT or MRI, where the exact coordinates defining the AVM and critical adjacent structures are established. The patient is then brought to the operating room, and anesthesia is induced with the frame still in place. In children it may be necessary to induce general anesthesia before placement of the frame, with anesthesia then being maintained during the CT or MRI procedure. The frame is removed at the conclusion of operation prior to emergence from anesthesia.

Until recently surgical treatment was only marginally successful, and most patients were obliged to live with their disorder until they died of a cerebral hemorrhage or the consequences of a seizure. The natural history of AVMs is that they bleed at a rate of about 2 to 3% per year, causing substantial mortality (6 to 30% with each bleed) or severe morbidity (15 to 80%).[11] Surgical excision is still the primary treatment for small AVMs, while larger lesions are treated with a combination of radiologic embolization, surgical excision, and Bragg peak proton beam therapy.[12] The essential feature of excision is occlusion of the arterial inflow before interfering with the venous outflow. In general, obliteration of an AVM must be complete; partial obliteration is seldom successful in preventing recurrent symptoms, signs, or hemorrhage. Surgical excision of large AVMs must be staged, with each operative period not to exceed about 6 to 7 hours. If surgery continues beyond that time, uncontrollable swelling and bleeding from the previously dry surgical excision site may occur suddenly and without warning. The cause of the breakthrough bleeding and swelling is not known, but may be related to the high concentration of thromboplastin and vasoactive amines in the brain. In experienced hands surgical mortality averages about 10%, and morbidity, primarily epilepsy, averages about 15%, with the remaining 75% of patients experiencing a complete and successful recovery.[12]

Revascularization Procedures

Revascularization of the ischemic brain is attempted with a variety of operations, the most common one being the creation of a surgical anastomosis between the external carotid circulation (usually the superficial temporal artery) and the internal carotid circulation (usually the middle cerebral artery). This is known as an extracranial-intracranial (EC-IC) bypass. The choice of internal anastomosis will depend upon several factors including area of ischemia, cortical arterial size, collateral circulation, etc. The intent is to increase blood flow to ischemic cortical tissue supplied by the anterior or middle cerebral arteries, or rarely to the occipital lobe or cerebellum via the occipital artery. If the external arterial circulation is not of sufficient size, length, or flow as determined by Doppler measurement to achieve satisfactory EC-IC bypass, neurosurgeons have recently attempted revascularization of a cerebral hemisphere using omentum, either as a free graft or as a pedicle graft tunneled subcutaneously from the abdomen to brain.

The indications for cerebral revascularization, regardless of the specific surgical technique, are highly controversial. In general, clinical results would suggest that it is not a very effective operation for treatment of a completed stroke or a stroke in evolution.[13] An international randomized trial also failed to demonstrate any benefit from EC-IC bypass in preventing strokes.[14] However, this study was strongly criticized by neurosurgeons because of its failure to evaluate the benefits of the operation in specific subsets of patients who are seemingly particularly susceptible to strokes, such as those with symptoms and signs of transient ischemic attacks, and angiographic evidence of focal, intracranial cerebral ischemia, or patients with a history of a completed stroke with continuing evidence of ischemia.[15,16] Patients with symptomatic moyamoya disease or bilateral carotid occlusion with reversible ischemic neurologic deficits would also appear to be particularly good candidates for this operation, especially considering there are no other forms of therapy that have proven to be effective. Flow studies using electromagnetic flowmeters or radioisotope techniques indicate that flow is generally increased by 15 to 20% (or 30 to 35 ml/min) following EC-IC bypass, although this percentage is extremely variable, and may change with time following operation.[13] Patency rates average 90% or better when vessels of 1 mm diameter or greater are anastomosed. If smaller vessels are used, patency rates decrease rapidly.

Carotid Endarterectomy

The incidence of occlusive or ulcerative lesions of the extracranial or intracranial vasculature increases with advancing years. Although occasionally found in young and middle-aged adults, these disorders are most commonly manifest after the age of 40 years.

A number of risk factors have been reported to be associated with the development of carotid artery disease. These include a history of smoking, diabetes, hypertension, and elevated serum lipid levels. Whereas males are more likely to develop carotid artery disease, females may have more severe disease.[17] There is a positive correlation between carotid artery disease and both coronary artery and peripheral vascular diseases.[18,19]

Occlusive or ulcerative lesions may be found anywhere in cerebral vessels, but they occur most frequently at sites of branching of cerebral vessels, such as the bifurcation of the common carotid artery into its internal

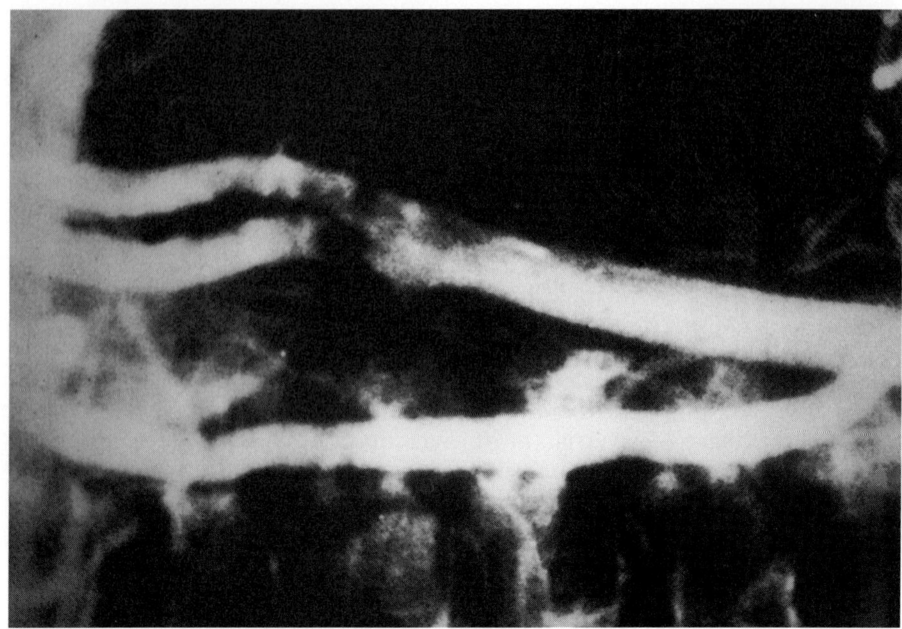

FIGURE **23–1.** Occlusive and ulcerative disease at the bifurcation of the internal carotid artery. (From Wylie EJ, Ehrenfeld WK (eds): Extracranial Occlusive Cerebrovascular Disease: Diagnosis and Management. Philadelphia, WB Saunders Co, 1970, with permission.)

and external branches (Fig. 23–1). While atherosclerosis is generally thought of as a diffuse vascular disease involving all arterial vessels uniformly, in this disease focal plaques accumulate at arterial branch points and cause progressive occlusion of the lumen of the vessels involved (Fig. 23–2). Generally these plaques do not cause any symptoms or signs from impaired CBF until the cross-sectional area of the lumen of the vessel is decreased by at least 50 to 70%.[20] The reason for this is that the cerebral vasculature has excellent collateral circulation, most importantly the circle of Willis (Fig. 23–3), but also the carotid-basilar anastomosis via the trigeminal artery and the extracranial-to-intracranial collateral flow via the ophthalmic artery or branches of the vertebral artery. Near total or total occlusion of one or both carotid arteries may not produce symptoms or signs in some patients if the collateral circulation is well developed.

The symptoms and signs of cerebrovascular insufficiency are due either to critical stenosis or occlusion of cerebral vessels, combined with inadequate collateral circulation, or to the development of ulcerative lesions at arterial branch points. The ulcerative lesions probably result either from degeneration of focal atherosclerotic plaques, or from destruction of the endothelium of the vessel and subsequent platelet aggregation and mural thrombus formation. The degenerative plaques or mural thrombi can break off from the vessel wall and are deposited into the arterial lumen where they travel among other places to terminal arterioles and capillaries in the cerebral circulation and cause focal ischemic lesions. Patients presenting for carotid endarterectomy will generally fall into one of three categories: transient ischemic attacks (TIAs), completed stroke, or asymptomatic bruit.

The relative risk of suffering a stroke is significantly different in patients who experience TIAs versus patients who are found to have asymptomatic bruits. The annual stroke risk rate in patients who develop TIAs is approximately 10% during the first year and then falls to an average of 5% in subsequent years.[19,21–25] Conversely, the stroke risk rate in patients with asymptomatic bruits is not only lower but varies in proportion to the degree

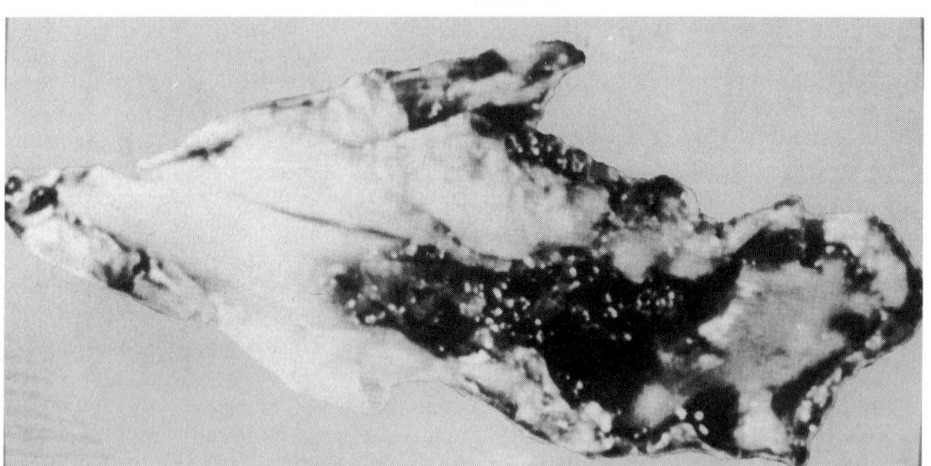

FIGURE **23–2.** Occlusion of the lumen at the point of arterial branching. (From Wylie EJ, Ehrenfeld WK (eds): Extracranial Occlusive Cerebrovascular Disease: Diagnosis and Management. Philadelphia, WB Saunders Co, 1970, with permission.)

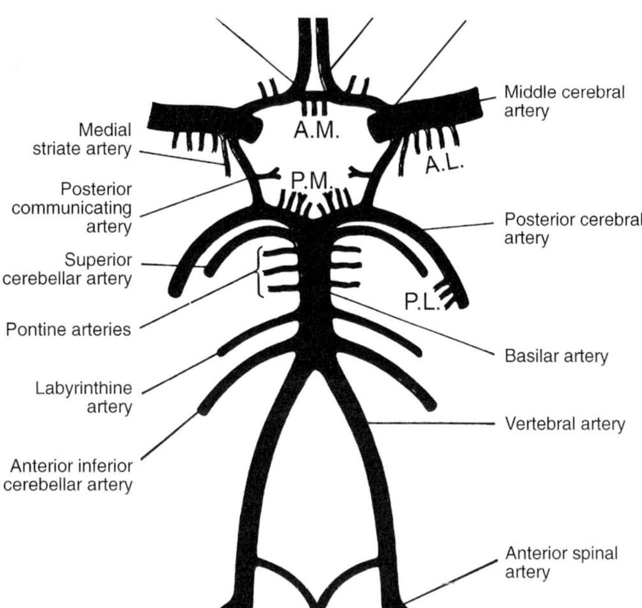

FIGURE **23–3.** Diagram of the arteries at the base of the brain, showing the constitution of the arterial circle. The arteries constituting this so-called arterial circle are commonly asymmetric and sometimes a constituent vessel is missing. AL, anterolateral central branches; AM, anteromedial central branches; PL, posterolateral central branches; PM, postermedial central branches. (From Gray's Anatomy, 38th ed. Edinburgh, Churchill Livingstone, 1995, with permission.)

of carotid stenosis. While patients with a stenosis greater than 75% experience a stroke risk of approximately 5% per year patients with carotid artery stenoses less than 75% experience an annual stroke risk rate of 1 to 2%.[19,25–33]

Transient Ischemic Attacks

These patients present with symptoms of TIAs that may be focal or generalized and include sensory deficits, motor weakness, speech disorder or monocular blindness if the lesion(s) is in the carotid vessels or vertigo, and ataxia or bilateral blurred vision if the lesion(s) is primarily in the vertebral vessels. TIAs generally resolve within 24 hours. Two recent clinical trials, one from North America[34] and the other from Europe,[35] clearly document that carotid endarterectomy is superior to medical management consisting of correction of hypertension, regulation of diet, cessation of smoking, and administration of platelet antiaggregation drugs in preventing the development of strokes in patients who are symptomatic from carotid stenosis of greater than 70%. Whether the same is true for patients who are symptomatic but have less than 70% stenosis is not yet documented.

Completed Stroke

These patients present with a history of a completed stroke, with or without a residual neurologic deficit. If the stroke is fresh (within 2 to 4 weeks), most surgeons will not operate on the patient for fear of converting an ischemic infarct into a hemorrhagic infarct. Angiographic evaluation following recovery from the acute stroke will demonstrate a stenotic and/or ulcerative lesion at the carotid bifurcation.

Asymptomatic Bruit

These are usually found on routine physical examination of the neck, and are of concern because they may signal the development of carotid stenosis. This population is not small, as evidenced by the Framingham Study in which the incidence was 3.5% among patients 44 to 54 years of age and 7% among patients 65 to 79 years of age.[29] There is no clear agreement about how these patients should be managed, since it is not known if the morbidity and mortality from endarterectomy exceeds the risk of a spontaneous stroke. Some studies indicate that the stroke rate is higher among those patients who do not receive an endarterectomy, but the Framingham Study indicated that an asymptomatic bruit is a nonfocal sign of advancing atherosclerotic disease rather than an indicator of local arterial stenosis which might later produce a cerebral infarction.

In a recent study from 11 Veterans Affairs medical centers, 444 men with asymptomatic carotid stenosis of 50% or more were randomly allocated to groups treated with medical therapy, aspirin, and carotid endarterectomy, or with just medical therapy and aspirin. These groups of patients were followed for up to 96 months (mean, 48 months).[36] The results indicate that ipsilateral neurologic events (TIAs or stroke) occurred in 8% of the surgical group and in 21% of the medical group. The incidence of stroke was 5% in the surgical group and 9% in the medical group, a difference that was not statistically significant. The overall incidence of stroke and death was not different in the two groups, suggesting that the operation itself did not decrease the death rate from strokes. The Asymptomatic Carotid Atherosclerosis Study in 1994 reported that surgery was superior to medical management in patients with a stenosis of 60% or greater, while others still recommend surgery for stenoses greater than 70%.[37–39] Indications for carotid endarterectomy in both the symptomatic and asymptomatic patients have recently been published.[40] Additional randomized trials must be completed to clarify the best management for this subset of patients with carotid disease.

Even more unclear is what the surgical and anesthetic management should be for patients with an asymptomatic bruit who require elective operations in which large fluctuations in blood pressure can be anticipated. Examples would be patients undergoing cardiac bypass surgery or major vascular surgery, or those in whom deliberate hypotension is desired. Questions always arise about how extensive the preoperative work-up for the bruit should be, and whether the patient can tolerate the hypotension. There is no clear answer to either of these questions, and in general local policy prevails. One approach would be to evaluate the patient by digital subtraction angiography, a safe, noninvasive study, and if this is normal to proceed with the planned operation. Support for this approach comes from studies such as that reported by Ropper et al.[41] in which they analyzed the incidence of strokes postoperatively in 104 patients with a carotid bruit preoperatively, most of whom were asymptomatic, as compared to 631 patients who did not have bruits. Although the number of patients with bruits was small, they found that the incidence of stroke postoperatively was no higher in these patients as compared to those without bruits.

Irrespective of the type of carotid lesion, percutaneous digital occlusion of the carotid arteries should not be performed at the time of preoperative evaluation. It is not a reliable test of tolerance to temporary circulatory occlusion, and it might endanger the patient by precipitating embolization from an ulcerative lesion or by inducing bradycardia and hypotension from activation of the carotid sinus reflex. However, it is desirable to position the patient's head in the operative position as a test of the effect of that position on CBF. Hyperextension and lateral rotation of the head may occlude vertebrobasilar flow by entrapment between the scalenus anticus and longus coli muscles and, if sustained, contribute to postoperative cerebral ischemia. Symptoms of dizziness or diplopia will emerge with this maneuver if CBF is compromised.

A variety of techniques are available for laboratory confirmation of the presence of extracranial or intracranial lesions,[42] but cerebral angiography remains the most informative and reliable method. Angiography will identify the type of lesion (ulcerative or stenotic), its exact location, and the extent of collateral circulation. Another technique for assessing the carotid circulation involves the intravenous injection of a contrast agent; through the use of computer reconstruction, a vascular image is formed. This method, called digital subtraction angiography, circumvents the need for arterial catheterization but does not give as clear or detailed an image as conventional angiography. More and more vascular surgeons are using noninvasive methods such as digital subtraction angiography or carotid duplex scanning as the initial study of the carotid circulation, reserving cerebral angiography for special circumstances where indirect evaluation is unsatisfactory.[43,44] As part of their preoperative evaluation, anesthesiologists can examine the angiograms of their patients so as to familiarize themselves with the type, location, and extent of the lesion.

Preoperative Preparation of Patients Undergoing Cerebral Vascular Surgery

Cardiovascular Function

In addition to the usual measures taken in preoperative evaluation of any patient undergoing anesthesia and surgery, there are special considerations that relate to patients who are to have cerebral vascular surgery. Most important among these is a careful evaluation of cardiovascular status, including a detailed history of cardiovascular function and serial determinations of blood pressure in both arms to establish the range of pressures that normally occur, and whether there are regional differences. Systolic blood pressure has been reported to vary by more than 20 mm Hg in over 20% of patients with peripheral vascular disease. The higher pressure was recorded in the right arm 60% of the time.[45] If the blood pressure is different in the two arms, it is desirable to measure it during surgery in the arm with the higher values. It is well to recognize that cerebral vascular disease may be a manifestation of systemic vascular disease, including coronary artery or renovascular disease, and perioperative outcome may benefit from careful preoperative evaluation and therapy for these systems.

Patients who have had a recent intracranial hemorrhage from leaking or rupture of a cerebral aneurysm are prone to develop systemic hypertension, hypovolemia,[46] and electrocardiographic abnormalities (especially in inferior leads and accompanying inferior wall motion abnormalities on echocardiogram [ECG].[47] The hypertension is thought to be due to autonomic hyperactivity, and is generally treated with antihypertensive medication, which should be continued up to the time of anesthesia and surgery. Why hypovolemia occurs following subarachnoid hemorrhage is not clear but may be due in part to cerebral vasospasm and to prolonged bed rest, which is known to decrease circulating blood volume. ECG abnormalities occur in 50 to 80% of patients who sustain an intracranial hemorrhage for unknown reasons. Appropriate preoperative preparation includes electrocardiographic characterization of the abnormality. If the patient has a history of ischemic heart disease, then echocardiographic and cardiac enzyme studies may be helpful in determining whether the ECG changes are due to primary heart disease or are secondary to the intracranial hemorrhage. Cardiac insufficiency is the cause of about half of the deaths following surgery in patients with cerebrovascular disease.[48] Chambers and Norris reported a significant correlation between carotid disease and coronary artery disease[19] (Figs. 23–4 through 23–6).

Careful evaluation of cardiovascular function is also important in patients undergoing carotid endarterectomy for two reasons. First, it is often necessary to administer vasoactive drugs to artificially regulate blood pressure during carotid endarterectomy, either to maintain it at a normal value, or sometimes to increase it as much as 20% above the highest resting pressure to maintain optimal collateral circulation during surgical carotid occlusion. Second, the incidence of perioperative myocardial

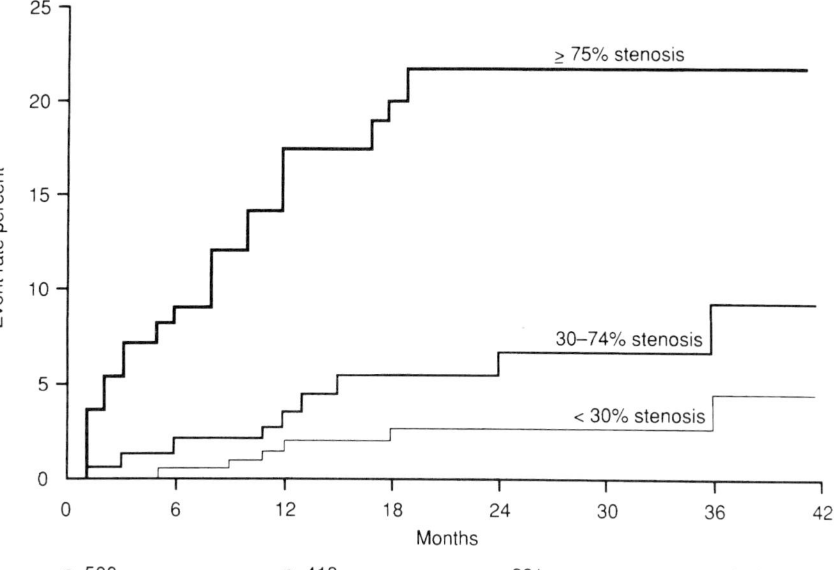

FIGURE **23–4.** Incidence of cerebral ischemic events (transient ischemic attack and stroke) in relation to severity of carotid artery stenosis. (From Chambers BR, Norris JW: Outcome in patients with asymptomatic neck bruits. N Engl J Med 315:860, 1986, with permission.)

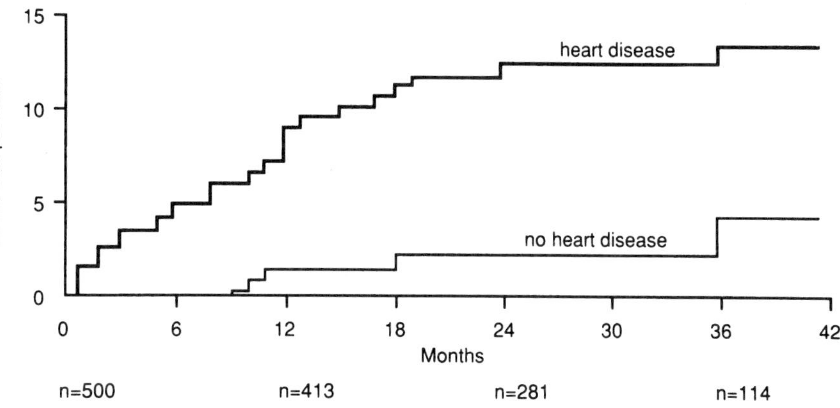

FIGURE **23–5.** Incidence of cerebral ischemic events (transient ischemic attack and stroke) in relation to pre-existing heart disease. (From Chambers BR, Norris JW: Outcome in patients with asymptomatic neck bruits. N Engl J Med 315:860, 1986, with permission.)

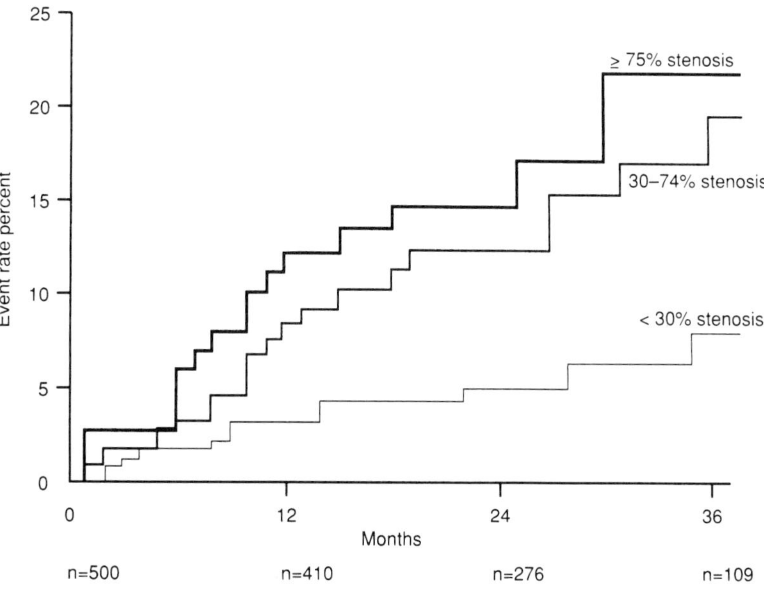

FIGURE **23–6.** Incidence of cardiac ischemic events in relation to the severity of carotid artery stenosis. (From Chambers BR, Norris JW: Outcome in patients with asymptomatic neck bruits. N Engl J Med 315:860, 1986, with permission.)

TABLE 23–1
Risk of Stroke in Patients with Symptomatic Carotid Occlusive Disease Undergoing Major Cardiovascular Surgery without Previous CEA*

Study	Characteristics	Type of Operation	No. of Patients	Risk of Stroke
Bower et al.,[50] 1993	Significant stenosis with transient ischemic attacks or recent ipsilateral stroke	Abdominal aortic repair	22	14%
Gerraty et al.,[51] 1993	Stenosis ≥50% with ipsilateral carotid territory cerebral ischemic symptoms	CABG Peripheral vascular surgery	49	8.2%
Hertzer et al.,[52] 1989	Signifiant stenosis with transient ischemic attacks or strokes	CABG	23	8.7%
Kartcher et al.,[53] 1982	Stenosis >60% with lateralizing neurologic symptoms	CABG Peripheral vascular surgery	41	17%

*From Wilke HJ II: Carotid Endarterectomy: Perioperative and Anesthesia Considerations. J Cardiol Vasc Anesth 10:928, 1996, with permission.
CEA, carotid endarterectomy; CABG, coronary artery bypass graft.

infarction in this surgical population is at least 1% and represents the most common, major postoperative complication from this operation. Except in the case of emergencies, anesthesia and operation should not proceed in the face of severe, uncontrolled hypertension, uncontrolled diabetes, or a myocardial infarction within the last 3 months.

The association between carotid artery disease and coronary artery disease presents a number of complex issues. If the patient has combined disease, which entity should be addressed first? The literature does not provide a clear answer to this question.[50–61] Tables 23–1 and 23–2 summarize the results of a number of studies that addressed the incidence of stroke in patients with either symptomatic or asymptomatic carotid disease who had undergone major cardiovascular surgery without prior carotid artery endarterectomy.[49] In patients with symptomatic carotid disease the stroke risk ranged from 8.2 to 17% compared to a stroke risk rate of 0.3 to 9.2% in patients with asymptomatic carotid disease. Conversely, the risk of a perioperative myocardial infarction following carotid endarterectomy ranged from 0 to 5% in patients known or suspected to have coronary artery disease compared to 0 to 2% in patients without coronary artery disease (Table 23–3).[49]

Some authors have recommended a combined operation in patients who have both coronary artery and carotid artery disease. Hertzer et al. reported a postoperative neurologic deficit rate of 8.1% and 10.0%, respectively, in patients with asymptomatic or symptomatic carotid artery disease following combined coronary artery and carotid artery surgery. The 5-year survival rate in patients having undergone a combined procedure was 83 ± 6% compared to 62 ± 13% in patients who had suspected coronary artery disease but had only undergone carotid artery surgery.[62] Craver et al. reported a stroke rate of 7.5% in patients undergoing combined carotid and coronary artery surgery.[63] Other authors have reported an operative mortality rate of as low as 2% and a neurologic complication rate as low as 3% in combined procedures.[64,65] In contrast, other series have reported perioperative mortality and stroke rates ranging

TABLE 23–2
Risk of Stroke in Patients with Asymptomatic Carotid Disease Undergoing Major Cardiovascular Surgery without Previous CEA*

Author/Year	Patient Characteristics	Type of Operation	No. of Patients	Risk of Stroke
Gerraty et al.,[51] 1993	Significant stenosis without ipsilateral carotid territory cerebral ischemic symptoms	CABG Peripheral vascular surgery	309	0.3%
Hertzer et al.,[52] 1989	Stenosis ≥70% without neurologic symptoms	CABG	58	6.9%
Reed et al.,[55] 1988	Carotid bruit	CABG	13	6.9%
Brener et al.,[56] 1987	Stenosis ≥50% without neurologic symptoms	CABG	153	9.2%
Schwartz et al.,[54] 1995	Stenosis >50% without neurologic symptoms	CABG	130	3.8%

*From Wilke HJ II: Carotid Endarterectomy: Perioperative and Anesthesia Considerations. J Cardiol Vasc Anesth 10:928, 1996, with permission.
CEA, carotid endarterectomy; CABG, coronary artery bypass graft.

TABLE 23-3
Risk of Perioperative Myocardial Infarction after CEA*

Study	No. of Patients	Basis for Determination of CAD	Risk of MI in Patients with Stable CAD	Risk of MI in Patients without Stable CAD	Overall Risk of MI in Entire Group of Patients	Overall Risk of Fatal MI in Entire Group of Patients
Urbinati et al.,[57] 1994	172	Clinical; thallium studies in selected cases	4%	0%	2%	2%
Urbanati et al.,[58] 1992	106	Clinical; thallium studies in selected cases	0%	0%	0%	0%
Rihal et al.,[59] 1992	177	Clinical	3%	2%	2.5%	0%
Mackey et al.,[60] 1990	614	Clinical	4.3%	0.7%	2.6%	0.3%
Yeager et al.,[61] 1989	224	Clinical	5%	1.5%	4.0%	0.4%
			3.2%**	0.84%**	2.2%**	0.54%**

*From Wilke HJ II: Carotid Endarterectomy: Perioperative and Anesthesia Considerations. J Cardiol Vasc Anesth 10:928, 1996, with permission.
**Average risk from all five studies.
CEA, carotid endarterectomy; CAD, coronary artery disease; MI, myocardial infarction.

from 8 to 40% in combined procedures.[66] There does not appear to be a clear approach to patients with combined disease. Each patient should be evaluated individually taking into account the severity of the two disease processes and institutional experience.

Respiratory Function

A history of moderate or severe pulmonary disease can be evaluated with spirometry, arterial blood gas determination, and chest roentgenogram. If there is evidence of pulmonary infection, appropriate antibiotic therapy should be instituted. If secretions are excessive, preoperative pulmonary physiotherapy including bronchodilator therapy may be indicated. Patients can be encouraged to stop smoking prior to anesthesia, even if only the night before. While cessation of smoking for such a short time will not lessen the volume of secretions appreciably or make the airways less irritable to a foreign body such as an endotracheal tube, it will provide sufficient time for the carbon monoxide levels in the blood to decrease, thereby enhancing the blood's oxygen-carrying capacity. And it may well lead to permanent cessation of smoking. Any patient who has sustained a neurologic deficit from an intracranial hemorrhage or cerebral ischemia from a carotid lesion is a candidate for pulmonary aspiration, which should be treated before proceeding with cerebrovascular surgery.

Neurologic Function

Neurologic function may be impaired either because of a prior hemorrhage and resultant neurologic deficits, or because of ischemia associated with inadequate cerebral perfusion. Control of blood pressure is particularly important in patients with a history of neurologic dysfunction. Any substantial increase in blood pressure may cause a serious rebleed, death, or permanent neurologic deficits; any substantial decrease in blood pressure may cause cerebral ischemia and infarction. As a consequence, consideration should be given to arterial catheterization and continuous beat-to-beat monitoring of blood pressure prior to induction of anesthesia in patients with aneurysms, AVMs, or potential cerebral ischemia because of extracranial or intracranial vascular occlusive disease.

Hematologic Function

Because many of these patients are taking anticoagulants or platelet-suppressive drugs such as aspirin, an analysis of hematocrit and platelet function should be considered before proceeding with operation. When desirable for surgical hemostasis (AVMs, aneurysms) these drugs can be discontinued a week prior to surgery. Failure to ensure adequate clotting prior to initiating intracranial surgery may result in difficulty controlling bleeding during operation or an intracranial hemorrhage postoperatively, both of which may result in disastrous neurologic consequences.

Premedication

Premedication is seldom necessary in adults; a detailed discussion with the patient and family about the anesthetic plan with appropriate reassurance is usually enough. Signs of an intracranial aneurysm leak or rupture, or of a new TIA or stroke occurring in the immediate preoperative period, may be difficult to distinguish from those associated with excessive responses to premedication. If medication is desired, small doses of a sedative-hypnotic such as midazolam 2 to 5 mg is preferable to opiates.

Intraoperative Considerations

Anesthetic Technique

In the developmental stage of carotid endarterectomy, regional anesthesia in the form of a superficial and deep cervical plexus block supplemented as needed by a local field block was used by most anesthesiologists and surgeons. Regional anesthesia was considered advantageous because it allowed the surgeon and anesthesiologist to evaluate cerebral function during surgical carotid occlusion. Once the carotid artery was exposed, a trial occlusion of 2 or 3 minutes was carried out. If the patient showed no adverse effects, the operation was completed under regional anesthesia. If the patient developed neurologic changes, a shunt was inserted or general anesthesia was induced and endotracheal intubation performed following which the operation was completed. However, in the 1970s regional anesthesia fell out of favor as the anesthetic technique of choice for both theoretical and practical reasons. Theoretically, regional anesthesia provides no protection to the brain should ischemia occur, while general anesthesia clearly does.[67,68] Practically, regional anesthesia presents several important problems. The conventional 2- or 3-minute trial of carotid occlusion does not always distinguish those patients who will or will not tolerate a period of surgical occlusion.[69] Patients may tolerate occlusion for 10 minutes or more before suddenly losing consciousness or developing a seizure. Once a carotid endarterectomy has begun under regional anesthesia, it is technically difficult and potentially hazardous to the patient to convert it quickly to a general anesthetic should the patient suddenly develop symptoms or signs of intolerance to the occlusion. Performing endotracheal intubation under the sterile surgical drapes to gain control of the airway with an open wound close by in a patient evidencing neurologic injury is not an event that most anesthesiologists want to experience more than once. Likewise, inserting a shunt under emergency conditions is not always uneventful. Finally, the incidence of operative (about 24%) and permanent postoperative (2.6%) neurologic complications including hemiparesis, monoparesis, and dysphasia can be relatively high[70] compared to those recommended by a committee of the Stroke Council of the American Heart Association.[71] Considering the caveats, it is somewhat surprising that regional anesthesia alone or in combination with infusions of propofol and fentanyl or other short-acting opiates has had a resurgence as an anesthetic technique for carotid endarterectomy, and the technique has an increasing number of advocates among anesthesiologists and surgeons.[66,69–77] Those centers continuing to use this technique claim that it more readily identifies patients who are at greater risk of developing permanent neurologic deficits, thereby decreasing the need to use a surgical shunt and avoiding the attendant complications of shunt insertion[70,74,76]; that because patients are alert during or immediately after operation it may permit more selective determination of which patients need postoperative intensive care unit (ICU) care[70]; that it decreases the length of stay in the ICU[71]; and that as an anesthetic technique it is well accepted by patients.[73]

The most common techniques for regional anesthesia frequently involve the use of a deep cervical plexus block that is often combined with a superficial cervical plexus block or a stellate ganglion block. Local infiltration and cervical epidurals are also described as effective techniques.[78–81] The deep cervical plexus block is performed with the intent of blocking nerves originating from C^2–C^4. Nerve root C^1 carries no sensory pathways and therefore block of this nerve root is not required.[82,83] The dermatone distribution of C^2–C^4 and methods to perform a superficial or deep cervical plexus block are depicted in Figures 23–7 through 23–9.[82,85] Relative and/or absolute contraindications to regional anesthesia include patient anticoagulation or clotting abnormalities, patient refusal, or infection at the site of the block. Possible complications include intravascular injection (including seizures following vertebral artery injection), total spinal anesthesia, spinal cord trauma, and/or phrenic nerve paralysis. Phrenic nerve paralysis is a major consideration in patients with limited pulmonary reserve such as those with advanced chronic obstructive pulmonary disease (COPD).

Despite its advocates, many anesthesiologists and surgeons have abandon regional anesthesia in favor of general anesthesia for this operation. General anesthesia offers both direct and indirect advantages for patients undergoing carotid endarterectomy. Recognizing that whether or not a surgical shunt is used there will be periods during the operation of potentially inadequate cerebral perfusion because of surgical carotid occlusion, general anesthesia offers the direct advantage of protecting ischemic brain by decreasing cerebral oxygen consumption and redistributing flow toward the potentially ischemic area. The indirect advantages are those of greater patient comfort and, more importantly, the ability to regulate arterial oxygen and carbon dioxide tensions and arterial blood pressure to maximize oxygenation and perfusion to potentially ischemic brain. This ability is important because the brain has a high rate of metabolism with essentially no storage capacity for oxygen. Consequently, any sustained interruption of CBF without a corresponding decrease in cerebral metabolism ($CMRO_2$) may produce neurologic sequelae. Normal values for cerebral variables are presented in Table 23–4.

Despite arguments favoring general anesthesia, recent studies comparing regional and general anesthesia suggest that there is no clear advantage of one technique over the other. In one retrospective study comparing regional and general anesthesia in 175 patients considered "high risk" for stroke because of contralateral carotid stenosis or occlusion, use of regional anesthesia decreased the need for surgical shunts because most patients did not evidence cerebral ischemia during surgical occlusion.[76] Furthermore, the incidence of stroke was no

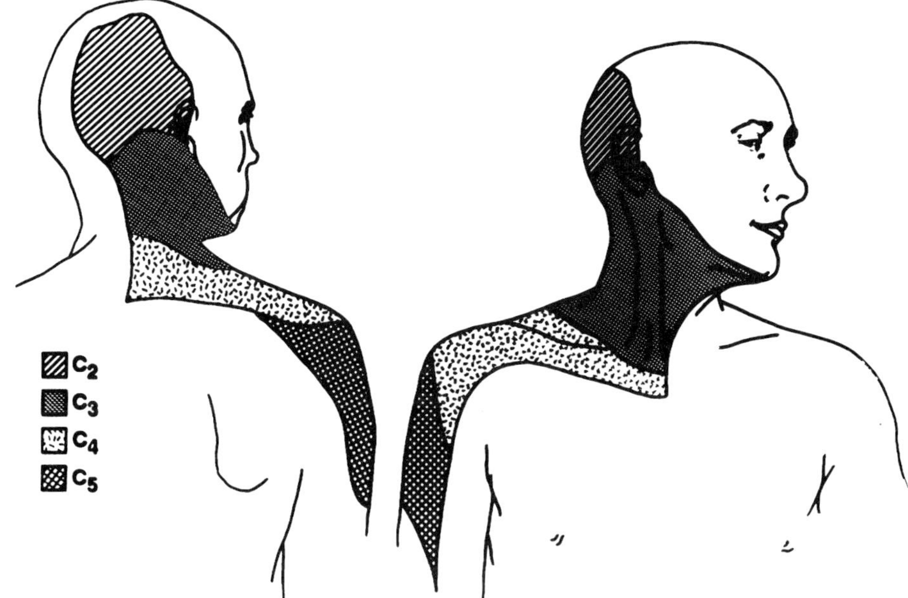

FIGURE **23–7.** Dermatome distribution of cervical nerves. (From Youngberg JA, Neely CF: Perioperative considerations for the carotid artery surgery patient. Adv Anesth 5: 291, 1988, with permission.)

greater in the regional than in the general group. In another retrospective study, 361 patients undergoing carotid endarterectomy received general anesthesia and 318 received regional anesthesia.[75] While the incidence of postoperative stroke (6% general, 4% regional), wound hematoma or infection (2% general, 1% regional), and death (4% general, 2% regional) were not significantly different between the two groups, the incidence of postoperative cardiovascular complications including arrhythmias, myocardial infarction, and blood pressure instability was significantly greater in the general group (8%) versus the regional group (4%). Considering all events, the postoperative complication rate was 16% in the general group and 9% in the regional group. Finally, the operating room time and length of hospital stay were significantly greater in the general group, resulting in a significant increase in hospital costs. Another retrospective review supports the conclusion that cardiovascular complications are more common in patients undergoing general anesthesia than regional anesthesia for carotid endarterectomy.[77] The incidence of postoperative ventricular dysrhythmias was 14% in 126 patients given general anesthesia and 6% in 140 patients given regional anesthesia, a significant difference. However, there were no significant differences in the incidence of postoperative death, myocardial infarction, or stroke. In a retrospective study of 1,000 patients undergoing carotid endarterectomy, Fiorani et al. reported no significant difference between regional and general anesthesia with respect to the incidence of cardiac complications; however, the stroke rate was 1.3% in the regional group compared to 3.2% in the general group (Table 23–5).[86] In summary, it would seem that either regional or general anesthesia is suitable when the anesthesiologists and surgeons are experienced in working with their technique of choice.

For all intracranial vascular surgery, general endotracheal anesthesia is preferred. The goals of anesthesia for intracranial vascular surgery are to (1) provide adequate surgical anesthesia; (2) maintain optimum cerebral perfusion pressure (CPP), which is cerebral arterial pressure minus cerebral venous or ICP, whichever is greater, but

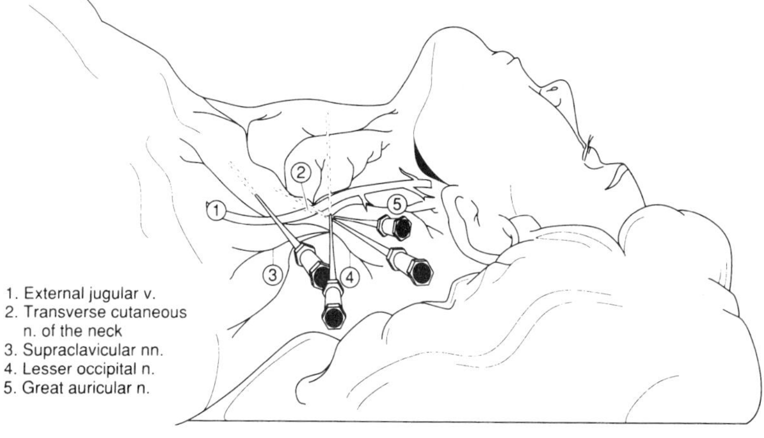

FIGURE **23–8.** Superficial cervical plexus block. v, vein; n, nerve. (From Youngberg JA, Neely CF: Perioperative considerations for the carotid artery surgery patient. Adv Anesth 5:291, 1988, with permission.)

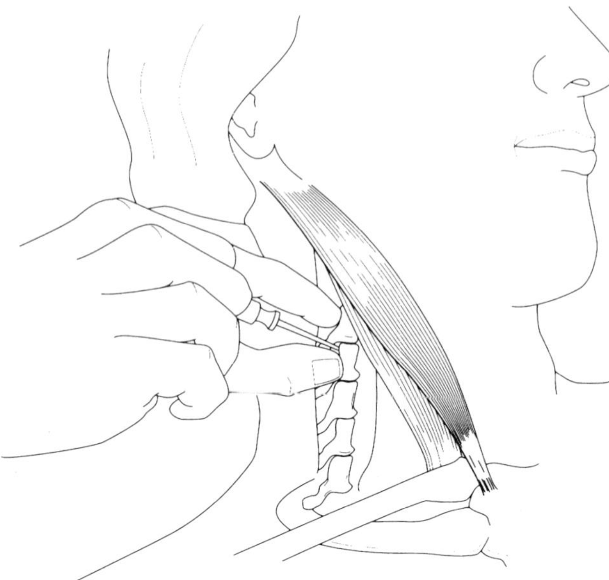

FIGURE **23–9.** Single-injection interscalene approach to the block of the cervical plexus. (From Winnie AB: Cervical plexus block simplified: A single injection technique. Anesth Analg 54:370, 1975, with permission.)

to be prepared to decrease CPP rapidly and profoundly if intracranial hemorrhage should occur during clipping of an aneurysm or excision of an AVM; (3) decrease intracranial volume (blood and tissue) to optimize the working space for the neurosurgeons within the cranial compartment, thereby minimizing the need for surgical retraction of brain tissue; and (4) minimize metabolic rate and $CMRO_2$ with the expectation that the brain will tolerate severe hypotension and ischemia if sudden decreases in systemic blood pressure and hence CPP should occur.

Induction of Anesthesia

Among the anesthetic drugs available for induction of anesthesia, both thiopental and propofol are suitable for achieving these goals. Arterial blood pressure, and hence CPP, will generally remain at acceptable levels during

TABLE **23–4**
Normal Values for Cerebral Variables

Variable	Value
Cerebral blood flow (CBF)	40–50 ml/100 g/min
Cerebral perfusion pressure (CPP) = MAP − ICP	80 mm Hg
Cerebral metabolic rate for oxygen ($CMRO_2$)	Adult 3–3.5 ml/100 g/min Child 5 ml/100 g/min Infant 2.5 ml/100 g/min
Cerebral metabolic rate for glucose (CMR gl)	1.28 μmol/g/min
Cerebral arteriovenous O_2 difference [$C(a\text{-}\bar{v})O_2$]	6.8 ml O_2/100 ml

TABLE **23–5**
Regional versus General Anesthesia for CEA

Study	Anesthesia	Outcome
Gableman et al.,[72] 1983	46 Gen vs. 54 Reg	4.3% MI vs. 0% MI
Allen et al.,[75] 1994	361 Gen vs. 318 Reg	N.S. difference
Ombrello et al.,[77] 1996	126 Gen vs. 140 Reg	N.S. difference
Fiorani et al.,[86] 1997	1,000 Patients total	3.2% stroke vs. 1.3% stroke

CEA, carotid endarterectomy; Gen, general; Reg, regular; MI, myocardial infarction; N.S., not significant.

induction with either of these agents, provided they are not given too rapidly and provided hypovolemia is treated with fluids prior to or during induction. Thiopental and propofol are also the most effective anesthetic drugs for decreasing $CMRO_2$. Finally, because of their ability to constrict normally reactive cerebral vessels, thiopental and propofol cause a redistribution of CBF toward potentially ischemic neurosurgical areas, thereby lessening the severity of neurosurgically induced ischemia. Propofol has the additional advantages of allowing the patient to emerge promptly from surgical anesthesia at the conclusion of the operation, as well as being a very good antiemetic.

One method for induction is to administer thiopental 10 mg/kg or propofol 3 to 5 mg/kg slowly by continuous infusion using a pump to allow time for assessment of cardiovascular responses. During induction the patient is instructed to breathe oxygen from a tight-fitting face mask attached to a circle anesthetic system with an oxygen inflow of 10 L/min. If there is concern about the possibility of hypotension from the use of thiopental or propofol, lidocaine 1.5 mg/kg intravenously can be combined with a lower doses of thiopental or propofol, recognizing that lidocaine is acting as a general anesthetic in the same manner as thiopental or propofol but without their myocardial depressant effects. Etomidate 0.3 to 0.5 mg/kg is also a suitable drug for induction of anesthesia especially for patients in whom there is concern about cardiovascular stability. Once consciousness is lost, a nondepolarizing muscle relaxant such as vecuronium 0.15 mg/kg, cisatracurium 0.1 to 0.2 mg/kg, or rocuronium 0.5 to 0.6 mg/kg is administered to provide muscle relaxation for tracheal intubation and positioning of the patient. During the induction phase, it is also appropriate to administer opiates for purposes of analgesia, the choice of drug being left to personal preference since they all have minimal effects on CBF or $CMRO_2$. Meperidine 2 to 3 mg/kg, fentanyl 2 to 5 μg/kg, or sufentanil 0.2 to 0.3 μg/kg may be given in divided doses or by continuous infusion during the first hour after the start of induction to minimize the cardiovascular responses to endotracheal intubation and application of the Mayfield headrest. Although not studied in patients undergoing neurovascular surgery, remifentanil given by continuous infusion may be an excellent opiate for these operations because of its rapid onset and recovery. Preliminary studies indicate that remifentanil has cerebrovascular effects that are similar to those for the other commonly used opiates.[87]

If the patient is in a stereotactic frame, endotracheal intubation is best accomplished before anesthesia is induced, because the frame partially occludes the mouth, making conventional laryngoscopy difficult. Oral fiberoptic intubation of the trachea is usually preferred over the nasal approach because it is generally easier and quicker, and is the more comfortable method for the patient. I (C.P.L.) will describe the technique that I use. Following moderate sedation with meperidine 0.5 to 1 mg/kg and midazolam 0.01 to 0.02 mg/kg, I spray the oropharynx vigorously three or four times over a span of 8 to 10 minutes using lidocaine 4% solution. Initially the spray is directed at the front of the tongue and gradually is directed further back in the throat until the entire oropharynx is numb. In reality, the lateral recesses of the oropharynx need not be topically anesthetized because during insertion both the fiberoptic laryngoscope and endotracheal tube should always be in the midline of the mouth. Then I administer a translaryngeal (transtracheal) injection of cocaine 4%, 2 to 3 ml using a 3-ml syringe and a 23-gauge 3/4-inch needle. To allow this injection to be made as rapidly as possible, it is important to use a small syringe, making certain that the connection between the syringe and needle is tight. Usually the injection is completed and the needle removed from the larynx before the patient begins to cough. However, since this is not always the case, it is important that the operator's hand be fixed firmly against the patient's skin at the time of injection to ensure that the full injection is made into the trachea. Once the injection is completed, the patient is urged to cough vigorously.

Once the mouth and trachea are anesthetized with local anesthetic, an oral airway with a central orifice (e.g., Tudor Williams, Patel) is placed in the midline of the mouth. I place a 7.0- to 7.5-mm orotracheal tube without the connector attached over a fiberoptic laryngoscope, and standing at the patient's side near the waist introduce the fiberoptic laryngoscope through the hole in the airway and advance it to the end of the airway. At this point the epiglottis should be visible. Passing the fiberoptic scope behind the epiglottis, I then flex the tip of the scope directly toward the patient's feet about 15 to 20 degrees, which usually brings the arytenoid cartilages and laryngeal opening into view. I then advance the scope slowly into the larynx visualizing tracheal rings and often a small blood spot from the site of injection of the cocaine. I then place the scope on the patient's chest, and holding it so that it does not advance further, slide the orotracheal tube gently into the trachea. To facilitate passage of the orotracheal tube past the arytenoid cartilages and into the larynx, it is often necessary to rotate the tube *counterclockwise* 90 or even as much as 180 degrees several times as it is being gently advanced. This rotational movement changes the plane of the bevel of the tube, directing it more toward the middle of the laryngeal opening, and obviates the need to ever push hard on the tube to position it in the larynx. Once the tube is in place, I remove the fiberoptic laryngoscope and oral airway, and attach a 15-mm connector to the tube. To verify that the tube is properly positioned, I attach a commercial device to the connector that will make a distinct whistle as the patient exhales. As one becomes more experienced with fiberoptic intubation, it is useful to be able to insert the fiberoptic scope into the larynx using external landmarks instead of relying entirely on visualization through the eyepiece of the scope. This technique is particularly useful in patients who have unusual anatomy because of prior oropharyngeal surgery or who have blood in the oropharynx. To do this I darken the operating room, and use the light reflecting from the scope through the skin over the oropharynx and sternal notch (similar to the technique for using a light wand) to direct the scope into the larynx. I then tape the orotracheal tube firmly in place at one side of the mouth. After anesthesia is induced I inflate the cuff on the tracheal tube and confirm its position near the sternal notch by ballottement. Standing at the patient's side rather than at the more conventional head of the bed or operating room table while performing fiberoptic laryngoscopy has three important advantages for the anesthesiologist, particularly when working alone: (1) rapid visualization of the patient and the monitors is easier, since the operator need only look up rather than turning sideways or walking around the bed or table; (2) the patient can be placed in a sitting or semirecumbant position rather than supine, which keeps the upper airway more open, making fiberoptic laryngoscopy easier; and (3) maintaining proper orientation of the fiberoptic scope is more likely, since the only motion required is flexion of the scope toward the patient's feet.

Maintenance of Anesthesia

Anesthesia may be maintained by a variety of agents. One satisfactory method for intracranial surgery is to continue to administer thiopental by continuous infusion to a total dose not to exceed about 20 to 25 mg/kg, and to be completed within 2 hours of induction. This dose provides additional amnesia, decreases cerebral blood volume, and maintains a lowered cerebral metabolism and oxygen consumption, all of which are the goals of cerebrovascular anesthesia. Propofol by continuous infusion at doses of 50 to 200 μg/kg/min may be used in place of thiopental for maintenance of anesthesia, since it has the same general pharmacologic effects on the brain. Unlike thiopental, propofol administration can be continued until the near conclusion of the operation because of its much more rapid biotransformation to inactive compounds by the liver. Isoflurane 1% or less inspired is usually administered either with oxygen or a mixture of nitrous oxide and oxygen. Some anesthesiologists prefer not to use nitrous oxide because of its potential for reversing the protective effects of thiopental from focal ischemia at light to moderate levels of barbiturate anesthesia.[88,89] Isoflurane in doses of 1% or less is thought to have cerebral protective effects from focal ischemia. Whether cerebral protection occurs at higher doses is controversial. Meyer and Muzzi[90] administered isoflurane to 2 to 2.5 minimal alveolar concentration (MAC) (2.4 o 3% concentration with oxygen) to produce electroencephalogram (EEG) isoelectricity in six patients undergoing cerebral aneurysm clipping. Phenylephrine was administered as needed to maintain normal cardiovascular function. Cerebral circulatory occlusion time varied from 20 to 135 minutes. All patients made an uneventful recovery, suggesting that isoflurane at high doses may be protective, perhaps through EEG suppression. Opiates such as fentanyl, alfentanil, or sufentanil can also be used by continuous infusion for maintenance of anesthesia. However, as drugs for maintenance, they provide analgesia but have none of the advantages of thiopental or propofol on cerebral volume or metabolism. While many neuroanesthesiologists administer nondepolarizing neuromuscular blocking drugs throughout anesthesia for neurovascular procedures because of their concern for patient movement or bucking on the endotracheal tube, these drugs are not necessary if adequate anesthesia is maintained. However, neuromuscular blocking drugs are advisable when cardiopulmonary bypass is to be used for clipping of a giant aneurysm.

One investigator has reported on the use of propofol as total intravenous anesthesia (TIVA) in 42 patients undergoing clipping of a cerebral aneurysm.[91] With a background infusion of fentanyl, anesthesia was induced with propofol 1.8 mg/kg, and maintained with 86 mg/kg/hr. Just prior to temporary clipping of the major feeding vessel, propofol 500 μg/kg/min was administered to produce burst suppression. Blood pressure was maintained using volume loading and dopamine 3 to 7 μg/kg/min. Postoperatively, 32 of 42 patients had Glasgow Coma Scale values of 13 or greater. This was regarded as an excellent outcome considering that in 35 of the 42 patients the cerebral aneurysm had hemorrhaged prior to surgery.

For carotid endarterectomy, isoflurane up to 1% inspired either alone or in combination with nitrous oxide 60% is satisfactory. Isoflurane is believed to be superior to either enflurane or halothane for this operation because of its relative protective effect in focal cerebral ischemia. Critical CBF, or blood flow below which EEG changes indicative of cerebral ischemia during carotid cross-clamp appear, is significantly lower (10 ml/100 g/min) for isoflurane than for halothane (20 ml/100 g/min) or enflurane (15 ml/100 g/min).[92] In addition, just prior to surgical cross-clamping of the carotid artery an additional dose of thiopental sufficient to produce burst suppression on the EEG (usually about 5 mg/kg) may be administered for its cerebral protective effects. Frawley et al. have suggested that thiopental adequately protects the brain during carotid endarterectomy, and that a surgical shunt is obsolete and never needed.[93] While under general anesthesia, 259 patients with carotid disease on one side and severe stenosis or occlusion on the other side were given sufficient thiopental to produce sustained burst suppression just prior to carotid occlusion. The total dose of thiopental administered averaged 1,350 mg (range, 600 to 3,000 mg). No shunt was used in any patient. The combined cerebral morbidity/mortality rate was 1.2%, which is similar to other studies. The only drawback to this anesthetic technique was the fact that the patients generally remained anesthetized for about 2 hours postoperatively.

Is inhalation anesthesia better than intravenous anesthesia for patients undergoing carotid endarterectomy? Mutch and colleagues[94] attempted to answer this question in a prospective study in 27 patients, 13 of whom received isoflurane in oxygen and a continuous infusion of alfentanil 30 μg/kg/hr, and 14 of whom received propofol 3 to 12 mg/kg/hr and alfentanil 30 μg/kg/hr for maintenance of anesthesia. Patients given isoflurane required a significantly higher dose of phenylephrine to maintain hemodynamic stability during the operation, but there was no difference in the two groups in terms of heart rate, blood pressure or ECG evidence of myocardial ischemia during the operation. However, on emergence from anesthesia patients given isoflurane evidenced significantly more hypertension and myocardial ischemia, and required significantly more vasodilator and/or β-blockade therapy to bring the heart rate and blood pressure under control. Despite the higher incidence of myocardial ischemia, the incidence of postoperative myocardial infarction was not different between the two groups, and no patients emerged from anesthesia with a new neurologic deficit. Unfortunately, this study does not answer the question whether a primary volatile anesthetic or a primary intravenous anesthetic is better for patients undergoing carotid endarterectomy.[95] However, it does clearly indicate that for whatever reason, isoflurane anesthesia is associated with more postoperative hemodynamic instability and myocardial ischemia that must be treated to avoid serious cardiac sequellae.

Monitoring

Monitoring of arterial pressure directly from a cannula placed in a radial or other convenient artery is considered essential by most anesthesiologists during cerebral vascular surgery. The marked fluctuations in blood pressure that may occur necessitating hypertensive or hypotensive drug therapy as well as the need for blood gas data make intra-arterial manometry desirable in most patients. If careful regulation of blood pressure is important, the arterial cannula can be placed before induction of anesthesia. If the patient is in a semisitting position, I place the transducer at the level of the head rather than the heart, since cerebral perfusion pressure is arterial pressure at the brain level, which might be substantially lower than that at the heart level in this position.

Monitoring of central venous pressure (CVP) via a right atrial catheter is considered desirable by anesthesiologists in most patients undergoing intracranial vascular surgery. The catheter is necessary to assess the adequacy of fluid therapy in the operative and postoperative periods as well as for infusion of vasoactive drugs, which are commonly used during and after neurovascular surgery. The ideal site for insertion of the catheter in order of preference is the right internal jugular, the right subclavian, and the right external jugular vein. Localization of the catheter may be determined by chest x-ray, by ECG tracing noting the P wave changes, or by pressure wave contour and values as the catheter is withdrawn from the right ventricle into the right atrium. If the patient has a high-flow AVM causing a large arteriovenous shunt, venous blood may appear arterialized or bright red during central venous catheterization suggesting wrongly that the operator has punctured an artery rather than a central vein. A CVP catheter is less necessary for a patient undergoing carotid endarterectomy. Vasoactive drugs can be given quickly and safely through a cannula placed in the upper arm.

Additional routine monitors include the ECG, urine output, ventilatory frequency, heart tones from a chest or esophageal stethoscope, and body temperature. Two additional monitors that are extremely valuable are an infrared carbon dioxide analyzer for monitoring end-tidal carbon dioxide (CO_2) tension, and a pulse oximeter for monitoring peripheral oxygen saturation. Once correlated with a simultaneously drawn arterial blood-gas sample, the end-tidal CO_2 analyzer provides a continuous indication of arterial carbon dioxide level because it generally maintains a constant relationship to arterial carbon dioxide even during long neurosurgical operations.[96] The relationship between CBF, blood pressure, $Pa{O_2}$ and $Pa{CO_2}$ is depicted in Figure 23–10.[97]

Monitoring for adequacy of cerebral perfusion is important during carotid endarterectomy even if a shunt is used, because temporary periods of occlusion of a major cerebral vessel are always necessary. There is no perfect monitor for use during general anesthesia which is why some surgeons strongly prefer to keep the patient awake during the operation. The "gold standard" for monitoring the adequacy of cerebral perfusion under general anesthesia is the measurement of regional cerebral blood flow (rCBF) using the washout of the radioisotope, xenon-133. Flows above 24 ml/min/100 g brain are regarded as satisfactory, and those below 18 ml/min/100 g brain are regarded as indicating the potential for cerebral ischemia. While ideal, the ability to make rCBF measurements in the operating room is limited to a few centers and is not generally practical for most institutions.

A more widely used method for assessing neurologic function is the EEG. Often, patients will have abnormal EEG tracings preoperatively, but such abnormalities do not predict the likelihood of cerebral ischemia during

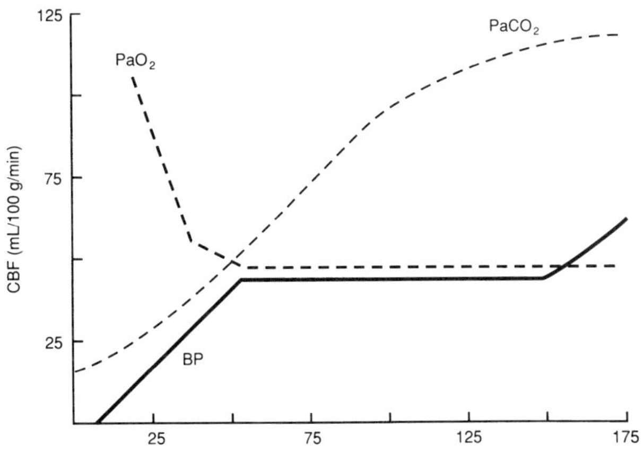

FIGURE **23–10.** Changes in cerebral blood flow (CBF) due to alterations in $Pa{CO_2}$, and blood pressure (BP). (From Shapiro HM: In Miller RM (ed): Anesthesia, 2nd ed. New York, Churchill Livingstone, 1986, with permission.)

carotid endarterectomy.[98] The relationship of EEG abnormalities to change in CBF and cerebral oxygenation is depicted in Figure 23–11.[97] With the development of spectral compression EEG techniques, on-line assessment of cerebral perfusion is possible. A variety of new instruments have recently emerged that will permit computerized EEG analysis in the operating room by the anesthesiologist. However, computerized analysis of spectral array density is not as good as conventional 16-channel EEG analysis for detecting mild cerebral ischemia.[99] The major disadvantages of conventional EEG analysis are four: namely, the EEG usually does not change until severe cerebral ischemia occurs, so it is not a good prodromal indicator of ischemia; the EEG may not identify small focal areas of ischemia; the depth of anesthesia and level of ventilation must be held stable or the EEG will not be interpretable; and there is a high incidence of false-positives and false-negatives, which makes interpretation of changes more difficult.[100] Monitoring of somatosensory evoked potentials (SSEPs) has been advocated by one group to determine adequacy of cerebral perfusion during temporary occlusion of a major cerebral artery such as the middle cerebral during aneurysm surgery.[101] Another group has not found SSEPs to be a reliable indicator of cerebral ischemia. In this study, 23 of 53 patients undergoing carotid endarterectomy under general anesthesia had evidence of cerebral ischemia by conventional EEG analysis, but only 10 of the 23 had an increase in SSEP latency, and only 1 of the 23 had a decrease in amplitude.[102]

Stump pressure (pressure distal to the carotid clamp, also sometimes called back-pressure) is used by some to evaluate the adequacy of cerebral perfusion during carotid surgery. Cerebral ischemia will rarely occur at stump pressures above 60 mm Hg, because of the excellent collateral circulation required to maintain that pressure. As the stump pressure decreases below that value, the chance for ischemia increases. However, since pressure is not identical to flow, it is possible to have stump pressures below 60 mm Hg and have adequate flow. The major criticism of stump pressure is the large number of false positives, that is, a stump pressure of less than 60 mm Hg and a rCBF of more than 24 ml/min/100 g brain. False-positives occur in about 33% of patients,[103] and often result in a shunt being placed when none is needed. Regardless of this criticism, the simplicity of the measurement and its validity when pressure exceeds 60 mm Hg still make it a useful clinical method for helping to ensure adequate perfusion during carotid endarterectomy.

One group of investigators has found transcranial Doppler scanning a useful method for detecting microemboli (air or particulate matter) during carotid endarterectomy.[104] They reported one case in which average velocity over the distribution of the middle cerebral artery on the operative side decreased suddenly after closure of the wound. Subsequent re-exploration revealed a thrombosis of the internal carotid artery at the operative site. Cerebral oximetry has also been used to evaluate cerebral perfusion during carotid endarterectomy.[105] Two cerebral oximeters whose light intensity is greater and bandwidth broader than that for conventional pulse ox-

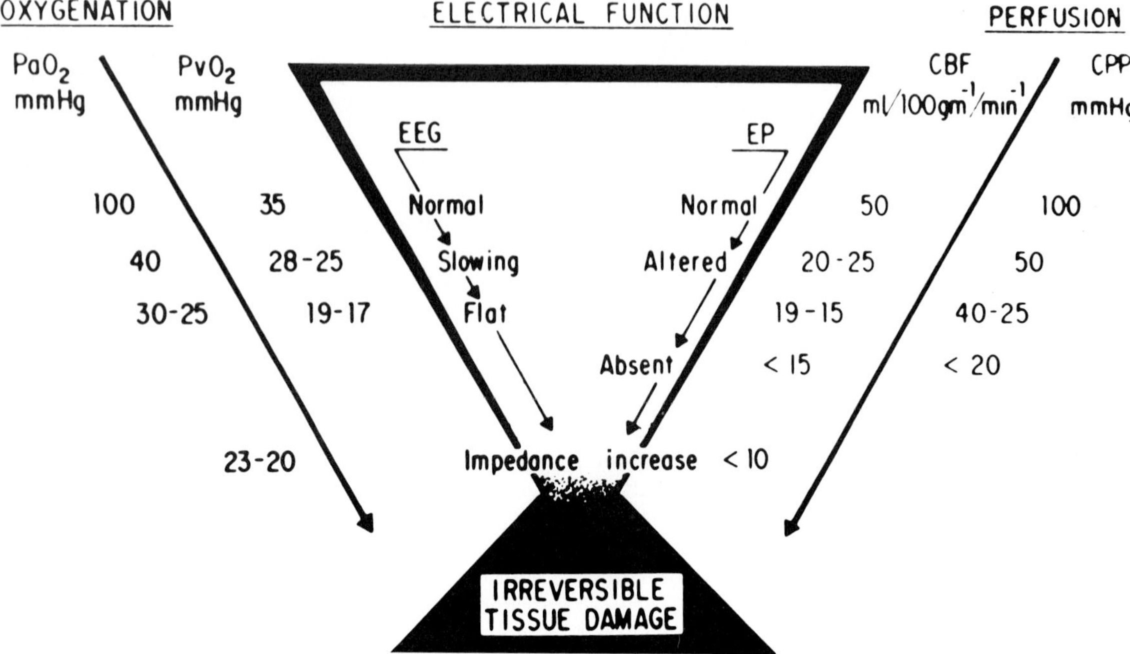

FIGURE **23–11.** Threshold for changes in cerebral electrical activity. The shaded area at the bottom of the triangle represents a deficiency in neuroelectric capabilities; that is, a gap exists between the last measurable electrical change and the development of irreversible tissue damage. During arterial hypoxia, brain oxygen extraction, cerebral blood flow (CBF), and cerebral perfusion pressure (CPP) are presumed to increase as a normal physiologic response to oxygen deprivation. Oxygen extraction also increases when CBF and CPP are reduced. PvO_2, venous oxygen pressure. (From Shapiro HM: In Miller RM (ed): Anesthesia, 2nd ed. New York, Churchill Livingstone, 1986, with permission.)

imetry, and housed in adhesive strips, are placed on the forehead on each side of the midline. In this position it is believed that the predominant measurement is blood flow through the frontal lobes. With carotid occlusion, ipsilateral oximetric values decreased but contralateral values did not. However, the oximetry values were extremely variable among patients both before and during carotid occlusion, and no correlation with cerebral ischemia could be made. Further studies will be needed before any conclusions can be drawn as to the value of transcranial Doppler scanning or cerebral oximetry for evaluating the adequacy of cerebral perfusion during carotid endarterectomy. Monitors employed to assess the adequacy of cerebral perfusion are summarized in Table 23–6.

Management of Ventilation

Ventilation is controlled with a mechanical ventilator from the completion of induction until the wound is closed. Tidal volume and frequency are adjusted so that mild to moderate hypocarbia is achieved (PaCO_2 between 25 and 30 mm Hg). Maintenance of a lower than normal PaCO_2 has several advantages, including decreasing cerebral vascular volume to give surgeons more space in which to work thus lessening the need for vigorous retraction of brain tissue. Hypocapnia also improves the regional distribution of CBF by preferentially diverting blood to potentially ischemic areas of the brain, better buffering of the brain lactic acid that may form as a result of focal ischemia, and decreasing the anesthetic requirement. The proposed hazards of this level of hypocarbia are either easily managed or strictly theoretical in nature. For example, the decrease in cardiac output that may occur with hyperventilation is readily managed by fluid therapy or administering a lower dose of anesthetic. The leftward shift in the oxyhemoglobin dissociation curve, and the increase in ventilation-perfusion abnormality are of theoretical concern only.

TABLE **23–6**
Monitors Reflecting Adequacy of Cerebral Perfusion

Stump pressure
Jugular venous oxygen saturation
Xexon washout measurement of cerebral blood flow
Unprocessed EEG
Processed EEG
Cerebral function monitor
Compressed spectral array
Density spectral array
Neurologic assessment under regional anesthesia
Near-infrared monitoring
Conjunctival oxygen tension
Doppler ultrasound
Ophthalmophlethysmography
Evoked potentials
Visual
Auditory
Somatosensory

Regulation of Blood Pressure

Control of blood pressure is critical to the successful outcome of most neurovascular procedures. For example, substantial increases in blood pressure will increase transmural pressure across an aneurysmal wall, thereby increasing the likelihood for rupture of the aneurysm. Likewise, substantial decreases in blood pressure may be necessary during clipping of an aneurysm to decrease transmural pressure and soften the aneurysmal sac. Close regulation of blood pressure during induction of anesthesia and prior to the start of excision of AVMs would appear to be less critical than for aneurysm surgery. In 1,000 patients with cerebral AVMs undergoing proton beam therapy, no patient experienced spontaneous cerebral hemorrhage despite marked increases in systolic and diastolic blood pressures.[106] However, once surgery is underway, close control of blood pressure is necessary to prevent excessive bleeding.

For all neurovascular surgery except carotid endarterectomy, blood pressure is generally regulated to the normal range or up to 20% below normal either with the anesthetic agents alone (e.g., increasing the dose of isoflurane) or in combination with a short-acting β-adrenergic blocking drug such as esmolol given by continuous infusion (i.e., 0.1 to 0.5 mg/kg/min) to decrease heart rate to a range of 50 to 60 bpm. If the desired blood pressure is not achieved with this combination, sodium nitroprusside 0.1 to 0.5 μg/kg/min may be added. If a vasoconstrictor is needed, a pure α-adrenergic stimulant, such as phenylephrine, is preferred because the evidence shows that it has minimal arrhythmogenic potential. If temporary occlusion of a major cerebral vessel is planned or becomes necessary because of uncontrolled bleeding, then blood pressure should be maintained at or above the normal range once the occlusion has occurred to better ensure that flow through collateral vessels is maintained. If an aneurysm should unexpectedly rupture, and bleeding is uncontrolled, blood pressure should be decreased immediately to whatever level (as low as 20 to 30 mm Hg) is necessary to permit control of bleeding, visualization of the bleeding site, and either clipping of the aneurysm or temporary occlusion of the parent vessel. Vigorous fluid replacement with crystalloid solution, albumin, and blood should accompany this transient period of induced hypotension to ensure cardiac filling and some cardiac output. Responses to vasoactive drugs are much easier to regulate if a normal blood volume has been established and maintained throughout the anesthetic period. More and more neurosurgeons are using temporary occlusion of feeding vessels and induced hypertension rather than induced hypotension to optimize conditions prior to aneurysmal clipping. While induced hypotension may not worsen outcome compared to normotension,[107,108] at least one study indicates that outcome is better when temporary occlusion rather than induced hypotension is used to control hemorrhage during cerebral aneurysm clipping.[109]

During carotid endarterectomy it is highly desirable to maintain systemic blood pressure at or slightly above the patient's highest recorded resting pressure while awake. The reason for this goal is that the occlusion of the carotid system that is necessary to perform the operation will often decrease distal perfusion pressure (stump pressure) below that required to maintain autoregulation (about 50 to 60 mm Hg). Also, the use of volatile agents such as isoflurane may induce some impairment of autoregulation. The consequences of these effects are that CBF distal to the surgical clamp or via collateral channels may be pressure dependent, and the higher the pressure, the more likely it is that cerebral perfusion will be adequate during surgical occlusion. Monitoring of the V_5 lead of the ECG or the short-axis view of the left ventricle on transesophageal echocardiography (TEE) will usually indicate if the increased blood pressure is causing myocardial ischemia.

Blood and Fluid Requirements

What fluid and how much depends on the patient's condition. If blood volume is normal, crystalloid fluid such as normal saline or lactated Ringer's solution should not exceed 10 to 15 ml/kg beyond that required to replace urine output, to lessen the possibility of postoperative cerebral edema. Whether the crystalloid solution should contain glucose remains controversial. Studies in the rat[110] and monkey[111] indicate that glucose worsens tolerance of the brain to *global* ischemia. In contrast, studies show that *focal* ischemia, which would correspond most closely to most neurovascular conditions, is not necessarily harmful, and may in fact be beneficial.[112,113] Furthermore, some evidence indicates that glucose values above about 225 mg/dl disrupt cerebral autoregulation. Because of the conflicting evidence, it would be prudent to avoid administering large volumes of glucose-containing solutions until this matter is resolved. Likewise, efforts to regulate blood glucose within very narrow normal ranges is also inappropriate. If blood volume is low for other reasons such as prolonged bed rest, albumin 5% and crystalloid solution can be given if the hematocrit is above 30%, or combinations of albumin or crystalloid solution and blood if the hematocrit is below that value. Hetastarch 6% is not recommended for most neurovascular surgical procedures, the exception being carotid endarterectomy, because of its potential for inducing a coagulopathy.[114] Even limiting the dose of hetastarch to less than 20 ml/kg does not eliminate the concern about its adverse effects on coagulation if excessive bleeding should occur during neurovascular surgery. Hetastarch is an appropriate fluid to maintain intravascular volume in patients undergoing carotid endarterectomy because it does stay in the intravascular compartment longer than crystalloid solutions.

Isovolemic hemodilution is used for those patients undergoing clipping of a giant aneurysm under femorofemoral cardiopulmonary bypass to lessen the risk of sludging of blood and thrombosis of vessels. Eight bottles of albumin 5% and four bags of normal saline are placed into a refrigerator at 4°C the night before operation to be used for cooling isovolemic hemodilution. After induction of anesthesia, about 1,000 ml of blood is removed from the patient into citrate-phosphate-dextrose bags, and replaced with an equal volume of cold albumin 5%. The "exchange" will usually result in a hematocrit of about 22 to 26%, the optimal range of hematocrit for isovolemic hemodilution. Frequent determinations of hematocrit during the operation are appropriate. In addition, I (CPL) administer cold normal saline 10 ml/kg plus a volume equal to urine output during the operation. The withdrawn blood is held at room temperature for reinfusion at the conclusion of operation. In addition, the perfusate from the cardiopulmonary bypass unit is spun down, and the packed cells are returned to the patient. If coagulation seems inadequate following reversal of the heparin, blood is sent for clotting studies, and platelets, fresh frozen plasma, and calcium gluconate are administered as needed.

Control of Brain Volume

Multiple methods are used to decrease brain volume during intracranial neurovascular procedures, thereby maximizing surgical visualization and minimizing need for brain retraction. These include:

1. Limitation of crystalloid fluid administration to 10 to 15 ml/kg above that volume needed to replace urine output.
2. Administration of thiopental or propofol.
3. Use of hyperventilation and hypocarbia to decrease intracranial blood volume.
4. Limitation of the dose of isoflurane to 1% inspired or less to minimize cerebral vasodilation.
5. Administration of mannitol 1 to 1.5 g/kg either alone or in combination with furosemide 0.3 mg/kg to produce an osmotic diuresis. The combination produces a faster diuresis than either drug alone, and prevents the transient increase in cerebral blood volume that occurs if mannitol is used alone.
6. Cerebrospinal fluid (CSF) drainage from a catheter inserted into the lumbar subarachnoid space after induction of anesthesia.
7. Avoidance of increases in ICP resulting from coughing or bucking on an endotracheal tube, increases in blood pressure or central venous pressure, or prolonged head-down positioning.
8. Use of mild hypothermia (32° to 34°C) (see below).

Whether all of these eight methods are used in a given patient will depend upon the condition of the patient and the surgery proposed. However, some of the eight are used in most patients owing to the fact that once brain volume increases from whatever cause, it is difficult to reverse, and may necessitate cancellation of the operation for fear the brain may herniate out of the wound if the dura is opened.

Positioning

For most neurovascular procedures the patient is positioned supine with the head turned laterally in three-point fixation (Mayfield headrest), with a roll under the shoulder on the side of operation. The anesthetic gas hoses and all monitoring and vascular catheter lines are directed to the patient's side or feet, where the anesthesiologist is positioned during the operation. In planning the anesthetic equipment to be used, the anesthesiologist must make sure that all of it will reach from the operating table to where the anesthesiologist will be positioned. TED hose and compression stockings are placed on the legs to minimize the development of venous thrombosis.

Patients are seldom placed in the seated position for neurovascular procedures, but if that should be necessary, special precautions are needed for the diagnosis and treatment of air embolism. Foremost among them is the placement of a Doppler flow probe on the chest along the right border of the sternum for continuous monitoring of heart sounds, and placement of a central venous catheter at the superior vena cava–right atrial junction for aspiration of air. In addition, continuous monitoring of end-tidal carbon dioxide and/or nitrogen with recording capabilities is highly desirable for documenting the onset and duration of the air embolism. TEE may also be used to detect venous air embolism. If air should be detected, the anesthesiologist should notify the surgeons immediately and attempt aspiration from the central venous catheter using a 10-ml syringe to confirm the diagnosis. Aspiration is faster and easier with a smaller syringe, and volumes of air that cannot easily be handled with a 10-ml syringe will seldom be encountered. If nitrous oxide is being used, it should be discontinued to avoid further expansion of the entrained air. Many believe that nitrous oxide should not be used when patients are in the seated position because it may convert an insignificant air embolism into a clinically dangerous one. Nitrous oxide 50% will double the size of an air bubble, and 70% will increase the size of an air bubble by fourfold. Additional, more extreme measures that can be taken if surgical flooding of the operative site and aspiration do not resolve the problem include placing the patient in a more head-down position to eliminate the negative pressure difference between the head and the heart, and make the bleeding site more obvious to the surgeons; applying bilateral jugular venous pressure or positive end-expiratory pressure (PEEP) up to 10 cm H_2O to stop further transfer of air from the head to the heart; and in extreme circumstances when cardiac output is impaired, placing the patient in left lateral decubitus in an attempt to float the air away from the pulmonary outflow tract; or initiating cardiopulmonary resuscitation.

Hypothermia

Mild hypothermia (core temperature of 32° to 34°C) is used in some centers during neurovascular surgery for two purposes: (1) to decrease brain metabolism and dependence on oxygen delivery and (2) to decrease brain size.[115] Cerebral metabolic oxygen consumption decreases about 7% for every degree decrease in brain temperature, so at 31°C cerebral metabolism is decreased about 40% below normal. From studies in animals it is generally believed that this level of hypothermia is beneficial,[116,117] although there are no studies in patients documenting decreased morbidity or mortality from its use. This level of hypothermia does not interfere appreciably with coagulation, nor is it generally associated with cardiac arrhythmias.

Surface cooling is begun as soon as induction of anesthesia is complete using a thermal blanket underneath the patient and ice packs on top of the patient, who is then covered with another thermal blanket that permits blowing of cold air over the patient (Bair Hugger, Augustine Medical, St. Petersburg, FL). With this combination the patient will cool at a rate of about 1°C per hour.[118] Rewarming is slower and it is often difficult to return the patient's temperature to above 35°C while still in the operating room, necessitating continued rewarming in the recovery room. At this temperature, some patients will shiver, so supplemental oxygen should be continued.

If more profound hypothermia (<20°C) is desired because circulatory arrest is planned for clipping of a giant aneurysm, cold fluids are infused as blood is removed to establish isovolemic hemodilution. In addition, thiopental or propofol is infused at rates sufficient to produce burst suppression on the EEG. Thiopental doses required to produce burst suppression range from 14 to 20 mg/kg/hr, while for propofol the doses are 200 to 300 μg/kg/min.[119] These agents are given in these doses in this special circumstance for their presumed ability to enhance the brain's tolerance to ischemia resulting from temporary circulatory arrest. Despite the large doses, both agents maintain satisfactory cardiovascular function in healthy patients undergoing this operation, although emergence from anesthesia is likely to be more rapid when propofol is used.[119,120] Once the neurosurgeons have exposed the giant aneurysm and determined that it cannot be clipped without resorting to CPB, systemic heparinization is established and the patient is placed on CPB using femorofemoral bypass and cooled to about 18°C. During the CPB cooling phase, the heart will usually fibrillate between 22° to 26°C. Once 18°C is reached, the CPB unit is shut off to deflate the aneurysm. The CPB unit may be activated and shut off several times during clipping to evaluate the adequacy of the surgical occlusion of the aneurysm, and to apply additional clips. Studies in rats suggest that intermittent reperfusion during prolonged circulatory arrest protects the brain from ischemia when compared to continuous arrest for the same time intervals.[121] The total circulatory arrest time should not exceed 45 minutes at this temperature.

Once the aneurysm is clipped, the AVM removed, or the revascularization completed, the patient is rewarmed by using a thermal blanket below and above the patient, warming the operating room, and using warming lights. If CPB has been used, it is resumed and warming instituted with it. Partial CPB is continued until normal cardiac rhythm is established and body temperature reaches about 36°C. Once partial CPB is discontinued, the patient will tend to cool unless vigorous efforts at rewarming are continued using the modalities noted above. Usually by the time the operation is completed, patient temperature is above 35°C and spontaneous ventilation is adequate, provided neurologic injury has not occurred or anesthetic drug therapy has not been excessive.

Emergence from Anesthesia

If the brain has not been injured by the surgical procedure, the patient usually awakens from the anesthetic within 30 minutes after cessation of isoflurane or propofol/opiate administration. As the patient is awakening, I (C.P.L.) ensure full reversal from neuromuscular blockade and close regulation of blood pressure. As recovery from anesthesia occurs, the patient's blood pressure will generally increase in response to the emergence stimuli. Tradition of β-adrenergic-receptor blocking drugs such as esmolol and/or vasodilators such as sodium nitroprusside can be initiated and the dose stabilized prior to transport to the ICU. If the patient begins to cough on the endotracheal tube, either remove the tube or suppress the cough reflex with lidocaine sprayed down the endotracheal tube. The patient is placed in bed in a 30-degree head-up position, and transported to the ICU breathing oxygen. With the techniques described, the patient will be sufficiently responsive within 30 minutes of the conclusion of the operation to permit gross neurologic evaluation and will not have any recall of the operative period.

Postoperative Complications

The major complications from neurovascular surgery include intracranial hemorrhage, stroke, cerebral edema and increased ICP, and cerebral vasospasm. Careful regulation of systemic blood pressure is essential to lessen the risk of intracranial hemorrhage. If any of these complications occur, it is likely that the patient's trachea will have to be reintubated and the patient transported to the CT scanner for radiologic evaluation and possible reoperation. Patients undergoing clipping of a giant aneurysm under CPB are also candidates for postoperative coagulopathy from the use of heparin and profound hypothermia, hypervolemia from excessive fluid therapy intraoperatively or postoperatively, and deep venous thrombosis or phlebitis, and resultant pulmonary embolism.

The major postoperative complications following carotid endarterectomy are circulatory instability with resultant myocardial infarction, loss of carotid body function, respiratory insufficiency, or stroke. Circulatory instability in the form of either hypotension or hypertension is common following carotid endarterectomy. Defining hypotension as a decrease and hypertension as an increase in systolic blood pressure of greater than 40 mm Hg below or above the usual pressure, we observed these changes in 47 of 100 patients following operation.[122] The mechanism for the hypotension is not known, but may be due to a variety of factors including hypovolemia, depression of circulation by anesthetic or other drugs, arrhythmias, or exposure of the baroreceptor mechanism to a new higher pressure causing an excessive reflex response. Some authors recommend the use of subcutaneously placed catheters at the operative site to provide for the instillation of local anesthetics to treat postoperative hypotension.[123,124]

The most attractive hypothesis to explain the hypertension is the loss of the normal carotid baroreceptor mechanism as a result of the operation. The carotid sinus is an integral part of the anatomy of the carotid bifurcation. Clamping above and below the sinus of denervation of the sinus in the dog causes a persistent fluctuant hypertension. We studied the baroreceptor reflex in patients before and after carotid endarterectomy using the standard Valsalva test and found that the reflex was outside the normal range before surgery and that it is further depressed by the operation.[122] Animal studies indicate that the carotid baroreceptor is a fragile structure and is easily damaged by surgery in the area. The potential complications from failure to control the hypertension include excessive bleeding at the operative site, increased myocardial oxygen consumption or arrhythmias and myocardial infarction, intracerebral hemorrhage, and increased intracranial pressure from cerebral edema.

Of equal importance to the loss of carotid baroreceptor function is the loss of carotid body function following carotid endarterectomy. Chemoreceptor function is lost in most patients after this operation, as evidenced by a loss of ventilatory and circulatory responses to hypoxia, and a modest increase in resting arterial $Pa{CO_2}$.[122] The loss may be temporary or permanent, and represents a potentially serious hazard to the patient. I recommend avoiding or obviating situations that are known to provoke hypoxemia. I augment the concentrations of oxygen the patient breaths postoperatively until fully conscious. Furthermore, special attention must be directed toward preventing serious atelectasis or other pulmonary or circulatory abnormalities that might cause arterial hypoxemia, to which the patient could only respond by further respiratory and circulatory depression, loss of consciousness, etc.

Acute respiratory insufficiency may occur early postoperatively because of hematoma formation with tracheal deviation, vocal cord paralysis from surgical traction on laryngeal nerves, or tension pneumothorax from dissection of air through the wound into the mediastinum and pleural space. Wound hematomas have been reported to occur in 2 to 2.8% of cases.[125,126] These three possibilities are thought of immediately when unexpected respiratory distress occurs postoperatively. In general, a hematoma causing respiratory distress should be evacuated *before endotracheal intubation is attempted.* Attempting oral or nasal intubation when the patient's airway is compressed and deviated is generally impossible and wastes valuable time. Likewise, a tension pneumothorax should be relieved immediately by needle evacuation if there is evidence of circulatory insufficiency. Hertzer et al. reported that the most common nerve injury was the recurrent (6%) followed by the hypoglossal (5%).[127] Wade et al. reported loss of carotid body function following bilateral carotid endarterectomies. This may result in a loss of respiratory response to hypoxemia.[122]

The mortality rate from carotid endarterectomy, including angiography should be less than 3%, while operative morbidity should not exceed 5%. The most serious complications are transient or permanent neurologic deficits and postoperative myocardial infarction. While most neurologic deficits first occur in the postoperative period, if a patient emerges from anesthesia for carotid endarterectomy with a new neurologic deficit, immediate cerebral angiography can be performed to determine if an intimal flap has formed at the site of operation. This flap is a surgically correctable lesion; if correction is performed immediately, the severity of the subsequent neurologic deficit may be lessened. Attention has been drawn to the relationship between heparin use in conjunction with protamine antagonism and the incidence of neurologic sequelae. Mauney et al. compared 193 patients who received protamine after heparin therapy to 155 patients who did not receive protamine. The stroke rate was 0 of 155 compared to 5 of 193 ($p < .045$). The incidence of hematoma requiring reexploration was 3 of 155 versus 2 of 193 ($p > .05$). Intraoperative shunts were used more frequently in the no-protamine group (84% vs. 67%; $p < .001$).[128] Trieman et al. reported that the use of protamine to antagonize heparin was not associated with an increase in stroke rate (6 of 328 patients vs. 10 of 369 patients who did not receive protamine). Significantly more patients experienced wound hematomas in the no-protamine group, however (6 of 328 vs. 24 of 369). The dose of protamine did not appear to be related to the incidence of neurologic sequelae.[129] The issue of protamine reversal and the incidence of neurologic sequelae and wound hematoma requires further investigation. Postoperative myocardial infarction occurs in about 1% of patients, a figure that is not surprising, since atherosclerosis is a generalized vascular disease usually involving the coronary as well as the cerebral circulation.

Summary

The anesthetic and surgical management of patients undergoing neurovascular surgical procedures has undergone substantial changes in recent years, with perhaps the most changes occurring with respect to carotid endarterectomy.[44] Because it is the most commonly performed vascular procedure, the trend has been toward simplifying the perioperative course, which includes greater use of indirect methods for evaluating carotid function, greater use of regional anesthesia, less use and reliance on monitors for evaluating adequacy of cerebral function, less use of surgical shunts, less use of ICU facilities, and earlier discharge from hospital.[43,44] These changes have decreased hospital costs for this operation by 40 to 50% without any documented increase in morbidity or mortality. In contrast, perioperative evaluation and care of patients with cerebral aneurysms and AVMs have become more complex in an effort to treat these diseases effectively regardless of size or location. Much of the surgical care has moved from the operating room to the neuroradiologic suite, but with no lessening of the need for anesthesia services. Anesthesiologists and surgeons continue to search for ways to protect the brain from ischemia during temporary interruption of its circulation.

References

1. Kassell NF, Torner JC: Epidemiology of intracranial aneurysms. In Varkey GP (ed): Anesthetic Considerations in the Surgical Repair of Intracranial Aneurysms. Boston, Little, Brown & Co, 1982, p 13.
2. Schievink WI, Michels VV, Piepgras DG: Neurovascular manifestations of heritable connective tissue disorders: A review. Stroke 25:889, 1994.
3. Schievink WI, Schaid DJ, Rogers HM, Piepgras DG: On the inheritance of intracranial aneurysms. Stroke 25:2028, 1994.
4. Schievink WI: Intracranial aneurysms. N Engl J Med 336:28, 1996.
5. Whittle IR, Dorsch NW, Besser M: Giant intracranial aneurysms: Diagnosis, management, and outcome. Surg Neurol 21: 218, 1984.
6. Samson D, Batjer HH, Bowman G, et al: A clinical study of the parameters and effects of temporary arterial occlusion in the management of intracranial aneurysms. Neurosurgery 34:22, 1994.
7. Silverberg GD, Reitz BA, Ream AK: Hypothermia and cardiac arrest in the treatment of giant aneurysms of the cerebral circulation and hemangioblastoma of the medulla. J Neurosurg 55: 337, 1981.
8. Silverberg GD: Giant aneurysms: Surgical treatment. Neurol Res 6:57, 1984.
9. Stein BM, Wolpert SM: Arteriovenous malformations of the brain. I: Current concepts and treatment. Arch Neurol 37:1, 1980.
10. Pool JL, Potts DG: Aneurysms and arteriovenous anomalies of the brain; diagnosis and treatment. New York, Harper & Row, 1965, p 326.
11. Wilkins RH: Natural history of intracranial vascular malformations: A review. Neurosurgery 16:421, 1985.
12. Steinberg GK: Multimodality treatment of intracranial vascular malformations: Embolization, helium-ion radiosurgery, microsurgical resection. In Yamada S (ed): Arteriovenous Malformation in Functional Brain Areas. Mt Kisco, NY, Futura Publishing Co, 1993.
13. Samson DS, Boone S: Extracranial-intracranial (EC-IC) arterial bypass: Past performances and current concepts. Neurosurgery 3:79, 1978.
14. The EC-IC Bypass Group: Failure of extracranial-intracranial arterial bypass to reduce the risk of ischemic stroke. Results of an international randomized trial. N Engl J Med 313:1191, 1985.
15. Ausman JI, Diaz FG: Critique of the extracranial-intracranial bypass study. Surg Neurol 26:218, 1986.
16. Day AL, Rhoton AL, Little JR: The extracranial-intracranial bypass study. Surg Neurol 26:222, 1986.
17. Homer D, Ingall TJ, Baker HL, et al: Serum lipids and lipoproteins are less powerful predictors of extracranial carotid artery atherosclerosis than are cigarette smoking and hypertension. Mayo Clin Proc 66:259, 1991.
18. Klop RB, Eikelboom C, Taks AC: Screening of the internal carotid arteries in patients with peripheral vascular disease by color-flow duplex scanning. Eur J Vasc Surg 5:41, 1991.
19. Chambers BR, Norris JW: Outcome in patients with asymptomatic neck bruits. N Engl J Med 315:860, 1986.
20. Wylie EJ, Ehrenfeld WK (eds): Extracranial Occlusive Cerebrovascular Disease: Diagnosis and Management. Philadelphia, WB Saunders Co, 1970.
21. Bauer RB, Meyer JS, Fields WS, et al: Joint study of extracranial arterial occlusion. III. Progress report of controlled study of long-term survival in patients with and without operation. JAMA 208:509, 1969.
22. Goldner JD, Whisnant JP, Taylor WF: Long-term prognosis of transient cerebral ischemic attacks. Stroke 2:160, 1971.
23. Cartlidge NEF, Whisnant JP, Elveback LR: Carotid and vertebral—basilar transient cerebral ischemic attacks: A community study, Rochester, MN. Mayo Clin Proc 52:117, 1977.
24. Muuronen A, Kask M: Outcome of 314 patients with transient ischemic attacks. Stroke 13:24, 1982.
25. Robinson RW, Demirel M, LeBeau RJ: Natural history of cerebral thrombosis nine to nineteen year follow-up. J Chronic Dis 21:221, 1968.
26. O'Holleran LW, Kennelly MM, McClurken M, et al: Natural history of asymptomatic carotid plaque. Am J Surg 154:659, 1987.
27. Meissner I, Weibers DO, Whisnant JP, et al: The natural history of asymptomatic carotid artery occlusive lesions. JAMA 258: 2703, 1987.
28. Bogousslavsky J, Despland PA, Regli F: Asymptomatic tight stenosis of the internal carotid artery: Long-term prognosis. Neurology 36:861, 1986.
29. Wolf PA, Kannel WB, Sorlie P, McNamara P: Asymptomatic carotid bruit and risk of stroke; the Framingham Study. JAMA 245:1442, 1981.
30. Wolf, PA, Kannel WB, Sorlie P, et al: Asymptomatic carotid bruit and risk of stroke. JAMA 245:1442, 1981.
31. Heyman A, Wilkinson W, Heydeu S, et al: Risk of stroke in asymptomatic persons with cervical arterial bruits. N Engl J Med 302:838, 1980.
32. Dixon S, Pais SO, Raviola C, et al: Natural history of nonstenotic, asymptomatic ulcerative lesions of the carotid artery. A further analysis. Arch Surg 117:1493, 1982.
33. Garraway WM, Akthar AJ, Smith DL, et al: The triage of stroke rehabilitation. J Epidemiol Community Health 35:39, 1981.
34. North American Symptomatic Carotid Endarterectomy Trial Collaborators: Beneficial effect of carotid endarterectomy in symptomatic patients with high-grade carotid stenosis. N Engl J Med 325:445, 1991.
35. European Carotid Surgery Trialists' Collaborative Group: MCR European carotid surgery trial: Interim results for systomatic patients with severe (70–99%) or with mild (0–29%) carotid stenosis. Lancet 337:1235, 1991.
36. Hobson RW, Weiss DG, Fields WS, et al, and the Veterans Affairs Cooperative Study Group: Efficacy of carotid endarterectomy for asymptomatic carotid stenosis. N Engl J Med 328:221, 1993.
37. Clinical Advisory: CEA for patients with asymptomatic internal carotid artery stenosis. Press release of the National Institutes of Neurological Disorders and Stroke, NIH, Bethesda, MD, September 28, 1994.
38. Endarterectomy for Asymptomatic Carotid Artery Stenosis: Executive Committee for the Asymptomatic Carotid Atherosclerosis Study. JAMA 273:1421, 1995.
39. European Carotid Surgery Trialists' Collaborative Group. Endarterectomy for modern symptomatic carotid stenosis: Interim results from the MCR European Carotid Surgery Trial. Lancet 347:1591, 1996.
40. Moore WS, Barnett HJM, Beebe HG, et al: Guidelines for carotid endarterectomy. A multidisciplinary consensus statement from the Ad Hoc committee, American Heart Association. Circulation, 91:566, 1995.
41. Ropper AH, Wechsler LR, Wilson LS: Carotid bruit and the risk of stroke in elective surgery. N Engl J Med 307:1388, 1982.
42. Bandyk DF, Thiele BL: Noninvasive assessment of carotid artery disease. West J Med 139:486, 1983.
43. Kraiss LW, Kilberg L, Critch S, Johansen KH: Short-stay carotid endarterectomy is safe and cost-effective. Am J Surg 169:512, 1995.
44. Mirko MK, Morasch MD, Burke K, et al: The changing face of carotid endarterectomy. J Vasc Surg 23:622, 1996.
45. Frank SM, Norris EJ, Christopherson R, Beattie C: Right and left arm blood pressure discrepancies in vascular surgery patients. Anesthesiology 75:457, 1991.
46. Brazenor GA, Chamberlain MJ, Gelb AW: Systemic hypovolemia after subarachnoid hemorrhage. J Neurosurg Anesth 2:42, 1990.
47. Andreoli A, dePasquale G, Pinelli G: Subarachnoid hemorrhage: Frequency and severity of cardiac arrhythmias. Stroke 18:558, 1987.
48. Fox JL: Microsurgical treatment of neurovascular disease. Neurosurgery 3:286, 1978.

49. Wilke HJ, Ellis JE, McKinsey JF: Carotid endarterectomy: Perioperative and anesthetic considerations. J Cardiothorac Vasc Anesth 7:928, 1996.
50. Bower TC, Merrell SW, Cherry KJ Jr, et al: Advanced carotid disease in patients requiring aortic reconstruction. Am J Surg 166:146, 1993.
51. Gerraty RP, Gates PC, Doyle JC: Carotid stenosis and perioperative stroke risk in symptomatic and asymptomatic patients undergoing vascular or coronary surgery. Stroke 24:1115, 1993.
52. Hertzer RN, Loop FD, Beven EG, et al: Surgical staging for simultaneous coronary and carotid disease: A study including prospective randomization. J Vasc Surg 9:455, 1989.
53. Kartcher MM, McRae LP: Carotid occlusive disease as a risk factor in major cardiovascular surgery. Arch Surg 117:1086, 1982.
54. Schwartz LB, Bridgman AH, Kieffer RW, et al: Asymptomatic carotid artery stenosis and stroke in patients undergoing cardiopulmonary bypass. J Vasc Surg 21:146, 1995.
55. Reed GL III, Singer DE, Picard EH, et al: A case control estimate of the risk from carotid bruits. N Engl J Med 319:1246, 1988.
56. Brener BJ, Brief DK, Alpert J, et al: The risk of stroke in patients with asymptomatic carotid stenosis undergoing cardiac surgery: A follow-up study. J Vasc Surg 5:269, 1987.
57. Urbinati S, DiPasquale G, Andreoli A, et al: Preoperative noninvasive coronary risk stratification in candidates for carotid endarterectomy. Stroke 25:2022, 1994.
58. Urbinati S, DiPasquale G, Andreoli, A, et al: Frequency and prognostic significance of silent coronary artery disease in patients with cerebral ischemia undergoing carotid endarterectomy. Am J Cardiol 69:1166, 1992.
59. Rihal CS, Gersh BJ, Whisnant JP, et al: Influence of coronary heart disease on morbidity and mortality after carotid endarterectomy: A population-based study in Olsted County, Minnesota 1970–1988. J Am Coll Cardiol 19:1254, 1992.
60. Mackey WC, O'Donnell TF, Callow AD: Cardiac risk in patients undergoing carotid endarterectomy: Impact on perioperative and long-term mortality. J Vasc Surg 11:226, 1990.
61. Yeager RA, Moneta GK, McConnell DB, et al: Analysis of risk factors for myocardial infarction following carotid endarterectomy. Arch Surg 124:1142, 1989.
62. Hertzer NR, Loop FD, Taylor PC, et al: Combined myocardial revascularization and carotid endarterectomy. Thorac Cardiovasc Surg 85:577, 1983.
63. Craver JM, Murphy DA, Jones EL, et al: Concomitant carotid and coronary artery reconstruction. Ann Surg 195:712, 1982.
64. Minami K, Sagoo KS, Breymann T, et al: Operative strategy in combined coronary and carotid artery disease. J Thorac Cardiovasc Surg 95:303, 1988.
65. Carrel T, Stillhard G, Turina M: Combined carotid and coronary artery surgery: Early and late results. Cardiology 80:118, 1992.
66. Chang BB, Darling RC, Shah DM, et al: Carotid endarterectomy can be safely performed with acceptable mortality and morbidity in patients requiring coronary artery bypass grafts. Am J Surg 168:94, 1994.
67. Smith A, Hoff J, Neilsen S, Larson CP: Barbiturate protection in acute focal cerebral ischemia. Stroke 5:1, 1974.
68. Michenfelder JD, Milde JH, Sundt TM: Cerebral protection by barbiturate anesthesia. Arch Neurol 33:345, 1976.
69. Shah DM, Darling RC, Chang BB, et al: Carotid endarterectomy in awake patients: Its safety, acceptability, and outcome. J Vasc Surg 19:1015, 1994.
70. Davies MJ, Mooney PH, Scott DA, et al: Neurologic changes during carotid endarterectomy under cervical block predict a high risk of postoperative stroke. Anesthesiology 78:829, 1993.
71. Moore WS: Carotid endarterectomy for prevention of stroke. West J Med 159:37, 1993.
72. Gabelman CG, Gann DS, Ashworth CJ, Carney WI: One hundred consecutive carotid reconstructions: Local versus general anesthesia. Am J Surg 145:477, 1983.
73. Davies MJ, Murrell GC, Cronin KC, et al: Carotid endarterectomy under cervical plexus block: A prospective clinical audit. Anaesth Intensive Care 18:219, 1990.
74. Benjamin ME, Silva MB Jr, Watt C, et al: Awake patient monitoring to determine the need for shunting during carotid endarterectomy. Surgery 114:673, 1993.
75. Allen BT, Anderson CB, Rubin BG, et al: The influence of anesthetic technique on perioperative complications after carotid endarterectomy. J Vasc Surg 19:834, 1994.
76. Anthony T, Johansen K: Optimal outcome for "high-risk" carotid endarterectomy. Am J Surg 167:469, 1994.
77. Ombrellaro MP, Freeman MB, Stevens SL, Goldman MH: Effect of anesthetic technique on cardiac morbidity following carotid artery surgery. Am J Surg 171:387, 1996.
78. Connolly JE: Carotid endarterectomy in the awake patient. Am J Surg 150:159, 1985.
79. Evans WE, Hayes JP, Waltke EA, et al: Optimal monitoring during carotid endarterectomy: Neurologic response under local anesthesia. J Vasc Surg 2:775, 1985.
80. Yared I, Martinis AG, Mack RM: Carotid endarterectomy under local anesthesia: A retrospective study. Am Surg 45:709, 1979.
81. Kainuma M, Shimado Y, Matsuura M: Cervical epidural anaesthesia in carotid artery surgery. Anaesthesia 41:1020, 1986.
82. Winnie AB: Cervical plexus block simplified: A single injection technique. Anesth Analg 54:370, 1975.
83. Moore DC: Regional Blocks. Springfield, IL, Charles C Thomas Publishers, 1965.
84. Adriana J (ed): Labat's Regional Anesthesia: Techniques and Clinical Applications. Philadelphia, WB Saunders Co, 1967.
85. Youngberg JA, Neely CF: Perioperative anesthetic considerations for the carotid artery surgery patient. Adv Anesth 5:291, 1988.
86. Fiorani P, Sbarigia E, Speziale F, et al: General anesthesia versus cervical plexus block and perioperative complications in carotid artery surgery. Eur J Vasc Endovasc Surg 13:37, 1997.
87. Warner DS, Hindman BJ, Todd MM, et al: Intracranial pressure and hemodynamic effects of remifentanil versus alfentanil in patients undergoing supratentorial craniotomy. Anesth Analg 83:348, 1996.
88. Hartung J, Cottrell JE: Nitrous oxide reduces thiopental-induced prolongation of survival in hypoxic and anoxic mice. Anesth Analg 66:47, 1987.
89. Warner DS, Zhou J, Ramani R, et al: Nitrous oxide does not alter infarct volume in rats undergoing reversible middle cerebral artery occlusion. Anesthesiology 73:686, 1990.
90. Meyer FB, Muzzi DA: Cerebral protection during aneurysm surgery with isoflurane anesthesia. J Neurosurg 76:541, 1992.
91. Ravussin P, deTribolet N: Total intravenous anesthesia with propofol for burst suppression in cerebral aneurysm surgery: Preliminary report of 42 patients. Neurosurgery 32:236, 1993.
92. Michenfelder JD, Sundt TM, Fode N, Shargrough FW: Isoflurane when compared to enflurane and halothane decreases the frequency of cerebral ischemia during carotid endarterectomy. Anesthesiology 67:336, 1987.
93. Frawley JE, Hicks RG, Gray LJ, Niesche JW: Carotid endarterectomy without a shunt for symptomatic lesions associated with contralateral severe stenosis or occlusion. J Vasc Surg 23:421, 1996.
94. Mutch WAC, White IWC, Donin N, et al: Haemodynamic instability and myocardial ischemia during carotid endarterectomy: A comparison of propofol and isoflurane. Can J Anaesth 42:577, 1995.
95. Archer DP, Tang TKK: The choice of anaesthetic for carotid endarterectomy: Does it matter? Can J Anaesth 42:566, 1995.
96. Sharma SK, McGuire GP, Cruise CJE: Stability of the arterial to end-tidal carbon dioxide difference during anaesthesia for prolonged neurosurgical procedures. Can J Anaesth 42:498, 1995.
97. Shapiro HM: Anesthesia effects upon cerebral blood flow, cerebral metabolism, electroencephalogram and evoked potentials. In Miller RD (ed): Anesthesia. New York, Churchill Livingstone, 1986. p. 1249.
98. Kearse LA Jr, Lopez-Bresnahan M, McPeck K, Zaslavsky A: Preoperative cerebrovascular symptoms and electroencephalographic abnormalities do not predict cerebral ischemia during carotid endarterectomy. Stroke 26:1210, 1995.
99. Kearse LA Jr, Martin D, McPeck K, Lopez-Bresnahan M: Computer-derived density spectral array in detection of mild analog electroencephalographic ischemic pattern changes during carotid endarterectomy. J Neurosurg 78:884, 1993.
100. Kresowik TF, Khoury MD: Limitations of EEG monitoring in the detection of cerebral ischemia accompanying carotid endarterectomy. J Vasc Surg 13:439, 1991.

101. Mooij JJ, Buchthal A, Belopavlovic M: Somatosensory evoked potential monitoring of temporary middle cerebral artery occlusion during aneurysm operation. Neurosurgery 21:492, 1987.
102. Kearse LA Jr, Brown EN, McPeck K: Somatosensory evoked potentials sensitivity relative to electroencephalography for cerebral ischemia during carotid endarterectomy. Stroke 23:498, 1992.
103. McKay RD, Sundt TM, Michenfelder JD: Internal carotid artery stump pressure and cerebral blood flow during carotid endarterectomy: Modification by halothane, enflurane, and innovar. Anesthesiology 45:390, 1976.
104. Gaunt ME, Ratliff DA, Martin PJ, et al: On-table diagnosis of incipient carotid artery thrombosis during carotid endarterectomy by transcranial Doppler scanning. J Vasc Surg 20:104, 1994.
105. Samra SK, Dorje P, Zelenock GB, Stanley JC: Cerebral oximetry in patients undergoing carotid endarterectomy under local regional anesthesia. Stroke 27:49, 1996.
106. Szabo MD, Crosby G, Sundaram P, et al: Hypertension does not cause spontaneous hemorrhage of intracranial arteriovenous malformations. Anesthesiology 70:761, 1989.
107. Inomata S, Mizuyama K, Sato S, et al: The effect of deliberate hypotensive anesthesia on the prognosis of patients who underwent early surgeries for ruptured cerebral aneurysm. Masui 41: 207, 1992.
108. Moss E: Cerebral blood flow during induced hypotension. Br J Anaesth 74:635, 1995.
109. Giannotta SL, Oppenheimer JH, Levy ML, Zelman V: Management of intraoperative rupture of an aneurysm without hypotension. Neurosurgery 28:531, 1991.
110. Pulsinelli WA, Waldman S, Rawlinson D, Plum F: Moderate hyperglycemia augments ischemic brain damage: A neuropathologic study in the rat. Neurology 32:1239, 1982.
111. Lanier WL, Stangland KJ, Scheithauer BW, et al: The effects of dextrose infusion and head position on neurologic outcome after complete cerebral ischemia in primates: Examination of a model. Anesthesiology 66:39, 1987.
112. Zasslow MA, Pearl RG, Shuer LM, et al: Hyperglycemia decreases acute neuronal ischemic changes after middle cerebral artery occlusion in cats. Stroke 20:519, 1989.
113. Kraft SA, Larson CP, Shuer LM, et al: Effect of hyperglycemia on neuronal changes in a rabbit model of focal cerebral ischemia. Stroke 21:447, 1990.
114. Cully MD, Larson CP, Silverberg GD: Hetastarch coagulopathy in a neurosurgical patient. Anaesthesiology 66:706, 1987.
115. Smith RM, Stetson JB: Therapeutic hypothermia. N Engl J Med 265:1097, 1961.
116. Berntman L, Welsh FA, Harp JR: Cerebral protective effect of low-grade hypothermia. Anesthiology 55:495, 1981.
117. Sano T, Drummond JC, Patel PM, et al: A comparison of the cerebral protective effects of isoflurane and mild hypothermia in a model of incomplete forebrain ischemia in the rat. Anesthesiology 76:221, 1992.
118. Baker KZ, Young WL, Stone JG, et al: Deliberate mild intraoperative hypothermia for craniotomy. Anesthesiology 81:361, 1994.
119. Stone JG, Young WL, Marans ZS, et al: Consequences of electroencephalographic-suppressive doses of propofol in conjunction with deep hypothermic circulatory arrest. Anesthesiology 85:497, 1996.
120. Stone JG, Young WL, Marans ZS, et al: Cardiac performance preserved despite thiopental loading. Anesthesiology 79:36, 1993.
121. Goldman MS, Anderson RE, Meyer FB: Effects of intermittent reperfusion during temporal focal ischemia. J Neurosurg 77:911, 1992.
122. Wade JG, Larson CP, Hickey RF, et al: Effect of carotid endarterectomy on carotid chemoreceptor and baroreceptor function in man. N Engl J Med 282:823, 1970.
123. Satiani B, Vasko JS, Evans WE: Hypertension following carotid endarterectomy. Surg Neurol 11:357, 1979.
124. Pine R, Avellone JC, Hoffman M, et al: Control of postcarotid endarterectomy hypotension with baroreceptor blockade. Am J Surg 147:763, 1983.
125. Corson JD, Chang BB, Shah DM, et al: The influence of anesthetic choice on carotid endarterectomy outcome. Arch Surg 122:807, 1987.
126. Welling RE, Ramadas HS, Gansmuller KJ: Cervical wound hematoma after carotid endarterectomy. Ann Vasc Surg 3:229, 1989.
127. Hertzer NR, Feldman BJ, Beven EG, et al: A prospective study of the incidence of injury to the cranial nerves during carotid endarterectomy. Surg Gynecol Obstet 151:781, 1980.
128. Mauney MC, Buchanan SA, Lawrence A, et al: Stroke rate is markedly reduced after carotid endarterectomy by avoidance of protamine. J Vasc Surg 22:264, 1995.
129. Treiman RL, Cossman DV, Foran RF, et al: The influence of neutralizing heparin after carotid endarterectomy on postoperative stroke and wound hematoma. J Vasc Surg 12:440, 1990.

CHAPTER 24

Peripheral Vascular Surgery

Jane Duggan, M.D.
Ira J. Isaacson, M.D.

Patients undergoing peripheral vascular surgery exhibit a wide range of pathophysiologic processes. In preparing a patient for surgery, physicians usually consider the host of diseases that accompany and exacerbate peripheral vascular disease and contribute to the complexity of each patient's anesthetic risk. Anesthesiologists face difficult choices: what tests constitute an appropriate preoperative evaluation? What hemodynamic monitors are useful and do they affect outcome? Does the choice of anesthetic change outcome? If so, why and in which patients?

Peripheral arterial occlusive disease is a common problem. An estimated 10% of patients over 65 years of age have chronic lower extremity arterial insufficiency, manifested by intermittent claudication. One to 2% of these elderly patients will develop limb-threatening ischemia. Approximately 90,000 amputations are performed each year in the United States because of acute or chronic arterial occlusive disease.[1]

Acute Arterial Disease

Peripheral vascular disease is seen in many forms. Arterial insufficiency (Table 24–1) may be acute or chronic. Acute limb ischemia is most frequently caused by intrinsic obstruction: clot or embolus (from the Greek word *embolos*, meaning plug or stopper).[4] The majority of emboli originate in the heart, with intermittent atrial fibrillation being the most frequent cause of emboli. Stasis of blood facilitates clot formation in a prominent left atrial appendage. Myocardial infarction is the next most frequent cause of emboli; a thrombus frequently is found at the apex of the heart after transmural anterior infarction.[4] Sixty to 70% of emboli travel to the lower extremities and lodge where vessels branch or taper, particularly in the common femoral, iliac, and popliteal arteries. Fifteen per cent of emboli travel to the upper extremity circulation. The brachial artery is the most common site in the upper extremity for an embolus to lodge, but emboli can also obstruct the subclavian or axillary vessels. Most of the remainder of emboli travel from the heart to the cerebral circulation, and a small percentage to visceral vessels.[1,2,4]

Embolization to smaller caliber vessels occurs when debris dislodges from a proximal aneurysm or plaque. If a plaque is degenerative, stenotic, irregular, or ulcerative, microemboli can shower the distal circulation. Most emboli are dislodged from arterial lesions located from the infrarenal aorta to the distal popliteal arteries. A common example of atheroembolism is the "blue toe syndrome," in which a toe is suddenly cool, painful, and cyanotic in the presence of palpable distal pulses.[5]

Extrinsic arterial obstruction is most frequently caused by blunt or penetrating injuries, such as knife or gunshot wounds. Iatrogenic injuries from arterial cannulation can also result in arterial obstruction. Secondary thrombosis can occur after an injury, especially in the presence of prolonged hypotension. Long-bone fractures and major joint disarticulation can cause arterial insufficiency, and soft tissue swelling frequently makes the diagnosis difficult. An infrequent cause of arterial insufficiency is venous outflow obstruction.[2]

In situ thrombosis of a diseased, stenotic artery can cause acute ischemia. The thrombotic occlusion of vascular bypass grafts is another cause of extremity ischemia. Thrombosis is favored in circumstances of low flow, such as hypotension, dehydration, and cardiogenic shock. Hypercoagulable states, such as antithrombin III deficiency or protein C or S deficiency, also predispose the patient to thrombosis.[1]

Ischemia is derived from the Greek words *ischō* (to keep back) and *haima* (blood) and is defined as local anemia due to mechanical obstruction of the blood supply. On a microscopic level, some cells are more susceptible to anoxia than others. Skeletal muscle and peripheral nerves are more vulnerable to hypoxia than skin is, for example. After 4 to 6 hours of acute arterial occlusion, irreversible changes occur in skeletal muscle and peripheral nerves. The ultimate outcome of ischemia depends on three factors: tolerance of different tissues to hypoxia, duration of ischemia, and reperfusion injury.[2]

Reperfusion of ischemic muscle is associated with significant further injury, which may be related to accumulation of oxygen free radicals, injury to microvascular endothelium and sequestration of activated white blood cells. Oxygen free radicals accumulate and may damage

TABLE 24–1
Causes of Peripheral Arterial Insufficiency

Acute
- Intrinsic sources
  - Embolus from heart, aneurysm, or atherosclerotic plaque
  - Thrombosis
- Extrinsic sources
  - Penetrating injury
  - Long-bone fracture or major joint dislocation
  - Venous outflow observation

Chronic
- Atherosclerosis
- Immune arteritis
- Thromboangiitis obliterans (Buerger's disease)
- Giant-cell arteritis
- Radiation arteritis
- Popliteal artery occlusive syndromes
- Homocysteinemia

Data from Seeger JM: Peripheral arterial occlusive disease. In Levine BA, Copeland EM, Howard RJ, et al (eds): Current Practice of Surgery. New York, Churchill Livingstone, 1993; Perry MO: Acute ischemia and its sequelae. In Rutherford RB (ed): Vascular Surgery, 3rd ed. Philadelphia, WB Saunders Co, 1989, p 541; and Harward TRS: Nonatherosclerotic peripheral vascular disease. In Levine BA, Copeland EM, Howard RJ, et al (eds): Current Practice of Surgery. New York, Churchill Livingstone, 1993.

cell membranes. Microvascular injury results in tissue edema and capillary plugging, which can limit reperfusion to ischemic tissue (the no-reflow phenomenon). White blood cells appear to play a major role in capillary plugging and are a source of oxygen free radicals. Animal studies have suggested that free radical scavengers and fibrinolytic agents may improve outcome. The applicability of these agents to humans is currently unproven.[1]

Acute arterial ischemia is usually a dramatic event characterized by the "five P's": pain, paralysis, paresthesia, pallor, and pulselessness. The pain is usually well localized to the affected extremity and quite severe, although good collateral circulation may diminish the prominence of this symptom. Paresis and paresthesia can help determine the extent of ischemic damage. For example, a patient may be unable to perceive light touch (carried by smaller nerve fibers, which are more susceptible to ischemia) while still able to sense pinprick pressure or temperature changes (transmitted by larger fibers, which are less susceptible to ischemia). Distal pulses are usually absent after acute arterial insufficiency, but detectable distal pulses do not rule out significant ischemia. Acutely ischemic extremities usually appear pale and cool. If palpation of the extremity reveals skeletal muscle with a thick, inelastic consistency, significant ischemia has already resulted in cellular swelling. As ischemia progresses, the muscle becomes stiff and firm, a sign of early necrosis. Surgical revascularization needs to be completed prior to this stage to have much success. Venous thrombosis may complicate matters, especially in patients where diagnosis is delayed.[2]

Chronic Arterial Disease

Chronic limb ischemia may be classified into two broad categories: intermittent claudication and limb-threatening ischemia. Claudication, derived from the Latin verb *claudicare*, meaning to limp, is defined as pain in the lower extremity, induced by exercise and relieved by rest. An obstruction in the arterial bed does not allow an exercise-induced increase in blood flow adequate to meet metabolic demands. The symptoms of claudication usually remain stable over years, with a minority of patients progressing to amputation. Cigarette smoking is the major risk factor for progression of ischemia. The severity of the initial arterial occlusive disease is another important risk factor.[6]

Limb-threatening ischemia occurs when blood flow is insufficient to meet the resting metabolic demands of the extremity. Ischemic rest pain is characterized as a burning pain, worse in the forefoot and toes, and worse at night when the patient is recumbent. Lowering the foot position improves blood flow by gravity and alleviates symptoms. Ulcers may evolve from small injuries and fail to heal because of inadequate blood supply. Gangrene is diagnosed when spontaneous necrosis occurs due to chronic inadequate perfusion.[6]

The causes of chronic arterial insufficiency are several (Table 24–1), but atherosclerosis is by far the most common etiology. Atherosclerosis is a disease of the intima of arteries from the size of the aorta down to 3 mm external diameter. Arteries are not affected uniformly; for example, while the internal mammary artery is usually spared, the coronary arteries are frequently involved. The process primarily involves lipid accumulation. Intimately intermingled within a connective tissue matrix, macrophages are the lipid-laden "foam cells" that enter the intima of arteries. In response to growth factors, smooth muscle cells synthesize collagen to form the matrix of the plaques, which evolve over years growing and obstructing the arterial lumen; thrombosis can occur over unstable plaques with resulting occlusion or distal embolization; medial atrophy can lead to aneurysm formation.[7,8]

Processes and risk factors modulate the progression of atherosclerosis. Genetic factors may determine the susceptibility of the arterial wall to injury, and the resulting response. Chronic tobacco use causes endothelial cell swelling and increases the filtration of large molecules, such as albumin, by the endothelium. Smoking thus increases the likelihood of vessel thrombosis. Hypertension may increase hemodynamic stress and therefore lead to medial smooth muscle hypertrophy and subsequent fibrosis. Elevated levels of serum low-density lipoprotein (LDL) cholesterol and low levels of serum high-density lipoprotein (HDL) cholesterol may be necessary for the development of atherosclerosis, since the disease is seen rarely in individuals whose serum total cholesterol has remained at less than 180 mg/dl throughout life, or whose HDL cholesterol is greater than 55 mg/dl.[1,7]

To a certain extent, arteries can adapt to occlusive changes. Initially the vessel dilates to maintain flow in response to plaque formation and luminal narrowing. The vessel diameter increases to maintain a nearly normal luminal diameter. The mechanism by which dilation occurs is unclear but may be related to sheer stresses. When the limits of dilatation are reached, collateral vessels develop from terminal, distribution branches of large- and medium-sized, arteries. The collateral vessels are not new, but are pre-existing pathways that enlarge when occlusion worsens. The process takes weeks to occur and the precise mechanism is unknown. Whereas collateral blood flow can mitigate the effects of chronic ischemia, it is usually inadequate to compensate for acute arterial occlusion.[1] While arterial narrowing is common in chronic and acute ischemia, vasoactive narrowing is often a final event in acute ischemia, if coronary ischemia is a valid model. Over 60% of myocardial infarctions occur in vessels with less than 50% fixed diameter reduction.[9]

The nonatherosclerotic etiologies of arterial insufficiency affect a small percentage of patients and are relatively few in number: immune arteritis; thromboangiitis obliterans; giant cell arteritis; fibromuscular dysplasia; radiation arteritis; popliteal artery occlusive syndrome; and homocysteinemia. Immune arteritis is a pattern reflected by multiple diseases that cause a necrotizing transmural inflammatory response. Immune complexes are deposited on the arterial endothelium, the complement cascade is activated, and white cells are attracted and release lysosomal enzymes with a resulting arterial wall injury and thrombosis. Surgical interventions, including sympathectomy, have not been found to be beneficial.[3]

Buerger's disease, or thromboangiitis obliterans, is another form of chronic arterial insufficiency to the extremities. The cause of Buerger's disease is unknown, but the pathophysiology is directly linked with tobacco use: all patients with the disease are smokers, and true nonsmokers never develop the disease. On a microscopic level, Buerger's disease is described as an inflammatory, occlusive disease of medium- and small-sized arteries of the extremity. Macroscopically, the occluded artery may appear tense and swollen, with the lumen obstructed by fresh thrombus. In later stages, the artery may appear contracted and indurated.[10]

Therapy for Buerger's disease includes cessation of smoking, first and foremost, then medical therapy: thrombolytic agents and anticoagulation, prostaglandin E, intra-arterial infusion, sympathectomy via epidural injection, and hyperbaric oxygen. Surgical interventions include direct arterial reconstruction, often difficult in the presence of multiple arterial obstructions. Surgical sympathectomy is a standard therapy and arrests progression of the ischemia. Unfortunately, debridement and amputation are the ultimate surgical requirements.[10]

Giant-cell arteritis can be divided into two separate entities with identical microscopic pathology: temporal arteritis and Takayasu's arteritis. Temporal arteritis is found most commonly in whites older than 55 years and in women (three times more frequently than in men). The chronic inflammatory process involves the aorta and its major branches. The diagnosis is made by history, elevated erythrocyte sedimentation rate, and temporal artery biopsy. The therapy is steroids, and surgery is contraindicated. Takayasu's arteritis is seen predominantly in young females. The arterial changes usually involve the aorta and/or renal arteries and lead to stenoses or aneurysmal dilatation. Although treatment regimens are not well defined, sometimes patients will present for aneurysm repair. This surgical selection is based on the same criteria as routine atherosclerotic aneurysms.[3]

Radiation therapy for neoplasms can cause severe pathologic changes in arteries. In the acute phase, the endothelium will slough, and the exposed thrombogenic surface can cause acute occlusion. In the long term, radiation results in accelerated atherosclerotic changes, and stiff arteries. The treatment is surgical revascularization.[3]

Popliteal artery occlusive syndrome includes both popliteal entrapment syndrome and adventitial cystic disease. Popliteal entrapment syndrome is a congenital abnormality where the popliteal artery takes an anomalous course under the gastrocnemius muscle. In early stages, surgical division of the entrapping muscle or fibrous band is indicated. Bypass grafting with an autogenous saphenous vein is the treatment of choice if permanent stenosis, poststenotic dilatation, and/or aneurysm formation has occurred. Adventitial cystic disease is caused by one or more ganglion-like, mucin-containing cysts in the subadventitial artery wall. The popliteal artery is most commonly affected, and it occurs in males in 80% of cases. Larger cysts require surgical excision and arterial bypass with autogenous saphenous vein graft. When unilateral claudication or arterial occlusion is noted in younger patients (< age 40), the differential diagnosis should include thromboangiitis obliterans, popliteal entrapment syndrome, and adventitial cystic disease.[3]

Homocysteinemia is an inborn error of metabolism that results in a variant of premature atherosclerosis. Excess homocysteine is converted by the liver to an atherogenic compound, homocysteine thiolactone, which alters the arterial wall and prostaglandin metabolism, and interferes with platelet activity. Although pharmacologic therapy can lower the homocysteine levels, no acute clinical benefits have been noted (chronic reduction in homocysteine levels by ferate [folic acid] is associated with dramatic reductions of the risks of those individuals with high homocysteine levels for developing coronary artery disease, carotid disease, and peripheral vascular disease).[11,12] Thus, symptomatic arterial occlusions are treated by standard surgical techniques of endarterectomy and/or bypass.[3]

Venous Disease

The pathophysiology of venous disease may be more complex than that of arterial disease. Whereas arteries are subject to two basic faults (obstruction and aneurysm formation), veins are subject to different ailments: obstruction, valvular insufficiency, intermittent flow, and low-pressure/low-flow states that engender thrombi. These thrombi can dislodge in the pulmonary circulation with unpredictable, life-threatening results.[13] Postoperative deep venous thrombosis (DVT) causes significant morbidity and mortality. The prevalence of DVT after surgery is striking: 10 to 40% of patients develop calf thrombosis after major abdominal or thoracic surgery; 2 to 8% develop iliofemoral thrombosis; and 1 to 8% will suffer a pulmonary embolism.[14] Pulmonary emboli cause 200,000 deaths a year.[15] Virchow's triad of stasis, en-

TABLE 24–2
Risk Factors for Deep Venous Thrombosis in Surgical Patients

Age greater than 40
Malignancy
Obesity
Pregnancy
Prior history of deep venous thrombosis or pulmonary embolism
Hip or knee surgery

Data from Sternbergh WC, Sobel M: Venous and lymphatic diseases. In Levine BA, Copeland EM, Howard RJ, et al (eds): Current Practice of Surgery. New York, Churchill Livingstone, 1986.

dothelial damage, and hypercoagulability provides the ideal milieu for development of a thrombus. DVT has been found to occur more frequently after surgery in certain groups of patients (Table 24–2).

When venous thrombosis is extensive, the outcome is likely to be poor. Phlegmasia cerulea dolens ("painful blue inflammation") is an uncommon and extreme example of venous thrombosis of the lower extremity. In this condition, the massive thrombosis and venous outflow obstruction in the leg prohibit the inflow of arterial blood. The etiologies fall into a few categories: malignancy and conditions promoting the stasis of blood, such as congestive heart failure, immobilization or trauma. The mortality rate for this disease is reported to be as high as 40%, with death stemming from either pulmonary emboli or the underlying disease process. Therapeutic choices depend on the extent of disease and include anticoagulation, thrombectomy, and amputation.[16,17]

Surgical Interventions

The goals of therapy for arterial occlusive disease are early enduring restoration of blood flow, confirmation of adequate perfusion, and management of the consequences of reperfusion. There are different methods to restore blood flow: thrombolysis, endovascular procedures (balloon angioplasty, atherectomy), surgical thromboembolectomy, and surgical arterial reconstruction. This overview will focus on lower extremity surgical bypass procedures. For correction of infrainguinal occlusive disease, an autogenous greater saphenous vein is the preferred vascular graft. The patency of saphenous vein grafts exceeds that of all types of synthetic grafts, such as polytetrafluoroethylene (PTFE) or Dacron grafts. The surgeon harvests the vein with great care to avoid ischemic or mechanical injury. The vein segment is distended with fluid (balanced crystalloid, albumin, or whole blood) under low pressure until ready for insertion. A long arm vein can be substituted if the greater saphenous is unsuitable. Commonly, heparin, 100 U/kg, is administered intravenously to prevent stasis during periods of arterial occlusion. The excised vein is removed from its bed and inverted so that the native proximal vein is anastomosed to the distal arterial site, and the native distal vein is sewn to the proximal arterial site—hence the term "reverse saphenous graft." The proximal arterial site of anastomosis is most frequently the common femoral artery, although other inflow sites can be used.[1,18]

Another technique for using the saphenous vein is the in situ graft. In this procedure, the surgeon dissects the saphenous vein; then, without removing the vein from its bed, the surgeon excises its valves with a valvulotome, and anastomoses proximal vein to proximal artery and distal vein to distal artery. Although some authors have suggested that this technique offers superior patency of the graft, prospective studies have not supported the notion. When veins are unsuitable, the alternative conduits include Dacron, umbilical vein, and PTFE grafts. The advantage of using these grafts is that no time is spent dissecting and preparing a vein graft, and no venous anatomy is distorted.[1,18] There are some circumstances in which prosthetic grafts are as good as or superior to vein grafts for long-term patency. For example, patency rates for above-knee femoropopliteal bypass grafts are similar.[1,19]

Preparing the Patient for Surgery

Once the need for surgery is decided, preoperative evaluation can proceed as thoroughly as possible, modified by the urgency of the situation. The in-hospital mortality for patients undergoing femoropopliteal bypasses ranges from 2 to 3%, and increases to 5 or 6% for distal tibial bypasses.[15] The long-term survival for these patients is limited by advanced age and complicated disease processes. The 5-year mortality after femoropopliteal grafts was reported by DeWeese and Rob to be 48%, and the 10-year mortality 73%.[20] Although the degrees of concomitant illness of some patients with limb-threatening ischemia might discourage some anesthesiologists and surgeons, patients undergoing revascularization may experience a better outcome than those undergoing amputation. In one investigation, revascularized patients had a significantly lower perioperative mortality rate (2.9% vs. 7.6%), shorter hospital stays, and improved long-term survival, compared to patients whose extremities were amputated.[21]

The major cause of perioperative and late postoperative mortality in patients with peripheral vascular disease is cardiac in origin.[15,20,22–26] Hertzer et al. evaluated 1,001 patients with peripheral vascular disease (cerebrovascular, aortic aneurysmal, or lower extremity occlusive disease) by coronary angiography. Only 10% of patients with lower extremity ischemia (n = 381) had normal coronary arteries. Mild to moderate coronary artery disease (CAD) was found in 33%; severe, correctable disease in 21%; and severe, inoperable disease in 7%. The usual screening tests, such as history, physical examination, and electrocardiogram (ECG), did not consistently predict the extent of the patient's CAD. For example, severe, correctable CAD was found in 19% of patients with no history of angina, and in 19% of the patients with normal ECGs.[25] (Details of preoperative risk and evaluation are found in Chapters 2 and 3 of this volume.)

These patients have multiple other disease processes to complicate evaluation and management. Hypertension is frequently found in patients with peripheral vascular disease, with a prevalence of 40 to 60%.[27] All arterial beds suffer the effects of longstanding, untreated hypertension. End-organ changes in the cerebral, myocardial, and renal vascular beds are especially important, and may render these patients more prone to perioperative cerebrovascular accidents, congestive heart failure, and renal insufficiency.[28,29] Antihypertensive therapy improves survival and lowers mortality in the general population,[30] yet, in the perioperative period, hypertension may[31] or may not[32] affect outcome. Routine use of β-adrenergic receptor blockade improves intermediate outcomes and improves 2-year survival from 79% to 90% in patients undergoing noncardiac surgery who were on average 68 years old at time of operation.[33–35] This improvement in outcome occurred irrespective of preoperative hypertensive state, and may relate to stabilization of the plaque. Exclusion criteria for this 50 mg twice daily oral dose of atenolol included severe LV or RV failure, and significant airway resistive disease.

Chronic obstructive pulmonary disease (COPD) is diagnosed in a significant fraction (one quarter to one half) of patients with peripheral vascular disease.[27] Patients with more advanced degrees of COPD may benefit from preoperative assessment and therapy to define the degree of pulmonary dysfunction as well as to maximize respiratory function. Although few patients require preoperative pulmonary function tests, findings may identify those patients at high risk for postoperative pulmonary complications, such as atelectasis, infection, cor pulmonale, or respiratory failure.[36] For example, if the forced expired volume in 1 second (FEV_1) is less than 1 L, or if the maximum breathing capacity is less than 50% of predicted, the patient is at high risk for postoperative respiratory sequelae.[37] Respiratory complications can also be predicted if the ratio of FEV_1 to forced vital capacity (FVC) is less than 65% and if the FVC is less than 70% of predicted,[38] or by diffusing capacity.[39,40]

Intraoperative management of patients with COPD raises additional questions. The effect of anesthetic choice on outcome will be discussed later in the chapter. Inherent in the choice of anesthesia is the method of postoperative pain control. Effective postoperative analgesia is critical in this population; the goals are minimal respiratory depression and maximum respiratory function to avoid atelectasis and pneumonia. Choice of monitoring may well include arterial cannulation to obtain baseline arterial blood-gas measurements as well as intraoperative partial pressures of oxygen and carbon dioxide. But in our experience, most patients with nonbronchospastic COPD can be treated with β-adrenergic receptor blocking drugs to decrease their risk of perioperative and 2-year cardiac events and death.

Diabetes mellitus is a pathophysiologic process frequently associated with peripheral vascular disease, with a reported incidence of 8 to 12%.[27] The disease process has far-reaching implications with regard to preoperative assessment and perioperative management. Coronary artery disease and silent ischemia are found more frequently in diabetics, as are other cardiac disorders, including cardiomyopathy and congestive heart failure. Diabetic nephropathy is a frequent finding with implications for perioperative management, such as preexisting renal dysfunction, hyperkalemia, and the potential for worsening renal insufficiency with hypovolemia or nephrotoxic agents.[41]

Hyperglycemia can escalate with the metabolic stress of surgery. Although intraoperative hypoglycemia can have grave neurologic consequences, hyperglycemia may contribute to neurologic injury in its own right, impair wound healing and leukocyte function, and increase wound infections. Hyperglycemia can also cause profound metabolic disturbances, such as electrolyte disturbances, osmotic diuresis, ketoacidosis, and hyperosmolar coma.[41]

Numerous regimens have been suggested for one of the major aspects of perioperative diabetic management, the control of glucose levels during the perioperative period. Yet blood glucose levels vary with each patient and depend on the severity of disease, the stress of surgery, and even the type of anesthesia. Therefore, each patient's insulin regimen could be tapered to individual needs. One proven and straightforward method of perioperative glucose control was tested by Watts et al.[42] In their protocol, intravenous fluids containing dextrose and an infusion of insulin (1.5 U/hr) are started on calibrated infusion pumps prior to surgery. Blood glucose is checked every 2 hours and the insulin infusion adjusted appropriately. Once the patient begins eating, the intravenous dextrose and insulin are discontinued, and appropriate subcutaneous doses of insulin restarted.[42] Of equal importance may be the need to search for the diabetic with autonomic neuropathy. These patients appear especially vulnerable to sudden life-threatening bradycardias in the postoperative period, and may be more at risk after regional anesthesia.[43]

Choice of Anesthetic

What is the best choice of anesthetic to optimize the outcome of lower extremity revascularization? This question defines the essence of this chapter and is the source of much debate. There are advantages and disadvantages to both regional and general anesthesia (Table 24–3). These facts are thoroughly described in the anesthesia literature; the factors most applicable to lower extremity revascularization will be discussed.

Studies comparing general and regional techniques (Table 24–4) are small in number, limited in size, and conflicting in their conclusions.[44–51] Only six studies were prospective,[41–44,47–51] and one of these was not randomized.[48] Several studies showed no difference in cardiac morbidity.[44,48–50] But two investigations[45,46] reported significantly more myocardial ischemia or infarction with regional anesthesia. Six of the eight studies reported no difference in mortality between general and regional anesthesia.[44,46–50] In contrast, mortality was much greater after regional in one study as reported in an abstract.[45]

TABLE 24–3
General and Regional Anesthesia

	Advantages	Disadvantages
General Anesthesia	Always works Duration—controlled Decreased MVO_2 Hemodynamic—controllable	Airway management Complication of intubation Decreased mucociliary flow Aspiration Malignant hyperthermia
Regional Anesthesia	Conscious patient Maintains own airway Monitor cerebral function Increased lower extremity blood flow Decreased thromboembolism Lowers stress response to surgery (cortisol, catecholamines, antidiuretic hormone, and corticotropin) Epidural analgesia can be continued into postoperative period	Hypotension Duration—not always controllable Local anesthesia toxicity Headache Hematoma Infection "Spotty" block

The reader should hesitate to conclude from any one study alone or even from the aggregate that anesthetic type (and not anesthesiologist and his/her knowledge and management of pathophysiology) makes the difference to outcome. The number of patients is too small to reach a statistically valid conclusion; the number of patients ranges from 19[47] to 213.[48] To detect a significant difference between groups—for example, a decrease in death from 5% to 2.5%—the design of the investigation with 80% power would require enrolling 715 patients in each group. No such study exists, nor will it exist until a multidisciplinary team of researchers, including anesthesiologists, vascular surgeons, cardiologists, and other specialists, are assembled from multiple institutions to undertake this formidable yet achievable task.

The influence of anesthetic technique on coagulation during the perioperative period may affect outcome (Table 24–5). In the early 1980s, investigators began to report fewer thromboembolic events with regional anesthesia than with general anesthesia, after hip surgery[52,53] and lower abdominal surgery.[54] In 1987, Yeager et al. published a well-publicized study, and reported the significantly improved outcome in high-risk patients who received epidural anesthesia and analgesia. Patients undergoing major vascular surgery were one subgroup that had a significantly lower mortality rate with regional added to a "light-general."[55] It is now clear that peripheral vascular surgery activates processes that result in a hypercoagulable state after surgery. Strategies that render such hypercoagulable state either nonexistent, or its effects on outcome will include regional anesthesia, sympatholysis, and anticoagulation.[56–58]

What are the proposed benefits of regional, especially epidural, analgesia for patients undergoing peripheral vascular procedures? If prolonged epidural analgesia can prevent thrombosis, then there is *less* potential for clots to occlude a new lower-extremity graft and coronary arteries, with resulting ischemia and infarction. In addition, deep venous thrombosis and pulmonary emboli may occur less frequently.

Several mechanisms are postulated by which regional analgesia may decrease thrombotic events. First, blood flow to the legs is improved by epidural analgesia.[59,60] As blood flow improves, stasis and resultant thrombosis become less likely. Hemorrheologic equilibrium changes after surgery, and is affected by blood viscosity and the balance between thrombosis and fibrinolysis.

The tendency toward decreased fibrinolysis has been noted in vascular surgery patients. Several studies have identified an increase in the serum levels of an inhibitor of fibrinolysis, plasminogen activator inhibitor 1.[61,62] On a macroscopic level, the incidence of deep venous thrombosis was significantly lower when epidural analgesia was used for hip surgery and for analgesia over the following 24 hours.[53]

Vascular surgery patients are known to be hypercoagulable before and after surgery. Thromboelastography showed larger alpha and MA values for these patients.[63] McDaniel and co-workers studied patients undergoing femorotibial bypass, and found postoperative increases in platelet reactivity and in factor VIII–related antigen. The increase in factor VIII–related antigen implied ongoing intravascular coagulation.[64] Also, levels of antithrombin III, a major circulating inhibitor of intravascular coagulation, were found to be decreased in these patients, thus theoretically predisposing them to thrombosis.[64,65]

How can the data regarding perioperative coagulation changes be summarized? There are no *large-scale* studies that conclusively show better outcomes when epidural analgesia is used for postoperative analgesia. However, more aggressive monitoring of coagulation changes may be in order. Some authors recommend the continued use of heparin in the week after surgery; the route of administration was not specified. Nonsteroidal, anti-inflammatory drugs were recommended if the fibrinogen exceeded 5 gm/L. Aspirin may be the preferred drug in those at risk of myocardial ischemia, as it seems to result in equal preventive and a much better therapeutic result if infarction occurs.[66,67] These authors also recommended

TABLE 24–4
Studies Comparing General and Regional Anesthesia in Patients Undergoing Lower-Extremity Revascularization

Study References	No. of Pts.		Description of		Mortality		Significant Results
	GA	REG	GA	Regional	GA	REG	
Cooke et al (1986)[38]	51	50	Fentanyl, thiopental, N_2O, halothane	SAB: cinchocaine	3/51 = 5.9%	1/50 = 2% *not diff.	GA Lost more blood More chest infections (35% vs 16%) SAB—more hypotension & bradycardia No difference in graft patency at 3 months Prospective No difference in mortality or cardiac morbidity
Underwood et al (1988)[39]	44	23	Etomidate, opioid, isoflurane	Epidural: 2-chloroprocaine	0	5/23 = 21.7%	3 regional patients sustained acute MIs immediately postoperatively and died All patients were >70 years old Retrospective Abstract only
Maniolo et al (1989)[40]	56	66 Epid 12 SAB	Not recorded	Not recorded	1 = 1.8%	3 = 3.9% *not diff.	12 patients demonstrated myocardial ischemia or infarction; 11/12 had regional anesthesia ($p = .015$) Retrospective
Damask et al (1990)[41]	10	9	Thiopental, N_2O, isoflurane, morphine	Epidural: 2-chloroprocaine	0*	0*	Epidural patients—more stable hemodynamics intraoperatively Prospective and randomized *No intraoperative deaths; study ends in PACU
Rivers et al (1991)[42]	117	96	Not recorded	Not recorded	4/117 = 3.4%	5/46 = 5.2% *not diff.	No difference in pulmonary complication, nonfatal perioperative MI, or other cardiac events Prospective, not randomized
Beattie et al (1993)[43]	51	49			3/51 = 5.9%	4/49 = 8.2% *not diff.	Very thorough study; continuous Holter monitoring No difference before groups in ischemia, infarction, or death Ischemia rate doubles with age >65, hypothermic ($t < 35.0$), and Hct <29% Mortality = Death within 6 months Reoperation for graft occlusion was significantly more common in GA (11) vs. Reg (2), and this finding led to termination of study
Bode et al (1996)[50]	138	149 = epidural 136 SAB	Thiopental, fentanyl, isoflurane or enflurane, N_2O	Epidural: lidocaine then bupivacaine SAB tetracaine	4/138 = 2.9%	5/139 = 3.4% 4/136 = 2.9% *not diff.	Through, prospective study No difference in any measure of mortality
Christoferson et al (1992)[51]	51	49	Thiamylal, fentanyl enflurane, N_2O, PCA	Epidural: bupivacaine	3/51	4/49 *not sign if	Significant difference in number requiring reoperation: 36% with general versus 12% with epidural

TABLE 24–5
Factors Affecting the Coagulation-Anticoagulation Balance

Factors that Oppose Clotting	Factors that Promote Clotting
Anticoagulants	Protamine
Heparin	Increased blood viscosity and fibrinogen
Warfarin	Increased platelet reactivity
Drugs that cause fibrinolysis	Increased factor VIII–related antigen
Streptokinase	Decreased antithrombin III
Urokinase	Decreased blood flow or stasis
Tissue plasminogen activator (t-PA)	
Drugs that decrease platelet function	
Nonsteroidal anti-inflammatory drugs	
Aspirin	
Dipyridamole	
Calcium channel blockers	
β-Blockers	
Antibiotics	
Dextran	
Hypothermia	

monitoring serial hematocrits and hemodilution, if necessary, to keep the hematocrit less than 35%.[62]

Another potential benefit of epidural anesthesia revolves around the concept of pre-emptive analgesia. If analgesics are given *before* surgical incision, sensitization of central neural functions may be decreased. With pre-emptive analgesia—local anesthetic plus opioid delivered to the epidural space prior to incision—patients have reported lower pain scores and required less postoperative analgesia.[68]

Now that the potential benefits of regional anesthesia and analgesia have been discussed, the risks should be acknowledged. Postoperative neurologic dysfunction, especially in anticoagulated patients, is a significant and potentially devastating complication. Several investigations have reported no evidence of neurologic dysfunction in patients receiving intraoperative anticoagulation.[69–71] Spinal cord hemorrhage with hematoma formation occurs,[72] and it has been reported to occur spontaneously,[73] with anticoagulants,[74,75] with neoplasms,[76] and with vascular anomalies of the spinal cord.[77,78] Thus, epidural and spinal hematoma can occur without epidural or spinal analgesia procedures; in fact, the data strongly suggest that the incidence of hematoma not caused by epidural or spinal instrumentation is many-fold greater than following it. Nonetheless, there are numerous reports of spinal cord hematoma following either epidural or subdural puncture and anticoagulation.[79–87] Although some patients may completely recover neurologic function, others suffer permanent deficits, including paraplegia or quadriplegia with respiratory failure and death.[73,74,79–87] The rapidity of diagnosis and evacuation of the hematoma after symptoms (often severe back pain with or without immediate peripheral decrements in neurologic motor and sensory function) appears crucial to restoring neurologic function.[88]

Rao and El-Etr published the largest examination of patients with regional anesthesia and subsequent anticoagulation. In their report of 3,164 epidural and 847 subdural catheter placements, they reported no neurologic consequences. However, they emphasized three important caveats: (1) proper patient selection (i.e., no history of leukemia, hemophilia, blood dyscrasias, thrombocytopenia, or preoperative anticoagulation therapy); (2) if the regional technique was traumatic or yielded a bloody tap, the patient's surgery was postponed and rescheduled for general anesthesia the following day; and (3) anticoagulation with heparin was closely monitored to keep the activated clotting time approximately twice the baseline value.[71]

A prevailing bias among physicians is that regional anesthesia is better than general anesthesia for patients with pulmonary dysfunction, but little outcome data support this notion. Although subarachnoid blocks to the midthoracic level in patients with COPD resulted in no impairment of quiet respiration, forced expiratory volumes were decreased. Thus, the ability to cough and to clear secretions was limited for a period of time.[89] General anesthesia and endotracheal intubation allow complete control of the airway, the ability to give bronchodilating agents, and the ability to suction secretions, thus maximizing pulmonary toilet.[90]

As with adverse postoperative cardiac events, postoperative management and interventions to treat pulmonary conditions are likely to have at least as great an impact on outcome as intraoperative management. Some studies report advantages of regional anesthesia, such as better Pa_{O_2} 1 hour,[91] and 1 to 3 days after surgery.[92] But does a higher postoperative Pa_{O_2} necessarily translate to a shorter intensive care unit (ICU) or hospital stay or to a lower hospital bill? Perhaps continued epidural analgesia over days makes a difference in pulmonary function. Yeager et al. found a difference in their high-risk population.[55] But does it matter for patients with healthy lungs? Jayr and colleagues found no reduction in pulmonary complications after intra-abdominal procedures and postoperative epidural analgesia (bupivacain and morphine), compared to parenteral morphine. One major difference was that the epidural patients were more comfortable after surgery.[93] Again, no large-scale outcome studies are available. To find a decrease in pulmonary complications from 26%[94] to 13%, a study with 80% power would need to enroll 114 (p = .05) patients in each group.

The Anesthetic Plan

The patient has been evaluated; preoperative therapies have been continued, and perhaps some such as β-blockade (atenolol 50 ng PO bid) added; the pros and cons of general and regional anesthesia are discussed. How does the clinician proceed in choosing an anesthetic for infrainguinal bypass procedures? The anesthesiologist can take into consideration the talents and desires of all the pertinent individuals; patient, surgeon, and anesthesiologist. If the anticipated duration of surgery exceeds reasonable limits of patient compliance with regional anesthesia, general anesthesia alone or in addition to regional anesthesia is clearly a superior choice. Longer surgical times may be expected if the surgery is technically difficult. Likewise, there are some surgeons who operate faster than others. Regional anesthesia is contraindicated (at least in some [but not all] experts' opinion) in the fully anticoagulated patient. When patients are particularly fearful or flatly refuse regional techniques, general anesthesia may be chosen. There are very few circumstances in which the anesthesiologist must insist on regional techniques. Regional anesthesia is a reasonable choice in circumstances other than those mentioned above.

At our hospital, the anesthesiology faculty has collectively chosen not to place epidural catheters prior to surgery in patients who will be anticoagulated. Therefore, the subarachnoid block is the technique of choice when regional anesthesia is chosen. If the patient who receives a single shot subarachnoid block will be monitored in the ICU after surgery, intrathecal morphine can be given with the local anesthetic, adding 18 to 24 hours of pain relief. In special circumstances (e.g., at the patient's specific request), an epidural catheter will be placed postoperatively after coagulation variables have been checked.

Intraoperative hemodynamic monitoring for a peripheral vascular procedure is chosen based on the patient's underlying diseases. American Society of Anesthesiologists (ASA) standard monitors alone can be employed in the relatively rare patient with no evidence of other systemic disease. If moderate blood loss is expected or the patient has a significant underlying medical disorder (such as uncontrolled hypertension or significant lung disease), continuous, invasive monitoring of arterial pressure may be indicated. At our institution, additional invasive hemodynamic monitors, such as central venous pressure or pulmonary artery pressure, are used only in unusual circumstances, such as the patient with renal failure or significantly compromised ventricular function who needs close monitoring of intravenous volume. Unfortunately, hemodynamic changes are poor indicators of myocardial ischemia.[95] Transesophageal echocardiography (TEE) may be the most sensitive monitor of myocardial ischemia. However, the value of TEE in vascular surgery patients remains uncertain. Although some researchers regard TEE as an "invaluable tool"[96] during vascular surgery, others decry its utility.[97]

The physiologic consequences of endoluminal surgery and its differences from conventional surgery are still evolving, and its physiologic trespass seems to diminish as surgical experience increases.[98,99]

Myocardial oxygen supply and demand may be in tenuous balance in the perioperative period. One important determinant of oxygen supply is hematocrit, and another is patient temperature. Anemia was found to be a risk factor for ischemia in one study of patients undergoing lower-extremity revascularization. A hematocrit of 29% was found to be a threshold point: patients with hematocrits below 29% on postoperative day 2 had significantly more ischemia than those with higher hematocrits.[100] We also believe that maintenance of normothermia in the postoperative period is important to outcome.

Whereas monitoring in the operating room is vigilant, with tight control of hemodynamic changes and other physiologic variables, the period immediately after surgery carries insidious risks. Many variables can contribute to the likelihood of postoperative myocardial ischemia: increased adrenergic activity can result from physical or emotional stress, withdrawal of analgesia, and altered vasomotor regulation. Hypothermia, hypoxemia, fluid shifts, and hypercoagulability may also contribute to ischemia.[101] Currently, because of the lack of data, it is impossible to know what the best postoperative methods are to improve outcome. For example, should patients be offered 3 or 4 days of continuous epidural analgesia to minimize stress, increase blood flow through the graft, and decrease hypercoagulability to some extent? Should each patient be partially or completely anticoagulated for the same period? In fact, how much does postoperative morbidity and mortality depend on coagulation? We do know that in those patients without exclusion criteria, a perioperative sympathectomy can be easily instituted with β-adrenergic receptor blocking drugs perioperatively, and improves 2-year survival rates significantly and substantially.[33–35,102] The answers require large outcome studies that by necessity will examine multiple variables.

Conclusion

Perhaps this review has raised more questions than it has answered, regarding anesthesia for peripheral vascular surgery. However, it is our hope that a clearer understanding of pathophysiology and the available choices will better serve the clinician and the patient.

References

1. Seeger JM: Peripheral arterial occlusive disease. In Levine BA, Copeland EM, Howard RJ, et al (eds): Current Practice of Surgery. New York, Churchill Livingstone, 1993.
2. Perry MO: Acute ischemia and its sequelae. In Rutherford RB (ed): Vascular Surgery, 3rd ed. Philadelphia, WB Saunders Co, 1989, p 541.
3. Harward TRS: Nonatherosclerotic peripheral vascular disease. In Levine BA, Copeland EM, Howard RJ, et al (eds): Current Practice of Surgery. New York, Churchill Livingstone, 1993.
4. Brewster DC, Chin AK, Fogarty TJ: Arterial thromboembolism. In Rutherford RB (ed): Vascular Surgery, 3rd ed. Philadelphia, WB Saunders Co, 1989, p 548.
5. Kaufman JL, Karmody AM, Leather RP: Atheroembolism and microthromboembolic syndromes (the blue toe syndrome and disseminated atheroembolism). In Rutherford RB (ed): Vascular Surgery, 3rd ed. Philadelphia, WB Saunders Co, 1989, p 565.
6. Taylor LM, Porter JM: Natural history and nonoperative treatment of chronic lower extremity ischemia. In Rutherford RB (ed): Vascular Surgery, 3rd ed. Philadelphia, WB Saunders Co, 1989, p 653.
7. Davies MJ, Woolf N: Atherosclerosis: What is it and why does it occur? Br Heart J suppl. 69:S3, 1993.
8. Badimon JJ, Fuster V, Chesebro JH, Badimon L: Coronary atherosclerosis—a multifactorial disease. Circulation (Suppl II): II-3, 1993.
9. Smith SC: Risk-reduction therapy: The challenge to change. Circulation 93:2205, 1996.

10. Shionoya S: Buerger's disease (thromboangiitis obliterans). In Rutherford RB (ed): Vascular Surgery, 3rd ed. Philadelphia, WB Saunders Co, 1989, p 207.
11. Pancharomitz N, Lewis CA, Sauberlah HE, et al: Plasma homocysteine, folate, and vitamin B12 concentrations and the risk for early onset coronary artery disease. Am J Clin Nutr 59:940, 1994.
12. Selhub J, Jacques PJ, Bostom AG, et al: Association between plasma homocysteine concentrations and extracranial carotid-artery stenosis. N Engl J Med 332:286, 1995.
13. Sumner DS: Hemodynamics and pathophysiology of venous disease. In Rutherford RB (ed): Vascular Surgery, 3rd ed. Philadelphia, WB Saunders Co, 1989, p 1483.
14. Sternbergh WC, Sobel M: Venous and lymphatic diseases. In Levine BA, Copeland EM, Howard RJ, et al (eds): Current Practice of Surgery. New York, Churchill Livingstone, 1986.
15. Smith RB, Perdue GD: Diseases of the peripheral arteries and veins. In Hurst JW, Schlant RC, Rackley CE, et al (eds): The Heart. New York, McGraw-Hill, 1990, p 1423.
16. Hirschmann JV: Ischemic forms of acute venous thrombosis. Arch Dermatol 123:933, 1987.
17. Weaver FA, Meacham PW, Adkins RB, Dean RH: Phlegmasia cerulea dolens: Therapeutic considerations. So Med J 81:306, 1988.
18. Bernhard VM: Bypass to the popliteal and infrapopliteal arteries. In Rutherford RB (ed): Vascular Surgery, 3rd ed. Philadelphia, WB Saunders Co, 1989, p 692.
19. Veith FJ, Gupta SK, Ascer E, et al: Six-year prospective multicenter randomized comparison of autologous saphenous vein and expanded polytetrafluoroethylene grafts in infrainguinal arterial reconstructions. J Vasc Surg 3:104, 1986.
20. DeWeese JA, Rob CG: Autogenous vein grafts ten years later. Surgery 82:775, 1977.
21. Ouriel K, Fiore WM, Geary JE: Limb-threatening ischemia in the medically compromised patient: Amputation or revascularization. Surgery 104:667, 1988.
22. Leather RP, Shah DM, Buchbender D, et al: Further experience with the saphenous vein graft used in situ for arterial bypass. Am J Surg 142:506, 1981.
23. Bunt TU: Aortic reconstruction versus extra-anatomic bypass and angioplasty. Arch Surg 121:1166, 1986.
24. Stoelting RK, Dierdorf SF, McCammon RL: Diseases of the nervous system. In Anesthesia and Co-Existing Disease, 2nd ed. New York, Churchill Livingstone, 1988, p 263.
25. Hertzer NR, Beven EG, Youns JR, et al: Coronary artery disease in peripheral vascular patients. Ann Surg 199:223, 1984.
26. Cooperman M, Pflug B, Martin EW, Evans WE: Cardiovascular risk factors in patients with peripheral vascular disease. Surgery 84:505, 1978.
27. Clark NJ, Stanley TH: Anesthesia for vascular surgery. In Miller RD (ed): Anesthesia, 3rd ed. New York, Churchill Livingstone, 1990, p 1693.
28. Hall WD: Mild and moderate hypertension. In Hurst JW (ed): Medicine for the Practicing Physician. Boston, Butterworths, 1988, p 391.
29. Breslow MJ, Lish M: Hypertension. In Breslow MJ, Miller CF, Rogers MC (eds): Perioperative Management. Washington, DC, CV Mosby Co, 1990, p 281.
30. Hypertension detection and follow-up program cooperative group: Five-year findings of the hypertension detection and follow-up program. JAMA 242:2562, 1979.
31. Prys-Roberts C, Green LT, Meloche R: Studies of anaesthesia in relation to hypertension. II: Haemodynamic consequences of induction and endotracheal intubation. Br J Anaesth 43:531, 1971.
32. Goldman L, Caldera DL: Risks of general anesthesia and elective operation in the hypertensive patient. Anesthesiology 30: 285, 1979.
33. Stone JG, Foex P, Sear JW, et al: Risk of myocardial ischemia during anaesthesia in treated and untreated hypertensive patients. Br J Anaesth 61:675, 1988.
34. Pasternack PF, Grossi EA, Baumann FG, et al: Beta blockade to decrease silent myocardial ischemia during peripheral vascular surgery. Am J Surg 158:113, 1989.
35. Mangano DT, Layug EL, Wallace A, Tateo I: Effect of atenolol on mortality and cardiovascular morbidity after noncardiac surgery. N Engl J Med 335:1713, 1996.
36. Benumof JL: Preoperative respiratory preparation. In Anesthesia for Thoracic Surgery. Philadelphia, WB Saunders Co, 1987, p 156.
37. Tisi GM: Preoperative identification and evaluation of the patient with lung disease. Med Clin North Am 71:399, 1987.
38. Gass CD, Olsen GN: Preoperative pulmonary function testing to predict postoperative morbidity and mortality. Chest 89:127, 1986.
39. Furguson MK, Little L, Rizzo L, et al: Diffusing capacity predicts morbidity and mortality after pulmonary resection. J Thorac Cardiovasc Surg 96:894, 1988.
40. Markos J, Mullan BP, Hillman DR, et al: Preoperative assessment as a predictor of mortality and morbidity after lung resection. Am Rev Respir Dis 139:902, 1989.
41. King LW, Snyder DS: Diabetes and other endocrine disorders. In Breslow MJ, Miller CF, Rogers MC (eds): Perioperative Management. Washington, DC, CV Mosby Co, 1990, p 292.
42. Watts NB, Gebhart SSP, Clark RV, et al: Postoperative management of diabetes mellitus: Steady-state glucose control with bedside algorithm for insulin adjustment. Diabetes Care 10:722, 1987.
43. Charlson ME, MacKenzie CR, Gold JP: Preoperative autonomic function abnormalities in patients with diabetes mellitus and patients with hypertension. J Am Coll Surg 179:1, 1994.
44. Cook PT, Davies MJ, Cronin KD, Moran P: A prospective randomized trial comparing spinal anesthesia using hyperbaric cinchocaine with general anesthesia for lower limb vascular surgery. Anaesth Intensive Care 14:373, 1986.
45. Underwood PS, Kepes E, Hollinger I: A comparison of epidural versus general anesthetic for elderly patients undergoing peripheral revascularization (Abstract). Anesthesiology 69:A105, 1988.
46. Maniolo TA, Beattie C, Christopherson R, et al: Regional versus general anesthesia in high-risk surgical patients: The need for a clinical trial. J Clin Anesth 1:414, 1989.
47. Damask MC, Weissman C, Todd G: General versus epidural anesthesia for femoral-popliteal bypass surgery. J Clin Anesth 2: 71, 1990.
48. Rivers SP, Scher LA, Sheehan E, Veith FJ: Epidural versus general anesthesia for infrainguinal arterial reconstruction. J Vasc Surg 14:764, 1991.
49. Beattie C: Personal communication of results of NIH grant GM 38177.
50. Bode RH, Lewis KP, Zarich SW, et al: Cardiac outcome after peripheral vascular surgery: Comparison of regional or general anesthesia. Anesthesiology 84:3, 1996.
51. Christopherson R, Beattie C, Frank SM, et al: Perioperative morbidity in patients randomized to epidural or general anesthesia for lower extremity vascular surgery. Anesthesiology 79:422, 1993.
52. Modig J, Borg T, Bagge L, Saldeen T: Role of extra-dural and of general anesthesia in fibrinolysis and coagulation after total hip replacement. Br J Anaesth 55:625, 1983.
53. Modig J, Borg T, Karlström G, et al: Thromboembolism after total hip replacement: Role of epidural and general anesthesia. Anesth Analg 62:174, 1983.
54. Bredbacka S, Blombäck M, Hagnevik K, et al: Pre- and postoperative changes in coagulation and fibrinolytic variables during abdominal hysterectomy under epidural or general anesthesia. Acta Anesthesiol Scand 30:204, 1986.
55. Yeager MP, Glass DD, Neff RK, Brinck-Johnsen T: Epidural anesthesia and analgesia in high-risk surgical patients. Anesthesiology 66:729, 1987.
56. Engleman E, Lipszyc M, Gilbart E, et al: Effects of clonidine on anesthetic drug requirements and hemodynamic response during aortic surgery. Anesthesiology 71:178, 1989.
57. Rosenfeld BA, Faraday N, Cambell D, et al: Perioperative platelet reactivity and the effects of clonidine. Anesthesiology 79: 255, 1993.
58. Ellis JE, Drijvers G, Pedlow S, et al: Premedication with oral and transdermal clonidine provides safe and efficacious postoperative sympatholysis. Anesth Analg 79:1133, 1994.
59. Cousins MJ, Wright CJ: Graft, muscle, and skin blood flow after epidural block in vascular surgical procedures. Surg Gynecol Obstet 133:59, 1971.
60. Poikolainen E, Hendolin H: Effects of lumbar epidural analgesia and general anesthesia on flow velocity in the femoral vein and

postoperative deep venous thrombosis. Acta Chir Scand 149: 361, 1983.
61. Gomez MJ, Carroll RC, Hansard MR, et al: Regulation of fibrinolysis in aortic surgery. J Vasc Surg 8:384, 1988.
62. Freyburger G, Janvier G, Dief S, Boisseau MR: Fibrinolytic and hemorrheologic alterations during and after elective aortic graft surgery: Implications for postoperative management. Anesth Analg 76:504, 1993.
63. Tuman KJ, McCarthy RJ, March RJ, et al: Effects of epidural anesthesia and analgesia on coagulation and outcome after major vascular surgery. Anesth Analg 73:696, 1991.
64. McDaniel MD, Pearce WH, Yao JST, et al: Sequential changes in coagulation and platelet function following femorotibial bypass. J Vasc Surg 1:261, 1984.
65. Flinn WR, McDaniel MD, Yao JST, et al: Antithrombin III deficiency as a reflection of dynamic protein metabolism in patients undergoing vascular reconstruction. J Vasc Surg 1:888, 1984.
66. Brown EJ, Kloner RA, Schoen FJ, et al: Scar thinning due to ibuprofen administration after experimental myocardial infarction. Am J Cardiol 51:877, 1983.
67. Pfeffer MA, Braunwald Z: Ventricular remodeling after myocardial infarction. Experimental observations and clinical implications. Circulation: 81:1161, 1990.
68. Katz J, Kavanagh BP, Sandler AN, et al: Preemptive analgesia: Clinical evidence of neuroplasticity contributing to postoperative pain. Anesthesiology 77:439, 1992.
69. Odoom JA, Sih IL: Epidural analgesia and anticoagulant therapy. Experience with one thousand cases of continuous epidurals. Anaesthesia 38:254, 1983.
70. Baron HC, LaRaja RD, Rossi G, Atkinson D: Continuous epidural analgesia in the heparinized vascular surgical patient: A retrospective review of 912 patients. J Vasc Surg 6:144, 1987.
71. Rao TLK, Ei-Etr AA: Anticoagulation following placement of epidural and subarachnoid catheters: An evaluation of neurologic sequelae. Anesthesiology 95:618, 1981.
72. Owens EL, Kasten GW, Hessel EA: Spinal subarachnoid hematoma after lumbar puncture and heparinization: A case report, review of the literature and discussion of anesthetic implications. Anesth Analg 65:1021, 1986.
73. Costabile G, Husag L, Probst C: Spinal epidural hematoma. Surg Neurol 21:489, 1984.
74. Bamford CR: Spinal epidural hematoma due to heparin. Arch Neurol 85:693, 1978.
75. Spurny OM, Rubin S, Wolf JW, Wu WQ: Spinal epidural hematoma during anticoagulant therapy. Arch Intern Med 114:103, 1964.
76. Prieto A, Cantu RC: Spinal subarachnoid hemorrhage associated with neurofibroma of the cauda equina. J Neurosurg 27:63, 1962.
77. Aminoff MJ, Logue V: The prognosis of patients with spinal vascular malformations. Brain 97:211, 1974.
78. Eastwood DW: Hematoma after epidural anesthesia: Relationship of skin and spinal angiomas. Anesth Analg 73:352, 1991.
79. Edelson RN, Chenik NL, Posner JB: Spinal subdural hematomas complicating lumbar puncture. Occurrence in thrombocytopenic patients. Arch Neurol 31:134, 1974.
80. Messer HD, Froshan VR, Brust JC, Hughes JEO: Transient paraplegia from hematoma after lumbar puncture. A consequence of anticoagulant therapy. JAMA 235:529, 1976.
81. Brem SS, Hafler DA, Van Uitert RL, et al: Spinal subarachnoid hematoma. N Engl J Med 303:1020, 1981.
82. Varkey GP, Brindle GF: Peridural anaesthesia and anticoagulant therapy. Can Anaesth Soc J 21:106, 1974.
83. Gingrich TR: Spinal epidural hematoma following continuous epidural anesthesia. Anesthesiology 29:162, 1968.
84. Helperin SW, Cohen DD: Hematoma following epidural anesthesia: A report of a case. Anesthesiology 35:641, 1971.
85. Butler AB, Green CD: Haematoma following epidural anaesthesia. Can Anaesth Soc J 17:635, 1970.
86. DeAngelis J: Hazards of subdural and epidural anesthesia during anticoagulant therapy: A case report and review. Anesth Analg 51:676, 1972.
87. Onishchuk JL, Carlsson C: Epidural hematoma associated with epidural anesthesia: Complications of anticoagulant therapy. Anesthesiology 77:1221, 1992.
88. Kroll DA, Caplan RA, Posner K, et al: Nerve injury associated with anesthesia. Anesthesiology 73:202, 1990.
89. Paskin S, Rodman T, Smith TC: The effect of spinal anesthesia on the pulmonary function of patients with chronic obstructive pulmonary disease. Ann Surg 169:35, 1969.
90. Blosser SA, Rock P: Asthma and chronic obstructive lung disease. In Breslow MJ, Miller CF, Rogers MC (eds): Perioperative Management. Washington, DC, CV Mosby Co, 1990, p 226.
91. McKenzie PJ, Wishart HY, Dewar KMS, et al: Comparison of the effects of spinal anaesthesia and general anaesthesia on postoperative oxygenation and perioperative mortality. Br J Anaesth 52:49, 1980.
92. Hole A, Terjensen T, Breivik H: Epidural versus general anaesthesia for total hip arthroplasty in elderly patients. Acta Anaesth Scand 24:279, 1980.
93. Jayr C, Mollie A, Bourgain MD, et al: Postoperative pulmonary complications: General anesthesia with postoperative parenteral morphine compared with epidural analgesia. Surgery 104:57, 1988.
94. Scott NB, Kehlet H: Regional anaesthesia and surgical morbidity. Br J Surg 75:299, 1988.
95. Urban MK, Grodon MA, Harris SN, et al: Intraoperative hemodynamic changes are not good indicators of myocardial ischemia. Anesth Analg 76:942, 1993.
96. Roizen MF, Ellis JE: Anesthesia for vascular surgery. In Barash PG, Cullen BF, Stoelting RK (eds): Clinical Anesthesia, 3rd ed. Philadelphia, JB Lippincott Co, 1992, p 1059.
97. Eisenberg MJ, London MJ, Leung JM, et al: Monitoring for myocardial ischemia during noncardiac surgery. JAMA 268:210, 1992.
98. Baker AB, Bookallil MJ, Lloyd G: Intentional asystole during endoluminal thoracic aortic surgery without cardiopulmonary bypass. Br J Anaesth 78:444, 1997.
99. Baker AB, Lloyd G, Fraser TA, et al: Retrospective review of 100 cases of endoluminal aortic-stent graft surgery from an anaesthetic perspective. Anaesth Intensive Care 25:378, 1997.
100. Christopherson R, Frank S, Norris E, et al: Low postoperative hematocrit is associated with cardiac ischemia in high-risk patients (Abstract). Anesthesiology 75:A99, 1991.
101. Massie BM, Mangano DT: Assessment of perioperative risk: Have we put the cart before the horse? J Am Coll Cardiol 21: 1353, 1993.
102. Roizen MF: Should we all have a sympathectomy at birth? Or at least preoperatively? (Editorial). Anesthesiology 68:482, 1988.

SECTION V

THORACIC ANESTHESIA

CHAPTER 25

Lung Isolation

Peter D. Slinger, M.D., F.R.C.P.C.

The routine isolation of one of the body's major paired organs, which is frequently necessary during lung surgery, is unique in medicine. Apart from the fascinating pathophysiologic changes that occur during lung isolation, the clinical usefulness of this separation is a cornerstone of thoracic anesthesia. The evolution of elective thoracic surgery was delayed more than half a century following the start of the modern era of anesthesia because anesthesiologists did not have (1) the technology to protect healthy lung regions from secretions and hemorrhage or (2) the ability to manage significant air leaks. In the mid-1930s several different practitioners pioneered the use of single-lumen endobronchial tubes,[1] bronchial blockers,[2] and double-lumen tubes[2] to achieve lung isolation. In spite of numerous modifications, these three methods have persisted to the present as the basis of modern lung isolation techniques.

All of these early methods required extensive clinical experience to achieve satisfactory positioning. The double-lumen endobronchial tube design introduced by Carlens[3] in 1949 (Figs. 25–1 and 25–2) for split lung function studies is a landmark in the development of thoracic anesthesia. The Carlens tube could be positioned reliably in the vast majority of cases without rigid bronchoscopy. The use of the Carlens and other derivative double-lumen tubes was soon advocated for all thoracotomies.[4]

Rationale for Isolation

Indications

The indications for the isolation of an entire lung, or an individual lobe or segment, from the rest of the tracheobronchial tree have traditionally been grouped into relative ("like to have it") and absolute ("really need it") categories. This division is somewhat arbitrary, since any relative indication may suddenly and unpredictably become an absolute indication if thoracic surgery is unable to continue, or if complications arise intraoperatively, during two-lung ventilation. Lung isolation is used in a wide spectrum of situations ranging from elective facilitation of surgery for pulmonary resections to emergency treatment of life-threatening massive hemoptysis. At all times, lung isolation is a therapy that must be based on a risk-benefit assessment for the individual case.

Initially, lung isolation was necessary in thoracic surgery because a high proportion of patients had "wet" lungs due to chronic untreated infectious processes (e.g., tuberculosis, bronchiectasis). Surgery in the lateral position could not be performed without potentially lethal soiling of healthy lung regions. These original indications for lung isolation still occur and include pulmonary hemorrhage, infected secretions, bronchial fistulae, and bullae ("blood, pus, and air").* However, in the vast majority of clinical situations, lung isolation is now used to facilitate the surgical exposure. The scope of potential one-lung operations has extended beyond pulmonary resections, to include surgery on all the main thoracic organ systems (Table 25–1). The use of lung isolation during anesthesia has increased, rather than decreased,[5] in spite of the decline in the number of surgical operations for infectious causes.

In addition to the nonpulmonary indications for lung isolation, there are several recently introduced or modified pulmonary procedures that require one-lung ventilation: lung transplantation,[6] and video-assisted thoracoscopic (VAT) surgery.[7] Also, lung isolation has become a proven therapeutic option in any patient requiring ventilatory support when there is a large discrepancy between the optimal gas exchange parameters of the two lungs. Such situations include predominately unilateral lung contusion or adult respiratory distress syndrome (ARDS), and also following pulmonary embolectomy.[8]

Contraindications

There are no absolute contraindications to isolating one lung or lobe from the rest of the respiratory system.

*This trio can be remembered as the same threesome responsible for complications from central line placement.

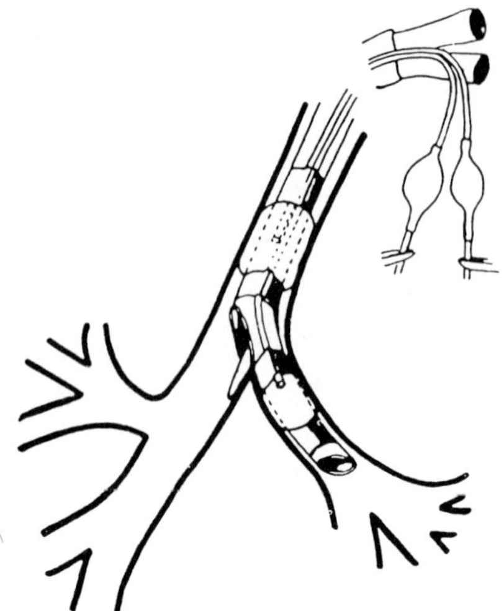

FIGURE 25–1. The double-lumen endobronchial tube designed by Carlens (circa 1950). Note the separate bronchial and tracheal lumens, the carinal hook protruding into the right mainstem bronchus, and the separate tracheal and bronchial cuffs. (From Mushin WW, Rendell-Baker L: The origins of thoracic anaesthesia. Wood Library. Museum of Anesthesiology, Park Ridge, IL, 1953, reprinted 1991, p 40, *and* Bjork VO, Conlons E: J Thoracic Surgery 20:151, 1950, with permission.)

There are contraindications to specific types of lung-isolation techniques in certain clinical situations. For example, the use of a left-sided double-lumen tube in the presence of a left endobronchial tumor would normally be contraindicated. Also, double-lumen tube placement can be hazardous in the presence of bronchial compression from a thoracic aortic aneurysm[9] or pulmonary artery compression from an anterior mediastinal mass.[10]

Emergency tracheobronchial intubation with a double-lumen tube is not contraindicated in a patient with a full stomach. However, it must be appreciated that the time required for initial placement is longer than for a single-lumen endotracheal tube and the theoretical risk of aspiration is somewhat increased. This potential increased risk must be weighed against the need for lung isolation in the particular case.

Similar considerations apply to lung isolation in patients who are initially hypoxemic or have abnormal coagulation.[11] Whether the need is for initial intubation or to change an in situ endotracheal tube, there is the potential for more hypoxemia or trauma during insertion of a double-lumen tube or bronchial blocker than during insertion of a single-lumen tube. However, these situations represent increased risks for lung isolation and are not contraindications.

Anatomy

Lung isolation requires a thorough knowledge of bronchial anatomy. Just as advances in invasive monitoring have mandated that anesthesiologists develop a more complete understanding of vascular anatomy in order to achieve reliable central vascular access, so has lung isolation necessitated detailed knowledge of bronchial anatomy. Minor variations in subsegmental anatomy are common. However, the anatomy of the lobar and segmental bronchi is consistent enough to be used as reference points for the positioning of endobronchial tubes and blockers.

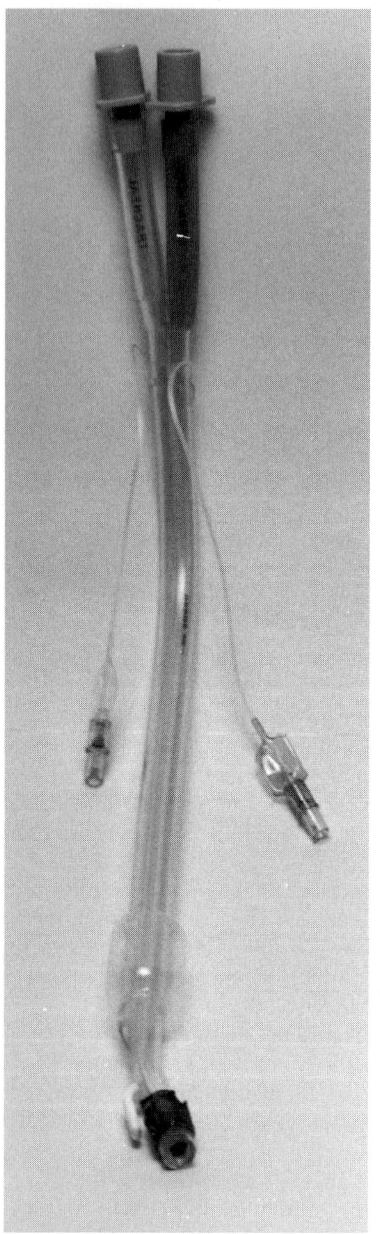

FIGURE 25–2. A modern polyvinyl chloride version of the double-lumen endobronchial tube based on the original design by Carlens (Rusch Inc., Duluth, GA). Note the small white carinal hook just proximal to the cuff of the bronchial lumen. The carinal hook was designed to facilitate bronchial positioning without bronchoscopy. However, these tubes are still frequently malplaced if positioned only with laryngoscopy and auscultation. The routine use of fiberoptic bronchoscopy to position endobronchial tubes eliminates the benefits of a carinal hook.

The mean (±SD) length of the adult trachea from vocal cords to carina is 12.4 ± 1.3 cm (females, 12.1 cm; males, 12.7 cm). This distance correlates with the height of the patient. However, the correlation is weak.[12] The trachea is commonly misconceived as a cylinder. In re-

TABLE 25–1
Potential Indications for Lung Isolation

Pulmonary
Resections: pneumonectomy, lobectomy, segment, wedge
Infection: abscess, empyema, bronchiectasis
Hemorrhage
Bullae, blebs
Lung transplantation
Lung biopsy
Thoracoscopy
Diagnostic
Video-assisted thoracoscopic surgery
Bronchial
Bronchopleural fistula
Bronchial sleeve resection
Bronchial tumor/injury
Cardiovascular
Thoracic aortic surgery
Pericardial: window, biopsy
Closed cardiac surgery
Cardiomyoplasty
Mediastinal
Biopsy
Mass excision
Digestive
Esophageal surgery
Hiatus hernia repair
Musculoskeletal
Thoracic vertebral column
Diaphragm repair
Chest wall surgery
Postoperative/ICU
Following pulmonary embolectomy
Unilateral contusion/ARDS
Following lung transplantation
Medical
Unilateral lung lavage

ICU, intensive care unit; ARDS, adult respiratory distress syndrome.

ality, its cross section is a modified D shape with an anterior semicircle of cartilage joined by a straight membranous posterior wall. With age or chronic bronchitis this posterior wall weakens and bulges anteriorly, creating a trachea with a modified C cross section, most noticeable during expiration (see Fig. 25–16). This bulging of the posterior tracheal wall can be severe enough to cause expiratory flow limitation.[13] The difference in shape of the anterior and posterior tracheal walls is a useful landmark for orientation during bronchoscopy, particularly when the patient is in the lateral position. Also useful as landmarks are the longitudinal elastic bundles that extend down the posterior wall of the trachea and branch into the posterior walls of the mainstem bronchi (see Figs. 25–10 and 25–11).

At the carina, the trachea divides into a larger (16-mm mean diameter) right mainstem bronchus and a smaller (13-mm diameter) left mainstem bronchus (Fig. 25–3). The left mainstem bronchus forms a larger angle with the midline than does the right mainstem bronchus (45 vs. 30 degrees). The mean length of the right mainstem bronchus in adults has been reported as 19 to 22 mm.[14] Not only is the right mainstem bronchus short, but its length is extremely variable (SD ± 8 mm). In 0.4% of patients the right upper lobe orifice exits above the carina in the trachea.[15] Thus, it is possible for any tube advanced on the right side to or beyond the carina to obstruct the right upper lobe.

Due to its size and angulation, the left mainstem bronchus is technically more difficult to enter with a tube or blocker than the right mainstem bronchus. However, the length of the left mainstem bronchus is estimated at 48 ± 8 mm. This gives a theoretical "margin of safety" of between 16 and 29 mm[14] for positioning left-sided tubes or blockers. Clinically, the margin of safety is rarely this large. This may be because during a right thoracotomy in the left lateral position, with the fall in functional residual capacity (FRC) of the dependent left lung,[16] there is a concomitant shortening of the left mainstem bronchus.

For proper positioning of endobronchial tubes or blockers it is necessary to understand segmental anatomy so that the orifices of the lobar bronchi can be identified. The lung has ten segments on the right and eight on the left (see Fig. 25–3). The superior segments of both lower lobes can also be referred to as the apical segments.[17] This provides the mnemonic "A PALM, A MAPL"[†] for the segments of the right lung in descending order. The mnemonic also can be applied on the left side with the modifications that the lateral and medial segments of the absent middle lobe become the superior and inferior segments of the left upper lobe lingula and there is no medial basal segment of the lower lobe due to the presence of the heart.

Note particularly that the superior segments of both lower lobes exit directly posteriorly and the right middle lobe takes off directly anteriorly from the bronchus intermedius (the section of the right mainstem bronchus distal to the orifice of the right upper lobe). These are very useful landmarks during bronchoscopic positioning of tubes or blockers (Fig. 25–4). Also, note that the longitudinal elastic bundles follow the posterior wall of the mainstem bronchi. On the left they extend to the posterolateral wall of the lower lobe.

Preoperative Assessment of Endobronchial Intubation

All anesthesiologists are familiar with the clinical assessment of the upper airway for ease of endotracheal intubation. In a similar fashion, each thoracic surgical patient must be assessed for the ease of endobronchial intubation.

At the time of the preoperative visit, there may be historical factors or physical findings that lead to suspicion of difficult endobronchial intubation (previous radiotherapy, infection, prior pulmonary or airway surgery). In addition, there is often a written bronchoscopy report with detailed description of anatomic features. However, fiberoptic bronchoscopy is not totally reliable for estimating potential problems with endobronchial tube positioning.[18] The single most useful predictor of difficult endobronchial intubation is the plain chest x-ray (Fig. 25–5).[19] The anesthesiologist should view the chest films prior to induction of anesthesia, since neither the

[†]I am indebted to Dr. D. Thomas for this mnemonic.

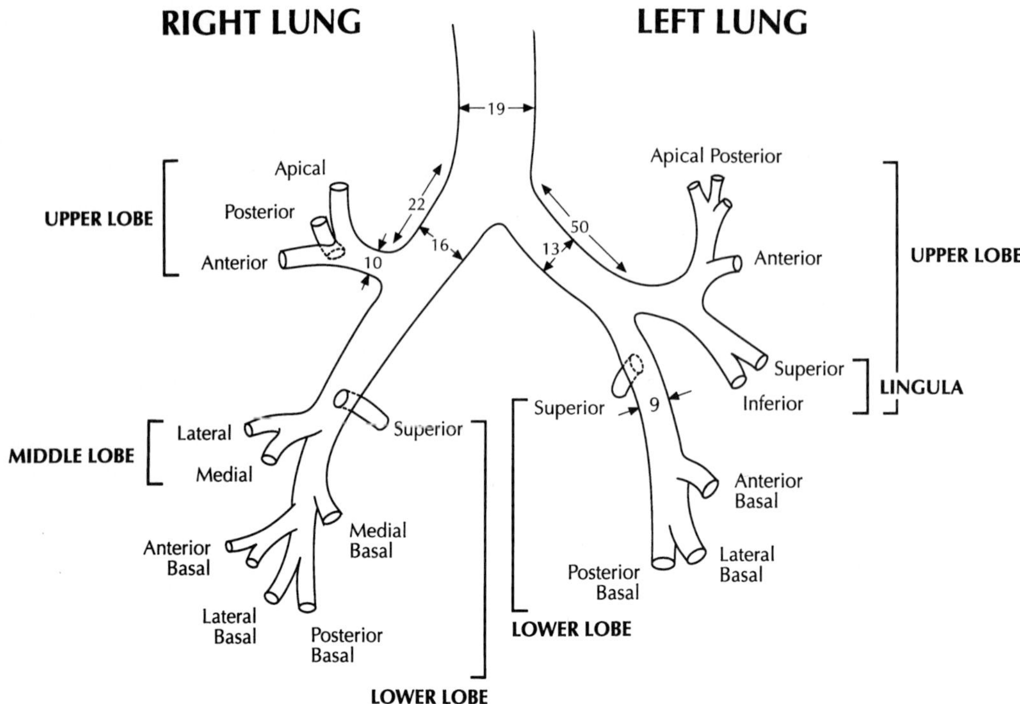

FIGURE **25–3.** Diagram of the tracheobronchial tree. Mean lengths and diameters are shown in millimeters. Note that the right middle lobe bronchus exits directly anteriorly while the superior segments of both lower lobes exit posteriorly. In a rostral to caudal direction the segmental bronchi of each lung give the mnemonic "A PALM A MAPL" (see text).

radiologist's nor the surgeon's report of the x-ray is made with the specific consideration of lung isolation in mind. A large portion of thoracic surgical patients will also have had a computed tomography (CT) scan done preoperatively. As anesthesiolgists have learned to assess chest x-rays, it is also worthwhile to learn to examine the CT scan. Endobronchial problems not evident on the plain chest film can sometimes be visualized on the CT scan.[20] Managing difficult endobronchial intubation is discussed in the section "Abnormal Airway Anatomy." The major factors in successful management are anticipation and preparation based on the preoperative assessment.

Fiberoptic Bronchoscopy

One of the major attractions of the Carlens double-lumen tube for thoracic anesthesia was that it could be positioned endobronchially using only laryngoscopy and auscultation. Subsequent double-lumen tube development with the design of the Robertshaw double-lumen tube[21] (eliminating the carinal hook) and the change from rubber to low-friction polyvinyl chloride have now created a situation where over 30% of all double-lumen tubes will be misplaced if positioned using traditional methods.[22]

The use of a pediatric fiberoptic bronchoscope to aid double-lumen tube placement was first described in 1982 by Shinnik.[23] Improvements in fiberoptic technology have led to the development of bronchoscopes that are specifically designed for anesthesiology (Table 25–2). The use of the fiberoptic bronchoscope for problematic placement or repositioning of endobronchial tubes has been universally accepted by the anesthesia community.[24] Also, it is now appreciated that placement of endobronchial blockers is difficult and potentially hazardous if done without direct bronchoscopic guidance.[25]

The use of bronchoscopy for routine double-lumen endobronchial tube positioning has been a subject of debate.[26] The arguments against routine bronchoscopic surveillance include equipment cost, increased anesthesia time, lack of attention to the whole patient, and the fact that it is usually possible to manage without direct endobronchial visualization. These are essentially the same arguments that have been advanced against any newly introduced intraoperative monitoring system (e.g., electrocardiogram, capnometry). However, during one-lung ventilation the incidence of hypoxemia is 10 to 20%,[27] and one of the major differential diagnoses of this hypoxemia is malplacement of an endobronchial tube or blocker. Routine bronchoscopy has now become the standard of practice.[28,29]

Irrespective of the clinical expertise of the anesthesiologist, if a double-lumen tube or blocker migrates during patient positioning or after the start of surgery and obstructs an upper lobe bronchus, it is extremely difficult to diagnose by auscultation. Both the double-lumen tube and the carina will move between the time of intubation, in the supine position, and the start of one-lung ventilation, especially in the lateral position with the nondependent hemithorax open.[30] It is impossible to avoid some movement of these structures no matter how careful the anesthesiologist is in stabilizing the endobron-

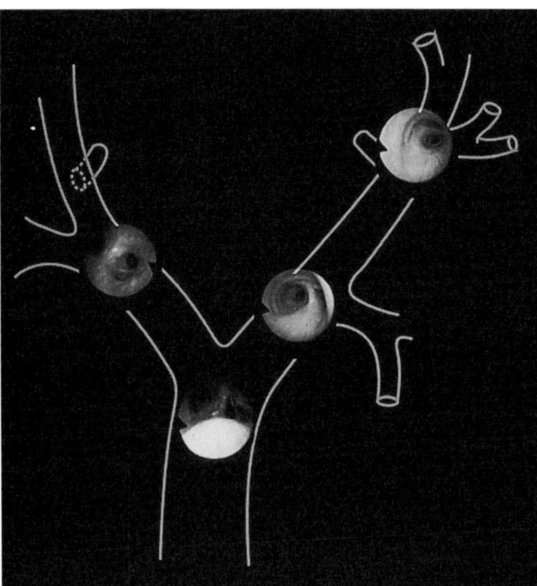

FIGURE **25–4.** Diagram of the tracheobronchial tree with inset photographs to demonstrate the bronchoscopic views of the primary and secondary carinae. The diagram is presented in the orientation most familiar to the anesthesiologist (i.e., standing at the head of a supine patient). In the photograph of the primary tracheal carina, there is a right-sided double-lumen tube in place. Important landmarks: note the tracheal carina in a 12- to 6-o'clock plane with the membranous posterior portion of the tracheal wall bulging anteriorly. In the photograph taken in the left main bronchus, note the secondary carina between the upper and lower lobes in a 2- to 8-o'clock plane while the narrow tertiary carina between the superior segment and the main portion of the left lower lobe lies distally in a 4- to 8-o'clock plane. In the right mainstem bronchus note the upper lobe orifice at 3 to 4 o'clock. In the right bronchus intermedius (distal to the upper lobe takeoff) note that the secondary carina between the right middle (anterior) and lower (posterior) lobes bisects the bronchus in a 3- to 9-o'clock plane. The orifices of all lobar bronchi should be identified every time a bronchial blocker or double-lumen tube is placed.

chial tube or blocker during positioning of the patient.[31] Significant secondary displacements of double-lumen tubes occur in over one third of patients.[32] Thus, the most important time to perform bronchoscopic surveillance of double-lumen tube or blocker position is after the patient has been fully positioned for surgery and, if possible, after the thorax has been opened (i.e., immediately prior to the initiation of one-lung ventilation).

Auscultation for double-lumen tube positioning is particularly unreliable in certain clinical situations: (1) bronchopleural fistula, (2) partial distal trachal lumen obstruction,[20] and (3) partial distal bronchial lumen obstruction due to improper angulation of the double-lumen tube in the left mainstem bronchus.

In cases of suspected abnormal airway anatomy, the fiberoptic bronchoscope should be used from the time of initial insertion to directly guide primary placement of a double-lumen tube.[24,33] Also, when there is significant risk to the patient from loss of lung isolation (e.g., bronchopleural fistula, abscess, bronchiectasis), bronchoscopy should be used at the time of initial intubation, then repeated after final patient positioning. In the majority of patients requiring lung isolation, double-lumen tubes can be positioned initially with auscultation; then the

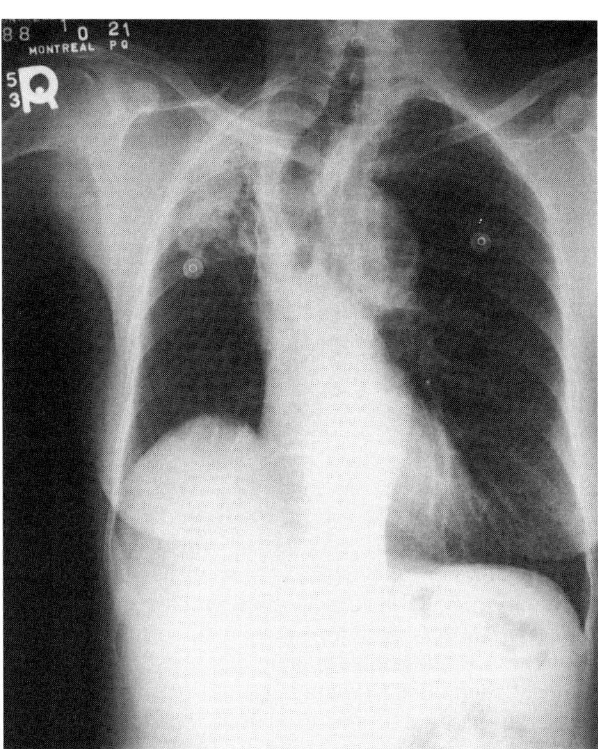

FIGURE **25–5.** Chest x-ray of a 69-year-old female with recurrent carcinoma of the right lower lobe (scheduled for right thoracotomy, possible completion pneumonectomy). The x-ray reveals a previous right upper lobectomy and tracheal deviation. The anticipated difficult left endobronchial intubation was managed with direct fiberoptic guidance via the bronchial side of a left double-lumen tube after induction of general anesthesia.

tube placement can be fined-tuned bronchoscopically after patient positioning.

To ensure adequate double-lumen tube or blocker placement, the tracheal carina and the orifices of all lobes should be verified each time the bronchoscope is used (see Fig. 25–4). It is important that both lumens of a double-lumen tube be examined bronchoscopically, since unilateral obstruction can occur in spite of normal auscultation and normal bronchoscopy of the other lumen.[34] Bronchoscopy via only one side of a double-lumen tube is equivalent to stopping at a railway crossing and looking only one way. The ability to use a fiberoptic bronchoscope to recognize normal and abnormal tube and blocker positions is a skill that all anesthesiologists who manage thoracic cases should possess.

TABLE **25–2**

Desirable Features of a Fiberoptic Bronchoscope for Management of Lung Isolation Procedures

Feature	Desirable Range
Bronchoscope diameter	≤4 mm
Range of motion of tip (in both flexion and extension)	>120 degrees
Working length	≥55 cm
Suction channel diameter	≥1.5 mm
Field of view	≥90 degrees

Like any skill, it is best learned under appropriate guidance in elective situations.

Lung Isolation Techniques

Double-Lumen Tubes

None of the features of the double-lumen endobronchial tube introduced by Carlens in 1949[3] was entirely new. There had been previous tubes with two lumens, tubes with bronchial and tracheal cuffs, and tubes with carinal hooks.[2] However, the unique combination of all of these factors in the Carlens tube resulted in an airway catheter that was far easier to use for lung isolation than any of its predecessors. In the late 1950s Robertshaw modified the Carlens tube for use during anesthesia.[21] These changes included: (1) wider D-shaped lumens with reduction in airflow resistance, (2) elimination of the carinal hook, and (3) design of a right-sided tube.

By the 1970s, double-lumen tubes had become the dominant method for producing lung isolation and were reported to be used in greater than 90% of thoracic cases in a multicenter study in Great Britain.[35] In the 1980s, the original red-rubber Robertshaw tube was displaced by polyvinyl chloride double-lumen tubes. This avoided the problems of reusing airway equipment and permitted the incorporation of high-volume low-pressure tracheal and bronchial cuffs, decreasing the potential for airway trauma. However, all modern polyvinyl chloride double-lumen tubes continue to be plagued by two design problems. First, the position of these tubes now must be monitored with bronchoscopy, since they are more prone to cause bronchial obstruction than the original Robertshaw tubes.[36] Second, the margin of safety in positioning these tubes in the short and variable right mainstem bronchus is very small.[14]

Since these tubes are oval shaped in cross section, it is not possible to size them simply according to internal or external diameter, as can be done for single-lumen tubes. Manufacturers follow the convention of French gauge (Fr) sizes for these tubes (this is based on a measurement of tube circumference and corresponds roughly to the tube circumference in millimeters). The appropriate size of double-lumen tubes for adults depends on the height and sex of the patient (Table 25–3). Polyvinyl chloride designs of double-lumen tubes that resemble the original Carlens tube, with a carinal hook, are available (Fig. 25–2). Although popular with some anesthesiologists,[37] these tubes have not met with widespread acceptance. They retain the problems associated with hooks (intraoperative repositioning for right pneumonectomy, potential laryngeal trauma at intubation) and still require bronchoscopic positioning, since malplacement occurs with unacceptable frequency if positioned blindly with auscultation.

TABLE 25–3
Suggested Sizes for Double-lumen Tubes in Adults

Sex	Height	Size of Tube (Fr)
Female	<160 cm (63 inches)	35
Female	≥160 cm	37
Male	<170 cm (67 inches)	39
Male	≥170 cm	41

For both right and left double-lumen tubes satisfactory initial endobronchial placement can be accomplished using standard laryngoscopy in the vast majority of patients. The bronchial limb is advanced with its distal curve concave anteriorly until the bronchial cuff passes the vocal cords using direct laryngoscopy as for a single-lumen tube. The double-lumen tube is then rotated 90 degrees (clockwise for a right-sided tube and counterclockwise for a left-sided tube) and the intubation stylet is removed from the bronchial lumen. The tube is then advanced using minimal pressure to a specific predetermined depth, provided no undue resistance is encountered. The depth of placement as indicated by the markings on the side of the tube depends on the height of the patient. The average tube depth markings at the central incisors will be 29 cm for an adult of medium height (170 cm [67 inches]) and will increase or decrease approximately 1 cm for each 10-cm increase or decrease in height.[38] Modern polyvinyl chloride double-lumen tubes are *not* designed to be advanced until resistance is encountered, as was formerly the case with the Carlens and Robertshaw tubes. Advancing polyvinyl chloride tubes until they "stop" results in a high percentage of accidental lobar bronchial intubation, lobar obstruction, and the potential for increased airway trauma.

After initial insertion to the appropriate depth, these tubes then need to be positioned to achieve adequate lung isolation. Many techniques have been advocated to aid in positioning of double-lumen tubes. Misting of the lumens with water vapor, end-tidal carbon dioxide,[39,40] and airway pressure changes (all of which occur with endobronchial intubation) have been advocated to aid positioning of double-lumen tubes. However, reliable positioning must be accomplished by two techniques used in tandem: auscultation and bronchoscopy. The simplest and safest routine for auscultation is outlined in Figure 25–6. The majority of significant malpositions will be quickly demonstrated by abnormal auscultation with this sequence (Fig. 25–7). However, lobar obstruction cannot be reliably detected by auscultation.[18]

Right-sided double-lumen tubes will usually enter the right mainstem bronchus without problem. With left-sided double-lumen tubes, 10 to 20% can be expected to initially enter the right mainstem bronchus.[22] Following inadvertent right mainstem bronchial intubation with a left-sided tube, it is reasonable to reattempt blind placement at least one time. Both cuffs should be deflated and the tube withdrawn until the distal bronchial lumen is above carina (~20 cm at the teeth). The patient's head is then rotated to the right 90 degrees and the tube is rotated a further 90 degrees counterclockwise so that the distal bronchial and tracheal lumens are correctly aligned with respect to the carina. The tube is advanced again to the correct depth and rechecked with auscultation. This maneuver of head rotation to the right

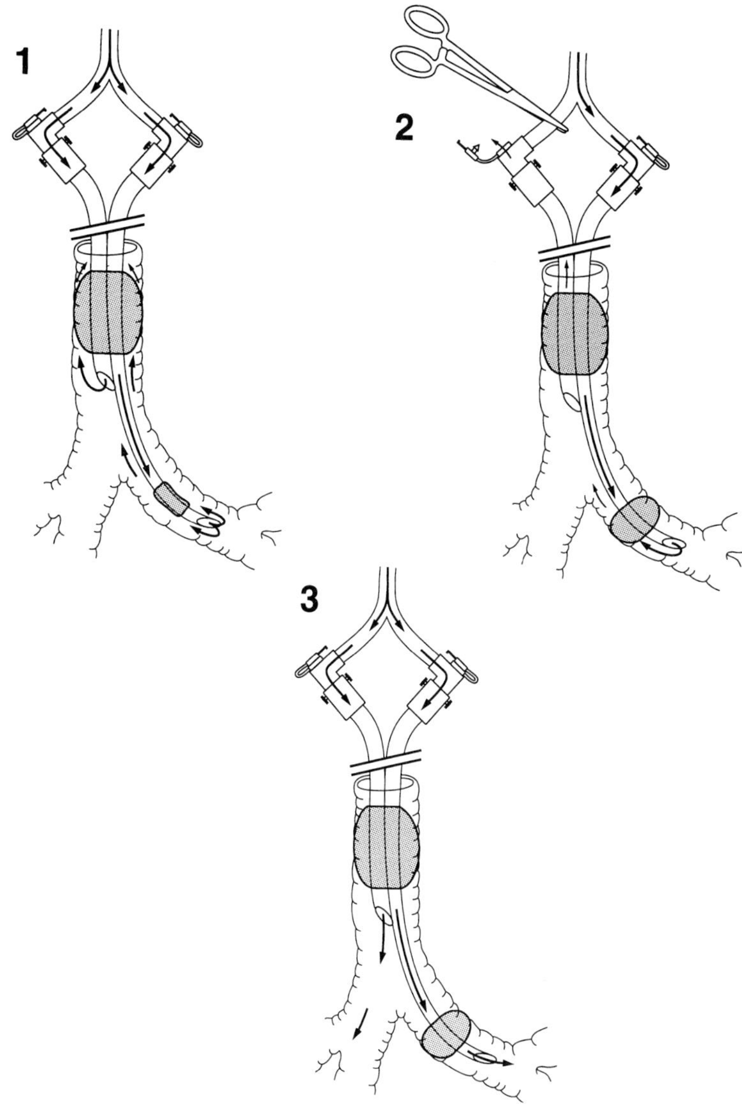

FIGURE **25–6.** The "three-step" method for auscultation to confirm double-lumen endobronchial tube positioning. *Step 1*, During bilateral ventilation the tracheal cuff is inflated to the minimal volume that seals the air leak at the glottis. Auscultate to confirm bilateral ventilation. *Step 2*, The tracheal lumen of the double-lumen tube is clamped proximally ("clamp the short side short") and the port distal to the clamp opened. During ventilation by the bronchial lumen, the bronchial cuff is inflated to the minimal volume that seals the air leak via the open tracheal port. Auscultate to confirm correct unilateral ventilation. *Step 3*, The tracheal lumen clamp is released and the port closed. Auscultate to confirm resumption of bilateral ventilation.

tends to lessen the angle to the left mainstem bronchus from the trachea and is frequently used for rigid bronchoscopy.[41] Some anesthesiologists perform this right head rotation maneuver at the time of initial intubation with a left double-lumen tube.

Another approach to accidental right mainstem bronchial intubation with a left-sided tube is to clamp the tracheal limb and withdraw the tube while gently ventilating manually until bilateral chest inflation can be appreciated. The patient's head is then rotated to the right and the tube advanced while continuing to ventilate via the bronchial limb.

If the double-lumen tube has lost its distal bronchial lumen curve due to prolonged storage, the metal stylet can be replaced and left in situ when the double-lumen tube is readvanced. If this fails to direct a left-sided tube into the left mainstem bronchus, the tube should again be withdrawn above the tracheal carina. Then, the fiberoptic bronchoscope should be passed via the bronchial lumen into the left mainstem bronchus and the double-lumen tube advanced over the bronchoscope, which serves as a guide. Ventilation via both the bronchial and tracheal lumens continues throughout positioning. In critical situations such as a bronchopleural fistula involving the proximal bronchi, where initial malplacement could produce additional trauma, fiberoptic techniques for placement should be used.[42]

The inflation pressure in the distal bronchial cuff required to ensure lung isolation will vary during thoracic surgery as the peak airway pressure changes. If lung isolation pressure is tested immediately after intubation in the supine position, often only 20 cm H_2O pressure in the bronchial cuff is required for isolation. After the patient is turned to the lateral position, the compliance of the dependent lung is decreased. If the same tidal volume is used during one-lung ventilation, a higher peak airway pressure results, and higher bronchial cuff isolation pressure is sometimes required. The compliance of the dependent lung improves markedly when the nondependent hemithorax is opened[16] and the bronchial cuff pressure required for lung isolation tends to return to its initial supine values.

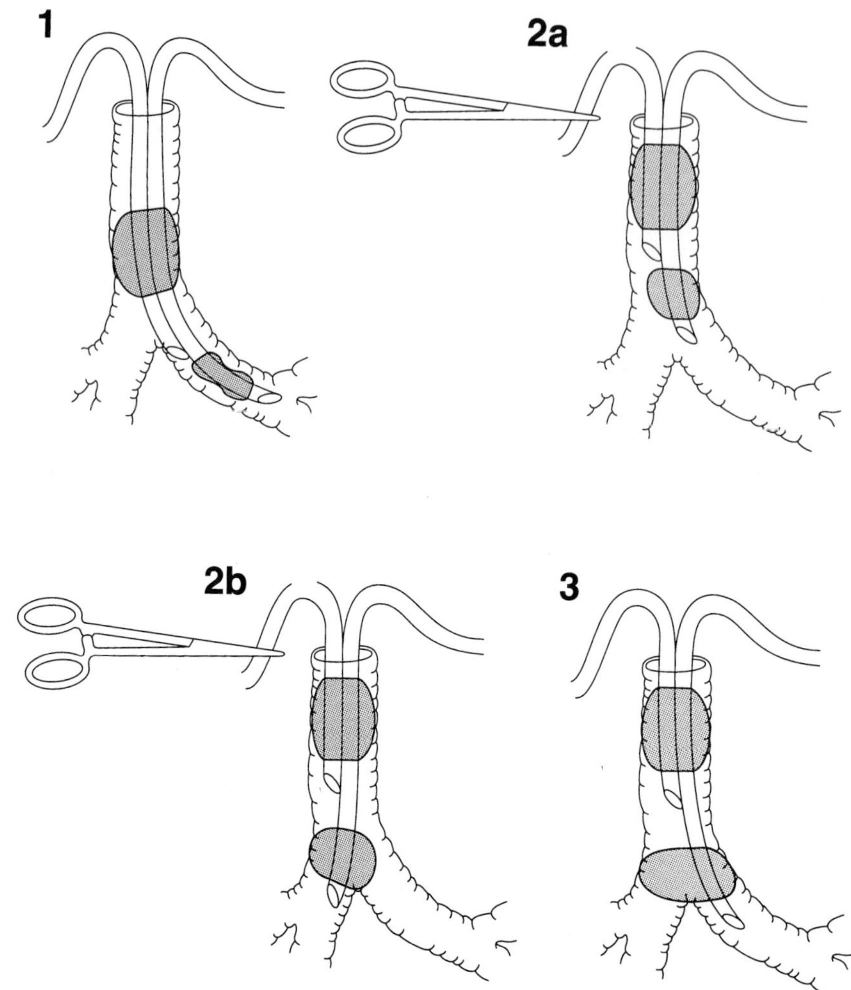

FIGURE **25–7.** The following common major initial malplacements of double-lumen endobronchial tubes will be detected sequentially during the "three-step" method (see Fig. 25–6) of auscultation. *Step 1*, Overly distal placement in either main bronchus. Revealed by unequal breath sounds. *Step 2a*, Overly proximal. Inability to achieve unilateral ventilation during ventilation by only the bronchial lumen. *Step 2b*, Incorrect side bronchial intubation. Unilateral breath sounds in the incorrect hemithorax. *Step 3*, Slightly too proximal. Appropriate isolation but unequal auscultation with resumption of bilateral ventilation.

Left Double-Lumen Tubes

The designs of the bronchial cuffs of the three most popular left double-lumen tubes in North America differ depending on the manufacturer (Fig. 25–8). The "rolling-pin" design of the Rusch (Duluth, GA) cuff and the "donut" design of the Mallinckrodt (Argyle, NY) cuff achieve bronchial isolation with lower cuff pressures than the "olive" shape of the Sheridan (Glens Falls, NY) cuff, both in vitro[43] and vivo[44] (Fig. 25–9). Modern left double-lumen tubes can achieve lung isolation with mean intracuff pressures in the range of 15 to 20 cm H_2O. This is well below a theoretical threshold cuff pressure at which ischemia is caused in the tracheobronchial mucosa (45 cm H_2O).[45] In the majority of cases, lung isolation can be achieved with bronchial cuff inflation volumes less than 2 ml. If greater than 3 ml is required, the tube position should be reassessed.

Fiberoptic positioning of left double-lumen tubes is demonstrated in Figures 25–10 through 25–13. It is usually most practical to perform the bronchoscopic surveillance of the tube position during the relatively stable period between patient positioning and the initiation of one-lung ventilation. The bronchoscope should be passed through the tracheal lumen first to ensure that the correct mainstem bronchus has been intubated. It is easier to get a general idea of the tube position with the wider field of view from the tracheal lumen. The tube position should be adjusted so that the bronchial cuff is barely visible in the left mainstem bronchus just below the carina (Fig. 25–10).[29] After confirmation of left endobronchial intubation, the right mainstem bronchus should be inspected (Fig. 25–11). Note that the takeoff of the right upper lobe bronchus lies at the 3 to 4-o'clock position (anterior = 12 o'clock, posterior = 6 o'clock). Note also the longitudinal submucosal elastic bundles that descend from the posterior (membranous) portion of

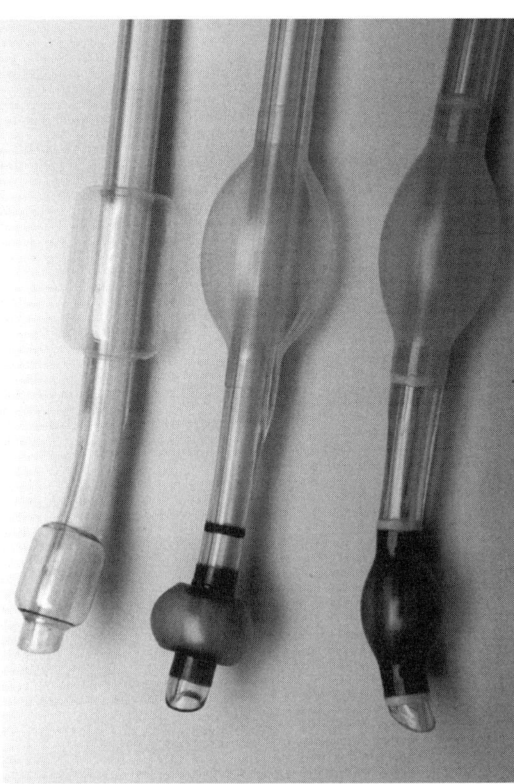

FIGURE **25–8.** Three different designs of left double-lumen tubes with tracheal and bronchial cuffs inflated: Rusch on the left, Mallinckrodt in the middle, Sheridan on the right. The difference in the shapes of the distal (bronchial) cuffs is evident. (From Slinger P, Chripko D: A clinical comparison of bronchial cuff pressures in disposable left double-lumen tubes. Anesth Analg 77:305, 1993, with permission.)

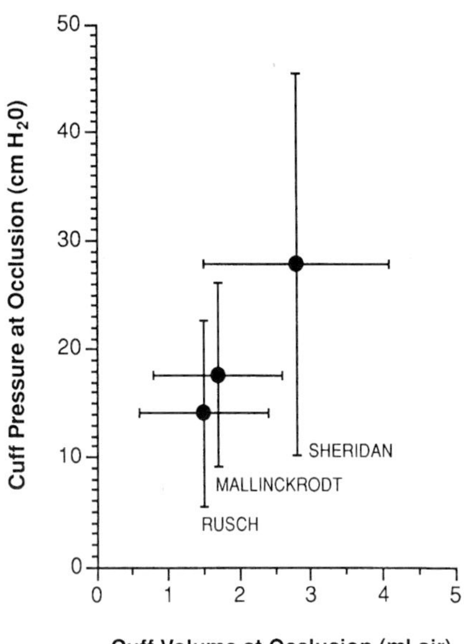

FIGURE **25–9.** The mean (±SD) bronchial cuff volumes and pressures for three designs of left-sided double-lumen tubes at the point of bronchial occlusion. (From Slinger P, Chripko D: A clinical comparison of bronchial cuff pressures in disposable left double-lumen tubes. Anesth Analg 77:305, 1993, with permission.)

the trachea and continue into the posterior wall of the right mainstem bronchus. The lateral bundles then lead to the right upper lobe orifice.

After proper initial positioning, the commonest significant malposition of left double-lumen tubes is left upper lobe obstruction due to entry of the distal bronchial lumen into the left lower lobe (Fig. 25–12). It is extremely important that the anesthesiologist be able to identify this malposition. If it occurs in midoperation, due to surgical manipulation, it can be extremely difficult to diagnose by other means. Note the difference in the bronchoscopy view between Figure 25–12, which shows the left lower lobe only, and Figure 25–13, which is a bronchial lumen view of both left upper and lower lobes. It is easy to confuse the secondary carina between the upper and lower lobes with the tertiary carina between the superior and basal segments of the left lower lobe. There are several useful landmarks to help make this clinically important distinction:

1. The shape and orientation of the secondary and tertiary carinae. The secondary carina is usually a fairly wide carina that runs in a 2- to 8-o'clock plane. The tertiary carina of the superior segment of the left lower lobe is normally a thin carina that lies in a 4- to 8-o'clock plane. Thus, the superior segment bronchus exits directly posteriorly from the tracheobronchial tree.
2. Within the left upper lobe bronchus when viewed from the bronchial lumen (not demonstrated in the photograph) there is normally only one tertiary carina visible, which divides the main portion of the left upper lobe from the lingula. In the main portion of the left lower lobe, when viewed from the bronchial lumen, the multiple tertiary carinae of the basilar segments are normally seen.
3. The longitudinal elastic bundles descend in the posterior wall of the left mainstem bronchus and divide, extending onto the posterolateral wall of the left lower lobe bronchus and the posteromedial wall of the left upper lobe. During bronchoscopic placement of endobronchial tubes or blockers it is important to always maintain orientation (anteroposterior and mediolateral) in the tracheobronchial tree, both in the supine and lateral positions.

Right Double-Lumen Tubes

The three most commonly used disposable right double-lumen tubes in North America vary greatly in design (Fig. 25–14) depending on the manufacturer. The Mallinckrodt design seems to be the most reliable. A new Rusch design is undergoing clinical trials (Fig. 25–15). All three designs include a ventilating side-slot in the lateral wall of the distal bronchial lumen for right upper lobe ventilation. Positioning this slot can be time consuming, and without fiberoptic guidance, up to 80% of these tubes will be malpositioned.[32]

When visualizing right-sided tubes with fiberoptic bronchoscopy, the bronchial cuff is often not seen at the carina even with a well-positioned tube (Fig. 25–16). This is particularly true for the Mallinckrodt tube due to its asymmetric bronchial cuff design. The key to posi-

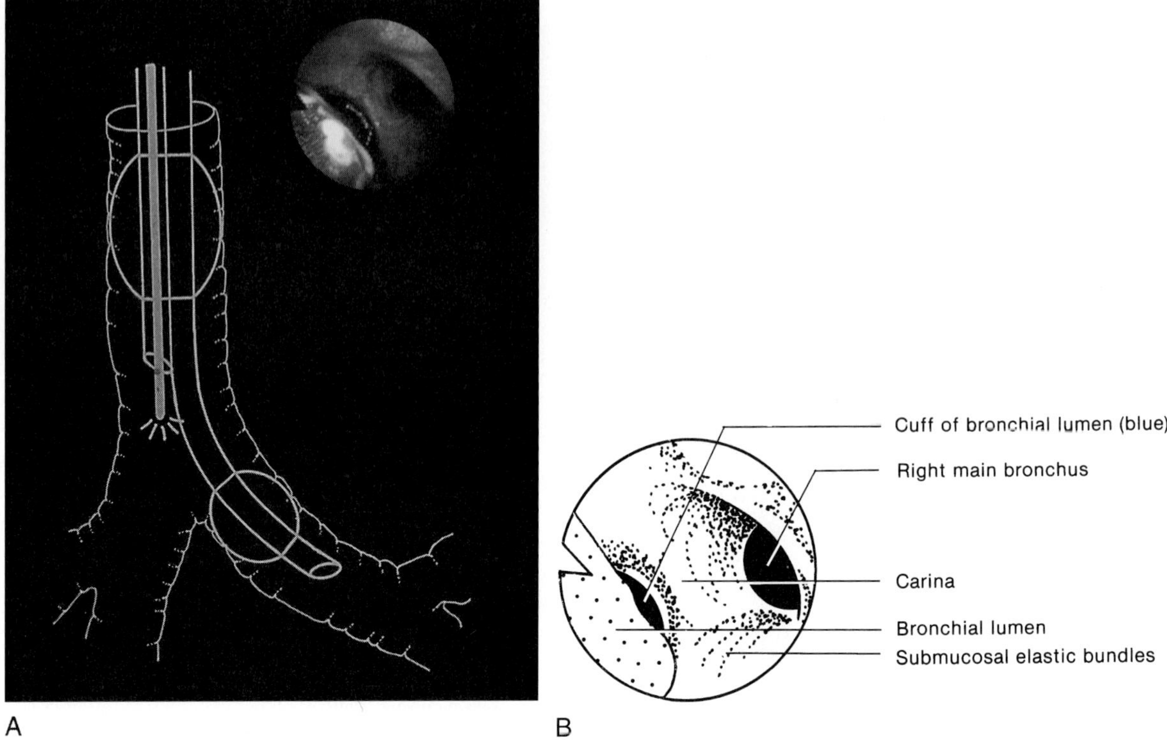

FIGURE **25–10.** In the upper right corner of the photograph (*A*) is the view from the fiberoptic bronchoscope when it is positioned as shown in the diagram of the airway. (*B*) Diagrammatic representation of what is seen in the bronchoscopic photograph. This illustration is an example of a well-positioned left-sided double-lumen tube as seen from the tracheal lumen. The view shows the carina seen from above. The exterior wall of the bronchial lumen of the double-lumen tube is seen entering the left main bronchus and is labeled "bronchial lumen." The proximal edge of the blue bronchial cuff can be visualized at the carina. The carina is normally aligned in the sagittal plane (12 to 6 o'clock) but may be angled up to 45 degrees from this plane. Note the longitudinal submucosal elastic bundles running in the posterior (membranous) tracheal wall and extending into the main bronchi. (From Slinger P: Fiberoptic bronchoscopic positioning of double-lumen tubes. J Cardiothorac Anesth 3:486, 1989, with permission.)

tioning the bronchial lumen lies in orienting the ventilating side-slot with the right upper lobe orifice. It is important to remember the bronchial anatomy. Note in Figure 25–17 (the photograph is rotated slightly counterclockwise relative to the supine position) that the longitudinal elastic bundles are in the posterior wall of the right mainstem bronchus and the secondary carina between the right middle and lower lobes extends in a plane from 3 to 9 o'clock. After orienting oneself via the distal bronchial lumen, the bronchoscope is withdrawn to reveal the ventilating side-slot in the lateral wall of the bronchial lumen (Fig. 25–18). Keeping the secondary carina between the middle and lower lobes visible, the right upper lobe orifice will be found on the lateral wall of the right mainstem bronchus at the 3- to 4-o'clock position. The tube can then be adjusted to reveal the entire right upper lobe orifice (Figs. 25–19 and 25–20).

Right double-lumen tubes require higher mean bronchial cuff pressures for lung isolation (40 to 50 cm H_2O)[46] than left double-lumen tubes (20 to 30 cm H_2O). However, this intracuff pressure is less than cuff pressures required by Univent[47] tubes or nondisposable double-lumen tubes.[48]

The benefits of double-lumen endobronchial tubes versus other methods of lung isolation relate primarily to two features (Table 25–4): (1) continuous easy access to both lungs for suctioning, application of continuous positive airway pressure (CPAP), and bronchoscopy; and (2) reliability of isolation, both initially and during subsequent surgical manipulations. The disadvantages of double-lumen tubes relate mainly to the fact that each tube has a fixed design with a predetermined distance between the orifices of the distal tracheal and bronchial lumens. These tubes often do not function well when dealing with either abnormal tracheobronchial anatomy or with a variant of normal anatomy.[15]

Spontaneous ventilation is occasionally necessary via a double-lumen tube (e.g., during weaning from mechanical ventilation, or during awake endobronchial intubation). The flow resistances of modern disposable double-lumen tubes are much lower than commonly appreciated. The airflow resistance of some commercial 37-Fr double-lumen tubes is actually less than that of a 7.5-mm internal diameter (ID) single-lumen endotracheal tube. However, the resistance due to the Y-connectors supplied with the tubes varies widely between different manufacturers. The narrow-lumen Y-connector of the

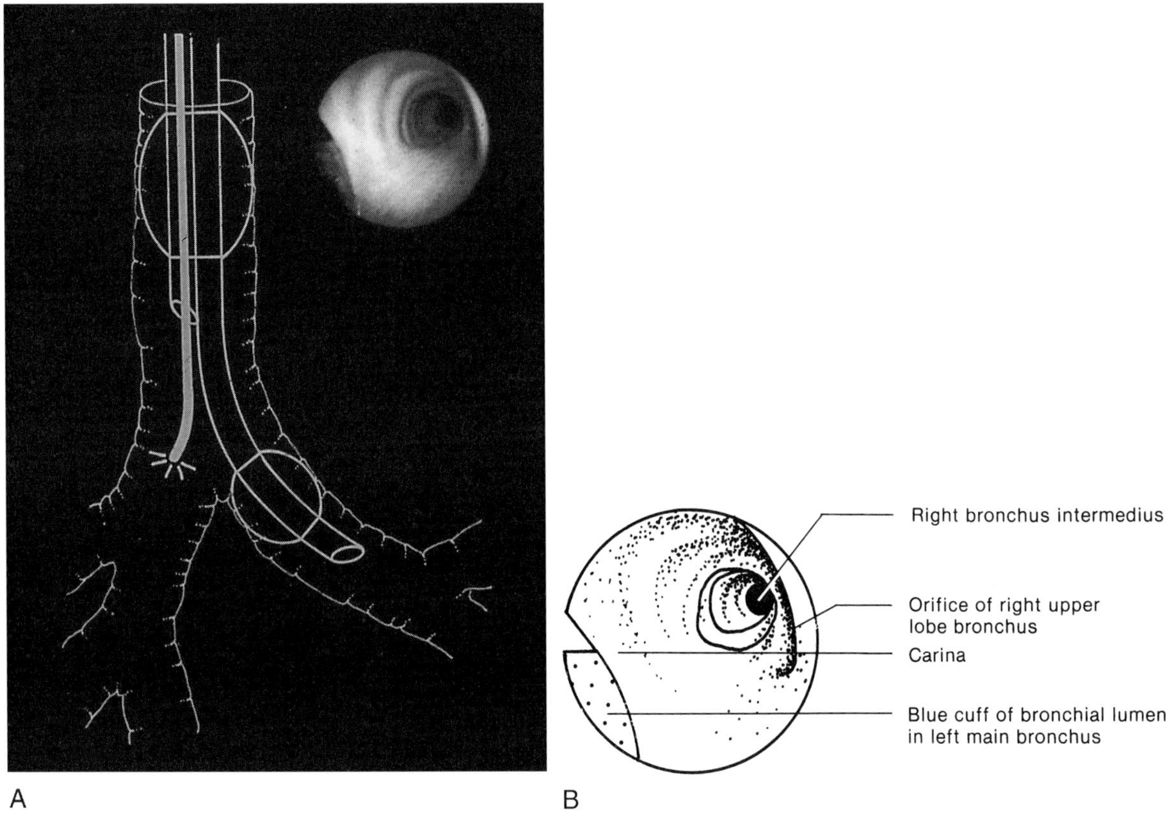

FIGURE **25–11.** *A*, View of the right mainstem bronchus from the tracheal lumen of a properly positioned left-sided double-lumen tube. *B*, Diagrammatic representation of what is seen in the bronchoscopic photograph. The rim of the blue bronchial cuff is just visible to the left of the carina. The orifice of the right upper lobe bronchus is barely visible on the right at 3 to 4 o'clock with a few longitudinal submucosal elastic bundles leading to it. The majority of the elastic bundles continue in the posterior wall to the bronchus intermedius, which leads to the right middle and lower lobe bronchi. (From Slinger P: Fiberoptic bronchoscopic positioning of double-lumen tubes. J Cardiothorac Anesth 3: 486, 1989, with permission.)

Mallinckrodt design causes much higher airflow resistance than that of either the Sheridan or Rusch double-lumen tubes.[48a]

In the exceptional case when it is difficult to achieve adequate positioning of a double-lumen tube either initially or after tube migration, the anesthesiologist should be aware that it is often very simple for the surgeon to aid in endobronchial positioning of a double-lumen tube or blocker by manually guiding the airway equipment into the appropriate bronchus when the chest is open.[49]

Univent Tube

The Univent tube was first described in 1982 by Inoue[50] for one-lung anesthesia. It consists of a single-lumen endotracheal tube with a separate internal channel on its concave surface housing a retractable 2-mm-diameter bronchial blocker (Fig. 25–21). Its applications have been extended from elective one-lung anesthesia to include most the indications for which double-lumen tubes are used.

Positioning the bronchial blocker of a Univent tube requires fiberoptic bronchoscopy. Tracheal intubation is done with simple laryngoscopy, as for any single-lumen tube with the concave surface anteriorly. Once the distal lumen of the Univent tube has passed the vocal cords, the tube is rotated 90 degrees to the side of the mainstem bronchus to be blocked (i.e., right mainstem bronchus: clockwise rotation; left mainstem bronchus counterclockwise rotation) then advanced and secured at the usual depth for a single-lumen tube (e.g., female, 20 cm; male, 22 cm at central incisors). After auscultation for bilateral ventilation and verification of end-tidal capnography, a fiberoptic bronchoscope is passed via the main lumen using a bronchoscopy connector. The bronchial blocker is then extended into the correct mainstem bronchus (Fig. 25–22*A* and *B*), and the blocker cuff is inflated and the chest auscultated to ensure lung isolation. The bronchial cuff is deflated until needed for one-lung ventilation. It is useful to leave the blocker partially extended in the mainstem bronchus prior to positioning the patient because after turning it can be difficult to get the bronchial blocker to re-enter the nondependent mainstem bronchus.

The bronchial blocker of the Univent is very stiff and occasionally will not enter the appropriate bronchus. This is particularly a problem on the left side. In these cases, the bronchial blocker can be withdrawn into the

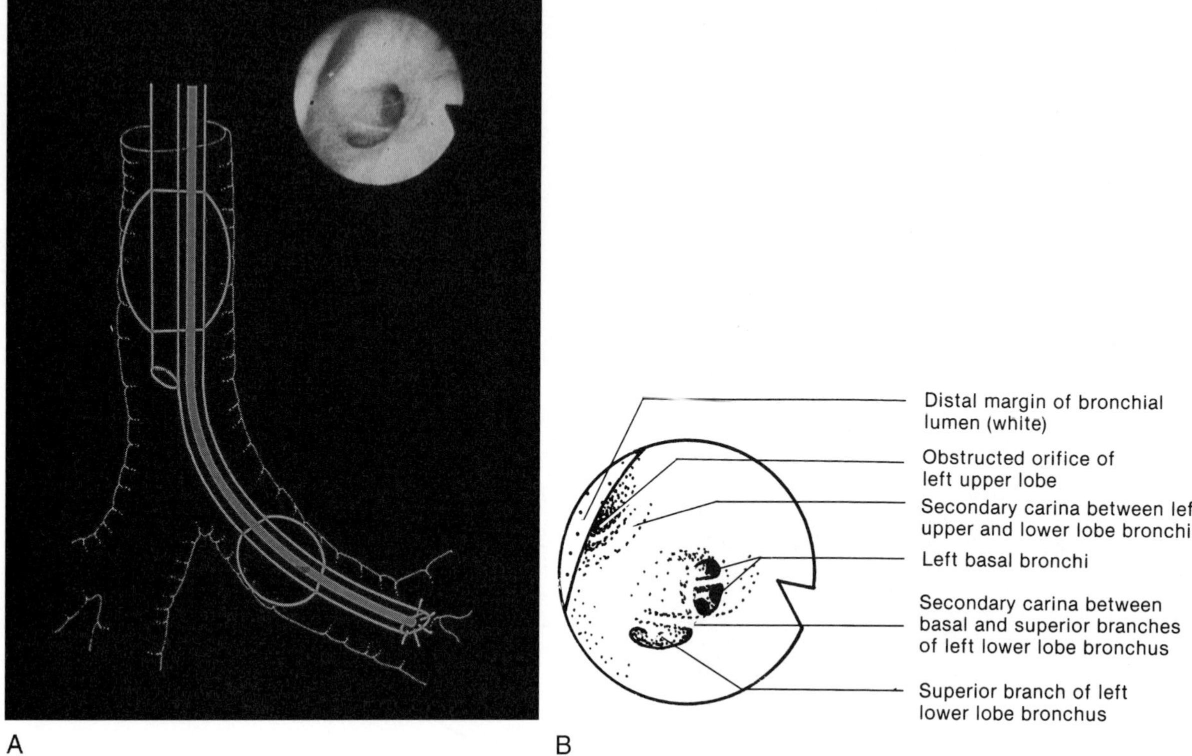

FIGURE **25–12.** *A*, View from the bronchial lumen of a left-sided double-lumen tube that is positioned too far distally. *B*, Diagrammatic representation of what is seen in the bronchoscopic photograph. This is a frequent and clinically important malposition. Intraoperatively, it can be detected reliably only by bronchoscopy. The center of the photograph shows only the orifice of the left lower lobe bronchus. Note the basal bronchi distally and the bronchus of the superior segment which exits posteriorly (inferiorly in this photograph). The edge of the orifice of the left upper lobe bronchus can be seen at the upper left of the photograph and is obstructed by the distal end of the bronchial lumen of the double-lumen tube. (From Slinger P: Fiberoptic bronchoscopic positioning of double-lumen tubes. J Cardiothorac Anesth 3: 486, 1989, with permission.)

Univent and the fiberoptic bronchoscope advanced into the correct mainstem bronchus. The fiberoptic bronchoscope then serves as a guide over which the Univent is advanced into the mainstem bronchus. Then the bronchial blocker is extended and left in the appropriate mainstem bronchus as the Univent is withdrawn into the trachea with fiberoptic bronchoscopic guidance (Fig. 25–23). The anesthesiologist must be aware that the external diameter of a Univent tube can exceed the diameter of the left mainstem bronchus (mean, 13 mm) in some patients.[51]

Inflation of the bronchial blocker of a Univent tube for lung isolation should be done in a controlled fashion so that the minimum volume and pressure required is used. This can be done with a positive-pressure ventilation leak test[52] by connecting the proximal hollow lumen of the bronchial blocker to an underwater drain. The bronchial blocker is then inflated until the underwater leak ceases from the nonventilated lung as the ventilated lung is held at a static inflation pressure (e.g., 30 cm H_2O). An alternative method is to connect the capnograph to the proximal blocker lumen and observe for the loss of respiratory fluctuations as the blocker is inflated.[53]

It requires larger volumes (4 to 8 ml) to seal the bronchial blocker of a Univent tube than a double-lumen tube (1 to 3 ml). The bronchial blocker of a Univent tube has high-pressure characteristics and cuff pressures during lung isolation are in the range of 200 to 250 mm Hg.[47] This far exceeds mean intracuff pressures in double-lumen tubes, but due to the high-pressure behavior of the Univent blocker the pressure transmitted to the bronchial wall will be significantly less than this.

The Univent has become popular because it can be left in situ as a single-lumen tube for postoperative ventilation when required without changing the tube.[50] Also, a larger size suction catheter can be used than with comparable size double-lumen tube. However, air flow resistance is a problem with the Univent, particularly the smaller size tubes. Flow resistance in a #7.5 Univent is much higher than in some comparable size double-lumen tubes (Fig. 25–24).

The size of Univent tubes is confusing due to the way the manufacturer has labeled them. They are labeled with a millimeter size (6 to 9) and their flow resistances correspond to single-lumen tubes with these internal diameters. They are also labeled with a French size since they are not circular in cross section. However, the French sizes marked on the tubes are inaccurate. These tubes are actually much larger than their labeling indicates and an anesthesiologist using these tubes needs to

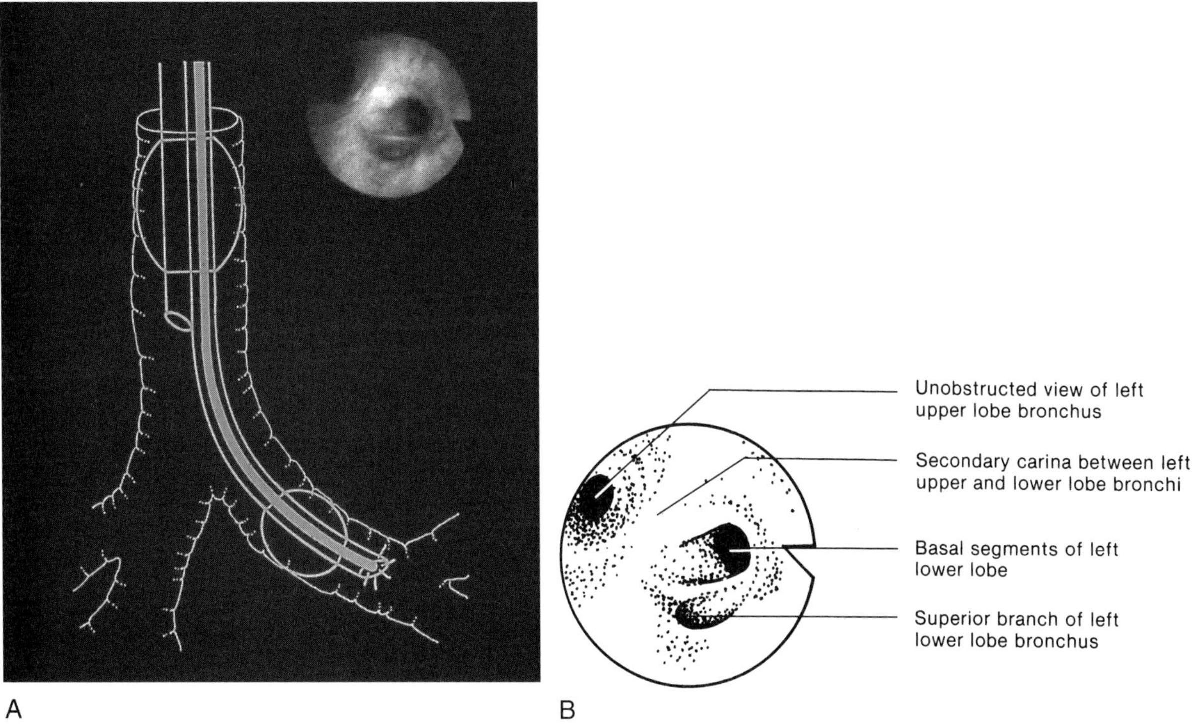

FIGURE **25–13.** *A*, View from the bronchial lumen of a properly positioned left-sided double-lumen tube (the tube in Fig. 25–12*A* has been withdrawn 2 cm). *B*, Diagrammatic representation of what is seen in the bronchoscopic photograph. The orifice of the left upper lobe bronchus can now be clearly seen. The secondary carina between the left upper lobe bronchus and the left lower lobe bronchus normally is angled from 2 to 8 o'clock across the anteroposterior plane (as in this photograph). The tertiary carina between the basilar and superior segments of the left lower lobe lies in a 4- to 8-o'clock plane and is narrower than the secondary carina. (From Slinger P: Fiberoptic bronchoscopic positioning of double-lumen tubes. J Cardiothorac Anesth 3:486, 1989, with permission.)

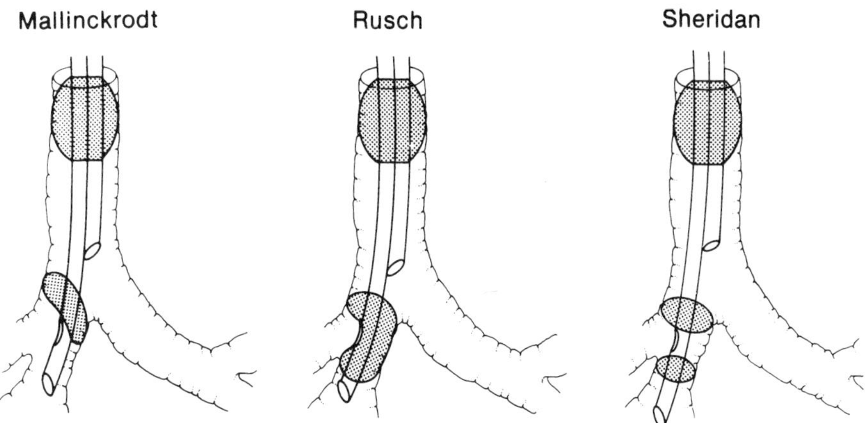

FIGURE **25–14.** Diagram of three different designs of disposable right-sided double-lumen tubes. All three designs incorporate a side-slot in the lateral wall of the bronchial lumen for ventilation of the right upper lobe. (From Slinger P, Triolet W: A clinical comparison of three different designs of right-sided double lumen tubes. Can J Anaesth 36:S59, 1989, with permission.)

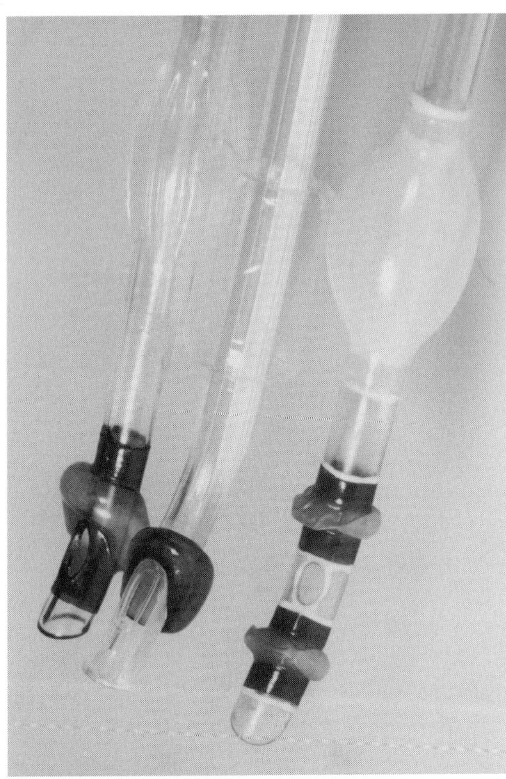

FIGURE **25–15.** Photographs of the bronchial cuffs of three designs of right double-lumen tube. Mallinckrodt on the left, Sheridan on the right. The Rusch design in the middle is a recently released modification.

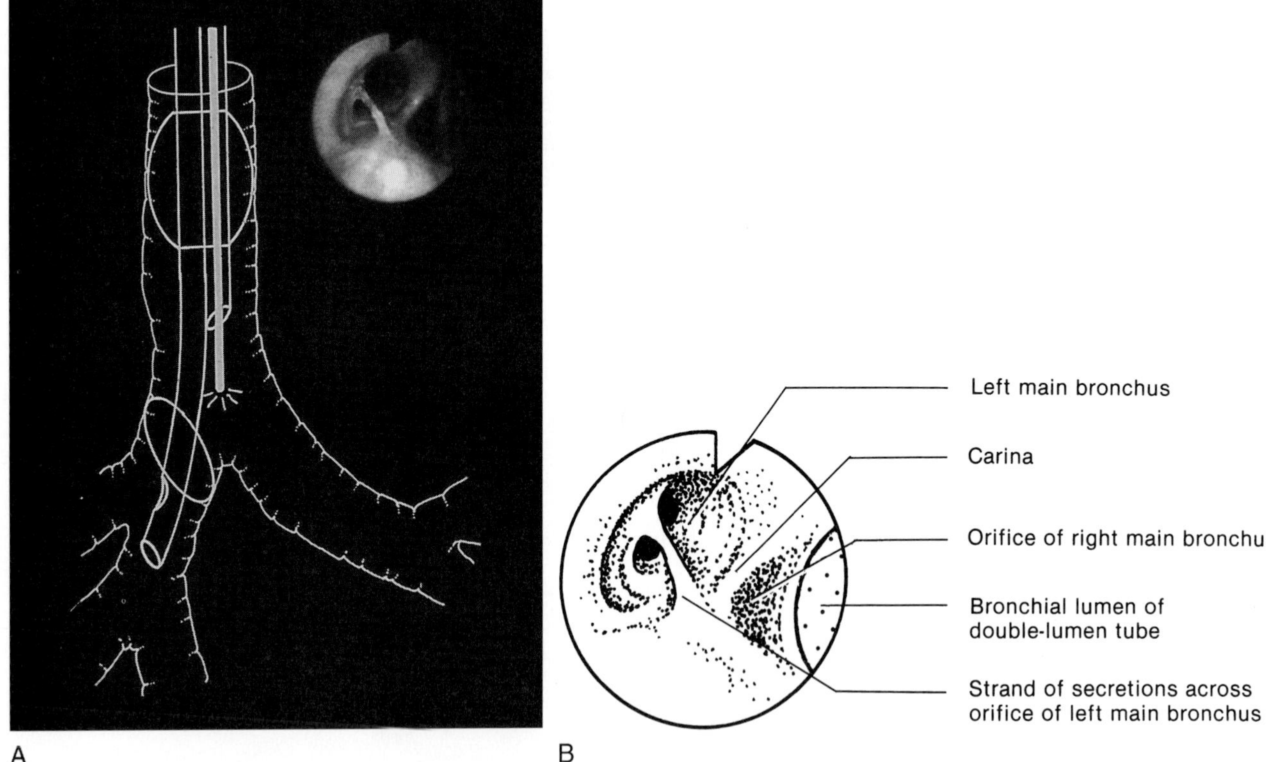

FIGURE **25–16.** *A*, Demonstration of a properly positioned Mallinckrodt right-sided double-lumen tube as seen from the tracheal lumen. *B*, Diagrammatic representation of what is seen in the bronchoscopic photograph. Note the bronchial lumen of the double-lumen tube entering the right main bronchus. This particular design of right-sided double-lumen tube has an eccentrically shaped bronchial cuff. The side ventilation slot of the bronchial lumen is distal to the cuff, not in the middle of the cuff, as in the original Robertshaw design. With the Mallinckrodt right-sided tube, the bronchial cuff is not normally visible at the carina when the tube is properly positioned. An incidental strand of secretions stretches across the orifice of the left main bronchus. Commonly, with chronic bronchitis, the posterior wall of the trachea is weakened and bulges anteriorly during expiration as seen in this photograph. (From Slinger P: Fiberoptic bronchoscopic positioning of double-lumen tubes. J Cardiothorac Anesth 3:486, 1989, with permission.)

A

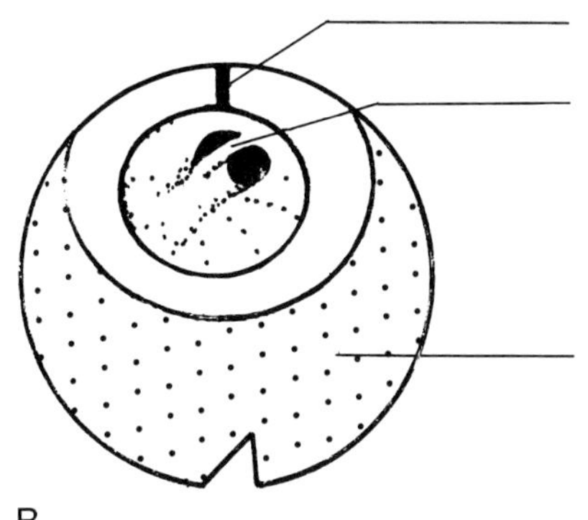

FIGURE **25–17.** *A*, View from the distal bronchial lumen of a right-sided Mallinckrodt double-lumen tube. The bronchoscope tip is within the blue bronchial cuff, and the right bronchus intermedius is seen through the distal lumen of the tube. The longitudinal submucosal elastic bundles are seen extending distally into the posterior wall of the bronchus intermedius. The secondary carina between the right middle lobe and right lower lobe can be seen distally. The radiographic marker at the distal tip of the bronchial lumen can be seen faintly at 12 o'clock. This marker is in line with the side ventilation slot in this design of right-sided double-lumen tube. The right upper lobe bronchus is normally on the lateral aspect of the right main bronchus (3 to 4 o'clock), just slightly posterior to the plane of the secondary carina between the right middle and lower lobes. Thus, this tube will have to be rotated clockwise approximately 45 degrees to find the right upper lobe bronchial orifice. *B*, Diagrammatic representation of fiberoptic photograph. (From Slinger P: Fiberoptic bronchoscopic positioning of double-lumen tubes. J Cardiothorac Anesth 3:486, 1989, with permission.)

be aware of this discrepancy (the manufacturer is now correcting this mistake).

Several complications have been reported with the Univent tube:

1. With early versions of the tube a portion of the distal bronchial blocker could detach and become a loose foreign body in the bronchus.[55]
2. Advancement of the bronchial blocker without continuous fiberoptic bronchoscope visualization can lead to bronchial perforation. The bronchial blocker can be advanced 8 cm beyond the tracheal lumen, far enough to produce lobar or segmental blockade. However, this is also far enough to perforate a tertiary or quaternary bronchus, since these have little cartilaginous support.[25]
3. Accidental inflation of the bronchial blocker during postoperative ventilation can lead to acute respiratory deterioration.[55]

Reviews of the Univent tube have not been consistent with respect to whether it is easier[56] or more difficult[57] to use than a double-lumen tube. Although its applications are not as widespread as the double-lumen tube (Table 25–4), the Univent has been used in anesthesia for cases involving trauma, hemoptysis, thoracoscopy, esophageal, mediastinal, thoracic aortic, and vertebral column surgery. The Univent blocker tends to be less stable intraoperatively than a double-lumen tube.[57]

Bronchial Blockers

The use of separate bronchial blockers has decreased since the introduction of modern double-lumen tubes. Bronchial blockers have a greater potential for instability during lung manipulation, particularly when placed in the short right mainstem bronchus. Migration of a bronchial blocker into the trachea intraoperatively can not

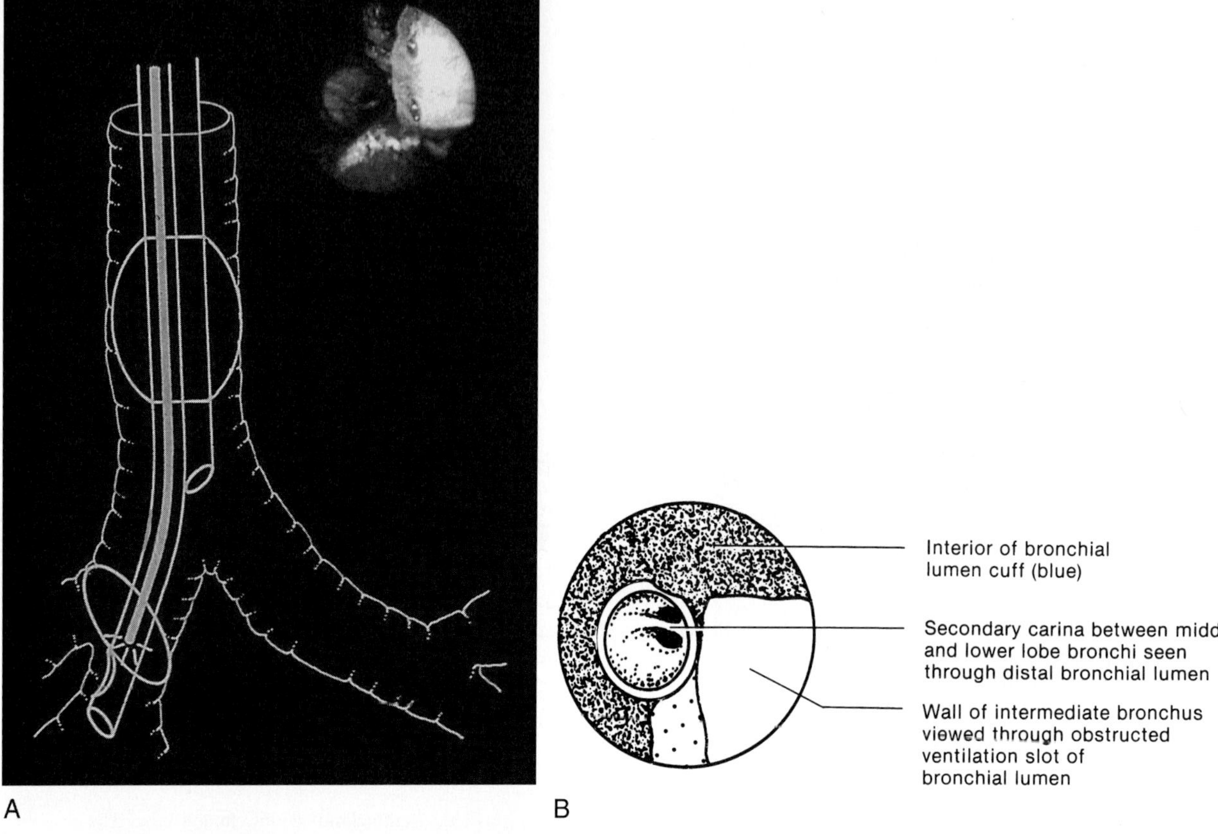

FIGURE **25–18.** *A*, View of the right-sided double-lumen tube from Figure 25–19, which has been rotated and the bronchoscope withdrawn and rotated until the side ventilation slot is visible. *B*, Diagrammatic representation of what is seen in the bronchoscopic photograph. This tube is positioned too far distally and only the lateral wall of the bronchus intermedius can be seen through the ventilation slot. The distal orifice of the double tube can be seen to the left of center in the photograph. The secondary carina between the right middle and lower lobes is visible through the distal orifice. (From Slinger P: Fiberoptic bronchoscopic positioning of double-lumen tubes. J Cardiothorac Anesth 3:486, 1989, with permission.)

only cause loss of lung isolation but may also severely interfere with ventilation due to obstruction of one or both mainstem bronchi. Deflation of the nonventilated lung occurs slowly as a result of absorption of trapped gas in the lung and is often facilitated by compression of lung by the surgeon.

However, bronchial blockers are still extremely useful in certain situations, such as for lobar or segmental obstruction versus entire lung isolation. Also, they permit production of lung isolation via a standard single-lumen endotracheal tube in situations where the need for lung isolation arises unforeseen intraoperatively. This is particularly helpful when it is impossible or dangerous to convert to a double-lumen tube. This scenario occasionally occurs in polytrauma.

Bronchial blockers specifically designed for anesthesiology are no longer widely available. Currently the most useful bronchial blocker is a Fogarty catheter (e.g., 8 to 10-Fr venous embolectomy catheter with a 4 to 10-ml balloon; American Hospital Supply Corporation, Irvine, CA). This can be passed through the vocal cords immediately prior to placing a single-lumen tube. It is important to create a 45-degree angulation in the distal 2 cm of the Fogarty catheter prior to insertion, to permit subsequent manipulation. Also, leaving the metal guidewire in the blocker aids initial placement. The bronchial blocker is positioned under direct vision with a fiberoptic bronchoscope passed via the single-lumen tube.

A Fogarty catheter is relatively stable when used in this fashion because it is held by the inflated cuff of the endotracheal tube. When necessary, the bronchial blocker and the fiberoptic bronchoscope can both be passed intraluminally in the endotracheal tube via a bronchoscopy swivel connector[58,59] (Fig. 25–25). After positioning, the fiberoptic bronchoscope is removed and an airtight seal can be achieved by closing the diaphragm of the bronchoscope connector with the blocker in situ. The major problem with bronchial blockers is that there is no access to the nonventilated lung for CPAP, suction, etc.

Endobronchial Tubes

The original technique for lung isolation was the distal placement of a single-lumen tube as an endobronchial

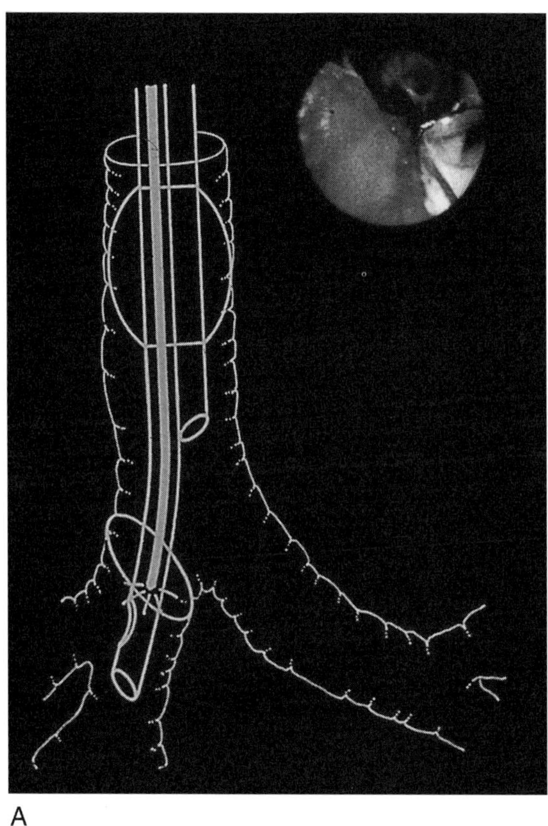

A

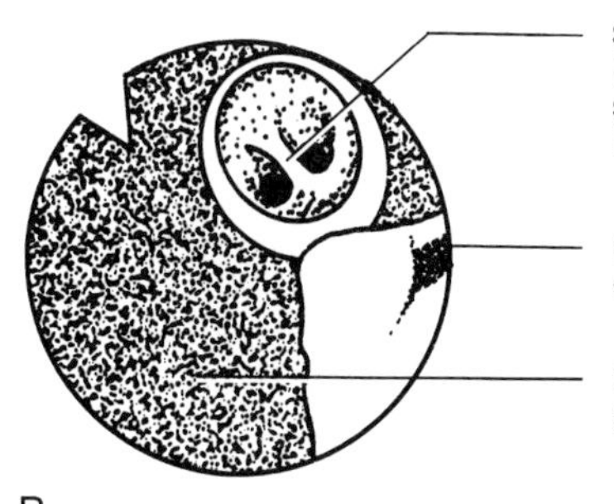

B

FIGURE **25–19.** *A*, The double-lumen tube in Figure 25–18 has been withdrawn until the orifice of the right upper lobe bronchus is partially visible through the ventilation slot. *B*, Diagrammatic representation of what is seen in the bronchoscopic photograph. Note the relationship between the plane of the secondary right middle/lower lobe carina and the orifice of the right upper lobe bronchus. (From Slinger P: Fiberoptic bronchoscopic positioning of double-lumen tubes. J Cardiothorac Anesth 3:486, 1989, with permission.)

tube as described by Gale and Waters.[1] Some anesthesiologists continue to use a standard 32-cm-long, 7.5-mm-ID, single-lumen tube as an endobronchial tube, in the majority of situations when lung isolation is required.[60] These tubes can be positioned with the usual adult size fiberoptic bronchoscopes (5- to 6-mm-diameter). Single-lumen endobronchial tubes will usually enter the right mainstem bronchus without problem. Left mainstem bronchus intubation can be achieved in more than 90% of cases by a combination of rotating the tube so that it is concave distally to the left (counterclockwise), while the patient's head is rotated 90 degrees to the right, prior to advancement.[61,62] This maneuver may be lifesaving during massive hemoptysis in an intubated patient, pending the availability of better equipment for lung isolation.

Endobronchial tubes are preferred by some surgeons for procedures involving the carina, since they are more flexible than double-lumen tubes and permit better mobilization and exposure of the carina.[63] A technique for managing distal tracheal trauma with bilateral endobronchial tubes has been described.[64]

An endobronchial tube in the right mainstem bronchus has a high risk of obstructing the right upper lobe orifice. Endobronchial tubes share with bronchial blockers the problems of lack of access to the nonventilated lung. Also, it is difficult to adequately survey endobronchial tube positioning with fiberoptic bronchoscopy. Economically, there is a strong advantage to the use of a simple single-lumen endobronchial tube versus a double-lumen tube or Univent tube (e.g., $3 per case vs. approximately $70 per case).

Management of Specific Indications

Specific indications for lung isolation will be discussed proceeding from clinically common to less frequent situations (Table 25–5).

Elective Pulmonary Resection: Right Lung

This is currently the most common adult indication for one-lung ventilation. The optimal choice is a left double-lumen tube (Fig. 25–26). A partial resection can proceed to a pneumonectomy, if required, without loss of lung isolation. There is continuous access to the nonventilated lung for suctioning, bronchoscopic monitoring, and

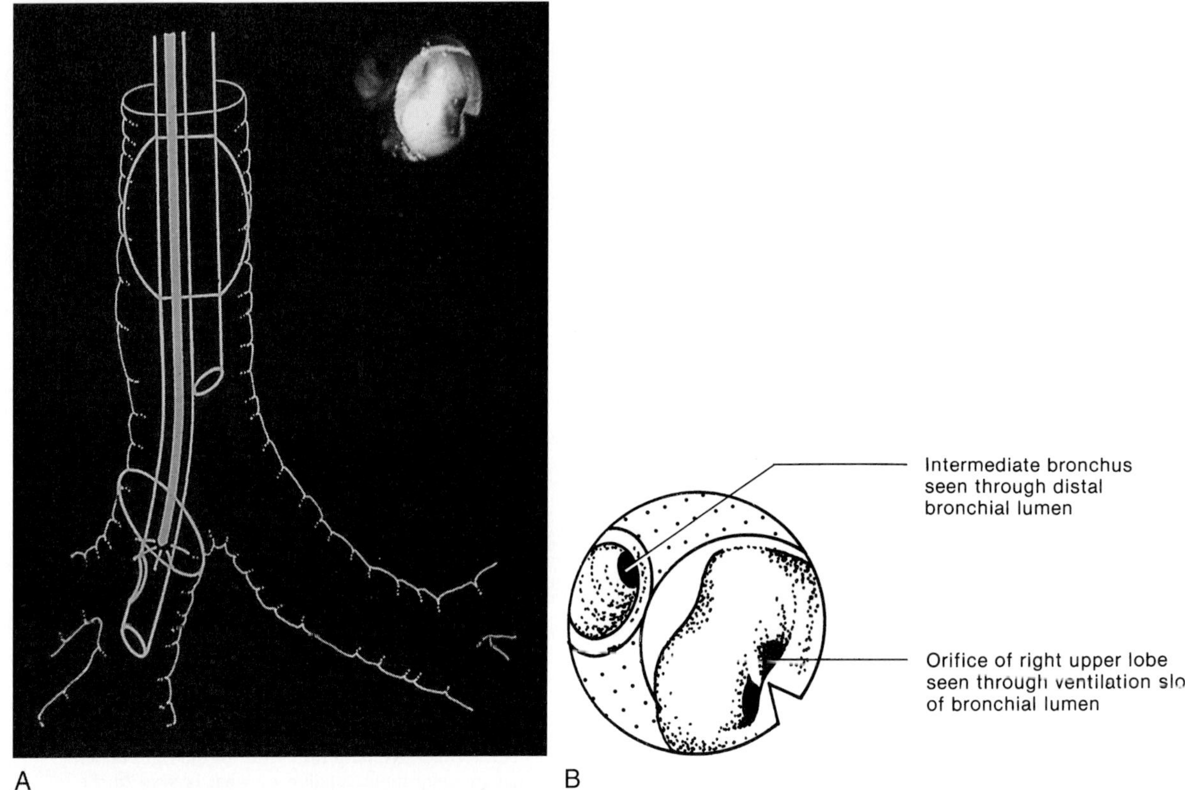

FIGURE **25–20.** *A*, View the entire orifice of the right upper lobe bronchus, which is visible through the ventilation slot of a right-sided double-lumen tube. The bronchoscope can now be passed out through the ventilation slot to inspect the right upper lobe bronchus. *B*, Diagrammatic representation of fiberoptic photograph. (From Slinger P: Fiberoptic bronchoscopic positioning of double-lumen tubes. J Cardiothorac Anesth 3:486, 1989, with permission.)

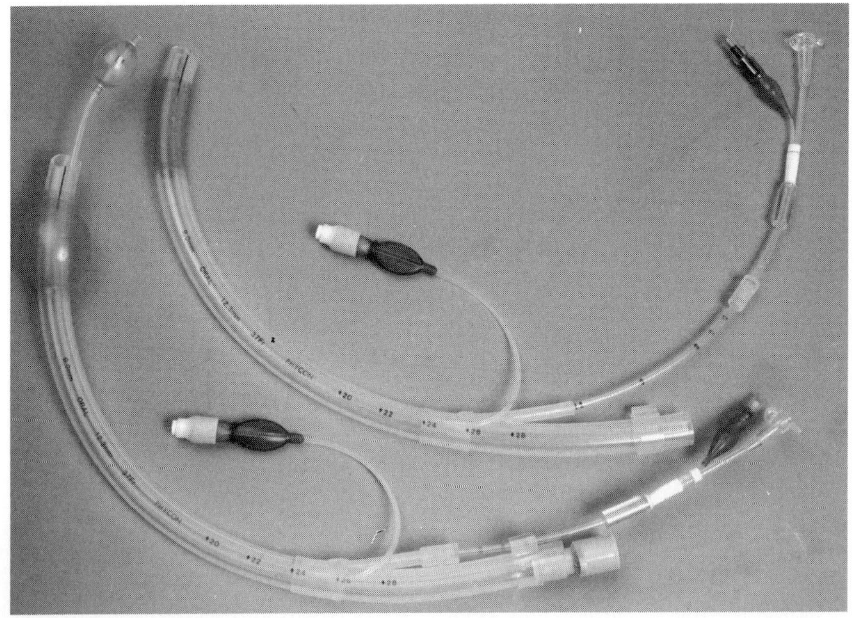

FIGURE **25–21.** The Univent tube (Fuji Systems, Tokyo, Japan) is a single-lumen endotracheal tube with a retractable bronchial blocker enclosed in a separate lumen.

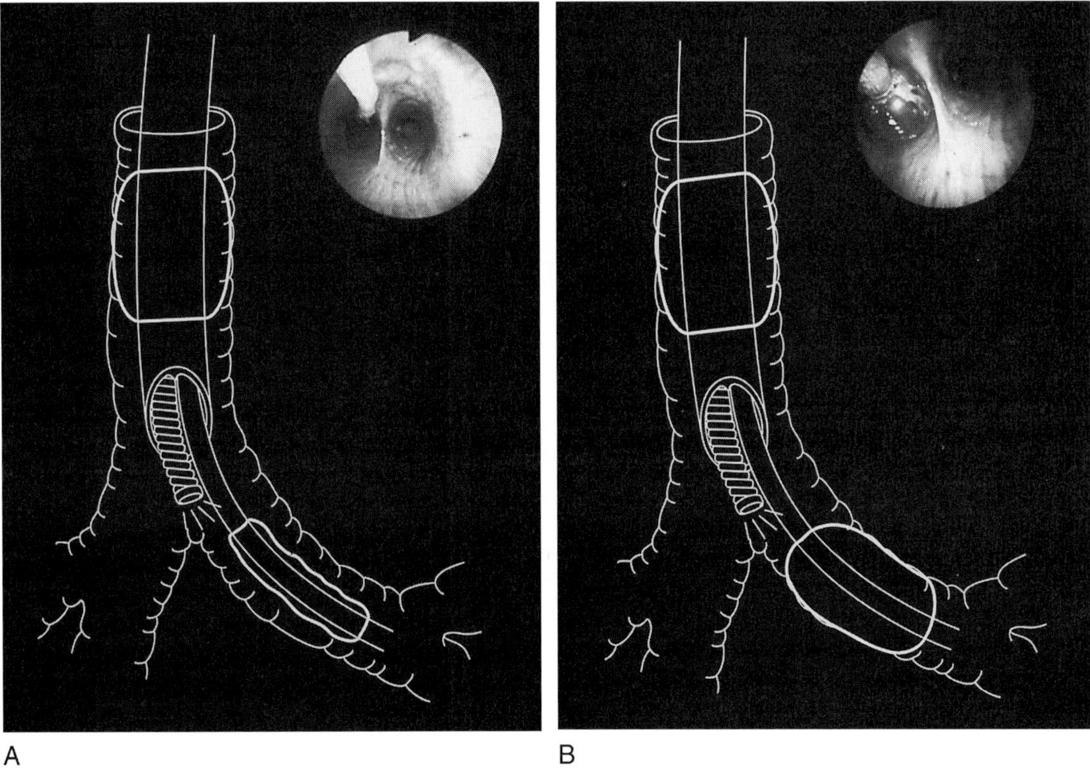

FIGURE **25–22.** *A*, Diagram and bronchoscopic photograph of the bronchial blocker of a Univent tube being passed into the left mainstem bronchus. The Univent tube has been rotated so that it is concave to the left. The blocker will then advance along the left lateral tracheal wall. *B*, Diagram and photograph of a well-positioned bronchial blocker of a Univent tube inflated to seal the left mainstem bronchus.

CPAP. The bevel of the bronchial orifice of current left double-lumen tubes (Fig. 25–8) facilitates left mainstem bronchus intubation but occasionally leads to partial obstruction of the bronchial lumen by the medial wall of the left mainstem bronchus. This often can be corrected with bronchoscopic adjustment, usually further advancement into the bronchus.

Alternative techniques for right lung resections are an endobronchial tube, Univent, or bronchial blocker. A right double-lumen tube can also be used but is more likely to create problems with isolation and will need repositioning for a pneumonectomy.

Elective Pulmonary Resection: Left Lung

The use of a left double-lumen tube for a left thoracotomy (Fig. 25–27) is a widely practiced technique. Rarely this is associated with obstruction of the tracheal lumen by the tracheal wall and subsequent problems with gas exchange in the ventilated lung.[20] Fiberoptic bronchoscopy often reveals that this is related to inadequate tube rotation such that the tracheal lumen tends to lie posteriorly against a bulging membranous tracheal wall. This is usually correctable simply by tube rotation with fiberoptic observation. A case of right tracheobronchial obstruction during left thoracotomy with a left double-lumen tube has been described that was alleviated by removal of the axillary roll.[65] Both a right double-lumen tube and a Univent tube are alternative choices. The Univent blocker may migrate into the trachea and require intubation with a double-lumen tube.[66]

Left Pneumonectomy

Lung isolation for a left pneumonectomy presents several challenges. Any left pulmonary resection may unforseeably become a pneumonectomy. If a left double-lumen tube is being used for one-lung ventilation, the tube can be withdrawn until the distal bronchial lumen is proximal to the carina (tube length <25 cm at the teeth). The bronchial cuff is then inflated and the bronchial lumen used as a single-lumen tube. It is usually possible to get a satisfactory seal in the distal trachea using only the bronchial cuff, which can inflate to a diameter of 22 mm. Alternatively, if adequate ventilation cannot be maintained with this method due to air leak around the bronchial cuff, the bronchial cuff can be deflated and the patient ventilated using both lumens. The distal tracheal orifice should be examined fiberoptically to ensure that it is beyond the vocal cords. It can be difficult to get a complete seal at the glottis, since the tracheal cuff lies between the vocal cords.

At present, the best technique of lung isolation when a left pneumonectomy is forseen is with a right-sided double-lumen tube. In more than two thirds of cases a right double-lumen tube can function adequately providing reliable lung isolation without obstruction and with

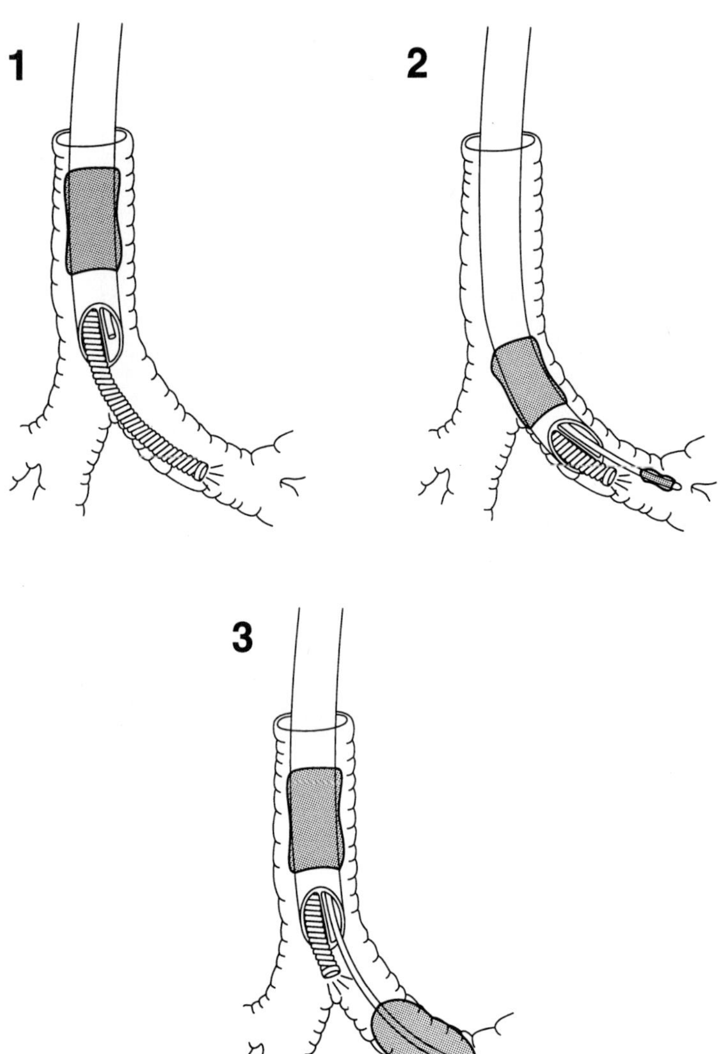

FIGURE **25–23.** In cases of problematic bronchial intubation with the blocker of a Univent tube the fiberoptic bronchoscope can be used to facilitate placement: *1*, The bronchoscope is passed via the main lumen of the Univent tube into the correct mainstem bronchus. *2*, The Univent tube is advanced over the bronchoscope, which serves as a guide. The blocker of the Univent tube is then extended into the distal portion of the main bronchus under direct vision. *3*, The blocker cuff is inflated and the Univent tube and bronchoscope are withdrawn leaving the blocker in situ.

acceptable bronchial cuff pressures.[46] A right double-lumen tube will permit the surgeon to palpate the left hilum during one-lung ventilation without interference from a tube or blocker in the left mainstem bronchus. This is useful when there is some question regarding the extent and resectability of a tumor.

The disposable right double-lumen tubes available in North America vary greatly in design depending on the manufacturer (Fig. 25–14). The most common problem with these tubes is that, due to the asymmetric designs of the bronchial cuffs, they may require greater than 50 cm H_2O bronchial cuff pressure to produce lung isolation.

Rarely, left lung isolation is impossible in spite of extremely high pressures in the bronchial cuff. In these cases, a Fogarty catheter can be passed into the left mainstem bronchus after estimation of the depth with a fiberoptic bronchoscope. The surgeon can then palpate the balloon of the Fogarty catheter in the bronchus to aid positioning. This avoids intraoperative replacement of the double-lumen tube.

For alternative methods of lung isolation during a left pneumonectomy, there is no clear preference among a left double-lumen tube, Univent, or other bronchial blocker. These all require repositioning intraoperatively. However, this is usually not a major problem. A right single-lumen endobronchial tube is almost certain to obstruct the right upper lung with an attendant increased risk of hypoxemia during one-lung ventilation.

Thoracoscopy

Although thoracoscopy is not a new procedure, advances in videoscopic technology in the past decade have permitted the current exponential growth in video-assisted thoracoscopic surgery (VATS). Thoracoscopy may become the commonest single indication for lung isolation (Table 25–6). VATS can be used for biopsy of lung, pleura, mediastinum, pericardium, or adrenal glands, and for sympathectomies.[67,68] VATS will probably become the procedure of choice for resection of blebs, bullae, and peripheral lung lesions, especially in patients with impaired pulmonary function.

Diagnostic thoracoscopies can be done without general anesthesia using a combination of sedation and re-

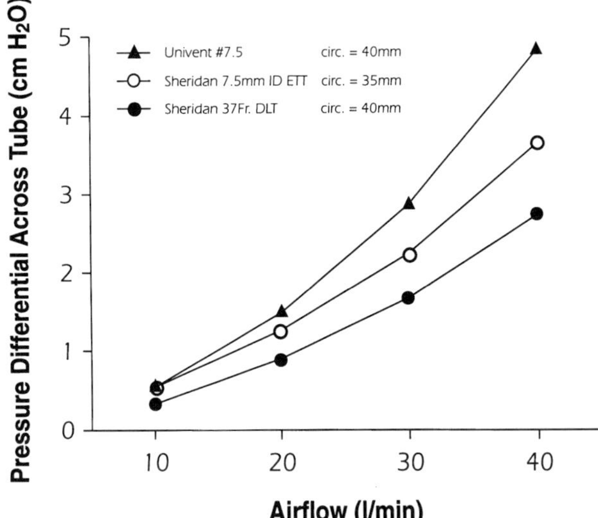

FIGURE **25–24.** A comparison of the flow resistances (measured as the pressure differential) at various airflow rates through a #7.5 Univent tube, a 7.5-mm-ID endotracheal tube (ETT), and a 37-Fr double-lumen tube (DLT). Although the Univent tube is labeled 31 Fr, its measured external circumference is 40 mm, approximately equivalent to a 37-Fr DLT (circumference, 40 mm). The circumference for the 7.5-mm ETT is 35 mm. Note that the airflow resistance of the DLT is less than that of the ETT and both are below that of the Univent. (From Slinger P, Lesiuk L: Flow resistances of disposable double-lumen, single-lumen and univent tubes. J Cardiothorac Vasc Anesth 12:133, 1998.)

gional/local anesthetic blocks. With spontaneous respiration the introduction of atmospheric pressure into the operative hemithorax causes the lung to collapse and facilitates surgical visualization. However, for resections or prolonged cases the procedure is usually better tolerated by the patient using general anesthesia. With general anesthesia, it is extremely difficult for the surgeon to visualize any intrathoracic structures unless the lung in the operative hemithorax is collapsed. When positive-pressure ventilation is used, lung isolation is necessary. During open thoracotomy the lung can be compressed by the surgeon to facilitate collapse prior to inflation of a bronchial blocker. This is not possible during thoracoscopy. Some surgeons insufflate carbon dioxide into the nondependent hemithorax to speed lung collapse. However, this technique is associated with hemodynamic instability in some cases due to the mass effect of the capnothorax.[69]

The use of a double-lumen tube is currently the optimal method of managing one-lung ventilation for VATS.[7] The rapid and complete deflation of the operative lung via the nonventilated lumen of the double-lumen tube obviates the need for carbon dioxide insufflation in the hemithorax. Particularly for right-sided VATS, the use of a bronchial blocker or Univent can cause problems. Minor movement of the blocker in the right mainstem bronchus secondary to positioning, cough, or surgical manipulation can lead to reinflation of the right upper lobe. It can then be a difficult exercise to get the right upper lobe to deflate again, since the bronchial orifice may be occluded by the blocker itself. A left double-lumen tube is the preferred method of lung isolation for VATS in either hemithorax.

It is possible to manage VATS during general anesthesia using a single-lumen tube with spontaneous ventilation and allowing the operative lung to collapse by introducing atmospheric pressure into the hemithorax when the initial incision for thoracoscopy port placement is made. This is a less controlled situation and requires particularly careful attention to monitoring oxygenation, ventilation, and hemodynamics.

Pulmonary Hemorrhage

Previously, life-threatening massive pulmonary hemorrhage was largely due to infectious diseases (e.g., tuberculosis, aspergillosis). Although these causes still occur, massive hemorrhage currently is usually secondary to a carcinoma or bronchiectasis. Bleeding is from bronchial arteries due to the increased vascularity associated with malignancy or inflammation. Since the bronchial circulation is a systemic-pressure system, blood can rapidly

TABLE **25–4**
Risks and Benefits of Various Methods of Lung Isolation

	Double-Lumen Endobronchial Tube (DLT)	Univent Single-Lumen Tube with Blocker	Bronchial Blocker with Single-Lumen Endotracheal Tube (BB)	Single-Lumen Endobronchial Tube (EBT)
Ease of positioning*	++	++	+	+
Reliability of lung isolation	++	+	+	+
Intraoperative stability	++	+	+	++
Continuous bilateral lung access	+++	+	0	0
Accidental lobar bronchial obstruction	+	0	0	+
Intentional lobar bronchial blockade†	+	++	+++	0
Lumen obstruction by tracheal or bronchial wall	+	0	0	0
Adaptability with abnormal airway anatomy	+	++	++	++
Postoperative two-lung ventilation	+	+	+++	+
Use in bronchial surgery	++	0	0	++
Iatrogenic trauma	++	+	+	+

*Fiberoptic guidance and/or surveillance of positioning.
†Bronchial blockade with DLT possible with combined use of blocker (see text).
+++, strong; ++, moderate; +, slight; 0, nil.

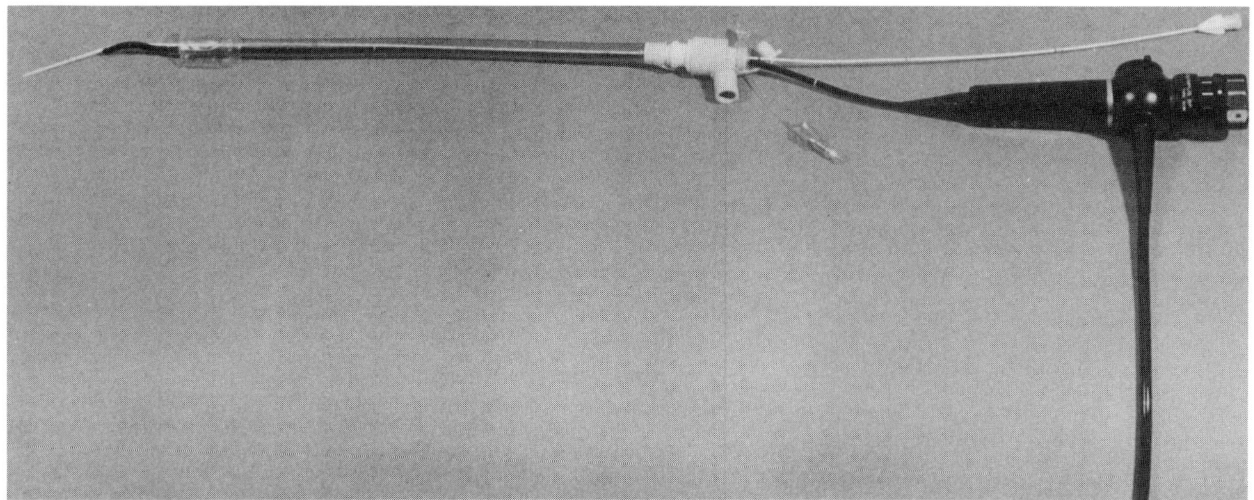

FIGURE 25–25. An 8-Fr Fogarty embolectomy catheter has been passed through a 7-mm-ID endotracheal tube beside a 4-mm-diameter fiberoptic bronchoscope via a bronchoscopy swivel connector. The Fogarty catheter can be positioned under direct vision as a bronchial blocker to achieve lung or lobe isolation via a standard single-lumen tube. After blocker positioning, the bronchoscope is removed and the plastic diaphragm of the swivel connector closed with the Fogarty catheter in place, to stabilize it. Note that the distal end of the Fogarty catheter has been angulated to aid intrabronchial manipulation. (From Zilberstein M, Katz RI, Levy A, et al: An improved method for introducing a bronchial blocker. J Cardiothorac Anesth 4:481, 1990, with permission.)

fill the tracheobronchial tree and cause death by asphyxiation before hypovolemia occurs.

Massive hemoptysis has been defined as 200 to 600 ml or more of blood in 24 to 48 hours.[70,71] These definitions are somewhat arbitrary. The important thing for the physician to recognize is that when the volume of hemorrhage exceeds the patient's ability to cough or the nursing staff's ability to suction the airway, the patient will die if left untreated. The mortality rate can be decreased to below 25%[72] with appropriate intervention. Management requires four sequential steps: lung isolation, resuscitation, diagnosis, and definitive treatment.

The anesthesiologist is often called to provide lung isolation for these patients outside of the operating suite: in the radiology department, emergency room, or intensive care unit. The initial method of lung isolation in each case will depend in part on the availability of appropriate equipment and trained accessory staff, and in part on the clinical scenario. There is no consensus on the best technique of lung isolation in these patients.

TABLE 25–5
Methods of Lung Isolation

Indication for Lung Isolation	Preferred Method(s)	Possible Alternative(s)
Pulmonary resection right side	Left DLT	EBT/Univent
Pulmonary resection left side		
Pneumonectomy unlikely	Left DLT/Univent	Right DLT/BB
Probable pneumonectomy	Right DLT	Univent/Left DLT/BB
Thoracoscopy (either side)	Left DLT	Univent/BB/Right DLT/EBT
Pulmonary hemorrhage	Left DLT	EBT/BB
Bronchopleural fistula		
Left mainstem bronchus	Right DLT	EBT
All others	Left DLT	EBT/BB
Purulent secretions (abscess, cyst, etc.)	BB and/or Left DLT	EBT/Univent
Bullae, blebs	Left DLT	Right DLT, Univent
Nonpulmonary surgery (thoracic aorta, esophagus, etc.)	Left DLT/Univent	BB/EBT/Right DLT
Bronchial surgery (tumor, trauma etc.)		
Left side	Right DLT	EBT
Right side	Left DLT	EBT
Upper airway abnormalities	Left DLT/EBT Univent/BB	Right DLT
Transplantation		
Double-lung	Left DLT	BB/Univent
Single right lung	Left DLT	Univent
Single left lung	Right DLT	Left DLT/Univent
Independent lung ventilation	Left DLT	Right DLT
Unilateral lung lavage	Left DLT	—

DLT, double-lumen tube; EBT, single-lumen endobronchial tube; BB, bronchial blocker.

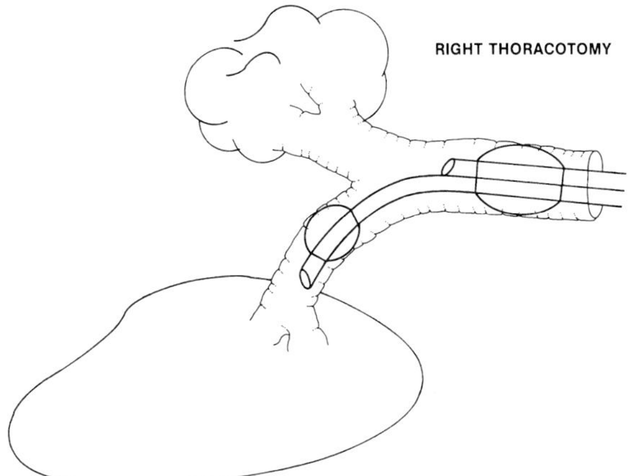

FIGURE **25–26.** A left-sided double-lumen tube is the most reliable method of producing one-lung ventilation for surgical procedures in the right hemithorax. Due to some telescoping of the left mainstem bronchus in the lateral position, the margin of safety for positioning the bronchial cuff and lumen is often small.

One option for the initial isolation method in these cases is a left double-lumen tube. With a double-lumen tube it is not necessary to know which lung is bleeding. Even if a left double-lumen tube is passed into the right mainstem bronchus, lung isolation will be achieved and the hypoxemia due to the obstruction of the right upper lobe is rarely significant. A case of left double-lumen tube insertion deliberately into the right mainstem bronchus as treatment for right upper lobe hemorrhage has been described.[73] The use of a double-lumen tube allows bilateral suctioning, thus both lungs can be cleared and the progress of further bleeding monitored.[74] In some cases, a fiberoptic bronchoscope can be passed via the double-lumen tube for diagnosis of the bleeding without loss of lung isolation.

The problems with using a double-lumen tube in these patients include the fact that the small-diameter suction catheters used with a double-lumen tube may not be adequate for a large-volume hemorrhage and clot may obstruct the narrow lumens of the tube. Also, insertion of a double-lumen tube is always somewhat more difficult than a single-lumen tube. This technical discrepancy between the two tubes is increased in a semiconscious patient coughing large quantities of blood. Furthermore, in the patient who is already intubated with a single-lumen tube, there is a risk of further aggravating hypoxemia during changing of the endotracheal tube, especially in the presence of the inevitable full stomach.

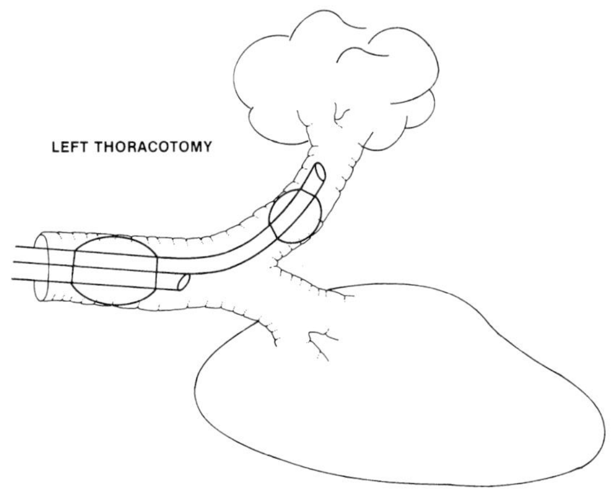

FIGURE **25–27.** A left double-lumen tube can be used for one-lung ventilation during a left thoracotomy. Partial obstruction of the distal tracheal lumen orifice from the tracheal wall can cause problems ventilating the dependent lung. This is usually due to malrotation of the tube such that the tracheal lumen lies posteriorly and is partially obstructed by the membranous portion of the trachea. The bronchial lumen of a left double-lumen tube would have to be withdrawn to a supracarinal position for a left pneumonectomy.

TABLE **25–6**
Potential Thoracoscopic Procedures

Pulmonary
Resections: wedge, lobectomy, pneumonectomy
Lung cancer staging
Bullae/bleb resections
Lung biopsy
Empyema, bronchopleural fistula
Chylothorax
Pleural disease
Biopsy
Sclerotherapy
Mediastinum
Biopsy/excision of cysts/masses
Esophageal
Esophagectomy
Myotomy
Cardiovascular
Pericardial biopsy/window
Cardiac surgery
Cardioverter/defibrillator implantation
Patent ductus arteriosus ligation
Skeletal
Thoracic outlet syndrome
Thoracic vertebral diskectomy/biopsy
Autonomic
Dorsal sympathectomy
Extrathoracic
Transdiaphragmatic adrenal biopsy

In these situations, advancement of a standard single-lumen tube for use as an endobronchial tube may be the best option, particularly if the site of bleeding can be surmised by history or chest x-ray. As described in the section "Endobronchial Intubation," the correct bronchus can be intubated blindly in most cases with a combination of head and tube rotation.[61] Single-lumen tubes can also be passed endobronchially with fiberoptic guidance, but this is often difficult until the airway can be adequately suctioned.

The use of bronchial blockers is also an option. However, blockers are difficult to place properly in the presence of ongoing massive hemorrhage. In a patient with hemoptysis and pulmonary hypertension, endobronchial blockade has been reported to lead to lobar rupture secondary to continued bleeding.[75]

It is often necessary to begin hemodynamic resuscitation at the same time as lung isolation. It must be appreciated that resuscitation in these patients is futile without lung isolation. After stabilization and correction of coagulation, diagnosis will require rigid bronchoscopy and/or bronchial or pulmonary angiography. Definitive therapy may require pulmonary resection or bronchial artery embolization depending on the clinical situation.

Management of iatrogenic pulmonary hemorrhage secondary to pulmonary artery perforation from a Swan-Ganz catheter is another situation that requires lung isolation. Catheter-induced pulmonary artery rupture is associated with peripheral catheter location, pulmonary hypertension, advanced age, anticoagulation, and hypothermia.[76,77] In patients outside the cardiac operating theater management involves the same basic principles as described above for other cases of pulmonary hemorrhage.

One half of the reported cases of catheter-induced pulmonary hemorrhage have occurred during weaning from cardiopulmonary bypass. In this situation, there are additional management options available (Fig. 25–28). Resumption of bypass ensures oxygenation while the tracheobronchial tree is adequately suctioned and then visualized with fiberoptic bronchoscopy. The use of a pulmonary artery vent may be required to decrease the pulmonary blood flow sufficiently to permit definition of the bleeding site (usually the right lower lobe). The pleural cavity is opened to assess the degree of lung parenchymal damage. Due to the high morbidity and mortality associated with pulmonary resection surgery in this setting, conservative management with a blocker or double-lumen tube should be considered if there is minimal lung damage.

A Fogarty catheter can be employed as a bronchial blocker to achieve lobar blockade. The adequacy of lung isolation is then observed through the bronchoscope placed just proximal to the inflated bronchial blocker during weaning from bypass and reversal of anticoagulation. A trial of Fogarty balloon deflation with direct fiberoptic bronchoscope surveillance can be undertaken after a stable period of 24 to 48 hours of postoperative ventilation.

If there is extensive parenchymal injury or if the visceral pleura is ruptured, pulmonary resection should be performed prior to discontinuing bypass. In patients with limited cardiorespiratory reserve, who may not tolerate a pulmonary resection, temporary pulmonary artery occlusion by a vascular loop has been reported.[78] This occlusion can then be released on the second postoperative day.

Hemoptysis can occur in cases of severe multiple trauma with blunt injury to the chest, such as from a motor vehicle accident. It is important for the anesthesiologist to appreciate that a certain amount of hemoptysis occurs in chest trauma due to alveolar rupture from

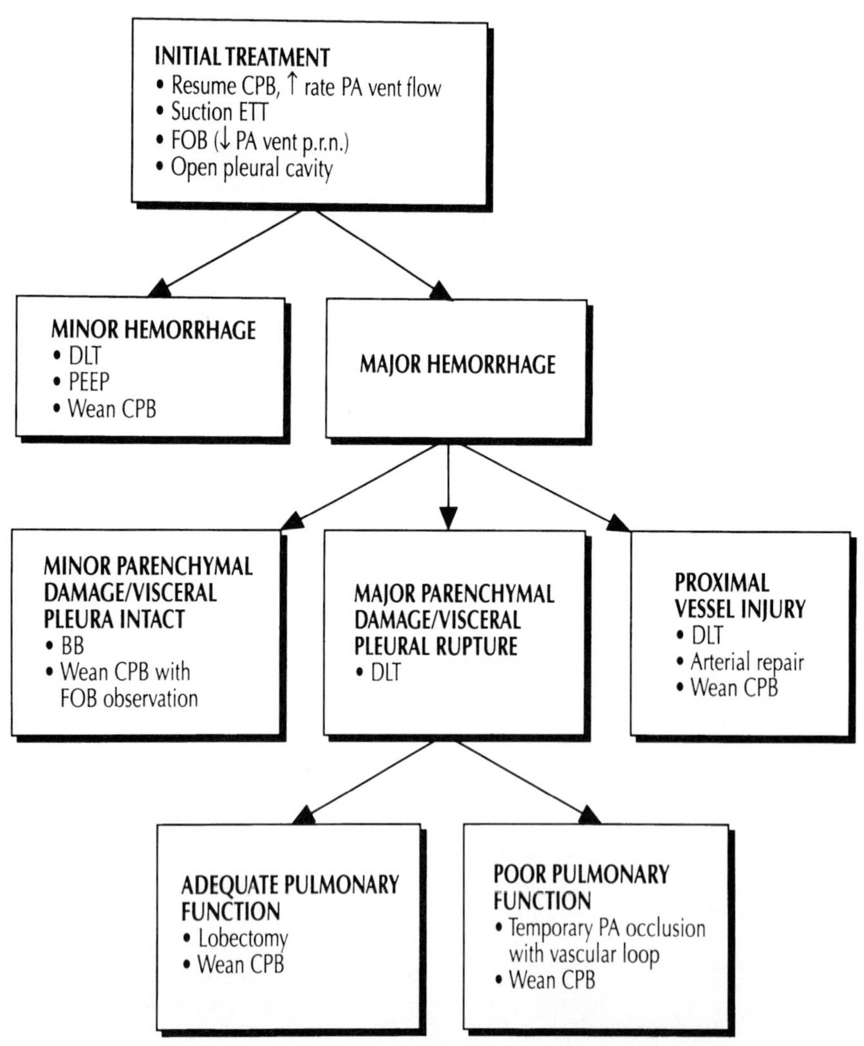

FIGURE **25–28.** Flow diagram for management of pulmonary hemorrhage due to pulmonary artery (PA) perforation by a PA catheter during weaning from cardiopulmonary bypass (CPB) (see text). DLT, double-lumen endobronchial tube; PEEP, positive end-expiratory pressure; FOB, fiberoptic bronchoscope; BB, bronchial blocker. (Based on Purut et al.[76] and Urschel and Myerowitz.[77])

rapid pulmonary parenchymal compression with subsequent intrapulmonary lacerations and alveolar hemorrhage.[79] This alveolar hemorrhage is rarely, in and of itself, life threatening. In a series of 208 such multiple trauma patients reported by Devitt et al., there were 13 cases of tracheobronchial hemorrhage,[80] 10 of which cleared with simple suctioning or fiberoptic bronchoscopy. Two required lung isolation and one patient who did not receive lung isolation died of asphyxiation due to hemorrhage. However, compared to the one death from hemorrhage-induced asphyxiation, there were 16 intraoperative deaths due to exsanguination in the series.

Lung isolation may be lifesaving in the treatment of hemoptysis due to multiple trauma, particularly if the hemorrhage persists after suctioning and fiberoptic bronchoscopy. In managing these situations several principles should be remembered: First, if assistance and equipment are limited, it is more useful to concentrate the anesthesiologist's efforts on resuscitation of the patient and to rely on single-lumen intubation and suction to treat pulmonary hemorrhage. Second, there may be a major tracheobronchial disruption and the distal airway must be inspected with bronchoscopy prior to any attempt at insertion of a double-lumen tube or bronchial blocker. Blind insertion of a double-lumen tube has the attendant risk of aggravating bronchial injury and loss of ability to ventilate these patients.

Bronchopleural Fistula

Bronchopleural fistulas occur in a wide variety of medical situations such as ARDS, pneumonia, lung abscess, and tuberculosis. The largest single cause of bronchopleural fistula is previous lung resection surgery.[81] Postpneumonectomy bronchopleural fistula is a particularly serious complication with a high mortality rate and poor chance of ultimate closure of the fistula. Factors predisposing to postpneumonectomy bronchopleural fistula are preoperative radiation therapy and postoperative empyema.[82]

The clinical presentation depends on the anatomy of the fistula itself, and the temporal relation to previous surgery. A major factor for the anesthesiologist to consider is whether the patient's mediastinum has become fixed: In patients who develop a fistula in the early postoperative period (<1 month) the mediastinum is mobile and tends to shift into the operated hemithorax with inspiration. These patients often present with a history of sudden massive expectoration of serosanguinous fluid and acute respiratory compromise due to either tension pneumothorax or mediastinal shift and soiling of the bronchial tree (Fig. 25–29).[83]

In chronic bronchopleural fistulas, the mediastinum is often fixed due to previous infection and fibrosis. These patients tend to present with persistent, minimally productive cough and fever. The importance in distinguishing between these two presentations of bronchopleural fistula is that the chronic group will usually tolerate spontaneous ventilation during induction of general anesthesia, while the acute group are at high risk for hypoxemia and hypoventilation with spontaneous ventilation during anesthesia. Bronchopleural fistulas following pulmonary resection will usually require some form of surgical correction: stapling, wedge resection, stump revision, thoracoplasty, etc.

Another subacute presentation is with a persistent air leak from a chest drain following either rupture of a bulla (this is an increasingly common presentation in patients with the acquired immunodeficiency syndrome)[84] or postoperatively. Although this presentation is not as dramatic as an acute bronchopleural fistula, the underlying pathophysiology is the same, since the mediastinum is mobile. If the parenchyma of the noninvolved lung is healthy, these patients will usually tolerate spontaneous ventilation during induction of anesthesia.

Anesthetic management for bronchopleural fistula involves three principles: (1) prevent soiling of healthy lung by secretions in the thorax distal to the fistula, (2) ensure adequate gas exchange in spite of loss of ventilatory volume via the fistula, and (3) avoid tension pneumothorax.

In order to respect these principles, prior to anesthesia, a chest tube must be placed in all bronchopleural fistula patients and as much fluid as possible evacuated from the thorax. A chest tube of sufficient caliber (>6 mm ID) should be used so that the potentially large volume of gas flow through the fistula can be effectively evacuated.[85]

The lung isolation method and anesthetic technique will depend on the clinical situation. In acute situations, such as dehiscence of a bronchial stump, the most secure method of lung isolation is a double-lumen tube. The safest management may be for the double-lumen tube to be placed in the awake patient using direct fiberoptic bronchoscope guidance.[33] This avoids the potential risks of trauma to the bronchial stump from the double-lumen tube, inability to ventilate prior to lung isolation, and aspiration of gastric contents in the patient with a full stomach.

However, in the patient who is already in respiratory decompensation, the risk of further deterioration during awake double-lumen intubation may outweigh the other risks. In these patients the optimal choice may be preoxygenation and rapid-sequence induction of general anesthesia with intravenous agents, muscle relaxants, and cricoid pressure.

A rapid-sequence endobronchial intubation requires two operators: the first operator performs the laryngoscopy and intubates the vocal cords with the double-lumen tube, which has a fiberoptic bronchoscope already positioned in the bronchial lumen with the tip of the fiberoptic bronchoscope flush with the distal bronchial lumen orifice. In effect, the fiberoptic bronchoscope replaces the usual metal stylet of the double-lumen tube. After the tip of the double-lumen tube passes through the vocal cords, the tube is rotated in a normal fashion. The first operator then advances the double-lumen tube the final 10 to 12 cm into correct endobronchial position as directed by the second operator, who is observing through the fiberoptic bronchoscope. The tracheal and bronchial cuffs are then inflated to prevent aspiration and soiling. After practicing on an intubation mannequin, this team procedure can be accomplished without adding

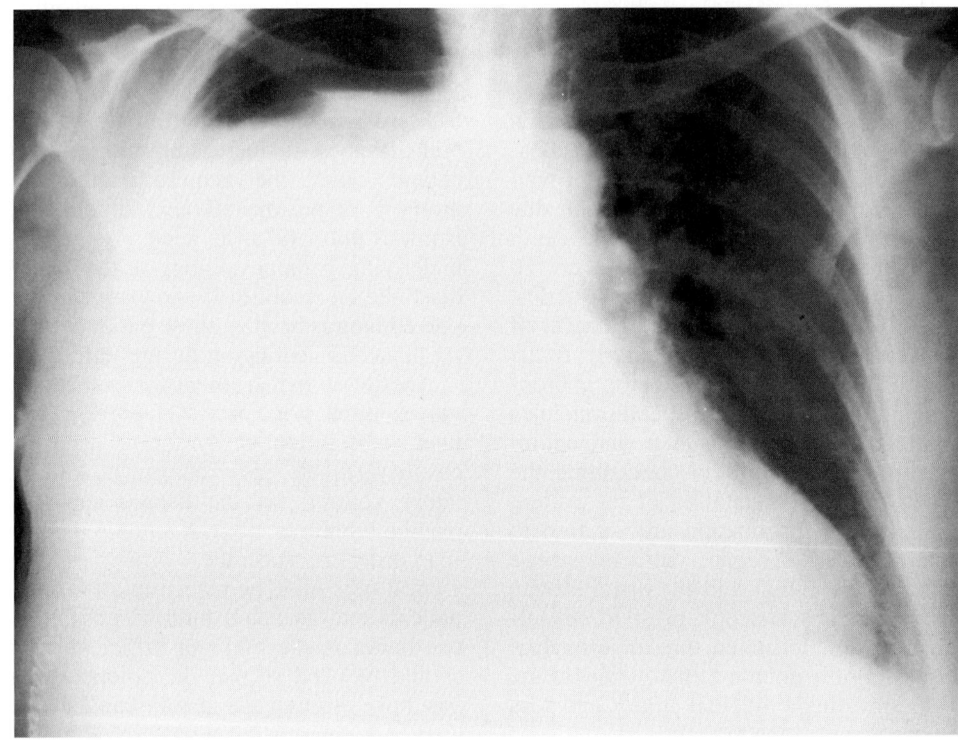

A

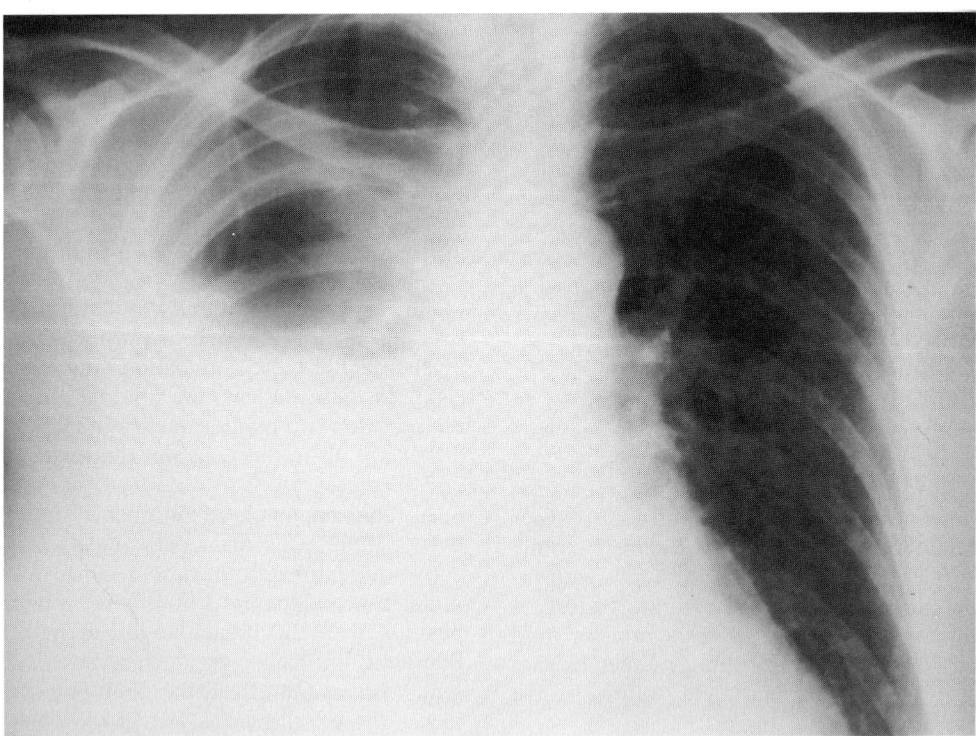

B

FIGURE **25–29.** *A*, Chest x-ray of a 70-year-old female on the fifth postoperative day following a right pneumonectomy. This is a typical postpneumonectomy film showing the gradual filling of the right hemithorax with serous fluid. *B*, Chest x-ray of the same patient taken on the seventh postoperative day after the sudden onset of dyspnea, desaturation, and cough productive of copious secretions. The fall in the fluid level in the hemithorax compared to the previous film, in combination with the clinical picture, is pathognomonic of an acute bronchopleural fistula due to dehiscence of the bronchial stump.

more than 30 seconds to the time taken for a routine rapid-sequence single-lumen intubation.

In patients with a chronic bronchopleural fistula, either of these techniques can be used for lung isolation. In this group it is also possible to induce general anesthesia while maintaining spontaneous ventilation.[86] The correct bronchus is then intubated with direct fiberoptic bronchoscope guidance via the double-lumen tube while gas exchange continues through the double-lumen tube. Nitrous oxide should be avoided in all patients with a bronchopleural fistula due to the risk of increasing the volume of a pneumothorax.

A bronchopleural fistula developing during mechanical ventilation of patients in the intensive care unit (ICU) is associated with significant mortality. This is particularly true if the air leak is large (>500 ml/breath).[87] These patients are not usually candidates for surgical repair of the bronchopleural fistula. Closure of the bronchopleural fistula may be aided by application of pleural sclerosing agents[88] or fiberoptic intrabronchial application of sealants to the fistula.[89] A series of ventilatory options have been developed for use in these patients, to permit adequate gas exchange in the face of loss of tidal volume via the bronchopleural fistula. These maneuvers include application of positive pressure to the chest drain during expiration to maintain lung FRC,[90,91] or synchronized intermittent closure of the chest drain during inspiration.[92]

Purulent Secretions

Patients with lung abscesses, hydatid cysts, bronchiectasis, pneumonitis distal to an obstructing carcinoma, and a variety of other diseases with infected intrathoracic secretions continue to present for surgery (Fig. 25–30). Anesthetic management has two major priorities in these patients: (1) restrict the spread of purulent material to the smallest possible region of lung parenchyma and (2) provide surgical access in the involved hemithorax.

Inability to isolate the lung or intraoperative loss of lung isolation in these cases is not merely a surgical inconvenience, but may be life threatening due to flooding or seeding of previously normal lung regions. The use of a left double-lumen tube has the highest probability of continuous adequate lung isolation but exposes the remainder of the lung on the involved side to contamination. This risk can be decreased by intraoperative surveillance, and suctioning of secretions in the nonventilated lung.

The Univent tube can be used for lobar blockade. This offers potential protection for ipsilateral lung regions but overall lung isolation is less secure. Manipulation of the relatively rigid Univent blocker into an individual lobe or segment can be difficult and time consuming.

In some cases, the optimal solution may be the combined use of a bronchial blocker and a double-lumen tube (Fig. 25–31). A Fogarty catheter can be passed through the vocal cords as a bronchial blocker then followed and directed into lobar/segmental position with direct fiberoptic bronchoscope guidance via a double-lumen tube. A blocker can also be positioned intraluminally with direct vision via the double-lumen tube.[93] This technique allows for easy surgical access in the infected hemithorax while protecting the uninvolved segments/lobes of the ipsilateral lung. As with any bronchial blocker, adequate positioning can be time consuming.

Bullae/Cysts

Patients with bullae may present for definitive resection of the bullae. Increasingly, this is being done with VATS.[94] The bullae may also be an incidental or concomitant finding, particularly in patients with chronic obstructive lung disease, presenting for any type of surgical procedure (Fig. 25–32).

Recent in vivo studies have revealed several important functional points about bullae.[95] First, the majority of bullae communicate slowly with the tracheobronchial tree. Second, the pressure in the bulla reflects the mean alveolar pressure averaged over the respiratory cycle. Thus, during normal spontaneous ventilation the intrabulla pressure at FRC is negative compared to the surrounding lung parenchyma. However, whenever positive-pressure ventilation is used, bullae will increase in size relative to the remainder of the lung.

Management of these patients, whether for thoracic or nonthoracic procedures, involves three principles:

1. Avoid agents such as nitrous oxide, which may increase the size of bullae.
2. With positive-pressure ventilation there is always a potential for rupture of the bulla and subsequent development of a tension pneumothorax.
3. When a chest drain is inserted in these patients (either to deal with a tension pneumothorax, or for any other reason) a bronchopleurocutaneous fistula may result in subsequent loss of the ability to ventilate the patient.

The anesthetic plan for these patients will always have to allow for the possible development and treatment of these complications and will, to a significant degree, depend on the intraoperative access to the patient's airway. Ideally, positive-pressure ventilation should be avoided. If the patient in Figure 25–32 required intraoperative positive-pressure ventilation for a laparoscopic cholecystectomy, there should still be adequate access to the airway to place a double-lumen tube, if required, in mid-operation for lung isolation. However, if bulla rupture were to occur during neurosurgery in the prone position, rapid access to the airway would be difficult and prophylactic placement of a double-lumen tube or blocker would be advisable. Prophylactic placement of a double-lumen tube does not rule out the possibility of using spontaneous ventilation during general anesthesia.

Patients with recurrent spontaneous pneumothoraces from rupture of blebs may present for blebectomy without a chest drain in situ. In some of these patients the maintenance of spontaneous ventilation after induction of general anesthesia until lung isolation is ensured may be an optimal method of management. This technique is a compromise between the time-consuming and generally unpleasant insertion of a double-lumen tube in the

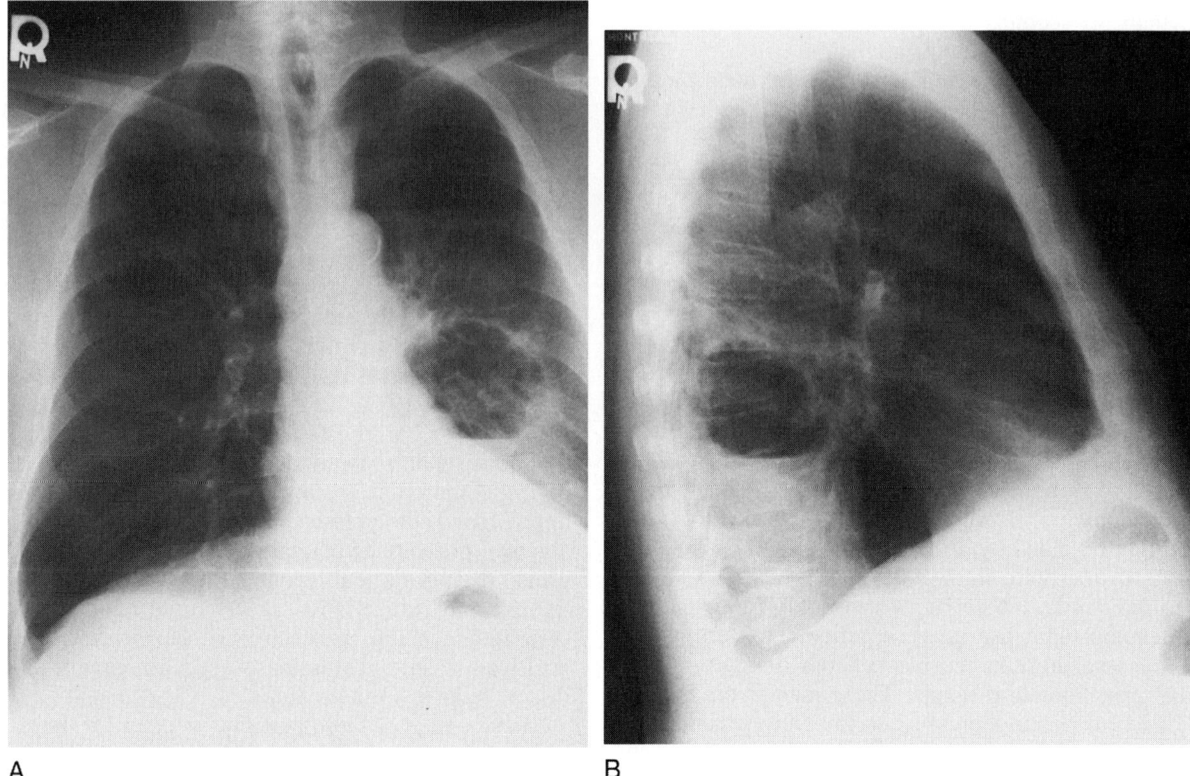

FIGURE 25–30. Chest x-rays (*A*, posteroanterior; *B*, lateral) of a 60-year-old male with an abscess cavity involving the superior and part of the posterobasal segments of the left lower lobe.

awake patient versus the potential inability to ventilate these patients when an intravenous anesthetic/muscle relaxant induction is employed. Propofol as an intravenous induction agent has been shown to be useful in similar patients when a priority is placed on maintenance of spontaneous ventilation.[96]

Nonpulmonary Intrathoracic Surgery

Lung isolation is used to facilitate surgical access to an increasing variety of intra- and extrathoracic structures. These include the heart, great vessels, esophagus, and vertebral column. Thus, lung isolation techniques may be required not only in the thoracic operating room, but also in the cardiac, vascular, general surgical, and orthopedic suites. There are two specific differences in one-lung anesthesia for nonthoracic surgical situations. First, the surgeon may be less accustomed to working with lung isolation and may not be as helpful in aiding positioning of a double-lumen tube or bronchial blocker by direct manipulation of the bronchus as a thoracic surgeon. Second, as a group, these patients tend to have better pulmonary function than patients presenting for pulmonary resection surgery. Paradoxically, nonpulmonary patients are at increased risk of desaturation during one-lung ventilation.[97,98] Also, the desaturation risk increases when the patient is in the supine or prone position due to the loss of the hydrostatic increase in perfusion to the dependent lung that occurs in the lateral position. Thus, it must be anticipated that maneuvers to increase saturation during one-lung ventilation will be required. The most useful of such maneuvers is the application of CPAP to the nonventilated lung.[99] This can be done via the lumen of a Univent bronchial blocker, but is technically easiest to apply and adjust via the nonventilated lumen of a double-lumen tube.[100] A left double-lumen tube is the optimal choice for lung isolation in most of these patients for surgery in either hemithorax. For left-sided surgery, a Univent is a viable alternative.

Bronchial Surgery

An intrabronchial tumor, bronchial trauma, or a bronchial sleeve-resection during a lobectomy requires that the surgeon have intraluminal access to the ipsilateral mainstem bronchus. Either a single-lumen endobronchial tube or a double-lumen tube in the contralateral bronchus is the lung isolation technique of choice. Some surgeons find the exposure easier with an endobronchial tube than with a double-lumen tube for this type of surgery due to the comparative rigidity of a double-lumen tube. The Wilson tube is a modified single-lumen tube for use as an endobronchial tube specifically for this type of surgery.[63] This topic is discussed in Chapter 28.

Upper Airway Abnormalities

Some of the most difficult problems faced by anesthesiologists managing thoracic surgical cases involve

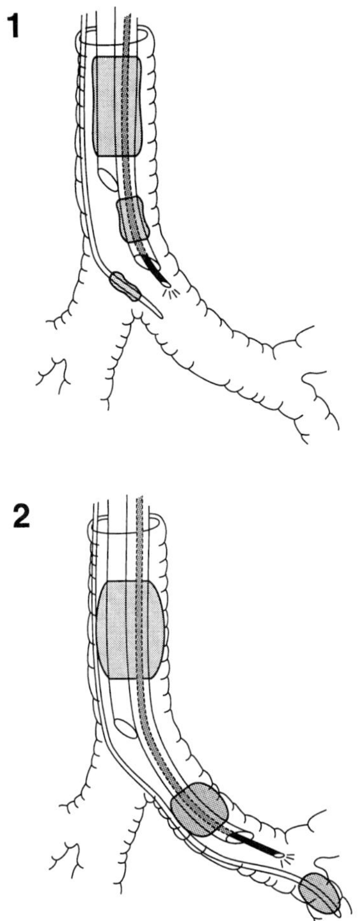

FIGURE **25–31.** A combination lung isolation technique with a double-lumen tube and a bronchial blocker can be used for patients such as the one shown in Figure 25–30. This technique facilitates surgical access in the left hemithorax while protecting the left upper lobe from purulent material in the lower lobe.

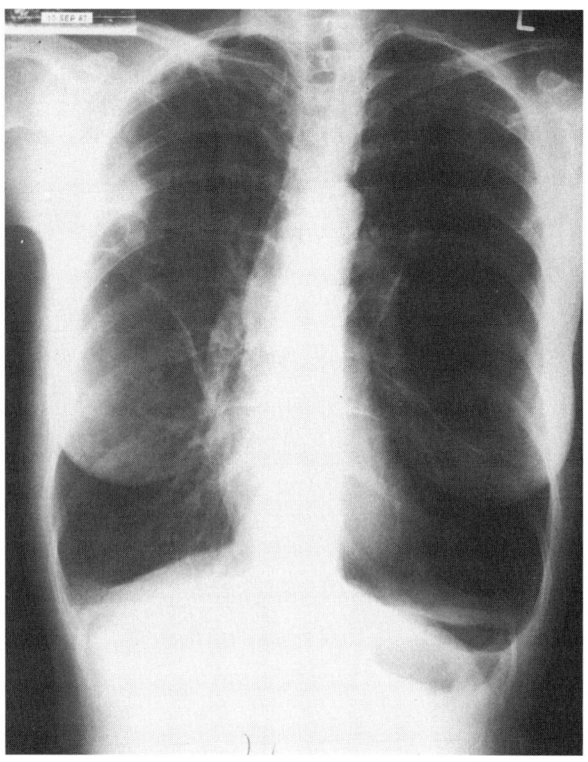

FIGURE **25–32.** Chest x-ray of a 55-year-old female with severe bilateral bullous emphysema and a carcinoma of the right upper lobe. Rupture of bullae with subsequent tension pneumothorax and bronchopleural fistula is a potential risk whenever positive-pressure ventilation is used in such a patient.

achieving lung isolation in the presence of abnormal upper airway anatomy. Previous upper airway surgery, trauma, or radiotherapy can cause distortions that preclude the use of normal techniques for lung isolation. Management first involves understanding the anatomy by assessment of x-rays, tomographs, CT scans, and awake fiberoptic bronchoscopy.

For patients in whom the airway assessment suggests that endotracheal intubation would be difficult (due to a proximal upper airway abnormality) but that the tracheobronchial anatomy distal to the glottis is normal, awake oral fiberoptic double-lumen intubation after thorough topical anesthesia can be performed.[33] Double-lumen intubation guided by a catheter or wire placed retrogradely through the cricothyroid membrane is also an option.[101] It is extremely helpful to soften a polyvinyl chloride double-lumen tube in hot water just prior to awake intubation.

In a patient with a tracheostomy, the simplest method of achieving one-lung isolation is to replace the tracheostomy tube with a standard oral double-lumen tube if there is unimpaired access from above (Fig. 25–33). Modified double-lumen tubes for insertion via a tracheostomy stoma have been described for use when the airway is not accessible above the tracheostomy.[102] These are not commercially available in North America. The smallest Univent tube, a #6, has approximately the same external diameter as a standard 8.5-mm-ID endotracheal tube and can be passed via the tracheal stoma or glottis in some of these patients. The measured external circumference of a #6 Univent is 34 Fr (in spite of the 26-Fr marking on the tube itself). Thus, it is not much smaller than the commonly used 35-Fr double-lumen tube.

Smaller double-lumen tubes (26, 28 and 32 Fr) are available. These smaller double-lumen tubes will not permit intraluminal passage of a fiberoptic bronchoscope of the diameter commonly used to monitor positioning (3.5 to 4.0 mm). An infant fiberoptic bronchoscope (2 mm) or a flexible ureteroscope can be used with these smaller double-lumen tubes to verify placement.

A single-lumen tube designed for microlaryngoscopy (5 to 6 mm ID and >30 cm length) can be used as an endobronchial tube, with fiberoptic bronchoscopic positioning. This is particularly useful in the left mainstem bronchus for right thoracotomies. For left thoracotomies, if the patient's upper airway will accept a 7.0-mm-ID endotracheal tube, a Fogarty catheter and a bronchoscope can be passed through the endotracheal tube for bronchial blockage (Fig. 25–25).

Patients with tracheobronchial compression due to a mediastinal mass present a difficult problem for safe induction of general anesthesia. Awake fiberoptic double-

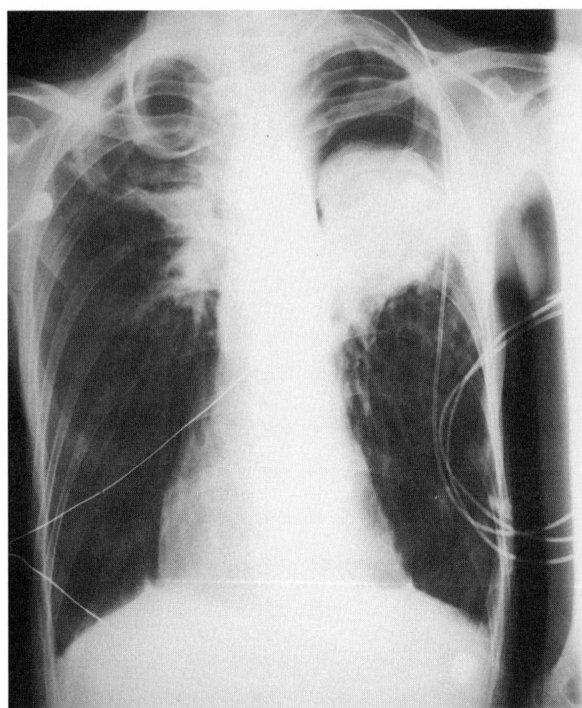

FIGURE **25–33.** Chest x-ray of a 50-year-old male with severe chronic obstructive pulmonary disease and a bronchopleural fistula in the left upper lobe secondary to an *Aspergillus* infection. The patient has a permanent tracheostomy placed following a previous right upper lobectomy. Lung isolation for left upper lobectomy was achieved with a left double-lumen tube placed orally after induction of general anesthesia with maintenance of spontaneous ventilation.

lumen intubation is a useful method of securing the airway in selected cases.[103]

The distances between the luminal orifices and cuffs of a double-lumen tube are fixed and are designed only to deal with the median of anatomic variance. For this reason, double-lumen tubes are often inappropriate in patients with distorted airway anatomy. Thus, anesthesiologists managing thoracic cases must remain familiar with the use of endobronchial tubes and bronchial blockers that permit more adaptability to deal with individual variation.

Replacing a double-lumen tube with a single-lumen tube or vice versa in a patient with an abnormal airway is a clinical challenge. Two recently described methods involve the use of a fiberoptic bronchoscope[104] or a tube exchanger[105] to manage this problem. The anesthesiologist should be aware that not all commercially available tube exchangers are long enough or narrow enough to accomplish this.

Lung Transplantation

A detailed discussion of the anesthetic management of lung transplantation is given in Chapter 31. The pathology, age, size, and complicating conditions of transplant recipients vary so widely that it is difficult to generalize about the best technique for lung isolation.

Independent Lung Ventilation

There are numerous potential indications for the use of independent lung ventilation in the intensive care setting whenever the ventilation and perfusion characteristics of the two lungs differ markedly. Such cases include predominantly one-sided chest trauma (Fig. 25–34), following single-lung transplant, following pulmonary embolectomy, and aspiration.[8] A double-lumen tube, preferably left-sided, is at present the only viable technique for lung isolation in these patients. Although position of the double-lumen tube can be visualized on the chest x-ray, it is best to perform bronchoscopic surveillance of double-lumen tube positioning initially and daily, since lobar obstruction is often a late radiographic finding. Bronchial and tracheal cuff pressures should be regularly monitored during prolonged double-lumen tube placement. The Mallinckrodt and Rusch designs of left double-lumen tube provide isolation with lower intrabronchial cuff pressures then the Sheridan design and are preferable for this indication.[44]

Patients should be appropriately sedated during independent lung ventilation with adequate muscle relaxation to ensure that patient movement does not cause double-lumen tube displacement or interfere with ventilation. Once the lungs are separated they can be ventilated in a synchronous or asynchronous fashion with as much variation of the ventilatory parameters to each lung (FIO_2, rate, tidal volume, PEEP) as required to maximize oxygen delivery and minimize lung trauma.

Lung isolation is maintained until it can be demonstrated that the ventilatory function of the two lungs has re-equilibrated to a degree that a trial of using the same ventilatory parameters via both sides of the double-lumen tube can be tolerated. At this point either replacement of the double-lumen tube with a single-lumen tube or weaning via the double-lumen tube are options. During the period of time that a patient has independent lung ventilation the anesthesia staff will need to maintain continuous contact with the medical and nursing staff of the ICU for ongoing advice and instruction on lung isolation.

Unilateral Bronchopulmonary Lavage

Although unilateral saline lavage of the bronchial tree has been performed in situations such as cystic fibrosis and asthma, it is generally of significant therapeutic benefit only in pulmonary alveolar proteinosis.[106] One other extremely rare indication is following the inhalation of radioactive dust.[107] Lung isolation is of pre-eminent importance, since these patients begin with extremely compromised respiratory function, and accidental flooding of the contralateral lung during unilateral lavage could be lethal.

These patients are best managed with a left double-lumen tube for lavage of either lung. After induction of general anesthesia and following patient positioning, double-lumen tube placement is confirmed by fiberoptic bronchoscopy. Then, isolation of the ventilated from the nonventilated lung must be meticulously checked. This

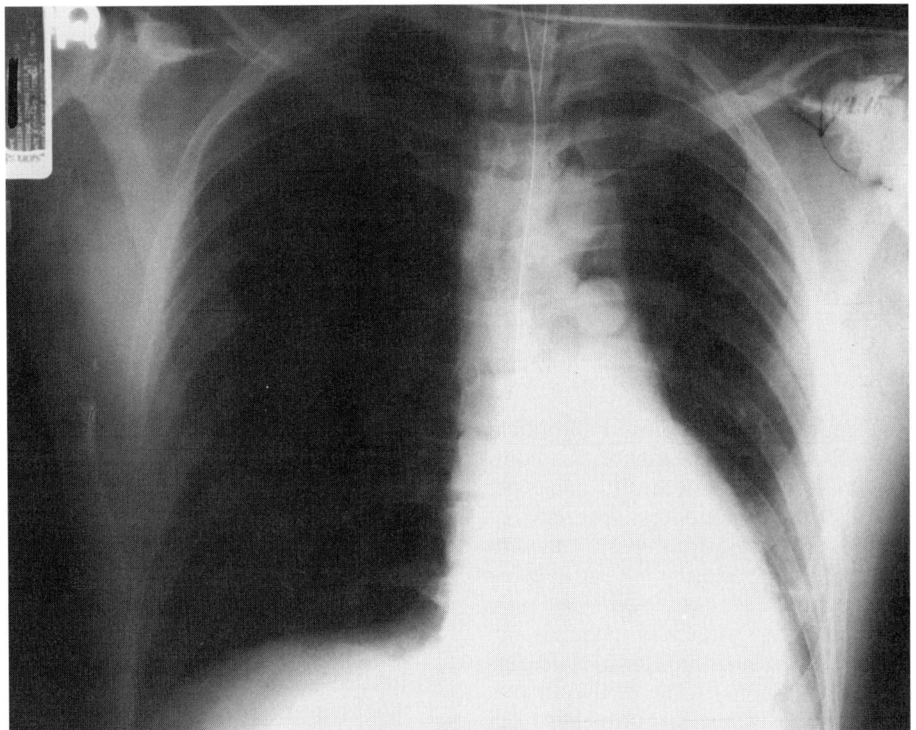

A

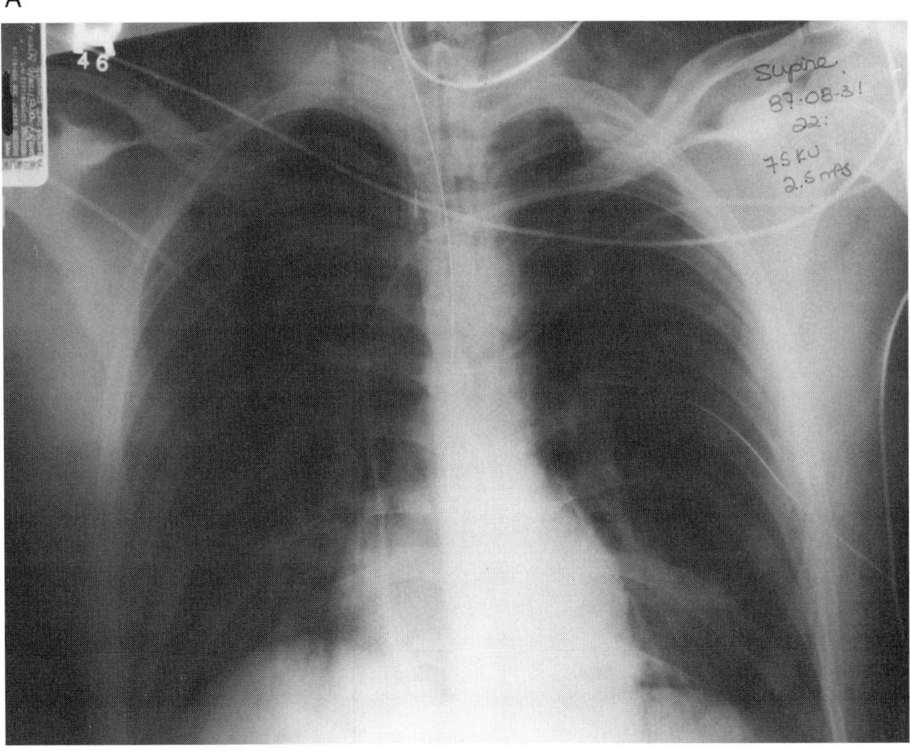

B

FIGURE **25–34.** *A*, Chest x-ray of a 27-year-old male with a left-sided pulmonary contusion, 24 hours after a motor vehicle accident. In spite of endotracheal intubation and ventilation with high levels of oxygen and PEEP, it was impossible to maintain acceptable arterial oxygenation. Note the hyperinflation of the healthy right lung with a shift of the mediastinum to the left. *B*, Chest x-ray of the same patient 12 hours later demonstrates that the single-lumen tube has been replaced by a left-sided double-lumen tube, which is in satisfactory position. Also, a left chest drain and pulmonary artery catheter have been placed. The patient received nonsynchronized independent lung ventilation with higher levels of PEEP to the left lung. Note the return of the mediastinum to a central position. Following 3 days of independent lung ventilation, the pulmonary function of the lungs had equilibrated, allowing reintubation with a single-lumen tube and subsequent weaning from mechanical ventilation.

is done by inflation of the bronchial cuff until the air leak via an underwater drain from the nonventilated lumen of the double-lumen tube is abolished during a static 50-cm H_2O inflation of the ventilated lung as described by Hannallah and Benumof.[52] Once lung isolation is ensured, neither the patient nor the double-lumen tube should be moved until the procedure is finished.

Complications of Lung Isolation

Airway Trauma

Tracheal or bronchial rupture is a recognized complication of double-lumen tubes. The frequency of this complication has been estimated to be between 0.5 and 2 per 1,000 cases.[108] The infrequent case reports with disposable double-lumen tubes have usually been attributed to using nitrous oxide as part of the anesthetic[109] or to using an inappropriately large tube.[110]

Tracheobronchial rupture due to airway catheters occurs most often at the junction of the posterior (membranous) and lateral (cartilaginous) walls of the airway. In the majority of reported cases, the diagnosis has been made intraoperatively and only rarely has the problem become evident postoperatively (Table 25–7). Intraoperative diagnosis necessitates immediate surgical repair. When the diagnosis is delayed until the postoperative period, conservative treatment with fiberoptic surveillance and antibiotic coverage is an option if the tracheobronchial wound is small, there are minimal symptoms, and the patient can be weaned from positive-pressure ventilation.

Several strategies should be followed to minimize the airway trauma due to endobronchial tubes and blockers (Table 25–8):

1. The majority of difficult endobronchial intubations can be predicted from viewing the chest x-ray (see Fig. 25–5). Pericarinal distortions due to tumor, previous surgery/infections, or other intrathoracic structures (especially the ascending aorta) are usually evident on the preoperative x-ray film. Alternatives to the standard practice of double-lumen tube placement via laryngoscopy will depend on the abnormal anatomy. Endobronchial intubation under direct vision using the fiberoptic bronchoscope as a guide is one alternative. Other possibilities include use of a double-lumen tube in the contralateral main bronchus (e.g., right instead of left double-lumen tube) or use of a bronchial blocker instead of a double-lumen tube.
2. Use of an appropriate size tube (see Table 25–3). Too small a tube will make lung isolation difficult. However, too large a tube is more likely to cause trauma. At all times, it is best to defer to direct fiberoptic bronchoscope airway assessment and use of a smaller size tube if undue resistance is encountered during intubation.
3. Avoid nitrous oxide as an anesthetic agent. Nitrous oxide will diffuse into the cuff of any airway tube/blocker that has been inflated with air. Nitrous oxide 70% can increase the bronchial cuff volume from 5 to 16 ml intraoperatively, a volume that has been demonstrated to be capable of rupturing the mainstem bronchus of a cadaver.[111] If nitrous oxide is used as part of the anesthetic, either inflate the bronchial cuff with the same nitrous/oxygen mixture, or use a continuous cuff inflation pressure-monitor/release-valve system.[112]
4. Inflate the bronchial cuff/blocker only to the minimum volume required for lung isolation. This minimal volume can be determined by observing for the cessation of leak from the nonventilated lumen of a double-lumen tube, or the central lumen of a Univent blocker, to a 1-cm underwater drain as the ventilated lung is held at a static inflation pressure (e.g., 30 cm H_2O).[52] Only in cases at exceptional risk for contamination of the ventilated lung (e.g., bronchopulmonary lavage, lung abscess) is a higher level of static inflation isolation-pressure (50 cm H_2O) required.
5. Since the risk of major contamination of the healthy lung with blood or pus occurs only in the minority of thoracic patients, in most thoracic cases, the bronchial cuff/blocker only needs to be inflated during the period when one-lung ventilation is required for surgical exposure. It is a false impression that inflating the bronchial cuff stabilizes the double-lumen tube position when the patient is turned to the lateral position.
6. The tracheobronchial mucosa is not firmly attached to its supporting cartilage and is susceptible to trauma from foreign bodies in the airway. Endobronchial intubation must be done gently. However, the majority of case reports of iatrogenic endobronchial trauma do not describe any difficulty in initial tube placement. A significant number of case reports are from cases

TABLE 25–7
Signs of Tracheobronchial Rupture from Endobronchial Tubes/Blockers

Intraoperative
Endobronchial tube/blocker cuff visible in operative field
Volume loss detected in anesthetic circuit
Pneumomediastinum
Difficulty to isolate one lung
Difficulty to ventilate one lung
Postoperative
Subcutaneous emphysema
Pneumomediastinum
Pneumothorax

TABLE 25–8
Avoiding Iatrogenic Trauma from Endobronchial Tubes/Blockers

Assess chest x-ray and CT scan before intubation
Use appropriate size of tube
Avoid nitrous oxide
Use minimal inflation volumes in cuff/blocker to isolate lung
Inflate bronchial cuff/blocker only when isolation required
Gentle manipulation of endobronchial equipment

of esophageal surgery.[108] In patients with malignancies, particularly in the area of the carina, the elastic supporting tissue may be weakened and predisposed to rupture from double-lumen tube placement.

The majority of airway catheter manufacturers recommend removing the guidewire from the bronchial lumen after the double-lumen tube tip has passed beyond the vocal cords, during intubation. However, leaving the guidewire in place has not been a factor in any of the recent reports of trauma due to double-lumen tubes.

Future Developments

The major foreseeable advance in lung isolation techniques will be the use of continuously monitored pressure-volume-flow information to diagnose misplacement of double-lumen tubes[32,113] (Fig. 25–35) and bronchial blockers intraoperatively. As anesthesiologists become familiar with this type of monitoring, it should be possible to detect not only complete lobar obstruction but also partial lobar or luminal obstructions. This will alert the anesthesiologist to the need for bronchoscopic reassessment and repositioning before desaturation occurs.

The design of double-lumen endobronchial tubes continues to be refined as the anatomy of the tracheobronchial tree is better appreciated. Several companies (Rusch and Mallinckrodt) have recently modified their left double-lumen tube designs based on the recommendations of Benumof.[114] Advances include elimination of the bevel on the distal bronchial orifice, increasing the angle of the distal bronchial lumen from 30 degrees to 45 degrees, and shortening of the bronchial cuff (Fig. 25–36).

The Fuji company plans to redesign the Univent tube with a high-volume low-pressure bronchial blocker. Also, the mislabeled circumferences will be corrected and smaller (potentially pediatric) sizes are to be developed (W. Stewart, Vitaid, Lewiston, NY, personal communication.)

Several designs of coaxial (tube-within-a-tube) systems for lung isolation have been recently developed.[115,116] These offer the possibility of independent lung ventilation after initial placement of a standard endotracheal tube. As yet there has not been widespread use of these techniques. The development of new materials for airway catheters[117] may permit the design of ultrathin-walled kink-resistant double-lumen tubes that could be placed in either the right or left mainstem bronchus.

The cost of double-lumen tubes and bronchial blockers represents a potential North American health care

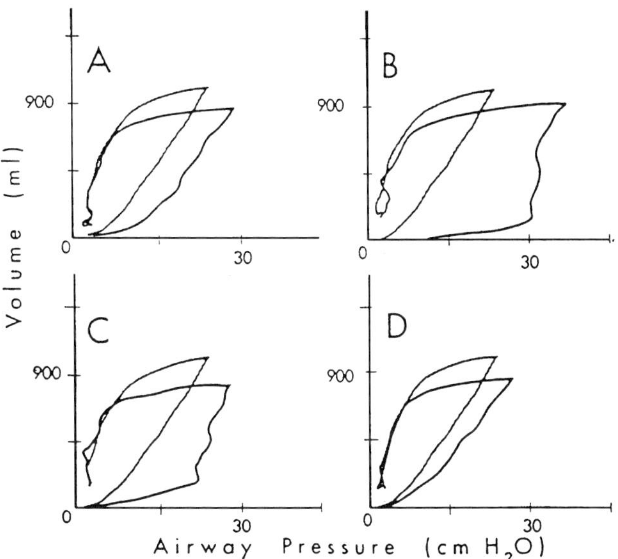

FIGURE **25–35.** Pressure-volume (PV) loops during two- and one-lung ventilation from a single patient at four different times (*A* to *D*) during a right thoracotomy with a left double-lumen tube. For all figures the one-lung loop lies shifted to the right of the initial two-lung loop (i.e., increased peak airway pressure and slight decrease in tidal volume during one-lung ventilation). Diagram *A* shows the normal two- and one-lung PV loops. Diagram *B* shows the intraoperative development of partial distal bronchial lumen obstruction by the medial bronchial wall (confirmed by bronchoscopy), with increased peak airway pressure and change in shape of the one-lung loop. Diagram *C* shows initial withdrawal of the tube, which partially relieved the obstruction. Although the peak airway pressure has decreased, the shape of the one-lung PV loop is still abnormal. Diagram *D* shows further repositioning of the double-lumen tube, which completely relieved the distal bronchial lumen obstruction. The change in shape of the one-lung loops between diagrams *C* and *D* is obvious. However, the variable bronchial obstruction would not be detected if only the airway pressure was monitored. (From Simon BA, Hurford WE, Alfille PH, et al: An aid in the diagnosis of malpositioned double-lumen tubes. Anesthesiology 76:862, 1992, with permission.)

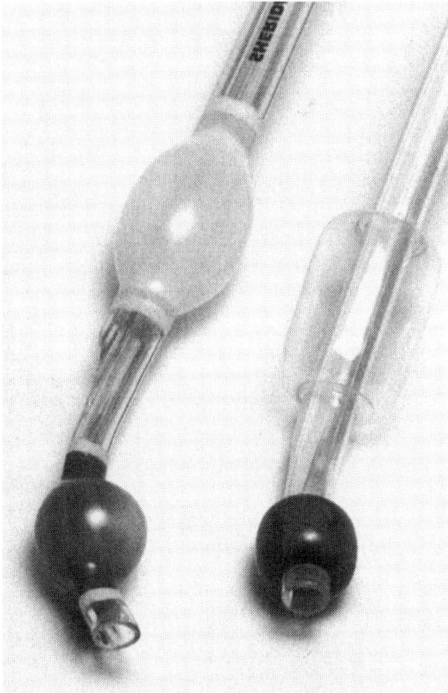

FIGURE **25–36.** A typical polyvinyl chloride left-sided double-lumen tube (Sheridan) on the left is compared to a recently modified left-sided double-lumen tube on the right (Rusch). Recent modifications include narrowing of the bronchial cuff (to increase the margin of safety for positioning in the left mainstem bronchus) and elimination of the bevel on the distal bronchial orifice (to decrease bronchial wall obstruction of the distal lumen). An increase in the angulation of the distal bronchial lumen from 30 degrees to 45 degrees has also been recommended.

cost of $10 million annually. There will be increasing pressure for anesthesiologists to provide lung isolation, when required, with less expensive techniques.

Summary

Although the incidence of cases with the original indications (blood/pus) for lung isolation has decreased, lung isolation is required with increasing frequency in an ever-widening spectrum of clinical situations. The preference of anesthesiologists has oscillated between bronchial blockers and double- or single-lumen endobronchial tubes for the past 50 years. At present, double-lumen tubes have the widest applications for providing lung isolation; however, each method has its strengths and weaknesses (see Table 25–4). The choice of the best technique of lung isolation for an individual case depends on an interplay of several factors, including the indication for lung isolation, concurrent patient problems, available equipment, and the skill/training of the anesthesiologist. All of these factors are continually evolving.

References

1. Gale JW, Waters RM: Closed endobronchial anesthesia in thoracic surgery: Preliminary report. Anesth Analg 11:283, 1932.
2. Mushin WW, Rendell-Baker L: The origins of thoracic anaesthesia. Wood Library. Museum of Anesthesiology, Park Ridge, IL, 1953, reprinted 1991.
3. Carlens E: A new flexible double-lumen catheter for bronchospirometry. J Thorac Surg 18:742, 1949.
4. Jenkins AV, Clarke G: Endobronchial anesthesia with the Carlens catheter. Br J Anaesth 30:13, 1958.
5. Silvay G, Desiderio D, Reich DL: Letter to the editor. J Cardiothorac Anesth 2:119, 1988.
6. Conacher ID: Isolated lung transplantation: A review of problems and guide to anaesthesia. Br J Anaesth 61:468, 1988.
7. Horswell JL: Anesthetic techniques for thoracoscopy. Ann Thorac Surg 56:624, 1993.
8. Adoumie R, Shennib H, Brown R, et al: Differential lung ventilation. J Thorac Cardiovasc Surg 105:229, 1993.
9. Cohen JA, Denisco RA, Richards TS, et al: Hazardous placement of a Robertshaw-type endobronchial tube. Anesth Analg 65:100, 1986.
10. Wells DG, Zelcer J, Podolakin W, et al: Cardiac arrest from pulmonary outflow tract obstruction due to a double-lumen tube. Anesthesiology 66:422, 1987.
11. Herenstein R, Russo JR, Moonka N, et al: Management of one-lung anesthesia in an anticoagulated patient. Anesth Analg 67: 1120, 1988.
12. Eagle CCP: The relationship between a person's height and appropriate endotracheal tube length. Anaesth Intensive Care 20: 156, 1992.
13. Fernandez R, Baigorri F, Blanchi L, et al: Auto-PEEP is favoured by weakness of the posterior wall of the trachea. Chest 102: 655, 1992.
14. Benumof JL, Partridge BL, Salvatierra C, et al: Margin of safety in positioning modern double-lumen endotracheal tubes. Anesthesiology 67:729, 1987.
15. Brodsky JB, Mark JBD: Bilateral upper lobe obstruction from a single double-lumen tube. Anesthesiology 74:1163, 1991.
16. Larsson A, Malmkvist G, Werner O: Variations in lung volume and compliance during pulmonary surgery. Br J Anaesth 59:585, 1987.
17. Sealy WC, Connally SR, Dalton ML: Naming the bronchopulmonary segments and the development of pulmonary surgery. Ann Thorac Surg 55:284, 1993.
18. Alliaume B, Coddens J, Deloof T: Reliability of auscultation in positioning of double-lumen endobronchial tubes. Can J Anaesth 39:687, 1992.
19. Saito S, Dohi S, Tajima K: Failure of double-lumen endobronchial tube placement: Congenital tracheal stenosis in an adult. Anesthesiology 66:83, 1987.
20. Bayes J, Slater EM, Hadberg PS, Lawson D: Obstruction of a double-lumen tube by a saber-sheath trachea. Anesth Analg 79: 186, 1994.
21. Robertshaw FL: Low resistance double-lumen endobronchial tubes. Br J Anaesth 34:576, 1962.
22. Klein U, Karzai W., Bloos F, et al: Role of fiberoptic bronchoscopy in conjunction with the use of double-lumen tubes for thoracic anesthesia. Anesthesiology 88:346, 1998.
23. Shinnick JP, Freedman ABP: Bronchofiberscopic placement of a double-lumen endotracheal tube. Crit Care Med 10:544, 1982.
24. Ehrenwerth J: Pro: Proper positioning of a double-lumen endobronchial tube can only be accomplished with endoscopy. J Cardiothorac Anesth 2:101, 1988.
25. Schwartz DE, Yost C, Larson MD: Pneumothorax complicating use of a Univent endotracheal tube. Anesth Analg 76:443, 1993.
26. Brodsky JB: Con: Proper positioning of a double-lumen endobronchial tube can only be accomplished with the use of endoscopy. J Cardiothorac Anesth 2:105, 1988.
27. Slinger P, Suissa S, Triolet W: Predicting arterial oxygenation during one-lung anesthesia. Can J Anaesth 39:1030, 1992.
28. Benumof JL: The position of a double-lumen tube should be routinely determined by fiberoptic bronchoscopy. J Cardiothorac Vasc Anesth 7:513, 1993.
29. Slinger P: Fiberoptic bronchoscopic positioning of double-lumen tubes. J Cardiothorac Anesth 3:486, 1989.
30. Saito S, Dohi S, Naito H: Alteration of double-lumen endobronchial tube position by flexion and extension of the neck. Anesthesiology 62:696, 1985.
31. Riley RH, Marples IL: Relocation of a double-lumen tube during patient positioning. Anesth Analg 75:1071, 1992.
32. Bardoczky GI, Levarlet M, Engelman E, et al: Continuous spirometry for detection of double-lumen endobronchial tube displacement. Br J Anaesth 70:499, 1993.
33. Patane PS, Sell BA, Mahla M: Awake fiberoptic endobronchial intubation. J Cardiothorac Anesth 4:229, 1990.
34. Asai T: Torsion of a double-lumen tube in the left bronchus. Anesthesiology 76:1064, 1992.
35. Pappin JC: The current practice of endobronchial intubation. Anaesthesia 34:57, 1979.
36. McKenna MJ, Wilson RS, Betelho R: Right upper lobe obstruction with right-sided double-lumen endobronchial tubes: A comparison of two tube types. J Cardiothorac Anesth 2:734, 1988.
37. Alfery DD: Increasing the margin of safety in positioning left-sided double-lumen endotracheal tubes. Anesthesiology 69:149, 1988.
38. Brodsky JB, Benumof JL, Ehrenworth J, et al: Depth of placement of left double-lumen endobronchial tubes. Anesth Analg 73:570, 1991.
39. Shafieha MJ, Sit J, Kartha R, et al: End-tidal CO_2 analyzers in proper positioning of double-lumen tubes. Anesthesiology 64: 844, 1986.
40. Shankar KB, Moseley HSL, Kumar AY: Dual end-tidal CO_2 monitoring and boule-lumen tubes. Can J Anesth 39:100, 1991.
41. Neustein SM, Cohen E, Kirschner PA: Intraopeative left endobronchial tube positioning. J Cardiothorac Vasc Anesth 5:101, 1991.
42. Riley RH, Wood BM: Induction of anaesthesia in a patient with a bronchopleural fistula. Anaesth Intensive Care 22:625, 1994.
43. Brodsky JB, Adkins MO, Gaba DM: Bronchial cuff pressures of double lumen tubes. Anesth Analg 69:608, 1989.
44. Slinger P, Chripko D: A clinical comparison of bronchial cuff pressures in disposable left double-lumen tubes. Anesth Analg 77:305, 1993.
45. Knowlson GTG, Bassett HFM: The pressures exerted on the trachea by endotracheal inflatable cuffs. Br J Anaesth 42:834, 1970.
46. Slinger P, Triolet W: A clinical comparison of three different designs of right-sided double lumen tubes. Can J Anaesth 36: S59, 1989.

47. Kelley JB, Gaba DM, Brodsky JB: Bronchial cuff pressures of two tubes used in thoracic surgery. J Cardiothorac Vasc Anesth 6:190, 1992.
48. Neto PPR: Bronchial cuff pressure: Comparison of Carlens and polyvinylchloride (PVC) double lumen tubes. Anesthesiology 66:255, 1987.
48a. Slinger P, Lesiuk L: Flow resistances of disposable double-lumen, single-lumen and univent tubes. J Cardiothorac Vasc Anesth 12:133, 1998.
49. Cohen E, Kirschner PA, Goldofsky S: Intraoperative manipulation for positioning of double-lumen tubes. Anesthesiology 68: 170, 1988.
50. Inoue H: New device for one lung anesthesia: Endotracheal tube with movable blocker. J Thorac Cardiovasc Surg 83:940, 1982.
51. Hannallah MS: Pneumothorax complicating the use of a Univent tube: A different mechanism. Anesth Analg 77:200, 1993.
52. Hannallah M, Benumof J: Comparison of two techniques to inflate the bronchial cuff of the Univent tube. Anesth Analg 75: 784, 1992.
53. Essig K, Freeman JA: Alternative bronchial cuff inflation technique for the Univent tube. Anesthesiology 76:978, 1992.
54. Arai T, Hatono Y: Yet another reason to use a fiberoptic bronchoscope to properly site a double-lumen tube. Anesthesiology 66:581, 1987.
55. Dougherty P, Hannallah M: A potentially serious complication that resulted from improper use of the Univent tube. Anesthesiology 77:835, 1992.
56. Gayes JM: Pro: One-lung ventilation is best accomplished with the Univent endotracheal tube. J Cardiothorac Vasc Anesth 7: 103, 1993.
57. Campos JH, Reasoner DK, Moyers JR: Comparison of a modified double-lumen endothacheal tube with a single-lumen tube with enclosed bronchial blocker. Anesth Analg 83:1268, 1996.
58. Zilberstein M, Katz RI, Levy A, et al: An improved method for introducing a bronchial blocker. J Cardiothorac Anesth 4:481, 1990.
59. Larson CE, Gasior TA: A device for endobronchial blocker placement during one-lung anesthesia. Anesth Analg 71:311, 1990.
60. El Baz N, Faber LP, Kettle F, et al: Bronchoscopic endobronchial intubation with a single-lumen tube for one-lung anesthesia. Anesthesiology 65:A480, 1986.
61. Kubota H, Kubota Y, Toyoda Y, et al: Selective blind endobronchial intubation in children and adults. Anesthesiology 67:587, 1987.
62. Bonica JJ, Hall WM: Endobronchial anesthesia for intrathoracic surgery. Anesthesiology 12:344, 1951.
63. Newton JR, Grillo HC, Mathiesen DJ: Main bronchial sleeve resection with pulmonary conservation. Ann Thorac Surg 52: 272, 1991.
64. Mitchell JB, Ward PM: The management of tracheal rupture using bilateral bronchial intubation. Anaesthesia 48:223, 1993.
65. Benumof JL, Harwood I, Pendelton S: Major obstruction of the right mainstem bronchus caused by placement of a right axillary roll. J Cardiothorac Vasc Anesth 7:200, 1993.
66. Scheller MS, Kriett JM, Smith CM, et al: Airway management during anesthesia for double-lung transplantation using a single-lumen endotracheal tube with enclosed bronchial blocker. J Cardiothorac Vasc Anesth 6:204, 1992.
67. The First International Symposium on Thoracoscopic Surgery. Ann Thorac Surg 56:609, 1993.
68. Mack MJ, Aronoff RJ, Acuff TE, et al: Thoracoscopic transdiaphragmatic approach for adrenal biopsy. Ann Thorac Surg 55: 772, 1993.
69. Peden CJ, Prys-Roberts C: Capnothorax: Implications for the anaesthetist. Anaesthesia 48:664, 1993.
70. Yeoh CB, Hubaytar RT, Ford JM, et al: Treatment of massive hemorrhage in pulmonary tuberculosis. J Thorac Cardiovasc Surg 54:503, 1967.
71. Garzon AA, Gourin A: Surgical management of massive hemoptysis. Ann Surg 187:267, 1978.
72. Crocco JA, Rooney JJ, Fankushen DS, et al: Massive hemoptysis. Arch Intern Med 121:495, 1968.
73. Carron H, Hill S: Anesthetic management of lobectomy for massive pulmonary hemorrhage. Anesthesiology 37:658, 1972.
74. Shivaram U, Finch P, Nowak P: Plastic endobronchial tubes in the management of life-threatening hemoptysis. Chest 92:1108, 1987.
75. Ravichandran PS, Kelley SP, Swanson JS: Thermodilution catheter-induced endobronchial hemorrhage with pulmonary hypertension. Ann Thorac Surg 52:1204, 1991.
76. Purut CM, Stewart SM, Parham JV, et al: Intraoperative management of severe endobronchial hemorrhage. Ann Thorac Surg 51:304, 1991.
77. Urschel JD, Myerowitz PD: Catheter-induced pulmonary artery rupture in the setting of cardiopulmonary bypass. Ann Thorac Surg 53:585, 1993.
78. Pellegrini RV, Marcelli G, DiMarco RF, et al: Swan Ganz catheter induced pulmonary hemorrhage. J Cardiovasc Surg 28:646, 1987.
79. Wagner RB, Crawford WO, Schimpf PP: Classification of parenchymal injuries of the lung. Radiology 167:77, 1988.
80. Devitt JH, McLean RF, Koch J-P: Anaesthetic management of acute blunt thoracic trauma. Can J Anaesth 38:506, 1991.
81. Baumann MH, Sahn SA: Medical management and therapy of bronchopleural fistulas in the mechanically ventilated patient. Chest 97:721, 1990.
82. Pomerantz AH, Derasari MD, Sethi SS, et al: Early postpneumonectomy bronchial stump fistula. Chest 93:654, 1988.
83. Hoier-Madsen K, Schulze S, Pedersen VM, et al: Management of bronchopleural fistula following pneumonectomy. Scand J Thorac Cardiovasc Surg 18:263, 1984.
84. Crawford BK, Galloway AC, Boyd AD: Treatment of AIDS-related bronchopleural fistula by pleurectomy. Ann Thorac Surg 54:212, 1992.
85. Rusch VW, Capps JS, Tyler ML, et al: The performance of four pleural drainage systems in an animal model of bronchopleural fistula. Chest 93:859, 1988.
86. Donnelly JA, Webster RE: Computer-controlled anaesthesia in the management of bronchopleural fistula. Anaesthesia 46:383, 1991.
87. Pierson DJ, Horton CA, Bates PW: Persistent bronchial air leak during mechanical ventilation. Chest 90:321, 1986.
88. Verschoof AC, Velde T, Greve LH, et al: Thoracoscopic pleurodesis in the management of spontaneous pneumothorax. Respiration 53:197, 1988.
89. Hartmann W, Rausch V: A new therapeutic application of fiberoptic bronchoscope. Chest 71:237, 1977.
90. Phillips YY, Lonigan RM, Joyner LR: A simple technique for managing a bronchopleural fistula while maintaining positive pressure ventilation. Crit Care Med 7:351, 1979.
91. Weksler N, Ovadia L: The challenge of bilateral bronchopleural fistula. Chest 95:938, 1989.
92. Gallagher TJ, Smith RA, Kirby RR, et al: Intermittent inspiratory chest tube occlusion to limit bronchopleural cutaneous air leaks. Crit Care Med 4:328, 1976.
93. Otruba Z, Oxorn D: Lobar bronchial blockade in bronchopleural fistula. Can J Anaesth 39:176, 1992.
94. Baker SJ, Clarke C, Trivedi N, et al: Anesthesia for thoracoscopic laser ablation of bullous emphysema. Anesthesiology 78: 44, 1993.
95. Morgan MDL, Edwards CW, Morris J, et al: Origin and behaviour of emphysematous bullae. Thorax 44:523, 1989.
96. Crofts SL, Hutchison GL: General anaesthesia and the undrained pneumothorax. Anaesthesia 46:192, 1991.
97. Kerr JH, Smith AC, Prys-Roberts C, et al: Observations during endobronchial anesthesia II: Oxygenation. Br J Anaesth 46:84, 1974.
98. Katz JA, Lavern RG, Fairley HB, et al: Pulmonary oxygen exchange during endobronchial anesthesia: Effect of tidal volume and PEEP. Anesthesiology 56:164, 1982.
99. Capan LM, Tundorf H, Chandkrakant P, et al: Optimization of arterial oxygenation during one-lung anesthesia. Anesth Analg 59:947, 1980.
100. Slinger P, Triolet W, Wilson J: Improving arterial oxygenation during one-lune anesthesia. Anesth Analg 59:847, 1980.
101. Alfery DD: Double-lumen endobronchial tube intubation using a retrograde wire technique. Anesth Analg 76:1374, 1993.
102. Brodsky JB, Tobler HG, Mark JBD: A double-lumen endobronchial tube for tracheostomies. Anesthesiology 74:387, 1991.

103. Younker D, Clark R, Coveler L: Fiberoptic endobronchial intubation for resection of an anterior mediastinal mass. Anesthesiology 70:144, 1989.
104. Gatell JA, Barst SM, Desiderio DP, et al: A new technique for replacing an endobronchial double-lumen tube with an endotracheal single lumen tube. Anesthesiology 73:340, 1990.
105. Hannallah M: Evaluation of tracheal tube exchangers for replacement of double-lumen tubes. Anesthesiology 77:609, 1992.
106. Cohen E, Eisenkraft JB: Bronchopulmonary lavage: Effects on oxygenation and hemodynamics. J Cardiothorac Anesth 4:609, 1990.
107. McClellan RO, Boyd HA, Benjamin RG, et al: Recovery of ^{239}Pn following bronchopulmonary lavage and DTPA treatment after an accidental inhalation exposure case. Health Phys 31:315, 1976.
108. Massard G, Rouge C, Dabbagh A. Tracheobronchial lacerations after intubation and tracheostomy. Ann Thorac Surg 61:1483, 1996.
109. Wagner DL, Gammage GW, Wong ML: Tracheal rupture following insertion of a disposable double-lumen endotracheal tube. Anesthesiology 63:698, 1985.
110. Burton NA, Fall SM, Lyons T: Rupture of the left main bronchus with a polyvinylchloride double lumen tube. Chest 83:928, 1983.
111. Peden CJ, Galizia EJ, Smith RB: Bronchial trauma secondary to intubation with a PVC double-lumen tube. J R Soc Med 85:705, 1992.
112. Willis BA, Lalto IP, Dyson A: Tracheal tube cuff pressure—clinical use of the Cardiff cuff controller. Anaesthesia 43:312, 1988.
113. Simon BA, Hurford WE, Alfille PH, et al: An aid in the diagnosis of malpositioned double-lumen tubes. Anesthesiology 76: 862, 1992.
114. Benumof JL: Improving the design and function of double-lumen tubes. J Cardiothorac Anesth 3:461, 1989.
115. Conacher ID: A coaxial technique for facilitating one-lung ventilation. Anaesthesia 46:400, 1991.
116. Trazzi R, Nazari S: Clinical experience with a new right-sided endobronchial tube in left main bronchus surgery. J Cardiothorac Anesth 3:461, 1989.
117. Kolobow T, Tsuno K, Rossi N, Aprigliano M: Design and development of ultrathin-walled non-kinking endotracheal tubes of a new "no pressure" laryngeal seal design. Anesthesiology 81: 1061, 1994.

CHAPTER 26

Pulmonary Resection

Hiroshi Chris Shibutani, M.D.

Pulmonary resection is the most commonly performed noncardiac major thoracic surgery done today. Particularly over the past decade the scope of procedures has grown to encompass a considerable range of variations in both magnitude and approach. In current practice, procedures range from a wedge resection of discrete parenchymal lesions to complex en bloc resection of tumors that have extensively invaded adjacent chest wall structures. In addition to "open" surgical techniques, technological advances coupled with a broadened enthusiasm for minimally invasive surgery have augured the increasing application of video-assisted endoscopic surgical techniques to the realm of pulmonary surgery. A continued increase in the frequency and complexity of procedures is ensured by a variety of factors including aging of the general population and the development of neoadjuvant treatment regimens for lung cancer. Anesthetic management requires an understanding of various fundamental clinical considerations, as well as a global appreciation for specific issues that impact on the overall perioperative management and outcome of the patient undergoing pulmonary resection.

Preoperative Considerations

Indications for Pulmonary Resection

The groundwork for pulmonary surgery was established in the 1930s with the development of surgical therapy for patients with pulmonary tuberculosis. As the availability of multiple drug regimens largely supplanted surgery as the primary mode of treatment for tuberculosis, the indications for pulmonary resection shifted to encompass a range of conditions of which neoplastic diseases predominant (Table 26–1).

Bronchogenic Carcinoma

By far the most common indication for pulmonary resection is bronchogenic carcinoma. Lung cancer accounts for 16% of all malignant tumors and 28% of cancer-related deaths worldwide. In the United States, it is the leading cause of cancer-related death in both men and women.[1] Lung cancer occurs most often between the ages of 40 and 70, with a peak incidence in the sixth or seventh decade. The association between cigarette smoking and the rising incidence of lung cancer has been well established.[2]

Bronchogenic carcinomas can be classified into four types: small cell, large cell, squamous cell, and adenocarcinoma. The histologic type governs the general outline of the clinical course and approach to treatment. Prognosis and treatment strategy are further delineated by the extent of disease as described by tumor stage. Four stages, each with various subdivisions, can be defined using the TNM classification scheme[3] (Table 26–2).

Though by definition tumor stage refers to the extent of disease at the time of presentation, in practice staging involves multiple steps. Following a thorough history and physical examination, standard evaluation includes a chest x-ray, and measurement of routine blood chemistries. The extent of disease may be further ascertained via noninvasive radiologic studies including computed tomography (CT) scan or magnetic resonance imaging (MRI) of the chest. A CT scan of the abdomen, particularly noting the liver and adrenal glands, and an MRI of the head may additionally be performed to evaluate possible metastatic spread of the primary disease. Histologic diagnosis and further staging information may then be obtained by a range of procedures including bronchoscopy, mediastinoscopy, and thoracoscopy. For a variable number of patients, diagnosis and tumor stage will not have been established prior to the patient's presentation for possible surgical resection.

In the context of surgical therapy, bronchogenic carcinomas are generally classified as either small cell or non–small cell type. For patients with non–small cell carcinoma of the lung, surgery is the most effective therapy. For patients with stage I disease, current 5-year survival for treatment by resection alone for small (T1) and larger (T2) tumors is 83 and 65%, respectively.[5] Overall survival rate following resection of stage II lesions is estimated at 40%; however, the rate of recurrence is

TABLE 26–1
Indications for Pulmonary Resection

Neoplastic disease
- Malignant tumors
  - Bronchogenic carcinoma
  - Carcinoid tumor
  - Malignant mesothelioma (primary pleural)
  - Metastatic lesions
- Benign lesions

Infectious disease
- Myobacterial
- Chronic lung abscess—bacterial, fungal

Chronic lung disease
Congenital anomalies
Vascular disease
Trauma

greater than with stage I disease.[6] For small cell carcinoma, surgery has traditionally been considered less beneficial, though advances in chemotherapy have encouraged a reappraisal of its adjunctive role. Patients with small cell carcinoma more commonly present at an advanced stage, with only 20% of cases presenting with limited disease. For patients with limited stage I disease, current data support the use of surgery to improve local control of disease, accompanied by perioperative chemotherapy and prophylactic cranial radiation therapy.[7,8]

Unfortunately, a majority of patients with lung cancer present for medical evaluation with relatively advanced disease. It is estimated that by the time a lesion has become radiographically apparent, it has on average been present for approximately 7 months, progressing through roughly three quarters of its natural history. Locally advanced (stage III) non–small cell lesions may be amenable to surgical therapy, typically as a component of a multimodality therapeutic approach including chemotherapy and radiation therapy. Surgery is not considered a primary mode of therapy for extensive (stage II and III) small cell carcinoma. For patients with unresectable disease, palliative procedures may be indicated in specific settings including massive hemoptysis, unremitting lung abscess distal to an obstructing tumor, or painful invasion of tumor into chest wall structures.

Benign Lesions

Compared with their malignant counterparts, benign lesions are rare, comprising approximately 5% of all bronchopulmonary neoplasms.[9] The most common benign lesion is a hamartoma (75%). Clinically, a majority of benign lesions are asymptomatic. Patients frequently present for evaluation with a history of an incidental lesion noted on routine chest film. If histology cannot be confirmed using endobronchial or percutaneous needle biopsy, patients may undergo limited resection for definitive diagnosis and treatment. Rarely, patients present with symptoms of bronchial obstruction from endobronchial extension of the lesion. In this setting, conservative resection with preservation of pulmonary parenchyma is the curative surgical treatment of choice.

Carcinoid Tumor

Bronchial carcinoids are slow growing, highly vascular tumors that arise from neuroendocrine (Kulchitsky) cells of the bronchial epithelium. A majority are centrally located lesions, growing in the wall of a subsegmental or larger bronchus. Clinical manifestations of bronchial carcinoids emanate from their intraluminal growth and the potential for some lesions to elaborate vasoactive compounds. These vasoactive agents, primarily serotonins, reach the systemic circulation without undergoing prior deamination in the liver, potentially resulting in a complex of symptoms referred to as the carcinoid syndrome. Specific manifestations include vasomotor disturbances (episodic flushing), intestinal hypermotility (cramping pain, diarrhea, nausea, and vomiting), and bronchoconstrictive attacks (cough, dyspnea, and wheezing resembling asthma). Most bronchial carcinoid tumors, however, do not have secretory activity and follow a relatively benign course for an extended period. Metastases occur in only 10% of cases, and the overall 5-year

TABLE 26–2
Staging of Bronchogenic Carcinoma

Stage	Percent*	Criteria
I	20	Primary tumor confined to the lung, located greater than 2 cm distal to the carina (T1 or T2); no regional lymph node involvement or metastases (NOMO)
II	10	Primary tumor confined to lung or bronchus (T2); with involvement of hilar or bronchopulmonary lymph nodes as the sole site of tumor spread (N1); no distant metastases (MO)
IIIa	45	Limited, circumscribed extrapulmonary extension of the primary tumor (T3); and/or lymphatic spread confined to ipsilateral mediastinal or subcarinal lymph nodes (N2); no distant metastases (MO)
IIIb	15	Primary tumor invading mediastinal structures, e.g., heart, great vessels, trachea, esophagus, vertebral body, or carina (T4); presence of malignant pleural effusion; spread to contralateral mediastinal lymph nodes (N2); no distant metastases (MO)
IV	10	Includes patients with distant metastatic disease (M1)—common sites include liver, brain, contralateral lung, adrenal, skeletal system, and kidney

*Refers to percentage presenting for surgical evaluation.[142]
T, site, size, and local extent of the tumor; N, presence and location of regional lymph node involvement; M, presence of distant metastases beyond the ipsilateral hemithorax.[4]

survival is better than 90%.[10] Surgical resection is indicated when tumor is recognized.

Malignant Mesothelioma

Pulmonary surgery may be indicated for selected patients with diffuse malignant mesothelioma, a primary malignancy of the pleura. Unfortunately, current therapeutic options for this aggressive disease are extremely limited. Regardless of treatment, median survival is only 6 to 14 months, with most patients ultimately dying of local complications rather than distant disease. At present, surgical interventions ranging from subtotal pleurectomy with gross tumor debulking to radical extrapleural penumonectomy may be performed primarily for palliative indications.[11] The appropriate therapeutic role of surgery for malignant mesothelioma remains to be defined.

Metastatic Disease to the Lung

The role of surgery in the treatment of pulmonary metastases continues to evolve, influenced by advances in understanding of the pathogenesis and natural history of malignant metastases. The lung is the most common site of metastases for all malignancies except those arising from the portal circulation.[12] Because of the distribution of pulmonary blood flow, metastases tend to develop in the periphery of the lung, and may thus be amenable to excision with a curative intent via limited procedures such as wedge resection and segmentectomy.

Minimum criteria for the selection of patients for whom resection of pulmonary metastases would be appropriate include adequate local control of the primary neoplasm, the absence of unresectable metastases to other organs, an acceptable operative risk, and adequate residual pulmonary function following resection of all metastatic lesions. Factors such as the number of lesions and the presence of bilateral disease do not necessarily exclude a patient from resection.[13]

Operability—The Assessment of Perioperative Risk

While surgical therapy offers the best chance for cure, particularly in patients with non–small cell bronchogenic carcinoma, the decision to proceed with a given procedure must incorporate an assessment of the patient's functional capacity, the stress in the immediate postoperative period, and ultimately benefit from the surgery. Pulmonary resection is associated with a relatively high rate of morbidity and mortality. Acute respiratory insufficiency, probably the most serious complication, occurs with an incidence of 4 to 5% following resection for carcinoma and is associated with a mortality rate of up to 50%. Overall perioperative mortality following pulmonary resection has been reported in most large series at 2.1 to 3.7%.[14–16] Major causes of death include pneumonia, respiratory failure, bronchopleural fistula, empyema, pulmonary embolism, and myocardial infarction.

A variety of factors have been associated with increased perioperative risk, including advanced age; patients over 70 years of age have an operative mortality rate five times greater than those under 60 years of age.[14] Another factor is the extensive nature and complexity of resection such as a pneumonectomy or bronchoplastic procedure.[17] However, perhaps the most significant factor contributing to perioperative risk among patients presenting for pulmonary resection is the prevalence of significant coexisting cardiac and pulmonary disease.

The approach to preoperative evaluation of cardiopulmonary function has traditionally included arterial blood-gas measurement, spirometry lung volume determination, and radionuclide ventilation-perfusion scanning. Data from pulmonary function tests often are combined with results obtained from split function ventilation-perfusion lung scanning in an effort to more precisely estimate the impact of pulmonary resection on residual cardiopulmonary function. Use of percent perfusion derived from split function ventilation-perfusion lung scans, when combined with forced expiratory volume in 1 second (FEV_1)-obtained from pulmonary function testing, have been found to correlate well with actual postoperative FEV_1 measured by spirometry following recovery from surgery.[18] Information obtained from these tests has thus been used to identify patients who could safely undergo pulmonary resection. Using primarily extrapolations of clinical data derived from various patient populations, specific criteria have been described in the literature for identifying patients for whom the increased risk is presumed to be prohibitive for proceeding with surgery.[19]

While the tests themselves are valid measures of physiologic function, the predictive value associated with a range of specific results is less well defined. For example, patients with abnormalities in preoperative arterial blood-gas measurements, including elevated $Paco_2$ and decreased Pao_2 have been classified as being at very high risk for postoperative respiratory complications.[20] However, these inferences derive primarily from anecdotal reports in the clinical literature relating to respiratory failure in patients with chronic lung disease. In fact, no study has specifically evaluated the predictive value of blood-gas abnormalities in patients undergoing pulmonary resection. Several recent investigations have failed to identify a consistent correlation between elevated Pco_2 and complicated postoperative course.[21]

While spirometry has long been recognized as a useful test of pulmonary function, studies have also yielded conflicting results regarding the use of preoperative pulmonary function tests as predictors of postoperative complications in patients undergoing pulmonary resection. Many of the criteria that have long been extolled as tolerance limits for pulmonary resection (Table 26–3) actually derive in part from data originally obtained on patients with pulmonary tuberculosis undergoing thoracoplasty.[22] The declaration of a predicted postoperative FEV_1 value of 800 ml as an accepted cutoff point did not arise in a study of a population of patients undergoing pulmonary resection, but derives from observations of the degree of respiratory impairment experienced by patients with severe chronic ob-

TABLE 26–3
Traditional Criteria for Identifying Patients at High Risk for Pulmonary Resection

Pulmonary function test criteria suggesting high risk in resective surgery
FVC <50% of predicted
FEV_1 <50% of FVC or <2 L
MVV <50% of predicted
RV/TLC ratio >50%
Diffusing capacity <50% of predicted
Minimum criteria for operability
Predicted postpneumonectomy FEV_1 value >0.800 L
Mean PAOP and exercise <35 mm Hg*
Systemic PaO_2

*Value on balloon occlusion and exercise >45 mm Hg.[18,19]
FVC, forced vital capacity; FEV_1, forced expiratory volume in 1 second; MVV, maximum voluntary ventilation; RV, residual volume; TLC, total lung capacity; PAOP, pulmonary artery occlusion pressure.

structive pulmonary disease (COPD). Subsequent studies have shown that patients with marked limitations in pulmonary function have tolerated limited resection with an acceptable risk.[23]

Conflicting study results and improvements in perioperative outcome, which have occurred as a result of advances in preoperative patient preparation,[24] operative techniques, and postoperative care, have promoted a reappraisal of previously established criteria for operability. In recent studies[21,25] predicted postoperative FEV_1, as opposed to preoperative FEV_1, of less than 1 L has been described as a valid predictor of postoperative complications. Predicted postoperative FEV_1 and forced vital capacity (FVC) can be calculated using a simple formula:

$$\text{Predicted postoperative } FEV_1 = \text{preoperative } FEV_1 * [1 - (S * .0526)]$$

where S = number of segments resected. Of note, this calculation assumes that each bronchopulmonary segment contributes equally to ventilatory function. In patients with severe atelectasis, hilar disease, or endobronchial involvement and significantly unequal ventilation or perfusion, quantitative ventilation-perfusion scanning may be more useful in predicting postoperative pulmonary function.

In an effort to improve preoperative risk assessment, additional investigative efforts have focused on the value of information obtained from tests of exercise capacity.[26] While studies have produced variable results, a reduction in maximum oxygen consumption (MVO_2) during exercise might be more sensitive than pulmonary function tests in detecting patients who can survive resective surgery.[27] Various studies have demonstrated that when peak oxygen consumption is below a certain threshold value, the risk of postoperative complications increases. In general, while patients with a MVO_2 greater than 20 ml/kg/min were found to be extremely unlikely to have complications, MVO_2 less than 15 ml/kg/min has been found to be associated with a higher likelihood of complications.[28,29] However, not all patients presenting for pulmonary resection are capable of exercising. For instance, patients with severe arthritis or other musculoskeletal problems, residual neurologic deficits from cerebrovascular accidents, severe peripheral vascular disease, or an inability to cooperate with the testing protocol may be unable to perform an exercise test even in the absence of significant cardiopulmonary disease. In these instances, it has been suggested that the inability to perform exercise in and of itself represents an independent risk factor for increased perioperative morbidity and mortality.[30]

Using routinely available clinical information, factors previously shown to correlate with increased risk of postoperative pulmonary complication were compiled into a multifactorial cardiopulmonary risk index to predict postoperative complications in patients undergoing resection for lung cancer[31] (Table 26–4). By combining a cardiac risk index as described by Goldman[32] and a pulmonary risk index, a nonweighted combined cardiopulmonary risk index (CPRI) has been described. The incidence of postoperative complications is greater with higher CRPI scores. Patients with a CPRI of 4 or greater were 22 times more likely to develop a complication, compared with a CRPI of less than 4.[31] The evaluation of prospective measures of risk specifically for patients undergoing pulmonary resection remains an area of active investigation.

Surgical Procedures for Pulmonary Resection

Following the pioneering efforts of Graham and Singer in 1933, pneumonectomy via thoracotomy was established as the standard surgical therapy for carcinoma of the lung.[33] By 1950, for carcinomas limited to a single lobe of the lung, lobectomy was demonstrated to yield an equal cure rate with less morbidity.[34] Subsequent developments in surgical techniques and advances in perioperative care permitted the exploration of more precise resections on high-risk patients, as well as more extensive procedures on patients with disease thought otherwise unresectable. In current practice, pulmonary resection is performed via a broad range of procedures that vary considerably in both extent and approach.

Limited Pulmonary Resection—Segmentectomy and Wedge Resection

Limited pulmonary resection is generally defined as removal of less than a single lobe of the lung. Individual lobes can be subdivided into bronchopulmonary segments, defined primarily by the anatomy of the blood supply. Removal of a lung segment, segmentectomy, requires precise anatomic dissection to define the bronchial and pulmonary vascular structures serving the lung parenchyma of the involved segment. A wedge resection, in contrast, is a nonanatomic resection involving the removal of a peripherally located portion of lung parenchyma containing a well-circumscribed lesion. A wedge resection may traverse segmental planes.

TABLE 26–4
Cardiopulmonary Risk Index*

Cardiac Risk Index

Variable	Points
Congestive heart failure	11
Myocardial infarction during previous 6 months	10
Greater than 5 PVC/min	7
Rhythm other than NSR or PACs	7
Age >70 years	5
Significant aortic valvular stenosis	3
Poor general medical condition	3

Cardiac Risk Index points = 3–27

CRI Score	Cardiac Risk Index
1	0–5 points
2	6–12 points
3	12–25 points
4	>25 points

Cardiac Risk Index score (CRI) = 0–4[32]

Pulmonary Risk Index

Variable	Points
Obesity (body mass index >27 kg/m^2)	1
Cigarette smoking within 8 weeks of surgery	1
Productive cough within 5 days of surgery	1
Diffuse wheezing/rhonchi within 5 days of surgery	1
FEV_1/FVC <70%	1
Pa_{CO_2} >45 mm Hg	1

Pulmonary Risk Index score (PRI) = 0–6
Cardiopulmonary Risk Index score (CPRI) = CRI + PRI = 1–10 points[31]

*Adapted from Epstein SK, Faling JL, Daly BD, et al: Predicting complications after pulmonary resection: Preoperative exercise testing vs. a multifactorial cardiopulmonary risk index. Chest 104(3): 694, 1993, with permission. Cardiac Risk Index adapted from Goldman L, Caldera DL, Nussbaum SR, et al: Multifactorial index of cardiac risk in noncardiac surgical procedures. N Engl J Med 297:845, 1977, with permission.

PVC, premature ventricular contraction; NSR, normal sinus rhythm; PAC, premature atrial contraction; FEV_1, forced expiratory volume in 1 second; FVC, forced vital capacity, Pa_{CO_2}, arterial partial pressure of carbon dioxide.

The primary advantage associated with limited resections, particularly in comparison with lobectomy and pneumonectomy, is the potential for decreased morbidity resulting from the conservation of lung tissue. Conservation of remaining lung tissue is particularly advantageous in patients who have undergone prior pulmonary resection, and in patients with metastatic lesions requiring bilateral or repeated thoracotomies.[37] For stage I disease, limited resection may also be considered for patients with significantly compromised cardiopulmonary function who are assessed to be at high risk for serious perioperative complications.[34,36] In otherwise healthy patients, however, limited resection is rarely considered an appropriate curative therapy for carcinoma. The potential advantage of reduced morbidity is mitigated by the greater possibility of inadequate resection and recurrent disease. Local recurrence within the remaining portion of the resected lobe is reported to occur in 10 to 15% of cases following limited resection.[38]

Prior to limited resection, fiberoptic bronchoscopy is typically performed to evaluate possible variations in segmental bronchial anatomy and to rule out tumor involvement of the segmental orifice, which would mandate performance of a more extensive procedure such as a lobectomy. Limited resections can be performed via thoracotomy or video-assisted thoracoscopy (VAT). If a thoracotomy is chosen, generally a smaller incision (so-called minithoracotomy) rather than a full posterolateral incision is usually sufficient. Intraoperatively, mediastinal, lobar, and segmental lymph nodes are carefully palpated and sampled for inspection by frozen section analysis. If there is evidence of microscopic metastatic disease and the patient is a suitable candidate, a larger resection such as lobectomy is indicated.

Lobectomy

In general, lobectomy remains the preferred method for the surgical therapy of peripheral lung cancer.[39] Removal of the right upper lobe is the most commonly performed pulmonary resection. From a surgical standpoint, performance of a lobectomy is characterized by several potential technical challenges. Two specific problems, the presence of adhesions (between visceral and parietal pleura) and incomplete fissures, are common to many patients undergoing lobectomy, especially when performed for inflammatory lesions or with the presence of a pleural effusion. The left upper lobe (LUL) is considered the most difficult lobe to resect. Inadvertent injury during division and ligation of the lingular and anterior segmental pulmonary arteries of the LUL can result in significant hemorrhage, compelling the surgeon to perform a pneumonectomy. The surgeon must also avoid injury to the recurrent laryngeal nerve at the aortopulmonary window. Interruption of the recurrent laryngeal nerve results in paralysis of the ipsilateral vocal cord in adduction. Partial airway obstruction, decreased ability to cough, and aspiration from an incompetent glottis may be seen postoperatively.

Pneumonectomy

Pneumonectomy remains an appropriate surgical therapy for centrally located lesions that cannot be adequately resected by lobectomy. Compared with lobectomy, pneumonectomy is associated with a greater risk of perioperative complications including dysrhythmias, pulmonary hypertension and right heart failure, pulmonary edema, and cardiac herniation. Removal of the right lung, which constitutes approximately 55% of total lung capacity, is associated with a greater incidence of complications than following a left pneumonectomy.

Surgical difficulty may be encountered when the tumor is located very proximal to the major pulmonary vessels. In this situation, it is usually necessary to expose the intrapericardial origins of the pulmonary vasculature to determine the extent and resectability of the tumor. When the pericardium is widely incised or removed, the position of the heart and mediastinum is partly maintained by the lungs on both sides. Following removal of lung from either side, the position of the heart shifts towards the operative side, increasing the risk for herniation of the heart through the pericardial defect. Cardiac herniation typically manifests abruptly. Kinking and compression of the venae cavae with a resultant acute decrease in systemic venous return results in acute severe hypotension and the potential for cardiac arrest and death. The risk of herniation is greatest in the immediate postoperative period, and is exacerbated by inadvertent placement of the patient in the lateral position with the operative side down, increased intrathoracic pressure on the nonoperative side from positive-pressure ventilation, and decreased intrathoracic pressure on the operative side.[40,41] Following a pneumonectomy, if chest tubes have been placed, they serve primarily to monitor hemostasis and potentially aid in the initial re-equilibration of intrathoracic pressure following chest closure. Suction must never be applied directly to chest tubes following a pneumonectomy.

Bronchoplastic Procedures ("Sleeve" Resections)

Bronchoplastic or "sleeve" resection refers to the en bloc removal of pulmonary parenchyma with a segment of major bronchus involved with tumor. The distinguishing feature of these procedures is that removal of a bronchial segment entails transient discontinuity of the airway, necessitating subsequent reanastomosis of proximal and distal bronchial margins (Fig. 26–1). In specific circumstances, bronchoplastic procedures may allow for either a more conservative resection with preservation of lung parenchyma (e.g., sleeve lobectomy as opposed to pneumonectomy) or a more radical resection (e.g., carinal resection for carcinoma located in the left or right mainstem bronchus encroaching on the carina.[42–44]

Pulmonary Resection with Chest Wall Involvement

Approximately 5% of primary lung tumors, most commonly peripherally located adenocarcinomas, extend into the parietal pleura or deeper structures including muscles, ribs, and neurovascular elements.[45] If extension of disease is limited to the pleura, pulmonary resection with parietal pleurectomy is considered adequate. However, in the absence of extrathoracic disease, with involvement of intercostal muscle and ribs, en bloc resection of the pulmonary lesion with involved segments of chest wall is the surgical requirement.

When a full-thickness chest wall resection is carried out, one normal rib above and below the area, plus a 5-cm margin on the involved rib, is resected. Reconstruction of the chest wall defect may be indicated for defects greater than 5 cm in diameter, particularly in regions where the remaining chest wall is not supported by the scapulae.[46] While invasion of the spine precludes complete resectability, removal of the tumor with reconstruction of the spine can afford considerable palliation.

Superior Sulcus Tumors

Superior sulcus tumors represent a subset of lung carcinomas invading the chest wall. The tumor is most commonly a non–small cell bronchogenic carcinoma located peripherally in the apex of the lung and extending superiorly into the thoracic outlet. Clinical presentation is notable for the general absence of pulmonary symptoms. Patients characteristically present with severe pain syndromes involving the shoulder region and back from invasion of chest wall structures including ribs and vertebrae. Invasion of the first and second thoracic and eighth cervical nerve roots as well as the brachial plexus may result in radicular pain and upper extremity weakness. About one third of patients will also present with Horner's syndrome (unilateral enophthalmos, ptosis, myosis, and anhidrosis of the face) from invasion of the stellate sympathetic ganglion. The entire symptom complex is often referred to as Pancoast's syndrome.[47]

Current standard therapy includes a combination of preoperative radiation therapy followed by radical en bloc resection of the carcinoma and chest wall. The involved lung is resected by either lobectomy or segmentectomy, with a radical dissection of hilar and mediastinal lymph nodes. The chest wall resection usually includes the entire first rib, posterior portions of the second and third ribs, portions of the first three thoracic

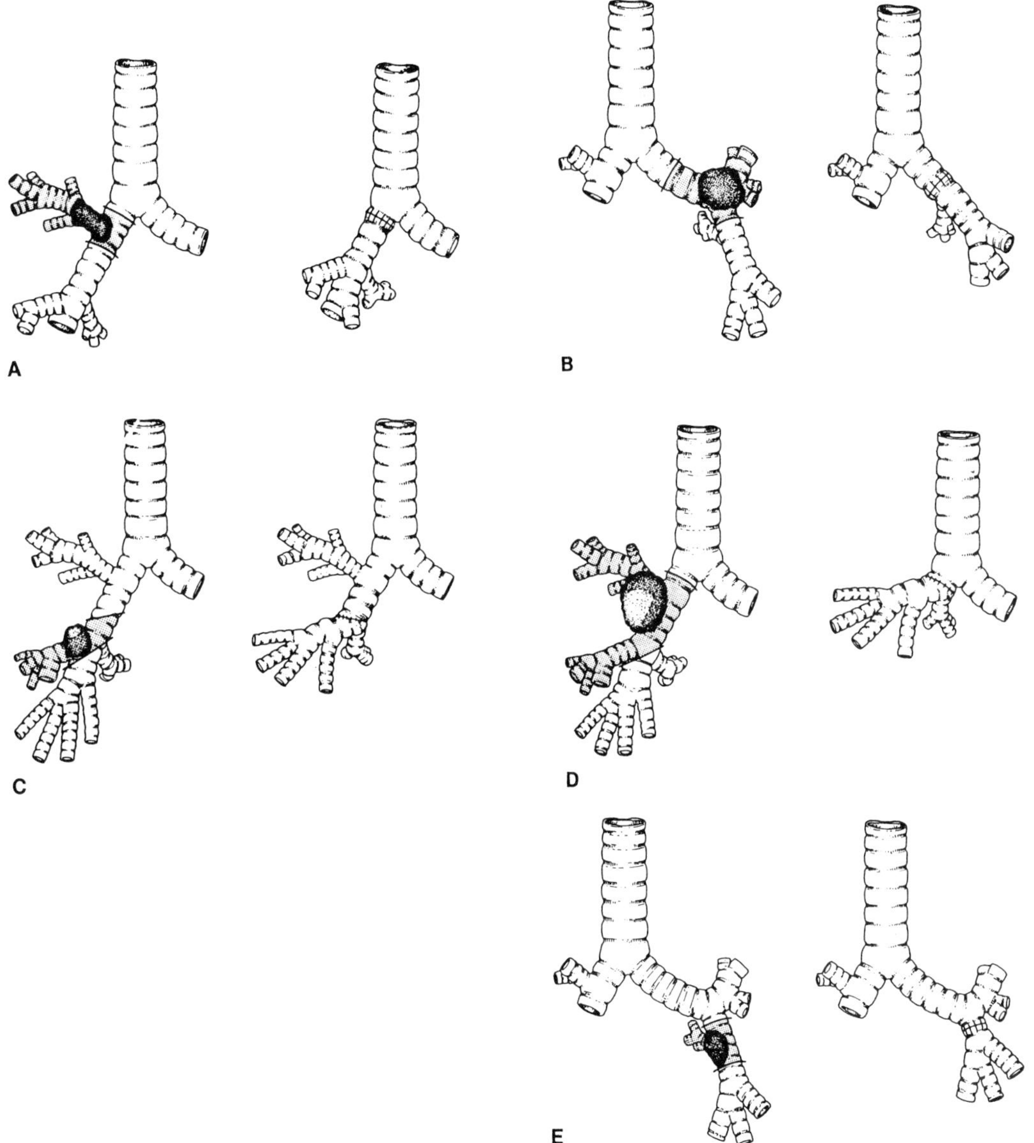

FIGURE **26–1.** *A*, Upper lobectomy on the right with bronchus sleeve. *B*, Upper lobectomy on the left with bronchus sleeve. *C*, Middle lobectomy with bronchus sleeve. *D*, Upper bilobectomy with bronchus sleeve. *E*, Resection of the apical lower lobe segment on the left with bronchus sleeve. (From Vogt-Moykopf I, Meyer G, Naunheim K, et al: Bronchoplastic techniques for lung resection. In Baue AE et al [ed]: Glenn's Thoracic and Cardiovascular Surgery, 6th ed., Vol 1. Norwalk, CT, Appleton & Lange, 1996, with permission.)

vertebrae including their transverse processes, the intercostal nerve roots together with the eighth cervical nerve root, the lower trunk of the brachial plexus, a portion of the stellate ganglion, and the dorsal sympathetic chain. Contraindications to resection include involvement of the subclavian vessels, vertebral bodies with or without cord compression, or widespread invasion of the major divisions of the brachial plexus.[48] Surgical resection in the vicinity of the subclavian vessels may incur significant blood loss, with the potential necessity of establishing surgical control of major vessel hemorrhage via clamping of the superior vena cava. The potential for such an event should be recognized, with early consideration of establishing large-bore intravenous access in a lower extremity vein.

Extrapleural Pneumonectomy

Perhaps the most radical pulmonary resection is the extrapleural pneumonectomy, which may be performed for patients with malignant mesothelioma. Extrapleural pneumonectomy involves en bloc resection of the lung, parietal and mediastinal pleura, pericardium, and diaphragm. Both the diaphragm and the pericardium are usually reconstructed with synthetic material. Unlike a majority of pulmonary resections, extrapleural pneumonectomy can be associated with the potential for considerable blood loss. Because of the relative high operative mortality (reported at 9%) and low survival rate (reported for 2 and 5 years at 24 and 6%, respectively), this procedure should be reserved for selected patients.[49]

Thoracoscopy

Video-Assisted Thoracoscopic Surgery

First introduced by Jacobaeus in 1910, operative thoracoscopies were performed in awake patients using a urologic cystoscope to inspect the pleural space. The artificial induction of pneumothoraces promoted the collapse and subsequent healing of tuberculous cavities. Its use, particularly in the United States, declined rapidly with the introduction of streptomycin in 1945. In Europe, however, it remained popular, and for several decades thoracoscopy was indicated primarily for diagnostic purposes in the setting of pleural disease. Using local anesthesia, spontaneously breathing patients were reported to tolerate brief thoracoscopic procedures without significant cardiorespiratory compromise.[50] Though traditional thoracoscopic techniques have virtually been abandoned in favor of video-assisted approaches, they remain a simple and effective option for brief procedures in the management of pleural disease. Its use under local, regional, and general anesthesia is well described.[51,52]

With the advent of video-assisted equipment, and the commensurate development of ancillary instrumentation, the indications and applications of thoracoscopy have broadened significantly. The general term video-assisted thoracoscopic surgery (VATS) encompasses diagnostic and therapeutic procedures in the management of a wide range of pulmonary, pleural, mediastinal, esophageal, and pericardial diseases (Table 26–5).

The increased popularity of thoracoscopy stems largely from its characterization as a minimally invasive technique. It is viewed as a sparing alternative to thoracotomy with a potential for reduced postoperative morbidity. Reductions in postoperative pain with VATS when compared to thoracotomy with concomitant improvements in postoperative pulmonary function have been reported.[54] In addition, it is speculated that VATS may be better tolerated than conventional thoracotomy in patients with severe underlying cardiopulmonary disease.[55] The asserted advantages of VATS relative to thoracotomy, based largely upon clinical impressions, warrant further prospective controlled evaluation.[56,58]

TABLE 26–5
Bronchogenic Carcinoma: Signs and Symptoms

Symptom	Nature of Tumor Involvement
Cough, wheezing, respiratory infection	Bronchial obstruction, irritation, or ulceration
Hemoptysis, stridor	Centrally located lesion
Hoarseness	Vocal cord dysfunction, potentially related to involvement of tumor or lymphadenopathy with recurrent laryngeal nerve (L>R)
Dyspnea	Pleural or pericardial effusion, paralysis of phrenic nerve
Dysphagia	Esophageal compression or erosion (tracheoesophageal fistula)
Pain	Localized—tumor involvement of chest wall (Pancoast tumor) Pleuritic—pleural effusion, extension of tumor beyond parietal pleura
Horner's syndrome	Pancoast tumor extending to thoracic inlet, involving sympathetic ganglia
Superior vena cava syndrome	Obstruction of lymphatic drainage and central venous return by extensive mediastinal involvement

VATS Instrumentation and Operative Techniques

The rapid emergence of VATS is largely a product of advances in videoendoscopic equipment which, similar to an open procedure, permit several operators to simultaneously view the surgical field. By using two monitors, the surgeon and assistants can view the procedure without looking away from the field. The uniquely enhanced view of the surgical field also affords the anesthesiologist the opportunity to integrate an awareness of surgical proceedings with airway and anesthetic management.

Standard components of VATS instrumentation include a range of thoracic instruments (e.g., lung clamps, retractors) that have been modified for endoscopic use. Access to the pleural space is established using a trocar cannula or "port." Compared with those designed for laparoscopy, trocars used for thoracoscopy are shorter and blunt tipped to reduce the potential for injury to underlying lung tissue. Endoscopic gastrointestinal anastomosis (GIA) staplers with 3-mm staples designed specifically for delicate pulmonary vascular structures have revolutionized the performance of VATS pulmonary resections. Yttrium-aluminum-garnet (YAG) lasers and ultrasound probes further supplement the armamentarium of accessory instrumentation for VATS.

Because VATS procedures, instrumentation, and surgical techniques are still evolving, there are variations on standard operative technique.[57] For most procedures, the video thoracoscope is inserted through a trocar placed in the midaxillary line in the seventh or eighth intercostal space. Instrument ports are established via two additional incisions made at approximately the fifth intercostal space in the anterior axillary line, and posteriorly about 2 to 3 cm away from the border of the scapula. A fourth port incision can be added to insert additional instruments, depending on the location of the lesion. VATS, as a general term, applies to both true video thoracoscopy as well as more complex video-assisted procedures that are distinguished by an additional small intercostal incision usually placed in the midaxillary line. This so-called minithoracotomy facilitates more extensive procedures, allowing for the use of nonendoscopic instruments and permitting direct access to lung tissue. Using retractors, limited exposure can be obtained without spreading the ribs. Video-assisted procedures thus represent a hybrid of minimally invasive and open approaches. In the event that a thoracoscopic procedure must be converted to an open thoracotomy, the port sites can be incorporated into the thoracotomy incision as well as sites for chest tube placement.

Preoperative Assessment and Patient Preparation

As specific criteria applicable to VATS have yet to be established, preoperative assessment of the patient scheduled to undergo VATS should essentially be the same as for thoracotomy. The decision for choosing VATS over thoracotomy in patients with significant underlying medical conditions is largely based upon the premise that VATS represents a potential for reduced perioperative morbidity. It must be recognized, however, that approximately one third of VATS procedures require intraoperative conversion to thoracotomy.[59] The decision to convert to thoracotomy is often based upon a variety of technical considerations including inadequate visualization due to pleural adhesions, difficulty localizing lesions, or the need for an extensive resection that cannot be readily accomplished by thoracoscopy. More acutely, unique complications such as hemorrhage from inadvertent injury to pulmonary vascular structures would necessitate immediate open thoracotomy and urgent resuscitation.

Future Role of VATS

While VATS has rapidly emerged in the therapy of a range of chest pathology, its role relative to open thoracotomy for pulmonary resection remains to be defined. Particularly within the realm of oncologic disease, including the resection of primary lung cancers and the treatment of pulmonary metastases, the role of VATS is controversial.[60,61] Inadequate nodal sampling or dissection can misguide decisions regarding the appropriate extent of pulmonary resection. Similarly, in patients with metastatic pulmonary disease, attainment of the ultimate goal of removing all gross disease in order to effect improved survival is challenged by the loss of bimanual palpation. While video capabilities have significantly improved visualization, and the introduction of ultrasound probes suggests a promising solution, palpation of the lung, the ultimate standard, is considered extremely limited with VATS.[61]

Among the factors that influence the role that VATS will play in thoracic surgery in a more global sense includes the cost-effectiveness of VATS relative to open thoracotomy. The potential benefits of shorter hospital stay, described in early evaluations, must be weighed against the significantly greater operative costs involving equipment, skilled personnel, and time. Comprehensive evaluations of this critical issue must consider the continual changes in instrumentation and an evolving level of clinician expertise.

Intraoperative Considerations

Patient Position

Patient position during thoracic surgery varies depending upon the nature of the procedure and site of incision.[62] Historically, operations for pulmonary tuberculosis or lung abscess were commonly performed with the patient in the prone position. Posterior or posterolateral incisions were favored, as this posture served to reduce the risk of contamination of the contralateral tracheobronchial tree. Correctly applied techniques of one-lung ventilation have largely obviated the advantage of this position. With the patient in the supine position, anterior, anterolateral, or median sternotomy incisions provide excellent access to the mediastinum, the main pulmonary arteries, and the superior pulmonary veins. Access to the major bronchi and the inferior pulmonary veins, particularly on the left, however, is considered less optimal. A transsternal bilateral thoracotomy, the so-called clamshell thoracotomy, provides access to both lungs and may be used during resection of multiple pulmonary metastases and during bilateral lung transplantation. Clinically, because fewer muscle groups are incised, anterior incisions are generally regarded as less painful than the more standard posterolateral approach, and may thus be better tolerated during the immediate postoperative period.

Most procedures, however, are done with the patient in the lateral (decubitus) position, which provides optimal access to one hemithorax with the least limitation to the extent of incision. The lateral approach is considered the safest when extensive dissection of hilar structures is required, as intrapericardial control of hilar vessels is possible. Posterolateral incisions, however, generally involve division or retraction of ribs and muscles of the chest wall, particularly the latissimus dorsi, which plays a vital role in the patient's efforts to cough. This clinically relevant disadvantage may be addressed when appropriate by the use of a muscle-sparing thoracotomy incision, which avoids transection of the latissimus muscle. In the lateral position, mechanical restriction of ventilation to the dependent lung may result from several mechanical factors including greater cephalad displacement of the dependent hemidiaphragm by the abdominal contents, downward displacement of the mediastinum, and restriction of chest wall movement by firm supports of the operating table beneath the patient. Compliance of the diaphragm and chest wall can be further impaired by improper positioning.

The Lateral Position—Recognition and Avoidance of Complications

A patient in the lateral position is at significant risk for injuries to soft tissue and neurovascular structures.[63] Inadequate padding or support, and inappropriate positioning can result in compression and stretch injuries. Significant functional impairment can persist postoperatively for varying durations with the potential for devastating consequences. The insidious nature by which most of these injuries develop mandates vigilant monitoring of patient position throughout the procedure.

Safe and effective positioning of the patient is a collaborative responsibility of the anesthesia, surgical, and nursing staffs. Effective communication as well as attention to detail are imperative. The anesthesiologist, primarily responsible for the airway, head, and neck regions, coordinates the initial change in position, with assistants positioned at the level of the patient's shoulders and hips. Prior to turning the patient, the anticipated dependent side arm should be abducted to 90 degrees from the body in order to avoid trapping this upper extremity and potentially dislodging arterial and venous catheters. Neutral alignment of the patient's head, neck, and torso must be maintained to minimize the risk of injury and the potential for displacement of the airway. Specifically, when turning the patient away from the anesthesia machine into the left lateral position, temporarily disconnecting the endotracheal tube from the circuit may reduce the risk of extubation or kinking. In the absence of cervical spine pathology, stability of the airway may be improved by a slight rotation of the patient's head toward the direction of the turn prior to moving the torso. Maintaining moderate inflation of the bronchial blocker balloon or the bronchial cuff of a double-lumen endotracheal tube may be considered in an attempt to further reinforce the position of the tube. Even when these precautions have been exercised during an apparently uneventful turn, it remains prudent to reconfirm the adequacy of endotracheal tube or bronchial blocker position using fiberoptic bronchoscopy.

Following confirmation of the adequacy of the patient's airway, appropriate support and position of the head and neck in the lateral position must be established. Neutral alignment of the cervical and thoracic spine must be achieved, with slight flexion of the neck preferable to extension. Prolonged deviations in position such as extreme lateral flexion can result in neurologic and cerebrovascular compromise. Complications that have been reported include obstruction to jugular venous drainage, occlusion of the vertebral artery with central nervous system (CNS) damage,[64] and Horner's syndrome from stretch of the cervical sympathetic chain.[65]

A donut- or C-shaped roll of gauze or foam serves well to support the side of the head and face. The dependent ear, placed within the "donut hole," should not be folded over, as dramatic deformities can result from compressive and ischemic injury. Excessive or prolonged pressure applied to the preauricular area can result in facial nerve dysfunction. The dependent eye is also at risk of damage. Permanent blindness from retinal artery thrombosis generated by external compression has been reported.[64] With compressive injury, the eyelids typically become edematous and the cornea may appear hazy. The affected pupil is dilated and reacts to consensual stimulation but not to direct light. The risk may be greater in diabetics and in circumstances that contribute to abnormal reductions in retinal perfusion such as prolonged hypotension.[66]

With several acceptable though not risk-free alternatives, establishing a satisfactory configuration for the upper extremities, with proper positioning of the nondependent "up" arm, is critical. From a surgical standpoint, optimal exposure is facilitated by pulling the scapula away from the site of the surgery. This typically involves flexing the elbow and extending the arm at the shoulder. However, abduction of the humerus greater than 90 degrees as well as pronation of the forearm should be avoided. Components of the brachial plexus, anchored in the neck at the transverse processes of the cervical vertebrae and in the upper arm by axillary fascia, particularly in the "up" arm are at risk for stretch and compression injuries.

The torso is inherently unstable in the lateral position and a variety of devices are available to provide support. A saety strap and/or adhesive tape, secured to the operating table, should also be placed across the hip to further stabilize the patient. A roll or pad is commonly placed beneath the patient to provide support to the upper part of the dependent rib cage. The purpose of this roll is to reduce pressure on the head of the dependent humerus, which can compress the axillary neurovascular bundle. Though often referred to as an axillary roll, the term "chest roll" is more appropriate, as improper placement of this roll into the axilla itself can cause harmful obstruction to both arterial perfusion and venous drainage of the dependent upper extremity.

Padding is required at bony prominences and between extremities to facilitate venous drainage and reduce the risk of compressive injury. The lateral malleolus of the dependent leg is particularly susceptible to the development of pressure sores to overlying skin. Flexion of the lower leg at both the hip and knee, with extension of the nondependent leg, both enhances patient stability and reduces the likelihood that bony prominences of the lower extremities are directly apposed. A pillow placed between the knees provides further protection and support.

Anesthetic Technique

The majority of procedures involving pulmonary resection are performed using general anesthesia. While VATS, similar to thoracoscopy, can be performed under monitored sedation, the complexity of most VATS procedures warrants the use of general anesthesia.[67,68] A variety of anesthetic agents using different approaches may be administered to provide satisfactory conditions for pulmonary resection. Numerous investigations comparing anesthetic agents within similar categories have resulted in recommendations for the use of specific approaches, particularly in the setting of one-lung ventilation.[69–72] The bases for such distinctions, however, are often subtle. In general, clinical evaluations have yet to reveal a specific drug or technique that can be uniquely advocated on the basis of its capacity to significantly improve anesthetic outcome.

Perhaps more relevant than the choice of agents is an appreciation for the overriding goals of perioperative management. As a majority of patients presenting for pulmonary resection have bronchogenic carcinoma, anesthetic management must incorporate an appreciation for the manifestations of the disease and its treatment. Patients with bronchogenic carcinoma may present with a range of clinical signs and symptoms that tend to characterize the nature and extent of disease (Table 26–6).

Appropriate selection of premedication must take into account the individual needs and medical condition of the patient. A short-acting benzodiazepine, such as diazepam or midazolam, may be indicated to reduce preoperative anxiety. Additional use of an anticholinergic for its antisialagogue effect reduces the volume of secretions generated in the course of repeated airway manipulations (e.g., multiple laryngoscopies for intubation

TABLE 26–6
Indications and Contraindications for VATS Procedures*

Diagnostic Indications
- Undiagnosed pleural effusion
- Indeterminate pulmonary nodule
- Undiagnosed interstitial lung disease
- Pulmonary infection in the immunosuppressed patient
- To define cell type in known thoracic malignancy
- To define extent of a primary thoracic tumor
- Nodal staging of a primary thoracic tumor
- Diagnosis of intrathoracic pathology to stage a primary extrathoracic tumor
- Evaluation of intrapleural infection

Therapeutic Indications
- Lung
  - Spontaneous pneumothorax
  - Bullous disease
  - Persistent parenchymal air leak
  - Benign pulmonary nodule
  - ? Resection of pulmonary metastases
  - ? Resection of a primary lung tumor
- Mediastinum
  - Drainage of pericardial effusion
  - Excision of bronchogenic or pericardial cyst
  - Resection of selected primary mediastinal tumors
  - Esophageal myotomy
  - Facilitation of transhiatal esophagectomy
  - ? Resection of primary esophageal tumors
  - ? Thymic resection
- Pleura
  - Drainage of a multiloculated effusion
  - Drainage of an early empyema
  - Pleurodesis
  - Ligation of the thoracic duct

Contraindications
- Extensive intrapleural adhesions
- Inability to sustain one-lung ventilation
- Extensive involvement of hilar structures
- Preoperative induction chemotherapy or chemoradiotherapy
- Severe coagulopathy

*From Rusch V: Thoracoscopy. Surgical technique supplement 2. Scientific American. Fall, 1993, with permission.

with a single-, then double-lumen endotracheal tube), thus facilitating visualization during both direct laryngoscopy and fiberoptic bronchoscopy. The intramuscular administration of glycopyrrolate (0.2 mg), 20 to 30 minutes prior to induction, produces a reliable reduction in oral and airway secretions, without considerable increases in heart rate.

Intraoperative goals of the anesthetic are to provide optimal conditions for the surgical manipulation of intrathoracic structures while maintaining adequate oxygenation and hemodynamic stability, particularly during one-lung ventilation. A specific concern is the potential for hyperreactivity of the airways, particularly in response to endobronchial intubation and surgical manipulation of the major conducting airways and pulmonary parenchyma. Inhalational anesthetics are particularly well suited to these clinical circumstances, as they induce relaxation of bronchial smooth muscle and depress airway reflexes. An additional advantage of the use of inhalational agents during pulmonary surgery is that they are readily eliminated at the conclusion of the procedure, thus providing for rapid emergence. The use of inhalational agents also permits the concomitant administration of a high FIO_2, which is particularly advantageous during one-lung ventilation. While nitrous oxide may be used during the procedure, both to reduce the requirement for volatile anesthetic and to facilitate a smoother emergence than with volatile agent alone, theoretically, the reduction in FIO_2 reduces a margin of safety for avoiding hypoxemia. A theoretical disadvantage associated with the use of a high FIO_2 is the development of absorption atelectasis. However, this can generally be compensated for by ventilation with appropriate tidal volumes and the judicious use of low levels of positive end-expiratory pressure (PEEP). The potential for the development of pulmonary toxicity secondary to perioperative oxygen administration is not a clinically significant concern, with the exception of patients who have previously been exposed to drugs associated with pulmonary toxicity, such as bleomycin and mitomycin.

Pulmonary toxicity secondary to bleomycin is relatively common, affecting approximately 10% of treated patients. An increased frequency of toxicity is associated with doses greater than 450 mg, age greater than 65 years, pre-existing chronic lung disease, and prior radiation therapy.[73,74] With supplemental oxygen administration, a dose-response pattern of increased risk for significant exacerbation of bleomycin-induced pulmonary toxicity has been described. While a high or even modestly elevated FIO_2 (>0.33) administered in the course of a general anesthetic has been implicated as a causative factor in postoperative respiratory failure and deaths,[75] the range of available clinical reports have provided conflicting results.[76] Several questions germane to anesthetic management, including the duration after bleomycin therapy that an increased risk persists, and the impact that duration of exposure to supplemental oxygen has on the risk of complications, remain unanswered. As data are available to support differing practices regarding oxygen administration during anesthesia, recommendations remain an area of controversy. Available evidence suggests that optimal management of patients who have received either bleomycin or mitomycin constitutes the delivery of the lowest FIO_2 compatible with adequate oxygenation.[77,78]

Muscle relaxants are used as an adjunct to inhalational anesthetics. The use of intermediate-acting relaxants to facilitate intubation, positioning, and chest wall incision are appropriate, as profound muscle relaxation is not required. A unique clinical circumstance that may impact upon the administration of muscle relaxants involves the association of bronchogenic carcinoma with paraneoplastic syndromes (pathophysiologic alterations in various extrathoracic organ systems that are not attributable to metastatic disease) affecting neuromuscular function. A myasthenic syndrome (Eaton-Lambert) has been described in association with all types of carcinoma, but is most commonly recognized with small cell lung carcinoma. This disorder is characterized by muscle weakness. In contrast to true myasthenia gravis, however, symptoms improve with exercise. The etiology is felt to be related to an autoimmune phenomenon in which antibodies to presynaptic calcium channels are produced, altering neuromuscular conduction. Intraoperative manifestations include a pronounced sensitivity to the effects of both depolarizing and nondepolarizing muscle relaxants.[79,80] It has also been described that antagonism of neuromuscular blockade with anticholinesterases may be inadequate.[81]

Pulmonary resection can be performed using a combined technique of general anesthesia with epidural anesthesia/analgesia. Narcotics and local anesthetics can be administered alone or in combination via an epidural catheter, usually placed within the thoracic region. A lumbar site may be chosen, though an increased volume and subsequent dose of drug may be required to achieve adequate levels for a thoracotomy incision.

The goal of the anesthetic approach at the end of the procedure is to have an awake, comfortable, and extubated patient. The advantage to prompt extubation includes avoiding the potentially disruptive effects of endotracheal intubation and positive-pressure ventilation on fresh bronchial suture lines. If an epidural catheter is present, a continuous infusion of narcotic (fentanyl 2 to 10 μg/ml) with or without a dilute local anesthetic that is relatively selective for sensory rather than motor nerve roots (e.g., bupivacaine, ropivacaine) can provide favorable postoperative analgesia with potentially fewer side effects when compared with the systemic administration of narcotics.[82] In the absence of an epidural catheter, intraoperative administration of parenteral narcotics is required to provide immediate postoperative analgesia. In addition to potentially undesirable sedation, however, the use of moderate or high doses of narcotics will reduce ventilatory drive. At the conclusion of the procedure, narcotics should thus be titrated carefully to minimize the necessity for postoperative ventilation. Narcotic analgesia may be potentiated by the concomitant administration of nonsteroidal anti-inflammatory drugs (NSAIDs).

Other methods including intrapleural catheters and intercostal blocks have been described as additional options for the management of postthoracotomy pain. This topic is addressed in Chapter 39.

Monitoring

The selection of monitors begins with consideration for the medical condition of the patient, and extent of the surgical procedure. Patients presenting for pulmonary resection are typically older adults with a relatively high incidence of significant cardiovascular and pulmonary disease. In addition, baseline chronic dysfunction of these systems may be acutely compromised by the disease process for which the procedure is indicated. Monitoring must thus focus on cardiovascular and pulmonary parameters.

Monitoring for all procedures begins with accepted standards of noninvasive techniques (Table 26–7). For pulmonary resection, additional, often invasive modes of monitoring are frequently indicated. The decision to incorporate invasive modalities must consider the risks and benefits to the patient not only during the procedure but also throughout the entire perioperative period.

TABLE 27–7
Standard Intraoperative Monitors

Precordial or esophageal stethoscope
Pulse oximeter
Oxygen analyzer
Capnometer
Airway pressure manometer
Continuous ECG
Device for noninvasive measurement of blood pressure
Temperature probe (oral or esophageal)
Peripheral nerve stimulator

Monitoring of Oxygenation and Ventilation

Intrathoracic procedures are associated with a significant potential for rapid and frequent alterations in oxygenation and ventilation. Combinations of standard available monitors fulfill the requirement for precise and continuous indicators of the patients status. While the adequacy of oxygenation and ventilation is most accurately characterized by arterial blood-gas sampling and analysis, the value of this mode is potentially limited by the availability and time required to obtain results. Technology introduced during the past decade, which proffered the possibility of continuous "on-line" arterial blood-gas measurements, have unfortunately not met expectations and requirements for reliability and practicality. The use of pulse oximetry throughout the perioperative period is thus an essential component of monitoring for pulmonary resection. Its value and reliability in the setting of one-lung ventilation has been well described.[83]

In view of both surgical and anesthetic manipulations of the patient's lungs and airway, a continuous assessment of the adequacy of ventilation is critical. Two useful monitors that are readily available as fundamental components of the anesthesia machine circuit include measurements of airway pressure and expired tidal volume. During changes from two-lung to one-lung ventilation, an increase in the peak inspiratory pressure of 5 to 15 cm H_2O pressure may be expected. Sudden changes, particularly acute or progressive increases in peak inspiratory pressure (PIP) during one-lung ventilation with unchanged tidal volumes, may result from alterations in the positioning of a double-lumen endotracheal tube, or the presence of secretions, blood, or tissue compromising the patient's airway. Either situation suggests the need to re-evaluate the patient's airway to ensure continued adequacy of ventilation.

Capnometry, the measurement of expired carbon dioxide, provides a reliable means to confirm the appropriate placement of an endotracheal tube following intubation. However, potential limitations must be recognized. While, excluding metabolic or therapeutic etiologies, progressive increases and elevations in P_{ETCO_2} are usually indicative of inadequate ventilation, particularly with the initial increase in shunt that occurs during one-lung ventilation, with a consequent increase in the A-a gradient, low or normal values for P_{ETCO_2} may not provide a reliable indication of adequate ventilation. Definitive confirmation is best obtained by intermittent arterial blood gas analysis.

Electrocardiogram

Perioperative arrhythmias are a common occurrence. In patients undergoing thoracic surgery, arrhythmias may occur in association with preanesthetic medications (e.g., digoxin), electrolyte abnormalities, and baseline cardiovascular disease (e.g., hypertension). Intraoperatively, arrhythmias may result from anesthetic agents (e.g., nodal rhythms in setting of high concentrations of inhalation agents) and surgical stimulation. Particularly common examples include supraventricular tachyarrhythmias, which are readily triggered during thoracic surgery by direct mechanical stimulation of the heart by the surgeon, and bradycardias secondary to vagal stimulation elicited by surgical dissection of the chest wall, particularly in the pericostal region. Though many of these dysrhythmias are usually benign, particularly in patients undergoing thoracotomy with known cardiac disease, the presence of arrhythmias in the perioperative period has been correlated with myocardial ischemia.[84] Furthermore, arrhythmias may occur in association with hypoxemia, hypercarbia, and hypothermia. Simultaneous monitoring of multiple electrocardiogram (ECG) leads (II, V_5) facilitates recognition of both arrhythmias as well as myocardial ischemia of the inferior and anterolateral wall.

Intravascular Pressure Monitoring—Arterial Line

Placement of an arterial line is particularly valued during thoracic surgery, as it provides a means to detect acute changes in blood pressure and readily permits sampling of arterial blood for blood-gas analysis. The advantage of an arterial line over standard noninvasive modalities is critically apparent in the setting of arrhythmias. Noninvasive automated blood pressure measurement devices are typically confounded by irregular or paroxysmal tachyarrhythmias (e.g., atrial fibrillation).

With regard to site of arterial line placement, with a patient in the lateral position, placement of the catheter in the radial artery of the dependent-side arm improves stability of the site and provides a means of monitoring inappropriate compromise of arterial flow to the dependent arm, which may result from malposition of supports or inappropriate displacement of the chest roll within the axilla. For the patient undergoing mediastinoscopy, placement of the catheter in the right arm may provide a means to detect inappropriate compromise of arterial flow to the upper extremity and possibly cerebral circulation by surgical manipulations of the mediastinoscope.[85]

Central Venous and Pulmonary Artery Catheterization

The indications for placement of a central venous or pulmonary artery catheter remain fundamentally unchanged from other major surgical procedures. Placement of a catheter into a central vessel provides a means of administering fluids, blood, and medications rapidly and directly into the central circulation. Standard indications for the placement of a pulmonary artery catheter (PAC) include significant coronary artery disease (as manifested by unstable angina or a recent myocardial infarction), significant valvular disease, myocardial dysfunction (congestive heart failure), and pulmonary hypertension (cor pulmonale).

For patients undergoing pulmonary resection with one-lung ventilation, several specific caveats apply. Regarding the selection of an appropriate site for insertion of a central venous or pulmonary artery catheter, it may be prudent to choose a site ipsilateral to the operative side to avoid injury (i.e., pneumothorax) to the lung on the side that will be relied upon during one-lung ventilation. The actual location of a pulmonary artery catheter within the pulmonary vasculature is a uniquely relevant consideration during pulmonary resection. Given the configuration of a standard pulmonary artery catheter and the distribution of blood flow, it has been described that the balloon-tipped catheter is most commonly located within the right lower lobe. However, the position of the catheter is subject to unpredictable changes in position, even between right and left pulmonary arterial systems. The reliability of standard radiologic means to confirm the location of the catheter may be inadequate.[86] Thus, particularly if a pneumonectomy is planned, gentle palpation of the pulmonary artery should be performed prior to ligation of the pulmonary artery, to exclude the presence of the catheter.

Potential limitations of pulmonary artery catheter measurements in patients with cardiac disease who are undergoing thoracic surgery have been described. In the setting of one-lung ventilation with the patient in the lateral position, if the catheter is located within the collapsed, nondependent lung, measurements of pulmonary artery pressure and cardiac output may be artifactually lower. This scenario reflects a specific circumstance in which measurements from the PAC may not accurately reflect left ventricular function. Measurements obtained should be interpreted with this understanding, and potentially viewed as primarily useful for their relative value and trend, rather than absolute value.[87]

Fluid Management

Perioperative management of fluid administration for the patient undergoing major pulmonary resection remains an area of controversy and ongoing investigation. The traditional practice of administering an extremely conservative fluid regimen stems largely from the concern that even moderate amounts of standard crystalloid solutions increase the risk for the development of pulmonary edema in the postoperative period.[88] Pulmonary edema is an uncommon but serious complication following major pulmonary resection. Though it has been described following lobectomy, it occurs more commonly following a pneumonectomy (right side four times more frequently than left), with an overall incidence of 2 to 4%. Clinically, during the first to fourth postoperative day, patients develop dyspnea that may progressively worsen to acute respiratory failure. Intubation and ventilatory support may be required to maintain adequate oxygenation. Treatment is primarily supportive as pulmonary edema in this setting is characteristically resistant to standard therapies. Mortality is high at greater than 50%.[89]

The pathophysiology of postpneumonectomy pulmonary edema (PPE) is not completely understood. It is postulated that intraoperative lung manipulation and collapse impairs lymphatic drainage during the early postoperative period. This altered homeostatic mechanism of the lung, in combination with resection of a significant portion of the pulmonary vascular bed, creates a nidus for the accumulation of excess fluid within the remaining lung. While fluid overload has been the most widely implicated contributing factor in the development of PPE,[90] a range of investigative efforts have failed to demonstrate a true cause-and-effect relationship between the volume of fluid administered and the occurrence of PPE.[91] Consistent with characteristic findings of a low pulmonary artery occlusion pressure (PAOP) and high-protein edema fluid, a role for alterations in pulmonary capillary endothelial permeability has been described as well.[92] The absence of a clearly identifiable mechanism suggests a multifactorial etiology and the need for further inquiry.

Regarding fluid requirements during pulmonary resection, in general, the majority of procedures are not typically associated with significant blood loss or large perioperative fluid shifts. During VATS in particular, minimal insensible fluid losses are incurred. Ultimately, perioperative management of fluid administration must consider an appropriate balance between efforts to reduce the potential for this complication, and the fundamental requirement to maintain a sufficient intravascular volume for adequate tissue perfusion.

One-Lung Ventilation

A fundamental component of anesthesia for pulmonary resection is the use of equipment and techniques to selectively isolate ventilation to a portion of the lungs. This most commonly involves separation of the two lungs and the use of one-lung ventilation (OLV). Though pulmonary resection is not considered an absolute indication for OLV, its routine use in this setting is associated with several significant advantages. Collapse of the operative lung facilitates exposure and provides a quiet surgical field. The risk of injury to the operative lung is reduced, as less retraction and compression of nonresected tissue is required. During the early stages of a lobectomy or limited resection, the capacity to variably inflate or deflate the operative lung may improve the definition of lobar fissures and segmental anatomy. Furthermore, during video-assisted thoracic surgery, OLV provides optimal visualization, which is essential for the safe introduction and manipulation of instrumentation.

Though a complete discussion of the equipment and techniques used to establish one-lung ventilation is presented in Chapter 25, unique issues arise with regard to management of one-lung ventilation during two specific procedures: pneumonectomy and bronchoplastic pulmonary resection.

During a pneumonectomy, optimal management of the airway requires particular attentiveness to surgical proceedings as manipulation of the operative side mainstem bronchus and adjacent structures can readily alter the proper positioning of a double-lumen endotracheal tube. Intraoperatively, during a left-sided pneumonectomy, if a left-sided double-lumen tube is used, prior to surgical clamping of the mainstem bronchus, the bronchial lumen of the tube should be withdrawn into the trachea. Ventilation then may continue to the nonoperative side lung via both lumens of the tube.

During a bronchoplastic resection, the fundamental consideration of intraoperative airway management is to establish appropriately isolated ventilation. Use of a standard double-lumen tube is usually sufficient and the most practical technique. In the event that one-lung ventilation is complicated by hypoxemia, the option exists to provide ventilation of the lung distal to the resected segment, using sterile endobronchial intubation and ventilation across the surgical field. Alternatively, jet ventilation may be provided to the distal pulmonary segment via a sterile catheter or conduit. At the conclusion of a bronchoplastic procedure, the double-lumen endotracheal tube (ETT) should be replaced with a single-lumen ETT through which immediate bronchoscopy is performed by the surgeon to examine the anastomosis. Inappropriate stenosis must be ruled out, as this can interfere with effective clearance of accumulated secretions. Subsequent suctioning of the airway and pulmonary toilet must be thorough yet cautious so as to avoid traumatizing the anastomosis.

The use of OLV, however, is associated with several risks and potential complications. The most serious concern is the maintenance of adequate oxygenation. During OLV, moderate to severe hypoxemia, defined as a PaO_2 less than 70 mm Hg, has been reported to occur in 15 to 35% of cases, despite the use of high inspired oxygen concentrations.[93–97] In addition to the various factors that can produce hypoxemia during any surgical procedure under general anesthesia, inadequate oxygenation during OLV results from several factors. These include (1) "mechanical" etiologies, (2) the presence of pre-existing abnormalities in pulmonary function, and (3) the overall relationship between ventilation and perfusion as defined by the extent of collapse of the operative lung, and the relative distribution of blood flow between the dependent and nondependent lungs.

"Mechanical" etiologies of hypoxemia are most frequently problems associated with the equipment and techniques used to establish OLV. Malposition of a double-lumen tube or endobronchial blocking device occurs in as many as 48% of cases and may acutely compromise ventilation, with the potential for collapse of one or more lobes of the ventilated lung, or total airway obstruction.[98,99] The lumen of the airway or ETT may also become obstructed from excessive secretions, blood, or tissue fragments. These common causes of inadequate ventilation and oxygenation must be considered early and corrected appropriately. A detailed discussion of the equipment and techniques used during OLV, including the use of flexible fiberoptic bronchoscopy, is presented in Chapter 25.

Baseline abnormalities in lung function also factor significantly in the patient's capacity to tolerate OLV. Characteristically, patients presenting for pulmonary resection are of advanced age and have a history of tobacco use and chronic lung disease. With increasing age, the mechanics of the lung are altered progressively such that the distribution of ventilation becomes more uneven and small airways close at smaller lung volumes. The progressive increase in the alveolar to arterial oxygen tension difference, or $P(A\text{-}a)O_2$, produces a predictable decrease in PaO_2 with age. This decrease in PaO_2 is exaggerated by smoking, obesity, and chronic pulmonary disease.[100] Ironically, it has been suggested that patients with obstructive lung disease may tend to have better PaO_2 values during OLV. The reasons for this observation are not known. Mechanisms that have been postulated include (1) a persistence of flow at end-expiration due to obstructive disease, or "intrinsic PEEP,"[101] which maintains dependent lung volume; and (2) an alteration in blood flow redistribution with the onset of one-lung ventilation due to unexplained differences in the hypoxic pulmonary vasoconstrictor response of patients with COPD.

The most significant factor contributing to the development of hypoxemia during OLV is the mismatch in the relationship between ventilation and perfusion. The extent to which perfusion continues to nonventilated regions of the operative lung (i.e., shunt flow) is the critical determinant of the degree to which the $P(A\text{-}a)O_2$ increases, and PaO_2 decreases. Alterations in the relationship between ventilation and perfusion result from a series of perturbations that occur during pulmonary surgery and OLV. Anesthetic management of OLV, including techniques to optimize oxygenation, derives from a fundamental understanding of the mechanisms that produce hypoxemia in this setting.

The occurrence of hypoxemia during OLV is often difficult to predict. The incidence has been observed to be greater in patients undergoing nonpulmonary as compared with pulmonary surgery.[102,103] This may be explained by compensatory changes in the distribution of ventilation and perfusion that occur chronically in response to focal lesions within the lung. Generally, patients with unimpaired blood flow to the collapsed lung are more likely to develop hypoxemia during one-lung ventilation than patients in whom pulmonary blood flow has chronically been decreased. A correlation between the side of surgery and PaO_2 during OLV has been observed. Because the smaller left lung normally receives 10% less perfusion than the right, PaO_2 during OLV when the patient is in the right lateral position is often higher.[104]

The extent to which oxygenation can potentially decrease during OLV may be estimated using preoperative ventilation-perfusion (V/Q) scans.[105] It has been described that hypoxemia during OLV is unlikely if less than one third of the cardiac output is perfusing the operative lung. Ten to 15% of patients with preoperative nondependent lung perfusion between 35 and 45% of cardiac output, and more than 30% of patients with perfusion greater than 45% of cardiac output, are considered at risk for the development of hypoxemia. An important limitation of V/Q scan data when viewed in the context of pulmonary resection is that perfusion scans are generally performed with the patient in the supine position, while patients undergoing surgery are typically in the lateral position.

The Effects of Position, General Anesthesia, and Thoracotomy

The distribution of ventilation is influenced by posture and the manner of ventilation. Under normal circumstances, in the awake, upright patient, a greater proportion of each tidal volume is distributed to the more numerous and compliant alveoli at the bases of the lungs. Blood flow within the pulmonary circulation, primarily influenced by gravity, is similarly distributed in greater proportion to the lung bases relative to the apex. With a change to the supine position, pressure from the abdominal contents causes cephalad displacement of the diaphragm into the thoracic cavity. Despite the consequent decrease in lung volumes, including functional residual capacity (FRC), in the awake patient, the lung bases continue to receive a greater proportion of each tidal breath as the diaphragm contracts more effectively in its higher position within the chest.[106] The distribution of blood flow remains essentially unchanged in the supine position, as the gravitational gradient from apex to base is replaced by the difference between anterior and posterior aspects.

With a change to the lateral position, the volume of the dependent lung becomes more diminished relative to the nondependent lung owing to both the greater extent of cephalad displacement of the diaphragm and by downward displacement of the overlying mediastinum. Dependent lung volume and compliance of the chest wall may be further compromised by inappropriate positioning and improper placement of operating table supports. Nonetheless, a greater proportion of each tidal breath is still delivered to the dependent lung owing to the more efficient contractions of the diaphragm on the dependent side. Primarily influenced by gravity, the dependent lung receives greater perfusion relative to the nondependent lung by roughly 5 to 25%.[107] Thus in the awake patient, with changes to the supine and lateral position, the distributions of ventilation and perfusion remain essentially well matched.

In the course of a surgical procedure, the first significant alteration in the distribution of ventilation and perfusion occurs with the administration of general anesthesia. Decreases in lung volumes, including FRC, which occurred in relation to patient position, become more pronounced as a result of greater cephalad displacement of the now flaccid diaphragm.[108] When the patient is turned to the lateral position, the paralyzed diaphragm is unable to counter the effects of the diminished lung volumes, and the delivery of positive-pressure ventilation favors the more compliant nondependent lung.[109,110] With opening of the chest wall and pleural cavity, loss of negative intrapleural pressure to a relatively more positive ambient pressure enables the full weight of the mediastinum to be transmitted to the dependent lung. The absence of restriction by an intact chest wall then favors the disproportionate distribution of ventilation to the nondependent lung.

With collapse of the operative lung and restriction of ventilation to the dependent lung, optimal oxygenation theoretically depends upon maximal alveolar recruitment in the dependent lung, and minimal blood flow to the atelectatic lung. During a thoracotomy in the lateral position, blood flow to the operative lung is decreased by several factors including gravity and to a limited extent by surgical manipulation.[111] However, the most important source of active regulation of the pulmonary circulation is hypoxic pulmonary vasoconstriction.

Hypoxic Pulmonary Vasoconstriction

Hypoxic pulmonary vasoconstriction (HPV) is an adaptive mechanism that describes the increase in pulmonary vascular resistance that occurs in response to a decrease in alveolar oxygen tension (PAO_2). Two distinct responses are observed with HPV is stimulated—a diversion of blood flow away from the hypoxic region and a generalized increase in pulmonary artery pressure. By shifting blood flow from poorly to better ventilated regions of lung, the relationship of ventilation and perfusion is improved, shunt is relatively decreased, and hypoxemia is reduced. In patients undergoing OLV in the lateral position, HPV is thought to play an important role in the reduction of blood flow to the atelectatic nondependent lung.[112]

The mechanism of hypoxic pulmonary vasoconstriction, first described by von Euler and Liljestrand in 1946[113] and widely characterized in a variety of scientific and clinical studies,[114–116] is not fully understood. In the past, various mediators, including catecholamines, histamine, serotonin, angiotensin II, neurotransmitters, and arachidonic acid metabolites, have been postulated to play a role. More recently, however, it has become apparent that the activity and regulation of endothelium-derived relaxing and constricting factors, including specifically nitric oxide, play an integral role in the regulation of the pulmonary vasculature. Elucidation of the precise mechanism of HPV, which appears to involve a complex cascade of biochemical modulators, remains an area of ongoing investigation.[117–119]

The predominant site of HPV is in the small muscular pulmonary arteries (35 to 50 μm) at the level of the terminal respiratory bronchioles.[120,121] The remaining small contribution to HPV arises from the pulmonary capillaries and pulmonary venous system. The increase in pulmonary vascular resistance occurs primarily in response to a decrease in PAO_2). An additional contribution to the initiation of the response comes from mixed venous oxygen ($P\bar{v}O_2$),[122] which is the stimulus for HPV in the atelectatic lung such as during one-lung ventilation.[123] In addition, there is increasing evidence that the bronchial circulation has an influence on HPV, regulating the tone of larger pulmonary arteries.[124] The threshold for vasoconstriction occurs at a PO_2 of approximately 60 mm Hg and progresses in a nonlinear fashion to a maximal response at a PO_2 of 30 mm Hg.

The HPV response is characterized by a rapid onset, beginning within seconds of alveolar hypoxia. A maximal response is attained within minutes, and can be sustained for hours.[125] Clinically, during OlV, the maximum intrapulmonary shunt is reached within the first 20 minutes.[96] The magnitude of the HPV response is dependent upon both the severity of alveolar hypoxia and the relative size of the hypoxic lung segment. If a very limited area (<20%) of lung is hypoxic, because the amount of blood flow diversion will be small, HPV will not influence PaO_2 to a significant extent. And in the setting where most of the lung is hypoxic, because of the absence of normoxic lung regions in which to divert blood flow to, the extent to which HPV will improve PaO_2 is also limited. Thus, when the extent of hypoxic lung is in the range of 30 to 70% as occurs during one-lung ventilation, there may be a significant improvement in PaO_2 based upon the contribution made by HPV. During one-lung ventilation, with roughly half of the total lung collapsed, the maximal flow reduction in the hypoxic segment is 50%.[126–128] The change in pulmonary artery pressure with HPV also varies according to the size of the hypoxic segment. Larger regions of lung hypoxia will produce greater elevations in pulmonary artery pressure.

CLINICAL SIGNIFICANCE OF HPV

The magnitude of the response as manifest in clinical settings is influenced by various physiologic factors, disease states, and drugs. Owing to the relative paucity and weakness of smooth muscle within the pulmonary vasculature, the HPV response is diminished in the setting of elevated intravascular pressure. Thus it is postulated that an altered HPV response may contribute to the abnormalities in ventilation and perfusion, and hypoxemia seen in conditions such as congestive heart failure and mitral valvular disease. Diminished or absent HPV responses have also been described in patients with cirrhosis, acute lung injury of various etiologies, sepsis, and pneumonia—particularly pneumococcal and granulomatous infections.[129] In patients with COPD, the response can be variable. In patients with advanced disease, proliferative changes and progressive constriction within the pulmonary vasculature is thought to diminish or alter the sensitivity of the HPV response.

HPV can be altered pharmacologically. Agents that blunt HPV include various classes of vasodilators—including calcium channel blockers, nitrates, nitroprusside, β_2-adrenergic agonist bronchodilators, nitric oxide, and inhaled anesthetics. Clinically, the influence of these agents on HPV, though often overlooked, is generally readily apparent. For example, when nitroprusside is used as a vasodilator, with normoxic ventilated lungs there is usually no appreciable effect on pulmonary vasculature. However, when nitroprusside is administered during collapse of one lung, there is a significant global decrease in pulmonary vascular resistance, resulting in an increase in intrapulmonary shunt, increased mismatch of ventilation to perfusion, and a reduction of PaO_2.[130]

THE EFFECTS OF ANESTHETICS ON HPV

Numerous investigations have been conducted on the influence of anesthetics on the HPV response. As demonstrated in both in vitro and in vivo studies, intravenous agents including barbiturates, Propofol,[131] benzodiazepines, narcotics, and muscle relaxants have no significant effect on the HPV response.[132] Regarding inhalational anesthetic agents, while in vitro studies demonstrate a depressant effect on HPV, variable and seemingly contradictory results have been reported during in vivo evaluations. The discrepancy between in vitro and in vivo studies of the effects of inhalational anesthetics on HPV can be explained by recognizing that in clinical settings, inhalational anesthetics have effects on other physiologic parameters, specifically cardiac output, which may influence oxygenation. During bilateral ventilation of normal lungs, changes in cardiac output have little effect on Qs/Qt or Pa_{O_2}. However, in the presence of regional atelectasis, changes in cardiac output can impact on oxygenation by altering shunt (Qs/Qt) and $P\bar{v}_{O_2}$).[133] A decrease in cardiac output results in a decrease in transmural pressure within alveolar vessels. During inspiration, for a given increase in alveolar pressure, a larger proportion of alveolar vessels in the dependent lung are compressed, favoring the redistribution of blood flow to the atelectatic nondependent lung. Assuming a steady state where oxygen demand remains relatively unchanged, a decrease in cardiac output, as may occur secondary to the administration of an inhalational agent, results in a decrease in $P\bar{v}_{O_2}$, which enhances the vasoconstrictor response in the collapsed lung. The relative distribution of blood flow is thus ultimately determined by the relative difference in vascular resistance between the dependent and nondependent lung. In the clinical setting, the myocardial depressant effect of inhalational agents, with their potential to decrease cardiac output, influences the overall effect of inhalational agents on HPV and oxygenation.

Management of One-Lung Ventilation—Conventional Approach

Management of OLV is based upon an understanding of the physiologic considerations discussed above, and involves a standard approach to basic ventilatory parameters, including F_{IO_2}, tidal volume, and respiratory rate. In a majority of cases, modest modifications of these variables combined with prompt attention to transient "mechanical" problems is sufficient to maintain adequate oxygenation and ventilation, and provide favorable surgical conditions.

F_{IO_2}

A high F_{IO_2} is routinely used during OLV, primarily to enhance the margin of safety against hypoxemia. In addition, delivery of a high F_{IO_2} produces pulmonary vasodilation, which favors perfusion of the dependent lung relative to the atelectatic nondependent lung of blood flow redistributed by HPV. Though hypoxemia may still occur, Pa_{O_2} values in the range of 150 to 210 mm Hg have generally been reported with the use of an F_{IO_2} of 1.0 during OLV.[93,96,103]

Tidal Volume and Respiratory Rate

During one-lung ventilation, ventilation and oxygenation are theoretically optimized under conditions in which ventilation to the dependent lung is minimally compromised. The term "alveolar recruitment" is frequently used in this setting to refer to the inflation and maintained patency of previously collapsed or compromised alveoli. Data obtained from studies comparing the use of different tidal volumes during OLV are notable for their demonstration of considerable variability between individual patients. The use of tidal volumes less than 8 ml/kg is inadequate to optimize alveolar recruitment and prevent atelectasis of the dependent lung. Oxygenation is decreased due to the decrease in ventilation and increased ventilation-perfusion mismatch. Conversely, excessive tidal volumes exceeding 12 to 15 ml/kg can increase intrathoracic pressures and secondarily increase pulmonary vascular resistance in the dependent lung, thus diverting blood flow into the nondependent lung. Thus, the reasonable recommendation is the use of dependent lung tidal volumes in the range of 8 to 12 ml/kg, which are very similar to those used during two-lung ventilation.[134] Typically, in transition from two-, to one-lung ventilation, peak airway pressures may increase roughly 10 to 15 cm H_2O.

Elimination of CO_2 is generally not a problem during OLV. As CO_2 is 20 times more diffusible than O_2, and the arterial-venous P_{CO_2} difference, or $P(a\text{-}v)_{O_2}$, is normally only 6 mm Hg, the increase in shunt that occurs during one-lung ventilation does not significantly impact on the elimination of CO_2. Thus, the minute ventilation required to maintain a normal Pa_{CO_2} is the same for one- and two-lung ventilation.

Hyperventilation with consequent hypocarbia should be avoided, as both may decrease Pa_{O_2}. With hyperventilation, the resultant increase in mean airway pressure may increase pulmonary vascular resistance within the dependent lung, diverting blood flow to the collapsed nondependent lung. In addition, hypocapnia may directly inhibit HPV within the nondependent lung, possibly by a direct vasodilator mechanism. In both instances, shunt may increase with a consequent decrease in Pa_{O_2}. Of additional note, variations in the inspiratory-expiratory ratio, and intermittent manual hyperventilation of the dependent lung have not been demonstrated to be beneficial in increasing Pa_{O_2} during one-lung ventilation.[135]

Management of One-Lung Ventilation—Supplementary Techniques

A variety of additional techniques involving the selective alterations in the manner of ventilation may be considered during the management of OLV in an effort to remedy conditions of inadequate oxygenation not otherwise responsive to standard approaches. While many of these approaches appear to be beneficial within a conceptual framework, in practice these techniques are frequently characterized by a narrow therapeutic window, and may even be associated with potentially significant disadvantages. Though these optional techniques have been extensively researched and described in the literature, in reality their use is seldom necessary.

PEEP to the Dependent Lung

As described earlier in this chapter, with the patient in the lateral position, volume of the dependent lung is decreased by a variety of factors including cephalad displacement of the diaphragm, compression by overlying mediastinal structures, and suboptimal positioning effects. Lung volume at end-expiration, by definition FRC, can be increased by the application of PEEP. An increase in FRC theoretically contributes to the prevention of airway and alveolar closure at end-expiration and to the recruitment of airways and alveoli during inspiration. With increased lung volume, compliance and ventilation are improved. The logical application of PEEP to the dependent lung, however, has variable effects on oxygenation.

Studies that have investigated the effects of PEEP applied to the dependent lung[136,137] have demonstrated that in a majority of patients, $Pa{O_2}$ either decreased or remained the same. In patients in whom $Pa{O_2}$ was improved by the application of 5 to 10 cm H_2O PEEP to the dependent lung, $Pa{O_2}$ prior to PEEP was less than 80 mm Hg. Patients with an initial $Pa{O_2}$ of greater than 80 mm Hg experienced either no significant change or even a decrease in $Pa{O_2}$ following the addition of PEEP to the dependent lung.

The mechanism for these responses can be explained by the opposing effects of positive airway pressure within the dependent lung on oxygenation. While increased positive pressure improves expansion of respiratory units, it has been demonstrated that intra-alveolar pressure can affect pulmonary vascular resistance (PVR), altering blood flow distribution. With an increase in PVR, blood flow is diverted to the nondependent lung, relatively increasing shunt and potentially further decreasing $Pa{O_2}$.[138] In patients who demonstrated an improvement in $Pa{O_2}$ with PEEP, presumably the dependent lung volume and FRC was low, with regions of atelectasis and low V/Q. Consequently, the beneficial effect of increased dependent lung volume predominated over the negative effect of increased PVR and shunt. Conversely, in patients who demonstrated either no change or a decrease in $Pa{O_2}$, the negative effect of increased shunt on oxygenation predominated. Shunt fraction will thus ultimately be determined by the sensitive balance between these two effects. These results suggest that the therapeutic range for the beneficial effects of PEEP is quite narrow.

The Nondependent Lung

Inadequate oxygenation and the increase in the $P(A\text{-}a)O_2$ gradient during one-lung ventilation is primarily due to the continued perfusion of the collapsed operative lung. Thus, manipulations of the nondependent lung are more likely to improve oxygenation than maneuvers on the ventilated lung. Available options are to reduce perfusion to atelectatic regions or to increase oxygen uptake by the perfusion that remains in the nondependent lung.

Vascular Manipulation

Occluding blood flow to the nondependent lung effectively eliminates a majority of shunt flow and significantly improves the matching of ventilation and perfusion. Surgical clamping of the delicate pulmonary arteries, however, is viewed with considerable caution. With the additional risk of complications stemming from pulmonary ischemia and infarction, vascular manipulations are generally not a first-line treatment for hypoxemia, and may be more appropriately reserved for a planned pneumonectomy. Even in this setting, the timing of this option is technically limited by the requisite surgical considerations. Occluding pulmonary blood flow by inflation of a pulmonary artery catheter balloon placed in the collapsed lung has been described and demonstrated to be effective in animal models.[135] Again, however, practical limitations as well as the risks associated with potential complications including pulmonary artery thrombosis and rupture preclude the routine application of this approach.

In the absence of clinically acceptable techniques to decrease nondependent lung blood flow, the corollary method remains to improve oxygen uptake by the nondependent lung. Oxygenation of blood perfusing the nondependent lung can occur without gross ventilatory movements that potentially interfere with the surgical field. The continuous insufflation of oxygen to the nondependent lung at low levels of continuous positive airway pressure (5 to 10 cm H_2O), to maintain the patency and continuity of conducting and respiratory units, has been demonstrated to be an effective means to increase $Pa{O_2}$ during one-lung ventilation.[96,136,137,139]

It is imperative that the application of continuous positive airway pressure (CPAP) to the nondependent lung be initiated during the deflation phase of a large tidal volume. In this way, expansion of the nondependent lung is more uniform and the critical opening pressures of distal airways and alveoli have been overcome. Without positive distending pressure, insufflation of oxygen to the nondependent lung has not been demonstrated to reliably improve oxygenation, as oxygen delivered remains primarily in the large conducting airways, inaccessible to gas-exchanging alveolar units. A variety of systems for providing nondependent lung CPAP are commercially available. All require a separate oxygen source and delivery system, as well as a means of measuring and regulating pressure.[140,141]

Based upon a similar concept, yet simpler to execute, periodic reinflation of the nondependent lung with moderate volumes (2 to 4 ml/kg) of oxygen is also a reliable treatment for hypoxemia if it can be conducted at appropriate times to minimize interference with the surgical procedure. It should be kept in mind, however, that a principal advantage of the use of OLV during pulmonary resection would be negated if the operative lung remained significantly distended throughout the procedure.

High-frequency ventilation (HFV) to the nondependent lung has also been investigated as a modality for treating hypoxemia during OLV. Results, however, have been variable. In addition to causing dilation of central airways, HFV is potentially an interference to the surgical resection. HFV may have a useful role in the setting of a pulmonary "sleeve" resection. During resection of the bronchial segment, in the event that hypoxemia develops prior to bronchial reanastomosis, ventilation to the distal lung parenchyma may be delivered using HFV.

References

1. Travis WD, Travis LB, Devesa SS: Lung cancer. Cancer 75(Suppl 1):191, 1995.
2. U.S. Surgeon General Reports on the Health Consequences of Smoking, 1964, 1979, 1982.
3. American Joint Committee for Cancer Staging and End Results Reporting: Clinical staging system for carcinoma of the lung. Chicago, 1973.
4. Mountain CF: A new international staging system for lung cancer. Chest 89(Suppl):S225, 1986.
5. Martini N, McCaughan BC, McCormack P, et al: Lobectomy for stage I lung cancer. In Kittle CF (ed): Current Controversies in Thoracic Surgery. Philadelphia, WB Saunders Co., 1986, p 171.
6. Martini N, Bains MS, McCormack P: Surgical treatment of non-small cell carcinoma of the lung: The Memorial Sloan-Kettering Experience. In Hoogstraten B, Addis BJ, Hansen HH, et al (eds): Lung Tumors: Lung, Mediastinum, Pleura, and Chest Wall. New York, Springer-Verlag, 1988, p 111.
7. Karrer K, Shields TW, Denck H, et al: The importance of surgery and multimodality treatment for small cell bronchial carcinoma. J Thorac Cardiovasc Surg 97:168, 1989.
8. Baker RR, Ettinger DS, Ruckdeschel JD, et al: The role of surgery in the management of selected patients with small-cell carcinoma of the lung. J Clin Oncol 5:697, 1987.
9. Clagett OT, Ellen TH, Payne WS, et al: The surgical treatment of pulmonary neoplasms—a ten-year experience. J Thorac Cardiovasc Surg 48:391, 1964.
10. Ranchod M, Levine GD: Spindle-cell carcinoid tumors of the lung: A clinicopathologic study of 35 cases. Am J Surg Pathol 4:315, 1980.
11. Deslauriers J, Beauchamp G, Desmeules M: Benign and malignant disorders of the pleura. In Baue AE (ed): Glenn's Thoracic and Cardiovascular Surgery, 5th ed., Vol 1. Norwalk, Appleton & Lange, 1991, p 459.
12. Willis RA: The Spread of Tumours in the Human Body, 3rd ed. London, Butterworth's, 1973.
13. McCormack PM, Bains MS, Beattie EJ Jr, et al: Pulmonary resection in metastatic carcinoma. Chest 73:163, 1978.
14. Ginsberg RJ, Hill LD, Egan RT, et al: Modern thirty-day operative mortality for surgical resections in lung cancer. J Thorac Cardiovasc Surg 86:654, 1983.
15. Deslauriers J, Ginsberg RJ, Dubois P, et al: Current operative morbidy associated with elective surgical resection for lung cancer. Can J Surg 32:335, 1989.
16. Wahi R, McMurtrey MJ, DeCaro LF, et al: Determinants of perioperative morbidity and mortality after pneumonectomy. Ann Thorac Surg 48:33, 1989.
17. Nakahara K, Ohno K, Hashimoto J: Prediction of postoperative respiratory failure in patients undergoing lung resection for cancer. Ann Thorac Surg 46:549, 1988.
18. Olsen GN, Block AJ, Tobias JA: Prediction of postpneumonectomy pulmonary function using quantitative macroaggregate lung scanning. Chest 66:13, 1974.
19. Olsen GN, Block AJ, Swenson EW, et al: Pulmonary function evaluation of the lung resection candidate: A prospective study. Am Rev Respir Dis 111:379, 1975.
20. American College of Physicians: Preoperative pulmonary function testing. Ann Intern Med 112:793, 1990.
21. Kearney DJ, Lee TH, Reilly JJ, et al: Assessment of operative risk in patients undergoing lung resection: Importance of predicted pulmonary function. Chest 105:753, 1994.
22. Gaensler EA, Cugell DW, Lindgren I, et al: The role of pulmonary insufficiency in mortality and invalidism following surgery for pulmonary tuberculosis. J Thorac Cardiovasc Surg 29:163, 1955.
23. Miller JI, Hatcher CR: Limited resection of bronchogenic carcinoma in the patient with marked impairment of pulmonary function. Ann Thorac Surg 44:340, 1987.
24. Tisi GM: Preoperative evaluation of pulmonary function. Validity, indications, and benefits. Am Rev Respir Dis 119:293, 1979.
25. Zeiher BG, Gross TJ, Kern JA, et al: Predicting postoperative pulmonary function in patients undergoing lung resection. Chest 108:68, 1995.
26. Olsen GN: The evolving role of exercise testing prior to lung resection. Chest 95:218, 1989.
27. Zibrak JD, O'Donnell CR, Marton K: Indications for pulmonary function testing. Ann Intern Med 112:763, 1990.
28. Smith TP, Kinasewitz GT, Tucker WY, et al: Exercise capacity as a predictor of post-thoracotomy morbidity. Am Rev Respir Dis 129:730, 1984.
29. Bechard D, Wetstein L: Assessment of exercise oxygen consumption as preoperative criteria for lung resection. Ann Thorac Surg 44:344, 1987.
30. Epstein SK, Faling JL, Daly BD, et al: Inability to perform bicycle ergometry predicts increased morbidity and mortality after lung resection. Chest 107:311, 1995.
31. Epstein SK, Faling JL, Daly BD, et al: Predicting complications after pulmonary resection: Preoperative exercise testing vs. a multifactorial cardiopulmonary risk index. Chest 104:694, 1993.
32. Goldman L, Caldera DL, Nussbaum SR, et al: Multifactorial index of cardiac risk in noncardiac surgical procedures. N Engl J Med 297:845, 1977.
33. Graham EA, Singer JJ: Successful removal of an entire lung for carcinoma of the bronchus. JAMA 101:1371, 1933.
34. Churchill ED, Sweet RH, Sutter L, et al: The surgical management of carcinoma of the lung. A study of cases treated at the Massachusetts General Hospital from 1930–1950. J Thorac Cardiovasc Surg 20:349, 1950.
35. Hoffman TH, Ransdell HT: Comparison of lobectomy and wedge resection for lung cancer. J Thorac Cardiovasc Surg 79:211, 1980.
36. McCormack PM, Martini N: Primary lung carcinoma. Results with conservative resection in treatment. NY State J Med 80:612, 1980.
37. McCormack P, Martini N: Secondary tumors in the lung. In Shields TW (ed): General Thoracic Surgery, 3rd ed. Philadelphia, Lea & Febiger, 1989, p 951.
38. Faber LP, Jensik RJ: Limited pulmonary resection. In Baue AE (ed): Glenn's Thoracic and Cardiovascular Surgery, 5th ed, Vol 1. Norwalk, Appleton & Lange, 1991, p 385.
39. Burt M, Martini N: Surgical treatment of lung carcinoma. In Baue AE (ed): Glenn's Thoracic and Cardiovascular Surgery, 5th ed., Vol 1. Norwalk, Appleton & Lange, 1991, p 355.
40. Maaijens PFJ, Hasenbos MA, Lacquet LK, et al: Cardiac herniation after pneumonectomy. Acta Anaesthesiol Scand 36:842, 1992.
41. Cassorla L, Katz JA: Management of cardiac herniation after intrapericardial pneumonectomy. Anesthesiology 60:362, 1984.
42. Lowe JE, Bridgman AH, Sabiston DC: The role of bronchoplastic procedures in the surgical management of benign and malignant pulmonary lesions. J Thorac Cardiovasc Surg 83:227, 1982.
43. Vogt-Moykopf I, Meyer G, Naunheim K, et al: Bronchoplastic techniques for lung resection. In Baue AE (ed): Glenn's Thoracic and Cardiovascular Surgery, 5th ed, Vol. 1. Norwalk, CT, Appleton & Lange, 1991, p 403.
44. Frist WH, Mathisen DJ, Hilgenberg AD, et al: Bronchial sleeve resection with and without pulmonary resection. J Thorac Cardiovasc Surg 93:350, 1987.
45. McCormack P Chest wall tumors. In Baue AE (ed): Glenn's Thoracic and Cardiovascular Surgery, 5th ed, Vol 1. Norwalk, Appleton & Lange, 1991, p 522.

46. McCaughan BC, Martini N, Bains MS, et al: Chest wall invasion of carcinoma of the lung: Therapeutics and prognostic implications. J Thorac Cardiovasc Surg 89:836, 1985.
47. Pancoast HK: Superior pulmonary sulcus tumor: Tumor characterized by pain, Horner's syndrome, destruction of bone and atrophy of hand muscles. JAMA 99:1391, 1932.
48. Paulson DL: Superior sulcus carcinomas. In Baue AE (ed): Glenn's Thoracic and Cardiovascular Surgery, 5th ed, Vol 1. Norwalk, Appleton & Lange, 1991, p 375.
49. DaValle MJ, Faber LP, Kittle CF, et al: Extrapleural pneumonectomy for diffuse, malignant mesothelioma. Ann Thorac Surg 42:612, 1986.
50. Faurschou P, Madsen F, Viskum K: Thoracoscopy: Influence of the procedure on some respiratory and cardiac values. Thorax 38:341, 1983.
51. Oldenburg FA Jr, Newhouse MT: Thoracoscopy: A safe, accurate diagnostic procedure using the rigid thoracoscope and local anesthesia. Chest 75:45, 1979.
52. Rusch VW: Thoracoscopy under regional anesthesia for diagnosis and management of pleural disease. Am J Surg 154:274, 1987.
53. Rusch V: Thoracoscopy. Surgical Technique Supplement 2. Scientific American. Fall, 1993.
54. Mulder DS: Pain Management principles and anesthesia techniques for thoracoscopy (Review). Ann Thorac Surg 56:630, 1993.
55. Barker SJ, Clarke C, Narendra T, et al: Anesthesia for thoracoscopic laser ablation of bullous emphysema. Anesthesiology 78: 44, 1993.
56. Daniel TM, Kern JA, Tribble, CG, et al: Thoracoscopic surgery for disease of the lung and pleura: Effectiveness, changing indications, and limitations. Ann Surg 217:566, 1993.
57. Landreneau RJ, Mack MJ, Hazelrigg SR, et al: Video-assisted thoracic surgery: Basic technical concepts and intercostal approach strategies. Ann Thorac Surg 54:800, 1992.
58. Ferson PF, Landreneau RJ, Dowling RD, et al: Comparison of open versus thoracoscopic lung biopsy for diffuse infiltrative pulmonary disease. J Thorac Cardiovasc Surg 106:194, 1993.
59. Landreneau RJ, Mack JM, Dowling RD, et al: The role of thoracoscopy in lung cancer management. Chest (Suppl 1):6S, 1998.
60. McCormack PM, Ginsberg KB, Bains MS, et al: Accuracy of lung imaging in metastases with implications for the role of thoracoscopy. Ann Thorac Surg 56:863, 1993.
61. Allen MS, Pairolero PC: Inadequacy, mortality, and thoracoscopy. Ann Thorac Surg 59:6, 1995.
62. Martin J: Positioning in Anesthesia and Surgery, 2nd ed. Philadelphia: WB Saunders Co, 1987, p 1147.
63. Courington FW: The role of posture in anesthesia. Clin Anesth 3:24, 1968.
64. Lincoln JR, Sawyer HP: Complications related to body positions during surgical procedures. Anesthesiology 22:800, 1961.
65. Jaffe TB, McLeskey CH: Position-induced Horner's syndrome. Anesthesiology 56:49, 1982.
66. Britt BA, Joy N, Mackay MB: Positioning trauma. In Orkin FK, Cooperman LH (eds). Complications in Anesthesiology. Philadelphia, JB Lippincott Co, 1983.
67. Horswell JL: Anesthetic techniques for thoracoscopy. Ann Thorac Surg 56:624, 1993.
68. Kraenzler EJ: Anesthetic considerations for video-assisted thoracic surgery. Semin Thorac Cardiovasc Surg 5:321, 1993.
69. Slinger P, Scott WAC: Arterial oxygenation during one-lung ventilation. A comparison of enflurane and isoflurane. Anesthesiology 82:940, 1995.
70. Benumof JL, Augustine SD, Gibbons JA: Halothane and isoflurane only slightly impair arterial oxygenation during one-lung ventilation in patients undergoing thoracotomy. Anesthesiology 67:910, 1987.
71. Rees DI, Gaines DY III: One-lung anesthesia: A comparison of pulmonary gas exchange during anesthesia with ketamine or enflurane. Anesth Analg 63:521, 1984.
72. Eisenkraft JB: Effects of anaesthetics on the pulmonary circulation. Br J Anaesth 65:63, 1990.
73. Batist G, Andrew J: Pulmonary toxicity of antineoplastic drugs. JAMA 246:1449, 1981.
74. Ginsberg SJ, Comis RL: The pulmonary toxicity of antineoplastic agents. Semin Oncol 9:34, 1982.
75. Goldiner PL, Carlon GC, Cvitkovic E, et al: Factors influencing postoperative morbidity and mortality in patients treated with bleomycin. Br Med J 1:1664, 1978.
76. La Mantia KR, Glick JH, Marshall BE: Supplemental oxygen does not cause respiratory failure in bleomycin-treated surgical patients. Anesthesiology 60:65, 1984.
77. Slevin BL: Cancer chemotherapy: Implications for the anesthesiologist. Anesth Analg 60:425, 1981.
78. Mathes DD: Bleomycin and hyperoxia exposure in the operating room. Anesth Analg 81:624, 1995.
79. Small S, Ali HH, Lennon VA, et al: Anesthesia for unsuspected Lambert-Eaton myasthenic syndrome with autoantibodies and occult small cell lung carcinoma. Anesthesiology 76:142, 1992.
80. Wise RP: A myasthenic syndrome complicating bronchial carcinoma. Anaesthesia 17:488, 1962.
81. Tellford RJ, Hallway TE: The myasthenia syndrome: Anaesthesia in a patient treated with 3,4 diaminopyridine. Br J Anaesth 64:363, 1990.
82. Temeck BK, Schafer PW, Park WY, Harmon JW. Epidural anesthesia in patients undergoing thoracic surgery. Arch Surg 124: 415, 1989.
83. Brodsky JB, Shulman MS, Swan M, Mark JBD: Pulse oximetry during one-lung ventilation. Anesthesiology 63:212, 1985.
84. Krowka MJ, Pairolero PC, Trastek V, et al: Cardiac dysrhythmia following pneumonectomy. Chest 91:490, 1987.
85. Petty C: Right radial artery pressure during mediastinoscopy. Anesth Analg 59:428, 1979.
86. Cohen E, Neustein M, Kirschner PA: Inadvertent transection of a pulmonary artery catheter during thoracic surgery. J Cardiothorac Vasc Anesth 7:337, 1993.
87. Benumof JL: "Monitoring" in Anesthesia for Thoracic Surgery. Philadelphia, WB Saunders Co, 1987, p 168.
88. Mathru M, Blakeman B: Don't drown the "down lung" (Editorial). Chest 103:6, 1993.
89. Shapira OM, Shahian DM: Postpneumonectomy pulmonary edema (Review). Ann Thorac Surg 56:190, 1993.
90. Zeldin RA, Normandin D, Landtwing D, et al: Post-pneumonectomy pulmonary edema. J Thorac Cardiovasc Surg 87:359, 1984.
91. Turnage WS, Lunn JJ: Postpneumonectomy pulmonary edema: A retrospective analysis of associated variables. Chest 103:1646, 1993.
92. Mathru M, Blakeman B, Dries DJ, et al: Permeability pulmonary edema following lung resection. Chest 98:1216, 1990.
93. Tarhan S, Lundborg RO: Carlens endobronchial catheter versus regular endotracheal tube during thoracic surgery: A comparison of blood gas tensions and pulmonary shunting. Can Anaesth Soc J 18:594, 1971.
94. Torda TA, McCullough CH, O'Brien HD, et al: Pulmonary venous admixture during one-lung anesthesia. Anaesthesia 29:272, 1974.
95. Aalto-Setala M, Heinonen J, Salorinne Y: Cardiorespiratory function during thoracic anaesthesia: A comparison of two-lung ventilation and one-lung ventilation with and without PEEP. Acta Anaesthesiol Scand 19:287, 1975.
96. Capan LM, Turndorf H, Chandrakant P, et al: Optimization of arterial oxygenation during one-lung anesthesia. Anesth Analg 59:847, 1980.
97. Katz JA, Laverne RG, Fairley HB, Thomas AN: Pulmonary oxygen exchange during endobronchial anesthesia—effects of tidal volume and PEEP. Anesthesiology 56:164, 1982.
98. Smith GB, Hirsch NP, Ehrenwerth J: Placement of double-lumen endobronchial tubes—correlation between clinical impressions and bronchoscopic findings. Br J Anaesth 58:1317, 1986.
99. McKenna MJ, Wilson RS, Botelho RJ: Right upper lobe obstruction with right-sided double-lumen endobrochial tubes: A comparison of two tube types. J Cardiothorac Anesth 2:734, 1988.
100. Wahba WM: Influence of aging on lung function—animal significance of changes for age twenty. Anesth Analg 62:764, 1983.
101. Slinger P, Hickey DR, Lenis SG, et al: Intrinsic PEEP during one-lung ventilation. Anesth Analg 68:S269, 1989.
102. Slinger P, Suissa S, Adam J, Triolet W: Predicting arterial oxygenation during one-lung ventilation with continuous positive airway pressure to the non-ventilated lung. J Cardiothorac Anesth 4:436, 1990.

103. Kerr LH, Smith AC, Prys-Roberts C, et al: Observations during endobronchial anesthesia II. Oxygenation. Br J Anaesth 46:84, 1974.
104. Nomoto Y: Preoperative pulmonary blood flow and one-lung anesthesia. Can J Anaesth 34:447, 1987.
105. Hurford WE, Kolker AC, Strauss W: The use of ventilation-perfusion lung scans to predict oxygenation during one-lung anesthesia. Anesthesiology 67:841, 1987.
106. Nunn JF: Applied respiratory physiology, 4th ed. London, Butterworth-Heinemann, 1993, p 143.
107. Kaneko K, Milic-Emili J, Dolovich MB, et al: Regional distribution of ventilation and perfusion as a function of body position. J Appl Physiol 21:767, 1966.
108. Bergman NA: Reduction in resting end-expiratory position of the respiratory system with induction of anesthesia and neuromuscular paralysis. Anesthesiology 57:14, 1982.
109. Froese AB, Bryan AC: Effects of anesthesia and paralysis on diaphragmatic mechanics in man. Anesthesiology 41:242, 1974.
110. Rehder K, Sessler AD, Rodarte JR: Regional intrapulmonary gas distribution in awake and anesthetized-paralyzed man. J Appl Physiol 42:391, 1977.
111. Miller FL, Chen L, Malmkvist G, et al: Mechanical factors do not influence blood flow distribution in atelectasis. Anesthesiology 70:481, 1989.
112. Friedlander M, Sandler A, Kavanagh B, et al: Is hypoxic pulmonary vasoconstriction important during single lung ventilation in the lateral decubitus position? Can J Anaesth 41:26, 1994.
113. Von Euler US, Liljestrand G: Observations on the pulmonary arterial blood pressure in the cat. Acta Physiol Scand 12:301, 1946.
114. Benumof JL: Mechanism of decreased blood flow to atelectatic lung. J Appl Physiol 46:1047, 1979.
115. Benumof JL: One lung ventilation and hypoxic pulmonary vasoconstriction: Implications for anesthetic management. Anesth Analg 64:821, 1985.
116. Bergman NA: Hypoxic pulmonary vasoconstriction. Semin Anesth 6:188, 1987.
117. Sprague RS, Thiemermann C, Vane JR: Endogenous endothelium-derived relaxing factor opposes hypoxic pulmonary vasoconstriction and supports blood flow to hypoxic alveoli in anesthetized rabbits. Proc Natl Acad Sci USA 89:8711, 1992.
118. McCormack DG, Crawley DE, Evans TW: New perspectives in the pulmonary circulation and hypoxic pulmonary vasoconstriction. Pulm Pharmacol 6:97, 1993.
119. Freden F, Wei SZ, Berglund JE, et al: Nitric oxide modulation of pulmonary blood flow distribution in lobar hypoxia. Anesthesiology 82:1216, 1995.
120. Kato M, Staub NC: Response of small pulmonary arteries to unilobar hypoxia and hypercapnia. Circ Res 19:426, 1966.
121. Marshall C, Marshall BE: Site and sensitivity for stimulation of HPV. J Appl Physiol 55:711, 1983.
122. Marshall C, Marshall BE: Influence of perfusate PO_2 on HPV in rats. Circ Res 52:691, 1983.
123. Domino KB, Wetstein L, Glasser SA, et al: Influence of mixed venous oxygen tension on blood flow to atelectatic lung. Anesthesiology 59:428, 1983.
124. Marshall BE, Marshall C, Magno M, et al: Influence of bronchial arterial PO_2 on pulmonary vascular resistance. J Appl Physiol 70:405, 1991.
125. Hauge A: Conditions governing the pressor response to ventilation hypoxia in isolated perfused rat lungs. Acta Physiol Scand 72:33, 1968.
126. Marshall BE, Marshall C: Continuity of response to hypoxic pulmonary vasoconstriction. J Appl Physiol 59:189, 1980.
127. Scanlon TS, Benumof JL, Wahrenbrock EA, Nelson WL: Hypoxic pulmonary vasoconstriction and the ratio of hypoxic lung to perfused normoxic lung. Anesthesiology 49:177, 1978.
128. Marshall C, Marshall BE: Site and sensitivity for stimulation of HPV. J Appl Physiol 55:711, 1983.
129. Cutaia M, Rounds S: Hypoxic pulmonary vasoconstriction: Physiologic significance, mechanism and clinical relevance. Chest 97:708, 1990.
130. Colley PS, Cheney FW: Sodium nitroprusside increases Qs/Qt in dogs with regional atelectasis. Anesthesiology 47:338, 1977.
131. Vann Keer L, Van Aken H, Vandermeersch E, Vermaut G: Propofol does not inhibit HPV in humans. J Clin Anesth 1:284, 1989.
132. Eisenkaft JB: Effects of anesthetics on the pulmonary circulation. Br J Anesth 65:63, 1990.
133. Cheney FW, Colley PS: The effect of cardic output on arterial blood oxygenation. Anesthesiology 52:496, 1980.
134. Katz JA, Larlane RG, Rairby HB, et al: Pulmonary oxygen exchange during endobronchial anesthesia: Effect of tidal volume and PEEP. Anesthesiology 56:164, 1980.
135. Khanam T, Branthwaite MA: Arterial oxygenation during one-lung anesthesia. Anaesthesia 23:280, 1973.
136. Alfery DD, Benumof JL, Trousdale FR: Improving oxygenation during one-lung ventilation in dogs: The effects of positive end-expiratory pressure and blood flow restriction to the nonventilated lung. Anesthesiology 55:381, 1981.
137. Cohen E, Eisenkraft JB, Thys DM, et al: Oxygenation and hemodynamic changes during one-lung ventilation. J Cardiothorac Anesth 2:34, 1988.
138. Hedenstierna G, Baehrendtz S, Klingstedt C, et al: Ventilation and perfusion of each lung during differential ventilation with selective PEEP. Anesthesiology 61:369, 1984.
139. Slinger P, Triolet W, Wilson J: Improving arterial oxygenation during one lung ventilation. Anesthesiology 68:291, 1988.
140. Thiagarajah S, Job C, Rao A: A device for applying CPAP to the non-ventilated lung during unilateral pulmonary ventilation. Anesthesiology 61:217, 1984.
141. Lylons TE: A simplified method of CPAP delivery to the non-ventilated lung during unilateral pulmonary ventilation. Anesthesiology 61:217, 1984.
142. Martini N: Preoperative staging and surgery for non-small cell cancer. In Aisner J (ed): Lung Cancer. New York, Churchill Livingstone, 1985, p 101.

CHAPTER 27

Anesthesia for Bronchoscopy and Mediastinoscopy

Roger S. Wilson, M.D.

Bronchoscopy

Bronchoscopy has been an important diagnostic and therapeutic procedure for the management of thoracic disease dating back to the turn of the century. For many years the standard approach to bronchoscopy employed the use of the rigid bronchoscope, as initially designed by Chevalier Jackson.[1] The rigid bronchoscope has been used for a wide variety of procedures including foreign body removal, pulmonary toilet, and the diagnosis and management of airway and pulmonary neoplasm. The technique of bronchoscopy was dramatically revolutionized in 1968, when Ikeda et al.[2] introduced the concept of a flexible bronchofiberscope. This device provided enhanced diagnostic and therapeutic utility associated with greater versatility, and the ability to perform this procedure in a more controlled and safer manner. The flexible bronchoscope, due to the ease of use and portability, moved the procedure from the operating room to a variety of other settings including outpatient and intensive care units. It also expanded the list of users to other physicians including anesthesiologists, critical care specialists, and pulmonologists. Contemporary bronchoscopy still relies on the utilization of both techniques—rigid and flexible—since both have decided roles and their own specific diagnostic and therapeutic indications.

Indications for Rigid Versus Flexible Bronchoscopy

Diagnostic and therapeutic bronchoscopy plays a significant role in the management of numerous pulmonary diseases. There are multiple clinical indications for performing bronchoscopy (Table 27–1). The choice of one technique over the other is dependent on many variables including availability of equipment, experience of the operator, and issues relating to patient safety and comfort. In some instances use of the flexible bronchoscope offers decided advantages over the rigid equipment. Under specific circumstances both techniques may be used concomitantly to either improve diagnostic yield or to facilitate a specific therapy.

Rigid Bronchoscopy

Rigid endoscopy generally is the preferred technique when issues of airway patency and control are paramount. This is especially true in situations where airways are occluded with foreign material, including massive hemoptysis, foreign body aspiration, aspiration of particulate material, and tumor invading the airway.[3–5] Moderate to massive hemoptysis is more efficiently managed using the rigid technique, since the operator has improved capability of suctioning and visualizing the potential source of bleeding when compared to use of the fiberoptic technique. The rigid bronchoscope provides an efficient means of packing and/or applying a topical vasoconstrictors to the bleeding site. Whereas small foreign bodies can be visualized and potentially grasped with fiberoptic techniques, the open rigid scope provides much more versatility in terms of types and size of forceps and improved ability to manipulate and remove the foreign body. In situations where the trachea or mainstem bronchi are occluded with various types of benign and malignant tumors the rigid approach provides distinct advantages. Airway management is facilitated, since the rigid scope can be passed distal to tumor, granulation tissue, or a strictured segment of the airway. Debulking of tumor with ability to biopsy larger specimens can be of decided therapeutic and also potentially diagnostic advantage.

Palliative therapies such as laser destruction of tumor and internal stenting of diseased airways frequently requires use of the rigid technique during some component of the procedure.[6] The rigid bronchoscope provides better depth perception and less distortion during evaluation of airway disease. It also provides a conduit for specific types of laser therapy and as a channel to manipulate simple or complex tracheal or tracheobronchial stints.

Endoscopic evaluation of the neonate or pediatric patient is often accomplished using the rigid technique, since it provides for better visualization and airway control when extremely small endotracheal tube size is required. In many cases it is the only available option due to the incompatibility of smaller flexible equipment and narrow lumen endotracheal tubes.

TABLE 27–1
Indications for Bronchoscopy

Massive hemoptysis
Airway obstruction/pathology
Neoplasm
Benign stricture
Foreign body
Inhalation injury
Trauma
Secretion removal and/or culture
Laser therapy
Endobronchial stinting
Endotracheal/tracheostomy tube positioning
Alveolar lavage

Flexible Fiberoptic Bronchoscopy

During the past 30 years the flexible fiberoptic bronchoscope has become the technique of choice for the vast majority of diagnostic and therapeutic endoscopic procedures. In comparison to the rigid bronchoscope, it enables visualization of more distal areas of the lung, provides better diagnostic and therapeutic yields and, when combined with video imaging using closed circuit systems, allows for visualization by other members of the team including the anesthesiologist. The majority of patients who present with both malignant and nonmalignant disease are generally assessed initially with fiberoptic techniques. This provides for excellent visualization of airway distortion, compression, and direct evasion from the tumor. Appropriate tissue samples are obtained either using small biopsy forceps and/or a brush technique. Modern fiberscopes with ample suction channels afford opportunity to remove secretions either for a diagnostic or therapeutic purpose. Hemoptysis, if mild in nature, can be adequately managed, provided that the blood in the airway does not obscure the light source and/or optics at the distal tip of the scope.

In general, patient comfort and safety are better served with the fiberoptic as opposed to the rigid technique. The procedure can be carried out either with or without use of an endotracheal intubation. As discussed in detail later in this chapter, the procedure may be performed with little to no sedation often with use of topical anesthesia or with general anesthesia. In cases where congenital defects, abnormal anatomy, trauma, or disease has involved the upper airway, the flexible scope may be simpler and safer when compared with the rigid method. In addition, use of the fiberoptic techniques provides anesthesiologists and critical care physicians the opportunity to confirm and/or reposition a variety of airway devices such as endotracheal tubes, double-lumen endobronchial tubes, and tracheostomy tubes. Stint placement and laser therapy may be managed with flexible equipment alone or in combination with rigid devices.

Equipment

Rigid Bronchoscopy

Rigid bronchoscopy requires several basic components of equipment in order to perform the procedure. As depicted in Figure 27–1, the components include the rigid

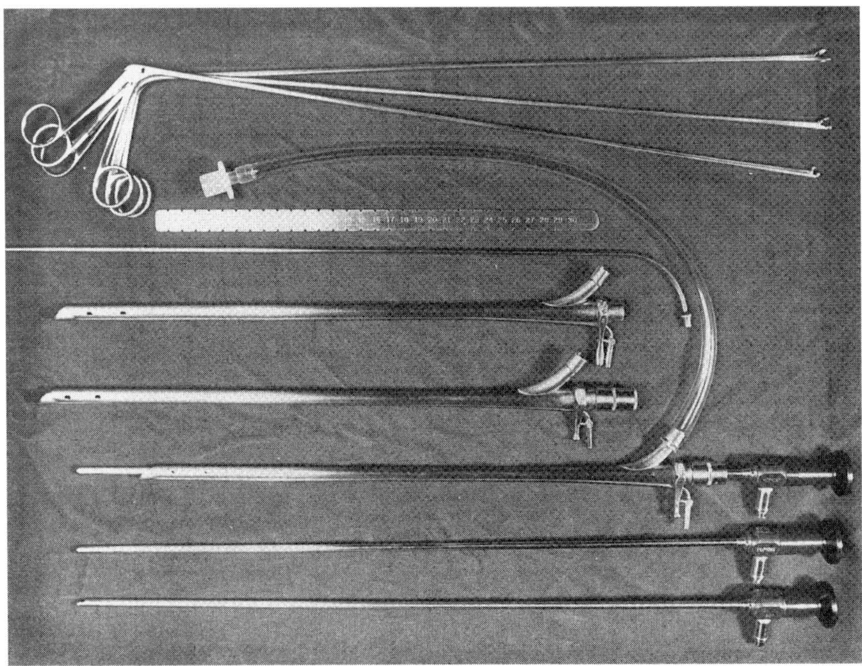

FIGURE **27–1.** Basic components for rigid bronchoscopy. Top to bottom: biopsy forceps, ruler, suction cannula, three bronchoscopes of different size (lower is fitted with a telescope and attachment for ventilation), and rigid (Hopkins) telescopes. (From Keshavjee S, Ginsberg RJ: Rigid bronchoscopy. In Pearson FG, et al [eds]: Thoracic Surgery. New York, Churchill Livingstone, 1995, p 190, with permission.)

bronchoscope, light source, suction device, forceps, and telescopes.

Bronchoscopes

Contemporary rigid bronchoscopes are all designed after the original type described by Jackson.[1] Adult scopes are generally 40 cm in length and vary from 6 to 9 mm in external cross-sectional diameter. Scopes of smaller diameter and of shorter length are available for use in pediatric patients and in adults where limited airway diameter, often seen with tumor and benign stricture, require downsizing of equipment. A light source is provided by a light carrier that is passed into a channel with the light tip located at the distal end of the scope. This is connected via a fiberoptic bundle to a cold halogen light source.

Accessories

Several devices are available to be in inserted through the scope depending on the intended purpose of the endoscopy. An important component of the equipment is a rigid suction cannula, which is designed to be long enough to protrude through the distal end of the scope. This suctioning device is essential to clear the airway of secretions, often during insertion of the scope, and to maintain a clear passage throughout the procedure. The suction cannula may incorporate a cautery tip used to coagulate specific sites of hemorrhage within the airway and used in conjunction with biopsy forceps during tumor debulking and/or biopsy. A wide variety of forceps are available for tissue biopsy and débridement, and to aid in the removal of foreign body and clotted blood. In general they are designed to provide deeper and more substantial biopsy specimens when compared to the smaller and finer design of forceps used with the fiberoptic technique. Telescopes are also designed to pass through the rigid bronchoscope. Modern telescopes provide outstanding optics and also afford ability to view beyond the "straight ahead" view afforded solely through the rigid scope. Designs include 0-, 30-, 60-, and 90-degree optics.

Fiberoptic Bronchoscopes

Several types of flexible fiberoptic bronchoscopes are currently available. Basic components include a fiberoptic light source, fiberoptic channel of imaging bundles, and one or more working channels for suctioning and insertion of ancillary equipment such as biopsy forceps, laser bundles, and culture devices. The configuration and variation of these components are a function of the external diameter moving from the smaller (3.5-mm) pediatric scopes to the larger (6.0-mm) adult types. Design features include the degree of flexibility of the distal tip and various components to equip the scope for video imaging. The proximal end of the scope is designed with features to provide attachment for suction from control for application of suction to the suction channel and individual ports to enable installation of saline for lavage and drugs such as local anesthetics.

Ventilation Techniques During Bronchoscopy

Rigid Bronchoscopy

As is true for any procedure, adequacy of ventilation to ensure oxygenation and carbon dioxide elimination is of prime importance. The method used to provide ventilation during rigid bronchoscopy is variable and dependent upon technical issues, objectives of the procedure, and the existent pulmonary pathology. In general Three techniques are available and include (1) spontaneous ventilation, (2) apneic oxygenation, and (3) positive-pressure ventilation. Spontaneous ventilation, although seldom used with rigid endoscopy, is an alternative. In selected cases, although rare, where rigid endoscopy is performed under topical anesthesia with or without supplemental sedation, spontaneous ventilation with supplemental inspired oxygen is feasible. Spontaneous ventilation during a general anesthetic, although possible, is less desirable due to the respiratory depression produced by either intravenous, inhalation, or combined techniques. Special conditions where this method of ventilation might be considered are circumstances concerning aspirated foreign body, especially when positive-pressure ventilation increases the risk of displacement and potential impaction of the foreign material into the more distal airway. During such circumstances, spontaneous ventilation may be utilized, especially at the initial part of the procedure, while the airway is being intubated and to the point where it can be ascertained as to where the foreign body resides. This is most important when movement of the foreign body with positive-pressure ventilation could occur.

Apneic oxygenation was first described by Fruman and colleagues in 1959.[7] Although seldom used in contemporary practice, it should be remembered that oxygenation, in the absence of ventilation, does provide safe operating conditions under certain circumstances and is a viable alternative. As initially described when using this technique, patients are denitrogenated either before or following induction of intravenous anesthesia and then treated with an appropriate neuromuscular blocking agent. The system must be designed such that oxygen can be delivered continuously into the conducting airway either through a catheter or some attachment within the bronchoscope. No attempt is made to provide ventilation and thus the rate of increase in alveolar and arterial carbon dioxide is a function of carbon dioxide production. Oxygenation is dependent on the integrity of lung volume, which is dictated by several variables including the initial functional residual capacity, the rate of absorption atelectasis, airway pressure (relative to atmospheric pressure), and other similar variables. Adequacy of oxygenation for periods of several minutes to approximately 1 hour has been described. The current practice of monitoring with pulse oximetry increases the feasibility and safety of this technique compared to the reliance on vital signs and observation of cyanosis when initially described.

The majority of rigid bronchoscopic procedures are carried out using some form of positive-pressure venti-

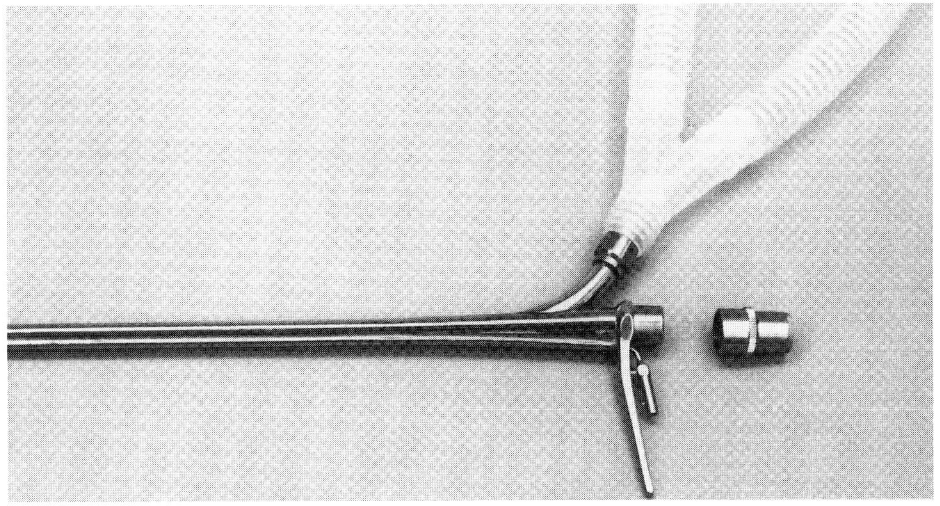

FIGURE **27–2.** Rigid bronchoscope with side-arm ventilation port attached to ventilation circuit. Optional eyepiece with lens can be used to close the distal end of the scope during use. (From Ehrenworth J, Brull SJ: Anesthesia for thoracic diagnostic procedures. In Kaplan JA [ed]: Thoracic Anesthesia, 2nd ed. New York, Churchill Livingstone, 1991, p 721, with permission.)

lation. This is accomplished either with traditional intermittent positive-pressure ventilation with hand-bag or mechanical ventilator or with use of a "jet" technique. Ventilating bronchoscopes with appropriate side ports, which can be attached directly to the anesthesia circuit, are technically the easiest to use. Intermittent digital occlusion of the proximal end of the bronchoscope or use of a glass-windowed port will provide a closed system for positive-pressure ventilation. The advantages of this technique is that it can be used with a wide variety of anesthetic agents, provides for optimization of lung volume, especially functional residual capacity (FRC), and provides for high concentrations of inspired oxygen. One limitation is the potential for excessive leakage around the bronchoscope through the glottic opening. This can be controlled by packing the posterior pharynx. Ventilation must be intercepted if the window is removed during use of suction cannula, biopsy forceps, or other similar devices. The latter results in potential loss of lung volume and egress of inhalation anesthetic agents into the operating room. Examples of rigid bronchoscopes equipped with ventilation side ports with or without telescopes are depicted in Figures 27–1 through 27–3.

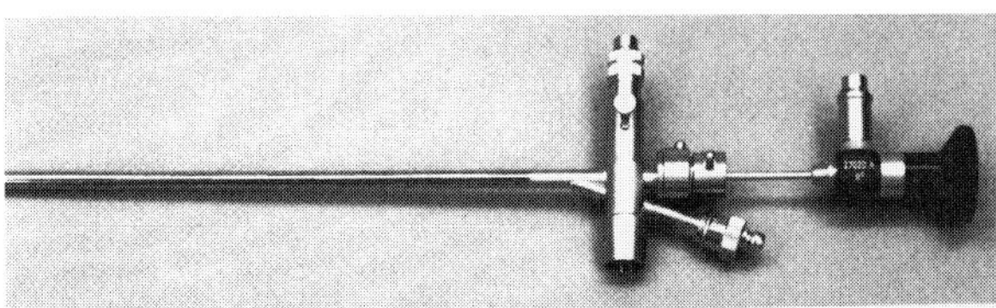

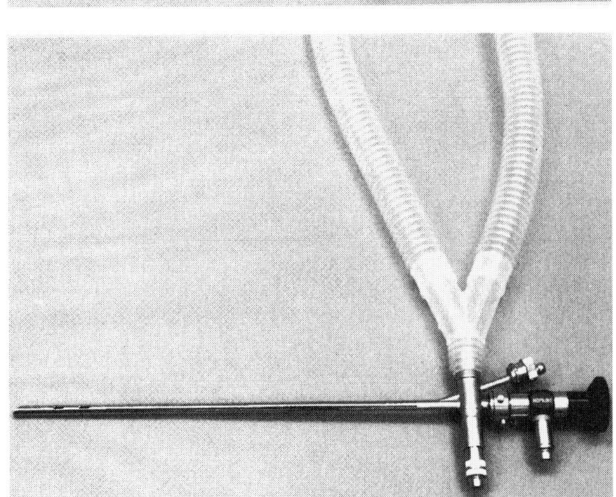

FIGURE **27–3.** Rigid ventilating bronchoscope with Hopkins telescope. (From Ehrenworth J, Brull SJ: Anesthesia for thoracic diagnostic procedures. In Kaplan JA [ed]: Thoracic Anesthesia, 2nd ed. New York, Churchill Livingstone, 1991, with permission.)

High-pressure jet or Venturi technique can also be used. A method described by Sanders[8] in 1967 employed a simple ventilating attachment for the bronchoscope. This device (Fig. 27–4) incorporates an injector fitted with an appropriate connection to supply intermittent positive pressure to the rigid bronchoscope (Fig. 27–5). The device incorporates the previously described adaptor attached to the bronchoscope, a high-pressure source with adjustable reducing valve and some form of triggering mechanism to intermittently connect the variable pressure oxygen source to the cannula attached to the proximal end of the bronchoscope. This system is dependent upon the Venturi principle. The high-pressure

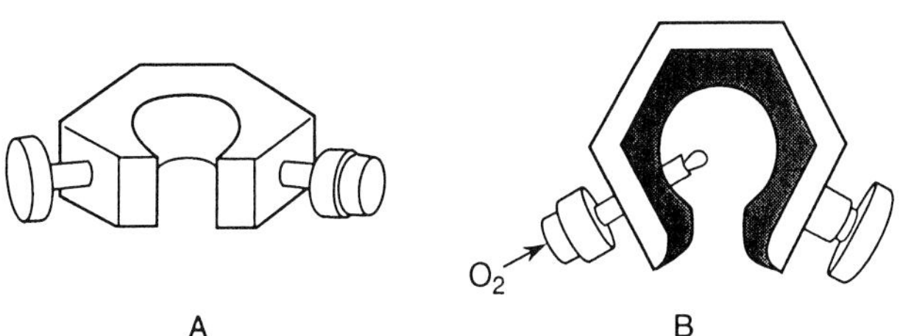

FIGURE **27–4.** Diagram of a Sanders injector attachment. *A*, Side view. *B*, Top view. (From Ehrenworth J, Brull SJ: Anesthesia for thoracic diagnostic procedures. In Kaplan JA [ed]: Thoracic Anesthesia, 2nd ed. New York, Churchill Livingstone, 1991, with permission.)

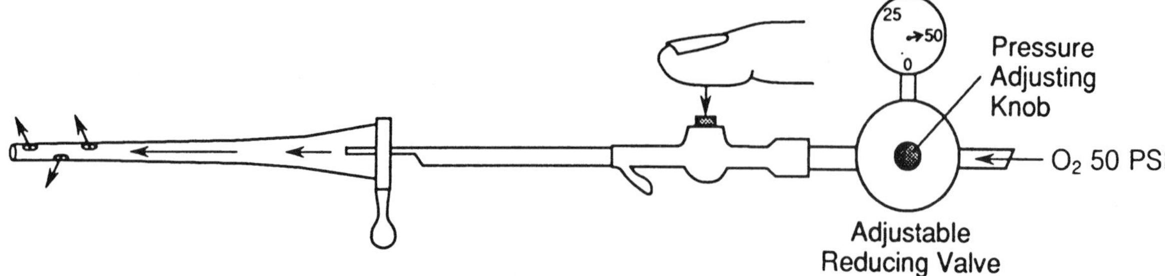

FIGURE **27–5.** Schematic of Sanders system. See text for details. (From Ehrenworth J, Brull SJ: Anesthesia for thoracic diagnostic procedures. In Kaplan JA [ed]: Thoracic Anesthesia, 2nd ed. New York, Churchill Livingstone, 1991, with permission.)

driving gas, in this case oxygen, jetted through the narrow orifice (Fig. 27–6) creates a negative pressure and thus entrains room air. Disadvantages include the limitations of inspired oxygen concentration due to dilution by room air and insufficient ventilation during conditions of reduced thoracic compliance. Carden et al.[9] described an important modification to this apparatus in 1973 (Fig. 27–7). This approach utilizes the side arm of the bronchoscope as the injector site. With the exception of the Venturi principle, lacking entrainment of room air, the system incorporates all of the other features previously described including high-pressure source, pressure-regulating device, and trigger mechanism. Advantages include the availability of high oxygen concentrations and the availability of higher driving pressures and hence more efficient ventilation in cases of decreased compliance. Other modifications could include incorporation of nitrous oxide during ventilation and an air/oxygen blender to control the inspired concentration of oxygen where reduced concentrations may be important due to factors during the use of laser techniques and/or past history of specific chemotherapeutic agents. Inherent dangers include potential for inadequate ventilation due to insufficient number of breaths, driving pressure, or technical problems and the potential for overdistention of the respiratory system resulting in cardiovascular compromise and potential for barotrauma. The latter, overdistention, is likely to occur where system problems or distal airway pathology create situations where there is inadequate cross-sectional diameter or inadequate time is allowed for exhalation.

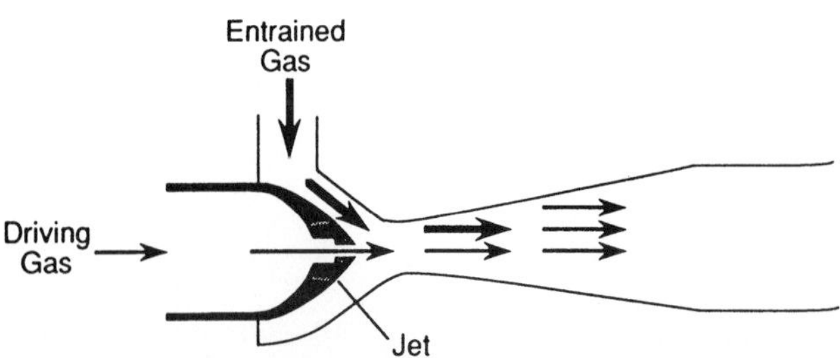

FIGURE **27–6.** Venturi principle. See text for details. (From Ehrenworth J, Brull SJ: Anesthesia for thoracic diagnostic procedures. In Kaplan JA [ed]: Thoracic Anesthesia, 2nd ed. New York, Churchill Livingstone, 1991, with permission.)

Commercially available and more sophisticated high-frequency jet ventilation systems can also be applied during rigid bronchoscopy.[10] They provide more versatility with respect to rate and aspects concerning the pattern of ventilation but also increase the complexity and cost of the system. Potential complications including overdistention and subsequent sequelae are similar to those previously described with these techniques.

Fiberoptic Bronchoscopy

The management of ventilation during use of the fiberoptic bronchoscopic technique is governed by several factors. In patients who are undergoing bronchoscopy without use of endotracheal intubation, spontaneous ventilation with supplemental oxygen is preferred. This can be achieved with use of a nasal cannula or using a modified commercially available face mask. In cases where endotracheal intubation with or without general anesthesia is used it is best to incorporate a commercially available right-angle swivel device (Fig. 27–8). Such a device facilitates passage of the bronchoscope into the respiratory system while maintaining the integrity and continuity of the anesthetic circle and hence ensuring potential adequacy of ventilation, oxygenation, and administration of volatile anesthetic if desired. One obvious limitation is the relationship of the internal diameter or cross-sectional area of the endotracheal tube and the external diameter of the fiberoptic bronchoscope. Careful selection, ensuring maximal endotracheal tube size and appropriate selection of the fiberoptic bronchoscope, will ensure adequacy of cross-sectional area around the bronchoscope to provide for sufficient inspired tidal volume and allow for passive exhalation. As previously described with jet techniques, either inadequacy of time or flow during exhalation and inappropriate timing of subsequent inspiration may result in progressive increase in lung volume, again leading to either cardiovascular compromise or barotrauma.

Anesthetic Techniques

The extent of preoperative assessment and preparation by the anesthesiologist, in part, depends on the nature of the pre-existing illness, presence of comorbid disease,

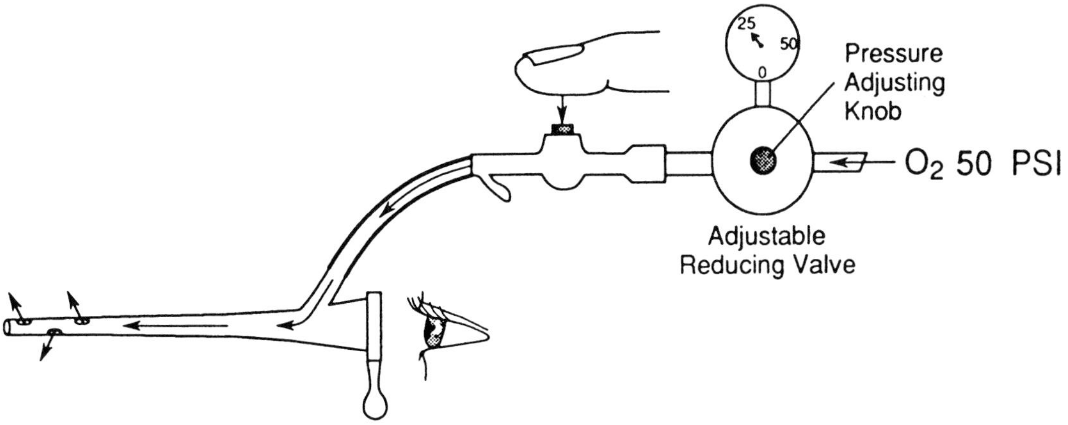

FIGURE **27–7.** Carden modification with side-arm ventilating bronchoscope. (From Ehrenworth J, Brull SJ: Anesthesia for thoracic diagnostic procedures. In Kaplan JA [ed]: Thoracic Anesthesia, 2nd ed. New York, Churchill Livingstone, 1991, with permission.)

the magnitude of the anticipated procedures beyond bronchoscopy, and the urgency for bronchoscopic evaluation. The majority of bronchoscopies are performed to diagnose disease in patients with nonspecific respiratory symptoms such as wheezing, stridor, or minor hemoptysis. Although such symptoms may be associated with early, potentially severe life-threatening pulmonary conditions, they also can be manifestations of chronic conditions such as bronchitis frequently associated with cigarette abuse. In many patients, diagnostic bronchoscopy is a component of work-up in clinical staging of lung cancer. Again, in the absence of significant comorbid disease involving the lung (e.g., chronic obstructive pulmonary disease [COPD], bronchospastic disease) or the cardiovascular system (e.g., coronary artery disease, peripheral vascular disease) the procedure in and of itself carries little known perioperative risk. The anesthetic assessment including laboratory and other diagnostic evaluations such as electrocardiogram (ECG) are based on institutional policies and individual preference. In many instances, because of the emergent nature of the procedure, such as aspiration of gastric material, foreign body, or life-threatening hemoptysis, minimal time will be available for any detailed evaluation.

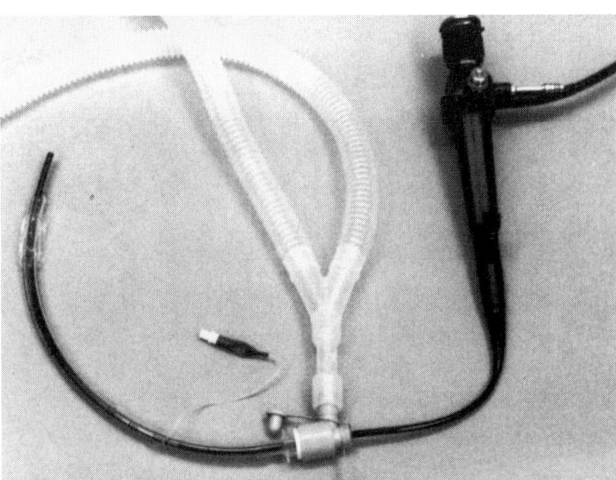

FIGURE **27–8.** Standard elbow attachment to an endotracheal tube providing ventilator circuit attachment and diaphragm seal for bronchoscope access. (From Ehrenworth J, Brull SJ: Anesthesia for thoracic diagnostic procedures. In Kaplan JA [ed]: Thoracic Anesthesia, 2nd ed. New York, Churchill Livingstone, 1991, with permission.)

Premedication

Selection of appropriate premedication is based on the patient's general state of health, the proposed surgical technique, and the operative setting (inpatient vs. outpatient). The objectives are similar to those for any other patient undergoing anesthesia. Included are analgesia; depression of reflexes, especially cough and vasovagal; diminution of oral and airway secretions; and the alleviation of anxiety. Combinations of narcotics, anticholinergics, and benzodiazepines are generally selected to achieve these objectives. It is obvious that the plan for premedication is somewhat dependent on the technique employed be it rigid or fiberoptic, the choice of local versus general anesthesia, and the extent of pre-existing pulmonary disease with potential for postprocedural complications.

Specific Considerations

The choice of anesthetic technique is dependent on bronchoscopic technique, intended procedure and concomitant surgery, patient preference, and significance of any pre-existing systemic disease. The use of the fiberoptic bronchoscopy provides conditions for the greatest versatility with respect to overall anesthetic care and management. Fundamental goals include amnesia, analgesia, and relaxation.

Topical anesthesia is frequently selected for reasonably healthy cooperative patients undergoing simple diagnostic or bedside procedures. Topical agents have traditionally included lidocaine, cocaine, or tetracaine.

Administration of the local anesthetic to pharyngeal and tracheobronchial structures must be done in a well-organized and precise fashion to achieve maximal effect. Drugs can be administered via nebulization with simple or ultrasonic nebulizers attached to a face mask, direct application of local anesthetics using bulb spray or commercially available atomizers, and direct application using cotton-tip applicators. Topical anesthesia provides sensory block but in most cases fails to attenuate the activity of pressure receptors thus leaving gag reflexes intact. Transtracheal injection of local anesthetic, generally 2 to 3 ml of 4% lidocaine, is easily and safely performed through transtracheal or cricothyroid membrane puncture. Various techniques have described use of small-gauge needles or intravenous catheters to minimize discomfort and potential trauma.

Nerve blocks are frequently used to supplement topical techniques. Glossopharyngeal nerve block can be accomplished orally with injection of local anesthetic into the lateral pharyngeal wall at the root of the tongue.[11] The technique has been described using 26- or 27-gauge needles with lidocaine often containing epinephrine. The superior laryngeal nerve block is performed using the superior thyroid cornu of the cricoid cartilage as a landmark. Use of these blocks will provide analgesia to sites superior to the glottis. Anesthesia to structures beneath the vocal cord is best accomplished through a transtracheal route. Although these topical and nerve block approaches are safe and inherently easy to perform, there is always potential for allergic reaction to the local anesthetic and for local trauma, and one must be aware of increased potential for aspiration of oral pharyngeal and gastric contents should motor or sensory components involved with laryngeal function and tracheal reflexes be altered.

The approach to general anesthesia includes selection of induction and maintenance agents, and consideration for the use of muscle relaxants. Selection of these agents in great part depends on the existence of systemic disease, the nature of the proposed surgical procedure, and the need to minimize the postprocedural recovery time. All intravenous induction agents including ketamine, thiopental, propofol, and etomidate are suitable. The choice depends on individual preference and other components of the anesthetic plan. Inhalation agents, often in combination with narcotic, barbiturate, or propofol bolus/infusion, provide adequate operating conditions. For many patients, the use of a short- to intermediate-acting nondepolarizer with or without succinylcholine for intubation facilitates a quiet operative field and potentially minimizes the need for high doses of inhalation or intravenous agents that would be necessary to maintain respiratory depression and attenuate gag and coughing during the procedure. Application of a local anesthetic to the pharyngeal mucosa and the trachea can also be used to supplement general anesthetics.

Although rarely done, rigid bronchoscopy can be accomplished with use of local anesthetics and topical or local anesthesia. Patient cooperation, experience of the operator, and the nature of the procedure dictate the potential use of this method. Passage of the rigid bronchoscope through the oral, posterior pharynx, and larynx requires that sufficient muscle relaxation and depression of vocal cord activity be provided to ensure optimal conditions. Most often this is accomplished with intravenous induction accompanied by use of depolarizing or nondepolarizing relaxants. The maintenance technique, be it inhalation or intravenous, is in great part dependent upon ventilation techniques used during the bronchoscopic procedure. Techniques using an open system with the previously described Sanders injector should preclude use of nitrous oxide and inhalation agents, making total intravenous anesthesia the technique of choice. Closed systems in which inhalation agents with or without nitrous oxide can be provided offer greater degrees of flexibility. Again, muscle relaxation is generally employed during the major component of diagnostic or therapeutic bronchoscopy, especially with the additional stimulation provided with use of rigid bronchoscope. Again, use of topical anesthesia involving pharyngeal and tracheal bronchial structures can play an important role in the overall anesthetic management.

Complications

In general, complications are a direct result of anesthetic technique and surgical manipulation (Table 27–2). Surgical complications, although rare, occur predominantly from trauma or biopsy. Reported death rates are less than 1% and complication rates are less than 10%.[12–14] Rigid techniques create the potential for trauma to any soft tissue or structure within the path of the distal tip of the bronchoscope. Dental injury, and trauma to oral and pharyngeal mucosa, laryngeal structures, and the integrity of the tracheal bronchial tree, can incur. Biopsy and/or destruction of airway lesions has potential to produce significant bleeding. Bleeding at biopsy sites is generally of minor significance, although destruction and attempted biopsy of intraluminal granulation tissue and/or tumor can lead to problematic and life-threatening hem-

TABLE 27–2
Complications

Surgical
Dental/oropharyngeal/laryngeal trauma
Airway disruption
Local tracheobronchial injury
Pneumothorax
Bleeding
Anesthetics
Inadequate ventilation
Hypoxemia
Hypercarbia
Sympathetic response
Hypertension
Hypotension
Arrhythmia
Bronchospasm
Awareness
Residual anesthetic agent effects
Combined
Local anesthetic reactions
Cardiopulmonary dysfunction

orrhage. Airway disruption, especially when unnoted, can lead to catastrophic, life-threatening tension pneumothorax. A timely diagnosis and immediate, appropriate therapy is essential. A high index of suspicion when otherwise unexplainable changes in cardiovascular function arise during the procedure is necessary. Flexible bronchoscopy potentially avoids the likelihood of soft tissue injury but still carries inherent risks of airway hemorrhage and disruption with invasive procedures. Other procedural complications as they relate to stint placement, laser therapy, and injury to the peripheral lung with transbronchial biopsy are self-evident and beyond the scope of this chapter.

Anesthetic complications, although varied, are usually related to either inadequacies of ventilation, results of autonomic system imbalance, or the result of excessive or insufficient anesthesia. Inadequacies of ventilation result in varying degrees of hypoxemia and hypercarbia depending on the nature of the mechanism and the presence of underlying cardiac and/or pulmonary disease. Awareness and vigilant monitoring should prevent the occurrence of significant problems. More problematic are the perturbations in cardiac rhythm. These occur frequently in the presence of inadequate anesthesia where reflex sympathetic tone may create potential for a variety of well-described arrhythmias, hypertension, or hypotension.[15] Although minor rhythm disturbances are frequent and do not require therapy, major arrhythmias are much less common, with a recorded frequency of 5 to 10%.[16,17] Unintentional anesthetic overdose, be it with inhalation or intravenous agents, always carries the potential for cardiovascular depression.

Awareness is always a potential problem. This problem always exists with potentially short yet stimulating procedures where focus may be directed to airway control, cardiovascular stability, and underlying disease rather than the adequacy of the anesthetic to eliminate auditory or somatic awareness.

Mediastinoscopy

Mediastinoscopy is used primarily in the staging of lung carcinoma to determine the potential for resectability. It is also used to biopsy mediastinal lymph nodes and other masses in order to establish a diagnosis of malignant and nonmalignant disease. Cervical mediastinal exploration was originally described by Harkens and associates in 1994.[18] The contemporary technique is fashioned after that described by Carlens in 1959[19] and expanded by Pearson in 1965.[20] This technique uses a specially designed mediastinoscope introduced through a suprasternal notch incision. It is designed to evaluate lymph node involvement in the superior mediastinum including nodes in the paratracheal areas. Lymph nodes located in the aortopulmonary window can be sampled by a slightly different approach, anterior mediastinotomy, first described by McNeil and Chamberland (1966).[21] Although this technique originally described use of a left parasternal incision it has been employed on the right side to explore disease in the anterior mediastinum, right hilum, and area of the superior vena cava. Extended cervical mediastinoscopy, described by Ginsberg and colleagues,[22] is an extension of the traditional mediastinoscopy and is used as an alternative to left anterior mediastinotomy.

Indications

As previously discussed, the primary indication for mediastinoscopy, as an adjunct to bronchoscopy, is to determine the potential resectability of patients presenting with carcinoma of the lung. Bronchogenic carcinoma that has metastasized to mediastinal lymph nodes (stage IIIa or IIIb) is likely not to benefit from surgical resection. Thus it is important to establish or rule out involvement of mediastinal lymph nodes in order to reduce the incidence of unnecessary thoracotomy. Mediastinoscopy can be performed either as a free-standing procedure, frequently preceded by bronchoscopy, or scheduled in conjunction with bronchoscopy and followed, during the same anesthetic, by thoracotomy and pulmonary resection. Mediastinal biopsies can be accurately evaluated by means of frozen section with the decision made to proceed or not during the course of single anesthetic. Noninvasive diagnostic studies such as computed tomography (CT) and magnetic resonance imaging (MRI), although useful as screening tests to detect the presence of enlarged or suspicious nodes within the mediastinum, have not been shown to date to be sensitive or specific enough to eliminate the need for mediastinoscopy in a large percentage of patients presenting with pulmonary tumors.[23]

There are relatively few absolute contraindications to performing mediastinoscopy. In general, those patients who should not be considered candidates include those with very peripheral pulmonary lesions or anterior mediastinal masses and individuals that are deemed nonresectable candidates for pulmonary resection based on other criteria. Absolute contraindications would basically be those that would preclude any other major surgical procedure such as marked debilitation, bleeding diatheses, and severe comorbid disease. The presence of ascending aortic aneurysm and/or aneurysmal dilatation of arch vessels should almost always be considered a contraindication for this procedure.

Cervical Mediastinoscopy

The procedure is carried out with the patient lying supine, generally with a bolster under the shoulder and the head extended. A small, 3- to 4-cm horizontal incision is used approximately one fingerbreadth above the suprasternal notch. Blunt dissection is then carried out in the midline separating strap muscles, retracting the thyroid out of the surgical field. Small vessels may either be electrocoagulated or tied off with fine sutures. The pretracheal fascia is exposed and entered with blunt dissection carried out along the anterior aspect of the trachea. The superior mediastinum is explored with a finger in order to attempt to palpate suspicious adenopathy. Once accomplished, a mediastinoscope is introduced anterior to the trachea; one should then attempt to visualize possible nodes for biopsy. Dissection of lymph nodes is often carried out using a suction cannula introduced through the mediastinoscope. Appropriate material is biopsied with a variety of forceps. If there is question as to the potential vascular nature of a structure, it is often aspirated with a fine needle and syringe prior to attempted biopsy. Once the appropriate material has been biopsied, the wound is checked for hemostasis and is then closed in an appropriate fashion.

Anterior Mediastinoscopy

As described, anterior mediastinoscopy is utilized to sample nodes in the subaortic and periaortic regions that are not accessible through the standard mediastinal approach. The procedure can use either a small incision through the second left intercostal space or, as originally designed, use a vertical parasternal incision to remove the second costal cartilage. Dissection proceeds much as described for mediastinoscopy using blunt dissection and digital exploration. Ultimately, a mediastinoscope is introduced through the incision in order to visualize appropriate nodes for biopsy.

Anesthetic Technique

Mediastinoscopy can be safely accomplished using either local or general anesthesia.[24,25] It would appear that the former, local anesthesia, although well described for this technique, is rarely used today. Selection is based on operator experience and patient choice and other scheduled, concomitant surgical procedures.

Preoperative evaluation differs little from any other similar procedure with the exception of the issues pertaining to symptomatology of mediastinal masses.[22] Significant issues with masses must consider their local effect with respect to displacement and compression of various structures including arteries, veins, and trachea. The potential for airway compression and associated difficulties with ventilation following any induction of general anesthesia is well described, especially in the pediatric population.[27] It is rarely problematic in the adult with the exception of extensively large masses especially involving the posterior aspect of the trachea. Potential for severe respiratory or cardiovascular compromise following induction and use of positive-pressure ventilation must be carefully considered in patients presenting with severe symptoms. Alternatives such as awake intubation, maintenance of spontaneous ventilation, and postural change must be considered.

Preparation

The use and choice of premedication is based on standard criteria. There are no special considerations when one is considering the patient's scheduled mediastinoscopy.

Positioning of the patient must be considered prior to preoperative placement of monitoring devices, as well as positioning of the anesthesiologist and anesthetic equipment during the procedure. Although approaches can vary, based on surgical preference, in most cases the surgeon will perform the procedure standing at the head of the table. The anesthesiologist and equipment can be appropriately placed at either the right or left side of the patient. Frequently, induction of anesthesia is carried out with the anesthesiologist in the customary position at the head. Once endotracheal intubation is established, the table is rotated 90 degrees for the surgical procedure. Occasionally, the anesthesiologist can be positioned at the head slightly off to the side with the surgeon working off the opposite shoulder.

Monitoring and vascular access must be tailored for the individual patient. In most cases vascular access with a single, adequately sized catheter (16 to 18 gauge) in an upper extremity is adequate. Arterial access is unnecessary for most cases. One caveat is consideration in placement of both blood pressure and pulse oximetry on the upper extremity.[28] The innominate artery crosses from left to right within the mediastinum and lends itself to compression during digital dissection and inspection, and following placement of the mediastinoscope. Such compression obviously could result in altered blood flow to the right hemisphere and right upper extremity. It has been advocated that continuous monitoring with pulse oximetry placed on the digit of the right hand alerts one to the possibility of compression. A standard method would be to use a blood pressure cuff on the left arm and pulse oximetry on the right in order to ensure measurement of blood pressures and to detect the potential for innominate artery compression. Under circumstances where the risk of significant vascular injury occurs, or with potential for venous bleeding, it is prudent to consider placement of a second intravenous in the lower extremity.

A wide variety of anesthetics can be used both for induction and for maintenance of anesthesia. It must be kept in mind that the procedure, although relatively brief in nature, also carries significant potential for stimulation. This is especially true during dissection of the superior mediastinum and compression of the trachea resulting in predictable cardiovascular response but also coughing and bucking. In most centers following use of standard induction agents the maintenance of anesthetic is performed with combinations of inhalation and supplemental agents such as narcotics or intravenous techniques with muscle relaxation. The latter is important to maintain a quiet surgical field, and to avoid coughing and bucking and the potential for increase in venous pressure with the potential for additional bleeding.

Complications

The complications of mediastinoscopy and mediastinotomy are extremely rare.[29,30] An incidence of 1 to 2% has been reported in several series that encompass thousands of patients. Complications include hemorrhage, nerve injury, or biopsy of adjacent structures including pleura and esophagus.

Major complications are most commonly found to be associated with procedures or biopsy at the tracheobronchial angle. The azygos vein and anterior pulmonary artery to the upper lobe are susceptible on the right side. The recurrent laryngeal nerve is most vulnerable at the left tracheobronchial angle. The most significant complication is massive bleeding associated with biopsy of a major vessel, arterial or venous. Venous bleeding is easily controlled with local pressure, either local digital compression or packing. Arterial bleeding obviously has more significant implications with respect to ultimate management.

Injury to other structures including the trachea, esophagus, or pleura are rare. Injury to the esophagus very often is recognized at a later stage when the patient develops mediastinitis, although frozen section may raise suspicion of esophageal biopsy. Tracheal bronchial injury, although rare, should be recognized during the procedure as evidenced by the presence of air bubbles in the surgical field or inability to maintain tidal volume or airway pressure with positive-pressure ventilation.

One must be aware of the potential for significant and potentially catastrophic injury, especially with respect to major blood loss. There always exists the potential for emergent exploration either through mediastinotomy or thoracotomy depending upon the suspected mechanism of injury. One must be prepared to establish additional venous access, especially involving the lower extremity if vascular injury involves vessels related to upper extremities.

Complications occurring from recurrent laryngeal nerve or phrenic nerve injury may pose problems during emergence. Vocal cord paralysis with stridor and airway compromise should be readily apparent and dealt with accordingly. Diaphragmatic dysfunction secondary to injury to the phrenic nerve may be more difficult to ascertain. Venous bleeding and/or pneumothorax leading to tension may occur into one fashion and be more difficult to diagnose. A high index of suspicion, diagnostic acumen, and appropriate evaluation in the postoperative period are most essential to avoid undesirable complications.

References

1. Boyd AD: Chevalier Jackson: The father of American bronchoesophagoscopy. Ann Thorac Surg 57:502, 1994.
2. Ikeda S, Yanain N, Ishikawa S: Flexible bronchofiberscope. Keio J Med 17:1, 1968.
3. Wedzicha JA, Pearson NC: Management of massive hemoptysis. Respir Med 84:9, 1990.
4. Weissberg D, Schwartz I: Foreign bodies in the tracheobronchial tree. Chest 91:730, 1987.
5. Hetzel MR, Smith STT: Endoscopic palliation of tracheobronchial malignancies. Thorax 46:225, 1991.
6. Cooper JD, Pearson FG, et al: Use of silicone stents in the management of airway problems. Ann Thorac Surg 47:371, 1989.
7. Frumin J, Epstein R, Cohen G: Apneic oxygenation in man. Anesthesiology 20:789, 1959.
8. Sanders RD: Two ventilating attachments for bronchoscopy. Del Med J 39:170, 1967.
9. Carden E: Positive-pressure ventilation during anesthesia for bronchoscopy: A laboratory evaluation of two recent advances. Anesth Analg 52:402, 1973.
10. Sjostrand U: High-frequency positive-pressure ventilation (HFPPV): Review. Crit Care Med 8:345, 1980.
11. Cooper M, Watson RL: An improved regional anesthetic technique for peroral endoscopy. Anesthesiology 43:372, 1975.
12. Credle WF Jr, Smiddy JF, Elliott RC: Complications of fiberoptic bronchoscopy. Am Rev Respir Dis 109:67, 1974.
13. Suratt PM, Smiddy JF, Gruber B: Deaths and complications associated with fiberoptic bronchoscopy. Chest 69:747, 1976.
14. Zavala DC: Complications following fiberoptic bronchoscopy: The "good news" and the "bad news." Chest 73:783, 1978.
15. Luck JC, Messeder OH, Rubenstein MJ, et al: Arrhythmias from fiberoptic bronchoscopy. Chest 74:139, 1978.
16. Elguindi AS, Harrison GN, Abdulla AM, et al: Cardiac rhythm disturbances during fiberoptic bronchoscopy: A prospective study. J Thorac Cardiovasc Surg 77:557, 1979.
17. Shrader DL, Lakshminarayan S: The effect of fiberoptic bronchoscopy on cardiac rhythm. Chest 73:821, 1978.
18. Harkens DE, Black H, Clauss R, Farrand RE: A single cervical mediastinal exploration for tissue diagnosis of intrathoracic disease. N Engl J Med 251:1041, 1954.
19. Carlens E: Mediastinoscopy: A method for inspection and tissue biopsy of the superior mediastinum. Chest 36:343, 1959.
20. Pearson FG: Mediastinoscopy: A method of biopsy in the superior mediastinum. J Thorac Cardiovasc Surg 49:11, 1965.
21. McNeil TM, Chamberlain JM: Diagnostic anterior mediastinotomy. Ann Thorac Surg 2:532, 1966.
22. Ginsberg RJ, Rice TW, Goldberg M, et al: Extended cervical mediastinoscopy: A single staging procedure for bronchogenic carcinoma of the left upper lobe. J Thorac Cardiovasc Surg 94:673, 1987.
23. McLoud TC, Bourgouin PM, Greenberg RW, et al: Bronchogenic carcinoma: Analysis of staging in the mediastinum with CT by correlative lymph node mapping and sampling. Radiology 182: 319, 1992.
24. Ward PH, Stephenson SE Jr, Harris PF: Exploration of the mediastinum under local anesthesia. Ann Otol Rhinol Laryngol 75: 368, 1966.
25. Selby JH Jr, Leach CL, Health BJ, Neely WA: Local anesthesia for mediastinoscopy: Experience with 450 consecutive cases. Am Surg 44:679, 1978.
26. Mackie AM, Watson CB: Anaesthesia and mediastinal masses. A case report and review of the literature. Anaesthesia 39:899, 1984.
27. Ferrari LR, Bedford RF: General anesthesia prior to treatment of anterior mediastinal masses in pediatric cancer patients. Anesthesiology 72:991, 1991.
28. Lee JH, Salvatore A: Innominate artery compression simulating cardiac arrest during mediastinoscopy: A case report. Anesth Analg 55:748, 1976.
29. Basca S, Czako Z, Vezendi S: The complications of mediastinoscopy. Panminerva Med 16:402, 1974.
30. Puhakka H: Complications of mediastinoscopy. J Laryngol Otol 103:312, 1989.

CHAPTER 28

Tracheal Surgery

Elizabeth C. Behringer, M.D.

Tracheostomy

Tracheostomy, a common surgical procedure, can be accomplished using several surgical techniques, including the percutaneous approach.[1–3] Indications for use includes (1) urgent airway access in cases of upper airway obstruction, (2) access for removal of pulmonary secretions, (3) route for administration of positive-pressure ventilation, and (4) airway protection from the aspiration of oropharyngeal or gastric contents.

Elective tracheostomy is frequently performed on intensive care unit (ICU) patients. The early institution of tracheostomy is proposed to decrease pulmonary morbidity as well as shorten time on ventilator, ICU, and hospital stay.[4] Tracheostomy improves patient comfort and suctioning of the airway, and perhaps facilitates weaning from mechanical ventilation.[5] Currently, elective tracheostomy can be accomplished in either of two settings: it is performed in the operating room or, alternatively, at the bedside. Each area has its relative merits. The elective tracheostomy in the operating room provides for a setting with adequate lighting, equipment, and personnel. One disadvantage is the added complexity and risk of transporting a critically ill ICU patient to the operating room. Morbidity during the transport of ICU patients has been reported.[6] A tracheostomy can be performed in the ICU using conventional or percutaneous endoscopic approach. Advantages include avoidance of patient transport and reduced procedural cost.[7] Disadvantages might include lack of adequate lighting and patient access. The reported rates of complication are similar for each approach.

Anesthesia for tracheostomy is accomplished using a variety of techniques. These include use of local anesthesia, monitored anesthesia care, and general anesthesia. The anesthetic requirement is based upon the level of patient awareness as well as coexisting disease. The level of monitoring selected depends on the patient's comorbid disease. Critically ill ICU patients generally require an approach similar to that used during their ICU care.

Surgical Procedure

Tracheostomy is carried out with the patient supine. The patient's neck should be extended by placing either a rolled towel or an inflated "thyroid bag" underneath the shoulders. Support the occiput with a gauze doughnut or a plastic head-dish. These maneuvers provide maximal exposure of the extrathoracic airway. A standard surgical approach is detailed in Figure 28–1. A short horizontal incision is made at the level of the second tracheal ring. The strap muscles are separated in the midline and the thyroid isthmus is divided and sutured as needed to obtain hemostasis. Tracheal rings are identified using the cricoid cartilage as a reference. The second and third rings are incised vertically in the midline for access to the trachea. The lateral wall of the trachea is retracted using thyroid pole retractors. An appropriate sized tracheostomy tube should be inserted as the endotracheal tube is slowly withdrawn to a more proximal position. The tracheostomy tube must be confirmed to rest within the trachea, following cuff inflation and connection to the anesthesia circuit. The standard methods of visual inspection of chest wall expansion and end-tidal carbon dioxide (P_{ETCO_2}) are used to confirm proper placement. The pre-existing endotracheal tube is now removed. The wound is approximated, and a skin suture is placed through the neck flange of the tube to secure it to the skin. A tie or trach tape can be used to provide additional support for the new tracheal appliance.

Several complications have been reported when a tracheostomy site is improperly positioned.[8] If the incision and tube placement is too cephalad, there may be resultant injury to the cricoid cartilage and adjacent structures. If the tracheotomy is caudad, then the tip of the tracheostomy tube and ifs cuff may impinge upon the carina or enter a bronchus. The innominate artery crosses the distal extrathoracic trachea anteriorly. A tracheoinnominate fistula can occur when the tracheostomy tube contacts and eventually erodes into this vessel. A tracheoesophageal fistula is possible secondary to injury to the posterior membranous wall by cuff or tube tip.

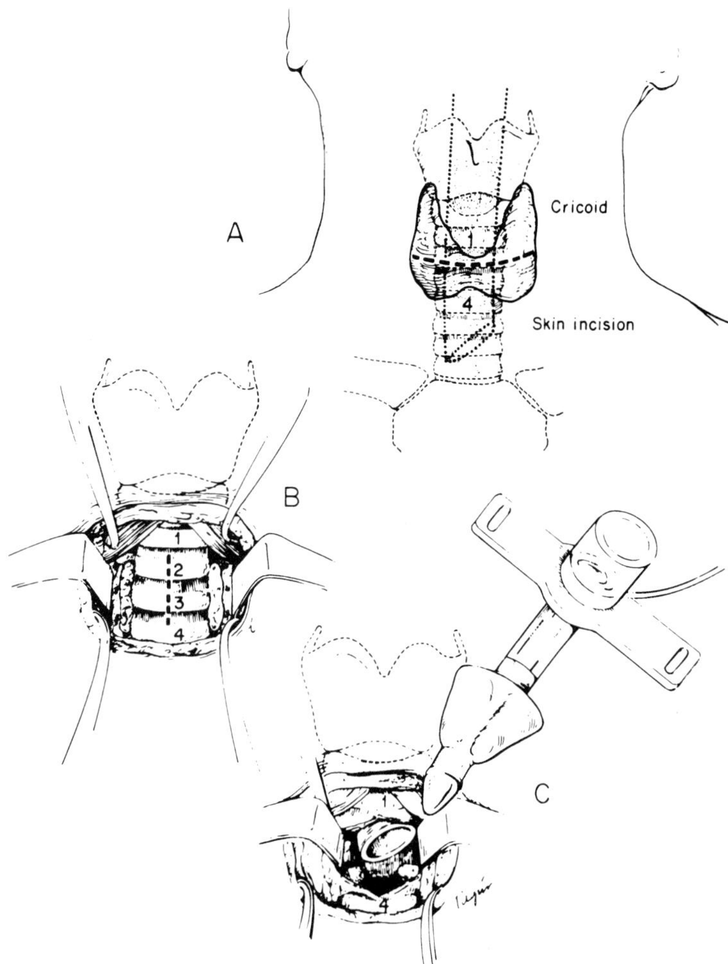

FIGURE **28–1.** Surgical technique. *A*, With an endotracheal tube in place, a horizontal skin incision is made 1 to 2 cm below the cricoid cartilage. *B*, Strap muscles are spread in the midline and the thyroid isthmus is divided. A vertical incision is made in the second and third cartilaginous rings. *C*, With the thyroid pole retractors holding back the cut edge of the trachea, the endotracheal tube is withdrawn and the tracheostomy tube is inserted.

Percutaneous endoscopic tracheostomy has gained acceptance as an alternative technique to the conventional open surgical tracheostomy.[3,9–11] It requires use of a flexible fiberoptic bronchoscope by an assistant positioned at the head of the bed. The patient is positioned and prepped in the fashion described for operative tracheostomy. The fiberoptic bronchoscope is introduced into the endotracheal tube and the tube is repositioned with the tip distal to the vocal cords. The thyroid cartilage, the cricothyroid membrane, and the tracheal rings are identified by palpation. The second tracheal ring is identified and a 2- to 2.5-cm transverse skin incision is made. The platysma is spread bluntly with a hemostat to avoid bleeding from local veins. A 16-gauge needle/catheter, attached to a 10-ml syringe, is inserted through the incision below the second tracheal ring. The exact position of the needle is confirmed by the aspiration of air and direct visualization with the bronchoscope. The needle is removed, leaving the catheter in situ. A guidewire is passed through the catheter into the distal trachea. Dilators of increase size are lubricated and passed sequentially into the trachea over the guidewire. Throughout the procedure, the bronchoscope is used to intermittently reconfirm the correct position of the dilator and guidewire. When dilation is completed, an appropriate size tracheostomy tube is passed over the 28-Fr dilator into the trachea. The dilator, obturator, and guidewire are then removed. Proper placement of the tracheostomy tube is confirmed in the standard fashion. Bronchoscopic visualization of the carina through the tracheostomy tube should be performed to confirm correct position. The inner cannula of the appliance is inserted, the cuff is inflated, and the patient is returned to mechanical ventilation. The tracheal appliance should be secured to the skin with two sutures and a trach tape placed around the patient's neck.

Complications

The complications arising from the performance of either an operative tracheostomy or percutaneous tracheostomy are well described.[12–16] Serious complications during and immediately following the procedure are rare.[17] Injury to a variety of adjacent structures has been documented as a result of tracheostomy. Injury to the recurrent laryngeal nerve or adjacent blood vessels and laceration of the posterior membranous wall of the trachea or the esophagus are possible. Inability to cannulate the trachea occurs with inadequate surgical exposure, an inordinately small incision, or selection of a tracheostomy tube that is too large for the tracheal stoma. Subcutaneous emphysema is indicative of false passage of the tracheostomy tube into the pretracheal space. Pneumomediastinum or pneumothorax occur with injury to the trachea, generally in the posterior membranous wall.

Tracheostomy Tubes

Tracheostomy tubes serve many purposes. A tracheostomy tube can provide a secure continuation of the airway as it passes through the soft tissues of the neck. It offers the possibility of positive-pressure ventilation, a route for pulmonary toilet, or a bypass of airway pathology. It provides airway protection against aspiration as well. Tracheostomy tubes remain the preferred method of prolonged airway maintenance.

Choosing a tracheostomy tube for a patient depends upon several factors. The material and design characteristics of each tracheostomy tube differ according to its intended use. They differ in rigidity, neck flanges, size, length, and cuff design. It is necessary to determine the mandatory and optional functions that the tracheostomy tube should provide for a patient prior to its insertion. Similarly, tracheostomy tubes should be changed in keeping with the patient's changing clinical status.

A standard tracheostomy tube has several design characteristics. Various materials such as silver, stainless steel, polyvinyl chloride (PVC), Silastic, or silicone can form tracheostomy tubes. Metal tracheostomy tubes are rigid and noncompliant. Increased rigidity may heighten the risk of mucosal trauma or tracheal wall perforation during tube insertion and maintenance. The most common material used is PVC. Plastic tracheostomy tubes offer varying degrees of rigidity based on their composition; therefore, they more readily conform to anatomic extremes. The silicone trach tube (Bivona Medical Technologies, Inc., Gary, IN) is flexible, improves patient comfort, and is associated with minimal skin irritation.

The neck flange or plate securely attaches to the tube to ensure maintenance of ideal tube position. It has openings to accommodate the tracheostomy ties. A variety of neck flanges are available. The neck flange can be a solid plate, adjustable, or swivel. The swivel flange allows the angle of the tube to change. The neck flange should be securely tied to avoid excessive tube movement and allow easy visualization of the stoma site.

In choosing the appropriate tracheostomy tube, the transmural distance needs to be approximated in each patient. This helps to ensure proper seating of the tube within the trachea. The transmural distance can be defined as the distance from the skin to the inner aspect of the anterior tracheal wall. Patients with normal airway anatomy are generally accommodated by standard tubes. Extra long tubes are manufactured by several companies, including Portex, Shiley, and Bivona. These devices are useful for obese patients, patients with short bull necks, and those with masses of the neck.

Today, most tracheostomy tubes have a large-volume, low-pressure cuff that is soft, thin-walled, and compliant. The maximum cuff length depends on the outer diameter of the tube. For example, an 8.0-mm internal diameter (IO) tracheostomy tube has a cuff 20 to 30 mm in length. Cuff length shortens as tube size decreases.

Cuffs can be cylindrical, round, or pear shaped. The cuff conforms to the shape of the trachea, achieving a seal with minimal lateral tracheal wall pressure. A low-pressure, high-volume cuff will have the ability to cause tracheal mucosal ischemia if it is overinflated. Cuff measurement is important to obtain as soon as a cuffed tracheostomy tube is placed. In a thin-walled, large-resting-diameter cuff, the intracuff pressure equals the pressure exerted against the lateral wall. The ideal cuff volume can be defined as the lowest possible volume and pressure required to maintain a cuff seal. Two techniques of cuff inflation are commonly in use, the minimal leak volume (ML) and minimum occlusion volume (MOV). Some studies indicate that the ML technique may cause less tracheal trauma than the MOV technique. However, the MOV technique may reduce the potential for aspiration around the cuff. Cuff pressure should not exceed 25 mm Hg to ensure that optimal tracheal blood flow is maintained. The frequency of cuff pressure monitoring should be every 4 to 8 hours, at the minimum. Cuff pressures can be obtained by connecting a manometer to the inflation line of the pilot balloon.

Tracheostomy tubes are sized according to their inner and outer diameter, expressed in millimeters. The size of a tube is located on the neck flange. The nominal length of a tracheostomy tube can be defined as the distance along a center line from the neck flange to the tip.

To ensure the proper fit of a tracheostomy tube, it is crucial to understand the relationship between tube size and length. The length varies in proportion with the size of the tube. The larger the internal diameter of the tube, the longer its length. The length of tracheostomy tubes varies among different manufacturers (Table 28–1).

Tracheostomy tubes are designed with a single or double cannula. Most have a removable and disposable inner cannula. The inner cannula can be cleaned or changed when removed with the outer cannula remaining in situ. This is particularly useful for patients with tracheostomies at home or with medical personnel inexperienced with tracheostomy care. The double-cannula system allows for fenestration of the outer cannula, an option permitting speech. A notable disadvantage of a double-cannula tracheostomy tube is the increased work of breathing accompanying insertion of the inner cannula. This may be significant in patients with marginal respiratory function. The inner cannula uses space normally available for air passage.

Several specialized tracheal appliances are available. The Kamen-Wilkinson "fome cuf" tracheostomy tube

TABLE 28–1
Tracheostomy Tube Length

Internal Diameter (mm)	Portex Standard (mm)	Portex Extra Length (mm)	Shiley Single Cannula (mm)	Shiley Double Cannula (mm)
5.0	67	NA	58	67
6.0	NA	NA	67	NA
7.0	73	84	80	78
8.0	78	95	88	84
9.0	84	106	99	NA
10.0	84	NA	105	84

(Bivona Medical Technologies, Inc., Gary, IN), has a large-resting-diameter silicone cuff filled with foam. This cuff is self-inflating. It inflates in a passive manner when the pilot balloon is opened to the atmosphere. Deflation is accomplished by withdrawing air with a syringe. This tube is used when the cuff pressures and volumes of standard tubes are excessive as seen commonly in patients with tracheomalacia. Over time the foam may lose its elasticity, and cuff leaks may occur. A patient with airway pressure greater than 45 cm H_2O per mechanical breath may develop a cuff leak. Bivona provides an auto control. A connector is inserted at the junction of the tracheostomy tube and ventilator connection with a pressure phase of mechanical ventilation to eliminate any leak. Air can be added in 1-ml increments to create an adequate seal. However, overinflation may cause cuff rupture, releasing foam into the airway.

The Rusch flexible armored tube with adjustable neck flange has several advantages. The wall of this tube is reinforced with a rigid spiral of material. This tube is very flexible. Practical uses of this tube include a patient who is status post total laryngectomy; patients with short, fat, or "bull" necks; and patients with mediastinal tracheal stoma.

Several kinds of extra-long tracheostomy tubes are manufactured in sizes 7 to 10 mm ID. Shiley manufactures a single-cannula, long tracheostomy tube. This tube has a relatively short distance from the flange to its circular bend. The Portex extra-long tracheostomy tube has an increased distance from the neck flange to its bend. It then drops vertically. Thus, it is helpful to ensure the proper fit in a patient with an increased transmural distance. Bivona provides an 8.0-mm ID tracheostomy tube fitted with an adjustable flange and shaft length of 130 mm.

Several categories of tracheal appliances exist that permit speech. Talking tracheostomy tubes permit vocalization with the cuff inflated. Positive airway pressure and airway protection are maintained. Several manufacturers provide talking tubes in sizes 7.0, 8.0, and 9.0 mm ID. These have a cuff inflation line and a speaking port. The speaking port is a small-bore tube set into the curvature of the tracheostomy stopping just above the cuff. The external end has a two-way connector. One is connected to compressed gas. When the other end is occluded, air flows into the trachea above the cuff and retrograde through the vocal cords, allowing vocalization. Common problems include poor voice quality and occlusion of the talk port with secretions. The compressed air flow may escape through the tracheal stoma or into the pretracheal tissue. Thus, it is advisable to wait 1 day after tube placement to permit the stoma to close down before the talking option is utilized.

Several types of fenestrated tubes exist. Portex, Shiley, and Boston Medical Products manufacture cuffed fenestrated tracheostomy tubes in sizes 5, 7, 8, and 9 mm ID. These double-cannula tubes permit speech with the cuff down and the inner cannula removed and the tube plugged. When the cuff is inflated and the inner cannula in place, positive-pressure ventilation and airway protection occur. Patients are considered candidates for a cuffed fenestrated tracheostomy tube when swallowing function is adequate. Patients should be able to protect their lower airway, clear secretions with minimal assistance, have only a modest amount of secretions, and breath spontaneously for at least a 2-hour period.

To ensure the proper alignment of fenestration within the tracheal lumen, either a lateral neck x-ray or bedside measurements should be obtained. At the bedside, the distances from the skin to the anterior and posterior tracheal walls are measured using sterile pipe cleaners. These maneuvers help to avoid plugging of the fenestrations with tracheal tissue by ensuring their proper position with the tracheal lumen.

Cuffless fenestrated tracheostomy tubes provide easy access for suctioning. They also serve as an airway stent for patients with underlying tracheal pathology. The fenestrations increase flow for vocalization in a compromised airway.

Tracheostomy buttons maintain stomal patency and provide easy access for suctioning or emergency ventilation. The Olympic tracheostomy button (Olympic Medical, Seattle, WA) is a hollow Teflon tube with distal flanges and is inserted through the stoma to the anterior tracheal wall. A solid plug is then inserted, spreading the distal flanges against the anterior wall of the trachea. The Montgomery Cannula (Boston Medical Products) is a silicone device, available in multiple sizes and lengths, which can be plugged or fitted with a one-way valve. A wide range of tube lengths, diameters, and spacing washers ensure an exact, secure fit of the Olympic button. The length of the stoma track should be determined for proper button size. A sterile pipe cleaner is inserted through the stoma and hooked on the anterior tracheal wall. The pipe cleaner is marked at the skin level and proper cannula length can be ascertained. The Montgomery silicone tracheal cannula and the Kistner cannula provide stomal patency and access for suctioning and emergency ventilation as well.

There are several types of one-way speaking valves. The Passy Muir one-way speaking valve fits on all tracheostomy tubes with a 15-mm hub adapter. It is ideal for use in patients who cannot tolerate plugging their deflected cuffed, fenestrated, or cuffless tubes. The valve opens with a minimal effort (-2 cm H_2O), and can be easily removed and cleaned. The inspiratory valve opens to allow air entry through the tube. The expiration valve closes and air is directed up into the trachea and upper airway, allowing speech.

Many tracheal appliances with various functions are currently manufactured. This brief overview is intended to serve as a guide for the clinician caring for the tracheostomized patient.

Care and Maintenance of a Tracheostomy

The routine care and maintenance of a patient following tracheostomy includes: (1) stomal care, (2) tracheostomy tube care, and (3) tracheostomy tube change. Stomal care focuses on cleansing the stoma and surrounding skin of accumulated secretions. The use of sterile gloves and a solution of hydrogen peroxide is advisable. Commercial kits for tracheostomy care are available. Tracheostomy dressings should be changed at least every 8 hours. Additional attention should be paid to the tracheostomy tapes, which can become soiled with secretions and merit subsequent change.

Tracheostomy tubes merit routine inspection for damage. Patients on "trach collar" must inspire humidified oxygen. The physiologic method of humidification is through the nasopharynx. This is bypassed in the tracheostomized patient. Humidification of oxygen is mandatory in these patients to avoid drying of pulmonary secretions and potential tube obstruction. Tracheostomy tubes with an inner cannula are unique. The inner cannula can be removed for cleaning, leaving the body of the tracheostomy tube in situ.

Tracheostomy tube change is merited for several reasons: (1) routine change to ensure stomal patency (every 4 to 6 weeks) and (2) elective change to a tracheal appliance with a special function (e.g., cuffless, talking). Elective tube changes should be made at least 5 days following initial surgical placement. This allows time for maturation of the stomal tract.

Elective tracheostomy tube change is a carefully monitored procedure. The patient should have the procedure explained to him/her in detail. If the patient requires mechanical ventilation, preoxygenation with 100% oxygen should occur for several minutes prior to tube removal. All necessary equipment should be set up and ready to go. This includes a tracheostomy changing kit, the new tracheostomy tube, sterile gloves, sterile lubricant, and a flashlight. Appliances to establish a translaryngeal airway should be available including a laryngoscope and suitable blade, and endotracheal tube, and an Ambu bag and mask. Initial tracheostomy change should be done with the patient supine. The neck should be extended in order to facilitate access to the tracheal appliance and stoma. The oropharynx and tracheostomy tube should be suctioned prior to tube change. This allows for ready visibility of the stoma and the avoidance of aspiration of oropharyngeal secretions. The tracheostomy tube cuff is deflated and the tube slowly withdrawn. In patients on trach collar oxygen or low levels of mechanical ventilatory assistance, a quick check of glottic function and tracheal integrity can be accomplished by gently occluding the stoma manually with a sterile sponge. The patient is asked to breathe slowly and phonate. The goal is to document lack of respiratory distress and stridor as well as adequate vocalization. Next, the stoma and tracheotomy incision are visualized with the aid of the flashlight. The tracheal appliance is introduced gently by advancing it through the tracheotomy incision and into the trachea. The cuff (if applicable) is inflated and the intratracheal placement confirmed by the standard methods of visual inspection, breath sounds, and P_{ETCO_2}.

Tracheostomy Under Special Conditions

Emergency Tracheostomy

Emergency airway access via tracheostomy, cricothyroidotomy, or needle cricothyroidotomy is occasionally warranted due to impending upper airway obstruction. The etiology is varied and includes trauma to the larynx or cervical trachea, angioneurotic edema, anaphylaxis, epiglottis, local infection or hematoma. A succinct review of the indications, contraindictions and methodology of these techniques can be found elsewhere.[18,19]

Minitracheostomy

Matthews and Hopkinson originally described the use of a minitracheostomy in 1984.[20] Minitracheostomy provides transtracheal access for pulmonary toilet and suctioning while preserving glottic function for vocalization and cough. A commercially available kit (Mini-Trach II, Portex, Concord, NH) contains a 4.0-mm-ID indwelling plastic cannula, guarded scalpel, guiding catheter, trach tape, as well as a 15-mm adapter. The minitracheostomy is placed percutaneously through the cricothyroid membrane under local anesthesia.[21] A series by Wain et al. described the use of this technique in 56 patients.[22] Indications for the placement of a minitracheostomy included excessive postoperative secretions, difficulty in "blind" endotracheal suctioning, preoperative secretions, and acute airway obstruction. The Mini-Trach can remain in situ for a prolonged period of time (e.g., >1 month). Complications of minitracheostomy placement include local hematoma, subcutaneous emphysema, hoarseness, and perforation of the posterior membranous wall of the trachea or the esophagus. Reported advantages of this technique include relative ease of insertion, ability to preserve glottic function, and favorable patient acceptance. The minitracheostomy has been described in the armamentarium of devices to establish emergency surgical airway access.[23]

Tracheal Resection and Reconstruction

The trachea, carina, and major bronchi are affected by many pathologic conditions that mandate surgical resection and reconstruction.[24–26] The anesthetic approach to surgery of the large airways requires knowledge of the airway pathology, the planned surgical approach, as well as the patient's comorbid disease.

Surgery involving the large airways was limited prior to 1960. Lesions of the cervical trachea were treated by permanent tracheostomy, while lesions of the distal trachea required serial dilations or, rarely, limited resection.[27] Since 1960, the diagnosis and medical, surgical, and anesthetic management of patients with large-airway pathology have undergone significant advancement resulting in successful primary resection and reanastomosis.

Several different multiple anesthetic approaches are summarized below.

1. *Placement of a standard orotracheal tube proximal to the lesion*: Used after the induction of general anesthesia.[28,29] This method is possible in only minor stenoses. Complete airway obstruction can occur if the orotracheal tube disrupts a stenotic or mass lesion.

Reanastomosis is technically difficult, since the endotracheal tube must remain in the surgical field.

2. *Intermittent jet ventilation*: Used through a small orotracheal tube or catheter positioned in the distal trachea or mainstem bronchus.[30–36] Oxygenation is maintained by the Venturi effect when the tube is positioned in the distal trachea. Performance of the surgical reanastomosis is possible when only a small catheter is present in the surgical field. Disadvantages of this technique include possible obstruction of the catheter or distal airway with pulmonary secretions and blood. Jet ventilators can cause serious barotrauma when care is not taken.
3. *High-frequency positive-pressure ventilation (HFPPV)*[37–44]: Tidal volumes of 50 to 200 ml combined with respiratory rates of 60 to 150 breaths/min are used with inspiratory pressures of 40 psi to provide adequate gas exchange. HFPPV provides uninterrupted ventilation, minimal movement of the mediastinal contents, as well as less frequent obstruction from blood and secretions.
4. *Cardiopulmonary bypass*[45,46]: The need for systemic anticoagulation predisposes patients to intrapulmonary hemorrhage due to lung retraction. This approach has been largely abandoned.
5. *Placement of a cuffed endotracheal tube into the open distal trachea*: This approach to resection remains the most frequently used and reliable technique for resection of the large airways.[27,47–55] This technique will be described in detail.

Etiology of Tracheal Lesions

Lesions of the trachea arise from a variety of pathologic etiologies (Table 28–2 and Fig. 28–2). These data are critical to the planned surgical and anesthetic approach.

Postintubation injury is the most common cause of tracheal stenosis.[56] Of 416 patients described by Grillo et al. undergoing primary tracheal resection and reconstruction for tracheal stenosis, 279 patients (67%) had postintubation lesions (Table 28–3). Of these, 263 patients (94%) had primarily stenotic lesions, while 6 patients (2.2%) had tracheomalacia. Ten patients (3.6%) had combination lesions. The locations of the reported postintubation lesions were varied. Nine patients sustained cricoid cartilage injury. Thirty-one patients sustained subglottic laryngeal injury Tracheoesophageal fistulas were found in 12 patients. One patient had a tracheoinnominate artery fistula as a result of a postintubation injury. Postintubation injuries of the trachea are located throughout the trachea. Lesions are a consequence of "traumatic" intubation or produced from use of endotracheal intubation or tracheostomy.[57]

The risk factors for significant tracheal mucosal injury and the subsequent development of tracheal stenosis are well known in intubated patients. Risk factors include prolonged hypotension, concurrent infection, prolonged intubation, as well as persistent elevation of endotracheal tube or tracheostomy tube cuff pressures.[58]

Tumors are the second leading cause for primary tracheal resection and reconstruction.[56] Grillo et al. described 56 patients with primary tumors of the trachea treated with primary resection and reconstruction.[56] The pathology of the lesions is varied. Squamous cell carcinoma was found in one third (19 patients), cystic adenomas in one third (18 patients), while the remaining one third (19 patients) had different types of rare tracheal tumors. This group included carcinoid adenomas, carcinosarcomas, pseudosarcomas, mucoepidermoid carcinomas, squamous papillomas, fibromas, hemangiomas, chondromas, and chondrosarcomas. A subsequent report of 198 patients with primary tracheal tumors detailed successful primary resection in 147 patients (74%).[59]

TABLE 28–2
Etiology of Tracheal Lesions

Congenital lesions
Tracheal agenesis/atresia
Congenital stenosis
Congenital chondromalacia
Neoplastic lesions
Primary neoplasms
Squamous cell carcinoma
Adenoid cystic carcinoma (cylindroma)
Carcinoid adenoma
Carcinosarcoma-chondrosarcoma
Secondary neoplasms
Bronchogenic carcinoma
Esophageal carcinoma
Tracheal carcinoma
Breast carcinoma
Head/neck carcinoma
Postintubation injuries
Laryngeal stenosis
Cuff injury
Ulceration/fistula
Granuloma formation
Posttracheostomy injury
Cuff lesions
Trauma
Penetrating
Blunt injuries
Cervical
Intrathoracic
Infection

Squamous cell carcinoma and adenoid cystic carcinoma together are the most common primary tumors of the trachea.[60,61] Squamous cell carcinoma of the trachea presents as a discrete exophytic or ulcerating lesion.[62] Adenoid cystic carcinomas are slow-growing tumors with two patterns of spread. Infiltration of the tracheal submucosa may occur. Highly malignant lesions can directly invade the lung parenchyma and pleura prior to diagnosis. Cure is optimized with early detection and wide resection margins at the time of initial surgical intervention.[63]

Secondary tumors of the trachea can be managed with tracheal resection and reconstruction. In Grillo's series 30 patients (7.2%) had secondary tumors of the trachea. Tumors of the thyroid, esophagus, lung, breast, thymus, as well as lymphomas and head and neck cancers can involve the trachea by direct extension and metastasis. Thyroid tumors, the most frequent in this group, cause symptoms of airway obstruction by extrinsic compression or by direct invasion. Thyroid tumors are the most amenable to palliation and cure.[64] Unfortunately, the ma-

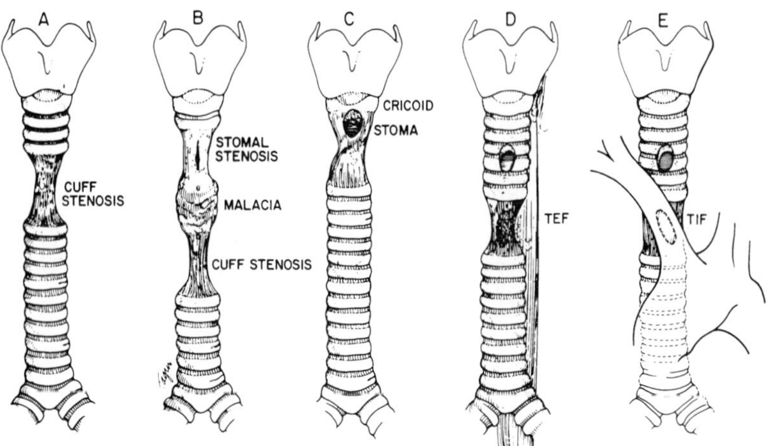

FIGURE **28–2.** Lesions associated with use of endotracheal and tracheostomy tubes. *A*, Cuff stenosis. *B*, Combined lesions including stenosis at the tracheotomy site, stenosis at the cuff, and area of malacia proximal to the cuff. *C*, Stomal stenosis with potential for laryngeal injury. *D*, Tracheal esophageal fistula. *E*, Tracheoinnominate artery fistula.

jority of secondary tumors of the trachea are not amenable to surgical treatment due to the advanced state of the underlying malignancy.

Penetrating or blunt trauma to the tracheobronchial tree may result in laryngotracheal stenosis.[65] Mathisen et al. reported a series of ten patients with acute laryngotracheal injury as a result of trauma.[66] Blunt trauma to the airway occurred in 50% of patients, penetrating trauma in 40%, while the remaining 10% of injuries occurred as a result of traumatic intubation. Blunt trauma to the head, neck, and chest were the most common coexisting injuries in these patients. The most frequent site of injury was the laryngotracheal junction (six patients). All ten patients underwent successful primary repair of their airway injuries.

Failure to recognize acute laryngotracheal injury can result in the development of progressive airway obstruction as stenosis ensues. Mathisen and Grillo reported a series of 17 patients with delayed traumatic laryngotracheal stenosis.[66] Blunt trauma to the airway as a result of motor vehicle accidents occurred in 11 patients. "Clothesline" injuries were seen in five patients. One patient had sustained prior penetrating injury to the airway. The location of these injuries was most frequently the laryngotracheal junction or the upper third of the trachea.

Vocal cord paralysis was a significant associated injury in 14 patients in this series. Seven patients had bilateral vocal cord paralysis. The remaining seven patients had unilateral vocal cord paralysis. It is mandatory to provide an adequate laryngeal airway prior to tracheal resection and reconstruction. Several procedures have been described in order to provide an adequate laryngeal airway in advance of tracheal resection.[66]

The initial evaluation and management of upper airway injuries in a population of trauma patients was recently reviewed.[68] Forty-six cases of upper airway injury admitted to a large trauma center were reviewed over a 4-year period. The diagnostic findings are illustrated in Table 28–4. In this series, the larynx sustained injury in 13 patients, the trachea in 24 patients, the cricoid cartilage in five patients, and multiple sites in four patients. The overall mortality rate was 24%. Mortality was not associated with age or mechanism of injury. Initial management depends upon rapid and accurate diagnosis.

Rarely, tracheal stenosis can be caused by infections such as typhoid, diphtheria, syphilis, or tuberculosis. Systemic lupus erythematosus, Wegener's granulomatosis, fibrosing mediastinitis, and amyloidosis can involve the trachea. Idiopathic tracheal stenosis is a well-recognized entity in previously healthy patients without a preceding history of intubation, tracheal trauma, or infection.[62]

Congenital lesions of the trachea occur infrequently.[62] Lesions such as tracheal agenesis are usually incompatible with life. Congenital tracheoesophageal fistulas are rarely associated with tracheal stenosis. Congenital tra-

TABLE **28–3**
Tracheal Resection and Primary Reconstruction

Type of Lesion	No. of Patients
Postintubation	279
Primary tumors	56
Adenoid cystic	18
Squamous	19
Other	19
Secondary tumors	30
Other	51
Total	416
Staged reconstruction	21

TABLE **28–4**
Diagnostic Findings in Patients with Airway Injuries

	Stab Wound (n = 9)	Gunshot Wound (n = 17)	Blunt Trauma (n = 20)
Radiographic soft tissue air	3 (33%)	9 (53%)	10 (50%)
Subcutaneous emphysema*	3 (33%)	4 (24%)	8 (40%)
Airway open into wound	5 (56%)	4 (24%)	1 (5%)
Computed tomography	0	1 (6%)	4 (20%)
Bronchoscopy	1 (11%)	1 (6%)	1 (5%)
Pneumothorax	0	2 (12%)	0
Sudden loss of airway	0	0	2 (10%)
Autopsy	0	0	1 (5%)

*All patients with subcutaneous emphysema also had soft tissue air present on radiography.

cheal stenosis occurs in several distinct patterns. Cantrell and Guild reviewed the three major kinds of congenital tracheal stenoses.[69] Generalized hypoplasia from the level of the cricoid cartilage to just above the carina can occur. Funnel-shaped narrowing of the trachea resulting in stenosis above the carina can occur. Segmental stenosis may occur throughout the trachea. Coexisting bronchial anomalies can be found as well. This includes takeoff of right upper lobe bronchus directly from the trachea. Web-like diaphragms are also found in the neonatal or pediatric trachea. The level of the trachea just distal to the cricoid is the most common site of webs.[62]

Congenital vascular anomalies are associated with congenital tracheal stenosis or compression. An aberrant left pulmonary artery may cause an associated congenital stenosis.[70] The tracheal rings are often completely circular.[71] The airway is corrected by repair of the pulmonary artery sling as well as the tracheal stenosis. Vascular ring or sling malformations can compress the neonatal trachea and esophagus, resulting in respiratory difficulty. Repair of the vascular lesion usually relieves the respiratory distress. Other vascular lesions such as an anomalous innominate artery, aberrant subclavian artery, double aortic arch, anomalous left carotid artery, or right aortic arch with a patent ductus arteriosis or ligamentum arteriosum may lead to tracheal compression.[72–74] Congenital tracheomalacia or congenital tracheobronchomegaly (Maunier-Kuhn disease) are extremely rare causes of congenital airway collapse.[62]

Congenital tumors and cysts resulting in laryngotracheal narrowing occur rarely.[74] Severe upper airway narrowing may result due to subglottic hemangiomas, laryngeal lymphangiomas, cystic hygromas, congenital cysts, and laryngoceles. Squamous papillomata or invasive papillary carcinoma of the trachea reportedly cause tracheal obstruction in children. Grillo and Zannini reported a series of 52 children, aged 7 weeks to 15 years, with obstructive disease of the trachea.[75] Six patients had congenital lesions, while the remaining 46 patients had acquired tracheal lesions. Thirty-two patients were treated conservatively with methods including serial observation, irradiation, cryotherapy, tracheostomy or tracheal T-tube. Twenty children, ages 5 to 15 years, underwent primary resection and reconstruction (Table 28–5).

TABLE 28–5
Tracheal Resection and Primary Reconstruction in Children*

		Results		
	No.	*Good*	*Failure*	*Death*
Congenital stenosis	3	2	—	1
Primary tumor	4	4	—	—
Posttraumatic stenosis	2	2	—	—
Idiopathic stenosis	1	—	1	—
Postintubation				
Stenosis	9	8	—	1
TEF	1	1	—	—
Total	20			

*Congenital patient needed reoperation for stenosis. One posttraumatic and the idiopathic patient had prior operative failures elsewhere.

Preoperative Evaluation

Preoperative evaluation of the patient with large-airway pathology includes a detailed history and physical examination, pulmonary function testing, roentgenographic evaluation, and diagnostic bronchoscopy. The extent of the diagnostic evaluation is dictated by the severity of the compromise to the airway. The patient presenting for elective repair warrants a detailed preoperative evaluation.[76] The patient with severely compromised life-threatening airway pathology may require surgical intervention after history and physical exam, and diagnostic bronchoscopy.

History and Physical Examination

Patients with a history of recent endotracheal intubation or tracheostomy must be considered to have an organic lesion unless proven otherwise. The signs and symptoms of large-airway obstruction depend upon several factors including the location of the lesion, the degree of obstruction, and the presence of comorbid cardiopulmonary disease. The symptoms of airway obstruction are detailed in Table 28–6. Adults are usually symptomatic when the cross-sectional diameter of the airway is reduced to roughly 50% of normal (5 to 6 mm). Physically active adults may have symptoms with less significant obstruction. Conversely, patients with significant cardiopulmonary disease may present with advanced lesions due to inactivity or misdiagnosis. Stridor at rest indicates severe narrowing of the airway to a value of 4 mm or less. The presence of stridor indicates a tenuous airway. Such patients warrant preoperative admission to an ICU for close observation. Hoarseness indicates pathology of the recurrent laryngeal nerve or the vocal cords. Direct or indirect examination of the larynx is warranted.

A careful physical examination of the airway is most important. Tracheal deviation or extrathoracic compression by a mass lesion should be sought by palpation. Stridor at rest or with maximal expiratory effort can often be elicited. Auscultation of the upper cervical airway may reveal high-pitched sounds characteristic of the air flow obstruction.

The range of motion of the patient's neck must be elicited preoperatively. In order to undergo successful resection, the patient should tolerate hyperflexion and hyperextension comfortably. Many disease states are associated with cervical spine instability (Table 28–7).[77] If the stability of the patient's cervical spine is questiona-

TABLE 28–6
Symptoms of Airway Obstruction

Dyspnea (especially effort-related)
Wheezing
Stridor
Persistent cough
Hoarseness
Difficulty clearing secretion
Inability to tolerate the supine position

TABLE 28–7
Syndromes Associated with Odontoid Hypoplasia and Conditions Associated with Atlantoaxial Subluxation

Morquio's syndrome
Klippel-Feil syndrome
Down's syndrome
Spondyloepiphyseal dysplasia
Dysproportionate dwarfism
Congenital scoliosis
Osteogenesis imperfecta
Neurofibromatosis
Conditions associated with atlantoaxial subluxation
- Congenital
  - Down's syndrome
  - Odontoid anomalies
  - Mucopolysaccharidoses
- Acquired
  - Rheumatoid arthritis
  - Still's disease
  - Ankylosing spondylitis
  - Psoriatic arthritis
  - Enteropathic arthritis
    - Crohn's disease
    - Ulcerative colitis
- Reiter's syndrome
- Trauma
  - Odontoid fracture
  - Ligamentous disruption

ble, radiographic evaluation should be undertaken electively.

If the patient has a tracheal appliance in situ preoperatively, its type and function must be clarified.[58] The relationship of the tracheal appliance to the tracheal lesion is crucial as well. The patient should be questioned concerning their ability to tolerate decannulation. The patient may require decannulation during radiologic examination of the airway as well as during the induction of anesthesia. The tracheal stoma should be examined for patency.

Diagnostic Studies

Pulmonary Function Testing

Standard spirometry may demonstrate a reduction in air flow throughout the respiratory cycle. The maximal expiratory or inspiratory flow is affected to a greater extent than the forced expiratory volume in 1 second (FEV_1). The ratio of peak expiratory flow to FEV_1 is a helpful index of airway obstruction. A ratio of 10:1 or greater suggests the presence of airway obstruction.

The flow-volume loop specifically diagnoses upper airway obstruction. The characteristic flow-volume loops of a variety of extrathoracic and intrathoracic lesions are found in Figure 23–3.[76–78] Extrathoracic lesions produce a characteristic plateau during inspiration, with little effect on expiratory flow. The converse is true of intrathoracic lesions.

Radiologic Examination of the Airway

Several radiographic studies are useful to demonstrate the extent and location of pathology involving the trachea.[79–81] Plain films are important to plan further radiographic studies, interpret tomograms and computed tomography (CT) scans, and visualize surrounding structures.[79] Posteroanterior and lateral chest films are standard preoperatively and will detail some pathology. Lateral cervical spine films help to elucidate the larynx and cervical trachea. Oblique views of the cervical spine often help to visualize defects of the entire trachea.

Fluoroscopy of the larynx allows visualization of vocal cord motion. Fluoroscopic views of the trachea can eliminate any superimposed bony structures when the patient is in the oblique position.[80] This technique is also an important approach used to demonstrate the presence of tracheomalacia.

Tomograms of the larynx and trachea are helpful in the presence of laryngeal tumors or in the investigation of the site and extent of tracheal stenosis.[79] Barium study

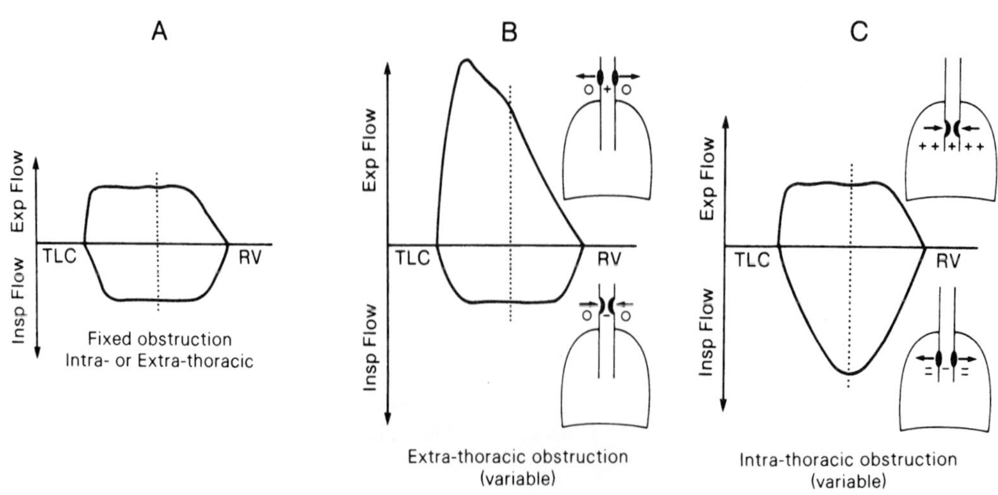

FIGURE **28–3.** Inspiratory and expiratory flow-volume curves. *A*, Fixed obstruction in either intra- or extrathoracic tracheal segments. *B*, Extrathoracic variable obstruction with schematic depicting pressure differences within and adjacent to trachea. *C*, Intrathoracic variable obstruction.

of the esophagus details the relationship of the thoracic trachea with the surrounding lymphatic and vascular structure.[79] Other specialized radiographic studies include angiography to define the vascular supply of tracheal tumors, xeroradiography, and contrast laryngotracheography.[79]

CT scans of the neck and chest evaluate mediastinal and laryngeal structures as well as the extent of tracheal stenosis. Tracheal deviation is often visualized. Magnetic resonance imaging (MRI) to date has been of limited use in the delineation of tracheal pathology. However, MRI has the ability to image directly in oblique planes. This is useful in evaluation of masses in relationship to the major bronchi.[82,83]

Anesthetic Management

The methods described in this chapter have been employed by Grillo and colleagues for resection and reconstruction of the large airways in several hundred patients since 1962.[24–26,85–88] One third to one half of the length of the adult trachea can undergo primary resection and reconstruction. The primary goal of this procedure is the maintenance of an adequate airway from the preoperative phase through induction anesthesia and well into the postoperative period. An adequate airway includes the maintenance of ventilation and oxygenation as well as the easy clearance of blood and pulmonary secretions. A thorough preoperative evaluation of the potential challenges involved in masking, laryngoscopy, and intubation is mandatory. Maintenance of the airway implies a detailed understanding of the nature and extent of the tracheal pathology as well as the surgical approach.

The airway management can be compromised during several critical stages of the operation. The first and often most important is during the induction of general anesthesia. The airway may also be tenuous during the resection period. This may occur for two main reasons: the distal airways may become obstructed with blood or secretions, and rarely, the distal trachea may withdraw into the mediastinum. Finally, the airway may be tenuous during the initial postoperative period due to the patient's hyperflexed position or edema at the anastomotic site. Knowledge of the primary goal of tracheal resection and reconstruction enables the anesthesiologist to plan a smooth and successful anesthetic.

Premedication

The degree of airway compromise governs the approach to premedication. A skilled preoperative anesthesiologist's visit serves to establish a rapport that can alleviate the need for sedative premedication.[89,90] Patients with significant tracheal narrowing (<5 to 6 mm in diameter) should not receive premedication until they are in the care of persons skilled in airway management. Oversedation and central respiratory depression must be avoided in these patients at all costs. Benzodiazepines have sedative as well as anxiolytic properties. Antisialagogues such as atropine and Robinul are potentially disastrous in the patient with tracheal stenosis. Viscous mucous plugs can cause near total obstruction of the airway. Premedication should be given sparingly and under the direct supervision of the anesthesiologist when the patient arrives in the operating room. Under special circumstances it may be prudent for the anesthesiologist and/or surgeon to travel with a patient with severe airway compromise from the ICU to the operating room.

Equipment

Specialized equipment should be readily available. A suggested list of equipment needed for tracheal resection and reconstruction is found in Table 28–8. An endotracheal tube individualized to the patient is chosen during rigid bronchoscopy and visualization of the airway. The type and size of the endotracheal tube depends upon the location of the airway lesion as well as the proposed surgical approach. Lesions of the proximal airway require an uncut (red rubber or PVC) endotracheal tube. Patients with an indwelling tracheostomy prior to surgery will require placement of a cuffed spiral wire tube prior to the induction of general anesthesia. A variety of tubes can be used during resection of the distal trachea or carina including jet ventilation catheters or single-lumen endobronchial tubes. Wilson tubes, which are constructed by joining a standard red rubber endotracheal tube with the cuff end cut off to the proximal end of a PVC endotracheal tube with a metal connector, have a long history of use.[55,91] High-frequency jet ventilation is required rarely during tracheal reconstruction. A ventilator capable of respiratory rates of 60 to 120 breaths/min with variable inspiratory-expiratory ratio and pressure settings is desirable.

Monitoring

General monitoring standards during anesthesia are well established.[92] Special monitoring techniques during tracheal resection and reconstruction are chosen based on specific patient problems. A monitoring approach for an uncomplicated patient is detailed in Table 28–9. A few specific points require explanation. Following intubation, an esophageal stethoscope provides useful information

TABLE 28–8
Equipment

Anesthesia machine with high-flow oxygen (up to 20 L/min)
Individualized mask and oral airways
Mask straps
Long bronchial sprayer with 4% topical lidocaine
Endotracheal tubes:
Uncut red rubber sizes 20–30 Fr
Cuffed and uncuffed uncut PVC tubes sizes 4.0–8.0 mm ID
20- to 34-Fr anode tubes, sterile and unsterile
Sterile anesthesia tubing and connectors
Single-lumen endobronchial tubes—Wilson tubes size 20–30 Fr
High-frequency jet ventilator
Jet catheters

TABLE 28–9
Monitoring for Tracheal Resection

2-lead electrocardiogram
Noninvasive blood pressure
Esophageal stethoscope
Pulse oximetry
End-tidal carbon dioxide
Left radial arterial catheter

concerning breath sounds and heart tones and serves as a guide for the surgical team to identify the esophagus in the surgical field. The preference for catheterization of the left radial artery is deliberate. The right radial artery may be lost due to compression or other deliberate sacrifice of the innominate artery.

The placement of a central venous or pulmonary artery catheter is dictated by the patient's history of cardiopulmonary disease. The location of central catheter placement must consider the operative approach. If the approach is via a cervical collar incision or via median sternotomy, the neck and clavicles are surgically prepped and included in the surgical field. Thus, central venous access is best accomplished through the antecubital or femoral vein. In the vast majority of resections, the intraoperative blood loss and fluid requirements are minimal.

Induction and Bronchoscopic Examination

The patient is positioned on the operating room table in a manner that maximizes comfort. A patient with extrinsic compression of the trachea or a critical airway lesion may prefer to sit upright. The anesthesiologist must be prepared to induce anesthesia, if possible, in the patient's position of preference. A stand may be required in order to gain adequate access to the patient. A deflated "thyroid bag" is placed under the patient's shoulders. All pressure points should be padded. Essential medical personnel and equipment should be present prior to the induction of general anesthesia in the patient with a critical airway lesion.

The conduct of the induction of general anesthesia depends upon the nature of the patient's airway. If the airway obstruction is of minor significance, due to a minor stenosis or the presence of a tracheal appliance, then usual intravenous induction agents such as thiopental or propofol are appropriate. If the stenosis is significant, an approach using a careful, controlled induction using volatile inhalation agents is preferred. Once the patient is denitrogenated with oxygen by face mask, the inhalational agent is gradually introduced as the patient continues to breathe spontaneously. The patient's breathing may be gently assisted with positive pressure to increase minute ventilation. The use of muscle relaxants should be avoided in patients with a critical airway stenosis and an unsecured airway, since the ability to visualize and intubate the trachea is not guaranteed. In addition, when airway obstruction is severe, it may be impossible to provide adequate gas exchange with a face mask and positive-pressure ventilation. Inhalation inductions may be very prolonged in patients with high-grade tracheal lesions.

Once the patient is adequately anesthetized, direct laryngoscopy is performed. Topical anesthesia (e.g., 4 or 10% lidocaine) is applied to the oropharynx and glottis. The face mask is reapplied and the inhalation agent–oxygen mixture continued. If the manifestations of light anesthesia are evident (e.g., tachycardia, hypertension, tearing), then induction continues to deepen the patient. When the patient is deep, a second laryngoscopy should be considered in order to topicalize the trachea by inserting the sprayer immediately below the vocal cords. If the anesthetic depth is deemed to be adequate, then rigid bronchoscopy may commence.

Rigid bronchoscopy serves several purposes. First, it allows the surgeon and the anesthesiologist to visualize the nature and extent of the airway lesion. Second, the type, size, as well as the potential difficulty in endotracheal tube placement can be judged. Third, it provides opportunity for tracheal dilation to provide an airway of adequate size. Fourth, it enables accurate measurements of diseased and normal trachea in order to judge resectability. Tracheal dilation is given careful consideration by the surgeon. The risks include airway damage, bleeding, as well as perforation into adjacent structures. Tracheal diameters that measure less than 5 mm should be considered for dilatation.[26,84] Tracheal dilation proceeds under direct vision using rigid pediatric bronchoscopes of graded size. These scopes are serially exchanged through the tracheal lesion, gently dilating it.

Airway manipulation of tumors should be undertaken with caution. Direct trauma to the tumor can ensue. The endotracheal tube can dislodge a portion of the tumor, leading to further airway obstruction or significant hemorrhage into the airway. Strictures of the anterior tracheal wall or tracheostomy stoma are generally dilated easily.

At the conclusion of rigid bronchoscopy, the patient is intubated with an appropriately sized endotracheal tube. In general, the patient is intubated in the sniffing position using direct laryngoscopy. The tube is passed into the airway, often through the area of tracheal stricture. Endotracheal placement is confirmed by the standard means of visual inspection, auscultation, as well as P_{ETCO_2} monitoring. Flexible fiberoptic bronchoscopy is useful to define precisely the location of the tube in relation to the airway lesion. The endotracheal tube is secured, the eyes protected, and an esophageal stethoscope positioned. Alternatively, if laryngoscopy has been difficult, the patient can be intubated by passing an airway exchange catheter through the rigid bronchoscope. The bronchoscope is removed and an endotracheal tube is passed over the in situ exchange catheter. Proper endotracheal placement is confirmed. It is important to pass an orogastric tube at this point. The stomach is emptied of gas as well as fluid, and the orogastric tube is removed.

Nitrous oxide may be used to supplement the inhalation agent–oxygen anesthetic in patients without significant pulmonary dysfunction or significant airway obstruction.

Positioning

Surgical approaches to lesions of the large airways are depicted in Figure 28–4. Lesions of the extrathoracic, cervical trachea are approached through an anterior collar incision. The patient is positioned supine with a thyroid bag inflated under the shoulders. The head is placed on a supporting doughnut. The back of the operating room table is elevated 10 to 15 degrees to position the cervical and sternal areas parallel to the floor when the head is extended fully. The arms are either tucked in at the sides or the left arm is extended on an arm board at a 45-degree angle to the trunk. The lesion is explored through the anterior collar incision. The sternum is divided if this is deemed necessary for surgical exposure.

Lesions of the distal trachea are approached via a right posterolateral thoracotomy in the fourth interspace or the bed of the fourth rib. The patient is placed in the standard left lateral decubitus position. The right arm may be draped and prepped into the surgical field. This allows the surgeon to manipulate the arm in order to gain access to the neck. A cervical collar incision is added if a laryngeal release procedure is warranted.

Reconstruction of the Cervical Trachea

As discussed previously, lesions of the cervical trachea are approached through a low cervical collar incision. Anterior dissection of the trachea is undertaken. Careful dissection around the innominate artery and other structures adjacent to the trachea occurs. Dissection around the posterior membranous wall of the trachea occurs inferior to the lesion. If the patient has not been intubated through the lesion, particular attention must be paid to the airway during this dissection. Total airway obstruction can occur with release of the external supporting structures of the trachea.

Anesthesia is maintained via the oral endotracheal tube. Prior to division of the trachea, nitrous oxide is eliminated from the inspired mixture, if present. Anesthesia is maintained with oxygen and an inhalation agent of choice. A surgical tape is placed around the trachea below the lesion. Lateral traction sutures are placed through the full thickness of the tracheal wall in the midline on either side at a point no more than 2 cm below the point of tracheal division. The endotracheal tube cuff is deflated prior to placement of these sutures to avoid inadvertent rupture. The trachea is transected below the level of the lesion (Fig. 28–5). The distal trachea is intubated surgically across the operative field using a flexible, sterile, wire-reinforced endotracheal tube. Sterile anesthesia tubing, consisting of corrugated tubing and a Y-piece, is passed to the anesthesiologist. This set of tubing is connected to the anesthesia circuit. The ability to ventilate the patient is ensured by manual positive-pressure ventilation. Surgical dissection continues to excise the tracheal lesion.

Once the adequacy of the tracheal lumen and extent of the tracheal resection is determined, the two free ends of the trachea are approximated. This is accomplished by traction sutures. The anesthesiologist assists the sur-

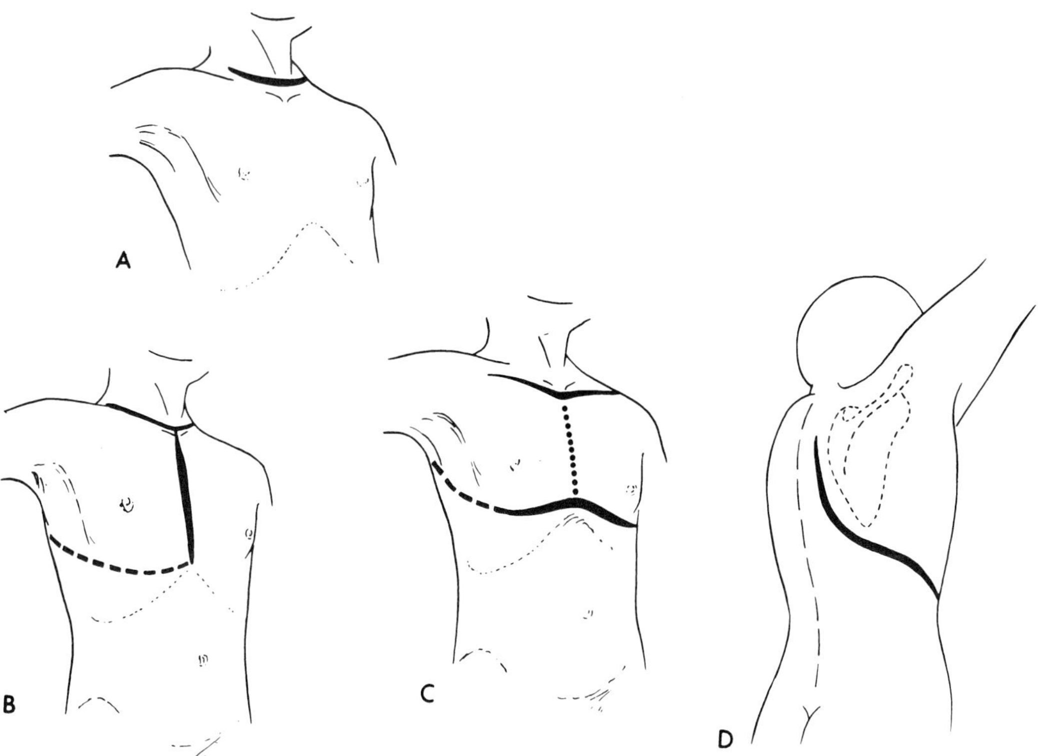

FIGURE **28–4.** Surgical approach. *A*, Collar incision. *B*, Collar incision with hemiclamshell. *C*, Clamshell. *D*, Posterolateral thoracotomy.

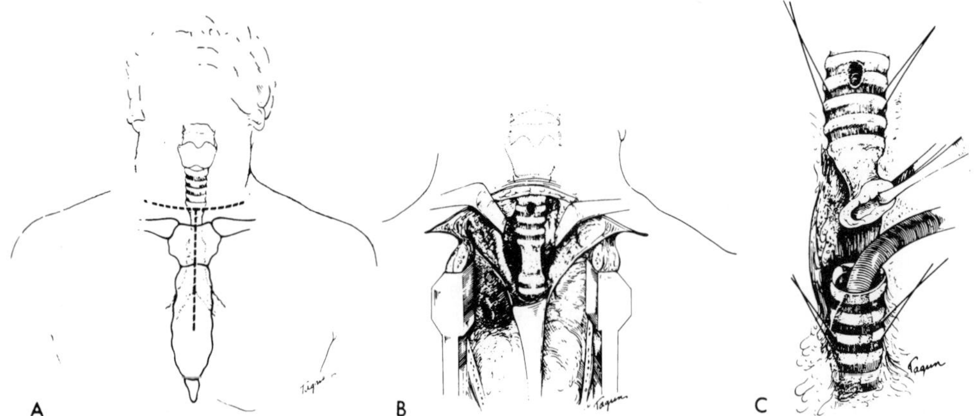

FIGURE **28–5.** Reconstruction of the upper trachea. *A*, Collar incision and extension for upper sternotomy. *B*, Dissection is carried down to isolate the damaged segment. *C*, Circumferential dissection is carried out immediately beneath the level of pathology. Traction sutures are in place and the distal airway intubated via the operating field.

geon by flexing the patient's neck and head from above. If the tracheal end can be anastomosed directly, intermittent sutures are placed through the trachea (Fig. 28–6). Anesthesia is maintained through the wire-reinforced endotracheal tube in the distal trachea. When it is not possible to bring the tracheal ends together directly due to undue tension on the anastomosis, a laryngeal release procedure is performed. Once all of the sutures have been placed, the distal wire-reinforced endotracheal tube is removed. The oral endotracheal tube, which has remained in the proximal portion of the trachea, is advanced carefully through the anastomosis and into the distal trachea under surgical observation. It should be noted that subsequent flexion of the neck to relieve anastomotic tension potentiates possible bronchial intubation. Prior to this final airway exchange, the airway is suctioned of blood and secretions. Anesthesia is administered through the oral endotracheal tube and original tubing. The sutures are secured to produce an airtight anastomosis. The anastomosis is checked for leaks with a sustained positive-pressure breath 30 mm Hg. Once all the sutures are in place, the patient's neck is flexed and

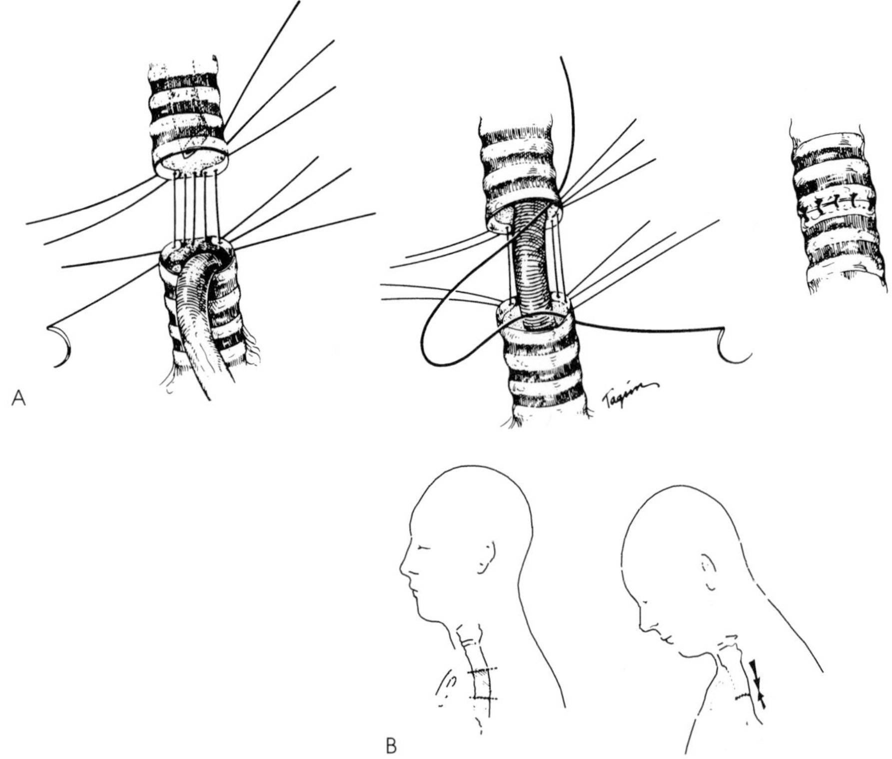

FIGURE **28–6.** Details of anastomotic technique. *A*, Original endotracheal tube positioned in the upper trachea with the distal trachea intubated. Once all sutures are in place, the endotracheal tube is advanced and the sutures are tied in serial fashion. *B*, With cervical flexion, the maximum amount of approximation is obtained.

the head is supported with additional pillows. The cervical collar incision is closed. A retention suture is placed from the chin to the skin above the sternum to maintain neck flexion and decrease tension on the surgical anastomosis.

The patient should be breathing spontaneously at the conclusion of the operation. Extubation should occur under awake circumstances. While the patient is emerging from anesthesia, the head and neck should be supported in the hyperflexed position to avoid excessive motion and undue tension on the anastomosis. It is prudent to extubate the patient in the operating room, where the airway can be assessed rapidly. A flexible, fiberoptic bronchoscope should be set up in the event that reintubation or diagnostic bronchoscopy is required. Reintubation may be required due to unanticipated airway pathology or edema. Given the patient's hyperflexed neck and new tracheal anastomosis, this is best achieved using direct vision with a flexible, fiberoptic bronchoscope. An oral or nasal endotracheal tube is positioned well above or below the anastomotic site. If the etiology of reintubation is due to significant edema of a high tracheal anastomosis, then a cuffless endotracheal tube is used to avoid cuff pressure on the new suture line.

Upper airway edema is the most common cause of respiratory distress in the immediate postoperative period. The replaced endotracheal tube acts as an airway stent. Reintubation remains an infrequent event after tracheal resection and reconstruction. Once the patient is awake and deemed to have a stable airway, transport to the ICU under appropriate monitoring proceeds. The patient should be transported with supplemental oxygen in place.

Reconstruction of the Distal Trachea and Carina

The preferred approach is via a right posterolateral thoracotomy. Several important management considerations for reconstruction of the distal trachea and carina deserve mention. These include the anesthetic plan, postoperative pain management, and tube selection and positioning.

The general principles governing airway management, as well as the induction and maintenance of anesthesia, are similar to those described for resection of the cervical trachea. The lateral thoracotomy incision has potential significant impact on negative postoperative pulmonary function.[93] Since the goal at the end of this procedure is an awake, comfortable patient with an adequate airway, pain control is paramount. A thoracic epidural catheter is placed prior to the induction of anesthesia.[94,95] After the patient is positioned in the left lateral decubitus position, the epidural may be bolused with solutions such as 2% lidocaine or 0.1% bupivacaine with 10 μg/ml fentanyl. The bupivacaine-fentanyl solution is also suitable as a continuous infusion in the postoperative period.[96]

Positive-pressure ventilation is employed during thoracotomy and surgical resection of the trachea. While it is preferable to maintain the patient's ability to spontaneously ventilate, this is not always possible. Muscle relaxants of intermediate duration should be used with appropriate train-of-four monitoring. Muscle relaxants should be fully and promptly reversed at the conclusion of the surgery.

It is helpful to have a tube that can enter either mainstem bronchus during reconstruction of the distal trachea or carina. A long tube (e.g., "Wilson tube") as described earlier provides flexibility at the tip and adequate length for bronchial intubation. This tube is initially placed through the larynx with the aid of a stylet. A flexible, fiberoptic bronchoscope is used to position the tube according to the location and extent of the lesion to be resected.

Initial resection is performed with the tube proximal to the airway lesion. Surgical exposure and resection are similar to the events described for cervical tracheal lesions. Once the trachea is divided, it is often too short to hold an endotracheal tube. The left mainstem bronchus is intubated from the operative field and one-lung ventilation is employed (Fig. 28–7). Attention to the progress of the surgery is essential, since the endobronchial tube may require frequent removal and reinsertion during resection of the lesion. If oxygenation is inadequate during these circumstances, several alternative methods can be employed in addition to standard means described elsewhere in this textbook.

A second endobronchial tube can be advanced into the right mainstem bronchus. Continuous positive airway pressure (CPAP) is employed with oxygen to the right lung. Several methods to deliver CPAP have been described.[97–99] However, the second endobronchial tube may make surgical access to the area of resection technically difficult.

HFPPV may be used to provide gas exchange in the right lung. A small sterile catheter is placed into the right mainstem bronchus from the surgical field. The proximal end of the catheter is passed to the anesthesiologist underneath the drapes. The jet ventilator is set to deliver modest inflation pressure to the right lung. Arterial oxygen saturation is monitored by pulse oximetry. HFPPV may be used in the left mainstem bronchus as an alternative to endobronchial intubation.

Lesions of the distal trachea, which do not involve the carina, proceed in the fashion described in the management of lesions of the cervical trachea. Upon completion of the anastomosis, the endotracheal tube is withdrawn into the proximal trachea. Ventilation proceeds through the area of the anastomosis. Position of the endotracheal tube is confirmed with the aid of a flexible fiberoptic bronchoscope.

Figure 28–8 depicts the variety of possible carinal resections. In general, the right mainstem bronchus is anastomosed to the distal trachea. The left mainstem bronchus is reimplanted in an end-to-side manner into the bronchus intermedius or the distal trachea. One-lung anesthesia is used commonly during such resections.

The anastomoses are completed, the adequacy of ventilation is ensured, and the surgical incision is closed. The patient should resume spontaneous ventilation at this point. In general, it is possible to extubate patients following thoracotomy and carinal resection. The process of extubation is similar to the approach described for resection of the cervical trachea. The patient is re-

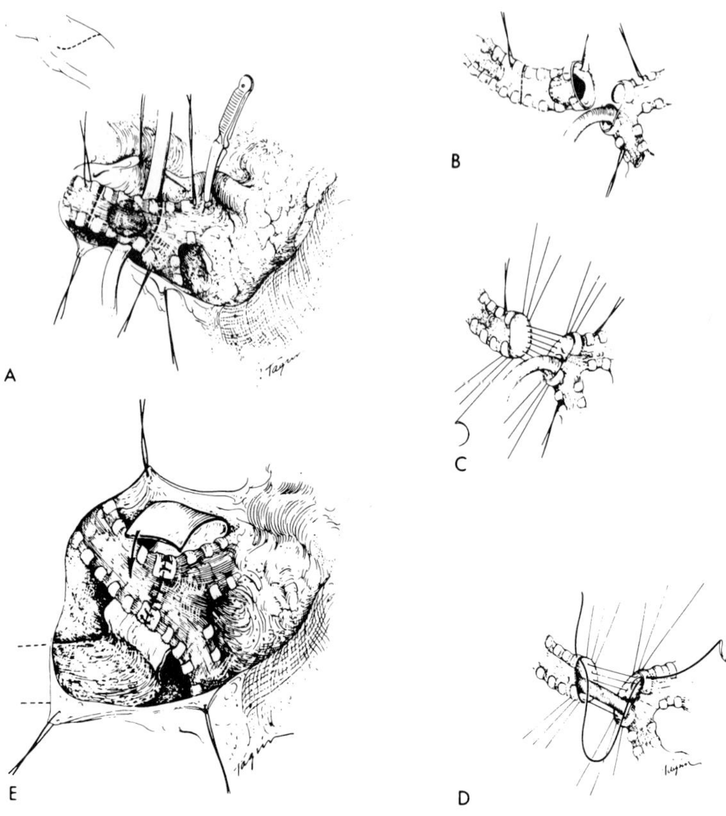

FIGURE **28–7.** Surgical approach to distal tracheal lesions. *A*, Distal trachea and carina are mobilized through a right thoracotomy. *B*, Trachea transected distal to the tumor and the left (dependent) lung is intubated as previously described. *C*, Sutures are placed circumferentially through the trachea. *D*, Endotracheal tube is advanced from the proximal trachea into the dependent lung. *E*, Sutures are secured and endotracheal tube is withdrawn into the proximal trachea.

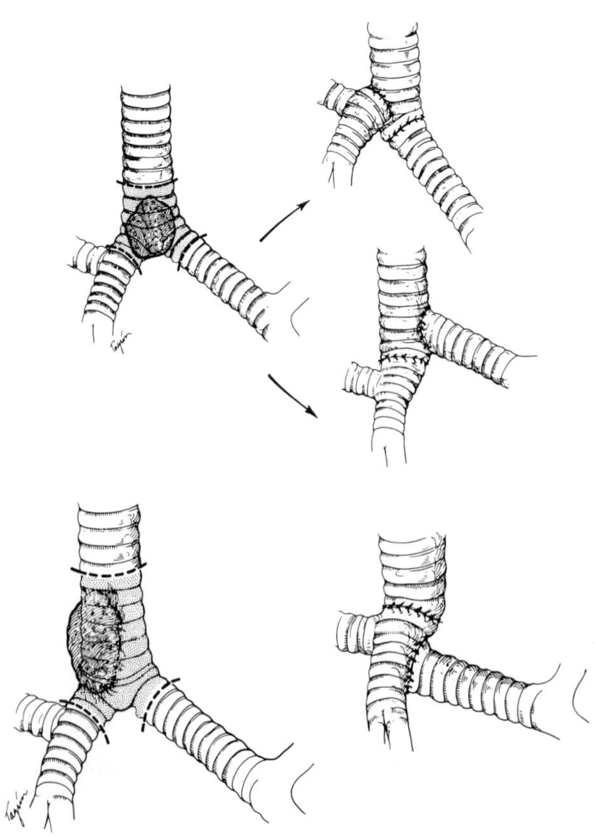

FIGURE **28–8.** Examples of tracheal bronchial anastomoses following carinal resection.

turned to the supine position for placement of the chin sutures. The patient, once extubated with a stable airway, is transported to the ICU under appropriate monitoring.

The most widely described anesthetic technique employs oxygen and a volatile anesthetic agent, with or without nitrous oxide. Inhalation anesthetics are potent bronchodilators ideally suited for patients with reactive airway disease and airway pathology. Inhalation agents can allow for a smooth, controlled mask induction maintaining spontaneous ventilation. Halothane, which is less pungent than isoflurane or sevoflurane, was used almost exclusively as an induction and maintenance agent. Isoflurane and sevoflurane are currently the induction and maintenance agents of choice in critical airway lesions for several reasons. Potential hepatotoxicity is avoided. Isoflurane and sevoflurane are less arrhythmogenic, as well. Halothane may potentiate arrhythmias in patients taking theophylline preparations, or β_2-agonists. Patients undergoing tracheal resection and reconstruction are prone to develop hypercarbia and respiratory acidemia during several points of the procedure. This can potentiate arrhythmias as well.

In patients with significant myocardial dysfunction, an inhalation-based anesthetic may not be appropriate. Anesthesia may be conducted in this case with oxygen, an intermediate-duration muscle relaxant, and a short-acting intravenous agent such as alfentanil or propofol.[100] The goals of the anesthetic management remain the same, albeit somewhat more challenging given the patient's cardiac and airway pathology.

Postoperative Care

Patients are candidates for postoperative ICU admission. The level of monitoring used in the operating room is duplicated in the ICU. A chest radiograph is obtained shortly after arrival in the ICU to exclude the presence of a pneumothorax. Oxygen is administered by a high-flow humidified system via face mask. This provides adequate oxygenation as well as thinning of secretions. The patient's head and neck are maintained in the flexed position by placing several pillows behind the occiput and the chest.

Chest physical therapy and routine nursing procedures are dictated by the nature of the patient's comorbid disease and the ability to maintain adequate gas exchange and pulmonary toilet. Blind nasotracheal suctioning is undertaken cautiously in patients with an inadequate cough reflex. Potential complications of this procedure include perforation of the anastomosis, tracheal and glottic irritation with subsequent edema, and airway obstruction, vomiting, and aspiration. If secretions are copious and frequent, then flexible, fiberoptic bronchoscopy is employed as an adjunct to pulmonary toilet. Following carinal resection, secretions tend to pool in the major bronchi without propulsion by the normal mechanisms of mucocilliary clearance. Flexible fiberoptic bronchoscopy is particularly useful in these patients. It is routinely used to examine the healing anastomosis as well.

Fortunately, reintubation after resection of the large airways is an uncommon event. In cases of respiratory distress or inadequate ventilation and oxygenation, reintubation is necessary with several caveats. If a patient is deemed to be at risk for reintubation, then the equipment needed for reintubation should be at the bedside. Due to the hyperflexed position and the new anastomosis, reintubation is best undertaken with the aid of a flexible fiberoptic bronchoscope. The patient's airway is topicalized and short-acting sedatives are given judiciously. An endotracheal tube is placed either orally or nasally with direct visualization of the larynx. The cuff is positioned either well above or below the anastomosis whenever possible. The potential for dehiscence of the anastomosis exists in the early postoperative phase under these conditions. Therapy is directed at minimizing positive pressure on the airway and the new anastomosis. Therapy is also directed at correction of the etiology for reintubation (e.g., abundant secretion, pneumonia, edema). Elective tracheostomy is considered when prolonged intubation is anticipated.

Laryngeal edema in the postoperative setting is another infrequent occurrence. It occurs most commonly after a high cervical reanastomosis or in patients with a prior history of laryngeal disease. Laryngeal edema presents as stridor or hoarseness in the postoperative setting. Therapy for patients with postoperative edema includes placement of the patient in the sitting position in order to promote venous and lymphatic drainage of the larynx and the limitation of fluid intake. Overzealous fluid administration will only exacerbate existing airway edema. Additional maneuvers include the use of inhaled racemic epinephrine. Racemic epinephrine, 0.5 ml of a 1:200 dilution in 2.5 ml of normal saline, is administered via nebulizer every 4 hours as needed. Heliox, a mixture of 80% helium and 20% oxygen, has gained acceptance in the temporizing treatment of postextubation stridor. Heliox is helpful in the treatment of upper airway obstruction due to its decreased density compared to mixtures of air-oxygen.[101] Heliox should be considered in the treatment of postoperative stridor in addition to the aforementioned modalities. Reintubation is, of course, indicated in patients with severe stridor and edema refractory to medical therapy.

Pain control in the postoperative period remains another important consideration.[102] The mode of pain control depends upon the location of the surgical incision and the patient's pain threshold and preoperative pulmonary function. After resection of a proximal tracheal lesion, parenteral, intramuscular, and patient-controlled analgesia (PCA) are viable methods for pain control.[102] Patients who required a thoracotomy or median sternotomy incision can achieve pain control with the use of epidural analgesia,[94-96] intrapleural analgesia,[103] intercostal blocks,[104,105] or PCA.[102]

Patients remain in the ICU overnight as dictated by the ability to discontinue cardiovascular monitoring, the need for frequent pulmonary toilet, as well as specialized nursing care. Once the patient is deemed to be stable, discharge to a general surgical or thoracic surgical floor is appropriate.

References

1. Heffner JE, Miller KS, Sahn SA: Tracheostomy in the intensive care unit. Part 1: Indications, technique management. Chest 90: 269, 1986.
2. Heffner JE, Miller KS, Sahn SA: Tracheostomy in the intensive care unit. Part 2: Complications. Chest 90:430, 1986.
3. Shrager JB, Sing RF, Anderson HL, et al: Percutaneous endoscopic tracheostomy. Surg Rounds 17:681, 1994.
4. Rodriguez JL, Steinberg SM, et al: Early tracheostomy for primary airway management in the surgical critical care setting. Surgery 108:655, 1990.
5. Plummet AL, Gracey DR: Consensus conference on artificial airways in patients receiving mechanical ventilation. Chest 101: 464, 1992.
6. Smith I, Fleming S, Cernaianu A: Mishaps during transport from the intensive care unit. Crit Care Med 18:278, 1990.
7. Barba CA, Angood PB, et al: Endoscopically guided percutaneous dilational tracheostomy: A safe, easy and cost-saving procedure. Crit Care Med 21(Suppl):S251, 1993.
8. Wilson RS: Tracheostomy and tracheal reconstruction. In Kaplan J (ed): Thoracic Anesthesia. New York, Churchill Livingstone, 1991, p 441.
9. Schachner A, Ovil Y, Sidi J, et al: Percutaneous tracheostomy —a new method. Crit Care Med 17:1052, 1989.
10. Ciaglia P, Firsching R, Synico C: Elective percutaneous dilational tracheostomy. A new simple bedside procedure: Preliminary report. Chest 87:715, 1985.
11. Marelli D, Paul A, et al: Endoscopic-guided percutaneous tracheostomy: Early results of a consecutive trial. J Trauma 30:433, 1990.
12. Astrachan DI, Kirchner JC, Goodwin WJ, Jr: Prolonged intubation vs. tracheotomy: Complications, practical and psychological considerations. Laryngoscope 98:1165, 1988.
13. Hutchinson RC, Mitchell RD: Life-threatening complications from percutaneous dilational tracheostomy. Crit Care Med 19: 118, 1991.
14. Stauffer J, Olson D, Petty T: Complications and consequences of endotracheal intubation and tracheotomy—a prospec-

tive study of 150 critically ill adult patients. Am J Med 70:65, 1981.
15. Dayal VS, El Masri W: Tracheostomy in intensive care setting. Laryngoscope 96:58, 1986.
16. Kirchner JA: Avoiding problems in tracheotomy. Laryngoscope 96:55, 1986.
17. Reilly PM, Anderson HL, Sing RF, et al: Occult hypercarbia—an unrecognized phenomenon during percutaneous endoscopic tracheostomy. Chest 107:1760, 1995.
18. Cicala RS, Grande CM, Stene JK, Behringer EC: Emergency and elective airway management for trauma patients. In Grande CM (ed): *Textbook of Trauma Anesthesia and Critical Care*. St Louis, CV Mosby Co, 1993, p 344.
19. Benumof JL: Management of the difficult airway. Anesthesiology 75:1087, 1991.
20. Matthews HR, Hopkinson RB: Treatment of sputum retention by mini-tracheostomy. Br J Surg 71:147, 1984.
21. Wain JC, Wilson DJ, Mathisen DJ: Clinical experience with mini-tracheostomy. Ann Thorac Surg 49:881, 1990.
22. Wain JC: Mini-tracheostomy. Perspect Crit Care 3:61, 1990.
23. Matthews HR, Fischer BJ, Smith BE, et al: Mini-tracheostomy: A new delivery system for jet ventilation. Thorac Cardiovasc Surg 92:673, 1986.
24. Grillo HC: The management of tracheal stenosis following assisted respiration. J Thorac Cardiovasc Surg 57:521, 1969.
25. Grillo HC: Reconstruction of the trachea. Experience in 100 consecutive cases. Thorax 28:667, 1973.
26. Grillo HC: Circumferential resection and reconstruction of the mediastinal and cervical trachea. Ann Surg 162:374, 1965.
27. Geffin B, Bland J, Grillo HC: Anesthetic management of tracheal resection and reconstruction. Anesth Analg 48:884, 1969.
28. Belsey R: Resection and reconstruction of the intrathoracic trachea. Br J Surg 38:200, 1950.
29. Kamvyssi-Dea S, Kritikon P, Exarhos N, et al: Anesthetic management of reconstruction of the lower part of the trachea. Br J Anaesth 47:82, 1975.
30. Macnaughton FI: Catheter inflation ventilation in tracheal stenosis. Br J Anaesth 47:1225, 1975.
31. Baraka A: Oxygen jet ventilation during tracheal reconstruction in patients with tracheal stenosis. Anesth Analg 56:529, 1977.
32. Clarkson WB, Davies JR: Anesthesia for carinal resection. Anaesthesia 33:815, 1978.
33. Ismail AB: Anaesthesia for tracheal resection. Modified use of the Carlen tube. Can J Anaesth 26:134, 1979.
34. Conacher ID, Paes ML, Morritt GN: Anaesthesia for carbon dioxide laser surgery on the trachea. Br J Anaesth 57:448, 1985.
35. Borland LM, Reilly JS, Smith SD: Anesthetic management of tracheal-esophageal fistula with distal tracheal stenosis. Anesthesiology 67:132, 1987.
36. Baraka A, Mansour R, Jaoude CA, et al: Entrainment of oxygen and halothane during jet ventilation in patients undergoing excision of tracheal and bronchial tumors. Anesth Analg 65:191, 1986.
37. Vourch G, Fischler M, Minchon F, et al: Manual jet ventilation versus high-frequency jet ventilation during laser resection of tracheo-bronchial stenosis. Br J Anesth 55:973, 1983.
38. Scamman FL, Choi WW: Low-frequency jet ventilation for tracheal resection. Laryngoscope 96:678, 1986.
39. Rogers RC, Gibbons J, Cosgrove J, et al: High-frequency jet ventilation for tracheal surgery. Anaesthesia 40:32, 1985.
40. Neuman GG, Asher AS, Stern SB, et al: High-frequency jet ventilation for tracheal resection in a child. Anesth Analg 63:1039, 1984.
41. Erikson I, Nilsson LG, Nordstrom S, et al: High-frequency positive-pressure ventilation (HFPPV) during transthoracic of tracheal stenosis and during perioperative bronchoscopic examination. Acta Anaesthesiol Scand 19:113, 1975.
42. El-Baz N, El-Ganzouri A, Gottschalk W, et al: One-lung high-frequency positive-pressure ventilation for sleeve pneumonectomy: An alternative technique. Anesth Analg 60:683, 1981.
43. El-Baz N, Holinger L, El-Ganzouri A, et al: High-frequency positive-pressure ventilation for tracheal reconstruction supported by tracheal T-tube. Anesth Analg 61:796, 1982.
44. El-Baz N, Jensik R, Fauer P, et al: One-lung high-frequency ventilation for tracheoplasty and bronchoplasty: A new technique. Ann Thorac Surg 34:564, 1982.
45. Woods F, Neptune W, Palatchi A: Resection of the carina and mainstem bronchi with extracorporeal circulation. N Engl J Med 264:492, 1961.
46. Coles JC, Doctor A, Lefcoe M, et al: A method of anesthesia for imminent tracheal obstruction. Surgery 80:379, 1976.
47. Young-Beyer P, Wilson RS: Anesthetic management for tracheal resection and reconstruction. J Cardiothorac Anesth 2:821, 1988.
48. Theman TE, Kerr JH, Nelems JM, et al: Carinal resection. A report of two cases and a description of the anesthetic technique. J Thorac Cardiovasc Surg 71:314, 1976.
49. Dodge TL, Mahaffey JE, Thomas JD: The anesthetic management of a patient with an obstructing intratracheal mass: A case report. Anesth Analg 56:295, 1977.
50. Akdikem S, Landmesser CM: Anesthesia for surgery of the intrathoracic portion of the trachea. Anesthesiology 26:117, 1965.
51. Lippman M, Mok MS: Tracheal cylindroma: Anesthetic management. Br J Anaesth 49:383, 1977.
52. Abou-Madi MN, Cuadrado L, Domb B, et al: Anaesthesia of tracheal resection: A new way to manage the airway. Can J Anaesth 26:26, 1979.
53. Boyan PC, Privitera PA: Resection of stenotic trachea: A case presentation. Anesth Analg 55:191, 1976.
54. Debrand M, Tseuda K, Browning SK, et al: Anesthesia for extensive repair of congenital tracheal stenosis in an infant. Anesth Analg 58:431, 1979.
55. Behringer EC, Wilson RS: Tracheal resection and reconstruction. In Cohen E (ed): The Practice of Thoracic Anesthesia. Philadelphia, JB Lippincott Co, 1995, p 531.
56. Grillo HC, Zannini P, Michelassi F: Complications of tracheal reconstruction. J Thorac Cardiovasc Surg 91:322, 1986.
57. Fryer ME, Marshall RD: Tracheal dilatation. Anaesthesia 31:470, 1976.
58. Wilson DJ: Airway appliances and management. In Kacmarek R, Stoller JK (eds): *Current Respiratory Care*. Philadelphia, BC Decker, 1988, p 80.
59. Grillo HC, Mathisen DJ: Primary tracheal tumors: Treatment and results. Ann Thorac Surg 49:69, 1990.
60. Hajdu SI, Huvas AG, Goodner JT, et al: Carcinoma of the trachea. Clinicopathologic study of 41 cases. Cancer 25:1448, 1970.
61. Houston H, Payne W, Harrison E: Primary cancers of the trachea. Arch Surg 2:123, 1969.
62. Grillo HC: Congenital lesions, neoplasms and injuries. In Sabiston DC Jr, Spencer FC (eds): Gibbon's Surgery of the Chest, 3rd ed. Philadelphia, WB Saunders Co, 1976.
63. Pearson FG, Thompson DW, Weissberg D, et al: Adenoid cystic carcinoma of the trachea. Experience with 16 patients managed by tracheal resection. Ann Thorac Surg 18:16, 1974.
64. Muehrcke DD, Suen HC, Mathisen DJ, et al: Surgical treatment of thyroid cancer invading the airway. Surg Rounds 17:669, 1994.
65. Grillo HC, Mathisen DJ, Wain JC: Laryngotracheal resection and reconstruction for subglottic stenosis. Ann Thorac Surg 53:54, 1992.
66. Mathisen DJ, Grillo HC: Laryngotracheal trauma. Ann Thorac Surg 43:254, 1987.
67. Mathisen DJ, Grillo HC: Laryngotracheal trauma—acute and chronic. In Grillo HC, Eschapasse H (eds): International Trends in General Thoracic Surgery, Vol 2: Major Challenges. Philadelphia, WB Saunders Co, 1987.
68. Cicala RS, Kudsk KA, Butts A, et al: Initial evaluation and management of upper airway injuries in trauma patients. J Clin Anesth 3:91, 1991.
69. Cantrell JR, Guild HG: Congenital stenosis of the trachea. Am J Surg 108:297, 1964.
70. Clarkson PM, Ritter DG, Rahimtoola SHI, et al: Aberrant left pulmonary artery. Am J Dis Child 113:373, 1967.
71. Jacobson JH, Morgan BC, Anderson DH, et al: Aberrant left pulmonary artery. J Thorac Cardiovasc Surg 39:602, 1960.
72. Gross RE: The Surgery of Infancy and Childhood. Philadelphia, WB Saunders Co, 1953.
73. Lincoln JCR, Deverall PB, Stark J, et al: Vascular anomalies compressing the esophagus and trachea. Thorax 24:295, 1969.
74. Maze A, Bloch E: Stridor in pediatric patients. Anesthesiology 50:132, 1979.
75. Grillo HC, Zannini P: Management of obstructive tracheal disease in children. J Pediatr Surg 19:414, 1984.

76. Kryger M, Bode F, Antic R, et al: Diagnosis of obstruction of the upper and central airways. Am J Med 61:85, 1976.
77. Crosby ET, Liu A: The adult cervical spine: Implications for airway management. Can J Anaesth 37:77, 1990.
78. Hyatt RE, Black LF: The flow-volume curve: A current perspective. Am Rev Respir Dis 107:191, 1973.
79. Momose KJ, Macmillan AS: Roentgenologic investigations of the larynx and trachea. Radiol Clin North Am 16:321, 1978.
80. Weber AL, Grillo HC: Tracheal tumors, a radiological, clinical and pathological evaluation of 84 cases. Radiol Clin North Am 16:227, 1978.
81. Weber AL, Grillo HC: Tracheal stenosis, an analysis of 151 cases. Radiol Clin North Am 16:291, 1978.
82. Gefter WB: Chest applications of magnetic resonance imaging. An update. Radiol Clin North Am 28:573, 1990.
83. Naidich DP: CT/MRI correlation in the evaluation of tracheobronchial neoplasia. Radiol Clin North Am 28:555, 1990.
84. Grillo HC: Surgical approaches to the trachea. Surg Gynecol Obstet 129:347, 1969.
85. Grillo HC: Terminal or mural tracheostomy in the anterior mediastinum. J Thorac Cardiovasc Surg 51:422, 1966.
86. Grillo HC: Tracheal tumors: Surgical management. Ann Thorac Surg 26:112, 1978.
87. Grilo HC: Surgical treatment of postintubation tracheal injuries. J Thorac Cardiovasc Surg 78:860, 1979.
88. Grillo HC, Mathisen DJ: Surgical management of tracheal strictures. Surg Clin Am 68:511, 1988.
89. Egbert LD, Battit GE, Turndorf H, et al: The value of the preoperative visit by an anesthetist. JAMA 185:553, 1963.
90. Leigh JM, Walker J, Janaganathan P: Effect of preanesthetic visit on anxiety. Br Med J 2:987, 1977.
91. Wilson RS: Tracheostomy and tracheal reconstruction. In Kaplan J (ed): Thoracic Anesthesia. New York, Churchill Livingstone, 1991, p 441.
92. Eichorn JH, Cooper JB, Cullen DJ, et al: Standards for patient monitoring during anesthesia at Harvard Medical School. JAMA 256:1017, 1986.
93. Cooper JD, Nelems JM, Pearson FG: Extended indication for median sternotomy in patients requiring pulmonary resection. Ann Thorac Surg 26:413, 1978.
94. James EC, Kolberg HL, Iwen GW, et al: Epidural analgesia for postthoracotomy patients. J Thorac Cardiovasc Surg 82:898, 1981.
95. Logas WG, El-Baz N, El-Ganzouri A, et al: Continuous thoracic epidural analgesia for postoperative pain relief following thoracotomy. A randomized prospective study. Anesthesiology 67: 787, 1987.
96. Fischer RL, Lubenow TR, Liceaga A, et al: Comparison of continuous epidural infusion of fentanyl-bupivacaine and morphine-bupivacaine in management of postoperative pain. Anesth Analg 67:559, 1988.
97. Cohen E, Eisenkraft JB, Thys C, et al: Oxygenation and hemodynamic changes during one-lung ventilation: Effects of $CPAP_{10}$, $PEEP_{10}$, and $CPAP_{10}/PEEP_{10}$. J Cardiothorac Anesth 2: 34, 1988.
98. Cook CE, Wilson RS: Dangers of using an improvised underwater seal for CPAP oxygenation during one-lung ventilation. Anesthesiology 66:707, 1987.
99. Scheller MS, Varvel JR: CPAP oxygenation during one-lung ventilation using a Bain circuit. Anesthesiology 66:708: 1987.
100. Steegers PA, Backx PJ: Propofol and alfentanil anesthesia during one-lung ventilation. J Cardiothorac Anesth 4:194, 1990.
101. Kemper KJ, Ritz RH, Benson MS, Bishop MS: Helium-oxygen mixture in the treatment of postextubation stridor in pediatric trauma patients. Crit Care Med 19:356, 1991.
102. Coleman DL: Control of postoperative pain: Non-narcotic and narcotic alternatives and their effect on pulmonary function. Chest 92:520, 1987.
103. Symreng T, Gomez MN, Ross N: Intrapleural bupivacaine vs. saline after thoracotomy—effects on pain and lung function—a double blind study. J Cardiothorac Anesth 3:144, 1988.
104. Woltering EA, Flye MW, Huntley S, et al: Evaluation of bupivacaine nerve blocks in the modification of pain and pulmonary function changes after thoracotomy. Ann Thorac Surg 30:122, 1980.
105. Toledo-Pereyra LH, DeMeester TR: Prospective randomized evaluation of intrathoracic intercostal nerve block with bupivacaine on postoperative ventilatory function. Ann Thorac Surg 27: 203, 1979.

CHAPTER 29

Esophageal Surgery

Anne C. Kolker, M.D.

Appropriate evaluation of a patient prior to esophageal surgery must consider the patient's pathology, pre-existing organ system disease, and the nature of the planned surgery. Although some esophageal procedures are of relatively short duration with minimal surgical manipulation, generally major procedures are complex, often requiring surgery in two body cavities. These patients can present significant preoperative challenges associated with nutritional depletion as well as chronic pulmonary problems due to recurrent aspiration. The postoperative course can be complicated not only by the pre-existing problems but also by life-threatening surgical complications.

Proper evaluation of a patient requiring esophageal surgery requires a complete understanding of esophageal anatomy and physiology. Most of the surgical procedures performed on the esophagus require a thoracotomy. However, adequate access may also include abdominal and cervical approaches. Therefore, the anesthesiologist involved in esophageal procedures must be knowledgeable in general thoracic anesthetic techniques and associated problems. When the esophagus is the focus of the surgical procedure, the anesthesiologist's awareness of possible reflux or motility problems should be heightened. The problem of gastroesophageal reflux, which can lead to aspiration, is often a significant concern. However, incident esophageal pathology should always be considered as part of a preanesthetic evaluation.

This chapter reviews basic anatomy and physiology of the esophagus, details pathology, and discusses the surgical management and complications. Since problems of swallowing, motility, and reflux may remain postoperatively, the management for airway protection is always a primary concern and is discussed in detail.

Esophageal Anatomy and Function

Development

The esophagus begins to develop embryologically by the third week of gestation.[1] It elongates and separates from the trachea by the 36th day. During the period from the sixth through the ninth week, the muscular layers and neuroblasts begin to be arranged and organized along the length of the tube. The fully developed esophagus extends from the pharynx at the level of the lower border of the cricoid cartilage to the diaphragm at the 11th or 12th thoracic vertebra, a total length of about 25 cm. Normal esophageal diameter is about 2 cm. There are three areas of constriction: (1) the narrowest portion (1.5 cm) at the cricopharyngeus, lies in the neck; (2) an area of compression behind the left bronchus; and (3) at the hiatus of the diaphragm. Arterial supply and venous drainage of the esophagus is via the inferior thyroid arteries and veins in the cervical region, the aorta, bronchial arteries, azygous and hemiazygous veins in the chest, and the left inferior phrenic and left gastric artery as well as the left gastric vein in the abdomen. Lymphatics arise in the mucosa and drain regionally to the inferior deep cervical, paratracheal, posterior mediastinal, and superior gastric nodes. Parasympathetic innervation arises from the recurrent laryngeal nerves and an esophageal plexus formed by the right and left vagus. Sympathetic innervation is derived from the thoracic sympathetic chain and from branches of the celiac plexus.

Position

In the neck the esophagus lies in the midline, posterior to the trachea. As it descends into the chest, it deviates to a position to the left of the trachea. Below the tracheal bifurcation it is posterior to the left atrium. In the region of the aortic arch, the esophagus returns to a midline position. Below the arch, the esophagus lies in the left chest and passes through the diaphragm to the left of midline. The right lateral border of the esophagus contacts the parietal pleura, while the left lateral border contacts the thoracic aorta (Fig. 29–1).

The anatomic relationships of the esophagus to adjacent structures dictate different surgical approaches to specific esophageal lesions as well as to potential perioperative complications. For purposes of conventional

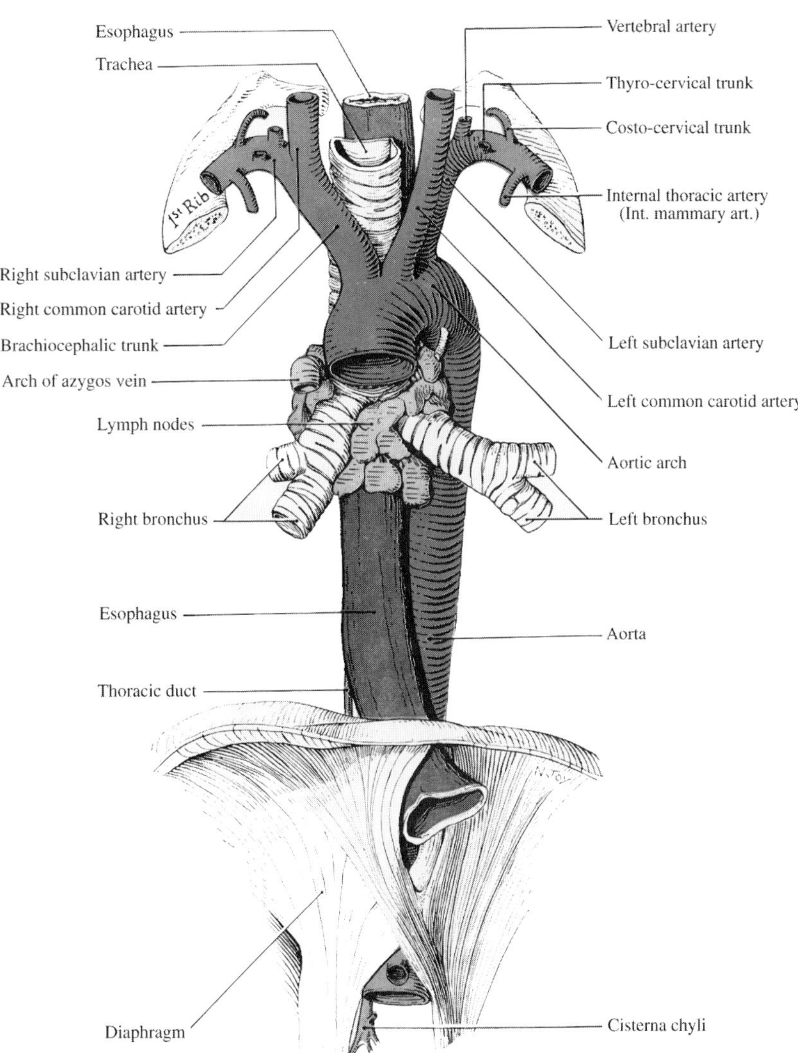

FIGURE **29–1.** Anatomic relationship of the esophagus to structures in the chest. (From Boileau Grant JC: An Atlas of Anatomy, 6th ed. Baltimore, Williams & Wilkins, 1972, p. 452, with permission.)

surgical discussion, the esophagus is divided into three segments; cervical, thoracic, and abdominal. The cervical portion of the esophagus extends from the cricopharyngeus muscles at the thoracic inlet (C6–T1). The intrathoracic portion begins at the lower edge of T1 and continues to the hiatus of the diaphragm at T10–T11. The abdominal esophagus begins at the level of the diaphragm and is 3 to 6 cm in length (Fig. 29–2).

Dynamic Function

The esophagus functions to actively propel materials from mouth to stomach. The oral cavity preparatory phase results in bolus formation. Swallowing begins with the tongue propelling the liquid or solid bolus posteriorly into the oropharynx. Once initiated via sensory input from the oropharynx and supraglottic larynx, swallowing is entirely reflex in nature. Simultaneously, the soft palate elevates to occlude the nasopharynx and the larynx elevates and pulls forward under the epiglottis and base of tongue. The vocal cords adduct and aspiration is prevented.

Opening of the hypopharynx secondary to laryngeal elevation results in negative pressure exerting a direct force on the bolus. The upper esophageal sphincter, the cricopharyngeus, reflexively relaxes to allow passage of the bolus, which is propelled into the thoracic esophagus both by posterior pharyngeal constriction and esophageal contractions aided by negative intrathoracic pressure. Within 0.5 second the cricopharyngeal pressure reaches approximately 30 mm Hg, thereby preventing reflux.

Once in the esophagus, food is propelled by orderly primary peristalsis over a pressure gradient ranging from −6 mm Hg in the intrathoracic portion to +6 mm Hg in the stomach. The lower third of the esophagus is the most important segment in pumping food across the pressure barrier. Although no distinct anatomic lower esophageal sphincter (LES) is definable in humans, a functional zone of intrinsic, high-pressure tone exists. The normal LES relaxes on swallowing, allowing passage of the bolus through the lower esophagus into the stomach. The gastroesophageal (GE) junction on the lesser and greater curvature of the cardia contracts to close the cardia once the bolus has passed. Diseases, medical conditions, and anatomic abnormalities can re-

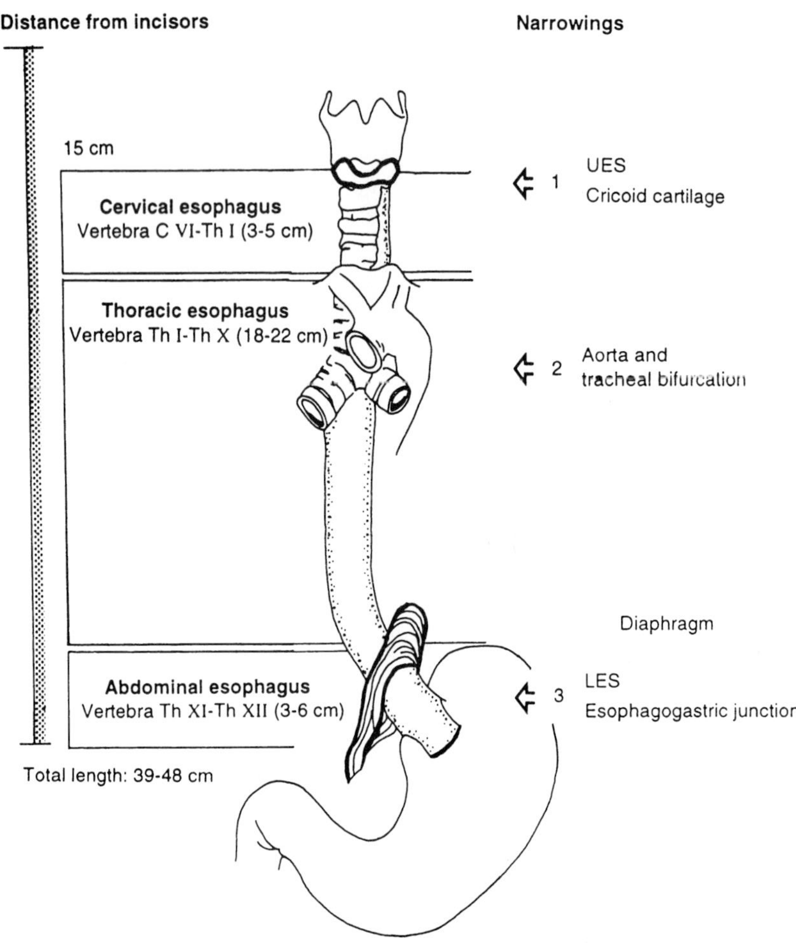

FIGURE 29–2. Division of the esophagus into cervical, thoracic, and abdominal segments. The three areas of narrowing are shown: UES (upper esophageal sphincter) at cricopharyngeus; aorta and tracheal bifurcation; LES (lower esophageal sphincter) at the diaphragmatic hiatus. (From Pearson FG (ed): Esophageal Surgery. New York, Churchill Livingstone, 1995, p. 2, with permission.)

sult in abnormal LES function or GE junction displacement leading to esophageal reflux.[2] Interestingly, myotomy can be performed along the length of the LES without resultant reflux. LES pressure is one of the many factors that are important in the intraoperative management of reflux. Also, many routinely used drugs increase or decrease LES pressure and impact on the ability to maintain a competent GE sphincter (Table 29–1).

The coordination of swallowing requires a highly ordered discharge of cranial nerves V, VII, IX, X, and XII as well as motor nerves C1 to C3. A variety of clinical disorders and neurologic disturbances can result in disruption of normal swallowing and peristalsis (Table 29–2). Many of these conditions are well suited for medical management.

TABLE 29–1
Drugs that Affect LES Pressure*

Increase	Decrease
Metoclopromide	Anticholinergics
Domperidone	Benzodiazepines
Succinylcholine	Opioids
Pancuronium	Thiopental
Neostigmine	Halothane
Edrophonium	Enflurane
Histamine	Nitrous oxide
Metoprolol	Dopamine
α-Adrenergic stimulants	Nitroprusside
	Nifedipine

*Drugs listed affect the esophagus in a standard dose-response manner. LES, lower esophageal sphincter, GE, gastroesophageal.

Diagnostic Evaluation

Noninvasive Techniques

Radiographic studies utilizing barium or gastrograffin may identify mucosal erosions, strictures, ulcerations, webs, diverticulae, neoplasms, or hiatus hernia. The most frequently performed diagnostic test for esophageal disease is the barium swallow. The double-contrast swallow, which utilizes heavy barium and carbon dioxide (CO_2) granules to outline the esophageal mucosa, best defines subtle mucosal abnormalities. If a perforation or leak is the problem being investigated, gastrograffin is used to study the esophagus, because a gastrograffin leak into the mediastinum is thought to be benign compared to barium. Barium is chosen for the patient at risk for aspiration due to swallowing difficulties or recurrent laryngeal nerve dysfunction. In this instance, barium is preferred over gastrograffin because aspiration of barium is benign, while aspiration of gastrograffin can poten-

TABLE 29–2
Clinical Disorders and Neurologic Disturbances that Can Result in Disruption of Normal Swallowing and Peristalsis

Mechanical obstruction
Tumors
Strictures
Lymph nodes
Bone spurs
Neurologic disease
Parkinsonism
Multiple sclerosis
Amyotrophic lateral sclerosis
Myasthenia gravis
Poliomyelitis
Stroke
Nerve injury
Neuropathy (diabetic, alcoholic)
Myogenic disorders
Achalasia
Diffuse esophageal spasm
Hypertensive LES
Medical conditions
Collagen vascular diseases
Metabolic (hypo-, hyperthyroidism)

LES, lower esophageal sphincter.

tially cause pulmonary edema due to the hypertonicity of the solution. Magnetic resonance imaging (MRI) and computed tomography (CT) are commonly used to identify enlarged lymph nodes or metastatic lesions from tumors.

Invasive Techniques

Rigid or flexible esophagoscopy is done to further elucidate disease or define small lesions and mucosal abnormalities not visible radiologically. Esophagoscopy allows not only for accurate location and measurement of the extent of an esophageal lesion, but also for biopsy to assess the pathology. Additional procedures include manometry for suspected motor abnormalities of the esophagus and a variety of pH studies, which can identify and analyze gastroesophageal reflux. Endoscopic ultrasound studies can also be used to evaluate local lymph nodes in determining tumor resectability.

While decisions regarding diagnostic evaluation are made by the surgeon, the anesthesiologist must understand the ramifications and results so as to plan for the ultimate surgical procedure. Following sections will consider the perioperative planning which is relevant for various surgical approaches and specific diseases.

Esophageal Disease

Esophageal surgery is indicated for a variety of benign and malignant conditions. Table 29–3 lists common diseases and conditions for which surgery is routinely performed.

While a full description of all surgical procedures and approaches is beyond the scope of this chapter, the following descriptions are intended to provide a basic understanding of what diseases and conditions require surgical intervention, followed by the basic rationale for surgical approach to specific areas of esophageal pathology, and highlight the common anesthetic considerations for esophageal procedures.

TABLE 29–3
Diseases and Conditions for Which Esophageal Surgery is Routinely Performed

Benign
Hiatal hernia
Strictures, webs, rings
Motility disorders
Diverticulae
Entrinsic compression
Congenital atresia-TE fistula/fistulae
Perforation
Chemical burns
Foreign bodies
Bleeding
Malignant
Carcinoma
Sarcoma
Melanoma

TE, tracheoesophageal.

Benign Disease

The majority of esophageal pathology is of a benign nature. The most common benign condition, hiatal hernia, is evident in 30 to 40% of upper gastrointestinal studies[2] (Fig. 29–3). The majority are asymptomatic. When symptomatic reflux occurs, patients are initially treated medically unless serious complications such as recurrent aspiration pneumonitis or esophageal stricture are presenting features. Occurrence of severe symptoms, refractory to medical management, ultimately requires surgical intervention.

Esophageal strictures can be separated into reflux- and nonreflux-related types. Reflux strictures are presumed

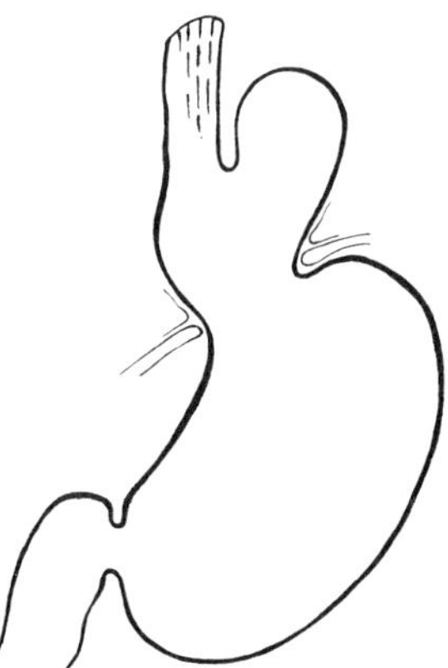

FIGURE 29–3. Schematic drawing depicting a hiatus hernia with both the esophagogastric junction and fundus of the stomach above the diaphragm. (From Baue AE, Naunheim KS: Hiatal hernia and gastroesophageal reflux. In Baue AE (ed): Glenn's Thoracic and Cardiovascular Surgery, 5th ed. Norwalk, CT, Appleton & Lange, 1991, p. 685, with permission.)

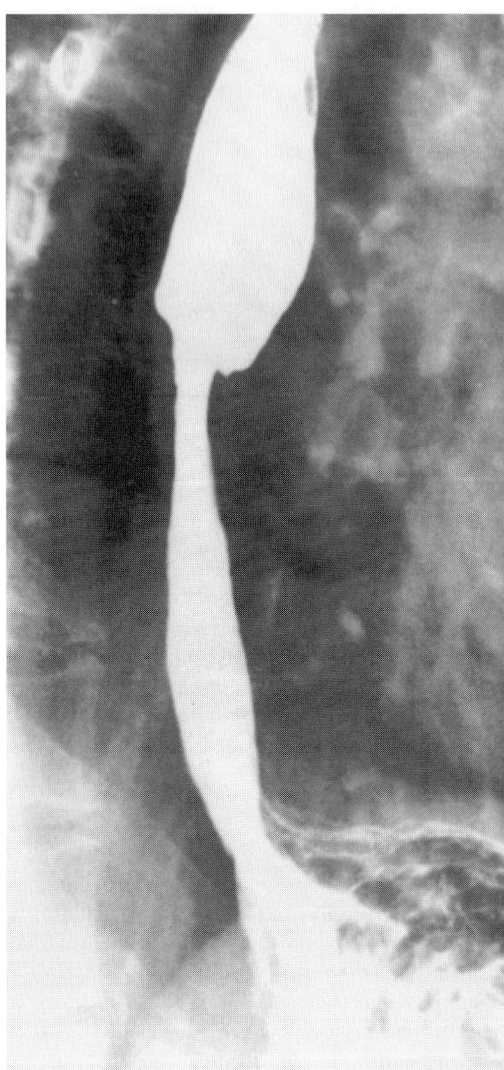

FIGURE **29–4.** Radiographic appearance of an esophageal stricture. (From Baue AE, Naunheim KS: Hiatal hernia and gastroesophageal reflux. In Baue AE (ed): Glenn's Thoracic and Cardiovascular Surgery, 5th ed. Norwalk, CT, Appleton & Lange, 1991, p. 703, with permission.)

to be due to repeated mucosal irritation causing scarring and contractures. Nonreflux-related strictures can be due to congenital webs or rings, infectious esophagitis, mechanical injury from caustic burns, prolonged nasogastric intubation, high-dose radiation to the chest, prior esophageal surgery, and medications that cause esophagitis (Fig. 29–4). Both types of strictures are initially treatable by dilatation. Ultimately, surgical repair may include one of several operations appropriate for hiatus hernia including esophagectomy.

Esophageal dysmotility can occur at several sites including the level of the oropharynx, the body of the esophagus, or at the lower esophageal sphincter. The etiology of resultant dysphagia generally determines the appropriateness of surgical intervention. As previously described, the initiation and coordination of swallowing requires intact cranial and somatic neural pathways as well as functional musculature. Oropharyngeal dysphagia can be due to mechanical obstruction, neurologic injury or disease, or neuromuscular disease. Mechanical obstruction due to tumors, strictures, webs, or bone spurs is often amenable to surgical management. Neurologic injury or disease is usually best managed medically. Cricopharyngeal myotomy, performed through a neck incision, may improve dysphagia caused by neuromuscular disorders. Dysphagia caused by primary disorders of the esophageal body (e.g., achalasia) and LES (hypertensive LES) are treatable by esophagomyotomy or in some cases esophagectomy.[3] Secondary disorders of the esophageal body such as collagen vascular diseases, diabetes, or neuromuscular disorders may respond to medical or surgical treatment.

Pulsion diverticulae are thought to be related to motility disorders. Zenker's diverticulae occur in the neck at the level of the inferior constrictor and cricopharyngeus muscles (Fig. 29–5). Symptoms of dysphagia, choking, regurgitation, aspiration, and even total obstruction can occur. Surgery is performed via a longitudinal neck incision accomplishing both cricopharyngeal myotomy and excision or suspension of the diverticulum. Lower esophageal or epiphrenic diverticulae are likely related to intermittent LES spasm. Symptoms are often secondary to associated esophageal dysmotility.

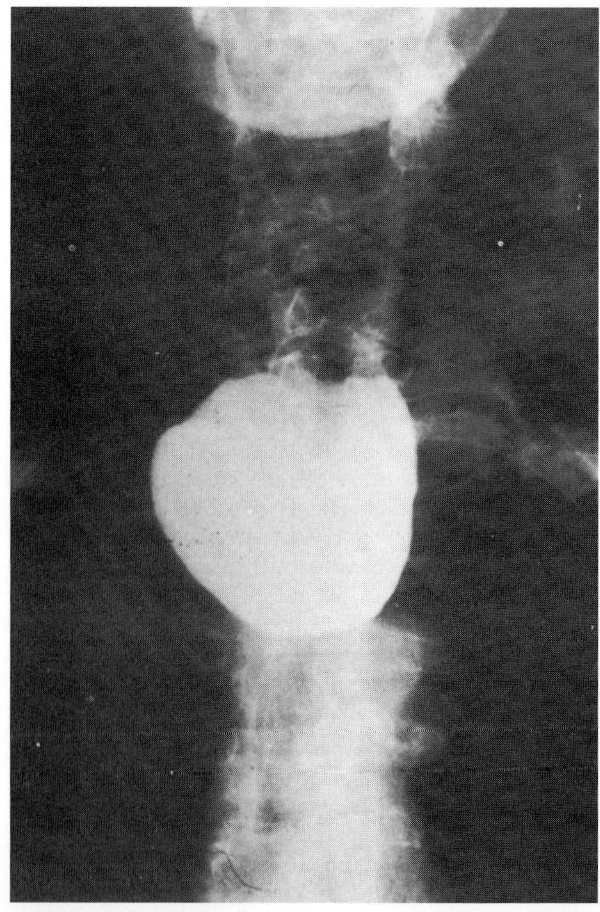

FIGURE **29–5.** A barium swallow showing a huge Zenker's diverticulum. (From Baue AE, Naunheim KS: Hiatal hernia and gastroesophageal reflux. In Baue AE (ed): Glenn's Thoracic and Cardiovascular Surgery, 5th ed. Norwalk, CT, Appleton & Lange, 1991, p. 751, with permission.)

Surgery, as described above, is the appropriate treatment in conjunction with excision of the diverticulum.

Extrinsic compression of the esophagus can occur as the result of anatomic abnormalities. The esophagus is normally indented by the descending aorta at the level of the tracheal bifurcation and any variation in aortic course or size may further impinge on the esophagus. Any structural change in the mediastinum including cardiac chamber enlargement, large tumors, or lymph nodes can present as dysphagia due to extrinsic compression. Treatment of the underlying problem usually relieves the esophageal symptoms. Placement of an internal esophageal stent can palliate a symptomatic patient.

Trauma, of a blunt or penetrating nature, produces injuries that include fistulae and perforation. The treatment of esophageal atresia and tracheoesophageal (TE) fistula as it pertains to pediatric surgery will not be considered for discussion. In adults, TE fistulae can develop as a consequence of advanced lung or esophageal tumors, or from mishaps relating to tracheal or esophageal injury, often occurring during diagnostic or therapeutic instrumentation.[4–6] The surgical approach to repair of a TE fistula depends on its location and the underlying cause. Esophageal tumor–related fistulae commonly occur in the distal trachea or at the level of the left mainstem bronchus. These fistulae can be palliated by positioning an esophageal stent within the defect. Traumatic fistulae need to be repaired either primarily or at a later date following an initial esophageal diversion.

Esophageal perforation can be iatrogenic, traumatic, or spontaneous, in the latter case usually associated with emesis. Although some patients may be managed conservatively by strict fasting and antibiotics, most perforations require emergent surgery to repair the defect and drain the surrounding area. The location of perforation will dictate the surgical approach used.

Ingestion of caustic substances, often alkaline cleaning agents, causes chemical burns. Acid ingestion causes minimal injury to the esophagus probably due to relative resistance of the squamous epithelium to acid. Acid produces a coagulation necrosis that limits penetration into deeper tissues. Endoscopic evaluation should be done to determine the extent of injury; emergency surgery is almost never indicated. Related injury to the larynx and trachea may complicate the induction of anesthesia. Ingestion of an alkaline substance causes liquefaction necrosis with extensive destruction of tissues, thrombosis of blood vessels, and deep tissue injury. If a full-thickness gastric injury occurs, resulting peritonitis can necessitate laparotomy and possible esophagogastrectomy. Once peritonitis has been excluded and oropharyngeal burns are absent or improved, endoscopy should be done to evaluate the extent of injury. When esophageal injury is extensive, strictures generally develop. In some cases, dilatation is not possible or not adequate to relieve symptoms. These patients may require esophagectomy with colon or jejunal replacement.

Foreign bodies and bleeding are also generally benign causes for esophageal surgery. The majority of esophageal foreign bodies are found in the pediatric population.[7] However, no matter what the age of the patient, the foreign bodies need to be removed to prevent aspiration into the airway or erosion and perforation of the esophagus. Most foreign bodies are found in the upper esophagus, which is the narrowest portion, although some may pass to the level of the aortic indentation or even the gastroesophageal junction. Foreign bodies are removed with rigid or fiberoptic endoscopy under general anesthesia or managed anesthesia care.

Esophageal bleeding may be caused by reflux esophagitis, Mallory-Weiss syndrome, or esophageal varices. Reflux esophagitis is treated medically. Mallory-Weiss tears due to vomiting are usually diagnosed endoscopically and treated medically. Rarely, a Mallory-Weiss tear will require surgical repair through a high abdominal approach to the gastroesophageal junction. Bleeding esophageal varices are often treated with endoscopic sclerotherapy.

Malignant Disease

The treatment of esophageal cancer depends on the extent of disease, the patient's medical status, and the patient's decision concerning various treatment options. At the present time, surgery with or without chemotherapy is the only possibly curative option, although surgery often results only in palliation of a previously unrecognized locally metastatic tumor. Patients who are unacceptable surgical risks or who have advanced disease may benefit from palliative radiation directed at the tumor site or placement of an internal esophageal stent to improve swallowing function.

Primary esophageal tumors are either squamous cell, arising from the squamous epithelium lining the esophagus, or adenocarcinomas of gastric glandular origin. Sarcomas and melanomas of the esophagus are rare. The location and extent of an esophageal cancer determines which surgical approach will be used. Since the division of the esophagus into segments is arbitrary and inclusion of esophagogastric tumors in some studies adds bias towards the lower third, it is difficult to compare reported frequencies of sites of cancer. However, middle and lower third lesions are the most common sites of esophageal malignancy (>70%). Upper third lesions are less common (10 to 25%), and cervical lesions are rare (3 to 8%).

Surgical Approaches to Esophageal Lesions

The following descriptions of various surgical procedures and approaches pertain to both esophageal cancers and benign conditions. The most common and easiest replacement of any resected segment of esophagus is with the stomach, which can be mobilized to reach into the neck if necessary.[8] Resection of an esophageal malignancy often requires removal of more than one half the esophagus so that adequate cancer-free margins are included in the specimen. The approach to a lower esophageal or GE junction lesion can be a midline abdominal incision. If resection can be accomplished with adequate margins via an abdominal approach, the surgery and concomitant anesthetic considerations are no different than for any abdominal procedure. However, if the lesion extends beyond what can be safely reached or adequately resected through the hiatus of the diaphragm, a transthoracic approach is required.[9] Once a thoracotomy is part of the planned procedure, it is often necessary to plan for single-lung ventilation during the thoracic portion of the surgery. Although it is possible to retract a ventilated lung away from the esophagus, a collapsed lung is less intrusive in the surgical field and likely to be less traumatized from retraction than an inflated one.

Thoracoabdominal

A thoracoabdominal approach that includes a left anterolateral thoracotomy extending obliquely across the costal margin into the abdomen is appropriate for lesions in the lower third of the esophagus (Fig. 29–6). Lesions in the middle and upper third of the esophagus are most easily approached via a right thoracotomy. Although the esophagus lies primarily in the left chest, a right-sided approach is indicated so that the proximal anastomosis can be accomplished at any level without hindrance from the aortic arch.

Thoracic and Abdominal (Ivor Lewis)

Resection of middle and upper third lesions may involve a combined but separate right thoracotomy and upper midline abdominal incision known as an Ivor Lewis esophagectomy.[10] First, the patient is explored (supine) through the abdominal incision to determine the extent of disease and in the case of malignancy to search for possible metastases that would preclude a surgical cure.

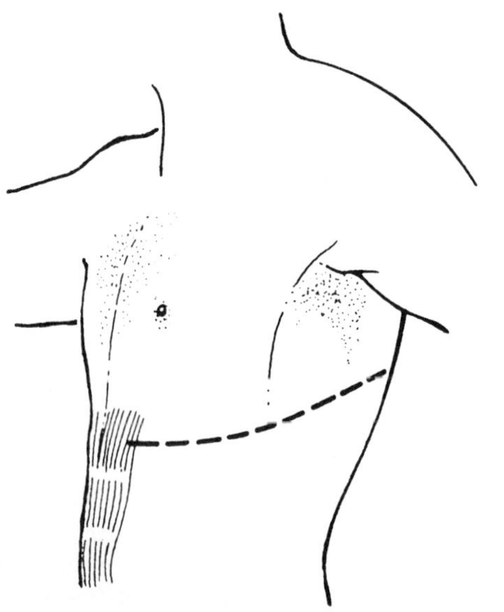

FIGURE **29–6.** The thoracoabdominal incision. (From Pearson FG (ed): Esophageal Surgery. New York, Churchill Livingstone, 1995, p. 659, with permission.)

The stomach is then mobilized so that it can be brought into the chest to substitute for the esophagus. The esophagus is then resected via a right thoracotomy (lateral position), and the stomach is pulled through the hiatus to be anastomosed at the level of the resected margin (Fig. 29–7). In high (upper third) esophageal lesions, a cervical anastomosis through a left neck approach may be required. Some surgeons prefer a cervical anastomosis without regard for the location of the lesion, although there are benefits and complications for either approach.[11–13]

Transhiatal

Esophagectomy can also be accomplished via a transhiatal approach without thoracotomy (Fig. 29–8). An upper abdominal incision is made to mobilize the stomach in a manner discussed above. The esophagus is then dissected free from above through the left neck and below through the diaphragmatic hiatus. Once the esophagus has been resected, the stomach is drawn through the posterior mediastinum to be anastomosed in the neck. The transhiatal approach avoids a thoracotomy and may therefore be preferable in patients with limited pulmonary reserve.[14] However, the period of esophageal dissection with the operator's hand compressing posterior mediastinal structures is often associated with profound cardiovascular decompensation and severe reduction in systemic perfusion.[15] Hypotension produced by this mechanism is not generally responsive to volume and/or pressors and, thus, a decrease in cardiac output and blood pressure must often be tolerated for at least short periods in order to perform the surgery. Additionally, blunt esophageal dissection can, on rare occasion, result in a tracheal tear usually in the membranous wall. In order to maintain ventilation in the event of a tracheal tear, it is prudent to use an *uncut* endodotracheal tube, which could be advanced past the tear, when the initial intubation is accomplished.

Interposition

The aforementioned procedures all require that the patient have an intact stomach unblemished by prior surgery or scarring. If the stomach is unsuitable, either colon interposition or jejunal transposition are viable alternatives. Both procedures add considerable technical complexity and increased operative time. In either case the patient must undergo preoperative angiography to define vascular supply to the bowel, and a full bowel preparation is required as with any elective bowel resection. Both angiography and bowel preparation will result in relative dehydration in a patient who may already have limited oral intake. Therefore, it is important to assess and treat volume replacement before and during the surgery.

Replacement of the esophagus by either colon or jejunum requires a laparotomy in addition to a thoracotomy. If the colon is utilized, either right or left colon can be suitable depending on the length of esophagus to

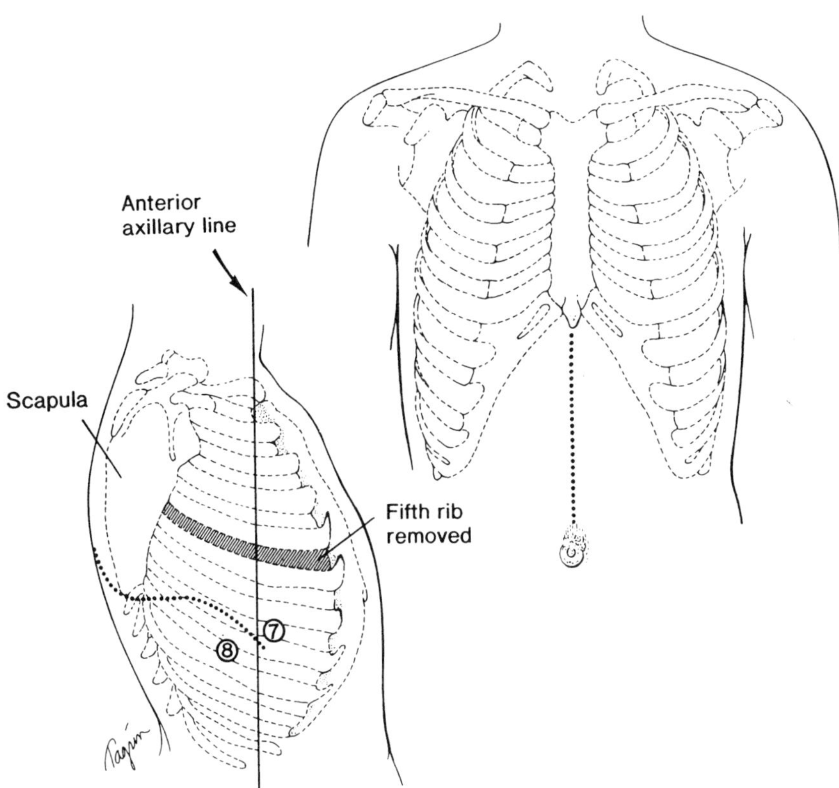

FIGURE **29–7.** The standard incisions for an Ivor Lewis esophagectomy. (From Pearson FG (ed): Esophageal Surgery. New York, Churchill Livingstone, 1995, p. 671, with permission.)

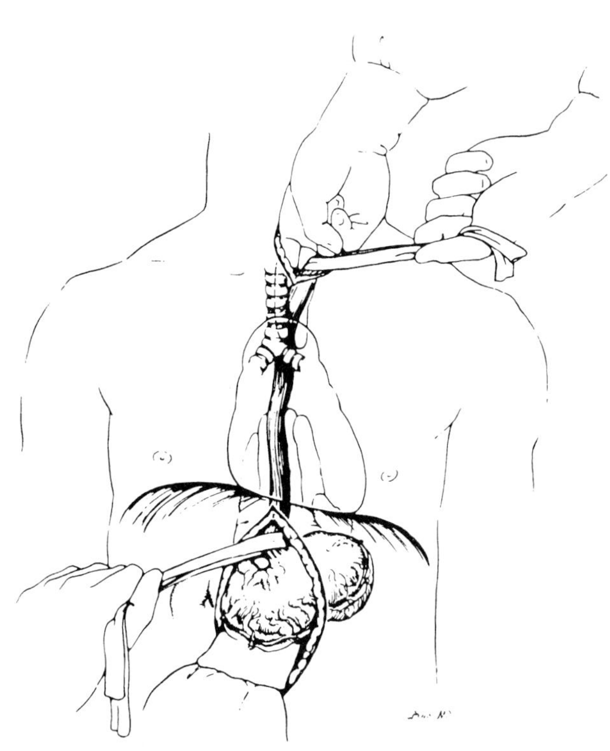

FIGURE **29–8.** The transhiatal approach dissects the stomach through an abdominal incision to be pulled up through the chest from above through a cervical incision. (From Pearson FG (ed): Esophageal Surgery. New York, Churchill Livingstone, 1995, p. 687, with permission.)

be replaced and the mesenteric vascular pedicle length. The colon can be positioned in a subcutaneous, substernal, or transpleural route, either anterior or posterior to the hilum of the lung (Fig. 29–9). Jejunal transposition is indicated primarily for replacement of the cervical esophagus. It involves transfer of a jejunal segment into or along the cervical esophageal bed as a free graft with subsequent microvascular anastomosis. The choice of colon versus jejunum may depend on prior intestinal surgery, suitable vascular supply to an appropriate segment of bowel, length of the reconstructed defect, and in the case of free graft, existence of a microvascular surgical team. Differences in caliber of lumen are relatively unimportant; segments can be positioned so as to maintain isoperistalsis, although gravity alone may be sufficient to effect swallowing. Intraoperative and postoperative volume requirements may be significant due to the lengthy bowel dissection and the large operative field exposed as well as pre-existing poor oral intake.

Stents

Patients who are not candidates for surgery because of advanced disease or coexisting medical conditions that would preclude their ability to tolerate surgery, can obtain temporary swallowing ability from placement of an internal stent. A TE fistula not surgically repairable for any reason may also be palliated with stenting. However,

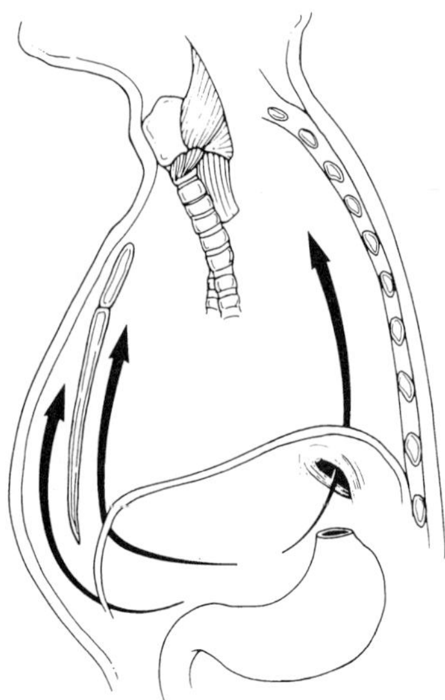

FIGURE **29–9.** The three routes for esophageal bypass shown schematically. (From Orringer MB: Surgical options for esophageal resection and reconstruction with stomach. Esophageal cancer. In Baue AE (ed): Glenn's Thoracic and Cardiovascular Surgery, 5th ed. Norwalk, CT, Appleton & Lange, 1991, p. 828, with permission.)

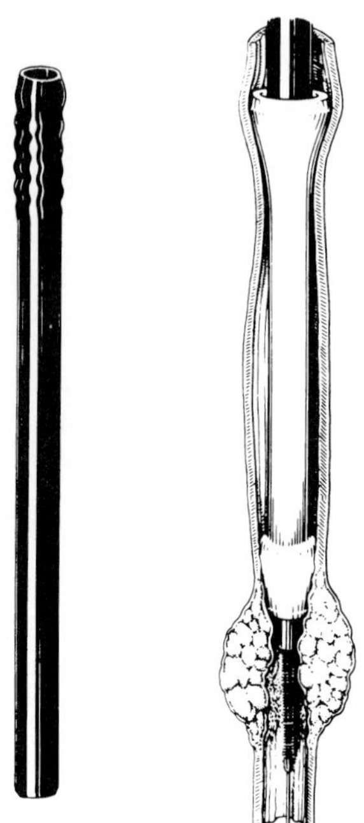

FIGURE **29–10.** An introducer (*left*) used to insert an esophageal stent shown in place (*right*). (From Orringer MB: Surgical options for esophageal resection and reconstruction with stomach. Esophageal cancer. In Baue AE (ed): Glenn's Thoracic and Cardiovascular Surgery, 5th ed. Norwalk, CT, Appleton & Lange, 1991, p. 832, with permission.)

an esophageal stent for a tumor-related TE fistula can compress the membranous trachea, thereby causing airway compromise once the patient is extubated.[16] It is therefore critical that the surgeon and anesthesiologist be prepared to emergently reintubate the trachea and remove the esophageal stent if required. Following tracheal extubation, a period of observation in the operating room should rapidly identify the patient with airway compromise. Stenting can be accomplished endoscopically from above using either a guidewire that has been passed through the narrowed esophagus or the endoscope to introduce and position the stent. Alternatively, the guidewire may be advanced into the stomach and located through a small laparotomy from where the stent may be pulled up into the narrowed esophagus (Fig. 29–10).

Nonthoracic

Surgery for some benign conditions already enumerated includes the approaches described above as well as a few other approaches and anesthetic problems worthy of consideration. Depending on the surgeon's preference as well as the patient's prior surgical history, the hiatus hernia repair can be accomplished via an abdominal incision (Nissen fundoplication, Hill repair)[17,18] in addition to the conventional transthoracic (Belsey Mark IV or V) approach.[19] The purpose of the surgery is to replace the lower esophageal sphincter and prevent reflux by creating a valve-like mechanism using plication around the esophagogastric junction.[18] Such surgery produces immediate results so that prior anesthetic concern for reflux should not be a major consideration at the time of emergence.

If surgery is required for benign stricture, the strictured portion of esophagus can be resected and replaced in any one of the previously described procedures for malignancy. Alternatively, the stricture can be dilated and an antireflux operation performed[20] when reflux is the precipitating factor in stricture formation. The relative merits of dilatation versus surgery are the subject of controversy due to surgical complications and failures. Dilatation with any one of a variety of weighted bougies or balloon catheters is usually sufficient to relieve the stricture albeit not permanently in all cases.

Patients with motility disorders should consume clear liquids for several days prior to a surgical procedure and may need esophageal lavage to remove debris immediately prior to induction of anesthesia. Surgical approach varies with the area involved. As with all instances of dysphagia, once the procedure is completed, the patient should emerge in a semierect position to a fully awake state prior to extubation to avoid possible aspiration.

The surgical approach to a benign TE fistula involving the upper portion of the esophagus, such as one due to prolonged tracheal intubation, is accomplished via a simple neck incision. Further exposure may require an upper median sternotomy or right thoracotomy to reach the carina.[6]

Retrieval of a foreign body from the esophagus can be accomplished using minimal intravenous sedation and flexible esophagoscopy whereby the foreign body is grasped with biopsy forceps and removed with direct continuous visualization. General endotracheal anesthesia should be reserved for patients who are unable to cooperate under sedation and for retrieval of sharp objects that require rigid endoscopy. Although a foreign body can totally obstruct the esophagus, aspiration precautions must be used with the induction of general anesthesia.

Anesthesia Care

Preoperative Evaluation

The three major areas of concern for any esophageal procedure are reflux as a risk for aspiration, pulmonary pathology, either secondary to reflux or tobacco abuse, and malnutrition with or without dehydration.

Aspiration

Problems with swallowing coordination due to any medical or surgical condition as well as incompetence of the LES resulting in reflux can lead to chronic aspiration. If aspiration is suspected, a pulmonary evaluation with appropriate treatment is required.

Gastroesophageal reflux is the most common condition requiring esophageal surgery. The nature and extent of reflux should be clearly identified. Often, clear-cut symptoms of reflux, including heartburn, substernal pain, or belching, are prominent and obvious findings. Less evident symptomatology may also exist. A patient may present with symptoms more consistent with what appears to be asthma, which is actually secondary to high-grade reflux and aspiration.[21] Difficulty swallowing or a sensation of solids sticking at a specific location is another prominent symptom associated with esophageal obstruction or motility disorders. Regurgitation may be associated with reflux, strictures, diverticulae, and obstructions from various causes. Patients often describe swallowing problems related to solids but not liquids. In all cases, one must maintain a high index of suspicion of either reflux, obstruction, or uncoordinated swallowing according to the presumptive diagnosis being investigated. Radiologic studies and endoscopic evaluation can help define the specific lesion accurately. The anesthesiologist must remember to include such information as part of the preoperative evaluation and use it accordingly. Any evidence of reflux symptoms requires either rapid sequence induction with cricoid pressure or awake fiberoptic intubation to provide maximal airway protection. Positioning the patient semiupright prior to and during induction also affords a slight advantage of gravity drainage.

Pulmonary Pathology

Patients requiring esophageal surgery commonly have significant associated pre-existing pulmonary disease,[22] particularly those with esophageal cancer who have an extensive tobacco history. A pulmonary evaluation including chest x-ray, standard pulmonary function testing, and arterial blood gases is often performed to assess the patient's baseline status. When the cause for pulmonary compromise is based on esophageal pathology, it is not always possible to fully treat an underlying pulmonary problem without correcting the precipitating esophageal factor as evidenced by recurrent aspiration or frank pneumonia. Thus, if requested, a pulmonary consultation should provide an approach to optimize the patient's pulmonary status in the face of continued esophageal dysfunction. Aggressive chest physical therapy, antibiotics, bronchodilator therapy and, on occasion, steroids may be required to improve the patient's preoperative pulmonary function. These are very important issues that are discussed in greater detail in Chapters 3, 4, and 5.

Nutritional Depletion

A further consequence of many esophageal pathologic states is nutritional depletion. Obstruction and swallowing difficulties may result in very limited oral intake with caloric limitations, concomitant weight loss, and the potential for dehydration. Malnourished patients are at increased risk for postoperative morbidity and mortality. Central venous access should be used both to assess hydration and to aid in parenteral nutrition when oral intake is severely limited by swallowing difficulties. In patients with benign disease, parenteral nutrition has been shown to be beneficial when given in the perioperative period. However, the efficacy of parenteral nutrition in cancer patients is equivocal at best.

Premedication

Selection of premedication is based on criteria used for any other surgical patient, but it must not obtund a patient who is at increased risk for aspiration. Therefore, if an anxiolytic agent is deemed necessary, the dose should be minimal (e.g., 2 to 3 mg of midazolam). Additionally, an antisialagogue (atropine, 0.4 mg, or glycopyrrolate, 0.2 mg given intramuscularly preoperatively) is necessary to limit secretions, since virtually all esophageal procedures include endoscopic evaluations, which induce increased secretions. Prophylaxis for acid aspiration should include premedication with an H_2 blocker (cimetidine or ranitidine) as well as Reglan to promote gastric emptying despite the fact that pre-existing esophageal pathology (dysmotility or obstruction) may limit the usefulness of such drugs. Any regimen that has been instituted for a pre-existing pulmonary problem should be continued with specific concern for stress steroid dosing in the patient who has recently received a course of steroid therapy.

Monitoring

Monitoring decisions are based on (1) pre-existing disease, (2) the planned procedure, and (3) expected perioperative events. Clinical experience with esophageal procedures is undoubtedly the best basis for monitoring decisions. Routine electrocardiogram leads, blood pressure cuff, and pulse oximeter probe should be placed as for any anesthetic. The patient should have at least one large-bore (16-gauge or larger) freely running intravenous line for all but the simplest (e.g., endoscopic) procedures. Blood loss varies, but rarely is transfusion a concern except perhaps in the patient who is anemic preoperatively. Additionally, invasive blood pressure monitoring is often clinically useful during periods of surgical manipulation in the chest, if one-lung ventilation is to be carried out for extended periods, or if the patient's cardiopulmonary status warrants appropriate intraoperative and postoperative monitoring. Clinical judgment can be used to decide whether a central line is needed to assess the patient's volume status, or the patient can be volume loaded with a crystalloid solution to maintain an adequate urine output (30 to 50 ml/hr for an average size adult). Central venous line placement allows for volume loading prior to surgical compression of the mediastinal structures, which often accompanies esophageal procedures, and for careful repletion of surgical losses. Pulmonary artery catheterization is dictated by existing cardiac disease.

Anesthesia for Endoscopy

Virtually all esophageal pathology other than dysmotility is evaluated with endoscopic visualization prior to surgical repair so that the exact location and extent of disease can be assessed. In cases of esophageal stricture, endoscopy, often performed with radiologic imaging for passing dilators, is therapeutic.

Minimal anesthesia (local and managed anesthesia care) is usually adequate for flexible endoscopic procedures that are brief and done for diagnostic evaluations. Excellent topical preparation of the oropharynx using 10% lidocaine spray (10 mg/spray) or 2% lidocaine gargle must be achieved to ensure patient comfort and cooperation. The patient is best positioned semiupright with the tongue extended and gently depressed with a tongue blade as the tonsilar pillars and posterior pharynx are sprayed with 10% lidocaine. After two or three sprays in each area, the patient should be instructed to swallow the liquid. Again with the patient's mouth open and tongue extended, the same areas should be sprayed while the tongue blade is slowly advanced toward the posterior pharynx both to improve visualization of the area and to test the adequacy of topical anesthesia. When 10% lidocaine spray is used, the total dose of lidocaine used must be monitored so as to avoid toxicity. If lidocaine gargle is used, the patient is given a small cup of viscous lidocaine and asked to gargle and swallow a mouthful of the liquid. The gargling process should be repeated several times to ensure coverage of the posterior pharynx. An emesis basin should be readily available, since patients often have difficulty swallowing the spray or the thick liquid. Once the patient tolerates a tongue blade being placed in the posterior pharynx, topicalization for endoscopy should be adequate. Patients treated with topical local anesthesia retain normal motility but have difficulty swallowing.[23] Therefore, while sedation is added to reduce anxiety and induce amnesia for the experience, the paramount consideration is that the patient remain conscious enough to follow commands and maintain airway protection. Titration of small (e.g., 0.5-mg) increments of midazolam and 10- to 20-mg boluses of propofol should be cautiously and slowly added to achieve the desired level of sedation. Constant verbal contact with the patient should serve to both reassure the patient and aid in assessing the patient's level of sedation.

Rigid endoscopy almost always requires general anesthesia as do procedures for which paralysis or total immobility is required, and for patients not suited to monitored anesthesia. A small endotracheal tube, placed to the left side of the mouth, will facilitate the surgical approach to the esophagus. Induction of general anesthesia must be planned so that the airway will be secured without mishap. The patient's anatomy should be carefully inspected to determine whether routine laryngoscopy will be successful. If there is any question as to the likelihood of easy intubation with laryngoscopy, the anesthesiologist can topicalize the mouth and pharynx as described above for monitored anesthetic procedures, then gently laryngoscope the patient to determine if the epiglottis or a portion of the larynx can be visualized. If visualization is possible, a standard rapid sequence induction can be accomplished. However, when the epiglottis or laryngeal structures cannot be visualized, a flexible fiberoptic bronchoscope should be used for awake intubation. Most of the topicalization required for an awake intubation will have already been accomplished.

Under ideal conditions, the rapid sequence induction secures the airway while minimizing risk of aspiration of gastric contents. When the decision to use rapid sequence induction with laryngoscopy is made, the anesthesiologist should be prepared for several possible problems. First, because intravenous induction must be rapidly administered, there may be wide swings in blood pressure, especially in patients who suffer from dehydration. The need to rapidly secure the airway may result in trauma to oropharyngeal structures. Also, there is the risk of failure to intubate despite evidence of what appears on clinical evaluation to be an anatomically normal airway. Alternatively, the fiberoptic intubation requires excellent topicalization so that gagging and regurgitation are not induced. Even with the bronchoscope in place in the trachea, it may be difficult to pass the endotracheal tube over the bronchoscope through the glottis.

It is important to remember that endoscopic procedures do not usually produce significant postoperative pain. Therefore, narcotics, if administered as part of the anesthetic, should be selected accordingly and given in minimal dosage. Regardless of anesthetic agents or techniques used, ultimately the patient must be fully awake at the termination of the procedure so that airway protection and handling of secretions is optimal. Positioning the patient semierect during or at the completion of the endoscopy may be helpful, particularly when reflux symptoms are prominent.

Anesthesia for Major Surgical Procedures

General anesthesia, with or without supplemental regional techniques, is required for surgical repair of the esophagus. The choice of specific anesthetic agents is based on the patient's preoperative evaluation as well as the type of surgical procedure, and the number and location of incisions. In cases where both an abdominal and thoracic incision are planned, or in patients at risk for pulmonary complications, placement of an epidural catheter prior to surgery for management of postoperative pain should be considered.[24,25] Advantages of a "combined" approach in this patient population has yet to be determined.

Prior to induction of anesthesia, one must determine whether reflux, dysmotility, or obstruction of the esophagus pose a risk for aspiration and therefore require appropriate precautions. Either awake fiberoptic bronchoscopy or rapid sequence induction as described above can be used if needed. If all or part of the surgery is performed through a thoracotomy incision, either a double-lumen endotracheal tube (DLT) or a single-lumen tube with a bronchial blocker can be used to allow for lung collapse. As previously noted, one-lung anesthesia is not absolutely indicated for esophageal surgery, but in most cases lung collapse affords the surgeon a quiet and unobstructed field in which to work without the need for lung retraction and thus improves operative conditions.

In choosing the initial tube and method to accomplish lung collapse, one must first consider the expected "success" of intubation. Commonly, esophageal procedures begin with an endoscopy under general anesthesia to make a final assessment of the pathology. If the initial intubation with a single-lumen endotracheal tube is deemed difficult, no attempt should be made to reintubate the patient with a DLT. A bronchial blocker can be placed either within or adjacent to the existing tube, and positioned with the visual aid of a fiberoptic bronchoscope. If no endoscopy precedes the surgery, one should consider the advisability and feasibility of both a rapid sequence induction and the intraoperative management of ventilation with a DLT or a bronchial blocker with a single-lumen tube (either a Univent tube or a single-lumen tube with a Fogarty venous occlusion catheter (8/14 Fr) used as a bronchial blocker).[26] The Univent tube incorporates a bronchial blocker in a separate channel within the endotracheal tube. The Univent blocker has a small channel that permits opening to atmosphere to allow for lung collapse. Alternatively, a Fogarty venous occlusion catheter can be placed in the trachea followed immediately by the endotracheal tube. In either case, the blocker can be manipulated with bronchoscopic guidance to occlude the mainstem bronchus of choice. Since airway protection is always a primary concern, proper endobronchial placement of a DLT or a bronchial blocker should be of minimal concern, at least initially. The tube position can always be adjusted after the airway has been secured, thereby limiting apneic time as well as risk of reflux and aspiration.

If fiberoptic intubation is planned, a DLT can be placed with excellent topical preparation of the airway as described for esophagoscopy. However, it may be difficult to pass a DLT over a small bronchoscope into the larynx. Therefore, it may become necessary to use a single-lumen tube with a bronchial blocker as an alternative. Intraoperative use of a DLT allows for rapid lung deflation and reinflation as well as easy lung separation and suctioning of secretions. Once positioned properly, DLTs move very little and rarely require adjustment of positioning.[27] A single-lumen tube using a bronchial blocker for lung isolation requires that lung deflation occur primarily by absorption atelectasis. Secretions are problematic, since they cannot be suctioned from the deflated lung. Additionally, a bronchial blocker can become dislodged into the trachea with resultant partial or complete airway obstruction. Nevertheless, if postoperative ventilation is planned or likely, the best choice might be to opt for a single-lumen tube with bronchial blocker so as to avoid the hazards of reintubation after a long procedure, particularly when the choice for initial intubation was to use a fiberoptic bronchoscope.

As with all thoracic surgical procedures, the anesthesiologist must be cognizant of the surgeon's activities on the field. Therefore, it is important to determine whether changes in ventilation or blood pressure are mechanical or physiologic in cause, particularly during esophageal resection in the mediastinum. Communication is obviously important and essential. Mechanical problems must be noted and may need to be tolerated for short periods of time to accommodate the surgical procedure. If ventilation becomes problematic, often due to mediastinal compression affecting the ventilating lumen of a DLT or causing repositioning of the bronchial blocker, the anesthesiologist must work with the surgeon so that compromise on both sides is limited and tolerable. Both the surgeon and anesthesiologist need to communicate during periods of hypotension to minimize the duration of a hypotensive episode and to avoid the misdiagnosis of bleeding, which could result in the inappropriate use of vasopressor therapy. Hypotension may also occur with mediastinal compression, especially with a closed transthoracic procedure.

Once the esophageal procedure is near completion, the anesthesiologist may be required to pass a nasogastric tube into the esophagus. Placement of a nasogastric tube through an anastomosis or repair requires careful guidance and secure taping so that it does not disrupt the surgical field and remains securely in place postoperatively.

Emergence from Anesthesia

Appropriate timing of extubation is a critical decision following esophageal surgery. In addition to meeting basic extubation criteria, the patient must often be considered at continuing risk for aspiration. The patient's state of awareness, as well as the ability to swallow secretions and cough, are of the utmost importance. Therefore, in deciding when to extubate the patient several factors need to be considered. The patient must be able to swallow and handle secretions. Pain control and muscle strength should be adequate in order to maximize the patient's ability to cough. Any prior respiratory compromise such as aspiration pneumonia should be resolved.

One must evaluate both the patient and the specifics of the surgical procedure so that the patient may either be safely extubated or remain intubated until extubation criteria are met. Assuming adequate preoperative pulmonary and nutritional status, most patients can be extubated immediately following endoscopic procedures, excision of diverticuli, myotomy, and hiatal hernia repair. Although motility problems may not be instantly alleviated, a patient who is fully awake, following commands, and semiupright should be capable of clearing secretions. In some cases where a TE fistula has been repaired, it may be desirable to leave the patient intubated so that the repair is protected and the airway stented for a short time. Surgical studies have found that swallowing, motility, and airway protection are abnormal after esophagectomy.[28-30] In addition, the LES is lost allowing free reflux. Although the advisability of early extubation has been considered,[31] most centers leave patients intubated for at least several hours postoperatively.[25,32,33] If a DLT has been used for the procedure, reintubation may be required if extubation is not planned or possible at the end of surgery.

Control of operative pain should be accomplished prior to extubation. As with all thoracic surgical procedures, patients need adequate pain control so that they may maintain ventilation and oxygenation without being under- or overmedicated. Although a single abdominal or thoracic incision would not routinely preclude extubation, some esophageal pathology is approached either via a left thoracoabdominal approach or a combined abdominal incision followed by a right thoracotomy. As previously mentioned, two surgical incisions may make initial pain control problematic such that postoperative ventilation affords time to make the patient comfortable. Additionally, pain from two significant surgical incisions can result in poor respiratory effort or overmedication leading to somnolence, both of which can lead to pulmonary compromise. Therefore, following esophageal resection, patients should be managed conservatively and extubated only when optimal pain control and an adequate level of sensorium have been achieved.[25] Many benign surgical conditions enumerated previously are treated with single-incision approaches and would therefore be considered for prompt extubation unless aspiration risk is considered to be significant, and the patient's state of arousal is judged to be inadequate.

Patients whose preoperative pulmonary status has been compromised by repeated aspiration pneumonia or underlying respiratory pathology may benefit from a more prolonged period of mechanical ventilation and pulmonary toilet in an attempt to optimize conditions for successful extubation. Patients who are severely nutritionally depleted may not have adequate muscle strength to maintain ventilation after a surgical procedure. When reintubation is planned, several factors must be considered. First, it is essential to review the events during the initial intubation. After several hours of surgery, often with the patient positioned lateral and somewhat head down, an initial "easy" intubation may become somewhat more difficult due to edema involving pharyngeal and laryngeal tissues. Direct visualization of laryngeal anatomy with direct laryngoscopy prior to any tube change could identify potential difficulties. If a straightforward laryngoscopy is planned, a second person should be present to assist and expedite tube exchange. The pharynx should be suctioned clear of secretions under direct vision so that with laryngoscopy the DLT is withdrawn and quickly replaced with a styletted single-lumen tube without loss of visualization of the larynx.

A nasogastric tube should be present to help identify the esophagus. Obviously, an esophageal intubation following esophageal surgery is to be avoided to avert direct trauma to the esophageal anastomosis and to avoid inflating the gastrointestinal tract with air, which could also traumatize the fresh surgical field.

In the event that some difficulty is anticipated, several techniques have been described to aid in changing from a double- to a single-lumen endotracheal tube. Only after denitrogenation, adequate paralysis, and sufficient anesthesia should tube exchange be performed. A tube exchanger (Cook Airway Exchange Catheter, 5 mm) can be inserted into the tracheal lumen of a DLT. Both cuffs are deflated and the DLT is quickly but gently withdrawn. An appropriate sized single-lumen tube is then threaded onto the tube exchanger and guided either with a hand in the pharynx or with some lift from laryngoscopy to aid in passage through the glottis. If difficulty is encountered and the oxygen saturation falls, the exchanger can be connected to a jet ventilator or an anesthesia circuit using the oxygen flush valve to provide ventilation while further maneuvers are attempted to achieve an intubation. Special care must be taken to ensure that the tube exchanger does not lodge distally into a bronchus, since when using jet ventilation or an oxygen flush valve, high pressures can build in distal airways and result in a pneumothorax. A similar technique uses a fiberoptic bronchoscope as an intubating stylette that allows for continuous visualization of the airway during extubation and reintubation.[34] However, continuous ventilation is not possible using the bronchoscope. In either case, both a bronchoscope and tube exchanger are thin and malleable so that re-entering the glottis may be difficult. If successful reintubation from a DLT is deemed unlikely, the tube may be left in place with the bronchial cuff pilot balloon removed so that the tube can be used safely for ventilation without the risk of tracheal obstruction by the bronchial cuff. Consideration of all the above issues, discussion with the surgeon, and careful preparation should result in an uneventful outcome.

Postoperative Complications

Following surgery, patients may suffer from a variety of complications, which can be classified as related to preexisting conditions, anesthesia, or surgery. The majority of complications are pulmonary in nature, and assignment to any of the above categories of complications is not always possible.

Pre-existing conditions associated with esophageal pathology are either pulmonary or nutritional. Both conditions can result in prolonged postoperative ventilation or eventual reintubation after initial extubation. As described earlier, severe reflux can present as asthma secondary to recurrent aspiration. High-grade obstruction with dysphagia or vocal cord paralysis, usually due to tumor involvement of the recurrent laryngeal nerve, can also lead to aspiration and airway compromise.[35] Pneumonias secondary to esophageal pathology often cannot be resolved without treatment of the underlying problem. If the patient's preoperative pulmonary status is borderline, the postoperative course may be prolonged and complicated by continuing specific treatment of pulmonary pathology. Failure to wean from mechanical ventilation can be attributable to depleted nutritional status with poor muscle strength.

Anesthesia-related complications are frequently pulmonary in nature and most often due to aspiration either at induction of anesthesia or after extubation. Extubation criteria require that the patient has adequate analgesia and is fully awake and able to clear secretions. When possible, patients should be extubated in the semierect position to allow for gravity drainage of the esophagus, particularly when a nasogastric tube is in place, thereby creating a pathway for free reflux. In addition, atelectasis with inability to clear secretions due to pain or limited cooperation can result in postoperative pneumonia requiring reintubation and ventilation.

Surgical complications vary according to the procedure. Strictures due to scarring can arise from any esophageal resection resulting in symptomatic dysphagia.[36] Strictures can often be easily treated with dilatations. If dilatation is inadequate, the anastomosis can be revised. Any endoscopic procedure including diagnostic and therapeutic (e.g., dilatation) can result in esophageal perforation. Following esophageal perforation, the patient is at risk for mediastinitis, which is potentially lethal. Perforations can be managed conservatively by maintaining NPO status and use of appropriate intravenous antibiotics. In extreme circumstances, the perforation can be treated with an esophagectomy. Failure of antireflux procedures is due to slippage of the plication with recurrent reflux or too tight a wrap causing bloating and inability to belch. Both problems usually require further surgery. Following esophagectomy with cervical anastomosis patients may suffer from dysphagia and aspiration due to lack of coordinated swallowing.[28,37] Any temporary damage or permanent loss of function of a recurrent laryngeal nerve prevents glottic closure with swallowing and thereby promotes aspiration.[29] Permanent recurrent laryngeal nerve damage can be treated with Teflon injection of the vocal cords or Silastic medialization.[29]

Esophageal resection for carcinoma is associated with a morbidity and mortality ranging from 15 to 40%.[38,39] The majority of complications associated with esophagectomy are pulmonary.[32,33,41] Transhiatal esophagectomy is associated with atrial arrhythmias, which are seen most often in patients with a prior history of cardiac disease.[41] The most morbid complication associated with esophageal resection and replacement is anastomotic leak, particularly when the anastomosis is in the chest and mediastinitis results. In one large series, the incidence of reoperation for complications was 2.7% with a 15% incidence of anastomotic leak.[42]

Anastomotic leak or loss of integrity of a resected area leading to spillage of esophageal contents can be life threatening, particularly if the leak occurs inside the chest. Suspected mediastinal leak is investigated by a gastrograffin swallow, and if confirmed, requires emergency surgery with drainage, esophageal diversion, and intensive antibiotic therapy. Even with appropriate and timely treatment, morbidity and mortality from resultant mediastinitis can be significant. Some authors advocate the use of a cervical anastomosis in esophageal resection so that any anastomotic breakdown can be easily treated by opening a neck incision.[43] Bowel or gastric ischemia in a transposed segment usually requires prompt removal.[44]

Single reports of complications abound in the surgical literature. A variety of unusual complications have been reported following esophagectomy including extrapericardial tamponade,[45] volvulus of the intrathoracic stomach,[46] and tracheal occlusion from an intrathoracic stomach.[47,48] Many complications require supportive care, usually ventilation and nasogastric suction to allow for resolution of symptoms. When a second surgical procedure is required, anesthesia considerations include those for the original procedure as well as precautions specific to the complication.

Progression of malignant disease may be evidenced by symptoms of recurrent dysphagia or vocal cord paralysis. Aspiration and pneumonia, which can commonly occur as a result of dysphagia, could also signify a tracheoesophageal fistula. Further attempts to alleviate complications of disease progression depend on the disease prognosis, the patient's wishes, and the willingness of surgeon and anesthesiologist to proceed.

Experience with esophageal surgical procedures affords the anesthesiologist an ability to anticipate problems in the perioperative period that may otherwise complicate the conduct of and recovery from anesthesia and surgery. In lieu of experience, knowledge of the pathology and planned procedure as well as communication with the surgical team throughout is essential.

References

1. Enterline H, Thompson J: The normal esophagus embryology, structure and function. In Pathology of the Esophagus. Berlin, Springer-Verlag Company 1984, p 1.
2. Baue AE, Naunheim KS: Hiatal hernia and gastroesophageal reflux. In Baue AE (ed): Glenn's Thoracic and Cardiovascular Surgery, 5th ed. Norwalk, CT, Appleton & Lange, 1991, p 683.
3. Waters PF, et al: Esophagectomy for complex benign esophageal disease. J Thorac Cardiovasc Surg 95:378, 1988.
4. Kron IL, Johnson AM, Morgan RF: Gastrotracheal fistula: A late complication after transhiatal esophagectomy. Ann Thorac Surg 47:767, 1989.
5. Grebenik CR: Anaesthetic management of malignant tracheo-oesophageal fistula. Br J Anaesth 63:492, 1989.
6. Hilgenberg AD, Grillo HC: Acquired nonmalignant tracheoesophageal fistula. J Cardiovasc Surg 85:492, 1983.
7. Little AG: Esophageal chemical burns, foreign bodies, and bleeding. In Baue AE (ed): Glenn's Thoracic and Cardiovascular Surgery; 5th ed. Norwalk, CT, Appleton & Lange, 1991, p 680.
8. Wang LS, Huang MH, Huang BS, Chien KY: Gastric substitution for resectable carcinoma of the esophagus: An analysis of 368 cases. Ann Thorac Surg 53:289, 1992.

9. Mathisen DJ, et al: Transthoracic esophagectomy: A safe approach to carcinoma of the esophagus. Ann Thorac Surg 45:137, 1988.
10. Lewis I: The surgical treatment of carcinoma of the oesophagus: With special reference to a new operation for growths of the middle third. Br J Surg 34:18, 1946.
11. Tilanus HW, et al: Esophagectomy with or without thoracotomy: Is there any difference? J Thorac Cardiovasc Surg 105:898, 1993.
12. Pac M, et al: Transhiatal versus transthoracic esophagectomy for esophageal cancer. J Thorac Cardiovasc Surg 106:205, 1993.
13. Lam KH et al: Anastomotic complications after esophagectomy. J Thorac Cardiovasc Surg 104:395, 1992.
14. Bains MS: Transabdominal esophagogastrectomy for the poor-risk patient. In Delarue NC (ed); International Trends in General Thoracic Surgery: Esophageal Cancer. St Louis, CV Mosby Co, 1988, p 222.
15. Yakoubian K, et al: Cardiovascular responses to manual dissection associated with transhiatal esophageal resection. J Cardiothorac Anesth 4:458, 1990.
16. Wiseman RS, Gravlee GP, Koufman JA, Kon ND: The perils of esophageal prosthesis placement in malignant tracheoesophageal fistula. J Clin Anesth 4:134, 1992.
17. Nissen R: Gastropexy and "fundoplication" in surgical treatment of hiatal hernia. Am J Dig Dis 6:954, 1961.
18. Hill LD, Aye RW, Ramel S: Antireflux surgery. Gastroenterol Clin North Am 19:745, 1990.
19. Orringer MB, Skinner DB, Belsey RHR: Long-term results of the Mark IV operation for hiatal hernia and analyses of recurrences and their treatment. J Thorac Cardiovasc Surg 63:25, 1972.
20. Little AG, Naunheim KS, Ferguson MK, Skinner DB: Surgical management of esophageal strictures. Ann Thorac Surg 45:144, 1988.
21. DeMeester TR, et al: Chronic respiratory symptoms and occult gastroesophageal reflux. Ann Surg 211:337, 1990.
22. Kendall AP, Lin E: Respiratory failure as presentation of achalasia of the oesphagus. Anaesthesia 46:1039, 1991.
23. Nasrallah SM, Hendrix E: The effect of topical pharyngeal anesthesia on esophageal motility. Am J Gastroenterol 82:523, 1987.
24. Tsui SL, et al: Postoperative analgesia for oesophageal surgery: A comparison of three analgesic regimens. Anaesth Intensive Care 19:329, 1991.
25. Watson A, Allen P: Influence of thoracic epidural analgesia on outcome after resection for esophageal cancer. Surgery 115:429, 1994.
26. Ginsberg RJ: New technique for one-lung anesthesia using an endobronchial blocker. J Thorac Cardiovasc Surg 82:542, 1981.
27. Desiderio DP, et al: The effects of endobronchial cuff inflation on double lumen endotracheal tube movement after lateral decubitus positioning. Anesth Analg 80:A141, 1995.
28. Heitmiller RF, Jones B: Transient diminished airway protection after transhiatal esophagectomy. Am J Surg 162:442, 1991.
29. Griffin SM, Chung SCS, Van Hasselt CA, Li AKC: Late swallowing and aspiration problems after esophagectomy for cancer: Malignant infiltration of the recurrent laryngeal nerves and its management. Surgery 112:533, 1992.
30. Shiraha S, et al: Motility studies of the cervical esophagus with intrathoracic gastric conduit after esophagectomy. Scand J Thorac Cardiovasc Surg 26:119, 1992.
31. Caldwell MTP, Murphy PG, Page R, et al: Timing of extubation after oesophagectomy. Br J Surg 80:1537, 1993.
32. Tsutsui S, et al: Multivariate analysis of postoperative complications after esophageal resection. Ann Thorac Surg 53:1052, 1992.
33. Nagawa H, Kobori O, Muto T: Prediction of pulmonary complications after transthoracic oesophagectomy. Br J Surg 81:860, 1994.
34. Gatell JA, et al: A new technique for replacing an endobronchial double-lumen tube with an endotracheal single-lumen tube. Anesthesiology 73:340, 1990.
35. Nishi M, Hiramatsu Y, Hioki K, et al: Pulmonary complications after subtotal oesophagectomy. Br J Surg 75:527, 1988.
36. Dewar L, Gelfand G, Finley RJ, et al: Factors affecting cervical anastomotic leak and stricture formation following esophagogastrectomy and gastric tube interposition. Am J Surg 163:484, 1992.
37. Hambraeus GM, Ekberg O, Fletcher R: Pharyngeal dysfunction after total and subtotal oesophagectomy. Acta Radio 28:409, 1987.
38. Ellis FH: Carcinoma of the esophagus. Cancer 33:264, 1983.
39. Postlethwait RW: Complications and deaths after operations for esophageal carcinoma: A critical review of surgery. J Thorac Cardiovasc Surg 85:827, 1983.
40. Vigneswaran WT, Trastek VF, Pairolero PC, et al: Transhiatal esophagectomy for carcinoma of the esophagus. Ann Thorac Surg 56:838, 1993.
41. Patti MG, Wiener-Kronish JP, Way LW, Pellegrini CA: Impact of transhiatal esophagectomy on cardiac and respiratory function. Am J Surg 162:563, 1991.
42. Matory YL, Burt M: Esophagogastrectomy: Reoperation for complications. J Surg Oncol 54:29, 1993.
43. Orringer MB: Surgical options for esophageal resection and reconstruction with stomach. Esophageal cancer. In Baue AE (ed) Glenn's Thoracic and Cardiovascular Surgery, 5th ed. Norwalk, CT, Appleton & Lange, 1991, p 806.
44. Cheng W, Heitmiller RF, Jones B: Subacute ischemia of the colon esophageal interposition. Ann Thorac Surg 57:899, 1994.
45. Granke K, Hoshal VL, Vanden Belt RJ: Extrapericardial tamponade with herniated omentum after transhiatal esophagectomy. J Surg Oncol 44:273, 1990.
46. Casson AG, Inculet R, Finley R: Volvulus of the intrathoracic stomach after total esophagectomy. J Thorac Cardiovasc Surg 100:633, 1990.
47. Anderson GB, Walsh TE, Swartz SE: Tracheal occlusion from an intrathoracic stomach. Chest 103:622, 1993.
48. Leite LP, Jones MD, Panasuk DB: Tracheal occlusion. Chest 105(6):1921, 1994.

CHAPTER 30

Lung Transplantation

Anastasios N. Triantafillou, M.D.
Paul M. Heerdt, M.D., Ph.D.
G. Alexander Patterson, M.D.

Although the first human lung allograft was performed in 1963,[1] transplantation of one or both lungs has only recently begun to truly emerge as a viable therapeutic option for patients with end-stage lung disease. In the St. Louis International Lung Transplant Registry (April 1996 report), 5,208 lung transplants, 243 double, 3,145 single, and 1,809 bilateral, had been reported (Fig. 30–1). Of these procedures, 2,880 have been performed in the last 3 years of data collection. Increased experience with lung transplantation (LTX) has rapidly led to refinement of technique, introduction of new procedures such as bilateral LTX (BLT) without cardiopulmonary bypass (CPB), and improved surgical management of postoperative complications. Concomitant with these surgical advances has been a rapid evolution of our approach to the anesthetic and intensive care management of the LTX recipient. Much of the information presented in this chapter reflects the clinical experience of the Washington University Lung Transplant Group, at Barnes Hospital in St. Louis, and it must be emphasized that, as with many facets of anesthetic care, institutional experience and bias are reflected in our management approach.

The criteria for selection as a potential lung recipient have also undergone considerable re-evaluation and evolution, particularly as more institutions initiate transplant programs. Current selection guidelines for the Washington University program are shown in Table 30–1. Noticeably absent are the previously published statements[2] denying eligibility to patients with the following:

1. History of recent steroid use (prednisone up to 20 mg/day) is now acceptable.
2. Previous intrathoracic surgery such as pleurodesis, pleurectomy, open lung biopsy, or lobectomy are no longer contraindications.
3. Ventilator dependence is now a relative contraindication. For example, patients who have been thoroughly evaluated and accepted for LTX, but later develop respiratory failure, while waiting, are still considered for transplantation.[3–5] However, patients who are referred because of ventilator-dependent respiratory failure are not considered for LTX.
4. Right ventricular failure.

Determination of the appropriate timing for LTX is also extremely important in order to ensure that the limited supply of organs is used in the most efficient manner. Guidelines used at Washington University to determine acuity are listed in Table 30–2. Alternatives to lung transplantation must always be utilized when available. This is especially important for patients with chronic obstructive lung disease (COPD) or α_1-antitrypsin-deficiency emphysema who under select circumstances may be better served by lung volume reduction surgery.[6]

Perioperative management of LTX recipients can represent a remarkable challenge to anesthesiologists, who find themselves confronted with the task of maintaining cardiopulmonary stability in patients with lung parenchymal and/or right ventricular function so poor that transplantation of one or both lungs is required. Due to marked differences in the pathophysiologic manifestations of the severe lung diseases precipitating transplantation, the approach to anesthetic management of the recipient cannot be easily standardized for single (SLT) or bilateral (BLT) transplants. The patient with COPD undergoing SLT, for example, requires different perioperative management—from premedication through postoperative ventilation—than does the patient receiving an SLT for pulmonary hypertension. Thus, we find it advantageous to categorize management strategies more by pathophysiology than procedure.

As noted in Figure 30–2, a substantial number of LTX reported to the registry were performed for restrictive lung diseases such as idiopathic pulmonary fibrosis. Reflecting a loss of lung parenchymal elasticity and compliance, end-stage restrictive disease is characterized by profoundly reduced lung volumes and diffusing capacity, but relative preservation of ventilatory flow rates. In a recent review of data from our institution, patients with idiopathic pulmonary fibrosis as the primary diagnosis demonstrated mean preoperative forced vital capacity

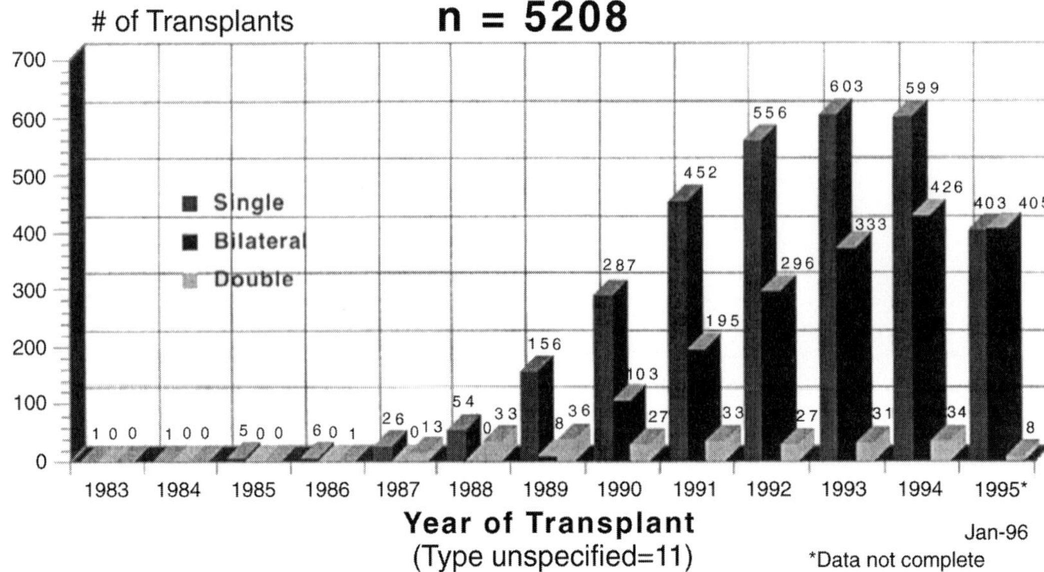

FIGURE **30–1.** Transplants reported to the St. Louis International Lung Transplant Registry as of January 1, 1996.

(FVC) and forced expiratory volume in 1 second (FEV_1) of 1.74 ± 0.9 and 1.5 ± 0.7, respectively. The underlying disease process also tends to obliterate pulmonary microvasculature, thus chronically increasing vascular resistance, producing pulmonary hypertension and predisposing to cor pulmonale.[7] Most patients with restrictive disease are candidates for an SLT procedure, since a native lung can usually be left intact without compromising the transplanted lung. We prefer a bilateral transplant in pulmonary fibrosis in two circumstances. First, patients with a cavitary component to their fibrosis are at risk of opportunistic infection in the native lung following transplant. These patients should have both native lungs resected. In addition, recipients of particularly large stature in comparison to the donor will obtain a better functional result with a bilateral transplant.

In contrast to restrictive lung disease, severe obstructive pulmonary disease is characterized by increased airway resistance, reduced expiratory flow rates (FEV_1 commonly below 20% predicted values), and high residual lung volumes. A spectrum of clinical pathologies produce obstructive pulmonary disease, with COPD, α_1-antitrypsin deficiency, and cystic fibrosis (CF) being the most common disorders in adults undergoing LTX (Fig. 30–2). At one time, concerns about mediastinal displacement and profound ventilation-perfusion mismatch secondary to hyperinflation of the remaining native lung prevented surgeons from attempting SLT for emphysema. However, clinical experience has demonstrated that many emphysemic patients can be successfully treated by SLT.[8–10] However, in patients of young age or larger stature, we prefer to utilize the bilateral procedure.

Pulmonary vascular disease leading to pulmonary hypertension (PH) and right ventricular dysfunction is a recent addition to the list of indications for LTX.[11] By definition,[12] pulmonary hypertension is present when pulmonary artery (PA) pressure exceeds 30/15 mm Hg or a mean over 18 to 20 mm Hg, at rest. Pathologically, severe pulmonary hypertension can result from proximal vascular processes, chronically increased pulmonary

TABLE **30–1**
Indications and Contraindications for Lung Transplantation at Washington University

Indications	Contraindications
Physiologically severe pulmonary disease with, medical therapy ineffective or unavailable	Significant and irreversible dysfunction of other vital organs
Substantial functional limitation in everyday living activities	Acute pulmonary or extrapulmonary infection
Predicted survival >18–24 mo	Ongoing medical noncompliance
Age: ≤60 yr for bilateral lung transplantation, ≤65 yr for single lung transplantation	Ongoing requirement for high-dose corticosteroid therapy
Satisfactory nutritional status	Uncured malignancy
Potential for rehabilitation/ambulation	Significant psychosocial problems
Patient's willingness	
Acceptable psychosocial support system	

TABLE 30–2
Timing of Lung Transplantation*

COPD and α_1-Antitrypsin-Deficiency Emphysema	Cystic Fibrosis
FEV_1 <25% PaO_2 <55–60 Hypercapnia Significant secondary pulmonary Hypertension	FEV_1 <30% PaO_2 <55 Hypercapnia
Clinical Course Determine rate of decline of FEV_1 Life-threatening excerbations	Clinical Course Exercise desaturation common Increasing frequency and severity of exacerbations Pneumothorax Hemoptysis Weight loss
Idiopathic Pulmonary Fibrosis VC, TLC <60% PaO_2 <60 Significant secondary pulmonary hypertension	
Primary Pulmonary Hypertension NYHA Class III or IV MPAP <25 mm Hg Cardiac index ≤2.5 L/min/m² Increasing vasodilator requirements Life-threatening clinical events (syncope)	

*Transplantation is potentially contraindicated if there is colonization with panresistant *Pseudomonas*, active *Aspergillus*, or mycobacteria infection.
COPD, chronic obstructive pulmonary disease; FEV, forced expiratory volume in 1 second; PaO_2, partial pressure of oxygen, arterial; VC, vital capacity; TLC, total lung capacity; NYHA, New York Heart Association; MPAP, mean pulmonary arterial pressure.

blood flow (i.e., Eisenmenger's syndrome from an atrial or ventricular septal defect), or pulmonary venous obstruction. Primary pulmonary hypertension, the most frequently encountered vascular disease in LTX recipients, produces sustained vasoconstriction and structural changes in the pulmonary circulation and may precipitate chronic hypoxemia if it is associated with a cardiac defect,[13] often presenting initially with shortness of breath or hemoptysis secondary to suprasystemic PA pressure (Fig. 30–3). The disease is more common in women than men, usually of idiopathic origin, and characterized by rapid progression and sudden death, despite

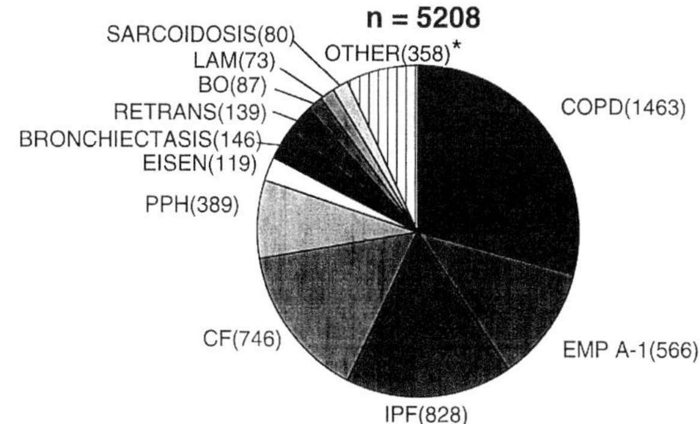

FIGURE **30–2.** Breakdown of the end-stage lung diseases leading to all transplants reported to the St. Louis International Lung Transplant Registry as of January, 1996. BO, bronchiolitis obliterans; CF, cystic fibrosis; COPD, chronic obstructive pulmonary disease; Eisen, Eisenmenger's syndrome; EMP A-1, α_1-antitrypsin deficiency; IPF, idiopathic pulmonary fibrosis; PPH, primary pulmonary hypertension; LAM, lymphangiomyomatosis; Retrans, retransplantation.

vasodilator therapy.[14] Prior to LTX, surgical treatment for this disease was limited to heart-lung transplantation. However, although replacement of both the heart and lungs has enjoyed considerable success, the shortage of heart-lung blocks, the complexity of the operation, and the development of bronchiolitis obliterans has imposed limitations on its widespread application. Furthermore, both laboratory and clinical studies have indicated reversibility of right ventricular dysfunction following the reduction of afterload in the setting of chronic, severe pulmonary hypertension, suggesting that replacement of the heart may not be always indicated. Since a native lung can usually be left intact without compromising a transplanted lung (which will receive the majority of blood flow), patients with pulmonary vascular disease may also be candidates for SLT with concurrent repair of any congenital cardiac anomalies. Unlike SLT for restrictive or obstructive disease, transplants for vascular pulmonary disease are often performed during partial normothermic CPB in order to protect the right ventricle from acute changes in afterload; however, SLT for pulmonary hypertension without CPB has been reported.[15] Following LTX and "unloading" of the RV, increased left ventricular filling and hemodynamic improvement are often immediate[16] (Fig. 30–4). To date, clinical data exist to indicate favorable perioperative morbidity and mortality as well as remarkable improvement in survival and New York Heart Association (NYHA) class following SLT for pulmonary hypertension.[17–20] In a recent study of a single institution's experience in 34 patients,[21] the authors presented a 91% overall discharge rate and 61% 3-year survival. In addition, a sustained improve-

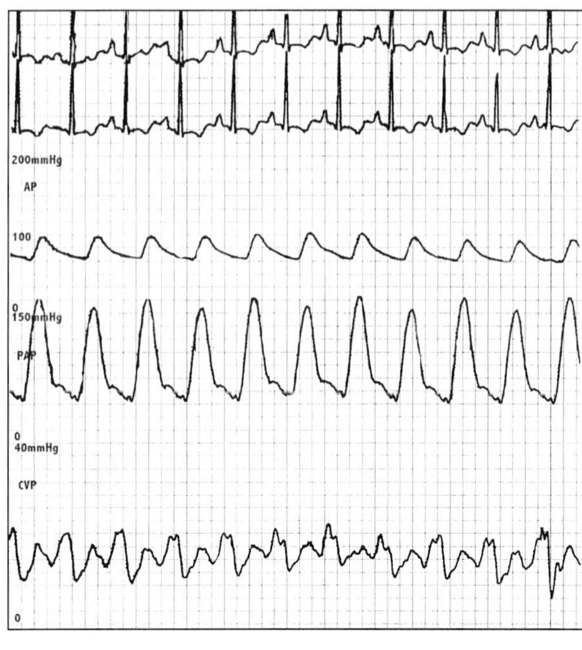

FIGURE 30–3. Hemodynamic parameters prior to induction of anesthesia in a patient with severe pulmonary hypertension and a history of hemoptysis.

ment over the 3-year period of pulmonary hypertension and right ventricular function was experienced in this group. Furthermore, assessing the efficiency of thoracic organ utilization, the authors noted that 31 donors provided organs for 82 thoracic organ transplants.

Nonetheless, the subject is controversial and other centers do not share this opinion. For example, Bando et al.[22] reviewed results from 11 single, 22 bilateral, and 24 heart-lung transplants. In this study, postoperative pulmonary artery pressures and cardiac index improved in all three allograft groups. However, the improvement was significantly superior in the BLT and heart-lung recipients. Accordingly, the authors concluded that BLT may be a more satisfactory option for patients with pulmonary hypertension and that heart-lung transplantation should be offered to selected patients. Likewise, other reports,[23,24] based primarily on increased mortality, have suggested that SLT may be suboptimal therapy in patients with pulmonary hypertension. Undoubtedly, long-term functional results from SLT versus BLT or even heart-lung must be carefully evaluated. For this reason we too have entered the field of BLT for pulmonary hy-

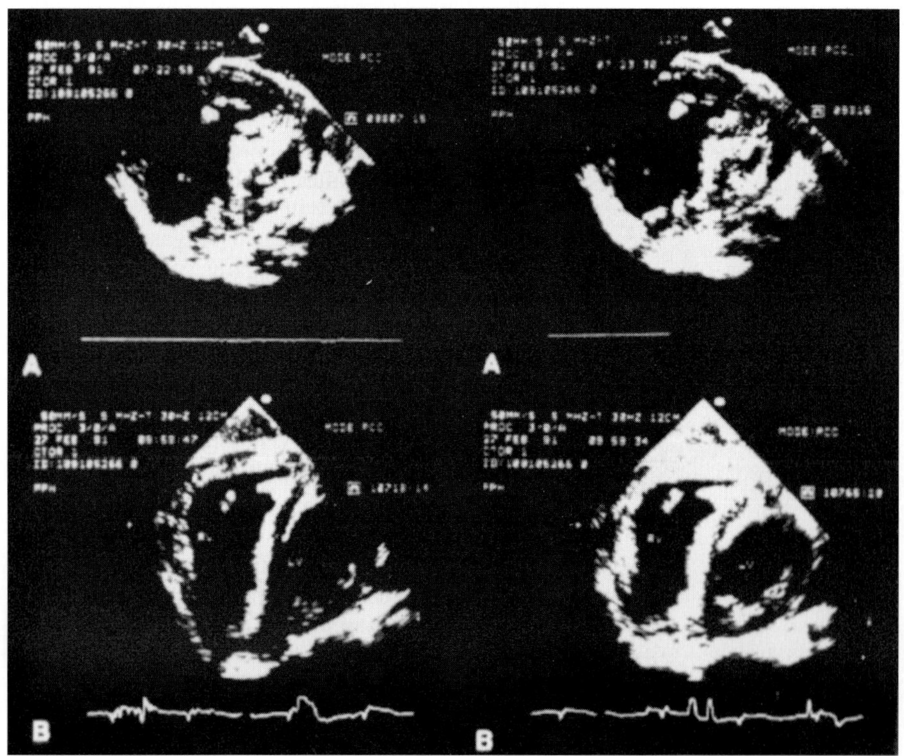

FIGURE 30–4. Transesophageal echocardiographic images of the right and left ventricles in a patient with primary pulmonary hypertension before and after reperfusion of a transplanted lung. *A*, End-diastole. *B*, End-systole. Note the increase of left ventricular filling after transplantation.

pertension but, at the present time, with an overall operative survival of 91% and a 61% 3-year survival (experience from 34 patients at Barnes Hospital) and given all the real problems with organ availability, we believe that SLT for pulmonary hypertension is still a very attractive solution.

Infectious lung disease such as cystic fibrosis is the most frequent indication for LTX in patients less than 18 years of age.[25] Due to potential infectious cross-contamination of the transplanted lung, chronic infectious disease represents a contraindication to SLT. There is anecdotal experience with SLT and contralateral pneumonectomy in cystic fibrosis, but no one considers this a realistic option.[26] Lung pathophysiology in cystic fibrosis is primarily obstructive in nature with increased airway reactivity. It is also characterized by chronic infection and the production of copious purulent secretions. As the disease progresses, the sputum often becomes colonized with mucoid strains of *Pseudomonas aeruginosa*.[27] Under most circumstances, residual volumes and functional residual capacity (FRC) are increased and bronchodilators have little effect on expiratory flow rates.

Preoperative Evaluation and Sedation

When the recipient is eventually admitted for the transplant procedure, time is often quite limited. Thus, it is advantageous to perform a detailed preoperative evaluation when the patient is first accepted into the transplant program. At most centers, an extensive physical examination, psychological evaluation, and numerous tests of cardiopulmonary function and reserve will have been performed prior to the anesthesiologist's preoperative assessment.[28,29] In addition to a standard history and physical examination, familiarity with pulmonary function tests; ventilation-perfusion scan results; and heart catheterization and echocardiographic data including evidence of intracardiac shunts, exercise tolerance, oxygen use, and dependence on continuous pulmonary vasodilator infusion (i.e., prostacyclin), is beneficial for formulating an anesthetic plan.

As with all surgical patients, considerations regarding preoperative sedation are governed primarily by the functional limitations imposed by the underlying disease. Since deterioration of respiratory and/or cardiac function between the preoperative evaluation and eventual transplantation is not unusual, careful reassessment of the patient's general condition and current arterial blood-gas data is warranted before ordering premedication. In severely compromised patients, often the best anxiolytic is calm discussion of preoperative events and premedication may be limited to an antisialagogue. When indicated, parenteral sedation is usually chosen due to insufficient time to effectively administer oral anxiolytics. Midazolam in titrated doses of 0.5 to 1.0 mg has been used safely in many patients. Diphenhydramine, 50 to 75 mg alone or in combination with midazolam, has also been found effective, and has the added benefit of potentially protecting the lung against drug-induced histamine release. Clinically, most patients with end-stage restrictive, obstructive, or infectious lung disease are tachypneic while breathing room air and cannot be aggressively sedated. In contrast, patients with primary pulmonary hypertension (PPH) and no intracardiac defect, presenting for LTX, often appear reasonably normal and will benefit from sedation because they may be prone to stress-related increases in pulmonary vascular resistance. Opioids should be used cautiously, however, due to the potentially adverse effects of respiratory depression and hypercarbia on right ventricular afterload. Alternatively, patients with pulmonary hypertension and significant right-to-left intracardiac shunting (i.e., Eisenmenger's physiology) are often cyanotic and cachectic, and may not tolerate sedation well.

Preoperative Vascular Access and Invasive Monitors

Monitoring of arterial oxygen saturation (SaO_2), electrocardiogram (ECG), and arterial pressure with a sphygmomanometer during placement of venous catheters and administration of parenteral sedation is often desirable. In patients with chronic infectious lung disease or a history of previous intrathoracic procedures, two large-bore intravenous catheters are advisable due to the potential for brisk blood loss during dissection of pulmonary adhesions. Additionally, since the arms are usually placed in a flexed position during both single and bilateral transplant procedures, it is often advantageous to place intravenous catheters in the wrist or forearm. Meticulous removal of air from venous infusion lines should be performed, particularly in patients with pulmonary hypertension and known or suspected right-to-left shunts.

Due to the possibility that the radial artery has been scarred by previous arterial punctures, it is often advantageous to attempt cannulation early in the course of preoperative preparation. This approach also facilitates blood sampling for preoperative tests. At some institutions, cannulation of a femoral artery instead of radial artery is performed under local anesthesia in the operating room.[30]

Profound changes in pulmonary and systemic hemodynamics are common both during and after LTX, thus preoperative placement of a PA catheter is advisable. Whether the catheter should be placed before or after induction of anesthesia is controversial. Clearly, obtaining central venous access can be exceptionally difficult, and the risk of venous air aspiration exists during spontaneous ventilation in many patients due to orthopnea and markedly negative intrathoracic pressures. On the other hand, since the transition from spontaneous to positive-pressure ventilation during induction of anesthesia often produces profound cardiovascular alterations, a PA catheter placed prior to induction may provide information that is, during this time, extremely valuable. Extensive efforts to place the PA catheter tip in the nontransplant branch of the pulmonary artery during SLT are probably not warranted. We have repeatedly observed that even when radiographically confirmed to be properly positioned, catheters frequently migrate to the operative side following lateral positioning. Thus, it is more efficient to simply remind the surgeon to palpate the pulmonary artery and withdraw the catheter if necessary before cross-clamping the vessel.

Epidural Catheter Placement

Pain control after LTX is a key part of the overall patient management. It can be critical in facilitating patient extubation and rehabilitation and may contribute to a successful outcome.[31] Earlier data suggested that epidural analgesia, following transplantation, is superior to intravenous opioids by improving postoperative pulmonary function, shortening extubation, and reducing intensive care unit (ICU) stay.[32] To date, there are no sufficient data indicating superiority of lumbar over thoracic epidural catheters; however, in one report thoracic epidural was found to be associated with a high interventional workload.[33] In our practice we place lumbar epidural catheters preoperatively in most patients except in those who are being anticoagulated preoperatively (such as patients with PPH). Review of the records of 120 transplant recipients revealed no adverse sequelae to preoperatively placed lumbar epidural catheters, including 18 patients who did require emergent heparinization and CPB for the completion of the procedure. Furthermore, review of indices of coagulation in 152 lung transplant recipients on admission to the ICU as well as on the first postoperative day demonstrated a coagulopathy—presumably dilutional and possibly exacerbated by immunosuppression—which, under most circumstances, would have challenged or precluded epidural catheter placement (Table 30–3). These data indicate that an epidural catheter can be safely placed before LTX, while coagulation status is normal, and that delaying its placement until the postoperative period may actually increase the risk of complications due to persistent coagulopathy.

Equipment and Intraoperative Monitoring

Special items we have found advantageous for LTX procedures include an anesthesia ventilator capable of delivering a wide range of inspiratory to expiratory (I:E) ratios and respiratory rates, a continuous positive airway pressure (CPAP) apparatus, and a CPB machine on standby. Additionally, it is advisable to keep a sterile circuit for the anesthesia machine in the room should the distal airway become disrupted or the endobronchial tube damaged necessitating direct bronchial intubation or jet ventilation on the surgical field.[34] Intraoperatively, hemodynamic and respiratory changes are often acute and profound, thus extensive monitoring is imperative. In addition to standard monitoring devices, we have used PA catheters capable of measuring right ventricular ejection fraction (RVEF) and mixed venous oxygen saturation ($S\bar{v}O_2$), in combination with two-dimensional transesophageal echocardiography (2D TEE) in an attempt to quickly and objectively assess right ventricular performance. Both these monitoring methods can be extremely helpful for management of LTX but are not without limitations. For example, TEE may be limited by poor visualization of the right ventricle in laterally positioned emphysemic patients. On the other hand, thermodilution ejection fraction measurements can be distorted by tricuspid regurgitation, a frequent conjugate of pulmonary hypertension.[35] In addition to cardiovascular monitoring, continuous measurement of pulmonary mechanics by sidestream spirometry may represent a valuable tool in early detection of reperfusion injury and graft dysfunction.[36]

TABLE 30–3
Coagulation Parameters Following LTX

	Mean	SD	Median
PT	15.6	3.3	15
PTT	44.3	25.6	36
PLT-POD #0	163.7	76.3	148
PLT-POD #1	111.2	49.9	99

LTX, lung transplantation; SD, standard deviation; PT, prothrombin time; PTT, partial thromboplastin time; PLT, platelet count; POD, postoperative day.

Induction and Maintenance of Anesthesia

A prolonged period of preoxygenation is advised, particularly in patients with high residual lung volumes secondary to obstructive disease. Since abrupt withdrawal of sympathetic tone in patients suffering from chronic hypoxia and hypercarbia can result in significant cardiovascular compromise—particularly during the transition from spontaneous to mechanical ventilation—induction of anesthesia can be eventful. In that most patients will have received little or no premedication, initial low-dose administration of a rapidly acting hypnotic agent to expedite airway management, prevent opioid-induced truncal rigidity, and provide amnesia has been found to be advantageous.[2,30,37] Thiopental (1 to 2 mg/kg), etomidate (0.1 to 0.2 mg/kg), and ketamine (0.5 to 1.0 mg/kg) have all been used safely. However, specific properties of each drug must be considered. Thiopental, for example, may not be desirable in patients with bronchospasm or pulmonary hypertension due to a propensity for histamine release. Alternatively, the sympathomimetic properties of ketamine may preclude use in the presence of pulmonary hypertension, while bronchodilating effects may be beneficial in patients with bronchospasm. After the administration of the hypnotic agent, either fentanyl (10 to 15 mg/kg) or sufentanil (1 to 2 mg/kg) are infused along with a nondepolarizing muscle relaxant. Due to the emergent nature of the procedure, a Sellick maneuver may be advisable.

Following induction of anesthesia, the trachea is usually intubated with a left endobronchial double-lumen tube for both SLT and BLT. Along with others,[31,37,38] we have also successfully used single-lumen endotracheal tubes with internal or external bronchial blocking catheters to provide lung isolation during transplant procedures. However, except for the fact that a double-lumen tube has to be exchanged for a single-lumen tube at some time in the postoperative period, we find left double-lumen tubes more desirable. Furthermore, a double-lumen endobronchial tube allows for many forms of differential lung ventilation if required either intraoperatively (see below) or postoperatively.

In patients with cystic fibrosis and thick tenacious secretions, there are distinct advantages to preoperative aggressive pulmonary toilet. We thus opt for initial tracheal intubation with a large-bore single-lumen tube followed by extensive lavage and suction, utilizing a large-channel fiberoptic bronchoscope and then replacement of the single-lumen endotracheal tube with a left endobronchial double-lumen tube prior to incision. In our experience, use of a double-lumen tube is preferable for two reasons: first, because spillover from an infected native lung to a new graft is still possible, when using a bronchial blocker; and second, because the ability to differentially ventilate the lungs is lost or compromised. Nevertheless, in some young, small-size patients with cystic fibrosis who would normally take a small-diameter double-lumen (35 Fr) tube (and in whom, therefore, each individual lumen of a double-lumen tube may be too narrow to allow effective intraoperative airway toilet), use of a regular tube with a bronchial blocker should be considered. Most pediatric lung transplant programs utilize a single-lumen tube and cardiopulmonary bypass for all bilateral transplants for cystic fibrosis.

The transition from spontaneous to mechanical ventilation invariably produces marked hemodynamic alteration due to acute changes in intrathoracic pressure, chest wall compliance, and expiratory flow dynamics. With obstructive lung disease, mechanical ventilation magnifies air-trapping leading to "pulmonary tamponade," (Fig. 30–5). Adjustment of the ventilatory pattern accordingly, using large I:E ratio (1:5 or greater) with moderate tidal volumes, often lessens circulatory compromise. Obviously, such a pattern, which requires high inspiratory flow, is likely to produce high peak inspiratory pressure (PIP); however, it should be kept in mind, that this pressure does not reflect true alveolar pressure.

Due to large residual volumes produced by severe obstructive lung disease, patients that have been preoxygenated for an extended period of time prior to induction of anesthesia will often tolerate prolonged apnea without arterial oxygen desaturation. Periods of permissive hypercapnia can thus often be safely used to maintain hemodynamic stability if mechanical ventilation becomes a burden. A summary of ventilatory management in 62 LTX recipients with obstructive lung disease during one- and two-lung ventilation is shown in Figure 30–6. During two-lung ventilation, with the respiratory rate adjusted to maintain hemodynamic stability, the average tidal volume delivered was 8.7 ml/kg, and under these conditions median $PaCO_2$ was 58 mm Hg with a median PaO_2 of 500 mm Hg. During one-lung ventilation, mean tidal volume was reduced to 7.6 ml/kg with minimal change in median $PaCO_2$ or PaO_2.

With restrictive disease, higher inflation pressures and positive end-expiratory pressure (PEEP) are often required. However, venous return may be compromised and pulmonary blood vessels mechanically compressed, subsequently decreasing cardiac output and increasing right ventricular afterload. Thus, optimal balance of ventilation with hemodynamic stability often necessitates tolerating a degree of hypoventilation and (permissive) hypercapnia. Acute hemodynamic compromise can usu-

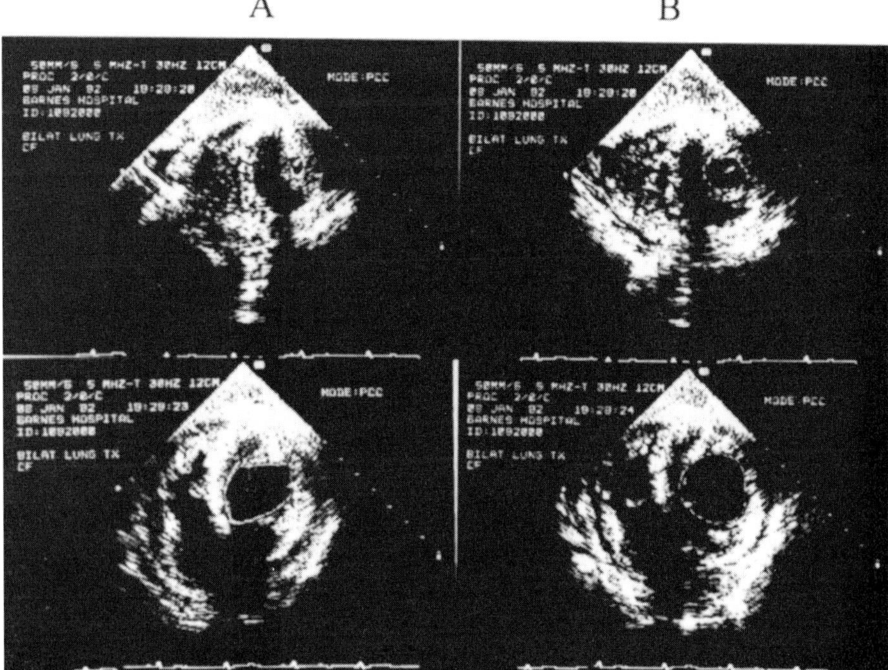

FIGURE 30–5. Transesophageal echocardiographic images of the right and left ventricles in a patient with cystic fibrosis during ventilation and a period of apnea. *A*, End-systole. *B*, End-diastole.

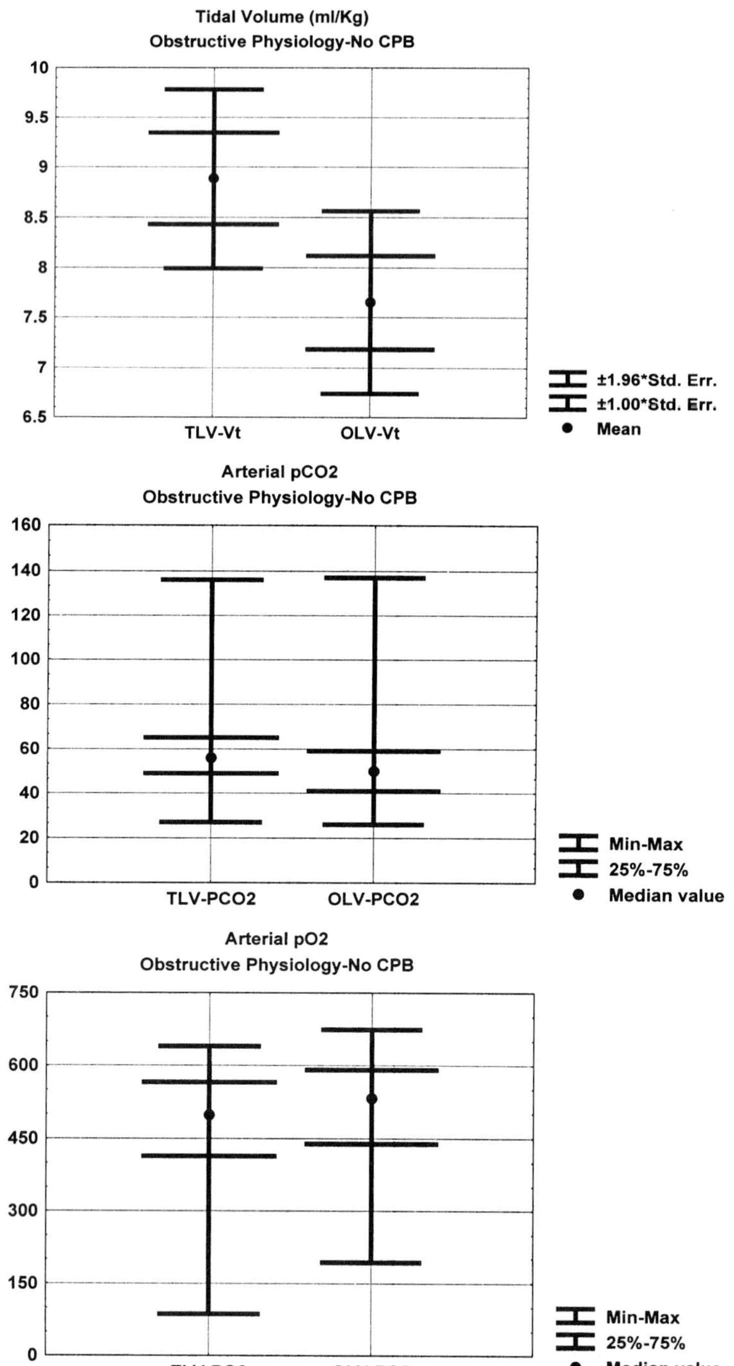

FIGURE **30–6.** Summary of delivered tidal volume along with arterial P_{O_2} and P_{CO_2} during two- (TLV) or one- (OLV) lung ventilation in 62 patients with obstructive lung disease undergoing lung transplantation in whom respiratory rate had been adjusted to maintain hemodynamic stability.

ally be treated successfully by decreasing intrathoracic pressure. In addition, increasing heart rate with vagolytics, increasing preload, and/or injection of sympathomimetics may be required. Often, periods of apnea interspaced with careful intermittent hand ventilation are required to restore cardiovascular stability until thoracotomy and cardiac decompression. In contrast, mechanical ventilation usually produces little physiologic change in patients with pulmonary vascular disease if caution is exercised not to increase pulmonary vascular resistance through hypoxia, hypercarbia, or lung hyperinflation.

After induction of anesthesia, tracheal intubation and initiation of mechanical ventilation, benzodiazepines, scopolamine, and/or volatile anesthetic agents are beneficial intraoperatively to promote amnesia. For maintenance of anesthesia and amnesia, isoflurane is our drug of choice, due to bronchodilating and positive chronotropic properties. Clearly, there are experimental and clinical data demonstrating inhibition of HPV by volatile anesthetics.[39,40] However, the clinical significance of these effects remains controversial[41,42] and we have not found volatile anesthetics to be deleterious in LTX patients.

Since most lung recipients have little pulmonary reserve, we favor ventilation with an FIO_2 of 1.0 intraoperatively. This approach is somewhat controversial due to concerns regarding oxygen toxicity to the transplanted organ.[31,43] To date, however, there are no data to support deleterious effects of transiently ventilating a transplanted lung with high FIO_2, and thus we prefer the margin of safety provided by high oxygen tension. High FIO_2 may also directly promote pulmonary vasodilatation and thus be beneficial in reducing right ventricular afterload.[44]

After transplantation and when hemodynamic and respiratory stability has been achieved, FIO_2 may be decreased.

It has been suggested that high-frequency jet ventilation (HFJV) is superior to conventional ventilatory modes in patients with severe pulmonary fibrosis.[45] However, we have not consistently found HFJV of both lungs to be more effective than conventional ventilation in transplant patients with restrictive disease and low FRC. In some cystic fibrosis patients, we have found that periodic jet ventilation during pneumonectomy may help to mobilize secretions and thus improve oxygenation. In many LTX procedures, particularly those for restrictive and infectious disease, some degree of hypoxemia may occur during one-lung ventilation. Multiple interventions have been employed to improve systemic oxygenation including administration of PEEP to the ventilated lung and oxygen insufflation, CPAP, and high-frequency ventilation of the nonventilated lung. Under most circumstances, adequate oxygenation can be maintained with these interventions.

This hypoxemia in most cases is related to persistent perfusion of the nondependent lung. Therefore, should profound, refractory hypoxemia occur, clamping of the pulmonary artery branch of the nondependent lung should usually and promptly reverse it. However, close monitoring of the right ventricle is necessary to reveal whether the abrupt increase of afterload can be tolerated. If hypoxemia persists or the right ventricle appears to distend, CPB may be required.

Surgical Technique and Intraoperative Management

It is extremely important that anesthesiologists be familiar with the surgical methods, since manipulation of the heart and lungs at specific points during the transplant can produce marked cardiopulmonary disturbances. Ideally, the anesthesiologist will anticipate these changes and adapt the anesthetic management accordingly.

Single-Lung Transplantation for Restrictive or Obstructive Disease

SLT is usually performed in the lateral decubitus position. In addition, we find it advantageous to fully extend the upper leg and tilt the pelvis to a semisupine angle to allow groin exposure for potential femoral cannulation and CPB. As with all surgical procedures, head, arm, and leg support and padding should be ensured to prevent compression injuries. Hemodynamic and ventilatory changes often occur during positioning; changes in venous return coupled with compression of the dependent lung by the mediastinum and diaphragm may promote systemic hypotension and ventilation-perfusion mismatch. Furthermore, pulmonary arterial pressure tends to rise following lateral positioning, probably due to gravity-induced shifts in pulmonary blood flow distribution, vascular congestion, and increased vascular resistance.

Isolated ventilation of the dependent lung is often accompanied by a marked increase in peak inspiratory pressure, necessitating compensatory changes in ventilation. Due to the beneficial effect of gravity on redistributing blood away from the nondependent, nonventilated lung, single-lung ventilation is often tolerated better from a respiratory standpoint by patients undergoing SLT in the lateral position than those undergoing BLT in the supine position. However, the impact of single-lung ventilation on right ventricular afterload may be more pronounced in the lateral position. Close monitoring of right ventricular performance during conversion to single-lung ventilation is thus extremely important. If the right ventricle becomes hypokinetic and distended, or ejection fraction falls, ventilation may have to be altered to minimize airway pressure while maintaining adequate minute ventilation. If right ventricular performance does not improve or persistent hypoxemia and/or hypercarbia result, heparinization and CPB may be required. Infusion of catecholamines, phosphodiesterase inhibitors, or pulmonary vasodilators, or administration of inhaled nitric oxide prior to initiating single-lung ventilation, may be beneficial in many patients by supporting the right ventricle and lessening the impact of acutely increased afterload.

The procedure is usually conducted through a standard fifth interspace posterolateral thoracotomy. However, for patients with emphysema, an anterolateral fourth interspace submammary incision provides acceptable exposure and less postoperative pain. Once stable single-lung ventilation is established, dissection for contralateral pneumonectomy is initiated with isolation of the ipsilateral main pulmonary artery. To assess the cardiopulmonary response to diverting the entire cardiac output through the contralateral lung, progressive occlusion of the vessel is first performed manually; if well tolerated, the vessel is then clamped and stapled. If occlusion is poorly tolerated, the vessel is unclamped and an inotropic infusion is begun or prostaglandin E_1 (PGE_1) is initiated or the dose increased, or inhaled nitric oxide is administered. Some authors advocate the routine infusion of dopamine at this point in the procedure.[43] Although we do not routinely infuse a catecholamine inotrope, when specifically indicated we prefer dobutamine due to a more predictable dose-response profile and less arrhythmogenicity. If severe respiratory or cardiovascular derangement persist following reclamping of the vessel despite pharmacologic intervention, heparin is administered and CPB instituted to avoid profound hypoxia or right ventricle (RV) failure. However, our experience has been that, for most patients, hypoxemia during one-lung ventilation and after PA clamping is rarely a problem and that RV performance can be maintained adequately, occasionally with some pharmacologic manipulation.

After PA ligation, the pneumonectomy is completed. The graft is placed in the chest and topical hypothermia maintained by crushed ice. Implantation of the graft begins with anastomosis of the airway. At some institutions, the bronchial anastomosis is wrapped with an omental pedicle, previously mobilized through a small abdominal incision, in an effort to improve blood supply to the airway and promote healing.[46] Other institutions now routinely use a "telescoping" bronchial anastomosis, which appears to remove the need for omental wrapping.[47,48] We employ an "end-to-end" technique with figure-of-8 sutures. The bronchial anastomosis is covered with local peribronchial nodal tissue and pericardium. The donor and recipient main pulmonary arteries are trimmed to size and connected in end-to-end fashion. The recipient left atrium is then clamped and the pulmonary veins opened to create a common left atrial cuff, which is then connected to the donor left atrial cuff. The implanted lung is then partially inflated, the left atrial cuff and pulmonary veins "de-aired," and circulation to the organ restored. Following reperfusion and subsequent ventilation of the new lung, PA pressures and arterial blood gases should be closely followed. Pulmonary artery pressure usually falls following reperfusion of the donor organ. However, if a substantial decrease is not observed, potential causes may include technical problems such as stenosis of the atrial cuff or the pulmonary artery anastomosis. Early reperfusion injury of the donor organ should also be suspected. Such injury may manifest itself with a progressive rise in PA pressure and/or the onset of pulmonary edema. Assessment of the pulmonary arterial and venous flow pattern by TEE can sometimes be of benefit in evaluating adequacy of the anastomoses.[49]

Single-Lung Transplantation for Vascular Disease

In the setting of chronic progressive pulmonary hypertension, the right ventricle has often been seriously compromised and may have little contractile reserve.[50] To avoid additional right ventricular stress, it is our practice to institute partial CPB during SLT for PPH, or in patients with severe pulmonary hypertension and right ventricular dysfunction, secondary to severe end-stage lung disease. Patients more likely to develop pulmonary hypertension and severely compromised right ventricular function are those with restrictive disease. The technical aspects previously used at our institution have been previously described[51] and involve femoral arterial and right atrial cannulation for CPB. However, over the last several years, the technique has been revised and now involves complete intrathoracic cannulation. For single-lung transplantation requiring CPB, we favor the right side. Intrathoracic cannulation of the ascending aorta and right atrium is much easier through the right chest than cannulation of the descending aorta and main pulmonary artery through the left chest. If simultaneous cardiac repair (e.g., ASD or VSD) is required, a left thoracotomy is contraindicated. Of course, median sternotomy provides acceptable exposure for single-lung transplantation on CPB. Implantation of the lung is otherwise performed in the same fashion as described above.

Double En Bloc Lung Transplantation

This technique, en bloc double LTX, was first described and performed by the Toronto Lung Transplant Group.[52] The procedure is performed via a median sternotomy using hypothermic CPB; cardioplegic cardiac arrest; and single-tracheal (or double-bronchial),[48] left atrial, and pulmonary artery anastomoses. However, although the procedure initially produced some encouraging results, considerable limitations related to its technical complexity, morbidity, mortality, and application to many patients with end-stage lung disease soon become apparent. Not surprisingly, the popularity of this procedure has declined sharply (Fig. 30–1), and has now been largely replaced by the BLT technique.

Bilateral Single-Lung Transplantation

After its introduction by Pasque et al.[52] in 1990, it appears to have become the surgical procedure of choice when replacement of both lungs is necessary. In contrast to SLT, BLT procedures are performed in the supine position. Technically the procedure involves bilateral anterior thoracotomies that extend from the midaxillary lines to meet in the center through a transverse sternotomy. For patients with emphysema it is occasionally possible to avoid sternal division. In general, the procedure can be regarded as having two phases. First, the most severely compromised lung (as determined by preoperative V/Q scanning) is removed during ventilation of the "good" contralateral lung. Implantation of the first lung is conducted as for single-lung transplantation. Removal and implantation of the second lung is then performed. There may be theoretical advantages to leaving the second pleural space closed until the first lung is implanted. First, because in obstructive lung disease, the most common pathology in BLT, mechanical ventilation of an emphysematous lung without the confines of the chest wall may promote gas trapping and cardiac compression. However, with appropriate attention to endotracheal tube placement and tidal volume administered, this is rarely a problem. Should it occur, it can be remedied immediately by disconnection of the ventilator. Second, air leaks may be created during dissection and compromise ventilation. This is also not a commonly encountered problem if appropriate care is taken during dissection. Furthermore, there are great advantages to opening both pleural spaces immediately. Usually, both lungs can be completely mobilized before the first lung is extracted. This greatly shortens ischemic time to the second lung.

Restoration of ventilation and perfusion to the first lung is usually followed by a dramatic decrease in PA pressure and peak inspiratory pressure. The second lung is then removed and transplanted during ventilation of the new lung alone. However, on occasion, reperfusion of the first lung is followed by a progressive increase in PA pressure and inspiratory pressures, coupled with hypoxia, hypotension and, even, pulmonary edema. This is an acute catastrophic event necessitating adjustment of ventilation, addition of PEEP, increased doses of vasopressors, inotropes, PGE_1, or nitric oxide administration. Should hemodynamic and ventilatory derangement be refractory to treatment, CPB or extracorporeal membrane oxygenation (ECMO) may be required. It has been postulated that reperfusion of an organ after lengthy ischemia may cause tissue damage or may unmask injury sustained during the ischemic period.[53,54] This phenomenon has been found to affect several organs including the lung, and it manifests itself by increased microvascular permeability.[55] In a recent review[56] this early catastrophic allograft dysfunction following reperfusion of the first lung was found to be the most common cause for emergent CPB during BLT. To date, refractory reperfusion injury has prompted the use of ECMO in 6 of 255 lung transplantations at Washington University. Whether this phenomenon is solely a result of cellular injury or related to the diversion of the entire cardiac output through the recently transplanted lung, leading to vascular engorgement and edema, is still unclear.

As with other LTX procedures, unless unilateral lung dysfunction is suspected and some form of differential lung ventilation indicated, the double-lumen endotracheal tube is removed and a single-lumen tube placed upon conclusion of the procedure. Flexible bronchoscopy confirms integrity of the bronchial anastomosis, and viability of donor bronchial mucosa and permits aspiration of any blood or secretion from the donor airway.

Intraoperative Fluid Management

Specific strategies for fluid management are not well defined, and clearly deserve extensive study. Due to disruption of pulmonary lymphatics, after LTX, there is always a concern regarding the amount of crystalloid that can be safely administered intraoperatively without adversely affecting graft function. Although all efforts are made to minimize fluid infusion intraoperatively, many patients undergoing both SLT and BLT require large amounts of fluid in order to maintain hemodynamic stability. Not uncommonly, patients display central venous and pulmonary capillary wedge pressures of 3 to 5 mm Hg immediately following a transplant despite infusion of large amounts of crystalloid and colloid and only moderate blood loss. A recent review of fluid management during 215 LTX,[57] revealed that intraoperative crystalloid administration varied widely (4 to 32 ml/kg/hr) with a mean of 13 ± 6 ml/kg/hr. Using Pa_{O_2}/F_{IO_2} on arrival in the ICU and time to extubation as indices of early graft function and initial outcome, respectively, this study showed no correlation between the amount of fluids administered and either of these indices, whether the data were combined or subdivided according to procedure (Fig. 30–7).

Hematologic Management

Prior to development of the BLT procedure, patients with a history of open lung or pleural procedures or infectious lung disease were not deemed acceptable candidates for en bloc double-lung transplantation because of the anticipated excessive bleeding associated with dissecting a scarred lung in an anticoagulated patient. Now, without the uniform requirement for heparinization, such patients are generally regarded as operative candidates, with intraoperative blood loss, in most recipients, only moderate and easily managed.

Review of intraoperative packed red cell use in all transplants performed to date at Washington University indicates an average of 0.75 ± 1.5 U/patient, in those who did not require CPB and an average of 2.6 ± 3.3 U/patient in those that did.

Although blood loss during LTX is generally modest, as with all surgical procedures, blood conservation is a concern. Preoperative hemodilution (whole blood drawn into a CPD bag and replaced with 3:1 crystalloid) has been performed in some polycythemic patients and may be particularly beneficial in those with pulmonary hypertension and right-to-left intracardiac shunt to initially reduce blood viscosity and improve cardiopulmonary function while also providing whole blood for reinfusion following CPB. Recently, continuous infusion of aprotinin has been proposed to reduce intraoperative bleeding during surgical procedures where the blood loss is anticipated to be excessive.[58,59] Limited use of this drug in patients with cystic fibrosis and/or history of previous intrathoracic surgery has, thus far, proved encouraging. However, detailed data from a large series of patients are lacking.

If blood products are to be used it is important, for the anesthesiologist, as with all transplant procedures, to be familiar with whether or not the patient has antibodies to cytomegalovirus (CMV), and to closely check blood products to confirm they coincide with the patient's status. Obviously the group to whom CMV status is critically important is the one where a CMV-negative patient is to receive a CMV-negative organ. On the other hand if a CMV-negative patient is to receive a CMV-positive organ, then CMV status of blood products is unimportant.

Cardiopulmonary Bypass

CPB during lung transplantation has generally been regarded as increasing blood loss and perioperative morbidity and mortality.[60–63] Correspondingly, as the indications for LTX have broadened, deciding whether CPB is necessary has complicated anesthetic management of

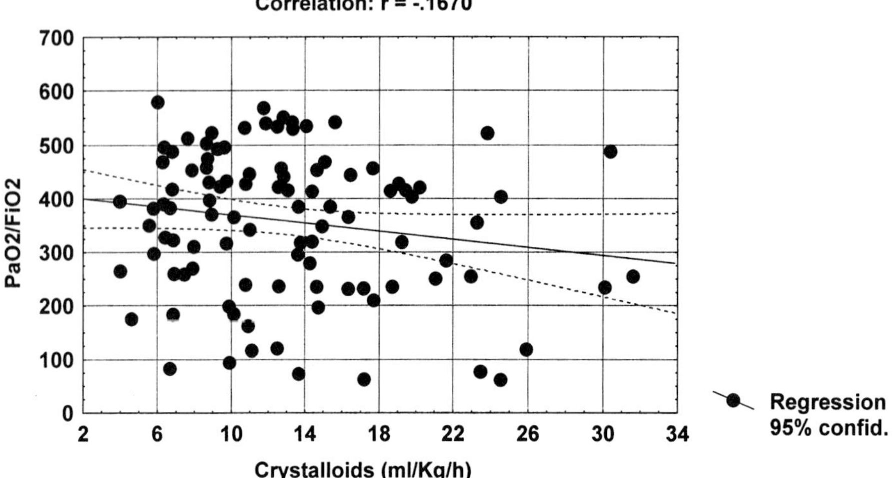

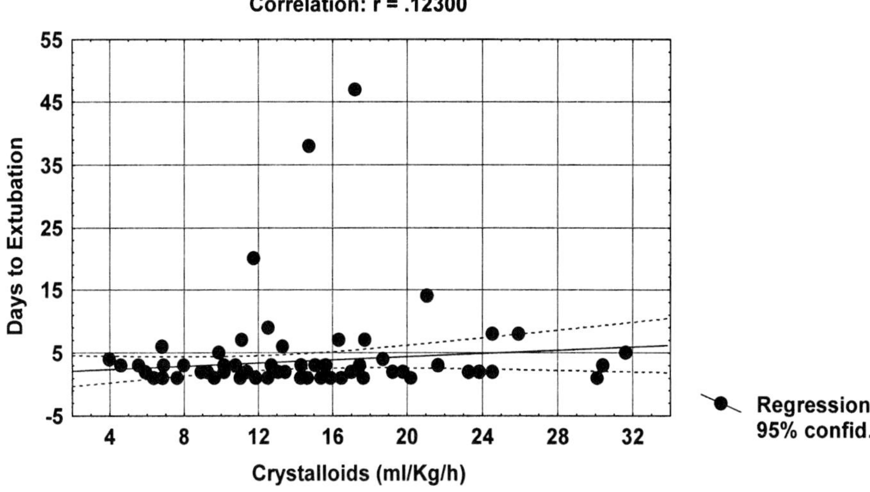

FIGURE 30–7. Correlation between intraoperative crystalloid infusion and PaO_2/FIO_2 ratio on admission to the intensive care unit, and the number of days to extubation.

these procedures. However, it must be emphasized that CPB should always be available and promptly employed if cardiorespiratory instability refractory to other interventions occurs intraoperatively. It has been our practice to have CPB capability on stand-by basis for all lung transplant procedures using a centrifugal pump that can be used intraoperatively or adapted for postoperative use as a right ventricular assist device or ECMO circuit.

As previously noted, for the en bloc double-lung transplantation technique total CPB was essential during the entire procedure. In contrast, when CPB is planned for SLT (i.e., patients with pulmonary vascular disease) or BLT, partial normothermic CPB is used with the nonoperative lung ventilated and the heart beating. For BLT cases in which CPB is planned or initiated prior to extraction or implantation of the first lung, our preference is to utilize total CPB with the heart empty and beating. Both native lungs are excised. The first lung is implanted, the clamps are left in place and the graft kept cold with topical crushed ice while the second lung is implanted. Each lung is then sequentially de-aired and reperfused. This strategy does lengthen ischemic time to the first lung. However, it avoids the uncontrolled perfusion of the first graft during partial bypass, which occurs with retraction necessary for the second implantation. Furthermore, it decreases the exposure time of the first lung to CPB. Having utilized many other strategies we have come to believe this technique provides superior results. In our experience, unplanned CPB has rarely proven necessary during SLT. During BLT, the need for CPB is highly variable, being unnecessary in many cases, and required in others for replacement of one or both lung. Raffin et al. have reported ten cases of bilateral lung transplantation of which one required bypass.[43]

TABLE 30–4
Unplanned Cardiopulmonary Bypass During BLT: Preoperative Predictors

	Bypass (n = 18)	Without Bypass (n = 50)
PAP_s	35.1 ± 9.6	34 ± 7.2 (p = N.S.)
PAP_d	18.8 ± 6.7	17.5 ± 4.7 (p = N.S.)
PAP_m	24.2 ± 7.4	23 ± 5.3 (p = N.S.)
$RAPo_2$	54.3 ± 12.1	55 ± 11.5 (p = N.S.)
Age	36.6 ± 15	41.5 ± 11 (p = N.S.)

BLT, bilateral lung transplantation; PAP, pulmonary arterial pressure in mm Hg; s, systolic; d, diastolic; m, mean; RA, room air; N.S., not significant.

More recently, Bando et al.[63] reported 39 SLT cases of which 4 required unplanned CPB, and nine BLT cases with two requiring CPB. De Hoyos et al.[64] have reported the Toronto experience and indicated that values of preoperative room air Pao_2 and pulmonary hemodynamics, as well as oxygen requirements, right ventricular function, and exercise capacity may serve as predictors for bypass requirements in SLT. In their experience nearly 50% of the SLT recipients required bypass. In another study, by Firestone et al., 36% (n = 20) of 55 SLT recipients were placed on CPB.[65] In this study, patients who required CPB have had higher pulmonary artery pressure and lower baseline Pao_2 than those who did not. Of the first 162 LTXs performed at Washington University, 56 patients required CPB.[56] Of these patients, CPB was planned in 37. In the remaining 19, CPB was used once, for correction of a surgical mishap, during SLT and instituted emergently in 18 BLT recipients, most frequently due to severe acute allograft dysfunction (n = 11). Possible predictors such as pulmonary preoperative arterial pressure and Pao_2 were not different between those who required bypass and those who did not (Table 30–4). In the same group of patients, however, CPB did not seem to affect outcome (Table 30–5). In contrast, in the series reported by Bando et al.,[63] all patients who required planned or unplanned CPB eventually died.

When CPB is used, gas flow across the oxygenator should be carefully adjusted to prevent relative hypocarbia and profound alkalosis, since many patients display chronic CO_2 retention and compensatory metabolic alkalosis preoperatively. Weaning from bypass is usually uneventful. However, it has been our practice to administer dobutamine and PGE_1 during and after the wean from bypass in patients with severe preoperative pulmonary hypertension. Should significant hemodynamic compromise persist, following CPB, with systemic hypotension limiting infusion of pulmonary vasodilators, infusion of α-adrenergic agonists via a left atrial line may be beneficial.

Many LTX patients, particularly those with CF, appear to respond to CPB differently than the conventional cardiac surgical patient. Marked reductions in systemic vascular resistance, which respond poorly to α-adrenergic agonists and necessitate high pump flows, have been observed. Etiology of this response is uncertain, but may result from loss of pulmonary metabolic function or initiation of cytokine-mediated processes such as stimulation of nitric oxide synthesis. Alternatively, it may be due to a systemic gram-negative bacteremia created during the vigorous and occasionally violent dissection necessary to extract these densely adherent septic lungs.

Postoperative Ventilatory Management

Usually a standard IMV ventilator is sufficient for postoperative ventilation. Following most procedures, we attempt to rapidly reduce the Fio_2 and initiate weaning from the ventilator as soon as the patient is warm, awake, and stable. An exception to this approach is the patient who has undergone single-lung transplantation for pulmonary hypertension. Due to a propensity for episodes of cardiopulmonary instability during the first 48 to 72 hours postoperatively, we have found it advantageous to keep these patients sedated, paralyzed, and ventilated during this period.

Postoperatively, V/Q mismatch and intrapulmonary shunt are often more pronounced in single than in double-lung recipients. Not surprisingly, following SLT, patients with restrictive disease often display the best pulmonary function, since the graft receives the majority of both ventilation and perfusion. Alternatively, following SLT the remaining native lung in emphysemic patients often receives a substantial portion of the tidal volume, and in patients with pulmonary hypertension, the native lung continues to be ventilated but receives very little blood flow.[66] Postural changes in arterial oxygen saturation are often prominent in SLT recipients. In general, patients who received a single lung for pulmonary hypertension or emphysema display better postoperative pulmonary function with the "transplant side up," whereas the opposite may be true in certain patients with restrictive lung disease.

TABLE 30–5
Unplanned Cardiopulmonary Bypass During BLT: Outcome Indicators

	Bypass (n = 18)	Without Bypass (n = 50)
Days to extubation	4.2 ± 3.1	2.8 ± 2.2 (p = N.S.)
Days in ICU	5.6 ± 3.8	5.2 ± 6.5 (p = N.S.)
Days to RA Po_2 <60 mm Hg	11.6 ± 10.4	9.2 ± 10 (p = N.S.)

BLT, bilateral lung transplantation; ICU, intensive care unit; RA, room air; N.S., not significant.

Postoperative Pain Management

Given the impact of postoperative pain on pulmonary mechanics and respiratory function,[67] planning postoperative analgesia is extremely important Our approach has been to initiate epidural opiate infusion immediately after admission to the ICU in patients that are hemodynamically stable. In a review of 119 transplant patients, we found that patients who received continuous infusion of morphine (0.3 to 1.0 mg/hr) via lumbar epidural catheters were extubated quicker and discharged from the ICU sooner than recipients treated with morphine patient-controlled anesthesia (PCA) devices.[32] As noted above, the only recipients who do not routinely have preoperative epidural catheters placed at our institution are those undergoing SLT for pulmonary hypertension.

Postoperative Complications Necessitating Anesthesia

Postoperative infection remains the leading cause of death following LTX, with the majority of fatal infections either viral or fungal in nature.[68,69] In general, complications requiring additional surgery can be regarded as early (i.e., bleeding, technical problems with vascular or bronchial anastomoses, profound reperfusion injury with graft failure necessitating retransplantation) or late (i.e., airway dehiscence, chronic rejection necessitating retransplantation). In our early experience, airway complications occurred in approximately 10 to 15% of cases. Multiple rigid and flexible bronchoscopies were required for laser therapy, dilatation, and stent placement. With evolution of techniques, better preservation, and more precise treatment of rejection and infection, the incidence of airway complications has decreased below 5%. Indeed, in our most recent 40 transplants, we have not had a single airway complication. In general, the immediate post-LTX patient can be treated like any other critically ill patient, as can the recipient with chronic airway compromise. Many recipients have undergone elective surgical procedures unrelated to their pulmonary disease following LTX, and have presented few anesthetic problems. Not surprisingly, differences in the compliance of a native and transplanted lung following SLT can result in alterations in intraoperative capnography.[71]

New Frontiers

Although not specifically addressed in this chapter, LTX in patients less than 18 years of age has experienced a remarkable increase in the last few years. The majority of these have been en bloc double or bilateral single transplants, with over 60% performed for cystic fibrosis. Actuarial survival at 12 months is approximately 85% for pediatric bilateral single lung.[25] Due to the extremely limited donor pool, use of adult lung lobes in pediatric transplantation is being utilized increasingly following the pioneering work at the University of Southern California (USC),[72] and the plausibility of xenografts is being investigated.

Other areas receiving considerable interest are the use of inhaled nitric oxide (NO) in the treatment of intraoperative pulmonary hypertension and postoperative reperfusion injury, and improved methods for monitoring right ventricular function. Numerous studies have demonstrated the cardiopulmonary benefit of the selective pulmonary vasodilation produced by inhaled NO, and early experience indicates similar benefits in some LTX recipients.[73] When compared to PGE_1 infusion, in 50 LTX recipients, NO inhalation was found to be equally effective as a pulmonary vasodilator, but in contrast to PGE_1 did not cause systemic vasodilation. Furthermore, only NO was found to significantly improve arterial oxygenation in a subset of patients that developed severe postoperative allograft dysfunction. Based on these findings, NO has been incorporated into our standard management of LTX recipients with early graft dysfunction. Interestingly, increased experience with the drug has now begun to suggest that in comparison to traditional treatment for early allograft dysfunction (i.e., diuretics, steroids, PEEP), NO inhalation not only improves oxygenation but may also lead to earlier extubation, reduced airway complications, and fewer deaths[74] (Table 30–6).

Another area that requires attention is whether SLT provides adequate long-term results. As shown in Figure 30–8, there is an abrupt decline of the SLT curve in the fourth posttransplant year and a significant advantage of BLT as compared to SLT. However, towards the middle of the fifth year the curves seem to meet together again and at the end of the year BLT still has an advantage but not as strong as a year before. Clearly, the number of patients qualifying for 5-year follow-up is rather small and outcome is heavily influenced by institutional dif-

TABLE 30–6
Nitric Oxide and Outcome in Patients With Early Allograft Dysfunction*

	Pao_2/Fio_2	Ext. Days	Airway Complications	Deaths
Group 1 (without NO) (*n* = 17)	81 ± 27	17 ± 5	3	4
Group 2 (with NO) (*n* = 15)	88 ± 30	123 ± 3	0	1

*Modified from Date H, Triantafillou AN, Trulock EP, et al: Inhaled nitric oxide reduces human allograft dysfunction. J Thorac Cardiovasc Surg 111:913, 1996, with permission.
Pao_2, partial pressure of oxygen, arterial; Fio_2, fraction of inspired oxygen; NO, nitric oxide.

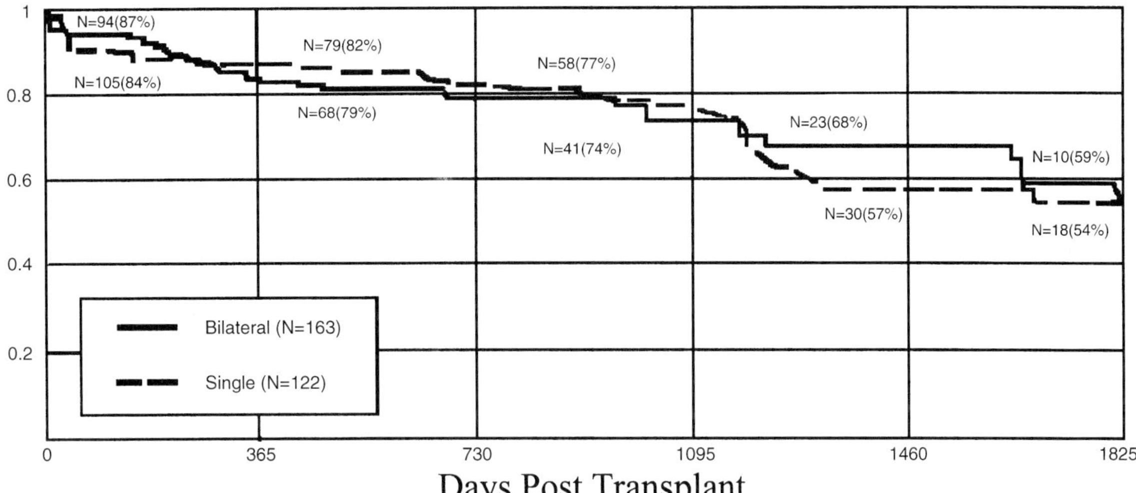

FIGURE **30–8.** Four-year actuarial survival of patients undergoing single and bilateral lung transplants at Washington University.

ferences in selection criteria, experience, and follow-up. Nevertheless, the security and "protection" from posttransplant events, such as infection and rejection, provided by two lungs may have long-term benefit. Of course, one might argue that the single-lung option enables conduct of double the number of transplants. This is true when both donor lungs are suitable as solitary grafts. This is often not the case. Our preference toward BLT enables our program to utilize many marginal lungs as bilateral grafts that would never be used as single lung grafts. Any conclusions regarding this very crucial issue are currently premature and longer survival and quality-of-life data should become available before an answer emerges.

Finally, the introduction of lung volume reduction surgery (LVRS) may change current thinking in relation to surgical treatment of severe obstructive lung disease. As noted previously, LVRS may now be an option offered to patients suffering from severe obstructive lung disease. The first report comparing LVRS versus either BLT or SLT was published recently.[70] From the results of this study it appears that LVRS resulted in an improvement of lung function which, although inferior to that of LTX, was satisfactory and achieved while avoiding immunosuppression or transplant-related complications. Furthermore, LVRS may be the only option for patients who have contraindications for LTX and, antithetically, LTX may be a further option for patients who have undergone LVRS when their improvement has faded.

Summary

Transplantation of one or both lungs continues to evolve as a valuable option for many patients with end-stage lung disease. As with most facets of anesthetic care, there are multiple ways to safely and effectively manage LTX recipients. In general, perioperative management of the transplant recipient requires the same skills as caring for any critically ill patient, but each patient presents a unique set of challenges and the approach to anesthetic management must be adapted to the pathophysiology of the underlying cardiopulmonary disease.

References

1. Hardy JD, Webb WR, Dalton ML, et al: Lung homotransplantation in man. JAMA 186:1065, 1963.
2. Triantafillou AN, Heerdt PM: Lung transplantation. Int Anesthesiol Clin 29:87, 1991.
3. Low D, Trulock EP, Kaiser LR, et al, and The Washington University Lung Transplantation Group: Lung transplantation in ventilator-dependent patients. Chest 101:8, 1992.
4. Flume PA, Egan TM, Westerman JH, et al: Lung transplantation for mechanically ventilated patients. J Heart Lung Transplant 13: 15, 1994.
5. Dennis C, Wallwork J: Mechanical ventilation and lung transplantation. J Heart Lung Transplant 13:22, 1994.
6. Cooper JD, Trulock EP, Triantafillou AN, et al: Bilateral pneumectomy (volume reduction) for chronic obstructive pulmonary disease. J Thorac Cardiovasc Surg 109:106, 1995.
7. Hinson KFW: Diffuse pulmonary fibrosis. Hum Pathol 1:825, 1970.
8. Mall H, Andreassin B, Fabrice P, et al: Unilateral lung transplantation in end-stage pulmonary emphysema. Am Rev Respir Dis 140:797, 1989.
9. Kaiser LR, Cooper JD, Trulock EP, et al, and The Washington University Lung Transplant Group: The evolution of single lung transplantation for emphysema. J Thorac Cardiovasc Surg 102: 333, 1991.
10. Low DE, Trulock EP, Kaiser LR, et al: Morbidity, mortality and early results of single versus bilateral lung transplantation for emphysema. J Thorac Cardiovasc Surg 103:1119, 1992.
11. Foweler NO, Westcott RN, Scott RC: Normal pressure in the right heart and pulmonary artery. Am Heart J 46:264, 1953.
12. Pasque MK, Kaiser LR, Dresler CM, et al: Single lung transplantation for pulmonary hypertension: Technical aspects and immediate results. J Thorac Cardiovasc Surg 103:475, 1992.
13. Voelkel NF, Weir EK: Etiologic mechanisms in primary pulmonary hypertension. In Weir EK, Reeves JT (eds): Pulmonary Vascular Physiology and Pathophysiology. New York, Marcel Dekker, 1989, p 513.

14. Glanville AR, Barke CM, Theodore J, et al: Primary pulmonary hypertension: Length of survival in patients referred for heart-lung transplantation. Chest 91:675, 1987.
15. Girard C, Mornex JF, Gamondes JP, et al: Single lung transplantation for primary pulmonary hypertension without cardiopulmonary bypass. Chest 102:967, 1992.
16. Triantafillou AN, Heerdt PM, Pasque MK, et al: Immediate improvement of pulmonary hemodynamics and right ventricular function after single lung transplantation for primary pulmonary hypertension. Circulation 84:1277, 1991.
17. Pasque MK, Trulock EP, Kaiser LR, Cooper JD: Single lung transplantation for pulmonary hypertension: Three-month hemodynamic follow-up. Circulation 84:2275, 1991.
18. Pasque MK, Kaiser LR, Dresler CM, et al: Single lung transplantation for pulmonary hypertension. Technical aspects and immediate hemodynamic results. J Thorac Cardiovasc Surg 130:475, 1992.
19. Globits S, Burghuber OC, Koller J, et al: Effect of lung transplantation on right and left ventricular volumes and function measured by magnetic resonance imaging. Am J Respir Crit Care Med 149(4 Pt 1):1000, 1994.
20. Levine SM, Gibbons WJ, Bryan CL, et al: Single lung transplantation for primary pulmonary hypertension. Chest 98:1107, 1990.
21. Pasque MK, Trulock EP, Cooper JD, et al: Single lung transplantation for pulmonary hypertension. Single institution experience on 34 patients. Circulation 92:2252, 1995.
22. Bando K, Armitage JM, Paradis IL, et al: Indications for and results of single, bilateral, and heart-lung transplantation for pulmonary hypertension. J Thorac Cardiovasc Surg 108:1056, 1994.
23. Levine SM, Jenkinson SG, Bryan CL, et al: Ventilation-perfusion inequalities during graft rejection in patients undergoing single lung transplantation for primary pulmonary hypertension [see comments]. Chest 101:401, 1992.
24. Bando K, Keenan RJ, Paradis IL, et al: Impact of pulmonary hypertension on outcome after single-lung transplantation. Ann Thorac Surg 58:1336, 1994.
25. Kaye MP: The Registry of the International Society for Heart and Lung Transplantation: Tenth Official Report–1993. J Heart Lung Transplant 12:541, 1993.
26. Shennib H, Massard G, Gauthier R, et al: Single lung transplantation for cystic fibrosis: Is it an option? J Heart Lung Transplant 12:288, 1993.
27. Rivera M, Nicotra MB: *Pseudomonas aeruginosa* mucoid strain. Its significance in adult chest disease. Am Rev Respir Dis 126: 833, 1982.
28. Morrison DL, Maurer JR, Grossman RF: Preoperative assessment for lung transplantation. Clin Chest Med 11:207, 1990.
29. Craven JL, Bright J, Lougheed Dear C: Psychiatric, psychosocial, and rehabilitative aspects of lung transplantation. Clin Chest Med 11:247, 1990.
30. Conacher ID: Isolated lung transplantation: A review of problems and guide to anesthesia. Br J Anaesth 61:468, 1989.
31. Thomas B, Slegel LC: Anesthetic and postoperative management of single-lung transplantation. J Cardiothorac Vasc Anesth 5:266, 1991.
32. Triantafillou AN, Heerdt PM, Hoque CW, et al: Epidural vs. intravenous morphine for postoperative pain management after lung transplantation. Anesthesiology 77:857, 1992.
33. Body S, Fanciullo G, Ferrante M, et al: Thoracic epidural analgesia after lung transplant. Anesthesiology 81:1285, 1994.
34. Panos L, Patterson GA, Demajo WA: The use of high-frequency jet ventilation during post-lung transplantation surgery. J Cardiothorac Vasc Anesth 7:202, 1993.
35. Konstam MA, Salem DN, Imner JM, et al: Vasodilator effect on right ventricular function in congestive heart failure and pulmonary hypertension. Am J Cardiol 54:132, 1984.
36. Bardoczky GI, de Franquen P, Engleman E, Capello M: Continuous monitoring of pulmonary mechanics with the side-stream spirometer during lung transplantation. J Cardiothorac Vasc Anesth 6:731, 1992.
37. Demajo WAP: Anesthetic technique for single lung transplantation. In Cooper DKC, Novitzky D (eds): The Transplantation and Replacement of Thoracic Organs. Boston, Kluwer Academic Publishers, 1990.
38. Scheller MS, Kriett JM, Smith CM, Jamieson SW: Airway management during anesthesia for double-lung transplantation using a single-lumen endotracheal tube with an enclosed bronchial blocker. J Cardiothorac Vasc Anesth 6:204, 1992.
39. Bjertnaes J, Hauge A, Torgrinson T: The pulmonary vasoconstrictor response to hypoxia: The hypoxia-sensitive site studied with a volatile inhibitor. Acta Physiol Scand 109:447, 1980.
40. Johnson D, Mayers I, To T: The effects of halothane in hypoxic pulmonary vasoconstriction. Anesthesiology 72:125, 1990.
41. Marshall BE: Anesthesia for one-lung ventilation (Letter). Anesthesiology 69:630, 1988.
42. Benumof JL: Anesthesia for one-lung ventilation (Reply to Letter). Anesthesiology 69:631, 1988.
43. Raffin L, Cherqui MM, Sperandio M, et al: Anesthesia for bilateral lung transplantation without cardiopulmonary bypass: Initial experience and review of intraoperative problems. J Cardiothorac Vasc Anesth 6:409, 1992.
44. Archer SL, McMurtry IF, Weir EK: Mechanisms of acute hypoxic and hyperoxic changes in pulmonary vascular reactivity. In Weir EK, Reeves JT (eds): Pulmonary Vascular Physiology and Pathophysiology. New York, Marcel Dekker, 1989, p 241.
45. Froese AB, Bryan AC: High frequency ventilation. Am Rev Respir Dis 135:1363, 1987.
46. Egan TM, Kaiser LR, Cooper JD: Lung transplantation. Curr Probl Surg 26:673, 1989.
47. Calhoon JH, Grover FL, Gibbons WJ, et al: Single lung transplantation. Alternative indications and technique. J Thorac Cardiovasc Surg 101:816, 1991.
48. Griffith BP, Magee MJ, Gonzalez IF, et al: Anastomotic pitfalls in lung transplantation. J Thorac Cardiovasc Surg 107:743, 1994.
49. Sarsam MA, Yonan NA, Beton D, et al: Early pulmonary vein thrombosis after single lung transplantation. J Heart Lung Transplant 12:17, 1993.
50. Heerdt PM, Pond CG, Kussman MK, Triantafillou A: Use of a Doppler pulmonary artery catheter for continuous measurement of right ventricular pump function and contractility during single lung transplantation. J Heart Lung Transplant 12:682, 1993.
51. Pasque MK, Cooper JD, Kaiser LK, et al: An improved technique for bilateral single lung transplantation: Rationale and clinical experience. Ann Thorac Surg 49:785, 1990.
52. Patterson GA, Cooper JD, Park JH, Jones MT: The Toronto Lung Transplant Group. Experimental and clinical double lung transplantation. J Thorac Cardiovasc Surg 95:70, 1988.
53. Jennische E: Post-ischemic calcification in skeletal muscle: A light microscopy study in rat. Acta Pathol Microbiol Immunol Scand [A] 92:139, 1984.
54. Majed Odeh: The role of reperfusion-induced injury in the pathogenesis of the crush syndrome N Engl J Med 324:1417, 1991.
55. Horgan MJ, Lum H, Malik AB: Pulmonary edema after pulmonary artery occlusion and reperfusion. Am Rev Respir Dis 140: 1421, 1989.
56. Triantafillou AN, Pasque MK, Huddleston CB, et al: Predictors, frequency, and indications for cardiopulmonary bypass during lung transplantation in adults. Ann Thorac Surg 57:1248, 1994.
57. Karanikolas MS, Triantafillou AN, Pond CG, et al: Outcome of lung transplantation in relation to fluid administration. Anesthesiology 81:1465, 1994.
58. Royston D: The serine antiprotease aprotinin (Trasylol): A novel approach to reducing postoperative bleeding. Blood Coagul Fibrinolysis 1:55, 1990.
59. Janssens M, Joris J, David JL, et al: High-dose aprotinin reduces blood loss in patients undergoing total hip replacement surgery. Anesthesiology 80:23, 1994.
60. Francalancia NA, Aeba R, Yousem SA, et al: Deleterious effects of cardiopulmonary bypass on early graft function after single lung allotransplantation: Evaluation of a heparin-coated bypass circuit. J Heart Lung Transplant 13:498, 1994.
61. Aeba R, Griffith BP, Kormos RL, et al: Effect of cardiopulmonary bypass on early graft dysfunction in clinical lung transplantation. Ann Thorac Surg 57:715, 1994.
62. Allinson RW, Limstrom SA, Sethi GK, Copeland JG: Central retinal vein occlusion after heart-lung transplantation. Ann Ophthalmol 25:58, 1993.
63. Bando K, Paradis IL, Yousem SA, et al: Comparison of outcomes after single and bilateral lung transplantation for obstructive lung disease. J Heart Lung Transplant 14:692, 1995.
64. de Hoyos A, Demajo W, Snell G, et al: Preoperative prediction

for the use of cardiopulmonary bypass in lung transplantation. J Thorac Cardiovasc Surg 106:787, 1993.
65. Firestone L, Carrera J, Firestone S, Rothfield K: Single lung transplants: Who needs bypass? Anesthesiology 78:A46, 1993.
66. Mannes GP, de Boer WJ, Meuzelaar JJ, Meinesz AF: Ventilation-perfusion inequalities in a patient with obliterative bronchiolitis after single-lung transplantation for primary pulmonary hypertension (Letter) [see comment]. Chest 103:1311, 1993.
67. Haimerl WE, Groh J, Briegel J, et al: Effect of intrapleural morphine on postoperative pain and pulmonary function. Br J Anaesth 69:637, 1992.
68. Dauber JH, Paradis IL, Dummer JS: Infectious complications in pulmonary allograft recipients. Clin Chest Med 11:291, 1990.
69. Maurer JR, Tullis DE, Grossman RF, et al: Infectious complications following isolated lung transplantation. Chest 101:1056, 1992.
70. Date H, Trulock EP, Arcidi JM, et al: Improved airway healing after lung transplantation. An analysis of 348 bronchial anastomoses. J Thorac Cardiovasc Surg 110:1424, 1995.
71. Williams EL, Jellish WS, Modica PA, et al: Capnography in a patient after single lung transplantation. Anesthesiology 74:621, 1991.
72. Starnes VA, Barr ML, Cohen RG, et al: Living-donor lobar lung transplantation experience: Intermediate results. J Thorac Cardiovasc Surg 112:1284, 1996.
73. Triantafillou AN, Pohl MS, Okayabashi K, et al: Effects of inhaled nitric oxide and prostaglandin E1 in the early postoperative management of patients following bilateral lung transplantation. Circulation 90:3432, 1994.
74. Date H, Triantafillou AN, Trulock EP, et al: Inhaled nitric oxide reduces human allograft dysfunction. J Thorac Cardiovasc Surg 111:913, 1996.
75. Gaissert HA, Trulock EP, Cooper JD, et al: Comparison of early results after volume reduction or lung transplantation for chronic obstructive pulmonary disease. J Thorac Cardiovasc Surg 111: 296, 1996.

S E C T I O N **VI**

GENERAL CONSIDERATIONS

CHAPTER 31

Dysrhythmias

Noel W. Lawson, M.D.
Joseph D. Tobias, M.D.

Dysrhythmias are among the most common perioperative cardiovascular events, regardless of age or gender. The term "dysrhythmia" is often used interchangeably with arrhythmia, but the choice depends upon your interpretation of Greek and whether the prefix "dys" (meaning bad) or "a" (meaning without, as in asystole) is more descriptive. The incidence of perioperative dysrhythmias also varies according to the surgical population; procedure; and the phase of anesthesia such as induction, intubation, and emergence.[1] In a recent multicenter study (n = 17,201), serious dysrhythmias accounted for 44% of 847 severe adverse outcomes.[2] The incidence of intraoperative dysrhythmias ranges between 60 and 80%; however, fewer than 2% are serious and require therapy. Excepting the known cardiac patient, serious dysrhythmias during anesthesia are usually of acute onset and unexpected. A serious dysrhythmia is defined as one that (1) results in a significant decrease in cardiac output, (2) impairs myocardial oxygen balance, or (3) predisposes to cardiac arrest.

Anatomy of the Cardiac Conduction System

Automaticity and rhythmicity are intrinsic properties of cardiac tissue. Pacemakers generate while conduction fibers distribute the cardiac electrical impulse so that the action of the heart is synchronized to produce a cardiac output appropriate to body needs. The surface electrocardiogram (ECG) is an integration of all the action potentials that occur in the myocardium. Conduction velocity (dromotropy) is the speed of transmission of a wave of depolarization through the myocardium. The cardiac conduction system is anatomically and functionally distinct from the working elements of the myocardium, and includes the sinoatrial (SA) node, atrial internodal tracts, atrioventricular (AV) node, bundle of His, right and left bundle branches, and subendocardial Purkinje fibers (Fig. 31–1).

The SA node is generously supplied with both sympathetic and parasympathetic nerves, with a predominance of parasympathetic innervation.[3,4] The sinus node artery, which arises with equal frequency from either the right or left circumflex coronary artery, nourishes the SA node. Two types of specialized muscle cells are found within the SA node: P (pacemaker) cells and T (transitional) cells. The P, or nodal cells, are the normal source of the cardiac impulse. T cells surround the SA node and probably serve both to organize impulses leaving the SA node and to hinder access of premature ectopic atrial impulses into the node. The T cells connect directly to internodal tracts that distribute the impulses to the atrial muscle.

Three internodal tracts and one interatrial tract rapidly distribute the SA impulse to the right and left atrium and AV node. The internodal pathways are the anterior, middle (Wenckebach's), and posterior (Thorel's) tracts. The anterior tract gives off a branch (Bachmann's bundle) to the left atrium. The three internodal tracts diverge as they move over the atrium and then reconverge as they approach the AV node. Internodal paths are not as anatomically discrete as the His bundle or Purkinje fibers, but their functional existence is proven. They form distinct pathways of least resistance with impulse condition velocities of about 1 m/sec.[5]

Extraneous internodal tracts, found in some hearts, are thought to represent vestiges of the fetal myocardium that persist into adult life. Three of these abnormal pathways have been identified and designated as the accessory bundle of Kent, James fibers, and Mahaim fibers. These vestigial tracts bypass the AV node and can thereby result in a more premature activation of the ventricles than if the impulse had reached the ventricles through the slower conducting pathway of the AV node. These accessory tracts are thought to be the mechanism by which anomalous ventricular excitation can occur. This can result in "ventricular pre-excitation." Dysrhythmias produced in this fashion range from simply shortened AV conduction to serious ventricular tachycardias orchestrated by atrial tachydysrhythmias such as fibrillation or flutter. The bundle of Kent is associated with the Wolff-Parkinson-White syndrome.

The AV node is abundantly supplied by autonomic nerves and receptors. The AV node is considered a trilaminar structure and has been divided into three areas

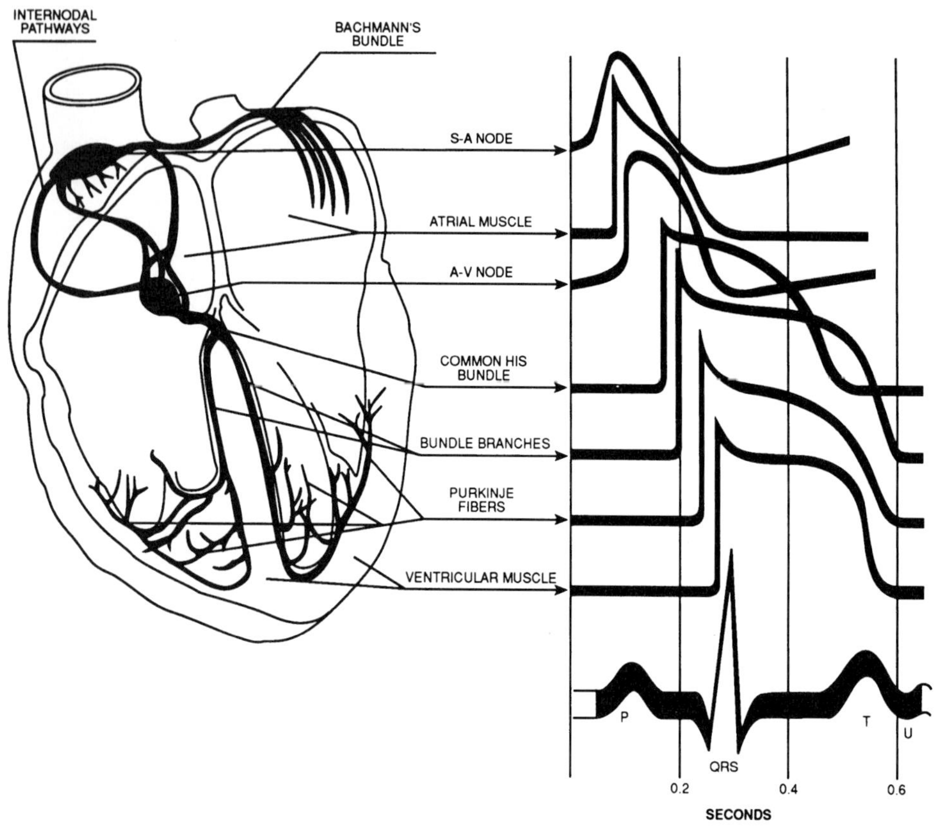

FIGURE **31–1.** The rate of spontaneous phase 4 depolarization and conduction velocity decreases as one descends from the SA node to the AV node and into the ventricle. This decremental inefficiency of conduction is, in large part, responsible for the orderly sequence of atrioventricular contraction. The delay from the SA node to the AV node is expressed as the PR interval on the ECG. Ventricular conduction is expressed as the width of the QRS.

designated as the: (1) A-N region, the transitional zone between atrium and the AV node; (2) the N region or midzone of the node; and (3) the N-H region, which is a transitional or penetrating zone where the AV node forms the bundle of His. The His bundle is the start of the ventricular conduction system.

The action potentials in the N region display slow automaticity via slow response potentials (see "Slow Action Potentials," later). The greatest conduction delay from the SA node occurs in the A-N and upper N regions, thus forming the PR interval on the ECG. This delay permits ventricular filling during atrial contraction. It also protects the ventricles from high rates of contraction when the atria are being depolarized at an abnormally high pace. The slowed conduction (0.02 to 0.1 m/sec) also permits the AV node to be a source of re-entry in pre-excitation syndromes. Retrograde conduction does occur.

The AV node is in close proximity to its nutrient artery.[3,4] The blood supply to the AV node is 90% of the time from the right coronary artery. In the remaining 10%, it comes from the left circumflex. The bundle of His, forming from the AV node, passes down the right side of the interventricular septum, dividing into the right and left bundle branches. Damage to the His bundle can cause AV conduction delay or complete AV block because it is the only normal route for the cardiac impulse from atria to ventricles. The upper portion of the interventricular septum is supplied by branches of both the anterior and posterior descending coronary arteries. This renders the penetrating portion of the AV bundle and bundle of His less vulnerable to ischemia or infarction. Coronary disease must be extensive to produce ischemic damage to the His bundle.

The right bundle is a direct extension of the His bundle, which proceeds down the right side of the interventricular septum. The left bundle branch arises almost perpendicularly from the bundle of His and perforates the interventricular septum. It divides into the thin left anterior division and the thicker left posterior division. Conduction blockade of either main bundle is known as a right or left bundle branch block. Blockade of the divisions of the left bundle branch is known as either a left anterior or left posterior hemiblock. These conduction defects produce characteristic ECG patterns.

The right and left bundles form a subendocardial network of Purkinje fibers that extend into the inner one third of the endocardium. These fibers have the largest diameter of any cells in the myocardium, accounting for their fast conduction velocity. The conduction velocity over the Purkinje fibers is the fastest of any tissue within the heart, traveling at 1 to 4 m/sec. This permits almost simultaneous activation of both right and left ventricular endocardial surfaces.[5,6]

Autonomic Innervation of the Heart

The heart is controlled by the balance between the antagonism of the sympathetic nervous system (SNS) and parasympathetic (PNS) nervous system. Autonomic innervation affects cardiac pumping in four ways: (1) by changing rate (chronotropy); (2) conduction velocity (dromotropy); (3) force of contraction (inotropy); and (4) modulating coronary blood flow. However, cardiac function is not dependent upon autonomic innervation for function, as witnessed by the success of the denervated heart in cardiac transplant patients.

Cardiac parasympathetic preganglionic neurons arise bilaterally in the medulla oblongata and enter the thorax via the recurrent laryngeal and thoracic vagus nerves. Vagal fibers to the heart merge with the sympathetic fibers from the stellate ganglia to form the cardiac vagus nerve. The thoracic vagus nerve to the heart is, therefore, a mixed nerve containing both PNS and SNS efferent fibers. The PNS vagal fibers are distributed mainly to the SA and AV nodes. They are distributed to a lesser extent to the atrial conduction pathways, and atrial myocardium via the coronary plexus along with the SNS fibers. Distribution of cholinergic vagal nerves to the ventricles is apparently sparse, but both ventricles do receive some cholinergic innervation.[7]

The main effect of vagal cardiac stimulation (muscarinic) to the conduction tissues is to produce negative chronotropism (rate) and dromotropism (conduction).[8] Vagal stimulation, particularly the right vagus, decreases the rate of SA automaticity and decreases excitability of the AV junction fibers, slowing impulse conduction to the ventricles. If the heart rate is slowed below a particular threshold, lower pacemakers with slower intrinsic automaticity may take over pacemaker function, producing a junctional (nodal) rhythm. A very strong vagal discharge can completely arrest SA node depolarization and block impulse conduction to the ventricles. A ventricular pacemaker may assume dominance, producing a ventricular escape beat. Strong vagal stimulation of the ventricular myocardium can also reduce inotropism as much as 10 to 20%. However, PNS stimulation is relatively unimportant in this regard compared to its predominant effect on heart rate.

Muscarinic blockade by atropine can double heart rate without altering contractility of the left ventricle.[9] However, muscarinic receptors are also found on presynaptic membranes of sympathetic nerve terminals in the myocardium and coronary vessels. These are referred to as adrenergic muscarinic receptors because of their location. Stimulation of these cholinergic (muscarinic) receptors inhibit norepinephrine (NE) release much like α_2-adrenergic receptor stimulation.

The first four or five thoracic spinal segments generate sympathetic preganglionic fibers that ascend in the neck to form three paired ganglia. These are the superior cervical, middle cervical, and stellate ganglia. These ganglia provide sympathetic innervation of the head, neck, upper extremities, heart, coronary arteries, and lungs. Sympathetic innervation to the ventricles follows the distribution of the coronary arteries from the base to apex. They course near the surface of the ventricle before projecting more deeply.[10] Afferent pain fibers also travel with these cervicothoracic nerves, accounting for the diffuse chest, neck, or upper extremity pain characteristic of myocardial ischemia.

NE is released at the cardiac neuroeffector junction, which activates the appropriate receptor in the myocardium and coronary vessels. Under stressful conditions, NE may be joined by hormonal epinephrine (EPI) to increase heart rate, conduction velocity, inotropism, preload, afterload, as well as dysrhythmias. The SNS has the same myocardial supraventricular distribution as the PNS, but with increased distribution to the ventricles. The right stellate ganglion distributes fibers to the SA node, anterior epicardial surface, and interventricular septum.[8] Right stellate stimulation increases heart rate and decreases systolic duration. The left stellate ganglion supplies the AV node as well as the posterior and lateral surfaces of both ventricles. Left stellate stimulation increases myocardial contractility without causing a significant change in heart rate. Stimulation of the left sympathetic fibers is more likely to produce a shift in pacemaker from the SA to AV junctional tissues.[5]

Myocardial Adrenoreceptors

There are three types (six subtypes) of adrenergic receptors that respond to the endogenous catecholamines: α- (α_1 and α_2) adrenergic, β- (β_1 and β_2) adrenergic, and dopaminergic (DA_1 and DA_2) receptors. Table 31–1 is a brief review of the function and location of some of the clinically important myocardial adrenergic receptors now known to exist.[11,12]

Only the α- and β-adrenergic receptors are important to myocardial inotropism, automaticity, and conduction. DA receptors have not been identified in the myocardium, but defining specific DA receptors has been difficult because DA also stimulates the α- and β-adrenergic receptors in a dose-related manner.[13] Dopamine is therefore as capable of causing dysrhythmias as is NE or EPI, although there are no proven DA receptors in the heart.

Adrenergic receptors are found at both presynaptic (prejunctional) and postsynaptic (postjunctional) sites (Fig. 31–2 and Table 31–1). Prejunctional receptors are innervated in that they are in the immediate vicinity of the neurotransmitter released by a sympathetic action potential. Postjunctional receptors can be innervated or noninnervated depending upon their proximity to the synaptic cleft.[14] Receptors located directly on postjunctional membranes are considered to be innervated. However, most postsynaptic α_1- and β_2-adrenergic receptors are extrasynaptic and considered noninnervated even though they are located in the vicinity of the postsynaptic membrane.[15] These receptors are influenced more by hormonal (circulating) catecholamines such as epinephrine and dopamine than by neurotransmitter catecholamines such as norepinephrine.

There is a large body of evidence documenting the presence of postsynaptic α_1- and α_2-adrenergic receptors in the mammalian myocardium and coronary arteries.[12] Stimulation of either postsynaptic α_1- and α_2-adrenergic receptors results in vasoconstriction. The presence of postsynaptic α-adrenergic receptors in the coronary arteries of man has not been established with certainty, but other mammalian models have demonstrated their pres-

TABLE 31–1
Myocardial Adrenergic Receptors

Receptor	Synaptic Site*	Anatomic Site	Action	LV Function and Stroke Volume
α_1-Adrenergic	Postsynaptic	Coronary arteries—epicardial Myocardium 30–40% of resting tone	Constriction Positive inotropism	 Improved
α_2-Adrenergic	Presynaptic	Coronaries?	Inhibits NE release Vasodilation?	
	Postsynaptic	Coronaries—endocardial	Constriction	Decreased
β_1-Adrenergic	Postsynaptic NE sensitive	Myocardium	Positive inotropism and chronotropism	Improved
		SA node Ventricular conduction	Increased conduction	Improved
β_2-Adrenergic	Presynaptic NE sensitive	Myocardium SA node Ventricular conduction	Accelerates NE release	Improved
	Postsynaptic (Extrasynaptic) (EPI sensitive)	Myocardium	Positive inotropism and chronotropism	Improved

*Dopamine is a nonselective, direct and indirect, dose-dependent agonist of α- and β-myocardial receptors
LV, left ventricular; NE, norepinephrine; SA, sinoatrial; EPI, epinephrine.

ence. There is a growing consensus that sympathetic stimulation causes coronary vasoconstriction, which is mediated more by postsynaptic α_2- than by α_1-adrenergic receptors.[16] The larger epicardial arteries possess mainly α_1-adrenergic receptors, while α_2-adrenergic receptors are present in the small coronary resistance vessels.[17] Epicardial vessels contribute only 5% to the total resistance of the coronary circulation; therefore, α_1-adrenergic agonists such as phenylephrine have little influence on coronary resistance.[18,19] Myocardial ischemia has been shown to increase receptor density in the coronary arteries and cause a reflex increase in sympathetic activity mediated by α_2-adrenergic mechanisms.[18,20] This cascade may further increase coronary vasoconstriction and reduce flow.

Postsynaptic α_1-adrenergic receptors are not dependent upon extracellular Ca^{2+} to constrict vessels, whereas the α_2-adrenergic constrictor response is highly dependent upon extracellular influx and exquisitely sensitive to calcium channel inhibitors.[21] This has important implications in the management of not only myocardial ischemia but ischemic dysrhythmias as well.

Recent studies have demonstrated the presence of postsynaptic, myocardial α_1-adrenergic receptors, which exert a facilitatory, positive inotropic effect on the myocardium (Table 31–1). Their contribution to malignant

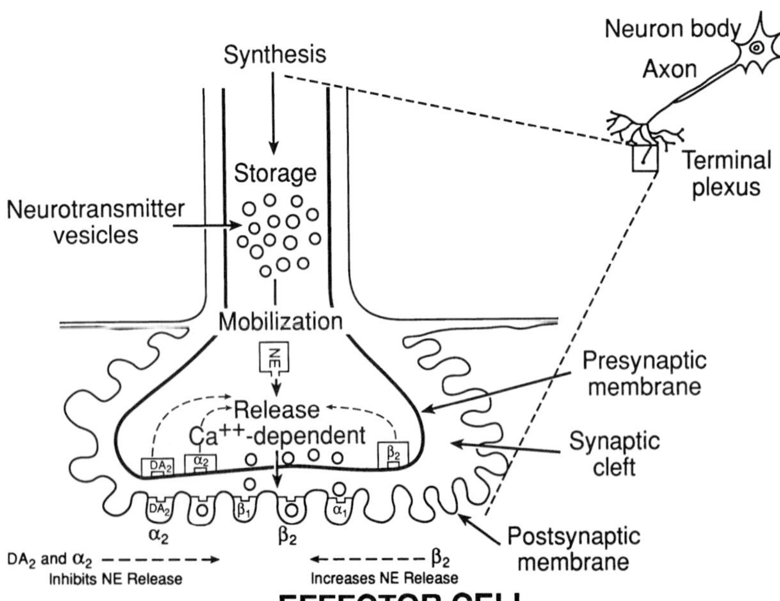

FIGURE 31–2. The anatomic loci of the adrenergic receptors on the sympathetic neuroeffector junction are demonstrated. Presynaptic DA_2 and α_2-adrenergic receptor agonists serve as negative feedback to the release of norepinephrine. Stimulation of these receptors inhibits norepinephrine release. Stimulation of presynaptic β_2-adrenergic receptors enhances norepinephrine release.

reperfusion dysrhythmogenesis has also been recognized.[22] Myocardial postsynaptic α_1-adrenergic receptors mediate as much as 30 to 50% of the basal inotropic tone of the normal heart.[23] These receptors play a more prominent inotropic role in the failing heart by serving as reserve to the normally predominant β_1-adrenergic receptors.[19,20] There is no down-regulation of α_1-adrenergic receptors in heart failure like that which occurs in β_1-adrenergic receptors.[24] The relative increase in myocardial α_1-adrenergic receptors may contribute to the positive inotropism seen during ischemia as well as to the malignant dysrhythmias that occur with reperfusion. The intracellular mobilization of cytosolic Ca^{2+} by the activated α_1-adrenergic myocardial receptors during ischemia appears to contribute to these dysrhythmias.[20] Drugs possessing potent α_1-adrenergic antagonism such as prazosin and phentolamine have been shown to possess significant antidysrhythmic activity, although they are of limited usefulness because of their effects on the peripheral vasculature (i.e., they lead to hypotension).[22] Enhanced α_1-adrenergic activity with myocardial ischemia may explain why the antidysrhythmic benefits of β-adrenergic antagonism in patients with myocardial infarction (MI) are far from certain.

Myocardial β-adrenergic receptors were originally classified as β_1-adrenergic receptors. Those in the vascular and bronchial smooth muscle were classified as the β_2-adrenergic subtype. However, radioligand studies have confirmed the coexistence of β_1- and β_2-adrenergic receptors in the myocardium and coronary arteries.[25] Both β_1- and β_2-adrenergic receptors are functionally coupled to the enzyme, adenylate cyclase, suggesting a similar involvement in the regulation of inotropism, chronotropism, and dysrhythmogenesis.

The β_2-adrenergic receptors have the same distribution as β_1-adrenergic receptors, but are found at both presynaptic and postsynaptic sites throughout the myocardium and coronary arteries. Activation of the presynaptic β_2-adrenergic receptor accelerates the release of NE into the synaptic cleft, whereas blockade inhibits NE release. Increased NE release increases inotropism via β_1-adrenergic agonism but also dilates the coronary and vascular smooth muscle. This action is diametrically opposed to those of the presynaptic α_2-adrenergic receptors (Table 31–1). The number of presynaptic β_2-adrenergic receptors is approximately 20 to 30% of the β-adrenergic receptors in the ventricular myocardium and up to 40% of those in the atrium. Postsynaptic β_2-adrenergic receptors, like the postsynaptic α_2-adrenergic receptors are considered noninnervated, extrasynaptic, hormonal receptors responding primarily to circulating EPI.

Selective β_1-adrenergic blockers are less effective in suppressing EPI-induced tachycardia than the nonselective β-adrenergic antagonist propranolol. Increased catecholamine levels associated with myocardial ischemia and heart failure lead to down-regulation of β_1-adrenergic receptor density with a relative sparing of the β_2-adrenergic subtype and an increase of the α_1-adrenergic subtype.[12,26,27] The β_2-adrenergic receptors increasingly mediate the inotropic, chronotropic, and conduction responses to catecholamines during heart failure and are facilitated by the α_1-adrenergic receptor.

Normal Electrophysiology of the Heart

There are two types of mycardial cells: (1) the pacemakers, which possess automaticity; and (2) the nonautomatic myocytes of the atria and ventricles. Depolarization and contraction of the latter do not normally occur without a stimulus. The automaticity of the pacemaker cells of the SA node is normally the source of the electrical impulse that depolarizes the remainder of the myocardium in a sequential manner. The SA node depolarizes more rapidly than the other pacemakers and controls the overall rate by overdrive suppression of other potential pacemakers. Cardiac impulses are rapidly conducted along the internodal tracts, resulting in the depolarization of the atria and the AV node.

The AV node also has automaticity, but at a slower intrinic rate than the SA node. It decreases the conduction velocity of the advancing wave of depolarization to ensure the delay of ventricular systole until after the atria have contracted. This results in the "atrial kick," which enhances presystolic ventricular filling, accounting for 25% of the normal stroke volume and up to 40% of the left ventricular end-diastolic volume in the presence of a hypertrophied ventricle such as is seen with aortic stenosis.[27] The impulse is transferred to the ventricular muscle via the Purkinje fibers.

Conductive tissue and contractile fibers possess distinctive action potentials: (1) slow-response action potential and (2) fast-response action potential (Fig. 31–3). The slow-response action potential is seen in the pacemakers and can be found throughout the conduction system of the heart. Fast-response action potentials are found in the working cardiac fibers of the atria and ventricles. However, the fast response action potential fibers can acquire pacemaker capability under abnormal conditions.

Fast-Response Action Potentials

A fast-response fiber at rest demonstrates a resting membrane electrical potential of approximately −90 mV inside the cell compared to the outside of the cell membrane (Fig. 31–3). With depolarization, a reversal of the membrane potential occurs to a value of around +20 mV. The fast-response action potential is divided into phases with numerical identification. Phase 0 is the stage of rapid depolarization followed by phases 1, 2, and 3, which represent stages of repolarization. It is important to emphasize that the phase 4 resting potential of the fibers possessing the fast-response action potentials does not change unless stimulated by a depolarizing current. The various phases of the fast action potential are due to changes in cell membrane permeability to the ions sodium, potassium, calcium, and magnesium (Fig. 31–4) (see Chapter 5).

Excitation of the membrane decreases the resting potential to a less negative level. When a specific level, the threshold potential, is reached, the membrane permeability to Na^+ increases more than 100-fold and depolar-

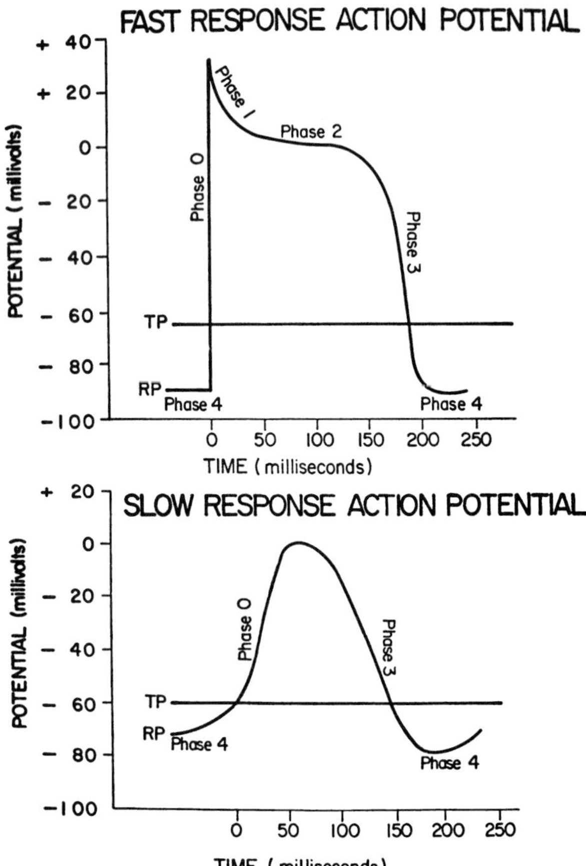

FIGURE **31–3.** The two main types of cardiac action potentials are demonstrated. The working muscles of the atria and ventricles possess the fast action potential. The slow action potential is characteristic of pacemakers. RP, resting membrane potential; TP, threshold potential.

ization (phase 0) of the fast-response potential occurs. Phase 0 is caused by a brief, explosive inward current of Na^+ through an ion-selective "fast" channel. Phase 0 corresponds to the QRS of the conventional ECG (Fig. 31–5). Although extracellular Na^+ has little influence on the resting membrane potential, it does determine the amplitude of the fast action potential. Another event is also initiated during this same instant. When the fast membrane voltage approaches −40 mV during phase 0, another inward current, the slow current, also develops. The rate of activation and inactivation of the slow inward current is several orders of magnitude slower than that of the fast Na^+ current. The slow inward current accounts for the plateau (phase 2) of the fast-response action potential (Fig. 31–4). The major ion traversing the membrane during the slow current is Ca^{2+}, although Na^+ also plays a small role. The membrane channels carrying the slow inward current are 100 times more selective for Ca^{2+} than for Na^+ or K^+. Therefore, the term "slow channels" and "Ca^{2+}" channels are often used interchangeably.

The phase 1 overshoot and decrease of voltage into phase 2 represents closing of the Na^+ channels. Phase 2, or the slow channel plateau, is important because it represents the inward flow of Ca^{2+}, making Ca^{2+} available for the intricate coupling of excitation with contraction. The rise in intracellular Ca^{2+} during phase 2 correlates with the development of a subsequent contraction. The QT interval on the ECG reflects extracellular Ca^{2+} status, with hypercalcemia being manifest as short QT intervals and hypocalcemia as long QT intervals.

Repolarization occurs with the efflux of K^+ from the cell and the return of the cell to its resting membrane potential. Repolarization of the ventricles is represented by the T wave on the ECG. The resting potential is determined chiefly by the concentration gradient of K^+ across the membrane and its relative permeability to other ions.[5] The permeability of the membrane to K^+ allows K^+ to move out of the cell, creating the imbalance of ions that determines the negativity of the resting potential. The negativity, or measure potential, varies inversely with the extracellular concentration of K^+.

The determinants of conduction velocity are (1) threshold voltage of the action potential, (2) rate of rise of the action potential (phase 0), and (3) the amplitude of the action potential.[28] The level of the resting membrane potential is an important determinant of conduction velocity in all myocytes. In general, the less negative the resting membrane potential, as seen in the pacemakers, the slower the velocity of impulse propagation regardless of the reason for the reduction of threshold level.[5] The stability and level of the resting membrane potential (phase 4) is maintained by the Na^+/K^+ pump, which involves active transport of Na^+ and K^+ against gradients to maintain this stability. Maintenance of this gradient at rest is an active process requiring oxidative energy metabolism (adenosine triphosphate [ATP]).

Excitability refers to the ability of a tissue to depolarize (i.e., open Na^+ gates). The refractory period is the phase of the action potential during which the cell cannot generate an action potential (i.e., Na^+ gates are closed). The potential excitability of a fast-response cardiac fiber is maximum at rest before depolarization occurs. Once depolarized, the membrane is absolutely refractory (AR) to further stimuli until repolarization returns to threshold (Fig. 31–5). This time is the effective refractory period (ERP). As threshold is reached during repolarization, the myocardium becomes relatively less refractory but capable of depolarizing with a greater than normal stimulus. This is known as the relative refractory period. During the latter stages of the relative refractory period, a vulnerable period occurs in which a less than normal stimulus, or repetitive stimuli, may cause another depolarization. This vulnerable period, though brief, often corresponds to, but is not limited to, the downstroke of the T wave (Fig. 31–5). The vulnerable period is the source of the dangerous electrocardiographic R on T phenomenon, where a premature depolarization may stimulate a re-entrant dysrhythmia such as ventricular fibrillation (VF) or sustained ventricular tachycardia (VT).

Slow-Response Action Potentials

There are two fundamental differences between the slow- and fast-response action potentials (Fig. 31–3).

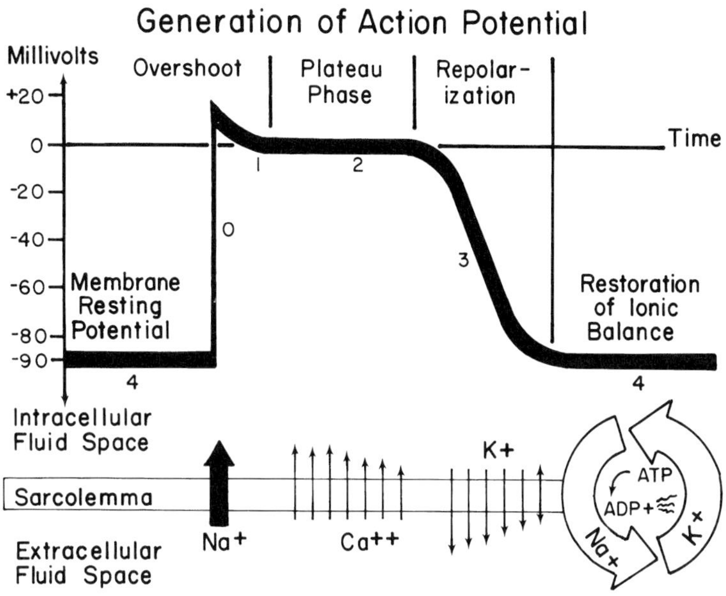

Generation of Action Potential

Millivolts
Overshoot
Plateau Phase
Repolar- ization
+20
0
-20
-40
-60
-80
-90
Time
1
2
0
3
Membrane Resting Potential
Restoration of Ionic Balance
4
4
Intracellular Fluid Space
Sarcolemma
Extracellular Fluid Space
Na+
Ca++
K+
ATP
ADP+
Na+
K+

FIGURE **31–4.** The generation of the fast action potential is a timed, ionic membrane event involving Na^+, K^+, Ca^{2+}, and Mg^{2+}. Stabilization of the resting membrane potential is energy dependent.

Pacemaker cells do not maintain a steady phase 4 resting potential and the spike of the fast or Na^+ channel is either absent or inoperative. The phase 4 membrane potential slowly decreases toward threshold, excitation results, and an action potential is initiated. Spontaneous depolarization (automaticity) of the slow action potential results from a steady decline of K^+ conductance, while actual depolarization results from the influx of Ca^{2+} through slow channels. These events closely resemble those that occur during phase 2 of the fast action potential. Pacemaker cells are, therefore, dependent upon Ca^+ influx through the slow or Ca^{2+} channels for automaticity, whereas working cardiac muscle is Na^+ dependent.

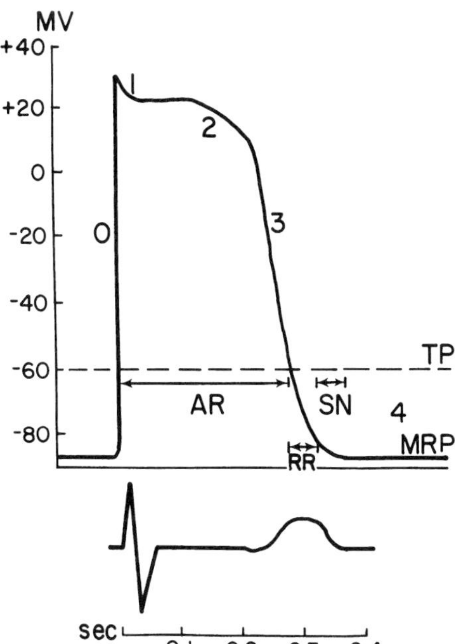

FIGURE **31–5.** Stages of cardiac excitability correlated to the ECG. AR, absolute or effective refractory period (ERP); RR, relative refractory period; SN, supernormal period; RMP, resting membrane potential; TP, threshold potential.

The slow action potentials differ from the fast action potential fibers in several other ways. The resting potential is closer to threshold with values of −50 to −65 mV as compared to −90 mV for the fast action cells (Fig. 31–3). The action potential rises more slowly and phase 2 is poorly developed, but there is still a plateau. The reduced threshold of the pacemaker cells makes them poor impulse conductors with conduction velocities of only 0.02 and 0.1 m/sec as compared to 1 to 4 m/sec for ventricular fibers. The rate of spontaneous phase 4 depolarization and conduction velocity decreases from the SA node to the AV node and into the ventricle. This decremental inefficiency of conduction is, in large part, responsible for the orderly sequence of atrial to ventricular contraction (Fig. 31–1). The delay from the SA node to the AV node results in the PR interval on the ECG. Ventricular conduction velocity determines the width of the QRS complex.

The Genesis of Dysrhythmias

Cardiac dysrhythmias are the consequence of disturbances in impulse formation (automaticity), impulse conduction (dromotropism), or both. The previous review of the mechanisms of the normal generation of the cardiac electrical impulse and its subsequent conduction suggest several mechanisms by which departure from the normal rhythm may occur. However, most dysrhythmias are ultimately attributed to a loss of membrane potential. That is, the maximum diastolic potential becomes less negative. As a result, it is very difficult to separate clinical dysrhythmias of automaticity from those of conduction. Some dysrhythmias may be initiated by one mechanism and sustained by another. A drug, normally effective in suppressing abnormal automaticity, may not terminate a conductive re-entry tachydysrhythmia, although it was initiated by a focus of abnormal automaticity.[28]

The term "proarrhythmia" is used to describe the phenomenon when any new or worsened dysrhythmia develops following the administration of an antidysrhythmic drug. The proarrhythmic action of antidysrhythmic agents was recognized in the early 1980s, with an incidence of 15 to 20% with some agents.[28] Four forms of proarrhythmias are recognized as a drug effect. These are (1) new or incessant ventricular tachycardia, (2) torsades de pointes, (3) new ventricular fibrillation, and (4) increased incidence of sudden death during treatment. The most perplexing of these is torsades de pointes. It should be distinguished from polymorphous ventricular tachycardia, which is more commonly seen in patients with ischemic disease or myocardiopathy. Torsades de pointes is literally a "twisting of the points" that appears as a rotation of the QRS axis around an isoelectric baseline (Fig. 31–6). This phenomenon is usually the result of iatrogenic disease and has the following features: (1) it is preceded by a marked prolongation of the QT interval and (2) associated with one or more of the following: the administration of antidysrhythmic drugs, hypokalemia, hypomagnesemia, bradycardia, and congenital long QT interval (i.e., Romano-Ward or Jervell-Lange-Nielsen syndrome); (3) it is initiated by ventricular ectopic beats (automaticity); (4) it is usually nonlethal and self-terminating; and (5) it responds to increasing heart rate and correction of electrolyte imbalances. Torsades de pointes has been reported with almost all antidysrhythmic drugs, but most frequently with quinidine and other agents of class IA and III (see "Antidysrhythmic drugs," later).

Disorders of Impulse Formation—Automaticity

Abnormal automaticity is a common source of intraoperative dysrhythmias. Abnormal automaticity may arise from sources that normally have pacemaker activity or from ectopic sites in the myocardium that normally do not have automaticity, but which have developed as a result of myocardial disease or damage. The simplest dysrhythmias of automaticity are those resulting from excessive speeding or slowing of normal pacemaker activity. The SA node normally blocks latent pacemaker activity by its faster rate of impulse formation (overdrive suppression). However, disease states can substantially alter the normal ionic resting potential of cells in the pacemakers or anywhere in the conduction system, which has latent pacemaker activity. These cells may increase their rate of automaticity and become the dominant pacemaker, overdriving the SA node. Ischemic Purkinje fibers are known to develop slow action potentials similar to those seen in the SA or AV nodes and initiate a higher rate of pacing to become the dominant pacemaker.

Abnormal automaticity may also come from myocytes that do not ordinarily possess automaticity. Under abnormal circumstances, nonautomatic fast-response myocardial fibers can be converted into slow-response pacemaker cells with their characteristics of automaticity and delayed conduction (Fig. 31–7). Hyperkalemia, myocardial stretch, catecholamines, hypoxemia, localized ischemia, and excessive concentrations of local anesthetics are all capable of inactivating the fast Na^+ channels or interfering with the energy-dependent membrane stability (Fig. 31–4). With the loss of the membrane stability, the membrane potential changes from the normal −90 mV to the range of −65 to −60 mV.[29] The action po-

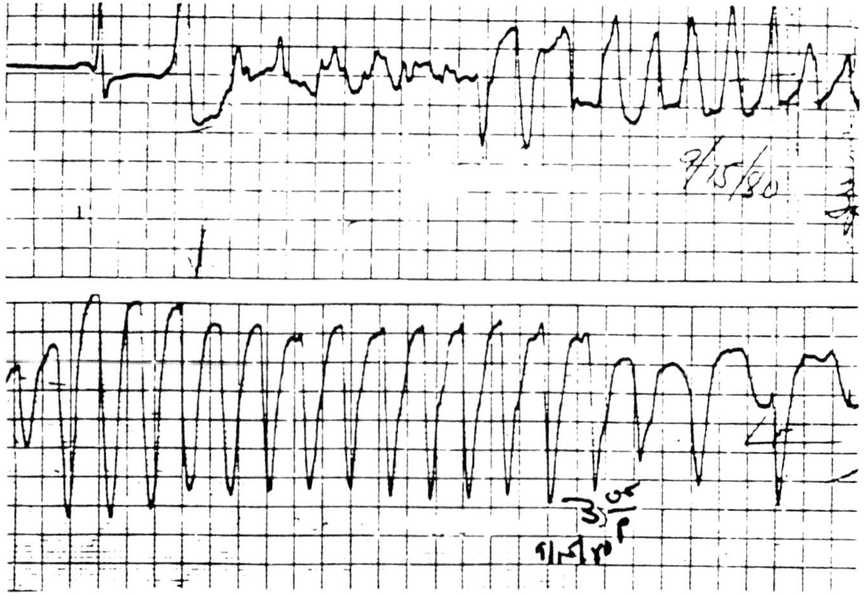

FIGURE 31–6. "Torsades de pointes" or "turning of the points" which can be seen following therapy with oral quinidine, diuretics, and hypokalemia.

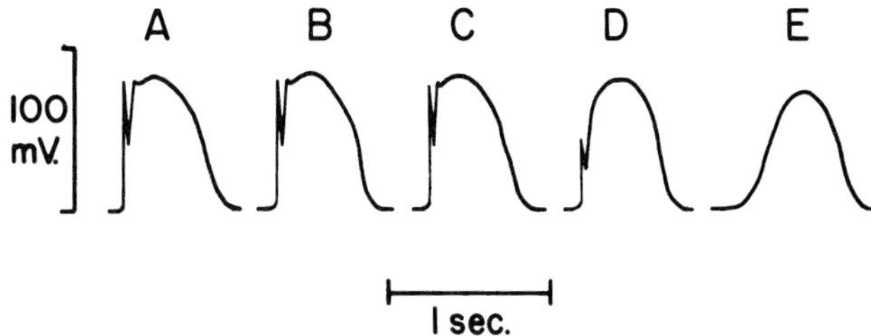

FIGURE **31–7.** Cardiac fibers with fast action potentials can be converted into cells with latent pacemaker activity by hypoxemia, stretch, hyperkalemia, and catecholamines. This conversion is thought to be an important source of dysrhythmia automaticity and delayed conduction with re-entry. Conversion is demonstrated here by activation of the Na^+ channels with tetrodotoxin. (From Berne RM, Levy MN: Control of the heart. In Berne RM, Levy MN [eds]: Cardiovascular Physiology. St Louis, CV Mosby Co, 1977, p 155, with permission.)

tentials resemble those of slow-response cells, but have "depressed fast responses," since the fast Na^+ channel is still marginally operative. Reduction of the resting potential from −90 to −60 mV also reduces the maximal rate of increase of phase 0 and reduces conduction velocity through that area as well.[30] If the membrane potential is depressed further to the range of −50 mV, the Na^+ channels are totally inactivated.[31,32] This phenomenon has been most extensively studied in regards to the effects of ischemia and infarction on the electrophysiology of the Purkinje system and ventricular muscle. Foci of enhanced ventricular automaticity can account for isolated premature ventricular contractions (PVCs), salvos of multifocal PVCs, or even runs of ventricular tachycardias.[33,34] However, these dysrhythmias of automaticity may not be distinguishable on the ECG from those produced by the more dangerous re-entry dysrhythmias (see "Re-entry," later).

Parasystole is another mechanism by which automaticity generates a dysrhythmia. Parasystole is the simultaneous existence of two independent pacemaker sites, which then compete to activate the myocardium. Parasystole also results in altered conductivity, but abnormal automaticity creates the abnormal parasystolic impulse. The second pacemaker is protected from overdrive suppression by the normal SA pacer by a "protection" block produced by the refractory period of the second pacer. This is thought to be the mechanism by which ventricular bigeminy or trigeminy occurs, depending upon the rate of discharge of the parasystolic site.[35]

Conterato suggests that the concept of triggered activity should be added to impulse formation and re-entry as a third source of dysrhythmias of automaticity.[34] Triggered activity includes the concepts of afterpotentials, oscillation, and incomplete repolarization.[36,37] Technically, these mechanisms are not true disorders of automaticity. True automaticity is the property of initiating a spontaneous impulse without need for prior stimulus. It should be self-generating. Most of these mechanisms require some degree of previous stimulus or afterdepolarizations to produce a source of automaticity.[38] Oscillation refers to multiple afterpotentials leading to repetitive afterdepolarizations. These complicated mechanisms usually occur in cells that are not ordinarily automatic. They are most often associated with events such as digitalis intoxication, hypercalcemia, Na^+-Ca^{2+} exchange, and catecholamine excess. These mechanisms are of more than academic interest because triggered automaticity closely resembles re-entrant dysrhythmias. However, the distinction can be difficult or impossible to make in the clinical setting.[28]

Disorders of Impulse Conduction: Re-entry

A delay or block of impulse conduction can result in either brady- or tachydysrhythmias. Disorders of impulse conduction can be further classified into either an anatomic block or a re-entry phenomenon. The anatomic blocks are more often responsible for bradydysrhythmias and are readily diagnosed by the ECG as first-, second-, or third-degree (complete) block. Escape or even ectopic beats may be seen with anatomic blocks when latent pacemakers distal to the block assume the next fastest rate of automaticity. In contrast to the anatomic block, the re-entry phenomenon is more often responsible for the majority of serious tachydysrhythmias, including ventricular tachycardia and fibrillation. The type of conduction delays causing re-entry are not the obvious major conduction blocks detectable by ECG, but rather electrically localized areas in which the conduction of a normal wavefront is altered.

A recycled cardiac impulse may errantly re-enter areas of adjacent normal repolarized myocardium because of localized conduction delays through the syncytium of myocardial fibers. The impulse re-enters and re-excites fibers through which it had previously passed[39] (Fig. 31–8). Re-entry can be ordered or random. Re-entrant circuits that follow definite anatomic conduction pathways are called ordered re-entry. These dysrhythmias are found originating anywhere within the conduction system and give rise to many of the supraventricular tachycardias such as Wolff-Parkinson-White (WPW) syndrome. Random re-entry is the result of fragmented impulses that are randomly delayed through islands of poorly conductive atrial or ventricular tissue without a specific anatomic pattern of distribution.[40] This form of re-entry is responsible for most atrial and ventricular fibrillation.

Two conditions must be met before re-entry can occur: (1) slowing of conduction and (2) a unidirectional block. The causes of the localized delay of conduction can be any mechanism that reduces the resting membrane potential (less negative). This is true for both types of cells (slow- or fast-response action potentials). Whenever the resting potential becomes less negative (i.e., −90 to −60 mV), the action potential rises more slowly and conduction velocity decreases. A unidirectional block means that at some point in the myocardial syncytium, the impulse is able to pass in one direction, but not in the other (Fig. 31–9). In the absence of unidirectional block, two wavefronts meeting head on in the syncytium, cancel out, or proceed. Likewise, a complete block in any, or all, of the branches of localized conduction also negates unidirectional block. However, the presence of a unidi-

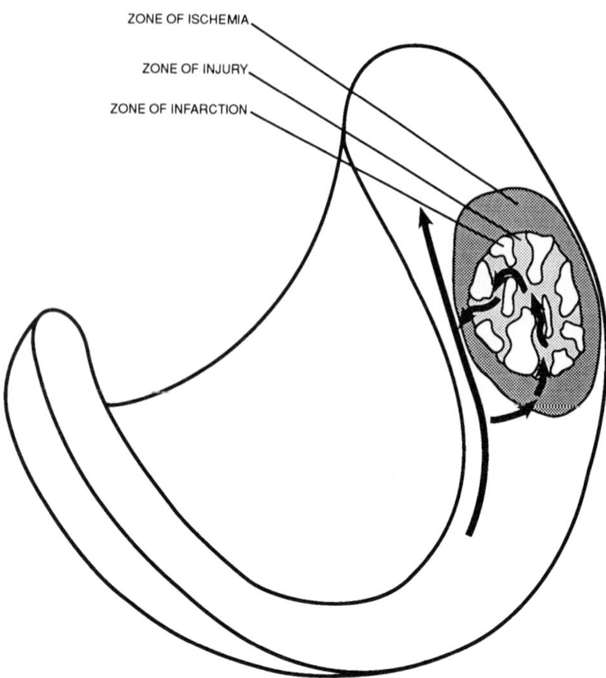

FIGURE **31–8.** A cardiac impulse may errantly re-enter areas of adjacent repolarized myocardium because of delayed localized conduction through the syncytium of myocardial fibers. The example here is that of a localized area of ischemia by which the impulse re-enters and re-excites fibers through which it had previously passed.

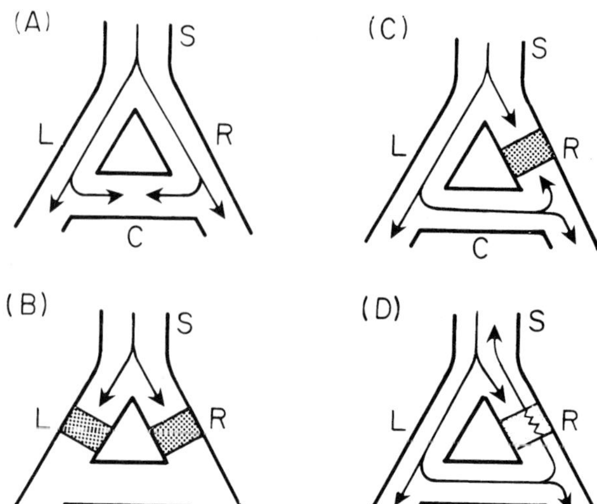

FIGURE **31–9.** Re-entry is explained by the development of a unidirectional block. *A*, Normal wavefronts traveling down a syncytium of fibers (S) continue down the left (L) and right (R) branches canceling each other out in the connecting bundle (C). *B* and *C*, Wavefronts are also canceled with the development of a complete block of one or both branches. A unidirectional block allows re-entry of a wavefront previously passed. (Redrawn from Berne RM, Levy MN: Control of the heart. In Berne RM, Levy MN [eds]: Cardiovascular Physiology. St Louis, CV Mosby Co, 1977, p 155, with permission.)

rectional slowing of conduction delays the propagated impulse long enough to allow the surrounding normal tissue to repolarize. An impulse entering an area of reduced conduction allows that wavefront, which having previously passed, to doubleback and re-enter the circuit to depolarize cells in a susceptible state of repolarization (Fig. 31–8). A minicircuit is established by which an atrial or ventricular tachydysrhythmia can be established and remain self-perpetuating. If this loop further fragments into enough random re-entry sites and muscle mass, fibrillation results. A single appropriately timed impulse can initiate fibrillation if that re-entrant wave lands on ventricular muscle in a vulnerable period of recovery and excitability.[41]

The phenomenon of re-entry has been most extensively studied in regards to the effects of ischemia and infarction on the electrical activity of the Purkinje system and ventricular muscle. These complex events in an island of ischemic ventricular muscle can be summarized as follows.[34,42] Acutely ischemic cardiac cells are unable to maintain their normal intracellular ion concentrations because of impairment of the ATPase pump. K^+ leaks out of the cell, and Na^+ accumulates within the cell. Hyperkalemia or Na^+ channel blockade would produce the same results. This reduces the stable resting membrane fast action potential from −90 mV toward a less negative potential (Fig. 31–7). A reduction of potential from −90 to −60 mV profoundly impairs, or even inactivates, the fast-response Na^+ channel current. The upstroke of depolarization is reduced in both velocity and amplitude accompanied by a reduced conduction velocity. Thus, under the conditions of ischemia, the nonautomatic fast response myocardial fibers can be converted into slow-response action potentials with all their characteristics of automaticity and delayed conduction. With this background, one can appreciate that dysrhythmias are the consequence of disturbances in impulse formation, conduction, or both.

Sources of Intraoperative Dysrhythmias

The sources of intraoperative dysrhythmias are not always clear. The etiology of dysrhythmias in patients undergoing cardiac, thoracic, or vascular surgery is similar to that in patients undergoing other surgical procedures. Some dysrhythmias are hazardous regardless of the clinical setting, whereas others are hazardous because of the clinical setting[43–47] (Fig. 31–10).

Halogenated Anesthetic Agents

The dysrhythmic and antidysrhythmic effects of halogenated volatile anesthetics have been well described.[48] Halothane is the agent most often implicated in producing dysrhythmias, especially in the presence of hypoxemia or hypercarbia. The effects of the halogenated agents on calcium channel activity have been clearly demonstrated, although no clear connection with specific dysrhythmias has been made.[39,49–51]

The most common halothane-induced dysrhythmias are: (1) SA or AV nodal bradycardias with variable degrees of block and (2) increased ventricular ectopic de-

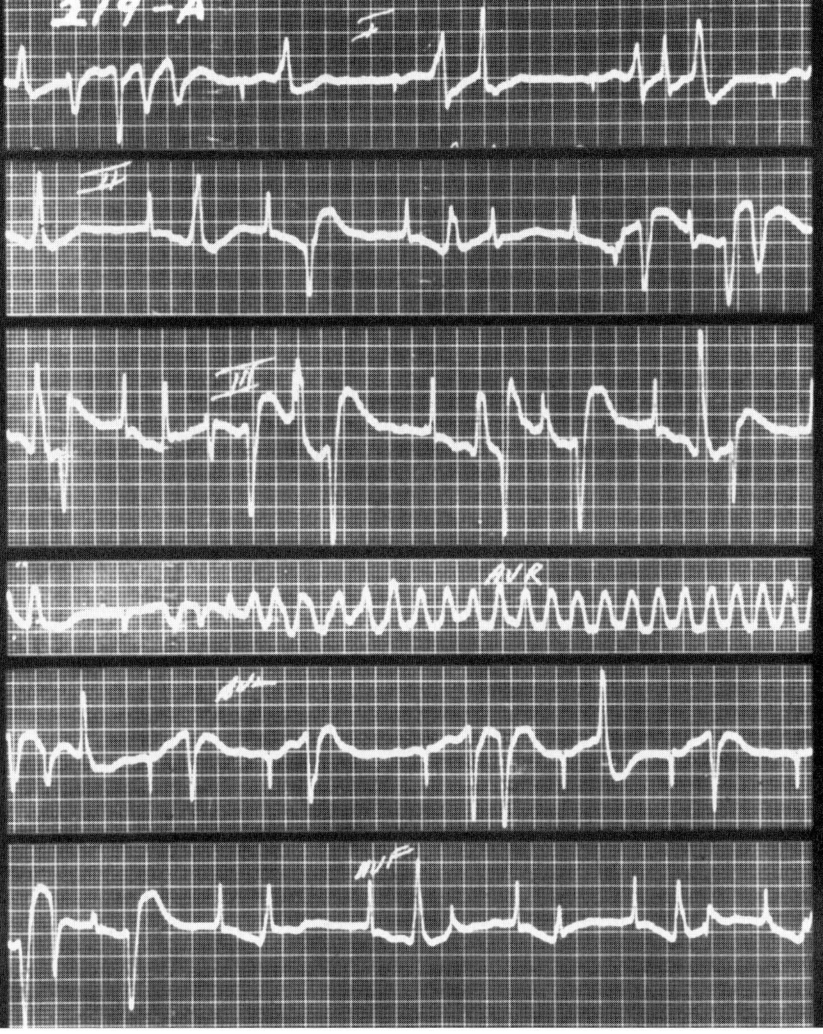

FIGURE **31–10.** Variables the anesthesiologist must consider in diagnosing and treating dysrhythmias are often quite different from those encountered by the cardiologist. This is a strip of dysrhythmias that developed during the manipulation of the cerebellopontine angle during neurosurgery. The dysrhythmias stopped upon cessation of manipulation. (Courtesy of Dr. John T. Martin.)

polarizations. Halothane decreases the rate and slope of phase 4 spontaneous depolarization in pacemaker cells accounting for decreased chronotropism.[52,53] Isoflurane also depresses phase 4 depolarization, but less so than halothane and is related to the fact that isoflurane has less effect on calcium influx than halothane.[55] Halothane also slows conduction through the AV node while equipotent concentrations of isoflurane do not. Halothane does not alter resting membrane potentials, but does decrease the threshold in pacemakers and the conduction system. This mechanism is, perhaps, the basis for the potentiating dysrhythmogenic effects of halothane with circulating catecholamines.[48] Epinephrine normally increases the rate of phase 4 depolarization in normal or ectopic pacemakers.

Both α_1- and β_1-adrenoceptors are also involved in the halothane-epinephrine dysrhythmia interaction. Maze and Smith demonstrated that both α_1- (prazocin) and β_1-adrenergic (metoprolol) blockade protected against catecholamine-induced dysrhythmias.[56,57] Dysrhythmia protection with α_1-adrenergic blockade was five times greater than with β_1-adrenergic blockade. Their study preceded the recent demonstration of the association of myocardial α_1-adrenoceptors and dysrhythmogenesis.[12,20,21] Kapur has also demonstrated that calcium channel blockade is equally effective as an antidysrhythmic agent in this circumstance.[58]

The potentiation of dysrhythmias of halogenated agents by catecholamines has been ascribed to a variety of mechanisms such as slowed conduction velocity, reduced refractory periods, reduced action potentials, and a disparity between refractory periods of the Purkinje fibers and ventricular muscle.[37] Taken in the context of electrophysiology, these mechanisms are probably all correct and related. The fact that most halogenated volatile anesthetics are slow channel depressants could also impart antidysrhythmic properties similar to the class IV antidysrhythmic agents: the calcium channel blockers. Both halothane and isoflurane have been reported to suppress reperfusion dysrhythmias.[48]

The incidence of catecholamine-induced dysrhythmias is greatest with halothane and least with enflurane.[59,60] Isoflurane holds an intermediate position, while dose-response curves have not yet been reported for sevoflurane or desflurane. Children seem to be more resistant to epinephrine-induced arrhythmias with halothane than adults.[61] However, the inhalation agents, particularly halothane, should be avoided when the need for a catecholamine infusion is anticipated for hemodynamic stability. The inhalation agents should also be used cautiously when infiltrating epinephrine with local anesthetic agents.[62] The subcutaneously injected dose of epinephrine necessary to produce ventricular cardiac dysrhythmias in 50% of patients anesthetized with a 1.25 minimum alveolar concentration (MAC) of a volatile agent was 2.1, 3.4, and 6.7 μg/kg during administration of halothane, enflurane, and isoflurane, respectively. The incidence of cardiac dysrhythmias was eliminated when this dose was halved.[59]

Other drugs that can produce dysrhythmias with halogenated agents are the methylxanthines such as aminophylline. These agents are phosphodiesterase inhibitors, which increase intracellular levels of cyclic adenosine monophosphate (cAMP), resulting in an adrenergic response. The specific phosphodiesterase III inhibitors, such as amrinone, have less effect on rate or rhythm and are less arrythmogenic. Dysrhythmias are the most common side effect with amrinone, but the incidence is only 3%. Increased catecholamine levels, combined with methylxanthines, may lead to synergistic dysrhythmic activity.[63] Methylxanthines such as aminophylline potentiate the halothane-epinephrine interaction, but not the interaction between isoflurane and epinephrine.[67]

Tricyclic antidepressants (TCA) can increase the risk of dysrhythmias because they block the reuptake of norepinephrine by the postganglionic sympathetic neurons.[8] However, recent studies have not confirmed this risk except with actual TCA overdose.[65,66] Death from TCA overdose is usually due to refractory ventricular dysrhythmias from a direct effect on the electrophysiologic function of the heart. TCAs also reduce the amount of epinephrine required to induce dysrhythmias with halothane. Edwards et al. have reported pancuronium-induced dysrhythmias in dogs pretreated with imipramine and anesthetized with halothane.[67]

The interaction of halothane with vagolytic drugs also produces significiant dysrhythmias. The cardiac conduction system has extensive parasympathetic innervation. Vagal stimulation of the pacemakers decreases the slope of phase 4 depolarization and increases the threshold potential (Fig. 31–11). Vagolytic drugs, such as atropine or pancuronium, decrease threshold and increase the slope and rate of phase 4 depolarization. If the more sensitive SA node is depressed by halothane, a junctional (nodal) tachycardia may be induced by these vagolytic agents.[68]

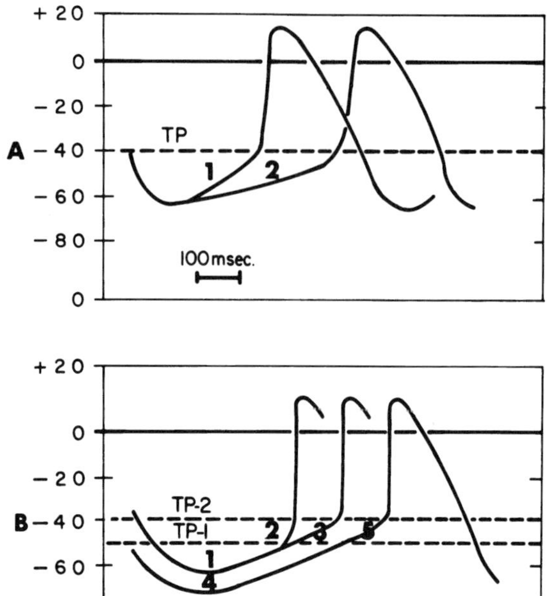

FIGURE **31–11.** *A*, Reduction in the slope of pacemaker potential from 1 to 2. β-Blockade could produce this reduction from the more steep slope of catecholamine stimulation. *B*, Concept of a decreased threshold (less negative) from TP-1 to TP-2. An increase in RMP (1 to 4) will also diminish frequency. (Redrawn from Berne RM, Levy MN: Control of the heart. In Berne RM, Levy MN [eds]: Cardiovascular Physiology. St Louis, CV Mosby Co, 1977, p 155, with permission.)

Local Anesthetics

Cocaine, like the TCAs, blocks the reuptake of norepinephrine and dopamine at neuronal synapses. This allows NE to accumulate producing vasoconstriction at the site. Overdose or systemic absorption can produce serious side effects such as hypertension, tachycardia, ventricular dysrhythmias, myocardial infarction, and death. Cocaine is detoxified by plasma cholinesterases. Patients with serious liver disease or cholinesterase deficiencies may be at increased risk for toxicity.[69]

The local anesthetic effects on cardiac electrophysiology have been extensively studied.[70] Most local anesthetics produce dose-related decreases in myocardial inotropism and conduction velocity. The exact effects and their severity vary according to the agent. Lidocaine, for example, does not change the resting membrane potential of cardiac muscle or conductive tissue, but does decrease the maximum rate of phase 4 depolarization in pacemakers. Lidocaine is believed to work by inhibiting conductance at the fast Na^+ channels. Bupivacaine has been found to markedly depress the rapid phase 4 depolarization and recovery compared to that seen with lidocaine.[69] Bupivacaine is approximately 70 times more potent than lidocaine in blocking cardiac conduction yet is only four times more potent in blocking nerve tissue than lidocaine.[71]

The local anesthetics may be capable of producing unidirectional block and re-entrant cardiac dysrhythmias. Lidocaine has no significant effect on slow inward Ca^{2+} currents in the region of the SA or AV node at the usual clinical doses employed. However, Josephson and Sperelakis[72] have reported that toxic doses of lidocaine, procaine, and tetracaine are capable of blocking slow channels in the myocardial sarcolemma. Blockade of spontaneous pacemaker activity resulting in sinus arrest and bradycardia with lidocaine had previously been reported in dogs.[73] Low concentrations of the Na^+ channel inhibitors are beneficial for prevention and treatment of dysrhythmias of automaticity,[74,75] but these actions appear to be biphasic. Higher concentrations of lidocaine and other local anesthetics may produce new dysrhythmias and cardiovascular collapse refractory to therapy related to the development of re-entry.[76,77] The administration of local anesthetics to patients who are already taking other Na^+ channel blockers for dysrhythmias may produce new dysrhythmias.[28,29]

Electrolyte Disturbances

Electrolyte disturbances are a frequent cause of rhythm disturbances. This is understandable when one considers the ionic events that occur during the action potential. There are no dysrhythmias directly associated with alterations of plasma Na^+. Lithium, used to treat psychiatric disorders, mimics Na^+ and can accumulate in the cardiac cell, causing the resting membrane potential to become less negative and closer to threshold. This can delay conduction velocity or increase automaticity.[78]

Hypo- and hyperkalemia are the electrolyte disturbances most often associated with dysrhythmias in the perioperative period.[79] However, this association may be more apparent than real. The ECG changes usually noted with hypo- or hyperkalemia are more related to the time over which the change occurs, and relative to the concentrations of other electrolytes responsible for cardiac action potentials (Na^+, Ca^{2+}, Mg^{2+}).[80] Chronic changes are less likely to provoke dysrhythmias than acute ones.[38,81,82]

The ratio of intracellular to extracellular K^+ determines most of the resting transmembrane potential. A decrease in extracellular K^+ increases the ratio of intracellular to extracellular K^+, producing a greater membrane electronegativity.[29] This causes hyperpolarization and increases the magnitude of the action potential. Hypokalemia also delays phase 3 repolarization time. Delayed repolarization allows a longer relative refractory period during which time the cells are vulnerable to repetitive stimulation. Thus, hypokalemia produces increased vulnerability to re-entrant dysrhythmias.[83]

The serious dysrhythmias most commonly associated with hypokalemia are atrial fibrillation and ventricular ectopy. Premature atrial contractions (PACs), paroxysmal atrial tachycardia (PAT), and other supraventricular tachycardias (SVT) have also been observed. Susceptibility to life-threatening ventricular tachycardia and/or fibrillation is a greater possibility in the presence of a hypoxic or failing myocardium.[84] Hypokalemia also enhances the toxicity of digitalis and increases the risk of ventricular arrhythmias.

Hypokalemia manifests on the ECG as delayed repolarization. This is seen as an apparent prolongation of the QT interval, flattening of the T wave and, with severe hypokalemia, the development of a U wave.[83] The increased QT interval is actually a fused QT-U interval. The ST segment may be depressed and ventricular ectopy may occur at serum levels of less than 3 mEq/L.

The conventional ECG is relatively insensitive to K^+ disturbances at the extreme ranges. The serious consequences of hypokalemia and hyperkalemia are not predictable on the basis of the serum levels of K^+ alone.[80] Electrolyte gradients determine the ECG and the relationships are relative. Hypokalemia is more likely to cause dysrhythmias if the serum Na^+ is normal or high. This same serum K^+ may pose no threat if the Na^+ is low. Likewise, hyperkalemia is potentiated by a low Na^+ but counteracted if high (Fig. 31–12). A serum K^+ of 4.5 mEq/L can produce the peaked T waves of hyperkalemia if a relative hyponatremia exists. Likewise, an isoelectric T wave can be seen with a combined hypokalemia and hyponatremia. Only 10% of those patients with a serum K^+ between 3.0 and 3.5 mEq/L will show typical changes of hypokalemia and in only 80% of those below 2.7 mEq/L will hypokalemia be evident.[29,84]

Despite the present therapeutic nihilism, the patient who is depleted of total body K^+ has multiple risks for morbidity during anesthesia and surgery.[81,82,85–88] Changes in acid-base balance affect heart rhythm through secondary changes in electrolytes and autonomic tone. Iatrogenic alkalosis, both metabolic and respiratory, has been implicated as an additional source of hypokalemia-induced dysrhythmias.[89,90] The proposed mechanism is an intracellular shift of K^+ associated with the alkalosis.[91] Regardless of the total body K^+ stores, it is primarily the extracellular moiety that is responsible for its electrophysiologic effects. Hypocarbic alkalosis has been noted to enhance the onset of supraventricular dysrhythmias, which are resistant to therapy, particularly in the presence of digitalis and previous diuretic therapy. Reducing ventilation may be effective in converting the dysrhythmias by resulting in an increase in serum K^+.[90]

Acute hypokalemia was once a frequent accompaniment of cardiopulmonary bypass resulting from hemodilution, diuresis, the alkalosis of lactate and citrate metabolism, catecholamines, and glucose-insulin relationships.[37] However, hyperkalemia is now more fre-

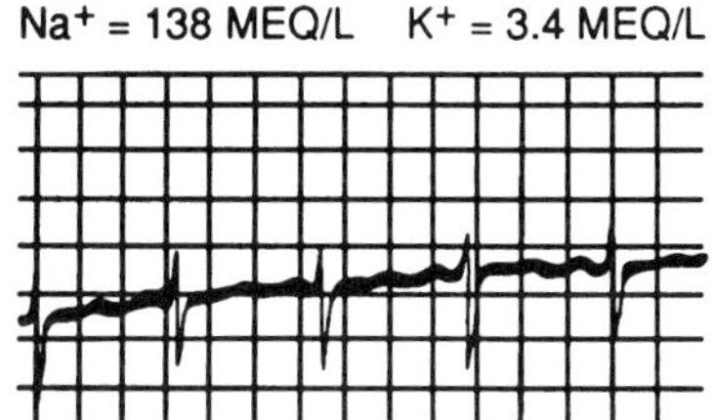

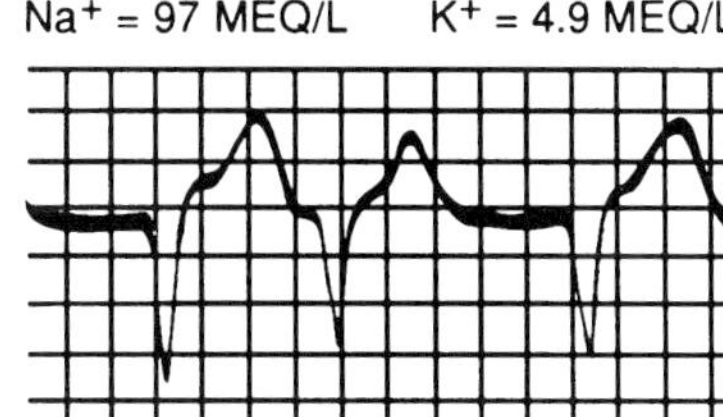

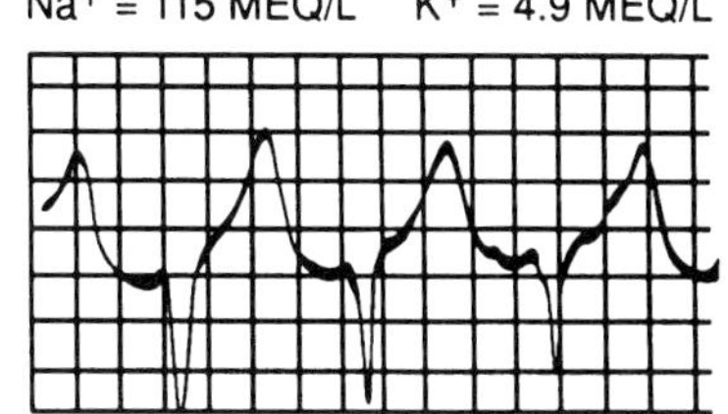

FIGURE **31–12.** This ECG demonstrates a relative hyperkalemia. The peaked T wave, characteristic of hyperkalemia, is present despite normal K^+. The patient is hyperkalemic relative to the serum Na^+ concentration. (From Ray CT: Water and electrolyte balance. In Sodeman WA, Sodeman WA Jr [eds]: Pathophysiologic Physiology. Philadelphia, WB Saunders Co, 1967, p 109, with permission.)

quent because of the hyperkalemic solutions used for cardioplegia. Other sources of hyperkalemia include the rapid administration of stored blood and limb or organ reperfusion.

Hyperkalemia produces the mirror image on the membrane potential as that of hypokalemia. The resting membrane potential is increased toward threshold, increasing slow channel automaticity. Increasing K^+ above 6 mEq/L increases K^+ permeability and repolarization is enhanced. The ST segment is shortened and the T wave of repolarization is peaked. Progressive widening of the QRS occurs with increasing hyperkalemia, which reflects slowing of conduction. Conduction blocks are common and ventricular asystole or fibrillation can occur. Fibrillation is possible due to delayed conduction and re-entry in the presence of repetitive stimuli as is common with the infusion of catecholamines.

Calcium and Magnesium

Disturbances of Ca^{2+} metabolism and dysrhythmias are well recognized but less common than those associated with K^+ disturbances.[37] Additionally, calcium disturbances are probably not as important in producing serious dysrhythmias except with large, acute changes. Increased availability of Ca^{2+} shortens phase 2 repolarization of slow channels resulting in a shortened QT interval. The rapid influx of extracellular Ca^{2+} does not appear to activate the contractile proteins. Instead, the influx of extracellular Ca^{2+} leads to the release of Ca^{2+} from the sarcoplasmic reticulum, which then binds to the muscle contractile proteins. Most of the myocardial energy is consumed in relaxing the heart, bringing the intracellular calcium concentration down from 10^{-5} to 10^{-7} mol via the ionic pumps. An ischemic heart that is in short energy supply is unable to power this sarcoplasmic pump. Extremely high intracellular hypercalcemia occurs and the heart stops in systole (stone heart).[86,93] The rigored heart was a common event in the early days of cardiac surgery when ischemic arrest was used to produce a quiescent heart.

Iatrogenic hypercalcemia is of no benefit to the patient immediately following cardiopulmonary bypass. Ca^{2+} should be given carefully in this situation and then only when the heart is not in oxygen debt.[8,94] The availability of the rapid measurement of serum ionized calcium allows the anesthesiologist to correct serum calcium when indicated. Alterations in the acid-base status such as overventilation with hypocapnia and an increased pH alters the protein binding of calcium and lowers the serum ionized calcium.

Dysrhythmias from hypocalcemia are usually due to conduction blocks and re-entrant ventricular fibrillation.[86] The ECG abnormality most often noted with hypocalcemia is a prolonged QT interval resulting from delayed phase 2 slow channel repolarization. This can be distinguished from the prolonged QT-U interval of hypokalemia by the absence of a U wave.

Recently, attention has been focused on the dysrhythmic potential of hypomagnesemia. Hypomagnesemia is a frequent occurrence in patients following cardiopulmonary bypass and may also occur with the use of diuretics, aminoglycoside antibiotics and chronic malnutrition. Recent attention has focused on the importance of normal magnesium homeostatis, and hypomagnesemia has been implicated in the genesis of serious ventricular dysrhythmias.[95,96] England[97] reported that 2 gm of Mg^{2+} over 30 minutes decreased the frequency of supraventricular and ventricular dysrhythmias following cardiopulmonary bypass.

The ECG manifestations of hypomagnesemia are nonspecific. The ECG pattern of hypocalcemia is exaggerated by low Mg^{2+} and corrected by hypermagnesemia.[98] The ECG pattern of hypomagnesemia alone is similar to that of hyperkalemia with tall, peaked T waves and a normal QT interval. Prolonged PR interval, widened QRS, and low T waves appear later.[99,100]

Hypermagnesemia is usually an iatrogenic problem. The effects of hypermagnesemia include a curare-like effect and asystole at serum levels of 25 mEq/L. However, muscle weakness and respiratory arrest occur at much lower levels. AV and intraventricular conduction blocks may be seen at Mg^{2+} levels as low as 5 mEq/L.[100] The neuromuscular effects of Mg^{2+} are related to its antagonistic effects of the inward movement of Ca^{2+} through the presynaptic membrane following axonal depolarization. This inward movement of Ca^{2+} is required for the release of acetylcholine and subsequent muscle contraction.

Autonomic Disturbances

Pacemakers are influenced by the relative tone of the autonomic nervous system, which alters the rate of spontaneous discharge. Heart rate can be altered by changing the slope of phase 4 depolarization, by changing the threshold potential, or by changing the resting potential (Fig. 31–11). Catecholamines cause a sinus tachycardia principally by increasing the slope of phase 4 in SA pacemaker cells. Vagal activity and the release of acetylcholine diminish heart rate by depressing the phase 4 slope and by increasing the resting potential. Acetylcholine (ACh) suppresses automaticity in the SA node by increasing K^+ conductance. This also reduces the velocity of conduction, setting up conditions necessary for reentrant dysrhythmias. Vagal stimulation may also evoke a pacemaker shift, wherein true pacemaker cells are inhibited more than some of the latent pacemakers in the atrium or AV node.[8] ACh has little effect on automaticity in Purkinje fibers because cholinergic fibers are sparse in the His-Purkinje system and Purkinje fibers have an intrinsic resistance to ACh. However, catecholamines enhance automaticity in all latent pacemakers such as in the Purkinje system.

Sympathetic stimulation with hypertension and tachycardia are common during intubation or surgical pain, anxiety, myocardial ischemia, and baroreflex activation with deliberate hypotension and the use of vasodilators. The parasympathetics may dominate during laryngeal and bronchial manipulations, traction or compression of the eyeball, abdominal or thoracic structures, carotid sinus pressure, sympathetic blockade with regional anesthesia, and some instances of inferior myocardial ischemia. Generalized tetanus, Guillain-Barré syndrome, and the autonomic dysfunction of diabetes are secondary disorders in which serious arrhythmias are common with wide swings in autonomic dominance.

Hypothermia

Moderate to deep hypothermia (33° to 17°C) is commonly used during cardiopulmonary bypass surgery for both adults and children. Both unattended and intentional hypothermia produce marked ECG changes. Unmedicated hypothermic patients develop an initial tachycardia with a 2°C decrease in core temperature because of the intense sympathetic response to hypothermia. The body will defend its temperature more intensely than volume loss if the two are in conflict. In contrast, patients receiving anesthesia and sympatholytics will show a progressive decline in heart rate proportional to the decline in temperature. The ECG reveals a progressive prolongation of the PR, QRS, and QT intervals.[101] A deflection at the end of the QRS complex called the J wave, Osborn wave, or camel hump may be seen as the core temperature approaches 30°C. Atrial tachydysrhythmias such as flutter or fibrillation are often seen in adults at that temperature level. Ventricular fibrillation may occur as the temperature decreases to 28°C. The ECG changes of decreasing temperature are similar to those seen with increasing doses of calcium channel blockers.[102] Considering that the slow channels are enzyme and voltage dependent, they will also be temperature dependent. Delayed conduction with re-entry from hypothermia is consistent with this observation. Recovery of myocardial electrical activity with rewarming follows the exact reverse sequence of that to the induction of hypothermia. Attempts to defibrillate a heart below 34°C are often difficult and futile. However, the myocardium of infants and children does not seem to follow the same rules as that of adults. Perhaps owing to a more even cooling of the myocardium obviating re-entry, dysrhythmias do not seem to be as frequent in children as in adults even with temperatures down to 17°C. Asystole occurs before fibrillation. Ventricular fibrillation in infants undergoing surface cooling for deep hypothermia is uncommon except with premature manipulation of the cooling myocardium.[101,103]

Antidysrhythmic Drugs

Antidysrhythmic drugs directly alter the electrophysiologic characteristics of individual cardiac myocytes. Other drugs, such as oxygen or atropine, while important in correcting precipitating factors or altering autonomic tone, are not direct antidysrhythmic agents.

Various schemes have been used to classify dysrhythmias.[104,105] The broad anatomic classification into either supraventricular or ventricular dysrhythmias is helpful, but does not indicate etiologic mechanisms. It is perhaps more appropriate when selecting antidysrhythmic therapy to consider dysrhythmias under two categories: tachy- or bradydysrhythmias.

Bradydysrhythmias are due to decreased automaticity of the SA node, reduced conduction velocity, or block somewhere in the AV conduction system with or without a latent pacemaker assuming dominance. Therefore, after excluding hypoxemia as the etiology, recognition of bradydysrhythmias would direct therapy towards pacing, either electrical or chemical. Drugs that enhance sympathetic tone, or reduce vagal tone, such as atropine or isoproterenol, may be useful until the source of the bradycardia is eliminated or electrical pacing is introduced.

Tachydysrhythmias, in contrast, occur on the basis of electrical instability due to enhanced automaticity or re-entry. Theoretically, re-entry can explain all tachydysrhythmias. The onset of a nonperfusing tachydysrhythmia may require immediate cardioversion, whereas a perfusing dysrhythmia may allow a more studied pharmacologic approach. Placed in context, most of the useful antidysrhythmic drugs are specific for tachydysrhythmias.

Vaughan Williams proposed a classification of these drugs into four functional classes based upon how the drugs affect the cardiac action potential. Table 31–2 lists the classes and the drugs currently available, some of which are in advanced stages of investigation. The Vaughan Williams classification, though useful, contains

TABLE 31–2
Vaughan Williams Classifications of Antiarrhythmic Drugs

Class	Action	Drugs
I	Sodium channel blockade Membrane stabilizers	
IA	Prolongs APD	Procainamide Quinidine Disopyramide Moricizine
IB	Shortens APD	Lidocaine Diphenylhydantoin Tocainide Mexiletine
IC	Normal APD	Aprindine Propafenone Encainide Flecanide
II	Antagonism of sympathetic nervous system: β-adrenergic blocking agents	Propranolol Esmolol Metoprolol Labetalol
III	Increased refractoriness Antifibrillatory agents	Bretylium Amiodarone Sotalol
IV	Calcium channel blockade	Verapamil Diltiazem
V	Chloride channel blockade	Alinidine
Unclassified	α_1-Blockade Increased PNS tone Slowing of AV conduction	Prazosin Digitalis Adenosine

APD, action potential duration; PNS, peripheral nervous system; AV, atrioventricular.

TABLE 31–3
Antiarrhythmic/Electrophysiologic Actions*

Drugs	Class I	Class II	Class III	Class IV	Other Action
Quinidine	++		++		α-Blockade
Procainamide	++		+		Ganglionic blockade
Lidocaine	+				
Disopyramide	++		+		Anticholinergic
Tocainide	+				
Mexiletine	+				
Flecainide	+++			+	K^+ channel blockade
Encainide	+++				
Propafenone	+++	+			
Bretylium			++		Sympathomimetic and sympatholytic
Amiodarone	++	++	++	+	α- and β-block, muscarinic block
Sotalol		++	+++		
Verapamil	+			++++	
Diltiazem				+++	

*From Woosley RL: Antiarrhythmic drugs. Ann Rev Pharmacol Toxicol 31:427, 1991. © 1991 by Annual Reviews, with permission.

caveats. Each class is a grouping of antidysrhythmic "drug action" and not a group of similar antidysrhythmic drugs.[28,106,107] Failure to respond to a drug in a given class does not predict a lack of response to other drugs in the same class. A drug may also possess electrophysiologic actions of more than one class (Table 31–3) and the metabolites of the drugs often have actions different from the parent drug. A class V category, not included in the Vaughan Williams classification, has been advocated to include a chloride channel blocker (alinidine) that produces negative chronotropism.[28,38] Likewise, α_1-blockers have been found useful in reperfusion dysrhythmias and may deserve a separate class like the β-blockers. Adenosine and digitalis are also important antidysrhythmic drugs that fall outside this electrophysiologic classification.

The pharmacokinetics of some of the drugs listed in Table 31–2 mitigate against their use for the treatment of the acute onset of dysrhythmias. Others, such as quinidine, have proven too toxic when given intravenously, while others must be given orally. In addition, the onset of action or elimination half-time of some of the drugs are too slow to be of benefit for the acute-onset dysrhythmias. All things considered, the antidysrhythmic agents useful to the anesthesiologist in the acute situation can be reduced to about ten drugs. Interestingly, most of the drugs useful to the anesthesiologists are those that were historically discovered to be antidysrhythmics rather than those designed to be antidysrhythmics. Drugs not ordinarily used by the anesthesiologist for the acute situation will be included for discussion because many patients coming to surgery are on chronic oral antidysrhythmic therapy. They may present special concerns for drug interactions and the development of new dysrhythmias (proarrhythmias).

Class I drugs, as a group, are called membrane stabilizers. They inhibit the fast Na^+ channel and act by slowing the rate of phase 0 depolarization. Quinidine is the prototype class I agent. However, there are three subclassifications in class I: A, B, and C, which are based on differences in potency and effects on repolarization. Class IA drugs increase, IB decrease, and IC have no effect on the duration of the action potential. Class II drugs are the β-adrenergic blockers, which competitively inhibit β-adrenergic receptors. They are antidysrhythmic because of the dysrhythmogenic role of the β-adrenergic receptors. Propranolol is the prototype class II drug. Class III agents, unlike other antidysrhythmic drugs, do not depress automaticity and their only effect is to prolong the action potential duration in normal ventricular and Purkinje fibers. Class III drugs include bretylium and amiodarone, which have antifibrillatory effects. The latter has recently been released as an intravenous preparation for the acute treatment of ventricular and supraventricular tachyarrythmias. Class IV drugs selectively act on the slow calcium channels and have their greatest effect on the SA and AV nodes where sodium channels are inactive. Verapamil is the prototype class IV drug.

Class I Drugs

The class I drugs have in common the ability to suppress phase 4 spontaneous depolarization (Figure 31–13). Automaticity in ectopic sites is usually extinguished at concentrations that exert only minimal effects on the automaticity of normal pacemakers. Thus, ectopic rhythms can be abolished without inducing asystole. However, all class I drugs can introduce bradycardia in the presence of a diseased SA node or perinodal fibers. Although reduction of abnormal automaticity is an important feature of the class I drugs, their efficacy is more likely due to the prevention of re-entry than suppression of automaticity. Altered conduction of the cardiac impulse (re-entry) rather than suppression of automaticity probably accounts for the majority of serious dysrhythmias. The electrophysiologic properties not shared by the class I drugs in this regard account for their further subclassification (IA, IB, IC). This class of drugs is usually re-

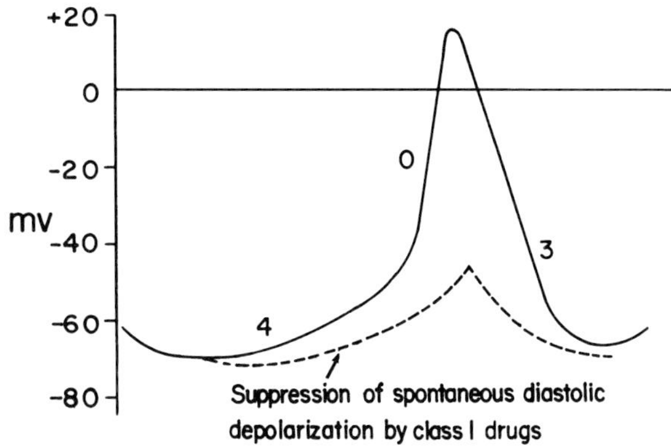

FIGURE 31–13. The ability to suppress spontaneous depolarization is a characteristic common to all class I drugs. Spontaneous ectopic foci are more sensitive to this action than are normal pacemakers.

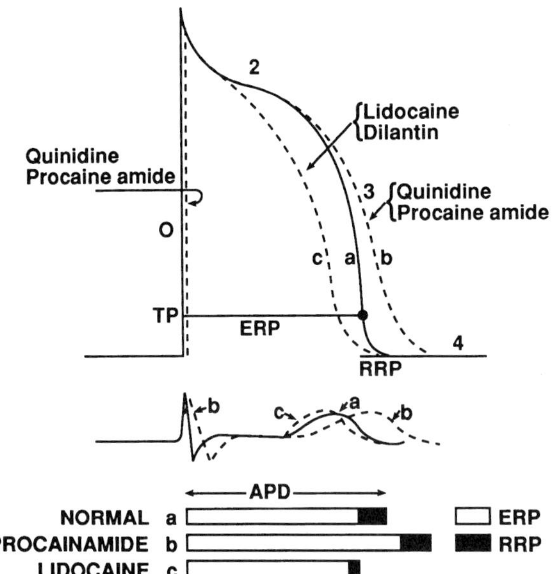

FIGURE 31–14. The effects of procainamide (IA) and lidocaine (IB) on the fast action potential are compared. Lidocaine (c) shortens the action potential difference (APD), whereas procainamide (b) lengthens it compared to normal. Procainamide toxicity widens the QRS and increases the QT interval giving potential to produce torsades de pointes. These differences account for their differing effects on the ECG with toxicity. Despite the contrasting effects on the APD, both drugs increase the effective refractory period (ERP) to relative refractory period (RRP) ratio.

ferred to as membrane stabilizers and includes the agents quinidine, procainamide, disopyramide, and moricizine.

Quinidine is of little use to the anesthesiologist because of its toxicity as an intravenous drug and its limitations as an oral agent. It may produce tachycardia and increase AV conduction to increase ventricular response to atrial flutter or fibrillation,[108] hence the use of routine administration of a drug such as digoxin to decrease AV conduction prior to instituting therapy with these agents. Quinidine also inhibits peripheral and myocardial α-adrenergic receptors and may produce hypotension. In addition, quinidine has a vagolytic effect through the direct blockade of muscarinic receptors. Bladder outlet obstruction resulting in urinary retention and gastrointestinal symptoms, seen with quinidine and disopyramide, are thought to be the result of their anticholinergic actions.

Procainamide is the prototype class IA drug for the anesthesiologist. The anticholinergic effects of procainamide are less than those of quinidine, while its electrophysiologic effects are similar. It inhibits the fast depolarizing influx of Na^+ during phase 0 depolarization and reduces K^+ efflux during rapid repolarization (phase 3). The effect on the action potential is to reduce the velocity of the phase 0 upstroke, and increase the absolute refractory period and the duration of the action potential (APD) (Fig. 31–14). It depresses both atrial and ventricular excitability by reduction of conduction velocity throughout the atria and His-Purkinje fibers. Therapeutic doses do not reduce the amplitude of depolarization; however, toxic doses intensify these changes. Therapeutic levels of procainamide may prolong the QRS duration by 5 to 10% as well as the PR and QT intervals. A widening of the QRS by 25% is a sign of early toxicity and a 50% increase is clearly toxic. Procainamide toxicity may also produce opposite effects on spontaneous depolarization and cause depolarization in Purkinje fibers and accelerate automaticity.

Metabolism of procainamide yields *N*-acetylated procainamide (NAPA), which is an active class III antidysrhythmic with a half-life of 6 to 8 hours. The latter may account for a significant portion of the therapeutic effect seen with procainamide and should be measured along with procainamide levels during therapy. Torsades de pointes is rare with procainamide, in contrast to the incidence reported with quinidine.

Procainamide is a broad-spectrum antidysrhythmic and is effective in both supraventricular and ventricular tachydysrhythmias, although it is more commonly used for the latter. It is an effective emergency treatment for ventricular dysrhythmias, particularly after failure of lidocaine. It is only modestly effective in converting atrial flutter and fibrillation to sinus rhythm. As with quinidine, it may accelerate AV node conduction and is generally used only after digoxin. Procainamide is effective in patients with WPW syndrome by slowing conduction velocity in the aberrant accessory pathways. It should be avoided in patients in whom dysrhythmias from digitalis toxicity is suspected. Procainamide can increase the toxic AV conduction block and initiate re-entry (Tables 31–4 and 31–5).

Disopyramide has electrophysiologic properties and clinical applications similar to quinidine and procainamide. The clinical applications are similar. It is available only in oral form in the United States and is not particularly useful in the acute situation.

Disopyramide has a half-life of 8 hours. Most of the undesirable side effects are related to its powerful anticholinergic effect. Disopyramide is 40 times more potent in its antimuscarinic effects than quinidine. Side effects such as urinary retention, constipation, dry mouth, and worsening of glaucoma have been reported in patients who are receiving the oral form of this drug. An unexplained side effect is negative inotropism[108] (see Tables 31–4 and 31–5).

TABLE 31–4
Antidysrhythmic Drugs for Ventricular Dysrhythmias

Class	Agent	Dose	Pharmacokinetics	Side Effects
IA	Quinidine	IV use not recommended. Oral dose: 200–600 mg q6h. Requires continuous monitoring of BP and ECG.	Excreted by liver. $t_{1/2}$ = 7–9 hr.	Potentiates nondepolarizing muscle relaxants. α-Blockade with hypotension and bradycardia when given IV. Monitor QRS, QT, serum K^+.
	Procainamide	100 mg IV over 2 min. Up to 20 mg/min to a maximum of 1 gm in 1 hr. Maintenance 2–6 mg/min.	$t_{1/2}$ = 3–5 hr. Hepatic or renal disease requires dose reduction.	Hypotension, heart block, torsades de pointes rare, but seen with class III combinations.
	Disopyramide	IV dose not available in U.S.	$t_{1/2}$ = 8 hr. Hepatic (50%) and renal (50%) excretion.	Hypotension, QRS or QT prolongation. Torsades de pointes with class III drugs. Strong anticholinergic effect. Negative inotropism.
	Moricizine	Oral only. 200–300 mg PO q8h.	$t_{1/2}$ = 1.5–3.5 hr. Reduced clearance with renal failure.	Enzyme inducer. Few interactions reported.
IB	Lidocaine	IV loading dose 1 mg/kg. May repeat q5min until CNS signs appear or total of 300 mg. Continuous infusion of 1–4 mg/min (20–50 μg/kg/min).	Therapeutic level 1.4–6 μg/ml. Toxic level 9 μg/ml.	Reduce with reduced liver flow, shock, β-blockade, cirrhosis, CHF.
	Diphenylhydantoin	50–100 mg IV slowly q5min for 1 gm.	$t_{1/2}$ = 24 hr. Hepatic or renal disease require dose reduction.	Hypotension, vertigo, enzyme inducer with cimetidine, lidocaine, mexiletine.
	Tocainide	PO 300–600 mg tid. IV 250 mg over 2 min, then 500 mg over 15 min, then 500 mg q6h for 48 hr. IV not approved in U.S.	$t_{1/2}$ = 14 hr.	Nausea, vomiting, cerebellar signs, pulmonary fibrosis.
	Mexiletine	PO loading dose of 400 mg followed by 300–1,200 mg in divided doses qd. IV not available in U.S.	$t_{1/2}$ = 7–15 hr.	Disorientation, tremor, nausea, bradycardia, hypotension.
	Aprindine	PO 100–150 mg qd.	$t_{1/2}$ = 20–60 hr.	Tremor, hallucinations, ataxia, vertigo.
	Propafenone	2 mg/kg followed by infusion at 2 mg/min (not approved in U.S.). PO: 150–300 mg tid. Slow onset of 2–4 hr. 3–4 days PO.	$t_{1/2}$ = 2–10 hr.	Limited to life-threatening ventricular dysrhythmias. May be used for supraventricular dysrhythmias including WPW syndrome. Negative inotropism and proarrhythmias.

IV, intravenous; BP, blood pressure; ECG, electrocardiogram; $t_{1/2}$, elimination half-life; tid, three times a day; U.S., United States; PO, orally; CNS, central nervous system; CHF, congestive heart failure; WPW, Wolff-Parkinson-White.

Moricizine is an oral drug that has recently been released by the U.S. Food and Drug Administration (FDA) for the treatment of life-threatening ventricular dysrhythmias. It has local anesthetic activity, but does not quite fit any of the usual subclasses of antidysrhythmic drugs. It most closely fits the class IA like quinidine or class IC like flecainide.[109] Moricizine suppresses abnormal automaticity and prolongs the PR and QRS intervals. Opie classifies moricizine as a IB/IC drug more like lidocaine. It is not of benefit in the treatment of acute dysrhythmias, as the full effect of an oral dose does not occur for about 10 to 14 hours. No interactions with digoxin, diuretics, β-blockers, calcium channel blockers, angiotensin converting enzyme (ACE) inhibitors, or anticoagulants have been reported, but proarrhythmic activity has been reported when used in conjunction with other local anesthetics.

The class IB drugs include lidocaine, diphenylhydantoin (DPH), tocainide, and mexilitine. Lidocaine, the prototype class IB drug, also appears to depress Na^+ influx during spontaneous diastolic depolarization, reducing automaticity. It does not alter ion exchange in the SA or AV nodes. Therapeutic doses have little effect on Na^+ influx during fast action potentials, but do enhance K^+ exit from the cells and hasten repolarization. As a result, neither the amplitude nor the velocity of the phase 0 upstroke is altered. In contrast to procainamide, lidocaine reduces both the ERP and the APD (Fig. 31–14). This effect is most prominent in the Purkinje fibers, where the action potential is longest. Lidocaine mini-

TABLE 31–5
Dosage Adjustments of Antidysrhythmic Drugs

Drug	Adjustment
Class IA	
Procainamide	Reduce dose with rental or hepatic disease; monitor plasma levels of procainamide and *N*-acetylated procainamide (class III metabolite); CHF Avoid with myasthenia gravis, heart block
Quinidine	Reduce dose with advanced age, cimetidine; class III drugs, digoxin Increase dose with phenobarbital, dilantin Avoid with long QT syndromes, hypokalemia, liver failure
Disopyramide	Reduce dose with renal and liver disease; no digoxin interaction Avoid with long QT syndromes, CHF, prostatism, glaucoma
Moricizine	Reduce dose with renal or liver insufficiency Avoid with clinical setting for proarrhythmias (hypokalemia, long QT)
Class IB	
Lidocaine	Reduce dose with CHF: reduce both loading and maintenance dose; cimetidine and β-blockers increase serum level; reduce dose in liver disease
Dilantin	Reduce dose with severe liver disease; variable effect with carbamazepine, disulfiram, isoniazid, sulphonamides
Mexiletine	Reduce dose with liver disease, reduced effectiveness in presence of enzyme inducers Avoid with heart block
Tocainide	Reduce dose with severe renal disease; no interactions known including digoxin Avoid with heart block, atrial flutter or fibrillation
Class IC	
Propafenone	Reduce dose with LV dysfunction, heart block, asthma Avoid with proarrhythmias common with other class I agents
Aprinidine	Reduce dose with calcium channel blockers; may interfere with slow channel activity Avoid with neurologic disease
Class II	
Propranolol	Reduce dose with liver disease Avoid with CHF, bronchospasm, sinus node disease, clonidine withdrawal, Raynaud's disease
Esmolol	Reduce dose with bronchospastic disease, renal dysfunction, warfarin; no interaction with succinylcholine Avoid with CHF, bradycardia
Metoprolol	Reduce dose with same precautions as with other β-blockers
Class III	
Amiodarone	Reduce dose with torsades de pointes with hypokalemia and class I drugs; warfarin
Bretylium	Reduce dose with renal disease, presence of digitalis Avoid with aortic stenosis, carotid obstruction, pulmonary hypertension, pheochromocytoma
Sotalol	Reduce dose with β-blockers; has combined class II and class III effects Avoid with hypokalemia; will prolong QT interval and risk torsades de pointes
Class IV	
Verapamil	Reduce dose with sinus or AV node dysfunction; β-blockers, digitalis, CHF Avoid with broad complex tachycardias; can be fatal if VT
Unclassified	
Digitalis	Reduce dose with quinidine therapy, advanced age, renal disease (digoxin), liver disease (digitoxin) Increase dose with dilantin therapy (digitoxin) Avoid with Wolff-Parkinson-White syndrome, diastolic dysfunction, obstructive cardiomyopathy, hypokalemia
Adenosine	Reduce dose with dipyramidole therapy Increase dose with methylxanthine therapy Avoid with asthma, COPD, second- or third-degree block; sick sinus syndrome

CHF, congestive heart failure; VT, ventricular tachycardia; AV, atrioventricular; COPD, chronic obstructive pulmonary disease; LV, left ventricular.

mizes differences in the APD that normally exist throughout the cardiac conduction system. This suggests that part of the antidysrhythmic action of lidocaine is a result of improved conduction velocity in ischemic areas.[110] Lidocaine does not induce automaticity in toxic concentrations as occurs with procainamide. It produces few systemic autonomic effects and hypotension is rarely seen except with the rapid administration of large doses.

Clinically, therapeutic concentrations of both procainamide and lidocaine increase the fibrillation threshold, reduce ventricular ectopy, and abolish re-entry.[111] Their contrasting effects on the ERP and fast action potential duration suggests that different cellular mechanisms are operative. Their contradictory effects on the absolute refractory period is a matter of relativity. Although lidocaine shortens the ERP, the ERP is actually increased relative to the time of the relative refractory period

(RFP) (Fig. 31–14). The greater part of the action potential is in absolute refraction reducing the relative time of exposure that the cell could be excited by a re-entrant wavefront. In contrast, procainamide produces both a real and relative increase in the ERP. The end result is the same: blockade of re-entry. Slowed conduction with a unidirectional block is a requirement for re-entry. Re-entry could, therefore, be abolished by either improving conduction through the block (lidocaine) or by converting the unidirectional block to a complete block (procainamide) (Fig. 31–15).

Lidocaine has been shown experimentally to improve conduction in ischemic cardiac tissue, but studies in humans have been inconclusive.[110,112,113] Lidocaine improves conduction when spontaneous depolarization occurs from a resting membrane potential (RMP) in the −80- to −60-mV range. As a result, the conduction velocity of an ectopic site would be improved and the unidirectional block removed (Fig. 31–15). This effect may be biphasic in that higher doses of lidocaine have also been shown to slow conduction in ectopic ischemic foci and decrease re-entrant ectopy after experimental infarction.[114] Lidocaine has not been effective as an antidysrhythmic on ventricular ectopy when spontaneous depolarization occurs in cells with an RMP in the −40- to −50-mV range.[115] Sodium channels are inoperative at this threshold but calcium channels are active. Calcium entry inhibitors thus hold some promise in treating some resistant ventricular dysrhythmias.[38,116] This would also explain why lidocaine has little effect on supraventricular dysrhythmias. Most ectopy and re-entry in this location starts with an RMP in the −50-mV range, where lidocaine would be ineffective.[107]

A major advantage of lidocaine is its lack of significant cardiac toxicity.[117,118] Therapeutic concentrations have little effect on myocardial contractility, blood pressure, or interventricular conduction. Toxicity is instead manifested by central nervous system (CNS) dysfunction including drowsiness, disorientation, muscle twitching, and convulsions. Thus, the ECG and vital signs may not be helpful in detecting early toxicity under anesthesia (Tables 31–4 and 31–6).

Lidocaine remains the first-line antidysrhythmic drug for the control and prevention of ventricular dysrhythmias and for increasing fibrillation threshold. It has a relatively wide margin of safety. If lidocaine fails, the cause of that failure should be determined before changing drugs. Are inotropes being given? Are there technical errors? Is the patient acidotic or alkalotic? Is hypokalemia or hypomagnesemia present? Hypokalemia and hypomagnesemia reduce the effectiveness of the class I drugs, while hyperkalemia augments their action. DPH (class IB) is the exception. If none of these factors are present, the infusion may either be cautiously increased or an alternative class I drug such as procainamide selected before resorting to bretylium (class III).

DPH shortens the action potential duration like lidocaine, but it also has a potential central sympatholytic action. It exerts its effect by increasing the ERP-APD ratio and by decreasing automaticity. It is particularly effective in abolishing afterpotentials seen with digitalis toxicity and hypokalemia. The primary use of DPH is to treat atrial or ventricular dysrhythmias produced by the cardiac glycosides digoxin and digitalis. It is not as effective against ventricular ectopy from other sources in adults. The drug has been reported to be particularly effective in the dysrhythmias seen in children following surgery for congenital heart disease.[119] The reason for this is unknown.[108] Rapid infusion of DPH at rates greater than 50 mg/min can cause a negative inotropic effect and conduction blockade, which may lead to cardiovascular collapse (Table 31–4). This has been related to the solvents propylene glycol and ethyl alcohol. The recent introduction of fosphenytoin, a water-soluble form of the drug, may eliminate this problem and allow a more rapid rate of administration.

Tocainide and mexiletine were developed specifically for oral administration,[120] but can also be given intravenously. They are analogues of lidocaine and have no proven advantages over it.[38] Both drugs are used to decreased the frequency of ventricular ectopy and tachycardia associated with MI. Tocainide is also effective against recurrent VT or VF. Both drugs are ineffective in the treatment of supraventricular dysrhythmias, and mexilitene may precipitate supraventricular tachycardias in patients with WPW syndrome. There are few interactions with anesthetic drugs (Table 31–4 and 31–5). Digitalis can be used with tocainide without changing drug levels. Tocainide has also been used with β-adrenergic blockers, other antidysrhythmic agents, and diuretics without evidence of interaction. Concurrent use of mexiletine with β-adrenergic blockers or disopyramide results in synergic negative inotropic effects.

Class IC drugs include propafenone, encainide, flecainide, and aprindine. These drugs, as all the class I drugs, suppress abnormal automaticity and stabilize membranes. They are powerful inhibitors of Na^+ channel conductance causing a marked reduction in the phase 0 upstroke of the fast action potential. They inhibit the velocity of His-Purkinje conduction fibers, but markedly shorten the action potential duration of the Purkinje fibers. The net result is no change in the duration of the fast action potential. The discrepancy in conduction velocities that these drugs produce perhaps explains their

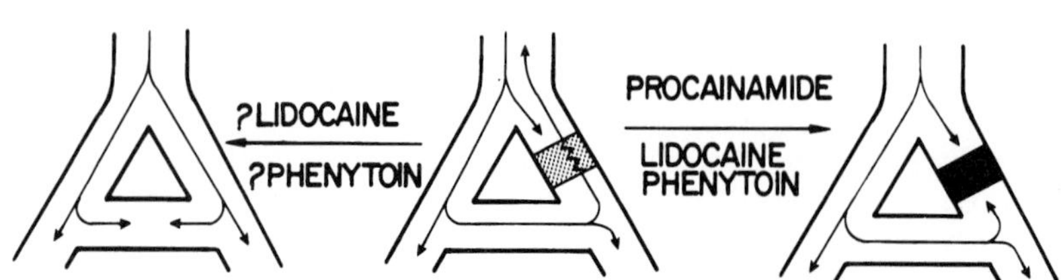

FIGURE **31–15.** Procainamide (IA) abolishes re-entry by increasing conduction block, whereas lidocaine (IB) may be biphasic in abolishing re-entry by either increasing conduction (low-dose) or increasing the block of unidirectional conduction delay (high-dose).

TABLE 31–6
Antidysrhythmic Drugs Useful for Supraventricular Dysrhythmias

Class	Agent	Dose	Pharmacokinetics	Side Effects
IA	Quinidine Procainamide	See Table 31–4. See Table 31–4.		
IB*				
IC	Propafenone	2 mg/kg followed by infusion of 2 mg/min (not approved in U.S.)		Useful for supraventricular tachycardias with WPW. Chronic recurring PSVT.
II	Propranolol	IV: 1 mg/2 min to total of 5–10 mg.	$t_{1/2}$ = 7 hr. Rapidly cleared by liver.	Best for PAT with emotion, excitement, thyrotoxicosis.
	Esmolol	IV loading: 100–500 μg/kg. Most respond to 150 μg/kg. Continuous infusion at 20–200 μg/kg/min.	$t_{1/2}$ = 9 min.	Transient hypotension, bradycardia, bronchospasm possible. Does not effect succinylcholine.
	Metoprolol	0.5–1.0 mg titrated to effect up to 0.1–0.15 mg/kg	$t_{1/2}$ = 3 hr.	β_2-Blocking effect is 1–2% propranolol. Reduced bronchoconstriction.
	Labetalol	5–10 mg IV in anesthetized patients. Titrated to effect.	α- and β-blockade in 1:7 ratio when given IV.	May increase heart failure. Antidysrhythmic effects untested.
III	Bretylium	IV: 5–10 mg/kg repeat to a maximum of 30 mg/kg. IV infusion 1–2 mg/min.	$t_{1/2}$ = 7 hr.	Hypotension, nausea, and vomiting in conscious patients. Sensitizes to other catecholamines. Effect reduced with tricyclic antidepressants.
IV	Verapamil	IV infusion: 1 mg/min to total of 10 mg. Maximum: 20 mg.	Hemodynamic effects last 3–20 min. Effect on AV node lasts 6 hr.	Caution with β-blocker or heart block, bradycardia, hypotension. Avoid with cardiomegaly, shock, or AV block.
Unclassified	Digoxin	IV: 0.25–0.5 mg in incremental doses to effect or toxicity.	Renal excretion, $t_{1/2}$ = 1.5 day.	May produce junctional dysrhythmias and heart block. Calcium potentiates toxicity. Hypokalemia increases toxicity.
	Adenosine	Rapid IV bolus of 6 mg, followed by 12-mg rapid bolus in 2 minutes if no effect. Repeat 12-mg bolus once.	$t_{1/2}$ = 9 sec.	Flushing, headache, dyspnea, chest pain. New dysrhythmias transiently 65% of time. Do not use in sick sinus syndrome. Good for WPW syndrome.

*No IB antidysrhythmic drugs are useful for supraventricular dysrhythmias. Dilantin may be the exception if the dysrhythmias are induced by digitalis and hypokalemia.
U.S., United States; WPW, Wolff-Parkinson-White; PSVT, paroxysmal supraventricular tachycardia; $t_{1/2}$, elimination half-life; IV, intravenous; PAT, paroxysmal atrial tachycardia; AV, atrioventricular.

propensity in certain circumstances to be "proarrhythmogenic," resulting in torsades de pointes and ventricular fibrillation.

Propafenone is a class IC antidysrhythmic drug.[108] A slow peak effect does not make it particularly suitable for acute-onset dysrhythmias (2 hours). The side-effect profile is also characteristic of IC drugs with proarrhythmic activity. It is used to suppress both supraventricular and ventricular dysrhythmias including those associated with WPW syndrome. Currently in the United States, it is approved only for life-threatening ventricular dysrhythmias. In addition to its class IC activity, it also has mild β-adrenergic blocking and Ca^{2+} channel antagonist activities. AV block, bundle branch block, and left ventricular (LV) dysfunction are relative contraindications.

Encainide and flecainide were generally assumed to be effective in patients with life-threatening or symptomatic ventricular dysrhythmias including ventricular tachycardia and fibrillation[121] without formal testing in placebo-controlled trials. The Cardiac Arrhythmia Suppression Trial (CAST) has recently demonstrated the potential lethal side effects of antidysrhythmic drugs.[122–124] Encainide and flecainide, after being approved for marketing, were removed from routine use after the CAST study demonstrated that the drugs were causing a two- to threefold increase in mortality compared to that in patients whose dysrhythmias were being treated by placebo. These drugs are recommended for use only when other more conventional therapies have failed.

Aprindine remains on the market for suppression of ventricular rate in patients with WPW syndrome.[38] It is limited to oral administration and has a high incidence of neurologic sequelae such as ataxia, vertigo, tremor, and hallucinations, which should not be attributed to complications of anesthesia.

Class II Drugs

The class II drugs include the β-adrenergic blocking agents such as propranolol, metoprolol, esmolol, and labetalol. The β-adrenergic blocking agents may be useful for antidysrhythmia therapy in the perioperative period because of the proarrythmogenic effects of increased catecholamines.

β_1- and β_2-adrenergic stimulation of the myocardium increases automaticity and conduction velocity and shortens the refractory period (see "Adrenoreceptors"). The primary antidysrhythmic action of propranolol and the other β-adrenergic antagonists is attributed to their competitive inhibition of β-adrenergic stimuli. In addition, these agents are able to suppress chronic ventricular dysrhythmias in the absence of β-adrenergic stimulation, suggesting a direct antidysrhythmic action at higher doses (Tables 31–4 and 31–5).

Propranolol is not a cardioselective β-blocker. It is an equipotent β_2-adrenergic blocker that can cause bronchoconstriction, pulmonary hypertension, and increased vascular resistance. The response to the β-blocking properties of propranolol is directly proportional to the degree of β-adrenergic stimulation. The response varies greatly depending on the underlying sympathetic tone and cardiovascular status. Propranolol produces little effect on dysrhythmias or heart rate in patients with normal sympathetic tone. Unusually large doses may be required to counter dysrhythmias characterized by excessive catecholamines, as with thyrotoxicosis. Conversely, small amounts of propranolol may produce profound hemodynamic changes when the heart condition and circulation are dependent upon β-adrenergic stimulation as a compensatory mechanism. Thus, the indiscriminate use of β-blockade to curb an "undesirable" tachycardia can have disastrous results.

The β-blocking activity of propranolol predominates at lower doses. It decreases the outward current of K^+. Changes in the ECG are primarily related to the reversal of the effects of β-adrenergic stimulation on conduction and automaticity. Inherent to the actions of propranolol is a tendency to decrease heart rate, decrease contractility, increase pulmonary artery pressure, and cause bronchoconstriction. It follows that the drug is relatively or absolutely contraindicated in the presence of heart failure, bradycardia, hypotension, pulmonary hypertension, asthma, or obstructive lung disease.[8] This limits its utility in the treatment of dysrhythmias if one or more of these conditions is present. Its myocardial depressant effects are a relative drawback with acute infarction. It does, however, decrease impulse conduction in acutely ischemic myocardium, but not in normal tissue.[108] Propranolol may be indirectly antidysrhythmic by reducing the metabolic requirements of the ischemic myocardium.

Propranolol is most effective against supraventricular dysrhythmias and dysrhythmias mediated by catecholamines (Table 31–6). It is used in the perioperative period specifically to control inappropriate sinus tachycardia, paroxysmal atrial tachycardia, and atrial fibrillation with fast ventricular response. β-Blockade may be used with the dysrhythmias of digitalis intoxication, but the coexistence of AV block usually makes DPH or lidocaine a better choice. Propranolol will stop the tachycardias of TCA overdose. The use of β-blocking agents alone in situations of catecholamine excess (pheochromocytoma, thyrotoxicosis, clonidine withdrawal, epinephrine administration) may cause severe hypertension due to unopposed α-mediated vasoconstriction. Such patients should receive an α-blocking agent or other vasodilator prior to giving a β-blocking agent to control the dysrhythmia or use labetalol. The β-adrenergic blocking agents are also commonly used to control the reflex tachycardia that occurs when direct-acting vasodilators such as sodium nitroprusside are used to control mean arterial pressure.

Excessive blockade may be corrected by intravenous atropine (1 to 2 mg), but glucagon is the drug of choice for severe toxicity (such as inadvertent or intentional overdose) because it stimulates formation of cAMP by a route that bypasses the occupied β-adrenergic receptor. Alternatively, dobutamine or isoproterenol may be given in sufficient dose to overcome the competitive blockade.

Although generally classified as a class II drug, propranolol shares some electrophysiologic effects with class IC agents. High doses of propranolol inhibit the inward Na^+ current, producing direct membrane-stabilizing effects, which are independent of its β-blocking action. It has the ability to suppress ventricular dysrhythmias in the absence of β-adrenergic stimulation similar to other class I drugs. This is often referred to as a quinidine-like effect.[104,105] This effect is noted on the ECG as an increased PR interval like that of procainamide, a shortened QT interval as with lidocaine, but the QRS is not altered. Hence, it is similar to other class IC drugs of the Vaughan Williams classification.

However, the membrane-stabilizing activity is not relevant to the clinical management of acute dysrhythmias in the operating room as a first-line antidysrhythmic agent. Other class I or class III agents are initially more appropriate. The propranolol concentrations required to produce membrane stabilization may be associated with excessive β-blockade. Effective β-blockade is seen at plasma levels of 100 to 300 ng/ml, whereas membrane stabilization requires levels of around 1,000 ng/ml.

Metoprolol is a relatively selective β_1-blocker, with a potency for β_1-blockade similar to that of propranolol.[125] It is available for oral or intravenous administration.[108] It produces less bronchoconstriction than propranolol, since it exhibits only 1 to 2% of the β_2-blockade of propranolol. The intravenous dosage is 0.5 to 1.0 mg, titrated to effect (Tables 31–4, 31–5, and 31–6).

Esmolol is an intravenous β-adrenergic blocker that has several uses in the perioperative period.[126,127] Its most unique feature is the ester group incorporated into its structure, which allows for rapid degradation by esterases in the red blood cells with a resultant pharmacologic half-life of 9 minutes.[128] The red cell esterase differs from the plasma cholinesterase and is not inhibited to a significant degree by physostigmine or echothiophate. There are no apparent important clinical interactions between esmolol and other ester-containing drugs. At the highest infusion rates (500 μg/kg/min), esmolol does not prolong neuromuscular blockade by succinylcholine.

The heart rate response to isoproterenol returns to control in 20 minutes.

Esmolol is β_1 cardioselective and has little effect on bronchial or vascular tone at doses that decrease heart rate in humans.[129] It has been used successfully in low doses in patients with asthma.

Esmolol has proven to be quite useful in the perioperative period because it is administered intravenously and has a short half-life.[130] These features allow it to be easily titrated by intravenous infusion and may permit a trial of β-adrenergic blockade in patients with relative contraindications.[131] Esmolol has been shown to blunt the response to intubation of the trachea, and is moderately effective in treating postoperative hypertension. The most beneficial approach seems to be a loading dose of 500 μg/kg followed by a continuous infusion of 50 to 300 μg/kg/min (Table 31–6). Peak blockade occurs within 5 minutes.

Labetalol is not usually thought of as an antidysrhythmic agent. It provides a combination of α- and β-adrenergic blockade, making it a good choice to treat catecholamine excess or catecholamine-anesthesia interactions leading to dysrhythmias. The relative α- and β-adrenergic blocking effects are dependent upon the route of administration. The ratio of α- to β-adrenergic blockade is 1:3 after oral administration and 1:3 to 7 with intravenous administration. The α-adrenergic effects are primarily α_1, and are roughly 10 to 15% that of an equivalent dose of phentolamine.[132] The β-adrenergic effects are nonselective and only 5 to 10% that of propranolol.

Reperfusion after temporary coronary occlusion produces malignant dysrhythmias by a mechanism different from that caused by prolonged coronary occlusion.[133] Reperfusion does not prolong conduction so re-entry is probably not a factor.[134] β-Blockade does not consistently prevent reperfusion dysrhythmias. However, the α-adrenergic blocking agents such as prazosin and phentolamine have been effective in preventing VF on release of coronary occlusion, but are of limited use because of hypotension.[22] Based on its α-adrenergic blocking properties, labetalol may have similar effects.[23]

The hemodynamic effects of labetalol consist primarily of decreased peripheral resistance and decreased or unchanged heart rate with little change in cardiac output. The elimination half-life after intravenous administration is 5.5 hours. The dosage schedule is shown in Tables 31–4 and 31–6. Another advantage of the drug is the ability to convert from intravenous (IV) to oral administration. Complications and contraindications are similar to those for the β-blockers. Labetalol should be used with caution in patients with compromised myocardial function because it may worsen heart failure. Also, it may induce bronchospasm in asthmatics because of its nonselective β-adrenergic antagonism.

Class III Drugs

The class III drugs, also known as the antifibrillatory agents, include bretylium, amiodarone, and sotalol. Little has been written on the prevention of VF by raising the ventricular fibrillation threshold (VFT). Most studies emphasize a drug's ability to eliminate PVCs or VT. However, 25% of deaths due to VF are associated with bradydysrhythmias, not VT.[145] This suggests that the threshold for VF may not always correlate with the threshold for VT and that the prevention of VF should be approached as a separate phenomenon from PVCs or even VT. Campbell[136] suggested the difference in threshold for VT and VF by demonstrating that while 16 of 17 episodes of VF were initiated by an R on T phenomenon, only 4 of 265 episodes of VT were initiated in this manner.

Nonuniformity of the refractory period in an area of the myocardium is thought to be the source of VF. Asynchronous refractory periods in adjacent cells leads to local re-entry and random, uncoordinated excitation waves. Anything that increases this temporal dispersion of the refractory state will lower the VF threshold and increase excitability. Delayed conduction velocity and ectopic impulses are also induced, but at different thresholds than for that of VF. Not all drugs work on both VF and VT equally well. For example, bretylium can prevent VF but not VT.[111,133] It is an excellent antifibrillatory drug, but a poor antiectopic agent.[137] The class III drugs are called antifibrillatory because of their effect on increasing the VF threshold.

Bretylium has direct effects on cardiac tissue but lacks most of the electrophysiologic properties associated with antidysrhythmic activity. Its only proven effect on action potentials is an increase in the APD and the refractory period in *normal* Purkinje and ventricular fibers. This will be noted on the ECG as a prolongation of the QT interval. Bretylium does not depress automaticity or contractility. These properties separate it from the class I drugs and account for its separate classification. The preferential prolongation of the refractory period in normal tissue surrounding a zone of ischemia could act to terminate re-entrant dysrhythmias by creating a conduction block in normal areas where re-entry would otherwise occur. This is distinctly different from the prevention of re-entry by the class I drugs, although the result is the same. However, the antidysrhythmic effects of bretylium cannot be fully explained by this electrophysiologic action.

Bretylium is primarily used for treatment of ventricular fibrillation to facilitate termination with electrical shock.[138] Unlike other antidysrhythmic drugs, bretylium can chemically reverse ventricular fibrillation when DC countershock has failed.[139] It increases the threshold to induce ventricular fibrillation and reduces the amount of current required to defibrillate. It is also highly effective in the treatment of recurrent ventricular dysrhythmias resistant to other drugs.[140] It can be used for the treatment of other ventricular dysrhythmias, but is not considered a first-line drug because hypotension may complicate its use (Table 31–4).

Aside from the direct cardiac effects of bretylium, it has a direct, biphasic effect on the SNS that is clinically important. Intravenous bretylium induces an initial release of NE from adrenergic nerve terminals that is clinically evident by an increase in arterial blood pressure and heart rate (1 to 2 minutes). This is transient and lasts approximately 20 minutes. Following this, bretylium blocks the release of NE, in effect producing a chemical sympathectomy. This results from an initial displacement of NE and then a selective accumulation of bretylium in sympathetic ganglia similar to the effects of guanethidine. The result is hypotension due to vasodilatation. Bretylium does not directly depress the myocardium as do some of the other antidysrhythmic agents. Bretylium has been shown to increase contractility. Hypotension, the major side effect, is unpredictable and occasionally severe enough to require fluids or vasopressors. Vasopressors should be given cautiously, since patients treated with bretylium may be extremely sensitive to catecholamines because of the adrenergic receptor sensitivity accompanying sympathetic denervation.

Norepinephrine release by bretylium may facilitate defibrillation in addition to its direct antidysrhythmic action. The timing of the NE release is consistent with observations that bretylium initially worsens ventricular tachycardia and ventricular ectopy but may chemically convert an established fibrillation.[140,141] The antidysrhythmic action of bretylium on ectopic dysrhythmias has been noted to be much slower (30 minutes to 2 hours) than its antifibrillatory action (1 to 2 minutes). The timing of these antidysrhythmic actions is also consistent with the onset of sympatholytic blockade and the later direct affect of bretylium on cardiac membranes. Bretylium is contraindicated in the treatment of digitalis-induced dysrhythmias because they are enhanced by NE.[105]

If bretylium is the initial drug given at the onset of ventricular fibrillation, other cardiotonic drugs are usually not necessary because of the initial inotropic action of bretylium. The administration of other antidysrhythmic drugs before bretylium may delay its effectiveness in converting ventricular fibrillation.[105,141]

Amiodarone is structurally related to thyroxine. The intravenous form of this drug has recently been released in the United States, thereby making it a recent addition to the armamentarium of the anesthesiologist for the acute treatment of dysrhythmias. The major electrophysiologic effects are to prolong both atrial and ventricular action potentials without significantly affecting the rate of rise of the action potential (phase 0).[142] It increases the VF threshold. Both α- and β-adrenergic receptors are blocked at therapeutic levels. Thus, amiodarone is a complex drug that shares some of the characteristics of all four classes of antidysrhythmics.[108]

Amiodarone depresses sinus node automaticity and slows conduction through the AV node and internodal pathways including the accessory pathway of the WPW syndrome.[142] With its recent introduction for intravenous administration, it may be considered a second-line agent when other conventional therapies fail for atrial and ventricular dysrhythmias. For chronic use, because of its toxicities, it is usually reserved for patients who are unresponsive to other modes of therapy. At least 50% of patients chronically treated with amiodarone experience one or more adverse effects.[39,40] Discontinuation of therapy will be necessary in approximately 8 to 10% of those treated. Complications include corneal deposits, visual disturbances, thyroid dysfunction, ataxia, pulmonary fibrosis, elevated liver enzymes, and proarrythmogenic effects including torsades de pointes. The sympatholytic effects of amiodarone may be enhanced by the volatile anesthetics, resulting in significant hypotension during intravenous administration. Interactions with halothane and lidocaine have been reported to produce sinus arrest.[105] Case reports have described hypotension and bradycardia that are resistant to ordinary doses of vasopressors that have developed during anesthesia.[143,144] Temporary pacing should be readily available in patients chronically receiving amiodarone who need a general anesthetic.

Amiodarone interferes with the metabolism of digitalis, warfarin, and several antidysrhythmic drugs such as quinidine, procainamide, and DPH. Amiodarone has an extremely long half-life of 25 to 110 days. Therapeutic levels are achieved only slowly with oral administration, averaging around 10 days.[105]

Sotalol is an orally administered antidysrhythmic drug that prolongs repolarization (class III) and has β-adrenergic blocking (class II) activity. It is used primarily for life-threatening ventricular dysrhythmias.[145] Although not approved for the treatment of supraventricular dysrhythmias, sotalol has been shown to suppress supraventricular tachycardias and atrial fibrillation. Sotalol is a nonselective β-blocker without intrinsic sympathomimetic or local anesthetic activity. It slows the heart rate and prolongs the QT interval with no effect on QRS duration.

Sotalol appears to be better tolerated than amiodarone. It has the usual contraindications to nonselective β-blockade and the same adverse effects including fatigue, bradycardia, dyspnea, and increased airway reactivity. The most serious complication is that of torsades de pointes, which can be seen in 5% of patients taking high doses. For this reason, diuretics that induce hypokalemia and drugs that prolong the QT interval should be used cautiously in patients taking sotalol. The concomitant administration of sotalol with phenothiazines, tricyclic antidepressants, and terfenadine (Seldane) has been associated with the development of torsades de pointes.

Class IV Drugs

The class IV drugs include the Ca^{2+} channel blockers. Ca^{2+} channel blockers, a heterogenous group of drugs with dissimilar structures, electrophysiologic properties, and pharmacologic properties, are not therapeutically interchangeable. Alteration of slow channel kinetics could be expected to produce vasodilation, depression of conduction velocity, contractility, and heart rate. All Ca^{2+} blockers tested do this but with varying degrees of potency in the intact human (Table 31–7). The Ca^{2+} channel blockers, of which there are many,[8,128] do not interact in the subcellular activity of Ca^{2+} but interact with cell membranes to inhibit the inward Ca^{2+} current. Extensive reviews of this valuable class of drugs are available.[146–148]

The pharmacologic and electrophysiologic properties of verapamil are strikingly different from the other antidysrhythmic drugs. Verapamil is the only Ca^{2+} channel inhibitor with significant antidysrhythmic activity that is

TABLE 31–7
Autonomic Effects of Calcium Entry Blockers in Intact Man

	Verapamil	Diltiazem	Nifedipine	Nicarpidine
Negative inotropic	+	0/+	0	0
Negative chronotropic	+	0/+	0	0
Negative dromotropic	++++	+++	0	0
Coronary vasodilation	++	+++	++++	++++
Systemic vasodilation	++	++	++++	++++
Bronchodilation	0/+	0	0/+	0

available intravenously. Other calcium channel antagonists are available for intravenous use (i.e., nicardipine) but are devoid of any useful antidysrhythmic activity and are primarily vasodilators. Diltiazem, although available for intravenous administration, has limited antidysrhythmic activity.

Verapamil does not alter the action potential upstroke in fibers whose RMP is more negative than −60 mV (i.e., fast action potentials).[116] It slows or prevents depolarization in cardiac tissue with an RMP less negative than −50 mV (i.e., calcium-dependent upstroke). The electrophysiologic effects of verapamil are seen predominantly in the SA and AV nodes in which phase 0 and spontaneous phase 4 depolarization are calcium dependent. Verapamil decreases the slope of spontaneous depolarization and reduces the action potential in the pacemakers. It prolongs conduction and increases the refractory period of the AV node. Verapamil prolongs the anterograde conduction velocity of the AV node, but has no effect on retrograde AV conduction.[105] Therefore, it has profound effects on pacemaker cells, which depend on the Ca^{2+} current for depolarization. A dose-dependent increase in the PR and AV interval is produced on the ECG, a quinidine-like effect similar to that produced by class IA drugs, which are also effective for supraventricular dysrhythmias. In contrast to procainamide, verapamil does not increase the QT interval, since it lacks activity on the sodium-dependent action potentials.

Verapamil is most effective in terminating supraventricular tachydysrhythmias (Table 31–5 and 31–6). Nearly all forms of supraventricular tachydysrhythmias are caused by re-entry using either the SA or AV node as part of the circuit.[96] Verapamil terminates these dysrhythmias by decreasing nodal conductivity and converting the unidirectional block of re-entry to a bidirectional block. In this regard, its action on supraventricular dysrhythmias is similar to that of procainamide on ventricular re-entry dysrhythmias. Verapamil has become a first-line drug for the rapid conversion of supraventricular tachydysrhythmias. The incidence of successful termination of PAT in adults approaches 90%. It is also effective in treating atrial fibrillation/flutter with conversion to a sinus rhythm (30%) or slowing of the ventricular response. The ventricular rate slows as a result of decreased conduction velocity through the AV node, even when conversion is not produced.

Caution must be exercised in treating patients when the underlying cause of the atrial tachycardia, fibrillation, or flutter is the WPW syndrome. An accessory bypass tract lying near the AV node participates in the re-entry of these tachydysrhythmias. Verapamil may terminate the tachydysrhythmia by its specific depressant effects on the AV node if the re-entrant conduction is anterograde from above through the AV node and retrograde via the accessory pathway. However, if the SVT is anterograde over the accessory pathway, in which verapamil has no effect, and retrograde through the AV node, verapamil may increase conduction velocity in the accessory tract and increase heart rate. This is particularly dangerous if atrial flutter or fibrillation is associated with the WPW syndrome, as ventricular fibrillation can be induced.[149]

Recent studies further support the hypothesis that Ca^{2+} participates directly in the genesis of ventricular dysrhythmias.[34,116,150] When sodium channels are inactivated by hypoxia, stretch, or hyperkalemia, the remaining Ca^{2+} current can produce a depolarizing current in these abnormal cells, especially in the presence of catecholamines. The conversion of a fast response cell to a cell with slow response characteristics provides all the necessary ingredients for the re-entry phenomenon: slow depolarization and delayed conduction. The resulting ventricular dysrhythmias can usually be terminated with one of the class I drugs as long as the RMP of the slow response is between −80 and −60 mV (Fig. 31–16). Verapamil has been effective in terminating ventricular tachycardias and premature depolarizations in about two thirds of the treatment trials when other drugs have failed. The RMP of these abnormal "slow response" foci has been postulated to be less negative than −60 mV; this is a range where lidocaine would be ineffective on the calcium current conduction and depolarization. More information is needed before recommendations can be made for verapamil in treating dysrhythmias other than supraventricular tachydysrhythmias. Other drugs remain significantly more effective for the initial treatment of ventricular dysrhythmias. Verapamil is not effective for most patients with sustained or recurrent VT and can be lethal in wide-complex VT[108] (see discussion of adenosine, below).

The important side effects of verapamil are directly related to its cardiovascular effects. Verapamil, valued for its specific antidysrhythmic activity, combines arteriolar dilatation with a direct negative inotropic effect. The hypotensive effects of intravenous verapamil peak at about 5 minutes, lasting for 10 to 12 minutes. However, its effects on nodal tissue can last for up to 6 hours.[106] It has also been shown to have local anesthetic activity slightly greater than that of procaine on an equimolar basis.[151] The significance of this observation in

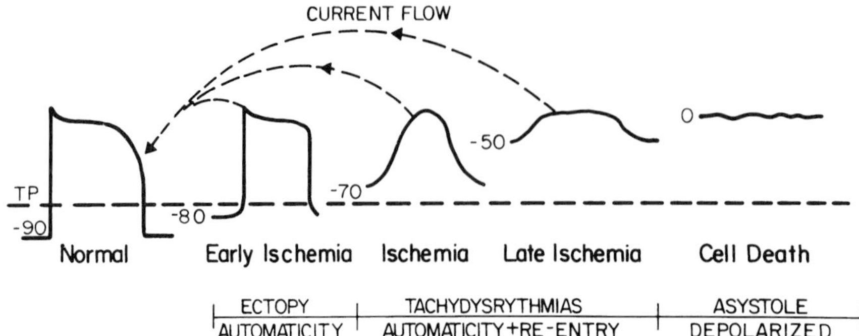

FIGURE **31–16.** Action potentials can undergo rapid degenerative transformation in a short period of time. The conventional ECG cannot determine the degree of degeneration, but only that a dysrhythmia is present. This may account for the varying degrees of success of a given drug for a given dysrhythmia. (From Lawson NW, Meyer DJ: Autonomic nervous system physiology and pharmacology. In Barash PG, Cullen BF, Stoelting RK [eds]: Clinical Anesthesia. Philadelphia, WB Saunders Co, 1996, p 253, with permission.)

man has not been established. It may produce unwanted AV conduction delays and bradycardia resulting in cardiovascular collapse.

Verapamil must be used cautiously in the presence of propranolol, since both inhibit Ca^{2+} influx. The combined effect can produce complete heart block and significant negative inotropic effects. It should be used carefully in digitalized patients for the same reason (synergistic negative dromotropic effects). Halothane also depresses slow channel conductance and may interact in a similar manner with verapamil.[8,102,152]

Verapamil has no adverse effects on bronchomotor tone and may be selected over propranolol in patients with altered airway reactivity. It should be avoided in patients with sick sinus syndrome, AV block, or heart failure. However, if the heart failure is the result of a supraventricular tachycardia, verapamil may be indicated.

Unclassified Antidysrhythmic Drugs

Although the digitalis glycosides have been used for over two centuries, their mechanism of action remains unclear. Digitalis enhances inotropy by inhibition of the membrane-bound Na^+/K^+–dependent ATPase. Inhibition of the Na^+ pump increases intracellular Na^+, which enhances Ca^{2+} influx, resulting in increased cytosolic Ca^{2+}. However, this mechanism does not explain all of the beneficial effects of digitalis. The autonomic nervous system is also involved in both the therapeutic and toxic effects of digitalis. Digitalis enhances the PNS and inhibits the sympathetic nervous system, resulting in sinus slowing and inhibition of AV nodal conduction.[108] It increases the slope of phase 4 depolarization and decreases the resting potential so that depolarization begins at a less negative RMP. The effect is to slow conduction velocity. Hypokalemia enhances the rate of phase 4 depolarization and automaticity.

Three forms of intravenous digitalis are available: digoxin, ouabain, and deslanoside. Digoxin is the most often used digitalis preparation for rapid digitalization. The three forms vary in their onset of action. Ouabain has the fastest onset of action (3 to 10 minutes), and a peak effect at 30 minutes following IV administration. Digoxin's onset is within 5 to 30 minutes after an IV dose. Deslanoside is the slowest, reaching a peak effect at 2 to 3 hours after an IV dose.

The principal uses of digitalis glycoside are (1) the treatment of congestive heart failure and (2) the control of ventricular rate secondary to supraventricular tachydysrhythmias. Digitalis enhances myocardial contractility and automaticity but slows impulse propagation through the conduction tissues. The most solid indication for chronic oral digitalis therapy is the combination of chronic congestive heart failure (CHF) with atrial fibrillation. In this setting, it may be used in combination with verapamil or β-adrenergic blocking agents. It remains useful in the operating room to control or convert supraventricular tachydysrhythmias that may or may not be related to heart failure. Historically, patients undergoing thoracic surgery were often digitalized because of the high frequency of cardiac dysrhythmias. Richie et al.[153] confirmed this observation and noted a 37% incidence of dysrhythmias after thoracic surgery and an even higher incidence after pneumonectomy. However, their study of 140 patients failed to show any benefit for prophylactic digitalization. The frequency of dysrhythmias was similar in digitalized and controlled patients.

Despite its efficacy in controlling the ventricular response in the presence of supraventricular tachyarrythmias, the indications for digitalis, particularly in the operating room, are decreasing.[154] Its therapeutic-toxicity ratio is very narrow. Better inotropic drugs are available for acute failure that are less toxic and may be stopped immediately if an untoward side effect should occur. The serum half-life of digoxin is 1.5 days compared to 2 minutes for dobutamine. The introduction of better diuretics and oral vasodilators has lessened the need for digitalis in heart failure with sinus rhythm. Verapamil, adenosine, or β-blockers are perhaps more efficacious for the acute treatment of supraventricular tachydysrhythmias not related to heart failure.

Prior to its use in the perioperative setting, the following factors should be considered:

1. Acute digitalization in the unstable patient may cause dysrhythmias.

2. Potassium balance in critically ill surgical patients is unstable. Therapeutic levels of digoxin may quickly become toxic.
3. Any dysrhythmia that ensues in the presence of digitalis must be considered to be related to digitalis toxicity until proven otherwise.
4. Digitalis dysrhythmias are more difficult to treat.
5. Reduced renal clearance can induce toxicity with "usual" doses.
6. Cardioversion is more likely to precipitate ventricular arrhythmias and fibrillation after acute digitalization.
7. Should initial digitalization fail, the use of alternative drugs may be more complicated because of interactions of these agents with digoxin.

Adenosine has been available for more than 50 years, but has been recognized only recently as a clinically useful drug (Table 31–6). It is a by-product of ATP, is found in every cell in the body, and is composed of adenine and a pentose sugar. Its production can be increased by stimuli such as hypoxia and ischemia.[155] It can combine with one, two, or three phosphates to form AMP, ADP, or ATP. This ubiquitous nucleoside has potent electrophysiologic effects in addition to having a major role in regulation of vasomotor tone. Adenosine is believed to have a cardioprotective effect by regulating oxygen supply and demand. The cardiovascular effects of adenosine depend upon which of two receptor sites are activated: $adenosine_1$ or $adenosine_2$.[155–157] The $adenosine_1$ receptors in the myocardial conduction system are the most sensitive and mediate SA node slowing and AV nodal conduction delay. The $adenosine_1$ receptor inhibits production of cAMP, whose formation is stimulated by β-adrenergic activity. The $adenosine_2$ smooth muscle receptor requires a higher concentration of adenosine for activation. It mediates systemic and coronary vasodilatation.

The $adenosine_2$ receptor directly increases the rate of formation of cAMP, functioning independently of β-adrenergic activity. Intravenous adenosine has significant negative chronotropic effects on the SA node as well as negative dromotropic effects on the AV node. Adenosine regulates atrial and ventricular rates independent of each other.

Adenosine hyperpolarizes atrial myocytes and decreases their action potential duration via an increase in outward K^+ current. These are the ACh-regulated K^+ channels.[156] Adenosine, like acetylcholine, has an extremely short plasma half-life of only seconds. Adenosine also antagonizes the inward Ca^{2+} current produced by catecholamines. This antidysrhythmic mechanism of Ca^{2+} channel blockade is thought to be an indirect effect and important only when β-adrenergic stimulation is present. This trait suggests a possible role in countering catecholamine-induced dysrhythmias. In this regard, adenosine exhibits some of the characteristics of a class IV antidysrhythmic. However, the primary antidysrhythmic effect of adenosine is to interrupt re-entrant AV nodal tachycardia through its effects on the K^+ current.

The major indication for adenosine is in the termination of supraventricular tachyarrythmias. Paroxysmal supraventricular tachycardia (PSVT) refers to a broad category of narrow-complex tachycardias with acute onset and cessation. The most common forms are AV nodal re-entry tachycardia and AV reciprocating tachycardia. PSVT accounts for about one third of all cases of perioperative dysrhythmias. Clinical studies support the use of adenosine for the treatment of tachycardias in WPW syndrome and other re-entrant tachycardias involving the AV node.[158]

The same characteristics that make adenosine an effective therapeutic agent may also make it an ideal agent for diagnosing other types of dysrhythmias. The incidence of incorrect diagnosis of supraventricular dysrhythmias has been reported to be as high as 15% using conventional means.[159] For example, a wide-complex tachycardia can either be a VT or an SVT with aberrant conduction. Verapamil can be fatal if the dysrhythmia is VT because the drug is long-lasting.[108,160] However, the fleeting action (9 to 10 seconds) of adenosine ensures that no harm will be done if the broad complex is of ventricular origin, providing a combined therapeutic and diagnostic test. Adenosine will stop SVT in 90% of cases in which the AV node forms one of the limbs of the re-entrant circuit, such as AV reciprocating tachycardia and AV nodal re-entry dysrhythmias.[157] However, adenosine has no effect on ectopic atrial dysrhythmias such as ectopic foci, multifocal SVT, or atrial flutter/fibrillation.[96] Approximately 10% of SVTs do not involve AV nodal re-entry. Adenosine will, nevertheless, slow AV nodal conduction in these cases, decrease the ventricular rate, and allow inspection of the P waves. Thus, adenosine may be useful in unmasking atrial fibrillation when fast ventricular responses are noted.

A number of side effects have been reported with adenosine including flushing, headache, dyspnea, bronchospasm, and chest pain. The majority of these are very brief (seconds) and not clinically significant. Transient, new dysrhythmias (65%) may be noted at the time of cardioversion. However, these are generally transient, disappearing within the half-life of the drug. Major hemodynamic changes are rare, but consist of hypotension and bradycardia. Adenosine should be given by a rapid intravenous bolus with a flush because of its extremely short half-life of less than 10 seconds. The initial adult dose is 6 mg (100 to 150 μg/kg in children). This can be followed by 12 mg within 1 to 2 minutes if the initial dose is without an effect.[159] The 12-mg dose may be repeated once. Higher doses may be required in patients receiving methylxanthines such as aminophylline, since these drugs are competitive antagonists at the adenosine receptors.

General Approach to the Management of Dysrhythmias

The recent literature on acute and chronic therapy of dysrhythmias indicates a high degree of uncertainty as well as a rapid evolution of knowledge in this area.[161,162] Dysrhythmia formation should be considered a dynamic event. Action potentials can rapidly undergo transformation ranging from normal, to increasing automaticity, to complete depolarization (asystole) in a short period of time (Fig. 31–16). The ECG in the operating room cannot determine the degree of degeneration of an action potential and only indicates that a particular dysrhythmia(s) is (are) present. Prior to instituting pharmacologic therapy, aggravating factors must be ruled out and treated including increased sympathetic or vagal stimulation from inadequate anesthesia, hypoxemia, hypercarbia, and myocardial ischemia. Electrolyte imbalances, especially hypokalemia and hypomagnesemia, should be treated.

The pharmacologic approach to dysrhythmia therapy remains empiric.[28] Drug selection depends upon the specific dysrhythmia, the usual response to that drug, the patient's condition, the urgency, and the circumstances in which the dysrhythmias occur.[38,104,105] Serious supraventricular tachycardias such as atrial fibrillation, flutter, and intra-atrial tachycardias are all re-entrant phenomena contained within the atria. Conduction of these arrhythmias through the AV node will alter the ventricular rate response, but will not affect the basic arrhythmia. Accessory pathways present another common form of macro re-entrant SVT. Typically, the re-entrant circuit is from the node and retrograde up the bypass tract (orthodromic). Less commonly, the circuit is retrograde or antidromic. Knowledge of the critical sites of abnormal impulse propagation for SVTs are not within the current capabilities of conventional operating room monitoring. However, class IA drugs slow atrial myocardial or accessory pathway conduction and class III agents are effective in treating re-entrant SVTs that use the atrial re-entrant circuit. Dysrhythmias originating or using the AV node as a limb of the re-entrant circuit are susceptible to the effects of class II (β-adrenergic blocking) agents and class IV agents (calcium channel blockers). Some class III agents are also useful in this type of dysrhythmia. Even if the dysrhythmia does not involve the AV node, β-adrenergic antagonists, calcium channel blockers, digitalis, and adenosine will slow the ventricular response to SVT even though they may not alter the primary dysrhythmia.

Combinations of antidysrhythmic agents are increasingly used in treating both supraventricular and ventricular dysrhythmias with the supposition that added potency may be achieved while minimizing the side effects of either drug.[108] This is a similar proposition to that of combining various vasodilators and inotropic agents to achieve hemodynamic fine tuning.[8] A useful guide in the acute situation is to avoid combining agents of the same class or subclass. The overlap of action by some drugs (Table 31–3), produces potentially additive side effects and should be combined with great care. An example would be the combination of a class IA drug with a class III drug, both of which prolong the QT interval increasing the susceptibility to torsades de pointes. These rules do not always apply, especially in the treatment of chronic dysrhythmias, which is outside the scope of this treatise. Antidysrhythmic "rule-breaking" combinations found useful in the chronic situation include the concomitant use of quinidine and procainamide, mexiletine with propranolol, and quinidine and verapamil, just to name a few.

References

1. Atlee JL: Cardiac dysrhythmias and anesthesia: Perspectives. In Atlee JL (ed): Perioperative Cardiac Dysrhythmias. Chicago, Year Book Medical Publishers, 1985, p 1.
2. Forrest JB, Rehder K, Cahalan MK, Goldsmith CH: Multicenter study of general anesthesia III: Predictors of severe perioperative adverse outcomes. Anesthesiology 76:3, 1992.
3. James TN: Anatomy of the human sinus node. Anat Rec 141: 109, 1961.
4. James TN: Cardiac innervation: Anatomic and pharmacologic relations. Bull NY Acad Med 43:1041, 1967.
5. Berne RM, Levy MN: Control of the heart. In Berne RM, Levy MN (eds): Cardiovascular Physiology. St Louis, CV Mosby Co, 1977, p 155.
6. Atlee JL: Normal electrical activity of the heart. In Atlee JL (ed): Perioperative Cardiac Dysrhythmias: Mechanisms and Recognition Management. Chicago, Year Book Medical Publishers, 1985, p 16.
7. DeGeest H, Levy MN, Zieske H, Lipman RI: Depression of ventricular contractility by stimulation of the vagus nerves. Circ Res 17:222, 1965.
8. Lawson NW, Meyer DJ: Autonomic nervous system physiology and pharmacology. In Barash PG, Cullen BF, Stoelting RK (eds): Clinical Anesthesia, 1996, p 253.
9. Flacke WE, Flacke JW: Cholinergic and anticholinergic agents. In Smith NT, Corbascio AN (eds): Drug Interaction in Anesthesia. Philadelphia, Lea & Febiger, 1986, p 160.
10. Herre JM, et al: Effect of transmural vs. non-transmural myocardial infarction on inducibility of ventricular arrhythmias during sympathetic stimulation in dogs. J Am Coll Cardiol 11:414, 1988.
11. Prys-Roberts C: New developments in adrenergic pharmacology. Curr Opin Anaesthesiol 4:111, 1991.
12. Prys-Roberts C: The changing face of adrenergic pharmacology. Curr Opin Anaesthesiol 5:113, 1992.
13. Goldberg LI: The role of dopamine receptors in the treatment of congestive heart failure. J Cardiovasc Pharmacol 14(Suppl 5): 521, 1989.
14. Van Zweiten PA: The role of adrenoreceptors in circulatory and metabolic regulation. Am Heart J 116(part 2):1384, 1988.
15. Insell PA: Structure and function of α-adrenergic receptors. Am J Med 87(Suppl):12S, 1989.
16. Moreland RS, Bohr DF: Adrenergic control of coronary arteries. Fed Proc 43:2857, 1984.
17. Cohen RA, Shepard JT, Vanhoutte PM: Effects of the adrenergic transmitter on epicardial coronary arteries. Fed Proc 43:2862, 1984.
18. Griggs DM, Chilian WM, Boatwright RB, et al: Evidence against significant resting α-adrenergic coronary vasoconstrictor tone. Fed Proc 43:2873, 1984.
19. Schmitz W, Kohl J, Neumann J, et al: On the mechanism of positive inotropic effects of alpha-adrenoreceptor agonists. Basic Res Cardiol 84(Suppl 1):23, 1989.
20. Corr PB, Heathers GP, Yamada KA: Mechanisms contributing to the arrhythmogenic influences of α_1-adrenergic stimulation in the ischemic heart. Am J Med 87(Suppl 2A):19S, 1989.
21. Timmermans PB, Van Zweiten PA: α_2-adrenoreceptors: Classification, localization, mechanisms and target for drugs. J Med Chem 25:1390, 1982.
22. Murdock CJ, Hickey GM, Hockings BE, et al: Effect of α_1-adrenoreceptor blockade on ventricular ectopic beats in acute myocardial infarction. Int J Cardiol 26:45, 1990.
23. Osnes JB, Aass H, Skomedal T: Adrenoreceptors in myocardial regulation: Concomitant contribution from both α- and β-adrenoreceptor stimulation to the inotropic response. Basic Res Cardiol 84(Suppl):9, 1989.
24. Bohm M, Diet F, Feiler G, et al: α Adrenoreceptors and α-adrenoreceptor-mediated positive inotropic effects in the failing human myocardium. J Cardiovasc Pharmacol 12:357, 1988.
25. Summers RJ, Molnaar P, Russell F, et al: Coexistence and localization of β_1- and β_2-adrenoreceptors in the human heart. Eur Heart J 10(Suppl B):11, 1989.
26. Prichard BNC, Owens CWI, Smith CCT, Walden RJ: Heart and catecholamines. Acta Cardiol (XLVI) 3:309, 1991.

27. Brodde OE: Pathophysiology of the beta adrenoreceptor system in chronic heart failure: Consequences for treatment with agonists, partial agonists, or antagonists? Eur Heart J 12(Suppl F): 54, 1991.
28. Woosley RL: Antiarrhythmic drugs. Ann Rev Pharmacol Toxicol 31:427, 1991.
29. Solomon RJ, Katz JD: Disturbances of potassium homeostasis. In Stoelting RK, Barash PG, Gallagher TJ (eds): Advances in Anesthesia. Chicago, Year Book Medical Publishers, 1986, p 169.
30. Zipes DP: Genesis of cardiac arrhythmias: Electrophysiological considerations. In Braunwald E (ed): Heart Disease. Philadelphia, WB Saunders Co, 1988, p 581.
31. Wit AL, Bigger JT Jr: Possible electrophysiological mechanisms for lethal arrhythmias accompanying myocardial ischemia and infarction. Circulation 52(Suppl 3):96, 1975.
32. Wit AL, Rosen MR, Hoffman BF: Electrophysiology and pharmacology of cardiac arrhythmias: Relationship of normal and abnormal electrical activity of cardiac fibers to the genesis of arrhythmias: Re-entry. Am Heart J 88:664, 1974.
33. Fozzard HA: Electrophysiology of the heart: The effects of ischemia. Hosp Pract 15:61, 1980.
34. Conterato JP, White RD: Mechanisms, diagnosis, and treatment of cardiac arrhythmias. In Tarhan S (ed): Cardiovascular Anesthesia and Postoperative Care. Chicago, Year Book Medical Publishers, 1989, p 439.
35. Zipes DP, Martins JB, Ruffy R, et al: Roles of autonomic innervation in the genesis of ventricular arrhythmias. In Disturbances of Neurogenic Control of the Circulation. Washington, DC, American Physiological Society, 1981, p 225.
36. Scherf D, Choi KH, Bahadori A, et al: Parasystole. Am J Cardiol 12:527, 1963.
37. Bigger JT: Electrical properties of cardiac muscle and possible causes of cardiac arrhythmias. In Dreifus LS, Likoff W (eds): Cardiac Arrhythmias. New York, Grune & Stratton, 1973, p 13.
38. Davis RF: Etiology and treatment of perioperative cardiac arrhythmias. In Kaplan J (ed): Cardiac Anesthesia. Philadelphia, WB Saunders Co, 1993, p 170.
39. Atlee JL: Abnormal electrical activity of the heart. In Atlee JL (ed): Perioperative Cardiac Dysrhythmias: Mechanisms, Recognition, Management. Chicago, Year Book Medical Publishers, 1990, p 57.
40. Lucas WJ, Maccioli GA, Mueller RA: Advances in oral antiarrhythmic therapy: Implications for the anaesthetist. Can J Anaesth 37:94, 1990.
41. Allessie MA, Bouke FIM, Schopman FJG: Circus movements in rabbit atrial muscle as a mechanism of tachycardia. Circ Res 41:8, 1977.
42. White RD: Mechanisms of cardiac dysrhythmias. EMT J 4:62, 1980.
43. Rogers M, Zakha KG, Nugent S, et al: Electrocardiographic abnormalities in infants and children with neurological injury. Crit Care Med 8:213, 1980.
44. Rogers M, Abildskov JA, Preston JB: Neurogenic ECG changes in critically ill patients: An experimental model. Crit Care Med 1:192, 1973.
45. Samra SK, Kroll DA: Subarachnoid hemorrhage and intraoperative electrocardiographic changes simulating myocardial ischemia: Anesthesiologist's dilemma. Anesth Analg 64:86, 1985.
46. Bedell SE, Aronson MD: Late development of electrocardiographic abnormalities after a stroke. South Med J 78:218, 1985.
47. Greenspahn BR, Barzilai B, Denes P: Electrocardiographic changes in concussion. Chest 74:468, 1978.
48. Katz RL: Epstein RA: The interaction of anesthetic agents and adrenergic drugs to produce cardiac arrhythmias. Anesthesiology 29:763, 1968.
49. Kroll DA, Knight PR: Antifibrillatory effects of volatile anesthetics in acute occlusion/reperfusion arrhythmias. Anesthesiology 61:657, 1984.
50. Atlee JL, Rusy BF: Halothane depression of AV conduction studied by electrograms of the bundle of His in dogs. Anesthesiology 36:112, 1972.
51. Lynch C, Vogel S, Sperelakis N: Halothane depression of myocardial slow-action potentials. Anesthesiology 45:360, 1981.
52. Bosnjak ZJ, Kampine JP: Effects of halothane on transmembrane potentials, Ca++ transients, and papillary muscle in the cat. Am J Physiol 251:H374, 1986.
53. Awalt CH, Frederickson EL: The contractile and cell membrane effects of halothane. Anesthesiology 25:A90, 1964.
54. Hauswirth O, Shaer H: Effects of halothane on the sino-atrial node. J Pharmacol Exp Ther 158:36, 1967.
55. Lynch C: Differential depression of myocardial contractility by halothane and isoflurane in the guinea pig papillary muscle. Anesthesiology 64:620, 1986.
56. Maze M, Smith CM: Identification of receptor mechanism mediating epinphrine-induced arrhythmias during halothane anesthesia in the dog. Anesthesiology 59:322, 1983.
57. Maze M, Hayward E, Gaba DM: Alpha-adrenergic blockade raises epinephrine-arrhythmia threshold in halothane anesthetized dogs in a dose-dependent fashion. Anesthesiology 63:611, 1985.
58. Kapur PA, Flacke WE: Epinephrine-induced arrhythmias and cardiovascular function after verapamil during halothane anesthesia in the dog. Anesthesiology 55:218, 1981.
59. Joas TA, Stevens WC: Comparison of the arrhythmic doses of epinephrine during isoflurane, halothane, and fluroxene anesthesia in dogs. Anesthesiology 35:48, 1971.
60. Johnston RR, Eger EI, Wilson C: A comparative interaction of epinephrine with enflurane, isoflurane, and halothane in man. Anesth Analg 55:709, 1976.
61. Karl HW, Swedlow DB, Lee KW, et al: Epinephrine halothane interactions in children. Anesthesiology 58:142, 1983.
62. Wood M: Drugs and the sympathetic nervous system. In Wood M, Wood AJ (eds): Drugs and Anesthesia. Baltimore, Williams & Wilkins, 1982.
63. Stirt JA, Berger JM, Ricker SM, et al: Arrhythmogenic effects of aminophylline during halothane anesthesia in experimental animals. Anesth Analg 59:410, 1980.
64. Stirt JA, Berger JM, Sullivan SF: Lack of arrhythmogenicity of isoflurane following administration of aminophylline in dogs. Anesth Analg 62:568, 1983.
65. Moir DC, Dingwall-Fordyce I, Weir RD: A follow-up study of cardiac patients receiving amitriptyline. Eur J Clin Pharmacol 6: 98, 1973.
66. Thompson TL, Moran MG, Nies AS: Psychotropis drug use in the elderly. N Engl J Med 308:194, 1983.
67. Edwards RP, Miller RD, Roizen MF, et al: Cardiac responses to imipramine and pancuronium during anesthetic with halothane or enflurane. Anesthesiology 50:421, 1979.
68. Atlee JL: Halothane. Cause or cure for arrhythmias? (Editorial). Anesthesiology 67:617, 1987.
69. Carpenter RL, Mackey DC: Local Anesthetics. In Barash PG, Cullen BF, Stoelting RK (eds): Clinical Anesthesia. Philadelphia, JB Lippincott Co, 1992, p 509.
70. Covino BG: Toxicity of local anesthetics. In Stoelting RK, Barash PG, Gallagher TJ (eds): Advances in Anesthesia. Chicago, Year Book Medical Publishers, 1986, p 37.
71. Clarkson CW, Hondeghen LM: Mechanism for bupivacaine depression of cardiac conduction. Anesthesiology 62:396, 1985.
72. Josephson I, Sperelakis N: Local anesthetic blockade of Ca^{++}-mediated action potentials in cardiac muscle. Eur J Pharmacol 40:201, 1976.
73. Sugimoto T, Schaal SF, Dunn NM, et al: Electrophysiologic effects of lidocaine in awake dogs. J Pharmacol Exp Ther 166: 146, 1969.
74. Dunbar RW, Boettner RB, Gatz RN, et al: The effect of mepivicaine, bupivicaine, and lidocaine on digitalis-induced ventricular arrhythmias. Anesth Analg 49:761, 1970.
75. Chapin JC, Kushins LG, Munson ES, et al: Lidocaine, bupivacaine, etidocaine, and epinephrine-induced arrhythmias during halothane anesthesia in dogs. Anesthesiology 52:23, 1980.
76. Albright GA: Cardiac arrest following regional anesthesia with etidocaine or bupivacaine. Anesthesiology 51:285, 1979.
77. Heavner JE: Cardiac dysrhythmias induced by infusion of local anesthetics into the lateral cerebral ventricle of the cat. Anesth Analg 65:133, 1986.
78. Tangedahi TN, Gan GT: Myocardial irritability associated with lithium carbonate therapy. N Engl J Med 287:867, 1972.
79. Springman SR, Atlee JL: The etiology of intraoperative arrhythmias. In Thomas SJ (ed): Diagnosis and Management of Intra-

operative Arrhythmias. Anesthesiol Clin of North Am 7:293, 1989.
80. Ray CT: Water and electrolyte balance. In Sodeman WA, Sodeman WA Jr (eds): Pathologic Physiology, 4th ed. Philadelphia, WB Saunders Co, 1967, p 109.
81. Hirsch IA, Tomlinson DL, Slogoff S, Keats AS: The overstated risk of preoperative hypokalemia. Anesth Analg 67:131, 1988.
82. Vitez TS, Soper LE, Wong KC, Soper P: Chronic hypokalemia and intraoperative dysrhythmias. Anesthesiology 63:130, 1985.
83. Surawicz B: The interrelationship of electrolyte abnormalities and arrhythmias. In Cardiac Arrhythmias: Their Mechanisms, Diagnosis and Management, 2nd ed. Philadelphia, JB Lippincott, 1987, p 96.
84. Solomon R: Ventricular arrhythmias in patients with myocardial infarction and ischemia: Relationship to serum potassium and magnesium. Drugs 28(Suppl 1):66, 1984.
85. Madias JE, Madia NE: Hypokalemia: New insights into ventricular ectopy. Hosp. Physician 12:53, 1986.
86. Zaloga GP, Chernow B: Calcium, magnesium and other minerals. In Chernow B, Lake CR (eds): The Pharmacologic Approach to the Critically Ill Patient. Baltimore, Williams & Wilkins, 1983, p 530.
87. Zaloga GP, Prough DS: Fluids and electrolytes. In Barash PG, Cullen BF, Stoelting RK (ed): Clinical Anesthesia. Philadelphia, JB Lippincott Co, 1992, p 203.
88. Busch EH, Ventura HO, Lavie CJ: Heparin-induced hyperkalemia. South Med J 80:1450, 1987.
89. Mokhtar S, et al: Fatal arrhythmias related to alkalosis in patients with acute myocardial infarction. Circulation 54(Suppl II): 132 1976.
90. Lawson NW, Butler GH, Ray CT: Alklosis and cardiac arrhythmias. Anesth Analg 52:951, 1973.
91. Edwards R, Winnie AP, Ramamurphy S: Acute hypocapneic hypokalemia: An iatrogenic anesthesia complication. Anesth Analg 56:786, 1977.
92. Surawicz B: Relationship between electrocardiogram and electrolytes. Am Heart J 73:814, 1967.
93. New W: Cellular mechanisms: A clinical view. In Ream AK, Fogdall R (eds): Acute Cardiovascular Management. Philadelphia, JB Lippincott Co, 1982, p 45.
94. Prielipp R, Zaloga GP: Calcium action and general anesthesia. Adv Anesth 8:241, 1991.
95. Wills MD: Magnesium and potassium: Interrelationships in cardiac disorders. Drugs 31(Suppl 4):121, 1986.
96. Kastor JA: Multifocal atrial tachycardia. N Engl J Med 322: 1713, 1990.
97. England MR, Gordon G, Salem M, Chernow B: Magnesium administration and dysrhythmias after cardiac surgery. JAMA 268:2395, 1992.
98. Gambling DR, Birmingham CL, Jenkins LC: Magnesium and the anaesthetist. Can J Anaesth 35:644, 1988.
99. Boriss MN, Papa L: Magnesium: A discussion of its role in the treatment of ventricular dysrhythmia. Crit Care Med 16:292, 1988.
100. Matz R: Magnesium: Deficiencies and therapeutic uses. Hosp Pract 28:79, 1993.
101. Ochsner JL, Lawson NW, Mills NL, et al: Technique of deep hypothermia and circulatory arrest in the neonate and infant. South Med J 69:607, 1976.
102. Lawson NW, Kraynack, BJ Gintautas J: Neuromuscular and electrocardiographic responses to verapamil in dogs. Anesth Analg 62:50, 1983.
103. Williams GD, Seifen AB, Lawson NW, et al: Pulsatile perfusion vs conventional high flow nonpulsatile perfusion for rapid core cooling and rewarming of infants for circulatory arrest in cardiac surgery. J Thorac Cardiovasc Surg, 1979.
104. Atlee JA: Management of specific cardiac dysrhythmias. In Atlee JA (ed): Perioperative Cardiac Dysrhythmias. Chicago, Year Book Medical Publishers, 1985, p 380.
105. Davies LK, Davis RF: Pharmacologic treatment of arrhythmias. In Thomas SJ (ed): Diagnosis and Management of Intraoperative Arrhythmias. Anesthesiol Clin North Am 7:421, 1989.
106. Vaughan Williams EM: Classification of cardiac antiarrhythmic drugs. In Sandoe E, Flensted-Jensen E, Olesen K (eds): Symposium on Cardiac Arrhythmias. Sodertalje, Sweden, AB Astra, 1970, p 449.
107. Vaughan Williams EM: A classification of antiarrhythmic actions reassessed after a decade of new drugs. J Clin Pharmacol 24: 129, 1984.
108. Opie LH: Antiarrhythmic Agents. In Opie LH (ed): Drugs for the Heart. Philadelphia, WB Saunders Co, 1991, p 180.
109. Abramowicz M: Moricizine for cardiac arrhythmias. Med Newslett 32:99, 1990.
110. Kupersmith J, Antman EM, Hoffman BF: In vivo electrophysiological effects of lidocaine in canine acute myocardial infarction. Circ Res 36:84, 1975.
111. Constant J: Preventing sudden death by raising the fibrillation threshold: A review (part I). Resident Physician 37:33, 1991.
112. Basset AL, Hoffman BF: Antiarrhythmic drugs: Electrophysiologic action. Annu Rev Pharmacol 11:143, 1971.
113. MacMahon S, Collins R, Peto R, et al: Effects of prophylactic lidocaine in suspected acute myocardial infarction. JAMA 260: 1910, 1988.
114. El-Sherif N, Scherlag BJ, Lazzara R, et al: Reentrant ventricular arrhythmias in the late myocardial infarction period. 4. Mechanism of action of lidocaine. Circulation 56:395, 1977.
115. Armengol RE, Graff J, Baerman JM, et al: Lack of effectiveness of lidocaine for sustained, wide QRS complex tachycardia. Ann Emerg Med 18:254, 1989.
116. Clusin WT, Bristor MR, Karaguezian HS, et al: Do calcium-dependent currents meditate ischemic ventricular fibrillation? Am J Cardiol 49:606, 1982.
117. Wesley RC, Resh W, Zimmerman D: Reconsideration of the route and preferential use of lidocaine in the emergent treatment of ventricular arrhythmias. Crit Care Med 19:1439, 1991.
118. King FG, Addetia AM, Peters SD: Prophylactic lidocaine for postoperative coronary artery bypass patients, a double blind, randomized trial. Can J Anaesth 37:363, 1990.
119. Garson A, Kugler JD, Gillette PC, et al: Control of late postoperative ventricular arrhythmias with phenytoin in young patients. Am J Cardiol 46:290, 1980.
120. Pottage A: Clinical profiles of new class I antiarrhythmic agents—tocainide, mexiletine, encainide, flecainide and lorcainide. Am J Cardiol 52:24C, 1983.
121. Horowitz LN, Morganroth J: Second generation antiarrhythmic agents: Have we reached antiarrhythmic nirvana? J Am Coll Cardiol 9:459, 1987.
122. CAST Investigators: 1989. Preliminary report. Effect of encainide and flecainide on mortality in a randomized trial of arrhythmia suppression after myocardial infarction. N Engl J Med 321: 406, 1989.
123. Goldstein S: Toward a new understanding of the mechanism and prevention of sudden death in coronary heart disease. Circulation 82:284, 1990.
124. Woosley RL: CAST: Implications for drug development. Clin Pharmacol Ther 47:553, 1990.
125. Kaplan JA: Role of ultrashort acting beta-blockers in the perioperative period. J Cardiothorac Anesth 2:683, 1988.
126. Reves J, Flezziani P: Perioperative use of esmolol. Am J Cardiol 56:57F, 1985.
127. Menkhaus P, Reves JG, Kissin I, et al: Cardiovascular effects of esmolol in anesthetized humans. Anesth Analg 64:327, 1985.
128. Gorczynski RJ: Basic pharmacology of esmolol. Am J Cardiol 56:3F, 1985.
129. Gray RJ, Bateman TM, Czer LCS, et al: Esmolol: A new ultrashort-acting beta-adrenergic blocking agent for rapid control of heart rate in postoperative supraventricular tachyarrhythmias. J Am Coll Cardiol 5:1451, 1985.
130. Merin RG: New drugs: Beta-adrenergic blockers. Semin Anesth 3:75, 1988.
131. Solomon DE, Rogers JN: Esmolol for the treatment of isorhythmic atrioventricular dissociation. J Cardiothorac Vasc Anesth 6:603, 1992.
132. Farmer JB, Kennedy I, Levy GT, et al: Pharmacology of AH5158: A drug which blocks both alpha- and beta-adrenoreceptors. Br J Pharmacol 45:660, 1972.
133. Constant J: Preventing sudden death by raising the fibrillation threshold: A review (part 4). Res Staff Phys 26:29, 1991.
134. Sheridan DJ, et al: Alpha adrenergic contribution to dysrhythmia during myocardial ischemia and reperfusion in cats. J Clin Invest 65:161, 1980.

135. Kempf FC, Josephson ME: Cardiac arrest recorded on ambulatory electrocardiograms. Am J Cardiol 53:1577, 1985.
136. Campbell RWF, et al: Ventricular arrhythmias in the first 12 hours of acute myocardial infarction: Natural history study. Br Heart J 46:351, 1981.
137. Anderson JL: Antifibrillatory versus antiectopic therapy. Am J Cardiol 54:7A, 1984.
138. Heissenbuttel RH, Bigger JT: Bretylium tosylate: A newly available antiarrhythmic drug for ventricular arrhythmias. Ann Intern Med 91:229, 1979.
139. Sanna G, Arcidiacono R: Chemical ventricular defibrillation of the human heart with bretylium tosylate. Am J Cardiol 32:92, 1973.
140. Lucchesi BR: Rationale of therapy in the patient with acute myocardial infarction and life-threatening arrhythmias: A focus on bretylium. Am J Cardiol 54:14A, 1984.
141. Nowak RM, Bodnar TJ, Droven S, et al: Bretylium tosylate as initial treatment for cardiopulmonary arrest: Randomized comparison with placebo. Ann Emerg Med 10:404, 1981.
142. Kreeger RW, Hammill SC: New antiarrhythmic drugs: Tocainide, mexilitine, flecainide, encainide, and amiodarone. Mayo Clin Proc 62:1033, 1987.
143. Buchser E, Chiolero R, Martin P, et al: Amiodarone-induced haemodynamic complications during anesthesia. Anaesthesia 38: 1008, 1983.
144. Gallagher JD, Lieberman RW, Meranze J, et al: Amiodarone-induced complications during coronary artery surgery. Anesthesiology 55:187, 1981.
145. Abramowicz M: Sotalol for cardiac arrhythmias. Med Newslett 35(issue 893), 1993.
146. Chelly JE, Wouters PF: Calcium channel blocking drugs. Semin Anesth 7:83, 1988.
147. Reves JG, Kissin I, Lell WA, et al: Calcium entry blockers: Uses and implications for anesthesiologists. Anesthesiology 57:504, 1982.
148. Snyder SH, Reynolds IJ: Calcium antagonist drugs. N Engl J Med 313:995, 1985.
149. Gulamhusein S, Ko P, Klein GJ: Ventricular fibrillation following verapamil in the Wolff-Parkinson-White syndrome. Am Heart J 106:145, 1983.
150. Fyke FE, Vlietstra RE, Danielson GK, et al: Verapamil for refractory ventricular fibrillation during cardiac operations in patients with cardiac hypertrophy. J Thorac Cardiovasc Surg 86: 108, 1983.
151. Kraynack BJ, Lawson NW, Gintautas J: Local anesthetic effect of verapamil in vitro. Reg Anesth 7:114, 1982.
152. Kapur PA, Flacke WE, Olewine SK: Comparison of effects of isoflurane versus enflurane on cardiovascular and catecholamine responses to verapamil in dogs. Anesth Analg 61:193, 1982.
153. Richie AJ, Bowe P, Gibbons JRP: Prophylactic digitalization for thoracotomy: A reassessment. Ann Thorac Surg 50:86, 1990.
154. Lewis RP: Digitalis: A drug that refuses to die. Crit Care Med 18:S513, 1990.
155. Belardinelli L, Linden J, Berne RM: The cardiac effects of adenosine. Prog Cardiovasc Dis 32:73, 1987.
156. Belardinelli L, Isenberg G: Isolated atrial myocytes: Adenosine and acetylcholine increase potassium conductance. Am J Physiol 244:H734, 1984.
157. Dimarco JP, Miles W, Akhtar M, et al: Adenosine for paroxysmal supraventricular tachycardia: Dose ranging and comparison with verapamil. Ann Intern Med 113:104, 1990.
158. Dreifus LS, Hessen SE: Supraventricular tachycardia: Diagnosis and treatment. Cardiology 77:259, 1990.
159. Rossi AF, Steinberg LG, Kipel G: Use of adenosine in the management of perioperative arrhythmias in the pediatric intensive care unit. Crit Care Med 20:1107, 1992.
160. Freilich A, Tepper D: Adenosine and its cardiovascular effects. Am Heart J 123:1324, 1992.
161. Woosley RL, Roden DM: Treatment of ventricular arrhythmias in acute myocardial infarction. In Francis GS, Alpert JS (eds): Modern Coronary Care. Boston, Little, Brown & Co, 1990, p 195.
162. Funck-Brentano C, Woosley RL: Current antiarrhythmic agents—clinical pharmacology. In El-Sherif N, Samet P (eds): Cardiac Pacing. Orlando, FL, Grune & Stratton, 1990, p 409.

Additional Reading

Belardinelli L, Lerman BB: Electrophysiological basis for the use of adenosine in the diagnosis and treatment of cardiac arrhythmias. Br Heart J 63:3, 1990.
Constant J: Preventing sudden death by raising the fibrillation threshold: A review (part 2). 37:29, 1991.
Davis RF: Etiology and treatment of perioperative cardiac arrhythmias. In Kaplan J (ed): Cardiac Anesthesia, 3rd ed. Philadelphia, WB Saunders Co, 1993, p 170.
De Mello WC, Hoffman BF: Potassium ions and electrical activity of specialized cardiac fibers. Am J Physiol 199:1125, 1960.
Edwards JD, Kishen R: Significance and management of intractable supraventricular arrhythmias in critically ill patients. Crit Care Med 14:280, 1986.
Firestone L: Heart transplantation. In Lebowitz PW (ed): Anesthesia and Organ Transplantation. Int Anesthesiol Clin 29:41, 1991.
Ganguly PK: Catecholamines and cardiovascular disorders: Pathophysiologic considerations. Am Heart J 118:868, 1989.
Kaplan JA, Wells PH: Electrocardiographic monitoring. In Ream AK, Fogdall RP (eds): Acute Cardiovascular Management. Philadelphia, JB Lippincott Co, 1982, p 163.
Kastor JA: Multifocal atrial tachycardia. N Engl J Med 322:24, 1990.
Stirt JA, Sullivan SF: Aminophylline. Anesth Analg 60:587, 1981.
Tarnow J, Muller RK: Cardiovascular effects of low-dose epinephrine infusions in relation to the extent of preoperative β-adrenoreceptor blockade. Anesthesiology 74:1035, 1991.
Vassalle M, Greenspan K, Jomain S, Hoffman BF: Effects of potassium on automaticity and conduction of canine hearts. Am J Physiol 207:334, 1964.

CHAPTER 32

Pacemakers

James R. Zaidan, M.D.

Anesthesiologists who attend patients with implanted pacemakers should have a sufficient level of sophistication to determine the impact of the pacemaker on anesthetic management. In addition, pacemaker technologic advancements complicate the functional evaluation of the generator and may lead to a greater possibility of intraoperative pacemaker failure.

Increasing complexity of implanted pacemakers requires a review of the basic knowledge associated with pacemaker operation and an acquaintance with the newest developments in technology of implanted generators. This chapter includes definitions and descriptions of different types of pacemakers, new pacemaker technology associated with rate responsiveness, evaluation of the patient with an implanted pacemaker, evaluation of the generator, and intraoperative management of patients for general surgical procedures or pacemaker implantation.

Definitions and Descriptions of Pacemakers

Anesthesiologists should be familiar with definitions associated with pacemakers, the system of naming them, and the basic designs of the generators.

Definitions

1. *Pacemaker*: The term "pacemaker" implies the complete, implanted or external system including the generator, the lead, and the electrode.
2. *Generator*: A generator is the device containing the electrical circuits and the energy supply that is usually implanted over the pectoralis muscle.
3. *Lead*: The lead is the insulated wire that extends from the generator to the electrode. It can be unipolar, implying that the negative electrode is in the heart and the positive electrode is in the generator, or it can be bipolar meaning that both electrodes are located 1 to 2 cm away from each other in the heart.

   The term "transvenous" is interchangeably used with the term "endocardial," both meaning that the lead extends through the innominate vein and superior vena cava to the right ventricular endocardium. The generator for a transvenous system is located over either pectoralis muscle just below the clavicle. An epicardial lead, rarely used today, implies that the lead has been tunneled in subcutaneous tissue from the generator located in the anterior abdominal wall at the waistline through the epicardium to the myocardium.
4. *Electrode*: The electrode is the metal portion of the lead that directly contacts the myocardium. An epicardial electrode extends through the epicardium to the myocardium, while an endocardial or transvenous electrode enters the myocardium through the right ventricular endocardium.

   The size of the electrode is very important. A large radius improves sensing capabilities through a reduction in electrode resistance and a reduction in polarization impedance.[1,2] A small-radius electrode improves the stimulation threshold by increasing current density at the metal/tissue interface.[3–5] The shape of the electrode is also important.[3,4] A smooth hemispheric design creates an even distribution of charge density, while an irregularly shaped electrode creates areas of high charge density that decreases the stimulation threshold. Recent designs combine a small-radius with a complex surface pattern to maintain lower stimulation thresholds and improve sensing.[4–6]
5. *Polarization*: During the generator's pulse, positive ions from the interstitial space surround the negative electrode. Eventually, negative ions surround the positive ions, forming a capacitor that retards the flow of current and increases impedence of the electrode. Decreasing pulse duration and increasing the surface area of the electrode will decrease the effect of polarization.
6. *Escape interval*: An escape interval is the time the generator takes to emit an impulse in the absence of an R wave. It can be the same as the automatic interval.

7. *Automatic interval*: The automatic interval is the time in milliseconds between successive pacemaker impulses. Divide this number into 60,000 to derive the heart rate. Most implanted pacemakers have an automatic interval of 846 msec set by the manufacturer that offers the patient a heart rate of 71 bpm. This feature is programmable.
8. *Hysteresis*: Hysteresis is the difference between the escape and automatic intervals that allows the patient's heart rate to decrease below the automatic interval before the pacemaker is activated (Fig. 32–1). Ten-beat hysteresis with an automatic rate of 75 bpm permits the patient's heart rate to decrease to 65 before initiating pacing at a rate of 75 bpm. This kind of pacing is useful in patients who have heart rates that approximate the automatic interval of the pacemaker and in patients who experience the pacemaker syndrome, a profound decrease in blood pressure with the loss of atrial kick secondary to VVI pacing.
9. *R-wave sensitivity*: R-wave sensitivity is the number of millivolts required to activate the sensing circuit and, in turn, inhibit the pacing circuit. The magnitude of the R wave measured by the analyzer must be greater than the R-wave sensitivity programmed in the pacemaker.
10. *Slew rate*: The slew rate is the rate of voltage change in the R wave of the ventricular electrogram. If the rate of change of a detected wave is too slow, usually defined as less than 0.5 V/sec, then the generator defines that wave as being something other than an R wave. T waves and the myopotentials associated with shivering can fall into this category.
11. *Triggered pacemaker*: A triggered pacemaker detects R waves and instantaneously triggers an impulse that appears exactly at the peak of every R wave on the surface electrocardiogram (ECG). This type of pacemaker is rarely, if ever, used.
12. *Inhibited pacemaker*: An inhibited pacemaker has a sensing circuit that detects R waves, compares those R waves to a programmed standard, and finally inactivates the pacing circuit if the R waves meet the standard. Included in the standards are the R wave's magnitude (usually >1.5 mV), slew rate (>0.5 V/sec), and frequency (usually occurring >70 bpm).
13. *Rate adaptive or rate responsive pacemaker*: This type of pacemaker varies its automatic interval (pacing rate) with the metabolic state or movement of the patient. It paces at a baseline rate and increases the rate if the patient exercises.
14. *Blanking period*: The blanking period occurs immediately after a paced or sensed event during which the pacemaker does not respond to any ECG wave. Essentially, the pacemaker turns off during this period so that it will not sense T waves.
15. *Pacemaker syndrome*: This problem occurs in some patients who have implanted ventricular inhibited pacemakers. Physiologically, the cardiac output decreases because of the loss of the atrial contribution to preload. The patient feels the result of the decreased cardiac output and blood pressure by becoming lightheaded or dizzy or, in the extreme, fainting (Fig. 32–2). The problem can be corrected by using a DDD pacemaker or in some instances by using a VVIR pacemaker. If the patient tolerates lower heart rates, then maintaining sinus rhythm at a lower rate by programming hysteresis might help the patient. In the operating room, this syndrome is characterized by a very marked decrease in blood pressure when the pacemaker turns on or when an external generator initially begins pacing.

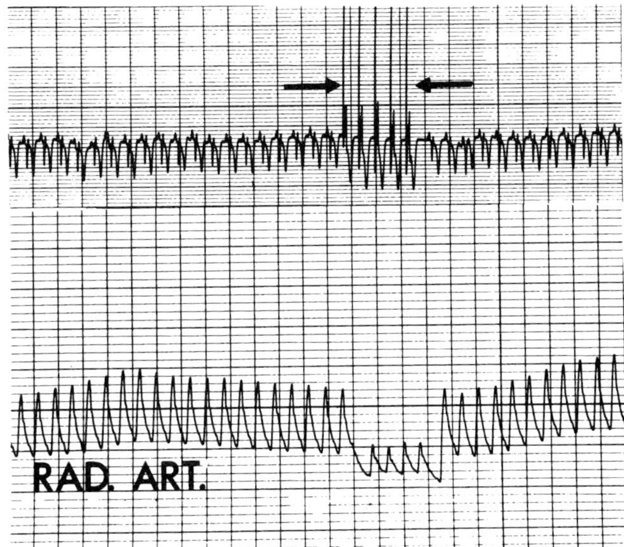

FIGURE **32–1.** The sudden decrease in blood pressure evident in this figure (between *arrows*) originates from the onset of ventricular pacing and the loss of atrial kick. Patients suffer from lightheadedness, dizziness, or even syncope and require hysteresis programmed into the VVI generator or DDD generator implantation.

Naming

Pacemakers are named according to pacing and sensing locations, mode of activity, programmability, and antitachycardia functions[7] (Table 32–1). The first letter signifies the *location* of pacing. The second letter reveals the pacemaker's *sensing location.* The third letter indicates the *mode of activity.* For instance, an "I" in the third position shows that the pacemaker turns off when it senses an R wave and therefore turns off. The fourth letter symbolizes *programmability.* A seldom used fifth letter indicates the ability of the pacemaker to *terminate tachycardias.* As examples, VVI pacemakers stimulate the ventricle, sense R waves, and, if it detects R waves, turns off. A DDD or fully automatic pacemaker includes atrial and ventricular pacing and sensing. It also has a mode of activity that is both inhibited and triggered, as follows: a sensed spontaneous P wave or the pacemaker's atrial output triggers an impulse to the ventricle if a spontaneous R wave does not occur; if a spontaneous R wave does occur, the ventricular pacing circuit turns off.

Essentially all implanted pacemakers are programmable. A letter in the fourth position indicates the extent of this programmability. The letter "P," usually not writ-

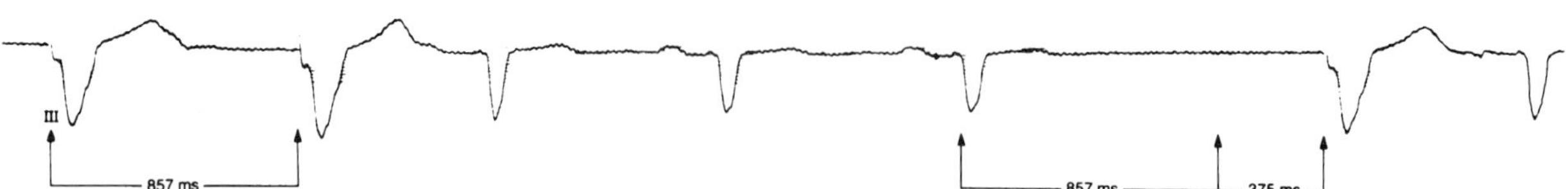

FIGURE 32–2. Hysteresis allows the patient's heart rate to slow below the pacing rate so that the pacemaker syndrome will not occur. In this figure, the automatic interval is 875 msec, resulting in a heart rate of 68.5. Since the escape interval is 1,250 msec, the heart rate will slow to 48 bpm before pacing occurs at the higher rate. (From Schuller H, Fahraeus T: Pacemaker Electrocardiograms–an Introduction to Practical Analysis, 1983. Solna, Sweden, Siemens-Elema AB, with permission.)

ten, suggests that the generator can be programmed for rate and output. Multiprogrammability indicated by the letter "M" suggests that other functions in addition to rate and output are programmable. An "R" in the fourth position reveals not only that the generator is multiprogrammable, but also that it is rate responsive. The R does not reveal the mechanism by which the rate changes.

Types of Pacemakers

Asynchronous

Although it is rarely used in implanted pacemakers, the asynchronous mode of activity remains an important intraoperative selection in an external generator. The VOO pacemaker cannot detect ventricular depolarizations; therefore, regularly spaced paced beats that are unrelated to the patient's heart rate appear on the ECG. The patient will experience an irregularly irregular pulse. Competition with the patient's own impulses can initiate ventricular tachycardia if a pacing impulse occurring on a T wave conducts a beat (Fig. 32–3).

Synchronous

To eliminate competition, engineers developed synchronous generators that contain sensing circuits. These circuits detect RR intervals, R-wave magnitudes, and slew rates and, after filtering, compare them to standards "memorized" by the sensing circuitry. The "memorized" standards comprise the program of the generator. If the comparison shows that the arriving impulse has the characteristics of an R wave, then the sensing circuit amplifies the signal, which travels to and then either inhibits or triggers the output circuit.

TABLE 32–1
Pacemaker Code

Position	Its Meaning	Letters
First	Pacing location	A, V, D
Second	Sensing location	A, V, D, O
Third	Mode of activity	T, I, D, O
Fourth	Programmability	P, M, R, C, O
Fifth	Antitachycardia function	P, S, D, O

From Zaidan JR: Practical Cardiac Electrophysiology for Advances in Anesthesia, vol 12. St. Louis, Mosby, 1995, with permission.

A, atrium; V, ventricle; D, dual or both; O, none; T, triggered; I, inhibited; P (fourth position), programmable for rate and output; M, multiprogrammable; R, rate adaptive; C, communicates; P (fifth position), pacing; S, shock; D (fifth position), pacing and shock.

Sequential Pacing

The addition of atrial pacing to the ventricular pacemaker offers the option of atrioventricular (i.e., sequential pacing). The advantage of sequential pacing, especially in patients who experience the pacemaker syndrome, lies in maintenance of normal AV contraction sequence. The external DVI generator senses R waves and paces both the atrium and the ventricle (Fig. 32–4). If an R wave is sensed, then the atrial and ventricular pacing circuits turn off. The implanted sequential pacemaker generally is a DDD that is programmable to other types such as a DVI, VVI, DOO, etc. (Figs. 32–5 and 32–6).

Automatic Implantable Cardioverter Defibrillator

Another kind of pacemaker is the automatic implantable cardioverter defibrillator (AICD). This generator is used in patients who experience arrhythmias that are poorly controlled by medications.[8] Indications for the use of the implanted defibrillator include recurring ventricular fibrillation or tachycardia that is refractory to antiarrhythmic drug therapy.

Sensing and stimulating electrodes are positioned in the heart.[9,10] When it senses changes in heart rate and contour of the ECG tracing signaling a ventricular arrhythmia, the AICD emits a cardioverting or defibrillating current of 23 to 28 J to terminate the arrhythmia. Approximately 5 to 15 seconds are required to charge the capacitors after a 5- to 20-second sensing period; therefore, after the onset of the arrhythmia, 10 to 35 seconds are required to shock the patient. The AICD will emit only four cardioverting or defibrillating shocks during any single arrhythmic episode. If the patient is cardioverted and experiences another arrhythmia, the AICD will sense and discharge four more times. The generator has enough stored energy to discharge approximately 100 times.

Rate Adaptive Pacing

Chronotropic incompetence, an important indication for a rate adaptive pacemaker, is the absence of a rate in-

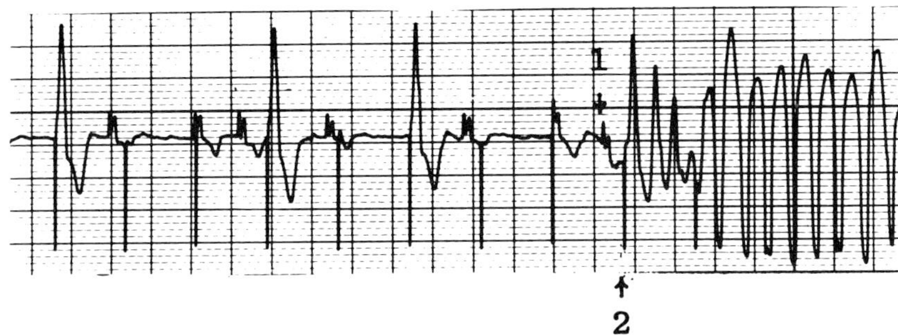

FIGURE **32–3.** Ventricular asynchronous pacing was imposed on this patient whose underlying rhythm was atrial fibrillation. *Arrow 1* signifies the last intrinsic beat and *arrow 2* locates the pacing impulse and paced beat that initiates ventricular tachycardia. Ventricular inhibited pacing might have avoided this complication of ventricular pacing.

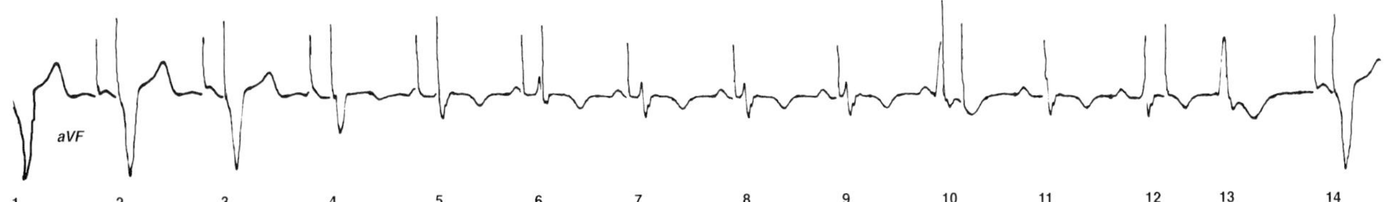

FIGURE **32–4.** DVI pacing can result in various ECG patterns, because the pacemaker looks for an R wave during both the atrial and ventricular escape intervals. The difference between these two intervals is the AV (PR) interval. Following is a beat-by-beat explanation. *2, 14*, Full sequential pacing occurred, because an R wave was not detected before the end of either the atrial or ventricular escape intervals. *3*, Atrial pseudofusion, ventricular pacing. *4, 5*, Atrial pseudofusion, ventricular fusion. *6*, The R wave was not sensed before the end of the atrial escape interval; therefore, the pacemaker emits an atrial impulse even though the P wave has already occurred. Ventricular pseudofusion also occurs. *7, 8, 9, 11*, Once again, the R wave was not detected by the end of the atrial escape interval; therefore, an atrial impulse was emitted after the P wave. The R wave was detected within the AV interval so that the ventricular impulse was not emitted. *10, 12*, The R wave occurs, but not in time to inhibit the atrial impulse. Since the pacemaker does not find the R wave within its AV interval, actually before the end of the ventricular escape interval, a ventricular pacing impulse occurs. *13*, A sensed R wave occurs that inhibits both the atrial and ventricular outputs of the pacemaker. (From Schuller H, Fahraeus T: Pacemaker Electrocardiograms–an Introduction to Practical Analysis, 1983. Solna, Sweden, Siemens-Elema AB, with permission.)

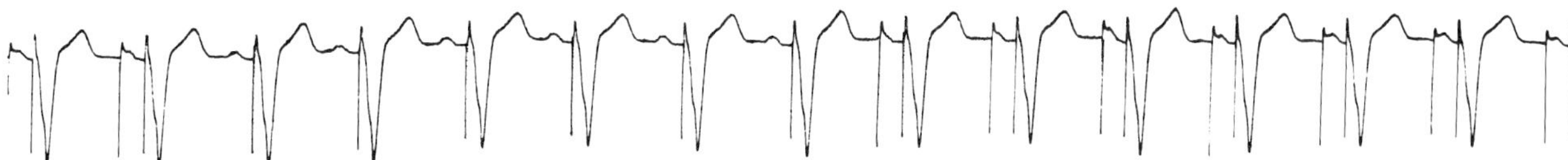

FIGURE **32–5.** DDD pacing in this patient results in consistent ventricular pacing with and without atrial pacing. (From Schuller H, Fahraeus T: Pacemaker Electrocardiograms–an Introduction to Practical Analysis, 1983. Solna, Sweden, Siemens-Elema AB, with permission.)

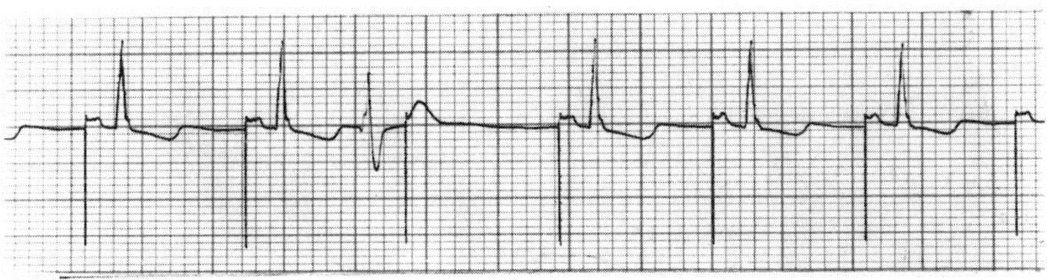

FIGURE **32–6.** This patient required atrial pacing from a DDD generator. The third R wave detected by the ventricular sensing circuit inhibits the ventricular output. However, because the pacemaker does not sense a P wave, an atrial pacing impulse is emitted into the atrium. On the surface ECG, the atrial pacing impulse occurs in the ST segment.

crease when the patient exercises or experiences stress.[11] Older models of pacemakers protect the patient only from bradycardias. Rate adaptation adds another dimension to pacing in that it increases heart rate to physiologic levels for a given level of exercise or stress. The VVIR and DDDR generators change their rates depending on the activity or the metabolic status of the patient. Unit increases in rate and level of activity necessary to change the rate are programmable.

General Description of Rate Adaptive Sensors

Rate adaptive sensors can be categorized according either to the physiologic parameter that they measure or to the technology that they use.[12]

Physiologic Category

Primary sensors respond to neural activity and endogenous catecholamines and are considered to be substitutes for the sinoatrial (SA) node. These types of experimental sensors are not yet available for clinical use. Secondary sensors respond to physiologic changes brought about by exercise. This group encompasses sensors that respond to changes in oxygen saturation, right ventricular pressure, central venous blood temperature, and electrocardiographic events. Several of these sensors are clinically available. Tertiary sensors have been in clinical use for several years and respond to vibrational or accelerational body movement.

Technologic Category

Another method of categorizing sensors is to group them according to how they work[13] (Table 32–2). Impedance has been used for many years to measure chest wall motion and is now used in pacemakers not only to sense changes in respiratory parameters associated with exercise but also to determine stroke volume and pre-ejection period. Impedance sensing is simple in design, but electrode motion artifacts occasionally cause oversensing.

Sensors measuring body movement use the piezoelectric effect, in which bending of a crystal is converted into an electric current. Although they function in similar fashion, they are classified according to their ability to sense vibration or acceleration of the casing of the generator.[14] If the piezoelectric crystal is directly attached to the pacemaker casing, then vibrations of the casing associated with body movement create an electrical current which, in turn, changes the pacemaker rate. If the crystal is attached to the circuit board of the pacemaker, but not directly to the casing, then a current begins in response to acceleration. Although these pacemakers have a very rapid onset of response, the rate change is lower than may be anticipated when the patient ascends an incline or walks up stairs. Also, their abrupt offset leaves the patient with a lower than required heart rate for the lingering metabolic demands. A programmed delay in the offset that slows the pacing rate over a period of several minutes allows heart rate to meet the metabolic demand.

A third group of sensors are those that detect intracardiac electrical events such as evoked QT interval and the ventricular gradient. It is possible to sense electrocardiographic events through the same electrodes that pace the heart; therefore, older electrodes can be used with technologically advanced generators. When a DDD or VVI generator is due for a change, it can be replaced with a DDDR or a VVIR pacemaker without the need to replace the pacing electrode.

The final group encompasses a wide variety of sensors that are located on specialized pacing leads. They include measurement of central body temperature, venous oxygen saturation, right ventricular dP/dt, pre-ejection period, tidal volume, and minute ventilation. These sensors are more complicated in that they require lead modification; however, once they are in place, they function with minimal input from the physician.

TABLE 32–2
Sensors Used in Rate Adaption

Technology	Sensed Parameter
Piezoelectric crystal	Vibration
	Acceleration
Impedance	Respiratory rate
	Minute volume
	RV pre-ejection period
Thermistor	RV temperature
ECG	Evoked QT interval
	Ventricular gradient
Pressure	RV dP/dt
Optical reflectance	Oxygen saturation

From Zaidan JR: Practical Cardiac Electrophysiology for Advances in Anesthesia, vol 12. St. Louis, Mosby, 1995, with permission.
RV, right ventricular; ECG, electrocardiogram.

Basic Design of Rate Adaptive Pacemakers

Rate adaptation requires that a sensor detect physical or physiologic change. The signal, modified by filtering, is compared to an algorithm to determine if rate modification is necessary. If rate modification is required, then the pacemaker responds by increasing or decreasing its automatic rate. Intermittent increases in the patient's intrinsic heart rate should inhibit rate adaptive pacing. That which is sensed must change in proportion to heart rate changes.[13] The sensor must be specific to the change and not respond to other signals. Changes in pacing rate should occur at the beginning of exercise without a prolonged lag period. Technically, sensors must be stable and not require excessive programming. They should be an appropriate size and not complicate lead design. Energy required by sensors that measure impedance or oxygen saturation should not excessively drain the pacemaker battery.

When the change in pacing rate reverses the physiologic effect that initiated the change, the pacemaker has a closed loop sensing system. For example, venous oxygen saturation decreases during exercise. An oxygen-saturation-sensing device located on the pacing lead would function through the algorithm to increase the pacing rate (decrease the automatic rate). Increased heart rate elevates cardiac output. More oxygen is delivered to the tissues and venous saturation increases, which in turn slows the pacing rate. Generally speaking, the physician must program only the lower and upper rates and the rate at which the pacemaker seeks the data.

An open loop system implies that the change in pacing rate does not reverse the signal that initiated the change. As an example, a sensor that detects motion through vibration or acceleration will induce an increase in pacing rate. In the open loop system, the increased heart rate will not negatively feed back to the amount of motion. An open loop requires more programming, because the algorithm will not inherently know the pacing rate required for a given level of exercise. The physician, therefore, must set not only the lower and upper pacing rates but also the sensitivity of the system and the rate at which the change occurs. This programming takes place during a graded series of exercises. The patient relates to the physician subjective feelings of shortness of breath and tiredness and the physician programs the pacemaker to a higher rate for that level of exercise.

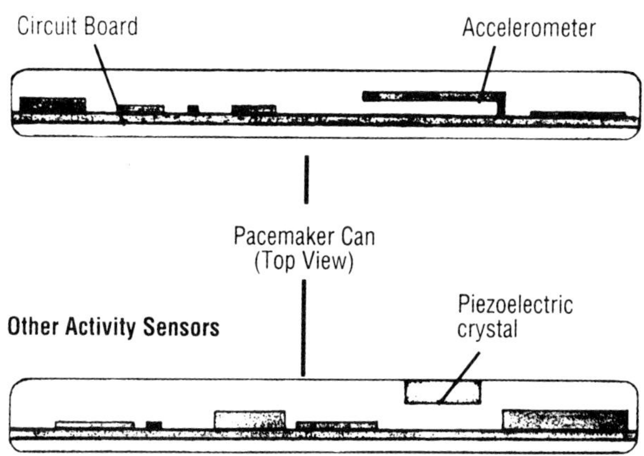

FIGURE **32–7.** This figure shows two types of motion-sensing pacemakers. In both designs, a piezoelectric crystal is used as the sensing device. When the crystal is deformed, the resulting electrical current enters the pacemaker's circuit and increases the rate. The *top picture* is an accelerometer. Note that it is not directly attached to the pacemaker container and deforms as the patient is accelerating. The *bottom picture* shows that the crystal is directly attached to the pacemaker container and therefore detects the body's vibrations that occur when the patient walks. (From Changing the Rate. Intermedics Inc, Angleton, Texas, with permission.)

Specific Rate Adaptive Sensors

Body Movement—Vibration

Movement sends vibrations with frequencies below 10 Hz throughout the body.[15,16] External interference usually has frequencies above 10 Hz.[15] Both types of vibrations are transmitted to the pacemaker casing (Fig. 32–7). A piezoelectric crystal attached directly to the generator's casing converts these vibrations into a signal that is processed and sent to the control section of the pacemaker. By working through the algorithm, the control section determines the final automatic interval and pacing rate of the pacemaker. The mass of the pacemaker casing and to some extent the build and clothing of the patient influence the mechanical vibrations received by the piezoelectric crystal. The sensor should face the patient's chest wall rather than subcutaneous tissue.

Almost all pacemakers are programmable for rate, output, and various other parameters. Activity-related, rate adaptive pacing is programmable also for upper and lower rate, activity threshold, rate response, acceleration time, and deceleration time. The upper and lower rates are the maximal and minimal rates that the pacemaker will use when determining the adaptation. Rates are usually programmed between about 60 and 120 to 170 pulses per minute (ppm). A circadian rhythm can be programmed to allow the pacemaker rate to decrease even more during the sleeping hours.

Activity threshold sets the ease with which the patient can activate rate adaptive pacing (Fig. 32–8). The pacemaker could require excessive activity or minimal activity to achieve a unit increase in rate. In some models of pacemakers, the number of peaks that pass a threshold are counted, while in other pacemakers, the signals are integrated rather than counting peak activity.

Rate response is the number of pacemaker impulses per minute that are in a unit increase in pacing rate (Fig. 32–9). The physician programs one of ten rate response curves with different slopes. The higher number gives the patient a higher number of ppm per unit increase. The pacemaker can cause a large increase in heart rate (rate response curve slope = 10) or a small increase in heart rate (rate response curve slope = 1) for a given level of exercise. Earlier models of activity-related rate adaptation used curvilinear response curves that made it difficult to reach the programmed upper rate. Newer pacemakers have straight-line response curves that allow the patient to reach the upper rate limit even if the rate response is set to a low number.

Acceleration time is the final parameter associated with an increase in pacing rate (Fig. 32–10). This setting determines how long the pacemaker should wait until it actually responds to the signal and allows the patient to perform minimal activity over a short time span without experiencing an increase in heart rate. Generally, 0.25, 0.50, and 1.0 minute are the three choices.

Once motion stops, the activity-related sensor will immediately stop sending signals to the control section and pacing rate will decrease to the lower rate. Since metabolic demand remains high for a few minutes, these pacemakers have another programmable feature called deceleration time. This feature tells the pacemaker how long it should take to lower the automatic rate. It is not related to metabolic demand, but allows the patient some time to recover from the exercise. Vibration-related sensors have limitations. Their rate adaptation is not related to metabolic demand. Rate is programmed by the subjective well-being of the patient during the programming phase after implantation. Sometimes the response is not well correlated with the activity.[17] Walking an incline results in lower paced rates than walking more quickly on level ground. Isometric exercise might not elicit a rate change. Direct pressure and tapping on the pacemaker casing can result in a higher pacing rate.[18] Some of these sensors use a frequency band of up to 70 Hz, which is

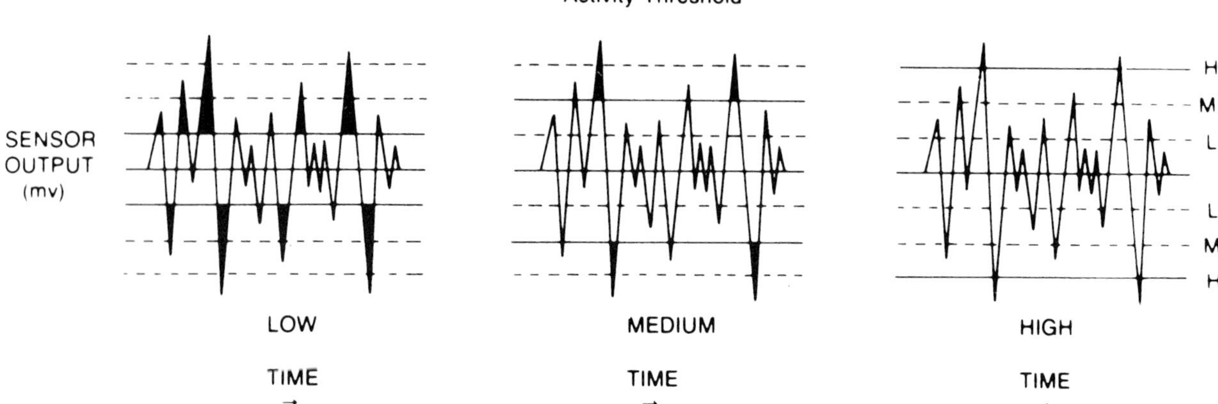

FIGURE **32–8.** One of the programmable parameters of the vibratory sensing pacemaker is the amount of activity (activity threshold) that is required to cause a unit increase in heart rate. This figure shows three different sensitivities and exactly the same amount of activity. In the example on the left, many peaks of activity (millivolts of sensor output) surpass the threshold (*solid horizontal lines*). This low activity threshold indicates that minimal activity will cause an increase in heart rate. In the example on the right, the peaks of activity barely reach the threshold. This patient's pacemaker will increase its rate only with a much higher level of activity. (Courtesy of Medtronic, Inc., Minneapolis, MN.)

far outside the range necessary to detect vibrations related to motion. This wide frequency band causes them to detect extraneous artifacts.[19]

One case report concerns intraoperative management of a patient with a vibration sensing pacemaker scheduled for a cesarean section. Paced heart rate appropriately responded to motion of the patient during moving to the operating room table, intubation, delivery of the fetus, and awakening. Aside from these increases, the paced rate remained at the lower rate limit.[20]

Body Movement—Acceleration

If the piezoelectric crystal is suspended from the circuit board and not directly attached to the pacemaker casing, the sensor is called an accelerometer (Fig. 32–7). In con-

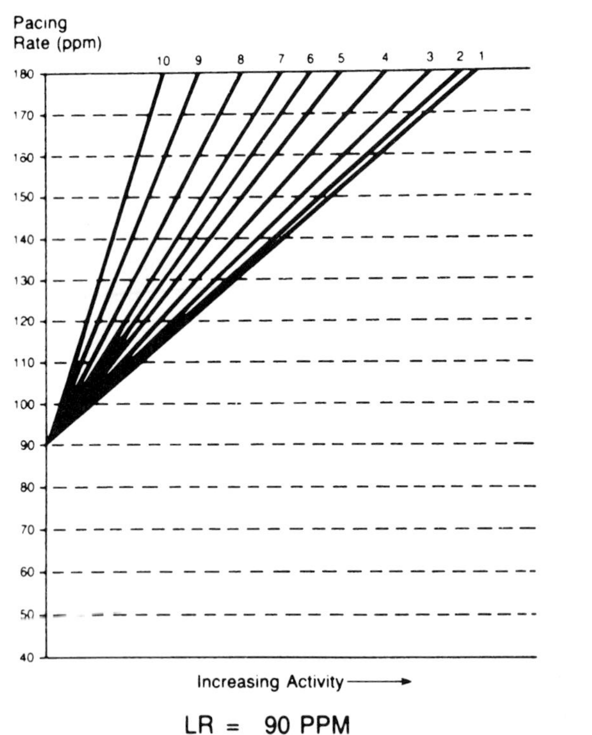

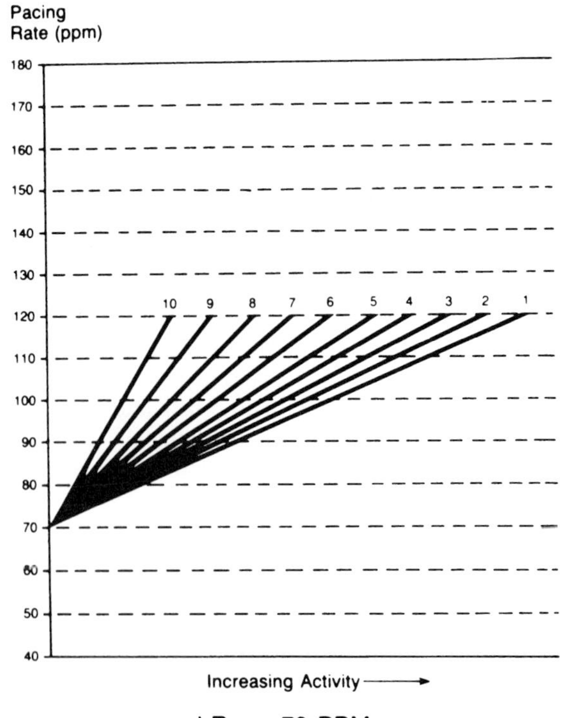

FIGURE **32–9.** Other programmable features of motion-sensing pacemakers are the lower/upper rate parameter and the slope of the response. The lower/upper rate parameters in this example are 90/180 and 70/120. Once the activity threshold is reached, the slope dictates the extent of the response. *Slope 7* is usually the default. *Slope 10* would offer a greater unit increase in heart rate than *slope 1* for the same amount of activity. These parameters are programmed by the cardiologist by exercising the patient while assessing the physical well-being of the patient. (Courtesy of Medtronic, Inc., Minneapolis, MN.)

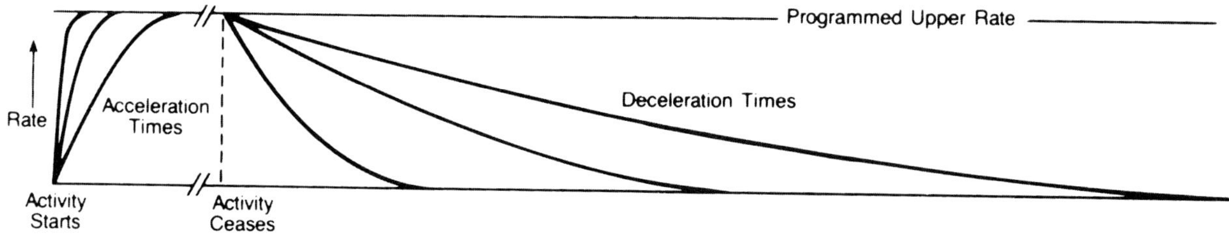

FIGURE **32–10.** One of the problems with a piezoelectric crystal is that its response is instant on and instant off. To offset this problem, acceleration and deceleration times are programmed. An acceleration time of 30 seconds means that the activity must continue for 30 seconds before the pacemaker responds. Slowing the deceleration time offers the patient a higher heart rate in the cool-down period of exercise. (Courtesy of Medtronic, Inc., Minneapolis, MN.)

trast to the vibration sensor, the accelerometer does not change pacing rate when direct pressure is applied to the casing. It is not affected by orientation, and it senses movement in the 4-Hz range. Acceleration-based pacemakers have a more physiologic response to graded treadmill exercise and descending stairs.

Pacemakers sensing acceleration have the same set of programmable features as the pacemakers using vibration sensors. One difference is the shape of the rate response curve (Fig. 32–11). It is a triphasic curve that allows a rapid increase in pacing rate early in the exercise period. If the exercise level remains constant, pacing rate does not further increase. The last part of the curve permits another increase in heart rate if the patient exercises at a higher level. As an example, the first increase in pacing rate would occur when a previously resting person starts to walk. The heart rate would remain at this level until the person begins to jog.

Impedance—Respiratory Rate and Minute Ventilation

Respiratory rate and minute volume proportionately increase in response to carbon dioxide (CO_2) production during exercise and can be used to alter heart rate.[21,22] In the earliest phase of exercise, tidal volume increases. At high levels of exercise, the respiratory rate begins to increase.[23,24] Pacemakers using respiratory rate might not respond as quickly to exercise as pacemakers that use minute volume as the parameter to increase heart rate.[24]

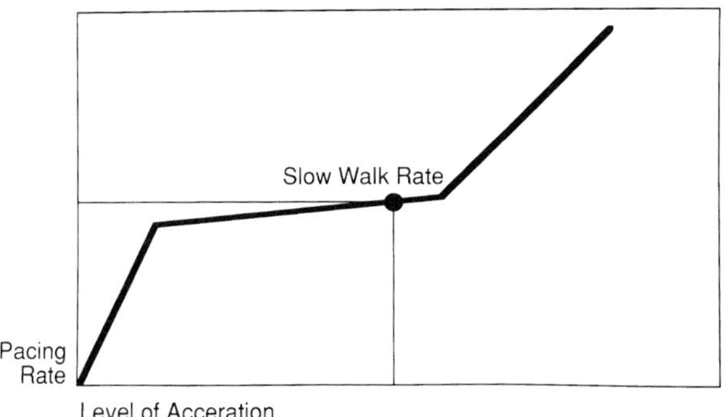

FIGURE **32–11.** Different phases of the response curve are shown above. This type of response curve allows the patient to assume a constant level of activity without reaching the highest heart rate. If activity increases above the first level, then the pacemaker responds by attaining the highest heart rate. (Courtesy of Intermedics Inc, Angleton, TX.)

These sensors work through a tripolar electrode system to detect changes in transthoracic impedance.[25] The pacemaker casing is used as the reference. A current of 1 mA with a pulse duration of 15 μsec is delivered every 50 msec from the distal electrode on the pacing lead. The resulting voltage at the proximal electrode in a bipolar pacing system or a special sensing electrode in a unipolar pacing system is used to calculate the transthoracic impedance. The magnitude of the changes in impedance are related to tidal volume, and the frequency of those changes is related to respiratory rate. Impedance is continuously stored and the measurement from the last minute is compared to the measurement over the last hour. By constantly comparing measurements from minute to hour, the pacemaker will not suddenly increase the pacing rate for short-duration respiratory changes such as a cough or sigh. Just as with activity-related sensors, respiratory controlled pacemakers are programmable for the ease with which the pacemaker initiates the change and the slope of the rate response.

Although this type of pacemaker has good correlation between pacing rate and ventilation, impedance sensors measuring respiratory parameters have several limitations. Arm movement can cause an unwanted rate increase.[26,27] This disadvantage can be utilized as an advantage, because patients with pacemakers that use respiratory rate for heart rate adaptation benefit by moving the right arm to initiate an increase in heart rate. During exercise, talking will decrease the maximal rate response, because talking initiates an irregular breathing pattern. Cheyne-Stokes breathing has been reported to cause a high pacing rate; however, the pacemaker described in the report was programmed to high rate response slope.[28] Decreasing the rate response slope would have decreased the pacing rate.[29] Impedance systems are susceptible to interference caused by electromagnetic interference and myopotentials.[30] Also, ECG monitors occasionally count the current impulses used to measure impedance and therefore falsely elevate the monitored heart rate (Fig. 32–12).

There are two case reports relating perioperative experiences with minute ventilation sensing pacemakers. In one case, during a Cesarean section, the paced rate

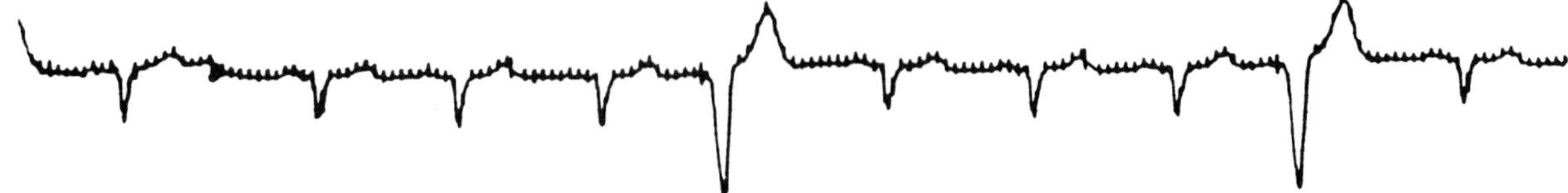

FIGURE **32–12.** The ECG in this figure reveals the electrical activity associated with an impedance-sensing pacemaker. Generally, these pacemakers measure respiratory parameters.

increased during hyperventilation to preoxygenate the patient.[31] The paced rate remained at the lower rate limit during surgery, but increased again as the patient was awakening. In another case, a patient undergoing a transurethral prostatic resection (TURP) experienced a heart rate increase during manual ventilation.[32] Decreasing the minute ventilation lowered the paced heart rate.

Electrocardiographic Events—Evoked QT Interval

QT interval shortens as heart rate increases. Several formulas have been recommended to normalize measured QT interval to heart rate. Bazett's formula is commonly used.[33] The fact that it does have a relationship to heart rate makes the QT interval measured from the pacing impulse to the point of maximum negative slope of the T wave useful in rate adaptive pacemakers. This possibility was first suggested by Rickards and Norman, who investigated the QT interval–heart rate relationship in three groups of patients.[34] One group of patients underwent exercise. Patients in the second group were atrially paced without exercise, and the last group were exercising patients who had third-degree block and permanent VVI pacemakers. In the first group, the QT interval decreased by 187 msec when the heart rate increased by 100 bpm. The second group experienced a 66-msec decrease in QT interval with the same increase in heart rate. The third group could not increase heart rate, but they still experienced a decrease in stimulus to T wave interval (evoked QT interval) associated with exercise. Ventricular rate by itself, therefore, is not the only determinant of QT interval. The authors suggested, later verified by other investigators, that QT interval during exercise is heavily influenced by catecholamines.[35,36]

With QT sensing, the pacemaker blanks for 200 msec after stimulating the ventricle. Then T wave sensing begins and persists for up to 450 msec. The algorithm sets the timing of the next pacing impulse depending on the duration of the preceding evoked QT interval. If the evoked QT interval is shorter, then the next pacing impulse will be delivered earlier. This pacemaker is actually measuring then correcting each QT interval to determine if the corrected QT correlates with heart rate. If the corrected QT interval is too short for the measured heart rate, then the pacemaker increases the heart rate.

Programmable features of this pacemaker include the rate response slope at the upper and lower rate limits, upper and lower rates, and the rate of decrease in pacing rate to the lower rate limit. A newer design permits autoprogramming of the rate response slope at the lower rate limit during sleeping hours and at the upper rate limit during exercise.[37]

As expected, this pacemaker has limitations. Some patients are not suitable candidates for evoked QT sensing. Patients receiving class IA or class III antiarrhythmics or who have repolarization abnormalities would not benefit, because the T-wave sensing could fall outside of the sensing duration of 450 msec and the pacemaker would function as a VVI generator. Patients with neuropathies that affect sympathetic stimulation of the heart do not vary their QT intervals, and would not benefit. A positive feedback loop is possible. Hedman et al. have reported that a shortened evoked QT interval can increase pacing rate that can, in turn, signal a further increase in pacing rate.[38]

Electrocardiographic Events—Paced Depolarization Integral

The depolarization gradient (i.e., the integral of the intraventricular electrogram) represents the area under the paced R wave (Fig. 32–13). In patients with complete heart block, the gradient decreases with exercise and increases again if the pacing rate is increased.[39] This finding allows the paced depolarization integral (PDI) to be used as a closed loop feedback system to increase the heart rate during exercise.[39] The sensor has the ability to change heart rate within about 10 seconds and, like evoked QT interval, increases pacing rate during periods of emotional stress.[40]

By modifying the pacing impulse to minimize electrode polarization, a unipolar electrode system can be used for pacemakers that utilize PDI sensing. Since this parameter must be measured during a paced beat, a patient with a slightly faster intrinsic rate that overrides the pacemaker will not benefit from rate adaptation. To circumvent this problem, the pacemaker emits one slightly premature impulse every fourth intrinsic beat and measures the PDI from the evoked response.

The PDI is related to ventricular mass and wall thickness.[41] Increases in ventricular mass and decreases in myocardial wall thickness decrease the PDI. Exercise at a fixed pacing rate will increase end-diastolic volume and decrease wall thickness. The result is a decreased PDI and a faster pacing rate. Lying down from a standing position has the same effect as exercise in the paced patient; therefore, this type of sensor causes paced rate to increase rather than decrease when the patient is supine.[42] Also, administration of β-blocking drugs can increase the paced rate by increasing end-diastolic volume and reducing wall thickness.[43]

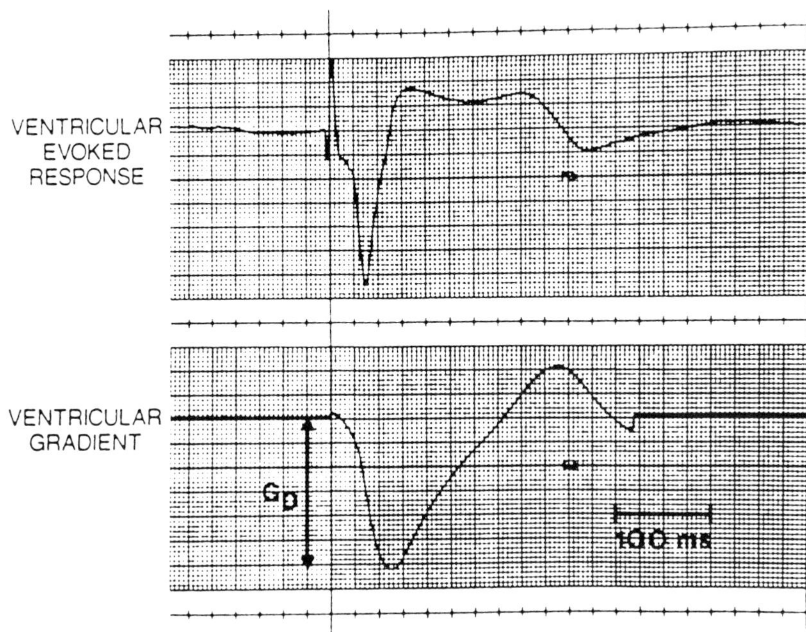

FIGURE **32–13.** One parameter used for rate adaptation is the ventricular gradient. A computer describes a curve that defines the area under the paced QRS complex (ventricular evoked response). The height of this curve is the gradient. It decreases with exercise and emotions and increases with an increase in heart rate. This finding permits a closed loop system around a baseline gradient. The gradient decreases as the patient exercises. The pacemaker senses this decrease and increases the heart rate to re-establish the baseline gradient.

Oxygen Saturation

Changes in oxygen saturation can be used as a closed loop sensing system to alter pacing rate during exercise. Exercise results in immediate increases in metabolic demand and extraction of oxygen from the arterial blood. This change is reflected in the venous blood as a decrease in oxygen saturation.[44] Normal subjects increase their heart rates to compensate for this increased metabolic demand. Patients with constant rate pacemakers cannot respond with an increase the heart rate.

The sensor has two light sources, which emit signals with wavelengths of 660 and 880 nm. The reflected light is collected by phototransistors, and the ratio of the reflected light is transferred to the timing circuit of the pacemaker. A dual light source has an advantage over light emitted at only 660 nm. Seifert et al. have shown that fibrous tissue layering of a dual light source does not affect the oxygen saturation recording, whereas a single light source responds with a falsely high saturation.[45] Emission of light requires energy from the battery that could be used for pacing in the non–rate-adaptive mode. To combat this loss of energy, the sensors are activated for only approximately 5 msec during diastole. Over a period of 5 years, the sensors, which are active for 100 hours, reduce the pacing life of the generator by 6 months.[46]

Central Venous Temperature

Metabolism associated with exercise generates not only mechanical energy but also heat that increases body temperature. Changes in temperature used to control pacing rate are variable from patient to patient.[47] In some patients, temperature decreases at the beginning of exercise as cool blood enters the central circulation, then rises to or above the baseline. Other patients have no initial drop in temperature, only an increase. Central venous blood temperature can cool either rapidly or slowly. The temperature response remains variable when the patient performs several, short, periods of exercise. All of these possibilities must be considered when developing an algorithm.

Temperature sensing requires a thermistor; therefore, a special lead is necessary. Thermistors are very reliable and are able to measure changes of as little as 0.004°C. Temperature is measured in the right ventricle several centimeters proximal to the negative electrode. Since a high impedance is required, breaks in the lead system result in loss of rate adaptive pacing.[47,48]

Several factors must be considered in the algorithm of temperature-controlled, rate adaptive pacing. Patients in heart failure experience decreases in temperature that will not necessarily increase during exercise.[49] Temperature also undergoes a circadian rhythm that the pacemaker's algorithm must consider before initiating a change in pacing rate. Environment plays an important role in that taking a hot shower or drinking hot liquids could increase the pacing rate. Also, exercising in an environment that facilitates dissipation of heat such as swimming potentially leads to an attenuated response.

Fever can affect pacing rate. These pacemakers are designed to review the temperature over a long period of time. Because the pacemaker eventually determines that the higher temperature is the baseline, prolonged fever will not maintain a high pacing rate. Acute-onset, short-duration bouts of fever will increase pacing rate.

The pacemaker responds by increasing the pacing rate to a predetermined value during the initial decrease in temperature. This initial increase in pacing rate allows the patient to experience a heart rate sufficient to begin exercising without waiting for the blood to warm. The rate will not further increase until the blood temperature has reached a specific, programmed value. At this temperature, the heart rate begins to track the changes in blood temperature according to a programmed response curve. When the patient has finished exercising, the pacing rate decreases as the temperature decreases. Commonly, temperature continues to rise for a few minutes after completing the exercise. If the patient begins a second exercise period immediately after the first, the blood temperature could decrease again. This time, the pacemaker erroneously could sense the temperature decrease as the end of exercise rather than the beginning and paradoxically decrease the pacing rate just when the patient requires a faster heart rate.[50]

Clinical Management

Preoperative Assessment of the Patient

The patient with an implanted pacemaker should receive the same attention afforded any other patient. Baseline history and physical examinations and laboratory evaluations are important. It is important to evaluate the underlying disease that led to the implantation. The patient should be specifically questioned about symptoms related to ischemic or valvular heart disease, diabetes mellitus, hypertension, and other medical illnesses.

Performing simple maneuvers such as determining pulse rate and blood pressure are important. A pulse rate that is slower than the pacemaker rate could indicate a failure of pacing capture, oversensing, or hysteresis. A loss in the volume of the peripheral pulse or a severe decrease in blood pressure when the generator initiates pacing could indicate that the patient suffers from the pacemaker syndrome. The chest and heart should be auscultated for signs of left ventricular failure and murmurs. Knowing that the patient has carotid bruits and hypertension becomes important, because even a short loss of pacing could lead to decreased cerebral perfusion. Listening for bruits also over the subclavian and femoral arteries and abdominal aorta will give an estimate of the extent of arterial disease. The physical examination must include the obvious, such as evaluation of the airway.

An extensive laboratory examination usually is unwarranted. Since these patients likely will be taking diuretics and digoxin, consider ordering serum electrolytes. Follow the usual guidelines for hemoglobin. A chest x-ray distinguishes between a unipolar and bipolar lead system, divulges the course of the lead, and pinpoints the location and possibly the identity of the generator. Comparing past and recent chest x-rays will help determine if the electrode has changed positions within the heart. A change in the position of the electrode could warn of changes in voltage threshold or sensing capabilities. An ECG discloses the patient's dependency on the pacemaker in addition to revealing pacemaker dysfunction. Aside from these suggestions, all other laboratory tests should be based on the individual patient's requirements.

Clinical Evaluation of the Pacemaker

The main reason to evaluate the pacemaker system is to determine if the system will continue to function normally throughout the perioperative period (Table 32–3). Anesthesiologists can perform this evaluation by noting the history and physical examination, by analyzing the ECG, and by placing the magnet over the pacemaker to determine if capture occurs. While taking the history, note the recurrence of symptoms that led to implantation of the pacemaker. These symptoms, which include syncope, lightheadedness, and dizziness, might be secondary to causes other than arrhythmias. Ask the patient about the date of the original implantation, any subsequent generator changes, and the results of the last telephone check of pacemaker function. Read the information on the patient's identification card, because it could offer at least the name of the manufacturer or the toll-free (1-800) telephone number. With that information, it might be possible to determine the pacemaker model. As noted above, the physical examination can offer some idea of pacemaker function. A heart rate lower than the pacemaker's programmed rate has several interpretations. The pacemaker could be abnormally functioning by oversensing ECG events. This problem is rectified by reprogramming to a less sensitive R-wave setting. Also, since the pacemaker's rate will decrease when the battery is nearing the end of its life, the battery could be depleted. The pacemaker also could be normally functioning during programmed hysteresis. During the initial moments of ventricular pacing, some patients experience the pacemaker syndrome. Hysteresis allows the patient's intrinsic heart rate to decrease to a rate lower than the pacing rate and therefore maintain sinus rhythm for longer periods of time.

TABLE 32–3
Evaluation of the Pacemaker

1. Ask patient about results of last telephone check.
2. Ask patient about location of pulse generator.
3. Ask patient to exercise muscles in area of generator. Observe for inhibition of pacing.
4. If patient cannot help with 1, 2, or 3, try to obtain ID card.
5. If 4 not possible, assume the patient has VVIR or DDDR, piezoelectric, vibratory-sensing pacemaker.
6. Observe chest x-ray for number and continuity of leads and location of electrodes.
7. Observe ECG for pacemaker dependency, failed capture, undersensing, and ventricular versus sequential pacing.
8. Apply magnet to check for pacing capture and for rate. If magnet rate is low (≤90), notify cardiologist.
9. In an emergency, proceed with the case. If the intrinsic heart rate is <50–60 and there are no impulses found on ECG, establish transcutaneous pacing.

From Zaidan JR: Practical Cardiac Electrophysiology for Advances in Anesthesia, vol 12. St. Louis, Mosby, 1995, with permission.

During the physical exam, ask the patient to exercise the muscles in the area of the generator to determine if muscle potentials will inhibit the pacemaker. Pressing the hands together will usually accomplish this task if the generator is located inferior to the clavicle. If inhibition occurs, it is possible that the pacemaker also could be inhibited during shivering.

The ECG discloses important information. Note the paced rate and compare it to the programmed rate. They should be the same. Observe for paced beats in relation to intrinsic beats. If the pacemaker is properly sensing, then pacemaker impulses and paced beats will not occur in the ST segment or on the T wave. Pacing impulses should be followed by a paced beat. If they are not, then the pacemaker might have lost pacing. In these instances, call the cardiologist.

If the patient's last telephone check was normal, the intrinsic heart rate is faster than the programmed rate, and there are no pacing impulses on the ECG, then the pacemaker is probably functioning normally. The only other necessary evaluation will determine if the pacemaker can emit impulses. Placing the magnet on the skin over the pacemaker should convert the generator to the VVI or VOO mode of activity and increase the pacing rate to approximately 90 to 100 impulses/min. When the magnet rate is similar to the pacing rate, then the battery could be low on energy and should be replaced. Also, the patient could perform a Valsalva maneuver to lower the intrinsic heart rate below the paced rate to determine if pacing impulses appear.

Monitoring

Monitoring must include standard devices such as blood pressure cuff, pulse oximeter, ECG, and end-tidal CO_2, and additional monitors when dictated by the patient's medical condition and surgical procedure. Pulmonary arterial catheterization requires consideration of the possible complications of inserting the catheter versus the benefits derived from the data. Complications include infection from a break in sterile technique and dislodgement of the pacemaker leads from the endocardial surface. The endocardial electrode's design suggests that it likely will not become dislodged while the catheter is being inserted. There are no data to determine if the catheter's withdrawal can dislodge the electrode. A central venous pressure (CVP) catheter can be inserted without difficulty; however, it is extremely important to maintain strict sterile technique.

Anesthetic Technique

General and regional anesthetic techniques can be used, provided that they take into account the patient's underlying medical illnesses, the patient's desires, and the planned surgical procedure. Volatile anesthetic agents have no apparent effect on voltage and current thresholds when added to a narcotic relaxant anesthetic technique.[51]

Anesthesia for Transvenous Pacemaker Implantation

Transvenous pacemakers are customarily implanted by the cardiologist using local anesthesia while the patient is in the electrophysiologic laboratory. Many older patients do not require sedation when they are cared for by experienced and gentle physicians. During implantation, monitor the patient with an ECG, a pulse oximeter, and a blood pressure cuff. Use end-tidal CO_2 monitoring when administering sedatives and narcotics. The anesthesiologist's hand on a peripheral pulse and verbal contact with the patient continue to be useful monitors. Epicardial electrodes are rarely used except in patients who are undergoing cardiac surgical procedures and require permanent pacemakers.

Testing Transvenous Electrode Function

Testing the function of the electrode is an important part of pacemaker implantation. Once the electrode is fluoroscopically located, a pacemaker analyzer is used to measure R-wave magnitude, impedence, and voltage and current thresholds (Table 32–4). Thresholds are determined by measuring the lowest voltage that will stimulate the ventricle and then reading the current threshold and the impedence. The analyzer turns off and becomes a sensing device to determine the number of millivolts in the R wave. The slew rate is another important measure of electrode function. The slew rate is the slope of an internal deflection of the ventriculogram. If the slope of this internal deflection is less than 0.5 V/sec, then the generator will not sense this deflection and will emit an impulse. As with measurement of the R-wave magnitude, testing the slew rate turns off the pacing circuit of the analyzer. Pacemaker-dependent patients who have third-degree block without an escape rhythm require temporary pacemakers and face obvious dangers when the analyzer is used as a sensing device. R-wave magnitude and slew rate evaluations are unnecessary in pacemaker-dependent patients, because the R waves are not present. Also, the analyzer would measure only falsely high readings from the temporary pacemaker's output.

Anesthesia for the Patient with an AICD

Cardiologists insert AICDs when the patient is in the electrophysiologic (EP) lab. When asked to participate

TABLE 32–4
Electrode Function at Implantation

Parameter Measured	Range
Voltage threshold	<1 V
Current threshold	2 mA
Impedance	500–750 Ω
R-wave magnitude	>5 mV
Slew rate	>0.5 V/sec

From Zaidan JR: Practical Cardiac Electrophysiology for Advances in Anesthesia, vol 12. St. Louis, Mosby, 1995, with permission.

in the more complex cases, anesthesiologists will be faced with patients who have poor left ventricular function and will have tried as many as four different antiarrhythmic drugs.[52] Almost 70% will have a history of coronary artery disease associated with several cardiac arrests. To facilitate induction of the arrhythmia, the patients' antiarrhythmic medication will be stopped at least a day before implantation. Patients can receive a sedative as long as oxygenation and ventilation remain normal.

If a patient with an AICD appears for general surgery, use the preoperative medications, monitoring, and anesthetic technique that are suitable for the patient's medical status. Continuing antiarrhythmic drugs until the time of surgery may help the patient maintain sinus rhythm. All types of anesthetic drugs have been successfully used in patients who have AICDs. The drugs used for anesthetic induction and maintenance should be based on the patient's preoperative cardiac status. Although volatile agents increase the fibrillation threshold in a canine model, no one knows the effect of these agents in humans.[53] The AICD should be programmed to a "no response" mode of activity for the duration of surgery by using the programming device. The patient should be in the operating room; monitored at least with a pulse oximeter, ECG, and blood pressure cuff; and prepped for surgery. Reprogramming the AICD while the patient is in the operating room allows it to function during transport to the postanesthesia care unit (PACU). The reader is referred to the discussion of electromagnetic interference for the deactivating and activating procedures in the section "Pacemaker Failure," below. Some clinicians advocate wearing gloves in the event that a defibrillating current is delivered to the patient when the AICD is active.

Pacemaker Failure

Intraoperative loss of pacing capture should be a rare event. Pacemakers lose capture during surgery mainly because of acute changes in potassium gradient across the cell membrane, electromagnetic interference, and muscle artifacts.

Acute Changes in Potassium Concentration

If potassium concentration acutely changes, the pacemaker impulse remains visible on the ECG; however, pacing capture fails. According to the modified Nernst equation, electromotive force (EMF) = $-62 \log ([K]_i/[K]_o)$ when $[K]_i$ is the potassium concentration inside the cell and $[K]_o$ is the potassium concentration outside the cell. Potassium concentrations on either side of the cell membrane normally are 150 mEq/L inside the cell and 5 mEq/L outside the cell, establishing a ratio of 30:1 and a typical resting membrane potential (RMP) of −90 mV. When this ratio acutely changes, the resting membrane potential either approaches or diverges from the threshold potential. As an extreme example, if the potassium concentration outside the cell suddenly became 1 mEq/L, then the membrane potential would change to −135 mV. The pacemaker's output would have to be increased to re-establish the charge density at the electrode-tissue interface and to stimulate the cells to threshold. Theoretically, this type of change in potassium concentration could occur if the patient were suddenly hyperventilated and potassium moved into the cell or if the patient suddenly received large quantities of potassium-free solutions that might be administered during massive volume resuscitation. If the opposite occurred and the potassium outside the cell suddenly increased to 15 mEq/L, then the RMP would become −62 mV. Less current would be required by the myocardial cells to reach threshold. A sudden change in the RMP in the positive direction could be caused by leakage of potassium from ischemic myocardial cells, by the bolus administration of potassium, or possibly by potassium release secondary to the administration of succinylcholine. These examples are extreme in nature and are meant only to reveal trends caused by acute changes in potassium concentrations.

Patients who are chronically potassium depleted potentially experience even greater problems with acute changes. Assume that a patient has a $[K]_i$ of 30 and a $[K]_o$ of 1. The ratio is 30:1 and the RMP is normal at −90 mV. If this patient receives enough potassium to raise the $[K]_o$ by 1 mEq/L, then a $[K]_o$ of 2 mEq/L creates a transmembrane ratio of 15 and an RMP of −73 mV. If a patient who is not depleted receives enough potassium to increase $[K]_o$ by 1 mEq/L, then the ratio becomes 150:6 or 25. In the normal patient, the RMP would change only to −87 mV. One would expect the depleted patient to experience more arrhythmias.

Changes in potassium concentration also effect variations in pacemaker sensing by changing the contour of the local R wave in the myocardium that surrounds the electrode. This local R wave is called the ventriculo-electrogram (VEG). Decreases in the slew rate, or slope, of the intrinsic deflection of the VEG and the magnitude of the VEG reduce the probability that the pacemaker will detect the patient's intrinsic cardiac electrical activity. The clinical result is a reduction in or loss of sensing with all of its attendant complications.

Electromagnetic Interference

Electromagnetic interference in the form of the electrocautery complicates anesthetic management. The asynchronous (VOO) generator will not be affected and will continue to emit impulses even while the electrocautery is in use. The ventricular inhibited nonprogrammable (VVIO) generator likely will be inhibited for one impulse then revert to VOO activity or to VVI activity at a different rate. It is reasonable to apply the magnet to the VVIO pacemaker while using the electrocautery to avoid any inhibition.

Programmable generators can reprogram, revert to VOO activity, or temporarily or permanently lose output.[54–57] If they are deliberately reset to VOO activity before the surgical procedure, they can still reprogram. Applying the magnet to a programmable pacemaker will increase the chance of a reprogram; however, the new program will not become manifest until the magnet is removed. Some manufacturers suggest not using the magnet. Always keep the patient fully monitored when removing the magnet. Avoiding the magnet will minimize the chance of a reprogram. If reprogramming occurs in the absence of a magnet, the new program will be instantly obvious if it involves change in rate or a decrease in output of the generator below the threshold.

Waiting until the patient is in the operating room before deactivating the AICD affords the patient arrhythmia protection during transport. If access to the generator is possible during the surgery, consider deactivating the AICD after prepping and draping the patient. "Deactivating" implies no response to the signal which would normally activate the AICD to charge and cardiovest. The AICD continues to record events, but it does not respond to the events. Apply disposable defibrillation pads for use during surgery. Reactivate the AICO before transport to the PACU, or use the disposable pads and transport the patient to the PACU with a portable defibillator.

Table 32–5 suggests guidelines for using the electrocautery in a patient with an implanted pacemaker. These guidelines will help to minimize the dangers of using the electrocautery, but they will not eliminate them. It is reasonable to program pacemakers to VOO activity to eliminate electrocautery-related inhibition. Programming to VOO will not reduce the likelihood of reprogramming to another set of parameters.

Magnetic Resonance Imaging

Implanted programmable pacemakers can revert to VOO activity, increase the ventricular rate above the high rate limit, or cease activity when they are subjected to strong magnetic fields such as that found in magnetic resonance imaging (MRI). Normal activity should resume after the magnetic field is eliminated. Pacemaker manufacturers recommend that patients with permanent pacemakers avoid MRI.

TABLE 32–5
Guidelines for Electrocautery Use

1. Never position the ground plate of the electrocautery such that the pacemaker generator is between the ground plate and the active electrode of the electrocautery.
2. Position the ground plate so that a line drawn between the two electrodes of the electrocautery are perpendicular to a line drawn between the pacemaker's electrodes.
3. Request that the surgeon not activate the electrocautery until ready to use it. The activated electrode does not have to touch the patient to affect the generator.
4. Use the smallest possible current.
5. Use the bipolar electrocautery.
6. Do not use the electrocautery within 5 inches of the pacemaker
7. Consider programming to VOO or DOO activity to eliminate inhibition of the pacemaker by the electrocautery. Remember that reprogramming out of VOO or DOO activity still can occur.
8. Consider programming to bipolar sensing if the pacemaker is using unipolar sensing. Although reprogramming can occur, bipolar sensing might reduce the possibility.
9. Apply the magnet if pacing stops (see text).

From Zaidan JR: Practical Cardiac Electrophysiology for Advances in Anesthesia, vol 12. St. Louis, Mosby, 1995, with permission.

Lithotripsy

It is possible for patients to undergo lithotripsy; however, the circuitry of the pacemaker including the piezoelectric crystal can be permanently damaged if it is at the focal point of the lithotripsy beam. For this reason, patients with piezoelectric, rate adaptive pacemakers implanted in the abdomen probably should not undergo lithotripsy. Some manufacturers suggest programming the pacemaker to a single-chamber, non–rate responsive mode of activity and ensuring that the focal point of the beam is more than 2 inches away from the generator. In a survey by Drach et al., 131 patients with pacemakers underwent 142 lithotripsies.[58] Only four patients had problems with the pacemakers. These problems were easily corrected. Celentano et al., in a case report, used isoproterenol to maintain the patient's heart rate and recommended that a cardiologist stand by to treat complications and that emergency pacing equipment be available.[59]

Myopotentials

Although they usually are outside the filtering limits and are too low in voltage to affect the pacing circuit or reprogram the generator, muscle potentials occasionally cause inhibition[60,61] (Fig. 32–14). To determine if inhibition occurs, ask the patient if exercising muscles in the area of the generator initiates prepacemaker symptoms. One case has been reported in which fasciculations associated with succinylcholine have inhibited a pacemaker.[62] Consider using a defasciculating dose of a neuromuscular blocking drug before administering succinylcholine.[63]

Severe shivering could have several effects depending on the type of pacemaker. VVIO pacemakers could be inhibited. Warming the patient would stop this inhibition. Movement-controlled VVIR and DDDR pacemakers may respond to shivering by increasing the rate. Warming the patient should slow the pacemaker rate to the baseline. Blood temperature– and oxygen saturation–controlled VVIR or DDDR pacemakers do not respond to shivering per se, but might increase their rates due to the physiologic changes associated with muscle activity. Their rates would remain high after shivering stopped until the metabolic effects of shivering dissipated.

Nitrous Oxide

Nitrous oxide used shortly after placement of a pacemaker and subcutaneous emphysema both have been reported as inhibiting unipolar pacemaker function.[64,65] Apparently, the ground electrode in the generator's casing did not have good contact with the tissue as the pocket around the pacemaker expanded with nitrous oxide. In these cases, applying pressure over the pacemaker reestablished pacing. Consider reprogramming to bipolar pacing.

Electrical Stimulators

Andersen et al. have described a method to ensure that dorsal column stimulators do not inhibit VVI pacemak-

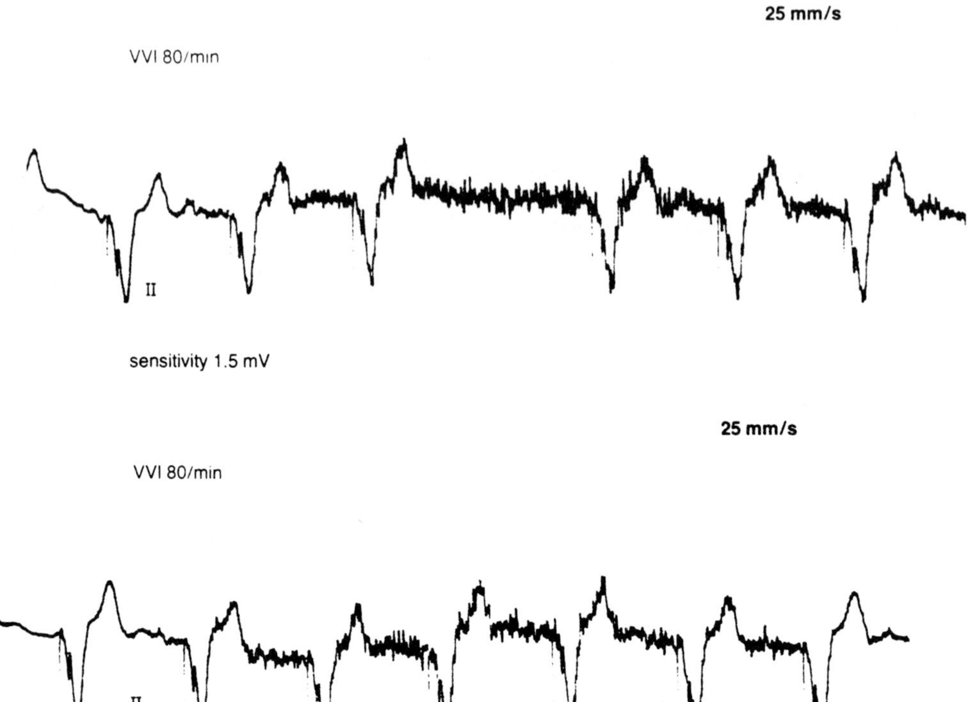

FIGURE **32–14.** The *upper figure* demonstrates myopotential inhibition of a pacemaker programmed to an R-wave sensitivity of 1.5 mV. In the center of the ECG, the patient pressed his hands together to cause the muscle activity. Notice the pause in pacing between the third and fourth paced beats. In the *lower figure*, programming the R-wave sensitivity to 2.4 mV corrected the problem. Notice that there is no pause in pacing associated with the lower sensitivity (higher number). (From Schuller H, Fahraeus T: Pacemaker Electrocardiograms–an Introduction to Practical Analysis, 1983. Solna, Sweden, Siemens-Elema AB, with permission.)

ers or convert VVI pacemakers to VOO activity.[66] Nerve stimulators have been applied directly over pacemaker generators purposely to inhibit the pacemakers.[67] This inhibition, which is possible even if the stimulator were used on the arm, could be used during surgery in patients who experience the pacemaker syndrome. By placing the electrodes over the pacemaker generator and artificially inhibiting the pacemaker, the patient's heart rate would decrease to lower levels without reprogramming and maintain sinus rhythm and higher blood pressure. The pacemaker would remain in the inhibited mode until the nerve stimulator is turned off even if the heart rate were unacceptably low.

Cross-Talk

Cross-talk, or far-field sensing of the atrial output by the R-wave sensing circuitry in a sequential pacemaker, is enhanced by very short blanking periods, very sensitive R-wave detection, and high atrial pacing outputs. The clinical outcome is accidental loss of ventricular pacing (Fig. 32–15). Engineers added additional sensing circuits to detect far-field signals. Signals detected during this special sensing period force ventricular pacing at a shorter than programmed AV interval rather than allowing inhibition. Therefore, it is possible for an implanted DDD or DDDR pacemaker to change its atrioventricular (AV) interval on a beat-to-beat basis. When using a DVI external generator in the operating room, it is possible to reduce the likelihood of cross-talk by setting the R-wave sensitivity to a higher number and decreasing the atrial output to the atrial pacing threshold plus 1 to 2 mA.

Myocardial Infarction

Myocardial infarctions (MIs) affect pacing and sensing. The radius of an electrode affects threshold. For a given current entering the electrode, a specific charge density that is related to the radius of the electrode develops at the electrode-myocardial interface. One cell reaches threshold and propagates the impulse throughout the myocardium. A healed myocardial infarction enlarges the radius of the electrode as scar tissue develops. If the radius of the electrode increases in size but the current remains the same, a smaller charge density occurs at the interface. Cells will not reach threshold and the pacemaker impulse will not pace the ventricle. This problem should not occur in the operating room. When it does occur, the cardiologist programs the pacemaker to a higher output.

A myocardial infarction can cause loss of sensing capabilities. For sensing to occur, a potential difference must develop between two electrodes. An acute myocardial infarction neighboring but not surrounding the electrode could alter the direction or the morphology of

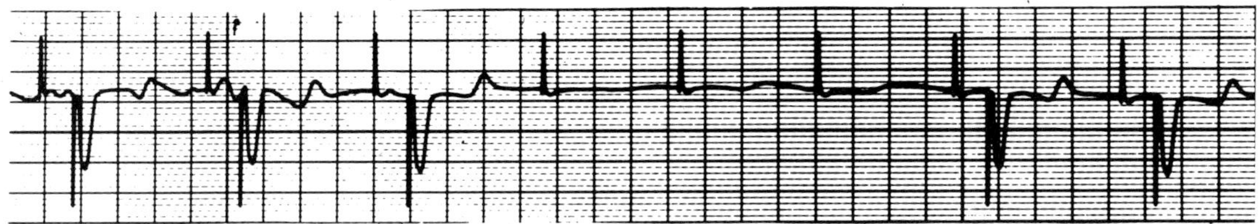

FIGURE **32–15.** Far field sensing, also called cross-talk, occurs at the fourth through sixth atrial pacing impulses. The atrial impulse inhibits the pacemaker's ventricular output. If this problem occurs in the operating room or in the intensive care unit, set the R-wave sensitivity to a higher number and decrease the atrial output of the generator.

the depolarization. A unipolar lead system lessens the chance that a change in the VEG will inhibit sensing, because its electrodes are separated by the entire length of the lead. Any depolarization passing the electrode in the heart will create a potential difference between the two electrodes. A bipolar system with its closely associated electrodes presents a different problem. A depolarization approaching bipolar electrodes parallel to the lead results in a large R wave, because the impulse will pass one electrode before reaching the other electrode and create a large potential difference between the two electrodes. A depolarization moving perpendicularly to the lead simultaneously approaches both electrodes. In this case, there will be no potential difference between the two electrodes, the pacemaker will not detect the depolarization, and the patient will experience loss of sensing.

Electrode Dislodgement

A well-placed, chronic electrode should not dislodge during the course of an operation. On the contrary, a temporary transvenous electrode can be dislodged from its initial location by motion of the ventricle or by accidental manipulation of the external portion of the lead. A sudden change in the size or direction of the pacing impulse or a sudden increase in threshold or loss of pacing diagnoses this problem. Increasing the output of the external generator might help to re-establish capture.

Treatment of Pacemaker Failure

Treatment of pacemaker failure depends on the patient's underlying rate and rhythm (Table 32–6). If the patient has a rate sufficient to maintain blood pressure and clinically assessed cardiac output, then continuous observation is reasonable. Bradycardia leading to compromise of cardiac output and blood pressure can be treated by administering atropine or isoproterenol or by using transcutaneous or transvenous pacing electrodes. Isoproterenol can be infused to increase the heart rate through its β_1-adrenergic effects. An infusion rate of approximately 0.01 μg/kg/min is a reasonable starting point. Transcutaneous electrodes should be applied over the sternum and between the scapulae. Begin pacing by setting the rate at approximately 70 impulses/min and then increasing the output of the external generator until pacing capture appears on the ECG and each paced beat creates a palpable pulse. The last choice is to insert a transvenous electrode, because it is difficult to position when the patient has a bradycardia or an arrest. Follow the usual basic and advanced cardiopulmonary resuscitation (CPR) guidelines if cardiac arrest occurs.

TABLE **32–6**
Treatment of Pacemaker Failure

Rate	Possible Treatment
Adequate to maintain blood pressure	1. Observe, oxygen 2. Atropine 3. Try magnet
Severe bradycardia, hypotension	1. Oxygen, airway control 2. Atropine 3. Isoproterenol 4. Try magnet 5. Transcutaneous pacing
No escape rhythm	1. CPR 2. Isoproterenol 3. Try magnet 4. Transcutaneous pacing

From Zaidan JR: Practical Cardiac Electrophysiology for Advances in Anesthesia, vol 12. St. Louis, Mosby, 1995, with permission.

Indications for Pacing

Permanent Pacemaker

The Committee on Pacemaker Implantation of the American College of Cardiology/American Heart Association Task Force on Assessment of Diagnostic and Therapeutic Cardiovascular Procedures developed guidelines for implantation of permanent pacemakers.[68] The indications listed in Table 32–7 are categorized according to the degree of agreement with the indication. These classifications are further modified by factors such as overall

TABLE **32–7**
Classification of Permanent Pacemaker Indications*

Class I	Conditions for which there is general agreement that permanent pacemakers or antitachycardia devices should be implanted
Class II	Conditions for which permanent pacemakers or antitachycardia devices are frequently used but there is divergence of opinion with respect to the necessity of their insertion
Class III	Conditions for which there is general agreement that pacemakers or antitachycardia devices are unnecessary.

*Modified from Dreifus LS, Fisch C, Griffin JC, et al: Guidelines for implantation of cardiac pacemakers and antiarrhythmia devices. ACC/AHA Task Force report. J Am Coll Cardiol 18:1, 1991, with permission.

physical and mental state of the patient, presence of associated underlying cardiac disease, presence of cerebrovascular disease, desire to drive a car, and distance to medical care.[68] Table 32–8 lists the indications that are further categorized into the three classes. To summarize the guidelines related to AV block, if symptoms including lightheadedness, dizziness, syncope or near syncope, marked exercise intolerance, or congestive heart failure are related to a bradycardia, then a permanent pacemaker is indicated. Pacemakers are not indicated if the patient experiences asymptomatic first-degree AV block or asymptomatic type I second-degree AV block within the AV node. If a patient is suffering from a myocardial infarction, then a permanent pacemaker is indicated only if type II second-degree AV block or complete AV block persists or if transient, advanced AV block occurs in the presence of bundle branch block.

Temporary Pacemaker

The indications for the placement of a temporary perioperative pacemaker are not as structured as the indications for permanent pacemakers.

Acute Myocardial Infarction

Sinus node dysfunction occurs in 5 to 30% of patients who have experienced a myocardial infarction.[69,70] Bradycardia does not require treatment unless there is evidence of worsening ischemia or the patient has symptoms. Atropine remains first-line therapy. Temporary pacing is the alternative if atropine or isoproterenol does not increase the heart rate or if the bradycardia is prolonged and continues to cause symptoms.

Atrioventricular blocks, especially first-degree, occur in up to 25% of patients with myocardial infarctions.[70,71] During an inferior infarction, third-degree block usually results in a narrow QRS complex and a stable, atropine-responsive rate of 50 to 60 bpm.[72,73] Temporary pacing generally is not necessary. Conversely, a first-degree block associated with an acute anterior myocardial infarction can quickly proceed to third-degree block, a wide complex, and a severe bradycardia.[74] Pacing is required in this clinical setting at the onset of the first-degree block. Patients with anterior myocardial infarctions and third-degree AV block suffer extensive damage often leading to congestive failure.

Bundle branch block below the AV node occurs more commonly after an anterior MI than after an inferior MI,[74] and once it develops, patients with a new bundle branch block (BBB) have a higher mortality rate.[75,76] It is recommended that patients who experience alternating BBB, first-degree AV block plus new bifascicular BBB, first-degree AV block plus old bifascicular BBB, or new bifascicular BBB have temporary pacemakers inserted.

Dysrhythmias

Torsades de pointes is one dysrhythmia that can be controlled with atrial or ventricular pacing even though it is not associated with AV or bundle branch block.[77,78] Some patients require temporary pacing while the cardiologist is finding the cause of and treating Torsades. If a patient is scheduled for emergency surgery and the cause of the torsades pattern is not known, then pacing will help control the dysrhythmia.

Rapid atrial pacing converts re-entrant supraventricular tachycardias (SVTs) to sinus rhythm. Occasionally, these dysrhythmias require repeated trials of rapid atrial pacing if cardioversion fails and drugs have not had time to reach therapeutic levels. Consider using atrial pacing to control the SVT during emergency surgery.

Perioperative

Inserting a temporary pacemaker specifically for the perioperative period should be a very rare occurrence. If a patient who is resolving an MI is scheduled for surgery, then the above recommendations for pacing during an MI should be followed with the help of the cardiologist. Occasionally, the anesthesiologist will encounter conduction blocks that the cardiologist will not treat with temporary pacing. In these instances, the anesthesiologist can modify the opinion by considering the extent and location of surgery, the possibility of blood loss and major fluid and electrolyte shifts, and the coronary anatomy with the possibility for extension of an inferior MI to an anterior MI.

A cardiologist's consult would be very helpful if the patient has a second-degree AV block plus bifascicular block. Also consider inserting a temporary pacemaker if the patient has evidence of a block on the ECG and just experienced a syncopal episode. As an example, a patient who fainted, fell, and fractured a hip might need a temporary pacemaker if the ECG reveals a complete LBBB. Although it would be a rare event, a patient who has a bifascicular block, is comatose, and is scheduled for evacuation of a subdural or epidural hematoma might benefit from a temporary pacemaker.

Commonly Used Pacing Modalities

Transcutaneous, transesophageal, and transvenous pacing are common forms of pacing the atrium and ventricle. Each modality is useful in the appropriate setting.

Transcutaneous Pacing

Transcutaneous pacing results in a hemodynamic picture similar to that of transvenous pacing either with simultaneous atrial and ventricular contraction or with retrograde ventriculoatrial conduction.[79,80] In its earliest form, transcutaneous pacing unfortunately caused discomfort from electrical stimulation and pectoralis muscle contraction.[81] Increasing both the surface area of the cutaneous electrodes and the pulse duration relieved these problems so that the technique is now far more acceptable to the patients.[82] Age, body habitus, and cardiac drug therapy seem not to affect the threshold; however,

TABLE 32–8
Indications for Permanent Pacing

Complete Heart Block Class I

1. Permanent or intermittent complete heart block associated with symptomatic bradycardia, medical conditions that require drugs that cause symptomatic bradycardia, congestive failure, documented asystole >3 seconds or heart rate. <40 in an asymptomatic patient, mental confusion that clears with temporary pacing, and post-AV junction ablation.
2. Symptomatic permanent or intermittent second-degree AV block.
3. Atrial fibrillation or atrial flutter associated with symptomatic bradycardia not caused by drugs.

Complete Heart Block Class II

1. Permanent or intermittent complete heart block associated with ventricular rates >40.
2. Permanent or intermittent asymptomatic type II second-degree heart block.
3. Asymptomatic type I second-degree AV block located within or distal to the bundle of His.

Complete Heart Block, Class III

1. First-degree AV block.
2. Asymptomatic type I second-degree AV block proximal to the AV node.

Bifascicular and Trifascicular Block, Class I

1. Bifascicular block in the presence of complete heart block and symptomatic bradycardia.
2. Bifascicular or trifascicular block with intermittent type II second-degree AV block without symptoms.

Bifascicular and Trifascicular Block, Class II

1. Bi- or trifascicular block associated with synscope of unidentified cause.
2. HV interval >100 msec.
3. Pacing-induced block distal to the bundle of His.

Bifascicular and Trifascicular Block, Class III

1. Fascicular block without AV block or with first-degree AV block without symptoms.

Sinus Node Dysfunction, Class I

1. Documented symptomatic bradycardia.

Sinus Node Dysfunction, Class II

1. Heart rate <40 in the presence of or absence of drug administration when the symptoms cannot unequivocally be related to the bradycardia.

Sinus Node Dysfunction, Class III

1. Asymptomatic bradycardia even when the heart rate is <40.
2. Symptoms that are clearly unassociated with bradycardia.

Hypersensitive Carotid Sinus, Class I

1. In the absence of medication that depresses the SA node, recurrent syncope caused by minimal stimulation of the carotid sinus.

Hypersensitive Carotid Sinus, Class II

1. Recurrent syncope in the absence of provocative events.
2. Syncope for which temporary pacing can benefit the patient during a provocative test.

Hypersensitive Carotid Sinus, Class III

1. Bradycardia without symptoms
2. Vague symptoms possibly related to carotid sinus stimulation.
3. No symptoms after carotid sinus stimulation.

Termination of Tachycardias, Class I

1. Medical failure of supraventricular tachycardias that are recurrent and symptomatic.
2. Drug-resistant, symptomatic, recurrent ventricular tachycardia following AICD implantation.

Termination of Tachycardias, Class II

1. An alternative to drug therapy.

Termination of Tachycardias, Class III

1. Tachydardias that are accelerated or converted to fibrillation by pacing.
2. An accessory pathway that rapidly conducts in an anterograde fashion regardless of the participation of that pathway in the tachycardia.

Indications for Acid Implantation, Class I

1. Repeated episodes of ventricular tachycardia or fibrillation when it is not feasible to use outpatient monitoring or electrophysiologic testing to determine the efficacy of drug therapy.
2. Repeated episodes of ventricular tachycardia or fibrillation when drug therapy has failed or when an effective drug was not tolerated.
3. Electrophysiologically inducible episodes of ventricular tachycardia or fibrillation in the presence of drug therapy or after surgery or catheter ablation when drugs have failed.

Indications for Acid Implantation, Class II

1. Documented ventricular tachycardia or fibrillation when electrophysiologic testing or monitoring is possible.
2. Syncope of undetermined origin in the presence of inducible ventricular tachycardia or fibrillation when there is no effective drug or a tolerated drug is not available or appropriate.

Indications for Acid Implantation, Class III

1. Syncope of undetermined origin when the patient does not have inducible arrhythmias.
2. Arrhythmias other than ventricular tachycardia or fibrillation.
3. Incessant ventricular tachycardia or fibrillation.

From Zaidan JR: Practical Cardiac Electrophysiology for Advances in Anesthesia, vol 12. St. Louis, Mosby, 1995, with permission.
AV, atrioventricular; AICD, automatic implantable cardioverter defibrillator.

air trapped in the pleural and mediastinal spaces after thoracic surgical procedures elevates the threshold.[82–84] Thresholds are also potentially elevated in patients who have emphysema or pericardial effusion or who require positive-pressure ventilation.[84–86]

The procedure to initiate pacing is as follows: position the negative electrode in the V_3 location and the positive electrode just to the left of the spine at the lower aspect of the scapula.[87] During a cardiac arrest, adjust the external generator to a pulse duration of 40 msec and an output of 120 mA. The pulse duration is usually 20 to 40 msec, and the threshold ranges from 40 to 120 mA.[84,88] Begin pacing in the asynchronous mode. Chest compressions can be performed over the anterior chest electrode.

Considering the possible complications associated with transvenous pacing and the recent technological refinements and unprecedented safety record for transcutaneous pacing, emergent situations now call for the use of transcutaneous pacing as the first therapeutic choice.[82,84,89,90]

Transvenous Pacing

Transvenous techniques provide both atrial and ventricular pacing in a manner that is easily accepted by the patient. Generally, pacing is reliable and stable over a long period of time.

Many of the temporary ventricular pacing catheters have a dual electrode configuration that permits the clinician to establish either unipolar or bipolar pacing. A balloon is commonly located at the tip of the catheter so that the catheter can be flow directed into the right ventricular endocardium (Fig. 32–16). The atrial lead usually assumes a J shape so that it can be directed into the right atrial appendage. During CPR, the right internal jugular vein approach allows the most rapid placement of a ventricular pacing catheter.[91]

Pacemakers used for temporary pacing have several controls with which the clinician should be familiar (Fig. 32–17). External generators have a "fool-proof" on-off switch that locks in the on position. Thresholds range from 2 to 4 mA, with a factory-set pulse duration of 1 to 2 msec. Overcome the loss of capture associated with positive-pressure ventilation by increasing the output of the generator. In order to determine the sensing threshold, increase the rate and output to ensure capture, then decrease the rate to 15% below the patient's heart rate. Starting with the R-wave sensitivity control at the lowest number, slowly increase the number (decrease the sensitivity) until pacing impulses reappear. The number indicated on the R-wave sensitivity control is the sensing threshold. Decrease the number once again to several millivolts below the threshold. If time does not permit this formal determination, adjust the R-wave sensitivity control to 5 mV so that the pacemaker will not sense shivering and possibly T waves but will sense R waves. The rate should be a physiologic value for the clinical situation. If sequential pacing is used, then the AV interval should be initially set at approximately 175 to 200 msec. Lengthening the AV interval in a patient who has

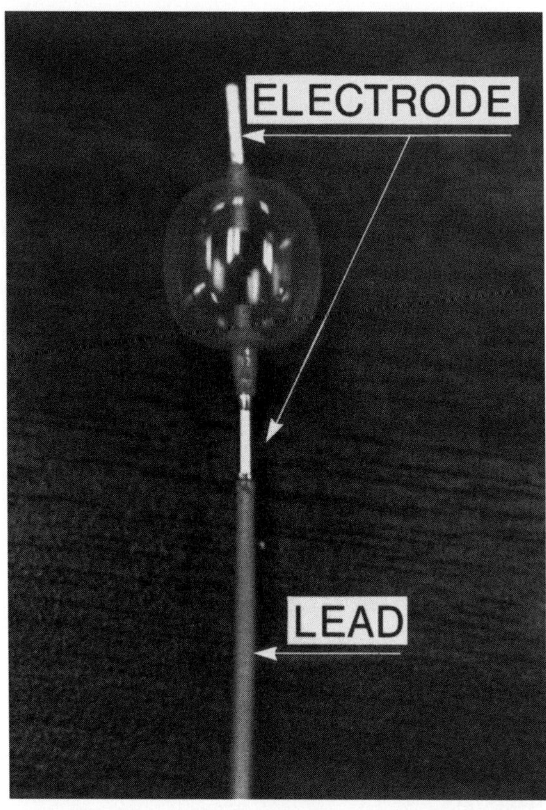

FIGURE **32–16.** A typical temporary, transvenous electrode for use in the right ventricle generally includes two electrodes. The distal electrode at the tip of the lead should be the negative or stimulating electrode. The balloon is inflated until the electrode enters the right ventricle. Once a ventricular tracing is noted on the ECG, the balloon is usually deflated and the lead slowly advanced until ST-segment elevation occurs.

a hypertrophic myocardium allows the atrium more time to fill the ventricle and increase the cardiac output.

A temporary, transvenous pacing lead can be positioned either by fluoroscopic control or by ECG analysis of the intracavitary electrogram. Figure 32–18 reveals the ECG configurations associated with the atrium, ventricle, and endocardium. To obtain the intracavitary ECG, connect the distal electrode to the chest lead and observe V_5, or connect the distal electrode to the left leg lead and the proximal electrode to the right arm lead and observe lead II. Keep the balloon inflated until the distal electrode enters the ventricle, then deflate the balloon and slowly advance the lead until ST-segment elevation appears. At this point, the electrode will be in contact with the endocardium. In an emergency, connect the generator to the pacing lead, set the generator to maximal output, asynchronous pacing and advance the lead until, it is hoped, ventricular pacing occurs.

Two complications that occur during transvenous pacing deserve comment. Ventricular arrhythmias can arise during insertion and manipulation of the electrode. It is appropriate either to administer lidocaine when the arrhythmias interfere with placement of the electrode, or to withdraw the electrode several centimeters to stop these arrhythmias.[92,93] A defibrillator should be present when inserting a transvenous pacing electrode. Apart

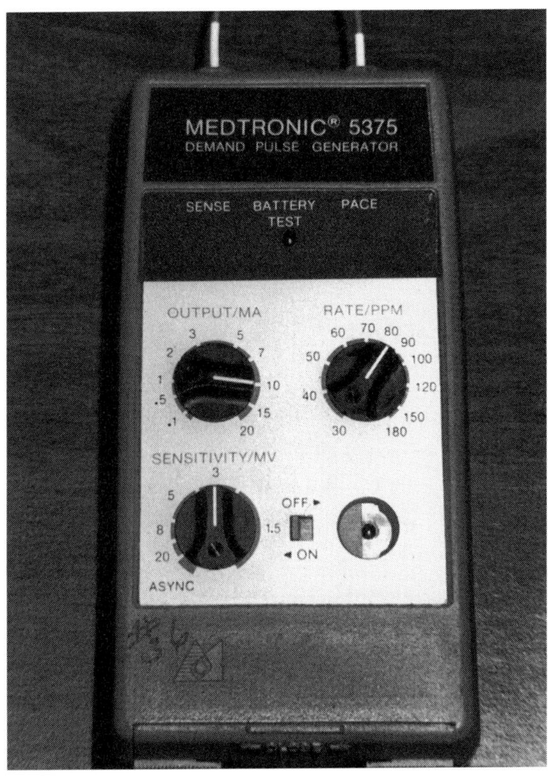

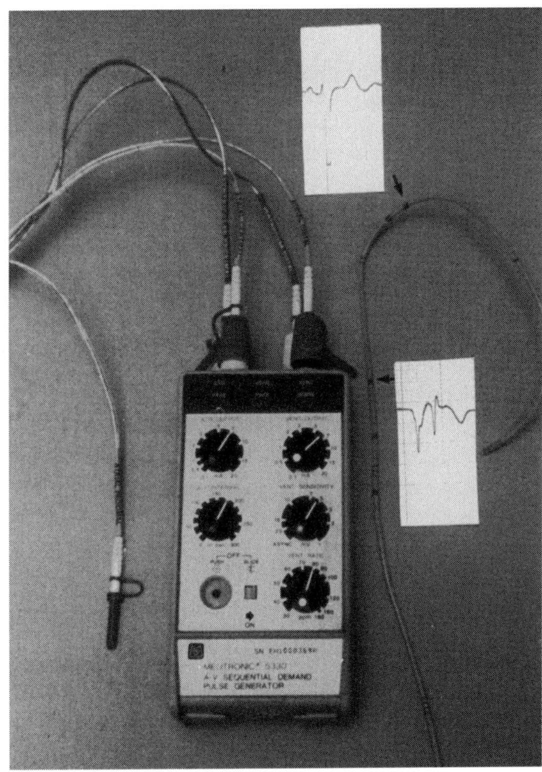

A B

FIGURE **32–17.** *A*, Three controls on the external VVI/VOO pacemaker are the output, the rate, and the R-wave sensitivity. *B*, In addition to the above controls, a DVI external generator includes controls for atrial output and AV interval. This figure reveals typical electrograms that should be recorded from the distal atrial and distal ventricular electrodes of a pacing pulmonary arterial catheter. (Courtesy of Medtronic, Inc., Minneapolis, MN.)

from mechanical stimulation, ventricular arrhythmias can occur also as an R on T phenomenon during ventricular pacing. Consistently sensing the R wave, stimulating with the negative electrode, and adjusting the output of the generator to no higher than twice the capture threshold should help to avert the arrhythmias.

Another complication of temporary, transvenous, ventricular pacing is perforation of the myocardium. This complication occurs in 2 to 20% of patients and, although clinical signs and symptoms can be absent, chest and shoulder pain and skeletal muscle or diaphragmatic pacing commonly occur[94,95]; 1% of the perforations lead to tamponade and 5% lead to pericarditis.[96] The chest x-ray should reveal an extracardiac location of the electrode. The surface ECG changes its configuration or axis, and ventricular arrhythmias occur. An intramyocardial electrode causes ventricular arrhythmias that have the same configuration as the paced beats.[96] Tamponade will require emergency aspiration of the pericardium and possibly surgery. Generally, the pacing lead can be withdrawn under ECG guidance and the patient placed under tamponade precautions.

Included in the design of the pacing pulmonary arterial catheter and the Paceport Swan-Ganz catheter are variations of the transvenous electrode (Figs. 32–18B and 32–19). Both of these catheters have a high degree of pacing success in clinical settings.[97,98] When using the pacing pulmonary arterial catheter, ensure that the tip is not in the permanent wedge position when the distal ventricular electrode reaches the ventricle. It might be necessary to withdraw the catheter several centimeters and lose ventricular pacing to avoid a permanent wedge. In this case, the ventricular electrodes can be used to pace the atrium. Figure 32–20 demonstrates simultaneous pressure and ECG recordings as the pacing pulmonary arterial catheter advances to its final position.

The Paceport Swan-Ganz catheter should be positioned as usual. At this point, transduce the right ventricular port to ensure a ventricular trace, then insert the electrode until the gray-green boundary on the lead is located exactly at the zero mark on the catheter. This zero position indicates that the tip of the electrode is located just at the opening of the right ventricular port. Inserting the lead farther will advance first the distal, negative electrode and then the more proximal, positive electrode toward the right ventricular endocardium. Generally, it is necessary to insert this catheter approximately 4 cm from the zero position to achieve low pacing thresholds. As the electrode is inserted, expect to notice ventricular contractions. This catheter is available with ventricular and atrial electrodes; however, the original catheter was not designed to accommodate atrial pacing.

Transesophageal Pacing

Transesophageal atrial pacing is feasible, because electrodes can be placed within 1.5 cm of the left atrium. In

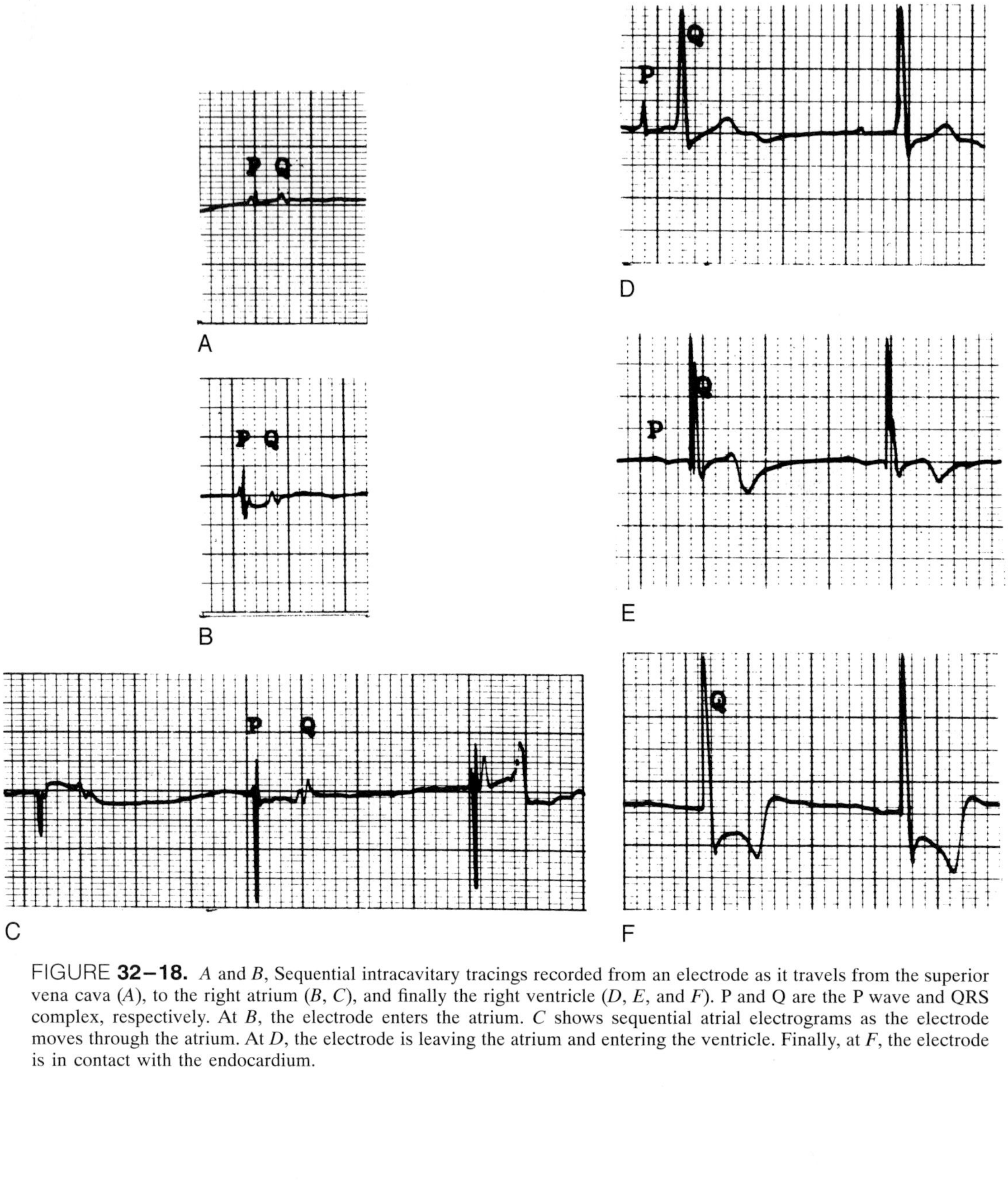

FIGURE **32–18.** *A* and *B*, Sequential intracavitary tracings recorded from an electrode as it travels from the superior vena cava (*A*), to the right atrium (*B*, *C*), and finally the right ventricle (*D*, *E*, and *F*). P and Q are the P wave and QRS complex, respectively. At *B*, the electrode enters the atrium. *C* shows sequential atrial electrograms as the electrode moves through the atrium. At *D*, the electrode is leaving the atrium and entering the ventricle. Finally, at *F*, the electrode is in contact with the endocardium.

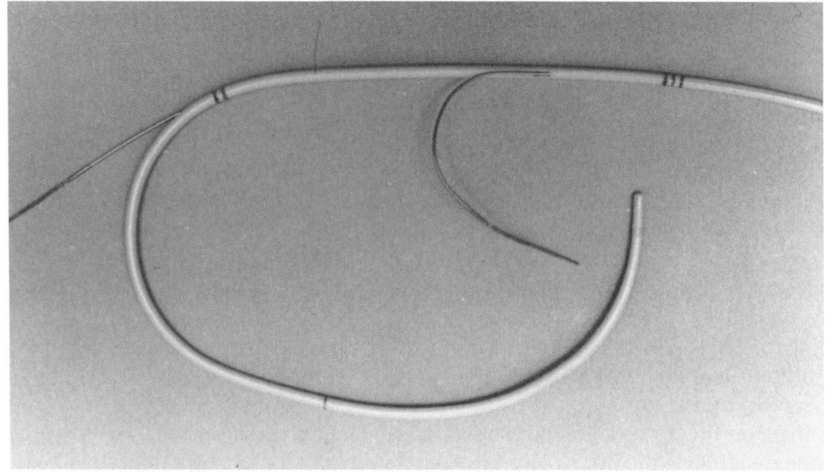

FIGURE **32–19.** A Paceport Swan-Ganz catheter is used as a routine pulmonary arterial catheter until pacing is required. The pacing probe is then inserted through the right ventricular port and extended from the opening in the catheter about 4 cm. A J-shaped atrial electrode is available.

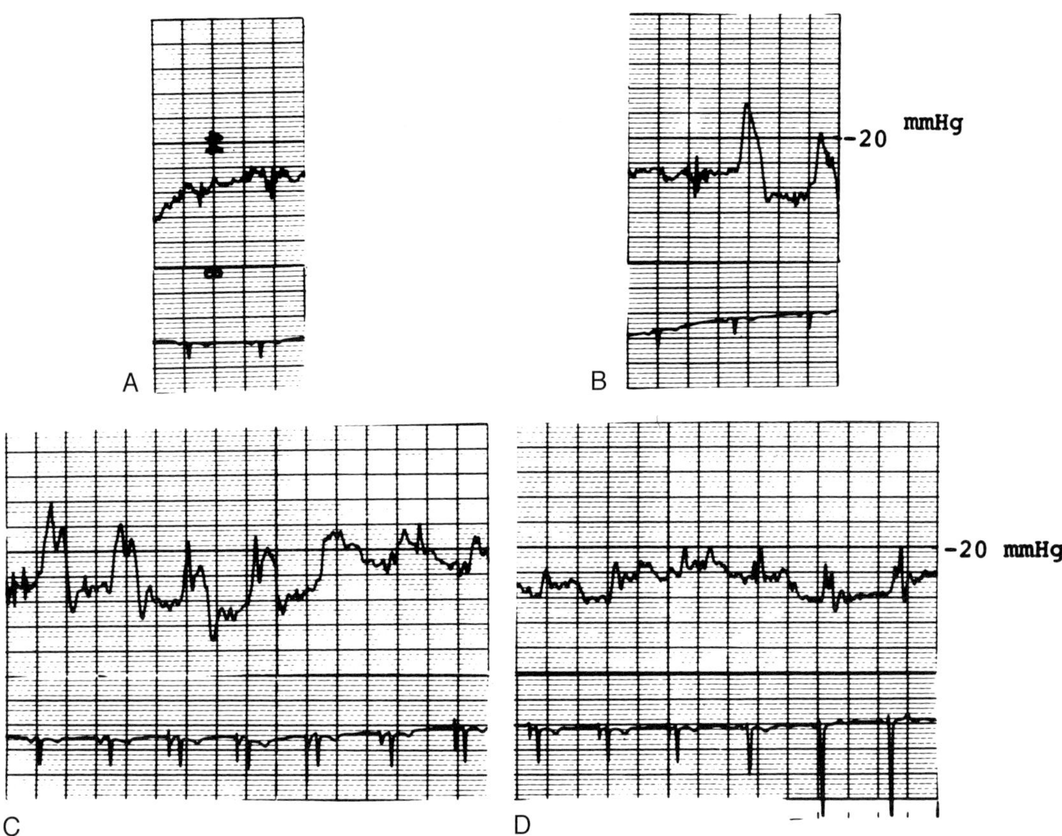

FIGURE **32–20.** *A* through *D*, Sequential and simultaneous tracings of a pacing pulmonary arterial catheter as it floats to the pulmonary artery and wedge positions. *A*, The catheter is recording pressure in the atrium (*upper pressure tracing*) and an electrogram in the SVC (*lower ECG*). *B*, The tip of the catheter reaches the right ventricle; however, the most distal ventricular electrode remains in the SVC. *C*, The pressure tracing shows movement of the catheter from the right ventricle through the outflow tract and into the pulmonary artery. At the same time, the electrode moves through the atrium as evidenced by the change in the P wave from a very small inverted deflection to a very deep inverted deflection and then to a biphasic wave. *D*, The pressure tracing reveals the wedge at the right margin and the electrode reaches the ventricle. Notice the large QRS complex with a small, almost nonexistent positive P wave.

an early form, esophageal electrodes were used to diagnose arrhythmias by simultaneously recording the esophageal atrial electrogram and the surface ECG. Other uses for this type of pacing include evaluation of sinus node function, assessment of AV nodal function, terminating supraventricular arrhythmias, terminating ventricular arrhythmias associated with bradycardia, and overriding sinus bradycardias.[99–101] Patients will experience a feeling of indigestion with generator outputs of 15 mA.[99] Intolerable burning occurs, especially above 30 mA.[102]

To position the esophageal electrodes in a normal sized adult, advance the probe approximately 35 cm from the teeth, connect the electrodes to an ECG, and finally manipulate the position until the atrial electrogram reveals the largest deflection[102,103] (Fig. 32–21). The lowest pacing threshold should be located within 3 cm of this point.[103] The incidence of atrial capture should approach 100% with thresholds of 8 to 14 mA.[99,100,104,105]

Esophageal ventricular pacing is not as easy to establish as atrial pacing.[105,106] Because the ventricles are located approximately 3 cm from the esophagus and the maximal current density at the electrode decreases with the cube of the distance from the source of the current, ventricles receive only 20% of the maximal current density.[99,107] Ventricular pacing thresholds, therefore, can reach 80 mA.[108] A suggested technique to establish emergency esophageal ventricular pacing in a patient with an esophageal probe in place is to insert the probe 2 to 4 more cm, increase the output of the generator, and observe for ventricular pacing.

Choosing a Pacing Modality

There are no data to suggest which type of pacing is best suited for an individual patient. The basic rule to remember is that ventricular pacing saves a life; therefore, in an emergent situation, it is best to establish ventricular pacing. Transvenous pacing is comfortable for the patient but requires time, is difficult to establish when the patient has a severe bradycardia or a complete arrest, and requires some expertise. Transesophageal electrodes are best for atrial pacing. If a patient arrests and the only means of pacing is through the esophagus, inserting the probe to approximately 40 cm and increasing the output might establish ventricular capture. Since transcutaneous pacing has few complications and all of the equipment is usually located with the defibrillator, it is reasonable

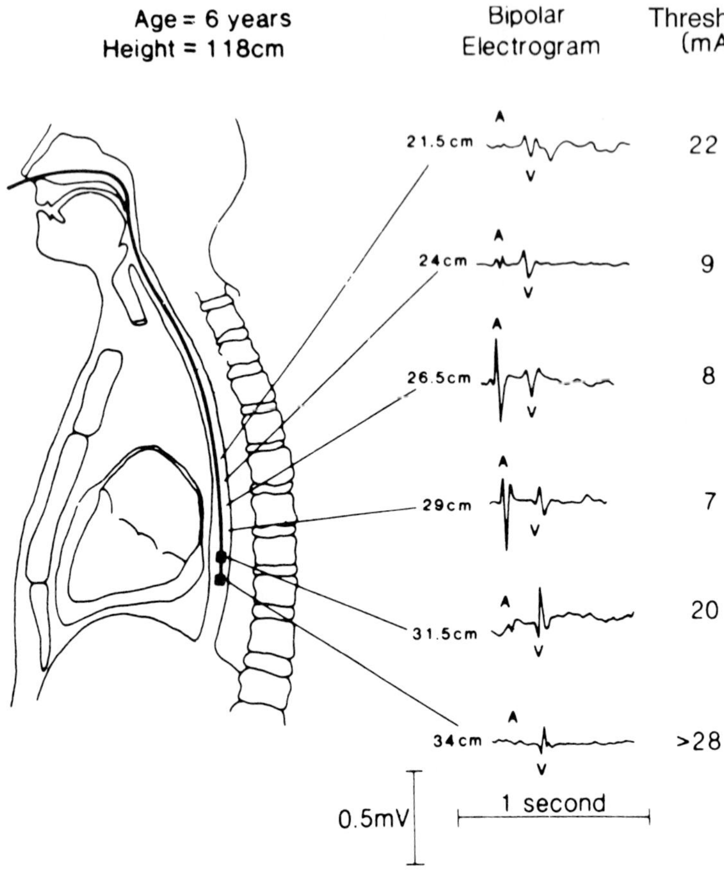

FIGURE **32–21.** This diagram shows the position of an esophageal electrode in the best position for pacing the atrium in a 6-year-old patient. The adult position would be approximately 35 cm. To pace the ventricle, insert the esophageal probe 4 cm more and expect to increase the output of the generator. (From Wood M, Ellenbogen K, Haines D: Temporary cardiac pacing. In Ellenbogen KA (ed): Cardiac Pacing, 1st ed. Cambridge, MA, Blackwell Publishing Co, 1992, p 199, with permission.)

to establish transcutaneous pacing when the patient requires emergency ventricular pacing.

References

1. Sinnaeve A, Willems R, Backers J, et al: Pacing and sensing: How can one electrode fulfill both requirements? PACE 10:546, 1987.
2. Kay GN: Basic aspects of cardiac pacing. In Ellenbogen KA (ed): Cardiac Pacing, 1st ed. Cambridge, MA, Blackwell Publishing Co, 1992, p 32.
3. Ripart A, Mugica J: Electrode-heart interface: Definition of the ideal electrode. PACE 6:410, 1983.
4. Irnich W: Comparison of pacing electrodes of different shape and material—recommendations. PACE 6:422, 1983.
5. Irnich W: The electrode myocardial interface. PACE 3:338, 1985.
6. Brandt J, Attewell R, Fahraeus T, Schuller H: Atrial and ventricular stimulation threshold development: A comparative study in patients with a DDD pacemaker and two identical carbon-tip leads. PACE 13:859, 1990.
7. Bernstein AD, Camm AJ, Fletcher RD, et al: The NASPE/BPEG generic pacemaker code for antibradyarrhythmia and adaptive-rate pacing and antitachyarrhythmia devices. PACE 10:794, 1987.
8. Mirowski M, Reid PR, Mower MM: Termination of malignant ventricular arrhythmias with an implanted automatic defibrillator in human beings. N Engl J Med 303:322, 1980.
9. Gaba D, Wyner J, Fish K: Anesthesia and the automatic implantable cardioverter/defibrillator. Anesthesiology 62:786, 1985.
10. Deutsch N, Hantler CB, Morady F, Kirsh M: Perioperative management of the patient undergoing automatic internal cardioverter-defibrillator implantation. J Cardiothorac Anesth 4:236, 1990.
11. Ellestad MH, Wan MKC: Predictive implications of stress testing: Follow-up of 2700 subjects after maximum treadmill stress testing. Circulation 51:363, 1975.
12. Gillette P: Critical analysis of sensors for physiological responsive pacing. PACE 7:1263, 1984.
13. Lau CP: Design of a rate adaptive pacing system: An overview of sensors and algorithms. In Lau CP (ed): Rate Adaptive Cardiac Pacing: Single and Dual Chamber, 1st ed. Mount Kisco, NY Futura Publishing Co, 1993, p 63.
14. Alt E, Matula M: Comparison of two activity-controlled rate-adaptive pacing principles: Acceleration versus vibration. Cardiol Clin 10:635, 1992.
15. Alt E, Matula M, Theres H, et al: The basis for activity controlled rate variable cardiac pacemakers: An analysis of mechanical forces on the human body induced by exercise and environment. PACE 12:1667, 1989.
16. Lau CP, Stott JR, Toff WD, et al: Selective vibration sensing: A new concept for activity-sensing rate-responsive pacing. PACE 11:1299, 1988.
17. Lau CP, Mehta D, Toff WD, et al: Limitations of rate response of an activity-sensing rate-responsive pacemaker to different forms of activity. PACE 11:141, 1988.
18. Lau CP, Tai YT, Fong PC, et al: Clinical experience with an activity sensing DDDR pacemaker using an accelerometer sensor. PACE 15:334, 1992.
19. Snoeck J, Berkhof M, Claeys M, et al: External vibration interference of activity based rate responsive pacemakers. PACE 15: 1841, 1992.
20. Andersen C, Oxhoj H, Arnsbo P, Lybecker H: Pregnancy and cesarean section in a patient with a rate-responsive pacemaker. PACE 12:386, 1989.
21. Rossi P, Plicche G, Canducci G, et al: Respiratory rate as a determinant of optimal pacing rate. PACE 6:502, 1983.
22. Rossi P, Plicche G, Canducci G, et al: Respiration as a reliable physiological sensor for controlling cardiac pacing rate. Br Heart J 51:7, 1984.

23. Cummin ARC, Iyawa VI, Mehta N, et al: Ventilation and cardiac output during the onset of exercise, and during voluntary hyperventilation in humans. J Physiol 370:567, 1986.
24. Vai F, Bonnet JL, Ritter PH, et al: Relationship between heart rate and minute ventilation, tidal volume and respiratory rate during brief and low level exercise. PACE 11:1860, 1988.
25. Nappholtz T, Valenta H, Maloney J, et al: Electrode configurations for a respiratory impedance measurement suitable for rate responsive pacing. PACE 9:960, 1986.
26. Webb SC, Lewis LM, Morris-Thurgood JA, et al: Respiratory-dependent pacing: A dual response from a single sensor. PACE 11:730, 1988.
27. Lau CP, Ritchie D, Butrous GS, et al: Rate modulation by arm movements of the respiratory dependent rate responsive pacemaker. PACE 11:744, 1988.
28. Scanu P, Guilleman D, Grollier G, et al: Inappropriate rate response of the minute ventilation rate responsive pacemaker in a patient with Cheyne-Stokes dyspnea (Letter). PACE 12:1963, 1989.
29. Kertes PJ, Mond HG: Patient with an implanted minute ventilation rate responsive pacemaker functioning at an upper rate during Cheyne-Stokes respiration (Letter; Comment). PACE 13: 948, 1990.
30. Lau CP, Linker NJ, Butrous GS, et al: Myopotential interference in unipolar rate responsive pacemakers. PACE 12:1324, 1989.
31. Lau CP, Lee CP, Wong CK, et al: Rate responsive pacing with a minute ventilation sensing pacemaker during pregnancy and delivery. PACE 13:158, 1990.
32. Madsen GM, Andersen C: Pacemaker-induced tachycardia during general anaesthesia: A case report. Br J Anaesth 63:360, 1989.
33. Bazett HC: An analysis of the time-relations of electrocardiograms. Heart 7:353, 1920.
34. Rickards AF, Norman J: Relation between QT interval and heart rate: New design of physically adaptive cardiac pacemaker. Br Heart J 45:56, 1981.
35. Fananapazir L, Bennett DH, Faragher EB: Contribution of heart rate to QT interval shortening during exercise. Eur Heart J 4: 265, 1983.
36. Jordaens L, Backers J, Moerman E, et al: Catecholamine levels and pacing behavior of QT-driven pacemakers during exercise. PACE 13:603, 1990.
37. Boute W, Gebhardt U, Begemann MJS: Introduction of an automatic QT interval drive rate responsive pacemaker. PACE 11: 1804, 1988.
38. Hedman A, Hjemdahl P, Nordlander R, et al: Effects of mental and physical stress on central hemodynamics and cardiac sympathetic nerve activity during QT interval-sensing rate-responsive and fixed rate ventricular inhibited pacing. Eur Heart J 11: 903, 1990.
39. Callaghan F, Vollmann W, Livingston A, et al: The ventricular depolarization gradient: Effects of exercise, pacing rate, epinephrine, and intrinsic heart rate control on the right ventricular evoked response. PACE 12:1115, 1990.
40. Singer I, Brennan AF, Steinhaus B, et al: Effects of stress and beta 1 blockade on the ventricular depolarization gradient of the rate modulating pacemaker. PACE 14:460, 1991.
41. Lau CP: The sensing of ventricular depolarization gradient and output pulse parameters. In Lau CP (ed): Rate Adaptive Cardiac Pacing: Single and Dual Chamber, 1st ed. Mount Kisco, NY Futura Publishing Co, 1993, p 142.
42. Paul V, Garrett C, Ward DE, et al: Closed loop control of rate adaptive pacing: Clinical assessment of a system analyzing the ventricular depolarization gradient. PACE 12:1896, 1989.
43. Lasaridis K, Paul VE, Katritsis D, et al: Influence of propranolol on the ventricular depolarization gradient. PACE 14:787, 1991.
44. Wirtzfeld AL, Goedel-Mienen L, Bock T, et al: Central venous oxygen saturation for the control of automatic rate responsive pacing. Circulation 64(Suppl IV):299, 1981.
45. Seifert GP, Moore AA, Graves KL, et al: In vivo and in vitro studies of a chronic oxygen saturation sensor. PACE 14:1514, 1991.
46. Lau CP: Central venous oxygen saturation and other sensors. In Lau CP (ed): Rate Adaptive Cardiac Pacing: Single and Dual Chamber, 1st ed. Mount Kisco, NY Futura Publishing Co, 1993, p 184.
47. Fearnot NE, Smith HJ, Sellers D, et al: Evaluation of the temperature response to exercise testing in patients with single chamber, rate adaptive pacemakers: A multicenter study. PACE 12:1806, 1989.
48. Arakawa M, Kambara K, Hiroyasu I, et al: Intermittent oversensing due to internal insulation damage of temperature sensing rate responsive pacemaker lead in subclavian venipuncture method. PACE 12:1312, 1989.
49. Shellock FG, Rubin SA, Ellrodt AG, et al: Unusual core temperature decrease in exercising heart-failure patients. J Appl Physiol 52:544, 1983.
50. Lau CP: Central venous temperature. In Lau CP (ed): Rate Adaptive Cardiac Pacing: Single and Dual Chamber. Mount Kisco, NY Futura Publishing Co, 1993, p 158.
51. Zaidan JR, Curling PE, Craver JM: Effect of enflurane, isoflurane, and halothane on pacing stimulation thresholds in man. PACE 8:32, 1985.
52. Echt DS, Winkle RA: Management of patients with automatic implantable cardioverter/defibrillator. Clin Prog 3:4, 1985.
53. Hunt GB, Ross DL: Comparison of effects of three anesthetic agents on induction of ventricular tachycardia in a canine model of myocardial infarction. Circulation 78:221, 1988.
54. Dresner DL, Lebowitz PW: Atrioventricular sequential pacemaker inhibition by transurethral electrosurgery. Anesthesiology 68:599, 1988.
55. Domino KB, Smith TC: Electrocautery-induced reprogramming of a pacemaker using a precordial magnet. Anesth Analg 62:612, 1983.
56. Mangar D, Atlas GM, Kane PB: Electrocautery-induced pacemaker malfunction during surgery. Can J Anaesth 38:616, 1991.
57. Levine PA, Balady GJ, Lazar HL, et al: Electrocautery and pacemakers: Management of the paced patient subject to electrocautery. Ann Thorac Surg 41:313, 1986.
58. Drach GW, Weber C, Donovan JM: Treatment of pacemaker patients with extracorporeal shock wave lithotripsy: Experience from two continents. J Urol 143:895, 1990.
59. Celentano WJ, Jahr JS, Nossaman BD: Extracorporeal shock wave lithotripsy in a patient with a pacemaker. Anesth Analg 74:770, 1992.
60. Echeverria HJ, Luceri RM, Thurer RJ, Castellanos A: Myopotential inhibition of unipolar AV sequential (DVI) pacemaker. PACE 5:20, 1982.
61. Iesaka Y, Pinakatt T, Gosselin AJ, Lister JW: Bradycardia dependent ventricular tachycardia facilitated by myopotential inhibition of a VVI pacemaker. PACE 5:23, 1982.
62. Finfer SR: Pacemaker failure on induction of anaesthesia. Br J Anaesth 66:509, 1991.
63. Sidhu VS: Interference with pacemaker function (Letter). Br J Anaesth 67:664, 1991.
64. Lamas GA, Rebecca GS, Braunwald NS, Antman EM: Pacemaker malfunction after nitrous oxide anesthesia. Am Cardiol 56:995, 1985.
65. Beaudoin M: An unusual case of failure to pace (Letter). Anaesth Intensive Care 17:235, 1989.
66. Andersen C, Oxhøl H, Arnsbo P: Management of spinal cord stimulators in patients with cardiac pacemakers. PACE 13:574, 1990.
67. Ducey JP, Fincher CW, Baysinger CL: Therapeutic suppression of a permanent ventricular pacemaker using a peripheral nerve stimulator. Anesthesiology 75:533, 1991.
68. Dreifus LS, Fisch C, Griffin JC, et al: Guidelines for implantation of cardiac pacemakers and antiarrhythmia devices. ACC/AHA Task Force report. J Am Coll Cardiol 18:1, 1991.
69. Parameswaran R, Ohe T, Goldberg H: Sinus node dysfunction in acute myocardial infarction. Br Heart J 38:93, 1976.
70. Rotman M, Wagner GS, Wallace AG: Bradyarrhythmias in acute myocardial infarction. Circulation 45:703, 1972.
71. DeGuzman M, Rahimtoola SH: What is the role of pacemakers in patients with coronary artery disease and conduction abnormalities? Cardiovasc Clin 13:191, 1983.
72. Tans AC, Lie KI, Durrer D: Clinical settings and prognostic significance of high degree atrioventricular block in acute inferior myocardial infarction: A study of 144 patients. Am Heart J 99:48, 1980.

73. Feigl D, Ashkenazy J, Kishon Y: Early and late atrioventricular block in acute inferior myocardial infarction. J Am Coll Cardiol 4:35, 1984.
74. Ellenbogen KA, Peters RW: Indications for permanent and temporary cardiac pacing in cardiac pacing. In Ellenbogen KA (ed): Cardiac Pacing. Cambridge, MA Blackwell Publishing Co, 1992, p 1.
75. Hauer RNW, Lie KI, Liem RL, Durrer D: Long-term prognosis in patients with bundle branch block complicating acute anteroseptal infarction. Am J Cardiol 49:1581, 1982.
76. Gann D, Balachandran PD, El-Sherif N, Samet P: Prognostic significance of chronic versus acute bundle branch block in acute myocardial infarction. Chest 67:298, 1975.
77. Khan MM, Logan KR, McComb JM: Management of recurrent ventricular tachyarrhythmias associated with QT prolongation. Am J Cardiol 47:1301, 1981.
78. Schwartz PJ: Idiopathic long QT syndrome: Progress and questions. Am Heart J 109:399, 1985.
79. Niemann JT, Rosborough JP, Garner D, et al: External noninvasive cardiac pacing: A comparative hemodynamic study of two techniques with conventional endocardial pacing. PACE 7: 230, 1984.
80. Falk RH, Ngai STA, Kumaki DJ, Rubinstein JA: Cardiac activation during external cardiac pacing. PACE 10(part 1):503, 1987.
81. Zoll PM: Resuscitation of the heart in ventricular standstill by external electric stimulation. N Engl J Med 247:768, 1952.
82. Kelly JS, Royster RL: Noninvasive transcutaneous cardiac pacing. Anesth Analg 69:229, 1989.
83. Klein LS, Miles WM, Heger JJ, Zipes DP: Transcutaneous pacing: Patient tolerance, strength-interval relations and feasibility for programmed electrical stimulation. Am J Cardiol 62:1126, 1988.
84. Zoll PM, Zoll RH, Falk RH, et al: External noninvasive temporary cardiac pacing: Clinical trials. Circulation 71:937, 1985.
85. Luck JC, Grubb BP, Artman SE, et al: Termination of sustained ventricular tachycardia by external noninvasive pacing. Am J Cardiol 61:574, 1988.
86. Hedges JR, Syverud SA, Dalsey WC, et al: Threshold, enzymatic, and pathologic changes associated with prolonged transcutaneous pacing in a chronic heart block model. J Emerg Med 7:1, 1989.
87. Falk RH, Ngai STA: External cardiac pacing: Influence of electrode placement on pacing threshold. Crit Care Med 14:931, 1986.
88. Geddes LA, Babbs CF, Voorhees WD, et al: Choice of the optimum pulse duration for precordial cardiac pacing: A theoretical study. PACE 8:862, 1985.
89. Abinader EG, Sharif D, Malouf S, Goldhammer E: Temporary transvenous pacing: Analysis of indications, complications and malfunctions in acute myocardial infarction versus noninfarction settings. Isr J Med Sci 23:877, 1987.
90. Voorhees WD, Foster KS, Geddes LA, Babbs CF: Safety factor for precordial pacing: Minimum current thresholds for pacing and for ventricular fibrillation by vulnerable-period stimulation. PACE 7(part 1):356, 1984.
91. Syverud SA, Dalsey WC, Hedges JR, Hanseits ML: Radiologic assessment of transvenous pacemaker placement during CPR. Ann Emerg Med 15:131, 1986.
92. Hynes JK, Holmes DR, Harrison CE: Five-year experience with temporary pacemaker therapy in the coronary care unit. Mayo Clin Proc 58:122, 1983.
93. Jowett MI, Thompson DR, Pohl JEF: Temporary transvenous cardiac pacing: A year's experience in one coronary care unit. Postgrad Med J 65:211, 1989.
94. Weinstein J, Gnoj J, Mazzara JT, Ayers SM, et al. Temporary transvenous pacing via the percutaneous femoral vein approach. Am Heart J 85:695, 1973.
95. Nathan DA, Center S, Pina RE, et al: Perforation during indwelling catheter pacing. Circulation 33:128, 1966.
96. Silver MD, Goldschlager N: Temporary transvenous cardiac pacing in the critical care setting. Chest 93:607, 1988.
97. Lumb PD: Atrioventricular sequential pacing with transluminal atrial and ventricular pacing probes inserted via a pulmonary artery catheter: A preliminary comparison with epicardial wires. J Clin Anesth 1:292, 1989.
98. Zaidan JR, Freniere S: Use of a pacing pulmonary artery catheter during cardiac surgery. Ann Thorac Surg 35:633, 1983.
99. Jenkins JM, Dick M, Collins S, et al: Use of the pill electrode for transesophageal atrial pacing. PACE 8:512, 1985.
100. Kerr CR, Chung DC, Wickham G, et al: Impedence to transesophageal atrial pacing: Significance regarding power sources. PACE 12:930, 1989.
101. Falk R, Werner M: Transesophageal atrial pacing using a pill electrode for the termination of atrial flutter. Chest 92:110, 1987.
102. Nishimura M, Katoh T, Hanai S, Watanabe Y: Optimal mode of transesophageal atrial pacing. Am J Cardiol 57:791, 1986.
103. Benson DW, Sanford M, Dunnigan A, Benditt DG: Transesophageal atrial pacing threshold: Role of interelectrode spacing, pulse width, and catheter insertion depth. Am J Cardiol 53:63, 1984.
104. Kerr CR, Chung DC, Cooper J: Improved transesophageal recording and stimulation utilizing a new quadripolar lead configuration. PACE 9:644, 1986.
105. Gallagher JJ, Smith WM, Kerr CR, et al: Esophageal pacing: A diagnostic and therapeutic tool. Circulation 65:336, 1982.
106. Lubell DL: Cardiac pacing from the esophagus. Am J Cardiol 27:641, 1971.
107. Dick M, Campbell RM, Jenkins JM: Thresholds for transesophageal atrial pacing. Cathet Cardiovasc Diagn 10:507, 1984.
108. Wood M, Ellenbogen K, Haines D: Temporary cardiac pacing. In Ellenbogen KA (ed): Cardiac Pacing, 1st ed. Cambridge, MA Blackwell Publishing Co, 1992, p 162.

CHAPTER 33

Coagulation and Coagulopathies

Norig Ellison, M.D.
Jan C. Horrow, M.D.

Normal Hemostasis

A knowledge of the normal hemostatic process is essential to understanding bleeding and its control during surgery. Bleeding is a normal accompaniment of surgery. Hemostasis is a tripartite function depending on vascular integrity, adequate number and function of platelets, and a normal coagulation mechanism. Bleeding represents a defect in one or more of these individual elements.

Vascular integrity will be disrupted during any surgical procedure. Restoration of hemostasis in major vessels is dependent on surgical ligation of the bleeding vessel as well as the normal hemostatic mechanisms in restoring vascular integrity. The importance of these mechanisms can perhaps best be appreciated by the fact that the majority of blood vessels are less than 1.0 mm in diameter. In vessels of this caliber platelets and coagulation factors play the major role in securing hemostasis. The hemostatic mechanisms alone will not be sufficient to restore vascular integrity in large defects where surgical ligation will be required.

Platelets are important because of their role in several phases of hemostasis. Platelets have been termed the "keystone" of hemostasis because they are involved in all phases from formation of the initial platelet plug through final clot retraction. When a vessel is damaged platelets adhere to the exposed collagen via their glycoprotein Ib receptors, with von Willebrand's factor as the molecular bridge between them. Subsequently, additional platelets are recruited to aggregate with the adherent platelets. Platelet adhesion is the affinity of platelets for nonplatelet surfaces. Platelet aggregation is the affinity of platelets for one another. Aggregation occurs at platelet glycoprotein receptor IIb/IIIa with fibrinogen as the molecular bridge. Adhesion and aggregation result in the formation of a platelet plug in the area of the damaged endothelium. Platelet activation accompanies platelet aggregation. Activation involves release of vasoactive substances that cause the injured vessel to constrict. It also provides the phospholipid surface on which coagulation factors assemble and interact (Fig. 33–1). Formation of a fibrin network within the platelet plug provides stabilization within the clot in order to prevent its dissolution. The final action of platelets is their role in clot retraction, caused by the platelet protein, thrombospondin.[1]

Activation of the coagulation cascade occurs, as is outlined in Figure 33–1. Factor X is activated by either the intrinsic or extrinsic system and initiates the final common pathway, which ultimately results in the formation of insoluble fibrin.[2] The intrinsic and extrinsic pathways are not mutually exclusive: a link occurs between them in that activated factor VII can directly activate factor IX. In fact, the majority of factor IX activation probably occurs in this way, rather than via the intrinsic coagulation factor XIa. Thrombin generation during surgery and cardiopulmonary bypass relate more to extrinsic pathway activation from released tissue factor than to contact activation on foreign surfaces.[3] The minimum levels of coagulation factors and platelets necessary for effective hemostasis are listed in Table 33–1.

Fibrinolysis is the body's mechanism for keeping the clotting mechanism localized to the area of bleeding. This mechanism, also called the plasminogen system, results in the dissolution of the fibrin network, which forms the fibrin-based clot. The fibrinolytic system is made up of enzymes, inhibitors, and activators, which are closely related to the enzymes, inhibitors, and activators involved in coagulation. This system acts to restore vascular patency and prevent widespread coagulation. Plasminogen binds to fibrinogen and fibrin at lysine residues, becoming incorporated into the cross-linked fibrin clot. Tissue plasminogen activator (t-PA), released from repaired endothelium, binds to fibrin and splits the fibrin-bound plasminogen to form plasmin. Plasmin then splits the locally available fibrin into its degradation products. Rarely, an overwhelming production of plasmin can achieve systemic activity. As such, it can digest circulating fibrinogen, factor V, and factor VIII. Therapeutic uses of the fibrinolytic pathway and the pathologic syndrome associated with excessive fibrinolysis are discussed below.

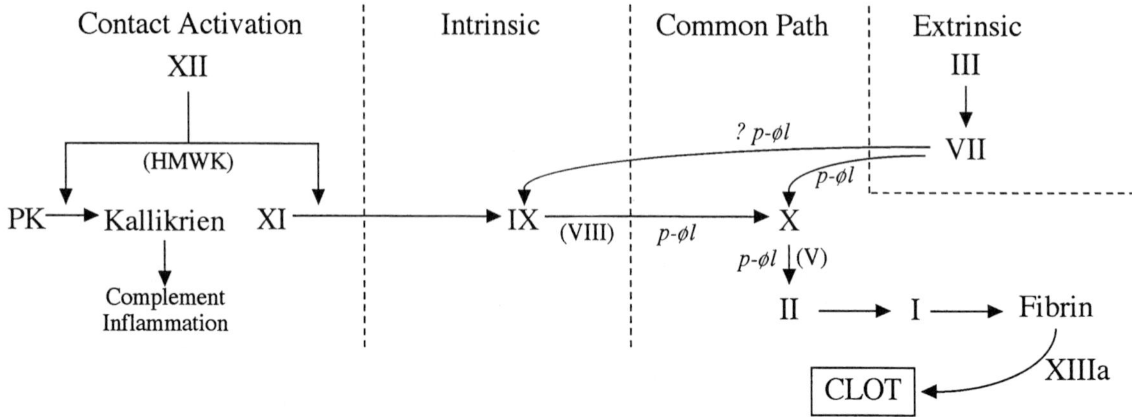

FIGURE **33–1.** The coagulation cascade with emphasis on the sites of platelet activity. PK, prekallikrein; HMWK, high-molecular-weight kininogen; *p-ϕl*, platelet phospholipid. (Modified from Horrow JC: Management of coagulopathy associated with CPB. In Gravlee GP, Davis RF, Utley JR [eds]: Cardiopulmonary Bypass. Principles and Practice. Baltimore, Williams & Wilkins, 1993, p 438, with permission.)

Preoperative Evaluation

Evaluation of hemostasis begins with the properly taken history and physical exam. Rarely will a pre-existing bleeding abnormality first manifest itself intraoperatively in a patient with a negative history.[4] Two important questions are often overlooked in taking a history: the hemostatic response to a prior surgical experience and a list of all drugs that the patient is taking. Specific questions regarding the bleeding tendency or excessive bleeding associated with previous surgery may suggest further laboratory evaluation. With respect to any history of bleeding episodes, their frequency and severity as well as the apparent cause should be ascertained. Family history of bleeding tendency should also be sought as a part of the preoperative evaluation. Equally important is the need to obtain a record of all medications the patient is taking. There are many drugs, including nonprescrip-

TABLE **33–1**

In Vivo Properties of Blood Clotting Factors and Platelets Necessary for Effective Hemostatis, Distribution, Half-Life, and Dosing Schedule*

Factor	Minimal Level for Surgical Hemostatis (% of Normal)	Apparent Volume of Distribution (× Plasma Volume)	In Vivo Half-Life	Therapeutic Agent	Dose (Per Kg Body Weight) Initial	Maintenance
I	100 mg/dl	2–5	3–6 days	Cryoprecipitate	Ppt from 100 ml	Ppt from 14–20 ml, qd
II	40 U/dl	1.5–2	2–3 days	Plasma	10–15 ml	5–10 ml, qd
V	10–15 U/dl	?	12 hr	Fresh or frozen plasma	10–15 ml	10 ml, qd
VII	5–10 U/dl	2–4	2–6 hr	Plasma	5–10 ml	5 ml, qd
VIII	30 U/dl	1–1.5	8–12 hr	Cryoprecipitate	Ppt from 70 ml	Ppt from 35 ml, bid
von Willebrand's	30 U/dl			Plasma (or cryoprecipitate)	10 ml (or Ppt from that amount)	10 ml, q 2–3 d
IX	10–40%	2–5	18–36	Plasma or II, VII, IX, X concentrate	60 ml variable	7 ml, qd
X	10–20%	1–2	2 days	Plasma	15 ml	10 ml, qd
XI	30%	1–1.33	3 days	Plasma	10 ml	5 ml, qd
XII	0	?		Not needed	If desired, use plasma 5 ml	5 ml, qd
XIII	1–5%	?		Plasma (or cryoprecipitate)	2–3 ml (or Ppt from that amount)	None
Platelets	50,000–100,000 cells/mm^3		6–10 days	Platelet concentrate	1–2 units per desired 10,000-increment in count	

*Adapted from Troianos CA, Ellison N: Hematological considerations in vascular surgery. In Kaplan JA (ed): Vascular Anesthesia. New York, Churchill Livingstone, 1991, p 549, with permission.

Ppt, precipitate; qd, every day; bid, twice daily.

TABLE 33–2
Baseline Screening Tests of Hemostatis*

Test	Comment
Activated coagulation time (ACT)	Can be done in OR; observe for clot retraction and lysis
Fibrinogen level	Decrease in consumptive coagulopathy
Prothrombin time (PT)	Prolonged in liver disease, vitamin K deficiency, Coumadin anticoagulation, consumptive coagulopathy
Activated thromboplastin time (aPTT)	Prolonged in factors V, VIII deficiency (massive transfusion), the hemophilias, or the presence of heparin
Platelet count	Diseased with dilutional thrombocytopenia, splanchnic sequestration, destruction syndromes, and consumptive coagulopathy
Bleeding time	Clinical test of platelet function; does not predict surgical bleeding[6]

*From Troianos CA, Ellison N: Hematological considerations in vascular surgery. In Kaplan JA (ed): Vascular Anesthesia. New York, Churchill Livingstone, 1991, p 549, with permission.
OR, operating room.

tion drugs, that can affect hemostasis by impairing platelet function as discussed later. Physical exam should focus on the presence of petechiae and ecchymoses, with the former suggesting a platelet or vascular defect and the latter more likely a coagulation factor defect.

Laboratory tests, in addition to serving as a screening tool, will help delineate the specific hemostatic defect. For screening purposes, determination of the prothrombin time (PT), activated partial thromboplastin time (aPTT), and platelet count is recommended. In the operating room, an activated clotting time (ACT) may be added to the list of baseline screening tests (Table 33–2). If screening tests are normal and the patient has a negative history and physical exam, it may reasonably be assumed that any intraoperative bleeding disorder is not due to a pre-existing defect.

In this era of cost containment the question of routinely obtaining screening tests must be addressed.[5,6] Repeated studies have suggested that false-positive tests that are ignored with potential medicolegal consequences are as much of a problem as failure to detect a hemorrhagic diathesis. Brent has argued that "a careful history and physical exam can identify nearly all patients with a risk of bleeding."[7] Indeed, the bleeding time as a screening test contributes little to the identification of pre-existing bleeding disorders or to the prediction of abnormal surgical bleeding.[6] Nevertheless, in cases where bleeding remains a potential problem, such as cardiac surgery, the preoperative screening tests will serve as a baseline for comparison to tests obtained intraoperatively should excessive bleeding develop.

Congenital Bleeding Disorders

Congenital bleeding disorders usually arise from the absence or decreased presence of a single coagulation factor. The three most common disorders are hemophilia A (classic hemophilia, factor VIII deficiency), hemophilia B (Christmas disease, factor IX deficiency), and von Willebrand's disease.

Hemophilia A, with an incidence of 1 in 10,000 live births, arises from a sex-linked autosomal recessive trait. The disease will prolong the aPTT, but leave the PT normal. Perioperative management aims at increasing factor VIII activity to near normal preoperatively, and maintaining concentrations of 30% or greater intraoperatively and for the duration of postoperative wound healing. This convalescent period can vary up to 10 days, depending on the magnitude of the surgical procedure (Table 33–3).[8] Cryoprecipitate or factor VIII concentrate are the blood products available for treatment of the coagulopathy due to hemophilia A. Factor VIII is now available in highly purified forms, providing increased safety against infectious diseases, but at higher expense. The determinants of the dose necessary for correction are listed in Table 33–4.

TABLE 33–3
Recommended Factor VIII Levels and Duration of Treatment for Surgical Procedure or Bleeding Condition*

		Treatment	
	Factor VIII Level (U/ml)	**Frequency (hr)**	**Duration (days)**
Hemarthrosis	0.30	Every 12	1
Dental (minor)	0.30	Every 12	1
Dental (extraction)	0.30	Every 8	1–2
All surgery	0.50	Every 8	2–10

*From Ellison N, Silverstein LE: Hemostasis in the perioperative period. In Stoelting RK, Barash PG, Gallagher TJ (eds): Advances in Anesthesia, Vol. 3. Chicago, Year Book Medical Publishers, 1986, p 67, with permission.

TABLE 33-4
Determinants of Dose of Blood Component Used to Correct Hemostatic Defect(s)*

Patient size
Initial level of deficient factor
Potency of preparation
Hemostatic level required
Magnitude of operation
Half-life of the factor
Redistribution
Metabolic rate

*From Troianos CA, Ellison N: Hematological considerations in vascular surgery. In Kaplan JA (ed): Vascular Anesthesia. New York, Churchill Livingstone, 1991, p 549, with permission.

In hemophilia B, an autosomal recessive trait, factor IX is deficient. Patients with hemophilia B demonstrate a prolonged PTT. Factor IX concentrate, a pooled product, carries a high risk of hepatitis as well as the potential to initiate consumptive coagulopathy because of the presence of activated forms of many coagulation factors. Factor IX concentrate also helps patients with factor VIII deficiency who have developed inhibitors. Factor IX concentrates with only minute amounts of other factors are now available at higher cost.[9]

Von Willebrand's disease, the most common inherited coagulopathy, results from decreased activity of the protein factor VIII:von Willebrand's factor (VIII:vWF), which plays an important role both in platelet function and factor VIII activity. The disease is classified according to the etiology of the defect. Type 1 involves a quantitative deficiency of factor VIII:vWF, while type 2 features normal quantities of defective molecules, and type 3 represents totally absent synthesis. The disease is inherited as either autosomal dominant (types 1 and 2), or very rarely, as an autosomal recessive trait (type 3). The disease results in defective platelet aggregation, manifested by a prolonged bleeding time, and decreased levels of factor VIII as manifested by a prolonged aPTT. Desmopressin acetate is effective in increasing endogenous release of factor VIII:vWF. It may also be provided through the administration of cryoprecipitate. Desmopressin acetate, administered the evening prior to surgery and the day of surgery, effectively neutralizes the defective platelet aggregation and increases factor VIII concentrations, thus benefiting patients with type I von Willebrand's disease.[8]

Acquired Bleeding Disorders

Unlike the congenital disorders, which are usually due to deficiencies of a single coagulation factor, the acquired bleeding disorders are usually multifactorial. The seven most common acquired bleeding disorders include vitamin K deficiency, anticoagulants, liver disease, platelet dysfunction, consumptive coagulopathy, massive blood transfusion, and inadequate surgical hemostasis.

Vitamin K Deficiency

Vitamin K is required for the production of factors II (prothrombin), VII, IX, and X. It acts via enzymatic addition of a γ-carboxyl group to the precursors of these factors. Because this process occurs in the liver, it requires adequate liver function in addition to adequate vitamin K absorption from the gastrointestinal (GI) tract. Without γ-carboxylation, these factors circulate in a dysfunctional state and cannot bind calcium, a cofactor in the coagulation process. Causes of vitamin K deficiency include malabsorption, "intestinal sterilization syndrome" (elimination of intestinal flora, a major source of vitamin K, through antibiotic therapy), Coumadin therapy which inhibits the action of vitamin K, and (rarely) a true dietary deficiency. Laboratory studies will initially reveal a prolonged PT with a normal aPTT, because factor VII is the most sensitive to vitamin K deficiency. As the vitamin K deficiency becomes greater, factors II, IX, and X become affected and then the aPTT is also prolonged (Fig. 33–2). Treatment depends on the urgency of correction because the administration of parenteral vitamin K requires 3 to 6 hours or longer to overcome a Coumadin effect, depending on the level of inhibition achieved and the adequacy of liver function. Plasma can correct the coagulopathy immediately, but carries all the risks of allogeneic blood transfusion. It should therefore be reserved for treatment of patients who are actively bleeding or undergoing emergency surgery. Although fresh frozen plasma (FFP) is usually used, stored plasma will suffice. This is because factors V and VIII, the only factors that decay in stored unfrozen plasma, remain normal in patients deficient in Vitamin K.

Anticoagulants

Patients scheduled for cardiovascular surgery are frequently treated with anticoagulants preoperatively. Thus Coumadin and heparin are other causes of acquired bleeding disorders. Heparin inhibits the action of the serine proteases factors IIa (thrombin), IXa, Xa, and XIa by its binding to the polypeptide antithrombin (AT). Heparin produces a conformational change in AT markedly enhancing the latter's inhibitory effects. Heparin potentiates the inhibitory action of antithrombin on thrombin by a factor of 2,000. It also potentiates antithrombin's inhibitory action on factor IXa by a factor of 10,000, and the action on factor Xa by a factor of 1,200.[11] The extreme sensitivity of factor IXa partially explains why small doses of heparin prolong the aPTT but not the PT, while larger doses prolong both tests.

Liver Disease

Liver disease leads to defects in coagulation by several mechanisms. Lack of bile salts creates malabsorption of fat-soluble vitamins, including vitamin K. Cirrhosis decreases the mass of hepatocytes available for synthesis of those coagulation factors made in the liver, which

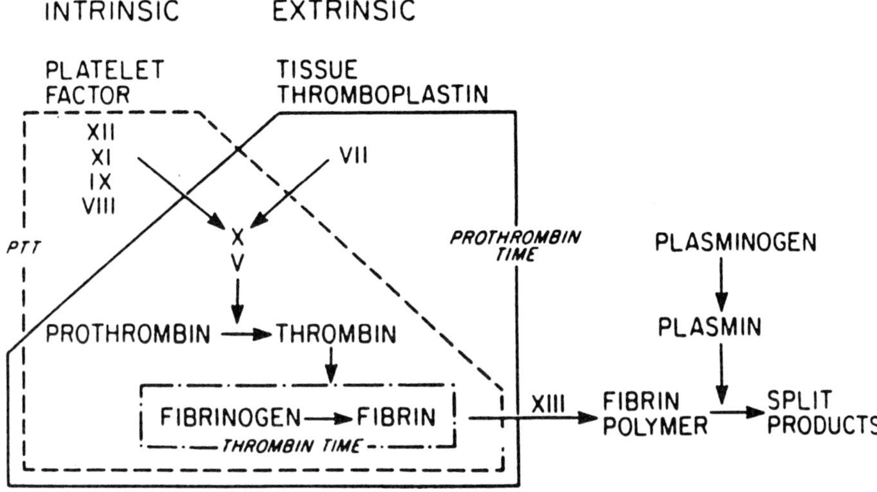

FIGURE **33–2.** The coagulation mechanism outlining the factors involved in the in vitro determination of prothrombin time, partial thromboplastin time (PTT), and thrombin time. (From Neerhout RC: Pediatr Clin North Am 16:681, 1969, with permission.)

include all but factor VIII and von Willebrand's factor. Pathologic liver synthesizes an abnormal fibrinogen, one that contains sialic acid residues, thus interfering with fibrinogen's function. Portal hypertension secondary to liver disease also leads to bleeding from esophageal varices or hypersplenism, which leads to destruction and sequestration of platelets.

Platelet Dysfunction

Platelet dysfunction can be qualitative or quantitative. Since the most common cause of bleeding due to platelet deficiency is one of number, a platelet count is the first step in evaluation. A decreased platelet count can be due to decreased production of platelets, increased destruction or loss, or excessive sequestration. Decreased production can occur during chemotherapy, while increased destruction can be idiopathic, related to certain disease states, or drug induced. Medications associated with thrombocytopenia from platelet destruction include heparin, quinine, quinidine, thiazide diuretics, and medications derived from sulfa.[12] Hypersplenism causes excessive platelet sequestration, also resulting in thrombocytopenia. The only medication shown consistently to irreversibly affect platelet function is aspirin.[13] Dozens of other substances may result in clinically significant platelet dysfunction, including but not limited to nonsteroidal anti-inflammatory drugs (NSAIDs), antihistamines, tricyclic antidepressants, dextran, aminoglycosides, protamine, certain local anesthetics, and α-adrenergic antagonists.[13,14] Certain foods and spices such as garlic, cloves, and tumeric have also been implicated. Other causes of platelet dysfunction include uremia and chronic liver disease.

Consumptive Coagulopathy

Consumptive coagulopathy, also known as disseminated intravascular coagulation (DIC), occurs rarely in the patient presenting for elective surgery, but may be seen in emergency cases in which the patient has suffered a catastrophic event or postoperatively in septic or hemodynamically unstable patients. Bleeding occurs as a result of a depletion of clotting factors and platelets by their consumption in the formation of fibrin clot within the circulation followed by secondary fibrinolysis. This digestion of fibrin, and less commonly fibrinogen, results in increased fibrin split products in the circulation that possess anticoagulant properties of their own. Laboratory findings reveal thrombocytopenia, prolonged PT and aPTT, decreased fibrinogen concentrations, and the presence of fibrin split products. Definitive treatment involves correcting the underlying problem causing DIC. When active bleeding and depletion of platelets or coagulation factors occurs, the administration of platelets and coagulation factors is indicated, in additon to treating the underlying problem. The use of heparin and/or antifibrinolytic drugs in this setting remains controversial and rarely indicated in the surgical patient.

Massive Blood Transfusion

Massive blood transfusion may be required for the patient who bleeds excessively as from a ruptured aortic aneurysm. Massive transfusion introduces dilutional hemostatic defects, the most important of which is dilutional thrombocytopenia. Dilution of clotting factors, especially the labile factors V and VIII, may also play a minor role in this acquired hemostatic defect. Treatment involves administration of platelets and FFP. The dilutional effects on the stable coagulation factors may be decreased by the administration of whole blood instead of packed red blood cells.

Inadequate Surgical Hemostasis

Inadequate surgical hemostasis, potentially occurring in every surgical procedure, is another acquired defect of hemostasis that must be considered. Inadequate surgical hemostasis may prolong postoperative bleeding. Administration of coagulation products cannot correct this defect, which requires surgical attention.

Hypercoagulable States and Venous Thrombosis

There is a balance in normal hemostasis between clot formation and thrombolysis. Derangements may produce excessive hemorrhage or thrombosis. Thrombotic disorders become evident with a history of repeated thromboembolic events, unexpected thrombosis, thrombosis in the face of anticoagulation, and perioperative thrombosis in the vascular surgical patient who has had a good surgical repair resulting in good blood flow through the repaired vessel.[10] Table 33–5 lists conditions that are associated with or may lead to thrombotic events. Most patients who present with thrombosis have one or more of these associated conditions. Less commonly, there exists a hereditary disorder predisposing the patient to thrombosis.

Clot formation is limited by the fibrinolytic system and by three plasma proteins: antithrombin, protein C, and protein S. Reduced amounts of these three proteins predispose patients toward excessive thrombosis.[15] In addition, disorders of the fibrinolytic system,[16] dysfibrinogenemias,[17] and the lupus anticoagulant[18] have been associated with an increased risk of thrombosis.

The risk of intravascular thrombus formation is further increased in the surgical patient when the vascular endothelium is damaged. Endothelial damage may result from obvious injury such as trauma or surgery, or from more subtle forms of injury such as hypertension or vascular distention. Exposure of the subendothelium promotes adhesion of platelets, release of vasoactive substances, and activation of the coagulation cascade. Whether a thrombus develops at this point depends on a number of factors. These include characteristics of blood flow and velocity, including diameter of the vessel, presense and concentration of coagulation factors, presence of coagulation inhibitors, platelet function, age of the patient, and activation of the fibrinolytic system. Venous thrombi tend to be red in color because they are formed in vessels with sluggish blood flow, resulting in a red cell–fibrin thrombus. Arterial thrombi, formed under high flow and shear conditions, tend to be white in color because they are "platelet rich" in their composition, with few red blood cells in their matrix.[19] Composition of a thrombus may be important in guiding therapy (i.e., antiplatelet vs. anticoagulant drugs).

For each surface, there is a critical velocity below which stasis becomes a significant factor in thrombosis and above which velocities provide adequate shearing forces to overcome the deposition of platelets and fibrin. Any deviation from normal laminar flow may lead to turbulence and to platelet aggregation. Whether this aggregation will lead to thrombosis depends not only on those physical factors, but the presence or absence of coagulation factors and inhibitors. The intact endothelial surface is rich in fibrinolytic activity. As this becomes disrupted, however, the fibrinolytic activity is overcome and thrombosis may develop. If a hypercoagulable state is superimposed, thrombosis is even more likely and may, in fact, involve a greater extent of the vessel.

TABLE 33–5
Clinical Conditions Associated with Thrombosis*

Trauma
Postoperative state, especially after orthopedic or other leg procedures
Advanced age
Prevent history of thrombosis
Immobilization
Paralysis
Obesity
Malignancy
Pregnancy
Estrogen or contraceptive therapy
Infusion of prothrombin concentrates
Myeloproliferative disorders
Nephrotic syndrome
Diabetes
Congestive heart failure
Smoking
Vasculitis
Heparin-induced thrombocytopenia
Homocystinuria
Polycythemia
Leukemia
Sickle cell disease
Hyperlipidemia
Thrombotic thrombocytopenic purpura

*From Troianos CA, Ellison N: Hematological considerations in vascular surgery. In Kaplan JA (ed): Vascular Anesthesia. New York, Churchill Livingstone, 1991, p 549, with permission.

Antithrombin Deficiency

AT is the primary inhibitor of thrombin (factor IIa) and other serine proteases in the coagulation cascade. The incidence of AT deficiency has been reported as high as 1 in 2,000. Congenital AT deficiency, inherited as an autosomal dominant trait, presents as both qualitative and quantitative AT defects. Patients with AT deficiency present with spontaneous thrombosis (36%), thrombosis during pregnancy or immediately after delivery (28%), and postoperatively (13%).[14] Acquired AT deficiency may occur in patients with nephrotic syndrome (enhanced protein elimination), liver disease (decreased production), and in patients with consumptive coagulopathy (increased consumption).

AT exerts its effect through an arginine group that covalently binds to the clotting factors via their serine group. In the absence of heparin, AT is a slow inhibitor of the serine proteases. In the presence of heparin, however, the arginine group is more accessible through a conformational change induced by heparin, thus enhancing its binding to clotting factors. In the absence of AT, heparin is ineffective as an anticoagulant.

Treatment of patients with mild AT deficiency who present with thrombosis requires the administration of heparin. If the deficiency is severe, AT concentrations must be increased through the administration of FFP or AT concentrates, where available.

Protein C Deficiency

Protein C, a vitamin K–dependent glycoprotein, proteolytically degrades the activated forms of factors V and VIII. It may inhibit factor Va activity on the platelet surface while inhibiting binding of factor Xa to the platelet surface. Protein C also has an effect on fibrinolysis by decreasing activity of plasminogen activator inhibitor type 1 (PAI-1), the circulating inhibitor of t-PA, permitting t-PA to activate plasminogen to plasmin unchecked.[14]

Clinical manifestations of protein C deficiency in heterozygotes include venous thrombosis and warfarin-induced skin necrosis. Massive and fatal neonatal thrombosis has been reported in neonates homozygous for protein C deficiency in which plasma levels of protein C were virtually absent.[20]

Acquired protein C deficiency can occur in consumptive coagulopathy, liver disease, adult respiratory distress syndrome, and following surgery.[20] Because it is a vitamin K–dependent protein, administration of Coumadin will worsen protein C deficiency. For this reason, treatment of acute thrombosis involves intravenous heparin administration first, while chronic therapy is initiated slowly with Coumadin. Initial large doses of Coumadin decrease protein C concentrations faster than decreasing factor X levels, thereby increasing the risk of thrombosis. Danazol, an anabolic steroid, has also been suggested as a treatment for protein C deficiency.[21] Danazol's mechanism of action is by increasing the synthesis of vitamin K–dependent proteins.

Protein S Deficiency

Protein S is a cofactor for the anticoagulant effects of activated protein C. While not possessing anticoagulant effects of its own, protein S markedly enhances the inhibitory effect of protein C on factor Va, and is required for the binding of activated protein C to platelets. Because protein S is a vitamin K–dependent cofactor, deficiency of protein S may be acquired in patients treated with Coumadin and in patients with liver disease. Protein S deficiency can also occur in consumptive coagulopathy, nephrotic syndrome, pregnancy, after an acute thrombotic event, and with systemic lupus erythematosus.[10] The usual clinical manifestation is venous thrombosis, although arterial thrombosis has also been reported in a patient with protein S deficiency.[22] Treatment includes intravenous heparin initially, followed by oral anticoagulants for chronic control of thrombosis.

Defects in Fibrinolysis

Thrombosis can also develop in patients with defects in fibrinolysis. These result from impaired synthesis or release of plasminogen activator, the presence of excess inhibitors of plasminogen activator, or a functionally abnormal fibrinogen molecule.[23] Long-term administration of antifibrinolytic therapy to patients with renal failure or neoplastic diatheses can cause thrombosis.[24] Short-term use, as for prophylaxis for surgical bleeding, appears safe in this regard.

Venous Thrombosis

Venous thrombosis is a problem that occurs in approximately 30% of general surgery cases,[19] and may be associated with significant morbidity with the development of the postthrombotic syndrome. It can be fatal if it results in pulmonary embolism. Surgical intervention may be necessary in patients who have failed medical therapy or in those patients who have a contraindication to anticoagulant therapy (Table 33–6). If the venous thrombosis is extensive or involves large veins, surgical removal may be required. Rarely, a patient will present for surgical removal of a pulmonary embolus if there is a contraindication to anticoagulant therapy in the face of repeated or massive pulmonary embolization.

The process of venous thrombosis begins with damage to the endothelial lining of the vessel wall. This leads to a vascular and platelet reaction resulting in stasis and the initiation of coagulation. The process may be acute or chronic, and may occur in visceral veins as well as those of extremities. It is termed thrombophlebitis when it is associated with an inflammatory process producing symptoms of pain, tenderness, and erythema. The majority of patients, however, lack any clinical manifestation of their disease.

Pulmonary embolism can be a fatal complication of venous thrombosis. The deep veins of the lower extremity are the source of 90% of pulmonary emboli. Patients with pulmonary embolism will present with an acute onset of dyspnea and tachycardia. If it is a large embolus, associated signs and symptoms may include chest pain, hypotension, central venous distention, and the manifestations of hypoxemia. Pulmonary angiography, echocardiography, or a "mismatch" of ventilation and perfusion seen on pulmonary radionuclide scan may secure the diagnosis of pulmonary embolism.

TABLE 33–6
Relative Contraindications to Anticoagulant Therapy*

Bleeding diathesis (except perhaps may be consumptive coagulopathy)
Ulcerative lesions of the gastrointestinal, genitourinary (especially prostate), or respiratory tract
Recent centeral nervous system or eye surgery
Severe hypertension
Recent cerebral hemorrhage
Subacute bacterial endocarditis or pericarditis
Uncooperative patient or inadequate laboratory control
Pregnancy, first trimester or near term (applies only to Coumadin)

*Adapted from Ellison N, Ominsky AJ: Clinical considerations for the anesthesiologist whose patient is on anticoagulant therapy. Anesthesiology 39:328, 1973; *and* Ellison N, Jobes DR, Schwartz AJ: Heparin therapy during cardiac surgery. In Ellison N, Jobes DR (eds): Effective Hemostatis in Cardiac Surgery. Philadelphia, WB Saunders Co, 1988, p 1, with permission.

Medical Therapy

Anticoagulants

Heparin

Heparin is a heterogenous mixture of straight chain anionic mucopolysaccharides, called glycosaminoglycans. These chains have a high degree of sulfation which imparts a negative charge that contributes to the anticoagulant activity through binding to AT. Heparin combines with AT in a 1:1 stoichiometric ratio and induces a conformational change in AT such that it will bind more readily to the serine proteases in the coagulation cascade.

Heparin therapy engenders a variable anticoagulant response. This variability among individuals may result from differences in endogenous concentrations of AT or antiheparin agents such as platelet factor 4. The desired effect of heparin and the degree of anticoagulation, therefore, need to be monitored. In particular, patients with antithrombin deficiencies may be quite resistant to anticoagulation. These patients include those who undergo prolonged therapy with heparin in whom concentrations of AT decrease with continued use. Other causes of "heparin resistance" are listed in Table 33–7. Although minidose heparin therapy minimally prolongs the aPTT, larger doses of heparin prolong the PT and ACT, as well as aPTT by inhibiting clotting factors in both intrinsic and extrinsic coagulation pathways. Minidose therapy works through its effect on factor IXa. Because factor IXa is necessary for the conversion of prothrombin to thrombin, minidoses of heparin inhibit the formation of thrombin with minimal effect on thrombin itself. Therefore, if thrombin formation has already occurred, minidose heparin will not be effective as an anticoagulant. Conventional dose heparin therapy, however, because it inhibits thrombin, will effectively anticoagulate even if thrombin formation has occurred. Inactivation of thrombin will prevent the conversion of fibrinogen to fibrin. Since heparin has no effect on fibrinolysis, heparin has no effect on an established thrombus, except to prevent its extension. Table 33–8 summarizes the three levels of heparin therapy.

The vascular surgical patient may receive heparin prior to surgery to treat venous thrombosis, pulmonary embolism, arterial embolism, as prophylaxis for these conditions. Patients with prosthetic heart valves receive heparin during conversion from Coumadin therapy. The goal of therapy is to prolong the aPTT time to 2 to 2½ times normal.[25] The intraoperative use of heparin will be discussed in a later section.

TABLE 33–7
Causes of Heparin Resistance*

Ongoing active coagulation
AT deficiency, congenital or acquired
Previous heparin therapy
Drug interaction as with oral contraceptives
Presence of other medical syndromes such as hypereosinophilia or coronary artery disease
Advanced age
Drug error in dose, route of administration, or product (not a true cause of heparin resistance, but must always be considered)

*Adapted from Ellison N, Jobes DR, Schwartz AJ: Heparin therapy during cardiac surgery. In Ellison N, Jobes DR (eds): Effective Hemostasis in Cardiac Surgery. Philadelphia, WB Saunders Co, 1988, p 1, with permission.
AT, antithrombin.

TABLE 33–8
Three Levels of Heparin Therapy

Dosage Level	Goal	Purpose
Minidose	Coagulation studies not prolonged	Prevent deep venous thrombosis
Conventional dose	Prolongation of aPTT 2.0 to 2.5 times the baseline	Anticoagulation Prevent thrombus formation
Maxidose	Total hemostatic paralysis	For institution of cardiopulmonary bypass

Coumadin

Coumadin interferes with the action of vitamin K in the synthesis of factors II, VII, IX, and X. The hemostatic defect produced by Coumadin is similar to vitamin K deficiency, described in a previous section.

Preoperatively, patients may be taking Coumadin for a number of indications as listed in Table 33–9. For elective surgery, patients receiving Coumadin may be converted to heparin and then have their Coumadin discontinued. Heparin can then be discontinued just prior to surgery. The question of discontinuing anticoagulation preoperatively, however, is controversial. As cardiac surgery demonstrates, patients can undergo surgery with an extreme degree of anticoagulation. Except for surgery involving the eye, central nervous system, and large raw surfaces (e.g., liver bed), most authorities agree that anticoagulation can be maintained intraoperatively.[25] The preoperative management of patients taking Coumadin is similar to patients with vitamin K deficiency and has been discussed previously. Similarly, the laboratory findings show a prolonged PT with a normal aPTT.

Patients treated with anticoagulants preoperatively present interesting dilemmas to the anesthesiologist. One concern involves initiation of invasive monitoring in an anticoagulated patient. The most conservative approach would be to neutralize heparin's effect with protamine,

TABLE 33–9
Indications for Coumadin Therapy*

Peripheral vascular disease
Deep venous thrombosis
Transient ischemic attacks
Atrial fibrillation
Prosthetic cardiac valves

*From Troianos CA, Ellison N: Hematological considerations in vascular surgery. In Kaplan JA (ed): Vascular Anesthesia. New York, Churchill Livingstone, 1991, with permission.

establish all the necessary invasive cannulations, and then reestablish anticoagulation with heparin. This approach introduces the potential risk of extending an established thrombus once the anticoagulant is neutralized. Another approach would be to initiate invasive monitoring while maintaining anticoagulation, and reversing the heparin only if complications arise, such as carotid puncture during attempted internal jugular cannulation, or repeated unsuccessful attempts leading to hematoma formation at the cannulation site.

Even greater controversy surrounds the question of administering spinal or epidural anesthesia to patients who are anticoagulated. Most anesthesiologists would avoid intraspinal techniques in patients whose blood is anticoagulated and consider abnormalities in blood clotting a contraindication to performing these techniques.[20,22–24] Odoom and Sih, however, reported a series of 1,000 epidural blocks performed on patients who were receiving anticoagulants preoperatively and they did not observe any side effects which could be related to epidural hematoma formation.[27] If traumatic needle insertion results in aspiration of blood during the needle insertion in a patient who will receive heparin intraoperatively, it may be prudent to delay surgery. A reasonable time period might be 24 hours.[28] The use of regional anesthesia in patients receiving minidose heparin preoperatively is another consideration. By definition, blood coagulation studies are not prolonged (Table 33–8), but the potential for epidural hematoma formation does exist.[29] Use of low molecular weight heparin contraindicates neuraxial block.[29a]

Platelet Inhibitors

There are a number of medications that interfere with platelet function, such as nonsteroidal anti-inflammatory drugs (NSAID) such as aspirin, and dipyridamole.[14] Aspirin interferes with platelet function by inhibiting cyclooxygenase, which is involved in the conversion of arachidonic acid to prostaglandin cyclic endoperoxides and thromboxane A_2. Since thromboxane A_2 is involved in platelet aggregation and vasoconstriction, interfering with its production will decrease platelet aggregation and prolong bleeding time. This inhibition is irreversible and persists for the life of the inhibited platelets, approximately 10 days. Therefore, it would be optimal if patients taking aspirin would discontinue the drug 2 weeks before elective vascular surgery, especially if major blood loss is anticipated.

Dipyridamole also interferes with platelet function. It is often prescribed in patients with vascular disease because of its synergistic effects with aspirin. Dipyridamole's mechanism of action, one different from that of aspirin, involves cyclic adenosine monophosphate (cAMP). A phosphodiesterase inhibitor, dipyridamole increases intracellular cAMP, resulting in decreased platelet aggregation and increased platelet survival time. Used as an adjunct to anticoagulants, dipyridamole prevents thromboembolic events. It aids long-term therapy of chronic angina pectoris. The use of regional anesthetic techniques in patients who are taking platelet inhibitors is controversial. While no evidence suggests that regional anesthesia must be avoided in these patients, an iatrogenic defect in the hemostatic system still exists.

Pentoxifylline

Pentoxifylline is a synthetic xanthine derivative used for symptomatic treatment of claudication in patients with peripheral vascular disease. Pentoxifylline increases the flexibility of red blood cells, allowing improvement in blood flow in the microcirculation, resulting in better tissue oxygenation. There is an associated decrease in blood viscosity and in total systemic vascular resistance.[30]

Pentoxifylline also has an inhibitory effect on platelet aggregation[26] via increases in concentrations of intracellular cAMP. This occurs by enhanced release and synthesis of prostacyclin, as well as through phosphodiesterase inhibition, both of which are effects of pentoxifylline.

Pentoxifylline also causes increased fibrinolytic activity and reduced fibrinogen concentrations. The reduction in fibrinogen level is reversible and has not been reported to cause an increased risk of bleeding. The enhanced fibrinolysis is thought to occur from increased levels of t-PA as well as from decreased antiplasmin activity.

Thrombolytic Agents

Thrombolytic therapy involves the activation of fibrinolysis in order to lyse a clot and may be administered for an acute vascular occlusion, such as coronary or peripheral artery thrombosis, pulmonary embolus, deep vein thrombosis, and occluded arteriovenous dialysis cannula. If emergent surgery is required after the administration of thrombolytic therapy, it is important to recognize the derangements in hemostasis that have been induced. Drugs that may be used as thrombolytic agents include recombinant t-PA, streptokinase, and urokinase. Each promotes fibrinolysis through the activation of plasminogen to plasmin, the serine protease that degrades fibrin; fibrinogen; and coagulation factors V, VIII, and XII (Fig. 33–3).[31]

Plasmin is inhibited by α_2-antiplasmin, α_2-macroglobulin, antithrombin, and α_1-antitrypsin. When these inhibitors are depleted, systemic activation of plasminogen leads to excessive amounts of circulating plasmin. Tissue plasminogen activator is selective in that it activates only fibrin-bound plasmin, while streptokinase and urokinase activate both fibrin-bound plasmin as well as freely circulating plasmin. This difference results in a more systemic fibrinolysis with streptokinase and urokinase, but t-PA can also produce systemic fibrinolysis during prolonged use or in large doses.

Preoperative bleeding may occur at sites of vascular access. Intramuscular injections should be avoided. Extreme care should be taken for the institution of new sites of vascular access. Preferably sites that are accessible to manual compression should be chosen for arterial and large-bore venous access. If uncontrollable bleeding

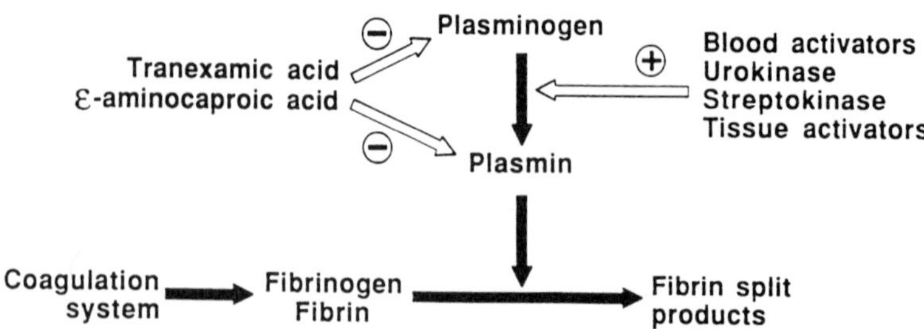

FIGURE 33–3. The thrombolytic pathway. (From Horrow JC: Management of coagulation and bleeding disorders. In Kaplan JA [ed]: Cardiac Anesthesia, 3rd ed. Philadelphia, WB Saunders Co, 1993, p 951, with permission.)

does occur, resource replacement with fresh frozen plasma or cryoprecipitate may be indicated in addition to packed red cells. Definitive therapy with an inhibitor of fibrinolysis such as ε-aminocaproic acid (EACA) will help.[32]

Antifibrinolytics

A recent re-examination of the role of antifibrinolytic drugs in limiting surgical blood loss has revealed that prophylactic administration of EACA, tranexamic acid, or aprotinin reduces postoperative blood loss by 30 to 40% in cardiac surgical populations.[33–35] This frequently translates to reduced exposure to allogeneic blood products.

Applications to noncardiac surgical populations support a wider role of such therapy, including liver transplantation, scoliosis surgery, major joint replacement, and major vascular surgery.

Despite isolated case reports and widespread concern that antifibrinolytic medications will engender thrombotic complications, prospective studies demonstrate safety.[33,34] However, studies properly powered to detect thrombotic complications have yet to be conducted.

The cost of antifibrinolytic agents varies widely despite nearly equivalent drug effects.[36]

Blood Loss and Replacement During Surgery

Over 50% of all transfusions of packed red blood cells (RBCs) occur in the perioperative setting and there is always the potential for significant blood loss in cardiovascular and thoracic surgery. In addition, these patients often have concomitant disease states, which may dictate that a higher level of hemoglobin be maintained, thus lowering the transfusion trigger for RBC administration. These disease states may include peripheral vascular disease, cerebrovascular disease, coronary artery disease, and impaired pulmonary and myocardial function. Although healthy individuals may tolerate hemoglobin levels of 7 gm/dl or lower, compromised patients are not likely to tolerate even higher levels before they have exhausted their ability to compensate for the anemia. Therefore, acceptable hemoglobin levels must be individualized for each patient, taking into account their ability to compensate, the additional blood loss expected, and the etiology of the anemia. Furthermore, as the hemoglobin level decreases, special attention should be given to minimizing the conditions that impair oxygen delivery to the tissues, such as alkalosis, hypothermia, or myocardial depressants, which may impair cardiac output. Postoperatively, conditions such as shivering and hyperthermia, which increase oxygen requirements, should be avoided.

For each individual patient and circumstance, the anesthesiologist must weigh the benefit of the transfusion against the risks. The risks are mainly associated with transmission of disease and transfusion reaction. The human hepatitis viruses are the most frequently transmitted infections. The incidences of hepatitis infections have decreased sharply in recent years owing to improved screening methods: 1 in 63,000 for hepatitis B and 1 in 34,000 for types B and C combined. The incidence of human immunodeficiency virus (HIV) infection via allogeneic blood is estimated at 1 in 493,000 with a lower limit confidence interval of 1 in 210,000.[37] Cytomegalovirus transmission, usually asymptomatic in immunocompetent patients, occurs in 1 in 103,000 exposures.[34]

Transfusion reactions occur in varying degrees. The most common reaction, consisting of fever, chills, and urticaria, occurs in 1 in 100 transfusions. Hemolytic transfusion reactions can be eliminated with compatibility testing but still occur on the order of 1 in 25,000 nonfatal and less than 1 in 1,100,000 fatal.[38,39] They are invariably due to a clerical error.

Transfusion of allogeneic blood can often be avoided if blood conservation measures are taken. These include (1) preoperative collection and storage of autologous blood concomitant with iron supplementation and erythropoietin administration; (2) the use of intraoperative hemodilution; (3) intraoperative blood salvage, washing, and return; and (4) intraoperative platelet pheresis with autotransfusion. Some of these techniques require that a certain degree of anemia be induced. That anemia can be minimized by prescribing iron supplementation. Recombinant erythropoietin may prevent the development of anemia during preoperative collection of autologous blood by stimulating erythropoiesis.[40]

Intraoperative fluid and blood loss begins with the surgical incision. As tissues become exposed, losses occur from evaporation and by a shift of extracellular fluid to the "third space" compartment as a result of the tissue trauma that occurs during surgery. The degree and rate of these losses depend on the extent of the incision and surgical exposure needed for the particular operation.

As blood loss ensues, there are resultant decreases in intravascular volume, hematocrit, clotting factors, and platelets. After replacement with clear fluids and RBCs has begun, the coagulation defect of dilutional thrombocytopenia may become apparent. When platelet count decreases below 50,000 to 100,000 cells/mm^3, platelet transfusion becomes necessary. Dilution of coagulation factors is usually not a problem until large quantities of blood have been replaced.

Heparin

The physical and pharmacologic properties of heparin have been discussed in a previous section. Heparin is used intraoperatively because of its immediate onset of action as a means of preventing intravascular clot formation while vessels are clamped. Commonly, intravenous doses such as 5,000 to 8,000 U are used in vascular surgery and 300 U/kg in cardiac surgery. In vascular surgery heparin is administered before the vessels are cross-clamped and a "top-off" dose may be usually administered subsequently every hour while the vessels remain clamped. In cardiac surgery it is essential that adequate heparin effect, commonly defined as prolongation of the ACT greater than 400 seconds, be achieved before starting cardiopulmonary bypass.[26]

Because of the variable response among patients to heparin, it is prudent to measure patient response to heparin with an ACT. A baseline ACT should be determined prior to the administration of heparin. For the dose of heparin used in vascular surgery (70 to 100 U/kg), the ACT becomes prolonged in the range of 250 to 300 seconds. Patients with AT deficiency, including those patients who have been receiving heparin therapy for an extended period of time preoperatively, will demonstrate heparin resistance, which is defined as the lack of prolongation of the ACT for a given dose of heparin (Table 33–7). These patients will require additional heparin. If the AT deficiency is severe, they may require administration of antithrombin concentrate or FFP in order to restore their levels of AT.

If surgical hemostasis has been achieved after the vascular reconstruction is completed, heparin may not need to be neutralized in vascular cases. However, if diffuse oozing persists and there is no surgical cause for bleeding, heparin is neutralized with protamine in a dose of 1.0 mg protamine per 100 U of heparin activity remaining. The ACT is again measured after neutralization with protamine in order to identify any residual heparin effect. For patients who are at risk for thrombotic events postoperatively, low-dose heparin may be continued until the patient can ambulate.

Although patients have been heparinized for cardiac surgery without having their heparin effect neutralized following termination of cardiopulmonary bypass, that practice is a rare event. Heparin-protamine dosing ratios vary greatly, but usually range from 1.0 to 3.0 mg protamine per 100 U of heparin. It is essential that a return to normal hemostasis be confirmed by measuring the ACT.

Rarely, patients will demonstrate a recurrence of heparin effect after complete heparin neutralization with protamine. This phenomenon, which is termed "heparin rebound," is usually seen several hours after surgery, is diagnosed by determining an increasing ACT or aPTT that had returned to normal after protamine administration, and is treated by administration of additional protamine.[41]

Heparin predictably degrades platelet function and number, with associated prolongation of the bleeding time, probably by binding at platelet membrane glycoprotein Ib. A more rare immune-mediated thrombocytopenia may also develop after prolonged exposure to heparin: the incidence is 1% after 7 days and 3% after 14 days of therapy. In this "type II" heparin-induced thrombocytopenia, antibodies to the heparin–platelet factor 4 complex activate platelets.[42]

When injured vascular endothelium exists, thrombosis may also occur, owing to presence of a site for aggregation of the activated platelets. Major morbidity and mortality occur in 15 to 30% of patients who develop this thrombotic form of heparin-induced thrombocytopenia. These patients often present for vascular surgery to restore circulation to limbs and vital organs.

Susceptible patients may respond adversely to heparin flush solution or heparin-bonded catheters. When suspected, all sources of heparin must be eliminated from the patient's environment. Caregivers must find suitable heparin substitutes for vascular surgery. Options include Ancrod, a snake venom that rapidly clears fibrinogen; low-molecular-weight heparins, which may cross-react with the antibodies to unfractionated heparin; plasmapheresis, which removes antibodies from the circulation; antiplatelet drugs, which may prevent platelet activation; dermatans, naturally occurring glycosaminoglycan polymers similar to heparin; and coumadin.

Protamine

Protamine sulfate is a cationic protein extracted from the sperm or mature testes of salmon. Because of its strongly basic property, protamine binds to the acidic heparin to form a stable salt. Protamine has a rapid onset of action, and dosage depends on the amount of heparin in the circulation. Doses of 1.0 to 3.0 mg of protamine per 100 U heparin administered are recommended. Since serum levels of heparin decrease rapidly after an intravenous injection of heparin, the amount of protamine required for neutralization also will decrease with time. Various methods have been described to determine the dose of protamine necessary for adequate heparin neutralization, including the ACT, dose-response curves, and protamine titration. Most important, however, is to monitor the adequacy of neutralization once a dose of protamine has been administered. Probably the most common, simplest, and most practical clinical method to determine an adequate protamine dose involves an estimation of an initial dose based on the amount of heparin administered, elapsed time since administration, and the ACT. After the initial dose of protamine is administered, a repeat measure of the ACT is obtained and further protamine therapy is guided by the results of the ACT. Essentially this is an in vivo protamine titration.

Protamine also has weak anticoagulant properties by affecting the function of thrombin. These in vitro anticoagulant effects, however, are not clinically important, as rather large doses of protamine have been administered with minimal effects on coagulation.[43,44]

Adverse effects of protamine range from mild systemic hypotension that is mostly a result of systemic vasodilatation through an anaphylactic/anaphylactoid reaction to catastrophic pulmonary vasoconstriction with severe, protracted hypotension.[45] It is important to identify patients at risk for serious reactions to protamine. These may include diabetic patients taking insulin, patients with prior exposure to intravenous protamine, patients with cross-reacting antigens (fish allergy, history of vasectomy), and patients with a previous history of catastrophic pulmonary vasoconstriction after administration.

Postoperative Bleeding and Reoperation

Bleeding in the postoperative period becomes apparent with a continued need for blood and fluid replacement as dictated by the patient's hemodynamics, urine output, laboratory studies, and ongoing blood loss. Retroperitoneal hemorrhage after aortic surgery can produce a distended and tense flank. The surgical causes of bleeding include leaking anastomoses, inadequately ligated vessels, or unrecognized laceration of major vessels during dissection. Immediate reoperation is indicated for excessive postoperative bleeding. Blood volume is replaced as rapidly as possible before induction of anesthesia unless blood loss is occurring so rapidly that attempting to replace the blood loss is futile. As the amount of blood replacement increases, the patient's own blood begins to take on characteristics of bank blood: low concentrations of 2,3-diphosphoglycerate (2,3-DPG), low activities of factors V and VIII, and a dilutional thrombocytopenia. While the surgeon is attempting to achieve surgical hemostasis, the anesthesiologist must continually evaluate the patient's hemostatic profile in order to recognize any new defects that must be treated.

The thrombin time, an underappreciated test, is prolonged in three conditions: (1) presence of even very small amounts of heparin, (2) too little or dysfunctional fibrinogen, and (3) presence of clinically significant concentrations of fibrin split products. A normal thrombin time safely rules out both consumptive coagulopathy and residual heparin as causes of bleeding.

Continued monitoring of activated clotting time, platelet count, fibrinogen level, and prothrombin and partial thromboplastin times should be carried out as long as active bleeding persists. These studies will aid in the identification of any nonsurgical cause for bleeding, such as heparin rebound, as well as a guide to therapy for the correction of the hemostatic defect.

References

1. Horrow JC: Management of coagulopathy associated with CPB. In Gravlee GP, Davis RF, Utley JR (eds): Cardiopulmonary Bypass. Principles and Practice. Baltimore, Williams & Wilkins, 1993, p 436.
2. Horrow JC: Management of coagulation and bleeding disorders. In Kaplan JA (ed): Cardiac Anesthesia, 3rd ed. Philadelphia, WB Saunders Co, 1993, p 951.
3. Boisclair MD, Lane DA, Philippou H, et al: Mechanism of thrombin generation during surgery and cardiopulmonary bypass. Blood 82:3350, 1993.
4. Salzman EW: Hemorrhagic disorders in the ACS Manual of Preoperative and Postoperative Care, Philadelphia, WB Saunders Co, 1983, p 153.
5. Suchman AL, Muslim AJ: How does the activated partial thromboplastin time predict postoperative hemorrhage? JAMA 256: 750, 1986.
6. Lind SE: The bleeding time does not predict surgical bleeding. Blood 77:2547, 1991.
7. Brent C: Bleeding abnormalities and the parturient, the anesthesiologist's responsibility. JAMA 260:1954, 1988.
8. Ellison N, Silberstein LE: Hemostasis in the perioperative period. In Stoelting RK, Barash PG, Gallagher TJ (eds): Advances in Anesthesia, Vol 3. Chicago, Year Book Medical Publishers, 1986, p 67.
9. Brettler DB, Levine PH: Clinical manifestations and therapy of inherited coagulation factor deficiencies. In Colman RW, Hirsh J, Marder VJ, Salzman EW (eds): Hemostasis and Thrombosis: Basic Principles and Clinical Practice. Philadelphia, JB Lippincott Co, 1994, p 169.
10. Troianos CA, Ellison N: Hematological considerations in vascular surgery. In Kaplan JA (ed): Vascular Anesthesia. New York, Churchill Livingstone, 1991, p 549.
11. Jordan RE, Oosta GM, Gardner WT, Rosenberg RD: The kinetics of hemostatic enzyme-antithrombin interactions in the presence of low molecular weight heparin. J Biol Chem 225:10,081, 1980.
12. Stoelting RK, Dierdorf SF: Anesthesia and Co-Existing Disease, 3rd ed. New York, Churchill Livingstone, 1993, p 415.
13. Kessler CM: The pharmacology of aspirin, heparin, coumarin, and thrombolytic agents. Implications for therapeutic use in cardiopulmonary disease. Chest 99:97S, 1991.
14. Jobes DR, Ellison N: Hemotherapy: Control of hemostasis and blood replacement. In Estafanous G, Barash P6, Reves JG (ed): Cardiac Anesthesia: Principles and Clinical Practice, Philadelphia, JB Lippincott Co, 1993, p 597.
15. Comp PC: Hereditary disorders predisposing to thrombosis. In Coller BS (ed): Progress in Hemostasis and Thrombosis, Vol 8. Orlando, FL, Grune & Stratton, 1986, p 71.
16. Aoki N, Moroi M, Sakata Y, et al: Abnormal plasminogen: A hereditary molecular abnormality found in a patient with recurrent thrombosis. J Clin Invest 61:1186, 1978.
17. Carrell N, Gabriel DA, Blatt PM, et al: Hereditary dysfibrinogenemia in a patient with thrombotic disease. Blood 62:439, 1983.
18. Mueh JR, Herbst KD, Rapaport SI: Thrombosis in patients with the lupus anticoagulant. Ann Intern Med 92:156, 1980.
19. Atik M: Venous thrombosis In Moore WS (ed): Vascular Surgery, A Comprehensive Review. Orlando, FL, Grune & Stratton, 1986, p 1043.
20. Seligsohn U, Berger A, Abend M, et al: Homozygous protein C deficiency manifested by massive venous thrombosis in the newborn. N Engl J Med 310:559, 1984.
21. Gonzalez R, Alberca I, Sala N, Vicente V: Protein C deficiency —response to danazol and DDAVP. Thromb Haemost 53:320, 1985.
22. Coller BS, Owen J, Jesty J, et al: Deficiency of plasma protein S, protein C, or antithrombin III and arterial thrombosis. Arteriosclerosis 7:456, 1987.
23. Schafer AI: The hypercoagulable states. Ann Intern Med 102: 814, 1985.
24. Naeye RL: Thrombotic state after a hemorrhagic diathesis, a possible complication of therapy with epsilon-aminocaproic acid. Blood 19:694, 1962.

25. Ellison N, Ominsky AJ: Clinical considerations for the anesthesiologist whose patient is on anticoagulant therapy. Anesthesiology 39:328, 1973.
26. Ellison N, Jobes DR, Schwartz AJ: Heparin therapy during cardiac surgery. In Ellison N, Jobes DR (eds): Effective Hemostasis in Cardiac Surgery. Philadelphia, WB Saunders Co, 1988, p 1.
27. Odoom JA, Sih IL: Epidural analgesia and anticoagulant therapy. Experience with one thousand cases of continuous epidurals. Anesthesia 38:254, 1983.
28. Bridenbaugh PO, Greene NM: Spinal neural blockade. In Cousins MJ, Bridenbaugh PO (eds): Neuronal Blockade in Clinical Anesthesia and Management of Pain. Philadelphia, JB Lippincott Co, 1988, p 244.
29. Parnass SM, Rothenberg DM, Fischer RL, Ivankovich AD: Spinal anesthesia and minidose heparin (Letter). JAMA 263:1496, 1990.
29a. American Society of Regional Anesthesia Consensus Statement: Neuraxial Anesthesia and Anticoagulations. Reg Anesthesia Pain Med 23(Suppl) 1, 1998.
30. Ward A, Clissold SP: Pentoxifylline. A review of its pharmacodynamic and pharmacokinetic properties, and its therapeutic efficacy. Drugs 34:50, 1987.
31. Marder VJ, Sherry S: Thrombolytic therapy, current status. N Engl J Med 318:1514, 1988.
32. Goldberg M, Colonna-Romano P, Babins N: Emergency coronary artery bypass surgery following intracoronary streptokinase. Anesthesiology 61:601, 1984.
33. DelRossi AJ, Cernaianu AC, Botros S, et al: Prophylactic treatment of postperfusion bleeding using EACA. Chest 96:27, 1989.
34. Horrow JC, Hlavacek J, Strong MD, et al: Prophylactic tranexamic acid decreases bleeding after cardiac operations. J Thorac Cardiovasc Surg 99:518, 1990.
35. Bidstrup BP, Roysten D, Sapsford RN: Reduction in blood loss and blood use after cardiopulmonary bypass with high dose aprotinin (Trasylol). J Thorac Cardiovasc Surg 97:364, 1989.
36. Horrow JC, Ellison N: Effective hemostasis in cardiac surgery. Can J Anesth 39:309, 1992.
37. Schreiber GB, Busch MP, Kleinman SH, Korelitz JJ: The risk of transfusion transmitted viral infections. The retrovirus epidemiology donor study. N Engl J Med 334:1734, 1996.
38. Sandler SG (ed): Increasing The Safety of Blood Transfusions. Washington, DC, American Red Cross, 1992.
39. Ellison N: A commentary on three NIH Consensus Development Conferences on Transfusion Medicine. Anesth Clin North Am 8: 609, 1990.
40. Kulier AH, Gamboltz H, Fuchs G: Subcutaneous recombinant erythropoietin and autologous blood donation before coronary artery bypass surgery. Anesth Analg 76:102, 1993.
41. Ellison N, Beatty CP, Blake DR, et al: Heparin rebound: Studies in patients and volunteers. J Thorac Cardiovasc Surg 67:723, 1974.
42. Amiral K, Bridley F, Dreyfus M: Platelet factor 4 complexed to heparin is the target for antibodies generated in heparin-induced thrombocytopenia (Letter). Thromb Haemostas 68:95, 1992.
43. Ellison N, Ominsky AJ, Wollman H: Is protamine a clinically important anticoagulant? Anesthesiology 35:621, 1971.
44. Kresowik TF, Wakefield TW, Fessler RD, Stanley JC: Anticoagulant effects of protamine sulfate in a canine model. J Surg Res 45:8, 1988.
45. Horrow JC: Protamine. A review of its toxicity. Anesth Analg 64:340, 1985.

CHAPTER 34

Thoracic Trauma

John K. Stene, M.D., Ph.D.

Chest injuries cause profound physiologic changes in the traumatized patient and thus cause some of the most difficult clinical challenges for the anesthesiologist managing trauma patients. Not only are these patients affected by direct life-threatening injury to the cardiopulmonary system, but they are also affected by indirect effects that complicate anesthetic care, such as shock and, occasionally, cerebral air embolism.

Although chest injuries cause one out of four trauma deaths in the United States, 90% of blunt chest trauma and 70 to 85% of penetrating chest trauma can be treated nonoperatively with simple measures of endotracheal intubation and tube thoracostomy (chest tube) insertion.[1] Trauma to the thorax may cause one of six immediately life-threatening chest injuries or one of six potentially life-threatening injuries. The six immediately life-threatening chest injuries are airway obstruction, tension pneumothorax, open pneumothorax, massive hemothorax, flail chest, and cardiac tamponade. The six potentially life-threatening chest injuries are pulmonary contusion, myocardial contusion, aortic disruption, traumatic diaphragmatic rupture, tracheobronchial disruption, and esophageal disruption (Table 34–1).

Because of the high rate of nonoperative treatment of chest injuries, anesthesiologists will be treating more patients with chest injuries in the emergency room than in the operating room. However, many patients with multiple injuries will have chest injuries and require operation for other associated injuries. In this chapter, we will discuss the effects of chest injuries on the anesthetic care of the trauma patient.

Although the majority of thoracic injuries can be adequately treated with simple, nonoperative maneuvers, an anesthesiologist will be involved in the care of the patient with thoracic injury in many ways including anesthetic induction to establish a patent artificial airway, surgical anesthesia for corrective operations, anesthesia to assist the surgeon in diagnostic tests, anesthesia for radiologic procedures, and finally, postinjury and/or postoperative analgesia and critical care.

Thoracic trauma commonly impairs the patient's gas exchange mechanisms (Table 34–2). Many patients require artificial mechanical ventilation to maintain appropriate alveolar and arterial blood-gas tensions. Endotracheal intubation to facilitate artificial ventilation in the patient with chest trauma is most easily achieved by direct laryngoscopy and orotracheal intubation following intravenous hypnotics and muscle relaxants.[2] Among the indications for intubation are the need to compensate for rib fractures, chest wall instability, and reduced respiratory muscle work secondary to hemorrhagic shock[3] and the need to control ventilation during surgery with an open chest (Table 34–3).

Patients with thoracic injuries frequently require ventilation for several days to stabilize the chest wall and provide adequate gas exchange via severely injured lungs. Prolonged analgesia and sedation are frequently required to optimize the critical care of patients with thoracic injuries both for endotracheal tube tolerance and to relieve pain from injuries. Combinations of opioids, benzodiazepines, and muscle relaxants are used to provide prolonged respiratory management in the critical care unit.

Regional anesthesia and patient-controlled analgesia (PCA) are useful for controlling the pain of thoracic injury in patients who do not require mechanical ventilation for maintenance of gas exchange. Continuous epidural analgesia through a catheter placed in the lumbar or thoracic epidural space has proved to be extremely effective for postthoracotomy as well as posttraumatic thoracic pain relief.[4,5] Epidural opioids with or without dilute local anesthetic solutions will allow high-level (to the cervical region) analgesia without major sympathetic nervous system blockade and muscle weakness. Appropriately applied anesthesia care can markedly enhance the management of the patient suffering from thoracic trauma (Table 34–4). Because many patients with blunt thoracic trauma can be treated nonoperatively without endotracheal intubation, intravenous opioids delivered by a PCA pump are very useful to provide low-level analgesia to these selectively managed patients.[6]

TABLE 34–1
The "Dirty Dozen" Chest Injuries

Injury	Treatment
Immediately life-threatening	
Airway obstruction	Relieve obstruction with endotracheal tube or tracheostomy
Tension pneumothorax	Chest tube drainage
Open pneumothorax	Close defect, drain pneumothorax with chest tube
Massive hemothorax	Chest tube to drain hemothorax, thoracotomy or VATS if hemorrhage continues
Flail chest	Analgesia to control splinting, endotracheal intubation and controlled ventilation
Cardiac tamponade	Pericardiocentesis followed by thoracotomy and repair of bleeding source
Potentially life-threatening	
Pulmonary contusion	Mechanical ventilation with PEEP, pulmonary toilet
Myocardial contusion	Observation, hemodynamic monitoring
Aortic disruption	Thoracotomy and grafting of aorta
Traumatic diaphragmatic rupture	Repair from thoracotomy or celiotomy
Tracheobronchial disruption:	
Larynx	Tracheostomy and repair chest tube for pneumothorax and surgical repair
Trachea	
Bronchus	Chest tube for pneumothorax, surgical repair
Esophageal disruption	Direct repair, or esophageal diversion in neck and gastrostomy

VATS, video-assisted thoracoscopic surgery; PEEP, positive end-expiratory pressure.

Direct Effects of Chest Injuries on Anesthetic Management

Chest Injuries

Pulmonary Contusion

Pulmonary contusion disrupts the alveolar capillary membrane and causes interstitial and alveolar hemorrhage. The contused area will alter the exchange of respiratory gases between the alveoli and blood.[7] If the contusion is small, these effects may have minimal impact on anesthetic management. However, large contusions will lead to marked impairment of oxygenation and carbon dioxide (CO_2) elimination. At the extreme, massive bilateral pulmonary contusion may require treatment with an extracorporeal membrane oxygenator.[8]

Classically, a contusion takes several hours to evolve fully on a chest x-ray, usually after fluid resuscitation restores cardiac output and pulmonary blood flow. The most prominent effect of lung contusion is to produce regions of low pulmonary ventilation to profusion ($\dot{V}/\dot{Q}$) ratio, frequently producing a $\dot{V}/\dot{Q}$ ratio of zero, right-to-left shunt or venous admixture.[9] Right-to-left shunts have marked effects on oxygenation as well as on the uptake of inhalation anesthetics. The poorly soluble anesthetic nitrous oxide (N_2O) will demonstrate an accelerated rise of its end-tidal to inspired concentration ratio and, therefore, a more rapid rise of alveolar concentration. This is because the pulmonary contusion also causes relative overventilation of other lung regions, especially during mechanical ventilation with a fixed tidal volume. However, the venous admixture effect of the contusion will retard the rate of rise of the arterial nitrous oxide concentration relative to alveolar concentration. The balance of more rapid alveolar rise with decreased arterial to alveolar ratio increase will be a slowing of the rate of change of anesthetic action. Isoflurane with a higher blood gas solubility than N_2O will also have an enhanced rate of rise of end-tidal to inspired concentration ratio as the alveolar concentration increases quickly secondary to the overventilation of the noncontused lung, but will have minimal retardation of the rise of arterial concentration relative to alveolar concentration secondary to venous admixture because each liter of mixed venous blood contains more isoflurane than N_2O. Thus, the induction of anesthesia with isoflurane may be

TABLE 34–2
Physiological Effects of Thoracic Trauma

Gas Exchange
Direct effects of injury
Hypoventilation
Airway obstruction
Regional $\dot{V}/\dot{Q}$ mismatch
Lung collapse
Indirect effects of injury
Shock
Pain with chest wall splinting
Posttraumatic ARDS
Sepsis
Cardiac Output
Direct effects of injury
Hemorrhage
Myocardial contusion
Great vessel disruption
Myocardial rupture
Pericardial tamponade
Indirect effects
Hypoxia
Hypercarbia
Sepsis

$\dot{V}/\dot{Q}$, ventilation-perfusion; ARDS, adult respiratory distress syndrome.

TABLE 34–3
Indications for Intubation in Thoracic Trauma

Indications	Therapy
Single-lumen endotracheal tube	
Respiratory distress	Pa_{CO_2} >50 i Pa_{O_2} <60 i with O_2 supplement Respiratory rate >35/min
Associated severe head inury	GCS score ≤8
Shock	Persistent hypotension with fluid administration
Double-lumen endobronchial tube	
Aortic disruption	Left endobronchial tube
Bronchial disruption	Use endobronchial tube in contralateral bronchus
Unilateral lung contusion	Left endobronchial tube for independent lung ventilation
Bronchopleural fistula with massive air leak	Left endobronchial tube for independent lung ventilation
Intrapulmonary hemorrhage	Preferably endobronchial lumen in hemorrhaging lung to prevent contamination of other lung

GCS, Glasgow Coma Scale.

only slightly delayed by pulmonary contusions or may actually be slightly enhanced.[10]

As lung contusions resolve, they frequently cause bullae or cyst formation in the lung.[11,12] These pulmonary cysts will act as dead space if they have bronchial connections, but will have no effect on gas exchange if they are not ventilated. However, posttraumatic pulmonary cysts may be particularly sensitive to rupture from ventilator barotrauma; therefore, the anesthesiologist must be careful to control ventilatory pressures in patients with such bullae.

Lung Laceration

Lung lacerations from either penetrating trauma (e.g., gunshot, stab wounds) or sharp edges of broken ribs complicate anesthetic management because of continued hemorrhage that can lead to hemorrhagic shock if not controlled. Significant lacerations of the lung cause both tension pneumothorax and massive hemothorax. A large bronchopleural fistula caused by a lung laceration will require increased inspired minute ventilation to compensate for loss of alveolar gas exchange. If the bronchopleural fistula diverts a significant portion of each tidal volume, independent lung ventilation with a double-lumen endotracheal tube will be lifesaving (Table 34–3). The nonlacerated lung can be ventilated with tidal volumes and rates high enough to compensate for poor CO_2 removal and oxygen (O_2) uptake from the lung with a large air leak. Unfortunately, the lacerated lung with the air leak will continue to cause an increased venous admixture despite independent lung ventilation. During thoracotomy, this situation can be surgically corrected by temporarily cross-clamping the pulmonary hilum to stop both ventilation and perfusion of that lung.

One of the worst complications of a pulmonary laceration is a bronchopulmonary venous fistula causing communication between the airways and pulmonary venules, leading to continuous entry of air into the pulmonary venous drainage and thus systemic air emboli.[13] Bronchopulmonary venous fistulae may occur following lung laceration from rib fragments, stab wounds, or gunshot wounds. Bronchopulmonary venous fistulae occasionally are also seen following sudden decompression in divers when alevolae rupture to form a continuous path of air entry into the pulmonary venous drainage. Treatment requires the discontinuation of both ventilation and perfusion to the lacerated lung. Again, a surgical clamp across the lung hilum will achieve this effect temporarily while the lung is being repaired. A double-lumen endotracheal tube can facilitate treatment by isolating and nonventilating the injured lung prior to surgical correction (see Chapter 25). Any neurologic damage from arterial air emboli can be improved by rapidly compressing the patient in a hyperbaric chamber, which will force the gas bubbles into solution in the bloodstream.

TABLE 34–4
Role of Anesthesiologist in Managing Patients with Thoracic Injuries

Patient Problem	Anesthesiologist's Solution
Airway obstruction	Intubation/mechanical ventilation
Respiratory distress	Intubation/mechanical ventilation
Cardiovascular instability	Intubation/mechanical ventilation
Associated severe head injury	Intubation/mechanical ventilation
Multiple rib fractures	Thoracic lumbar/epidural
Chest wall pain without gas exchange impairment	PCA
Massive chest trauma with impaired gas exchange	ECMO

PCA, patient-controlled anesthesia; ECMO, extracorporeal membrane oxygenation.

Chest Wall Injury

The most common chest injury is a rib fracture, which is most prevalent in the elderly. Multiple rib fractures during thoracic trauma frequently causes instability of the chest wall secondary to either flail chest or an open pneumothorax (sucking chest wound). Multiple rib fractures destabilize the chest wall (flail chest) so that it becomes difficult for the patient to generate enough negative pleural pressure for ventilation. (At least three adjacent ribs must be broken in two places to produce a flail segment.) If the rib fractures are unilateral, the ventilation will tend to shift to the lung in the intact hemithorax. However, blood flow will not be diverted away from the lung in the unstable hemithorax; therefore, the patient will develop marked venous admixture. During blunt trauma, the energy transfer that fractured the ribs usually also produces contusion of the underlying lung. This contused lung will become less compliant than the normal lung and will further aggravate relative hypoventilation within the injured hemithorax. The sharp ends of fractured ribs frequently lacerate underlying lung parenchyma and may also penetrate the skin, leading to an open pneumothorax.

Penetrating thoracic injuries cause both lung laceration and some degree of open pneumothorax. If the defect in the chest wall is greater than two thirds the diameter of the trachea and is open to atmosphere, the pleural space will be ventilated preferentially to the trachea. If the resistance to air flow through the open pneumothorax is less than the resistance to air flow through the trachea and bronchus to that hemithorax, the underlying lung will collapse rapidly as changes in interpleural pressure cause ventilation of the pleural space—not the tracheal bronchial tree. Open pneumothoraces must be covered with air-tight dressings (taped on three sides) and treated with chest tubes inserted to evacuate pleural air. If the air-tight dressing is taped on four sides, a tension pneumothorax may develop, as pleural air cannot escape prior to chest tube insertion.

The treatment of an unstable chest wall requires intubation or tracheostomy and mechanical ventilation to splint the ribs while they heal. This treatment, described by Avery in 1956,[14] revolutionized the management of patients with flail chest. Prior to this treatment technique, attempts to operatively fixate the rib fractions were successful in stabilizing the ribs but frequently increased the patient's morbidity; however, this operative fixation of rib fractures is regaining some favor.[15]

Not all patients with multiple rib fractures and lung contusion will require endotracheal intubation and mechanical ventilation.[6] Excellent analgesia from continuous thoracic epidural analgesia will allow many patients to maintain adequate pulmonary toilet with a natural airway and spontaneous ventilation. Avoiding chest wall splinting and consequent hypoventilation from the pain of multiple rib fractures will allow many patients to heal their chest wall without a mechanical ventilator.[4,5,16–18] Patients with massive chest-wall and/or multiple injuries will probably still need to be maintained with mechanical ventilation for a period of time following their injury, but the use of continuous regional anesthesia via an epidural, intercostal, or interpleural approach appears to be promising in the management of chest wall injuries[4,5,11–13,16–18] (Tables 34–5 and 34–6).

TABLE 34–5
Continuous Regional Analgesia for Thoracic Trauma

Technique	Advantages
Continuous spinal catheter	Very small doses of opioids (i.e., 0.25 mg of morphine) provide prolonged analgesia
Continuous lumbar epidural catheter	Simple to insert: chest wall analgesia can be achieved with higher volumes of drugs
Continuous thoracic epidural catheter	Excellent chest wall analgesia with small volumes of drug
Continuous intercostal catheter	Good unilateral analgesia: large volume can provide bilateral analgesia

TABLE 34–6
Choice of Anesthesia for Patients with Thoracic Trauma

Anesthetic Technique	Advantages
General anesthesia	Provides positive-pressure ventilation to manage impaired gas exchange; allows operations with an open hemithorax Optimum cardiovascular control during shock resuscitation
Regional anesthesia	Provides excellent long-term analgesia postoperatively either with or without mechanical ventilation
Monitored anesthesia care	Minimal physiologic trespass for operations in isolated regions

Cardiac and Great Vessel Injuries

Myocardial Contusion

Blunt trauma to the anterior chest wall can easily cause myocardial contusion.[19,20] The myocardial pathophysiology is characterized by disrupted capillaries and a hematoma (bruise) surrounding the cardiac myocytes.[21] A large transmural contusion will frequently lead to cellular disruption with necrosis of the cardiac myocytes and hemodynamically mimic a transmural myocardial infarction. This can occur with release of intracellular enzymes into the bloodstream and regional myocardial dyssynergia. However, the contused myocardium is not surrounded by a zone of relative ischemia, as is the case with infarcted myocardium.

A small epicardial contusion will frequently cause only transient arrhythmias by acting as an irritable focus.[22] Large transmural contused areas lead to dyssynergia of the ventricular wall and can impair stroke volume and cardiac output. The worst complication from a large myocardial contusion is disruption of the papillary muscles with acute mitral valve regurgitation.[21] Acute traumatic mitral regurgitation following contusion through the left ventricular papillary muscles is frequently fatal unless it is possible to perform an immediate mitral valve replacement.

The natural history of myocardial contusion and the best method of treatment are still controversial.[7,23–25] Because it is so difficult to diagnose small myocardial contusions, it has been very difficult to identify patients with myocardial contusions and follow them to ascertain the natural history of the contusion as well as the best forms of treatment. Although ventricular arrhythmias are the most common abnormality associated with myocardial contusion, the presence of arrhythmias is too nonspecific to be diagnostic for myocardial contusion. Intracellular enzymes such as MB band creatine phosphokinase (MBCPK) are released from large contusion areas of the myocardium. However, diagnostic levels of serum MBCPK are extremely difficult to determine because other injured tissues also can release MBCPK. Echocardiography, which reveals areas of myocardial dyssynergia is the best technique to diagnose hemodynamically significant myocardial contusion.[25]

Some traumatologists feel that a patient with a myocardial contusion must be treated as if he/she had a myocardial infarction (i.e., with rest and oxygen for several days). However, a patient with a contused myocardium does not need pharmacologic manipulations to decrease the zone of relative ischemia around the infarction. Patients with myocardial contusions seem to tolerate anesthesia very well unless the contusion is large enough to cause dyssynergia of the left ventricle and hemodynamic impairment. Because the majority of contusions apparently affect the right ventricle, such hemodynamic impairment is rare. However, a patient who has a large transmural contusion should be monitored intraoperatively with a pulmonary artery (Swan-Ganz) catheter and treated appropriately to continuously optimize his/her hemodynamic status.

The anesthesiologist managing a patient with thoracic trauma must have a high index of suspicion to diagnose myocardial contusion by identifying patients at risk because of blunt trauma in the region of the heart, identifying arrhythmias on electrocardiogram (ECG) and regional wall motion abnormality on echocardiography.[25] Transesophageal echocardiography (TEE) has become increasingly used and will probably become the diagnostic instrument of choice for myocardial contusion.[26,27]

Cardiac Rupture/ Pericardial Tamponade

More serious injuries to the myocardium are lacerations secondary to either penetrating trauma or chamber rupture from blunt trauma.[19] Large lacerations frequently are rapidly fatal. However, some patients can survive ventricular laceration especially because right ventricular muscle edges of the laceration reapproximate as interchamber and extrachamber interpericardial pressures equilibrate. These patients are salvageable with rapid intraoperative repair. Penetrating trauma to a coronary artery will lead to both ischemia of the myocardium distal to the injury and pericardial hemorrhage. If the patient has relatively good collateral flow to this area of myocardium, the ischemic damage may be minimal. However, lacerated coronary arteries frequently bleed briskly into the pericardium, leading to hemopericardium with cardiac tamponade.

Pericardial tamponade can also be caused by a massive interstitial pulmonary air leak that leads to pneumomediastinum with air actually dissecting into the pericardium, causing pneumopericardium. Classically, tamponade of the pericardium is diagnosed by Beck's triad: elevated venous pressure, decline in arterial pressure, and muffled heart tones. If a pulmonary artery catheter has been inserted, both the central venous pressure (CVP) and the pulmonary capillary wedge pressure (PCWP) will be elevated and numerically equal and the cardiac output will be decreased. Echocardiography will demonstrate an enlarged pericardial space and small ventricular volumes during tamponade. Tamponade must be relieved rapidly to allow the heart to function normally. Frequently, resuscitation of the patient with chest injuries must proceed before an echo can be obtained. In the patient in persistent shock following direct trauma, needle pericardiocentesis may be formed both diagnostically and, by relieving tamponade, therapeutically for suspected hemopericardium or pneumopericardium. If there is any question about pericardial tamponade reaccumulating, the patient should receive a pericardial window to vent the pericardium. The pericardiocentesis catheter should be left in situ until the pericardial effusion can be surgically relieved. The anesthetic management of a patient with pericardial tamponade is organized around the maintenance of a rapid heart rate to minimize the ventricular filling time and the avoidance of drugs that depress the myocardium.[28] Furthermore, intravenous fluids should be administered to increase cardiovascular preload to maximize cardiac performance. Useful drugs in these patients include benzodiazepines, such as midazolam, to induce unconsciousness and amnesia. In the absence of a closed head injury, ketamine hydrochloride can be very useful in this situation because it tends to promote a tachycardia and accentuates sympathetic stimulation to the myocardium. Judiciously utilized opioids can maintain the patient's level of analgesia without depressing myocardial contractility and venous return.

Aortic Disruption

Blunt chest trauma from a high-speed deceleration injury can rupture the thoracic aorta thus causing an acute traumatic thoracic aortic aneurysm. These aneurysms frequently rupture completely with resulting exsanguination and death. A majority of patients with this injury die at the scene. However, the hemorrhage may be controlled temporarily by adventitial hematoma formation that allows the patient time to receive definitive medical therapy. Local hematoma formation associated with an aortic injury will cause the upper mediastinum to be widened on an upright chest x-ray. Definitive diagnosis requires arteriography.[7] Because of the high potential for the aneurysm to completely rupture and lead to sudden death, these patients need to undergo immediate surgical repair of the aortic injury. Aneurysms distal to the left subclavian takeoff may be surgically managed with short-term cross-clamping and resection followed by repair with a tube graft. Ventricular venting or partial bypass from the left ventricle to the distal aorta may be used to reduce the afterload stress on the left ventricle during the repair.

More proximal aneurysms, including the ascending aorta and the aortic arch, will require cardiopulmonary bypass (CPB) for complete repair. The anesthetic management of the trauma patient who requires CPB for aortic repair is similar to that used for the patient requiring anesthesia for cardiac surgery. For the patient whose distal thoracic aortic aneurysm is repaired without CPB, the anesthetic management is designed to maintain cardiac preload and venous return during cross-clamping, with potent arterial vasodilators used to minimize the acute afterload effects on the left ventricle. Consideration must be given to the trade-offs of reducing afterload by systemic vasodilatation and associated loss of perfusion pressure and blood flow to the spinal cord. Close communication and cooperation between the surgeon and anesthesiologist are crucial to successful management of circulation requirements in such cases.

Renal protection is attempted with diuresis prior to aortic cross-clamping. Aggressive replacement of the patient's blood volume must be undertaken to prevent profound hypotension following release of the aortic cross-clamp. Both mannitol and furosemide are useful to stimulate diuresis—for example, mannitol 12.5 gm, just prior to cross-clamping and repeated 15 minutes later. Systemic metabolic acidosis will occur as the ischemic vascular bed is reperfused following release of the cross-clamp. Prophylactic hyperventilation will help buffer the effect of the metabolic acidosis. Intravenous buffers, such as bicarbonate or tromethamine, may be used to treat the metabolic acidosis. Patients with ruptured thoracic aortas should be monitored with intra-arterial catheters, preferably in the right radial artery, because cross-clamping will decrease pressure in the femoral and left radial arteries. If the patient's condition is sufficiently stable, a pulmonary artery catheter should be placed preoperatively to monitor cardiac output and the hemodynamic effects of cross-clamping. While still a controversial modality, a lumbar subarachnoid catheter (spinal) has been reported to be experimentally useful to reduce ischemia of the spinal cord during aortic cross-clamping.[29] Aortic cross-clamping leads to increased pressure in the carotid arteries proximal to the cross-clamp. Increased carotid arterial pressure will be transmitted to the intracranial cerebrospinal fluid (CSF), which is in continuity with the spinal cord CSF. At the same time the pressure in the distal spinal cord CSF is raised, the arterial perfusion pressure to the spinal cord is reduced by the aortic cross-clamp. If the mean arterial pressure in the spinal cord is reduced too much while CSF pressure rises, the perfusion of the spinal cord will be impaired and infarction may occur, especially in the watershed regions of spinal cord perfusion. Draining CSF through a continuous lumbar spinal catheter will reduce the rise in spinal cord CSF pressure and may help maintain adequate spinal cord perfusion pressure. Postoperatively, local anesthetics and opioids may be administered through a spinal catheter just as they are through an epidural catheter. A subarachnoid (spinal) catheter may be used safely up to 48 hours postoperatively. The doses of drugs administered directly to the CSF are 10 to 20% of the doses used with an epidural catheter.

Indirect Effects of Chest Injury on Anesthesia

Hemorrhagic Shock

Hemorrhagic shock complicates the anesthetic management of trauma patients with or without chest trauma. Anesthesiologists must be careful to use drugs to provide adequate hypnosis, amnesia, and analgesia while optimizing cardiovascular homeostasis when anesthetizing trauma patients[2] (Table 34–7). Many anesthetic drugs are myocardial depressants. These drugs must be either avoided or used in very small, judiciously titrated doses during hemorrhagic shock. Ketamine stimulates release of catecholamines, which increases heart rate and blood pressure. However, the patient in shock may be unable to further increase catecholamine secretion and the direct myocardial depressant effects of ketamine are unmasked.

TABLE 34–7
Choice of Anesthetic Drugs for Anesthesia in Patients with Chest Trauma

Drugs	Effects
Induction	
Thiopental	Myocardial depressant; titrate in small doses
Propofol	Myocardial depressant; titrate in small doses
Etomiodate	Titrate to effect in hypovolemic patient
Midazolam	Long acting; vasodilating in large doses; titrate to effect
Ketamine	Elevates intracranial pressure; increases heart rate and blood pressure
Muscle Relaxation	
Succinylcholine	Hyperkalemia, increased intraocular and intracranial pressure
Vecuronium	Need large doses and thus long duration to achieve rapid onset
Atracurium	Histamine release and vasodilation
Rocuronium	Need large doses for rapid onset
Pancuronium	Tachycardia
Analgesia	
Fentanyl	Vasodilating
Sufentanil	Potent analgesia, vasodilator
Morphine	Vasodilating, relatively long acting
Hydromorphone	Useful for epidural use

Furthermore, ketamine should be avoided in patients with closed head injuries. Drugs such as thiopental, etomidate, propofol, fentanyl, or sufentanil are highly lipophilic and will rapidly cross the blood-brain barrier. If these drugs are injected intravenously into a patient with a blood volume reduced from hemorrhagic shock, the concentration achieved in the bloodstream will be much higher than in a euvolemic patient. Therefore, very small doses of these drugs can be used to achieve the desired hypnosis or analgesia while cardiovascular depression can be avoided by carefully monitoring the patient's response. Nitrous oxide should be avoided because it tends to accumulate in closed air spaces such as pneumothoraces. Furthermore, nitrous oxide and opioid combinations tend to decrease cardiac output, but may maintain arterial pressure with an elevated systemic vascular resistance (SVR).[30] Therefore, air should be used instead of N_2O to keep the FIO_2 below 1. Although isoflurane is a myocardial depressant and vasodilator, in low concentrations it will improve the hypnosis and analgesia of intravenous agents with minimal cardiac depression. An advantage of an inhalationally delivered drug is that if the patient shows excessive cardiovascular depression from the anesthetic, the drug can be eliminated rapidly through the lungs. Although pulmonary contusion will slow the change of inhalational gas tensions in the blood stream as described above, the change in anesthetic depth is still more rapid with inhalation drugs than with intravenous drugs.

Shock must be treated by restoring the intravascular fluid volume. Shock treatment priorities are to (1) restore the circulating volume, (2) restore hemoglobin concentration to a level adequate for oxygen consumption, and (3) restore coagulation. Initially, asanguinous fluids are used to establish open intravenous lines and to rapidly restore circulating volume. Colloidal resuscitation fluids (albumin, hetastarch) are more effective in rapidly restoring circulating volume than crystalloid resuscitation fluids (Ringer's, saline, Normosol). However, all patients will need a large enough volume of crystalloid infusion following trauma to replace water lost to the extravascular interstitial compartment (third space). Water is lost both in hemorrhagic blood loss and in edema that occurs in the region of traumatized tissues.

Experimental animal preparations and some human experiments have demonstrated the superior capability of colloid resuscitation to rapidly restore circulating volume as well as cardiac output and oxygen consumption.[31,32] Since hypoperfusion of vascular beds during shock states leads to total obstructin of capillaries and a no-reflow phenomenon following resuscitation, it may be advantageous to rapidly restore circulating volume with colloidal fluids to prevent widespread intravascular sludging in the microcirculation and capillary obstruction. (Experiments with tissue perfusion corroborate the value of this approach.[33]) Hemoglobin concentration must be maintained at levels adequate to support oxygen delivery and required oxygen consumption. Since increased velocity of microcirculatory blood flow compensates for the loss of hemoglobin, hemoglobin and hematocrit levels do not have to be restored to normal values to maintain adequate tissue oxygen exchange. Although the optimum postresuscitation hemoglobin concentration is unknown, it is known that a mild degree of hemodilution can enhance microvascular perfusion.

The value of forcing higher than normal oxygen delivery in the immediate postresuscitation period has recently been demonstrated by Fleming et al. in trauma patients[34] and Boyd et al. in high-risk surgical patients.[35] The need to repay oxygen debt accumulated during shock was demonstrated in animals by Crowell and Smith[36] in 1964 and has intrigued traumatologists for years. Measurements of oxygen fluxes in survivors and nonsurvivors of traumatic injury[37,38] suggested that survivors maintained elevated oxygen consumptions and oxygen deliveries relative to nonsurvivors. Therefore, it was postulated that maintaining a high oxygen delivery would force patients to maintain elevated oxygen consumption. Although Fleming and Boyd's groups have shown the value of maintaining high oxygen delivery through the maintenance of hemoglobin concentration and an elevated cardiac index, others have suggested titrating oxygen delivery to the point that oxygen consumption is no longer dependent on oxygen delivery[38] (Table 34–8).

Air Embolism

Air embolism was discussed above as a result of penetrating injuries to the lung. Nitrous oxide should be avoided at all costs in patients in whom systemic gas embolism is suspected, since it will rapidly diffuse into air bubbles and cause them to expand in volume. Ventilation with 100% O_2 may help reduce the size of the embolic air bubbles because it will lead to an increased gradient for nitrogen and other insoluble gases to diffuse air out of the air bubble into solution in the blood. An unsuspected arterial air embolism from a penetrating lung injury can lead to intraoperative neurologic dysfunction and even to the failure of the patient to wake up at the end of an anesthetic.

Adult Respiratory Distress Syndrome

Prolonged hypoperfusion associated with traumatic tissue injury can lead to the adult respiratory distress syndrome (ARDS). ARDS is characterized by excessive pulmonary interstitial edema with normal intravascular pressures. Excessive edema is the result of large leaks

TABLE 34–8
Oxygenation Indices for Posttrauma Care

Parameter	Posttrauma Resuscitation Goals
Cardiac index (CI)	≥4.5 L/min/m²
Oxygen delivery index ($\dot{D}O_2$) (CI × arterial O_2 content)	≥670 ml/min/m²
Oxygen consumption index ($\dot{V}O_2$) (CI × arterovenous O_2 content)	≥166 ml/min/m²
Slope of the $\dot{V}O_2$ vs. $\dot{D}O_2$ graph	Parallel to the $\dot{D}O_2$ axis*

*When the $\dot{V}O_2$ vs. $\dot{D}O_2$ graph is parallel to the $\dot{D}O_2$ axis, oxygen delivery is in excess of oxygen demand and increasing $\dot{D}O_2$ will have no effect on $\dot{V}O_2$.

in pulmonary capillary membranes, which allow fluid to escape into the pulmonary interstitium. The prolonged presence of interstitial pulmonary edema provides a focus for collagen to be laid down, leading to fibrotic areas of the lung. As the lung develops interstitial fibrosis, alveoli are disrupted, with a loss of the alveolar epithelium. The alveolar epithelium is replaced by proliferation of the type II pneumocytes that are sparsely represented in the normal lung. These cells secrete surfactant into the normal alveolus and also appear to be embryonic alveolar cells. If the patient survives the hypoxia of ARDS and the cause of lung injury is removed, the lung will begin to heal, and the type II pneumocytes will differentiate into the normal alveolar epithelium.

Since one cause of ARDS is neutrophils stimulated by a generalized inflammatory state, damaging the pulmonary endothelium (leading to leaky capillaries), ARDS frequently heralds further inflammatory damage to other organs. In patients who had prolonged ischemia secondary to hemorrhagic shock, ARDS frequently heralds a progressive multisystem organ dysfunction. The appearance of ARDS in a trauma patient who was recovering uneventfully frequently heralds systemic sepsis. Respiratory failure is often followed by renal, hepatic, and bone marrow failure, accompanied by loss/injury of the epithelial barrier in the intestine, which frequently leads to patient death in the full multisystem organ failure syndrome.[39] Prevention of ARDS and multisystem organ failure requires rapid restoration of both circulating volume and adequate oxygen delivery to meet cellular demands during resuscitation. Presumably, this rapid resuscitation reduces systemic inflammation. Mechanical ventilation of the lungs with relatively large tidal volumes and positive end-expiratory pressure (PEEP) set high enough to prevent large areas of alveolar collapse also seems to help prevent ARDS, probably because the lung maintained in the well-ventilated state with normal anatomic relationships of alveoli and capillaries will not develop intravascular areas of relative hypoxia to aggravate the inflammatory attack on the capillary endothelium. Once ARDS occurs, efforts must be made to prevent further damage to the lung. The maintenance of euvolemia will help prevent excessive fluid from leaking through the injured pulmonary capillaries. Ventilation with a high FIO_2 should be avoided because oxygen directly damages the lung and also causes absorption atelectasis in poorly ventilated regions. If the patient can be supported until the capillary endothelium stops excessive fluid leaking, then supportive care (maintaining oxygenation and ventilation with a mechanical ventilator) will usually lead to survival. Although the lungs that have been insulted by ARDS take a long time to completely heal, many of these patients will return to relatively normal pulmonary function.

Analgesia

Epidural

Patients with multiple rib fractures and injuries to the chest wall benefit greatly from continuous epidural analgesia (Table 34–5). Epidural catheters can be placed into the epidural space at the cervical, thoracic, or lumbar level of the cord. Cervical epidural catheters are difficult to insert and have a high potential for complications; therefore, they are of little use in managing the patient with chest trauma. Thoracic or lumbar level epidural catheters, however, are quite useful in managing such patients. Both local anesthetics and preservation-free opioids can be injected through the catheter to provide analgesia. Because the spread of analgesia tends to be equally cephalad and caudad from the level of the tip of the catheter, it is particularly advantageous to use thoracic level epidural catheters in patients with chest trauma. Thoracic catheters will provide a band of anesthesia throughout the thoracic dermatomes while minimizing the effects on the patient's lower extremities. Local anesthetic solutions can anesthetize motor, sensory, and autonomic neurons in the spinal cord, whereas epidurally administered opioids bind to enkephalinergic receptors in the dorsal columns of the spinal cord and thus provide only sensory analgesia. Opioids and the local anesthetics appear to work synergistically when injected together into the epidural space.[17,40] However, the anesthesiologist must be careful when injecting the local anesthetic solution epidurally to avoid sympathetic nervous system paralysis with a high (above T4) block. Very dilute solutions of bupivacaine (0.0625 to 0.125%) have been used to provide synergistic analgesia with opioids and to avoid profound sympathetic nervous system paralysis. Opioids can be used to achieve high levels of epidural analgesia without sympathetic paralysis. However, one must be careful with opioids; if they are given in a volume that extends the blockade above the servical cord into the brainstem, profound respiratory depression will result.[41] Furthermore, the systemic vascular absorption of the opioids (especially fentanyl) will lead to appreciable blood levels following epidural injection, which may cause the patient to be excessively sedated.

Subarachnoid (spinal) opioids also provide prolonged analgesia. Very small amounts, (i.e., $\leq$1 mg) of morphine sulfate injected into the lumbar CSF will provide analgesia up to cervical levels of the spinal cord with almost no systemic absorption. Although subarachnoid catheters are useful in draining off CSF to reduce the lumbar CSF pressure during thoracic aortic cross-clamping, this form of continuous analgesia is more limited than epidural analgesia following chest trauma. A percutaneous catheter into the lumbar subarachnoid space can be used for up to 48 hours with minimal risk of CSF infection. However, leaving the catheter in place longer than 48 hours places the patient at risk for meningitis. Epidural catheters dwell in a space relatively resistant to infection and may be left in place for prolonged periods (at least 5 days) with minimal risk of systemic or local infection.

Another continuous regional anesthetic technique useful for thoracic trauma is the use of a continuous intercostal catheter—an epidural catheter placed in the subcostal neurovascular space.[42] An intercostal catheter is inserted just caudad to the edge of the rib approximately 7 cm lateral to the midline through a Tuohy needle walked off the caudal surface of the rib and passed centrally into the neurovascular groove on the caudad surface of the rib. Large volumes (30 ml) of local anesthetics injected through an intercostal catheter will result in bilateral chest wall analgesia. For a patient with one or two isolated rib fractures, such a catheter may be more useful than an epidural catheter. Other investigators report great success by passing the catheter through the pleural membrane so that it terminates in the pleural space and then injecting large doses of local anesthetics that again spread across the pleura and can even provide bilateral chest wall analgesia.[43]

Patient-Controlled Analgesia

For the patient who is alert and has moderate to minimal pain following chest trauma, an intravenously administered PCA device is ideal. This device allows the patient to control the rate at which intravenously administered opioids are received. To prevent inadvertent overdose, the physician sets the limit on the maximum rate of opioid injection that the patient can receive each hour. It has been demonstrated many times that patients use fewer milligrams of morphine with a PCA pump than when the drug is given on demand by the nurses. Furthermore, patients with PCA pumps receive a more constant level of analgesia than they do when they have to demand injections from the nurses every 3 or 4 hours.[44]

Summary

Carefully administered anesthetic care for the patient with serious chest trauma will improve his/her outcome. The anesthesiologist must ensure the patient has an adequate airway, receives adequate ventilation, and is capable of adequate gas exchange despite the traumatic alterations to pulmonary physiology. The anesthesiologist also must ensure that the patient can maintain adequate cardiac output to meet homeostatic needs despite direct injury to the myocardium or great vessels. Anesthetic drugs must be administered carefully to avoid excessive cardiovascular depression and to allow monitoring of potential neurologic damage from thoracic trauma. Finally, posttraumatic/postoperative pain relief can be maintained by continuous regional anesthesia techniques or continuous patient-controlled analgesia administration.

References

1. American College of Surgeons Committee on Trauma: Advanced Trauma Life Support Program, Chicago, American College of Surgeons, 1993, p 111.
2. Stene JK: Anesthesia for the critically ill trauma patient. In Siegel JH (ed): Trauma: Emergency Surgery and Critical Care. New York, Churchill Livingstone, 1987, p 843.
3. Peters RM: Fluid resuscitation and oxygen exchange in hypovolemia. In Siegel JH (ed): Trauma: Emergency Surgery and Critical Care. New York, Churchill Livingstone, 1987, p 157.
4. Ullman DA, Fortune JB, Greenhouse BB, et al: The treatment of patients with multiple rib fractures using continuous thoracic epidural narcotic infusion. Reg Anaesth 14:43, 1989.
5. MacKersie RC, Shackford SR, Hoyt DB, Karagianes TG: Continuous epidural fentanyl analgesia: Ventilatory function improved with routine use in treatment of blunt chest injury. J Trauma 27:1207, 1987.
6. Richardson JD, Adams L, Flint LM: Selective management of flail chest and pulmonary contusion. Ann Surg 196:481, 1982.
7. Jackimczyk K: Blunt chest trauma. Emerg Med Clin North Am 11:81, 1993.
8. Snider MT, Campbell DB, Kofke WA, et al: Venovenous perfusion of adults and children with severe acute respiratory distress syndrome. Trans Am Soc Artif Intern Organs 34:1014, 1988.
9. Craven KD, Oppenheimer L, Wood LDH: Effects of contusion and flail chest on pulmonary perfusion and oxygen exchange. J Appl Physiol 47:729, 1979.
10. Eger EI II: Anesthetic Uptake and Action. Baltimore, Williams & Wilkins, 1974.
11. Grenning R, Kynette A, Hodes PJ: Unusual pulmonary changes secondary to chest trauma. AJR 77:1059, 1957.
12. Cochlin DL, Shaw MRP: Traumatic lung cysts following minor blunt chest trauma. Clin Radiol 29:151, 1978.
13. Graham JM, Beall AC Jr, Mattox KL, Vaughan GD: Systemic air embolism following penetrating trauma to the lung. Chest 72:449, 1977.
14. Avery EE, Morch ET, Benson DW: Critically crushed chests: A new method of treatment with continuous mechanical hyperventilation to produce alkalotic apnea and internal pneumatic stabilization. J Thorac Surg 32:291, 1956.
15. Rodriguez A: Injuries of the chest wall, the lungs and the pleura. In Turney SZ, Rodriguez A, Cowley RA (eds): Management of Cardiothoracic Trauma. Baltimore, Williams & Wilkins, 1990, p 155.
16. Abouhatem R, Hendrickx P, Titeca M: Thoracic epidural analgesia in the treatment of rib fractures. Acta Anaesthesiol Belg 35(Suppl):271, 1984.
17. Rankin APN, Comber REH: Management of fifty cases of chest injury with a regimen of epidural bupivacaine and morphine. Anaesth Intensive Care 12:311, 1984.
18. Worthley LIG: Thoracic epidural in the management of chest trauma. Intensive Care Med 11:312, 1985.
19. Getz BS, Davies E, Steinberg SM, et al: Blunt cardiac trauma resulting in right atrial rupture. JAMA 255:761, 1986.
20. Sutherland GR, Calvin JE, Driedger AA, et al: Anatomic and cardiopulmonary responses to trauma with associated blunt chest injury. J Trauma 21:1, 1981.
21. Saunders CR, Doty DB: Myocardial contusion. Surg Gynecol Obstet 144:595, 1977.
22. Dolara A, Morando P, Pampaloni M: Electrocardiographic findings in 98 consecutive non-penetrating chest injuries. Dis Chest 52:50, 1967.
23. Doty DB, Anderson AE, Rose EF, et al: Cardiac trauma: Clinical and experimental correlations of myocardial contusion. Ann Surg 180:452, 1974.
24. Brantigan CO, Burdick D, Hopeman AR, Eiseman B: Evaluation of technetium scanning for myocardial contusion. J Trauma 18: 460, 1978.
25. King RM, Mucha P, Seward JB, et al: Cardiac contusion: A new diagnostic approach utilizing two-dimensional echocardiography. J Trauma 23:610, 1983.
26. Shapiro MJ, Yanofsky SD, Trapp J, et al: Cardiovascular evaluation in blunt thoracic trauma using transesophageal echocardiography (TEE). J Trauma 31:835, 1991.
27. Liu N, Bouilhaguetf, Amich A, et al: Quantitative texture analysis in transesophageal echocardiography allows the diagnosis of acute myocardial contusion in trauma patients. Eur J Emerg. 7: 40, 1994.
28. Lake CL: Anesthesia and pericardial disease. Anesth Analg 62: 431, 1983.
29. Hollier LH: Protecting the brain and spinal cord. J Vasc Surg 5: 524, 1987.
30. Eisele JH: Cardiovascular effects of nitrous oxide. In Eger EI II (ed): Nitrous Oxide/N_2O. New York, Elsevier, 1985, p 125.
31. Hankeln K, Radel C, Beez M, et al: Comparison of hydroxyethyl starch and lactated Ringer's solution on hemodynamics and oxygen transport of critically ill patients in prospective crossover studies. Crit Care Med 17:133, 1989.

32. Schott U, Lindbom LO, Sjostrand U: Hemodynamic effects of colloid concentration in experimental hemorrhage: A comparison of Ringer's acetate 3% dextran-60, and 6% dextran-70. Crit Care Med 16:346, 1988.
33. Gelin L-E, Dawidson I: Plasma expanders and hemodilution in the treatment of hypovolemic shock. In Cowley RA, Trump BF (eds): Pathophysiology of Shock, Anoxia and Ischemia. Baltimore, Williams & Wilkins, 1982, p 454.
34. Fleming A, Bishop M, Shoemaker W, et al: Prospective trial of supranormal values as goals of resuscitation in severe trauma. Arch Surg 127:1175, 1992.
35. Boyd O, Grounds RM, Bennett ED: A randomized clinical trial of the effect of deliberate perioperative increase of oxygen delivery on mortality in high-risk surgical patients. JAMA 270:2699, 1993.
36. Crowell JW, Smith EE: Oxygen deficit and irreversible hemorrhagic shock. Am J Physiol 206:313, 1964.
37. Shoemaker WC, Appel PL, Kram HB: Tissue oxygen debt as a determinant of lethal and nonlethal postoperative organ failure. Crit Care Med 16:1117, 1988.
38. Pasquale MD, Cipolle MD, Cerra FB: Oxygen transport: Does increasing supply improve outcome? Respir Care 38:800, 1993.
39. DeCamp MM, Demling RH: Posttraumatic multi-system organ failure. JAMA 260:530, 1988.
40. Olsson GL, Leddo CC, Wild L: Nursing management of patients receiving epidural narcotics. Heart Lung 18:130, 1989.
41. Etches RC, Sandler AN, Daley MD: Respiratory depression and spinal opioids. Can J Anaesth 36:165, 1989.
42. Murphy DF: Intercostal nerve blockage for fractured ribs and postoperative analgesia. Reg Anaesth 8:151, 1983.
43. Reiestad F, Stromskag KE, Holmqvist E: Interpleural administration of bupivacaine in postoperative management of pain. Anesthesiology 65:A204, 1986.
44. Harmer M, Rosen M, Vickers MD: Patient-controlled analgesia. Oxford, Blackwell Scientific Publications, 1985.

SECTION VII

POSTOPERATIVE CONSIDERATIONS

CHAPTER 35

Cardiac Complications

Avner Sidi, M.D.
Nikolaus Gravenstein, M.D.

Complications and Outcome

Morbidity and Mortality—The Outcome Questions

Coronary artery disease (CAD) continues to be a significant public health problem worldwide. A substantial amount of clinical research in anesthesiology is focused on CAD in an attempt to identify the factors affecting perioperative morbidity. The morbidity and mortality associated with vascular surgery (e.g., aortic aneurysm repair) has decreased significantly over the last 30 years as a result of improved anesthetic management, surgical techniques, and postoperative management.[1-9] Despite these improvements, perioperative adverse outcome in these procedures remains substantial. The greatest cause of morbidity and mortality among vascular surgery patients is myocardial ischemia, myocardial infarction (MI),[1,4,5,9,10] and associated cardiovascular dysfunction. The frequent occurrence of other major systemic diseases in these patients places them at a substantial risk for postoperative complications. Perioperative cardiovascular morbidity rates associated with vascular surgery are as high as 40 to 100% (Table 35–1).[4,11] This high rate results from perioperative stresses superimposed on a population with a high frequency of coexisting cardiac disease (Table 35–2).

The anesthesia literature is replete with studies detailing the interactions of specific pharmacologic agents used for anesthesia and the physiologic changes for many clinical or experimental cardiovascular disease models. Yet the most important question, which was stated a decade ago, "What does it do to outcome?"[12] is only now being systematically approached. This void is not unique to anesthesiology. Major outcome studies of the risks of coronary artery and valvular surgery appeared only after the operative procedures were well established. Unfortunately, many failed to report the variables of intraoperative anesthetic management.[13-15] In this chapter we analyze the anesthetic management—avoiding, recognizing, and treating cardiac complications—of cardiovascular surgical patients, including monitoring and interventions; and, where possible, focus on available outcome data to support a given practice.

Anesthetics and Outcome

The perioperative period is one of significant physiologic stress. Whether the specific anesthetic agent(s) or technique utilized exerts a positive, negative, or neutral influence on overall outcome following surgery has not been established. Experimentally, some volatile anesthetics provide increased coronary vascular reserve by decreasing severity and increasing tolerance to myocardial ischemia.[16-20] Yet the same anesthetics may change coronary blood flow and autoregulation, promote coronary steal, and induce ischemia.[21-27] In order to correctly interpret such disparate results, the question "Does it really matter?" becomes integral and essential.[28] Among the numerous studies on anesthetics and outcome, to date only one[29] reported a difference in outcome between general anesthetic agents. Unfortunately, most studies were retrospective, with the attendant incomplete and nonstandardized data collection. Of the few prospective studies that measured cardiac outcome thoroughly, only one used random multiple anesthetic assignment.[30]

More than a decade ago, *narcotic* and *inhalational* anesthetics in patients undergoing cardiac surgery were compared by analyzing data from five previous studies.[31] Although substantial differences were found in the physiologic responses to induction and surgery (including surgical blood loss) with halothane and morphine or fentanyl, no difference in morbidity or mortality was noted. Although one of these studies[32] demonstrated a difference in lactate production, neither opioid nor inhalation anesthesia could be recommended as a superior agent for coronary surgery. Few additional clinical outcome studies have been published. One study in patients undergoing abdominal or thoracoabdominal aortic reconstruction demonstrated significantly less postoperative renal insufficiency and heart failure when sufentanil instead of isoflurane was used. However, no explanation

TABLE 35–1
Cardiovascular Morbidity and Mortality in Vascular Surgical Patients*

Procedure	% Mortality of Total Population	% Mortality Due to Cardiac Events	% of Total Patients Having Cardiac Events
Abdominal aortic aneurysm			
Elective	0.9–7.9	33–100	2.7–15
Emergency	26–52	8–45	15–26
Descending thoracic aortic aneurysm	9–12	26	3
Aortoiliac disease	2.3–3.8	50–74	2.9
Lower extremity revascularization and femorofemoral bypass	1.4–3.3	52	N/A
Carotid endarterectomy	0–2	0–60	0–4
Renal vascularization	0–1.4	0–44	N/A

*From Boggs DP, Davis RF: Postoperative cardiovascular complications and management. In Kaplan JA (ed): Vascular Anesthesia. New York, Churchill Livingstone, 1991, p 588, with permission.

or relation to any physiologic or metabolic changes explained the observed protective effect of sufentanil.[33]

It is also difficult on the basis of outcome data to recommend a particular inhalational agent (halothane, isoflurane, enflurane) for use during aortocoronary bypass (ACB) surgery: none were superior in minimizing myocardial damage, defined by electrocardiogram (ECG) and enzymes.[34] Even in a series of investigations performed in one institution by the same group using similar methodology for different agents (halothane, isoflurane, enflurane),[32,35,36] myocardial lactate production was the only metabolic difference detected (higher with isoflurane and enflurane) and no difference in morbidity or mortality was noted.

The adverse effect of isoflurane on CAD patients has been attributed to its vasodilation properties with regional flow redistribution away from ischemic regions ("coronary steal"). This effect has been shown experimentally in a canine model,[37] but represents the only demonstration of coronary steal with any anesthetic, despite the observation that 23% of patients presenting for ACB surgery have "steal-prone" anatomy. Another issue is that the use of "equi-MAC" anesthetic concentrations in that study instead of titration using their effect—equal levels of hemodynamic depression—is in dispute. Other animal studies failed to demonstrate flow redistribution or exacerbation of ischemia with isoflurane, and even showed decreased myocardial infarct size with isoflurane.[20]

Since 1989, three large prospective clinical studies of anesthetic technique and outcome in patients who had ACB surgery have been published.[30,38,39] These studies are large—examining 1,012, 1,024, and 1,178 patients. The results of the first two studies[30,38] support the hypothesis that anesthetic choice has little influence on outcome in the patient with CAD. They also appear to validate the position that isoflurane, when used as a primary or secondary anesthetic, is not deleterious in CAD patients if hemodynamic function is controlled. However, both studies have limitations and pose unanswered questions, such as the incidence of ischemia,[30] anesthetic randomization with a large number of different anesthetic combinations,[38] and outcome measurement.[30,38] These unresolved questions preclude resolution of the issue of anesthetic choice, particularly regarding isoflurane, even in patients who undergo ACB surgery.

These studies show that outcome may be related to multiple factors that are not directly under the anesthesiologist's control (e.g., prolonged time for aortic cross-clamping, recent MI, preinduction and intraoperative equivalent of "silent ischemia," preoperative congestive heart failure, unstable angina, and severe arrhythmias). In the third study,[39] lack of randomization and standardization of patients and anesthetic techniques limit the significance of the finding that isoflurane negatively influenced outcome. The authors did not study differences in hemodynamics, intraoperative ischemia, or surgical factors. It is perhaps wisest to view all of these studies

TABLE 35–2
Coexisting Disease in Vascular Surgical Patients*

Procedure	Type of Disease (%)†				
	CAD	COPD	CRI	DM	HTN
Abdominal aortic aneurysm	41–66	7–49	5–17	6–7	24–68
Thoracic aortic aneurysm	17	25	21	N/A	69
Carotid endarterectomy	41–75	N/A	N/A	17–33	59–75
Aortoiliac disease	37–47	N/A	N/A	12	53
Lower extremity revascularization	48	N/A	N/A	25–35	50–65

*From Boggs DP, Davis RF: Postoperative cardiovascular complications and management. In Kaplan JA (ed): Vascular Anesthesia. New York, Churchill Livingstone, 1991, p 588, with permission.
†Reported range of incidence (%) among various categories of vascular patients.
CAD, coronary artery disease; COPD, chronic obstructive pulmonary disease; CRI, chronic renal insufficiency; DM, diabetes mellitus; HTN, hypertension; N/A, not applicable.

as forerunners to a series of randomized, prospective outcome investigations addressing this issue. Controversies regarding the effects of anesthetics on coronary blood flow, myocardial ischemia, and cardiac outcome need to be resolved.

Recent evidence suggests that the inhalation anesthetic technique, rather than choice of anesthetic, can influence outcome in patients undergoing carotid endarterectomy.[40] In this study using "light" (low concentration; sufficient to maintain anesthesia, yet just enough to maintain blood pressure) anesthesia to maintain hemodynamic function was associated with a reduced incidence of intraoperative myocardial ischemia, but not perioperative MI or unfavorable neurologic outcome; no difference between halothane and isoflurane was noted. This limited evidence suggests that the choice of anesthetic affects outcome less if hemodynamic stability is maintained.

Among the analgesics and dissociative drugs, a comparative randomized study between morphine and ketamine reported the same frequency of postoperative complications and mortality in ACB patients, even though morphine produced fewer adverse physiologic changes.[41] No similar comparisons are available for the opioid analgesics morphine, fentanyl, and sufentanil, as used in cardiac anesthesia, nor are such comparisons available among the common sedative/hypnotic drugs used for anesthetic induction. However, sufentanil is associated with more rapid emergence and earlier extubation than morphine or fentanyl.[42] Although patients with early extubation (regardless of agent used) were reported to have less cardiopulmonary morbidity,[43] the direct outcome effect was not answered.

The choice between agents is often arbitrary and based on the predicted physiologic effect and the goal of maintaining hemodynamic stability and physiologic normality. Given this limitation, with the goal of preserving supply-demand ratio, can monitoring of the physiologic changes and intervention when necessary change outcome? In the following section, we consider ECG monitoring to detect ischemia, and pulmonary artery (PA) pressure monitoring with cardiac output measurement to assess cardiac function and complications in the perioperative period.

Monitoring and Outcome

Electrocardiography

The ECG supplies an enormous amount of information regarding the status of the coronary circulation.[44] The importance of detecting myocardial ischemia has been highlighted by several studies[45,46] in which the amount of ST-segment depression was directly related to the incidence of postoperative MI. Using a calibrated ECG in the diagnostic mode employing leads V_5 and II simultaneously, 96% of ischemic events can be detected.[44] When intraoperative myocardial ischemia was localized by continuous 12-lead ECG, sensitivity of single-lead was greatest for V_5 (75%) and the sensitivity of two-lead combinations was highest for V_4 and V_5.[47] Also, note that the combined two-lead sensitivity is considerably greater than any single lead (Fig. 35–1). During angioplasty, more ischemia is detected by a 12-lead (rather than a three-lead) system, but this is not practicable in the operating room.[48] Hemodynamic monitoring may provide earlier detection for ischemia.[49]

Most investigators use one or a combination of the ECG signs listed in Table 35–3 as indicating ischemia[48]: ischemia cannot, however, be accurately assessed by ECG in patients who have left bundle branch block, pacemakers, or left ventricular (LV) strain. In fact, not all perioperative ECG changes signify increased risk,[50] or represent ischemia and may instead represent nonspecific changes. Oscilloscopic presentation[51] and comput-

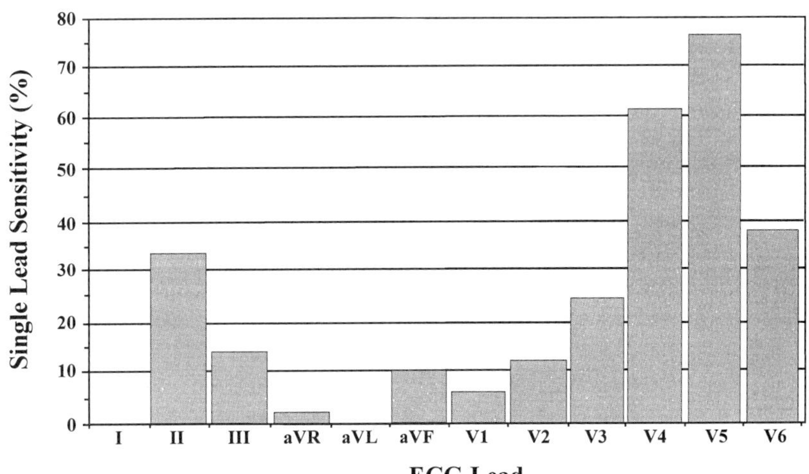

FIGURE **35–1.** The distribution of ischemic ST-segment changes in each of the 12 leads considered individually in a group of 105 coronary artery disease patients during anesthesia is shown. The number of ST-segment changes in each lead has been summed. The estimated sensitivity was calculated from the number of changes in a single lead as a percentage of the total number of episodes. Sensitivity was highest in lead V_5 (75%). (From London MJ, Hollenberg M, Wong MG, et al: Intraoperative myocardial ischemia: Localization by continuous 12-lead electrocardiography. Anesthesiology 69:232, 1988, with permission.)

TABLE 35–3
Electrocardiographic Signs Indicating Ischemia*

>1-mm ST-segment depression
>1-mm J-point depression
>1-mm ST-segment elevation
Inverted T waves
Pseudopolarization of T waves
Onset of new arrhythmias

*From Wohlgelernter D, Cleman M, Highman HA, et al: Regional myocardial dysfunction during coronary angioplasty; evaluation by two-dimensional echocardiography and 12 lead electrocardiography. J Am Coll Cardiol 7:1245, 1986. Copyright American College of Cardiology, with permission.

erized continuous ST-segment analysis[52] have improved our ability to detect intraoperative ST-segment changes.

Pulmonary Artery Catheterization

Does the use of the PA catheter (PAC) lead to less morbidity and mortality in cardiac surgical patients? Changes in pulmonary capillary wedge pressure (PCWP), cardiac output, and the presence of "ac" waves are indicators of reduced LV compliance and myocardial ischemia in some situations.[44,53] However, the detection of ischemia with the PAC is limited and its major application is in the evaluation of hemodynamic responses to guide pharmacologic and fluid therapy. In one intraoperative study, physicians were blinded to PAC data and were unaware of 65% of the severe hemodynamic abnormalities in a group of patients undergoing ACB surgery.[54]

Measuring mixed venous O_2 saturation ($S\bar{v}O_2$) may further enhance care,[55,56] since abrupt and serious decreases in $S\bar{v}O_2$ sometimes occur without corresponding decreases in other hemodynamic parameters. A randomized intensive care unit (ICU) study showed that PAC monitoring combined with pharmacologic therapy to achieve a given hemodynamic end point results in a significant improvement in cost-benefit ratio.[57] The use of such monitoring, in conjunction with appropriate pharmacologic therapy and intensive care, significantly reduces postoperative MI.[58]

Although PCWP and cardiac output data serve as important hemodynamic landmarks for guiding diagnosis and therapy, a number of limitations arise. These may have an important impact on patient care: most importantly, LV end-diastolic volume correlates poorly with LV end-diastolic pressure or PCWP measured by the PAC.[59] Thus, where LV compliance is reduced, PCWP may be a poor indicator of LV end-diastolic volume. Furthermore, PCWP may not correlate with LV end-diastolic pressure in mitral stenosis in the presence of elevated airway pressure.

The intermittent versus continuous nature of conventional thermodilution cardiac output measurements and catheter-related complications are important parts of the "monitoring equation."[60] While investigating the question of outcome, with or without the use of a PAC in ACB patients, one group found no difference in mortality.[61] The overall mortality rate and incidence of MI in this group of patients without the use of PAC was comparable to data from a multicenter collaborative study in coronary artery surgery using PACs.[14] This study can be used as a rationale for clinical safety of central venous pressure (CVP) monitoring in elective ACB patients without significant preoperative myocardial dysfunction.

Another prospective study, not randomized for anesthetic technique, examined the effect of PAC monitoring on outcome in aortic aneurysm patients with similar risk classifications and also found no difference in outcome.[62] This prospective study suggested that pulmonary artery catheterization does not play a major role in influencing outcome after cardiac surgery, that high-risk patients may be safely managed with CVP monitoring, and that delaying pulmonary artery catheterization until clinically necessary does not influence outcome, but may have an important impact on cost savings. An outline and general model for determining the efficacy of medical technology can be adopted from the six-tiered model for evaluation of diagnostic technology.[63] The six levels of efficacy are: technical, diagnostic, diagnostic thinking, therapeutic, patient outcome, and societal. Only four level-five studies comparing pulmonary artery catheterization with CVP monitoring during cardiac surgery have been attempted; these are reviewed in Table 35–4.[61,62,64,65] There has been no prospective, randomized study reporting outcome-related benefit with routine PA catheter use in cardiac surgery patients.[66] Part of the problem is the lack of consistency in data interpretation and standardization of the clinical expertise using this tool[67]; increased use in complicated and severely ill patients also affects data analysis (Table 35–5).[58,62,68–76]

The theoretical evaluation of the cost-effectiveness of pulmonary artery catheterization in patients undergoing ACB surgery may help us to evaluate future adaptations, including some that measure continuous cardiac output.[63] However, there is still the question of how such analyses should be placed in perspective. In other words, what is the likelihood that the use of pulmonary artery catheterization (as opposed to CVP monitoring) results in incremental mortality improvement in the range of 0.2% (or 2 lives saved per 1,000 patients), which can be deduced or assumed (Fig. 35–2) from the cost-effectiveness studies. The answer to this question depends partially on bias, because the actual result is unknown. It may also depend on preoperative risk to the patient, because healthier patients would be expected to receive less benefit from pulmonary artery catheterization. It is possible that the use of pulmonary artery catheterization may actually cause increased overall mortality,[66] but this view is not widely accepted.[67]

Transesophageal Echocardiography

Despite the effort and cost involved, intraoperative transesophageal echocardiography (TEE) is widely used. Few investigators have addressed the issue of whether it truly makes a difference in terms of patient management and outcome. Anesthesiologists are interested in monitoring regional LV wall motion as a marker for myocardial ischemia and infarction.[77,78] TEE shows that patients with-

TABLE 35–4
Outcome Studies of PAC Versus CVP*

Authors	Type of Study	No. of Patients	Conclusions	Weaknesses
Moore et al. (1978)[68]	Retrospective, historical controls	48	Mortality reduced from 20% to 3.5% using PAC and hemodynamic interventions	Historical controls; role of PAC not differentiated from role of hemodynamic interventions
Bashein et al. (1985)[61]	Retrospective, historical controls	698	Low incidence of morbidity and reduced cost without PAC	Retrospective, historical controls
Tuman et al. (1989)[62]	Prospective, nonrandomized	1,094	No difference in morbidity between CVP and PAC; PAC patients had longer ICU stays	Possible selection bias
Pearson et al. (1989)[67]	Prospective, randomized	226	No outcome differences between groups; PAC more costly	Selection bias; small sample size; group crossover

*From Spackman TN: A theoretical evaluation of cost-effectiveness of pulmonary artery catheters in patients undergoing artery surgery. J Cardiothorac Vasc Anesth 8(5):571, 1994, with permission.
PAC, pulmonary artery catheter; CVP, central venous pressure; ICU, intensive care unit.

out regional wall motion abnormalities almost invariably do well, while patients with new and persistent abnormalities have an increased risk for perioperative MI. However, most patients in this latter category also have a favorable outcome. Even if TEE can predict adverse cardiac outcome in immediately postoperative ACB patients,[78] whether prompt application of appropriate therapeutic interventions can improve outcome remains unproven.

The value of TEE and color flow Doppler imaging has also been examined in adult patients undergoing valve surgery.[79] In this population, TEE can be used for intraoperative decision-making to reduce valvular insufficiency and dysfunction following bypass and to guide "de-airing" of the heart, which are often associated with adverse outcome. Transesophageal echocardiography has become standard for mitral valve repair in many institutions.[80]

Hemodynamic Control or Drug Intervention and Outcome

The impact of prophylactic treatment for prevention of myocardial ischemia must be examined, since perioperative ischemia is accepted as a risk factor for adverse outcome. Commonly used prophylactic antianginal drugs include nitrates, calcium channel blockers, and β-adrenergic blockers. β-Adrenergic blockers are more protective against ischemia than calcium channel blockers, largely because they are more effective at preventing tachycardia.[81] However, as much as 75% of perioperative ischemia occurs without hemodynamic abnormalities.[82] Thus, while tight hemodynamic control is a desirable goal, it is not a panacea. Recently, Mangano et al. showed in a randomized, double-blind, multicenter study, that β-blocker treatment influenced outcome. Treatment with atenolol before and immediately after surgery in patients with CAD reduced cardiovascular complications and mortality, as long as 2 years following surgery.[83] In another multicenter study, treatment with purine nucleoside (acadesine) before and afer ACB surgery reduced early cardiac death, MI, and combined adverse cardiovascular outcomes.[84]

Nitroglycerin and other organic nitrates are used frequently to reverse ECG signs of intra- or perioperative ischemia.[85] Prophylactic perioperative use of nitroglycerin likely does not reduce morbidity or mortality significantly. Even a double-blind, randomized study in patients who underwent ACB using prophylactic nitroglycerin failed to show significant differences between groups for ECG-detected perioperative ischemia,[86] although data for incidence of postoperative complications or mortality were not reported.

Complications

Myocardial Ischemia and Infarction—Diagnosis

Postoperative MI is the single most important cause of morbidity and mortality in cardiac and vascular surgery patients. Control of the determinants of oxygen (O_2) supply and demand, and the ratio of myocardial oxygen supply and demands may help to prevent ischemia. Not only myocardial demand (MVO_2), but also supply and oxygenation, are dependent on changes that can lead to a significant risk for postoperative myocardial ischemia.[87] Ischemia has a definite association, intra- and postoperatively, with subsequent adverse cardiac events including MI and congestive heart failure in cardiovascular surgical patients.[88,89] Also, ischemia may lead to cardiac dysfunctions that continue even after the initial ischemic event has been removed.[90] The timing of post- or perioperative MIs is variable. Some reports show the most frequent occurrence to be on postoperative days 3 to 5, while others demonstrate occurrence within the first 3 days in patients with a history of prior MI or abnormal ECG.[91–94] Although evidence exists for earlier occurrences,[95,96] most studies depend on signs and symptoms rather than on more systematic and sensitive diagnosis. When the diagnosis is made by daily ECGs and serial creatine kinase measurements, there is more evidence that MI has actually occurred on the operative day.[97]

Asymptomatic myocardial ischemia and infarct, in most cases, occur postoperatively and may be asymp-

TABLE 35–5
Controlled Studies of Pulmonary Artery Catheterization with Clinical Outcomes*†

Study	Location	N‡	Clinical Setting	Study Design	Significant Clinical Outcomes§	Comments
General Surgery						
Shoemaker et al. (1988)[68]	Los Angeles, CA	146	General surgery in high-risk patients	RCT; groups = CVP, PAC normal, PAC supranormal	Postoperative mortality, mean ICU stay, ventilator use lower in PAC supranormal group	Small sample size, poor control for confounding, uncertain case mix
Rao et al. (1983)[58]	Maywood, IL	733/364	Noncardiac surgery in patients with prior myocardial infarction	Obs-historical controls; 1977–1982 cohort vs. 1973–1976 cohort	Lower perioperative reinfarction and mortality rates in study cohort	Historical controls, nonrandom selection, uncertain case mix, role of hemodynamic monitoring unclear
Cardiac Surgery						
Pearson et al. (1989)[64]	Iowa City, IA	226	Elective cardiac surgery	RCT; groups = CVP, PAC, PAC with mixed venous oxygen	None	Small sample size, significant crossover between groups
Tuman et al. (1989)[62]	Chicago, IL	1,094	Elective coronary artery bypass graft surgery	Controlled prospective cohort	Mean ICU stay greater in PAC high-risk group than CVP group	Nonrandom selection, uncertain case mix
Moore et al. (1978)[55]		28/20	Surgery for left main coronary artery stenosis	Obs-historical controls; study cohort vs. previous year	Lower rates of perioperative myocardial infarction, ventricular fibrillation, deaths in PAC vs. CVP	Historical controls, nonrandom selection, statistical significance not reported
Aortic Reconstruction						
Joyce et al. (1990)[71]	Toronto, Canada	40	Abdominal aortic aneurysm repair	RCT; groups = CVP, PAC; comparison group of 11 high-risk patients	ICU stay longer in CVP and high-risk patients (combined) than PAC	Small sample size, comparison of CVP and PAC ICU stay not reported
Isaacson et al. (1990)[70]	Atlanta, GA	102	Abdominal aortic reconstruction	RCT; groups = CVC, PAC	No difference in morbidity, mortality, ICU, or hospital stay	Possible type II error

Hesdorffer et al. (1987)[72]	Johannesburg, South Africa	61/87	Abdominal aortic aneurysm repair	Obs-historical controls; 1983–1984 cohort vs. 1980–1982 cohort	Lower perioperative hypotensive episodes and mortality in study cohort than historical controls	Historical controls, nonrandom selection, does not compare PAC use, inconsistent data, uncertain attrition, statistical significance not reported
Hemodynamic Disorders						
Gore et al. (1987)[73]	Worcester, MA	3,263	Acute myocardial infarction	Retrospective cohort analysis of community-based population	Higher-in hospital case fatality rate and hospital stay in PAC	Uncertain case mix
Zion et al. (1990)[74]	Jerusalem, Israel	5,841	Acute myocardial infarction	Prospective cohort	Higher in-hospital mortality in PAC	Uncertain case mix; adjustment for case mix by authors suggests association between PAC use and severity of illness
Bush et al. (1989)[75]		345	Medical ICU	Retrospective chart review	Higher mortality and severity of illness in PAC	Published only as abstract, uncertain case mix, selection process not described, mortality rates unreported
Reynolds et al. (1988)[76]	Detroit, MI	100/112	Septic shock	Obs-historical controls; study year vs. prior year	Lower mortality rate in study cohort	Historical controls, nonrandom selection, did not compare PAC use
Peripheral Vascular Surgery						
Berlauk et al. (1991)[69]	Minneapolis, MN	89	Vein graft arterial bypass for limb salvage	RCT; groups = PAC 12 and 3 hr before surgery, no preoperative PAC	Fewer intraoperative hemodynamic disorders and postoperative graft thromboses	Uncertain group assignment methods, discrepancies in data reporting regarding cardiac morbidity

*Modified from Task Force on Guidelines for Pulmonary Artery Catheterization: Practice guidelines for pulmonary artery catheterization. Anesthesiology 78:380, 1983; and International Anesthesiology Research Society Executive Summary, San Francisco, CA, 1993, p 13, with permission.

†See text of original reference for results of uncontrolled studies and case series.

‡In observational studies with historical controls, sample size of study group and historical cohort reported.

§Does not include outcomes for which no significant benefit was observed.

RCT, randomized controlled trial (composition of randomized groups described); Obs-historical, observational study with historical controls; PAC, patients monitored by pulmonary artery catheter; CVP, patients monitored by central venous pressure measurements; ICU, intensive care unit.

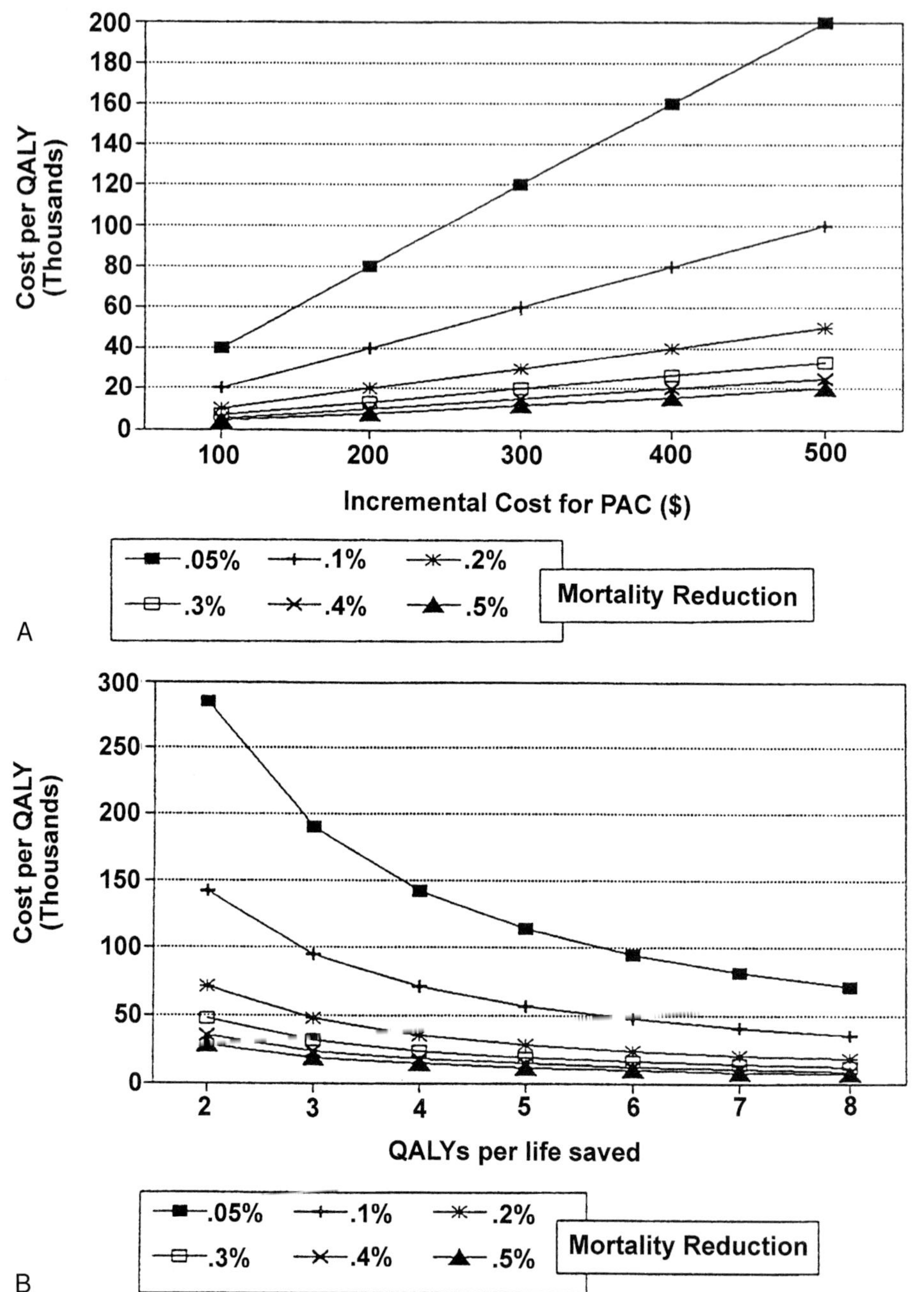

FIGURE 35–2. *A*, Cost per quality-adjusted life years (QALY) for different catheter costs with the assumption that for each incremental life saved by use of the PAC, 5 QALYs result. Each line represents a level of incremental lives saved. For example, 0.1% represents the line if the benefit is assumed to be 1 incremental life saved per 1,000 CABG operations done with use of a PAC. Thus, the graph shows that for an incremental cost of $300 or less and for 5 QALYs per life saved, any reduction in mortality greater than 0.1% results in the cost per QALY of less than $60,000. *B*, Changes in cost per QALY if the incremental cost per catheter is assumed to be $285 and different levels of benefit and different QALYs per life saved are chosen. It shows that for QALYs per life saved greater than 3, the cost per QALY is less than $50,000 for a benefit of 0.2% or more. (From Spackman TN: A theoretical evaluation of cost-effectiveness of pulmonary artery catheters in patients undergoing coronary artery surgery. J Cardiothorac Vasc Anesth 8[5]:570, 1994, with permission.)

tomatic because of residual anesthetic effects, analgesic and sedative distraction by surgical pain, and a large number of silent ischemia episodes.[98]

Electrocardiographic changes are only 73% sensitive for MI, although their specificity is high.[99] ST-segment changes are the most sensitive indicators of postoperative MI in asymptomatic patients.[95] New Q-wave development is associated with MI in only 65% of cases, but new T-wave changes do not appear to predict subsequent ischemic events.[50] Using pulmonary artery waveform changes to detect ischemia is less sensitive than TEE,[77,100] even though the role of TEE in the postoperative period is less well evaluated and much more cumbersome.[100–102] Transesophageal echocardiography can detect ischemia intraoperatively without ECG or PA waveform changes,[101] may be superior to the ECG in detecting ischemia predictive of infarction,[77] and allows direct functional evaluation of therapeutic interventions.[102]

Measurement of cardiac isoenzymes, especially creatine kinase, is a very sensitive indicator of postoperative MI. The suspicion of MI is strong when total creatine kinase is elevated and the creatine kinase level is greater than 3 to 5% of the total.[99,103] Enzyme diagnosis of MI is retrospective, since enzyme release follows myocardial cell death. However, MI is often a dynamic process and early diagnosis may allow protective measures to be taken to treat areas "at risk" (viable but not yet infarcted) before infarction ensues.

The preoperative use of β-adrenergic blocking agents in ACB patients correlates with reduced postoperative incidence of MI, in contrast to calcium channel blockers.[81] Preoperative treatment with calcium channel blockers alone is associated with a higher incidence of prebypass ischemia.[104] Preoperative β-blockade is effective in reducing perioperative MI and myocardial ischemia, which correlates with postoperative MI.[89,105] Though a tight hemodynamic control (with or without β-blockers) is not free of possible ischemia, intraoperative monitoring of ECG and hemodynamics has an incremental value for predicting postoperative MI. ECG changes (ST-segment changes, conduction defects), duration of hypotension, and duration of CPB can be independent predictors of perioperative MI.[106] The use of perioperative β-blockers reduced cardiovascular complications, death from cardiac causes, and overall mortality.[83] Nitroglycerin infusion (1.0 μg/kg/min) may decrease intraoperative ischemia[107] and prevent decreases in ejection fraction immediately after extubation in CAD patients.[108] The role of antianginal drugs in the prevention of myocardial ischemia and MI postoperatively has not yet been determined. As a rule, any "effective" antianginal treatment given preoperatively should be continued throughout the perioperative period.

Treatment for acute MI should begin with interventions directed to maximize O_2 delivery and minimize MVO_2 (Table 35–6). Thus, supplemental O_2 in order to maintain an $S\bar{v}O_2$ above 80% and a PaO_2 between 300 and 500 mm Hg improves myocardial oxygenation and perhaps decreases ischemia.[109,110] In order to achieve these goals, ventilatory support, including mechanical ventilation, may be required. Treatment of ventricular arrhythmias starts with lidocaine.[111] Procainamide should be considered as an additional drug when ventricular arrhythmia is refractory to maximal lidocaine treatment (4 mg/min followed by 1- to 1.5-mg/kg bolus). Magnesium supplements (2 to 4 gm IV) can decrease the incidence of lethal arrhythmia with an acute MI.[112]

β-Blockers reduce infarct size experimentally[113] and lower mortality clinically by decreasing MVO_2.[114,115] The usual relative contraindications must be considered: bronchoconstriction, bradycardia, heart block, and congestive heart failure. In such cases, a short-acting β_1-cardioselective β-blocker with equally efficacious results (such as esmolol)[116] should be considered in order to minimize unwanted side effects, such as bronchospasm.[117]

Nitroglycerin increases coronary blood flow, reduces preload and afterload, and decreases infarct size[118,119] and mortality[120,121] in acute MI. The recommended starting dose is 0.5 μg/kg/min which should be titrated according to chest pain, ST-segment changes, blood pressure, and heart rate.

Several other agents have been shown to be effective, probably by reducing overall demand and consumption due to changes in contractility, preload, or afterload. Diltiazem reduces reinfarction incidence in the immediate postinfarction period.[122] Diuretics may cause an exaggerated effect, with decreased ventricular compliance, and low filling pressures, causing systemic blood pressure to drop. They should be used with extreme caution with congestive heart failure due to MI. Amrinone improves LV performance, increasing regional myocardial blood flow without worsening regional metabolic effects during experimental ischemia.[123] It also successfully treats perioperative low cardiac output syndrome associated with ischemia.[124] However, it should be used with caution because it vasodilates vascular beds and can cause hypotension.

TABLE 35–6
Principles of Treating Perioperative Ischemia

Principle	Goals	Action
Increase oxygen supply	Keep $S\bar{v}O_2$ >80%	Ventilatory support
	Keep PaO_2 >300 mm Hg	Supplemental oxygen
	Increase coronary blood supply	Support blood pressure
		Thrombolysis
		Percutaneous transluminal coronary angioplasty
Decrease oxygen demand	Avoid/treat arrhythmia	Lidocaine
		Procainamide
		Magnesium
	Reduce myocardial load	
	Contractility	β-Blockers
		Calcium channel blockers
	Afterload	Amrinone, sodium nitroprusside
	Preload	Nitroglycerin

$S\bar{v}O_2$, mixed venous oxygen saturation; PaO_2, oxygen pressure in arterial blood (mm Hg).

Streptokinase and tissue plasmogen activator mechanically promote coronary flow and lysis of coronary thrombosis, but are only indicated more than 10 days postoperatively because of their potential to cause bleeding in the surgical site if given within 1 hour of infarction.[125–128] In any case, the potential side effect of bleeding due to thrombolytic therapy should be weighed against the possible improvement in coronary flow. Even intracoronary, lesion-directed administration of thrombolytic agents resulted in a 40% chance of severe bleeding, morbidity of 7% MI, and 11% recurrent ischemia, when the revascularization success was 89%.[129] On the other hand, systemic intraoperative fibrinolytic therapy may cause bleeding in the treated site, even if there is no evidence of systemic fibrinolysis or systemic hemorrhage.[130] Also, postoperative percutaneous transluminal coronary angioplasty has a potential benefit following MI, but its role is not clearly defined.

Ventricular conduction blocks may develop following acute MI in 20 to 30% of patients,[131,132] and should be treated with pacing in cases of third-degree (complete), second-degree (Mobitz type II), and bifascicular blocks.[133–135]

Cardiac Arrhythmias

Cardiac arrhythmias are the most frequent perioperative cardiovascular abnormalities, with a reported incidence of 20 to 80%.[136] A higher incidence (84%) can be recorded with Holter-type monitoring systems.[137] The incidence of serious perioperative arrhythmia is less than 1%.[138]

Previous classification systems (Table 35–7) were not fully satisfactory for understanding the mechanisms and differences between various antiarrhythmic drugs. These systems used to depend on membrane action (class I), sympatholysis (class II), prolonged repolarization (class III), and calcium channel blockers (class IV). To provide a better operational framework for antiarrhythmic drugs that will stimulate research and development and encourage their use (while at the same time considering their molecular targets, mechanisms, and clinical applications), a new approach to classification was developed, the "Sicilian Gambit."[139] The system is so named to represent a gambit, an opening move that provides a variety of aggressive options, on the part of investigators who met in 1991 in Sicily. A new classification of drug action based on modification of vulnerable parameters was suggested (Table 35–8). A summary of the potentially most important action of drugs on membrane channels, receptors, and ionic pumps in the heart is represented in Figure 35–3.

Bradycardia

Sinus bradycardia with resulting hypotension due to baroreceptor dysfunction is seen postoperatively after carotid endarterectomy.[140] It can be prevented or treated with the intraoperative local anesthetic blockade of the carotid sinus nerve.[141] Postoperative bradycardia can be caused by excess vagal tone, acetylcholinesterase inhibitors, residual narcotics, β-adrenergic or calcium channel blockers, digitalis, or sinus node dysfunction. Adequacy of perfusion should be the guide for treatment, since therapy may cause tachycardia. Atropine (0.2 to 0.4 mg, up to 0.02 mg/kg) can be given, but in low doses can cause a paradoxical slowing. Thus, atropine and glycopyrrolate should be titrated until the desired heart rate (50 to 70 bpm) is reached. When bradycardia is resistant to parasympatholytic treatment, β-stimulation with isoproterenol (5- to 10-μg bolus and 0.01- to 0.02-μg/kg/min infusion) titrated to heart rate response or until the onset of ventricular ectopy often will resolve bradycardia. However, isoproterenol increases MVO_2, decreases diastolic coronary perfusion pressure, and aggravates ischemia. Thus, it should be exchanged for pacing, as soon as feasible. Atrioventricular (AV) dissociation causing bradycardia also responds to isoproterenol, but when practical, ventricular or AV-sequential pacing is preferred.

TABLE 35–7
Vaughan Williams Classification of Antiarrhythmic Drugs*

Class I	Class II	Class III	Class IV
Drugs with direct membrane action (Na channel blockade) Ia. Depress phase 0 Slow conduction Prolong repolarization Ib. Little effect in phase 0 in normal tissue Depress phase 0 in abnormal fibers Shorten repolarization Ic. Markedly depress phase 0 Markedly slow conduction Slight effect on repolarization	Sympatholytic drugs	Drugs that prolong repolarization	Calcium channel–blocking drugs

*From Task Force of the Working Group on Arrhythmias of the European Society of Cardiology: The Sicilian Gambit: A new approach to the classification of antiarrhythmic drugs based on their actions on arrhythmogenic mechanisms. Circulation 84:1832, 1991, with permission.

TABLE 35–8
Classification of Drug Actions on Arrhythmias Based on Modification of Vulnerable Parameter*

Arrhythmia	Mechanisms	Vulnerable Parameter	Representative Drugs
Automaticity			
Inappropriate sinus tachycardia	Enhanced normal	Phase 4 depolarization (decrease)	β-Adrenergic–blocking agents
Some idiopathic ventricular tachycardias	Enhanced normal		Sodium channel–blocking agents
Ectopic atrial tachycardia	Abnormal	Maximum diastolic potential (hyperpolarization) or phase 4 depolarization (decrease)	M_2 agonists, adenosine Calcium or sodium channel–blocking agents, M_2, agonists, adenosine
Accelerated idioventricular rhythms	Abnormal	Phase 4 depolarization (decrease)	Calcium or sodium–channel blocking agents
Triggered Activity			
Torsades de pointes	EAD	Action potential duration (shorten) or EAD (suppress)	β-Agonists, vagolytic agents (increase rate), calcium channel–blocking agents, Mg^{2+}; β-adrenergic blockers
Digitalis-induced arrhythmias	DAD	Calcium overload (unload) or DAD (suppress)	Calcium channel–blocking agents, sodium channel–blocking agents
Certain autonomically mediated ventricular tachycardias	DAD	Calcium overload (unload) or DAD (suppress)	β-Adrenergic–blocking agents, calcium channel–blocking agents, adenosine
Re-entry (Sodium Channel–Dependent)			
Atrial flutter type I	Long excitable gap	Conduction and excitability (depress)	Atrium: sodium channel–blocking agents (except lidocaine, mexiletine, tocainide)
Circus movement tachycardia in WPW	Long excitable gap	Conduction and excitability (depress)	Sodium channel–blocking agents (except lidocaine, mexiletine, tocainide)
Sustained monomorphic ventricular tachycardia	Long excitable gap	Conduction and excitability (depress)	Ventricle: sodium channel–blocking agents
Atrial flutter type II	Short excitable gap	Refractory period (prolong)	Potassium channel blockers
Atrial fibrillation	Short excitable gap	Refractory period (prolong)	Potassium channel blockers
Circus movement tachycardia in WPW	Short excitable gap	Refractory period (prolong)	Amiodarone, sotalol
Polymorphic and sustained monomorphic ventricular tachycardia	Short excitable gap	Refractory period (prolong)	Quinidine, procainamide, disopyramide
Bundle branch re-entry	Short excitable gap	Refractory period (prolong)	Quinidine, procainamide, disopyramide
Ventricular fibrillation	Short excitable gap	Refractory period (prolong)	Bretylium
Re-entry (Calcium Channel–Dependent)			
AV nodal re-entrant tachycardia		Conduction and excitability (depress)	Calcium channel–blocking agents
Circus movement tachycardia in WPW		Conduction and excitability (depress)	Calcium channel–blocking agents
Verapamil-sensitive ventricular tachycardia		Conduction and excitability (depress)	Calcium channel–blocking agents

*Modified from Task Force of the Working Group on Arrhythmias of the European Society of Cardiology: The Sicilian Gambit: A new approach to the classification of antiarrhythmic drugs based on their actions on arrhythmogenic mechanisms. Circulation 84:1842, 1991, with permission.
EAD, early afterdepolarization; DAD, delayed afterdepolarization; WPW, Wolff-Parkinson-White syndrome; M_2, muscarinic subtype 2.

Ectopy

Extrasystoles with premature atrial beats can also cause significant hemodynamic effects and precede the onset of atrial-type arrhythmia (flutter or fibrillation). They may be due to metabolic imbalance, such as hypo- or hyperkalemia, hypoxia, acidosis, or alkalosis, or hemodynamic abnormalities, such as atrial distention. Simple premature atrial beats with stable hemodynamics need not be treated; however, if necessary, treatment should correct the basic imbalance or abnormality. Antiarrhythmic drugs previously classified as class I (lidocaine) are not usually effective, but class II (β-adrenergic blockers) and class IV (calcium channel blockers) drugs are useful for pharmacologic therapy (Table 35–8).

Tachycardia

Postoperative sinus tachycardia is usually due to inadequate analgesic and anesthetic level, volume status (fluid overload, deficit, or anemia), or metabolic disorders (fever, hypercarbia, or hypoxia). The initial treatment is aimed at correcting the underlying cause, and only afterward to control heart rate. Postoperative supraventri-

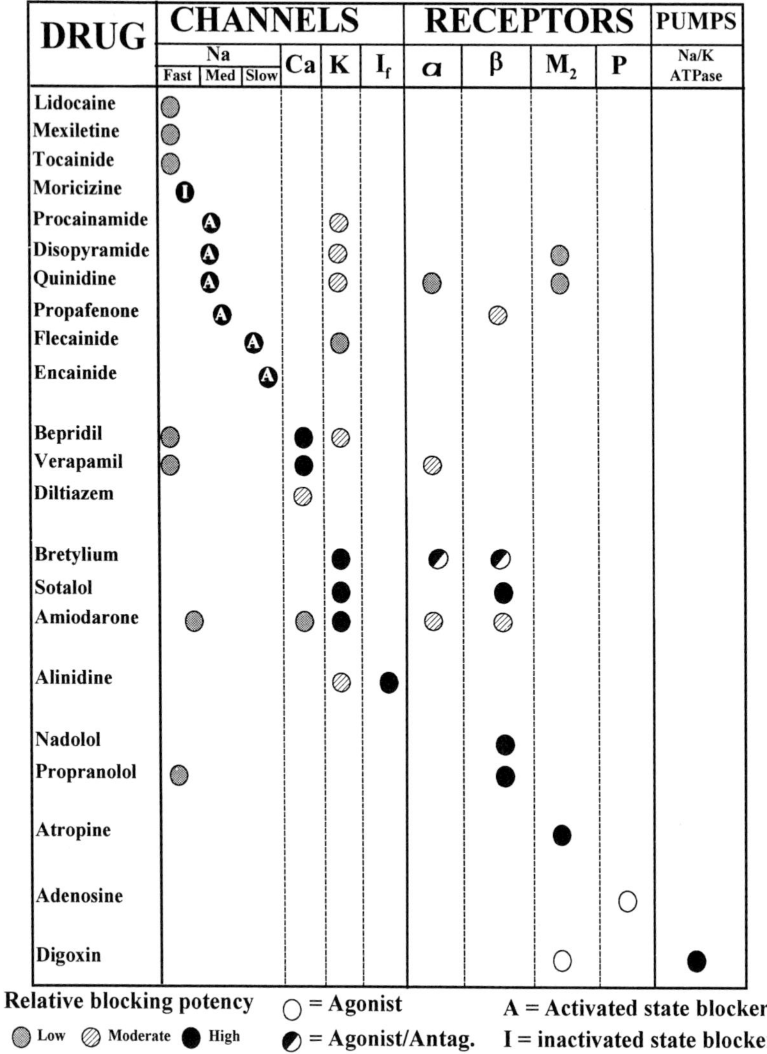

FIGURE **35–3.** Summary of the potentially most important actions of drugs on membrane channels, receptors, and ionic pumps in the heart. Included are examples of drugs used to modify cardiac rhythm. Most are already marketed as antiarrhythmic agents, but some are not yet approved for this purpose. The drugs (rows) are ordered in a fashion similar to the columns so that generally the entries for their predominant action(s) form a diagonal. Drugs with multiple actions (e.g., amiodarone) depart strikingly from the diagonal trend. The actions of drugs on the sodium, calcium, potassium (I_k), and I_f channels are indicated. Sodium channel blockade is subdivided into three groups of actions characterized by fast (<300 msec), medium (Med) (200–1,500 msec), and slow (>1,500 msec) time constants for recovery from block. This parameter is a measure of use dependence and predicts the likelihood that a drug will decrease conduction velocity of normal sodium-dependent tissues in the heart and perhaps the propensity of a drug for causing bundle branch block or proarrhythmia. The rate constant for onset of block might be even more clinically relevant. Blockade in the inactivated (I) or activated (A) state is indicated. Information on the state dependency of the block caused by moricizine, propafenone, encainide, and flecainide is especially limited and may be altered with additional research. Drug interaction with receptors (α, β, muscarinic subtype 2 [M_2], and A_1 purinergic [P]) and drug effects on the sodium/potassium pump (Na/K, ATPase) are indicated. *Filled circles* indicate antagonist or inhibitory actions; *unfilled circles* indicate direct or indirect acting agonists or stimulators. The darkness of the symbol increases with the intensity of the action. *Half-filled circles* for bretylium indicate its biphasic action to initially stimulate α- and β-adrenergic receptors by release of norepinephrine followed by subsequent block of norepinephrine release and indirect antagonism of these receptors. (From Task Force of the Working Group on Arrhythmias of the European Society of Cardiology: The Sicilian Gambit: A new approach to the classification of antiarrhythmic drugs based on their actions on arrhythmogenic mechanisms. Circulation 84:1831, 1991, with permission.)

cular tachycardia responds well to adenosine because it primarily affects supraventricular tissues, but it also blocks conduction at the atrioventricular (AV) node.[142] Carotid sinus massage may be effective; however, it probably should be avoided in vascular surgery patients because of the potential for thromboembolism. When treating a patient with supraventricular tachycardia, it is ideally approached by selecting drugs based on their primary site of action (see the "Sicilian Gambit" in Table 35–8). Knowledge of the critical sites and mechanisms of abnormal impulse generation or propagation is essential.

Drugs that slow atrial or accessory pathway conduction, such as those previously classified as class I (quinidine, procainamide) or class III (amiodarone), are effective in treating re-entrant rhythms that use those structures as the limb of a re-entrant circuit. Drugs that blunt AV nodal function including class II (β-blockers) and class IV (calcium channel blockers) drugs, as well as some class III, are helpful in suppressing arrhythmias that originate from AV node or utilize this structure as a limb of a re-entry circuit. Although β-blockers, calcium channel blockers, cardiac glycosides, and purinergic agonists (adenosine) slow ventricular response to atrial tachycardia, they usually do not modulate these tachycardias primarily (Table 35–8 and Fig. 35–3).

Atrial Flutter and Atrial Fibrillation

Atrial flutter and fibrillation can have significant hemodynamic effects due to decreased diastolic filling caused by rapid heart rate and loss of coordinated atrial systole. They can be precipitated by metabolic disorders, drugs, and vascular accidents. When the ventricular rate is increased, β-blockade using propranolol (0.5-mg increments up to 0.1 mg/kg), or esmolol (starting dose 0.25 mg/kg followed by infusion starting at 50 μg/kg/min and titrated to effect) is the treatment of choice. Another option is the calcium channel blocker verapamil (titrated doses up to 0.15 mg/kg). Atrial pacing that overrides the supraventricular arrhythmia with brief, 5- to 10-second episodes of fast heart rate, 400 to 800 bpm, can convert the rhythm to sinus. If the dysrhythmia fails to convert pharmacologically or with pacing, or an emergency situation exists with hypotension, synchronized cardioversion is recommended. Prevention of postoperative supraventricular arrhythmia can be achieved in many cases by prophylactic perioperative digitalization prior to surgery in lung resection patients,[143] but this observation has not been documented in cardiovascular procedures.

The use of adenosine (6- to 12-mg IV bolus) in the treatment of arrhythmias or tachycardia is indicated in (1) supraventricular tachycardia or paroxysmal atrial tachycardia involving sinus node, atrial muscle, or AV node; (2) Wolf-Parkinson-White syndrome; or (3) re-entrant arrhythmia involving the AV node (narrow complex type). It is not indicated, but may be diagnostic in (1) supraventricular tachycardia when the AV node is not part of the circuit (i.e., atrial flutter or fibrillation); or (2) ventricular tachycardia that is a wide complex type. These arrhythmias may be associated with myocardial ischemia and a variety of metabolic disorders such as hypokalemia, hypoxia, acidosis, hypothermia, digitalis toxicity, and hypomagnesemia (Table 35–9 and Fig. 35–4). A 12-lead ECG (including any precordial lead) can help to distinguish between supraventricular and ventricular arrhythmias. Adenosine can aid in the diagnosis and treatment by making AV dissociation more evident. Ventricular tachycardia should be suspected in any case of hemodynamic instability[144] and can be treated initially with lidocaine. When ventricular tachycardia is associated with hypotension, it requires synchronized electrical cardioversion; treatment of ventricular fibrillation is immediate unsynchronized direct current shock.

Ventricular and Atrial Arrhythmias

A clear understanding of the physical and chemical factors that may alter the formation and conduction of an impulse will lead to appropriate therapy and, more importantly, to a decision of whether treatment is necessary. Instead of treating ECG manifestations of arrhythmia, treatment of the disturbed physiology (e.g., hypoxia or acidosis) is preferable. The causes include depth of analgesia, level of ventilation, drug side effects, or metabolic disorders. Arrhythmias caused by congestive heart failure are better treated with cardiac glycosides and diuretics than antiarrhythmic drugs alone; excessive vagal activity should be treated with anticholinergic compounds, and hypotension with α-adrenergic agonists.

Considerable disagreement exists concerning which arrhythmias require treatment. Atrial arrhythmias that interfere with adequate ventricular function should be treated to restore ventricular rate. If the atrial disturbance is chronic, digitalis or β-blockers may be used. If the atrial disturbance is acute, cardiotonic vasopressor and vagotonic agents, such as neostigmine, or DC cardioversion may be used. "R on T" ventricular arrhythmias should be considered the most dangerous, since the ectopic electrical activity may re-enter the Purkinje system during the supernormal conduction period, causing a disorganized depolarization and leading to ventricular fibrillation. Treatment consists of correcting the abnormalities leading to the ectopic impulse formation with antiarrhythmia therapy (lidocaine). Other ventricular activity that requires immediate and similar treatment includes multiform ectopic beats, which may lead to ventricular fibrillation; ventricular ectopic beats that occur in "series," which may lead to ventricular tachycardia or ventricular fibrillation (Fig. 35–4); and ventricular ectopic beats at frequencies greater than five per minute.

Pacemakers

Failure of pacemaker lead-pulse generator system may occur with (1) myocardial ischemia at the site of electrode attachment or in the conduction pathways around the electrode (increasing generator output may correct this kind of failure); (2) hypokalemia or hyperkalemia and failure to capture due to increased threshold for pacing (these effects are increased with hypoventilation, acidosis, potassium overload, and potassium shift to the extracellular compartment); and (3) postoperative shivering that causes myopotential interference with pacemaker output generation. In suspected pacemaker failure, heart rate should be determined from palpation of the pulse, arterial waveform analysis, or oximetry, not through the ECG. Most pacemakers can be converted from synchronous to a fixed or asynchronous mode by placing a magnet over them. However, a programmable pacemaker may require a programming transceiver, and magnet application may cause unpredictable resetting.

The indications for temporary transvenous, transcutaneous, or transesophageal pacing are (1) failure of a permanent pacemaker, (2) symptomatic heart block, (3) bifascicular block during acute anterior MI, and (4) all cases in which the indication for a permanent pacemaker

TABLE 35–9
Ventricular Arrhythmias: Diagnosis and Treatment*

Abnormality[†]	Causes/Risk Factors	Mechanism	Diagnostic Features	Management
Monomorphic VT after MI	1. MI 2. History of sustained monomorphic VT. The re-entry circuit remains unless ablated. Antiarrhythmic drugs may suppress recurrences but drug effects can be reversed by sympathetic stimulation. 3. Large infarction, typically LV ejection fraction <0.4. 4. Nonreperfused infarction, thrombolysis reduces late VT.	Slow conduction velocity through surviving bands of ventricular muscle in the fibrous scar tissue allow re-entry.	1. Sudden onset 2. QRS duration >0.12 (rarely less). 3. AV dissociation discernable in approximately 30%. a. Fusion beats. b. Dissociation p waves. 4. Often produces hemodynamic collapse, but can be well tolerated if relatively "slow" (e.g., <180/min) with good ventricular function. IV adenosine or verapamil fail to terminate VT, but may make AV dissociation more evident. 5. In any precordial lead with an RS complex—onset of R wave to the nader of S wave >0.1 sec favors VT rather than SVT.	1. Electrical cardioversion, QRS synchronized reduces VF. 2. Remove precipitating factors: hypokalemia, hypoxia, sympathetic stimulation, ectopy induced in intracardiac catheters or pacing wires, ischemia. 3. Intravenous antiarrhythmic drugs (e.g., lidocaine, procainamide, bretylium). 4. Proarrhythmia, occasionally an antiarrhythmic drug increases VT recurrences or makes VT incessant.
Polymorphic VT—general (torsades de pointes)	Anything that delays ventricular repolarization: a. Hypokalemia, hypocalcemia, hypomagnesemia. b. Antiarrhythmics: quinidine, procainamide, NAPA, disopyramide, sotalol, amiodarone. c. Other drugs: phenothiazines, erythromycin, pentamidine, terfenadine. d. Severe bradycardia. e. CNS injury, subarachnoid hemorrhage. f. Congenital long QT syndrome.	Early afterdepolarizations, QT prolongation.	1. QT >0.46 sec, often >0.56 sec in beats preceding VT. 2. Usually initiated by a long-short sequence of RR intervals, QT prolongation after the long RR interval 3. Waxing and waning QRS amplitude, may appear monomorphic for several beats in a single ECG lead. 4. Initiation is favored by slow heart rates.	1. Cardioversion/defibrillation of sustained episodes. 2. Remove precipitating causes. 3. $MgSO_4$ 1–2 gm IV over 1–2 min, continuous infusion if ectopy continues. 4. Overdrive atrial or ventricular pacing. 5. Isoproterenol infusion—increases heart rate, shortens QT (contraindicated in congenital long QT). 6. Drugs unlikely to aggravate torsades de pointes, but usually not beneficial (e.g., lidocaine, bretylium?, digoxin, nitroglycerin, atropine).
Polymorphic VT due to acute ischemia	Ischemia	"Random re-entry" in the ischemic zone, circulating re-entry wavelets.	1. Often degenerates rapidly to VF. 2. In contrast to torsades de pointes. a. Not necessarily preceded by QT prolongation. b. Aggravated by rapid heart rates. c. May or may not start with long-short RR intervals. d. Favored by high sympathetic tone.	1. Defibrillation of sustained episodes. 2. Intravenous lidocaine. 3. Reduce ischemia—nitroglycerin, β-adrenergic blockers if tolerable, magnesium? 4. Intra-aortic balloon counterpulsation.

*Modified from Levi R: The cardiovascular physiology and pharmacology of adenosine. In 15th Annual Meeting Program. Society of Cardiovascular Anesthesiologists, 1993, p 93, with permission.
[†]See Figure 35–1 for VT configuration—monomorphic and pleomorphic.
MI, myocardial infarction; NAPA, *N*-acetyl procainamide; CNS, central nervous system; QT, interval in ECG; VT, ventricular tachycardia; LV, left ventricular; QRS, complex in ECG; AV, atrioventricular; SVT, supraventricular tachycardia; ECG, electrocardiogram; VF, ventricular fibrillation.

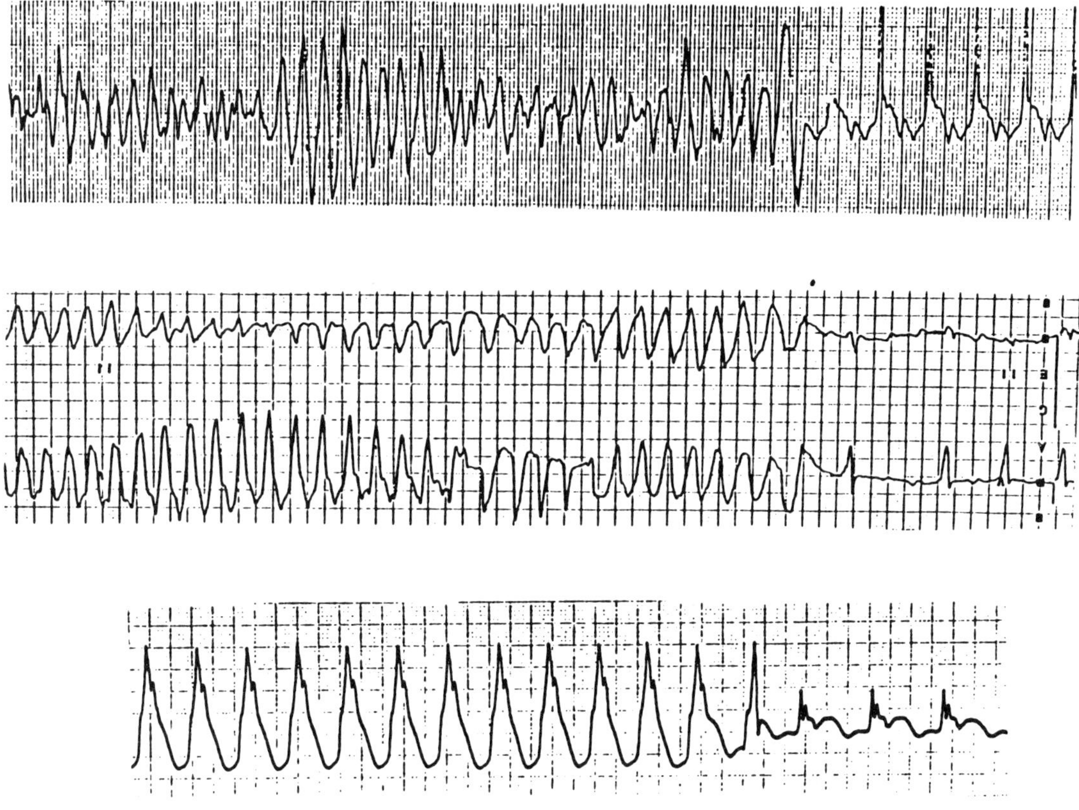

FIGURE **35–4.** Monomorphic ventricular tachycardia late after myocardial infarction (*top*); torsades de pointes (*middle*); polymorphic ventricular tachycardia due to acute ischemia (*bottom*). (From Levi R: The cardiovascular physiology and pharmacology of adenosine. In 15th Annual Meeting Program. Society of Cardiovascular Anesthesiologists, 1993, p 93, with permission.)

exists but timing is a problem. Prophylactic pacemaker use in the perioperative period to prevent progression to complete heart block is debatable, especially in cases of pre-existing conduction system disease. Data do not support prophylactic pacemaker insertion in asymptomatic patients with a combination of low (first-degree) block with bundle-branch block (complete right, incomplete left, left anterior, or posterior hemiblock), or certain bundle-branch combination blocks (incomplete right and complete left).[133] However, when these conditions exist with signs and symptoms of decreased perfusion, a permanent pacemaker is indicated.

Temporary pacing can be achieved by transvenous, transcutaneous, or transesophageal approaches. Transcutaneous pacing devices are easy, effective, and fast to use.[145] Transvenous insertion is easily done through the jugular into the right ventricle, and can be achieved using a PA catheter with its pacing port situated within the right ventricle cavity and a bipolar pacing electrode advanced to the endocardial surface contact (Paceport, Edwards Laboratory, Inc.).

Blood Pressure Changes

Hypertension

Postoperative hypertension is often due to pain, hypercarbia, hypoxemia, or fluid overload. The etiology should be investigated, diagnosed, and treated. Preoperative withdrawal of antihypertensive medication should be considered as a possible cause of postoperative hypertension. Severe hypertension can lead to LV failure, MI, or arrhythmias due to a sharp increase in MVO_2. Acute hypertension may also precipitate acute pulmonary edema or cerebral hemorrhage. Hypertension occurs after cardiopulmonary bypass in 15 to 60% of patients,[146,147] increasing the risk of postbypass ischemia and bleeding. The cause of hypertension after ACB is not clear, but may involve several mechanisms (some easily treatable) such as pain, hypoxia, hypoventilation, and hypothermia.

If clinically apparent etiologies are corrected and significant hypertension still exists, specific pharmacologic treatment is indicated. The speed and degree of arterial pressure control should be decided based on the degree of hypertension and its potential clinical consequences.

Acute pharmacologic therapy of postoperative hypertension consists of vasodilators such as nitroprusside, nitroglycerin, or hydralazine[148,149]; adenosine[150]; α- or β-adrenergic receptor blocking agents, such as phentolamine or propranolol, and esmolol, respectively; and mixed α- and β-antagonists, such as labetalol. Calcium channel blockers can also be used as antihypertensive agents. Which agent to use depends not only on its availability as an intravenous preparation but on its titratability and direct autonomic or compensatory side effects, which may cause bradycardia or tachycardia.

Hypotension

Hypotension in the recovery phase of anesthesia and surgery results from two basic processes: decreased preload and reduced myocardial contractility. Preload reduction occurs as a result of intravascular volume depletion, vasodilation, or blockage of flow. Reductions in myocardial contractility occur because of drugs, perioperative MI, ischemia, or pre-existing dysfunction. Prompt diagnosis and treatment are extremely important, since prolonged hypotension can result in hypoperfusion and ischemia of the vital organs.

Postoperative fluid administration should be guided by direct hemodynamic assessment rather than by specific protocol. In this regard, the evaluation of data trends are more useful than a single isolated measurement. The effect of ventilation on hemodynamic function is an important element in diagnosis and treatment.[151] Fluid administration according to these criteria should come before the use of diuretics. However, aggressive fluid administration, which is administered on the basis of oliguria, risks fluid overload. In a study of aneurysm repairs, almost 10% of patients were clinically overloaded postoperatively when fluids were given on the basis of oliguria.[152] If hypotension persists despite attempts at fluid replacement, the state of ventricular preload should be further assessed. During this time, a vasopressor should be administered to prevent prolonged hypotension while diagnosis is established and correct treatment is chosen.

Crystalloids and Colloids

The choice between crystalloid and colloid solution administration for volume replacement is still controversial in cardiovascular patients.[153] In a small, randomized, prospective study in patients undergoing surgery for aortic aneurysm repair, intraoperative colloid (5% albumin) use was associated with smaller alveolar-arterial oxygen (O_2) difference, greater intravascular volume, and higher serum colloid-oncotic pressure.[154] Another study in patients undergoing surgery for abdominal aorta repair compared postoperative fluid management. The albumin-treated group demonstrated a faster return to baseline values of O_2 consumption and cardiac output and less increase in alveolar-atrial O_2 difference and ventilation-perfusion mismatch.[155] Crystalloid resuscitation, the investigators argued, results in an increase in pulmonary wedge pressure and a decrease in colloid-oncotic pressure.

A colloid-oncotic/pulmonary wedge pressure gradient less than 4 mm may[156] or may not[157,158] correlate with pulmonary edema. However, colloids can also leak extravascularly, thereby increasing interstitial colloid-oncotic pressure in hemorrhagic shock and other conditions with increased protein permeability, predisposing to pulmonary edema. Individualization of therapy seems indicated, considering the desired end point for treatment. Crystalloid solutions are the logical choice to rehydrate the interstitium, and colloid solutions may be advantageous in filling the intravascular space.

Hypertonic saline solution for perioperative fluid management of trauma or cardiovascular patients has been investigated. Intraoperative or perioperative administration of hypertonic saline (3.5 to 7.5%, 400 to 1,500 ml) decreases overall fluid requirement needed to maintain systemic hemodynamic and renal performance.[159,160]

Blood products should be used only when specifically indicated for blood loss, low hemoglobin, coagulation factor deficit, and thrombocytopenia. They are not indicated for volume expansion alone. Ultimately, the choice of a resuscitation solution may revolve around its cost. Colloid and blood fractions can be 100 or more times more expensive than an equally effective crystalloid.[161]

Cardiac Arrest and Resuscitation

The incidence of cardiac arrest in the cardiovascular population is not well documented, but the incidence in the overall surgical population was 1 in more than 3,000[162] over 30 years ago. Within the last 20 years, it has increased to 1 in approximately 1,000[163,164] despite improved monitoring and anesthetic techniques, probably because of the increasing numbers of patients with increased risk factors who are subjected to anesthesia and surgery. Survival after perioperative cardiac arrest is 41 to 50%, depending upon whether aggravating factors such as hypoxia, hemorrhage, metabolic imbalance, and pulmonary embolism were present.[164,165]

Cardiac arrest is usually diagnosed by the absence of palpable pulse or blood pressure. The objective of cardiopulmonary resuscitation is to prevent cerebral anoxia. Current standards for cardiopulmonary resuscitation have been established by the American Heart Association.[166] The standards include the familiar **A**irway, **B**reathing, **C**irculation steps.

True cardiac arrest involves either asystole or ventricular fibrillation. In asystole the therapeutic objective is to initiate electrical activity, either by inducing ventricular fibrillation with drugs or by promoting ventricular contractions with electrical pacing. Drugs commonly used for asystolic cardiac arrest are epinephrine, isoproterenol, calcium chloride, and sodium bicarbonate. The latter three agents are not recommended in the latest resuscitation guidelines except in very limited and specific circumstances.[166] When ventricular fibrillation is observed, defibrillation is indicated.

Combining the new recommendations issued by the American Heart Association[166] with those of the European Resuscitation Council, new directions and concepts have been established and adapted[167]:

- **A**irway control.
- **B**reathing time for filling the lungs should be limited to 2 seconds in order to decrease the likelihood of gastric insufflation.
- Resuscitation drugs can be administered via the tracheal route to establish **C**irculation, but with higher doses and dilution.

- In pulseless adults, initial dose of epinephrine remains unchanged, 1 mg IV, and lidocaine should be infused at a rate of 1.5 mg/kg.
- Sodium bicarbonate and calcium are not recommended routinely, and atropine should be limited to the maximal dose of 0.04 mg/kg.
- Hypomagnesemia (recurrent and refractory ventricular fibrillation) should be corrected with 1 to 2 gm of magnesium sulfate IV.
- Thrombolytic agents are classified as useful and effective in the treatment of acute MI.
- Glucose-containing fluids are discouraged in resuscitation efforts.

Embolization Syndromes

Air Embolism

Complications that may occur in cardiac operations include those associated with establishing and maintaining cardiopulmonary bypass. The introduction of air into the arterial circulation, including the coronary vessels, through the aortic cannula is a serious complication of cardiopulmonary bypass that can cause instant death.[168] Air can also come from the heart or pulmonary veins as a consequence of an open procedure or venting the left ventricle.

Atheroembolism

Atheroemboli or abnormalities consistent with atheroemboli can be identified in 22% of patients undergoing myocardial revascularization or valve operations.[169] Atheroembolism from the ascending aorta is an emerging problem in cardiac surgery because the age of patients undergoing cardiac operations has increased. The prevalence of atherosclerotic disease increased dramatically from 4.5% in 1982 to 48.3% in 1989. Most patients have multiple atherosclerotic sites, including brain, spleen, and kidney. Atheroemboli are common in patients undergoing ACB (26.1%) and valve procedures (8.9%),[170] and there is a high incidence of complications with severe atherosclerosis of the ascending aorta.

Ultrasonic scanning and epigastric echocardiography are sensitive methods of detecting atherosclerotic changes in the ascending aorta and aortic arch.[171,172] In a group of patients undergoing a variety of cardiac operations, early death, primarily from cardiogenic shock and arrhythmia, occurred in patients with mild and moderate to severe atherosclerosis (58 and 60%, respectively).[172]

Techniques for management of an atherosclerotic ascending aorta during cardiac operations include femoral artery catheterization, use of intraluminal balloon catheter instead of aortic clamping, hypothermic fibrillatory arrest, ascending aorta endarterectomy, and graft replacement with hypothermic circulatory arrest.[172] Most patients who need the latter technique may have complex and combined cardiac operations, including ACB, aortic valve replacement, LV aneurysmectomy, and carotid endarterectomy.

Risks and Complications

Thoracic Surgery

Thoracic and upper abdominal procedures have the highest incidence of cardiopulmonary complications, including respiratory failure, MI, cardiac arrhythmia, pneumonia, atelectasis, pulmonary embolism, and death. Patients with chronic obstructive pulmonary disease (COPD) have a high incidence (42 to 66%) of perioperative pulmonary complications, which are correlated with the degree of respiratory dysfunction preoperatively.[173,174] Aggressive preoperative pulmonary preparation using antibiotics, bronchodilators, and physiotherapy can reduce the incidence of complications. Outcome can be improved by identifying and treating those patients at increased risk.

Preoperative, prophylactic use of digitalis in patients undergoing thoracic surgery is controversial. The incidence of postoperative arrhythmias is 20% (14 to 37%)[175-177] in patients undergoing thoracic surgery, and is even higher in older patients.[175] The mechanism for these arrhythmias may be associated with pulmonary resection and distention of the right heart chambers. Digitalis may prevent these arrhythmias or slow the ventricular response; it reduced the incidence from 14% to 2.7% in one study.[176] The period of maximum risk is the first 24 hours postoperatively.[177] Preoperative prophylactic digitalis does not change the postoperative arrhythmia incidence. Indications for digitalis treatment in patients with cor pulmonale are more clear-cut. Withholding the drug for 24 hours preoperatively may be indicated in order to decrease the chance of digitalis toxicity, since these patients are prone to hypercarbia, hypoxia, and acidosis.

Appropriate baseline pulmonary function testing includes spirometry, indices of air flow obstruction, and diffusing capacity measurements, all of which are standardized and related to evaluation of increased risk (Table 35–10).[178-186] Determination of risk and prediction of postoperative status[182,183] in candidates for lung surgery begins with baseline pulmonary function testing.

TABLE 35–10
Pulmonary Function Criteria and Increased Risk*

Indicator	Absolute Value Indicating Increased Risk	% Normal Value = Increased Risk
FVC	1.7–2.0 L	≤70%
FEV	1.2 L	
	<2.0 L	<50%
FEV_1/FVC		35–50%
MEFR	200 L/min	
$FEF_{25-75\%}$	1.6 L/min	
RV	RV/TLC	≥50%
$\dot{D}$CO		≤50%
MVV	45 L/min	50–55%

*From Boysen PG: Preoperative assessment of the patient undergoing noncardiac thoracic surgery. In Mangano DT (ed): Preoperative Cardiac Assessment. Philadelphia, JB Lippincott Co, 1990, p 125, with permission.

FVC, forced vital capacity; FEV_1, forced expiratory volume in 1 second; MEFR, maximum expiratory flow rate; $FEF_{25-75\%}$, forced expiratory flow between 25–75%; RV, residual capacity; $\dot{D}$CO, diffusing capacity using carbon monoxide; MVV, maximal voluntary ventilation.

Failure to meet the criteria in Table 35–10 indicates increased risk.

Patients identified to be at risk should undergo split lung function testing using bronchospirometry or radionuclide scanning.[187] Once split lung function data are acquired, resectability and operability can be determined.[182] Pulmonary arterial hypertension often accompanies inadequate pulmonary reserve in COPD and postpneumonectomy patients,[188] resulting in decreases in cardiac output, cross-sectional area of the pulmonary vascular bed, and exercise capacity. Vascular catheterization studies can estimate the postoperative effects of pneumonectomy during temporal and reversible flow alteration and exercise. Pulmonary artery pressure above 35 mm Hg or arterial O_2 saturation less than 80% during flow occlusion indicates inoperability.[188–191] Increased pulmonary vascular resistance can indicate that a patient will not tolerate lung resection.[192] Exercise tolerance testing also provides information on cardiac, pulmonary, and muscular performance, and cellular function.[192–195] Although a relationship between maximal MVO_2 and postoperative pulmonary complications has been established (Fig. 35–5),[196] conclusive assessment using these techniques is not yet possible because of the wide variability of test results.[197]

No data currently define whether a particular anesthetic technique improves cardiac outcome; anesthetic management is developed primarily to facilitate the surgical procedure.[197] Intraoperative fluid management is crucial. Overhydration may decrease lung compliance, cause pulmonary edema, and increase work of breathing. Lung resection decreases pulmonary reserve, compromises right ventricular function, and may stretch the right atrium and contribute to arrhythmias, as mentioned previously. However, although it demonstrated a relationship between radiographic appearance of pulmonary edema and survival, a retrospective study of pneumonectomy patients failed to establish a relationship between perioperative fluid administration and survival.[198] The authors suggested restricting fluid administration to less than 2 L perioperatively, and to 75% of the calculated maintenance level after that.

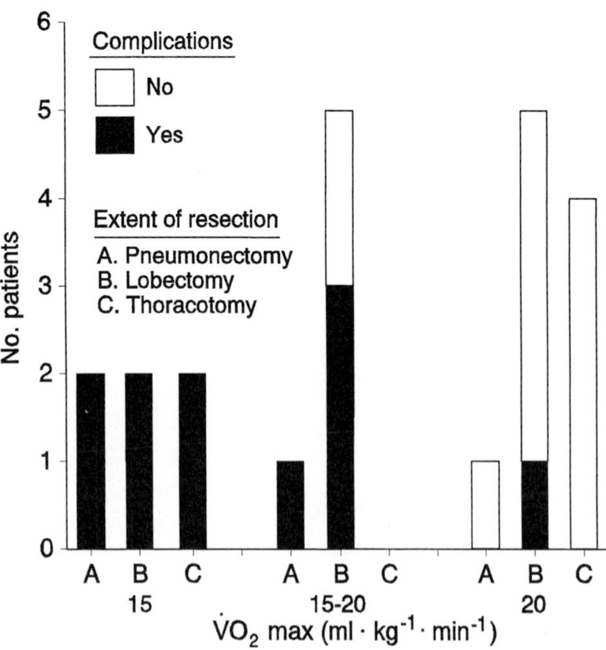

FIGURE 35–5. Preoperative $\dot{V}O_{2max}$ during exercise with the extent of resection and predicted postoperative complications. (From Eugene J, Brown SE, Light RW, et al: Maximum oxygen consumption: A physiology guide to pulmonary resection. Am Rev Respir Dis 125:604, 1982. © American Lung Association, with permission.)

Separation of the two lungs by means of a double-lumen tracheobronchial tube provides the selective bronchial intubation that is indicated for certain thoracic procedures. Placement of such a tube carries some risk for tracheobronchial rupture[199] and death.[200] However, with fiberoptic bronchoscopy used to verify correct positioning, the procedure can be safe and relatively easy.[201]

Intraoperative pulse oximetry is expected to add safety to anesthesia for thoracic surgery, although this fact has not been proven. Desaturation in these procedures can occur rapidly, and may be detectable only by oximetry. Unfortunately, at low levels of arterial saturation, the pulse oximeter can be inaccurate.[202,203]

Atelectasis and the resultant hypoxemia is a frequent complication following thoracic procedures. Postoperative pain contributes to atelectasis, since it interferes with the patient's ability to breathe deeply and cough. Various methods of analgesia have been used after thoracotomy: systemic analgesics, intercostal nerve blocks, and spinal and epidural analgesia with local anesthetics of opioids. Respiratory mechanics after thoracotomy in patients receiving epidural morphine may be superior compared to systemic opioids.[204] A retrospective study in postthoracotomy patients receiving a combination of general and epidural anesthesia demonstrated reduced morbidity and mortality, but this study provided no control data.[205] There is no evidence that suggests that pain control, including epidural opioids, decreases morbidity or mortality. Furthermore, some alterations in diaphragmatic function are not correctable, even with total relief of pain.

Ischemic Heart Disease Patients: Risk Factors

Ischemia

Little information is available regarding the interaction of perioperative management and clinical outcome in patients undergoing cardiovascular and cardiothoracic surgery. Most data are derived from patients with ischemia undergoing ACB procedures and are extrapolated to other groups. However, there are almost no data in other surgery groups.

Almost 20 years ago, Goldman and others analyzed more than 1,000 patients who underwent major noncardiac surgery.[91] Using multivariate analysis, they identified nine preoperative variables that independently correlated with postoperative cardiac complications. Although the patient population was "noncardiac," the Goldman Cardiac Risk Index became popular because of the relative weight or value assigned to each factor, which facilitated calculation of "overall cardiac risk."

TABLE 35–11
Prospective Evaluation of the Goldman Index in Abdominal Aortic Surgery Patients*

Goldman Class	No. of Patients	Goldman Prediction of Number of Events†	Actual Events Found†
1	56	0–1 (1%)	4 (7%)
2	35	2–3 (7%)	4 (11%)
3	8	1 (14%)	3 (38%)

*From Jeffrey CC, Kunsman J, Cullen DJ, Brewster DC: A prospective evaluation of cardiac risk index. Anesthesiology 58:462, 1983, with permission.
†Numbers in parentheses are the percentage of patients for each Goldman class who suffered a cardiac event.

Eventually this index was used to quantitate preoperative cardiac recommendations.

The scientific validity of this index was eventually questioned,[206] as was its prediction for adverse cardiac outcome in comparison to the American Society of Anesthesiologists (ASA) physical status classification for noncardiac surgery.[207] The latter work actually showed that patients undergoing abdominal aortic aneurysm surgery were at higher risk for cardiac complications than the Goldman index suggested. Another study specifically investigated the utility of this index in vascular surgery,[208] and found that more cardiac events occurred than it could have predicted (Table 35–11). Thus, as a tool to plan perioperative management, the original Goldman index failed in the cardiovascular patient population.

Another prospective assessment of the index was conducted by Detsky and colleagues in patients undergoing noncardiac surgery (Table 35–12).[209,210] Changes in the index were proposed to improve its accuracy. The modified index added risk factors such as angina, pulmonary edema, and old MI, and deleted risk factors of major surgery. The likelihood ratios presented in Table 35–13 convert a given pretest probability of complications into the posttest probability or change in risk, based on points assigned by the Detsky Index. A likelihood ratio of greater than 1 denotes an incremental risk over the pretest probability that a high point score impacts a given procedure.[209]

Although good predictive accuracy was found, independent verification is lacking. Even though these frequently utilized indices of cardiac risk assessment appear to be most reliable in identifying those at highest risk, a low score does not guarantee that a patient will be free from cardiac events, but merely that he or she is a lower risk. Also, the reliability of each of these indices must be considered in assessing the score, since both the Goldman and the Detsky scales utilize physical examination as the only tool determining LV function. Measured ejection fraction has not been included as an independent component in multifactorial risk indices, even though evidence suggests that the degree of LV dysfunction predicts outcome in noncardiac surgery.[211] Thus, the cardiac risk indices remain imperfect but useful tools for determining perioperative risk for cardiac events. Additional cardiac tests should be routinely employed in determining the individual patient's current risk status. Goldman himself in an editorial entitled "To Everything There is a Season" recognized that new techniques and information changed the methods for preoperative evaluation.[212] The first breakthrough was the actual use of biostatistical analysis; the second was using sophisticated evaluation such as echocardiography and scintigraphy to deal with the less-well-defined middle-risk group. The next breakthrough may be in the utilization of randomized control trials, a methodologic rather than a technologic breakthrough. Work is ongoing by different investigators (including a new study by Goldman[213]) to continuously update the cardiac risk indices, which remain important in the current era. Estimating an updated probability, it is quite possible that the risk indices derived on general patient populations may not be accurately or perfectly applicable to more selected patient samples (such as for cardiac or aortic surgery). By integrating the patient's score on a risk index with the prior

TABLE 35–12
Detsky's Modified Multifactorial Index*

Variables	Points
Coronary artery disease	
Myocardial infarction within 6 mo	10
Myocardial infarction more than 6 mo	5
Canadian Cardiovascular Society angina	
Class 3	10
Class 4	20
Unstable angina within 3 months	10
Alveolar pulmonary edema	
Within 1 wk	10
Ever	5
Valvular disease	
Suspected critical aortic stenosis	20
Arrhythmias	
Sinus plus atrial premature beats or rhythm other than sinus on last preoperative electrocardiogram	5
More than 5 ventricular premature beats at any time prior to surgery	5
Poor general medical status†	5
Age >70 years	5
Emergency operation	10

*From Detsky AS, Abrams HB, McLaughlin JR, et al: Predicitng cardiac complications in patients undergoing noncardiac surgery. J Gen Intern Med 1:211, 1986; and Detsky AS, Abrams HB, Forbath N, et al: Cardiac assessment for patients undergoing noncardiac surgery, a multifactorial clinical risk index. Arch Intern Med 146:2131, 1986, with permission.
†Oxygen partial pressure, <60 mm Hg; carbon dioxide partial pressure, >50 mm Hg; serum potasium, <3.0 mEq/L (<3.0 mmol/L); serum bicarbonate, <20 mEq/L (<20 mmol/L); serum urea nitrogen, >50 mg/dl (>18 mmol/L); serum creatinine, >3 mg/dl (>260 mmol/L); asparate aminotransferase, abnormal; signs of chronic liver disease; and/or bedridden from noncardiac causes.

TABLE 35–13
Likelihood Ratios of Perioperative Cardiac Complications by Points in the Detsky Index*

Class (Points)	Major Surgery	Minor Surgery	All Surgery
I (0–15)	0.42	0.39	0.43
II (15–30)	3.58	2.75	3.38
III (>30)	14.93	12.20	10.60

*From Detsky AS, Abrams HB, McLaughlin JR, et al: Predicting cardiac complications in patients undergoing noncardiac surgery. J Gen Intern Med 1:217, 1986, with permission.

probability of major complications in a large population of similar patients, the resulting "risk estimate" may be superior to the prior probability or the old risk index alone (Table 35–14).

Prior Myocardial Infarction

Prior MI long has been associated with increased perioperative risk and cardiac complications, particularly reinfarction. Twenty to 30 years ago, the connection between prior MI and increased risk of postoperative MI was established.[207,214] Further work at the Mayo Clinic found a reinfarction rate of about 30% if the MI was 0 to 3 months old, and 15% if the MI was 3 to 6 months old.[93,215] Later data, however, found a reinfarction rate of approximately 8% if the MI was 0 to 3 months old and approximately 3% if the MI was 3 to 6 months old.[58] This improved incidence may have been achieved because of invasive monitoring coupled with the aggressive use of medications to control rhythm and hemodynamics. Unfortunately, no "control" group can ever be concurrently available. The improved results are still considered preliminary, because the much higher figures came from larger groups of patients.

The history of MI is the most constant finding in all of the studies examining cardiac risk factors. Mortality from perioperative reinfarction after noncardiac surgery remains 50% and is expected to be at least as high for cardiac or cardiothoracic surgery (higher than that expected from reinfarction without surgery). Why recent MI markedly increases surgical risk is unclear, as is the reason for reduced risk after 6 months. Perhaps that is the time needed for scarring or healing to mature, and for the development of sufficient collateral circulation.[206]

Congestive Heart Failure

Congestive heart failure has been recognized for years as a risk factor for anesthesia and surgery. Perioperative cardiac functional capacity is perhaps the most sensitive predictor of morbidity and mortality.[91,216] This relationship is emphasized when patients undergo more stressful surgery.[216] Patients not requiring digitalis and diuretics for congestive heart failure tolerate surgery better.[216,217] Even mild signs of congestive heart failure can be associated with the development of postoperative pulmonary edema.[218] Despite invasive monitoring, pharmacologic agents, and aggressive care, preoperative congestive heart failure remains a significant risk factor.[58] Clinical evaluation for congestive heart failure is an important supplement to thallium-dipyridamole tests in predicting postoperative cardiac outcome in vascular surgery[219,220] as well as noncardiac surgery.[217]

Age

Elderly patients have increased risks for adverse cardiovascular and pulmonary events perioperatively during noncardiac[221,222] and thoracic surgery.[223] Major perioperative cardiac complications have been reported in 14% of elderly patients. However, the ASA classification provides similar sensitivity and supports the management strategies suggested by the aforementioned studies.[221,223] Thus, the ASA classification should provide reasonable risk assessment in these patients.

Hypertension

Available data suggest little relationship between hypertension and adverse cardiac outcome.[207] Past history of either treated or untreated hypertension was not associated with increased risk of postoperative MI or cardiac death (Table 35–15).[224,225] However, patients with pre-

TABLE 35–14
Potential Use of the Original Multifactorial Cardiac Risk Index to Estimate the Probability of Cardiac Complications in Different Types of Patients

Type of Patient	Approximate Baseline Risk of Major Cardiac Complications (%)	Approximate Risk of Major Cardiac Complications as Adjusted Using Multifactorial Index (%)*			
		Class I (0–5 Points)	Class II (6–12 Points)	Class III (13–25 Points)	Class IV (≥26 Points)
Minor surgery	1	0.3	1	3	19
Unselected consecutive patients more than 40 yr old who have major noncardiac surgery	3	1	3.5	10	45
Patients with known high-risk characteristics, such as patients undergoing abdominal aortic aneurysm surgery	10	3	10	30	75

*Calculated using data from Goldman L, Caldera DL, Nussbaum SR, et al: Multifactorial index of cardiac risk in noncardiac surgical procedures. N Engl J Med 297:845, 1977; Jeffrey CC, Kunsman J, Cullen DJ, Brewster DC: A prospective evaluation of cardiac risk index. Anesthesiology 58:462, 1983; Detsky AS, Abrams HB, McLaughlin JR, et al: Predicting cardiac complications in patients undergoing noncardiac surgery. J Gen Intern Med 1:211, 1986; and more than 4,300 patients using the original multifactoral cardiac-risk index on various types of patients.

TABLE 35–15
Correlation of Preoperative Hypertension to Adverse Cardiac Outcomes*

Hypertension Characteristics			No. of Patients	Postoperative Incidence (%)	
Existence	Treatment	Response		Infarction	Cardiac Death
No	No	No	661	2	2
Yes	Yes	Yes	127	4	3
Yes	No	No	90	1	2
Yes	Yes	No	61	0	2

*From Goldman L, Caldera DL, Southwick FS, et al: Cardiac risk factors and complications in noncardiac surgery. Medicine 57:357, 1978, with permission.

operative hypertension were more likely to develop intraoperative or postoperative hypertension. Hypertensive episodes are reported in about 75% of vascular surgery patients, particularly those having abdominal aortic aneurysm or carotid endarterectomy surgery. Nevertheless, preoperative hypertension is not an independent predictor for postoperative cardiac complications.

Angina

There is no strong relationship between angina pectoris and risk for postoperative cardiac complications,[93] even though patients with this symptom could have other diseases such as carotid artery or cerebrovascular disease that place them at increased risk. Some studies show an increased risk with angina, but the risks are minimal (~10%)[207,226] compared with other risk factors.[227]

Valvular Heart Disease

Relatively few outcome data exist concerning the perioperative risk of valvular heart disease patients, probably because specific perioperative criteria are not easy to obtain in this group. Acute hypertension (which results in accentuated v wave and mitral regurgitation), tachycardia-induced hypotension with aortic stenosis, and oliguria/hypovolemia with aortic regurgitation are potential perioperative episodes that can be transient and treatable, without changing severity and potential risk status. Without objective data, one can only extrapolate known risk factors for perioperative cardiac morbidity and complications in valvular heart disease patients to the ischemic or noncardiac surgical patients.[91,216]

For patients with all forms of valvular heart disease, the perioperative risk of developing or aggravating congestive heart failure was reported to be about 20%.[207] Perioperative symptoms confirmed by physical examination were the only independent predictor of postoperative congestive heart failure in valvular heart disease patients. Aortic stenosis, the only form of valvular heart disease found to be an independent risk factor for perioperative cardiac complications in patients with or without congestive heart failure, resulted in a 14-fold higher postoperative mortality. Mitral valve regurgitation, grade 2/4 or above, was also associated with a higher mortality, but was not identified as an independent risk factor. In fact, even the increase in mortality with mitral valve regurgitation can be attributed to its association with other independent risk factors such as S_3 gallop, jugular venous distention, and recent MI.[91]

Signs and symptoms of congestive heart failure that are accurate indicators for depressed contractility in ischemic heart disease patients may not correlate with the underlying contractile state in valvular heart disease patients, particularly those with aortic and mitral stenosis. These symptoms in valvular heart disease patients often indicate imbalance between ventricular loading and the inotropic state rather than inotropic dysfunction, particularly in uncorrected mitral valve regurgitation or mitral stenosis with ventricular failure and end-stage pulmonary hypertension.

Aortic valvular disease was the most prominent identified risk factor in patients undergoing more extensive intrathoracic or intra-abdominal surgery.[216] Aortic "critical" stenosis that presents with symptoms such as syncope with exertion is a significant indicator for limited survival.[210]

Vascular Procedures

Carotid Endarterectomy

Extracranial cerebral vascular disease patients have a high incidence of coexisting disease (Table 35–2). The two main causes of morbidity and mortality postoperatively for carotid endarterectomy patients are cerebral vascular accident and MI. Overall mortality following carotid endarterectomy is 2%; MI risk is 4%, with an associated 20 to 66% mortality.[10,228–240] Patients who undergo ACB prior to vascular surgery have a lower mortality rate (0.3%) for carotid endarterectomy. However, the overall mortality of ACB and subsequent carotid endarterectomy was not different from carotid endarterectomy without protective ACB.[10] The management of patients with carotid disease who require ACB remained controversial in the mid and late 1990s.[241–245] Recent studies have demonstrated that only with older age and more advanced coronary disease in patients undergoing simultaneous carotid endarterectomy and ACB was long-term outcome and perioperative morbidity and mortality worse, compared to the outcome of carotid endarterectomy alone.[241] Concomitant carotid endarterectomy and ACB can be performed with acceptably low operative risk (3.5% mortality), and good long-term freedom from coronary (81%) and neurologic (92%) events.[242] Both early cardiac complications and neurologic complications were less frequent in patients who underwent the combined procedure than the staged (carotid endarterectomy followed later by ACB) procedure, or ACB alone.[243] However, there are recent data that demonstrate the simultaneous procedure is associated with increased neurologic morbidity (14.3% vs. 3.4% in staged procedure) and higher cardiac complications and morbidity rate.[244] Another study reviewed data from 512 patients and found that only after the mid 1980s, the simultaneous procedure had outcome data similar to the staged procedure, presumably due to advances in myocardial protection and perioperative hemodynamic management.[245]

Hypertension and hypotension are common complications following carotid endarterectomy.[228-232,246-248] Hypotension, which is associated with bradycardia, has been attributed to baroreceptor hyperactivity and occurs postoperatively in 10 to 50% of carotid endarterectomy patients.[228-230,247-249] Following plaque removal, the carotid sinus wall is more distended and less compliant. These factors, along with increased nerve activity after carotid endarterectomy, all correlate with hypertension.[247] Carotid endarterectomy–induced hypotension can be prevented by surgical denervation[250] or by local application of lidocaine.[229,247,248] Decreased activity of the carotid sinus nerve may result from intraoperative injury to the nerve or vessel wall baroreceptors.[247] Postoperative hypotension following carotid endarterectomy, even though it may be brief, has been associated with neurologic deficits.[228,232,233]

According to one study, surgical nerve division may cause hypertension. Lidocaine may decrease the incidence of hypertension by 10%, but may increase hypotension by 50%.[229] Postoperative hypertension is expected to vary from 60 to 75% (Table 35–2) and has been reported more frequently in patients who had preoperative hypertension (especially uncontrolled); however, its presence is not necessarily an accurate predictor.[230,246] This group is also prone to develop new neurologic deficits postoperatively.[228,230,234,246,251] Postoperative hypertension has been implicated in postoperative intracerebral bleeding, but it is not clear if it is a cause or an effect.[251] Neurologic deficits after carotid endarterectomy are commonly described as primarily embolic in nature, and not due to blood pressure changes.[229,233,246]

Another complication after carotid endarterectomy is airway obstruction due to cervical wound hematoma. This complication has been associated with postoperative hypertension and the perioperative use of antiplatelet drugs, but it also may be related to difficult tracheal intubation.[252] In any case, when airway obstruction is developing, early intubation is recommended before the airway is compromised. In case of obstruction, the wound should be opened using local anesthesia to evacuate the hematoma and decompress the airway and facilitate intubation.

Abdominal Aortic Aneurysm Repair

Mortality for elective abdominal aortic aneurysm repair ranges from 0.9 to 7.9%[1,4,11,253-260]; however, the mortality for emergency repair is reported to be much higher, 25 to 50% (Table 35–1).[2,5,8,9,256] Myocardial infarction, congestive heart failure, and arrhythmias are the major causes for mortality, followed by renal and respiratory complications.[2,5,7,256,257,259] Overall perioperative mortality from cardiac complications ranges from 33 to 100% and the incidence of MI in this group is 3 to 15% (Table 35–1).[2,5-7,65,253,255-259] The incidence of congestive heart failure is 8.9 to 37%, and that of treated arrhythmia 10.5 to 14%.[5,257]

The relationship between preoperative data and perioperative complications reveals that the occurrence of adverse cardiac events correlates with age, history of congestive heart failure, and ECG changes that are consistent with previous MI.[257] Perioperative MI is associated with age, angina, and prolonged aortic cross-clamp time. The incidence of arrhythmias is related to pre-existing arrhythmia and is increased with postoperative mechanical ventilation longer than 48 hours, perioperative angina, and COPD. Perioperative congestive heart failure is associated with ischemic ECG changes and COPD.

Postoperative hypertension after abdominal aortic aneurysm repair may be due to fluid overload, vasoconstriction, or increased renin activity, and may be correlated with preoperative hypertension.[260] Pulmonary hypertension after abdominal aorta aneurysm repair may also occur and possibly is related to thromboxane A_2 release following aortic declamping.[261]

Apart from myocardial ischemia, other organ ischemia may be related to low output or flow and become apparent postoperatively. Ischemic spinal cord injury has a reported incidence of 0.15 to 0.25% after abdominal aortic repair,[257,262] probably due to interference with cord blood flow through the lumbar arteries. Ischemia of the colon occurs in up to 1.1% and presents with abdominal pain, metabolic acidosis, and sepsis. Ischemic colitis diagnosed by colonoscopy can occur in as many as 7.5% of patients.[263] Ischemic damage to the kidneys with acute renal failure occurs in 0.6 to 7% of patients[5,256,257,259] and is associated with high preoperative creatinine, suprarenal aortic cross-clamping, or renal vein ligation. Intraoperative treatment with mannitol, which maintains intravascular volume, cardiac output, and renal artery flow, and also scavenges free radicals, can reduce the incidence of renal failure.[8,254]

Peripheral Vascular Disease

Repair of aortoiliac occlusive disease is associated with 2.3 to 3.8% mortality, and 40 to 75% is secondary to MI.[11,264,265] The mortality rate for lower extremity vessel reconstruction is similar, 1.1 to 3.3%,[11,265-267] and perioperative MI has a mortality rate of 33 to 66%.

Renal revascularization surgery combined with other aortic procedures has a mortality of 5 to 12%, compared to a mortality rate of 1% for isolated renal lesions.[268-271] Myocardial infarction is the primary cause of death in 33 to 44%, and occurs mainly in atherosclerotic ischemic heart disease patients.[268,269] Mortality is also increased with azotemia, peripheral vascular disease, abnormal ECG, and combined aortic and visceral arterial lesions.[268]

Postoperative hypotension can result from renal revascularization or from the residual effect of antihypertensive drugs and low intravascular volume.

Evaluating Cardiac Risk—The ACC/AHA Guidelines and Algorithm

During the last two decades, mortality related to cardiovascular disease has decreased significantly, due to surgical and nonsurgical coronary interventions and improved use of medications.[4–9] During the same time, improvements in anesthetic and surgical techniques and life-support methods have helped to reduce the risk of operation. In the past, when diagnostic technology and therapeutic interventions were limited, the physician had to identify clinical factors that could be anticipated and controlled in order to reduce overall stress and risk. In recent years, however, the development of better noninvasive techniques to determine cardiac function and the application of these techniques to coronary therapy have helped to reduce cardiac risk and complications. However, these same techniques have also caused concern and created confusion for physicians as they prepare patients for cardiac and noncardiac surgery. In order to deal with those concerns and confusion, the American College of Cardiology and American Heart Association published in 1996 guidelines for perioperative cardiovascular evaluation and risk assessment.[272–273] These guidelines provide a framework of cardiac risk in noncardiac surgery patients and various operative situations. However, these guidelines can also be applied to patients undergoing major cardiac or vascular surgery. The guidelines strive to incorporate the most current information on perioperative risk and how this information can be used to treat individual patients.

The methods used to develop these guidelines are described in Tables 35–16 through 35–19. The preoperative risk evaluation should be determined according the following guidelines.

CLINICAL PREDICTORS OF INCREASED PERIOPERATIVE RISK (Table 35–16)

These include the potentially serious cardiac disorders including (1) CAD (prior MI, angina), (2) CHF, and (3) electrical instability. Also, defining disease severity, stability, and prior treatment is essential. Other clinical factors that help determine cardiac risk include: (1) functional capacity (Table 35–17); (2) age; (3) comorbid conditions (diabetes mellitis, peripheral vascular disease, renal dysfunction, and chronic lung disease); and (4) type of operation (Table 35–18)—aortic and major vascular procedure, prolonged procedures associated with large fluid shifts and/or blood loss, such as complicated thoracic procedures, and emergent major operations, particularly in the elderly, are considered higher risk.

FURTHER PREOPERATIVE TESTING TO ASSESS CARDIAC RISK

These include (1) resting LV function with special attention to LV ejection fraction less than 30% and severe diastolic dysfunction; (2) exercise-stress testing to identify ischemia, with or without nuclear (myocardial) perfusion imaging or echocardiography, which may cause functional incapacity, ischemic symptoms, or electrical instability; and (3) pharmacologic stress testing with dipyridamole or adenosine with thallium (or comparable radiopharmaceutical). Myocardial perfusion imaging has a high sensitivity and specificity for perioperative coronary events. Also, pharmacologic testing involving echocardiography (with dobutamine) has also emerged as a promising method, which provides information and safety similar to the imaging technique.

In certain patients at high risk, proceeding directly to coronary angiography is indicated. The indications for angiography are similar to those in the nonoperative setting (Table 35–19). First, it is essential to ensure that management with percutaneous transluminal coronary angioplasty (PTCA) or coronary artery bypass grafting (CABG) surgery is a viable option. Second, angiography should be reserved for patients at high risk, especially those suspected of having left-main or three-vessel CAD.

Although both exercise and pharmacologic stress testing provide useful information for risk prediction, no prospective study has firmly established that the cost-effectiveness or efficacy of either exercise or pharmacologic testing improves perioperative or long-term outcome. The lack of adequately controlled or randomized clinical trials to determine the optimal evaluation strat-

TABLE 35–16
Clinical Predictors of Increased Perioperative Cardiovascular Risk (Myocardial Infarction, Congestive Heart Failure, Death)

Major
Unstable coronary syndromes
Recent myocardial infarction* with evidence of important ischemic risk by clinical symptoms or noninvasive study
Unstable or severe† angina (Canadian Cardiovascular Society Class III or IV)‡
Decompensated congestive heart failure
Significant arrhythmias
High-grade atrioventricular block
Symptomatic ventricular arrhythmias in the presence of underlying heart disease
Supraventricular arrhythmias with uncontrolled ventricular rate
Severe valvular disease
Intermediate
Mild angina pectoris (Canadian Cardiovascular Society Class I or II)
Prior myocardial infarction by history or pathologic waves
Compensated or prior congestive heart failure
Diabetes mellitis
Minor
Advanced age
Abnormal electrocardiogram (left ventricular hypertrophy, left bundle branch block, ST-T abnormalities)
Rhythm other than sinus (e.g., atrial fibrillation)
Low functional capacity (e.g., unable to climb one flight of stairs with a bag of groceries)
History of stroke
Uncontrolled systemic hypertension

*The American College of Cardiology National Database Library defines *recent myocardial infarction* as greater than 7 days but less than or equal to 1 month (30 days)
†May include "stable" angina in patients who are unusually sedentary.
‡Campeau L: Grading of angina pectoris. Circulation 54:522, 1976.

TABLE 35–17
Estimated Energy Requirements for Various Activities*

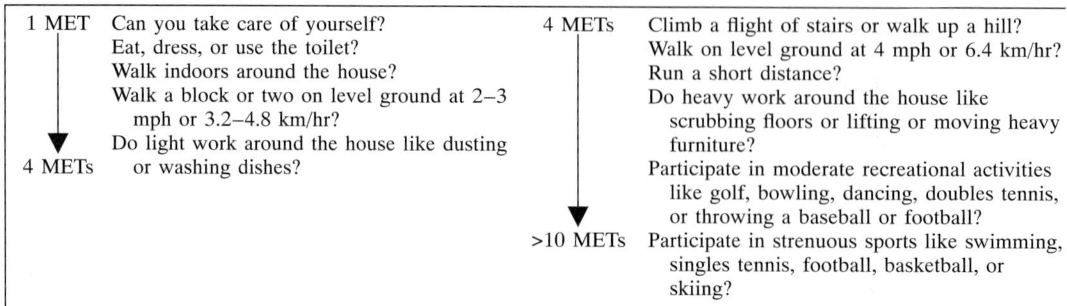

METs	Activity	METs	Activity
1 MET ↓ 4 METs	Can you take care of yourself? Eat, dress, or use the toilet? Walk indoors around the house? Walk a block or two on level ground at 2–3 mph or 3.2–4.8 km/hr? Do light work around the house like dusting or washing dishes?	4 METs ↓	Climb a flight of stairs or walk up a hill? Walk on level ground at 4 mph or 6.4 km/hr? Run a short distance? Do heavy work around the house like scrubbing floors or lifting or moving heavy furniture? Participate in moderate recreational activities like golf, bowling, dancing, doubles tennis, or throwing a baseball or football?
		>10 METs	Participate in strenuous sports like swimming, singles tennis, football, basketball, or skiing?

*Adapted from Hlatky MC, Boineau RE, Higginbotham MB, et al: A brief self-administered questionnaire to determine functional capacity (the Duke Activity Status Index). Am J Cardiol 64:651, 1989; and Fletcher FG, Balady G, Froelicher VF, et al: Exercise standards: A statement for healthcare professionals from the American Heart Association. Circulation 91:580, 1995, with permission.

egy has led to a proposed algorithm based on collected observational data and expert opinion. A stepwise bayesian strategy is built on the following clinical markers: prior coronary evaluation and treatment, functional capacity, and surgery-specific risk. These markers are outlined and correlated with the information in Tables 35–16 through 35–19. This stepwise algorithm format is a framework that determines cardiac risk and those patients that are candidates for cardiac testing or angiography.[272–274]

Special Effects on Postoperative Cardiovascular Complications

Pulmonary Effect on Cardiovascular Function

Postoperative mechanical ventilation may adversely affect cardiovascular function when airway pressure manipulation decreases the effective cardiac filling volume or increases pulmonary vascular resistance. Decreased cardiac output with positive end-expiratory pressure is attributed to decreased venous return to the right heart chamber, increased pulmonary resistance with increased right-side afterload, and decreased LV filling.[275] Intravascular volume expansion can correct decreased right and LV filling, but may also aggravate lung water accumulation and increase pulmonary venous admixture. Pulmonary vasodilators can decrease right-side afterload, but may further increase shunt fraction and decrease oxygenation.[276] Positive end-expiratory pressure appears to establish the level that provides the best balance between pulmonary and hemodynamic responses to establish optimum pulmonary and cardiac function. Airway pressure therapy may have adverse hemodynamic effects, and its use should not be focused on pulmonary effects alone.

TABLE 35–18
Cardiac Event Risk* Stratification for Noncardiac Surgical Procedure

High
(Reported cardiac risk often >5%)
Emergent major operations, particularly in the elderly
Aortic and other major vascular
Peripheral vascular
Anticipated prolonged surgical procedures associated with large fluid shifts and/or blood loss
Intermediate
(Reported cardiac risk generally <5%)
Carotid endarterectomy
Head and neck
Intraperitoneal and intrathoracic
Orthopedic
Prostate
Low†
(Reported cardiac risk generally <1%)
Endoscopic procedures
Superficial procedures
Cataract
Breast

*Combined incidence of cardiac death and nonfatal myocardial infarction.
†Further preoperative cardiac testing is not generally required.

Effect of Postoperative Anemia on Cardiovascular Function

Within the physiologic range of hematocrit and intravascular volume, maintenance of normovolemic status is more important to systemic O_2 delivery than is hemoglobin concentration.[277] However, in cardiovascular patients, the increased cardiac output required to maintain O_2 delivery with reduced hemoglobin concentrations may not be well tolerated. Hematocrit above 32% is recommended to maintain O_2 delivery and ensure patient survival.[278] However, other factors to be considered are overall metabolic status and transfusion risks. Minor reactions occur in 1 in 100 of transfusions, and more serious complications in 1 in 6,000 to 10,000. The risk for posttransfusion hepatitis, however, can be as high as 1 to 7% in certain surgical groups.[279]

Effect of Postoperative Hypothermia and Shivering on Cardiovascular Function

Postoperative hypothermia with shivering increases MVO_2 up to 500%.[280] Its incidence is 5% in noncardiac

TABLE 35–19
Indications for Coronary Angiography in Perioperative Evaluation Before (or After) Noncardiac Surgery*†

Class I:‡ Patients with suspected or proven CAD
High-risk results during noninvasive testing
Angina pectoris unresponsive to adequate medical therapy
Most patients with unstable angina pectoris
Nondiagnostic or equivocal noninvasive test in a high-risk patient (Table 35–16) undergoing a high-risk surgical procedure (Table 35–18)
Anticipated prolonged surgical procedures associated with large fluid shifts and/or blood loss
Class II‡
Intermediate risk results during noninvasive testing
Nondiagnostic or equivocal noninvasive test in a lower-risk patient (Table 35–1) undergoing a high-risk noncardiac surgical procedure (Table 35–3)
Urgent noncardiac surgery in a patient convalescing from acute MI
Perioperative MI
Class III‡
Low-risk noncardiac surgery (Table 35–3) in a patient with known CAD and low-risk results on noninvasive testing
Screening for CAD without appropriate noninvasive testing
Asymptomatic after coronary revascularization, with excellent exercise capacity (≥7 METs)
Mild stable angina in patients with good LV function, low-risk noninvasive test results because of concomitant medical illness
Patient is not a candidate for coronary revascularization because of concomitant medical illness
Prior technically adequate normal coronary angiogram within previous 5 years
Severe LV dysfunction (e.g., ejection fraction <20%) and patient not considered candidate for revascularization procedure
Patient unwilling to consider coronary revascularization procedure

CAD, coronary artery disease; MI, myocardial infarction; MET, metabolic equivalent; LV, left ventricular.
*Adapted from ACC/AHA Guidelines for Coronary Angiography. (JACC 10: 935, 1987; and Circulation 76:963A, 1987, with permission.)
†If results of coronary angiography will affect management.
‡Class I: Conditions for which there is evidence for and/or general agreement that a procedure be performed or a treatment is of benefit. Class II: Conditions for which there is a divergence of evidence and/or opinion about the treatment. Class III: Conditions for which there is evidence and/or general agreement that the procedure is not necessary.

procedures,[281] and it may be higher in cardiac procedures that involve cooling and rewarming. Hypothermia can also cause vasoconstriction, increased afterload, and hypertension. Treatment should include warm humidification of respiratory gases if intubated, warming blankets, radiant warming devices and forced air warmers[281]; the latter are superior in maintenance of body temperature.[282] Effective treatment for shivering without reducing MVO_2 can be achieved with meperidine (12.5 to 25 mg),[283] while muscle activity can be stopped using muscle relaxants in mechanically ventilated patients. Even though the effect of meperidine is transient, shivering tends not to recur. Postoperative shivering can also occur after regional anesthesia, when motor and sensory function return, and should be treated to decrease MVO_2.

Effect of Cardiac Surgery with Cardiopulmonary Bypass on Cardiovascular Function

Establishing and maintaining cardiopulmonary bypass can be associated with cardiovascular problems.[284] Confirming the location of the perfusion cannula tip is important in order to reduce the likelihood of complications. During cardiopulmonary bypass, damage to the coronary artery can result from the improper use of intraluminal cardioplegia perfusion cannulae, surgical dissection of the myocardium retractors and clamps, and other manipulations.

Technical problems in ACB surgery can damage the myocardium and influence its survival. Small anastomoses have a 50% incidence of occlusion within the first year.[285] Any interruption of the inflow of the coronary artery may increase the risk for thrombus formation, wall dissection, and graft failure. Aortic and myocardial anastomotic sites are prone to many complications. In addition, subadventitial hematoma and, rarely, true aortic dissection may originate at the proximal site. Graft occlusion can appear early (within the first month) or late (after the first year) (see Table 35–20).[284] Internal mammary arteries have a patency rate of over 90%. However, their use may lead to increased postoperative bleeding, graft occlusion with large respiratory inflation volumes, and respiratory failure due to the opened pleural cavity.[286]

Hypotension and low cardiac output may occur in patients in whom significant ischemic areas remain after cardiopulmonary bypass grafting, or in whom myocardial metabolic imbalance occurs from hyperkalemia and acidosis. Low-output syndrome is characterized by low cardiac output, vasoconstriction, hypotension, and acidosis, resulting also in low perfusion to the extremities

TABLE 35–20
Mechanism of Perioperative Myocardial Infarction Due to Surgical Factors*

Event	Coronaries	Contractility	Surgical Factors
Severity of preoperative myocardial ischemia	Diffuse multiple vessel coronary artery disease 1. Technical difficulties with anastomosis 2. Prolonged cross-clamp time 3. Prolonged CPB 4. Incomplete revascularization Left main coronary disease	Depressed preoperative ejection fraction Elevated preoperative left ventricular end-diastolic pressure (LVEDP)	Reperfusion injury Localized trauma to coronary arteries from clamps or snares Endarterectomy Intramyocardial dissection

*Modified from Conahan TJ III: Complications of cardiac surgery. In Kaplan JA (ed): Cardiac Anesthesia, 2nd ed, Vol. 2. Orlando, FL, Grune & Stratton, 1987, p 1105, with permission.

and kidneys. Parallel right and left filling pressures without response to controlled fluid challenge can help to detect and treat the syndrome.

General guidelines for treatment include ensuring maximal O_2 delivery (O_2 administration, maintenance of hemoglobin, ensuring adequate diastolic perfusion time) and correction of metabolic disorders. Pharmacologic therapy is directed at increasing contractility (catecholamines, amrinone), decreasing afterload (nitroprusside, nitroglycerin), and increasing substrate delivery (glucose, insulin, potassium solution).[287] When pharmacologic support is not enough, mechanical circulatory support must be added. The need for an intra-aortic balloon pump varies 2 to 5% between centers.[288] Use of an intra-aortic balloon pump is associated with an 11 to 23% incidence of complications. Successful insertion may occur in only 70% of patients. Damage to the femoral/iliac artery, aortic dissection, distal ischemia of the leg, peripheral neuropathy, and local hematoma or infection can occur.[289]

The risk of perioperative MI following cardiopulmonary bypass is about 6%.[290,291] Factors associated with this complication are summarized in Table 35–20. The severity of preoperative coronary disease and cardiopulmonary bypass duration are associated with an increased incidence of MI; however, the clinical implications of this observation are less clear.[284] Long-term survival is decreased when the MI is complicated by congestive heart failure, cardiogenic shock, arrhythmia, ventricular tachycardia, or cardiac arrest.[290]

Surgical relief of valve incompetence does not always result in immediate cardiac function improvement. Replacement of an insufficient valve may suddenly force a marginally functioning ventricle to increase work against a higher afterload. Also, chronic pulmonary problems due to longstanding valvular disease can complicate the postoperative course.

Technical aspects of the operation can also affect outcome. Thrombus formation in the left atrium, especially with atrial fibrillation, can be a source of emboli, especially in the prebypass period. Most open-valve surgery procedures are performed with the heart arrested using hypothermia and cardioplegia for myocardial protection. For some valvular disease patients, myocardial preservation is less effective due to severe ventricular hypertrophy. Different cardiac valve prostheses may cause different complications: flow obstruction, valve incompetence, thrombogenicity, hemolysis, endocarditis, or certain anatomic problems.[292] Removal of the damaged valve can also cause problems such as the forcing of debris into the left atrium, LV, or coronary arteries. Extensive removal of calcium from mitral anulus may cause disruption of the AV junction—almost always fatal—and damage to the bundle of His and the AV node.[293]

Pericardial closure after cardiac operations to prevent adhesions and protect grafts may force graft repositioning, compromise flow, cause ischemia, and create conditions for tamponade in case of postoperative bleeding. All filling pressures are elevated and tend to equalize, reflecting increased intrapericardial pressure and reduced cardiac output due to underfilled LV. Reflex tachycardia will further decrease diastolic filling time and myocardial ischemia will be inevitable. Rapid reopening of the periocardium with support of the circulation are essential.[294]

Acknowledgment

The authors wish to thank R.F. Davis for his crucial part in initiating this work and laying the foundation for the gathering of related information.

References

1. DeBakey ME, Crawford CS, Cooley DA, et al: Aneurysm of abdominal aorta: Analysis of results of graft replacement therapy one to eleven years after operation. Ann Surg 160:622, 1964.
2. Falkenberg M, Gabel H, Gothman B, et al: Abdominal aortic aneurysm: An interhospital study of 171 surgically treated patients. Scand J Thorac Cardiovasc Surg 9:271, 1975.
3. Szilagyi DE, Smith RF, DeRusso FJ, et al: Contribution of abdominal aortic aneurysmectomy to prolongation of life. Ann Surg 164:678, 1966.
4. Young AE, Sandberg GW, Couch NP: The reduction of mortality of abdominal aortic aneurysm resection. Am J Surg 134:585, 1977.
5. Thompson JE, Hollier LH, Patman RD, et al: Surgical management of abdominal aortic aneurysms: Factors influencing mortality and morbidity—a 20-year experience. Ann Surg 181:654, 1975.
6. Hicks GL, Eastland MW, DeWeese JA, et al: Survival improvement following aortic aneurysm resection. Ann Surg 181:863, 1975.
7. Fedde CW, Hobson RW, Rich NM: Surgical management of 100 consecutive abdominal aortic aneurysms. Am J Surg 129:506, 1975.
8. Scobie TK, Masters RG: Changing factors influencing abdominal aortic aneurysm repair. J Cardiovasc Surg 23:309, 1982.
9. Crawford ES, Saleh SA, Babb JW, et al: Infrarenal abdominal aortic aneurysm: Factors influencing survival after operation performed over a 25-year period. Ann Surg 193:699, 1981.
10. Yeager RA, Moneta GL, McConnell DB, et al: Analysis of risk factors for myocardial infarction following carotid endarterectomy. Arch Surg 124:1142, 1989.
11. Jamieson WRE, Janusz MT, Miyagishima RT, et al: Influence of ischemic heart disease on early and late mortality after surgery for peripheral occlusive vascular disease. Circulation 66(Suppl I):I-92, 1982.
12. Roizen MF: But what does it do to outcome. Anesth Analg 63:789, 1984.
13. Miller DC, Stinson EB, Oyer PE, et al: Discriminant analysis of the changing risks of coronary artery operations: 1971–1979. J Thorac Cardiovasc Surg 85:197, 1983.
14. Kennedy JW, Kaiser GC, Fisher LD, et al: Clinical and angiographic predictors of operative mortality from the collaborative study in coronary artery surgery (CASS). Circulation 63:793, 1981.
15. Christakis GT, Kormos RL, Weisel RD, et al: Morbidity and mortality in mitral valve surgery. Circulation 72(Suppl II):II-120, 1985.
16. Verrier ED, Edelist G, Consigny PM, et al: Greater coronary vascular reserve in dogs anesthetized with halothane. Anesthesiology 53:445, 1980.
17. Bland JH, Lowenstein E: Halothane-induced decrease in experimental myocardial ischemia in the non-failing canine heart. Anesthesiology 45:287, 1976.
18. Tarnow J, Markschies-Hornung A, Schulte-Sasse U: Isoflurane improves the tolerance to pacing-induced myocardial ischemia. Anesthesiology 64:147, 1986.
19. Davis RF, DeBoer LW, Rude RE, et al: The effect of halothane anesthesia on myocardial necrosis, hemodynamic performance, and regional myocardial blood flow in dogs following coronary artery occlusion. Anesthesiology 59:402, 1983.
20. Davis RF, Sidi A: Effect of isoflurane on the extent of myocardial necrosis and on systemic hemodynamics, regional myocar-

dial blood flow, and regional myocardial metabolism in dogs after coronary artery occlusion. Anesth Analg 69:575, 1989.
21. Hickey RF, Sybert PE, Verrier ED, Cason BA: Effects of halothane, enflurane, and isoflurane on coronary blood flow autoregulation and coronary vascular reserve in the canine heart. Anesthesiology 68:21, 1987.
22. Priebe H-J: Differential effect of isoflurane on right and left ventricular performances, and on coronary, systemic, and pulmonary hemodynamics in the dog. Anesthesiology 66:262, 1987.
23. Sill JC, Bove AA, Nugent M, et al: Effects of isoflurane on coronary arteries and coronary arterioles in the intact dog. Anesthesiology 66:273, 1987.
24. Buffington CW, Romson JL, Levine A, et al: Isoflurane induces coronary steal in a canine model of chronic coronary occlusion. Anesthesiology 66:280, 1987.
25. Lowenstein E, Foex P, Francis CM, et al: Regional ischemic ventricular dysfunction in myocardium supplied by a narrowed coronary artery with increasing halothane concentration in the dog. Anesthesiology 55:349, 1981.
26. Reiz S, Balfors E, Sorensen MB, et al: Isoflurane—a powerful coronary vasodilator in patients with coronary artery disease. Anesthesiology 59:91, 1983.
27. Becker LC: Is isoflurane dangerous for the patient with coronary artery disease? Anesthesiology 66:259, 1987.
28. Mangano DT: Anesthetics, coronary artery disease, and outcome: Unresolved controversies. Anesthesiology 70:175, 1989.
29. Rao TK, Jacobs KH, El-Etr AA: Reinfarction following anesthesia in patients with myocardial infarction. Anesthesiology 59: 499, 1983.
30. Slogoff S, Keats AS: Randomized trial of primary anesthetic agents on outcome of coronary bypass operations. Anesthesiology 70:179, 1989.
31. Roizen MF: Does choice of anesthetic (narcotic versus inhalational) significantly affect cardiovascular outcome after cardiovascular surgery? In Estafanous FG (ed): Opioids in Anesthesia. Boston, Butterworth, 1984, p 180.
32. Moffitt EA, Sethna DH, Bussell JA, et al: Myocardial metabolism and hemodynamic responses to halothane or morphine anesthesia for coronary artery surgery. Anesth Analg 61:979, 1982.
33. Benefiel DJ, Roizen MF, Lampe GH, et al: Morbidity after aortic surgery with sufentanil vs. isoflurane anesthesia (Abstract). Anesthesiology 65:A516, 1986.
34. Reves JG, Samuelson PN, Lell WA, et al: Myocardial damage in coronary artery bypass surgical patients anesthetized with two anaesthetic techniques: A random comparison of halothane and enflurane. Can Anaesth Soc J 27:238, 1980.
35. Moffitt EA, Imrie DD, Scovil JE, et al: Myocardial metabolism and haemodynamic responses with enflurane anaesthesia for coronary artery surgery. Can Anaesth Soc J 31:604, 1984.
36. Moffitt EA, Barker RA, Glenn JJ, et al: Myocardial metabolism and hemodynamic responses with isoflurane anesthesia for coronary arterial surgery. Anesth Analg 65:53, 1986.
37. Buffington CW, Romson JL, Levine A, et al: Isoflurane induces coronary steal in a canine model of chronic coronary occlusion. Anesthesiology 66:22, 1987.
38. Tuman KJ, McCarthy RJ, Spiess BD, et al: Does choice of anesthetic agent significantly affect outcome after coronary artery surgery? Anesthesiology 70:189, 1989.
39. Inoue K, Reichelt W, El-Banayosy A: Does isoflurane lead to a higher incidence of myocardial infarction and perioperative death than enflurane in coronary artery surgery? Anesth Analg 71:469, 1990.
40. Smith JS, Roizen MF, Cahalan MK, et al: Does anesthetic technique make a difference? Augmentation of systolic blood pressure during carotid endarterectomy: Effects of phenylephrine vs. light anesthesia and of isoflurane vs. halothane on the incidence of myocardial ischemia. Anesthesiology 69:846, 1988.
41. Reves JG, Lell WA, McCracken LE Jr, et al: Comparison of morphine and ketamine anesthetic technics for coronary surgery: A randomized study. South Med J 71:33, 1978.
42. Stanford TJ Jr, Smith NT, Dec-Silver H, et al: A comparison of morphine, fentanyl, and sufentanil anesthesia for cardiac surgery: Induction, emergency, and extubation. Anesth Analg 65: 259, 1986.
43. Quasha AL, Loeber N, Feeley TW, et al: Postoperative respiratory care: A controlled trial of early and late extubation following coronary-artery bypass grafting. Anesthesiology 52:135, 1980.
44. Barash PG: Monitoring myocardial oxygen balance: Physiologic basis and clinical application. American Society of Anesthesiologists. Refresher Courses in Anesthesiology 13:21, 1985.
45. Slogoff S, Keats AS: Further observations on perioperative myocardial ischemia. Anesthesiology 5:539, 1986.
46. Slogoff S, Keats AS: Does perioperative myocardial ischemia lead to postoperative myocardial infarction? Anesthesiology 62: 107, 1985.
47. London MJ, Hollenberg M, Wong MG, et al: Intraoperative myocardial ischemia: Localization by continuous 12-lead electrocardiography. Anesthesiology 69:232, 1988.
48. Wohlgelernter D, Cleman M, Highman HA, et al: Regional myocardial dysfunction during coronary angioplasty; evaluation by two-dimensional echocardiography and 12 lead electrocardiography. J Am Coll Cardiol 7:1245, 1986.
49. Kaplan JA, Wells PH: Early diagnosis of myocardial ischemia using the pulmonary arterial catheter. Anesth Analg 60:789, 1981.
50. Breslow MJ, Miller CF, Parker SD, et al: Changes in T-wave morphology following anesthesia and surgery: A common recovery-room phenomenon. Anesthesiology 64:398, 1986.
51. Biagini A, L'Abbate AL, Testa R, et al: Unreliability of conventional visual electrocardiographic monitoring for detection of transient ST segment changes in coronary care unit. Eur Heart J 5:784, 1984.
52. Kotrly K, Kotter GS, Mortara D, Kampine JP: Intraoperative detection of myocardial ischemia with ST segment trend monitoring system. Anesth Analg 63:343, 1984.
53. Kaplan JA, Wells PH: Early diagnosis of myocardial ischemia using the pulmonary artery catheter. Anesth Analg 60:789, 1981.
54. Waller JL, Johnson SP, Kaplan JA: Usefulness of pulmonary artery catheters during aortocoronary bypass surgery. Anesth Analg 61:221, 1982.
55. Baele PL, McMichan JC, Marsh HM, et al: Continuous monitoring of mixed venous oxygen saturation in critically ill patients. Anesth Analg 61:513, 1982.
56. Waller JL, Kaplan JA, Bauman DI, Carver JM: Clinical evaluation of a new fiberoptic catheter oximeter during cardiac surgery. Anesth Analg 61:676, 1982.
57. Shoemaker WC, Appel PL, Kram HB, Lee TS: Comparison of two monitoring methods (central venous pressure versus pulmonary artery catheter) and two protocols as therapeutic goals (normal values versus values of survivors) in a prospective randomized clinical trial of critically ill surgical patients. Crit Care Med 13:304, 1985.
58. Rao TLK, Jacobs KH, El-Etr AA: Reinfarction following anesthesia in patients with myocardial infarction. Anesthesiology 59: 499, 1983.
59. Hansen RM, Viquerat CE, Matthay MA, et al: Poor correlation between pulmonary arterial wedge pressure and left ventricular end diastolic volume after coronary artery bypass graft surgery. Anesthesiology 64:764, 1986.
60. Katz JD, Coronau LH, Barash PG, Mandel SD: Pulmonary artery flow-guided catheters in the perioperative period. Indications and complications. JAMA 237:2832, 1977.
61. Bashein G, Johnson PW, Davis KB, et al: Elective coronary bypass surgery without pulmonary artery catheter monitoring. Anesthesiology 63:451, 1985.
62. Tuman KJ, McCarthy RJ, Spiess BD, et al: Effect of pulmonary artery catheterization on outcome in patients undergoing coronary artery surgery. Anesthesiology 70:199, 1989.
63. Spackman TN: A theoretical evaluation of cost-effectiveness of pulmonary artery catheters in patients undergoing coronary artery surgery. J Cardiothorac Vasc Anesth 85(5):570, 1994.
64. Pearson KS, Gomez MN, Moyers JR, et al: A cost benefit analysis of randomized invasive monitoring for patients undergoing cardiac surgery. Anesth Analg 69:336, 1989.
65. Moore CH, Lombardo R, Allums JA, Gordon FT: Left main coronary artery stenosis: Hemodynamic monitoring to reduce mortality. Ann Thorac Surg 26:445, 1978.
66. Robin ED:Death by pulmonary artery flow-directed catheter. Chest 92:727, 1987.

67. Task Force on Guidelines for Pulmonary Artery Catheterization: Practice guidelines for pulmonary artery catheterization. Anesthesiology 78:380, 1993.
68. Shoemaker WC, Appel PL, Kram HB, et al: Prospective trial of supranormal values of survivors as therapeutic goals in high-risk surgical patients. Chest 94:1176, 1988.
69. Berlauk JF, Abrams JH, Gilmour IJ, et al: Preoperative optimization of cardiovascular hemodynamics improves outcome in peripheral vascular surgery: A prospective randomized clinical trial. Ann Surg 214:289, 1991.
70. Isaacson IJ, Lowdon JD, Berry AJ, et al: The value of pulmonary artery and central venous monitoring in patients undergoing abdominal aortic reconstructive surgery: A comparative study of two selected, randomized groups. J Vasc Surg 12:754, 1990.
71. Joyce WP, Provan JL, Ameli FM, et al: The role of central haemodynamic monitoring in abdominal aortic surgery: A prospective randomised study. Eur J Vasc Surg 4:633, 1990.
72. Hesdorffer CS, Milne JF, Meyers AM, et al: The value of Swan-Ganz catheterization and volume loading in preventing renal failure in patients undergoing abdominal aneurysmectomy. Clin Nephrol 28:272, 1987.
73. Gore JM, Goldbert RJ, Spodick DH, et al: A community-wide assessment of the use of pulmonary artery catheters in patients with acute myocardial infarction. Chest 92:721, 1987.
74. Zion MM, Balkin J, Rosenmann D, et al: Use of pulmonary artery catheters in patients with acute myocardial infarction: Analysis of experience in 5,841 patients in the SPRINT Registry. Chest 98:1331, 1990.
75. Bush HS, Taylor RW, Thoi L, et al: Does invasive hemodynamic monitoring improve survival in a medical intensive care unit? (Abstract). Crit Care Med 17:S137, 1989.
76. Reynolds NH, Haupt MT, Thill-Baharozian MC, Carlson RW: Impact of critical care physician staffing on patients with septic shock in a university hospital medical intensive care unit. JAMA 260:3446, 1988.
77. Smith JS, Cahalan MK, Benefiel DJ, et al: Intraoperative detection of myocardial ischemia in high-risk patients: Electrocardiography versus two-dimensional transesophageal echocardiography. Circulation 72:1015, 1985.
78. Leung JM, O'Kelly B, Browner WS, et al: Prognostic importance of post-bypass regional wall motion abnormalities in patients undergoing coronary bypass graft surgery. Anesthesiology 71:16, 1989.
79. Sheikh KH, deBruijn NP, Rankin JS, et al: The utility of transesophageal echocardiography and Doppler color flow imaging in patients undergoing cardiac valve surgery. J Am Cell Cardiol 15:363, 1990.
80. Clements F: The evolution of the anesthesiologist-echocardiographer. In deBruijn NP, Clements FM (eds): Intraoperative Use of Echocardiography. Philadelphia, JB Lippincott Co, 1991, p 1.
81. Slogoff S, Keats AS: Does chronic treatment with calcium entry blocking drugs reduce perioperative myocardial ischemia? Anesthesiology 68:676, 1988.
82. Knight AA, Hollenberg M, London MJ, et al: Perioperative myocardial ischemia: Importance of the preoperative ischemic pattern. Anesthesiology 68:861, 1988.
83. Mangano DT, Layug EL, Wallace A, Tateo I: Effect of atenolol on morbidity after noncardiac surgery. Multicenter study of perioperative ischemia research group. N Engl J Med 335:1713, 1996.
84. Mangano DT: Effects of acadesine on myocardial infarction, stroke, and death after surgery. A meta-analysis of 5 international randomized trials. The multicenter study of perioperative ischemia (McSPI) research group. JAMA 277:325, 1997.
85. Kaplan JA, Dunbar RW, Jones EL: Nitroglycerin infusion during coronary-artery surgery. Anesthesiology 45:14, 1976.
86. Thomson IR, Mutch WAC, Culligan JD: Failure of intravenous nitroglycerin to prevent intraoperative myocardial ischemia during fentanyl-pancuronium anesthesia. Anesthesiology 61:385, 1984.
87. Mangano DT: Perioperative cardiac morbidity. Anesthesiology 72:153, 1990.
88. Ouyang P, Gerstenblith G, Furman WR, et al: Frequency and significance of early postoperative silent myocardial ischemia in patients having peripheral vascular surgery. Am J Cardiol 64:1113, 1989.
89. Pasternack PF, Grossi EA, Baumann FG, et al: The value of silent myocardial ischemia monitoring in the prediction of perioperative myocardial infarction in patients undergoing peripheral vascular surgery. J Vasc Surg 10:617, 1989.
90. Braunwald E, Kloner RA: The stunned myocardium: Prolonged postischemic ventricular dysfunction. Circulation 66:1146, 1982.
91. Goldman L, Caldera DL, Nussbaum SR, et al: Multifactorial index of cardiac risk in noncardiac surgical procedures. N Engl J Med 297:845, 1977.
92. Tarhan S, Moffitt EA, Taylor WF, et al: Myocardial infarction after general anesthesia. JAMA 220:1451, 1972.
93. Steen PA, Tinker JH, Tarhan S: Myocardial reinfarction after anesthesia and surgery. JAMA 239:2566, 1978.
94. von Knorring J: Postoperative myocardial infarction: A prospective study in a risk group of surgical patients. Surgery 90:55, 1981.
95. Pasternack PF, Imparato AM, Bear G, et al: The value of radionuclide angiography as a predictor of perioperative myocardial infarction in patients undergoing abdominal aortic aneurysm resection. J Vasc Surg 1:320, 1984.
96. Diebel LN, Lange MP, Schneider F, et al: Cardiopulmonary complications after major surgery: A role for epidural analgesia? Surgery 102:660, 1987.
97. Charlson ME, MacKenzie CR, Ales K, et al: Surveillance for postoperative myocardial infarction after noncardiac operations. Surg Gynecol Obstet 167:407, 1988.
98. Cohn PF: Silent myocardial ischemia. Ann Intern Med 109:312, 1988.
99. Lott JA, Stang JM: Serum enzymes and isoenzymes in the diagnosis and differential diagnosis of myocardial ischemia and necrosis. Clin Chem 26:1241, 1980.
100. Haggmark S, Hohner P, Ostman M, et al: Comparison of hemodynamic, electrocardiographic, mechanical, and metabolic indicators of intraoperative myocardial ischemia in vascular surgical patients with coronary artery disease. Anesthesiology 70:19, 1989.
101. Roizen MF, Beaupre PN, Alpert RA, et al: Monitoring with two-dimensional transesophageal echocardiography: Comparison of myocardial function in patients undergoing supraceliac, suprarenal-infraceliac, or infrarenal aortic occlusion. J Vasc Surg 5:607, 1987.
102. Gewertz BL, Kremser PC, Zarins CK, et al: Transesophageal echocardiographic monitoring of myocardial ischemia during vascular surgery. J Vasc Surg 5:607, 1987.
103. Lott JA: Serum enzyme determinations in the diagnosis of acute myocardial infarction: An update. Hum Pathol 15:706, 1984.
104. Chung F, Houston PL, Cheng DCH, et al: Calcium channel blockade does not offer adequate protection from perioperative myocardial ischemia. Anesthesiology 69(3):323, 1988.
105. Pasternack PR, Grossi EA, Baumann FG, et al: Beta blockade to decrease silent myocardial ischemia during peripheral vascular surgery. Am J Surg 158:113, 1989.
106. Jain U, Laflamme CJ, Aggarwal A, et al: Electrocardiographic and hemodynamic changes and their association with myocardial infarction during coronary artery bypass surgery. A multicenter study. Multicenter study of perioperative ischemia (McSPI) research group. Anesthesiology 86:576, 1997.
107. Coriat P, Daloz M, Bousseau D, et al: Prevention of intraoperative myocardial ischemia during noncardiac surgery with intravenous nitroglycerin. Anesthesiology 61:193, 1984.
108. Coriat P, Mundler O, Bousseau D, et al: Response of left ventricular ejection fraction to recovery from general anesthesia: Measurement by gated radionuclide angiography. Anesth Analg 65:593, 1986.
109. Maroko PR, Radvany P, Braunwald E, Hale S: Reduction of infarct size by oxygen inhalation following acute coronary occlusion. Circulation 52:360, 1975.
110. Shnier CB, Cason BA, Horton A, et al: Hyperoxemic reperfusion does not increase myocardial infarct size. Am J Physiol 260:H-1307, 1991.
111. Lie KI, Wellens HJ, van Cappelle FJ, et al: Lidocaine in the prevention of primary ventricular fibrillation: A double-blind, randomized study of 212 consecutive patients. N Engl J Med 291:1324, 1974.
112. Abraham AS, Rosenmann D, Kramer M, et al: Magnesium in

the prevention of lethal arrhythmias in acute myocardial infarction. Arch Intern Med 147:753, 1987.
113. Peterson JE, Emmot WW: Therapies to limit infarct size. Timing, dosage, and effectiveness. Postgrad Med 86:54, 1989.
114. ISIS-1 (First International Study of Infarct Survival) Collaborative Group: Randomised trial of intravenous atenolol among 16,027 cases of suspected acute myocardial infarction: ISIS-1. Lancet 2:57, 1986.
115. Yusuf S, Peto R, Lewis J, et al: Beta-blockade during and after myocardial infarction: An overview of the randomized trials. Prog Cardiovasc Dis 26:335, 1985.
116. Morganroth J, Horowitz LN, Anderson J, et al: Comparative efficacy and tolerance of esmolol to propranolol for control of supraventricular tachyarrhythmia. Am J Cardiol 56:33F, 1985.
117. Steck J, Sheppard D, Byrd RC, et al: Pulmonary effects of esmolol—an ultra short-acting beta adrenergic blocking agent (Abstract). Clin Res 33:472A, 1985.
118. Bussmann WD, Passek D, Seidel W, et al: Reduction of CK and CK-MB indexes of infarct size by intravenous nitroglycerin. Circulation 63:615, 1981.
119. Jaffe AL, Geltman EM, Tiefenbrunn AJ, et al: Reduction of infarct size in patients with inferior infarction with intravenous glyceryl trinitrate: A randomised study. Br Heart J 59:452, 1983.
120. Flaherty JT, Becker LC, Bulkley BH, et al: A randomized prospective trial of intravenous nitroglycerin in patients with acute myocardial infarction. Circulation 68:576, 1983.
121. Yusuf S, Collins R, MacMahon S, et al: Effect of intravenous nitrates on mortality in acute myocardial infarction: An overview of the randomised trials. Lancet 1:1088, 1988.
122. Gibson RS, Boden WE, Theroux P, et al: Diltiazem and reinfarction in patients with non-Q-wave myocardial infarction. Results of a double-blind, randomized, multicenter trial. N Engl J Med 315:423, 1986.
123. Sidi A, Pool JM, Rush W: Early administration of amrinone does not impair regional metabolism of O_2 or lactate and, by improving myocardial performance, preserves myocardial blood flow in the ischemic canine heart. Anesth Analg 76:1201, 1993.
124. Fita G, Gomar C, Jimenez MJ, et al: Amrinone in perioperative low cardiac output syndrome. Acta Anaesthesiol Scand 34:482, 1990.
125. Rutherford JD, Braunwald E: Thrombolytic therapy in acute myocardial infarction. Chest 97(Suppl 4):136S, 1990.
126. Second International Study of Infarct Survival Collaborative Group (ISIS-2): Randomized trial of intravenous streptokinase oral aspirin, both, or neither among 17,187 cases of suspected acute myocardial infarction. ISIS-2. Lancet 2:349, 1988.
127. Wilcox RG, von der Lippe G, Olsson CG, et al: Trial of tissue plasminogen activator for mortality reduction in acute myocardial infarction. Lancet 2:525, 1988.
128. Spann JF, Sherry S: Coronary thrombolysis for evolving myocardial infarction. Drugs 28:465, 1984.
129. Gurbel PA, Navetta FI, Bates ER, et al: Lesion-directed administration of altepase with intracoronary heparin in patients with unstable angina and coronary thrombus undergoing angioplasty. Cathet Cardiovasc Diagn 37:382, 1996.
130. Law MM, Gelabert HA, Colburn MD, et al: Continuous postoperative intra-arterial urokinase infusion in the treatment of no reflow following revascularization of the acutely ischemic limb. Ann Vasc Surg 8:66, 1994.
131. Atkins JM, Leshin SJ, Blomqvist G, et al: Ventricular conduction blocks and sudden death in acute myocardial infarction: Potential indications for pacing. N Engl J Med 288:281, 1973.
132. Gann D, Balachandran PK, Sherif NE, et al: Prognostic significance of chronic versus acute bundle branch block in acute myocardial infarction. Chest 67:298, 1975.
133. Zaiden JR: Pacemakers. Anesthesiology 60(4):319, 1984.
134. Lindsay BD, Cain ME: Cardiac arrhythmias. In Orland MJ, Saltman RJ (eds): Manual of Medical Therapeutics, 25th ed. Boston, Little, Brown & Co, 1986.
135. Lown B, Kosowsky BD: Artificial cardiac pacemakers (first of three parts). N Engl J Med 283:907, 1970.
136. Katz RL, Bigger JT Jr: Cardiac arrhythmias during anesthesia and operation. Anesthesiology 33:193, 1970.
137. Bertrand CA, Steiner NV, Jameson AG, et al: Disturbances of cardiac rhythm during anesthesia and surgery. JAMA 216:1615, 1971.
138. Vanik PE, Davis HS: Cardiac arrhythmias during halothane anesthesia. Anesth Analg 47:299, 1968.
139. Task Force of the Working Group on Arrhythmias of the European Society of Cardiology: The Sicilian Gambit: A new approach to the classification of antiarrhythmic drugs based on their actions on arrhythmogenic mechanisms. Circulation 84: 1831, 1991.
140. Bove EL, Fry WJ, Gross WS, et al: Hypotension and hypertension as consequences of baroreceptor dysfunction following carotid endarterectomy. Surgery 85:633, 1979.
141. Cafferata HT, Merchant RF, DePalma RG: Avoidance of postcarotid endarterectomy hypertension. Ann Surg 196:465, 1982.
142. Levi R: The cardiovascular physiology and pharmacology of adenosine. In 15th Annual Meeting Program. Society of Cardiovascular Anesthesiologists, 1993, p 93.
143. Deutsch S, Dalen JE: Indications for prophylactic digitalization. Anesthesiology 30:648, 1969.
144. Wellens HJJ, Bar FWHM, Lie KI: The value of the electrocardiogram in the differential diagnosis of a tachycardia with a widened QRS complex. Am J Med 64:27, 1978.
145. Berliner D, Okun M, Peters RW, et al: Transcutaneous temporary pacing in the operating room. JAMA 254:84, 1985.
146. Estafanous FG, Tarazi RC: Systemic arterial hypertension associated with cardiac surgery. Am J Cardiol 46:685, 1980.
147. Salerno TA, Henderson M, Keith FM, et al: Hypertension after coronary operation. J Thorac Cardiovasc Surg 81:396, 1981.
148. Davis RF: Acute perioperative hypertension. In Barash PG (ed): Refresher Courses in Anesthesiology, Vol 17. Chicago, American Society of Anesthesiologists, 1989, p 59.
149. Flaherty JT, Magee PA, Gardner TL, et al: Comparison of intravenous nitroglycerin and sodium nitroprusside for treatment of acute hypertension developing after coronary artery bypass surgery. Circulation 65:1072, 1982.
150. Owall A, Gorden E, Lagerkranser M, et al: Clinical experience with adenosine for controlled hypotension during cerebral aneurysm surgery. Anesth Analg 66:229, 1987.
151. Perel A, Pizov R, Cotev S: Systolic blood pressure variation is a sensitive indicator of hypovolemia in ventilated dogs subjected to graded hemorrhage. Anesthesiology 67:498, 1987.
152. Cohn LH, Powell MR, Seidlitz L, et al: Fluid requirements and shifts after reconstruction of the aorta. Am J Surg 120:182, 1970.
153. Rackow EC, Falk JL, Fein IA: Fluid resuscitation in circulatory shock. Crit Care Med 11:839, 1983.
154. Skillman JJ, Restall DS, Salzman EW: Randomized trial of albumin vs electrolyte solutions during abdominal aortic operations. Surgery 78:291, 1975.
155. Boutros AR, Ruess R, Olson L, et al: Comparison of hemodynamic, pulmonary, and renal effects of use of three types of fluids after major surgical procedures on the abdominal aorta. Crit Care Med 7:9, 1979.
156. Rackow EC, Fein IA, Siegel J: The relationship of the colloid osmotic-pulmonary artery wedge pressure gradient to pulmonary edema and mortality in critically ill patients. Chest 82:433, 1982.
157. Metildi LA, Shackford SR, Virgilio RW, et al: Crystalloid versus colloid in fluid resuscitation of patients with severe pulmonary insufficiency. Surg Gynecol Obstet 158:207, 1984.
158. Gallagher TJ, Banner MJ, Barnes PA: Large volume crystalloid resuscitation does not increase extravascular lung water. Anesth Analg 64:323, 1985.
159. Davies LK, Kirby RR: Shock and resuscitation of the trauma patients. Semin Anesth 8:187, 1989.
160. Shackford SR, Sise MJ, Fridland PH, et al: Hypertonic sodium lactate versus lactated Ringer's solution for intravenous therapy in operations on the abdominal aorta. Surgery 94:41, 1983.
161. McGouch E, Kirby RR: Fluids and electrolytes. In Kirby RR, Gravenstein N (eds): Clinical Anesthesia Practice. Philadelphia, WB Saunders Co, 1994, p 715.
162. Pierce JA: Cardiac arrests and deaths associated with anesthesia. Anesth Analg 45:407, 1966.
163. Jude JR, Bolooki H, Nagel E: Cardiac resuscitation in the operating room: Current status. Ann Surg 171:948, 1970.
164. McLure JN, Skardasis GM, Brown JM: Cardiac arrest in the operating area. Am Surg 38:241, 1972.
165. Minuck M: Cardiac arrest in the operating room—part I (1965–1974). Can Anaesth Soc J 23:357, 1976.

166. Emergency Cardiac Care Committee and Subcommittee, American Heart Association: Standards for cardiopulmonary resuscitation and emergency cardiac care. JAMA 1992:2171, 1992.
167. Prengel AW, Lindner KH, Geravis HW: What's new in cardiopulmonary resuscitation? Anesthetist 43(5):309, 1994.
168. Mills NL, Ochsner JL: Massive air embolism during cardiopulmonary bypass. J Thorac Cardiovasc Surg 80:708, 1980.
169. Blauth CI, Cosgrove DM, Webb BW, et al: Atheroembolism from the ascending aorta. J Thorac Cardiovasc Surg 103:1104, 1992.
170. Ohteki H, Tsuyoshi I, Natsuaki M, et al: Intraoperative ultrasonic imaging of the ascending aorta in ischemic heart disease. Ann Thorac Surg 50:539, 1990.
171. Karalis DG, Chandrasekaran K, Victor MF, et al: Recognition and embolic potential of intraaortic atherosclerotic debris. J Am Coll Cardiol 17:73, 1991.
172. Wareing TH, Davila-Roman VG, Barzilai B, et al: Management of the severely atherosclerotic ascending aorta during cardiac operations. A strategy for detection and treatment. J Thorac Cardiovasc Surg 103:453, 1992.
173. Stein M, Cassara EL: Preoperative pulmonary evaluation and therapy for surgery patients. JAMA 211:787, 1970.
174. Stein M, Cassara EL: Preoperative pulmonary evaluation and therapy for surgery patients. JAMA 211:787, 1970.
175. Silvay G, Weinreich AI, Eisenkraft JB: Anesthesia for pulmonary surgery. In Kaplan JA (ed): Thoracic Anesthesia. New York, Churchill Livingstone, 1983, p 347.
176. Shields TW, Vjiki GT: Digitalization for prevention of arrhythmias following pulmonary surgery. Surg Gynecol Obstet 136: 743, 1968.
177. Ritchie AJ, Bowe P, Gibbons JRP: Prophylactic digitalization for thoracotomy: A reassessment. Ann Thorac Surg 50:86, 1990.
178. Gaensler EA, Cusell DW, Lindgren I, et al: The role of pulmonary insufficiency in mortality and invalidism following surgery for pulmonary tuberculosis. J Thorac Cardiovasc Surg 29: 163, 1955.
179. Mittman C: Assessment of operative risk in thoracic surgery. Am Rev Respir Dis 84:197, 1961.
180. Boushy SF, Billig DM, North LB, et al: Clinical course related to preoperative and postoperative pulmonary function in patients with bronchogenic carcinoma. Chest 59:383, 1971.
181. Miller JI, Grossman GD, Hatcher CR: Pulmonary function test criteria for operability and pulmonary resection. Surg Gynecol Obstet 153:893, 1981.
182. Markos J, Mullan BP, Hillman DR, et al: Preoperative assessment as a predictor of mortality and morbidity after lung resection. Am Rev Respir Dis 139:902, 1989.
183. Olsen GN, Block AJ, Swenson EW, et al: Pulmonary evaluation of the lung resection candidate: A prospective study. Am Rev Respir Dis 111:379, 1975.
184. Ali ML, Mountain CF, Ewer MS, et al: Predicting loss of pulmonary function after pulmonary resection for bronchogenic carcinoma. Chest 77:337, 1980.
185. Latimer RG, Dickman M, Day WC, et al: Ventilatory patterns and pulmonary complications after upper abdominal surgery determined by preoperative and postoperative computerized spirometry and blood gas analysis. Am J Surg 122:622, 1971.
186. Candler L: Physiologic assessment and management of the preoperative patient with pulmonary emphysema. Am J Cardiol 12: 324, 1963.
187. Kristersson S, Lindell SE, Svanberg L: Prediction of pulmonary function loss due to pneumonectomy using ^{133}Xe-radiospirometry. Chest 62:694, 1972.
188. Harrison RW, Adams WE, Long ET, et al: The clinical significance of cor pulmonale in the prediction of cardiopulmonary reserve following extensive pulmonary resection. J Thorac Surg 36:352, 1958.
189. Degraff AC, Taylor HF, Ord JW, et al: Exercise limitation following extensive pulmonary resection. J Clin Invest 44:1514, 1965.
190. Uggla LG: Indication for and results of thoracic surgery with regard to respiratory and circulatory function tests. Acta Chir Scand 111:197, 1956.
191. Stein M, Koots GM, Simon M, Frank EA: Pulmonary evaluation of surgical patients. JAMA 181:756, 1962.
192. Fee JH, Holmes EC, Gerwitz HS, et al: Role of pulmonary vascular resistance measurements in preoperative evaluation of candidates for pulmonary resection. J Thorac Cardiovasc Surg 75: 519, 1975.
193. Reichel J: Assessment of operative risk of pneumonectomy. Chest 62:570, 1972.
194. Colman NC, Schraufrasel DE, Rivington RN, et al: Exercise testing in evaluation of patients for lung resection. Am Rev Respir Dis 125:604, 1982.
195. Smith TP, Kinasewitz GT, Tucker WY, et al: Exercise capacity as a predictor of post-thoracotomy morbidity. Am Rev Respir Dis 129:730, 1984.
196. Eugene J, Brown SE, Light RW, et al: Maximum oxygen consumption: A physiology guide to pulmonary resection. Am Rev Respir Dis 125:604, 1982.
197. Boysen PG: Preoperative assessment of the patient undergoing noncardiac thoracic surgery. In Mangano DT (ed): Preoperative Cardiac Assessment. Philadelphia, JB Lippincott Co, 1990, p 125.
198. Alfille PH, Hurford WE: Upper airway injuries. J Clin Anesth 3(2):88, 1991.
199. Cuernelli N, Bragaglia RB, Briccoli A, et al: Tracheobronchial ruptures due to cuffed Carlens tubes. Ann Thorac Surg 28:66, 1979.
200. Newman RW, Finer GE, Downs JE: Routine use of the Carlens double-lumen endobronchial catheter. An experimental and clinical study. J Thorac Cardiovasc Surg 42:327, 1961.
201. Benumof JL: Anesthesia for Thoracic Surgery, 1984. Annual Refresher Course Lectures. Park Ridge, IL, American Society of Anesthesiologists, 1984, p 214.
202. Sidi A, Rush W, Gravenstein N, et al: Pulse oximetry fails to accurately detect low levels of arterial hemoglobin oxygen saturation in dogs. J Clin Monit 3:257, 1987.
203. Severinghaus JW, Naifeh KH, Koh SO: Errors in 14 pulse oximeters during profound hypoxia. J Clin Monit 5:72, 1989.
204. Shulman M, Sandler AN, Bradley JW, et al: Postthoracotomy pain and pulmonary function following epidural and systemic morphine. Anesthesiology 61:569, 1984.
205. Temeck BK, Schafer PW, Park WY, et al: Epidural anesthesia in patients undergoing thoracic surgery. Arch Surg 124:415, 1989.
206. Ross AF, Tinker JH: Cardiovascular disease. In Brown DL (ed): Risk and Outcome in Anesthesia. Philadelphia, JB Lippincott Co, 1988, p 39.
207. Schoeppel SL, Waters J, Wilkinson C, et al: Effect of myocardial infarction on perioperative cardiac complications. Anesth Analg 62(5):493, 1983.
208. Jeffrey CC, Kunsman J, Cullen DJ, Brewster DC: A prospective evaluation of cardiac risk index. Anesthesiology 58:462, 1983.
209. Detsky AS, Abrams HB, McLaughlin JR, et al: Predicting cardiac complications in patients undergoing noncardiac surgery. J Gen Intern Med 1:211, 1986.
210. Detsky AS, Abrams HB, Forbath N, et al: Cardiac assessment for patients undergoing noncardiac surgery, a multifactorial clinical risk index. Arch Intern Med 146:2131, 1986.
211. Foster ED, Davis KB, Carpenter JA, et al: Risk of noncardiac operation in patients with defined coronary disease: The coronary artery surgery study (CASS) registry experience. Ann Thorac Surg 41:42, 1986.
212. Goldman L: Perioperative myocardial ischemia: To everything there is a season (Editorial). Anesthesiology 76:331, 1992.
213. Goldman L: Cardiac risk in noncardiac surgery: An update. Anesth Analg 80:810, 1995.
214. Tinker JH: Perioperative myocardial infarction. Semin Anesth 1: 253, 1982.
215. Sundt TM, Sandok BA, Whisnant JP: Carotid endarterectomy. Complications and preoperative assessment of risk. Mayo Clin Proc 50:301, 1975.
216. Skinner JF, Pearce ML: Surgical risk in the cardiac patient. J Chronic Dis 17:57, 1964.
217. Mangano DT, Browner WS, Hollenberger M, et al: Association of perioperative myocardial ischemia with cardiac morbidity and mortality in men undergoing noncardiac surgery. N Engl J Med 323:1781, 1990.
218. Goldman L: Cardiac risks and complications of noncardiac surgery. Ann Intern Med 98:504, 1983.

219. Eagle KA, Singer DE, Brewster DC, et al: Dipyridamole-thallium scanning in patients undergoing vascular surgery. JAMA 257:2185, 1987.
220. Eagle KA, Coley CM, Newell JB, et al: Combining clinical and thallium data optimizes preoperative assessment of cardiac risk before major vascular surgery. Ann Intern Med 110:859, 1989.
221. Gerson MC, Hurst JM, Hertzberg VS, et al: Cardiac prognosis in noncardiac geriatric surgery. Ann Intern Med 103:832, 1985.
222. Del Guercio LRM, Cohn JD: Monitoring operative risk in the elderly. JAMA 243:1350, 1980.
223. Gerson MC, Hurst JM, Hertzberg VS, et al: Prediction of cardiac and pulmonary complications related to elective abdominal and noncardiac thoracic surgery in geriatric patients. Am J Med 88: 101, 1990.
224. Goldman L, Caldera DL, Southwick FS, et al: Cardiac risk factors and complications in noncardiac surgery. Medicine 57:357, 1978.
225. Goldman L, Caldera DL: Risks of general anesthesia and elective operation in the hypertensive patient. Anesthesiology 50: 285, 1979.
226. Cooperman M, Pflug B, Martin EW, Evans WE: Cardiovascular risk factors in patients with peripheral vascular disease. Surgery 84:505, 1978.
227. Shah KB, Kleinman BS, Rao TLK, et al: Angina and other risk factors in patients with cardiac diseases undergoing noncardiac operations. Anesth Analg 70:240, 1990.
228. Bove EL, Fry WJ, Gross WS, et al: Hypotension and hypertension as consequences of baroreceptor dysfunction following carotid endarterectomy. Surgery 85:633, 1979.
229. Cafferata HT, Merchant RF, DePalma RG: Avoidance of postcarotid endarterectomy hypertension. Ann Surg 196:465, 1982.
230. Asiddao CB, Donegan JH, Whitesell RC, et al: Factors associated with perioperative complications during carotid endarterectomy. Anesth Analg 61:631, 1982.
231. Riles TS, Kopelman I, Imparato AM: Myocardial infarction following carotid endarterectomy: A review of 683 operations. Surgery 85:249, 1979.
232. Owens ML, Wilson SE: Prevention of neurologic complications of carotid endarterectomy. Arch Surg 117:551, 1982.
233. Steed DL, Peitzman AB, Grundy BL, et al: Causes of stroke in carotid endarterectomy. Surgery 92:634, 1982.
234. White JS, Sirinek KR, Root HD, et al: Morbidity and mortality of carotid endarterectomy: Rates of occurrence in asymptomatic and symptomatic patients. Arch Surg 116:409, 1981.
235. Kirshner DL, O'Brien MS, Ricotta JJ: Risk factors in a community experience with carotid endarterectomy. J Vasc Surg 10: 178, 1989.
236. Sutherland GR, Barr HWK: Postoperative complications following carotid endarterectomy and their management. Int Anesthesiol Clin 22:165, 1984.
237. Hertzer NR, Young JR, Beven EG, et al: Coronary angiography in 506 patients with extracranial cerebrovascular disease. Arch Intern Med 145:849, 1985.
238. Prough DS, Scuderi PE, Stullken E, et al: Myocardial infarction following regional anaesthesia for carotid endarterectomy. Can Anaesth Soc J 31:192, 1984.
239. Peitzman AB, Webster MW, Loubeau JM, et al: Carotid endarterectomy under regional (conductive) anesthesia. Ann Surg 196: 59, 1982.
240. Gabelman CG, Gann DS, Ashworth CJ, et al: One hundred consecutive carotid reconstructions: Local versus general anesthesia. Am J Surg 145:477, 1983.
241. Mackey WC, Khabbaz K, Bojar R, O'Donnell TF Jr: Simultaneous carotid endarterectomy and coronary bypass: Perioperative risk and long term survival. J Vasc Surg 24:58, 1996.
242. Akins CW, Moncure AC, Daggett WM, et al: Safety and efficacy of concomitant carotid and coronary artery operations. Ann Thorac Surg 60:311, 1995.
243. Carrel T, Stillhard G, Turina M: Conbined carotid and coronary artery surgery: Early and late results. Cardiology 80:118, 1992.
244. Giangola G, Migaly J, Riles TS, et al: Perioperative morbidity and mortality in combined vs. staged approaches to carotid and coronary revascularization. Ann Vasc Surg 10:138, 1994.
245. Takach TJ, Reul GJ Jr, Cooley DA, et al: Is an integrated approach warranted for concomitant carotid and coronary artery disease? Ann Thorac Surg 64:16, 1997.
246. Towne JB, Bernhard VM: The relationship of postoperative hypertension to complications following carotid endarterectomy. Surgery 88:575, 1980.
247. Angel-James JE, Lumley JSP: The effects of carotid endarterectomy on the mechanical properties of the carotid sinus and carotid sinus nerve activity in atherosclerotic patients. Br J Surg 61:805, 1974.
248. Pine R, Avellone JC, Hoffman M, et al: Control of postcarotid endarterectomy hypotension with baroreceptor blockade. Am J Surg 147:763, 1984.
249. Wade JG, Larson CP, Hickey RF, et al: Effect of carotid endarterectomy on carotid chemoreceptor and baroreceptor function in man. N Engl J Med 282:823, 1970.
250. Tarlov E, Schmidek H, Scott RM, et al: Reflex hypotension following carotid endarterectomy: Mechanism and management. J Neurosurg 39:323, 1973.
251. Caplan LR, Skillman J, Ojemann R, et al: Intracerebral hemorrhage following carotid endarterectomy: A hypertensive complication? Stroke 9:457, 1978.
252. Kunkel JM, Gomez ER, Spebar MJ, et al: Wound hematomas after carotid endarterectomy. Am J Surg 148:844, 1984.
253. Yeager RA, Weigel RM, Murphy ES, et al: Application of clinically valid cardiac risk factors to aortic aneurysm surgery. Arch Surg 121:278, 1986.
254. Whittemore AD, Clowes AW, Hechtman HB, et al: Aortic aneurysm repair: Reduced operative mortality associated with maintenance of optimal cardiac performance. Ann Surg 192:414, 1980.
255. Brown OW, Hollier LH, Pairolero PC, et al: Abdominal aortic aneurysm and coronary artery disease: A reassessment. Arch Surg 116:1484, 1981.
256. Diehl JT, Cali RF, Hertzer NR, et al: Complications of abdominal aortic reconstruction. Ann Surg 197:49, 1983.
257. Johnston KW: Multicenter prospective study of nonruptured abdominal aortic aneurysm. Part II. Variables predicting morbidity and mortality. J Vasc Surg 9:437, 1989.
258. McCann RL, Wolfe WG: Resection of abdominal aortic aneurysm in patients with low ejection fractions. J Vasc Surg 10:240, 1989.
259. Bickerstaff LK, Hollier LH, VanPennen HJ, et al: Abdominal aortic aneurysm repair combined with a second surgical procedure: Morbidity and mortality. Surgery 95:487, 1984.
260. Grindlinger GA, Vegas AM, Williams GH, et al: Independence of renin production and hypertension in abdominal aortic aneurysmectomy. Am J Surg 141:472, 1981.
261. Paterson IS, Klausner JM, Pugatch R, et al: Noncardiogenic pulmonary edema after abdominal aortic aneurysm surgery. Ann Surg 209:231, 1989.
262. Szilagyi DE, Hageman JH, Smith RF, et al: Spinal cord damage in surgery of the abdominal aorta. Surgery 83:38, 1978.
263. Ernst CB: Prevention of intestinal ischemia following abdominal aortic reconstruction. Surgery 93:102, 1983.
264. Crawford ES, Bomberger RA, Glaeser DH, et al: Aortoiliac occlusive disease: Factors influencing survival and function following reconstructive operation over a twenty-five-year period. Surgery 90:1055, 1981.
265. Tomatis LA, Fierens EE, Vergrugge GP: Evaluation of surgical risk in peripheral vascular disease by coronary arteriography: A series of 100 cases. Surgery 71:429, 1972.
266. von Knorring J, Lepantalo M: Prediction of perioperative cardiac complications by electrocardiographic monitoring during treadmill exercise testing before peripheral vascular surgery. Surgery 99:610, 1986.
267. Hertzer NR: Fatal myocardial infarction following lower extremity revascularization: Two hundred seventy-three patients followed six to eleven postoperative years. Ann Surg 193:492, 1981.
268. Lawrie GM, Morris GC, Soussou ID, et al: Late results of reconstructive surgery for renovascular disease. Ann Surg 191: 528, 1980.
269. Dean RH, Keyser JE, DuPont WD, et al: Aortic and renal vascular disease: Factors affecting the value of combined procedures. Ann Surg 200:336, 1984.
270. Stanley JC, Whitehouse WM, Graham LM, et al: Operative therapy of renovascular hypertension. Br J Surg 69(Suppl):S63, 1982.

271. Stoney RJ, Skoldebrand CG, Ovarfordt PG, et al: Juxtarenal aortic atherosclerosis: Surgical experience and functional result. Ann Surg 200:345, 1984.
272. Committee on Perioperative Cardiovascular Evaluation for Noncardiac surgery: Guidelines for Perioperative Cardiovascular Evaluation for Noncardiac Surgery: Report of the American College of Cardiology/American Heart Association Task Force on Practice Guidelines. J Am Coll Cardiol 27:910, 1996.
273. Committee on Perioperative Cardiovascular Evaluation for Noncardiac surgery: Guidelines for Perioperative Cardiovascular Evaluation for Noncardiac Surgery: Report of the American College of Cardiology/American Heart Association Task Force on Practice Guidelines. Circulation 93:1278, 1996.
274. Guidelines for Perioperative Cardiovascular Evaluation for Noncardiac Surgery: An Abridged version of the Report of the American College of Cardiology/American Heart Association Task Force on Practice Guidelines. Mayo Clin Proc 72:524, 1997.
275. Dorinsky PM, Whitcomb ME: The effect of PEEP on cardiac output. Chest 84:210, 1983.
276. Bergman N: Hypoxic pulmonary vasoconstruction. Semin Anesth 6:188, 1987.
277. Allen JB, Allen FB: The minimum acceptable level of hemoglobin. Int Anesthesiol Clin 20:1, 1982.
278. Czer LSC, Shoemaker WC: Optimal hematocrit value in critically ill postoperative patients. Surg Gynecol Obstet 147:363, 1978.
279. Aach RD, Kuhn RA: Post-transfusion hepatitis: Current perspectives. Ann Intern Med 92:539, 1980.
280. Bay J, Nun JF, Prys-Roberts C: Factors influencing arterial PO_2 during recovery from anaesthesia. Br J Anaesth 40:398, 1968.
281. Sharkey A, Lipton JM, Murphy MT, Giesecke AH: Inhibition of post-anesthetic shivering with radiant heat. Anesthesiology 66(2):249, 1987.
282. Kurz A, Kurz M, Pieschl G, et al: Forced air warming maintained intraoperative normothermia better than circulating water mattresses. Anesth Analg 77:89, 1993.
283. Macintyre PE, Pavlin EG, Dwersteg JF: Effect of meperidine on oxygen consumption, carbon dioxide production and respiratory gas exchange in postanesthesia shivering. Anesth Analg 66:751, 1987.
284. Conahan TJ III: Complications of cardiac surgery. In Kaplan JA (ed): Cardiac Anesthesia, 2nd ed, Vol 2. Orlando, FL, Grune & Stratton, 1987, p 1105.
285. Campeau L, Lesperance J, Bourassa MG: Natural history of saphenous vein aortocoronary bypass grafts. Mod Concepts Cardiovasc Dis 53:59, 1984.
286. Loop FD, Lytle BW, Cosgrove DM, et al: Influence of the internal mammary artery graft on 10-year survival and other cardiac events. N Engl J Med 314:1, 1986.
287. Goldstein RA, Byrnes TJ, Geraci SA: Pharmacologic therapy of low output syndromes after cardiac surgery. Arch Int Physiol Biochem 92:S21, 1984.
288. McGee MG, Zillgitt SL, Trono R, et al: Prospective analyses of the need for mechanical circulatory support after cardiopulmonary bypass. Am J Cardiol 46:135, 1980.
289. Pennington DG, Swartz M, Codd JE, et al: Intraaortic balloon pumping in cardiac surgical patients: A nine-year-experience. Ann Thorac Surg 36:125, 1983.
290. Schaff HV, Gersh BJ, Fisher LD, et al: Detrimental effect of perioperative myocardial infarction on late survival after coronary artery bypass. J Thorac Cardiovasc Surg 88:972, 1984.
291. Roberts AJ: Perioperative myocardial infarction and changes in left ventricular performance related to coronary artery bypass graft surgery. Ann Thorac Surg 35:208, 1983.
292. McClung JA, Stein JH, Ambrose JA, et al: Prosthetic heart valves: A review. Prog Cardiovasc Dis 26:237, 1983.
293. Smith GH: Complications of Cardiopulmonary Surgery. London, Bailliere Tindall, 1984, p 123.
294. Reedy S, Curtiss EI, O'Toole JD, et al: Cardiac tamponade: Hemodynamic observations in man. Circulation 58:265, 1978.

CHAPTER 36

Central Nervous System Complications

Brad Hindman, M.D.

Incidence and Outcome

When severe, neurologic injuries occurring in association with cardiac surgery can render meaningless an otherwise successful operation. Despite a vast literature, many reports regarding the incidence and outcome of these complications cannot be considered reliable, primarily because of retrospective design. Sotaniemi, a neurologist, examined 100 patients before and after valve replacement (aortic and/or mitral).[1] Postoperatively, 35 of 96 survivors (36%) had some new neurologic abnormality. Seven of the affected patients had deficits which the author considered so severe as to be "obvious." Nevertheless, only four of these seven deficits (57%) were noted by any other physician. Overall, detection of new neurologic signs by nonneurologists was 4 of 35 (11%). Similarly, in Silverstein's series of 55 patients, only 40% of postoperative neurologic deficits were noted by nonneurologists.[2] These studies demonstrate the necessity of qualified examiners and prospective evaluation in studies of neurologic outcome. Retrospective chart reviews, which comprise the majority of the literature, likely underreport the incidence of neurologic complications of cardiac surgery, even those that are major.

Another difficulty in interpreting incidence data arises from inconsistencies in the method of neurologic evaluation. Some studies employ clinical neurologic exams; others neuropsychological testing[3]; and still others biochemical variables,[4] electroencephalography,[5] and, more recently, imaging studies.[6] It is often impossible to know how an abnormality detected by one modality relates to any other, or how a given abnormality affects the functional status of patients. Furthermore, only a few reports describe temporal aspects of neurologic injuries (i.e., their onset and resolution over time). This shortcoming is becoming more important, as several studies now indicate 20 to 40% of neurologic deficits occurring in association with cardiac surgery occur well into the postoperative period.[7-12] The pathophysiology and management of these events may differ considerably from those occurring intraoperatively. Of available prospective reports, only a handful have complete descriptions of operative, anesthetic, and cardiopulmonary bypass management, or have any follow-up. Consequently, from most reports it is impossible to discern when neurologic deficits were first noted, what may have contributed to their occurrence, and to what extent patients were disabled. Also, as operative, anesthetic, and cardiopulmonary bypass techniques have evolved, many early reports are probably irrelevant to current practice. Finally, to identify neurologic complications that are unique to cardiac surgery patients, and to provide insight into their mechanisms, comparisons between cardiac and noncardiac surgery patients, and nonoperative patients may be necessary. Thus, ideally, incidence and outcome studies should include an appropriately matched noncardiac surgery control group.

With the above considerations in mind, the following discussion will focus upon a series of reports by Shaw et al. concerning neurologic injuries occurring in association with coronary artery bypass grafting (CABG).[7,13-17] These reports are probably the best of the current literature because of their large study population, prospective design, qualified examiners, standard evaluative procedures, detailed reporting, long-term follow-up, and the inclusion of a noncardiac surgery control group. Although derived from patients undergoing CABG only, the findings are in general agreement with those that include other types of adult cardiac surgery.

Clinical Neurologic Findings

Shaw (a neurologist) and co-workers examined 312 patients prior to CABG.[7,13-16] Follow-up neurologic examinations were performed 7 days after surgery, and again 6 months later. Anesthesia was maintained with fentanyl, droperidol, and nitrous oxide, supplemented with a "volatile agent." "Moderate hemodilution" and hypothermia (28°C) were employed during cardiopulmonary bypass (1.6 to 2.4 L/m^2/min), and both membrane and bubble oxygenators without arterial filtration, and both pulsatile and nonpulsatile cardiopulmonary bypass were used. There is no description of arterial pressure or acid-base management during cardiopulmonary bypass.

Preoperatively, 109 of 312 (35%) patients had detectable neurologic abnormalities, most often consisting of peripheral nerve lesions, abnormal tendon reflexes, or primitive reflexes. Although, at first, this seems like an extraordinarily high incidence of pre-existing neurologic abnormalities, other prospective studies report comparable incidences (13 to 57%).[9,18,19] The control group consisted of 50 patients having major vascular surgery (abdominal aortic aneurysm repair, aortofemoral bypass). The control group was well matched to the CABG group in terms of age, history of heart disease, hypertension, pre-existing neurologic symptoms, type of anesthesia, operative duration, intensive care unit (ICU) duration, and postoperative inotrope use.[15] New neurologic abnormalities were present in 191 of 308 (62%) patients surviving CABG versus 9 of 49 (18%) patients surviving vascular surgery (Table 36–1). Most notably, of 308 patients surviving CABG, one suffered a fatal hypotensive global ischemic event (0.3%) and definite stroke occurred in 15 patients (5%). Possible mild strokes occurred in nine additional patients (3%). In stark contrast, new neurologic findings in vascular surgery patients were limited almost exclusively to peripheral neuropathies.

Of CABG patients suffering a definite stroke, 58% still had a deficit 6 months postoperatively, leaving more than half with a "significant functional disability." Possible minor strokes, noted initially in nine patients, uniformly resolved by 6 months. New visual field defects, present in eight patients (3%) at first follow-up, persisted in 57% of the cases at 6 months. Primitive reflexes, considered to indicate diffuse cortical injury, and noted in 123 patients postoperatively (39%), persisted in approximately 50% of patients at 6 months. At 6 months, ten patients (4% of those evaluable) had functionally important deficits, preventing return to work in four (2%). Thus, it is clear CABG patients had a much greater incidence, severity, and diversity of neurologic injury when compared to noncardiac surgery patients and, although there was improvement over time, 2 to 4% were permanently and significantly disabled.

Neuropsychologic Alterations

Impairment of cognition, memory, and psychomotor coordination are commonly noted postoperatively, often in patients who would, on first appearance, seem normal. For example, Slogoff et al. reported 25% of patients appearing neurologically normal after cardiac surgery had impaired neuropsychologic performance.[20] A number of studies indicate standard neurologic examination can, at times, be remarkably insensitive to cortical injuries. For example, Sellman et al., comparing pre- and post-CABG magnetic resonance imaging (MRI) images, found new (large) cerebral infarctions in 2 of 29 (7%) patients who were without any overt sign of neurologic injury.[6] The current consensus is that marked impairment of neuropsychologic performance following cardiac surgery is *probably* due to subclinical brain injury, *probably* occurring during surgery and/or cardiopulmonary bypass. Nevertheless, as will be discussed, the relationship between perioperative events and long-term neuropsychologic dysfunction is not yet definitively established.

One of the principal difficulties in neuropsychologic testing is controlling for the numerous possible determinants of performance. In other words, to what degree is a change in performance due to practice, motivation, illness, drugs,[21] mood,[22,23] etc., and how much is due to actual organic brain injury? More important, and even more difficult to determine, is the degree to which, in a given patient, a performance change is functionally "significant." For example, decreased fine motor skill might not be important to one person, but might be disabling to a musician. For this reason, studies of neuropsychologic performance are, preferably, based on *individual* performance, rather than upon group performance. In the study by Shaw et al., ten neuropsychologic tests were administered preoperatively and at follow-up examinations.[14,16] A change in an individual's performance was considered "significant" if the change exceeded the standard deviation of the group performance. Although arbitrary, this level of change is probably "significant," in that an individual's performance would have to change his/her percentile rank approximately 33%. As shown in Table 36–2, at 7 days postoperatively, CABG patients had markedly greater incidence and severity of

TABLE 36–1
Neurologic Status at 7 Days Postoperatively*

New Neurologic Findings	CABG	(*n* = 308)	Peripheral Vascular (*n* = 49)
Fatal cerebral injury	1	(0.3%)	0
Depressed consciousness >24 hr	10	(3%)	0
Definite stroke	15	(5%)	0
Reversible ischemic deficit	9	(3%)	0
Ophthalmologic disorders[†]	78	(25%)	0
Primitive reflexes	123	(39%)	2 (4%)
Psychosis	4	(1%)	0
Peripheral neuropathy	37	(12%)	7 (14%)

*Data from Shaw P, Bates D, Cartlidge NEF, et al: Early neurological complications of coronary artery bypass surgery. Br Med J 291:1384, 1985 and Shaw PJ, Bates D, Cartlidge NEF, et al: Neurologic and neuropsychological morbidity following major surgery: Comparison of coronary artery bypass and peripheral vascular surgery. Stroke 18:700, 1987.

[†]Ophthalmologic disorders include visual field defects, retinal infarction, retinal emboli, and reduced acuity.
CABG, coronary artery bypass grafting.

TABLE 36–2
Neuropsychologic Status Compared to Preoperative Baseline at 7 Days Postoperatively*

Severity of Deterioration	CABG	(*n* = 298)	Peripheral Vascular (*n* = 48)
None	63	(21%)	33 (69%)
Mild†	164	(55%)	15 (31%)
Moderate‡	57	(19%)	(0%)
Severe§	14	(5%)	(0%)
Symptomatic	89	(30%)	(0%)
Disabled	23	(8%)	(0%)

*Data from Shaw PJ, Bates D, Cartlidge NEF, et al: Neurologic and neuropsychological morbidity following major surgery: Comparison of coronary artery bypass and peripheral vascular surgery. Stroke 18:700, 1987.
†Deterioration in one to two out of ten tests.
‡Deterioration in three to four out of ten tests.
§Deterioration in five or more out of ten tests.
CABG, coronary artery bypass grafting.

deterioration in neuropsychologic performance relative to their preoperative baseline as compared to vascular surgery patients. Approximately 79% of CABG patients had a performance decrement in at least one of ten tests, and 24% had a decrement in at least three tests. Contrast this with the vascular surgery patients, in whom 69% had no significant decrement in any test, and no patient had a decrement in more than two tests. Cognitive abilities that deteriorated most were psychomotor speed, attention and concentration, new learning ability, and auditory short-term memory. Nearly 1 out of every 12 CABG patients (8%) was so intellectually impaired as to be overtly disabled in routine postoperative hospital activities! Thus, as was the case with conventional neurologic signs, CABG patients had a far greater incidence and severity of acute neuropsychologic deterioration than did other surgical patients.

The results of 6-month follow-up testing in CABG patients are shown in Table 36–3. One group of patients (20% of the cohort) had no significant decrement in neuropsychologic performance relative to their preoperative baseline at 7 days after surgery. Hence, there was no evidence of brain injury due to CABG. Another group of patients (31% of the cohort), who had significant performance decrements 7 days after operation, either returned to or exceeded preoperative performance 6 months postoperatively. Thus, whatever caused early neuropsychologic impairment had apparently resolved. Another group of patients (17% of the cohort) had impaired performance relative to preoperative baseline at first follow-up, and had impairment 6 months postoperatively, although on *different* tests (in other words, if impaired in tests, A, B, and C at 7 days, they were impaired on tests D, E, and F at 6 months). Although declining in their neuropsychologic status, it is difficult to confidently conclude cardiac surgery was directly causative. A fourth group of patients (32% of the cohort) had impaired performance at 7 days compared to their preoperative baseline, and continued impairment in the *same* tests 6 months later, although usually not to the same degree (if impaired in tests A, B, and C at 7 days, they were *still* impaired in tests A, B, and C at 6 months). Almost certainly, this group, nearly a third of the evaluable patients, sustained some form of subtle neurologic injury that had its origin in the perioperative period.

Of all patients having measurable decrements in neuropsychologic performance at 6 months (~50% of the total cohort), most had, in fact, improved over time. Only about a third of these patients (~15% of the cohort) reported any noticeable symptoms, usually problems with memory and concentration. Only three of the evaluable patients (~1%) had seriously disabling impairment of cognitive function at 6 months, and all had had major perioperative strokes.

Although this study indicates cardiac surgery patients are uniquely at risk of neuropsychologic deterioration, not all studies concur. In a recent report from England, Treasure et al. did *not* detect differences in neuropsychologic status between patients undergoing cardiac and noncardiac surgery.[21] In the latter study, the incidence of neuropsychologic deterioration in cardiac surgery patients was comparable to that reported by Shaw et al.,[14,16] but, in contrast, noncardiac surgery patients had equally severe and sustained neuropsychologic deterioration. Thus, impairment of neuropsychologic performance following cardiac surgery is probably not *exclusively* due to brain injury occurring during surgery and cardiopulmonary bypass. Nevertheless, because numerous studies find associations between early neuropsychologic impairment and perioperative factors, there is probably some "organic" basis to these defects. Prior investiga-

TABLE 36–3
Neuropsychologic Performance Compared to Preoperative Baseline in 252 Patients Tested at Both 7 Days and 6 Months After CABG*

7 Days	6 Months	*n* (%)
Normal	Impaired	19 (8%)
Normal	Normal	31 (12%)
Impaired	Normal	78 (31%)
Impaired	Impaired (different tests)	43 (17%)
Impaired	Impaired (same tests)	81 (32%)

*Data from Shaw PJ, Bates D, Cartlidge NEF, et al: Long-term intellectual dysfunction following coronary artery bypass graft surgery: A six month follow-up study. Q J Med 62:259, 1987.
CABG, coronary artery bypass grafting.

tions have found bypass duration[9,21,24,25] multiple valve replacement,[24,26] age,[9,21] and hypotension during bypass[21] to be associated with early neuropsychologic impairment. In Shaw's study, moderate and severe deterioration in neuropsychologic performance at 7 days (Table 36–3) correlated with (1) a preoperative history of stroke/transient ischemic attack (TIA); (2) postoperative hypotension; (3) a large decrease in hemoglobin concentration perioperatively; (4) the presence of concurrent peripheral vascular disease; and (5) ICU duration.[17] This hypothesis is further supported by the findings of Sotaniemi et al., wherein neuropsychologic outcome 5 years after valve replacement correlated with bypass duration.[27] Patients having a bypass duration greater than 2 hours had long-term impairment of neuropsychologic performance relative to patients having lesser bypass times. On the other hand, two recent studies have been unable to identify *any* perioperative factor as being associated with longer term (2 to 6 months) neuropsychologic outcome.[17,21] Were long-term neuropsychologic changes due to organic brain injury occurring during surgery and cardiopulmonary bypass, one would expect *some* association with *some* perioperative factor. Shaw et al. found only a preoperative history of congestive heart failure and poor ejection fraction to be associated with long-term impairment in neuropsychologic function.[17] Thus, although intuition suggests deterioration of neuropsychologic performance following cardiac surgery and cardiopulmonary bypass is almost certainly the result of some subtle form of brain injury, only circumstantial evidence exists. A definitive link between structural neuronal damage and neuropsychologic deterioration remains elusive.

Summary

Current reports indicate that between 2 and 6% of adult cardiac surgery patients sustain unequivocal focal neurologic injury (stroke) in the perioperative period.[9,28–31] In a recent study, CABG patients having neurologic complications had three times longer ICU stay (9 ± 11 days vs. 3 ± 3 days) and nine times greater perioperative mortality (36% vs. 4%) than patients free of neurologic injury.[31] Similarly, patients having neurologic complications following CABG have significantly longer hospital stay than those who do not (21 ± 18 vs. 9 ± 10 days, respectively).[32] Although patients with focal deficits often (~75%) make a good functional recovery,[13,18,19,31] 20 to 30% of those having a stroke have permanent neurologic disability.[13,18,19] Patients who fail to regain consciousness after surgery (i.e., are comatose) have a much worse prognosis.[5,7,11] In the first postoperative week, more subtle neurologic abnormalities and/or neuropsychologic alterations are noted in 30 to 60% of adult cardiac surgery patients.[7,9,14,30,33,34] Although improving over time, about 30 to 50% of patients have measurable decrements in neuropsychologic performance 6 months postoperatively,[16,22,34] although only about 10 to 15% report any change in mental abilities. Thus, there is significant neurologic morbidity associated with cardiac surgery, with increased perioperative mortality, length of ICU and hospital stay, and, in some patients, long-term neurologic and cognitive impairment. A reduction in the incidence and/or severity of these injuries could significantly improve the quality of life for many thousands of patients each year.

Risk Factors and Mechanisms of Injury

The Patient

Ascending Aortic Atherosclerosis

Due to the difficulties associated with the possible pathogenesis of postoperative neuropsychologic dysfunction (see above), subsequent discussion will be limited to neurologic abnormalities detected by conventional clinical neurologic examination. These findings can be reasonably assumed to result from focal, multifocal, or global cerebral ischemia and infarction.

To gain insight on the possible mechanisms of injury, Shaw et al. used multivariate analysis, correlating clinical variables with the occurrence of new neurologic signs.[17] The results of their analysis are shown in Table 36–4. Signs of systemic arteriosclerosis stand out as the most consistent risk factors for the development of neurologic abnormalities in association with cardiac surgery. Why?

TABLE 36–4
Risk Factors for Development of New Postoperative Neurologic Signs*

New Neurologic Findings	Risk Factors
Depressed consciousness >24 hr	Subclavian bruit, prior TIAs, difficulty terminating bypass, large decrease in hemoglobin concentration
Definite stroke	Peripheral vascular disease, congestive heart failure
Retinal emboli	BP difference between arms, prior stroke
New palmomental reflex	Large decrease in hemoglobin concentration
New snout reflex	Subclavian bruits, mean arterial pressure <40 mm Hg
Severe neuropsychologic change	Peripheral vascular disease, large decrease in hemoglobin concentration

*Data from Shaw PJ, Bates D, Cartlidge NEF, et al: An analysis of factors predisposing to neurological injury in patients undergoing coronary bypass operations. Q J Med 72:633, 1989.
TIAs, transient ischemic attacks; BP, blood pressure.

Recent transcranial Doppler studies demonstrate cerebral embolization commonly occurs during both aortic cannulation and initiation of bypass.[35–37] When the aorta is manipulated, cannulated, or cross-clamped, atheromatous material can be dislodged and embolized. Similarly, atheromas can be "sand-blasted" off the lumen of the aorta by the high flow of arterial perfusate exiting the aortic perfusion cannula.[38] It is, therefore, not surprising that severe atherosclerosis of the ascending aorta (present in 10 to 30% of adult cardiac surgery patients)[38–42] is emerging as the principal risk factor for the development of focal neurologic injury in adult cardiac surgery patients[12,38,43–46] (Fig. 36–1).

Human autopsy studies show atheromatous emboli arising from the aorta usually occlude arteries 100 to 150 μm or smaller.[47–49] Most often the result is focal infarction in the terminal ("watershed" or arterial boundary zone) distribution of the middle and posterior cerebral artery.[45,48–52] Watershed areas are usually considered to be at risk of infarction via hypotension or hypoperfusion because of limited collateral perfusion.[53,54] However, for the same reason, these areas are especially susceptible to embolic infarction. The pattern of infarcted tissue may mimic the arterial boundary zone distribution of cerebral hypoperfusion.[54] Certainly, however, larger emboli can result in large areas of infarction.

In a recent autopsy series of 221 adults dying in hospital after cardiac surgery, Blauth et al. found atheroemboli in 37% of patients who had severe atherosclerosis of the ascending aorta versus 2% in patients free of significant ascending aortic disease ($p < .001$).[55] Brain was the organ most frequently embolized. Multivariate risk factors for the presence of ascending aortic atherosclerosis were (1) concomitant peripheral vascular disease, (2) increasing age, and (3) hypertension. These risk factors are strikingly similar to risk factors identified by Shaw et al. (subclavian bruits, peripheral vascular disease, and blood pressure asymmetries) for the development of stroke, retinal emboli, primitive reflexes, and severe neuropsychologic deficits following CABG.[17] Recently, Mills et al. observed a 79% incidence of concomitant carotid disease in patients having severe ascending aortic calcification.[44] Likewise, Katz et al. found a strong association between the presence of carotid bruits and severe atheromatous disease of the aortic arch.[38] Thus, the presence of carotid disease may also serve as a marker of aortic disease (more below).

There are only a few reports of the consequences of "routine" cannulation and clamping of aortas recognized as being severely diseased. Stroke incidence in each report was 50%.[38,39,44] A potentially very important advance was recently described by Wareing et al., wherein intraoperative ultrasound was used to locate ascending aortic abnormalities.[40] Moderate or severe ascending aortic disease was identified in 60 of 500 (14%) adults undergoing cardiac operation. Aortic palpation alone identified only a third of these patients. When significant disease was identified, the procedure was modified to avoid manipulation, cannulation, or clamping of the atherosclerotic segment. Using these techniques, these investigators, and other groups,[38,42] report perioperative neurologic complications that are no more frequent in patients with ascending aortic atherosclerosis than in those free of aortic disease (~1.5%). In the presence of severe verrucous disease or circumferential calcification, more aggressive techniques such as aortic endarterectomy or aortic replacement are advocated by some.[38,39,41] Transesophageal echocardiography (TEE), especially with a biplane probe, may also be a useful tool to localize ascending aortic irregularities. Using this technique, Katz et al. identified severe atheromatous disease in the aortic arch in 18% of patients age 65 or greater.[38] In agreement with other studies, palpation alone did not identify these high-risk patients.

Cerebrovascular Disease

The role of coexisting cerebrovascular disease in the development of perioperative neurologic injury has been an issue of longstanding concern. Carotid artery atherosclerosis is present in 5 to 15% of adult cardiac surgery patients[56–59] and is considered by many to increase risk of neurologic complications.[10,60–62]

Prospective studies of cardiac surgery patients report an incidence of asymptomatic carotid bruits of 6 to 16%.[56–58,63–65] When evaluated as a risk factor for the development of perioperative stroke, asymptomatic carotid bruits have consistently failed to be a reliable pre-

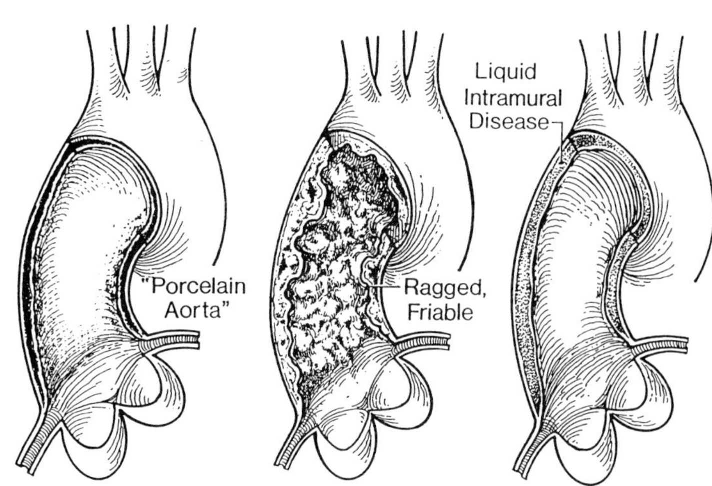

FIGURE **36–1.** Forms of ascending aortic atherosclerosis. (From Mills NL, Everson CT: Atherosclerosis of the ascending aorta and coronary artery bypass. J Thorac Cardiovasc Surg 102:546, 1991, with permission.)

dictor.[57,58,63,65] The most likely reason for this observation is that carotid bruits are neither a sensitive nor a specific sign of cerebrovascular disease. Studies of Balderman et al.,[56] Barnes et al.,[57] and Ivey et al.[63] each show that only 25 to 35% of carotid bruits are associated with a significant carotid stenosis. Conversely, when Barnes et al. prospectively identified 40 cardiac surgery patients as having carotid "obstruction" using Doppler screening (12% of the cohort), only 27% of patients so identified had an audible bruit.[57] Hence, the presence or absence of a carotid bruit is poorly correlated with the presence or absence of carotid stenosis. A recent retrospective study reported the presence of carotid bruits increased perioperative stroke risk almost 400%.[8] Notably, strokes did not correlate with the side of the bruit. In light of the fact that carotid bruits are not reliable indicators of hemodynamically significant carotid stenoses, this finding suggests carotid bruits may act as a marker for other processes contributing to perioperative stroke (i.e., ascending aortic atherosclerosis; see above).

Controversy surrounds the management of cardiac surgery patients with known carotid *stenoses*. The principal concern is that carotid stenoses will limit cerebral blood flow (CBF) during cardiopulmonary bypass (where arterial pressure is often far lower than normal), and that stroke will be the result. Thus, the principal justification for carotid endarterectomy (CEA) in these patients has been the *presumption* that CEA would protect the brain from hypoperfusion during bypass, and thereby reduce the incidence of stroke. On the one hand, some studies indicate asymptomatic carotid stenoses do not either (1) limit CBF during bypass[66–68] or (2) confer increased risk for acute perioperative stroke.[57,59,69,70] On the other hand, there are a sufficient number of reports indicating that carotid stenoses *are* a risk factor for the development of stroke with cardiac surgery, that the issue cannot be entirely dismissed. The key question to be asked is the following: In the presence of known carotid stenoses, is the incidence of stroke after cardiac surgery less in those patients who have undergone CEA (either before or during the cardiac surgery) as compared to patients who have not undergone CEA? In other words, is CEA protective?

An interesting study, albeit retrospective and nonrandomized, is that of Brener et al.[60] Over a 7-year period, the author's practice changed. Initially, all patients with asymptomatic carotid stenoses had combined CEA/cardiac surgery. Over time, the authors phased out this practice such that eventually, no patient with asymptomatic carotid disease had CEA before or during cardiac surgery. The results of their retrospective review are shown in Table 36–5. Although the presence of carotid disease did significantly increase the risk of perioperative stroke/TIA as compared to patients with normal carotids (by a factor of 5), CEA *did not* appear to reduce the risk of acute perioperative stroke. A similar conclusion can be drawn from the report of Hertzer et al., concerning 274 CABG patients who had at least one carotid stenosis (≥70% diameter reduction).[61] Acute perioperative stroke following CABG occurred in 9 of 193 (5%) patients undergoing CEA prior to or simultaneous with CABG (i.e., "protected") versus 6 of 81 patients (7%) undergoing CABG without CEA (i.e., unprotected). Thus, CEA did not convincingly provide neurologic protection in this series. Finally, a recent meta-analysis of existing studies reports the overall incidence of acute perioperative stroke following cardiac surgery in patients with known carotid stenoses to be approximately 5.6% (range, 0 to 10%) for those who underwent combined carotid and coronary revascularization (i.e., "protected") versus approximately 5.2% (range, 0 to 17%) in patients undergoing CABG only (i.e., "unprotected").[62] Thus, there is little evidence, *especially in the absence of symptoms*, that CEA protects patients from acute perioperative stroke in association with cardiac surgery. The association between carotid disease and atherosclerosis of the ascending aorta[38,44] may explain why "prophylactic" CEA does not appear to reduce the incidence of acute perioperative stroke in patients with carotid stenoses. Quite simply, stroke following heart surgery in patients with asymptomatic carotid bruits/stenoses may be more likely the result of cerebral emboli from an atherosclerotic aorta than from hemispheric hypoperfusion.

TABLE 36–5
Postoperative Stroke/TIA in Cardiac Surgery Patients with Asymptomatic Carotid Stenosis*

Carotid Disease	Perioperative Stroke/TIA
Normal carotids	74/3,894 (2%)
Unilateral stenosis	
Simultaneous CEA	2/35 (6%)
No CEA	3/49 (6%)
Bilateral stenosis	
Simultaneous CEA	0/15 (0%)
No CEA	0/10 (0%)
Stenosis/occlusion	
Simultaneous CEA	3/7 (43%)
No CEA	1/5 (20%)

*Data from Brener BJ, Brief DK, Alpert J, et al: The risk of stroke in patients with asymptomatic carotid stenosis undergoing cardiac surgery: A follow-up study. J Vasc Surg 5:269, 1987.
TIA, transient ischemic attack; CEA, carotid endarterectomy.

However, this is not the end of the story. Several studies indicate that in the days,[10] weeks,[71] and months[70] after CABG, patients with significant carotid stenoses are at much greater risk of new neurologic symptoms (TIA/stroke) than are patients without cerebrovascular disease, and possibly those who underwent CEA at time of CABG.[70] These data are consistent with the findings of Roederer et al., who found a dramatic increase in neurologic symptoms when previously asymptomatic carotid stenoses (first detected as carotid bruits) exceeded 80% reduction in luminal diameter.[72] Hence, all patients, including cardiac surgery patients, having a high-grade carotid stenosis must be considered at high risk of acute neurologic symptoms (TIA/stroke). The unanswered question is whether overall long-term neurologic morbidity and mortality is reduced in patients with coexisting carotid and coronary disease by performance of simultaneous CABG/CEA or whether better outcome will result from staged procedures.

With occasional exceptions,[29,73] most studies agree that prior neurologic symptoms (stroke/TIA) and/or signs markedly increase the risk of neurologic complications with heart surgery.[8,12,17,31,43,74,75] Presumably, neurologically symptomatic patients have either more severe cerebral atherosclerosis, and/or regions with impaired autoregulation, and/or poor collateral perfusion, rendering them more susceptible to cerebral ischemia. It is now established that CEA improves long-term neurologic outcome in *symptomatic* patients with carotid stenoses greater than or equal to 70%.[76,77] Thus, neurologically symptomatic patients scheduled for nonemergent heart surgery deserve carotid examination and, if significant carotid disease exists, they should be considered candidates for CEA. Decisions regarding simultaneous versus staged procedures should be decided individually, based on the acuity/severity of both the carotid and cardiac disease. There are, as yet, no definitive studies as to which approach results in the best overall morbidity and mortality.

Other Patient-Related Risk Factors

Advanced age is a consistent risk factor for the development of neurologic complications, although exactly why this is, remains unknown. Recently, however, Stump et al. showed patients older than 60 years have more embolic events during cardiac surgery than those who are younger.[78] Presumably this reflects the increasing incidence of aortic atherosclerosis with advancing age.

Recent studies indicate poor preoperative ventricular function is also a risk factor for the development of neurologic and/or neuropsychologic complications.[8,16,17,29,33] Presumably, poor ventricular function is associated with low postoperative systemic pressure and perfusion, factors linked with worse neurologic outcome.[12,17,19,20,31,33]

Left ventricular thrombi are also recognized as a potential source of emboli.[12,79] Breuer et al. reported the occurrence of 15 perioperative strokes in 155 cardiac surgery patients in whom left ventricular thrombi were seen on preoperative cardiac catheterization. The incidence of perioperative stroke in this group (10%) exceeded that of a comparable group of 421 patients (2 to 5%) who were free of left ventricular thrombi.[80] Harrison et al. in a study of approximately 1,000 cardiac surgery patients found that up to 30% of perioperative strokes could be potentially attributed to left ventricular thrombi.[81] Thus, although only a small percentage of patients presenting for cardiac surgery will have intracardiac thrombi, disruption or mobilization of thrombi during surgery will place these patients at risk of embolic stroke.

The Procedure

The literature is fairly evenly divided as to whether or not open procedures (e.g., valve, ventricular aneurysm) have a greater incidence of neurologic complications versus closed procedures (e.g., CABG), although recent work cannot detect a difference.[22,29] A retrospective study from Japan indicates that now, perhaps due to increasing age and incidence of vascular disease in CABG patients, neurologic complications may occur more frequently in CABG patients as compared to valve patients.[74] In general, open procedures have been suggested as having a higher incidence of neurologic injury because of greater embolization of air,[37,82] clot, or valve fragments.[29] For this reason, some authors advocate using TEE as a means to monitor and document clearance of intraventricular microbubbles prior to resumption of ejection,[83,84] presuming this will decrease neurologic injuries. However, Topal et al. found that although valve replacement patients had a much greater incidence and severity of intracardiac microbubbles compared to CABG patients, neurologic outcome was indistinguishable between groups.[85] Thus, at least in Topal's study, intracardiac microbubbles, as detected by TEE, did not clearly affect neurologic outcome. Microbubbles from the field, following standard air evacuation maneuvers, and as detected by TEE, *may* not be a problem, due perhaps to their small size. This conclusion is suggested from transcranial Doppler studies wherein most patients are noted to have at least some cerebral gas emboli during cardiac surgery, and yet overt neurologic sequelae are not obvious.[37,66] Transcranial Doppler studies during CEA also detect a high incidence of cerebral gas microemboli without apparent neurologic sequelae.[86]

It is not the author's intent to suggest care should not be taken to clear as much air from the heart as possible prior to resumption of ejection. Recent studies demonstrate large (milliliters) air pockets ("pooled air") can be present after open procedures, despite routine air clearance techniques.[87] Instead, the author's intention is to show that, although intuitive, a direct cause-and-effect relationship between the presence of intraventricular microbubbles and neurologic/neuropsychologic complications has yet to be established.

The Pump

Increasing bypass duration, especially greater than 2 hours, continues to be associated with poor neurologic outcome, presumably because of progressive cerebral embolization. It is well established that cardiopulmonary bypass can introduce a wide variety of material into the systemic circulation. Material may include air; antifoaming agents[88–91]; fat[92,93]; fibers[94] and plastic chips[95]; and aggregates of leukocytes,[96] platelets,[97] and fibrin.[98–101] The suspicion that microemboli created by bypass systems are a major cause of perioperative neurologic injury has been pervasive in the literature since the earliest days of its use. Controversies have centered on which bypass and oxygenator systems create the smallest number of microemboli, the utility of filtration in removing these contaminants, and whether neurologic outcome is improved when microparticulate embolization is decreased.

Studies have repeatedly shown membrane oxygenators produce fewer numbers of microscopic gas emboli than bubble oxygenators.[102–107] Some studies suggest membrane oxygenators produce fewer platelet and fibrin emboli as well.[98,100,108] Microbubbles produced by bubble oxygenators appear to range from 70 to 150 μm in diameter as assessed by studies employing ultrasonic detectors.[96,105,109,110] Membrane oxygenators produce emboli that are rarely larger than 50 μm.[98,105] Factors that increase release of microbubbles from bubble oxygenators include: (1) increasing the ratio of gas flow to blood flow,[105,109–111] (2) low levels of blood in the oxygenator,[109–111] and (3) agitation of the oxygenator.[109–111]

Cardiotomy suction, which returns scavenged blood from the operative field to the bypass circuit, is a major source of embolic debris.[93] Solis, in two reports, found the level of particulate microemboli in cardiotomy return line blood to be as much as 16 times the level found in blood from the defoaming chamber of a bubble oxygenator![92,108] Particles varied in size, with about half being less than 32 μm. The remaining particles, 32 to 80 μm, approximated the size of platelet aggregates. Fat globules were also identified. A Dacron wool filter removed 89% of all microparticles, whereas a 40-μm polyester mesh filter removed about 60%. These findings have recently been confirmed by Liu et al.[107] Solis et al. suggested filtration of cardiotomy return blood would be sufficient to remove the majority of embolic material created by bypass systems. In support of this conclusion, a number of reports showed filtration of cardiotomy return blood appeared to improve overall perioperative mortality and decreased the incidence of nonfat cerebral emboli (fibrin-platelet aggregates and refractile bodies) seen at autopsy.[112–114] Cardiotomy blood contains a high level of microparticulates due to a turbulent air/blood interface created at the sucker tip. As the ratio of aspirated air to blood increases, greater degrees of hemolysis and platelet aggregation are observed.

An important aspect of cardiopulmonary bypass, often ignored when discussing microparticle formation, is adequacy of anticoagulation. Young et al., studying rhesus monkeys, assessed anticoagulation during bypass using the whole blood activated clotting time (ACT).[115] Animals in which the ACT decreased below 400 seconds had abundant fibrin and platelet debris on the oxygenator filter mesh. Animals in which the ACT was greater than 400 seconds had little debris on oxygenator filters as well as higher postbypass platelet counts and fibrinogen levels. Similarly, Abts et al., using an ultrasonic particle counter, found microparticles 150 μm or larger increased in number as the ACT decreased.[105] These studies indicate that inadequate anticoagulation during bypass (ACT <400 seconds) will result in creation of a greater number of fibrin and platelet aggregates which, if not removed by arterial filtration, will be delivered to the patient.

Using fluoroescein angiography, Blauth et al. recently observed retinal vascular occlusions in 21 of 21 patients undergoing cardiopulmonary bypass with a bubble oxygenator.[116] Occlusions occurred in 50-μm vessels (arterioles) and 4 of 21 (19%) had focal leakage of fluoroescein during bypass, indicating loss of vascular integrity. Companion studies in dogs showed the occlusions to be due to platelet-fibrin microaggregates 20 to 70 μm in diameter. Although there appeared to be partial reperfusion 30 minutes after bypass in about 80% of cases, 2 of 16 (13%) patients had persistently occluded retinal vessels 8 days postoperatively and new "cotton-wool spots, indicative of focal retinal ischemia, were seen in 2 of 21 (10%) patients. It is reasonable to think that a similar process almost certainly occurs in the cerebral vasculature, resulting in diffuse multifocal microinfarcts. It is also reasonable to propose that diffuse microinfarcts might be responsible for the commonly observed neuropsychologic disturbances following bypass (see above). Thus, it would seem that a decrease in the incidence or severity of these lesions, either by arterial filtration or use of membrane oxygenation, might lead to a decrease in the severity of neuropsychologic deterioration. Unfortunately, Blauth et al. found neither to be the case. Inclusion of a 40-μm arterial filter into the bypass circuit did not appear to reduce the incidence of retinal vascular occlusions.[116] (However, a filter of this size would not efficiently remove particles <50 μm.) Membrane oxygenation reduced, but did not eliminate, retinal vascular occlusions (100% of patients with bubble oxygenators vs. 47% of patients with membrane oxygenators).[117] Despite this reduction, neuropsychologic status was no better in patients having membrane oxygenation as compared to those having bubble oxygenation.

Based on transcranial Doppler studies, which can detect particles *at least* in the 30- to 50-μm range,[35,36] there is no doubt membrane oxygenation and/or arterial filtration do reduce the embolic challenge to the brain during bypass.[35,36,82,117] Nevertheless, clinical evidence of better neurologic or neuropsychologic outcome with membrane oxygenation or arterial filtration remains either unconvincing[35] or, in fact, does not support the hypothesis.[17,30,117] For example, Pugsley et al. randomized 40 patients undergoing bypass with bubble oxygenators to receive a 40-μm arterial filter or no filter.[35] Although nonfiltered patients had a cerebral microembolic rate during bypass *40 times greater* than that of filtered patients, there was no significant difference in neurologic or neuropsychological outcome. These findings are consistent with larger studies that report no difference in neurologic and/or neuropsychologic outcome between patients undergoing filtered versus nonfiltered bypass,[30] or membrane versus bubble oxygenation.[17] Thus, although again intuitive, it is not yet definitively established that microparticles (either gas or particulate) originating from the cardiopulmonary bypass circuit play a major role in the genesis of neurologic or neuropsychologic complications of cardiac surgery. (See "Massive Cerebral Gas Embolism" below.)

Controversies in Anesthetic and Cardiopulmonary Bypass Management

In day-to-day practice, the pathogenesis of most neurologic injuries is rarely obvious, although cerebral ischemia—focal or global, transient or permanent—is almost certainly the final common mechanism. Thus, a parallel approach to the problem of perioperative neurologic injury has been to try to establish anesthetic and cardiopulmonary bypass techniques that "optimally" maintain cerebral physiology and/or minimize damage secondary to a cerebral ischemic insult.

Glucose Management

With normal levels of CBF, PaO_2, and serum glucose concentration, the brain extracts 35 to 45% of the available oxygen, but only 10 to 15% of the available glucose. Accordingly, even when CBF is inadequate to support aerobic glucose oxidation and adenosine triphosphate (ATP) generation (ischemia), there is usually sufficient glucose to permit continued anaerobic metabolism. Anaerobic glucose metabolism results in intracellular lactic acidosis. Intracellular acidosis is known to be associated with loss of neuronal ion and cell volume control, lactate clearance, and mitochondrial ATP generation.[118] In fact, several studies have found the severity of intracellular acidosis to be an important negative correlate of neuronal metabolic and functional recovery[119–121] and postischemic reperfusion.[122] Hyperglycemia, by providing more glucose for anaerobic metabolism, increases the severity of intracellular acidosis under ischemic conditions.[123] Thus, hyperglycemia is associated with worse neurologic outcome in both animal[124–127] and human[128] studies of cerebral ischemia and infarction. In order to avoid exacerbation of neurologic injuries associated with cardiac surgery, avoidance of hyperglycemia during bypass has been recommended.[129]

Nevertheless, two recent human studies challenge the supposition that hyperglycemia during bypass should negatively affect neurologic outcome. Metz and Keats reported no neurologic injury in 54 patients undergoing CABG managed with glucose-containing fluids (serum glucose ~700 mg/dl during bypass) versus 1 stroke and 1 case of encephalopathy in 53 patients in whom glucose was avoided during CABG (glucose ~200 mg/dl).[130] This report can be faulted for its lack of sensitive monitors of neurologic outcome and its small sample size relative to the stroke rate. Nevertheless, a more detailed study of postoperative neuropsychologic performance found no correlation between serum glucose level during bypass (103 to 379 mg/dl) and subsequent neuropsychologic deterioration.[131]

In each of the above studies, cardiopulmonary bypass was conducted with moderate hypothermia. Lundgren et al. recently showed that even mild hypothermia (32° to 33°C) markedly attenuates the detrimental effects of hyperglycemia in rats undergoing to 10 to 15 min of cerebral ischemia.[132] Thus, perhaps the lack of detrimental effect of hyperglycemia in human cardiopulmonary bypass studies can be ascribed to the use of hypothermia. Nevertheless, it is this author's opinion, based upon the preponderance of convincing animal data, that avoidance of hyperglycemia during periods of potential neurologic injury (bypass) still appears prudent.

Hemodilution

Hemodilution is employed during cardiopulmonary bypass to compensate for hypothermia-induced increases in blood viscosity, to reduce blood utilization and, supposedly, to improve tissue oxygen delivery. Both human[133] and animal[134] studies indicate brain oxygen supply-demand relationships are preserved with hematocrit (Hct) levels in the mid-20s during cardiopulmonary bypass at 27°C. Many centers, in an attempt to avoid transfusion, now accept Hct's in the 20s in the early postoperative period. At issue is whether postbypass hemodilution of this magnitude might adversely affect neurologic outcome in patients who sustain a neurologic insult before or during cardiopulmonary bypass.

Hemodilution has been shown to increase blood flow in areas of cerebral ischemia, presumably via reduction of blood viscosity.[135,136] For this reason, hemodilution has been investigated as a possible treatment modality for stroke. In animal studies, hemodilution to an Hct of 30% appears to provide a moderate degree of neurologic benefit,[137–139] although, in one study, reduction in infarct size was critically dependent upon maintenance of normal arterial pressure.[137] Similarly, in few small studies of human stroke patients, hemodilution to an Hct of approximately 30% also appears to confer modest neurologic benefit.[140,141] Despite these encouraging reports, other trials have failed to demonstrate any neurologic benefit with hemodilution in nonsurgical human stroke patients (Hct decreased from ~43% to ~36%).[142–145]

The normal cerebrovascular response to hemodilution is to increase both cerebral blood flow and oxygen extraction[146] (Fig. 36–2). In this way, brain oxygen (O_2) delivery and consumption are maintained at normal levels. For hemodilution to confer neurologic benefit in *ischemic* tissue, Hct must be reduced to a level where increases in CBF more than compensate for decreased arterial O_2 content, such that net cerebral O_2 delivery in the ischemic region actually *increases*. This flow-content balance is delicate. Thus, inadequate hemodilution is unlikely to confer benefit (perhaps the case in the human

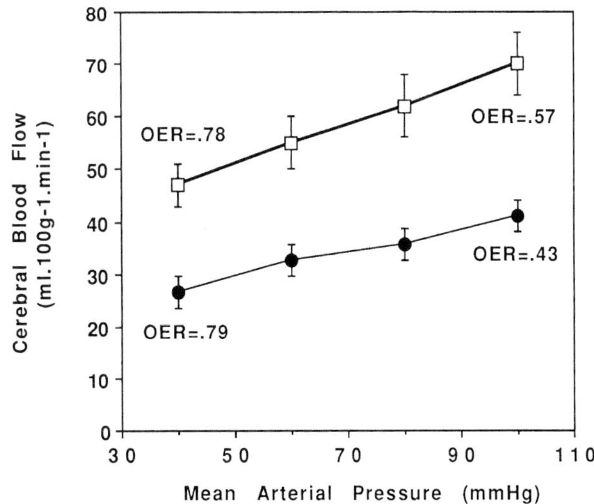

FIGURE **36–2.** Cerebrovascular responses to hemodilution. *Solid circles*, Hct = 40%; *open squares*, Hct = 20%; OER, oxygen extraction ratio. (Modified from Maruyama M, Shimoji K, Ichikawa T, et al: The effects of extreme hemodilutions on the autoregulation of cerebral blood flow, electroencephalogram and cerebral metabolic rate of oxygen in the dog. Stroke 16:675, 1985, with permission.)

multicenter trials[142–145]), and conversely, excessive hemodilution could be detrimental. For example, Nagao et al. showed in normal baboons that hemodilution to an Hct below 15% resulted in evoked potential changes suggestive of cerebral oxygen deprivation.[147] Areas of cerebral ischemia, having little vasodilatory or oxygen extraction reserve, would seem likely to be compromised at a significantly greater Hct value than normal regions.

Thus, when it comes to neurologic outcome, Hct's in the low 30s, with maintenance of blood pressure and cardiac output would seem unlikely to be detrimental, and may *possibly* be beneficial to patients sustaining neurologic injury during surgery or bypass. On the other hand, there is the possibility that Hct's in the 20s after bypass are *not* helping neurologic outcome. Savagaeu et al. reported neuropsychologic impairment 9 days after operation was associated with Hct below 30 in the first 12 hours after operation.[33] More recently, Shaw et al. reported acute neurologic and neuropsychologic outcome to be significantly worse in patients having the greatest perioperative reductions in Hct.[17] Thus, perhaps we are reaching the lower tolerance limits for hemodilution. Use of oxygen-carrying hemodilutants, such as cross-linked or recombinant hemoglobin, hold real promise in the future treatment and management of acute cerebral ischemia.[138]

Moderate Hypothermia

Hypothermia has long been considered to provide a measure of "cerebral protection" during cardiopulmonary bypass. Within limits, as temperature decreases, the brain's tolerance to ischemia increases. By reducing cerebral metabolic rate, hypothermia slows the rate of high-energy phosphate depletion[148–151] and the development of intracellular acidosis during cerebral ischemia.[149–151] In this way, hypothermia is thought to delay or prevent neuronal energy failure and terminal membrane depolarization during an ischemic period.[152,153] Thus, brain protection has been traditionally considered to be directly related to the degree of cerebral metabolic suppression afforded by hypothermia.

Croughwell et al., studying 41 adults during cardiopulmonary bypass at 27°C, found cerebral metabolic rate for oxygen ($CMRO_2$) was reduced to a value of approximately 36% of the normothermic value (1.4 ± 0.3 vs. 0.5 ± 0.2 ml/100 gm/min).[154] In this and comparable adult studies, the $CMRO_2$ ratio over a 10°C interval, referred to as Q_{10}, ranges from 2.4 to 2.8.[155–157] The suppressive effect of hypothermia upon cerebral metabolism may be somewhat greater in children than in adults. Greeley et al., studying cerebral blood flow and metabolism in 46 children during cardiopulmonary bypass, found $CMRO_2$ to decrease logarithmically with decreasing temperature to values of approximately 36% and 12% of normothermic values at 28°C and 19°C, respectively[158] (Fig. 36–3). In this study Q_{10} ranged between 3.3 and 3.6. Based on these Q_{10} values, one would predict that, at 27°C, the brain would tolerate ischemia about three times longer than it would at 37°C. Likewise, at 17°C, the brain might be expected to tolerate ischemia about nine (3 × 3) times longer than it would at 37°C.

Until recently, metabolic suppression was considered to be the only mechanism of hypothermic cerebral protection.[159] New evidence indicates hypothermia can con-

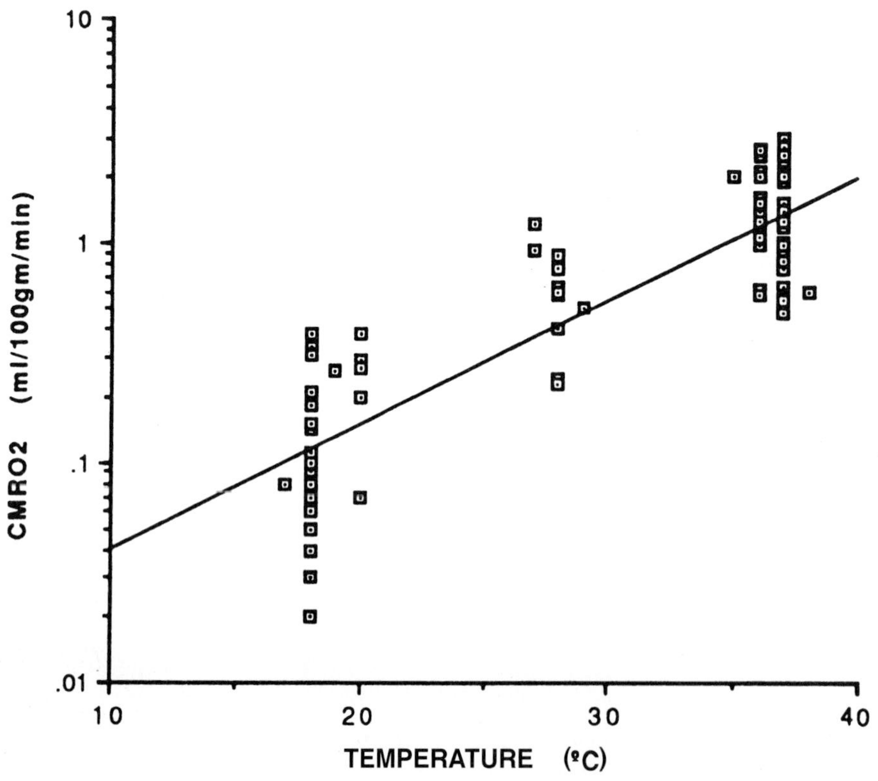

FIGURE **36–3.** Cerebral metabolic rate for oxygen ($CMRO_2$) versus temperature in children undergoing cardiopulmonary bypass. (From Greeley WJ, Kern FH, Ungerleider RM, et al: The effect of hypothermic cardiopulmonary bypass and total circulatory arrest on cerebral metabolism in neonates, infants and children. J Thorac Cardiovasc Surg 101:783, 1991, with permission.)

fer cerebral protection even when cellular energy failure occurs[148,160–162] via modulation of intra- and postischemia (reperfusion) phenomena.[163] Most notable is the discovery that hypothermia attenuates peri-ischemic excitatory neurotransmitter release.[164–167] Release of excitatory amino acids (e.g., glutamate, aspartate) are thought to produce neuronal injury by, among other actions, activation of *N*-methyl-D-aspartate (NMDA) receptor-gated calcium channels, which result in a massive increase in intracellular calcium concentration.[168] Increased intracellular calcium triggers a pathologic cascade that includes free fatty acid release, free radical production, and the uncoupling of mitochondrial oxidative metabolism.[168] Hypothermia, by limiting or preventing glutamate release, lessens or prevents neurologic injury. Hypothermia has also been shown to attenuate postischemic edema and leukotriene formation.[169] The "neuroprotective" effect of mild to moderate hypothermia (30° to 35°C) appears to be mediated primarily via attenuation of these intra- and postischemic phenomena.[159,163]

Although hypothermia clearly provides a measure of neurologic protection in the face of temporary cerebral ischemia,[160,162,170] it is less clear how much hypothermia protects brain in the presence of a permanent lesion (e.g., atherosclerotic embolus). Using nonbypass rat models of permanent focal cerebral ischemia, Ridenour et al. found mild hypothermia (2 hours at 33°C) did not reduce the extent to cerebral infarction,[171] whereas Onesti et al. found deep hypothermia (~1 hour at 24°C) did.[172] At the intermediate temperature of 30°C, Morikawa et al. observed a strong trend (but not statistically significant) toward a reduction in cerebral infarction.[173] Thus, laboratory evidence suggests conventional moderately hypothermic bypass (27° to 28°C) might provide some measure of brain protection when compared to normothermic bypass, even for permanent lesions (e.g., atheroemboli).

Recently, there has been great interest in the use of normothermic ("warm") cardioplegia along with normothermic bypass.[174,175] At issue is whether neurologic outcome, in the absence of hypothermia, might be worse with "warm bypass" as compared to conventional moderately hypothermic bypass. If predominant mechanisms of neurologic injury are related to temporary hypoperfusion when the brain is "usually" cold (low arterial pressure and/or [perhaps] microscopic gas emboli during bypass) neurologic outcome should be worse with warm bypass. If, on the other hand, major mechanisms are permanent embolic lesions (atherosclerotic plaque) or temporary hypoperfusion when the brain is "usually" warm (low pressure before/after bypass) outcome should be essentially unaffected. To date, only one study addressing this issue has been published. Wong et al. randomized 34 patients undergoing CABG to normothermic (34.7° ± 0.5°C) versus hypothermic (27.8° ± 2.0°C) bypass, with each patient undergoing neuropsychologic testing before and after operation as an index of neurologic status.[176] Bypass duration, anesthetic management, and arterial pressure during bypass were comparable between groups. No patient suffered a focal stroke and neuropsychologic scores did not differ between groups. This indicates that hypothermia did not confer protection. Nevertheless, small group sizes relative to the occurrence rate (0% stroke) and the small temperature differences between groups (~6°C) may have resulted in insufficient statistical power to detect neurologic outcome differences between "cold" and "warm" bypass. This finding, if confirmed by others, indicates that much of the neurologic and neuropsychologic morbidity associated with cardiac surgery is not the result of temporary cerebral ischemia during hypothermic bypass but, rather, is more likely the result of permanent lesions (e.g., atherosclerotic emboli or fibrin/platelet microemboli) or events occurring during *normothermic* phases of the perioperative period (see "Hemodynamics," below). Because *hyperthermia* (even 2°C greater than normal) markedly exacerbates the severity of injury secondary to an ischemic insult,[177,178] "overheating" of the brain should be avoided during warming.

Hypothermic Acid-Base Management (The α-Stat vs. pH-Stat Controversy)

When hypothermic, poikilotherms and hibernators tend to use two very different acid-base strategies, α-stat and pH-stat, respectively (see below). Because humans are neither poikilotherms nor hibernators, nor do humans normally become hypothermic, it is unclear which hypothermic acid-base strategy might be more "physiologically appropriate" for humans during hypothermic cardiopulmonary bypass. To date, the α-stat versus pH-stat controversy has focused on the brain because, as will be discussed, hypothermic acid-base management has been shown to influence cerebral physiology.

Before discussing the clinical implications of the α-stat versus pH-stat controversy, a review of the underlying physiology is necessary. Electrochemical neutrality is defined as the point where $[H^+]$ is equal to $[OH^-]$. At 37°C, the $[H^+]$ at neutrality is 1.58×10^{-7} mol/L, giving a neutral pH (pN) of 6.80.[179,*] When aqueous solutions are cooled, both $[H^+]$ and $[OH^-]$ decrease because of a reduction in the spontaneous dissociation of water. For example, at 17°C, the $[H^+]$ at neutrality approximates 0.7×10^{-7} mol/L, giving a pN of 7.14. Thus, with anaerobic cooling of aqueous solutions (including blood) pN spontaneously increases, following the relationship: $\Delta pN/\Delta T \cong -0.017$ pH units/°C.[180] With some exceptions,[180,181] poikilotherms tend to maintain intracellular pH near pN over a wide range of body temperatures. Simultaneously, they maintain extracellular pH at more alkalotic values, keeping a fairly constant intra- to extracellular pH gradient of 0.5 to 0.7 pH units.[179] Thus, at 37°C, intracellular pH is about 6.8 and extracellular (blood) pH is about 7.4. As poikilotherms cool, both intra- extracellular pH increase in a manner virtually identical to the anaerobic cooling of water: $\Delta pH/\Delta T \cong -0.017$ pH units/°C.[182] Reeves observed the pK of the histidine imidazole group also varies with temperature in a fashion almost identical to that of water: $\Delta pK/\Delta T$ is $\cong -0.016$ pK units/°C.[183] By maintaining intracellular

* Although we tend to think of "neutral" pH (pN) = 7.00, this is true only at 25°C, where $[H^+] = [OH^-] = 1 \times 10^{-7}$.

TABLE 36–6
α-Stat Versus pH-Stat Acid-Base Management*

In vivo Temperature	Measured and Reported at 37°C				Corrected to in vivo Temperature			
	pH		P_{CO_2} (mm Hg)		pH		P_{CO_2} (mm Hg)	
	α-stat	*pH-stat*	*α-stat*	*pH-stat*	*α-stat*	*pH-stat*	*α-stat*	*pH-stat*
37°C	7.40	7.40	40	40	7.40	7.40	40	40
33°C	7.40	7.34	40	47	7.44	7.40	35	40
30°C	7.40	7.30	40	54	7.50	7.40	29	40
27°C	7.40	7.26	40	62	7.55	7.40	26	40
23°C	7.40	7.21	40	74	7.60	7.40	22	40
20°C	7.40	7.18	40	84	7.65	7.40	19	40
17°C	7.40	7.14	40	96	7.69	7.40	17	40

*Corrections for temperature taken from Andritsch et al.[184]

pH near pN, poikilotherms maintain the ionization state of histidine imidazole (called α) at a constant level, despite changing body temperature. Hence, the name α-stat. The α-stat hypothesis contends that the *histidine imidazole ionization state is the primary determinant of both the charge state and pH-dependent function of many of the body's key functional proteins.*[180] Thus, during hypothermia with α-stat management, changing body temperature alters neither pN nor histidine ionization. Consequently, protein charge state, structure, and function remain near normal, and poikilotherms can remain active over a wide range of body temperatures.

Poikilotherms achieve this by appearing to anaerobically cool their blood. As poikilotherms cool, both intracellular and extracellular (blood) pH increase as described above. Simultaneously, because gas solubility increases with decreasing temperature, the partial pressure of carbon dioxide (CO_2) decreases,[†] although total blood CO_2 content does not change. Thus, poikilotherms establish what appears to be a respiratory alkalosis when blood gases are corrected to actual in vivo temperature, "worsening" with deepening hypothermia relative to normothermic blood-gas values. α-Stat management is approximated during human hypothermic cardiopulmonary bypass by maintaining arterial pH at 7.40 and P_{CO_2} at 40 mm Hg as measured at 37°C, regardless of the patient's actual in vivo temperature (blood gases are not temperature-corrected). When corrected to in vivo temperature, α-stat management is seen to result in a respiratory alkalosis (low P_{CO_2}, high pH), a consequence of the spontaneous shift of pH and P_{CO_2} with decreasing temperature (Table 36–6). α-Stat proponents suggest that,[179,185,186] as with poikilotherms, this respiratory alkalosis is, in fact, physiologically appropriate, and will better preserve intracellular electrochemical neutrality and normal cellular structure and function. This assumes of course, that the key functional group in all human tissues (including brain) is histidine imidazole; however, it may not be.

[†]Henry's law states that the amount of a gas in solution is proportional to its partial pressure. Therefore, $[CO_2] = P_{CO_2} \times \sigma$, where $[CO_2]$ = concentration of CO_2 in solution (mmol/L), σ = temperature-dependent solubility coefficient of CO_2 in aqueous solution (mmol/L/mm Hg), P_{CO_2} = partial pressure of CO_2 (mm Hg). This equation can be rewritten as $P_{CO_2} = ([CO_2]/\sigma)$. With hypothermia, σ increases, therefore P_{CO_2} decreases.

The other hypothermic acid-base strategy, referred to as "pH-stat," approximates that used by hibernators; pH-stat management attempts to maintain arterial pH at 7.40 and P_{CO_2} at 40 mm Hg as measured at, or corrected to, the subject's actual in vivo temperature (i.e., blood gases are temperature-corrected). As discussed above, anaerobic cooling of blood results in a shift of pH to more alkaline values and a reduction of P_{CO_2}. In order to maintain fixed (temperature-corrected) values of pH and P_{CO_2} during cooling, H^+ (CO_2) must be added. Thus, with pH-stat management, it is necessary to increase the total CO_2 content of blood as temperature is reduced. As shown in Table 36–6, pH-stat management produces a relative hypercarbia and acidemia compared to α-stat management, increasing in magnitude as temperature decreases. Most enzyme reaction rates are pH-dependent, and many enzymes have pH optima that follow the predictions of α-stat theory.[187,188] Because pH-stat management creates a relatively acidic intracellular environment, this would be expected to decrease enzyme reaction rates, ATP consumption, and, consequently, metabolic rate. In fact, this process has been proposed as the mechanism by which hibernating species, which follow pH-stat acid-base strategy, reduce oxygen consumption in nonessential organs to lowest possible values.[188–190]

To date, there has been limited work on whether hypothermic blood-gas management (α-stat vs. pH-stat) might influence cerebral metabolism during human hypothermic cardiopulmonary bypass. The existing data are limited to adults during moderate hypothermia and are contradictory. Prough et al. measured $CMRO_2$ in 25 adults during cardiopulmonary bypass at 27°C over a Pa_{CO_2} range that encompassed both α-stat and pH-stat conditions.[191] These investigators found $CMRO_2$ decreased with increasing P_{CO_2}. $CMRO_2$ values under pH-stat conditions were approximately 50% that of α-stat values (0.2 ± 0.1 vs. 0.4 ± 0.1 ml/100 gm/min, respectively). Similarly, Rogers et al. measured $CMRO_2$ in adults during cardiopulmonary bypass at 27°C, finding pH-stat patients to have $CMRO_2$ values about 20% less than α-stat patients.[192] In contrast, Murkin et al.[156] and Stephan et al.[193] reported $CMRO_2$ values in patients having either α-stat or pH-stat management (~27°C) that were indistinguishable. In agreement with the latter authors, we found no apparent difference in $CMRO_2$ between α-stat and pH-stat management in our rabbit model of cardiopulmonary bypass at 27°C.[134] Thus, at moderate hypothermia (≥27°C), the weight of current evidence indicates $CMRO_2$ is minimally affected by choice of blood-gas management. Inspection of Table 36–6 suggests pH and P_{CO_2} differences between these techniques are, really, fairly modest at temperatures of 27°C or higher and would seem unlikely to affect $CMRO_2$.

Cerebral blood flow, like $CMRO_2$, decreases during hypothermic cardiopulmonary bypass. Nevertheless, the cerebral vasculature retains its responsiveness to changing Pa_{CO_2}.[194–197] Consequently, the relative hypercarbia of pH-stat management is believed to induce cerebral vasodilation, resulting in: (1) greater CBF relative to α-stat patients; and (2) impairment of cerebral autoregulation. A highly illustrative study was that of Murkin et al., wherein 38 adults underwent cardiopulmonary bypass at approximately 26°C under either α-stat or pH-stat management[156] (Fig. 36–4). As shown in Figure 36–4, CBF appeared to be independent of perfusion pressure under α-stat conditions (i.e., cerebral autoregulation was intact). In contrast, under pH-stat conditions, CBF appeared to vary with perfusion pressure (i.e., cerebral autoregulation was absent). Other studies in adults during moderately hypothermic cardiopulmonary bypass have been consistent with these findings.[198–203] Because in Murkin's study $CMRO_2$ did not differ between α-stat or pH-stat patients, it was clear pH-stat management resulted in a greater $CBF/CMRO_2$ ratio than did α-stat management.[156] At issue was whether the "luxury perfusion" afforded by pH-stat management: (1) provided some margin of safety during hypotensive periods on bypass; or (2) alternatively, resulted in unnecessary cerebral hyperperfusion.

As can be seen in Figure 36–4, as cerebral perfusion pressure decreases, CBF differences between α-stat and pH-stat diminish. In the range of perfusion pressures often used during cardiopulmonary bypass (~45 to 60 mm Hg), CBF differences between α-stat and pH-stat are often, actually, fairly small.[204] As arterial pressure decreases, the curves converge. Lundar et al., using transcranial Doppler to measure CBF velocity in humans during hypothermic bypass, found the cerebral vasodilatory effect of CO_2 varied with arterial pressure. CBF responses to CO_2 decreased when mean arterial pressure (MAP) was less than about 60 mm Hg.[200] There comes a point (~30 mm Hg) where autoregulatory cerebral vasodilation (afforded by α-stat management) is equivalent to CO_2-induced cerebral vasodilation (afforded by pH-stat management). Cerebral vasodilation is maximized at this point. Therefore, should perfusion pressure fall below this level, CBF will decrease with either technique. Consequently, pH-stat management would seem incapable of providing substantively greater CBF than α-stat management in the presence of hypotension during bypass.[205]

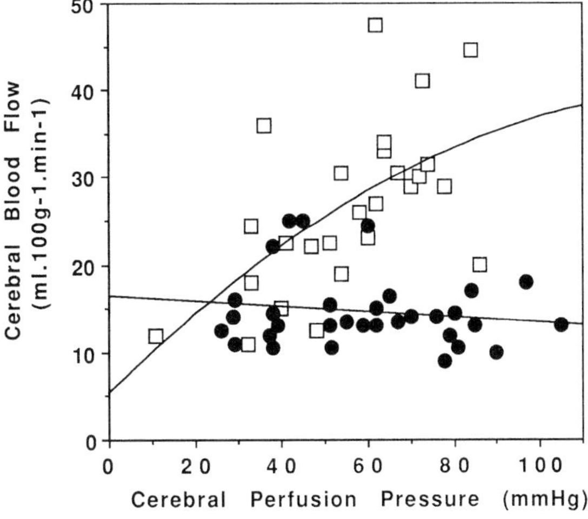

FIGURE **36–4.** Cerebral blood flow versus mean cerebral perfusion pressure in adults undergoing cardiopulmonary bypass (26° to 28°C). *Solid circles*, α-stat; *open squares*, pH-stat. (Modified from Murkin JM, Farrar JK, Tweed A, et al: Cerebral autoregulation and flow/metabolism coupling during cardiopulmonary bypass: The influence of PaCO2. Anesth Analg 66:825, 1987, with permission.)

The cerebral oxygen extraction ratio (OER),[‡] the ratio of oxygen consumption relative to oxygen delivery, is approximately 0.40 during normothermic cardiopulmonary bypass.[154–157,206] During bypass at 27°C, OER is approximately 0.25 with α-stat management[154–156,191,192,206] and approximately 0.10 to 0.15 with pH-stat management.[156,157,191,192] These findings suggest CBF is, in fact, in excess of metabolic demand with *both* techniques, but most especially with pH-stat management. *Thus there is no evidence that the lesser CBF of α-stat management results in global cerebral hypoperfusion.* In fact, some authors speculate the "excess" CBF produced by pH-stat management might be potentially harmful by increasing the amount of emboli delivered to the brain during bypass. The fact that cerebral OER during moderate hypothermia is less than normothermic values, even with α-stat management, implies hypothermia is somehow altering the normal relationship between brain metabolism and blood flow.

To recapitulate, at moderate hypothermia (~27°C) $CMRO_2$ differences between α-stat and pH-stat management appear minimal. Likewise, over a fairly broad range of cerebral perfusion pressure, CBF differences are also fairly small. Because of the small differences in CBF and $CMRO_2$ between techniques, one might anticipate neurologic outcome would be minimally affected, if at all, by choice of blood-gas management. The first study to address this issue supported that hypothesis. Bashein et al., randomly allocated 86 adults undergoing cardiac surgery to either α-stat or pH-stat management.[3] Cardiopulmonary bypass was conducted at approximately 30°C with an unfiltered bubble oxygenator with MAP ranging from 50 to 60 mm Hg. Neuropsychologic testing, used as an index of neurologic integrity, was conducted preoperatively, and at 7 days and 6 months postoperatively. In this study CBF and $CMRO_2$ were not measured. Both short- and long-term neuropsychologic status were unaffected by choice of hypothermic acid-base management. In a more recent study, Stephan et al.

‡ Oxygen extraction ratio (OER) = [cerebral O_2 consumption ÷ cerebral O_2 delivery] = [{CBF × (brain arterial-venous O_2 content difference)} ÷ {CBF × (arterial O_2 content)}].

randomly allocated 65 adults to α-stat or pH-stat management during cardiopulmonary bypass at 26°C.[193] These investigators used a filtered membrane oxygenator with MAP ranging from 55 to 85 mm Hg. As expected, at these higher perfusion pressures, CBF was considerably greater in pH-stat patients as compared to α-stat patients, but $CMRO_2$ did not differ between groups. New neurologic deficits were more common in pH-stat patients (10 of 35) as compared to α-stat patients (2 of 30) ($p = .04$). This study indirectly supports the notion that, somehow, "excess" CBF during cardiopulmonary bypass is disadvantageous. Thus, the weight of current evidence indicates there is no neurologic disadvantage to α-stat management during continuous cardiopulmonary bypass at moderate hypothermia, and *perhaps* is an advantage. That similar studies arrived at different conclusions regarding α-stat versus pH-stat management and neurologic outcome suggests hypothermic acid-base management is but one of many aspects of the conduct of cardiopulmonary bypass that can, at times, influence neurologic outcome.

Hemodynamics

Cerebral metabolic demands are lowered during cardiopulmonary bypass by the institution of hypothermia and the action of various anesthetics. However, at the same time cerebral oxygen delivery may be compromised by hemodilution, hypotension, or hypoperfusion. Hence, the safe lower limits of arterial pressure and systemic perfusion during cardiopulmonary bypass are unpredictable and a matter of particular interest and controversy.

A classic and often cited study is that of Stockard et al., in which perioperative neurologic outcome was correlated with changes in intraoperative blood pressure and electroencephalography (EEG).[207] Hypothermia (28° to 32°C) was *not* consistently induced during bypass, but rather, "employed during lengthy procedures." The report does not state whether $Paco_2$ was corrected for temperature, nor does it state the degree to which hemodilution was employed. During bypass, flow was maintained at 2.2 L/m^2/min, *irrespective of pressure*. The authors proposed an index of hypotension, referred to as the tm50, as a predictor of perioperative neurologic dysfunction:

$$tm50 = \int [50 - MAP\ (mm\ Hg)] \cdot \partial t\ (min)$$

The authors found six of seven patients with a tm50 greater than 100 mm Hg/min had abnormal intraoperative EEG patterns and "generalized" postoperative neurologic deficits. Presumably patients with a tm50 above 100 mm Hg/min had cerebral hypoperfusion. Only 2 of 16 patients with tm50 below 100 mm Hg/min had transient postoperative deficits that could be attributable to intraoperative events. None of these 16 patients had intraoperative EEG abnormalities. The authors proposed that (1) MAP should be at least 50 mm Hg during bypass, and (2) a tm50 above 100 mm Hg/min was predictive of irreversible EEG changes and postoperative neurologic dysfunction, presumably on an ischemic basis.

Stockard's study can be criticized in that patients having neurologic deficits were significantly older and had longer bypass times that those patients who suffered no deficits. Furthermore, and more importantly, it is not clear which patients were hypothermic and which were normothermic (the paper suggests most were normothermic), so conclusions and recommendations made by Stockard et al. may not apply to hypothermic bypass. On the other hand what's "comfortable" about their conclusions is: (1) tm50 is consistent with clinical intuition (a little hypotension for a little while is better tolerated than a lot of hypotension for a long time); (2) tm50 gives us a numeric threshold for action; and (3) tm50 is consistent with 50 mm Hg being the lower limit of cerebral autoregulation.

However, this comfort and this intuition may be wrong; in the 20 years subsequent to Stockard's report, the great majority of studies have not found an association between MAP and/or tm50 during bypass and neurologic injury. How is that possible? During hypothermic bypass, Govier et al.[198] and Murkin et al.[156] found CBF to be independent of MAP between approximately 30 and 100 mm Hg. Also, Feddersen et al. found that, although CBF decreased at MAPs below 30 mm Hg during hypothermic bypass, increased brain oxygen extraction preserved cerebral metabolism at normotensive levels.[155] These findings are supported by the recent reports of Slogoff et al.[29] and Bashein et al.,[3] wherein no correlation between neurologic impairment and tm50, either as a continuous or dichotomous variable, could be demonstrated. Govier also found CBF to have little dependence on systemic perfusion between the ranges of 1.0 to 2.0 L/m^2/min.[198] Although Soma et al., using pH-stat management, demonstrated a dependence of CBF upon systemic perfusion, jugular venous saturations remained high (86%) even at the lowest bypass flow rate (40 ml/kg/min).[208] Likewise, Slogoff et al. found no correlation between periods of systemic hypoperfusion (<40 ml/kg/min) and neurologic outcome during hypothermic bypass.[29] Thus, *when hypothermic*, the brain appears very tolerant to low MAP and systemic perfusion. In total, these studies indicate that for the majority of adult patients, cerebral blood flow and oxygen delivery are adequately maintained with MAP is 40 mm Hg or higher and systemic flow is 40 or more ml/kg/min during hypothermic bypass. In fact, systemic pressure and flow may be even lower than these values for varying periods of time without adversely affecting neurologic outcome.

During normothermic bypass this "rule of thumb" should not be considered reliable. Hypotension (systolic blood pressure <80 mm Hg), low cardiac output, and the need for hemodynamic support in the weaning, postbypass, and ICU phases has been clearly associated with adverse neurologic outcome.[12,17,19,29,31] Recent studies report jugular venous saturation decreases significantly during warming.[133,209] For example, Croughwell et al., using a jugular bulb catheter, found 31 of 133 (23%) patients had jugular venous saturations less than or equal to 50% during rewarming.[133] Thus, the brain would seem most vulnerable (oxygen supply-demand relationship least favorable) during the warming, separation, and postbypass phases of the operation (low arterial pressure, low Hct, warm brain). Nevertheless, the normal brain usually has sufficient extraction and vasodilatory reserves to maintain aerobic metabolism, and postoperative neuropsychologic deficits cannot be readily ascribed to this imbalance.[133] In contrast, the brain that has just suffered an acute ischemic insult will be *far less* tolerant of disturbances of oxygen delivery (see "Hemodilution," above). Tranmer et al. recently showed, in monkeys undergoing middle cerebral artery occlusion, that CBF in the ischemic region, in contrast to the nonischemic region, was exquisitely sensitive to changes in cardiac output.[210] Thus, it makes perfect sense that hemodynamic instability following bypass and in the ICU could contribute to neurologic morbidity.

Barbiturates

When given in sufficient dose, anesthetic barbiturates suppress spontaneous neuronal synaptic activity, producing a flat (isoelectric) EEG. With an isoelectric EEG, cerebral metabolic demands are approximately halved. Residual metabolic demands are due to processes vital to neuronal viability, such as maintenance of transmembrane ion gradients, protein synthesis, and other basal homeostatic processes. These latter processes are unaffected by barbiturates.[152,211–213] In general, as long as CBF (oxygen delivery) is sufficient to maintain basic neuronal homeostatic processes, neurons remain viable.

It has long been postulated that barbiturate-induced cerebral metabolic suppression might increase the tolerable duration of cerebral ischemia. By eliminating the synaptic component of cerebral metabolic rate, neuronal ATP stores could go toward maintenance of basal homeostatic processes. However, under conditions of ischemia severe enough to induce a flat EEG, barbiturates do not affect cerebral metabolic rate. Hence, in this circumstance, there is no metabolic or energetic benefit to barbiturate administration. In addition, once ATP stores are exhausted and/or CBF decreases below that needed to maintain homeostatic metabolism, neurons depolarize and die, unaffected by the presence of barbiturates.[152,214] Thus, at best, barbiturate-induced metabolic suppression can only "buy time." In "no-flow" or "low-flow" states, recent studies indicate metabolic suppression delays onset of neuronal depolarization by *only 1 to 2 minutes*.[159,215] One can imagine that in many settings, this rather small amount of "protection" could easily be rendered inconsequential.

Indeed, in models of global cerebral ischemia in dogs[216] and primates,[217] neither pentobarbital[216] nor thiopental[217] confer neurologic benefit. Similarly, use of thiopental after cardiac arrest in humans (a global cerebral injury) has also been found to be without neurologic benefit.[218] in contrast to these disappointing results, high-dose barbiturates have been found to be effective in attenuating neurologic injury in numerous animal models of *focal* cerebral ischemia.[219–223] In focal ischemic injury, barbiturates may be protective by creating an "inverse steal" cerebral circulatory state.[214,224] If a region of brain that is *nonischemic* is made isoelectric by the use of barbiturates, the resulting decrease in metabolic demand causes local vasoconstriction. (Flow in the nonischemic area decreases in response to decreased metabolic need: flow/metabolism coupling.) If an ischemic and a nonischemic region are supplied by a common or collateral arterial system, then CBF, which is no longer going to the vasoconstricted nonischemic area, can be diverted to the vasodilated ischemic area. Hence, perfusion (oxygen delivery) to the ischemic area can be improved, potentially to the point where homeostatic metabolic requirements can be satisfied. In this way, cerebral infarction can be averted, and barbiturates provide neurologic protection.

However, one cannot administer barbiturates forever. Eventually, they must be discontinued. Thus, again, barbiturates can only buy time. If the lesion causing the reduction in CBF is still present at the time barbiturates are discontinued, then infarction is likely to proceed. Consequently, barbiturates have been found to be far more effective in protecting the brain from *temporary* focal ischemia than from *permanent* focal ischemia. Selman et al. studied the effects of temporary versus permanent middle cerebral artery (MCA) occlusion in baboons treated with barbiturates.[223] In control groups (no barbiturates), animals undergoing permanent occlusion had better neurologic outcome than those that underwent temporary (6 hours) occlusion, suggesting a detrimental effect of reperfusion. However, animals sustaining temporary occlusion had far superior neurologic outcome compared to control animals if they were given barbiturates. In fact, barbiturates provided near complete protection in animals subjected to temporary MCA occlusion. In contrast, animals undergoing permanent occlusion with barbiturate treatment had the worst outcome of any group. These investigators concluded barbiturates were effective in treating temporary, but not permanent, focal ischemic states. With the preceding discussion as a background, studies of barbiturate "cerebral protection" in the setting of cardiac surgery will be reviewed.

Nussmeier et al. randomly allocated 182 patients undergoing open cardiac procedures to receive either standard anesthetic/surgical management or thiopental in addition to standard management.[225] Thiopental was given by constant infusion in the pre- and intrabypass period at doses sufficient to maintain a flat EEG (40 ± 8 mg/kg). Perfusion pressure was maintained at equal levels in both groups. Bypass was maintained at normothermia (≥34°C) with a bubble oxygenator without arterial filtration. At 10 days postoperatively, patients receiving thiopental had a lower incidence of neuropsychiatric abnormalities (0 of 89, 0%) than those who had not received thiopental (7 of 89, 7.5%; $p < .025$). In stark contrast, Zaidan et al. found no evidence of neurologic benefit with thiopental in 300 patients undergoing CABG.[28] Similar to the Nussmeier study, thiopental was given to maintain EEG burst-suppression throughout the procedure (30 ± 11 mg/kg). Zaidan's study differed in that a membrane oxygenator, arterial filtration, and systemic hypothermia (28°C) were used during bypass. Strokes occurred in 5 of 149 (3%) of patients receiving thiopental versus 2 of 151 (1.3%) receiving placebo. Although thiopental did not affect neurologic outcome, patients receiving thiopental had an 80% greater need for inotropes after bypass, required 50% longer to regain consciousness, and required postoperative ventilation approximately 30% longer. How can one resolve these directly opposing conclusions regarding the neurologic benefit of thiopental?

As discussed above, barbiturates are most likely to be protective under conditions of temporary, rather than permanent, focal ischemia. In the Nussmeier study, patients were perfused with an unfiltered bubble oxygenator, a circumstance known to introduce a large number of microscopic gas emboli to the cerebral circulation.[35] To a certain extent, microscopic gas emboli act as temporary lesions.[226–229] Microbubbles are cleared in only a few minutes, and capillary flow is restored. Accordingly, the "lesions" created in Nussmeier's study were those most amenable to barbiturate therapy, especially so because Nussmeier's patients were nearly normothermic (i.e., there was no protection being afforded by hypothermia). Had microscopic gas emboli been avoided (by use of membrane oxygenators and/or arterial filters) or hypothermia used, barbiturate therapy might not have resulted in neurologic benefit. That, in fact, is what Zaidan et al. observed. Zaidan's patients were at low risk of cerebral gas microemboli (membrane oxygenator and arterial filter) and, in addition, had a pre-existing degree of protection from hypothermia. Patients suffering stroke in Zaidan's study had documented focal lesions on computed tomography (CT) scan, suggestive of a permanent focal lesion (atheromatous plaque?) where, as discussed above, short-term barbiturate therapy is unlikely to be of benefit.

Thus, barbiturates *may* be of benefit for temporary focal lesions (gas emboli from bypass pump or open chamber) if metabolic suppression is not being achieved by hypothermia. But under "usual" conditions (membrane oxygenator, and/or arterial filter, and/or hypothermia) these insults are either not created or are fairly well tolerated. Barbiturates do not protect the brain against permanent embolic lesions. Thus, the effectiveness of thiopental in reducing neurologic and neuropsychologic sequelae of cardiac surgery must be seriously questioned and its use balanced against some clear disadvantages, namely, cardiac depression, and prolonged emergence and ventilatory requirements.

Profound Hypothermia and Circulatory Arrest

Profound hypothermia (14° to 19°C) is the principal means of neurologic protection during surgical procedures that require markedly reduced systemic perfusion and/or circulatory arrest. Such procedures include repair of some congenital heart defects in children[230–233] and some forms of thoracic aortic disease in adults.[234–236] Animal studies show that at 13° to 20°C, hypothermic circulatory arrest (HCA) is tolerated for 60 to 75 minutes without subsequent histologic or behavioral evidence of neurologic injury.[237–240] Nevertheless, clinically, hypothermic brain protection appears less effective. Clinical studies report 10 to 30% of children[241–244] and an equal percentage of adults[245–247] have some form of acute perioperative neurologic injury following HCA. Choreoathetosis is a rare but potentially catastrophic complication of profound hypothermia and HCA that seems unique to children.[248–250]

Because hypothermic brain protection is graded, with increasing protection as brain temperature decreases,[251,252] achievement of desired brain temperature prior to arrest is a critical determinant of the effectiveness of the technique. Recent studies suggest brain cooling may, in fact, often be incomplete. Bellinger et al. reported that the duration of prearrest perfusion cooling affected postoperative developmental outcome in 28 infants undergoing HCA.[253] Infants cooled on bypass for less than 20 minutes had lower postoperative developmental scores than those who, undergoing equivalent periods of arrest, had greater durations of prearrest cooling. The authors suggested that despite achievement of desired rectal temperatures, brain cooling may have been incomplete in infants with the shorter cooling periods. In support of that conclusion, Kern et al. found 6 of 17 (35%) children cooled on bypass for 7 to 10 minutes to have comparatively low jugular bulb saturations in the immediate prearrest period.[254] The authors similarly interpreted this finding as indicating that, despite desired tympanic temperatures, brain cooling was probably incomplete in these children. Thus, a key issue in the application of HCA is the duration of cooling needed to ensure brain temperature equilibration. To address this issue, our group developed a mathematical model of human brain heat transport. The model allowed us to determine the factors that have the greatest effect upon the rate and the completeness of brain cooling during cardiopulmonary bypass.[255] Using this model, a computer simulation of cooling the infant brain from 37°C to 17°C indicated that 22 to 26 minutes are required before brain temperature equilibration is complete. This prediction is consistent with the findings of the above studies and suggests that, in many clinical protocols, inadequate time is given to brain cooling.

More recently, Jonas et al. reported postoperative developmental outcome in children undergoing HCA appeared to be better in those who received pH-stat management as compared to those who received α-stat management.[256] The authors noted the prearrest cooling duration in their population was somewhat short, 14.5 ± 6.2 minutes. They hypothesized better postoperative development outcome in the (hypercarbic) pH-stat patients was due to greater CBF during prearrest cooling, resulting in more complete brain cooling. α-Stat patients were proposed as having lesser CBF and, consequently, to have had incomplete brain cooling prior to arrest. Indeed, some animal studies suggest ventilatory gas mixtures containing 7 to 10% CO_2 may increase the rate of brain cooling during cardiopulmonary bypass, presumably because of increased CBF.[257,258] On this basis, many groups report adding CO_2 to their ventilatory gas mixtures during cooling (achieving concentrations of 2.5 to 10%).[232,241,243,259] Although no comparative human data exist, recent animal studies do support this hypothesis. Using a rabbit model of cardiopulmonary bypass, our group found no difference in the rate of brain cooling to 27°C between groups managed with either α-stat or pH-stat strategies.[260] Watanabe et al., ventilating dogs with either 5% CO_2/95% O_2 (pH-stat conditions) or 100% O_2 (α-stat conditions), observed no difference in the rate of brain cooling to 20°C.[258] Finally, Aoki et al., cooling piglets to 18°C, also found no difference in the rate of brain cooling between α-stat and pH-stat management.[261] Thus, despite differences in $Paco_2$ between α-stat and pH-stat management, CBF differences may not be sufficiently great as to affect the rate of brain cooling.

An alternative explanation for the developmental outcome differences observed by Jonas et al.[256] is that pH-stat management might have some "neuroprotective" effect. The existing literature on this issue is contradictory. One study is that of Watanabe et al., wherein recovery of brain Po_2 and brain pH following HCA was more complete in animals with α-stat management as compared to pH-stat management.[258] In contrast, Aoki et al. recently observed more rapid normalization of brain pH and ATP following HCA with pH-stat management.[261] As of now, it is far from clear which hypothermic acid-base strategy (α-stat vs. pH-stat) provides the optimal neurologic outcome for patients undergoing HCA.

In a series of reports, Greeley et al. demonstrated HCA alters CBF and $CMRO_2$ in the postarrest period. Children undergoing cardiac surgery with continuous bypass, with either moderate (28°C) or profound (18°C) hypothermia, had restoration of CBF and $CMRO_2$ to prebypass levels upon warming and separation from bypass.[158,262,263] In contrast, children undergoing HCA at 18°C (39 ± 17 minutes) were found to have significantly lower $CMRO_2$, brain oxygen extraction, and CBF in the warming and postbypass periods. Greeley's work clearly shows even when the duration of HCA is well within the clinically "safe" period, the brain sustains a significant insult and its physiology is disordered for some time afterward. On this basis, some authors advocate continuous "low-flow" bypass over HCA whenever possible.[264]

Recent animal studies by Swain et al., using ^{31}P nuclear magnetic resonance techniques, show that during HCA progressive intracellular acidosis develops in the brain, as well as ATP and creatine phosphate depletion.[265] Although these biochemical changes could be prevented by maintaining systemic flow at only 10 ml/kg/min, 5 ml/kg/min was inadequate. HCA with an intermittent period of reperfusion, sometimes used when prolonged HCA is necessary, did not support brain biochemistry as well as continuous low-flow bypass. These investigators also found intermittent perfusion of the cerebral circulation with a cold (4°C) crystalloid solution ("cerebroplegia") during HCA, maintained intracellular pH and energy state far better than HCA alone, with a shorter latency to EEG recovery upon warming (36 ± 6 minutes vs. 117 ± 23 minutes, respectively; $p < .05$).[266] Animals receiving cerebroplegia were found to have better neurologic outcome following 2 hours of HCA, than a group undergoing HCA alone.[267] Interestingly, neurologic outcome was also significantly improved in a group that simply had their heads packed in ice during the arrest period (the HCA-alone group did not). Thus, "cerebroplegia" may exert much of its beneficial effect by simply maintaining cerebral hypothermia during the arrest interval.

Indeed, many studies have shown that during HCA, brain temperature drifts toward ambient room temperature. By decreasing skull temperature, packing the head in ice reduces the temperature gradient for conductive heat gain[255] and helps maintain cerebral hypothermia during HCA. In animals models, simply packing the head in ice significantly improves neurologic tolerance to HCA.[267,268]

Until recently, delayed recovery of CBF, $CMRO_2$, and electrophysiology following HCA was not clearly associated with poor clinical neurologic outcome. Indeed, in Greeley's studies, neurologic outcome in the HCA and continuous flow groups were indistinguishable. However, a randomized prospective trial of HCA versus low-flow bypass in 171 children undergoing repair of D-transposition suggests neurologic outcome may be superior with low-flow bypass.[269] In this study, patients undergoing HCA were more likely to have postoperative seizures, as defined clinically or electroencephalographically, and had a greater release of brain isoenzyme of creatine kinase (CK-BB). The incidence of seizures and magnitude of CK-BB release both correlated with HCA duration. Although overall neurologic outcome did not differ between groups at discharge, results of long-term follow-up are not yet available. Thus, the evidence is mounting, but is not yet conclusive, that neurologic outcome is superior with "low-flow" bypass.

The work of Swain and others shows that a critical level of systemic flow is necessary to prevent brain biochemical deterioration during profound hypothermia. And yet, what that value is clinically, is unknown. In fact, the critical perfusion level likely varies from patient to patient. Recently, Burrows et al. demonstrated the feasibility of monitoring CBF during low-flow bypass via transcranial Doppler.[270] In 17 of 22 (77%) children undergoing low-flow bypass, the Doppler blood flow signal became undetectable, indicating that CBF was, in fact, near zero. In 5 of 17 (29%) patients losing the CBF signal, CBF responses upon restoration of full flow resembled those of patients undergoing HCA. Thus, despite the maintenance of continuous systemic flow, a certain percentage of low-flow patients appeared physiologically equivalent HCA patients. Thus, transcranial Doppler may be useful as a monitor whereby systemic pressure and flow during low-flow bypass can be maintained at a level that maintains cerebral perfusion.

Massive Arterial Gas Embolism

Massive arterial gas embolism is a rare but disastrous complication. In 1980, two studies reported massive arterial gas embolism occurred in 0.1 to 0.2% of all cardiac surgery cases.[271,272] Twenty to 30% of affected patients died immediately, with another 30% having transient and/or nondebilitating neurologic deficits. Circumstances commonly contributing to gas embolism were (1) inattention to the blood level in the reservoir (i.e., they pumped air), (2) reversal of left ventricular vent flow, or (3) unexpected resumption of ejection of an opened heart. Rupture of pulsatile assist devices[273] or intra-aortic balloon pumps[274] may also introduce gas into the arterial circulation.

The pathophysiology of cerebral gas embolism (both macro- and microscopic) is incompletely understood. Many studies have not controlled for factors likely to affect outcome, such as (1) gas composition,[109] (2) bubble size,[227,275] or (3) total volume of gas delivered.[276] Tissue damage following gas embolization is thought to be initiated from simple mechanical blockage of blood vessels by bubbles.[228,229] Although gas emboli may be absorbed or pass through the capillary circulation within 1 to 5 minutes,[226–229] the local reaction of platelets and proteins to the blood-gas interface and/or endothelial damage[277–279] results in blood-brain barrier disruption, edema formation,[279] and a delayed and sustained decrease in cerebral blood flow.[226] Areas of marginal perfusion, such as arterial boundary zones, do not clear gas emboli as rapidly as well-perfused zones,[228] producing a pattern of ischemia or infarction that can be difficult to distinguish from hypotension or embolization of solid particles.[280]

Intraoperative management of massive arterial gas embolism uniformly includes (1) immediate cessation of bypass with aspiration of as much gas as possible from the aorta and heart, (2) clearance of air from the arterial perfusion line, (3) assumption of the Trendelenburg position, (4) implementation of hypothermia (18° to 27°C) during completion of the operation, (5) clearance of gas from the coronary circulation prior to emergence from bypass, and (6) the administration of glucocorticoids (0.5 to 25 mg/kg dexamethasone) in an attempt to minimize cerebral edema.[272,273,281–284] In experimental models, hypotension increases the residence time of cerebral air emboli as well as the severity of resulting ischemia.[285] Hence, maintenance of moderate hypertension intraoperatively and postoperatively seems reasonable. Mills and Oshsner suggested retrograde cerebral perfusion as a method to clear gas emboli.[272] Retrograde perfusion via the superior caval cannula at 1.2 L/min at 20°C for 1 to 2 minutes was used in five of eight patients sustaining massive gas embolism. None of the patients so treated had evidence of neurologic injury. Other groups have also reported successful use of this technique.[284,286–289] However, Hendriks et al., in an animal model of venoarterial perfusion, found only 50% of injected gas (nitrogen) could be recovered from the aorta[290]; 98% of the removable gas was collected from the aorta in the first 7 to 10 minutes of retrograde perfusion. Although no animal appeared to sustain neurologic injury, the authors concluded that venoarterial perfusion did not completely remove embolized gas, and that hyperbaric therapy remained the treatment of choice (see below).

Postoperative management consists of general "neurosupportive" care, such as treatment of cerebral edema (hyperosmotic agents, steroids) and maintenance of normal glucose levels. In a number of case reports, seizures were observed and patients were treated with anticonvulsants.[277,282,283,288] Because seizures after an ischemic insult are associated with poor outcome (due perhaps to their hypermetabolic effects), prophylactic use of phenytoin in this setting seems reasonable. Some authors report dramatic neurologic recovery with the use of hyperbaric oxygenation, even when started many hours after the initial event.[273,281–284,291,292] There are several mechanisms by which hyperbaric oxygenation is thought to confer benefit in this setting. High pressure results in a reduction of bubble diameter, such that bubbles may be more easily cleared. High oxygen tensions produce a large diffusion gradient, favoring absorption of nitrogen within the bubble. High oxygen tensions also increase the blood-to-tissue oxygen diffusion gradient, such that tissue oxygenation may improve in areas of low cerebral blood flow. Nevertheless, spontaneous recovery from air emboli has been reported[272,293,294] and, to date, no prospective study of hyperbaric therapy in the cardiac surgery setting has been performed.[295] Thus, the superiority of hyperbaric oxygenation over general neurosupportive care has yet to be confirmed. Unfortunately, few institutions performing cardiac surgery have an appropriately equipped and staffed compression chamber to allow rapid initiation of hyperbaric therapy. Nonetheless, immediate transfer is often possible and should be seriously considered.

References

1. Sotaniemi KA: Cerebral outcome after extracorporeal circulation. Comparison between prospective and retrospective evaluations. Arch Neurol 40:75, 1983.
2. Silverstein A, Krieger HP: Neurologic complications of cardiac surgery. Arch Neurol 5:601, 1960.
3. Bashein G, Townes BD, Nessly ML, et al: A randomized study of carbon dioxide management during hypothermic cardiopulmonary bypass. Anesthesiology 72:7, 1990.
4. Åberg T, Ronquist G, Tyden H, et al: Release of adenylate kinase into cerebrospinal fluid during open-heart surgery and its relation to postoperative intellectual function. Lancet ii:1139, 1982.
5. Sotaniemi KA: Clinical and prognostic correlates of EEG in open-heart surgery patients. J Neurol Neurosurg Psychiatry 43: 941, 1980.
6. Sellman M, Hindmarsh T, Ivert T, Semb BKH: Magnetic resonance imaging of the brain before and after open heart operations. Ann Thorac Surg 53:807, 1992.
7. Shaw P, Bates D, Cartlidge NEF, et al: Early neurological complications of coronary artery bypass surgery. Br Med J 291:1384, 1985.
8. Reed GL, Singer DE, Picard EH, DeSanctis RW: Stroke following coronary-artery bypass surgery. N Engl J Med 319:1246, 1988.
9. Carella F, Travaini G, Contri P, et al: Cerebral complications of coronary bypass surgery. A prospective study. Acta Neurol Scand 77:158, 1988.
10. Faggioli GL, Curl GR, Ricotta JJ: The role of carotid screening before coronary artery bypass. J Vasc Surg 12:724, 1990.
11. Bojar RM, Najafi H, DeLaria GA, et al: Neurological complications of coronary revascularization. Ann Thorac Surg 36:427, 1983.
12. Lynn GM, Stefanko K, Reed JF, et al: Risk factors for stroke after coronary artery bypass. J Thorac Cardiovasc Surg 104: 1518, 1992.
13. Shaw PJ, Bates D, Cartlidge NEF, et al: Neurological complications of coronary artery bypass graft surgery: Six month follow-up study. Br Med J 293:165, 1986.
14. Shaw PJ, Bates D, Cartlidge NEF, et al: Early intellectual dysfunction following coronary bypass surgery. Q J Med 58:59, 1986.
15. Shaw PJ, Bates D, Cartlidge NEF, et al: Neurologic and neuropsychological morbidity following major surgery: Comparison

of coronary artery bypass and peripheral vascular surgery. Stroke 18:700, 1987.
16. Shaw PJ, Bates D, Cartlidge NEF, et al: Long-term intellectual dysfunction following coronary artery bypass graft surgery: A six month follow-up study. Q J Med 62:259, 1987.
17. Shaw PJ, Bates D, Cartlidge NEF, et al: An analysis of factors predisposing to neurological injury in patients undergoing coronary bypass operations. Q J Med 72:633, 1989.
18. Sotaniemi KA: Brain damage and neurological outcome after open-heart surgery. J Neurol Neurosurg Psychiatry 43:127, 1980.
19. Breuer AC, Furlan AJ, Hanson MR, et al: Central nervous system complications of coronary artery bypass graft surgery: Prospective analysis of 421 patients. Stroke 14:682, 1983.
20. Slogoff S, Girgis KZ, Keats AS: Etiologic factors in neuropsychiatric complications associated with cardiopulmonary bypass. Anesth Analg 61:903, 1982.
21. Treasure T, Smith PLC, Newman S, et al: Impairment of cerebral function following cardiac and other major surgery. Eur J Cardiothorac Surg 3:216, 1989.
22. Townes BD, Bashein G, Hornbein TF, et al: Neurobehavioral outcomes in cardiac operations. A prospective controlled study. J Thorac Cardiovasc Surg 98:774, 1989.
23. Newman S, Klinger L, Venn G, et al: Subjective reports of cognition in relation to assessed cognitive performance following coronary artery bypass surgery. J Psychosom Res 33:227, 1989.
24. Åberg T, Kihlgren M: Cerebral protection during open-heart surgery. Thorax 32:525, 1977.
25. Smith PLC, Newman SP, Ell PJ, et al: Cerebral consequences of cardiopulmonary bypass. Lancet i:823, 1986.
26. Åberg T, Åhlund P, Kihlgren M: Intellectual function late after open-heart operation. Ann Thorac Surg 36:680, 1983.
27. Sotaniemi KA, Mononen H, Hokkanen TE: Long-term cerebral outcome after open-heart surgery. Stroke 17:410, 1986.
28. Zaidan JR, Klochany AI, Martin WM, et al: Effect of thiopental on neurologic outcome following coronary artery bypass grafting. Anesthesiology 74:406, 1991.
29. Slogoff S, Reul GJ, Keats AS, et al: Role of perfusion pressure and flow in major organ dysfunction after cardiopulmonary bypass. Ann Thorac Surg 50:911, 1990.
30. Aris A, Solanes H, Camara ML, et al: Arterial line filtration during cardiopulmonary bypass. J Thorac Cardiovasc Surg 91:526, 1986.
31. Tuman KJ, McCarthy RJ, Najafi H, Ivankovich AD: Differential effects of advanced age on neurologic and cardiac risks of coronary artery operations. J Thorac Cardiovasc Surg 104:1510, 1992.
32. Weintraub WS, Jones EL, Craver J, et al: Determinants of prolonged length of hospital stay after coronary bypass surgery. Circulation 80:276, 1989.
33. Savageau JA, Stanton BA, Jenkins CD, Klein MD: Neuropsychological dysfunction following elective cardiac operation. I. Early assessment. J Thorac Cardiovasc Surg 84:585, 1982.
34. Sotaniemi KA, Juolasmaa A, Hokkanen ET: Neuropsychologic outcome after open-heart surgery. Arch Neurol 38:2, 1981.
35. Pugsley W, Klinger L, Paschalis C, et al: Microemboli and cerebral impairment during cardiac surgery. Vasc Surg 24:34, 1990.
36. Padayachee TS, Parsons S, Theobold R, et al: The detection of microemboli in the middle cerebral artery during cardiopulmonary bypass: A transcranial Doppler ultrasound investigation using membrane and bubble oxygenators. Ann Thorac Surg 44:298, 1987.
37. van der Linden J, Casimir-Ahn H: When do cerebral emboli appear during open heart operations? A transcranial Doppler study. Ann Thorac Surg 51:237, 1991.
38. Katz ES, Tunick PA, Rusinek H, et al: Protruding aortic atheromas predict stroke in elderly patients undergoing cardiopulmonary bypass: Experience with intraoperative transesophageal echocardiography. J Am Coll Cardiol 20:70, 1992.
39. Ribakove GH, Katz ES, Galloway AC, et al: Surgical implications of transesophageal echocardiography to grade the atheromatous aortic arch. Ann Thorac Surg 53:758, 1992.
40. Wareing TH, Davila-Roman VG, Barzilai B, et al: Management of the severely atherosclerotic ascending aorta during cardiac operations. A strategy for detection and treatment. J Thorac Cardiovasc Surg 103:453, 1992.
41. Wareing TH, Davila-Roman VG, Baily BB, et al: Strategy for the reduction of stroke incidence in cardiac surgical patients. Ann Thorac Surg 55:1400, 1993.
42. Bar-El Y, Goor DA: Clamping of the atherosclerotic ascending aorta during coronary artery bypass operations. Its cost in strokes. J Thorac Cardiovasc Surg 104:469, 1992.
43. Gardner TJ, Horneffer PJ, Manolio TA, et al: Major stroke after coronary artery bypass surgery: Changing magnitude of the problem. J Vasc Surg 3:684, 1986.
44. Mills NL, Everson CT: Atherosclerosis of the ascending aorta and coronary artery bypass. J Thorac Cardiovasc Surg 102:546, 1991.
45. McKibbin DW, Bulkley BH, Green WR, et al: Fatal cerebral atheromatous embolization after cardiopulmonary bypass. J Thorac Cardiovasc Surg 71:741, 1976.
46. Parker FB, Marvasti MA, Bove EL: Neurologic complications following coronary artery bypass. The role of atherosclerotic emboli. Thorac Cardiovasc Surg 33:207, 1985.
47. Harris LS, Kennedy JH: Atheromatous cerebral embolism. A complication of surgery of the thoracic aorta. Ann Thorac Surg 4:319, 1967.
48. Price DL, Harris J: Cholesterol emboli in cerebral arteries as a complication of retrograde aortic perfusion during cardiac surgery. Neurology 20:1209, 1970.
49. Soloway HB, Aronson SM: Atheromatous emboli to central nervous system. Arch Neurol 11:657, 1964.
50. Winter WJ: Atheromatous emboli; a cause of cerebral infarction. Arch Pathol 64:137, 1957.
51. Sturgill BC, Netsky MG: Cerebral infarction by atheromatous emboli. Arch Pathol 76:85, 1963.
52. David NJ, Klintworth GK, Friedberg SJ, Dillon M: Fatal atheromatous cerebral embolism associated with bright plaques in the retinal arterioles. Neurology 13:708, 1963.
53. Gravlee GP, Hudspeth AS, Toole JF: Bilateral brachial paralysis from watershed infarction after coronary artery bypass. J Thorac Cardiovasc Surg 88:742, 1984.
54. Brierley JB, Graham DI: Hypoxia and vascular disorders of the central nervous system. In Adams JH, Corsellis JAN, Duchen LW (eds): Greenfield's Neuropathology, 4th ed. New York, John Wiley & Sons, Inc, 1984, p 123.
55. Blauth CI, Cosgrove DM, Webb BW, et al: Atheroembolism from the ascending aorta. An emerging problem in cardiac surgery. J Thorac Cardiovasc Surg 103:1104, 1992.
56. Balderman SC, Gutierrez IZ, Makula P, et al: Noninvasive screening for asymptomatic carotid artery disease prior to cardiac operation. J Thorac Cardiovasc Surg 85:427, 1983.
57. Barnes RW, Liebman PR, Marszalek PB, et al: The natural history of asymptomatic carotid disease in patients undergoing cardiovascular surgery. Surgery 90:1075, 1981.
58. Turnipseed WD, Berkoff HA, Belzer FO: Postoperative stroke in cardiac and peripheral vascular disease. Ann Surg 192:365, 1980.
59. Breslau PJ, Fell G, Ivey TD, et al: Carotid arterial disease in patients undergoing coronary artery bypass operations. J Thorac Cardiovasc Surg 82:765, 1981.
60. Brener BJ, Brief DK, Alpert J, et al: The risk of stroke in patients with asymptomatic carotid stenosis undergoing cardiac surgery: A follow-up study. J Vasc Surg 5:269, 1987.
61. Hertzer NR, Loop FD, Beven EG, et al: Surgical staging for simultaneous coronary and carotid disease: A study including prospective randomization. J Vasc Surg 9:455, 1989.
62. Rizzo RJ, Whittemore AD, Couper GS, et al: Combined carotid and coronary revascularization: The preferred approach to the severe vasculopath. Ann Thorac Surg 54:1099, 1992.
63. Ivey TD, Strandness DE, Williams DB, et al: Management of patients with carotid bruit undergoing cardiopulmonary bypass. J Thorac Cardiovasc Surg 87:183, 1984.
64. Mehigan JT, Buch WS, Pipkin RD, Fogarty TJ: A planned approach to coexistent cerebrovascular disease to coronary artery bypass candidates. Arch Surg 112:1403, 1977.
65. Ropper AH, Wechsler LR, Wilson LS: Carotid bruit and the risk of stroke in elective surgery. N Engl J Med 307:1388, 1982.
66. von Reutern GM, Hetzel A, Birnbaum D, Schlosser V: Transcranial Doppler ultrasonography during cardiopulmonary bypass

in patients with severe carotid stenosis or occlusion. Stroke 19: 674, 1988.

67. Gravlee GP, Roy RC, Stump DA, et al: Regional cerebrovascular reactivity to carbon dioxide during cardiopulmonary bypass in patients with cerebrovascular disease. J Thorac Cardiovasc Surg 99:1022, 1990.
68. Johnsson P, Algotsson L, Ryding E, et al: Cardiopulmonary perfusion and cerebral blood flow in bilateral carotid artery disease. Ann Thorac Surg 51:579, 1991.
69. Furlan AJ, Craciun AR: Risk of stroke during coronary artery bypass graft surgery in patients with internal carotid artery disease documented by angiography. Stroke 15:797, 1985.
70. Schultz RD, Sterpetti AV, Feldhaus RJ: Early and late results in patients with carotid disease undergoing myocardial revascularization. Ann Thorac Surg 45:603, 1988.
71. Barnes RW, Nix ML, Sansonetti B, et al: Late outcome of untreated asymptomatic carotid disease following cardiovascular operations. J Vasc Surg 2:843, 1985.
72. Roederer GO, Langlois YE, Jager KA, et al: The natural history of carotid arterial disease in asymptomatic patients with cervical bruits. Stroke 15:605, 1984.
73. Beall AC, Jones JW, Guinn GA, et al: Cardiopulmonary bypass in patients with previously completed stroke. Ann Thorac Surg 55:1383, 1993.
74. Kuroda Y, Uchimoto R, Kaieda R, et al: Central nervous system complications after cardiac surgery: A comparison between coronary artery bypass grafting and valve surgery. Anesth Analg 76:222, 1993.
75. Branthwaite MA: Neurological damage related to open-heart surgery. Thorax 27:748, 1972.
76. Mayberg MR, Wilson SE, Yatsu F, et al: Carotid endarterectomy and prevention of cerebral ischemia in symptomatic carotid stenosis. JAMA 266:328, 1991.
77. NASCE Trial Collaborators: Beneficial effect of carotid endarterectomy in symptomatic patients with high-grade carotid stenosis. N Engl J Med 325:445, 1991.
78. Stump DA, Tegeler CH, Newman SP, Wallenhaupt S: Older patients have more emboli during coronary artery bypass graft surgery (Abstract). Anesthesiology 77:A52, 1992.
79. Hartman RB, Harrison EE, Pupello DF, et al: Characteristics of left ventricular thrombus resulting in perioperative embolism. J Thorac Cardiovasc Surg 86:706, 1983.
80. Breuer AC, Franco I, Marzewski D, Soto-Velasco J: Left ventricular thrombi seen by ventriculography are a significant risk factor for stroke in open-heart surgery (Abstract). Ann Neurol 10:103, 1981.
81. Harrison EE, Sheldon S, Pupello DF, et al: Cerebrovascular accidents as an immediate complication of coronary bypass surgery or ventricular resection (Abstract). Stroke 8:4, 1977.
82. Padayachee TS, Parsons S, Theobold R, et al: The effect of arterial filtration on reduction of gaseous microemboli in the middle cerebral artery during cardiopulmonary bypass. Ann Thorac Surg 45:647, 1988.
83. Oka Y, Moriwaki KM, Hong Y, et al: Detection of air emboli in the left heart by m-mode transesophageal echocardiography following cardiopulmonary bypass. Anesthesiology 63:109, 1985.
84. Oka Y, Inoue T, Hong Y, et al: Retained intracardiac air. Transesophageal echocardiography for definition of incidence and monitoring removal by improved techniques. J Thorac Cardiovasc Surg 91:329, 1986.
85. Topol EJ, Humphrey LS, Borkon AM, et al: Value of intraoperative left ventricular microbubbles detected by transesophageal two-dimensional echocardiography in predicting neurologic outcome after cardiac operations. Am J Cardiol 56:773, 1985.
86. Spencer MP, Thomas GI, Nicholls SC, Sauvage LR: Detection of middle cerebral artery emboli during carotid endarterectomy using transcranial Doppler ultrasonography. Stroke 21:415, 1990.
87. Orihashi K, Matsuura Y, Hamanaka Y, et al: Retained intracardiac air in open heart operations examined by transesophageal echocardiography. Ann Thorac Surg 55:1467, 1993.
88. Ehrenhaft JL, Claman MA, Layton JM, Zimmerman GR: Cerebral complications of open-heart surgery: Further observations. J Thorac Cardiovasc Surg 42:514, 1961.
89. Lindberg DAB, Lucas FV, Sheagren J, Malm JR: Silicone embolization during clinical and experimental heart surgery employing a bubble oxygenator. Am J Pathol 39:129, 1961.
90. Brierly JB: Neuropathological findings in patients dying after open-heart surgery. Thorax 18:291, 1963.
91. Orenstein JM, Sato N, Aaron B, et al: Microemboli observed in deaths following cardiopulmonary bypass surgery: Silicone antifoam agents and polyvinyl choride tubing as sources of emboli. Hum Pathol 13:1082, 1982.
92. Solis RT, Noon GP, Beall AC, DeBakey ME: Particulate microembolism during cardiac operation. Ann Thorac Surg 17:332, 1974.
93. Clark RE, Margraf HW, Beauchamp RA: Fat and solid filtration in clinical perfusions. Surgery 77:216, 1975.
94. Dimmmick JE, Bove KE, McAdams AJ, Benzing G: Fiber embolization — a hazard of cardiac surgery and catheterization. N Engl J Med 292:685, 1975.
95. Reed CC, Romagnoli A, Taylor DE, Clark DK: Particulate matter in bubble oxygenators. J Thorac Cardiovasc Surg 68:971, 1974.
96. Dutton RC, Edmunds LH: Measurement of emboli in extracorporeal perfusion systems. J Thorac Cardiovasc Surg 65:523, 1973.
97. Guidoin RG, Awad JA, Laperche Y, et al: Nature of deposits in a tubular membrane oxygenator after prolonged extracorporeal circulation. J Thorac Cardiovasc Surg 69:479, 1975.
98. Dutton RC, Edmunds LH, Hutchinson JC, Roe BB: Platelet aggregate emboli produced in patients during cardiopulmonary bypass with membrane and bubble oxygenators and blood filters. J Thorac Cardiovasc Surg 67:258, 1974.
99. Allardyce DB, Yoshida SH, Ashmore PG: The importance of microembolism in the pathogenesis of organ dysfunction caused by prolonged use of the pump oxygenator. J Thorac Cardiovasc Surg 52:706, 1966.
100. Ashmore PG, Svitek V, Ambrose P: The incidence and effects of particulate aggregation and microembolism in pump-oxygenator systems. J Thorac Cardiovasc Surg 55:691, 1968.
101. Hill JD, Aguilar MJ, Baranco A, et al: Neuropathological manifestations of cardiac surgery. Ann Thorac Surg 7:409, 1969.
102. Carlson RG, Lande AJ, Ivey LA, et al: The Lande-Edwards membrane oxygenator for total cardiopulmonary support in 110 patients during heart surgery. Surgery 72:913, 1972.
103. Carlson RG, Lande AJ, Landis B, et al: The Lande-Edwards membrane oxygenator during heart surgery. J Thorac Cardiovasc Surg 66:894, 1973.
104. Kessler J, Patterson RH: The production of microemboli by various blood oxygenators. Ann Thorac Surg 9:221, 1970.
105. Abts LR, Beyer RT, Galletti PM, et al: Computerized discrimination of microemboli in extracorporeal circuits. Am J Surg 135: 535, 1978.
106. Yost G: The bubble oxygenator as a source of gaseous microemboli. Med Instrum 19:67, 1985.
107. Liu JF, Su ZK, Ding WX: Quantitation of particulate microemboli during cardiopulmonary bypass: Experimental and clinical studies. Ann Thorac Surg 54:1196, 1992.
108. Solis RT, Kennedy PS, Beall AC, et al: Cardiopulmonary bypass, microembolization and platelet aggregation. Circulation 52:103, 1975.
109. Patterson RH, Kessler J: Microemboli during cardiopulmonary bypass detected by ultrasound. Surg Gynecol Obstet 129:505, 1969.
110. Gallagher EG, Pearson DT: Ultrasonic identification of sources of gaseous microemboli during open heart surgery. Thorax 28: 295, 1973.
111. Loop FD, Szabo J, Rowlinson RD, Urbanek K: Events related to microembolism during extracorporeal perfusion in man: Effectiveness of in-line filtration recorded by ultrasound. Ann Thorac Surg 21:412, 1976.
112. Aguilar MJ, Gerbode F, Hill JD: Neuropathologic complications of cardiac surgery. J Thorac Cardiovasc Surg 61:676, 1971.
113. Osborn JJ, Swank RL, Hill JD, et al: Clinical use of a Dacron wool filter during perfusion for open-heart surgery. J Thorac Cardiovasc Surg 60:575, 1970.
114. Hill JD, Osborn JJ, Swank RL, et al: Experience using a new Dacron wool filter during extracorporeal circulation. Arch Surg 101:649, 1970.

115. Young JA, Kisker CT, Doty DB: Adequate anticoagulation during cardiopulmonary bypass determined by activated clotting time and the appearance of fibrin monomer. Ann Thorac Surg 26:231, 1978.
116. Blauth CI, Arnold JV, Schulenberg WE, et al: Cerebral microembolism during cardiopulmonary bypass. J Thorac Cardiovasc Surg 95:668, 1988.
117. Blauth CI, Smith P, Newman S, et al: Retinal microembolism and neuropsychological deficit following clinical cardiopulmonary bypass: Comparison of a membrane and a bubble oxygenator. Eur J Cardiothorac Surg 3:135, 1989.
118. Siesjö BK: Pathophysiology and treatment of focal cerebral ischemia. Part II: Mechanisms of damage and treatment. J Neurosurg 77:337, 1992.
119. Rehncrona S, Rosén I, Siesjö BK: Excessive cellular acidosis: An important mechanism of neuronal damage in the brain? Acta Physiol Scand 110:435, 1980.
120. Rehncrona S, Rosén I, Siesjö BK: Brain lactic acidosis and ischemic cell damage: 1. Biochemistry and neurophysiology. J Cereb Blood Flow Metab 1:297, 1981.
121. Welsh FA, Ginsberg MD, Rieder W, Budd WW: Deleterious effect of glucose pretreatment on recovery from diffuse cerebral ischemia in the cat. II. Regional metabolite levels. Stroke 11: 355, 1980.
122. Ginsberg MD, Welsh FA, Budd WW: Deleterious effect of glucose pretreatment on recovery from diffuse cerebral ischemia in the cat. I. Local cerebral blood flow and glucose utilization. Stroke 11:347, 1980.
123. Anderson RV, Siegman MG, Balaban RS, et al: Hyperglycemia increases cerebral intracellular acidosis during circulatory arrest. Ann Thorac Surg 54:1126, 1992.
124. Lanier WL, Stangland KJ, Scheithauer BW, et al: The effects of dextrose infusion and head position on neurologic outcome after complete cerebral ischemia in primates: Examination of a model. Anesthesiology 66:39, 1987.
125. de Courten-Myers G, Kleinholz M, Wagner K: Effect of hyperglycemia on infarct size after cerebrovascular occlusion in cats. Stroke 21:357, 1990.
126. Chew W, Kucharczyk J, Moseley M, et al: Hyperglycemia augments ischemic brain injury: In vivo MR imaging/spectroscopic study with nicardipine in cats with occluded middle cerebral arteries. AJNR Am J Neuroradiol 12:603, 1991.
127. Dietrich WD, Alonso O, Busto R: Moderate hyperglycemia worsens acute blood-brain barrier injury after forebrain ischemia in rats. Stroke 24:111, 1993.
128. Pulsinelli WA, Levy DE, Sigsbee B, et al: Increased damage after ischemic stroke in patients with hyperglycemia with or without established diabetes mellitus. Am J Med 74:540, 1983.
129. Lanier WL: Glucose management during cardiopulmonary bypass: Cardiovascular and neurologic implications (Editorial). Anesth Analg 72:423, 1991.
130. Metz S, Keats AS: Benefits of a glucose-containing priming solution for cardiopulmonary bypass. Anesth Analg 72:428, 1991.
131. Frasco P, Croughwell N, Blumenthal J, et al: Association between blood glucose level during cardiopulmonary bypass and neuropsychiatric outcome (Abstract). Anesthesiology 75:A55, 1991.
132. Lundgren J, Smith ML, Siesjö BK: Influence of moderate hypothermia on ischemic brain damage incurred under hyperglycemic conditions. Exp Brain Res 84:91, 1991.
133. Croughwell ND, Frasco P, Blumenthal JA, et al: Warming during cardiopulmonary bypass is associated with jugular bulb desaturation. Ann Thorac Surg 53:827, 1992.
134. Hindman BJ, Dexter F, Cutkomp J, et al: Hypothermic acid-base management does not affect cerebral metabolic rate for oxygen ($CMRo_2$) at 27°C. A study during cardiopulmonary bypass in rabbits. Anesthesiology 79:580, 1993.
135. Cole DJ, Drummond JC, Shapiro HM, et al: The effect of hypervolemic hemodilution with and without hypertension on cerebral blood flow following middle cerebral artery occlusion in rats anesthetized with isoflurane. Anesthesiology 71:580, 1989.
136. Korosue K, Heros RC: Mechanism of cerebral blood flow augmentation by hemodilution in rabbits. Stroke 23:1487, 1992.
137. Cole DJ, Drummond JC, Osborne TN, Matsumura J: Hypertension and hemodilution during cerebral ischemia reduce brain injury and edema. Am J Physiol 259:H211, 1990.
138. Cole DJ, Schell RM, Drummond JC, Reynolds L: Focal cerebral ischemia in rats. Effect of hypervolemic hemodilution with diaspirin cross-linked hemoglobin versus albumin on brain injury and edema. Anesthesiology 78:335, 1993.
139. Tu YK, Heros RC, Karacostas D, et al: Isovolemic hemodilution in experimental focal cerebral ischemia. Part 2: Effects on regional cerebral blood flow and size of infarction. J Neurosurg 69:82, 1988.
140. Koller M, Haenny P, Hess K, et al: Adjusted hypervolemic hemodilution in acute ischemic stroke. Stroke 21:1429, 1990.
141. Goslinga H, Eijzenbach V, Heuvelmans JHA, et al: Custom-tailored hemodilution with albumin and crystalloids in acute ischemic stroke. Stroke 23:181, 1992.
142. Italian Acute Stroke Study Group: Haemodilution in acute stroke: Results of the Italian hemodilution trial. Lancet i:318, 1988.
143. Scandinavian Stroke Study Group: Multicenter trial of hemodilution in acute ischemic stroke. I. Results in the total patient population. Stroke 18:691, 1987.
144. The Hemodilution in Stroke Study Group: Hypervolemic hemodilution treatment of acute stroke. Results of a randomized multicenter trial using pentastarch. Stroke 20:317, 1989.
145. Mast H, Marx P: Neurological deterioration under isovolemic hemodilution with hydroxyethyl starch in acute cerebral ischemia. Stroke 22:680, 1991.
146. Maruyama M, Shimoji K, Ichikawa T, et al: The effects of extreme hemodilutions on the autoregulation of cerebral blood flow, electroencephalogram and cerebral metabolic rate of oxygen in the dog. Stroke 16:675, 1985.
147. Nagao S, Roccaforte P, Moody RA: The effects of isovolemic hemodilution and reinfusion of packed erythrocytes on somatosensory and visual evoked potentials. J Surg Res 25:530, 1978.
148. Sutton LN, Clark BJ, Norwood CR, et al: Global cerebral ischemia in piglets under conditions of mild and deep hypothermia. Stroke 22:1567, 1991.
149. Berntman L, Welsh FA, Harp JR: Cerebral protective effect of low-grade hypothermia. Anesthesiology 55:495, 1981.
150. Chopp M, Knight R, Tidwell CD, et al: The metabolic effects of mild hypothermia on global cerebral ischemia and recirculation in the cat: Comparison to normothermia and hyperthermia. J Cereb Blood Flow Metab 9:141, 1989.
151. Michenfelder JD, Theye RA: The effects of anesthesia and hypothermia on canine cerebral ATP and lactate during anoxia produced by decapitation. Anesthesiology 33:430, 1970.
152. Astrup J, Skovsted P, Gjerris F, Sorensen HR: Increase in extracellular potassium in the brain during circulatory arrest: Effects of hypothermia, lidocaine, and thiopental. Anesthesiology 55: 256, 1981.
153. Bering EA: Effects of profound hypothermia and circulatory arrest on cerebral oxygen metabolism and cerebrospinal fluid electrolyte composition in dogs. J Neurosurg 39:199, 1974.
154. Croughwell N, Smith LR, Quill T, et al: The effect of temperature on cerebral metabolism and blood flow in adults during cardiopulmonary bypass. J Thorac Cardiovasc Surg 103:549, 1992.
155. Feddersen K, Aren C, Nilsson NJ, Radegran K: Cerebral blood flow and metabolism during cardiopulmonary bypass with special reference to effects of hypotension induced by prostacyclin. Ann Thorac Surg 41:395, 1986.
156. Murkin JM, Farrar JK, Tweed A, et al: Cerebral autoregulation and flow/metabolism coupling during cardiopulmonary bypass: The influence of PaCO2. Anesth Analg 66:825, 1987.
157. Stephan H, Sonntag H, Lange H, Rieke H: Cerebral effects of anaesthesia and hypothermia. Anaesthesia 44:310, 1989.
158. Greeley WJ, Kern FH, Ungerleider RM, et al: The effect of hypothermic cardiopulmonary bypass and total circulatory arrest on cerebral metabolism in neonates, infants and children. J Thorac Cardiovasc Surg 101:783, 1991.
159. Todd MM, Warner DS: A comfortable hypothesis reevaluated. Cerebral metabolic depression and brain protection during ischemia (Editorial). Anesthesiology 76:161, 1992.
160. Busto R, Dietrich WD, Globus MYT, et al: Small differences in intraischemic brain temperature critically determine the extent of ischemic neuronal injury. J Cereb Blood Flow Metab 7:729, 1987.

161. Natale JE, D'Alecy LG: Protection from cerebral ischemia by brain cooling without reduced lactate accumulation in dogs. Stroke 20:770, 1989.
162. Welsh FA, Sims RE, Harris VA: Mild hypothermia prevents ischemic injury in gerbil hippocampus. J Cereb Blood Flow Metab 10:557, 1990.
163. Ginsberg MD, Sternau LL, Globus MYT, et al: Therapeutic modulation of brain temperature: Relevance to ischemic brain injury. Cerebrovasc Brain Metab Rev 4:189, 1992.
164. Globus MYT, Busto R, Dietrich WD, et al: Effect on ischemia on the in vivo release of striatal dopamine, glutamate, and gamma-aminobutyric acid studied by intracerebral microdialysis. J Neurochem 51:1455, 1988.
165. Globus MYT, Busto R, Dietrich WD, et al: Intra-ischemic extracellular release of dopamine and glutamate is associated with striatal vulnerability to ischemia. Neurosci Lett 91:36, 1988.
166. Busto R, Globus MYT, Dietrich WD, et al: Effect of mild hypothermia on ischemia-induced release of neurotransmitter and free fatty acid in rat brain. Stroke 20:904, 1989.
167. Baker AJ, Zornow MH, Grafe MR, et al: Hypothermia prevents ischemia-induced increases in hippocampal glycine concentrations in rabbits. Stroke 22:666, 1991.
168. Siesjö BK: Pathophysiology and treatment of focal cerebral ischemia. Part I: Pathophysiology. J Neurosurg 77:169, 1992.
169. Dempsey RJ, Combs DJ, Maley ME, et al: Moderate hypothermia reduces postischemic edema development and leukotriene production. Neurosurgery 21:177, 1987.
170. Sano T, Drummond JC, Patel PM, et al: A comparison of the cerebral protective effects of isoflurane and mild hypothermia in a model of incomplete forebrain ischemia in the rat. Anesthesiology 76:221, 1992.
171. Ridenour TR, Warner DS, Todd MM, McAllister AC: Mild hypothermia reduces infarct size resulting from temporary but not permanent focal ischemia in rats. Stroke 23:733, 1992.
172. Onesti ST, Baker CJ, Sun PP, Solomon RA: Transient hypothermia reduces focal ischemic brain injury in the rat. Neurosurgery 29:369, 1991.
173. Morikawa E, Ginsberg MD, Dietrich WD, et al: The significance of brain temperature in focal cerebral ischemia: Histopathological consequences of middle cerebral artery occlusion in the rat. J Cereb Blood Flow Metab 12:380, 1992.
174. Lichtenstein SV, Ashe KA, El Dalati H, et al: Warm heart surgery. J Thorac Cardiovasc Surg 101:269, 1991.
175. Christakis GT, Koch JP, Deenar KA, et al: A randomized study of the systemic effects of warm heart surgery. Ann Thorac Surg 54:449, 1992.
176. Wong BI, McLean RF, Naylor CD, et al: Central-nervous-system dysfunction after warm or hypothermic cardiopulmonary bypass. Lancet i:1383, 1992.
177. Minamisawa H, Smith M-L, Siesjö BK: The effect of mild hyperthermia and hypothermia on brain damage following 5, 10, and 15 minutes of forebrain ischemia. Ann Neurol 28:26, 1990.
178. Dietrich WD, Busto R, Valdes I, Loor Y: Effects of normothermic versus mild hyperthermic forebrain ischemia in rats. Stroke 21:1318, 1990.
179. Rahn H, Reeves RB, Howell BJ: Hydrogen ion regulation, temperature, and evolution. Am Rev Respir Ds 112:165, 1975.
180. Nattie EE: The alphastat hypothesis in respiratory control and acid-base balance. J Appl Physiol 69:1201, 1990.
181. Hickey PR, Hansen DD: Temperature and blood gases: The clinical dilemma of acid-base management for hypothermic cardiopulmonary bypass. In Tinker JH (ed): Cardiopulmonary Bypass: Current Concepts and Controversies. Philadelphia, WB Saunders Co, 1989, p 1.
182. Malan A, Wilson TL, Reeves RB: Intracellular pH in cold-blooded vertebrates as a function of body temperature. Respir Physiol 28:29, 1976.
183. Reeves RB: An imidazole alphastat hypothesis for vertebrate acid-base regulation: Tissue carbon dioxide content and body temperature in bullfrogs. Respir Physiol 14:219, 1972.
184. Andritsch RF, Muravchick S, Gold MI: Temperature correction of arterial blood-gas parameters: A comparative review of methodology. Anesthesiology 55:311, 1981.
185. White FN: A comparative physiological approach to hypothermia. J Thorac Cardiovasc Surg 82:821, 1981.
186. Swan H: The importance of acid-base management for cardiac and cerebral preservation during open heart operations. Surg Gynecol Obstet 158:391, 1984.
187. Somero GN, White FN: Enzymatic consequences under alphastat regulation. In Rahn H, Prakash O (eds): Acid-Base Regulation and Body Temperature. Boston, Martinus Nijhoff Publishing, 1985, p 55.
188. Somero GN: Protons, osmolytes, and fitness of internal milieu for protein function. Am J Physiol 251:R197, 1986.
189. Malan A: Acid-base regulation during hibernation. In Rahn H, Prakash O (eds): Acid-Base Regulation and Body Temperature. Boston, Martinus Nijhoff Publishing, 1985, p 33.
190. Malan A, Mioskowski E: pH-temperature interactions on protein function and hibernation: GDP binding to brown adipose tissue mitochondria. J Comp Physiol B 158:487, 1988.
191. Prough DS, Rogers AT, Stump DA, et al: Hypercarbia depresses cerebral oxygen consumption during cardiopulmonary bypass. Stroke 21:1162, 1990.
192. Rogers AT, Prough DS, Roy RC, et al: Cerebrovascular and cerebral metabolic effects of alterations in perfusion flow rate during hypothermic cardiopulmonary bypass in man. J Thorac Cardiovasc Surg 103:363, 1992.
193. Stephan H, Weyland A, Kazmaier S, et al: Acid-base management during hypothermic cardiopulmonary bypass does not affect cerebral metabolism but does affect blood flow and neurological outcome. Br J Anaesth 69:51, 1992.
194. Prough DS, Stump DA, Roy RC, et al: Response of cerebral blood flow to changes in carbon dioxide tension during hypothermic cardiopulmonary bypass. Anesthesiology 64:576, 1986.
195. Johnsson P, Messeter K, Ryding E, et al: Cerebral vasoreactivity to carbon dioxide during cardiopulmonary perfusion at normothermia and hypothermia. Ann Thorac Surg 48:769, 1989.
196. Kern FH, Ungerleider RM, Quill TJ, et al: Cerebral blood flow response to changes in arterial carbon dioxide tension during hypothermic cardiopulmonary bypass in children. J Thorac Cardiovasc Surg 101:618, 1991.
197. Hindman BJ, Funatsu N, Harrington J, et al: Cerebral blood flow response to $PaCO_2$ during hypothermic cardiopulmonary bypass in rabbits. Anesthesiology 75:662, 1991.
198. Govier AV, Reves JG, McKay RD, et al: Factors and their influence on regional cerebral blood flow during nonpulsatile cardiopulmonary bypass. Ann Thorac Surg 38:592, 1984.
199. Lundar T, Lindegaard KF, Froysaker T, et al: Dissociation between cerebral autoregulation and carbon dioxide reactivity during nonpulsatile cardiopulmonary bypass. Ann Thorac Surg 40: 582, 1985.
200. Lundar T, Lindegaard KF, Froysaker T, et al: Cerebral carbon dioxide reactivity during nonpulsatile cardiopulmonary bypass. Ann Thorac Surg 41:525, 1986.
201. Johnsson P, Messeter K, Ryding E, et al: Cerebral blood flow and autoregulation during hypothermic cardiopulmonary bypass. Ann Thorac Surg 43:386, 1987.
202. Rogers AT, Stump DA, Gravlee GP, et al: Response of cerebral blood flow to phenylephrine infusion during hypothermic cardiopulmonary bypass: Influence of PaCO2 management. Anesthesiology 69:547, 1988.
203. Brusino FG, Reves JG, Smith LR, et al: The effect of age on cerebral blood flow during hypothermic cardiopulmonary bypass. J Thorac Cardiovasc Surg 97:541, 1989.
204. Prough DS, Stump DA, Troost BT: PaCO2 management during cardiopulmonary bypass: Intriguing physiologic rationale, convincing clinical data, evolving hypothesis? (Editorial). Anesthesiology 72:3, 1990.
205. Hindman BJ, Funatsu N, Harrington J, et al: Differences in cerebral blood flow between alpha-stat and pH-stat management are eliminated during periods of decreased systemic flow and pressure. Anesthesiology 74:1096, 1991.
206. Woodcock TE, Murkin JM, Farrar JK, et al: Pharmacologic EEG suppression during cardiopulmonary bypass: Cerebral hemodynamic and metabolic effects of thiopental or isoflurane during hypothermia and normothermia. Anesthesiology 67:218, 1987.
207. Stockard JJ, Bickford RG, Schauble JF: Pressure-dependent cerebral ischemia during cardiopulmonary bypass. Neurology 23: 521, 1973.
208. Soma Y, Hirotani T, Yozu R, et al: A clinical study of cerebral

circulation during extracorporeal circulation. J Thorac Cardiovasc Surg 97:187, 1989.

209. Nakajima T, Kuro M, Hayaski Y, et al: Clinical evaluation of cerebral oxygen balance during cardiopulmonary bypass: Online continuous monitoring of jugular venous oxyhemoglobin saturation. Anesth Analg 74:630, 1992.
210. Tranmer BI, Keller TS, Kindt GW, Archer D: Loss of cerebral regulation during cardiac output variations in focal cerebral ischemia. J Neurosurg 77:253, 1992.
211. Astrup J, Sorensen PM, Sorensen HR: Inhibition of cerebral oxygen and glucose consumption in the dog by hypothermia, pentobarbital, and lidocaine. Anesthesiology 55:263, 1981.
212. Astrup J, Sorensen PM, Sorensen HR: Oxygen and glucose consumption related to Na^+-K^+ transport in canine brain. Stroke 12: 726, 1981.
213. Michenfelder JD: The interdependency of cerebral functional and metabolic effects following massive doses of thiopental in the dog. Anesthesiology 41:231, 1974.
214. Branston NM, Hope T, Symon L: Barbiturates in focal ischemia of primate cortex: Effects on blood flow distribution, evoked potential and extracellular potassium. Stroke 10:647, 1979.
215. Verhaegen MJ, Todd MM, Warner DS: A comparison of cerebral ischemic flow thresholds during halothane/N_2O and isoflurane/N_2O anesthesia in rats. Anesthesiology 76:743, 1992.
216. Steen PA, Milde JH, Michenfelder JD: No barbiturate protection in a dog model of complete cerebral ischemia. Ann Neurol 5: 343, 1979.
217. Gisvold SE, Safar P, Hendrickx HHL, et al: Thiopental treatment after global brain ischemia in pigtailed monkeys. Anesthesiology 60:88, 1984.
218. Brain Resuscitation Clinical Trial I Study Group: Randomized clinical study of thiopental loading in comatose survivors of cardiac arrest. N Engl J Med 314:397, 1986.
219. Hoff JT, Smith AL, Hankinson HL, Nielsen SL: Barbiturate protection from cerebral infarction in primates. Stroke 6:28, 1975.
220. Michenfelder JD, Milde JH: Influence of anesthetics on metabolic, functional and pathological responses to regional cerebral ischemia. Stroke 6:405, 1975.
221. Michenfelder JD, Milde JH, Sundt TM: Cerebral protection by barbiturate anesthesia. Arch Neurol 33:345, 1976.
222. Moseley J, Laurent JP, Molinari GF: Barbiturate attenuation of the clinical course and pathologic lesions in a primate stroke model. Neurology 25:870, 1975.
223. Selman WR, Spetzler RF, Roessmann UR, et al: Barbiturate-induced coma therapy for focal cerebral ischemia: Effect after temporary and permanent MCA occlusion. J Neurosurg 55:220, 1981.
224. Feustel PJ, Ingvar MC, Severinghaus JW: Cerebral oxygen availability and blood flow during middle cerebral artery occlusion: Effects of pentobarbital. Stroke 12:858, 1981.
225. Nussmeier NA, Arlund C, Slogoff SL: Neuropsychiatric complications after cardiopulmonary bypass: Cerebral protection by a barbiturate. Anesthesiology 64:165, 1986.
226. Helps SC, Meyer-Witting M, Reilly PL, Gorman DF: Increasing doses of intracarotid air and cerebral blood flow in rabbits. Stroke 21:1340, 1990.
227. Feinstein SB, Shah PM, Bing RJ, et al: Microbubble dynamics visualized in the intact capillary circulation. J Am Coll Cardiol 4:595, 1984.
228. Fritz H, Hossmann KA: Arterial air embolism in the cat brain. Stroke 10:581, 1979.
229. Kort A, Kronzon I: Microbubble formation: In vitro and in vivo observation. J Clin Ultrasound 10:117, 1982.
230. Castaneda AR, Mayer JE, Jonas RA, et al: The neonate with critical congenital heart disease: Repair—a surgical challenge. J Thorac Cardiovasc Surg 98:869, 1989.
231. Bailey LL, Takeuchi Y, Williams WG, et al: Surgical management of congenital cardiovascular anomalies with the use of profound hypothermia and circulatory arrest. Analysis of 180 consecutive cases. J Thorac Cardiovasc Surg 71:485, 1976.
232. Barratt-Boyes BG, Simpson M, Neutze JM: Intracardiac surgery in neonates and infants using deep hypothermia with surface cooling and limited cardiopulmonary bypass. Circulation 43(Suppl I):I-25, 1971.
233. Bender HE, Fisher RD, Walker WE, Graham TP: Reparative cardiac surgery in infants and small children. Five years experience with profound hypothermia and circulatory arrest. Ann Surg 190:437, 1979.
234. Sweeney MS, Cooley DA, Reul GH, et al: Hypothermic circulatory arrest for cardiovascular lesions: Technical considerations and results. Ann Thorac Surg 40:498, 1985.
235. Coselli JS, Crawford ES, Beall AC, et al: Determination of brain temperatures for safe circulatory arrest during cardiovascular operation. Ann Thorac Surg 45:638, 1988.
236. Mahfood S, Qazi A, Garcia J, et al: Management of aortic arch aneurysm using profound hypothermia and circulatory arrest. Ann Thorac Surg 39:412, 1985.
237. O'Connor JV, Wilding T, Farmer P, et al: The protective effect of profound hypothermia on the canine central nervous system during one hour of circulatory arrest. Ann Thorac Surg 41:255, 1986.
238. Mujsce DJ, Towfighi J, Vannucci RC: Physiologic and neuropathologic aspects of hypothermic circulatory arrest in newborn dogs. Pediatr Res 28:354, 1990.
239. Fessatidis IT, Thomas VL, Shore DF, et al: Brain damage after profoundly hypothermic circulatory arrest: Correlations between neurophysiologic and neuropathologic findings. An experimental study in vertebrates. J Thorac Cardiovasc Surg 106:32, 1993.
240. Mezrow CK, Sadeghi AM, Gandsas A, et al: Cerebral blood flow and metabolism in hypothermic circulatory arrest. Ann Thorac Surg 54:609, 1992.
241. Tharion J, Johnson DC, Celermajer JM, et al: Profound hypothermia with circulatory arrest. Nine years' clinical experience. J Thorac Cardiovasc Surg 84:66, 1982.
242. Ferry PC: Neurologic sequelae of cardiac surgery in children. Am J Dis Child 141:309, 1987.
243. Brunberg JA, Reilly E, Doty DB: Central nervous system consequences in infants of cardiac surgery using deep hypothermia and circulatory arrest. Circulation 49(Suppl II):II-60, 1974.
244. Ferry PC: Neurologic sequelae of open-heart surgery in children. An 'irritating question.' Am J Dis Child 144:369, 1990.
245. Davis EA, Gillinov AM, Cameron DE, Reitz BA: Hypothermic circulatory arrest as a surgical adjunct: A 5-year experience with 60 adult patients. Ann Thorac Surg 53:402, 1992.
246. Griepp RB, Ergin MA, Lansman SL, et al: The physiology of hypothermic circulatory arrest. Semin Thorac Cardiovasc Surg 3:188, 1991.
247. Svensson LG, Crawford ES, Hess KR, et al: Deep hypothermia with circulatory arrest. Determinants of stroke and early mortality in 656 patients. J Thorac Cardiovasc Surg 106:19, 1993.
248. DeLeon S, Ilbawi M, Arcilla R, et al: Choreoathetosis after deep hypothermia without circulatory arrest. Ann Thorac Surg 50:714, 1990.
249. Wical BS, Tomasi LG: A distinctive neurologic syndrome after induced profound hypothermia. Pediatr Neurol 6:202, 1990.
250. Robinson RO, Samuels M, Pohl KRE: Choreic syndrome after cardiac surgery. Arch Dis Child 63:1466, 1988.
251. Gillinov AM, Redmond JM, Zehr KJ, et al: Superior cerebral protection with profound hypothermia during circulatory arrest. Ann Thorac Surg 55:1432, 1993.
252. Haneda K, Sands MP, Thomas R, et al: Prolongation of the safe interval of hypothermic circulatory arrest: 90 minutes. J Cardiovasc Surg 24:15, 1983.
253. Bellinger DC, Wernovsky G, Rappaport LA, et al: Cognitive development of children following early repair of transposition of the great arteries using deep hypothermic circulatory arrest. Pediatrics 87:701, 1991.
254. Kern FH, Jonas RA, Mayer JE, et al: Temperature monitoring during CPB in infants: Does it predict efficient brain cooling? Ann Thorac Surg 54:749, 1992.
255. Dexter F, Hindman BJ: Computer simulation of brain cooling during cardiopulmonary bypass. Ann Thorac Surg 57:1171, 1994.
256. Jonas RA, Bellinger DC, Rappaport LA, et al: Relation of pH strategy and developmental outcome after hypothermic circulatory arrest. J Thorac Cardiovasc Surg 106:362, 1993.
257. Payne WS, Theye RA, Kirklin JW: Effect of carbon dioxide on rate of brain cooling during induction of hypothermia by direct blood cooling. J Surg Res 3:54, 1963.
258. Watanabe T, Miura M, Inui K, et al: Blood and brain tissue gaseous strategy for profoundly hypothermic total circulatory arrest. J Thorac Cardiovasc Surg 102:497, 1991.

259. Di Eusanio G, Ray SC, Donnelly RJ, Hamilton DI: Open heart surgery in first year of life using profound hypothermia (core cooling) and circulatory arrest. Experience with 134 consecutive cases. Br Heart J 41:294, 1979.
260. Hindman BJ, Dexter F, Cutkomp J, et al: Cerebral blood flow and metabolism do not decrease at stable brain temperature during cardiopulmonary bypass in rabbits. Anesthesiology 77:342, 1992.
261. Aoki M, Nomura F, Stromski ME, et al: Effects of pH on brain energetics after hypothermic circulatory arrest. Ann Thorac Surg 55:1093, 1993.
262. Greeley WJ, Ungerleider RM, Smith LR, Reves JG: The effects of deep hypothermic cardiopulmonary bypass and total circulatory arrest on cerebral blood flow in infants and children. J Thorac Cardiovasc Surg 97:737, 1989.
263. Greeley WJ, Ungerleider RM, Kern FH, et al: Effects of cardiopulmonary bypass on cerebral blood flow in neonates, infants, and children. Circulation 80(Suppl I):I-209, 1989.
264. Greeley WJ: Deep hypothermic circulatory arrest must be used selectively and discretely (Editorial). J Cardiothorac Vasc Anesth 5:638, 1991.
265. Swain JA, McDonald TJ, Griffith PK, et al: Low-flow hypothermic cardiopulmonary bypass protects the brain. J Thorac Cardiovasc Surg 102:76, 1991.
266. Robbins RC, Balaban RS, Swain JA, et al: Intermittent hypothermic asanguineous cerebral perfusion (cerebroplegia) protects the brain during prolonged circulatory arrest. A phosphorus 31 nuclear magnetic resonance study. J Thorac Cardiovasc Surg 99: 878, 1990.
267. Crittenden MD, Roberts CS, Rose L, et al: Brain protection during circulatory arrest. Ann Thorac Surg 51:942, 1991.
268. Mault JR, Ohtake S, Klingensmith ME, et al: Cerebral metabolism and circulatory arrest: Effects of duration and strategies for protection. Ann Thorac Surg 55:57, 1993.
269. Newberger JW, Jonas RA, Wernovsky G, et al: A comparison of the perioperative neurologic effects of hypothermic circulatory arrest versus low-flow cardiopulmonary bypass in infant heart surgery. N Engl J Med 329:1057, 1993.
270. Burrows FA, Bissonnette B: Cerebral blood flow velocity patterns during cardiac surgery utilizing profound hypothermia with low-flow cardiopulmonary bypass or circulatory arrest in neonates and infants. Can J Anaesth 40:298, 1993.
271. Stoney WS, Alford WC, Burrus GR, et al: Air embolism and other accidents using pump oxygenators. Ann Thorac Surg 29: 336, 1980.
272. Mills NL, Ochsner JL: Massive air embolism during cardiopulmonary bypass. Causes, prevention, and management. J Thorac Cardiovasc Surg 80:708, 1980.
273. Tomatis L, Nemiroff M, Riahi M, et al: Massive arterial air embolism due to rupture of pulsatile assist device: Successful treatment in the hyperbaric chamber. Ann Thorac Surg 32:604, 1981.
274. Haykal HA, Wang AM: CT diagnosis of delayed cerebral air embolism following intraaortic balloon pump catheter insertion. Comput Radiol 10:307, 1986.
275. Meyer JS, Gotoh F, Tazaki Y: Circulation and metabolism following experimental cerebral embolism. J Neuropathol Exp Neurol 21:4, 1962.
276. Hekmatpanah J: Cerebral microvascular alterations in arterial air embolism. Adv Neurol 20:245, 1978.
277. Menkin M, Schwartzman RJ: Cerebral air embolism. Arch Neurol 34:168, 1977.
278. Warren BA, Philp RB, Inwood MJ: The ultrastructural morphology of air embolism: Platelet adhesion to the interface and endothelial damage. Br J Exp Pathol 54:163, 1973.
279. Garcia JH, Klatzo I, Archer T, Lossinsky AS: Arterial air embolism: Structural effects on the gerbil brain. Stroke 12:414, 1981.
280. Graham DI: The pathology of brain ischaemia and possibilities for therapeutic intervention. Br J Anaesth 57:3, 1985.
281. Steward D, Williams WG, Freedom R: Hypothermia in conjunction with hyperbaric oxygenation in the treatment of massive air embolism during cardiopulmonary bypass. Ann Thorac Surg 24:591, 1977.
282. Lar LW, Lai LC, Ren LW: Massive arterial embolism during cardiac operation: Successful treatment in a hyperbaric chamber under 3 ATA (Letter). J Thorac Cardiovasc Surg 100:928, 1990.
283. Armon C, Deschamps C, Adkinson C, et al: Hyperbaric treatment of cerebral air embolism sustained during an open-heart surgical procedure. Mayo Clin Proc 66:565, 1991.
284. Toscano M, Chiavarelli R, Ruvolo G, et al: Management of massive air embolism during open-heart surgery with retrograde perfusion of the cerebral vessels and hyperbaric oxygenation. Thorac Cardiovasc Surg 31:183, 1983.
285. Furlow TW: Experimental air embolism of the brain: An analysis of the technique in the rat. Stroke 13:847, 1982.
286. Stark J, Hough J: Air in the aorta: Treatment by reversed perfusion. Ann Thorac Surg 41:337, 1986.
287. Bayindir O, Paker T, Akpinar B, et al: A 58-year-old man had a massive air embolism during cardiopulmonary bypass. J Cardiothorac Vasc Anesth 5:627, 1991.
288. Brown JW, Dierdorf SF, Moorthy SS, Halpin M: Venoarterial cerebral perfusion for treatment of massive arterial air embolism. Anesth Analg 66:673, 1987.
289. Watanabe T, Shimasaki T, Kuraoka S, et al: Retrograde cerebral perfusion against massive air embolism during cardiopulmonary bypass (Letter). J Thorac Cardiovasc Surg 104:532, 1992.
290. Hendriks FFA, Bogers AJJC, de la Riviere AB, et al: The effectiveness of venoarterial perfusion in treatment of arterial air embolism during cardiopulmonary bypass. Ann Thorac Surg 36: 433, 1983.
291. Peirce EC: Specific therapy for arterial air embolism. Ann Thorac Surg 29:800, 1980.
292. Kol S, Ammar R, Weisz G, Melamed Y: Hyperbaric oxygenation for arterial air embolism during cardiopulmonary bypass. Ann Thorac Surg 55:401, 1993.
293. Voorhies RM, Fraser RAR: Cerebral air embolism occurring at angiography and diagnosed by computerized tomography. J Neurosurg 60:177, 1984.
294. Meldrum BS, Papy JJ, Vigouroux RA: Intracarotid air embolism in the baboon: Effects on cerebral blood flow and the electroencephalogram. Brain Res 25:301, 1971.
295. Layton AJ: Hyperbaric oxygen treatment for cerebral air embolism — where are the data? (Editorial). Mayo Clin Proc 66: 641, 1991.

CHAPTER 37

Respiratory, Renal, and Gastrointestinal Complications

Christopher L. Campese, M.D.
Philip D. Lumb, M.B., B.S., F.C.C.M.

Respiratory Complications

Thoracic Surgery

Preoperative Evaluation and Preparation

The preoperative period remains the most efficient and proper setting for a thorough evaluation of a patient's baseline pulmonary status and for prediction/prevention of many common postoperative complications. Obtaining a set of complete pulmonary function tests prior to surgery can often be extremely helpful in the prediction of postoperative morbidity and mortality, and this information should be used routinely in patients who are to undergo major pulmonary and chest wall resections.[1,2]

Additionally, the preoperative course should be utilized as the time in which to optimize the patient's medical condition. It has been well documented that the incidence of postoperative respiratory complications is two to six times greater in smokers than in nonsmokers. However, there remains much debate regarding the pulmonary effects of acute smoking cessation preoperatively and the time frame required for true beneficial effects to appear. Mucocilliary clearance, in a great number of smokers, returns to baseline after several months of abstinence, while only 1 week of abstinence was shown to provide no significant improvements. Similarly, pulmonary tests of small airways function have only been shown to improve after 1 to 6 months' cessation of smoking. It is also during this period that the larger bronchial airways become hyperreactive and episodes of bronchospasm become more likely in the asthmatic population. Other potential abnormalities that may occur due to preoperative smoking abstinence include a possibly increased risk for deep venous thrombosis and marked psychological effects including increased anxiety, irritability, and sleep disorders. Most recent clinical studies have shown a decrease in the postoperative pulmonary complication rate only when smoking cessation has occurred at least 6 to 8 weeks prior to surgery, while abstaining for a shorter period prior to surgery is potentially associated with an increase in postoperative respiratory morbidity.[3–6]

Proper treatment of any underlying pulmonary infection, especially in the patient with chronic obstructive pulmonary disease (COPD), can be an important factor in the prevention of postoperative pneumonia and atelectasis. Finally, an aggressive regimen of chest physiotherapy and exercise, as well as deep breathing maneuvers are among the more useful strategies that may be employed preoperatively to maximize postoperative benefits.[7]

Postoperative Complications

ATELECTASIS

The most frequent respiratory complication encountered following thoracic surgery is atelectasis. Its incidence, however, remains the subject of much debate, with most authors reporting significant occurrence rates in the range of 20 to 30% of patients following thoracotomy.[8,9]

The classic model used to explain the development of atelectasis was that of small airway obstruction by mucous plugs resulting in the resorption of distal trapped air causing total alveolar collapse.[10,11] More recent investigations have shown, however, that the causes of alveolar collapse are multifaceted and include bronchospasm, prolonged shallow respirations as a result of postoperative pain and splinting, pneumothorax, hemothorax and other volume-occupying states, absorption atelectasis, and compression of lung tissue due to surgical retraction.[12] Additionally, any disease process that decreases surfactant production and thereby increases lung surface tension, such as sepsis, adult respiratory distress syndrome (ARDS), lung parenchymal injury, or malnutrition, will also increase the likelihood of developing pulmonary atelectasis. Patients with significant atelectasis often present with hypoxia, tachycardia, tachypnea, and fever. The physiologic changes seen with this process include a decrease in vital capacity as well as functional residual capacity (FRC) and lung compliance. These reductions in critical lung volumes often present for up to 1 week postoperatively.[13]

Blood clots, thick mucous secretions, and bronchospasm are the most common causes of airways obstruction following pulmonary resection. It has long been thought that the proper use of a double-lumen endotracheal tube during surgery aids in preventing these types of complications.[14] Postoperative fluid balance is also a significant consideration, as dehydration tends to thicken mucous secretions, making them much more difficult to remove. The patient with airway obstruction may present with tachypnea, wheezing, rhonchi, hypoxia, and decreased breath sounds over the affected areas. Chest physiotherapy and aggressive postoperative suctioning are mandatory for these patients, especially those who have had a left upper lobectomy. In these patients, elevation of the left lower lobe to fill the now empty left upper hemithorax causes a torsion of the left bronchus as it passes under the aortic arch and makes the elimination of secretions more difficult.

DEAD SPACE EFFECT

A number of significant postoperative complications are related to the dead space effects of the postresection intrapleural cavity. There are several physiologic mechanisms of compensation that occur after the removal of lung tissue. These include hyperexpansion of the remaining lung tissue, mediastinal shift towards the involved hemithorax, narrowing of intercoastal spaces, and elevation of the involved hemidiaphragm.[15] The postresection cavity does not usually cause major postoperative deficits, and most can be managed conservatively and resolve spontaneously over time. In a small percentage of patients (6% in one study), the postresection space does not resolve spontaneously, but remains large, thick-walled, and fluid filled, and eventually becomes infected.[16,17] These patients usually present with fever, elevated white blood cell counts, and poor respiratory function. In the most severe cases, chest tubes or open drainage may be required to remove accumulated fluid.[18] A thorough preoperative evaluation may be useful in identifying those patients with the highest risk for developing this complication. Those with a history of inflammatory disease of the lungs, prior pulmonary resections, or radiation to the chest should alert the anesthesiologist to the increaseed likelihood that a potential postresection space will develop. In any patient with a residual postoperative space, it is crucial to maximize the clearance of retained secretions in the residual lung tissue by aggressive chest physiotherapy, suctioning, and even bronchoscopy. Increasing chest tube suctioning, and evaluation of persistent air leaks and the possible need to maintain postoperative ventilatory support should be considered. In the most severe cases, surgical re-exploration and treatment is often required.

AIR LEAKAGE

The problem of postoperative pulmonary air leak is often a challenging one for the anesthesiologist. The generally accepted consensus is that any air leak presenting/persisting 7 or more days after a thoracotomy is termed persistent and requires treatment. The majority of air leaks arise from the transected small bronchioles and alveoli and, with proper chest tube drainage, do not pose a significant risk for postoperative complications. In patients with increased risks (i.e., persons with marked emphysema), several postoperative maneuvers including continued mechanical ventilation and even high-frequency jet ventilation have been studied and found to provide possible benefits in their management.[19,20] In some cases, discontinuing the chest tube suction may provide relief from a persistent air leak by eliminating the increased negative intrapleural pressure created by suction. It is essential to follow these patients with chest radiographs to document the size of the related pneumothorax and to rule out any increased development within the chest.

Bronchopleural fistula, while not the major postoperative complication it was in the past, remains a problem that, if present, is associated with a mortality of over 20%.[21–23] Bronchopleural fistulae have often been described as occurring early or late in the postoperative course and both systemic and local factors have been implicated in their formation. Typically, early bronchopleural fistulae present within the first 48 to 72 hours following surgery while those seen later become evident between 7 and 14 days. The early dehiscence of a bronchial stump is often attributed to poor closure, while later on inadequate blood supply, local infection, or the presence of malignancy in the stump itself is often the cause. These patients exhibit a persistent and notably elevated air leak via chest tube and an increased pneumothorax on the involved side. In addition, a persistent cough, fever, and even hemoptysis may be present. Bronchoscopy followed by prompt re-exploration to evaluate the integrity of the transected stump and closure of the fistula is necessary. If the patient's condition is compromised, immediate reoperation may not be feasible. In these situations, chest tube drainage should be maintained until the patient's status has improved and the surgery can be attempted safely.

The use of a double-lumen endotracheal tube in patients who are returning for operative therapy of a bronchopleural fistula is strongly indicated for several reasons. Patients with this complication have a much greater incidence of pleural infection and empyema and are often maintained with the operated side down to prevent spillage of contaminated pleural fluid into the remaining lung via the tracheobronchial tree. Using a double-lumen tube to isolate and avoid infection of the contralateral lung is therefore recommended.

PULMONARY INFARCTION

Another serious postoperative pulmonary complication is that of lobar torsion and subsequent pulmonary infarction. When the remaining lung is re-expanding to occupy the newly created intrapleural cavity, it is possible for the vessels of a segment or lobe to become twisted. The low-pressure pulmonary veins collapse and the bronchial and pulmonary arteries remain open, causing engorgement and, ultimately, infarction and gangrene.[24] Most commonly, the right middle lobe is affected following a right upper lobectomy. These patients must be identified and treated quickly to prevent serious consequences. Chest radiography is often useful as is flexible bronchoscopy in identifying segments or lobes at risk. Patients may often lack any notable clinical signs until the situation has progressed to infarction or gangrene. At that stage, blood-tinged sputum; purulent and foul-smelling chest drainage; and fever, chills, and other signs of sepsis are often encountered.[25] An immediate thoracotomy should be performed if there is a strong suspicion that a torsion is present, with derotation or removal of the involved tissue and drainage of the affected pleura.

PLEURAL EFFUSION

In all postoperative pulmonary patients, the significant fluid collections in the pleural space should remain high on the list of causes for concern. When a persistent effusion or drainage is noted along with clinical signs of sepsis, the presence of empyema should be suspected. The possible sources for empyema should include a chest wall infection, untreated preoperative pulmonary infection, operative contamination, bronchopleural fistula, or even communication with the gastrointestinal tract. In all cases, tube drainage of the empyema should begin immediately[26] and in the most severe cases open pleural drainage followed by thoracoplasty may be required.

Chylothorax is another possible complication, especially following a left pulmonary resection.[27] When the thoracic duct or its branches are transected, the leaking chyle may collect in the pleural space. Although chyle is a poor medium for the growth of bacteria, it may complicate a patient's postoperative course by causing a marked loss of fat and fat-soluble vitamins. In these cases, chyle drainage should be limited by diet control with hyperalimentation supplements, but surgical closure of the leaking thoracic duct is usually required.[28]

POSTOPERATIVE HEMORRHAGE

Sustained postoperative bleeding is usually not encountered following thoracotomy and, when present, inadequate hemostasis is the most common cause. Blood losses via chest drainage should generally not exceed 500 ml. In 24 hours following thoracotomy, and continued pleural drainage in excess of 200 ml of blood per hour over a 4- to 6-hour period is an indication to re-explore the chest to achieve hemostasis surgically.[29] In addition, the patient in whom intrathoracic bleeding is suspected should undergo chest radiography and a complete set of coagulation studies. Most postoperative bleeding occurs from the high-flow, high-pressure systemic circulation, especially from chest wall or mediastinal vessels. While rare, the possibility of low-pressure, high-flow pulmonary vessel bleeding should be considered, and if suspected, quickly controlled with emergency thoracotomy and surgical repair.[30] In all patients, serial chest radiographs may elucidate important changes such as fluid accumulations, mediastinal shift, etc. Fluid and blood replacement should be aggressive in these patients and continuous hemodynamic monitoring is essential. Major postoperative bleeding can be a severe complication, with emergency thoracotomy indicated in 3% of all patients and an associated mortality of over 20%.[31] In patients who are greater than 24 hours postthoracotomy, the incidence of persistent bleeding is very low but, when present, usually requires emergency thoracotomy for control.

Cardiac Surgery

The postoperative effects of cardiopulmonary bypass (CPB) on the pulmonary system can range from mild to severe. The most common complications following CPB are pleural effusion, atelectasis, pneumonia, and pneumothorax. In addition, many alterations in pulmonary function are seen, including a large alveolar-arterial oxygen difference [$D(A-a)O_2$], increased physiologic shunt and decreased total lung volumes.[32] The alveolar-arterial gradient is maximal at 48 hours postoperatively and then returns towards baseline values. It has been found that the physiologic changes noted correlate directly with the length of CPB.

Mechanical complications are important to consider when evaluating the post-CPB patient with poor pulmonary function. The clinician must check the endotracheal tube for proper positioning and evaluate the patient for pneumothorax or hemothorax immediately if a problem is suspected. All pneumothoraces, regardless of size, should be treated with chest tubes while the patient is mechanically ventilated. A tension pneumothorax can develop quickly in the postoperative ventilated patient and can cause major hemodynamic compromise.[33] Hemothorax likewise is possible given the state of heparin-induced systemic anticoagulation during CPB. Any trauma to the upper airway, trachea, or lungs themselves can lead to an increased risk of airway bleeding. The resultant respiratory insufficiency, alveolar collapse, atelectasis, and hypoxemia can cause significant morbidity or mortality.

Pulmonary edema, especially of noncardiogenic origin, is a rare but potentially severe complication of cardiopulmonary bypass. If pulmonary capillary permeability is altered and intravascular fluids and proteins shift into the pulmonary interstitium and alveoli, patients experience respiratory distress and hypoxia associated with decreased pulmonary compliance. In contrast to cardiogenic pulmonary edema caused by raised capillary hydrostatic pressure secondary to depressed left ventricular function, noncardiogenic pulmonary edema is noted for decreases in left atrial pressures and an exudative fluid that has a composition similar to plasma.[34] There are several theories that have attempted to explain the etiology of noncardiogenic pulmonary edema. These include the use of the pump oxygenator, use of fresh frozen plasma, leukocyte reactions, endotoxins, and even protamine reactions. Blood contact with pump oxygenators has, in particular, been noted to activate the complement pathways with subsequent formation of anaphylatoxins.[36] With the development of newer membrane oxygenators, many of the problems seen in the older bubble oxygenators have been eliminated. Indeed, as the entire CPB circuit has become more sophisticated, the incidence of "pump lung" (as the postreperfusion

ARDS-like syndrome was classically termed) has decreased notably. Many of the advancements such as improved filters, materials, and pumps themselves have essentially eliminated the problems caused by particulate matter, platelet aggregates, and thromboemboli in otherwise healthy cardiac patients.

The management of a postoperative cardiac surgical patient with pulmonary edema can be quite challenging. Mechanical ventilation with positive end-expiratory pressure (PEEP) is usually mandatory in treating this condition, and the physiologic shunt may increase to 40% or greater.[37] Aggressive suctioning is also required to remove the increased volume of pulmonary edema. The combination of high peak inspiratory pressures, increasing hypoxia, PEEP, and noncompliant pulmonary tissues can cause significantly depressed cardiac outputs with resultant severe metabolic acidosis. One less commonly required therapy is extracorporeal membrane oxygenation, which has been used to treat critical cases of noncardiogenic pulmonary edema in the postbypass period.[38]

Vascular Surgery

Major vascular surgery, like its thoracic and cardiac counterparts, has a significant potential for pulmonary complications and requirements for postoperative respiratory support. Mechanical ventilation may be required following vascular surgical procedures for anesthetic reasons (e.g., in cases where residual narcotics or prolonged neuromuscular blockage is an issue[39] or for preexisting medical reasons necessitating postoperative critical care management).

The major components of pulmonary function to be considered following major vascular surgery are (1) the patient's age, (2) the effects of intra-abdominal and especially upper abdominal surgery on postoperative pulmonary activity, and (3) baseline respiratory status. The majority of patients in this surgical population are elderly, and the predictable changes of pulmonary function secondary to the aging process may have clinical relevance in the postoperative period.[40] These changes include decreased chest wall complaince, decreased elastic recoil of lung parenchyma, reduced strength and endurance of respiratory muscles, and a relative decrease in the size of the intervertebral spaces. When combined, these changes effect a measurable amount of closure of the small airways that is associated with reduced vital capacity (VC), increases in FRC, and an overall increase in residual volume (RV).[41] The closing capacity often exceeds FRC, and there is a notable decrease in the arterial partial pressure of oxygen in the elderly patient.[42]

Effects of Surgery

Compounding these changes are the often severe effects of abdominal surgery on respiratory function; for example, forced vital capacity (FVC) can be reduced to approximately 40% preoperative levels and can take up to 10 days to return to baseline. In addition, FRC is reduced up to 75% of preoperative values, and can also take several days to return to normal. Finally, pulmonary compliance, tidal volume, peak expiratory flow, and forced expiratory volume in 1 second (FEV_1) are similarly reduced after vascular surgery. Several studies have documented the effects of postoperative pulmonary function in the vascular surgery population. One, in particular, found that the overall incidence of postoperative pulmonary complications in all patients was 37% and the incidence of major respiratory complications (atelectasis, postoperative pneumonitis, prolonged mechanical ventilation for 12 to 48 hours, or pleural effusion) was 15%.[43] These numbers are much greater in patients undergoing abdominal aortic surgery via the transabdominal approach, with a total incidence of respiratory complications over 50% and major complications affecting about 25% of patients. Several other risk factors associated with an increased incidence of respiratory complications, including any recent episodes of bronchitis, chest wall deformities, prolonged surgical time, and a preoperative decrease in the FEV_1/FVC ratios were identified.

Emergency or Elective Surgery

There seems to be a direct correlation between emergency or elective aortic repair and the incidence of postoperative complications. In one study, the incidence of postoperative pneumonia and respiratory insufficiency approached 15 to 20% for the patients who underwent elective aortic reconstruction; this number rose to approximately 40 to 45% for patients undergoing emergent repair of the aorta.[44] Other studies confirm that other respiratory complications, notably atelectasis and respiratory insufficiency with prolonged ventilatory support, are more numerous in patients presenting for repair of ruptured aortic aneurysm.[45] Surgical approach may also play an important role in the prevention of postoperative pulmonary complications. Leather et al. examined a series of 299 aortic replacements and found a lower incidence of pulmonary complications and an almost 50% reduction in the duration of postoperative intubation in patients with a retroperitoneal approach when compared to the standard transabdominal approach.[46]

Anesthetic Effects on Pulmonary Function

Several studies have attempted to evaluate the potential effects of varied anesthetic techniques on the incidence of postoperative pulmonary complications.[47–49] While there is some disagreement amongst researchers regarding the superiority of epidural anesthesia versus general anesthesia with parenteral narcotic analgesia or inhalational agents, it is important to recognize that postoperative deterioration in pulmonary function occurs regardless of the technique employed. One important study by Mankikian et al. demonstrated a significant impairment in postoperative function after intra-abdominal vascular surgery that was most likely due to an impairment in phrenic nerve activity.[50]

Alterations such as this, along with other important considerations of postoperative analgesia, its effects on gas exchange, and respiratory effort, all suggest that a combined technique of epidural analgesia added to a standard postoperative narcotic regimen appears to have the greatest likelihood to improve respiratory function in the early postoperative period.[51,52]

Renal Complications

Cardiac Surgery

Renal complications following cardiopulmonary bypass present in a variety of ways. The incidence of significant renal failure following open heart surgery is quite variable, with most studies placing it in a range of 2 to almost 30%.[53,54] It remains an important and often severe complication, leading to an overall mortality of 65 to 70% in the postoperative period. Acute renal failure (ARF) after cardiac surgery appears to occur more commonly in elderly patients and in those persons with preoperative abnormalities in cardiac output, renal perfusion and/or function, and urine output.[55] The primary cause of post–coronary artery bypass graft (CABG) renal failure is believed to be associated with a low perfusion state secondary to decreased cardiac output. Urine output remains one of the most sensitive indicators of cardiac output in the postoperative period. Urine output of less than 0.5 ml/kg/hr is highly suggestive of the presence of oliguric acute tubular necrosis (ATN). ATN is a significant postoperative complication of cardiopulmonary bypass and has been linked to an overall increase in mortality rates.[56] It is believed to occur following episodes of decreased perfusion that ultimately result in a decrease in renal cortical blood flow and nephron damage. The nonpulsatile perfusion from the cardiopulmonary bypass apparatus has long been suggested as a major component of the hypoperfusion states that are seen during cardiac surgery.[57]

However, research by Hilberman et al. and Slogoff et al. documented that the conditions of CPB are not solely responsible for the development of ARF or ATN and that this condition is multifactorial in its causes and presentation.[58,59] Other possible causes include the use of renal or peripheral vasoconstrictors, episodes of hypotension, and microembolic events. Modern techniques of CPB such as the use of adequate perfusion rates, pulsatile flows, hemodilution, filtration systems, diuresis during bypass, and maintenance of an alkaline urine have helped to reduce the overall incidence of postoperative renal failure.

Oliguric ATN: Diagnosis and Treatment

Oliguric ATN is recognized to have a much poorer prognosis than nonoliguric ATN. The treatment plan for oliguric ATN in the postoperative cardiac patient involves maintenance of fluid and electrolyte balance and the prevention of further renal damage. Diuretics are often used to maintain urine volume postoperatively but have never been shown to be protective of ATN development.[60] Indeed, the presence of high urine volumes postoperatively does not ensure that either oliguric or nonoliguric ATN will not occur. When urine outputs fall to less than 0.5 ml/kg/hr, oliguric ATN should be suspected. A trial of diuretics combined with adequate replacement of intravascular fluid volume should help to determine the presence or absence of renal function. Persistent oliguria with the presence of muddy, granular casts, epithelial cells in the urine, high urine sodium levels, and a fluid osmolality approximating serum osmolality substantiates the diagnosis of oliguric ATN.

Increases in cardiac output are beneficial in treating ATN. However, use of drugs such as epinephrine and dopamine can, when given in excessive doses, cause renal vasoconstriction and decrease renal cortical perfusion. Similarly, all drugs that require good renal function for excretion or are known nephrotoxins should be discontinued. Extrarenal fluid losses should be replaced and electrolytes such as sodium bicarbonate, potassium, creatinine, and blood urea nitrogen (BUN) carefully followed. Peritoneal dialysis is sometimes required to treat the complications of uremia, hyperkalemia, acidosis, fluid accumulation, and even encephalopathy that can accompany acute renal failure. Some researchers have found that early institution of dialysis (within the first 24 hours of oliguria) can help to reduce overall mortality rates from ARF to about 10%.[61]

Cardiac Surgery in Patients with Renal Failure

Cardiac surgery is now more frequently performed in patients with end-stage renal disease requiring hemodialysis or peritoneal dialysis.[62,63] These patients usually undergo dialysis within 24 hours prior to their operation and then renal dialysis is performed during the cardiopulmonary bypass. This is accomplished by placing a dialysis filter within the CPB circuit for ultrafiltrate. This aids in maintaining normal potassium levels and favorable fluid balance throughout the procedure.[64]

Vascular Surgery

Renal Complications

The anesthesiologist must be aware of the multiple etiologies of acute renal failure and the wide variety of clinical presentations in order to provide aggressive and timely prevention and treatment. ARF is the major renal complication following vascular surgery. It results from insufficient renal perfusion, persisting for a sufficiently long duration. Vascular surgery compromises blood flow to the kidneys in a variety of ways.[65] Major vascular procedures, including aortic aneurysm repair and renal revascularization, often involve periods of direct renal ischemia or altered renal perfusion due to suprarenal or infrarenal aortic cross-clamping and/or partial occlusion of the renal arteries.[66,67]

In addition, many vascular procedures are of considerable duration and involve not only extensive tissue manipulation but also occasional massive blood loss with associated fluid shifts between the intravascular, interstitial, and intracellular compartments. Hemorrhage can compromise renal perfusion by substantial intravascular volume depletion.

Preoperative Evaluation and Treatment

The preoperative period is important in the genesis of ARF in susceptible patients. ARF is a well-known complication of the large doses of radiographic contrast material needed during angiographic procedures prior to vascular surgery.[68] It is most important to consider whether the patient has any pre-existing renal dysfunction prior to angiography. One study by Martin-Paredero et al. showed an incidence of ARF of over 40% in these patients, while the occurrence of acute renal dysfunction in patients without known pre-existing renal disease was just over 10%.[69] Additionally, the renal effects of angiography often are an unknown variable to be considered at the time of vascular surgery. The osmotic load from contrast agents can cause significant diuresis, intravascular volume deficits, and fluid shifts that can complicate anesthetic management and intraoperative hemodynamic balance. For this reason, it has been suggested that a 24- to 48-hour waiting period be instituted between angiography and aortic resection in the elective surgical patient population,[70] during which aggressive hydration is accomplished.

The cornerstone of management of acute renal failure lies in prevention of its occurrence rather than treatment. While advances in surgical technique, hemodynamic monitoring, and understanding of renal physiology have all helped to contribute to an overall decline in the incidence of perioperative ARF, the mortality from established disease remains in the range of 50 to 90%.[71–74] This rate has remained essentially unchanged over the last three decades in spite of many advances in supportive care and treatment, including intensive dialysis therapy.[75,76]

The incidence of acute renal failure in patients undergoing major vascular surgery depends most significantly on the site of aortic cross-clamping. Renal perfusion decreases approximately 90% during thoracic aortic cross-clamping and the overall incidence of ARF following this procedure is in the range of 3 to 13%.[77–80] Other studies have shown an incidence of renal failure after repair of extensive aorto-occlusive disease or suprarenal aneurysms to be in the range of 10 to 30%.[81–83] Patients at greatest risk for developing renal failure were those who had a renal ischemic time greater than 30 minutes, pre-existing heart disease, need for reoperation, or who experienced postoperative respiratory insufficiency.[84]

When the aorta is cross-clamped below the renal arteries, there is still a significant alteration in renal hemodynamics that occurs, including a decrease in renal blood flow of at least 40%.[85] One study, by Green et al., showed that when infrarenal cross-clamping was not possible, and supraceliac versus immediate suprarenal clamping were compared, the incidence of ARF that required dialysis was 3% in the supraceliac group and 23% in the suprarenal clamp category. This increase was attributed to several factors, including aortic and renal artery trauma, as well as atheromatous plaque dislodgement causing a partial but permanent loss in functioning nephron mass.[86,87] Other studies have examined serum creatinine elevations in patients undergoing infrarenal aortic cross-clamping, finding an increase of 0.5 mg/dl or greater in approximately 15%.[88]

The overall incidence of renal dysfunction after aortic aneurysmectomy is significant, ranging from 1 to 8%, and remains an important cause of mortality during elective aortic surgery. Following emergency aortic aneurysm repair, the incidence of ARF rises to 8 to 46%.[88,90] Some studies have reported a lower overall mortality if aggressive medical management is quickly initiated, while other series continue to note a generally poor prognosis in the critically ill population.[91–93] If renal revascularization is combined with aortic surgery, fewer than 10% of patients develop ARF, which is only slightly greater than the incidence noted when a previously identified renal stenosis is not surgically repaired.[94]

The mainstay of renal protection during major vascular and especially aortic surgery remains the maintenance of adequate cardiac output, which should maximize renal perfusion throughout the perioperative period. Aggressive hemodynamic management and preload optimization should be performed using a pulmonary artery catheter (PAC) to most closely assess left ventricular filling pressures and to aid in cardiac output determinations.[95–98] Fluid management plays an especially important role in the postoperative period, where treatment of suspected or diagnosed oliguric ARF requires the preservation of appropriate cardiovascular hemodynamics to eliminate prerenal etiologies of oliguria before progression to ARF. Prerenal causes of oliguria include hypovolemia as a result of third spacing, excessive blood loss, and possible inappropriate diuretic therapy and/or hypothermia-induced renal tubular dysfunction.[99] The indications for use of a PAC might also include the ability to distinguish congestive heart failure from hypovolemia as a prerenal cause of oliguria. If treatment with inotropes, diuretics, preload, and/or afterload augmentation is indicated for a low-output state in a patient with congestive heart failure (CHF), a PAC should be used to provide the hemodynamic information necessary to make optimal therapeutic decisions. Hypovolemia as a cause of diminished renal perfusion is best treated by volume infusion adjusted to optimal cardiac output and pulmonary artery occluded pressures.[100]

In the postoperative intensive care unit setting, the most common form of ARF is the nonoliguric type with resultant urine production of greater than 15 ml/hr. It is crucial to recognize and diagnose this situation as quickly as possible so that appropriate fluid volume and hemodynamic management can begin and any possible use of nephrotoxic medications can be avoided. Measurement of a creatinine clearance from a 2-hour urine collection can often help to quantify renal function in patients with nonoliguric renal dysfunction.

Postoperative ARF is routinely managed by artificial means including hemodialysis, peritoneal dialysis, continuous arteriovenous hemodialysis (CAVHD), venovenous hemofiltration, and continuous arteriovenous hemofiltration (CAVHF). Depending on the patient's clinical situation, a specific method of renal replacement therapy can be employed and tailored to maintain and improve fluid and/or electrolyte balance as well to treat conditions such as uremia.[101] It is important to note that the vascular surgery patient has certain limitations that cause one or more forms of renal therapy to be ill advised. An example is that the use of arteriovenous cannulation with continuous heparinization as required by CAVHF is contraindicated. Similarly, peritoneal dialysis may be successfully used in the postabdominal aortic surgical patient provided the patient has not received a celiotomy. In each of these situations, the benefits and requirements of each form of renal replacement therapy must be considered within the context of the vascular surgery patient and the special conditions presented throughout this postoperative course.

Gastrointestinal Complications

Major gastrointestinal (GI) complications following cardiac and thoracic surgical procedures are seen rarely. The incidence of gastrointestinal complications requiring therapeutic intervention is approximately 1 to 3% with an associated mortality of greater than 65%.[102–104] The spectrum of GI complications is large and includes gastroduodenal ulcer (the most common); gastritis; acute pancreatitis or cholecystitis; intestinal ischemia; perforation or hemorrhage; thromboembolic events; and nonthrombotic mesenteric infarction, ileus, and jaundice. A recent study by Huddy et al. showed the overall risk of GI complications increased fourfold if the heart is opened during the surgical procedure, and that cardiac transplant patients had a 20% risk of significant postoperative GI complications.[105] Major risk factors include elderly patients (age >70 years), female gender, prior history of GI disorders, use of vasopressor drugs, emergency surgical procedures, and prolonged cardiopulmonary bypass (CPB) time with nonpulsatile perfusion and aortic cross-clamp time. In addition, it has been shown that GI complications occur more frequently in combined CABG-valve procedures than for CABG operations alone.[106,107]

Preoperatively, all patients should have a thorough clinical evaluation to identify those at increased risk to develop postoperative gastrointestinal problems. Appropriate therapeutic management should be instituted throughout the perioperative period, and should include preoperative H_2 antagonists and avoidance of aspirin and other nonsteroidal anti-inflammatory drugs (NSAIDs). Recognizing patients at risk and employing presumptive radiographic and endoscopic diagnostic techniques may be of benefit in avoiding severe and possibly life-threatening postoperative GI sequelae by early therapeutic intervention.

The most common GI complication following cardiac surgery is bleeding requiring transfusion, which generally occurs within the first month postoperatively.[108,109] In the majority of patients, bleeding occurs in the gastroduodenal area. Most patients with postoperative GI bleeding had significant associated postoperative dysfunction of multiple organ systems. There may be a wide range of causative factors for these findings, including a prior history of peptic ulcer disease, the use of high-dose anticoagulant therapy during the surgical procedure, lack of effective antacid or H_2 blockade, and the overall physiologic stress of the operation.[110] Several studies have shown that maintaining an elevated gastric pH (>4.0) is effective in preventing gastric mucosa erosion.[111,112] Acute cholecystitis remains the second most common GI complication after CPB, with some researchers reporting mortality rates of up to 50% occurring in this population.[113,114]

Mesenteric ischemia and intestinal infarction are also noted to be a significant cause of GI complications postoperatively, although the clinical presentation can be quite variable. The causes may be embolic in nature, or in the majority of cases, of a nonocclusive etiology. Initial symptoms can be mild and the complete syndrome may not fully present until the patient is acutely ill. A high index of suspicion is required to make the proper diagnosis early and institute appropriate aggressive management.[115]

Several authors have noted an increased incidence of pancreatitis following cardiac surgery.[116–119] In one postmortem study, the incidence of unexplained pancreatitis was approximately 16% and, of these, 7% were recognized to be severe cases. Their overall mortality has been shown to be as high as 85% percent.[117] Some possible etiologies include shock, hypovolemia, associated multisystem organ failure, splenic vasoconstriction, hypercalcemia and the use of calcium chloride intraoperatively, thromboembolic events, operative trauma, and the use of chlorothiazide diuretics.[118,119]

Hyperbilirubinemia or "postpump jaundice" has been found by researchers to occur at varying rates between 0.06 and 20%[120,121] and may be associated with significantly increased mortality. Several theories have been advanced to explain the occurrence of elevated bilirubin levels, including longer CPB times, increased requirements for blood and blood products, and operations for multiple valve replacements. However, it has been noted that hyperbilirubinemia can occur in even the most uncomplicated surgical procedures.

Large and small bowel lesions present rarely following CPB and require different theories to explain their occurrence. These lesions, including acute diverticulitis, ileus, cecal perforation, appendicitis, and bowel infarction, have been thought to be due to ischemia or tissue hypoxia while on cardiopulmonary bypass, which leads to a breakdown of the mucosal barrier. However, no true cause-and-effect relationship has ever been proven.[122]

While no single therapeutic intervention has been completely effective in preventing these complications, it seems reasonable that maintaining adequate cardiac output and tissue perfusion is a crucial factor in improving patient outcome. Clearly, most authors agree that early aggressive management, including surgical intervention for bleeding that fails to respond rapidly to appropriate conservative medical therapy, is most important in reducing the incidence of potentially disastrous gastrointestinal complications.[123,124]

References

1. Gass GD, Olsen GN: Preoperative pulmonary function tests to predict postoperative morbidity and mortality. Chest 89:127, 1986.

2. Stein M, Cassara EL: Preoperative pulmonary evaluation and therapy for surgery patients. JAMA 211:780, 1970.
3. Warner MA, Offord K, Warner ME, et al: Role of preoperative cessation of smoking, and other factors in postoperative pulmonary complications: A blinded prospective study of coronary artery bypass patients. Mayo Clin Proc 64:609, 1989.
4. Buisst AS, Sexton GV, Nagy JM, et al: The effects of smoking cessation and modification of lung function. Am Rev Respir Dis 123:149, 1981.
5. Jones RM: Smoking before surgery: The case for stopping smoking. Br Med J 290:1763, 1985.
6. Pearce AC, Jones RM: Smoking and anaesthesia: Preoperative abstinence and perioperative morbidity. Ann Surg 290:1763, 1985.
7. Pearce AC, Jones RM: Smoking and anaesthesia: Preoperative abstinence and perioperative morbidity. Anesthesiology 61:576, 1984.
8. Nagasaki F, Flehinger BJ, Martini N: Complications of surgery in the treatment of carcinoma of the lung. Chest 82:25, 1982.
9. O'Donohue WJ: National survey of the usage of lung expansion modalities for the prevention and treatment of postoperative atelectasis following abdominal and thoracic surgery. Chest 87:76, 1985.
10. Lewis FR: Management of atelectasis and pneumonia. Surg Clin North Am 67:1391, 1980.
11. Marini JJ: Postoperative atelectasis: Pathophysiology, clinical importance, and principles of management. Respir Care 29:516, 1984.
12. Bartlett RH: Pulmonary pathophysiology in surgical patients. Surg Clin North Am 60:1323, 1980.
13. Stock MC, Downs JB, Gauer PK: Prevention of postoperative pulmonary complications with CPAP, incentive spirometry, and conservative therapy. Chest 87:151, 1985.
14. Carlens E: A new flexible double lumen catheter for bronchospirometry. J Thorac Cardiovasc Surg 18:742, 1949.
15. Brooks JW: Complications following pulmonary lobectomy. In Cordell RA, Ellison RG (eds): Complications of Intrathoracic Surgery. Boston, Little, Brown & Co, 1979, p 235.
16. Kirsh MM, Rotman H, Behrendt DM, et al: Complications of pulmonary resection. Ann Thorac Surg 20:215, 1975.
17. Silver AW, Espiras EE, Byron FX: The fate of the post-resection space. Ann Thorac Surg 2:311, 1966.
18. Backer WL, Langston HT, Naffah P: Post-resectional thoracic spaces. Ann Thorac Surg 2:299, 1966.
19. Bjork VO, Engstrom CG: The treatment of ventilatory insufficiency after pulmonary resection with tracheostomy and prolonged artificial ventilation. J Thorac Cardiovasc Surg 30:356, 1955.
20. Roth MD, Wright JW, Bellamy PE: Gas flow through a bronchopleural fistula. Measuring the effects of high frequency jet ventilation and chest tube suction. Chest 93:210, 1988.
21. Williams NS, Leus CT: Bronchopleural fistula: A review of 86 cases. Br J Surg 63:530, 1976.
22. Lawrence GH, Ristroph R, Wood JA, et al: Methods for avoiding a dire surgical complication. Bronchopleural fistula after pulmonary resection. Am J Surg 144:136, 1982.
23. Hankins JR, Miller JE, Attar S, et al: Bronchopleural fistula: Thirteen year experience with 77 cases. J Thorac Cardiovasc Surg 76:755, 1978.
24. Schuler JG: Intraoperative lobar torsion producing pulmonary infarction. J Thorac Cardiovasc Surg 65:951, 1973.
25. Mullin MJ, Zumbro GL, Fishbach ME, et al: Pulmonary lobar gangrene complicating lobectomy. Ann Surg 175:62, 1972.
26. Adler RH, Plaut ME: Post pneumonectomy empyema. Surg 71: 210, 1972.
27. Bessone LN, Fergueson TB, Burford TH: Chylothorax. Ann Thorac Surg 12:527, 1971.
28. Milsom JW, Kron IL, Rheuban LS, Rodgers BM: Chylothorax: An assessment of current surgical management. J Thorac Cardiovasc Surg 89:211, 1985.
29. Pairoleno RC, Payne WS: Postoperative Care and Complications in the Thoracic Surgical Patient. In Glenn, Baue, Geha, Hammond, Cales (eds): Thoracic and Cardiovascular Surgery, 4th ed. Norwalk, CT, Appleton-Century-Crofts, 1983, p 344.
30. Peterffy A, Henze A: Hemorrhagic complications during pulmonary resections: A retrospective review of 1428 resection with 113 hemorrhagic episodes. Scand J Thorac Cardiovasc Surg 17: 28, 1983.
31. Parker DJ, Karp RB, Kirklin JW, et al: Lung water and alveolar and capillary volumes after intracardiac surgery. Circulation 45(Suppl I):I-139, 1972.
32. Edmunds LH, Alexander JA: Effects of cardiopulmonary bypass on the lungs. In Fishman AP (ed): Pulmonary Diseases and Disorders. New York, McGraw-Hill, 1980, p 1733.
33. Bitto T, Mannion J, Stephenson LW, et al: Pneumothorax during positive pressure ventilation. J Thorac Cardiovasc Surg 89:585, 1985.
34. Culliford AT, Thomas S, Spencer FC: Fulminating non-cardiogenic pulmonary edema. J Thorac Cardiovasc Surg 80:868, 1980.
35. Maggart M, Stewart S: The mechanisms and management of non-cardiogenic pulmonary edema following cardiopulmonary bypass. Ann Thorac Surg 43:231, 1987.
36. Tamiya T, Yamisaki M, Maeo Y, et al: Complement activation in cardiopulmonary bypass with special reference to anaphylatoxin production in membrane and bubble oxygenators. Ann Thorac Surg 4:47, 1988.
37. Conahan TJ: Complications of cardiac surgery. In Kaplan J (ed): Cardiac Anesthesia, 3rd ed. Philadelphia, WB Saunders Co, 1993, p 1249.
38. Katz NM, Buckholz BJ, Howard E, et al: Venovenous extracorporeal circulation for noncardiogenic pulmonary edema after cardiopulmonary bypass. Ann Thorac Surg 46:462, 1988.
39. Roberts KW, Lumb PD: Complications of vascular surgery. In Kaplan JA (ed): Vascular Anesthesia. New York, Churchill Livingstone, 1991, p 664.
40. Wabba WM: Influence of aging on lung function-clinical significant of changes from age twenty. Anesth Analg 62:764, 1983.
41. Craig DB: Postoperative recovery of pulmonary function. Anesth Soc J 60:46, 1981.
42. Desmeules H, Fournier L, Trembly PR: Systemic changes in the elderly patient and their anesthetic implications. Can Anesth Soc J 32:184, 1985.
43. Vodinh J, Bonnet F, Touboul C, et al: Risk factors of postoperative pulmonary complications after vascular surgery. Surgery 105:360, 1989.
44. Cappellier W, Ramierez H, Kortman H: Abdominal aortic aneurysms: Risk factors and complications and their influence or indications for operation. J Cardiovasc Surg 30:572, 1989.
45. Diehl J, Cali R, Hertzer N, Beven E: Complications of abdominal aortic reconstruction: An analysis of perioperative risk factors in 557 patients. Ann Surg 197:49, 1983.
46. Leather R, Shah D, Kaufman J, et al: Comparative analysis of retroperitoneal and transperitoneal aortic replacement for aneurysm. Surg Gynecol Obstet 168:387, 1989.
47. Cuschien RJ, Morran CG, Howie DC, McArdle CJ: Postoperative pain and pulmonary complications: comparison of three analgesic regimens. Br J Surg 72:495, 1985.
48. Jayr C, Mollie A, Bourgain JL, et al: Postoperative pulmonary complications: General anesthesia with postoperative parenteral morphine compared with epidural analgesia. Surgery 104:57, 1988.
49. Yeager MP, Glass DD, Neff RK, Brinck-Johnsen T: Epidural anesthesia and analgesia in high risk surgical patients. Anesthesiology 66:729, 1987.
50. Mankikian B, Cantineau JP, Bertrand M, et al: Improvement of diaphragmatic function by thoracic extradural block after upper abdominal surgery. Anesthesiology 68:379, 1988.
51. Dureuil B, Viires N, Cantineau JP, et al: Diaphragmatic contractility after upper abdominal surgery. Appl Physiol 61:1775, 1986.
52. Spence AA, Smith G: Postoperative analgesic and lung function: A comparison of morphine with extradural block. Br J Anesth 43:144, 1971.
53. Hilberman M, Myers BD, Camer BJ, et al: Acute renal failure following cardiac surgery. J Thorac Cardiovasc Surg 77:880, 1979
54. Baht JB, Glude NC, Lowenstein J, et al: Renal failure after open heart surgery. Ann Intern Med 84:677, 1976.

55. Corwin HL, Sprague SM, DeLaria GA, et al: Acute renal failure associated with cardiac operations. J Thorac Cardiovasc Surg 98: 1107, 1989.
56. Abel RM, Buckley MJ, Austen WG, et al: Incidence and prognosis of renal failure following cardiac operations. J Thorac Cardiovasc Surg 71:323, 1976.
57. Kron IL, Joob AW, Van Meter C: Acute renal failure in the cardiovascular surgical patient. Ann Thorac Surg 39:590, 1985.
58. Slogoff S, Ruel G, Keats A, et al: Role of perfusion pressure and flow in major organ dysfunction after cardiopulmonary bypass. Ann Thorac Surg 50:911, 1990.
59. Hilberman M, Myers BD, Carrier BJ, et al: Acute renal failure following cardiac surgery. J Thorac Cardiovasc Surg 77:880, 1979.
60. Bolman RM, Anderson RW, Molina JE, et al: Cardiac operations in patients with functioning renal allografts. J Thorac Cardiovasc Surg 88:537, 1984.
61. Goilunas P, Chawla R, Lazares JM, et al: Acute renal failure following cardiac operations. J Thorac Cardiovasc Surg 79:241, 1980.
62. Bolman RM, Anderson RW, Molina JE, et al: Cardiac operations in patients with functioning renal allografts. J Thorac Cardiovasc Surg 88:241, 1980.
63. Monson BK, Wickstrum PH, Haglin JJ, et al: Cardiac operations and end stage renal disease. Ann Thorac Surg 30:267, 1980.
64. Wiggins EL, Dearing PD: Simultaneous cardiopulmonary bypass and dialysis. J Extracorp Technol 17:117, 1985.
65. Castronuouvo J, Flanigan D: Renal failure complicating vascular surgery. In Bernard V, Towne J (eds): Complication in Vascular Surgery. Orlando, FL, Grune & Stratton, 1986.
66. Gamulin Z, Forster A, Morel D, et al: Effects of infrarenal aortic cross clamping on renal hemodynamics in humans. Anesthesiology 61:394, 1984.
67. Gamulin Z, Forster A, Simonet F, et al: Effect of renal sympathetic blockade on renal hemodynamics in humans. Anesthesiology 65:688, 1988.
68. Alexander R, Berkes S, Abuelo G: Contrast media-induced oliguric renal failure. Arch Intern Med 138:381, 1978.
69. Martin-Paredero V, Dixon S, Baker J, et al: Risk of renal failure after major angiography. Arch Surg 118:1417, 1984.
70. Shenaq S: Anesthesia for repair of aortic aneurysm. In Estafanous F (ed): Anesthesia and the Heart Patient. Boston, Butterworth, 1985.
71. Hou S, Bushinsky DA, Wish JB, et al: Hospital acquired renal insufficiency: A prospective study. Am J Med 74:243, 1983.
72. Gillum DM, Dixon BS, Yanover MJ, et al: The role of intensive dialysis in acute renal failure. Clin Nephrol 25:249, 1986.
73. Bullock ML, Umen AJ, Finkelstein M, Keane WF: The assessment of risk factors in 462 patients with acute renal failure. Am Kidney Dis 5:97, 1985.
74. Corwin HL, Bonventre JV: Acute renal failure in the intensive care unit. Part 1. Intensive Care Med 14:10, 1988.
75. Camron JS: Acute renal failure in the intensive care unit today. Intensive Care Med 12:64, 1986.
76. Conger JD: A controlled evaluation of prophylactic dialysis in post-traumatic acute renal failure. J Trauma 15:1056, 1975.
77. Gelman S, Reves J, Fowler K, et al: Regional blood flow during cross clamping of the thoracic aorta and infusion of sodium nitroprusside. J Thorac Cardiovasc Surg 85:287, 1983.
78. Crawford E, Walter H, Salch S, Norman H: Graft replacement of aneurysm in descending thoracic aorta: Results without bypass or shunting. Surgery 89:73085, 1981.
79. Carlson DE, Karp RB, Kouchoukos NT: Surgical treatment of aneurysms of the descending thoracic aorta: An analysis of 85 patients. Ann Thorac Surg 35:58, 1983.
80. Najafi H, Havid H, Hunter, et al: Descending aortic aneurysmectomy without adjuncts to avoid ischemia. Ann Thorac Surg 30:326, 1980.
81. Spargo P, Crosse M: Anesthetic problems in cross clamping of the thoracic aorta. Ann R Coll Surg 70:64, 1988.
82. Casthely P, Ryman P, Abrams L, et al: Thoracoabdominal aortic aneurysm repair—an analysis of postmorten morbidity. Arch Surg 123:871, 1988.
83. Hollier L, Symmonds H, Pairolero P, et al: Anesthesia for aortic arch aneurysm repair: Experience with 17 patients. Can Anesth Soc J 132:23, 1985.
84. Robert KW, Lumb PD: Complications of vascular surgery. In Kaplan JA (ed): Vascular Anesthesia. New York, Churchill Livingstone, 1991, p 644.
85. Gamulin Z, Foster A, Morel D, et al: Effects of infrarenal aortic cross-clamping on renal hemodynamics in humans. Anesthesiology 61:394, 1984.
86. Green R, Ricotta J, Ouriel K, De Weese J: Results of supraceliac aortic clamping in the difficult elective resection of infrarenal abdominal aortic aneurysm. J Vasc Surg 91:124, 1989.
87. Pitts RF: Physiology of the Kidney and Body Fluids, 3rd ed. Chicago, Year Book Medical Publishers, 1974, p 167.
88. Alpert RA, Roizen MF, Hamilton WK, et al: Intraoperative urinary output does not predict postoperative renal function in patients undergoing abdominal aortic revascularization. Surgery 95:707, 1984.
89. Gornule CC Jr, Kjellstrand CM: Acute renal failure complicating aortic aneurysm surgery. Nephron 35:145, 1983.
90. Abbott W: Acute renal failure complicating vascular surgery. In Bernard V, Towne J (eds): Complications in Vascular Surgery. Orlando, FL, Grune & Stratton, 1980.
91. Sapir DG, Dandy WE Jr, Whelton A, Cooke CR: Acute renal failure after ruptured abdominal aortic aneurysm. An improved clinical prognosis. Crit Care Med 7:59, 1979.
92. Sinicrope RA, Serra RM, Engle JE, et al: Mortality of acute renal failure after rupture of abdominal aortic aneurysms. Am J Surg 141:240, 1981.
93. Bartlett RH, Mault JR, Dechert RE, et al: Continuous arteriovenous hemofiltration: Improved survival in acute surgical renal failure? Surgery 100:400, 1986.
94. Sterpetti AV, Schultz, RD, Feldhaus RJ, Peetz DJ Jr: Aortic and renal atherosclerotic disease. Surg Gynecol Obstet 163:54, 1986.
95. Bush H, Huse J, Johnson W, et al: Prevention of renal insufficiency after abdominal aortic aneurysm resection by optimal volume loading. Arch Surg 116:1517, 1981.
96. Clark N, Stanley T: Anesthesia for vascular surgery. In Miller R (ed): Anesthesia, 2nd ed. New York, Churchill Livingstone, 1986.
97. Roizen M: Anesthesia for vascular surgery. In Barasch P, Cullen B, Stoelting R (eds): Clinical Anesthesia. Philadelphia, JB Lippincott Co, 1985.
98. Whittemore A, Clowes A, Hechtman H, Mannick J: Aortic aneurysm repair: Reduced operative mortality with maintenance of optimal cardiac performance. Ann Surg 192:414, 1980.
99. Reuler J: Hypothermia: Pathophysiology, clinical settings and management. Ann Intern Med 89:519, 1979.
100. Hertzer N, Beven E, Young J, et al: Coronary artery disease in peripheral vascular patients: A classification of 1000 coronary angiograms and results of surgical management. Ann Surg 199: 223, 1984.
101. Garcia J, Pagini E: Acute renal failure: Etiology, diagnosis and therapy. In Estafanous F (ed): Anesthesia and the Heart Patient. Boston, Butterworth, 1989.
102. Rosemurgy AS, McAllister E, Karl RC: The acute surgical abdomen after cardiac surgery involving extracorporeal circulation. Ann Surg 207:323, 1988.
103. Pinson CW, Alberty RE: General surgical complications after cardiopulmonary bypass surgery. Am J Surg 146:133, 1983.
104. Krasna MJ, Flanobaun L, Trooskin ZS, et al: Gastrointestinal complications in 4473 patients who underwent cardiopulmonary bypass surgery. Surgery 104:733, 1988.
105. Huddy SPJ, Joyce WP, Pepper JR: Gastrointestinal complications in 4473 patients who underwent cardiopulmonary bypass surgery. Br J Surg 8:293, 1991.
106. Leitman MI, Paull DE, Barie PJ: Intraabdominal complication of cardiopulmonary bypass operations. Surg Gynecol Obstet 165:251, 1987.
107. Krasna MJ, Flanobaun L, Trooskin ZS, et al: Gastrointestinal complications after cardiac surgery. Surgery 104:733, 1988.
108. Hanks JB, Curtis SE, Hanks BB, et al: Gastrointestinal complications after cardiopulmonary bypass. Surgery 92:394, 1982.
109. Ohri S, Desai J, Gaer J, et al: Intraabdominal complications after cardiopulmonary bypass. Ann Thorac Surg 52:826, 1991.
110. Sutherland AD, et al: The effect of preoperative oral fluid and ranitidine in gastric fluid volume and pH. Can J Anesth 34:117, 1987.

111. Priebe HJ, Skillman JJ: Methods of prophylaxis in stress ulcer disease. World J Surg 5:323, 1981.
112. Zinner MJ, Zuidema GD, Smith PL, et al: The prevention of upper gastrointestinal tract bleeding in patients in an intensive care unit. Surg Gynecol Obstet 153:214, 1981.
113. Pinson CW, Albert RE: General surgical complications after cardiopulmonary bypass surgery. Am J Surg 146:133, 1983.
114. Hanks JB, Curtis SE, Hanks BB, et al: Gastrointestinal complications after cardiopulmonary bypass. Surgery 92:394, 1982.
115. Long WB: Abdominal complications of cardiopulmonary bypass. In Utlery JR (ed): Pathophysiology and Techniques of Cardiopulmonary Bypass, Vol 2. Baltimore, Williams & Wilkins, 1983, p 715.
116. Feiner H: Pancreatitis after cardiac surgery. A morphologic study. Am J Surg 131:684, 1976.
117. Rose DM, Ranson JHC, Cunningham JN, et al: Patterns of severe pancreatic injury following cardiopulmonary bypass. Ann Surg 199:168, 1984.
118. Anderson IDR, Stephenson LW, Edmunds LH: Management of complications of cardiopulmonary bypass: Complications of organ systems. In Waldhausen, Orriger (eds): Complications in Cardiothoracic Surgery. St Louis, Mosby Year Book, 1991, p 53.
119. Ferrandy Del Castillo C, Harringer W, Warslaw A, et al: Risk factors for pancreatic cellular injury after cardiopulmonary bypass. N Engl J Med 325:382, 1991.
120. Collins JD, Bassendine MF, Ferner R, et al: Incidence and prognostic importance of jaundice after cardiopulmonary bypass surgery. Lancet 1:1119, 1983.
121. Hanks JB, Curtis SE, Hanks BB, et al: Gastrointestinal complications after cardiopulmonary bypass. Surgery 92:394, 1982.
122. Arnata GV, Pickleman J, Pitarri R, et al: The reasons for gastrointestinal consultation after cardiac surgery. Ann Surg 50:301, 1984.
123. Taylor PC, Loop FD, Hermann RE: Management of acute stress ulcer after cardiac surgery. Ann Surg 178:1, 1973.
124. Shockett E, et al: Gastroduodenal perforation after open heart surgery. Am J Surg 134:643, 1977.

CHAPTER 38

Continuous Quality Improvement in Cardiac and Thoracic Anesthesia

Allen J. Hinkle, M.D.
Paul E. Stensrud, M.D.
David L. Brown, M.D.

The application of the principles of continuous quality improvement to medical practice is still in its infancy in the United States. To a large extent the growth of managed care has been responsible for the wide interest in the implementation of quality improvement efforts in medicine.

Currently there are very few examples of comprehensive continuous quality improvement efforts in anesthesia practice. Cardiothoracic anesthesia is an exception and these will be discussed later in this chapter.

The first section of this chapter will describe the basics of continuous quality improvement. Both the principles and tools will be discussed. Then outcome studies in cardiothoracic and vascular anesthesia will be reviewed. As we will see, studies in anesthesiology have tended to focus on the immediate clinical effects of drugs and anesthetic techniques rather than overall outcome.[1] Finally, examples of quality improvement in cardiothoracic surgery that include cardiothoracic anesthesia contributions will be examined. The difference between anesthesia outcomes studies and the multidisciplinary approach to quality improvement work will be emphasized. The goals of this chapter are to educate the reader in continuous quality improvement and to encourage the formation of multidisciplinary quality teams in your institution.

History of Continuous Quality Improvement

The management philosophy of continuous quality improvement (CQI) or total quality management (TQM) is synonymous with the name Dr. W. Edwards Deming. Dr. Deming is considered to be the father of the modern quality improvement movement. When the United States entered World War II, Dr. Deming got the opportunity to apply his statistical methods to the process of manufacturing war materials. By 1945 it is estimated that he educated some 30,000 technical workers and engineers about CQI methods.[2] Despite his great success in reducing scrap and rework in the war materials manufacturing process, there was little appreciation for how his knowledge could be applied to the management of United States businesses.

In the early 1920s Dr. Walter Shewhart, a statistician, was working at Bell Laboratories where he was developing and applying the use of control charts to measure process variation. Shewhart's control charts were based on a combination of probability theory and practical experience. While managers and engineers at Bell Laboratories knew of his work, his methods were regarded as technical and therefore were not used in industry.

Finally, Drs. Deming and Shewhart began working together at Western Electric in the early 1930s. It is the melding together of their works that resulted in CQI as we know it today.

After World War II, Dr. Deming traveled to Japan to help the Department of War with census surveys and other studies.[3] This was the beginning of his long friendship with Japan, and Dr. Deming found an audience there that was eager to learn his methods. Much of modern Japan's production of high-quality manufactured goods and its robust economy are the result of Dr. Deming's contributions.

Eventually Deming's CQI principles and techniques found their way back into the United States manufacturing industry. Seeing the improvements that resulted in manufacturing, the service industry quickly adopted CQI as well. With the dramatic changes occurring in health care, it is not surprising that a new management approach such as CQI is being applied to health care improvement efforts. Efforts are underway nationwide to apply the CQI principles to improving the health care system as well as improving clinical processes.

Total Quality Management

Total quality management, or continuous quality improvement, represents a new set of principles for transforming traditional Western style management practices.

The centerpiece of TQM is Deming's 14 Points for Management (Table 38–1).

Rosander has concentrated on the specific application of Deming's 14 points to service industries.[5] Hospitals frequently confuse quality control measures such as institutional quality, quality performance of professionals, and patient service quality. Medical services primarily exist to serve the patient. The institution, professionals, and other personnel are supportive to delivering the highest quality patient service. Although applying all of Deming's 14 points to anesthesia practice reform is important, breaking down barriers between staff areas presents a particular challenge. The perioperative nature of anesthesia requires close interactions between multiple areas of the patient critical pathway, including the preoperative clinic, same day unit, emergency room, operating room (OR), postanesthesia care unit (PACU), intensive care units, and inpatient units.

By embracing and applying Deming's 14 points within a system of profound knowledge, the principles of TQM can lead the necessary transformation. By linking Deming's four elements of a system of profound knowledge with our professional knowledge (i.e., anesthesia knowledge), we can continuously improve our component of the health care system.

Deming's System for Profound Knowledge[6]:

- Knowledge of a system
- Knowledge of variation
- Knowledge of psychology
- Theory of knowledge

By using Deming's improvement knowledge and our professional health care knowledge, Nolan[7] instructs us as to how the PDSA (Plan-Do-Study-Act) cycle (Fig. 38–1) offers an effective model for guiding our improvement efforts. The PDSA cycle will help us develop tests of change and, by repeatedly using these change cycles, we can build the knowledge necessary to improve the process. As an example, if our aim is to decrease OR time for cardiac surgical patients, one PDSA cycle may concentrate on decreasing the "ready for surgeon to surgical incision" time component of total OR time. A test of change might be that the surgeon physically arrives in the OR simultaneously with the patient!

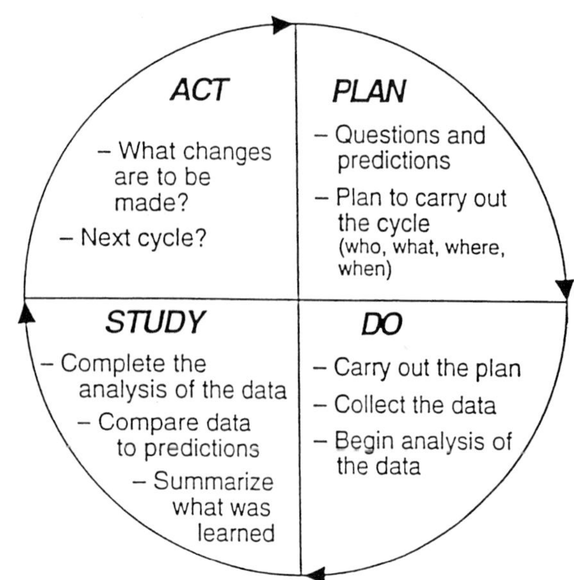

FIGURE **38–1.** The PDSA cycle for learning and improvement.

Gaining knowledge of a system is an important first step in achieving Deming's profound knowledge. From a TQM perspective, a system is a network of interdependent components that work together to try to accomplish the aim of the system. To be a system, an organization must have an aim that is clear to everyone in the system, includes plans for the future, is a value judgment, and emphasizes purpose. Within a system reside a multitude of processes. It is the continuous improvement of these processes that is the core of TQM. Flowcharting provides a very powerful tool to define a process, which is the first step in improvement work. Once the process is understood, Paul Batalden, M.D. (Center for Evaluative Clinical Sciences, Dartmouth Medical School, 1995) offers his ten secrets for improving the process, which can be quite valuable for any quality improvement team (Fig. 38–2). In addition, flowcharting the process can aid in constructing the membership of the quality improvement team. Those persons closest to the process need to own the improvement efforts in order for them to be effective.

Initial efforts to ensure quality in medical care (often termed "quality assurance" programs) focused on structure and process, as these variables are more easily defined and measured. Determination of the adequacy of such components of structure as the physical plant, personnel credentialing and policies, and maintenance of available equipment can be easily documented and monitored. Structure in most anesthesiology departments across the United States is uniform following the imple-

TABLE 38–1
Deming's 14 Points for Management*

1. Create constancy of purpose for improvement of product and service.
2. Adopt the new philosophy.
3. Cease dependence on mass inspection.
4. End the practice of awarding business on the basis of price tag alone.
5. Improve constantly and forever the system of production and service.
6. Institute training.
7. Adopt and institute leadership.
8. Drive out fear.
9. Break down barriers among staff areas.
10. Eliminate slogans, exhortations, and targets for the work force.
11. Eliminate numerical quotas for the work force and numerical goals for people in management.
12. Remove barriers that rob people of pride of workmanship.
13. Encourage education and self-improvement for everyone.
14. Take action to accomplish the transformation.

*From Scherkenbach WW: The Deming Route to Quality and Productivity. Milwaukee, ASQC Quality Press, 1986, with permission. Reprinted from *Out of the Crisis* by W. Edwards Deming by permission of MIT and The W. Edwards Deming Institute. Published by MIT, Center for Advanced Educational Services, Cambridge, MA 02139. Copyright 1986 by The W. Edwards Deming Institute.

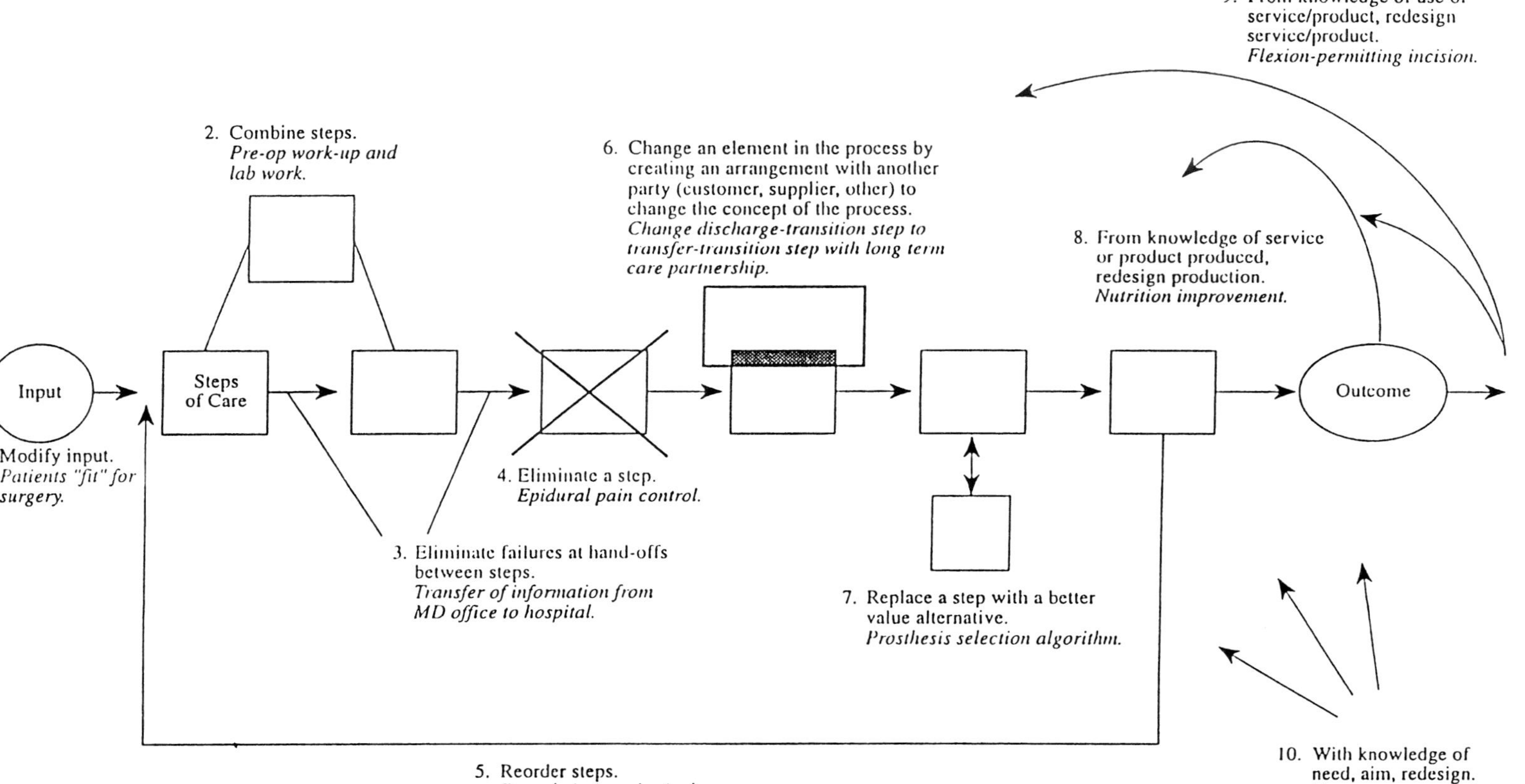

FIGURE **38–2.** A process flowchart of total hip arthroplasty with ten secrets of managing care for improved value. Examples of improvements in the value of hip joint replacement are shown in italics. (Courtesy of P. Batalden.)

mentation of guidelines for monitoring and similar initiatives. Anesthetic process is less easily analyzed. Analysis of process has been dependent on internal and external "peer review" of medical records by independent practitioners who must judge adequacy of care.[8] The peer review process obviously entails many real and potential problems and the accuracy of peer review has been called into question. Goldman analyzed 12 studies of peer review and demonstrated poor agreement among physician reviewers regarding quality of care.[9] Caplan et al. demonstrated that severity of adverse outcomes influenced the opinion of reviewers regarding quality of care; that is, if permanent adverse outcome occurred, the reviewer was more apt to determine that quality of care was inadequate as opposed to the situation in which the same care was delivered with only a temporary adverse outcome.[10] There may be an assumption on the part of some reviewers that adverse outcome implies poor quality of care, despite the many other variables affecting outcome. Modification of peer review may provide at least a partial solution to these problems, but the modifications proposed entail their own difficulties.[9] Multiple reviewers could be used and more objective review procedures might be developed. Higher standards for reviewers than mere possession of a medical license could be instituted. These changes would be costly and could prove cumbersome. Provision of practice guidelines would provide a framework for reviewers to assess quality of care, but more outcome data would need to be gathered to ensure that optimal care was included in such guidelines. Furthermore, practice guidelines should only be instituted as part of a wider program of quality improvement, in order to increase the impact of the guidelines on physician behavior.[11] Further studies of techniques to analyze medical process must be undertaken.

The assumption underlying analyses of structure and process is that good structure combined with good process must result in good medical outcome. This assumption may be false. Indeed, medical outcome may be more dependent on the patient's underlying medical condition than on the delivery of extremely high quality care, as opposed to adequate care. In other words, poor patient outcome may occur despite the presence of excellent medical structure and process.[12] Conversely, poor structure and process do not necessarily result in poor outcome, although intuitively the likelihood of poor outcome would seem to be increased in this situation, and reliance on the resilience of the patient is imprudent. This is not to say that structure and process are not important to the delivery of high-quality medical care, only that they must be analyzed concurrently with medical outcome and not be considered in isolation.

The success of quality improvement efforts relies heavily on using the right data that are displayed in a useful format. Therefore, it is not surprising to read Deming's work and find that it is replete with Shewhart's understanding that data analysis through the use of control charts provides the robust tools needed for process improvement. Just as TQM provides the new thinking required for transforming an organization, statistical process control (SPC) provides the new tools for gaining insight into the data that emanate from processes that can be used to lead improvement initiatives and we will review SPC later.

Principles of Continuous Quality Improvement

Before embarking on a CQI project it is important to understand some of the basic principles that define CQI. While each of these principles is critical for a successful CQI effort, having all of the principles integrated into improvement work is a necessity.

Customer-Driven

In anesthesia practice understanding our many customers does not typically get high priority. In CQI work the improvement efforts must be customer-focused. Frequently this means learning who your various customers might be in anesthesia practice. In cardiac anesthesia some customers may be:

- the patient
- the patient's family
- referring primary care physician
- same day surgery staff
- OR staff
- ICU staff
- surgeons
- cardiologists

Understanding who your customers are and then using feedback from them to continuously improve care is fundamental to CQI.

System Optimization and Alignment

Any given health care organization is made up of many interdependent parts that come together to form a system. Cardiothoracic anesthesia is an example of such a part that is interdependent with cardiac surgery, yet both contribute to the success of the XYZ Medical Center System.

Organizations strive to improve the performance of the whole system, not just one of the interdependent parts. Within the system there must be alignment of mission, values, processes, policies, and people.

Continual Improvement and Innovation

The multiple processes within a system should be continually improved in a systematic and scientific manner. This requires process definition, measurement, data collection, and analysis, which leads then to process improvement. It becomes a never-ending pursuit of further improvement and higher service quality.

New services that delight customers also contribute to improvement. Percutaneous transluminal coronary angioplasty rather than coronary artery bypass grafting may be such an example for the cardiac patient. Likewise the use of continuous thoracic epidural analgesia for postthoracotomy pain management was an innovative improvement for thoracic surgical patients.

Continual Learning

In order to effectively apply CQI in an organization there must be a commitment to continual learning. Senge best describes how to become and maintain a learning organization.[13] Resources for learning must be made available in the organization and learning from experience is required.

Management Through Knowledge

A learning organization uses data to continuously improve. Understanding variation and statistical thinking are key attributes of a successful CQI program.

Collaboration and Mutual Respect

The organization instituting a CQI program must respect the many contributors to improvement work. To effectively improve any process requires collaboration with all of those involved in the process.

For cardiac anesthesiologists this means collaborating and respecting the contributions of surgeons, OR nurses, perfusionists, ICU nurses, and many other team members. The process of providing anesthesia services for cardiac or vascular surgery patients is a complex one and anesthesiologists cannot effectuate significant improvement in the care process of their patients without collaborating with nonanesthesia personnel.

Statistical Process Control

Dr. Walter Shewhart is regarded as the grandfather of SPC and control charts. It was his understanding of the existence of two kinds of variation—common cause and special cause variation—that contributed immeasurably to our knowledge. He identified two mistakes that are frequently made when attempting to improve a process, both of which add avoidable costs.

Mistake 1: To react to an outcome as if it came from a special cause when it actually came from common cause variation.

Mistake 2: To treat an outcome as if it came from common cause variation when it actually came from special cause.

When a process is measured, the data that are collected over time can be displayed on a control chart. The control chart can assure us of the continued stability of the process and allow us to predict the future performance of that process. However, an unstable process (i.e., a control chart with special cause variation) is unpredictable. An unstable process must be brought into stability first, and it is only then that the process can be further improved. Once the process is brought into statistical control (i.e., only common cause variation), improvement efforts can focus on minimizing the variation within the process, shifting the average closer to the ideal position whether it be higher or lower or both of these goals. Of course, the economic advantage of the improvement must make sense with regard to the anticipated cost of the improvement.

Although control charts are key tools in the quality improvement tool kit, they can primarily help us achieve what Deming meant when he said, "If I had to reduce my message for management to just a few words, I'd say it all had to do with reducing variation."[14] It is interesting that, quite often, we pride ourselves in medicine on the variation in clinical practice as an asset. However, we should not lose sight of Shewhart's fourth foundation for control charts: "Control charts are effective only to the extent that the organization can use, in an effective manner, the knowledge gained from the charts."[15] Shewhart was warning us not to let TQM and SPC become disconnected during improvement work. Although we may have the tools of SPC in hand and understand them, it is the principles of TQM that will determine where and how we use these tools (i.e., the data will be meaningless if removed from their context).

In health care improvement work, most collected data are typically individual values. For this reason, the XmR control chart is the most common control chart used for displaying data (Fig. 38–3). The X values are plotted in appropriate time sequence on the top graph while the moving ranges (mR) are plotted on the lower chart. The moving range is a measure of the variation or absolute difference between one data point and the next on the X chart. Together, these two charts define an XmR control chart. The X portion of the XmR chart also contains the average or central line for X (Cl_x), the upper natural process limit for X ($UNPL_x$), and the lower natural process limit for X ($LNPL_x$). The mR portion of the XmR chart contains the average mR or the central line for R(CL_r), and the upper control limit for the range (UCL_r). When the data reside between these limits of the XmR chart and do not display any out-of-control patterns, the process being measured is stable or functioning as best it can as currently designed. In other words, the variation is from common causes inherent in the process. If any of the rules of detection for special cause variation (Fig. 38–4) apply, the process is unstable and out of control and needs our attention. In such a situation, removing special cause variation should be the first order of business in order to bring stability into the process.

Introduction to XmR Control Charts

The XmR control chart is a simple yet powerful statistical tool used to analyze data that emanate from a pro-

X Chart (observed data)

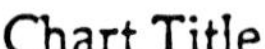

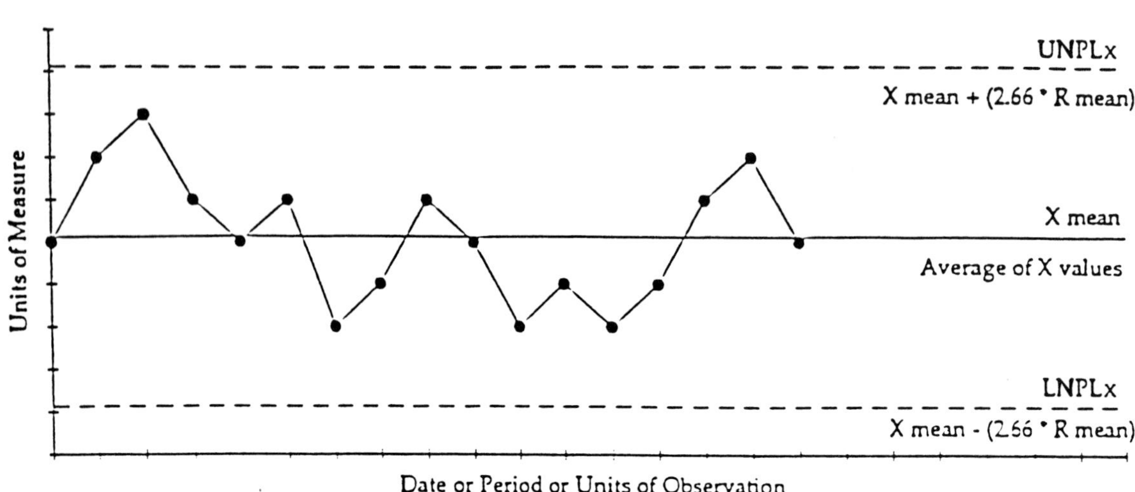

Date or Period or Units of Observation

Moving Range (mR) Chart

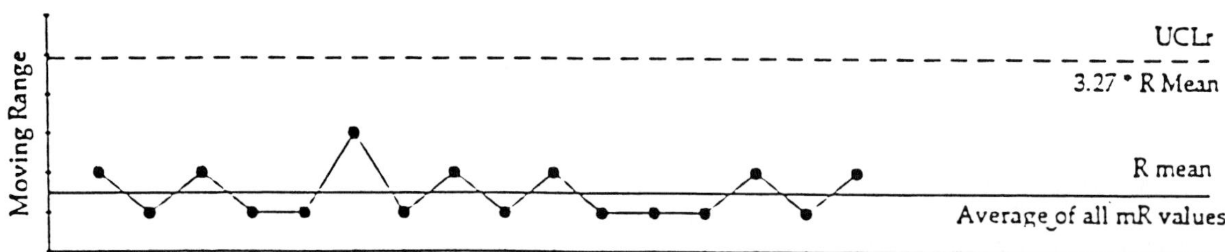

Date or Period or Unit of Observation

FIGURE **38–3.** The anatomy of an XmR control chart, $UNPL_x$, upper natural process for x; $LNPL_x$, lower natural process for x; UCL_r, upper control limit for the moving range; R mean, average of all the moving range values, X mean, average of all the x values.

cess over time. It can be used to monitor the effects of intentional process improvement efforts, to diagnose process performance, or to predict future process performance.

The XmR control chart consists of two time-series graphs. The top portion of the chart is referred to as the X chart, which contains the variable that is measured over time. These observed data points are referred to as the "*x*" values. The bottom portion of the chart is referred to as the moving range chart and contains the values which represent the difference from one *x* variable to the next. Such differences are referred to as the moving range or "*mR*" values. The limits for each chart are calculated from this simple set of data and when put together, the X and mR charts are called an XmR control chart.

Constructing an XmR Control Chart

1. The first step in constructing an XmR control chart is to enter the x values into the cells typically provided at the top of the chart. The time sequence of these values is critical for accurate interpretation of the data, so be sure that the data points are in historical time order (Step 1) (Fig. 38–5*A*).
2. The second step is to calculate the mR values, which are simply the difference from one successive x value to the next. It is important to note that the first cell in the moving range row will always be an empty cell. Thus, the moving range values will always contain one less data point than the x values (Step 2) (Fig. 38–5*B*).
3. The third step is to plot the x and mR values as data points onto the corresponding chart. At this point, the data are simply displayed in the form of trend charts (Step 3) (Fig. 38–5*C*).
4. The fourth step is to calculate the mean for the x and the mR values. To calculate the mean for the x values, add the x values together and divide by the total number of x values. The resulting value is the central line for the x values, also referred to as the CLx. To calculate the mean for the mR values, add the mR values together and divide by the total number of mR values. Remember, the total number of mR values that you divide by will be one data point less than the total

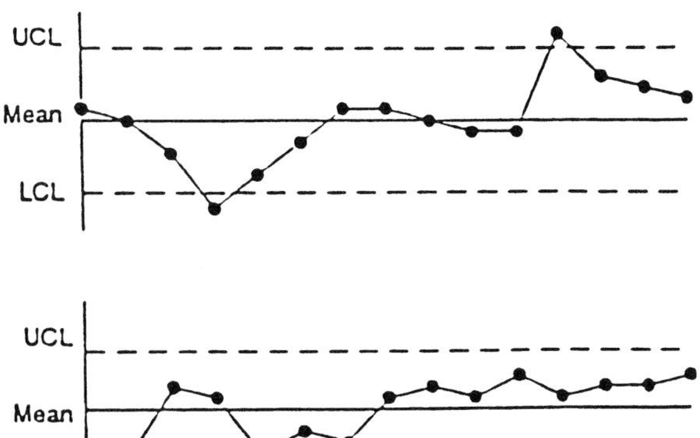

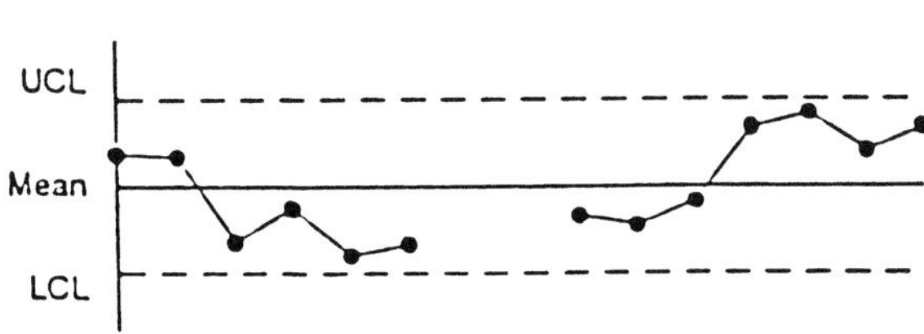

FIGURE **38–4.** The rules for detecting special cause variation on the x portion of an XmR control chart. *Top*, One or more points outside the control limits. *Middle*, Eight or more successive values on the same side of the central line. *Bottom*, Three of four consecutive points that are closer to one of the limits than to the central line.

number of x values. The result is the central line for the mR values, also referred to as the CLr. Draw the calculated means on the corresponding chart as a horizontal line and label accordingly, as either CLx or Clr (Step 4) (Fig. 38–5*D*).

5. The fifth step is to calculate the upper and lower natural process limits for the x values, referred to as UNPLx and LNPLx, respectively. To obtain the value for the UNPLx, simply add the product of 2.66 times the mean for the moving range (2.66 × CLr) to the mean of the x values (CLx). To obtain the value for the LNPLx, simply subtract the product of 2.66 times the mean for the moving range (2.66 × CLr) from the mean of the x values (CLx). Draw the calculated limit lines on the x chart as horizontal lines and label accordingly, as either UNPLx or LNPLx (Step 5) (Fig. 38–5*E*).
6. The sixth step is to calculate the upper control limit for the moving range, also referred to as the UCLr. This is calculated by multiplying the mean of the mR values (CLr) by a constant of 3.27 (3.27 × CLr). Draw the calculated value for the upper control limit as a horizontal line and label accordingly, as UCLr (Step 6) (Fig. 38–5*F*).
7. The seventh step is to analyze the data and evaluate the process performance.

As you begin to construct an XmR control chart, you start to observe the behavior of the data over time. Even without the central lines or limits, you can start to see that something is happening. The data begin to come alive. Once you add the central line, you should notice that the data has a central tendency around that line if the process is stable. You then add the limits to both charts. You should observe the data moving around the central line in a random fashion, visiting either side of the central line, moving slightly away from the center line, but not too far, and not spending too much time on one side of the line, such as eight in a row, or getting too close to the limits or certainly not migrating outside of one of the natural process limits.

Notice that when the difference from one successive x value to the next is excessive, the average variation for the moving range increases as a result of this excessive moving range value and the natural process limits widen, since the average moving range increases. However, if the difference from one successive x value to the next is small, the average moving range decreases and the natural process limits begin to narrow. To understand and interpret the XmR control chart and analyze the process being measured in more detail, you will need to understand the following four rules of detection (Fig. 38–6). When one of the four rules of detection come into play in an XmR control chart, the process has become unstable and is being subjected to special cause variation.

Interpreting the XmR Control Chart Using the Four Rules of Detection

The four rules of detection are used to identify signals within a process that are the result of some special cause and justify investigation on an economic basis. The first three rules apply to the X chart and the fourth applies to the mR chart.

When we observe one of the rules of detection occurring in a process, Shewhart teaches us that it makes economic sense to go in and understand why the process has become unstable. There is potential for us to improve the process and it is worth our while to understand what has contributed to the special cause variation and then fix it if necessary. Remember, too, that a special cause variation may also occur because we are trying to intentionally change the process. In fact, we may be looking to create special cause variation in a process as we seek to improve the process.

Separating Signals from Noise

Unlike the tabular form of presenting data, control charts allow us to filter out the noise so that we can identify and then interpret signals. The upper and lower limits for the individual x values are referred to as the natural process limits and serve to help us define the voice of the process. These limits also define the capability of the "current" process as long as the process is stable. The random variation that occurs within these limits can be described as the noise of the process, often referred to as common cause variation. A nonrandom pattern of the data or a data point that resides outside any of the limits (UNPLx, LNPLx, or UCLr) is interpreted as a signal, and often referred to as special cause variation. When this occurs, something in the process has changed and should be understood. Such a signal may be indicative

Hour	1	2	3	4	5	6	7	8	9	10	11	12	13	14	15	16	17	18	19	20	21	22	23	24
mm (x)	**44**	**44**	**44**	**43**	**45**	**44**	**44**	**43**	**44**	**33**	**44**	**31**	**45**	**29**	**46**	**32**	**46**	**34**	**29**	**26**	**21**	**23**	**24**	**18**
Moving Range																								

Millimeters (mm)
60
50
40
30
20
10
0
1 2 3 4 5 6 7 8 9 10 11 12 13 14 15 16 17 18 19 20 21 22 23 24
Hour

Moving Range (mR)
25
20
15
10
5
0
1 2 3 4 5 6 7 8 9 10 11 12 13 14 15 16 17 18 19 20 21 22 23 24

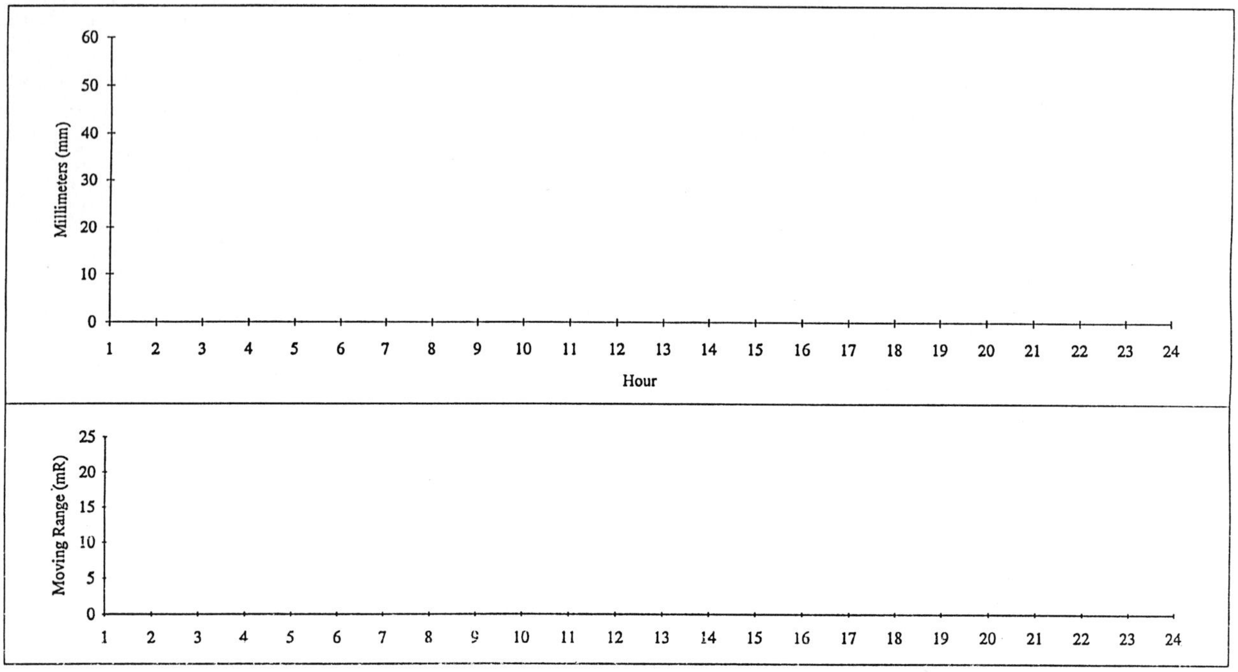

A

Hour	1	2	3	4	5	6	7	8	9	10	11	12	13	14	15	16	17	18	19	20	21	22	23	24
mm (x)	44	44	44	43	45	44	44	43	44	33	44	31	45	29	46	32	46	34	29	26	21	23	24	18
Moving Range		**0**	**0**	**1**	**2**	**1**	**0**	**1**	**1**	**11**	**11**	**13**	**14**	**16**	**17**	**14**	**14**	**12**	**5**	**3**	**5**	**2**	**1**	**6**

Moving Range = Difference between successive data values
E.g., value of data point 2 - value of data point 1 = 44 - 44 = 0

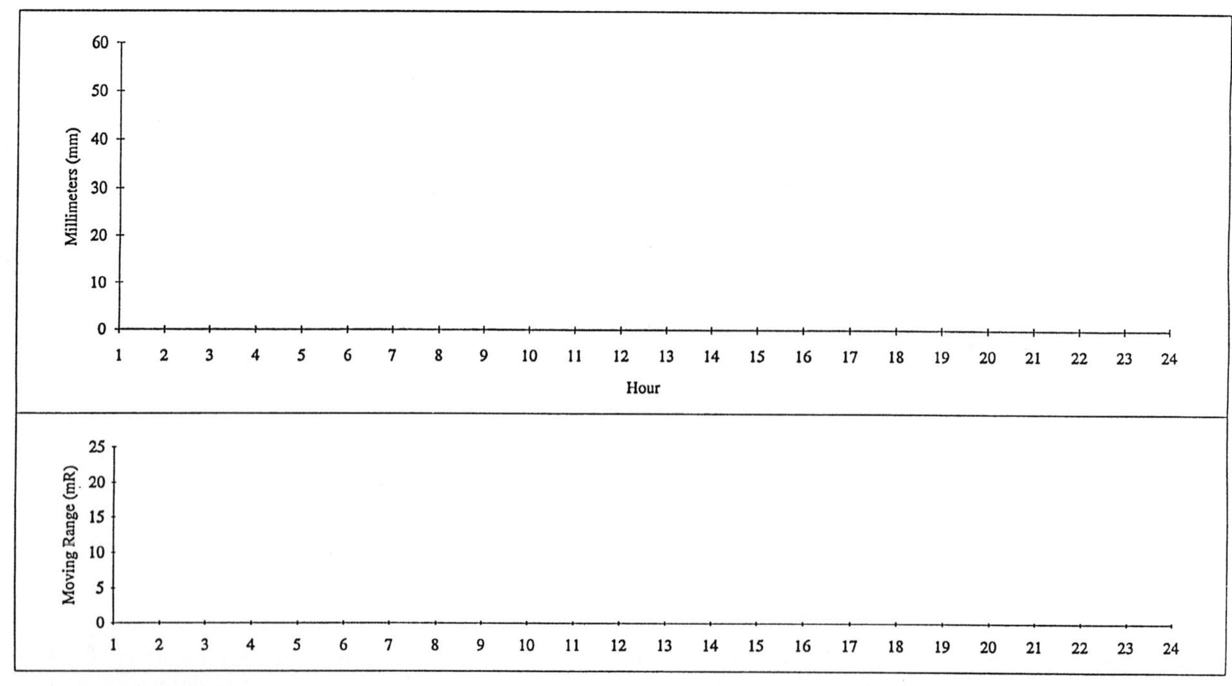

B

FIGURE **38–5.** *A*, Step 1: Enter x values. *B*, Step 2: Calculate mR values. *C*, Step 3: Plot x and mR values on chart. *D*, Step 4: Calculate mean for x and mR values. *E*, Step 5: Calculate $UNPL_x$ and $LNPL_x$. *F*, Step 6: Calculate UCL_r. *Illustration continued on opposite page*

Hour	1	2	3	4	5	6	7	8	9	10	11	12	13	14	15	16	17	18	19	20	21	22	23	24
mm (x)	44	44	44	43	45	44	44	43	44	33	44	31	45	29	46	32	46	34	29	26	21	23	24	18
Moving Range		0	0	1	2	1	0	1	1	11	11	13	14	16	17	14	14	12	5	3	5	2	1	6

Moving Range = Difference between successive data values = E.g., value of data point 2 - value of data point 1 = 44 - 44 = 0

Millimeters (mm)
Hour
Moving Range (mR)

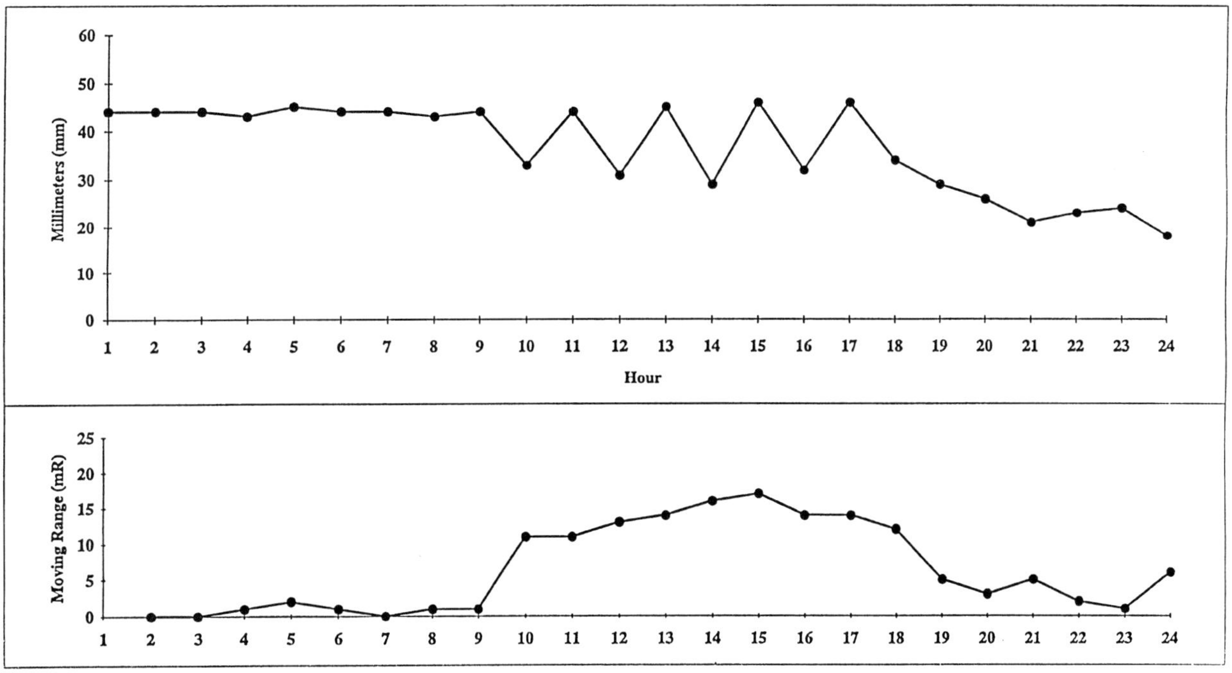

C

Hour	1	2	3	4	5	6	7	8	9	10	11	12	13	14	15	16	17	18	19	20	21	22	23	24
mm (x)	44	44	44	43	45	44	44	43	44	33	44	31	45	29	46	32	46	34	29	26	21	23	24	18
Moving Range		0	0	1	2	1	0	1	1	11	11	13	14	16	17	14	14	12	5	3	5	2	1	6

Moving Range = Difference between successive data values = E.g., value of data point 2 - value of data point 1 = 44 - 44 = 0

CLx = Mean x = Average of all x values = sum of all x values/number of values = 876 / 24 = 36.5

CLr = Mean r = Average of all mR values = sum of all mR values/number of values = 150 / 23 = 6.5

(note there is one less mR value than x values)

Millimeters (mm)
CLx
36.5
Hour
Moving Range (mR)
CLr
6.5

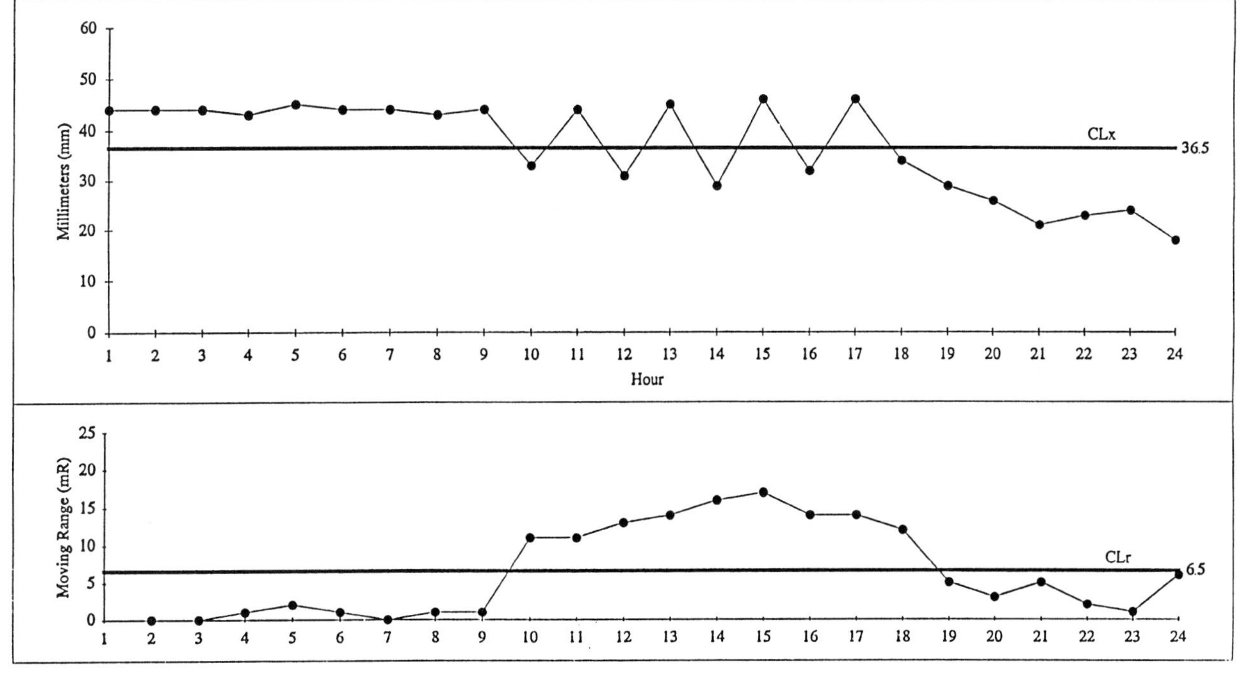

D

FIGURE **38–5.** *Continued on following page*

Hour	1	2	3	4	5	6	7	8	9	10	11	12	13	14	15	16	17	18	19	20	21	22	23	24
mm (x)	44	44	44	43	45	44	44	43	44	33	44	31	45	29	46	32	46	34	29	26	21	23	24	18
Moving Range		0	0	1	2	1	0	1	1	11	11	13	14	16	17	14	14	12	5	3	5	2	1	6

Moving Range = Difference between successive data values = E.g., value of data point 2 - value of data point 1 = 44 - 44 = 0

CLx = Mean x = Average of all x values = sum of all x values / number of values = 876 / 24 = 36.5

CLr = Mean r = Average of all mR values = sum of all mR values / number of values = 150 / 23 = 6.5 (note there is one less mR value than x values)

UNPLx = UCLx = CLx + (2.66 * CLr) = 36.5 + (2.66 * 6.5) = 53.8

LNPLx = LCLx = CLx - (2.66 * CLr) = 36.5 - (2.66 * 6.5) = 19.2

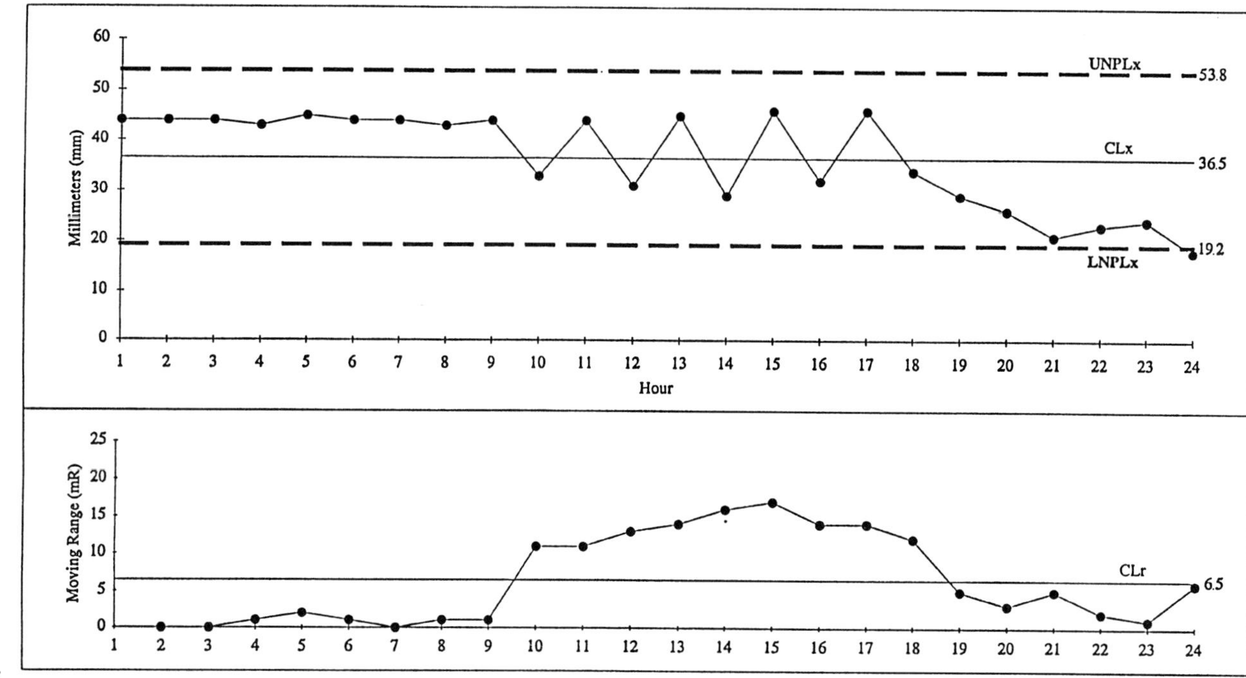

E

FIGURE **38–5.** *Continued on opposite page*

of a problem in the process that needs to be remedied, or it may be occurring as a result of a PDCA test of change that is moving the process in an improved and intended direction.

The Unstable Process

When we observe one or more signals occurring in a process using the rules of detection, we have special cause variation and, thereby, refer to it as an unstable process. As a result, the process is also unpredictable, since one can never be sure whether the next data point will be common cause or special cause variation. The first step that we need to take when observing an unstable process is to understand why it has become unstable and then work to bring it back into statistical control. Signals are opportunities crying out for improvement. But you must remember that special cause variation may also result because we are proactively trying to change a process. In fact, we may be looking to create special cause variation as evidence of improvement efforts, or perhaps even a breakthrough.

The Stable Process

When we do not observe special cause variation taking place in a process, but only random variation occurring within the limits and no rules of detection are being violated, we refer to this as a stable process. As a result, the process is predictable. It now becomes possible to predict the next data point by using the average variation (CLr) in the process and not allowing any of the rules of detection to occur. One can then conclude that the process is performing in the best manner that it can or behaving in the way it was designed. What it doesn't tell you is whether you are pleased with its performance. Is the amount of variation that is occurring in the process what you desire? Do you like where the process is centered? If not, the process may need a complete redesign effort.

Commonly Asked Questions About XmR Control Charts

1. *When do I have enough data points to construct my limits?* This is the most frequently asked question. It is particularly relevant when you are beginning to collect data prospectively and you would like to set the limits and then look for the introduction of special cause variation into the process you are measuring. If you read the manufacturing literature with regard to this issue, you will frequently hear the recommendation that once you have 20 data points you can

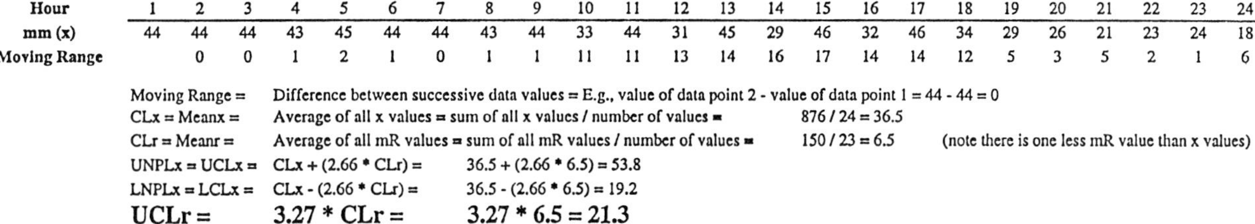

Hour	1	2	3	4	5	6	7	8	9	10	11	12	13	14	15	16	17	18	19	20	21	22	23	24
mm (x)	44	44	44	43	45	44	44	43	44	33	44	31	45	29	46	32	46	34	29	26	21	23	24	18
Moving Range		0	0	1	2	1	0	1	1	11	11	13	14	16	17	14	14	12	5	3	5	2	1	6

Moving Range = Difference between successive data values = E.g., value of data point 2 - value of data point 1 = 44 - 44 = 0
CLx = Meanx = Average of all x values = sum of all x values / number of values = 876 / 24 = 36.5
CLr = Meanr = Average of all mR values = sum of all mR values / number of values = 150 / 23 = 6.5 (note there is one less mR value than x values)
UNPLx = UCLx = CLx + (2.66 * CLr) = 36.5 + (2.66 * 6.5) = 53.8
LNPLx = LCLx = CLx - (2.66 * CLr) = 36.5 - (2.66 * 6.5) = 19.2
UCLr = 3.27 * CLr = 3.27 * 6.5 = 21.3

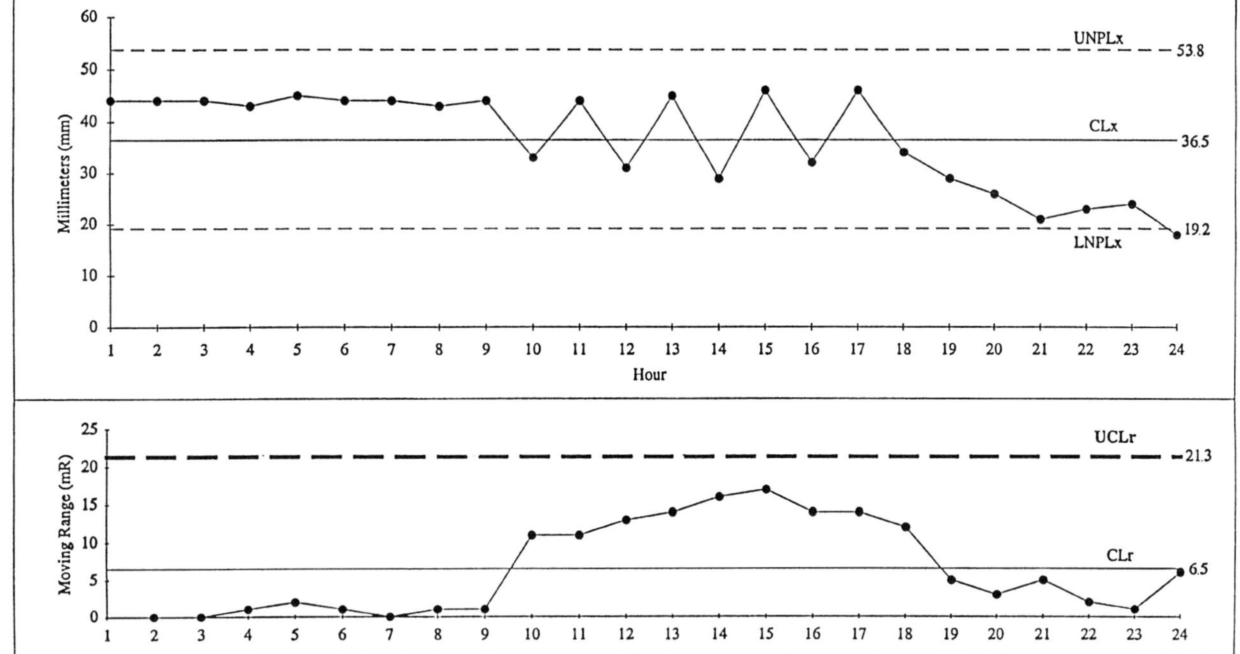

F

FIGURE **38–5.** *Continued*

calculate the limits. The service industry and, in particular, the health care industry, might be measuring monthly data or data from other time frequencies that make waiting for 20 data points impractical.

In general, it is fine to include each new data point in these instances into the calculation of the control limits. Thus, as each successive data point is added, simply recalculate the limits including the most recent data point. As you look at your developing XmR control chart, make a determination as you examine the data dispersion pattern over time whether the pattern is diverging or converging (Fig. 38–7). If the pattern is a nondiverging pattern, it is acceptable to hold the limits and continue to plot the data using those limits. Even if you use successive data points to calculate revised limits at each point, special cause variation will still remain detectable.

In health care, sometimes it is helpful to redesign your data collection method. For instance, if you are measuring monthly days/1,000 in managed care, the monthly measure may not be adequate enough for process improvement. A redesign of this process might result in implementing a daily inpatient census process. The daily census becomes a proxy measure for inpatient days/1,000. Now you have daily data points and a more valuable database to lead CQI efforts around inpatient care.

2. *When should I make a break in the process and recalculate control limits?* In general, it is best to let the data dictate that the process has changed because of an occurrence of one of the rules of detection. However, it is important to understand why the signal has occurred before recalculating new limits. If a PDCA improvement effort is driving the onset of a new process, then a break should be made once the result of the improvement effort has produced the demonstrable presence of a new process, as evidenced by the presence of one of the rules of detection occurring on the control chart.

If special cause variation occurs that is due to an unintended activity, then the limits do not need to be revised. However, you may want to remove the out-of-control point from your limit calculations. An example would be the measurement of daily emergency room visits. Suddenly, a severe hurricane hits and emergency room visits increase 20-fold for 1 day. There is no need to revise the limits in this situation, but excluding the "hurricane day" would be advisable. It is most important that you expend energy in understanding the cause of the special cause variation and not dwell on revising limits.

Remember that once you make a process break on a control chart, you will lose the signal or rule of detection that caused you to make a process break.

Rule One: One or more data points reside above the upper natural process limit (UNPLx) or below the lower natural process limit (LNPLx).

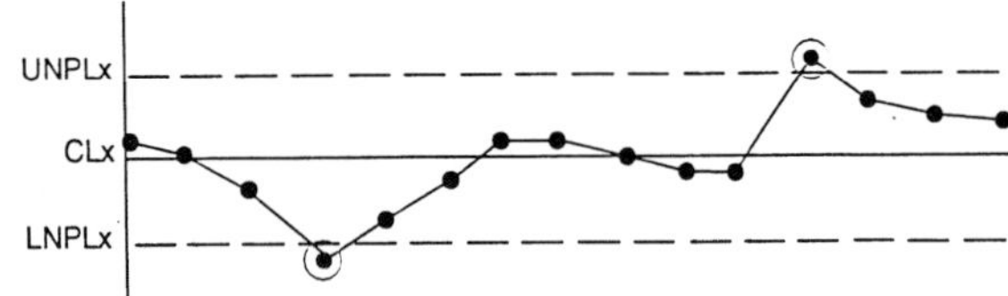

Rule Two: Eight or more successive data points reside on the same side of the central line (Clx).

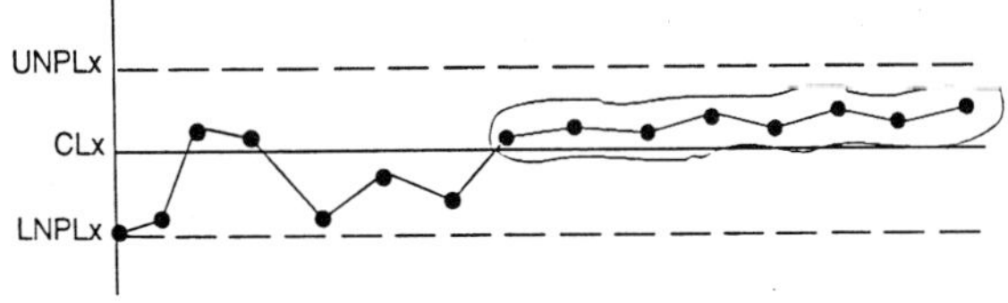

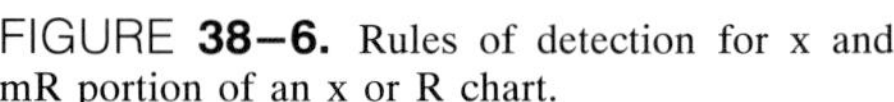
FIGURE **38–6.** Rules of detection for x and mR portion of an x or R chart.

Rule Three: Three out of four consecutive data points reside closer to one of the natural process limits (UNPLx or LNPLx) than to the central line (CLx). The midway lines can help you apply this rule.

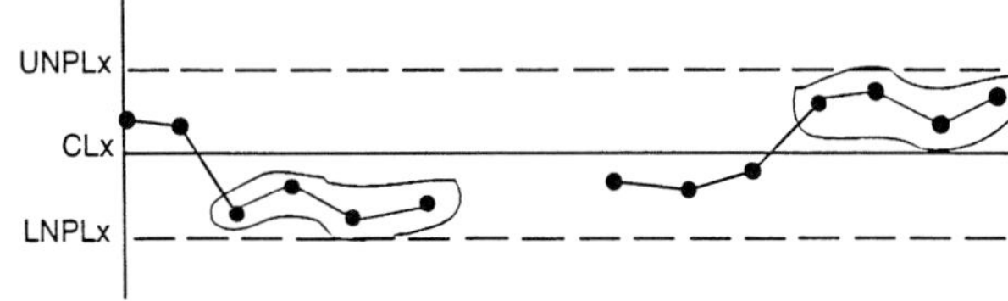

Rule Four: One or more data points reside above the upper control limit for the moving range (UCLr).

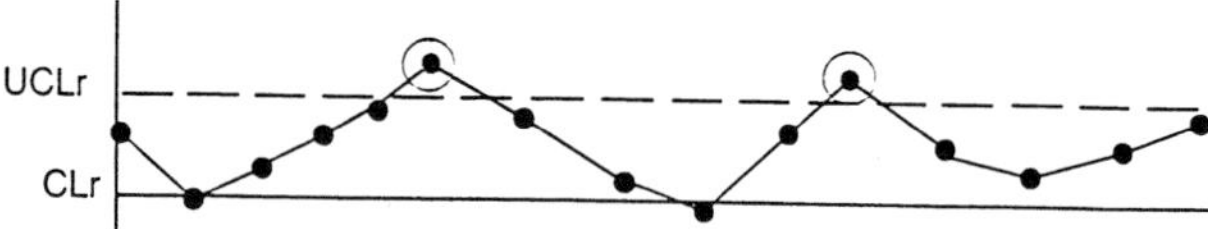

Be sure to make notes on the control chart to indicate the reason for the recalculation of limits.

3. *Should I be using XmR control charts since I am a front-line health care worker or should I leave it to management?* The XmR control chart is simple to use and its value is enhanced in an organization where those closest to the process are using the charts. Shewhart intended the control chart for front-line people. Owning the process that you work in is the ultimate in empowerment for you.
4. *Are there control charts other than XmRs?* Yes, there are many other types of control charts; however, the XmR control chart is widely applicable for health care. It will answer most of your needs; the other types of control charts are more applicable to the manufacturing industry where they were developed.

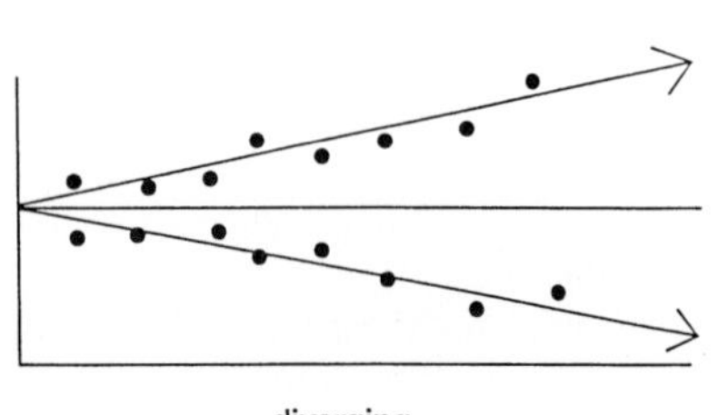

converging

FIGURE **38–7.** Diverging and converging patterns.

The XmR control chart is particularly useful for health care measures.

Outcome Studies in Anesthesia

Historically, studies of anesthetic outcome have used three primary designs. The study may be epidemiologic, measuring the prevalence of a specific outcome in a patient population, such as the studies by Beecher and Todd or Tiret.[16,17] Studies may be based on a collection of cases with adverse outcomes (e.g., "closed-claims" analysis), such as those by Eichhorn et al. and the American Society of Anesthesiologists.[18,19] Finally, the frequency of some critical or "sentinel" event may be reported. All of these study designs have limitations, but practical considerations dictate that most prospective studies be performed within these limitations.

The problem of determining the "efficacy" versus the "effectiveness" of anesthetic procedures must be addressed in studies of anesthetic outcome. Efficacy has been defined as the outcome resulting from application of specific medical technology to a well-defined population under ideal conditions. Effectiveness refers to the outcome resulting from application of this medical technology to the general patient population by average practitioners.[20] Studies of efficacy are the most common means of evaluating new procedures or technologies, whereas information relating to effectiveness is more relevant to patients, practitioners, and third-party payers.

Outcome studies must study large patient populations (provide sufficient statistical "power") in order to draw valid conclusions in regard to outcomes which have a relatively rare incidence. One group of investigators studying the effect of anesthetic agents on perioperative outcomes, including myocardial infarction and death, included 17,201 patients in their study and noted that due to the relative safety of anesthetic care, more than 1 million patients would need to be studied in a similar fashion to demonstrate a 50% reduction in death rate.[21] Outcome studies must also integrate the multiple variables that affect patient outcome, analyze outcome longitudinally over time, and precisely define outcome indices, some of which may be qualitative and difficult to measure.

Let's briefly discuss examples of outcome studies that have been performed in the areas of cardiac, vascular, and thoracic anesthesia and indicate some new directions for future study.

Cardiac Anesthesia

A number of large, prospective studies of anesthetic technique and outcome in coronary artery bypass patients have been performed. Fewer studies relating to anesthetic technique have been performed in patients undergoing valvular surgery, patients requiring repeat cardiac surgery, or patients undergoing repair of congenital cardiac defects because it is difficult to study adequate numbers of similar patients in these categories, whereas it is easier to study adequate numbers of patients who are to undergo primary coronary artery bypass. Slogoff and Keats found no significant difference in incidence of intraoperative ischemia, perioperative myocardial infarction, or mortality in over 1,000 patients randomized to enflurane, isoflurane, halothane, or sufentanil as primary anesthetics.[22] Tuman et al. reported on over 1,000 patients receiving fentanyl, sufentanil, diazepam and ketamine, or halothane as primary anesthetics.[23] No difference was found in incidence of perioperative myocardial infarction, low cardiac output state, arrhythmias, or mortality. Inoue et al. did find a significantly higher incidence of myocardial infarction, need for inotropic support (an intermediate outcome), and in-hospital mortality in patients receiving isoflurane versus those receiving enflurane.[24] This study, however, has been criticized, as it contained a significant number of patients who received no cardioplegia and thus may have had inadequate myocardial protection, patients received much lower doses of narcotic agents to supplement the volatile anesthetics, and the investigators did not report hemodynamic variables. Multiple factors undoubtedly determine outcome following coronary artery bypass, and anesthetic technique is merely one of these factors. Evidence that anesthetic technique does have an impact on outcome is provided by the finding of Slogoff and Keats that tachycardia, hypertension, and intraoperative ischemia was much more common in patients anesthetized by a specific anesthesiologist participating in a further study.[25] This finding is supported by the work of Merry et al., who found that the incidence of postoperative myocardial damage as indicated by enzyme assay on postoperative day 1 was related to the anesthesiologist caring for the patient.[26] Bypass time, coronary anatomy, coexisting disease, preoperative medical regimen, and many other factors may be significant determinants of outcome in coronary artery surgery patients. Study design incorporating multivariate analysis of patient and anesthetic variables similar to Goldman et al. and the Coronary Artery Surgery Study (CASS) may allow more precise prediction of the relationship of anesthetic care to outcome in coronary surgery patients.[27,28] Knowledge that clinical anesthetic care influences outcome in these patients is not enough: we must understand the specific aspects of this care that affect outcome in order to improve overall anesthetic care.

The Cooperative Cardiovascular Project of the HCFA may further define patient, surgical, and anesthetic variables that significantly affect outcome in coronary surgery patients and allow improved outcome prediction and allocation of resources.[29] Nevertheless, the applicability of these data to anesthetic care will need to be analyzed before practice changes are recommended. Further assessment of the impact on patient outcome of invasive hemodynamic monitoring, transesophageal echocardiography, and diverse anesthetic techniques on coronary artery bypass and other types of cardiac surgery, such as valvular repair or replacement needs to be performed to better define the proper application of costly technologies in these patient groups. Furthermore, studies need to address other areas of cardiac anesthetic practice such as transfusion guidelines, optimal use of antifibrinolytic and other agents used to reduce bleeding, optimum flow and blood pressure on bypass, early extubation techniques, and many other areas. However, due to the limited numbers of comparable patients in these populations, probably only larger, multicenter study designs will provide the statistical power necessary to draw meaningful conclusions relating to anesthetic techniques. These studies must, however, control for differences in results between institutions. An example of one such study is discussed later in this chapter.

Vascular Anesthesia

Alternative anesthetic choices are available and widely used in patients undergoing vascular surgery. For example, major vascular surgery can be performed during general anesthesia alone, or combined regional and general anesthesia, with the regional anesthetic potentially continued into the postoperative period. Peripheral vascular surgery can be performed during either regional or general anesthesia. It has been proposed that combined regional-general anesthesia for patients undergoing abdominal aortic surgery results in a more stable intraoperative course and lower morbidity postoperatively.[30] The precise mechanism of this difference has not been elucidated. This study has been criticized for its relatively small sample size and high rates of some complications relative to other reported series. The safety of placing epidural catheters in vascular surgical patients, many of whom are anticoagulated or develop a coagulopathy intraoperatively, was examined by Rao et al., who found no instances of permanent neurologic damage related to the epidural catheters in over 4,000 patients.[31] In peripheral vascular surgery, regional anesthesia does appear to offer advantages in minimizing early morbidity, specifically, a reduced incidence of graft occlusion.[32,33] As the accompanying editorial pointed out, further questions remain that will require larger study groups to provide sufficient statistical power to determine whether cardiac and pulmonary morbidity is affected by anesthetic technique in these patients.[34] In thoracic aortic surgery, cerebral spinal fluid drainage via a lumbar intrathecal catheter has been proposed as a means to decrease postoperative incidence of paraplegia by increasing the spinal cord perfusion pressure. A recent study of this technique did not support this hypothesis.[35] Baron et al. have examined the use of regional versus general anesthesia in peripheral vascular surgery, with varying results in terms of effects on coagulation and morbidity and mortality.[36] As in cardiac anesthesia, studies of anesthesia outcome in this patient population are ongoing, and may better define optimal anesthetic technique for these patients.

Thoracic Anesthesia

Anesthetic practice for thoracic surgery has evolved over the past two decades, with increasing use of invasive and noninvasive monitoring, selective ventilation, various positive-pressure ventilation modes, and ICU monitoring.[37] Studies have examined relative morbidity related to options for single-lung ventilation such as selective intubation, double-lumen endotracheal tubes, and various types of bronchial blockers. Recent editorials have highlighted the fact that the "best" method of providing single-lung ventilation is yet to be determined, and, indeed, that there may be no one best method of providing one-lung ventilation in all patients.[38,39] Postoperative analgesia in patients who have undergone thoracotomy can be provided by intravenous or epidural opioids, either continuously or intermittently. There is evidence of some decrease in the hormonal response to surgery with continuous epidural fentanyl relative to continuous intravenous fentanyl.[40] The optimal method of providing postoperative analgesia in these patients is yet to be defined.

Continuous Quality Improvement in Cardiothoracic Anesthesia

With an understanding of the principles of continuous quality improvement and the techniques of statistical process control it is easy to understand the difference between anesthesia outcome activity and the more comprehensive nature of quality improvement. Continuous quality improvement aims to improve clinical processes that transcend one clinical specialty. Lowering patient mortality may be an overall aim of improvement work, but to accomplish improvement requires a complex team approach that takes into account many participants in the patient's care.

A good example of continuous quality improvement in cardiothoracic surgery and anesthesia is the Northern New England Cardiovascular Disease Study Group (NNECVDSG).

The Northern New England Cardiovascular Disease Study Group

In 1987 a consortium called the NNECVDSG was formed for the purpose of providing information pertaining to the management of cardiovascular disease in the northern New England states of New Hampshire, Maine, and Vermont. Multiple institutions joined together on a voluntary basis to work on improving medical and surgical care for the cardiac surgical patient.

Cardiothoracic surgeons, interventional cardiologists, anesthesiologists, scientists, and administrators from five medical centers agreed to work together to "improve continuously the quality, safety, effectiveness and cost of medical interventions in cardiovascular disease."[41] This group has demonstrated the need to assemble multidisciplinary teams in order to continuously improve the clinical aspects of health care. Cardiac anesthesiologists were key members of this group and had they decided to work alone on improvement work they would have accomplished very little. The complexities of caring for cardiothoracic or vascular surgery patients obviate this team approach.

Improving Hospital Mortality Rate for CABG

The NNECVDSG studied the effectiveness of using CQI in a regional cardiac care model. Three interventions were used to improve mortality rates:

1. Feedback of outcome data—each cardiac surgeon received three outcome reports, their own data, their medical center data, and the regional outcomes data.
2. CQI training—training sessions were conducted for the group about the thinking and tools of CQI.
3. Site visits—teams made site visits to review the entire CABG system (from cardiac catheterization to postoperative care). The processes at each site were defined and then they were shared amongst the various sites.

After instituting the above interventions, 6,488 patients underwent CABG surgery. The mortality rate dropped 24% as a result of these interventions (Fig. 38–8). Some of the changes made in clinical care included:

- Changed to a dedicated OR staff for the cardiac surgery program
- Implemented an informal internal review of all deaths with cardiologist, cardiac surgeons, nurses, perfusionists, and anesthesiologists participating
- Switched from cold to warm cardioplegia
- Implemented a shorter time for extubation protocol
- Adopted a reduced flow technique when hypotension is needed rather than turning the pump off
- Instituted a same-day admission program

The cardiac anesthesiologists had a direct role in many of these interventions. In particular, CQI efforts to decrease intubation time post-CABG can contribute to reducing overall length of stay for the procedure.

CQI in the Post-CABG ICU Patient

Institution of a protocol that moved away from the practice of administering very-high-dose narcotic for CABG surgery has resulted in more rapid extubation in the ICU. In Figure 38–9, the first improvement in intubation time was the result of such an intervention. As a result of the opiate dosing reduction intervention, a significant process improvement occurred resulting in the first process break in Figure 38–9. The second improvement inter-

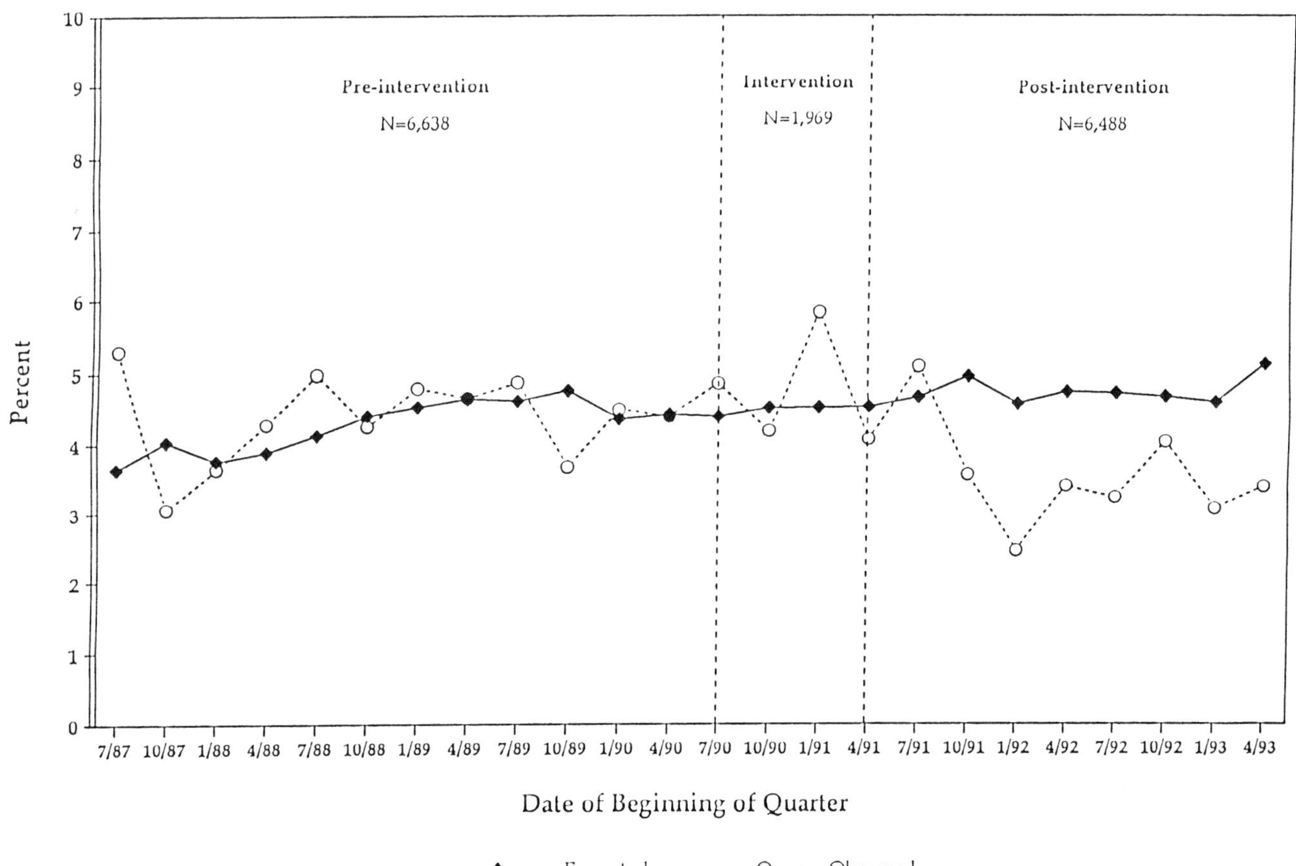

FIGURE **38–8.** Expected/observed mortality post CABG, all patients (n = 15,095). (Courtesy of S. Plume NNECVDS6.)

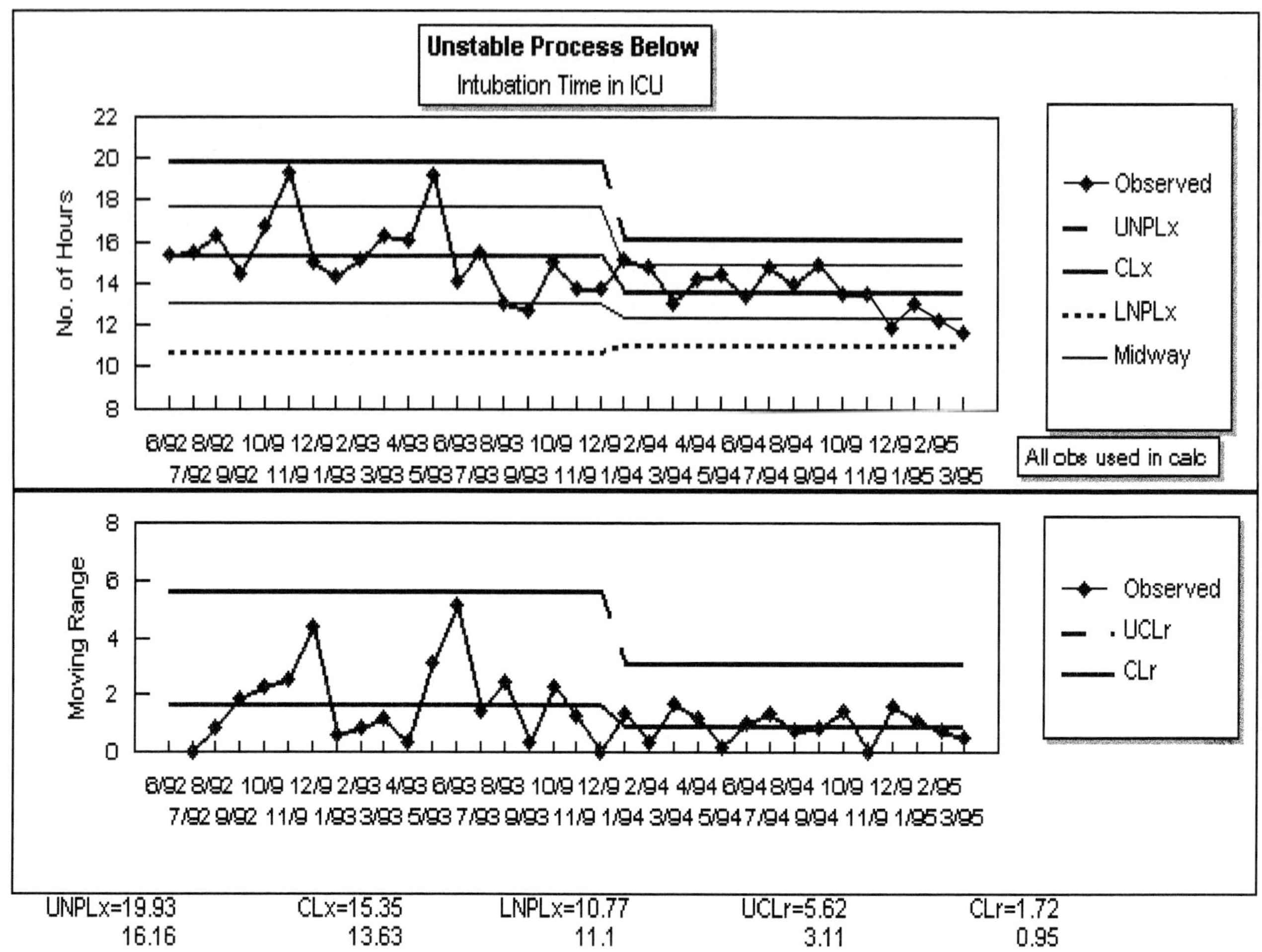

FIGURE **38–9.** Post-CABG intubation time in the ICU. Opiate dosing reduction started 1/94.

vention was implemented by the respiratory therapists and consisted of more frequent suctioning of the endotracheal tube and instituting a strict protocol related to changing the patient's position from partial right or left chest-up and supine position. As a result of this second intervention, average monthly intubation time in the ICU post-CABG is further reduced.

Earlier extubation improvement work has contributed to an overall reduction in average length of stay for CABG surgery. In Figure 38–10, the postoperative length of stay has had two significant improvement reductions from 8.64 days to 6.64 days. In addition, the percentage of CABG patients discharged in less than five days has increased from 30% to 50% (Fig. 38–11).

While anesthesiologists certainly contributed directly to these achievements, it was the work of a multidisciplinary team that made it happen and will be responsible for holding the gains. Unless process changes are maintained and continually improved, all of the gains will be lost. It is always possible that the results of a CQI effort can be reversed if an unexpected source of variation enters the improved process. If efforts are appropriately directed towards continual improvement, any such variation should be detected early on and managed accordingly.

Sternal Complication Improvement Project

After median sternotomy for CABG surgery, there is a risk of such sternal complications as sternal infection or sternal dehiscence. A high rate of sternal complications could be the stimulus for the formation of a clinical quality improvement team aimed at reducing sternal complications. Such was the case at a cardiac surgical service in the southern United States.

In Figure 38–12 there are high quarterly complication rates in October 1993 of 4.0% and in October 1994 of 5.1%. A quality improvement team included OR nurses, infectious disease specialists, surgeons, and anesthesiologists. The anesthesiologists' contribution centered on the timing of antibiotic administration management before and after bypass. Providing adequate antibiotic blood levels before sternotomy and appropriate redosing during and after bypass were important interventions to reduce sternal complications.

For the last six months, the average complication rate is 0.86%. Using a control chart to track the quarterly complication rate, this team is hoping to produce special cause variation indicating the effectiveness of their quality improvement interventions.

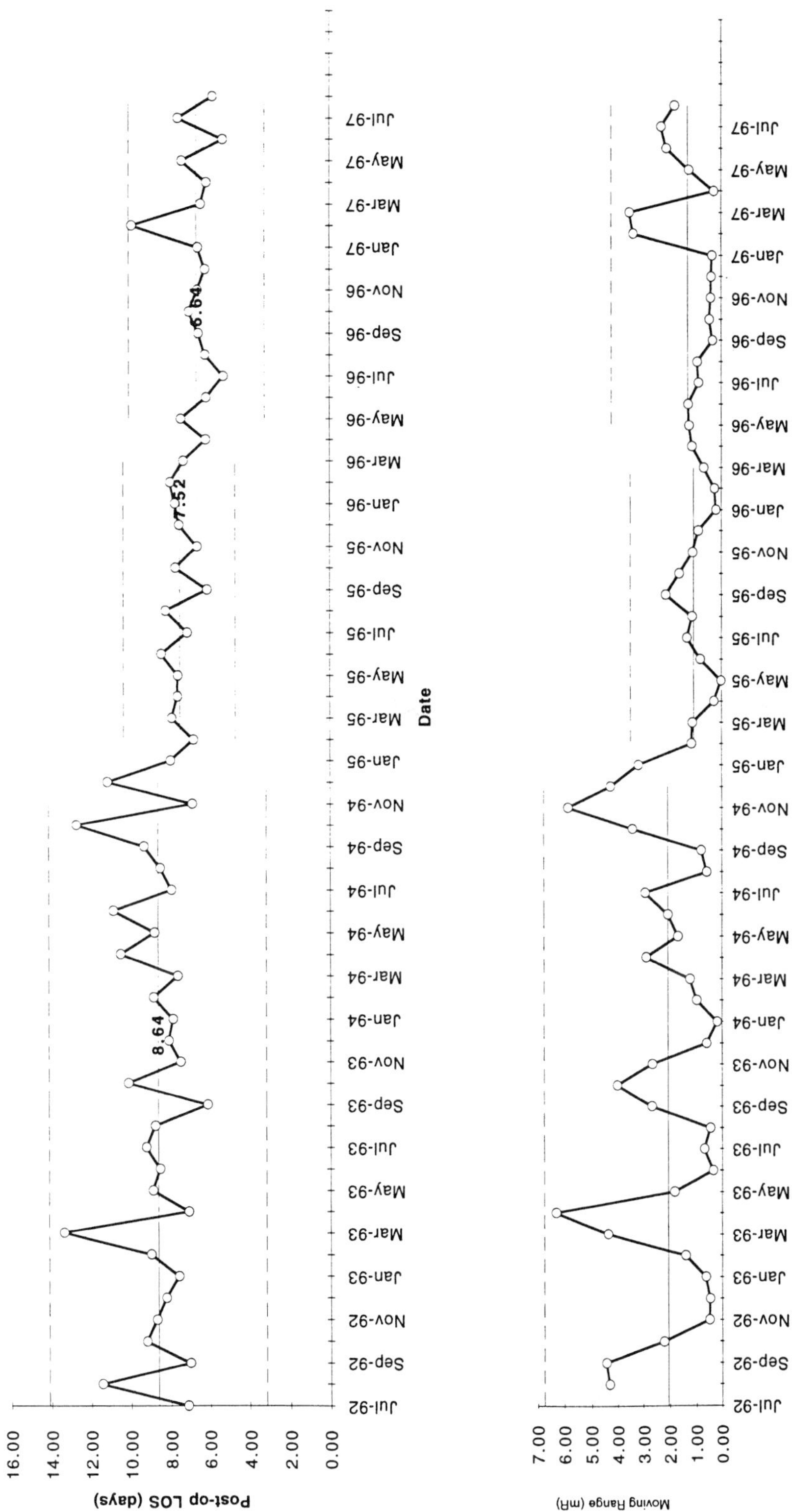

Control limits calculated on first 20 points, recalculated 2x due to 8 points in a row below central line

FIGURE 38–10. Postoperative LOS (mean) for all isolated CABG procedures. (Courtesy of S. Plume.)

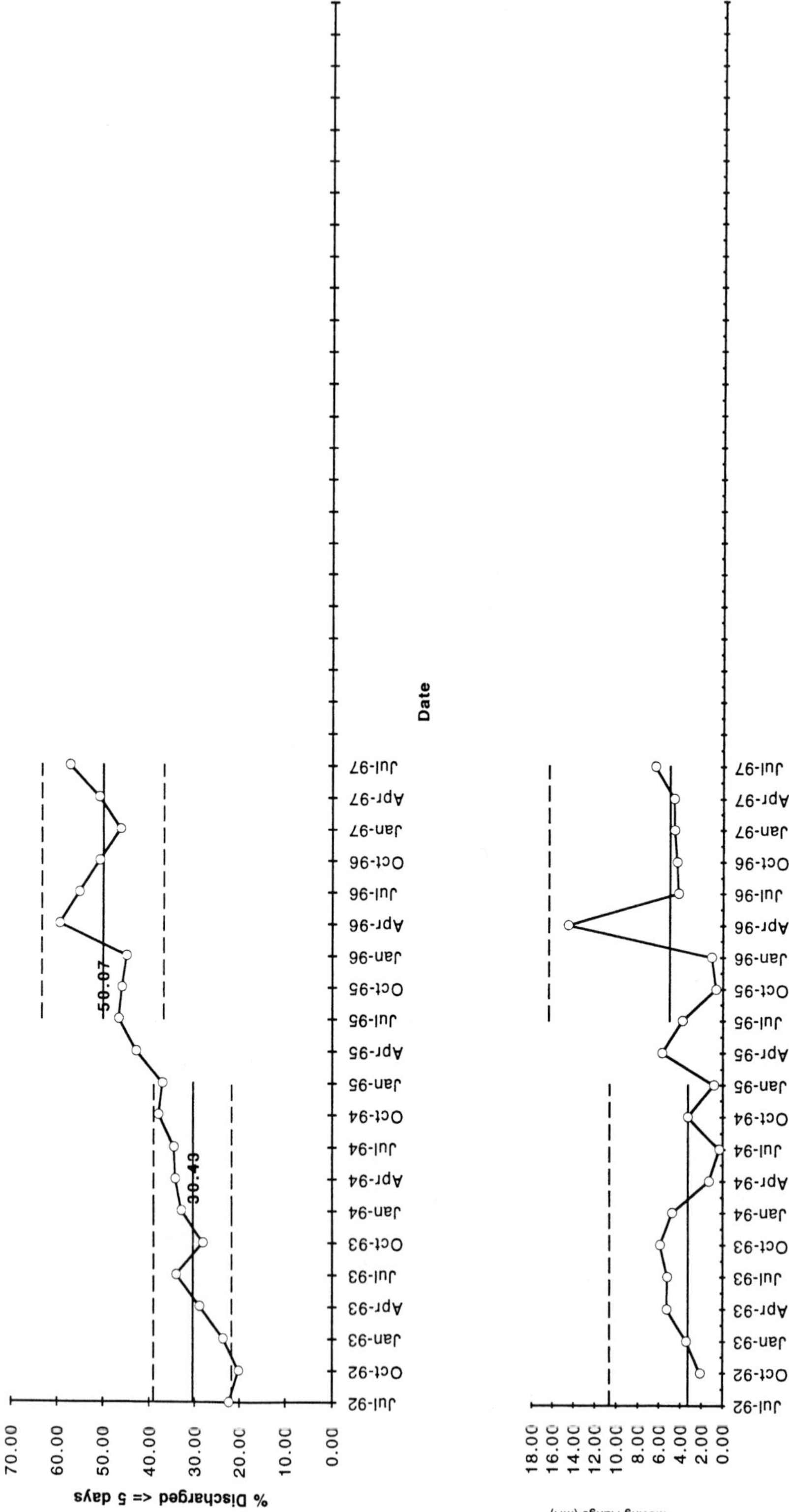

Control limits calculated on first 20 points, reduced to 11 and recalculated because of points > UCL

FIGURE 38–11. Discharges ≤5 days for isolated CABG procedures. (Courtesy of S. Plume.)

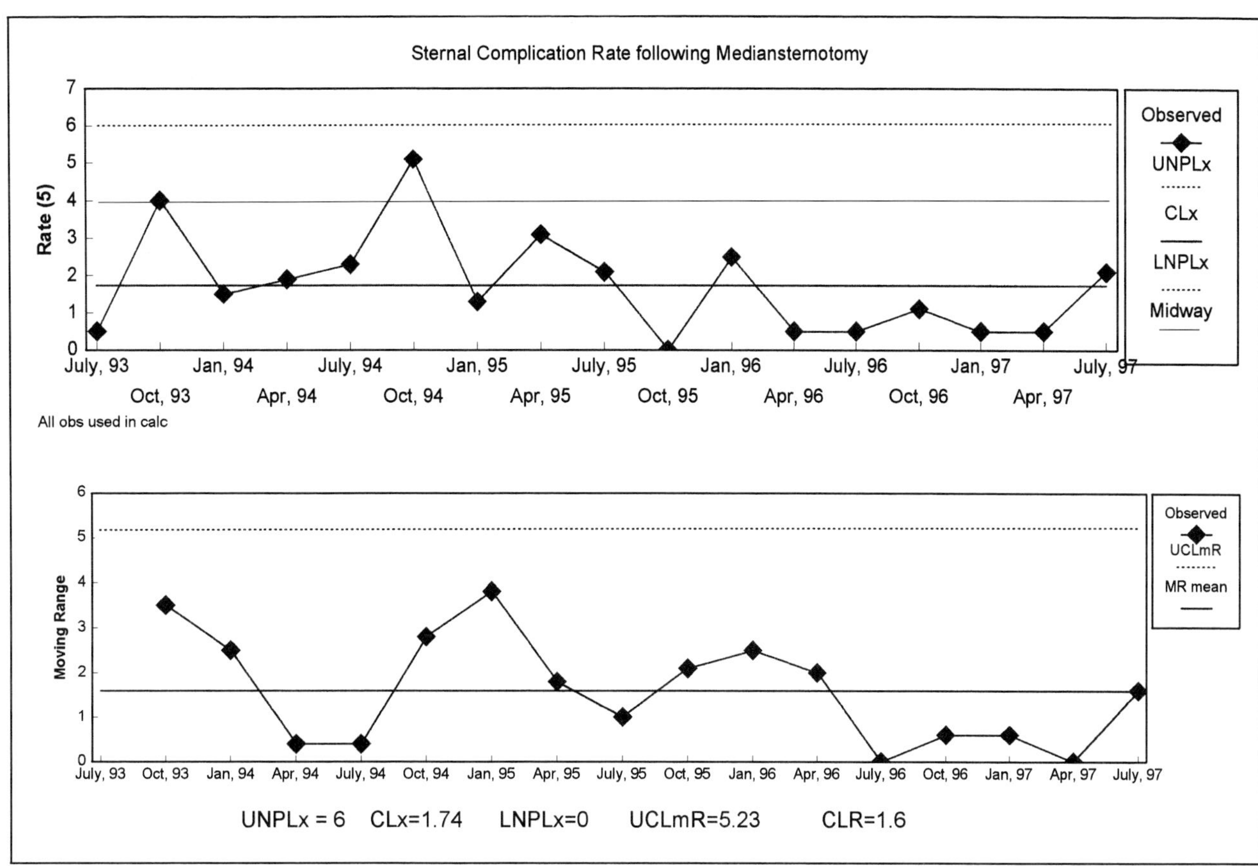

FIGURE **38–12.** Sternal complication rate following median sternotomy.

Re-exploration for Bleeding Improvement Project

After successfully completing CABG surgery, it is frustrating to return to the OR due to excessive postoperative bleeding. Maintaining a low re-exploration rate is a measure of the quality of care. The reasons for excessive bleeding after CABG surgery are numerous. Inadequate heparin reversal, prolonged bypass time, and surgical technique are only a few of the possible causes.

At one cardiac surgical center they were tracking quarterly re-exploration rates and after looking at their rates, they formed a quality improvement team to reduce the rate of this complication. In Figure 38–13 the April 1994 re-exploration rate of 6.5% was the final impetus to change.

Once quality improvement efforts were put in place in July 1994, the overall re-exploration rate was decreased by 27%. In addition, as depicted in Figure 38–12, the quarter-to-quarter variation of re-exploration rates has been minimized as seen on the lower moving range portion of this control chart. The interventions were multiple, including a protocol for the optimal use of antifibrinolytic agents.

Summary

Much of the current outcomes research in cardiothoracic and vascular anesthesia has focused on improving care within the anesthetic process. More improvement work needs to be done by multidisciplinary teams collaborating to improve the more global care of cardiothoracic and vascular patients. In this chapter, the thinking and tools of continuous quality improvement have been presented to stimulate the continuation of ongoing efforts to improve the care of surgical patients. Anesthesiologists are involved in the most important component of the critical pathway—the intraoperative process. Because of our significant role in the operating room, we are positioned to lead and improve the intraoperative process and thereby contribute to the overall care of the patient's total hospital experience.

The most important word in the phrase continuous quality improvement is "continuous." Improving clinical care should be a never-ending activity. By continually measuring the process outcomes, opportunities to implement new interventions aimed to further improve the care process will be evident. Ultimately, our patients

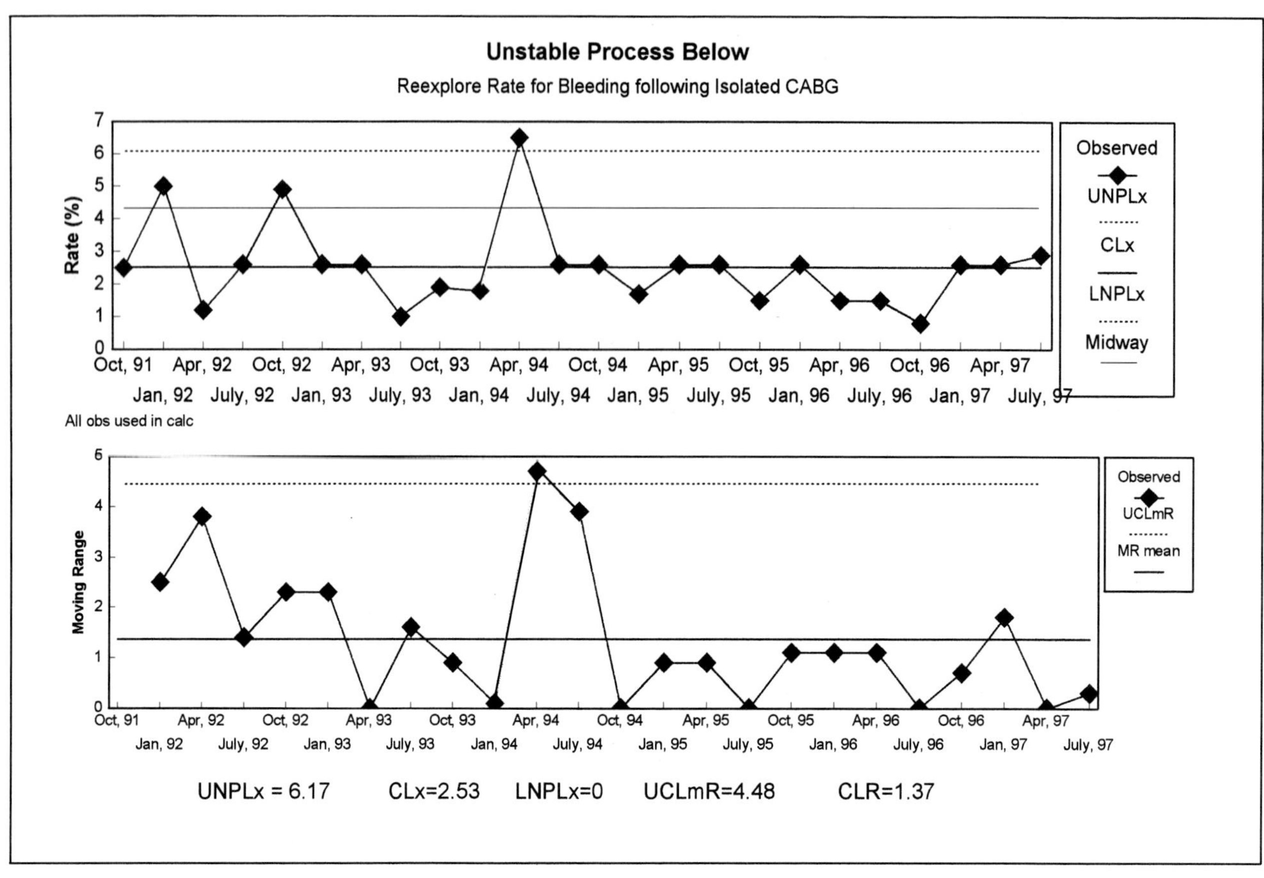

FIGURE **38–13.** Re-explore rate for bleeding following isolated CABG.

will benefit from our dedication to the continuous improvement of clinical quality.

References

1. Lanier WM, Warner MS: New frontiers in anesthesia research: Assessing the impact of practice patterns on outcome, health care deliver, and cost. Anesthesiology 78:1001, 1993.
2. Wheeler DJ: Advanced Topics in Statistical Process Control. Knoxville, SPC Press, 1995.
3. Deming WE: Out of the Crisis. Cambridge, MIT CAES Press, 1986.
4. Scherkenbach WW: The Deming Route to Quality and Productivity. Milwaukee, ASQC Quality Press, 1986.
5. Rosander AC: Deming's 14 Points Applied to Services. Milwaukee, ASQC Quality Press, 1991.
6. Deming WE: The New Economics for Industry, Education, Government. Cambridge, MIT CAES Press, 1993.
7. Langley GJ, Nolan KM, Nolan TW: The Foundation of Improvement. Quality Progress 81–86, 1994.
8. Goran MJ, Roberts JS, Kellogg M, et al: The PSRO hospital review system. Med Care 13(Suppl 4):1, 1975.
9. Goldman RL: The reliability of peer assessments of quality of care. JAMA 267:958, 1992.
10. Caplan RA, Posner KL, Cheney FW: Effects of outcome on physician judgments of appropriateness of care. JAMA 265:1957, 1991.
11. Lomas J, Anderson GM, Dommick-Pierre K, et al: Do practice guidelines guide practice? The effect of a consensus statement on the practice of physicians. N Engl J Med 321:1306, 1989.
12. Schroeder SA, Kabcenell AI: Do bad outcomes mean substandard care? JAMA 265:1995, 1991.
13. Serge PM: The Fifth Discipline. Doubleday Currency, New York, 1990.
14. Wheeler DJ, Chambers DS: Understanding Statistical Process Control. Knoxville, SPC Press, 1986.
15. Wheeler DJ: Understanding Variation. Knoxville, SPC Press, 1993.
16. Beecher HK, Todd DP: A study of the deaths associated with anesthesia based on a study of 599,548 anesthesias in ten institutions, 1948–1952, inclusive. Ann Surg 140:2, 1954.
17. Tiret L, Desmonts JM, Hatton F, Vourc'h G: Complications associated with anaesthesia: A prospective survey in France. Can Anaesth Soc J 33:336, 1986.
18. Eichhorn JH: Prevention of intraoperative anesthesia accidents and related severe injuries through safety monitoring. Anesthesiology 70:572, 1989.
19. Caplan RA, Posner K, Ward RJ, Cheney FW: Adverse respiratory events in anesthesia: A closed claims analysis. Anesthesiology 72:828, 1990.
20. Brook RH, Lohr KN: Efficacy, effectiveness, variations, and quality: Boundary-crossing research. Med Care 23:710, 1985.
21. Forrest JB, Cahalan MK, Rehder K, et al: Multicenter study of general anesthesia. II. Results. Anesthesiology 72:262, 1990.
22. Slogoff S, Keats AS: Randomized trial of primary anesthetic agents on outcome of coronary artery bypass operations. Anesthesiology 70:179, 1989.
23. Tuman KJ, McCarthy RJ, Spiess BD, et al: Does choice of anesthetic agent significantly affect outcome after coronary artery surgery? Anesthesiology 70:189, 1989.
24. Inoue K, Reichelt W, El-Banayosy A, et al: Does isoflurane lead to a higher incidence of myocardial infarction and perioperative

death than enflurane in coronary artery surgery? Anesth Analg 71: 469, 1990.
25. Slogoff S, Keats AS: Further observations on perioperative myocardial ischemia. Anesthesiology 65:539, 1986.
26. Merry AF, Ramage MC, Whitlock RML, et al: First-time coronary artery bypass grafting: The anaesthetist as a risk factor. Br J Anaesth 68:6, 1992.
27. Goldman L, Caldera D, Nussbaum SR, et al: Multifactorial index of cardiac risk in non cardiac surgical procedures. N Engl J Med 197:845, 1977.
28. CASS principal investigators and their associates: Coronary artery surgery study (CASS): A randomized trial of coronary artery bypass surgery; survival data. Circulation 68:939, 1983.
29. Jencks SF, Wilensky GR: The health care quality improvement initiative: A new approach to quality assurance in Medicare. JAMA 268:900, 1992.
30. Yeager MP, Glass DD, Neff RK, Brinck-Johnsen T: Epidural anesthesia and analgesia in high risk surgical patients. Anesthesiology 66:729, 1987.
31. Rao TLK, El-Etr AA: Anticoagulation following placement of epidural and subarachnoid catheters: An evaluation of neurologic sequelae. Anesthesiology 55:618, 1981.
32. Christopherson R, Beattie C, Frank SM, et al: Perioperative morbidity in patients randomized to epidural or general anesthesia for lower extremity vascular surgery. Anesthesiology 79:422, 1993.
33. Rosenfeld BA, Beattie C, Christopherson R, et al: The effects of different anesthetic regimens on fibrinolysis and the development of postoperative arterial thrombosis. Anesthesiology 79:435, 1993.
34. Gelman S: General versus regional anesthesia for peripheral vascular surgery: Is the problem solved? Anesthesiology 79:415, 1993.
35. Murray MJ, Bower TC, Oliver WC, et al: Effects of cerebrospinal fluid drainage in patients undergoing thoracic and thoracoabdominal aortic surgery. J Cardiothorac Vasc Anesth 7:266, 1993.
36. Baron J, Bertrand M, Barré E, et al: Combined epidural and general anesthesia versus general anesthesia for abdominal aortic surgery. Anesthesiology 75:611, 1991.
37. Saidman LJ: A step forward. In Benumof JL (ed): Anesthesia for Thoracic Surgery. Philadelphia, WB Saunders Co, 1987, p vii.
38. Gayes JM: Pro: One-lung ventilation is best accomplished with the Univent endotracheal tube. J Cardiothorac Vasc Anesth 7:103, 1993.
39. Slinger P: Con: The Univent tube is not the best method of providing one-lung ventilation. J Cardiothorac Vasc Anesth 7:108, 1993.
40. Salomaki TE, Leppaluoto J, Laitinen JO, et al: Epidural versus intravenous fentanyl for reducing hormonal, metabolic, and physiologic responses after thoracotomy. Anesthesiology 79:672, 1993.
41. O'Connor GT, Plume SK, Olmstead EM, et al: A regional intervention to improve the hospital mortality associated with coronary artery bypass graft surgery. JAMA 275:841, 1996.

C H A P T E R 39

Postoperative Pain Management

Steven D. Bell, M.D.
Joseph L. Seltzer, M.D.
Mclvin C. Gitlin, M.D., F.A.C.P.M.

While those caring for patients with postoperative pain have always tried to relieve pain for humanitarian reasons, it has now become apparent that adequate postoperative analgesia has additional important implications in the care of the surgical patient. The importance of adequate postoperative pain management has recently been highlighted by the publication of *Acute Pain Management: Operative or Medical Procedures and Trauma.*[1] This document represents the first "clinical practice guidelines" issued by the United States Department of Health and Human Services' Agency for Healthcare Policy and Research. Postoperative analgesic requirements are thoroughly covered and eight recommendations are made (Table 39–1). These recommendations emphasize the right of the patient to receive adequate postoperative analgesia and to be informed in advance of this right. The guidelines require that a record be kept in the patient's chart of the adequacy of the pain relief achieved. Each institution is directed to have a plan that reviews patient pain intensity and relief levels and allows for modifications in treatment to occur. Clinically, the quality assurance committees of the hospital should randomly review selected charts of patients who have had surgery within the previous 72 hours to determine the adequacy of the patient's pain relief. The guidelines suggest, unless it is contraindicated, that all patients should receive around-the-clock nonsteroidal anti-inflammatory drugs (NSAIDs), as well as opioids as necessary. The guidelines also recommended that "rescue" doses of opioids be available if the usual regimen is not providing adequate relief. The guidelines go on to recommend that any hospital in which abdominal or thoracic surgery is routinely performed should have available for its patients postoperative regional anesthesia, spinal opioids, and patient-controlled analgesia (PCA) infusions under the supervision of an acute pain service. Nonpharmacologic interventions such as cognitive and behavioral based regimens should also be available. Finally, there should be a regular review of the pain services as part of the institution's quality assurance procedures.

Techniques such as epidural regional analgesia, spinal opioids, PCA, intrapleural analgesia, and transcutaneous electrical nerve stimulation (TENS) have now been studied extensively and have been reported to ameliorate the patient's postoperative course. When intravenous and intramuscular morphine were compared to epidural bupivacaine, the patients who had received epidural bupivacaine had significantly greater analgesia and were able to maintain higher oxygen levels. The epidural group's improved oxygenation remained significantly higher than the morphine group for the first 3 postoperative days. There were also significant decreases in atelectasis and positive postoperative sputum cultures in patients receiving epidural bupivacaine.[2] Comparisons of intravenous to epidurally administered morphine demonstrated that the epidural route provided superior pain relief during the first 8 hours postoperatively.[3] Pulmonary function as measured by forced vital capacity (FVC) and forced expiratory volume at 1 second (FEV_1) were superior in the epidural morphine group, although no significant difference in arterial blood pressure was shown between the two groups. Patients receiving intravenous morphine had significantly higher heart rates at 24 hours postoperatively.[3] Not all studies have reported superiority of regional versus parenteral administration of opioids when evaluating pulmonary complications. In a group of patients who had undergone abdominal surgery and received epidural bupivacaine plus morphine, superior pain relief was obtained when compared to a control group receiving parenteral morphine alone. The epidural bupivacaine plus morphine group showed less decrease in vital capacity on the first postoperative day, and arterial oxygen tensions were higher when compared to the parenteral morphine group. The incidence of pulmonary complications and chest x-ray abnormalities were similar between both groups.[4] In a study evaluating the postoperative stress response to surgery, epidural administration of morphine and bupivacaine resulted in lower pain scores and in lower plasma cortisol, epinephrine, and norepinephrine levels. The authors concluded

TABLE 39–1
U.S. Department of Health and Human Services Clinical Practice Guidelines Recommendations*

1. Promise patients attentive analgesic care
2. Chart and display assessment of pain and relief
3. Define pain and relief levels to trigger a review
4. Survey patient satisfaction
5. Nonopioid and opioid analgesic use should comply with several basic principles
6. Specialized analgesic technologies should be made available†
7. Nonpharmacologic analgesic interventions should be available
8. Efficacy of pain treatment should be monitored

*From Acute Pain Management Guideline Panel: Acute pain management: Operative or medical procedures and trauma. Clinical practice guideline. AHCPR Pub. No. 92-0032. Rockville, MD, Agency for Health Care Policy and Research, Public Health Service, U.S. Department of Health and Human Services. Feb. 1992.
†Applies to hospitals routinely performing abdominal and thoracic operations.

that adequate pain relief was an important factor in modifying the surgical stress response.[5] Opioid requirements following thoracotomy have been reduced by the use of TENS.[6] The use of TENS resulted in less depression of arterial oxygenation, functional residual capacity, and FVC, thus minimizing pulmonary complications.[6] In high-risk surgical patients receiving epidural analgesia postoperatively, pulmonary and endocrine responses were compared to patients receiving parenteral opioids. The overall outcomes of the two groups were evaluated based on the length of intensive care unit (ICU) stay, the length of hospital stay, and overall hospital costs. There were 55 patients enrolled in the study: a group of 28 patients received postoperative epidural analgesia, and a second group of 27 patients received parenteral opioids for analgesia for 48 to 79 hours. Nine of the 28 patients treated with epidural analgesia developed postoperative complications (cardiovascular, respiratory, renal, hepatic, major infections) compared to 19 of 27 patients who received parenteral opioids. The rate of cortisol production was significantly lower in the epidural group during the first 24 hours. The epidural group required 6 hours of mechanical ventilation compared to 81 hours for those receiving parenteral opioids.[5,7] Fewer intensive care days as well as a shorter length of hospital stay was noted in the epidural group. These differences, however, did not reach statistical significance. The hospital costs for those patients receiving epidural analgesia postoperatively were significantly less.[7] Other investigators subsequently confirmed a decreased incidence of postoperative complications as well as duration of intensive care stay in patients receiving postoperative epidural analgesia.[8] Other workers, however, were able to corroborate neither the decrease in incidence of pulmonary complications nor a decreased length of stay in patients receiving epidural analgesia and cautioned against the risk of episodic hypotension, which may exist in patients receiving epidural local anesthetic agents.[4]

The American Society of Anesthesiologists' (ASA) guidelines for acute pain management in the perioperative setting were published in 1995.[9] This work reiterated the possibility of adverse outcome resulting from the undertreatment of postoperative pain. Thromboembolic and pulmonary complications, prolongation of ICU and hospital stay, as well as reduced patient satisfaction are potential sequelae of undermanaged pain. A review of the literature performed by the ASA task force members revealed that the performance of PCA with systemic opioids; epidural or intrathecal analgesia with opioids or epidural opioid/local anesthetic mixtures; and various regional techniques such as intercostal neural blockade, neural plexus infusions, and local anesthetic perineural infiltrations had no greater incidence of adverse events than less effective techniques of alleviating postoperative pain. Adequate postoperative analgesia was also recommended for special populations such as pediatric, geriatric, and ambulatory surgery patients. The consequences of suboptimal postoperative pain control and suggestions for effective management have been previously well described in suggested guidelines prepared by a task force of the International Association for the Study of Pain.[10]

A survey of acute pain management in American hospitals concluded that despite a growing trend of the availability of postoperative pain management programs, additional education is required to reduce the incidence and magnitude of postoperative pain[11]; 77% of adults responded that they believed it was appropriate to experience some pain postoperatively. Interestingly, 57% of patients who have had surgery acknowledged the potential for postoperative pain as their primary preoperative concern. Seventy-seven per cent of the adults reported postoperative pain; significantly, 80% of this group of patients reported experiencing moderate to extreme pain. The provision of adequate acute postoperative pain management and lay and professional education remains a formidable challenge.

Mechanism of Pain

Tissue injury results in painful stimuli that originate from specific nerve endings known as nociceptors. Several types of nociceptors exist and their classification is based on the receptors' response to noxious mechanical and heat stimuli. Mechanical heat receptors associated with C fibers are referred to as CMH receptors, while those associated with A fibers are referred to as AMH receptors. High-threshold mechanical receptors known as HTM receptors react only to very intense stimuli and are located in both myelinated and unmyelinated fibers. Muscle fibers also contain nociceptors that are divided into very small myelinated group III muscle afferents and those found in unmyelinated group IV muscle afferents. Joints also have a distinct nociceptor. Nociceptors may be associated with small myelinated A delta group fibers or unmyelinated C fibers afferents. The different nociceptors are distinguished from one another both by the nerve fiber with which they are associated and the type of stimulus that activates them.[12]

Impulses from nociceptors enter the spinal cord at the dorsal root. The reception of repetitive stimuli may alter the neurochemistry of the dorsal horn and alter pain sensitivity thresholds.[13] The term "windup" is used to describe a progressive increase in action potential discharge in the spinal cord resulting from repetitive stimulation of primary afferent fibers. This may produce a prolonged increase in the excitability of the spinal cord neurons. Central sensitization refers to the phenomenon of altered pain due to changes in receptive fields of spinal neurons that may follow an increase in excitability produced by the input of peripheral nociceptors. There is hyperexcitability of subsequent stimuli. Additionally, stimuli that may have been previously perceived as innocuous are now interpreted as painful. *N*-methyl-D-aspartic acid (NMDA) has been reported to mediate the increase in excitability, while NMDA antagonists may block the response.[14]

Painful stimuli ascend through the spinal cord in the spinothalamic tracks. Descending tracks originating in the brain's periaqueductal gray matter, the brain stem, and the reticular formation modify the afferent impulses at the dorsal horn.

In addition to NMDA, numerous other transmitters exist in the spinal cord. Substance P, a peptide, is associated with primary afferent tracks and has been reported to be found in the terminals of small-diameter fibers in the substantia gelatinosa of the dorsal horn. Substance P excites neurons in the spinal cord.[15–17] When opioids are injected into the cerebrospinal fluid, there is a suppression of substance P release.[17] Clonidine activates both the pre- and postsynaptic α_2-adrenergic receptors in the spinal cord and inhibits substance P release. When administered epidurally, clonidine has a significant analgesic effect.[18] Serotonin is also associated with painful stimuli and appears to be a neurotransmitter in the spinal cord pain pathway.[19] There are two major serotonin receptors, which have been labeled D receptors and M receptors. The M receptors have been divided into three subtypes. It is one of these M subtypes of receptors that is reported to be associated with the mediation of pain.[20] Additionally, serotonin has been demonstrated to sensitize nociceptors in the muscles to painful responses to bradykinins.[21]

Psychological factors play a large role in the patient's perception of painful stimuli. Patients' anxiety levels prior to surgery have been evaluated and correlated to the patient's perception of postoperative pain.[22–24] Acute preoperative fear should be differentiated from chronic anxiety. Chronic anxiety rather than acute preoperative fear correlates with increased postoperative pain. The patient's emotional status is important in planning the analgesic needs postoperatively. Patients with a history of chronic pain as well as those suffering from depression tend to report a greater intensity of pain following surgical procedures.[22] A higher patient educational level has been reported to be correlated with a lessened self-reported postoperative pain score.[22] Preoperative patient education may have a positive effect on the patient's postoperative perception of pain. Patients tend to report levels of pain that are equivalent to what they anticipated. One study has shown that providing information regarding the upcoming surgery has correlated with higher pain scores,[24] while another has challenged this concept, maintaining that the better informed patients have less postoperative pain.[23] Adequately educating the patient about what to expect in the postoperative period, including the types of analgesic techniques to be used postoperatively, may be beneficial to the patient.

Pre-emptive Analgesia

Basic research has demonstrated that following tissue injury, an increased sensitivity to pain occurs in the area of the injury and in adjacent undamaged tissue. This increased sensitivity appears to occur for two reasons: (1) local inflammatory reactions result in an increase in sensitivity of the nociceptors and (2) there is increased activity seen within the dorsal horn cells of the spinal cord.[13,25,26] The etiologic phenomena are referred to as peripheral and central sensitization.[26] NMDA receptors have been shown to be directly involved with the development of central sensitization.[14,29] The central sensitization is stimulated by C afferent fibers, and experimental evidence indicates that fibers originating in muscle have a much greater effect than fibers that are cutaneous in origin.[27,28] NMDA antagonists have been shown to inhibit the occurrence of central sensitization.[30] Ketamine is the only drug presently clinically available that has NMDA antagonistic properties.[30] Other attempts to prevent central sensitization from occurring have been directed toward blocking the afferent input to the dorsal horn.

Pre-emptive analgesia is based on the theory that if central excitation can be suppressed before an injury, the resultant pain might be reduced. Pre-emptive analgesia is an attempt to forestall the amplification of postoperative pain through a potential suppression of altered sensory processing.[31] The concept of pre-emptive analgesia is not recent and is attributed to George Crile in 1913.[32] Crile suggested that by blocking nociceptive input to the brain by multiple routes one might be able to prevent "painful scars" that might lead to an enhancement of postoperative pain.[32] Use of regional anesthesia or opioids before surgery has been studied to determine if pre-emptive analgesia can be obtained in man (Table 39–2).

A large series of patients undergoing various orthopedic procedures compared patients receiving a combination of opioid premedication and a local anesthetic block to patients receiving neither an opioid premedication nor a local anesthetic block. Opioid premedication increased the time to the first request for postoperative analgesia. Local anesthetic block produced a further sig-

TABLE 39–2
Approaches to Pre-emptive Analgesia

Opioid premedication
Intraoperative opioids
Low-dose ketamine
Ketamine anesthesia
Regional nerve block
Infiltration of the wound with local anesthetic
Epidural opioids and/or local anesthetics
Subarachnoid opioids and/or local anesthetics

nificant increase and the combination of opioid premedication with local anesthetic block produced the longest time to first request for postoperative analgesia.[33] The use of bupivacaine prior to tonsillectomy decreased pain scores on the second, fifth, and tenth postoperative days.[34] In a well-conducted study of pain relief following inguinal herniorrhaphy in patients who received general anesthesia, patients who also received local infiltration prior to incision had less pain at 24 and 48 hours and 10 days when compared to patients who received general anesthesia or spinal anesthesia alone. Spinal anesthesia alone significantly decreased pain at 24 and 48 hours as well.[35] While the pre-emptive analgesic effect of local infiltration prior to incision appears to have been confirmed,[36] other investigators have challenged this concept secondary to inability to demonstrate any pre-emptive analgesic effect when employing an inguinal field block.[37] Patients undergoing posterolateral thoracotomy who were administered an epidural bolus of 4 μg/kg of fentanyl in 20 ml of saline before surgical incision had superior pain relief when compared to patients who received an identical dose of fentanyl 15 minutes after incision.[38] A similar study using 7 ml of bupivacaine with 2 mg of morphine administered epidurally followed by a bupivacaine/morphine infusion 40 minutes prior to an incision for abdominal surgery compared to a group of patients receiving the same drug regimen beginning at the closure of the surgical wound did not demonstrate any significant difference in the request for additional morphine or visual analogue pain scales in the postoperative period.[39] Similar results were obtained in patients undergoing abdominal hysterectomy who had received 15 ml of 0.5% bupivacaine epidurally 15 minutes before surgery versus those who received the same dose at the conclusion of surgery.[40] The use of regional anesthesia utilizing 0.5% bupivacaine for shoulder surgery significantly decreased VAS scores and opioid use at 24 and 48 hours postoperatively; this is long after the anticipated resolution of the block.[41] In a separate study, 142 patients scheduled for major abdominal surgery were randomized into three groups. Group one received intramuscular diclofenac, intravenous metamizole, and epidural mepivacaine plus morphine prior to skin incision. Group two patients received the same regimen before skin closure. Group three patients did not receive any of the study substances. Each group received the same general anesthetic regimen. The authors found that the preoperative provision of this balanced pre-emptive analgesic protocol led to pronounced postoperative opioid-sparing effects.[42]

Stimulation of NMDA receptors in the spinal cord produces prolonged excitability. Ketamine, a currently available NMDA receptor antagonist, has been studied as a pre-emptive analgesic. Twenty-two female patients undergoing open cholecystectomy were divided into a ketamine group and a control group. The ketamine group received the same anesthetic technique as the control group except for the addition of a single 0.15 mg/kg dose of ketamine 5 minutes before the incision. The patients receiving ketamine had lower postoperative morphine requirements.[43] Patients undergoing transabdominal hysterectomy were divided into three groups: a 5 μg/kg fentanyl group followed by a 0.02 μg/kg/min infusion; a 2 mg/kg ketamine bolus, followed by 20 μg/kg/min ketamine infusion group; and a control group receiving only thiopental and isoflurane. The fentanyl and ketamine groups showed significantly less postoperative wound hyperalgesia at 48 hours postoperatively than the controls.[44]

While it is well accepted that central sensitization can be demonstrated in laboratory preparations, clinical attempts at preventing this phenomenon employing pre-emptive analgesic techniques have yielded mixed results. While further well-controlled studies will be necessary to finally resolve this question, it appears reasonable to consider the administration of regional anesthesia and/or spinal opioids before surgical incision when general anesthesia is being used concomitantly. It is interesting to note that while spinal opioids and regional anesthetics appear to be effective in providing pre-emptive analgesia, high concentrations of potent inhalational agents only produce a modest modification of the central effect of a painful stimulus.[45]

It has been suggested that the term "pre-emptive analgesia" may not have been used in a rigorous enough fashion, thereby creating the possibility for misinterpretation of study results.[31,46] Antinociceptive interventions provided preoperatively differ from those that are targeted at preventing the development of central sensitization through continued administration throughout the operative period including the postoperative one.[31] The importance of prolonged blockade in pre-emptive analgesia models has been reported.[47] Ongoing investigation should aid us in discerning the true value of pre-emptive analgesia in modulating postoperative pain.

Patient-Controlled Analgesia

PCA is an effective method for delivering postoperative analgesia.[48] Traditional parenteral analgesia administered every 3 to 4 hours will yield an adequate serum analgesia concentration for only 35% of the time. Peak concentrations vary three- to fivefold and the time to reach peak serum levels varies three- to sevenfold in different patients.[49] In addition, the minimum serum drug concentration needed for adequate analgesia varies significantly from patient to patient.[50]

With wide variability in patients' requirements and drug levels, standard regimens of intramuscular opioid administration may prove unsatisfactory secondary to the long lag time between patient recognition of analgesia need and the attainment of analgesic effect. The patient in the typical intramuscular dosing scheme must ask the nurse for an opioid analgesic. The nurse must obtain the medication from a locked narcotic cabinet, record it in the appropriate record, and then take it to the patient's room.[51] After administration, the time required to reach peak analgesic effect with morphine is approximately 60 to 90 minutes.[52] Excessive serum drug levels may be produced at peak serum concentrations thus potentially leading to patient oversedation and respiratory depression. There are inherent inadequacies in the intramuscular dosing schedules that do not take into account patients' individual needs, with drug dosages being prescribed either empirically or according to body weight. Another cause of inadequate analgesia is that health care workers not infrequently underestimate the intensity of the patient's pain; nurses tend to give the lowest amount of a dosing schedule.[53]

The psychological makeup of an individual may have significant impact on the serum concentrations required to produce adequate analgesia. This is especially true in patients with heightened anxiety and those suffering from neurotic personality disorders.[17,49,54] Patients' emotional states vary greatly. Increased anxiety will make pain less tolerable, with the state of anxiety being a linear predictor of postoperative pain.[49] Furthermore, pain enhances anxiety.

Intravenous administration of opioids has been shown to provide superior analgesia when compared to intramuscular (IM) administration of the same opioid.[47] There are major disadvantages to the intravenous route of administration. Serum levels of intravenous opioid administered as a bolus decline rapidly. When serum levels fall, central nervous system levels consequently fall and pain ensues. This can be overcome by using larger doses; however, higher doses are associated with a greater incidence of side effects such as nausea, vomiting, sedation, and respiratory depression.[55] While the frequent administration of small boluses would overcome this problem, it is impractical for nursing staffs to repeatedly administer small intravenous doses of analgesics to a large postoperative surgical population.

PCA was first introduced in 1970 as an alternative to intramuscular analgesia.[56] PCA is an analgesic system that is designed to maintain optimal serum analgesia levels throughout the postoperative period. The initial PCA infusion pumps utilized only a single injection mode and the patient received a specified bolus dose of opioid on demand.[56–58] This delivery system worked well during the day but sometimes functioned suboptimally at night, potentially resulting in inadequate analgesia and interrupted sleep.

Newer PCA devices consist of an infusion pump integrated with a timing unit. These devices deliver a continuous baseline infusion known as the basal mode. Additionally, there is a demand mode that delivers a preset bolus of the selected analgesic when the patient triggers the device by depressing a button. The timing unit prevents overdosage by interposing an inactivation period, called the lockout time, between the patient-initiated doses. Despite the frequency with which a patient may press the bolus button, actual drug delivery will only occur at preset intervals, thus preventing self-overdosing. The total dose administered is determined by the rate of the basal infusion and by the size and frequency of the bolus dose.

For PCA therapy to be successful, the physician, nurse and patient must understand the PCA concept. Patient education is usually accomplished in the preoperative period, either as an inpatient or in the outpatient evaluation center. It is advisable to inform patients that PCA therapy will modulate but not totally eradicate their pain; however, the patient must be encouraged to utilize the device to optimize analgesia, especially during early ambulation and maneuvers for pulmonary toilet. Patients must understand that the physicians and nurses are not using this device to avoid patient care interactions but rather to afford them the opportunity to "fine tune" their own analgesic requirements thereby attempting to minimize under- or overmedication. The perfect dosing scheme would have the basal level set at a level where the patient has minimal to no discomfort when lying in bed. The bolus mode would be utilized only to yield additional analgesia when incident pain might be produced by various activities. Recently, it has been reported that not all patients require a basal infusion.[59] Other studies have reported improvement in postoperative pain therapy and sleep when both basal and bolus modes are employed.[60–62] It is the authors' practice to assess the type of surgery that the patient has undergone and the pain tolerance exhibited by the patient and individualize the PCA regimen to that particular patient.

Table 39–3 displays possible bolus and basal infusion dosages and lockout intervals for a wide variety of analgesics. Most opioids provide satisfactory analgesia at rest. A study that compared morphine, meperidine, and oxymorphone reported oxymorphone to have the fastest onset but was also associated with the highest incidence of nausea and vomiting. In the same study, the meperidine-treated patients were most likely to report severe pain when they moved, while morphine produced the most sedation and pruritus.[63]

Over a 30-minute period, patients are intravenously administered a loading dose of the selected analgesic until they are comfortable. Dosages in adult patients generally range from 2 to 10 mg of morphine or 25 to 100 mg of meperidine. Once this initial level of comfort is achieved, the clinician must decide if the basal infusion rate mode is to be utilized. If so, the basal infusion rate is generally set to deliver 1 mg/hr morphine or 10 mg/hr meperidine in adult patients. The bolus rate is set to deliver 1 mg morphine or 10 mg meperidine. Generally, the basal infusion rate should equal the low bolus dose range. The lockout interval is set at 10 minutes. Under the above conditions, the patient would receive a total hourly dose of 7 mg morphine or 70 mg meperidine. If the bolus-only mode is utilized, an initial starting point in adult patients may be to set the bolus rate at 1 to 2 mg of morphine or 10 to 20 mg of meperidine and the lockout interval at 10 minutes. Analgesia usually occurs at lower opioid doses than sedation.[65] Peak central nervous system drug levels occur rapidly, resulting in sedation and interfering with the patient's triggering of the device. A lockout time of 10 minutes should aid in guarding against accumulation of the analgesic. Studies have reported that patients can effectively treat themselves without overmedication.[57,63,66–68] Some investigators report that most patients prefer to tolerate some pain in order to maintain a clear sensorium.[57]

Adjusting the Dose

Fine adjustments of the analgesic dosages are determined by examining and talking with the patient (Table

TABLE 39–3
Basal and Bolus Infusion Dosages and Lockout Intervals for Analgesics*

	Basal Dose	Bolus Dose	Lockout Interval
Agonist			
Morphine	1.0–2.0 mg/hr	0.5–3.0 mg	5–20 min
Meperidine	10–20 mg/hr	5–30 mg	5–15 min
Methadone	1.0 mg/hr	0.5–3.0 mg	5–15 min
Hydromorphone	0.2 mg/hr	0.1–0.5 mg	5–15 min
Fentanyl	50–75 μg/hr	15–75 μg	3–10 min
Sufentanil	2–7 μg/hr	2–10 μg	3–10 min
Agonist/antagonist			
Pentazocine	5 mg/hr	5–30 mg	5–15 min
Nalbuphine	1 mg/hr	1–5 mg	5–15 min
Bupremorphine	None given	0.03–0.2 mg	5–20 min

*Modified from White PF: Use of patient-controlled analgesia for management of acute pain. JAMA 259:243, 1988, with permission.

39–4). If the patient has resting pain, the basal infusion rate may be increased 50%. If analgesia needs are greater with activity, the dosage of the bolus dose may be increased by 50%. If the patient becomes sedated, the infusion rate and bolus doses are often decreased by 50%. If a patient receiving only a bolus-mode infusion is comfortable during the day but has awakened frequently at night, the clinician might consider adding a basal infusion. Infusions of morphine are usually begun in the range of 1 mg/hr; however, infusion rates ranging from 0.9 to 5.1 mg/hr have been reported to be necessary for adequate postoperative analgesia.[55] This wide analgesic range has also been reported to occur when fentanyl[67] or meperidine[69] are used. If institutional policy allows all physicians to prescribe PCA, upper limits of therapy should be defined. If these upper limits are reached, the acute pain service should be consulted. Adjustment in basal infusion rates may be necessary, as diurnal variation in patients' requirements have been demonstrated. Following abdominal surgery, the peak times for morphine use have been reported to be 9 AM and 8 PM.[70] The clinician must remember that in a continuous infusion system, the weight or mass of a patient is not a variable. Once the body compartments are saturated with a drug, the plasma concentration depends on the amount of drug given and the elimination of the drug; redistribution is no longer a factor. Investigators have reported a balance between the intake and steady-state blood level that provided adequate analgesia.[69,71] There was no accumulation in these patients and steady-state blood concentrations were far below the maximum blood level that could have been reached had the patient utilized the maximum dosage the PCA device would have allowed. Because of the use of frequent small doses in the bolus-only mode, the clinician can equate the bolus-only mode as a steady-state infusion.

PCA is usually safe; however, there are scattered reports of respiratory depression in the literature.[72,73] Respiratory depression may be theoretically minimized or eliminated by routine excellent nursing care and careful monitoring of the postoperative patient on the surgical wards. The use of morphine or meperidine may further

TABLE 39–4
PCA Schematic

	Awake From Surgery	
	2-mg IV morphine bolus Repeat 2–3 minutes until minimal at rest	
	Basal infusion 1.0 mg/hr Bolus 1.0 mg Lockout 10 min	
Comfortable at rest Comfortable with activity Maintain infusion rate	Comfortable at rest Uncomfortable with activity Maintain basal infusion Maintain lockout Increase bolus by 0.5 mg Re-evaluate every 30 minutes until comfortable	Uncomfortable at rest Uncomfortable with activity Increase basal infusion mg/hr Maintain lockout Maintain bolus infusion Re-evaluate every 30 minutes until comfortable
	Comfortable Awake	
Sedated or somnolent		Become uncomfortable Re-evaluate as above
	Monitor for respiratory depression (Consider naloxone [100 μg] for severe respiratory depression)	
Temporarily stop infusion or Decrease both basal and bolus infusion rates		

increase safety, as these are the analgesics with which surgical nurses are most familiar.[65]

There have been numerous studies supporting the analgesic efficacy of PCA and its superiority to intramuscular injections,[55,57,65,74] while other investigators have failed to demonstrate a distinct difference between pain relief attained when comparing intramuscular opioids and PCA systems.[67,68] In a study comparing PCA morphine to IM morphine, 92% of the patients who received PCA characterized their postoperative state as comfortable or mildly uncomfortable versus 58% of the patients who received IM injections.[55] Not only was PCA associated with superior pain scores when compared to intramuscular administration, PCA also was the much preferred technique.[55] An early study reported lower total dosages of analgesics used with PCA when compared to the intramuscular route.[57] This study utilized only bolus infusions. A later study reported no significant differences in the amount of analgesic used when the two techniques were compared.[62] Other investigators have demonstrated that the combination of basal and bolus infusions doses increases the total amount of opioid used.[59] Studies on the effect of PCA on pulmonary function are varied, with some authors reporting no improvement in pulmonary function and oxygenation when compared to the intramuscular route,[68] and others demonstrating significant improvement in FVC, and peak expiratory flow rates (PEFR).[75] In addition, when PCA fentanyl is compared to epidural bupivacaine after peripheral arterial surgery, both techniques were equally effective in providing adequate analgesia without respiratory depression.[66] To the authors' knowledge, there are no definitive long-term outcome studies in relation to pulmonary function or other factors such as length of ICU or hospital stay.

In summary, PCA is effective, beneficial, and usually safe. PCA provides safe, efficient analgesia with minimal sedation and improved pulmonary function with minimal side effects. Optimal analgesic dosage can be achieved with the ability to alter doses to match the changing demands of the patients. PCA allows for individualization of therapy. The lag time for nursing response is eliminated. This decreased dependence on the nursing staff may allow for greater spontaneous patient activity. Both nursing and patient acceptance is high.[68]

Local Anesthetics

Local anesthetics have been used to relieve pain for over a century. Clinically available drugs can be divided into one of two groups: esters or amides. Chloroprocaine, tetracaine, procaine, and cocaine are ester local anesthetics. Lidocaine, prilocaine, mepivacaine, bupivacaine, ropivacine and etidocaine are amides. Amides undergo hepatic metabolism, while esters are hydrolyzed into inactive forms.

Local anesthetics prevent nerve impulse conduction in several ways. The normal resting potential of a nerve is −70 mV. An impulse or action potential is transmitted along the nerve by a progressive depolarization process. This process involves the opening of sodium channels allowing sodium ions to pass into the nerve cell and changing the resting membrane potential to +40 mV.[76] Local anesthetics progressively lower the amplitude of the action potential, which retards the rate of rise and elevates the firing threshold. The velocity of the impulse conduction is thus slowed. The refractory period is lengthened. The site of action of local anesthetics appears to be at the sodium channel's internal openings. The nondissociated or nonionized form of the local anesthetic diffuses through the nerve membranes. Once inside the nerve, the local anesthetics must become dissociated or enter into an ionized form in order to effectively block the sodium channel.[76]

The maximum dose of local anesthetic that may be given varies with the site of injection as well as the specific characteristics of the drug. Signs of toxicity vary according to the individual agent. The classic signs of toxicity seen with older anesthetic agents such as lidocaine often present first with a subjective feeling of lightheadedness, numbness and tingling of the lips, and tinnitus. As toxic levels are approached, drowsiness ensues, which may progress to confusion, slurred speech, twitching, generalized muscle tremors, and then overt seizures. Local anesthetic toxicity-related seizures may not be lethal if proper cardiorespiratory support is given. As higher blood levels are reached, cardiac arrest can occur. With the newer local anesthetics such as bupivacaine and etidocaine, cardiac arrest can occur without the prodrome described above. Cardiac resuscitation has been reported to be extremely difficult following bupivacaine overdoses.[77–80] Close attention to proper dosing and techniques is important when employing these agents.

Local anesthetics are useful in providing postoperative pain relief. Potentially augmenting the use of local anesthetics for peripheral nerve, intrapleural, plexus, and epidural blockade are simple techniques such as intermittent injection or continuous perfusion of surgical wounds with local anesthetics. The latter techniques have been shown to reduce postoperative pain and opioid requirements.[81] Intravenous infusions of 2 mg/min of lidocaine have significantly lowered pain scores and reduced opioid requirements.[82]

Epidural and Spinal Local Anesthetics

Epidural blockade has been used extensively for postoperative analgesia and is especially effective when combined as part of an operative anesthetic technique utilizing an appropriately placed catheter. By placing the catheter in the middle of the dermatome segments to be anesthetized, the clinician may achieve optimal blockade with minimal drug dosage.

Since the duration of action of all local anesthetics is shorter than the desired time of postoperative analgesia, one of two techniques may be utilized to maintain pain relief: (1) intermittent bolus technique or (2) continuous infusion technique. The intermittent bolus or "top-up" technique involves reinjecting the catheter when pain returns. It is essential that the reinjection be done quickly, since regression of analgesia may be very rapid. The top-up volume and concentration vary with the site of the catheter.[83]

The duration of analgesia depends upon which local anesthetic is used, its concentration, and its volume. Virtually any local anesthetic may be utilized; however, studies demonstrate that lidocaine 1.0% and etidocaine 1.5%, tetracaine 0.15% and 0.25%, bupivacaine 0.25% and 0.50%, and etidocaine 0.5% and 1.0% are the most effective concentrations.[84] Generally, top-up doses are initiated at 4 to 6 ml and are increased as indicated. Tachyphylaxis is defined as a diminution of intensity, duration, and extent of block with repeated injections of local anesthetics. Tachyphylaxis occurs when local anesthetic drugs are given repeatedly at the same site and occurs more rapidly and to a greater degree when pain is allowed to recur. For this reason some authors have advocated empiric top-up dosing of drugs to avoid the return of pain.[85] Toxicity should always be a concern when local anesthetics are utilized. Studies involving obstetric patients report a very slow rise in serum bupivacaine peak plasma levels with the top-up technique.[86] When additional local anesthetics are administered, the patient should be placed in the supine position prior to injections. Blood pressure, pulse, and signs of toxicity should be monitored closely for 20 to 30 minutes following injection.

The continuous-infusion method involves infusing the local anesthetic at a rate equal to that at which the drug is removed from the epidural space. This technique seeks to avoid the period of pain that may be seen with the top-up dose technique. Lidocaine 0.5% or 1.0% and bupivacaine 0.125%, 0.25%, or 0.5% are the most commonly used drugs and concentrations. Infusion rates vary depending on the concentrations of drug used.[84] Toxicity is potentially less of a problem, since the continuous-infusion technique avoids the peaks in plasma local anesthetic concentrations seen when the top-up dose is given. A steady state in plasma levels appears in approximately 40 to 48 hours.[87] There is always the potential of catheter migration into a blood vessel during the continuous infusion.

The side effects of epidural local anesthetic blockade may be significant. A hyperdynamic state exists when the cardiac output increases up to 40% with a concomitant decrease in total systemic vascular resistance and mean arterial pressure. Heart rate and stroke volume are increased while cardiac work remains constant. With pain, cardiac output, mean arterial pressure, and cardiac work increase. The level of blockade and the presence or absence of epinephrine in the anesthetic solution affect the cardiovascular responses. The degree of hypotension is also affected by the preload and overall condition of the cardiovascular system, with some patients experiencing minimal changes and others experiencing very severe decreases in blood pressure.[88,89] There are few data with regard to the high-risk elderly patient.

The effects on renal function are essentially those of a reflection of the integrity of the cardiovascular system. While the kidney is capable of adjusting for minor cardiovascular alterations, large decreases in mean arterial pressure are accompanied by similar decreases in the glomerular filtration rate and renal plasma flow.[90]

Following vascular surgery in the thorax or abdomen, there is a significant decrease in FVC, FEV_1, and functional residual capacity (FRC).[91] It initially was concluded that pain was the primary explanation for the pulmonary dysfunction.[92–94] However, when pain is totally eradicated, pulmonary parameters do not return to preoperative values.[3,6] Studies comparing epidural local anesthetics and intramuscular morphine have reported that epidural local anesthetics are superior in maintaining FVC,[95] although there was no significant difference in effect on FRC.[96] The effect on PaO_2 was variable depending on the study, with most showing no significant difference.[97–99] To the authors' knowledge, there have been no long-term patient outcome studies.

The quality of epidural analgesia with local anesthetic agents is generally perceived to be excellent with any of the drugs used in appropriate concentrations. There are no data that clarify whether the top-up technique or continuous-infusion technique is superior. Disadvantages of epidural local anesthetic techniques are the potential for motor blockade, which may make ambulation difficult or impossible, and sympathetic blockade, which may result in cardiovascular instability.

The provision of continuous spinal analgesia was potentially facilitated by the development of microcatheters.[100] Continuous spinal analgesia with local anesthetics could offer theoretical advantages. The use of very low doses of a drug without epinephrine might be administered in a continuous manner to provide constant analgesia.[101]

Use of continuous spinal analgesia with microcatheters for postoperative pain relief has been hampered by potential problems of neurotoxicity associated with the use of this technique. Multiple cases of cauda equina syndrome were reported with the use of small-bore-catheter intraspinal delivery of 5% lidocaine with 7.5% dextrose.[102] This led to a decision to withdraw these catheters from the market for this indication.[103] An obvious theoretical impediment to the use of continuous spinal analgesia is the potential for motor blockade which might develop, thereby adversely impacting on the ability of the patient to ambulate.

Intercostal and Intrapleural Nerve Blocks

Intercostal nerve blocks represent a technique providing analgesia in a relatively simple fashion. Intercostal nerve blocks have been used extensively for postoperative analgesia.[104,105] When used for thoracotomy incisions, adequate pain relief requires the blockade of the affected dermatomes and two to three dermatomes above and below the incision. The areas through which chest tubes and drains are placed should also be blocked. When performing intercostal nerve blocks, the injection should be made as proximal as possible to ensure blockade includes the posterior divisions of the nerve. Midline abdominal incisions usually require bilateral intercostal nerve blocks. Intercostal blocks are superior to intramuscular opioids after abdominal surgery when pulmonary function tests such as FVC and forced expiratory flow rate (FEFR) are measured. Whether intercostal nerve blocks are effective in improving hypoxemia is controversial as variable results have been reported.[104,106,107]

While all local anesthetic agents may be utilized for intercostal nerve blocks, the longer acting ones, 0.5% etidocaine and more popularly 0.5% bupivacaine with epinephrine, are commonly used. A duration of action between 5 and 11 hours may be expected when employing these agents.[84] A disadvantage of provision of postoperative analgesia with the technique of intercostal blockade is that the patient may require reinjection several times a day in order to obtain continuous analgesia. Frequent reinjections are not only work-intensive for the practitioner but also not very well tolerated by some patients. Intercostal nerve block is associated with the highest serum drug levels of any regional anesthetic technique.[108] Since the half-life of both etidocaine and bupivacaine are quite long, the risk of accumulation and toxicity exists when they are used for repeated intercostal nerve blocks. Some anesthesiologists are of the opinion that local anesthetics with epinephrine should never be used in patients with coronary artery disease.[86] If epinephrine were to be omitted, then even higher blood levels might be attained with intercostal block.

Lidocaine has been used for continuous intercostal nerve block. Widespread intercostal nerve block has been demonstrated following insertion of a catheter into the intercostal space and intermittent injections of local anesthetic to provide satisfactory analgesia in patients with multiple rib fractures and after cholecystectomy and cardiac surgery.[109] The effectiveness and potential side effects of a continuous infusion of lidocaine after lateral thoracotomy were studied.[110] An indwelling catheter was placed in an appropriate intercostal space before thoracotomy closure. A bolus of 3 mg/kg of 1.5% lidocaine with epinephrine followed by a continuous infusion of 1% lidocaine without epinephrine at the rate of 1 mg/kg/hr was administered. Lowering of pain scores and complete cutaneous analgesia to pinprick over a median of three thoracic dermatomes was seen. Partial analgesia spreading over six to nine dermatomes was demonstrated. When steady-state infusion conditions were met, the maximum plasma concentrations of lidocaine were 5 μg/ml. The authors concluded that the use of a continuous infusion of lidocaine utilizing a single-catheter technique might provide effective analgesia following thoracotomy.

The technique of intrapleural block has been described. An epidural catheter is placed percutaneously into the posterior aspect of the thoracic cavity. Most studies report the use of 0.5% bupivacaine as the anesthetic agent of choice. Volumes injected have ranged from 20 to 30 ml with epinephrine.[111–116] Intrapleural blockade has been reported to provide analgesia for unilateral incision[111,112,114–116]; however, intrapleural blockade has not been demonstrated to be effective in providing adequate postoperative pain relief for patients having undergone thoracotomy.[113,117,118] Serum bupivacaine levels following intrapleural injection have been reported to range from as low as 0.3 μg/ml to as high as 3.27 μg/ml.[112,114,119–121] Blood levels as low as 2.3 μg/kg of bupivacaine have been associated with seizure activity.[122] Intrapleural injections provide adequate analgesia for an average of 3 to 5 hours.[112,114,123] To be useful for an abdominal incision, bilateral blocks are necessary. There is only one report describing the use of bilateral blocks, and the blocks were not performed for postoperative pain relief.[124] Additional studies will be necessary to demonstrate the safety of bilateral intrapleural nerve blocks before this technique can be widely applied.

Intrathecal Opioids

Since 1979 the use of spinal opioids for postoperative pain relief has increased dramatically.[125] A number of studies now document the superiority of spinal or centrally acting opioids as analgesics for the treatment of severe postoperative pain.[126–128] The advantages of effective, long-acting, selective analgesia are partially offset by the side effects of early and late respiratory depression, nausea, vomiting, pruritus, and urinary retention.[129] Opioids act centrally at the substantia gelatinosa of the dorsal horn of the spinal cord.[130] A selective blockade of pain conduction may inhibit both presynaptic and postsynaptic neuronal afferent transmission. Used independently, centrally acting opioids do not produce sufficient anesthesia for intraoperative pain; they do, in many instances, though, provide effective postoperative analgesia.[126–128]

There are significant differences between the analgesic effects of local anesthetics and opioids when administered centrally.[130] Although the chemical properties of opioids and local anesthetics are similar in many ways, their effects differ markedly. Spinal opioids have minimal effect on myocardial contractility, heart rate, and systemic vascular resistance. Sympathetic reactivity is preserved. Motor blockade is obviated. Respiratory depression, although rare, does occur when opioids are used intrathecally. The temporal sequence in which respiratory depression occurs depends upon the technique and drug used. The potential for sedation varies from nonexistent to marked depending upon the drug used and its dosage. Nausea, vomiting, pruritus, and urinary retention occur; the frequency of these effects are dependent upon drug, dosage, and technique.[129] There is a close relationship between lipid solubility and the onset and duration of analgesia.[131] The more lipid soluble the drug, the quicker the onset and the shorter the duration of analgesia.[119]

The first successful use of intrathecal opioids in humans was performed in patients with chronic pain secondary to malignancies. Intrathecal morphine was subsequently used for postoperative analgesia in patients who had undergone herniorrhaphies.[133] The effectiveness of this route of administration was confirmed by a multitude of studies reporting similar results. A central rather than systemic explanation for the analgesia resulting from intrathecal opioid administration was suggested by study of serum morphine levels.[134] Visual analog pain scores were low in all studies, indicating excellent analgesia.[135,136]

Highly ionized drugs such as morphine remain in the cerebrospinal fluid (CSF), since they are unable to easily diffuse across membranes into spinal cord receptor sites due to their low lipid solubility.[131,137,138] This hydrophilic characteristic explains the relatively slow onset of action of intrathecal morphine analgesia. CSF elimination half-life for morphine is approximately 3 hours.[138] Since morphine is minimally absorbed by the spinal cord or surrounding tissue, CSF concentrations remain elevated for relatively long periods of time. This differs pharmacodynamically from the situation after an intravenous injection of the drug. The morphine may, however, diffuse rostrally in the CFS after intrathecal administration.

Lipophilic drugs such as meperidine and fentanyl are quickly taken up by the spinal cord. Compared to the hydrophilic agents, lipophilic drugs have a more rapid onset but a shorter duration of action.[131] CSF levels of the lipophilic agents are low because they rapidly penetrate the spinal cord; therefore, there is little drug available for cephalad diffusion. Morphine is the most frequently administered drug for intrathecal analgesia. Fentanyl has been added to morphine to enhance the onset of action. Intrathecal opioids may have significant side effects. Respiratory depression is certainly a significant side effect of intrathecal opioid administration and was first reported in 1979.[139,140] Since morphine is not taken up quickly by the cord due to its low lipid solubility, it slowly diffuses cephalad and thereby may produce delayed respiratory depression. Doses of 0.5 to 1.0 mg of morphine have been commonly used.[141] Doses above these are associated with a much higher incidence of all side effects including respiratory depression.[139] Intrathecal doses up to 4 mg of morphine have been reported to have been used without respiratory depression; however, all of these patients had a history of significant prior parenteral utilization.[142,143] The onset of respiratory depression following intrathecal morphine is quite variable. It usually occurs within 6 to 20 hours; it may occasionally be delayed even longer. A return to normal respiration may require up to 23 hours after the onset of respiratory depression.[135,140,144–146] The risk of respiratory depression from intrathecal morphine injection is increased with advanced age[135] and higher doses.[139] The incidence of delayed respiratory depression from intrathecal morphine injection ranges from 0.26 to 0.9%.[126]

The reported incidence of nausea and vomiting following intrathecal opioid administration ranges from 14 to 100%[117] and the range of urinary retention is also variable. The side effects of intrathecal morphine can be antagonized with naloxone. Respiratory depression from intrathecal morphine may require repeated doses of naloxone up to 1.2 mg followed by a continuous naloxone infusion titrated to effect.[147,148]

The clinician will observe the onset of action of intrathecal morphine in 15 to 45 minutes with doses ranging from 0.5 to 1.0 mg. The onset of action may be shortened by 5 minutes by adding 25 μg of fentanyl to 0.25 mg of morphine.[149] The duration of the analgesia following intrathecal morphine administration ranges from 18 to 24 hours depending upon the dose. Obviously, a limitation of this technique is the finite nature of the postoperative pain relief. Repeated subarachnoid injections would be subsequently required for the maintenance of postoperative analgesia in the absence of an indwelling intrathecal catheter.

Almost all efficacy studies have reported marked superiority in the degree of postoperative analgesia produced by intrathecal morphine as compared to intramuscular and intravenous opioids.[133,141] A double-blind, placebo-controlled study investigated the efficacy of intrathecal fentanyl administered through microcatheters in patients having undergone thoracotomy. A control group received 0.9% saline through the catheters. All patients received morphine PCAs. The authors reported a more rapid onset of action, significantly lower pain at rest and incident pain scores, and higher peak expiratory flow rates in the intrathecal fentanyl group. Neither early nor delayed respiratory depression was observed.[150] Large-dose intrathecal morphine has been reported to provide reliable postoperative analgesia but not to reliably attenuate the stress response during and after cardiac surgery.[151]

Epidural Opioids

The use of epidural opioids in humans was reported in 1979.[152] Morphine was initially studied; experience with other opioids was subsequently attained. Compared to the intrathecal route, epidural administration is more complex because of the need for the opioids to diffuse through the CSF. Evaluation of the effects of epidural opioids is complicated, since significant serum concentrations may result from this route of administration. The pharmacokinetics and pharmacodynamics of the short-acting lipophilic drugs and the long-acting hydrophilic drugs differ.[153]

Morphine and meperidine have been extensively studied.[154–157] Although both morphine and meperidine produce significant blood levels, the onset and degree of analgesia appear to be related to drug levels.[129,158] In several studies, patients did not achieve sufficient drug serum levels to explain analgesia, yet reported significant and intense pain relief; this has been interpreted as support for the concept of a central site of action.[134,159] In addition, the duration of analgesia of epidurally injected opioids lasted far longer than the elevation of the plasma drug levels.[134,159] When injected, opioids diffuse through the dura into the CSF. This may be accomplished by direct dural membrane penetration or by diffusion through the arachnoid granulations in the dural cuff region.[160,161] Some investigators have proposed uptake of the drug by the vascular system and transfer of the drug via the posterior radicular artery, which has branches that directly penetrate the dorsal horn region.[129] The exact mode of entry into the central nervous system remains unclear. The analgesic effect of epidurally administered morphine appears to be independent of morphine-6-glucuronide (M6G) concentrations. Recent work has demonstrated that neither the transport of M6G across the blood-brain barrier nor the metabolism of spinal morphine to M6G contributes to acute morphine analgesia.[162]

As with subarachnoid injections, there is selectivity of the epidural opioid blockade. The sympathetic nervous system is not altered; vasodilation, vasoconstriction, and increases in heart rate are able to occur appropriately. Motor activity, equilibrium, touch, and perception are unimpaired.[129] Individuals who have received epidural opioids are usually able to ambulate postoperatively without difficulty.

There is a difference in the incidence and degree of severity of side effects when the long-acting versus short-acting opioids are compared. Respiratory depression is the most potentially dangerous of the side effects. The incidence of respiratory depression from epidural morphine is very low, ranging from 0.09 to 0.90%.[126,154,163] The ventilatory response to CO_2 is reduced maximally within the first 6 hours after injection.[159] It appears that debilitated individuals, elderly patients, and larger doses of opioids predispose to respiratory depression. Prior chronic opioid exposure from any route tends to make patients very tolerant to intrathecal or epidural opioid-induced respiratory depression even with utilization of large doses. One case of delayed respiratory depression with meperidine was reported in a series of 9,000.[164] Both epidural fentanyl and sufentanil may cause acute respiratory insufficiency due to their rapid uptake by both the CSF and the systemic circulation.[165,166] However, to the authors' knowledge, delayed respiratory depression from fentanyl has not been reported. This apparent lack of significant respiratory depression is presumably attributable to fentanyl's high lipid solubility, which allows most of the drug to diffuse out of the CSF prior to possible ascension to the brain stem. Opioid withdrawal symptoms may occur in those patients who chronically have received large doses of parenteral agonist opioids and were subsequently given a mixed agonist-antagonist opioid epidurally for postoperative analgesia.[167] Patients with prior exposure to large doses of opioids may need significantly larger doses of epidural narcotics to achieve adequate analgesia.[168]

Nausea and vomiting are real and distressing side effects of epidurally administered opioids.[154] The reported incidence of nausea and vomiting ranges from 15 to 50% for morphine and from 10 to 50% for fentanyl. The incidence and severity of these side effects is somewhat lower than reported with intrathecal opioids.[154,169] Nausea and vomiting associated with morphine is dose dependent, with the larger doses producing a higher incidence.[154] The severity of nausea and vomiting with fentanyl is less than that experienced with morphine and frequently abates in 1 to 2 hours without treatment. Pruritus occurs in 10 to 100% of patients receiving either morphine or fentanyl.[126,153] The pruritus with fentanyl is usually transient and rarely requires treatment.[170] As with intrathecal opioids, the side effects are respiratory depression, nausea, vomiting, and pruritus.[154] Nalbuphine 10 mg subcutaneously has been reported to significantly decrease the intensity of pruritus following epidural fentanyl administration.[171] Many practitioners, therefore, prefer to administer continuous naloxone infusions of 0.2 to 0.4 mg over several hours to potentially prevent the occurrence of nausea, vomiting, or pruritus. The use of naloxone may require increasing the opioid dose to maintain a steady level of analgesia. Urinary retention is another side effect of epidural opioids.[154,172] Obviously, if a patient has a urinary bladder catheter the problem of urinary retention is obviated. If a patient does not have a urinary bladder catheter, however, the possibility of urinary retention must be considered when devising postoperative care plans.

Morphine and meperidine have been commonly used epidurally. Hydromorphone, fentanyl, sufentanil, and alfentanil are also used.[173] The authors are of the opinion that preservative-free solutions should be utilized. Four to 6 mg of morphine is the usual dosage for upper abdominal and thoracic pain[154] (Table 39–5). This dose represents a compromise between rapid onset and intensity, and the incidence and severity of side effects. Detectable onset is approximately 15 to 30 minutes, with complete pain relief in 1 hour. Duration of action is 12 to 18 hours, with additional boluses given as needed.[154,174]

Dosing of Opioids

Epidural morphine may be given as a bolus (0.03 mg/kg) followed by a continuous infusion (0.2 to 1.0 mg/hr) (Fig. 39–1). This technique has been reported to produce superior analgesia on postoperative days 1 and 2 when compared to bolus dosing alone. There were no significant differences in pulmonary function tests or side effects between the groups.[175] Morphine combined with bupivicaine has been reported to be effective for postoperative analgesia and to be superior to parenterally administered morphine. The degree of postoperative pulmonary dysfunction was not altered.[176]

Meperidine, administered as a 50-mg bolus, has an onset time of 5 to 10 minutes, with complete pain relief achieved in 30 minutes. The duration of action of meperidine is 5 to 7 hours.[155] Fentanyl can be administered as a 100-μg bolus with an onset of 5 to 10 minutes and a peak action at 20 minutes.[155,177] The duration of action of fentanyl is approximately 3 hours.[155,177]

Both butorphanol and nalbuphine have been studied. Butorphanol provided equivalent postoperative analgesia when epidural administration and intravenous administration were compared.[178] Nalbuphine given epidurally (10- and 20-mg boluses) was not found to provide ade-

TABLE 39–5
Indications for Acute Pain Management Service Consultation in Hospital Where PCA May Be Prescribed By All Physicians

History of drug abuse
History of chronic pain prior to the acute pain episode
History of prior use of large doses of opioid analgesics
Uncontrolled pain with maximal PCA doses
>2 mg of morphine (or equivalent) bolus dose
>1.5 mg of morphine (or equivalent) bolus in presence of basal infusion of 1 mg/hr morphine (or equivalent)
>8 mg of morphine consistently per hour

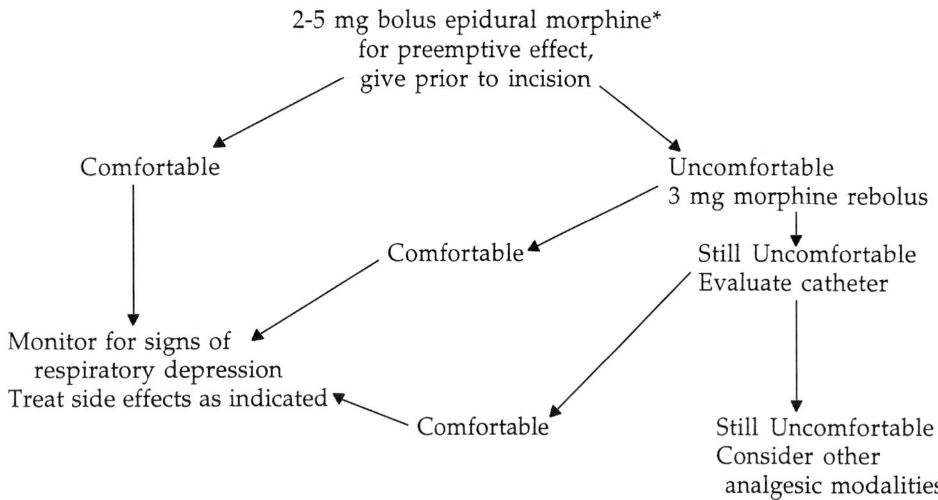

FIGURE **39–1.** Epidural morphine schematic. *Depends on catheter placement: 2 to 3 mg for thoracic placement; 5 mg for lumbar placement. †Consider infusion of 0.4 mg naloxone/liter IV fluids.

quate postoperative analgesia in thoracotomy patients.[179] Ketamine combined with continuous-infusion epidural morphine was reported to improve analgesia and respiratory function postoperatively when compared to morphine alone.[180]

Fentanyl is frequently administered as a continuous infusion due to its short duration of action. Continuous infusion of epidural fentanyl was reported to produce superior analgesia when compared to cryoanalgesia.[181] Lumbar versus thoracic administration of fentanyl was compared with the degree of analgesia being found to be equivalent. The total amount of drug needed to produce adequate analgesia was greater in the lumbar group.[182] Multiple studies have been performed comparing epidurally administered fentanyl to intravenously administered fentanyl. The consensus of investigators demonstrates that analgesia is equivalent at rest[183–187] and at ambulation.[188] Plasma fentanyl levels were also equivalent when studied.[184,185,188] Equivalent analgesia with thoracic epidural fentanyl infusions and lumbar epidural infusions was obtained when these infusions were compared to intravenous fentanyl infusions; however, the plasma fentanyl concentrations were lower in the thoracic and lumbar epidural infusion groups.[186,187] Epidural fentanyl infusions versus PCA intravenous morphine in postthoracotomy patients produced significantly better pain scores.[189]

Sufentanil is generally given as a bolus technique. The commonly employed doses utilized are 15 to 50 μg.[166,190–192] The onset of action is 7 minutes with a peak effect of 15 to 20 minutes. The duration of action of sufentanil is 5 to 6 hours. Little has been published on continuous infusions of sufentanil. One technique of a 50-μg bolus followed by a 0.5 μg/kg/hr continuous infusion of sufentanil demonstrated satisfactory results.[192] There have not been adequate studies to evaluate the safety and proper dosage of repeated bolus or continuous-infusion sufentanil.

Efficacy studies of most opioids administered epidurally have been performed.[126,154,155] All narcotics tested are reported to relieve pain. Epidural morphine, meperidine, fentanyl, and sufentanil have been demonstrated to be superior to intramuscularly administered opioids. Epidural morphine has been shown to produce marked improvement in FEV_1 and in PEFR when compared to intramuscular morphine.[128,193] After cholecystectomies, epidural morphine provides superior analgesia when compared to intercostal local anesthetic blockade.[194] When epidural morphine and epidural bupivacaine were compared to intramuscular morphine, they were shown to improve the FEV_1 and PEFR.[195] Analgesia was comparable in the two groups; however, the side effects of sympathectomy were not evident in the epidural morphine group. The incidence of hypertension is decreased with epidural morphine administration.[196] Compared to intramuscular morphine, patients who received epidural opioids had better outcomes defined as shorter ICU stays and hospital stays than those who received more conventional analgesia techniques.[7]

Ketamine has been injected into the epidural space for the purpose of providing postoperative analgesia. The most effective dose after abdominal surgery appears to be 30 mg of ketamine in 10 ml of saline. This dose provided excellent analgesia in all patients studied. The duration of effect was 9½ hours, with a range of 6 to 24 hours. Although only a small group of patients were studied, there was no cardiovascular instability, respiratory depression, urinary retention, or neurologic deficit. No patients reported hallucinations or abnormal dreams. Ketamine was theorized to be an agonist at central nervous system receptors.[197] The efficacy of ketamine as an epidural analgesic is controversial. While some authors report efficacy with this technique,[198,199] others do not.[200,201] Recent work has demonstrated that although the epidural administration of ketamine may not independently provide analgesia, ketamine does potentiate the analgesia effect of epidurally administered morphine.[202] A recent study has demonstrated that the immediate preoperative administration of epidural morphine and ketamine to patients undergoing upper abdominal surgery was more effective in reducing their postoperative pain when compared to those patients who received the same combination of epidural morphine and ketamine intraoperatively.[203] However, further study is needed to ensure the safety of epidural ketamine administration.[204]

Clonidine, an α_2-adrenergic agonist, has been evaluated for postoperative analgesia. Clonidine produces analgesia after epidural administration by acting on spinal α_2-adrenergic receptors. This is a mechanism that differs from both opioids and local anesthetics.[205] Epidural clonidine has been used successfully to provide relief of pain in both malignant and nonmalignant models.[206,207] Clonidine produced satisfactory analgesia in the postoperative period in patients undergoing abdominal, orthopedic, or perineal surgery. Doses of 100 to 900 μg have been employed. The duration of action of clonidine was 3½ to 5 hours depending on the dosage used. Clonidine was associated with a 15% decrease in mean blood pressure and a 10 to 30% decrease in heart rate in patients who received epidural treatment.[18,208] The addition of clonidine to an epidural opioid enhances the opioid's analgesic effect, which not only provides prolonged analgesia but also potentially lowers the opioid dose and may reduce risk of respiratory depression.[205]

The optimal position of the epidural catheter in terms of proximity to the site of incision and mechanism of action of some administered opioids has been controversial. The position of the epidural catheter has been considered to be important when local anesthetics and/or lipophilic opioids have been utilized; the position of the epidural catheter has been deemed to be less important when the hydrophilic agents have been employed. After thoracotomy, a retrospective analysis found that lumbar epidural morphine provided postoperative analgesia that was indistinguishable from that provided by thoracic epidural morphine with respect to dosage, duration, and quality of analgesia.[209] There have been similar reports concerning fentanyl.[155,156,170,182,209] One group of investigators believe, however, that the lipophilic opioids exert their activities at peripheral receptor sites and that epidural administration offers no benefit over intravenous administration of the drug.[183–188,212] Other investigators believe that the lipophilic opioids have a spinal effect similar to that of morphine. The epidural administration of fentanyl after thoracotomy has been reported to provide only marginal benefit over intravenous or lumbar epidural administration.[213] Other authors, however, have advocated that when the catheter site is considered a spinal analgesic effect is certainly discernible.[214,215]

There is no doubt that continuous epidural infusion of fentanyl produces significant blood levels that are capable of producing analgesia.[218] However, there is a question as to whether they also exert some action centrally, since equivalent analgesia was obtained with lower plasma fentanyl concentrations in the epidural group.[186,187,217] Others contend that the predominant mode of action of epidural fentanyl infusions is achieved by its systemic absorption.[216]

Controversy exists whether an epidural catheter should be placed in a patient who will soon receive heparin and if surgery should be delayed if a "bloody tap" occurs when attempting to perform the epidural. One argument states that if a "bloody tap" were to occur, heparinization should then be postponed until the following day due to the possibility of epidural hematoma formation. The other argument contends that if the catheter is placed preoperatively, even if a bloody tap were to occur there would be ample time for clot formation before heparin administration. Heparin has little effect on an already formed clot; therefore, it would be safe to proceed with the proposed surgical procedure. Two large series were reported on vascular patients in whom epidural or intrathecal catheters were inserted.[210,211] One group of patients was heparinized after catheter insertion and the other group of patients had received oral anticoagulants prior to catheter insertion. The two groups totaled 4,161 patients; there were no patients who experienced catheter-related sequelae. The importance of careful monitoring of the extent of anticoagulation and removal of the catheter when heparin activity is at its lowest was emphasized.[211] Two reviews of large numbers of patients who received central blockade while receiving low-molecular-weight heparins reported no epidural hematomas.[219,220]

However, Vandermeulen et al reported special concerns with regard to low molecular weight heparin usage in regional anesthesia.[221] Vandermeulen recommended that regional anesthesia should not be initiated within 10 to 12 hours of low molecular weight heparin administration and that an epidural catheter should not be removed within 10 to 12 hours of the administration of low molecular weight heparin. Additionally, it was recommended that low molecular weight heparin should not be administered within 2 hours of the performance of a regional anesthetic or placement of an epidural catheter. The longer half-life of low molecular weight heparin appears to be associated with a far greater incidence of epidural hematoma in association with regional anesthesia.

Albeit the very small risk of the development of spinal or epidural hematomas in patients who undergo central regional techniques while concurrently receiving antiplatelet drugs or anticoagulant therapies, the authors nonetheless emphasize that potentially devastating neurologic consequences may ensue.[211,222]

Whether opioids are administered epidurally or spinally, patients tend to be very sensitive to any other opioids or sedatives administered peripherally. The authors advise that other opioids and sedatives generally not be administered when a central acting narcotic is being utilized. If another central nervous system depressant drug is to be utilized, the dosage should be decreased and the patient should be carefully observed for exaggerated effects.

Transdermal Therapeutic Systems

There have been a number of recent developments in transdermal therapeutic systems (TTS) enabling the use of this delivery system with drugs such as nitroglycerin, clonidine, nicotine, and estrogen. Fentanyl transdermal therapeutic systems have been used for postoperative pain relief.[223] The goal of TTS is to obtain a constant and effective plasma concentration of the drug in the blood, thereby eliminating the peak-and-valley effect seen with intramuscular injections,[224] thus yielding a consistent level of analgesia.[225–228] Fentanyl transdermal patches are currently available in 25, 50, 75, and 100-μg/hr modalities.

The TTS consists of a small patch that is applied to an area of thoroughly cleansed skin. The upper chest is the site most frequently chosen, but the forearm has also been used. The TTS system has several compartments: (1) a reservoir in which the drug is stored, (2) a semi-synthetic porous rate-limiting membrane that allows the release of the drug at a constant rate, (3) an adhesive layer that enables the TTS to adhere to the skin with a minimum of pressure and which subsequently permits removal from the skin, and (4) a release liner that serves as a protective material and is peeled away prior to use. The patches are changed every 72 hours.

The fentanyl TTS is applied to the skin; the stratum corneum layer is the principal barrier to fentanyl's diffusion.[229] The fentanyl must diffuse through this part of the dermis to reach the vascular supply. In addition to providing relatively constant serum fentanyl concentrations, the TTS has been reported to offer analgesia lasting up to 3 days with a single patch application.[226] The doses reported to be most effective for major surgery are TTS systems delivering 75 μg/hr and 100 μg/hr.[224–227,230]

With a TTS, the diffusion rate of a drug is essentially equal to the infusion rate of an intravenous delivery system.[229] Continuous infusions or TTS differ from an intramuscular opioid injection in which the diminution of analgesia results mainly from redistribution. Fentanyl is a very lipid-soluble drug and thus diffuses rapidly through the skin.[231] The TTS fentanyl system functions similarly to a continuous intravenous infusion of fentanyl. As in a continuous-infusion system, the severity of the pain and individual patient needs are the determining factors for drug dosage.[229]

Numerous studies have reported that the time for the fentanyl TTS to reach a peak steady serum concentration may be in excess of 24 hours.[224–228] This peak serum concentration correlates with the time required for fentanyl to saturate body compartments. The gradual rise in serum concentration results from redistribution and diffusion resistance prior to saturation. The results are unacceptably low serum concentrations of fentanyl for pain relief for the first 4 to 8 hours. To augment the serum levels during this time, intravenous loading doses ranging from 100 to 300 μg of fentanyl must be given. Comparison between intravenous fentanyl and TTS fentanyl have reported comparable serum drug levels. The serum fentanyl concentrations associated with both analgesia and acceptable respiratory function ranges between 1 and 3 μg/ml.[232] Continuous intravenous administrations of 125 μg/hr of fentanyl have resulted in unacceptable respiratory depression in some patients.[233] Based on this information, 50, 75, and 100-μg/hr TTS fentanyl systems were tested. The 50-μg/hr system did not produce adequate pain relief. The 75-μg/hr TTS fentanyl system provided adequate analgesia and yielded a serum fentanyl concentration of approximately 1.0 μg/ml when used for 24 hours and 1.5 μg/ml when left in place for 72 hours.[226,234] The 100-μg/hr TTS fentanyl yielded a serum concentration of 1.91 ± 2.15 μg/ml after 24 hours.[226,227] When the 75-μg/hr TTS fentanyl system was replaced daily for 3 days, the serum fentanyl plasma levels rose to 2.7 ± 2.05 μg/ml, which was associated with a higher risk of respiratory depression.[225] Intramuscular morphine has been compared to fentanyl TTS for postoperative pain relief after abdominal surgery. Those patients who had received fentanyl TTS had lower pain scores and patient satisfaction was high. Ninety per cent of the patients in this study who had previous surgery felt that the TTS system provided superior analgesia to intramuscular opioids they had received in the past.[225,226]

Morphine augmentation may be required upon emergence from anesthesia, but the total morphine dose may be reduced when compared to those patients without a TTS system. The average patient with a fentanyl TTS patch in place prior to abdominal surgery required 11.5 mg morphine in the first 24 hours, 11.2 mg in the second 24 hours, and 10.6 mg in the third.[225,226] A review of similar cases without TTS fentanyl revealed a morphine requirement of approximately 30 mg/day during each of the first 3 postoperative days. Patient satisfaction is high, with 80 to 90% of patients rating this technique superior to intramuscular morphine.[226] A study evaluating possible adverse respiratory effects of fentanyl TTS reported that the 100-μg/hr system posed a risk for respiratory depression and recommended that it not be used for routine postoperative pain relief.[235] A randomized, placebo-controlled, double-blind study of 81 patients undergoing total abdominal hysterectomy studied postoperative analgesia provided by 25, 50, 75, and 100-μg/hr fentanyl TTS and found a depression of respiratory rates with the higher dosage systems.[236]

Even though the TTS system has been reported to be efficacious, there are several potential limitations to the widespread use of this modality for postoperative pain relief. First, a long time is required to reach steady-state serum concentrations.[228] Second, once a steady-state serum level is achieved, a fixed serum drug level results that will decrease very slowly when the patch is removed. Thus, if this drug level were to cause adverse pharmacodynamic effects, the time to reach a nontoxic level might be prolonged. This limitation is compounded by the fact that analgesic needs vary significantly from day to day in the postoperative state. With other techniques available, it would seem that TTS fentanyl as presently available might be a suboptimal choice for postoperative pain control.

Epidural PCA

PCA has been extended to include this modality in conjunction with epidurally administered drugs. A wide variety of agents have been successfully employed for a wide variety of surgical procedures. PCA-E (patient controlled analgesia-epidurally) utilizing hydromorphone in general surgery patients was reported to offer equivalent analgesia with lower total dosage requirements when compared to continuous epidural infusions.[237] PCA-E was compared with continuous epidural infusion utilizing bupivicaine 0.125% with fentanyl 1 μg/ml. Analgesia and dosage uses were equivalent.[238] PCA-E has been studied in labor and delivery patients and has been reported to be effective.[239,240] Bupivicaine 0.125% alone[239] and bupivicaine 0.125% with fentanyl 2 μg/ml[240] were administered with PCA-E and compared to standard continuous infusions. Analgesia was deemed equivalent; however, the PCA-E group utilized less drug to achieve the same degree of analgesia.

Transcutaneous Electrical Nerve Stimulation

TENS has been employed to provide postoperative analgesia. Electrodes are placed along each side of the surgical incision. Electrical current is then delivered through the electrodes. Once the patient is awake and able to communicate, electric current can be adjusted until the patient is comfortable. Patients describe a feeling of tingling in the area of the incision during stimulation. Generally, electrodes are left in place for 48 to 72 hours.[241] TENS is a low-risk, nontoxic treatment.

The mechanism of TENS analgesia is unknown. TENS may interfere with small-fiber nociceptive input by activating larger fiber input to the spinal cord.[241,242] It may also augment the activity of descending pain inhibitory pathways and increase levels of naturally occurring analgesics such as enkephalins and β-endorphins.[6]

The effectiveness of TENS for postoperative analgesia has been investigated in a study in which a control group did not receive TENS, a second group had electrodes placed as a sham stimulus, and a third group received TENS after upper abdominal surgery.

The TENS group demonstrated a significantly lessened requirement for opioid analgesics in the postoperative period than did patients in the other groups. Additionally, superior pulmonary functions were measured and less hypoxia was noted in the patients who had received TENS.[6] Thoracotomy patients who had received TENS therapy reported lower pain scores in the first 24 hours postoperatively and had shorter recovery room stays and tolerated chest physiotherapy better than those patients in whom sham stimulators were applied.[243] Another study involving thoracotomy patients compared TENS with intercostal nerve cryoanalgesia. The TENS-treated patients had significantly better pulmonary function studies on the first postoperative day. Both methods were considered to have some analgesic efficacy.[244] The role of TNS therapy for the management of postthoracotomy pain has been deemed to be uncertain.[245] A recent study evaluated the efficacy of TENS for the provision of postoperative thoracotomy pain in a series of 324 patients who had undergone various types of surgical procedures. The patients were divided into three groups: control, TENS, and placebo TENS. The results indicated the efficacy of TENS treatment only for mild to moderate pain. TENS, in this series, was not deemed to be an effective modality for the treatment of severe postoperative thoracotomy pain.

Acute Pain Services

Acute pain services have been developed in many hospitals to expedite the provision of the more complex postoperative pain entities such as epidural opioids and PCA as well as in recognition of the benefits of such services.[11] While many models exist to fulfill the needs of individual institutions, in general, acute pain management pain services exist to provide consultative, educational, clinical, and administrative resources. In many institutions, PCA pumps are available for use by the entire medical staff. The authors suggest the establishment of guidelines formulated by appropriate contributors prior to the initiation of such unlimited utilization of PCA technology. The acute pain service might assist in the care of patients whose pain control is found to be suboptimal following these suggested guidelines and protocols. The acute pain service might additionally offer assistance in the care of difficult patients such as those with a history of a drug abuse or addiction disorder.

The hospital's nursing service must be an integral component of the pain team. Without the full commitment of the nursing services, the program will not be successful. The authors suggest that nursing representatives work closely with directors of the acute pain service to develop educational programs that will promote the successful utilization of PCA, peripheral and central analgesic techniques, as well as other indicated modalities. We suggest that this education include but not be limited to study of appropriate aspects of anatomy, nociceptor pathways, spinal opioid actions, and side effects and complications of the various techniques to be utilized. The nursing staff is invaluable in caring for acute pain management service patients by assessing the effectiveness of an analgesic regimen as well as monitoring them to potentially forestall the emergence of adverse consequences of treatment. Some authors consider an untrained nursing staff to be a contraindication to the use of epidural opioids and PCA.[246]

Additional valuable members of the acute pain service are clinical nurse specialists, physician assistants, pharmacists, and administrators. Commonly a physician member of the team, usually an anesthesiologist, joined by other members of the pain service will see patients on a daily basis to review their care and change dosages and techniques as deemed necessary. If patients are receiving PCA or intraspinal opioids, the acute pain service should be responsible for all analgesic and sedative orders to optimize patient safety. Under most protocols, once therapy prescribed by the acute pain service is discontinued, care of the patient returns to the referring physician. It has been suggested that this transition may occur when the patient obtains satisfactory pain relief with the utilization of oral analgesics.[10] Therefore, it is necessary that excellent communication exists between the referring physician and the acute pain service so that the transition of analgesic care will be facilitated. Another suggested approach is for the referring surgeon to write analgesic orders at the conclusion of the operation that are to take effect once the acute pain service is no longer involved in the patient's care.[246]

Standard protocols for the various types of analgesic agents and techniques to be utilized should be available to individuals involved in the patient's care. These protocols should discuss the responsibility of the acute pain service as well as the attending surgeon. Nursing protocols must be included. These should address the importance of frequent, ongoing observation of the patient. The patient's level of pain relief as well as their level of sedation are extremely important to document at the time of each nursing visit. Good nursing observation of the patient has been reported to be superior to the use of apnea monitors in detecting respiratory depression.[73,247] Sedation has been noted to be a warning sign for the potential development of respiratory depression when intrathecal opioids are used.[248] Protocols should clearly outline criteria for discontinuing treatment and for administering antagonists. Anesthesiologists who are to be responsible for the intraoperative care of the patient should take the postoperative pain management plan into consideration when planning intraoperative anesthetic management. Finally, a determination should be made of which areas of the hospital are appropriate for the administration of the various acute pain management techniques. While some institutions still require patients receiving epidural opioids to be patients in an intensive care unit or intermediate intensive care unit, many are now allowing these patients to be cared for on general surgical floors. A recent study has reiterated the desirability of protocol establishment when planning for the provision of acute pain management services.[163] Excellent reference sources are available to facilitate such planning.[1,9,10]

References

1. Acute Pain Management Guideline Panel: Acute pain management: Operative or medical procedures and trauma. Clinical practice guideline. AHCPR Pub. No. 92-0032. Rockville, MD, Agency for Health Care Policy and Research, Public Health Service, U.S. Department of Health and Human Services. Feb. 1992.
2. Cuschieri RJ, Morran CG, Howie JC, McArdle CS: Postoperative pain and pulmonary complication: Comparison of three analgesic regimens. Br J Surg 72:495, 1985.
3. Shulman M, Sandler AN, Bradley JW, et al: Postthoracotomy pain and pulmonary function following epidural and systemic morphine. Anesthesiology 61:569, 1984.
4. Jayr G, Thomas H, Rey A, et al: Postoperative pulmonary complications: Epidural analgesia using bupivacaine and opiates vs. parenteral opiates. Anesthesiology 78:666, 1993.
5. Rutberg H, Hakanson E, Anderberg B, et al: Effects of extradural administration of morphine, or bupivacaine, on the endocrine response to upper abdominal surgery. Br J Anaesth 56:233, 1984.
6. Ali J, Yaffe CS, Serrette C: The effects of transcutaneous electric nerve stimulation on postoperative pain and pulmonary function. Surgery 89:507, 1981.
7. Yeager MP, Glass DD, Neff RK, Brinck-Johnsen T: Epidural anesthesia and analgesia in high risk surgical patients. Anesthesiology 66:729, 1987.
8. Turman K, McCarthy R, March R, et al: Effects of epidural anesthesia and analgesia on coagulation and outcome after major vascular surgery. Anesth Analg 73:696, 1991.
9. Practice Guidelines for Acute Pain Management in the Perioperative Setting: A Report by the American Society of Anesthesiologists Task Force on Pain Management, Acute Pain Section. Anesthesiology 82:1071, 1995.
10. Ready BL, et al: Management of Acute Pain: A Practical Guide. IASP Publications, Seattle, WA, 1992.
11. Warfield CA, Kahn CH: Acute pain management programs in U.S. hospitals and experiences and attitudes among U.S. adults. Anesthesiology 83:1090, 1995.
12. Raja SN, Meyer RA, Campbell JN: Peripheral mechanisms of somatic pain. Anesthesiology 68:571, 1988.
13. Woolf C: Evidence for a central component of post-injury pain hypersensitivity. Nature 306:686, 1983.
14. Woolf C, Thompson S: The induction and maintenance of central stimulation is dependent on N-methyl-D-aspartic acid receptor activation: Implications for treatment of post-injury pain hypersensitivity status. Pain 44:293, 1991.
15. Go VLW, Yaksh TL: Release of substance P from the cat spinal cord. J Physiol 391:141, 1987.
16. Piercey MF, Schroeder LA, Folkers K, et al: Sensory and motor functions of spinal cord substance P. Science 214:1361, 1981.
17. Jessell TM, Iversen LL: Opioid analgesics inhibit substance P release from rat trigeminal nucleus. Nature 286:549, 1977.
18. Eisenach JC, Lysak SZ, Viscomi CM: Epidural clonidine analgesia following surgery: Phase I. Anesthesiology 71:640, 1989.
19. Hammond DL, Tyce GM, Yaksh TL: Efflux of 5-hydroxytryptamine and noradrenaline into spinal cord superfusates during stimulation of the rat medulla. J Physiol 359:151, 1985.
20. Richardson BP, Engel G, Donatsch P, Stadler PA: Identification of serotonin M-receptor subtypes and their specific blockage by a new class of drugs. Nature 316:126, 1985.
21. Mense S: Sensitization of group IV muscle receptors to bradykinin by 5-hydroxytryptamine and prostaglandin E2. Brain Res 225:95, 1981.
22. Taenzer P, Melzack R, Jeans ME: Influence of physiologic factors on postoperative pain, mood and analgesic requirements. Pain 24:331, 1986.
23. Wallace LM: Surgical patients' expectations of pain and discomfort: Does accuracy of expectations minimize post-surgical pain and distress? Pain 22:363, 1985.
24. Scott LE, Clum GA, Peoples JB: Preoperative predictors of postoperative pain. Pain 15:283, 1983.
25. Dahl JB, Kehlet H: The value of pre-emptive analgesia in treatment of postoperative pain. Br J Anaesth 70:434, 1993.
26. Woolf CJ, Chung MS: Preemptive analgesia—treating postoperative pain by preventing the establishment of central sensitization. Anesth Analg 77:362, 1993.
27. Woolf CJ, Wall PD: Relative effectiveness of C primary afferent fibers of different origins in evoking a prolonged facilitation of the flexor reflex in the rat. J Neurosci 6:1433, 1986.
28. Wall PD, Woolf CJ: Muscle but not cutaneous C-afferent input produces prolonged increases in the excitability of the flexion reflex in the rat. J Physiol 356:443, 1984.
29. Davies SN, Lodge D: Evidence for involvement of N-methyl aspartate receptors in "wind-up" of class 2 neurones in the dorsal horn of the rat. Brain Res 424:402, 1967.
30. Dubner R: Pain and hyperalgesia following tissue injury: New mechanisms and new treatments. Pain 44:213, 1991.
31. Kissin I: Preemptive analgesia—why its effect is not always obvious. Anesthesiology 84:1015, 1996.
32. Crile GW: The kinetic theory of shock and its prevention through anoci-association (shockless operation). Lancet 185:7, 1913.
33. McQuay HJ, Carroll D, Moore RA: Postoperative orthopaedic pain—the effect of opiate premedication and local anaesthetic blocks. Pain 33:291, 1988.
34. Jebeles JA, Reilly JS, Gutierrz JF, et al: The effect of pre-incisional infiltration of tonsils with bupivacaine on the pain following tonsillectomy under general anesthesia. Pain 47:305, 1991.
35. Tverskoy M, Cozacov C, Ayache M, et al: Postoperative pain after inguinal herniorrhaphy with different types of anesthesia. Anesth Analg 70:29, 1990.

36. Ejlersen E, Andersen HB, Eliasen K, Mogensen T: A comparison between preincisional and postincisional lidocaine infiltration and postoperative pain. Anesth Analg 74:495, 1992.
37. Dierking GW, Dahl JB, Kanstrup J, et al: Effect of pre- vs postoperative inguinal field block on postoperative pain after herniorrhaphy. Br J Anaesth 68:344, 1992.
38. Katz J, Kavanagh B, Sandler A, et al: Preemptive analgesia: Clinical evidence of neuroplasticity contributing to postoperative pain. Anesthesiology 77:439, 1992.
39. Dahl JB, Hansen BL, Huortso NC, et al: Influence of timing on the effect of continuous extradural analgesia with bupivacaine and morphine after major abdominal surgery. Br J Anaesth 69: 4, 1992.
40. Pryle B, Vanner R, Enriquez N, Reynolds F: Can pre-emptive lumbar epidural blockade reduce postoperative pain following lower abdominal surgery? Anaesthesia 48:120, 1993.
41. Seltzer J, Greek R, Maurer P, et al: The preemptive analgesic effect of regional anesthesia for shoulder surgery. Anesthesiology 79:A815, 1993.
42. Rockemann MG, Seeling W, Bischof C, et al: Prophylactic use of epidural mepivacaine/morphine, systemic diclofenac, and metamizole reduces postoperative morphine consumption after major abdominal surgery. Anesthesiology 84:1027, 1996.
43. Roytblat L, Kurotkoruchko A, Katz J, et al: Postoperative pain: The effect of low-dose ketamine in addition to general anesthesia. Anesth Analg 77:1161, 1993.
44. Tverskoy M, Oz Y, Osakson A, et al: Preemptive effect of fentanyl and ketamine on postoperative pain and wound hyperalgesia. Anesth Analg 78:205, 1994.
45. Abram S, Yaksh T: Morphine, but not inhalation anesthesia blocks postinjury facilitation. Anesthesiology 78:713, 1993.
46. Carr DB: Preemptive analgesia implies prevention. Anesthesiology 85:1499, 1996.
47. Pederson JL, Crawford ME, Dahl JB, et al: Effect of preemptive nerve block on inflammation and hyperalgesia after human thermal injury. Anesthesiology 84:1020, 1996.
48. Bennett RL, Batenhorst RL, Graves D, et al: Morphine titration in postoperative laparotomy patients using patient controlled analgesia. Curr Ther Res 32:45, 1982.
49. Austin KL, Stapleton JV, Mather LE: Multiple intramuscular injections: A major source of variability in analgesic response to meperidine. Pain 8:47, 1980.
50. Austin KL, Stapleton JV, Mather LE: Relationship between blood and meperidine concentrations and analgesic response: A preliminary report. Anesthesiology 53:460, 1980.
51. Vache E: Inadequate treatment of pain in hospitalized patients. N Engl J Med 307:55, 1982.
52. Woodsmith FG, Stewart HC, Butterworth HC: Drugs in Anesthetic Practice. London, 1962, p 97.
53. Cohen FL: Post-surgical pain relief: Patient's status and nurses' medication choices. Pain 9:265, 1980.
54. Lim AT, Edis G, Kranz H, et al: Postoperative pain control: Contribution of psychologic factors and transcutaneous electrical stimulation. Pain 17:179, 1983.
55. Bennett RL, Batenhorst RL, Bivins BA, et al: Patient controlled analgesia: A new concept in postoperative pain relief. Ann Surg 195:700, 1982.
56. Forrest WH, Smethurst PW, Kienitz ME: Self-administration of intravenous analgesics. Anesthesiology 33:336, 1970.
57. Sechzer PH: Studies in pain with the analgesic-demand system. Anesth Analg 50:1, 1971.
58. Keeri-Szanto M: Apparatus for demand analgesia. Can Anaesth Soc J 18:581, 1971.
59. Parker RK, Holtman B, White PF: Patient controlled analgesia: Does a concurrent opioid infusion improve pain management after surgery? JAMA 266:1947, 1991.
60. MacKenzie R, Rudy T, Tantisura B: Comparison of PCA and PCA with continuous infusion on pain relief and quality of sleep. Anesthesiology 73:A787, 1990.
61. Vinik HR, Hammonds W, Kissin LI: Patient controlled analgesia combined with continuous infusion. Anesth Analg 70:S418, 1990.
62. Sinatra R, Chung KS, Silverman DG, et al: An evaluation of morphine and oxymorphone administered via patient controlled analgesia or PCA basal infusion in post caesarean delivery patients. Anesthesiology 71:502, 1989.
63. Sinatra RS, Lodge K, Sibert K, et al: A comparison of morphine, meperidine, and oxymorphone as utilized in patient-controlled analgesia following cesarean delivery. Anesthesiology 70:585, 1989.
64. White PF: Use of patient-controlled analgesia for management of acute pain. JAMA 259:243, 1988.
65. Graves DA, Foster TS, Batenhorst RL, et al: Patient-controlled analgesia. Ann Intern Med 99:360, 1983.
66. White WD, Pearce DJ, Norman J: Postoperative analgesia: A comparison of intravenous on-demand fentanyl with epidural bupivacaine. Br Med J 2:166, 1979.
67. Rosenberg H, Heino A, Scheinin B: Comparison of intramuscular analgesia, intercostal block, epidural morphine and on-demand-iv-fentanyl in the control of pain after upper abdominal surgery. Acta Anaesthesiol Scand 28:603, 1984.
68. Wheatley RG, Somerville ID, Sapsford DJ, Jones JG: Postoperative hypoxaemia: Comparison of extradural, I.M., and patient-controlled opioid analgesia. Br J Anaesth 64:267, 1990.
69. Tamsen A, Hartvig P, Fagerlund C, Dahlstrome B: Patient-controlled analgesia therapy, Part 2: Individual analgesic demands and analgesic plasma concentrations of pethidine in postoperative pain. Clin Pharmacokinet 7:164, 1982.
70. Burns JW, Hodsman NBA, McLintock TTC, et al: The influence of patient characteristics on the requirements for postoperative analgesia: A reassessment using patient-controlled analgesia. Anaesthesia 34:2, 1989.
71. Tamsen A, Hartbig P, Dahlstrome B, et al: Patient controlled analgesic therapy in the early postoperative period. Acta Anaesth Scand 23:462, 1979.
72. White PF: Mishaps with patient controlled analgesia. Anesthesiology 66:81, 1987.
73. Hammonds WD, Hord HA: Additional comments regarding an anesthesiology-based postoperative pain service. Anesthesiology 69:139, 1988.
74. Bennett RL, Batenhorst RL, Graves AD: Variations in postop analgesia requirements in the morbidly obese following gastric bypass surgery. Pharmacotherapy 2:43, 1982.
75. Bennett RL, Batenhorst RL, Foster TS, et al: Postoperative pulmonary function with patient controlled analgesia. Anesth Analg 61:171, 1982.
76. DeJong RH: Physiology and Pharmacology of Local Anesthetics. Springfield, IL, Charles C Thomas, 1970, p 14.
77. DeJong RH, Ronfeld RA, DeRosa RA: Cardiovascular effects of convulsant and superconvulsant doses of amide local anesthetics. Anesth Analg 61:3, 1982.
78. Prentiss JE: Cardiac arrest following caudal anesthesia. Anesthesiology 50:51, 1979.
79. Albright GA: Cardiac arrest following regional anesthesia with etidocaine or bupivacaine. Anesthesiology 51:285, 1979.
80. Marx GF: Cardiotoxicity of local anesthetics—the plot thickens. Anesthesiology 60:3, 1984.
81. Thomas DFM, Lambert WG, Lloyd Williams K: The direct perfusion of surgical wounds with local anesthetic solution: An approach to postoperative pain? Ann R Coll Surg Engl 65:226, 1983.
82. Cassuto J, Wallin G, Hogstrom S, et al: Inhibition of postoperative pain by continuous low dose intravenous infusion of lidocaine. Anesth Analg 64:971, 1985.
83. Galindo A, Hernandes J, Benavides O, et al: Quality of spinal extradural anesthesia: The influence of the spinal nerve root diameter. Br J Anaesth 47:41, 1975.
84. Buckley FP, Simpson BR: Acute traumatic and postoperative pain management. In Cousins MJ, Bridenbaugh PO (eds): Neuronal Blockade in Clinical Anesthesia and Management of Pain. Philadelphia, JB Lippincott Co, 1980, p 586.
85. Bromage PR, Pettigrew RT, Crowell DE: Tachyphylaxis in epidural anesthesia: I. Augmentation and decal of local anesthetics. J Clin Pharmacol 9:30, 1969.
86. Reynolds F, Taylor G: Maternal and neonatal blood concentrations of bupivicaine. A comparison with lignocaine during continuous extradural analgesia. Anaesthesia 25:14, 1970.
87. Renck H, Edstrom H: Thoracic epidural analgesia III—prolongation in the early postoperative period by intermittent injections of etidocaine with adrenalin. Acta Anaesthesiol Scand 20:104, 1976.

88. Stanton-Hicks M: Cardiovascular effects of extradural anaesthesia. Br J Anaesth 47:253, 1975.
89. Bonica JJ, Akamatsu TJ, Berges PU, et al: Circulatory effects of peridural block: II. Effects of epinephrine. Anesthesiology 34: 514, 1971.
90. Kennedy WF, Sawyer TK, Gerbershagen HU, et al: Systemic cardiovascular and renal hemodynamic alterations during peridural anesthesia normal man. Anesthesiology 31:414, 1969.
91. Craig DV: Postoperative recovery of pulmonary functions. Anesth Analg 60:46, 1981.
92. Diament ML, Palmer KN: Postoperative changes in gas tensions of arterial blood and in ventilatory function. Lancet 2:180, 1966.
93. Pecora DV: Predictability of the effects of abdominal and thoracic surgery upon pulmonary function. Ann Surg 170:101, 1969.
94. Egbert LD, Laver MB, Benedixen HH: Surg Gynecol Obstet 115:295, 1962.
95. Simpson BR, Parkhouse J, Marshall R, Lambrechts W: Extradural analgesia and the prevention of postoperative respiratory complications. Br J Anaesth 33:628, 1961.
96. Drummund GB, Littlewood DG: Respiratory effects of extradural analgesia after lower abdominal surgery. Br J Anaesth 49: 999, 1977.
97. Spence AA, Smith G: Postoperative analgesia and lung dysfunction: A comparison of morphine with extradural block. Br J Anaesth 43:144, 1971.
98. Holmdahl MH, Modig J: The role of regional block versus parenteral analgesics in patient management with special emphasis on the treatment of postoperative pain. Br J Anaesth 47:264, 1975.
99. Pflug AE, Murphy TM, Butler SH, Tucker GT: The effects of postoperative peridural analgesia on pulmonary therapy and pulmonary complications. Anesthesiology 41:8, 1974.
100. Hurley RJ, Lambert DH: Continuous spinal anesthesia with a micro-catheter technique: Preliminary experience. Anesth Analg 70:97, 1990.
101. Underwood RJ: Continuous spinal anesthesia in fiscal status group IV patients. Anesth Analg 47:18, 1968.
102. Rigler ML, Drasner K, Krajcie TC, et al: Cauda equina syndrome after continuous spinal anesthesia. Anesth Analg 72:276, 1992.
103. FDA Safety Alert: Cauda equina syndrome associated with use of small-bore catheters in continuous spinal anesthesia. May 29, 1992, Dept. of Health and Human Services, Food and Drug Administration, Rockville, MD 20857.
104. Kaplan JA, Miller ED, Gallagher EG: Postoperative analgesia for thoracotomy patients. Anesth Analg 54:773, 1975.
105. Galway JE, Caves PK, Dundee JW: Effect of intercostal nerve blockade during operation on lung function and the relief of pain following thoracotomy. Br J Anaesth 47:730, 1975.
106. Delilkan AE, Lee CK, Yong NK, Ganendran A: Postoperative local anesthesia for thoracotomy with direct bupivacaine intercostal blocks. Anaesthesia 28:561, 1973.
107. Faust RJ, Nauss LE: Post thoracotomy intercostal block comparison of its effect on pulmonary functions with those of intramuscular meperidine. Anesth Analg 55:542, 1976.
108. Braid DP, Scott DB: The systemic absorption of local analgesic drugs. Br J Anaesth 37:394, 1965.
109. Baxter AD, Jennings FO, Harris RS, et al: Continuous intercostal blockade after cardiac surgery. Br J Anaesth 59:162, 1987.
110. Safran D, Kuhlman G, Orhant EE, et al: Continuous intercostal blockade with lidocaine after thoracic surgery: Clinical and pharmacokinetic study. Anesth Analg 70:345, 1990.
111. Reiestad F, Stromskag KE: Interpleural catheter in the management of postoperative pain. A preliminary report. Reg Anesth 11:89, 1986.
112. Seltzer JL, Larijani GE, Goldberg ME, Marr AT: Intrapleural bupivacaine—a kinetic and dynamic evaluation. Anesthesiology 67:798, 1987.
113. Rosenberg PH, Scheinin BA, Lepantalo MJ, Lindfors O: Continuous intrapleural infusion of bupivacaine for analgesia after thoracotomy. Anesthesiology 67:811, 1978.
114. Brismar B, Pettersson N, Tokics L, et al: Postoperative analgesia with intrapleural administration of bupivacaine-adrenalin. Acta Anaesthesiol Scand 31:515, 1987.
115. Frank ED, McKay W, Gallo JP, Rocco A: Interpleural bupivacaine for postoperative analgesia following cholecystectomy: A randomized prospective study. Reg Anesth 15:26, 1990.
116. VadeBoncouer TR, Riegler FX, Gautt RS, Weinberg GL: A randomized double blind comparison of the effects of interpleural bupivacaine and saline on morphine requirements and pulmonary functions after cholecystectomy. Anesthesiology 71:339, 1989.
117. Seltzer JL, Bell SD, Moritz H, Cantillo J: A double blind comparison of intrapleural bupivacaine and epidural fentanyl for post thoracotomy pain. Anesthesiology 71:A665, 1989.
118. Raffin L, Fletcher D, Sperandio M, et al: Interpleural infusion of 2% lidocaine with 1:200,000 epinephrine for postthoracotomy analgesia. Anesth Analg 79(2):328, 1994.
119. Kambam JR, Handte RE, Parris WC, Hammon J: Intrapleural anesthesia for post thoracotomy pain relief. Reg Anesth 12:106, 1987.
120. Chan EW, Arthur GR, Ferrante FM: Intrapleural bupivacaine administration for pain relief following thoracotomy. Reg Anesth 13:70, 1988.
121. Symreng T, Gomez MN, Rossi N: Intrapleural bupivacaine v saline after thoracotomy—effects of pain and lung function—a double blind study. J Cardiothorac Anesth 3:144, 1989.
122. Ryan DW: Accidental intravenous injection of bupivacaine: A complication of obstetrical epidural anesthesia. Br J Anaesth 45: 907, 1983.
123. Stromskag KE, Reiestad F, Holmqvist EL, Ogenstad S: Intrapleural administration of 0.25%, 0.375%, and 0.5% bupivacaine with epinephrine after cholecystectomy. Anesth Analg 64:430, 1988.
124. Aguilar JL, Llamazares JF, Montero A, Lopez FV: Bilateral interpleural injection of local anesthetics. Reg Anesth 14:93, 1989.
125. Wang JK, Nauss LE, Thomas JE: Pain relief by intrathecally applied morphine in man. Anesthesiology 50:149, 1979.
126. Rawal N, Arner S, Gustafsson LL, Allvin R: Present state of extradural and intrathecal opioid analgesia in Sweden. A nationwide follow-up survey. Br J Anaesth 59:791, 1987.
127. Lanz E, Theiss D, Riess W, Sommer U: Epidural morphine for postoperative analgesia: A double blind study. Anesth Analg 61: 236, 1982.
128. Shulman M, Sandler AN, Bradley JW, et al: Post thoracotomy pain in pulmonary function following epidural and systemic morphine. Anesthesiology 61:569, 1984.
129. Cousins MJ, Mather LE: Intrathecal and epidural administration of opioids. Anesthesiology 61:276, 1984.
130. Yaksh TL: Spinal opiate analgesia: Characteristics and principles of actions. Pain 81:293, 1981.
131. Sjostrom S, Tamsen A, Persson MP, Hartvig P: Pharmacokinetics of intrathecal morphine and meperidine in humans. Anesthesiology 67:889, 1987.
132. McQuay HJ, Sullivan A, Smallman K, Dickenson A: Intrathecal opioids, potency and lipophilicity. Pain 36:111, 1989.
133. Katz J, Nelson W: Intrathecal morphine for postoperative pain relief. Reg Anesth 6:1, 1981.
134. Chauvin M, Samii K, Schermann JM, et al: Plasma pharmacokinetics of morphine after IM, extradural and intrathecal administration. Br J Anaesth 54:843, 1982.
135. Gjessing J, Tomlin PJ: Postoperative pain control with intrathecal morphine. Anaesthesia 36:268, 1981.
136. Cousins MJ, Mather LE, Glynn CJ, et al: Selective spinal analgesia. Lancet 1:1141, 1979.
137. Moore A, Bullingham R, McQuay H, et al: Spinal fluid kinetics of morphine and heroin. Clin Pharm Ther 35:40, 1984.
138. Nordberg G, Hedner T, Mellstrand T, Dahlstrom B: Pharmacokinetic aspects of intrathecal morphine analgesia. Anesthesiology 60:448, 1984.
139. Glynn CJ, Mather LE, Cousins MJ, et al: Spinal narcotics and respiratory depression. Lancet 2:356, 1979.
140. Liolios A, Andersen FH: Selective spinal anesthesia. Lancet 2: 357, 1979.
141. Gray JR, Fromme GA, Nauss LE, et al: Intrathecal morphine for post thoracotomy pain. Anesth Analg 65:873, 1986.
142. Samii K, Chauvin M, Viars P: Postoperative spinal analgesia with morphine. Br J Anaesth 53:817, 1981.

143. Sidi A, Davidson JT, Behar M, Olshwang D: Spinal narcotics and central nervous system depression. Anaesthesia 36:1044, 1981.
144. Davies GK, Cleaver CL, James TL: CNS depression from intrathecal morphine. Anesthesiology 52:280, 1980.
145. Davies GK, Cleaver CL, James TL: Respiratory depression after intrathecal narcotics. Anaesthesia 35:1080, 1980.
146. Odoom JA, Sih IL: Respiratory depression after intrathecal morphine. Anesth Analg 61:70, 1982.
147. Brookshire GL, Shnider SM, Abboud TK, et al: Effects of naloxone on the mother and neonate after intrathecal morphine for labor analgesia. Anesthesiology 59:A417, 183.
148. Dailey PA, Brookshire GL, Shnider SM, et al: The effects of naloxone associated with intrathecal use of morphine in labor. Anesth Analg 64:658, 1985.
149. Leighton BL, DeSimone CA, Norris MC, Ben-David B: Intrathecal narcotics for labor revisited: Fentanyl 25 mcg and morphine 0.25 mg provide rapid, profound analgesia. Anesthesiology 69.A680, 1988.
150. Sudarshan G, Browne BL, Mathews JN, Conacher ID: Intrathecal fentanyl for post-thoracotomy pain. Br J Anaesth 75(1):19, 1995.
151. Chaney MA, Furry PA, Fluder EM, Slogoff S: Intrathecal morphine for coronary artery bypass grafting and early extubation. Anesth Analg 84:241, 1997.
152. Behar M, Olshwang D, Magora F, Davidson JT: Epidural morphine in the treatment of pain. Lancet 1:527, 1979.
153. Sjostrom S, Hartvig P, Persson P, Tamsen A: Pharmacokinetics of epidural morphine and meperidine in humans. Anesthesiology 67:877, 1987.
154. Stensseth R, Sellevold O, Breivik H: Epidural morphine for postoperative pain: Experience in 1,085 patients. Acta Anaesthesiol Scand 29:148, 1985.
155. Torda TA, Pybus DA: Comparison of four narcotic analgesics for extradural analgesia. Br J Anaesth 54:291, 1982.
156. Rutter DV, Skewes DG, Morgan M: Extradural opiates for postoperative analgesia. A double blind comparison of pethidine, fentanyl and morphine. Br J Anaesth 53:915, 1981.
157. van den Hoogen RH, Colpaert FC: Epidural and subcutaneous morphine, meperidine (pethidine), fentanyl and sufentanil in the rat: Analgesic and other in vivo pharmacologic effects. Anesthesiology 66:186, 1987.
158. Tamsen A, Sjostrom S, Hartvig P, et al: CSF and plasma kinetics of morphine and meperidine after epidural administration. Anesthesiology 54:A196, 1983.
159. Bromage PR, Camporesi EM, Durant PA, Nielsen CH: Influence of epinephrine as an adjunct to epidural morphine. Anesthesiology 58:257, 1983.
160. Glynn CJ, Mather LE, Cousins MJ, et al: Peridural meperidine in humans: Analgesic response, pharmacokinetics, and transmission into CSF. Anesthesiology 55:520, 1981.
161. Moore RA, Bullingham RE, McQuay HJ, et al: Dural permeability to narcotics: In vitro determination and application to extradural administration. Br J Anaesth 54:1117, 1982.
162. Kalman S, Metcalf KM, Eintrei C: Morphine, morphine-6-glucuronide, and morphine-3-glucuronide in cerebrospinal fluid and plasma after epidural administration of morphine. Reg Anesth 22(2):131, 1997.
163. Rawal N, Allvin R: Epidural and intrathecal opioids for postoperative pain management in Europe—a 17 nation questionnaire study of selected hospitals. Euro Pain Study Group on Acute Pain. Acta Anaesthesiol Scand (9):1119, 1996.
164. Brownridge P: Epidural and intrathecal opiates for postop pain relief. Anaesthesia 38:74, 1983.
165. Klepper ID, Sherrill DL, Boetger CL, Bromage PR: Analgesic and respiratory effects of extradural sufentanil in volunteers and the influence of adrenalin as an adjunct. Br J Anaesth 59:1147, 1987.
166. Whiting WC, Sandler AN, Lau LC, et al: Analgesic and respiratory effects of epidural sufentanil in patients following thoracotomy. Anesthesiology 69:36, 1988.
167. Weintraub SJ, Naulty JS: Acute abstinance syndrome after epidural injection of butorphanol. Anesth Analg 64:452, 1985.
168. Leon-Casasola OA, Myers DP, Donapharthi S, et al: A comparison of postoperative epidural analgesia between patients with chronic cancer taking high doses of oral opioids versus opioid naive patients. Anesth Analg 76:302, 1993.
169. Reiz S, Westberg M: Side effects of epidural morphine. Lancet 2:203, 1980.
170. Welchew EA, Thornton JA: Continuous thoracic epidural fentanyl. A comparison of epidural fentanyl with intramuscular papaberetum for postoperative pain. Anaesthesia 37:309, 1982.
171. Davies GG, From R: A blinded study using nalbuphine for prevention of pruritis induced by epidural fentanyl. Anesthesiology 69:763, 1988.
172. Thompson WR, Smith PT, Hirst M, et al: Regional analgesic effect of epidural morphine in volunteers. Can Anaesth Soc J 28:530, 1981.
173. de Leon OA, Lema MJ: Postoperative epidural opioid analgesia: What are the choices? Anesth Analg 83:867, 1996.
174. Torda TA, Pybus DA: Extradural administration of morphine and bupivacaine; a controlled comparison. Br J Anaesth 56:141, 1984.
175. Rauck BL, Raj PP, Knarr DC, et al: Comparison of the efficacy of epidural morphine given by intermittent injection or continuous infusion for the management of pain. Reg Anesth 19:316, 1994.
176. Jayr C, Thomas H, Rey A, et al: Postoperative pulmonary complications: Epidural analgesia using bupivacaine and opioids versus parenteral opioids. Anesthesiology 78:666, 1993.
177. Wolfe MJ, Davis GK: Analgesic action of extradural fentanyl. Br J Anaesth 52:357, 1980.
178. Camann WR, Loferski BL, Fanciullo GJ, et al: Does epidural administration of butorphanol offer any clinical advantage over the intravenous route? Anesthesiology 76:216, 1992.
179. Etches RC, Sandler AN, Lawson SL: A comparison of the analgesic and respiratory effects of epidural nalbuphine or morphine in postthoracotomy patients. Anesthesiology 75:9, 1991.
180. Edwards ND, Fletcher A, Cole JR, Peacock JE: Combined infusions of morphine and ketamine for postoperative pain in elderly patients. Anaesthesia 48:124, 1993.
181. Gough JP, Williams AM, Vaughan RS, et al: The control of postthoracotomy pain. A comparative evaluation of thoracic epidural fentanyl infusions and cryo-analgesia. Anaesthesia 43:780, 1988.
182. Coe A, Saginson R, Smith MW, et al: A randomized double-blind comparison of lumbar versus thoracic epidural fentanyl. Anaesthesia 45:918, 1991.
183. Glass PSA, Estok P, Ginsburg B, et al: Use of patient-controlled analgesia to compare the efficacy of epidural to intravenous fentanyl administration. Anesth Analg 74:345, 1992.
184. Ellis DJ, Millar WL, Reisner LS: A randomized double-blind comparison of epidural versus intravenous fentanyl infusion for analgesia after cesarean section. Anesthesiology 72:981, 1990.
185. Sandler AN, Stringer D, Panos L, et al: A randomized, double-blind comparison of lumbar epidural and intravenous fentanyl infusion for post thoracotomy pain relief. Anesthesiology 77: 626, 1992.
186. Salomaki TE, Laitinen JO, Nuutinen LS: A randomized double-blind comparison of epidural versus intravenous fentanyl infusion for analgesia after thoracotomy. Anesthesiology 75:790, 1991.
187. Grant RP, Dolman JF, Harper JA, et al: Patient-controlled lumbar epidural fentanyl compared with patient controlled intravenous fentanyl for post-thoracotomy pain. Can J Anaesth 39:214, 1993.
188. Loper KA, Ready BL, Downey M, et al: Epidural and intravenous fentanyl infusions are clinically equivalent after knee surgery. Anesth Analg 70:72, 1990.
189. Benson HT, Wong HU, Belvac AM, et al: A randomized double-blind comparison of epidural fentanyl infusion versus patient-controlled analgesia with morphine for postthoracotomy pain. Anesth Analg 76:316, 1993.
190. Verborgh C, van der Aauwera D, van Droogenbroek E, Camu F: Epidural sufentanil for post surgical pain relief. Eur J Anaesth 3:313, 1986.
191. Donadoni R, Rolly G, Noorduin H, Vanden Bussche G: Epidural sufentanil for postoperative pain relief. Anaesthesia 40:634, 1985.
192. Madej TH, Watson NC, Martin BC: Large dose epidural sufentanil. Management of postoperative pain with few side effects. Anaesthesia 42:1204, 1987.
193. Rybro L, Schurizek BA, Petersen TK, Wernberg M: Postoperative analgesia and lung function: A comparison of intramuscular with epidural morphine. Acta Anaesthesiol Scand 26:514, 1982.

194. Rawal N, Sjostrand UH, Dahlstrom B, et al: Epidural morphine for postoperative pain relief: A comparison study with epidural narcotics and intercostal nerve block. Anesth Analg 61:93, 1982.
195. Modig J, Paalzow L: A comparison of epidural morphine and epidural bupivacaine for postoperative pain relief. Acta Anaesthesiol Scand 25:437, 1981.
196. Breslow MJ, Jordan DA, Christopherson R, et al: Epidural morphine decreases postoperative hypertension via attenuating sympathetic nervous system hyperactivity. JAMA 261:3577, 1989.
197. Naguib M, Adu-Gyamfi Y, Absood GH, et al: Epidural ketamine for postop analgesia. Can Anaesth Soc J 33:116, 1986.
198. Islas JA, Astorga J, Laredo M: Epidural ketamine for control of postoperative pain. Anesth Analg 64:1161, 1985.
199. Chung SK, Chan KH, Lee TY, et al: Epidural ketamine for postoperative pain relief. Anesth Sinic 24:251, 1986.
200. Ravat F, Dorne R, Baechle JP, et al: Epidural ketamine or morphine for postoperative analgesia. Anesthesiology 66:819, 1987.
201. Auwera VD, Verborgh C, Camu F: Epidural ketamine for postoperative analgesia. Anesth Analg 66:1340, 1987.
202. Wong CS, Liaw WJ, Tung CS, et al: Ketamine potentiates analgesic effect of morphine in postoperative epidural pain control. Reg Anesth 21(60):534, 1996.
203. Choe H, Choi YS, Kim YH, et al: Epidural morphine plus ketamine for upper abdominal surgery: Improved analgesia from preincisional versus postincisional administration. Anesth Analg 84:560, 1997.
204. Yaksh TL: Epidural ketamine: A useful, mechanistically novel adjuvant for epidural morphine? Reg Anesth 21(6):508, 1996.
205. Eisenach JC: Three novel spinal analgesics: Clonidine, neostigmine, amitriptyline. Reg Anesth 21(6S):81, 1996.
206. Rauck RL, Eisenach JC, Jackson K, et al: Epidural clonidine study group. Epidural clonidine treatment for refractory reflex sympathetic dystrophy. Anesthesiology 79:1163, 1993.
207. Eisenach JC, DuPen S, Duboois M, et al: Epidural clonidine analgesia for intractable cancer pain. Pain 61:391, 1995.
208. Bonnet F, Boico O, Rostaing S, et al: Postoperative analgesia with extradural clonidine. Br J Anaesth 63:465, 1989.
209. Fromme GA, Steidl LJ, Danielson DR: Comparison of lumbar and thoracic epidural morphine for relief of post thoracotomy pain. Anesth Analg 64:454, 1985.
210. Odoom JA, Sih IL: Epidural analgesia and anticoagulation therapy. Experience with 1,000 cases of continuous epidurals. Anaesthesia 38:254, 1983.
211. Rao TK, El-Etr AA: Anticoagulation following placements of epidurals and subarachnoid catheters: An evaluation of neurologic sequellae. Anesthesiology 55:618, 1981.
212. Loper KA, Ready LB, Sandler AN, et al: Epidural and intravenous fentanyl infusions are clinically equivalent following knee surgery. Anesthesiology 71:A1149, 1989.
213. Guinard JP, Mavrocordatos P, Chiolero R, et al: A randomized comparison of intravenous versus lumbar and thoracic epidural fentanyl for analgesia after thoracotomy. Anesthesiology 77: 1108, 1992.
214. Salomaki TE, Laitinen JO, Nuutinen LS: A randomized double-blind comparison of intravenous versus lumbar and epidural fentanyl for analgesia after thoracotomy. Anesthesiology 75:790, 1991.
215. Grant RP, et al: Fentanyl compared with patient-controlled intravenous fentanyl for postthoracotomy pain. Can J Anaesth 39: 214, 1992.
216. Loper KA, et al: Epidural and intravenous fentanyl infusions are clinically equivalent after knee surgery. Anesth Analg 70:72, 1990.
217. Welchew EA, Breen DP: A comparison of patient controlled on-demand fentanyl delivered epidurally or intravenously. Anaesthesia 46:438, 1991.
218. Badner NH, Sandler AN, Colmenares ME: Lumbar epidural fentanyl infusions for post thoracotomy patients. Anesthesiology 71:A667, 1989.
219. Bergqvist D: Review of clinical trials of low molecular weight heparins. Eur J Surg 158:67, 1992.
220. Schwander D, Bachmann F: Heparin and spinal or epidural anaesthesia: Clinical decision making. Ann Fr Anesth Reanim 10: 284, 1991.
221. Vandermeulen EP, Van Aken H, Vermylen J: Anticoagulants and spinal-epidural anesthesia. Anesth Analg 79:1165, 1994.
222. Rauck RL: The anticoagulated patient. Reg Anesth 21(6S):51, 1996.
223. Caplan RA, et al: Transdermal fentanyl for postoperative pain. JAMA 261:1036, 1989.
224. Nimmo WS, Duthie DJ: Plasma fentanyl concentrations after transdermal or IV infusion of fentanyl. Anesthesiology 65:A559, 1986.
225. Bell SD, Larijani GE, Goldberg ME, et al: Evaluation of transdermal fentanyl for multiday analgesia in postoperative patients. Anesthesiology 69:A362, 1988.
226. Bell SD, Goldberg ME, Larijani GE, et al: Evaluation of transdermal fentanyl for multiday analgesia in postoperative patients. Anesth Analg 68:S22, 1989.
227. Caplan RA, Ready LB, Oden RB, et al: Transdermal fentanyl for postoperative pain management: A double blind placebo study. JAMA 260:1036, 1989.
228. Varvel JR, Shafer SL, Hwang S, et al: Absorption characteristics of transdermally applied fentanyl. Anesthesiology 70:928, 1989.
229. Nairn JG: Transdermal therapeutic systems: Some fundamental considerations. Can J Hosp Pharm 41:85, 1988.
230. Rowbotham DJ, Wyld R, Peacock JE, et al: Transdermal fentanyl for the relief of pain after upper abdominal surgery. Br J Anaesth 63:56, 1989.
231. Sabel PS, Barrett CW, Kirk CJ, Heykants J: Transdermal absorption of fentanyl and sufentanil in man. Eur J Clin Pharmacol 32:529, 1987.
232. Duthie JR, Rowbotham DJ, Wyld R, et al: Plasma fentanyl concentrations during transdermal delivery of fentanyl to surgical patients. Br J Anaesth 60:614, 1988.
233. Holley FO, Van Steennis C: Postoperative analgesia with fentanyl: Pharmacokinetics and pharmacodynamics of constant rate IV and transdermal delivery. Br J Anaesth 60:608, 1988.
234. Plezia PM, Linford J, Kramer TH, et al: Transdermal therapeutic systems (fentanyl) for postoperative pain: An efficiency toxicity and pharmacokinetic trial. Anesthesiology 65:1986.
235. Bulow HH, Linnemann M, Bertg H, et al: Respiratory changes during treatment of postoperative pain with high dose transdermal fentanyl. Acta Anaesthesiol Scand 39(6):835, 1995.
236. Broome IJ, Wright BM, Bower S, Reilly CS: Postoperative analgesia with transdermal fentanyl following lower abdominal surgery. Anaesthesia 50(4):300, 1995.
237. Marlowe S, Engstrom R, White PF: Epidural patient controlled analgesia (PCA): An alternative to continuous epidural infusions. Pain 37:97, 1989.
238. Nolan JP, Dow ACC, Para MJA, et al: Patient controlled epidural analgesia following post-traumatic pelvic reconstruction. Anaesthesia 47:1037, 1992.
239. Gambling PR, Yu P, Cole C, et al: A comparative study of patient controlled epidural analgesia (PCEA) and continuous infusion epidural analgesia (CIEA) during labour. Can J Anaesth 35:249, 1988.
240. Ferrante RM, Lu L, Jamison S, Datta S: Patient-controlled epidural analgesia: Demand dosing. Anesth Analg 73:547, 1991.
241. Tyler E, Caldwell C, Ghia JN: Transcutaneous electrical nerve stimulation: An alternative approach to the management of postoperative pain. Anesth Analg 61:449, 1982.
242. Melzack R, Wall PD: Pain mechanisms: A new theory. Science 150:971, 1965.
243. Warfield CA, Stein JM, Frank HA: The effect of transcutaneous electrical nerve stimulation on pain after thoracotomy. Ann Thorac Surg 39:462, 1985.
244. Rooney SM, Jain S, McCormack P, et al: A comparison of pulmonary function test for post thoracotomy pain using cryoanalgesia and transcutaneous nerve stimulation. Ann Thorac Surg 41:204, 1986.
245. Kavanagh BP, Katz J, Sandler AN: Pain control after thoracic surgery: A review of current techniques. Anesthesiology 81:737, 1994.
246. Ready LB, Oden R, Chadwick HS, et al: Development of anesthesiology-based postoperative pain management service. Anesthesiology 68:100, 1988.
247. Bromage PR: A postoperative pain management service. Anesthesiology 69:435, 1988.
248. Brodsky JB, Brose GW, Vivenzo K: A postoperative pain management service. Anesthesiology 70:719, 1989.

CHAPTER 40

Postoperative Ventilatory Support

Robert M. Kacmarek Ph.D., R.R.T.

The development of pulmonary complications following thoracic or cardiac surgery is well established. As early as 1943, Maier and Cournard[1] described the presence of some degree of arterial hypoxemia for as long as a week following thoracic surgery. One primary reason for the hypoxemia is the decrease in functional residual capacity (FRC) that accompanies cardiac/thoracic surgery,[2] increasing the likelihood of postoperative atelectasis.[3] Essentially, a restrictive deficit in pulmonary function persisting for more than 2 weeks is present.[4] The precise reasons for this level of pulmonary dysfunction are still unclear but are believed to include the inhibitory effects of general inhalational anesthetics on hypoxic pulmonary vasoconstriction[5] and the diminution of the hypoxic and hypercapnic ventilatory drives that occurs when intravenous narcotics are used for induction.[6] These issues coupled with the increased frequency that major cardiac/thoracic surgery is performed on patients with significant underlying chronic pulmonary disease has increased the probability that ventilatory support will be required in the postoperative period.

The focus of this chapter is to describe the rationale, purpose, and problems associated with the various approaches used to provide ventilatory support in the postoperative period. Specific focus will be placed on approaches to total and partial ventilatory support, applied positive end-expiratory pressure (PEEP), and auto-PEEP, as well as ventilator-induced lung injury. Specific emphasis will be placed on managing the patient with obstructive and restrictive lung disease.

Ventilatory Targets

Application of mechanical ventilation in any mode can be approached from two different perspectives: volume targeting, or pressure targeting.[7] Simply stated, the clinician selects either a specific volume that is delivered with each positive-pressure breath or a specific peak airway pressure that is established but not exceeded with each breath. Selection of the ventilatory target establishes the primary variable of concern when ventilatory support is applied: maintenance of ventilation with volume targeting and avoidance of high airway pressure (induced lung injury) when pressure targeting is selected.[8]

Volume Ventilation

Modes of ventilation that are volume targeted terminate the inspiratory phase when a preset tidal volume is delivered. This approach to cycling also defines the variables that must be set when adjusting the mechanical ventilator. The specific set of variables adjusted is dependent upon manufacturer design; either VT, peak flow and flow waveform are selected, or VT, flow waveform and inspiratory time are adjusted.[7] With some ventilators, minute volume, inspiratory-expiratory (I:E) ratio, and flow waveform need to be selected. Regardless of specific ventilator design, the clinician must select parameters that define volume delivered, time it takes to deliver the volume, and the flow waveform used during volume delivery.[9] What is not programmed by the clinician is a pressure target. When volume targeted ventilation is selected, volume delivery and thus level of ventilation (Pa_{CO_2}) is controlled but peak airway and peak alveolar pressure are allowed to vary on a breath-by-breath basis.[10]

Figure 40–1 illustrates the pressure, flow, and volume waveforms established during typical volume-targeted assist/control mode ventilation with a square waveflow pattern. Note that both pressure and volume linearly increase throughout the entire inspiratory phase. Since the flow pattern is square wave, the peak airway pressure reflects the amount of pressure necessary to overcome both compliance and resistance.[11] To identify peak alveolar pressure, an end-inspiratory hold (Fig. 40–2) must be programmed after the actual tidal volume delivery. The end-inspiratory plateau pressure is equal to peak alveolar pressure if system gas flow rate is zero for sufficient time to allow pressure to equilibrate (~1 to 2 seconds).[9,12] Figure 40–3 also illustrates volume-targeted ventilation, but with a decelerating flow pattern and an end-inspiratory hold. Note the difference between the

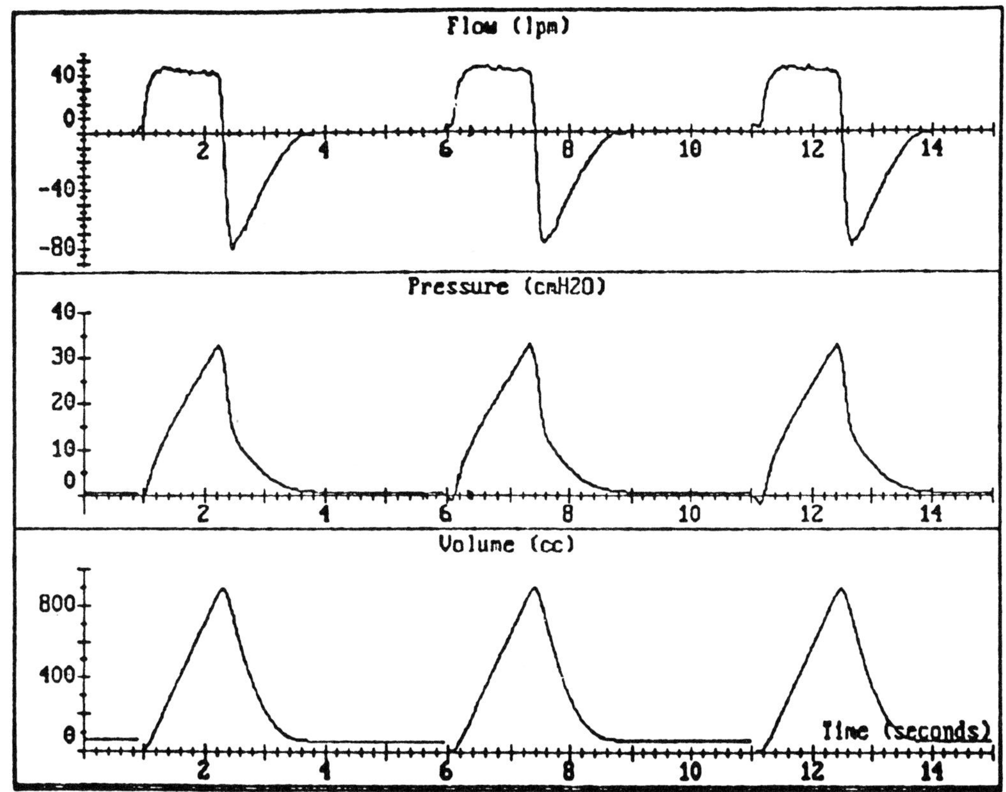

FIGURE **40–1.** Pressure, flow, and volume versus time waveforms during volume-targeted assist/control ventilation. (From Kacmarek RM, Hess D, Stoller JD [eds]: Monitoring in Respiratory Care. Chicago, Mosby-Yearbook Medical Publishers, 1993, with permission.)

pressure, volume, and flow waveforms in Figures 40–1 and 40–3 during the active gas delivery (before the end-inspiratory hold) phase. With decelerating flow, the majority of the tidal volume is delivered early in the inspiratory phase, thus the airway pressure pattern is more of a square wave. For the same tidal volume, inspiratory time, ventilatory rate, and I:E ratio, a decelerating flow pattern demonstrates a lower peak airway pressure and higher mean airway pressure than a square waveflow pattern, in spite of the fact that peak flow must be higher with decelerating flow than square flow.[13] However, the peak alveolar pressure will be the same if the same volume is maintained in the airway at zero flow. In Figure 40–3 peak alveolar pressure is equal to the end-inspiratory plateau pressure established just before exhalation. There is evidence that gas exchange is improved with a decelerating flow pattern as compared to other flow patterns (square, sign, accelerating).[14,15] In fact, provided appropriate inspiratory time is maintained,

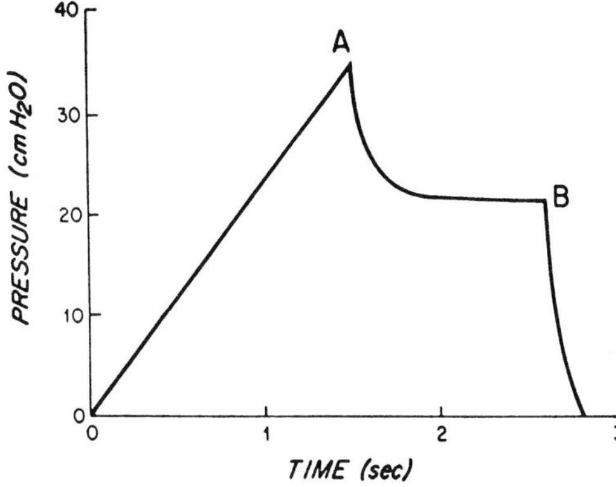

FIGURE **40–2.** Airway pressure waveform versus time during square waveform volume-targeted ventilation with an end-inspiratory plateau. *A*, Peak airway pressure; *B*, End-inspiratory plateau pressure (equivalent to peak alveolar pressure). (From Kacmarek RM, Hess D, Stoller JD [eds]: Monitoring in Respiratory Care. Chicago, Mosby-Yearbook Medical Publishers, 1993, with permission.)

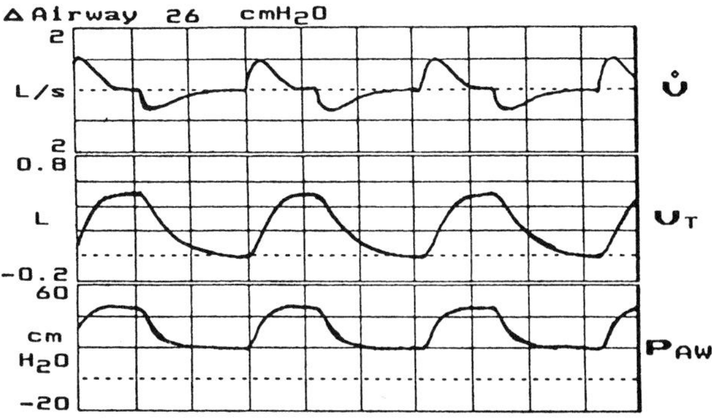

FIGURE **40–3.** Airway (PAW), flow ($\dot{V}$), and volume (VT) waveforms during volume-targeted controlled ventilation, incorporating a decelerating flow waveform and inflation hold. (From Kacmarek RM, Hess D, Stoller JD [eds]: Monitoring in Respiratory Care. Chicago, Mosby-Yearbook Medical Publishers, 1993, with permission.)

none of the other inspiratory flow patterns show an advantage over the decelerating pattern.[16,17]

Pressure Ventilation

Figure 40–4*A* and *B* depicts typical pressure-targeted, control mode ventilation. Note the similarities between Figures 40–3 and 40–4*B*. With pressure-targeted ventilation the clinician sets the target pressure and inspiratory time or I:E ratio.[10] Since pressure is the target, tidal volume may vary from breath to breath. However, peak alveolar pressure does not exceed the targeted pressure. Pressure-targeted ventilation, although appearing similar to volume-targeted, decelerating flow ventilation, does differ from it in some fundamental aspects. With pressure control, the ventilator is designed to deliver enough gas flow at the onset of inspiration to rapidly pressurize the system to the target level,[7] after which the flow decreases, frequently exponentially, to maintain the target pressure. If inspiratory time is long enough and the impedance (resistance and compliance) of the system high enough, flow rate will reach zero before the end of the inspiratory phase (Fig. 40–4*B*). If this occurs the pressure target is equal to the peak alveolar pressure.[7] When pressure-targeted ventilation is selected, precise control over peak alveolar pressure is the goal; however,

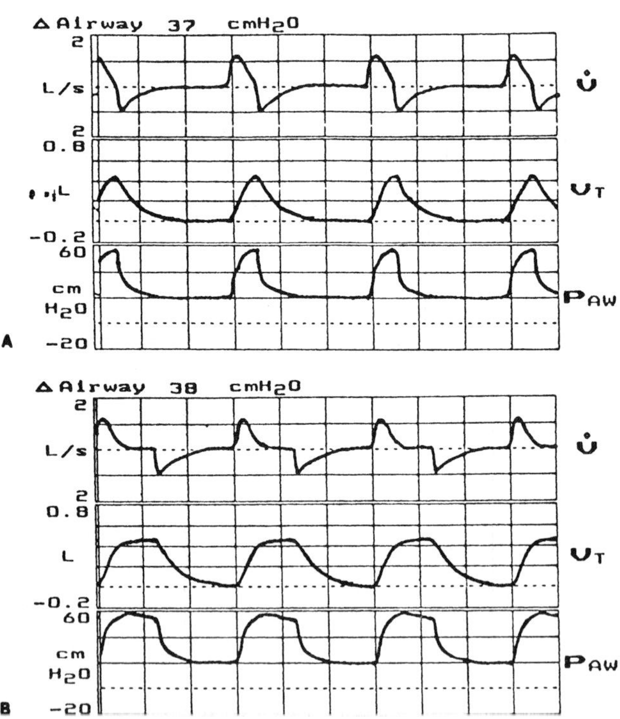

FIGURE **40–4.** *A*, Airway pressure (PAW), flow (V̇), and (VT) waveforms during pressure-control ventilation. Note that inspiratory time is inadequate; flow rate has not returned to zero, nor is an inflation hold (zero-flow period) observed. *B*, Results of increasing inspiratory time. Now flow returns to zero about midway through the inspiratory time period. The remaining inspiratory time illustrates an end-inspiratory hold. (From Kacmarek RM, Hess D, Stoller JD [eds]: Monitoring in Respiratory Care. Chicago, Mosby-Yearbook Medical Publishers, 1993, with permission.)

TABLE **40–1**
Factors Affecting Tidal Volume During Pressure-Targeted Ventilation

Pressure target level
Applied PEEP
Rate (auto-PEEP)
Patient/ventilator system compliance
Patient/ventilator system resistance
Inspiratory time (I:E ratio, auto-PEEP)

PEEP, positive end-expiratory pressure; I:E, inspiratory to expirator.

tidal volume and, as a result, Pa_{CO_2} may vary dependent upon changes in system impedance.[14]

Tidal volume delivered in pressure-targeted ventilation is dependent upon many variables. Any variable that affects the inspiratory pressure gradient or impedance of the system can alter VT (Table 40–1). As illustrated in Figure 40–4*A*, whenever inspiratory flow is greater than zero at the end of inspiration, lengthening of the inspiratory time has the potential of increasing tidal volume (Fig. 40–4*B*). The only setting where tidal volume would not increase is if lengthening inspiratory time caused air trapping (auto-PEEP) to develop. If there is a zero-flow period at the end of inspiration (Fig. 40–4*B*), lengthening of the inspiratory time will not increase VT, but may result in a decrease in VT, if air trapping develops.[10] Development of auto-PEEP during pressure-targeted ventilation always decreases VT, since the ventilator applies the pressure-targeted level above circuit baseline pressure (atmosphere or applied PEEP).[18] Since auto-PEEP is not recognized on a breath-to-breath basis by the ventilator, its presence results in system pressure immediately increasing to the auto-PEEP level, essentially decreasing the applied inspiratory pressure gradient by a level equal to the auto-PEEP.[19] The result is always a decrease in VT. There is an optimal inspiratory time in all patients where tidal volume delivery with pressure ventilation is maximal.[20] This inspiratory time period is dependent upon the compliance and resistance of the system. The more compliant and more resistant the lung, the greater likelihood for the development of auto-PEEP, whereas the less compliant and less resistant the system, the less likely the development of auto-PEEP. Generally, with obstructive lung disease auto-PEEP can develop with shorter inspiratory times than seen in patients with acute restrictive lung disease.[20]

Increasing ventilatory rate with pressure-targeted ventilation may increase or decrease minute ventilation dependent upon the development of air trapping and auto-PEEP. If an increase in the ventilatory rate causes auto-PEEP, VT and minute ventilation may decrease increasing Pa_{CO_2}.

Applied PEEP in pressure-targeted ventilation may increase or decrease VT depending upon whether it recruits lung units, improving compliance, or it overdistends lung units, decreasing compliance. In general during pressure-targeted ventilation, any factor that increases impedance (decreased compliance/increased resistance) to ventilation, decreases VT, and any factor that decreases impedance increases VT.

Pressure Versus Volume Ventilation

Considerable data have accumulated comparing pressure- and volume-targeted ventilation.[21–28] The early data indicated that pressure-targeted ventilation was superior to volume-targeted ventilation in reference to gas exchange and pulmonary mechanics; however, all of these early studies[21–23] were uncontrolled case series many of which were retrospective. More recently, numerous well-controlled prospective animal[24] and human[25–28] studies have demonstrated no difference in gas exchange or pulmonary mechanics when pressure and volume control were compared with total PEEP[23,25,27] (applied plus auto) or mean airway pressure[24] kept constant.

The decision to use either pressure or volume targeting is dependent on which of the following is of primary concern: (1) maintenance of VT and Pa_{CO_2} despite airway and alveolar pressure increases, or (2) maintaining a limit on peak alveolar and airway pressure, but allowing VT and Pa_{CO_2} to vary as system impedance varies. Table 40–2 compares volume- and pressure-targeted ventilation. As illustrated in Figures 40–3 and 40–4*B* airway pressure, flow, and volume waveforms can be set identically with pressure and volume ventilation.[29] Again the primary difference between the two approaches is the targeting of tidal volume or system pressure. If volume control is selected, careful monitoring of peak airway pressure must be maintained, whereas with pressure targeting, careful monitoring of VT/minute volume is required.

With pressure targeting it is more difficult to identify acute changes in impedance than volume targeting. A decrease in impedance during volume ventilation normally results in high-pressure alarms being activated, and if the change in impedance is progressive as with a tension pneumothorax, the peak airway pressure alarm continues to activate as pressure continues to increase. With pressure targeting, an equilibrium between the peak airway pressure and the pressure inside the pneumothorax eventually occurs, limiting the change in impedance. Frequently, pneumothorax with pressure control is not identified until routine chest x-ray or by concern over acutely altered blood gases.

Volume and pressure ventilation are available on most intensive care unit (ICU) ventilators. Either is available in assist (A), assist/control (A/C), control (C), intermittent mandatory ventilation (IMV), synchronized intermittent mandatory ventilation (SIMV), and mandatory minute ventilation (MMV).[30]

TABLE 40–2
Pressure Versus Volume-Targeted Ventilation

	Volume Target	Pressure Target
Peak airway pressure	Variable	Constant
Peak alveolar pressure	Variable	Constant
Tidal volume	Constant	Variable
Minimum rate	Preset	Preset
Inspiratory time	Preset	Preset
Peak flow	Constant	Variable
Flow pattern	Preset	Decelerating

Mode of Ventilatory Support

The primary modes of ventilatory support available with volume- and pressure-targeted ventilation are summarized in Tables 40–3 and 40–4. Historically, modes of mechanical ventilation have been classified as C, A/C, A, IMV, or SIMV. During control ventilation, regardless of whether it is pressure or volume targeted, the patient is unable to interact with the ventilator. The clinician determines all aspects of gas delivery. With A/C, the patient is able to control the initiation of the mechanical breath, provided it is at a rate greater than that programmed. However, all other aspects of gas delivery are programmed by the clinician. As recently demonstrated by Cinnella et al.,[31] pressure ventilation (pressure control [PC]) can be used in the assist/control modes the same as volume ventilation. The key is appropriate setting of the inspiratory time. In some patients inspiratory time settings of as short as 0.7 second have been used to ensure patient ventilator synchrony. Normally with volume ventilation the assist mode is never used, whereas with pressure-targeted ventilation, the assist mode is pressure support, which is commonly used.

Pressure Support Ventilation

This form of pressure-targeted ventilation, although similar to other modes of pressure ventilation, does have features that make it unique (Fig. 40–5). As indicated above it is a pure assist mode of ventilatory support.[32] As a result, an intact ventilatory control capability is assumed whenever pressure support (PS) is used. Only one variable is set with pressure support; the inspiratory pressure level.[33] The onset of the inspiratory phase is initiated by patient effort and inspiration is normally terminated by a decrease in peak flow delivery to a preset level.[32,33] As a result, ventilatory rate, inspiratory time, I:E ratio, peak inspiratory flow, and tidal volume are patient controlled and may change on a breath-to-breath basis. With some ventilators both the inspiratory rise time and the end-inspiratory flow trigger can be preset.[34] The rise time (Fig. 40–6) is the speed with which pressure rises from baseline to the set pressure support level. Dependent upon the ventilator or the setting of the rise time, the target pressure can be met rapidly (≤100 msec), or with other ventilators, the targeted pressure may not be met until the end of the inspiratory phase.[34,35] Proper settings of the rise time is dependent upon patient demand.[34] If pressure at the onset of the breath exceeds the set level (Fig. 40–6, *B1*), the rise time is set to fast, whereas if flows are less than the patient's demand, a very slow (concave) rise to set pressure may occur. During pressure support inspiration ends when delivered flow decreases to a predetermined level, either manufacturer set (e.g., liters per minute) or a percentage of the achieved peak flow (e.g., 25%).[7] Secondary triggers to

TABLE 40–3
Volume-Targeted Modes*

Mode	Description	Advantages	Disadvantages
Volume control	Complete control of ventilation; patients unable to interphase with machine; VT constant; peak pressure variable; FVS only	Control over minute volume and method of delivery	Patient unable to interact with machine; requires sedation, sedation/paralysis, or hyperventilation; spontaneously breathing patient fights ventilator; peak airway pressure variable
Volume A/C	Volume control; however, spontaneous breathing can increase rate; VT constant; peak pressure variable; FVS only	Patients may determine rate over set level; control over minimum minute volume and delivery methodology; can provide volume control with J sedation, sedation/paralysis, or hyperventilation	May cause respiratory alkalosis, air trapping, auto-PEEP, cardiovascular compromise with high rates; peak airway pressure variable
IMV	Volume control with continuous flow in between control breaths allowing spontaneous breathing; PVS to FVS	Able to provide any level of ventilatory support; at low levels patient able to breathe spontaneously; air trapping, auto-PEEP, and patient-induced respiratory alkalosis less likely than in volume A/C; can provide volume control with sedation, sedation/paralysis, or hyperventilation; less cardiovascular compromise than volume control or A/C	Stacking of mechanical breaths on spontaneous breaths; increased work of breathing at low IMV mandatory rate; may cause respiratory alkalosis, air trapping, auto-PEEP at rapid spontaneous respiratory rates; peak airway pressure variable
SIMV	Volume A/C with demand spontaneous breathing in between A/C breaths; PVS to FVS	No stacking of mechanical breaths on spontaneous breaths; same as IMV	Same as IMV
MMV	Ventilator maintains minimum minute volume, may provide volume control, total spontaneous breathing, or anything in between dependent on patient's spontaneous minute ventilation; PVS to FVS	Allows some patients to wean themselves	Rapid shallow breathing when setting of MMV is low may prevent mandatory volume A/C breaths; increased WOB at low mandatory rate; requires clinician to decrease MMV if weaning is to continue; peak airway pressure variable

*From Pierson DJ, Kacmarek RM (eds): Foundations of Respiratory Care. New York, Churchill Livingstone, 1992, p 957, with permission.
VT, tidal volume; FVS, full ventilatory support; PEEP, positive end-expiratory pressure; A/C, assist/control; PVS, partial ventilatory support; IMV, intermittent mandatory ventilation; MMV, mandatory minute ventilation; WOB, work of breathing.

exhalation with pressure support include an increase in pressure over target by 2 to 3 cm H_2O or a prolongation of inspiration time (≥3 seconds).[7] Of concern is when the patient elects to exhale before the trigger to exhalation is met. This causes the end-inspiratory pressure to exceed the set level (Fig. 40–6, *D1*).[34–36] If this is occurring, the patient is activating accessory muscles of exhalation in order to oppose the pressure support breath and cycle to exhalation.[37] This increased effort tends to stimulate ventilatory drive and increase patient-ventilator dyssynchrony (Fig. 40–7).[37] In chronic obstructive pulmonary disease (COPD) patients this is a common occurrence if the trigger to exhalation in pressure support is a low flow (i.e., 5 L/min), since in many COPD patients inspiratory flows do not decrease to zero toward the end of the inspiratory phase but remain high.[37] If an end-inspiratory trigger sensitivity is available it should be adjusted to eliminate the rise in pressure above set level at end-inspiration.

Of all the available modes of ventilation, pressure support has been the most extensively studied.[38–47] In general, it is the mode that affords the patient the most flexibility in interacting with the ventilator. Pressure support can be used at high levels to apply near-total ventilatory support[42,43] or it can be used at low levels (5 to 12 cm H_2O) to unload the work of breathing imposed by the ventilator demand system and artificial airway.[44–46] Titration of pressure support level is generally performed to produce a ventilatory pattern that is consistent with that expected following extubation.[47] Brochard et al.[41] has recommended titrating PS to the level that eliminates activation of accessory muscles of respiration, primarily the sternocleidomastoid muscle.[41] Titration to this level coincides with a reduction of work of breathing to levels seen following extubation.[41,44] Many have proposed adjusting PS to produce a ventilatory pattern in which the rate is 25 or fewer breaths/min and the VT is greater than 7 ml/kg.[43,46] Pressure support can also be used in

TABLE 40–4
Pressure-Targeted Modes*

Mode	Description	Advantages	Disadvantages
Pressure control	Complete control of ventilation; peak airway pressure constant, VT variable; FVS only	Control over method of delivery except VT, which may vary from breath to breath	Generally requires sedation, sedation/paralysis, or hyperventilation; spontaneously breathing patient may fight gas delivery
Pressure A/C	Pressure control; however, patient may increase rate of ventilation; pressure constant, VT variable; FVS only	Patient may determine rate over set level; peak pressure constant; pressure control available with sedation, sedation/paralysis, or hyperventilation	May cause respiratory alkalosis, air trapping, auto-PEEP, cardiovascular compromise with high rates; VT variable
Pressure support	Peak pressure set, otherwise all aspects of ventilation controlled by patient; PVS to FVS	Patient has control over process of ventilation; machine responds to patient demands; gas is delivered in response to patient desires; peak airway pressure set	VT variable; no backup rate, continuous nebulizer therapy may cause hypoventilation; air trapping, auto-PEEP possible if rate high
Airway pressure release ventilation	Delivery of two levels of CPAP using continuous flow system; normally I:E ratio inversed; spontaneous breathing at each CPAP level possible; designed for use via artificial airway; PVS to FVS	Simple setup; airway pressure controlled; spontaneous breathing	VT variable; increased WOB at inspiratory CPAP level, no alarms, no patient monitors
Bilevel pressure ventilation	Delivery of PS or press A/C with PEEP; designed for use via nasal mask; normal I:E ratio, patient can control rate, length of inspiration; PVS to FVS	Commercially available; airway pressure controlled; patient controls all aspects of ventilation except pressure level; designed for noninvasive use	VT variable; no alarms, no patient monitors
MMV pressure limited	Ventilator maintains minimum minute volume by varying PSV level in response to patient's ability to maintain MMV level; PVS to FVS	Allows some patients to wean themselves; peak airway pressure maintained within specified range	Rapid shallow breathing can defeat goal of MMV; requires clinician to decrease MMV level if weaning is to continue; VT variable

*From Pierson DJ, Kacmarek RM (eds): Foundations of Respiratory Care. New York, Churchill Livingstone, 1992, p 956, with permission.
VT, tidal volume; FVS, full ventilatory support; A/C, assist/control; PEEP, positive end-expiratory pressures; PVS, partial ventilatory support; CPAP, continuous positive airway pressure; WOB, work of breathing; I:E, inspiratory to expiratory; MMV, mandatory minute ventilation.

conjunction with SIMV to support the spontaneous breaths.[45] Used in this setting, Hurst et al.[45] demonstrated dramatic improvement in gas exchange, hemodynamics, and ventilatory pattern in a group of trauma patients weaning from ventilatory support.

Intermittent Mandatory Ventilation

This approach to ventilatory support is a combination of control ventilation with spontaneous breathing (Fig. 40–8) and was initially introduced as a means of ventilatory support in infants[48,49] and to facilitate weaning in adults.[50] It can be applied with both volume- and pressure-targeted approaches.[7] With IMV, a continuous flow of gas is maintained to allow spontaneous inspiration and periodically a mandatory breath is delivered.[30] SIMV is a variation of IMV now used exclusively in place of IMV.[7] In SIMV, the mandatory breaths are assist/control breaths and the spontaneous breaths activate demand flow (Fig. 40–8).[30] As a result, pressure support can be used in conjunction with either pressure- or volume-targeted SIMV.[30] Of major concern with IMV or SIMV is dyssynchrony as a result of differing gas delivery patterns (i.e., mandatory breaths interspersed between spontaneous breaths).[51] Some patients poorly tolerate IMV/SIMV especially at lower SIMV rates[52] (four to ten breaths/min dependent on total respiratory rate). In addition, the work of breathing at low IMV/SIMV rates may be overwhelming and necessitate the addition of pressure support or a change of mode.[52]

Mandatory Minute Ventilation

This mode is a variation of SIMV where in addition to the normal settings in either pressure or volume targeting, a minimal minute ventilation is also set.[7] Generally, with volume-targeted MMV, the mandatory rate is adjusted to ensure a minimum minute volume, whereas in pressure-targeted MMV, the pressure support or pressure control level is adjusted.[53] As a result total ventilatory support, partial ventilatory support or no ventilatory support may be provided dependent upon the patient's abil-

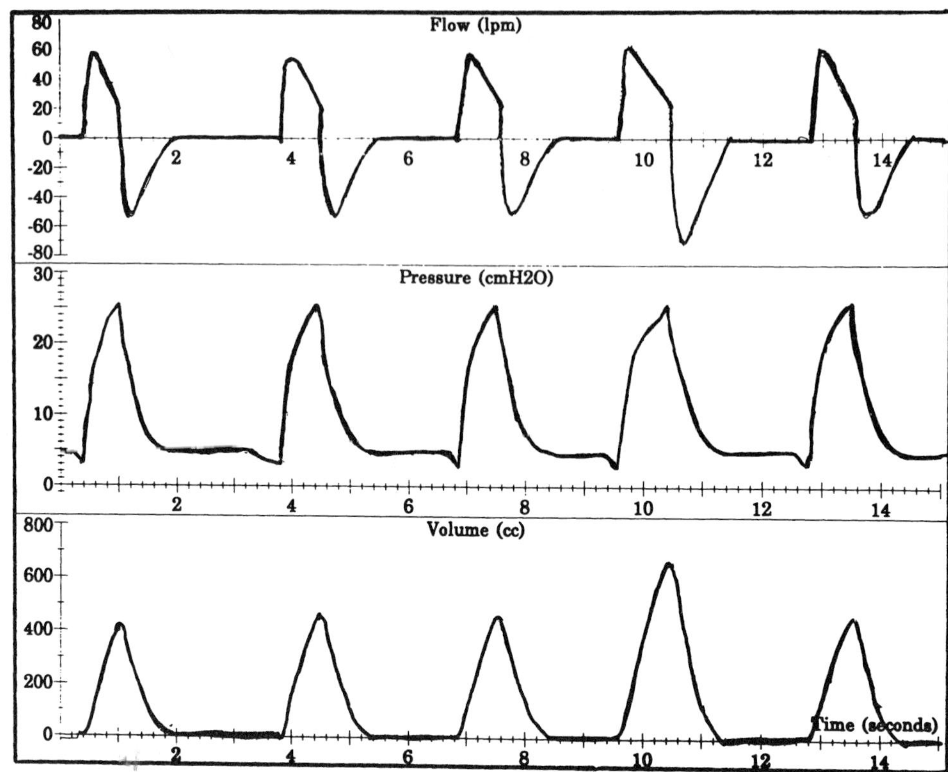

FIGURE **40–5.** Flow, pressure, and volume waveforms during pressure-support ventilation. Note that each breath is patient triggered and that inspiratory time and volume vary with each breath. (From Kacmarek RM, Hess D: Basic principles of ventilatory machinery. In Tobin MJ [ed]: Principles and Practices of Mechanical Ventilation. New York, McGraw-Hill, 1994, p 65, with permission.)

ities and desire to breathe spontaneously. This modification of SIMV was introduced to allow patients to "wean themselves,"[54] however, it has not performed as expected. Patients can satisfy the minute volume requirement by an unacceptably rapid and shallow breathing pattern.[55] Unfortunately no data are available to date to support the use of MMV. The concept of MMV appears to be sound; however, considerable refinement in the algorithms used are necessary before improved efficacy can be expected.

Airway Pressure Release Ventilation and Bilevel Pressure Ventilation

These are very similar modes of pressure-targeted ventilation (Fig. 40–9) and both can be considered a variation of pressure-targeted A/C ventilation. One of the major differences between airway pressure release ventilation (APRV), bilevel pressure ventilation (BiPAP) and typical pressure-targeted ventilation is that a continuous flow of gas is maintained across the airway with both APRV and bilevel pressure ventilation.[7]

Currently, bilevel pressure ventilation is only available on portable home mechanical ventilation units.[36,56] It is essentially pressure support with continuous positive airway pressure (CPAP). The patient may control all aspects of gas delivery except pressure levels and an A/C minimum rate (optional). With some units control ventilation can also be provided. APRV, on the other hand, is similar to IMV, patients are allowed to inspire spontaneously between mandatory increases in system pressure, but also can inspire while at the mandatory pressure level (Fig. 40–9). APRV has been described as bilevel CPAP with spontaneous breaths allowed at each CPAP level. Bilevel pressure ventilation is designed to be used at patient selected I:E ratios,[57] whereas APRV is intended to be used at inverse ratios.[58–61] APRV is currently available on the Drager Evita Ventilator. However, most centers using APRV have developed "homemade" systems.[58]

The indications for APRV and bilevel pressure ventilation diverge along grossly different clinical routes. Proponents of APRV believe it is best used in intubated patients with mild to moderate acute ventilatory failure.[58–61] By contrast, bilevel pressure ventilation has been designed for noninvasive ventilatory support through a nasal mask.[57,62] Its primary use is in patients with chronic ventilatory failure who require nocturnal ventilatory muscle rest. However, bilevel pressure ventilation has also been used to reverse acute ventilatory failure in patients with chronic ventilatory insufficiency,[63] and as a transition from invasive mechanical ventilation.[64]

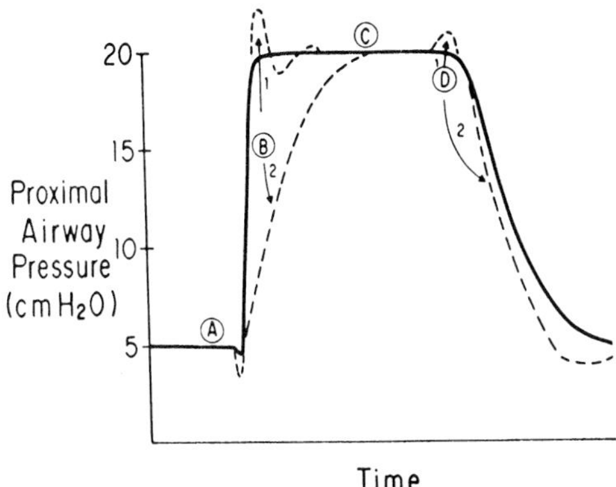

FIGURE **40–6.** Design characteristics of a pressure-supported breath. In this example, baseline pressure (i.e., PEEP) is set at 5 cm H_2O and pressure support is set at 15 cm H_2O (PIP 20 cm H_2O). The inspiratory pressure is triggered at *point A* by a patient effort resulting in an airway pressure decrease. Demand valve sensitivity and responsiveness are characterized by the depth and duration of this negative pressure. The rise to pressure (*line B*) is provided by a fixed high initial flow delivery into the airway. Note that if flows exceed patient demand, initial pressure exceeds set level (*B1*), whereas if flows are less than patient demand, a very slow (concave) rise to pressure can occur (*B2*). The plateau of pressure support (*line C*) is maintained by servo control of flow. A smooth plateau reflects appropriate responsiveness to patient demand; fluctuations would reflect less responsiveness of the servo mechanisms. Termination of pressure support occurs at *point D* and should coincide with the end of the spontaneous inspiratory effort. If termination is delayed, the patient actively exhales (bump in pressure above plateau) (*D1*); if termination is premature, the patient will have continued inspiratory efforts (*D2*). (From McIntyre N, Nishimuron M, Usada Y, et al: The Nagoya Conference on system designs and patient-ventilator interactions during pressure support ventilation. Chest 97:1463, 1990, with permission.)

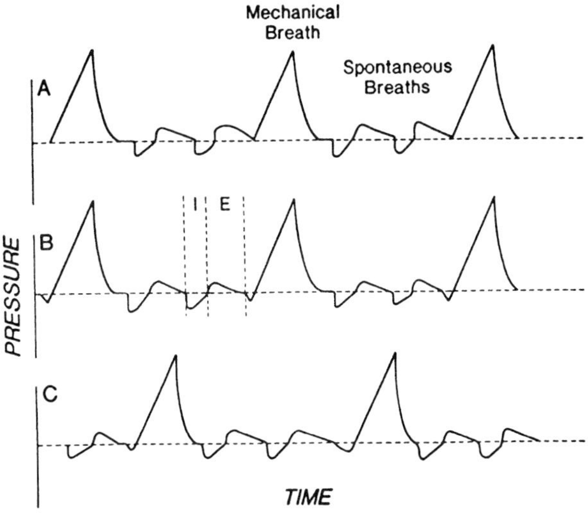

FIGURE **40–8.** Pressure versus time waveforms during (*A*) IMV, (*B*) SIMV, and (*C*) volume-controlled MMV positive-pressure ventilation. Note each spontaneous breath occurs between volume-targeted breaths. With IMV, mandatory volume breaths are controlled, while with SIMV, they are patient triggered. MMV pressure waveforms are exactly the same as SIMV. Defections below baseline are created by patient inspiratory efforts. I, spontaneous inspiration; E, spontaneous expiration. (From Pierson DJ, Kacmarek RM [eds]: Foundations of Respiratory Care. New York, Churchill Livingstone, 1992, with permission.)

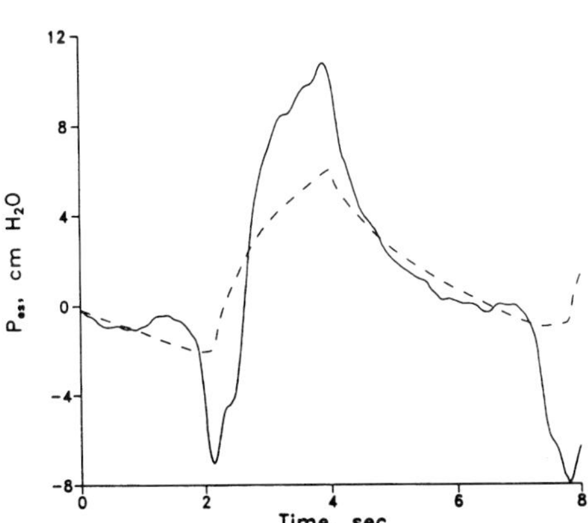

FIGURE **40–7.** Esophageal pressure (Pes, continuous line) and estimated recoil pressure of the chest wall (Pes_{CW}, interrupted line) tracings in a patient receiving pressure support ventilation of 20 cm H_2O. Pressure tracings have been superimposed so that Pes_{CW} is equal to Pes at the onset of the rapid fall in Pes during late expiration. The presence of expiratory muscle activation during late inspiration is illustrated by the rise in Pes above Pes_{CW}. (From Jubran A, Van de Graaf WB, Tobin MJ: Variability of patient-ventilatory interaction with pressure support ventilation in patients with chronic obstructive pulmonary disease. Am J Respir Crit Care Med 152:129, 1995. Copyright American Lung Association, with permission.)

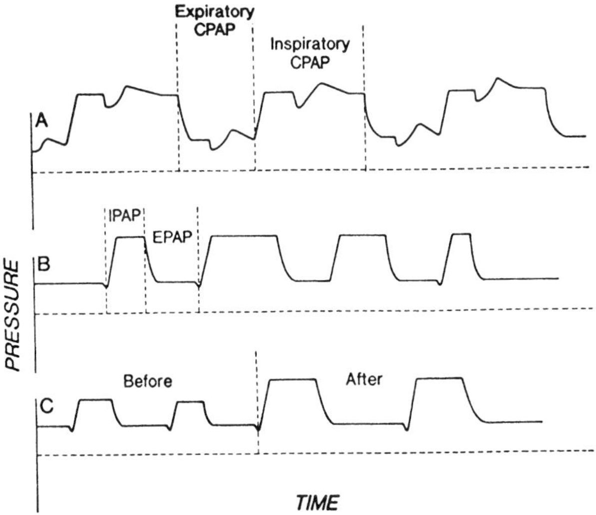

FIGURE **40–9.** Pressure versus time waveforms during (*A*) airway pressure release ventilation (APRV), (*B*) bilevel CPAP, and (*C*) pressure-limited MMV. By design, APRV is usually adjusted with the inspiratory time longer than expiratory time and it is expected that patients will superimpose a spontaneous breath at both the inspiratory and expiratory CPAP levels. With bilevel CPAP, normal application is via the timed/spontaneous mode (A/C), in which the patient is allowed to control all aspects of gas delivery except the inspiratory positive airway pressure (IPAP) level and expiratory positive airway pressure (EPAP). In pressure limited MMV, the PSV level is periodically adjusted to ensure MMV. PSV levels are depicted before and after adjustment. (From Pierson DJ, Kacmarek RM [eds]: Foundations of Respiratory Care. New York, Churchill Livingstone, 1992, with permission.)

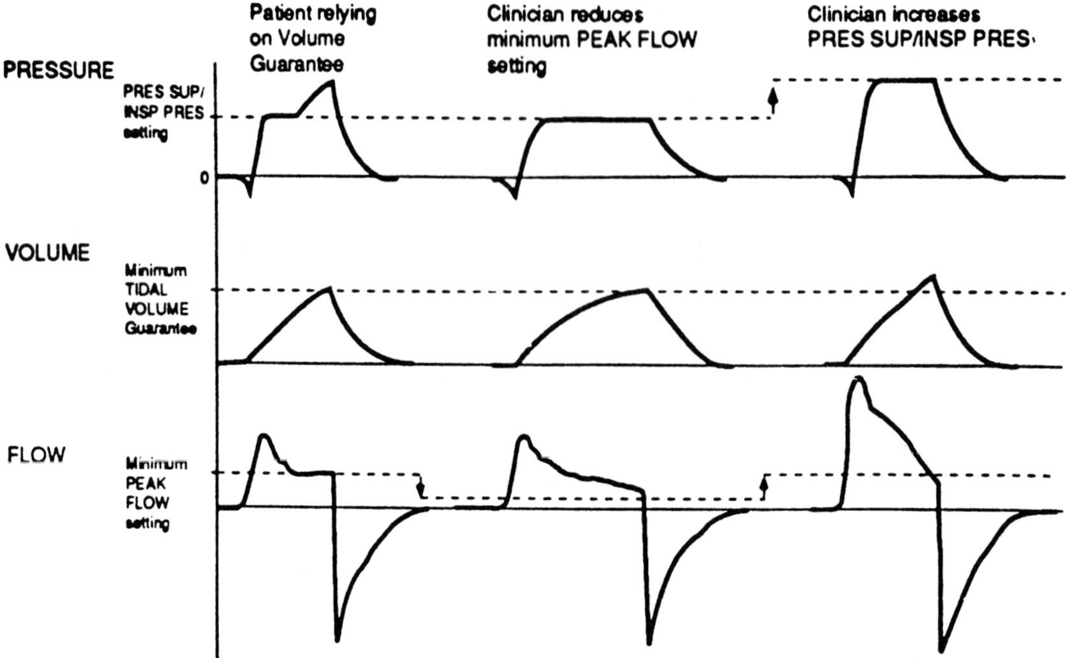

FIGURE **40–10.** A minimum tidal volume is guaranteed during pressure augmentation. Note that the minimum tidal volume is delivered despite a decrease in patient demands or changes in resistance and compliance. With an increase in patient demand, the pressure and flow waveforms approximate those seen with pressure-support ventilation. (From Bear product literature, with permission.)

Combined Pressure/Volume Modes

As is obvious from the previous discussion, regardless of whether pressure or volume targeting is selected there are positives and negatives to each approach. More recently, a number of newer modes have been introduced that combine the beneficial effects of pressure and volume ventilation. Amato et al.[65] very nicely demonstrated that patient effort could be greatly reduced and patient-ventilation synchrony increased if demand flow was added to standard square wave flow, volume-targeted ventilation. This approach has been referred to as volume-assured pressure support or pressure augmentation and is now available on a number of ventilators. As illustrated in Figure 40–10 the gas delivery pattern is dependent upon patient demand.[66] If patient demand is low, gas delivery resembles normal volume ventilation, whereas if demand increases, gas delivery is similar to pressure support. With this mode, target VT, rate, and square wave gas flow are set, but as patient demand increases set peak flow, VT and rate can be exceeded.[7]

A similar approach to combining pressure and volume targeting is available on the Servo 300 ventilator (Fig. 40–11).[7] Volume support and pressure-regulated volume

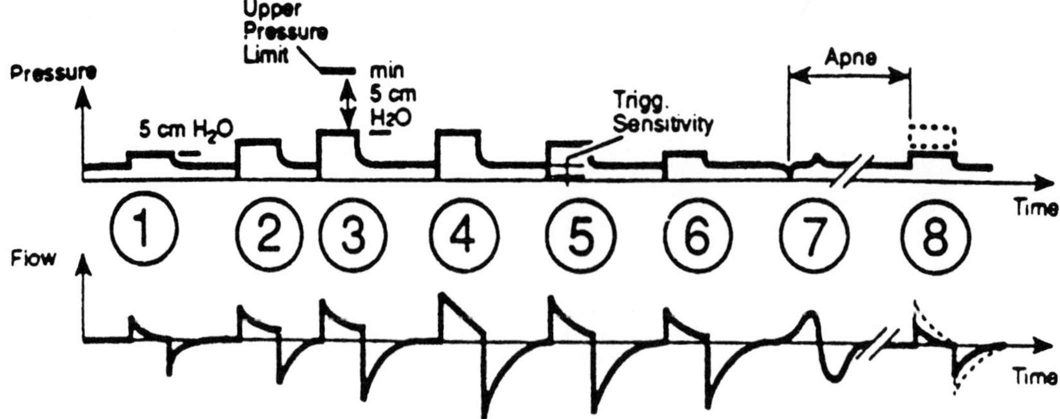

FIGURE **40–11.** Pressure and flow waveforms during volume support. *1*, Test breath. *2* to *5*, Adjustment of pressure target to ensure delivered tidal volume. *5* and *6*, Pressure limit decreased to maintain tidal volume at target level. *7*, Period of apneic ventilation. *8*, Ventilator switches to pressure-regulated control modes. (From Siemens product literature, with permission.)

control both are combined pressure- and volume-targeted modes. With both of these modes a volume target and maximum pressure limit are set. Each mode initially delivers a test breath at 5 cm H_2O pressure from which compliance is calculated and pressure needed to deliver 75% of the targeted V_T is estimated. After the delivery, three additional test breaths at the 75% level are delivered, and the PS or PC level is then increased by up to 3 cm H_2O per breath until the target V_T is delivered. Readjustment of the set pressure level to reach the target V_T occurs on a breath-by-breath basis. This mode functions similar to the MMV mode; however, pressure can only be decreased to zero if the patient is capable of spontaneously breathing the target tidal volume. The only difference between volume support and pressure-regulated volume control is the setting of inspiratory time and back-up rate. There is limited literature supporting the use of either of these modes of ventilatory support.[67]

Full Versus Partial Ventilatory Support

Controversy has long existed regarding the optimal mode of ventilation to employ during various phases of acute ventilatory failure. However, regardless of the mode selected, ventilatory support can be categorized into two general approaches: full ventilatory support (FVS) and partial ventilatory support (PVS).[68] During FVS, the mechanical ventilator provides all or nearly all the effort required to maintain gas exchange. As noted below, many of the commonly available modes of ventilation can provide FVS, provided they are appropriately set and the patient is properly sedated.[69] FVS may also be provided in patients triggering the ventilator, as long as the adjustment of gas delivery is consistent with patient demands.[30,70]

Most patients requiring ventilatory support for acute respiratory failure present with hypercarbia, hypoxemia, acidosis, and either ventilatory muscle dysfunction or fatigue, and are commonly exhausted.[68] For these reasons, FVS techniques are recommended during the first 24 to 72 hours of ventilatory support.

During partial ventilatory support, the patient provides a significant percentage of the effort required to maintain gas exchange. Partial ventilatory support can be provided by IMV, SIMV, PSV, APRV, MMV, and any of the combined pressure- and volume-targeted modes.[30] Each of these approaches allows the clinician to titrate the level of support provided by the ventilator.[68] With IMV, SIMV, or MMV, the frequency of the predetermined pressure- or volume-targeted breath can vary, allowing the patient to breathe spontaneously between the mandatory breaths.[7] By contrast, PSV, APRV, and bilevel pressure ventilation allow the clinician to select the level of ventilatory effort required of the patient for each breath by varying the pressure limit selected.[7] Each of these modes (IMV, SIMV, PSV, MMV, APRV, bilevel pressure ventilation and the combined pressure- and volume-targeted modes) allow various levels of patient-ventilator interaction from almost completely spontaneous ventilation to FVS.

Partial ventilatory support is a more physiologic approach to mechanical ventilation and the recommended approach to managing patients once they are past the acute phase of respiratory failure.[10,68,69] Allowing patients to play a more significant role in the process of ventilation normally improves $\dot{V}/\dot{Q}$ matching, decreases hemodynamic compromise and may prevent further deterioration of diaphragmatic function.[41,68] The key to appropriate application of PVS techniques is to titrate the level of patient-machine interaction so that active patient involvement is present but sufficient support is provided to prevent deterioration of ventilatory muscle function and overall cardiopulmonary status.[33,35,41] Because of the delicate balance required, FVS is generally easier to employ appropriately than PVS, with clinical judgment being the key to the optimal titration of PVS.

Patient-Ventilatory Synchrony

It is difficult in the acutely ill patient to select the mode of ventilation and to appropriately set the ventilator to overcome the imposed loads of the artificial airway/ventilator system and to meet the changing ventilatory demands of patients during partial ventilatory support. If the ventilator is set improperly or an inappropriate mode is selected, patient-ventilatory dyssynchrony frequently results.

Technical Factors Affecting Ventilatory Load

Table 40–5 lists those primary technical variables that can increase ventilatory load during partial ventilatory support. Although all are potential problems in a given patient, most can be compensated for by the selection of the appropriate equipment and settings of the ventilator.

Artificial Airways

In the operating room few patients experience difficulty with the selection of type and size of the artificial airway, since patients are sedated and receive controlled ventilatory support and few of the total population of patients undergoing anesthesia have chronic pulmonary disease. This is generally not true for patients requiring ventila-

TABLE 4–5 Technical Factors Affecting Ventilatory Load

Artificial airways
Demand gas delivery systems
Ventilator triggering
Humidification devices
Peak flow setting
Mode of ventilation

tory support for longer than 12 to 48 hours postoperatively. Most patients have underlying cardiopulmonary disease and many are managed with partial ventilatory support. In this setting the artificial airway may impose a considerable ventilatory load.[71–73] Figure 40–12 is from a study performed by Shapiro et al.[71] on young healthy volunteers who breathed through varying sized endotracheal tubes via a mouthpiece/nose clip with a pneumotachograph and with an esophageal balloon in place. When asked to maintain tidal volume constant using visual feedback but to increase respiratory rates, all achieved fatiguing workloads with a 6-mm internal diameter (ID) endotracheal tube as their minute volumes exceeded 15 L/min. Figure 40–13 is from Wright et al.[72] where resistance to flow through an 8-mm ID endotracheal tube was evaluated at different peak flows both in vitro and in vivo. The in vivo evaluation resulted in larger variations in resistance to flow and greater resistance than observed in vitro. These data clearly illustrate the fact that an 8-mm ID endotracheal tube in vivo may actually have the physical characteristics of a 7-mm tube or less if its contour is changed as it passes the upper airway or has secretions adhering to its inner walls. Of particular concern in spontaneously breathing patients is nasotracheal intubation. Generally, this route requires a small-sized tube, and the acute angle the tube must traverse in some patients as it passes through the nasal pharynx may markedly decrease the effective inner diameter.[74] In patients requiring partial ventilatory support, a large-sized oral endotracheal tube is the airway of choice despite the difficulties securing the airway, providing oral hygiene, and avoiding stimulation of upper airway reflexes.[74]

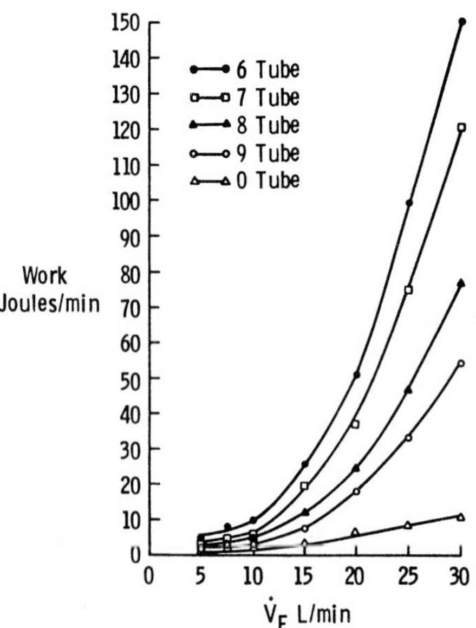

FIGURE **40–12.** Relationship between work of breathing and increasing minute ventilation ($\dot{V}_E$) of volunteers breathing through different sized endotracheal tubes. (From Shapiro W, Wilson RK, Casar G, et al: Work of breaths through different sized endotracheal tubes. Crit Care Med 14:1028, 1986, with permission.)

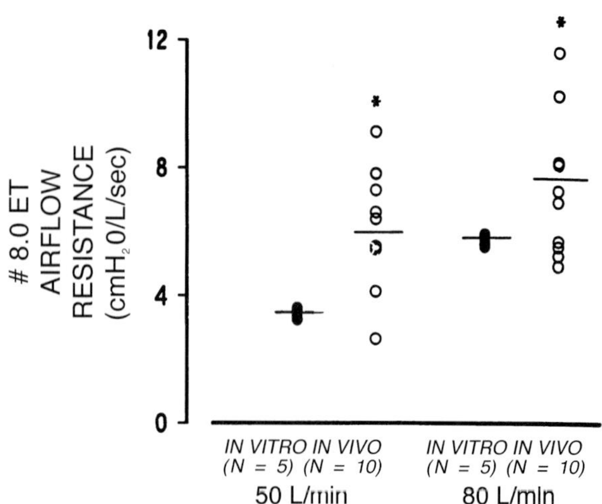

FIGURE **40–13.** Comparison of the calculated endotracheal tube resistance in vitro (average of inspiratory and expiratory resistance) with measurements made in vivo. Resistance was higher when measured in vivo than in vitro at both flow rates. (*$p < .05$ in vivo vs. in vitro.) *Horizontal lines* indicate mean values. (From Wright PE, Marini JJ, Bernard GR: In vitro versus in vivo comparison of endotracheal tube airflow resistance. Am Rev Respir Dis 142:10, 1939. Copyright American Lung Association, with permission.)

Ventilatory Triggering

Regardless of mode of ventilation or the application of CPAP, spontaneously breathing patients must trigger the ventilator each breath to activate gas delivery.[7] Depending on the ventilator, type of triggering mechanism used, and its actual setting, ventilator triggering may impose a significant ventilatory load.[74]

Most ventilators historically used a pressure trigger to activate breath delivery.[7] With most of the newest ventilators, variable flow triggering has been added as an option or a replacement for pressure triggering.[75–77] As illustrated in Figure 40–14, during CPAP and pressure triggering up to a total of 250 msec delay can occur from patient activation of inspiratory effort to actual delivery of flow sufficient to meet patient demand (return system pressure to baseline[75]). Much of this delay can be eliminated by the use of flow triggering during CPAP. With appropriately set flow triggering (Fig. 40–15) pressure change to trigger and time delay in flow delivery can be markedly reduced.[75] With many of the flow-triggered systems time delay is less than 100 msec.[78,79]

With CPAP, flow triggering is much more efficient than pressure triggering and ideally should always be used if available.[74] However, with assisted ventilation, flow triggering does not seem to possess the same advantage over pressure triggering.[76,80] As recently demonstrated by Goulet et al.,[80] properly set flow and pressure triggers resulted in the same time delay and pressure change required to trigger during pressure support. The difference between CPAP and pressure support in regard to triggering effort and time delay is associated with the posttrigger period (Fig. 40–16).[80] With partial ventilatory support modes, the posttrigger period is dependent on the ventilator algorithm to achieve pressure or volume target. With CPAP and pressure triggering the ventilator targets a system pressure at the sensitivity setting (e.g.,

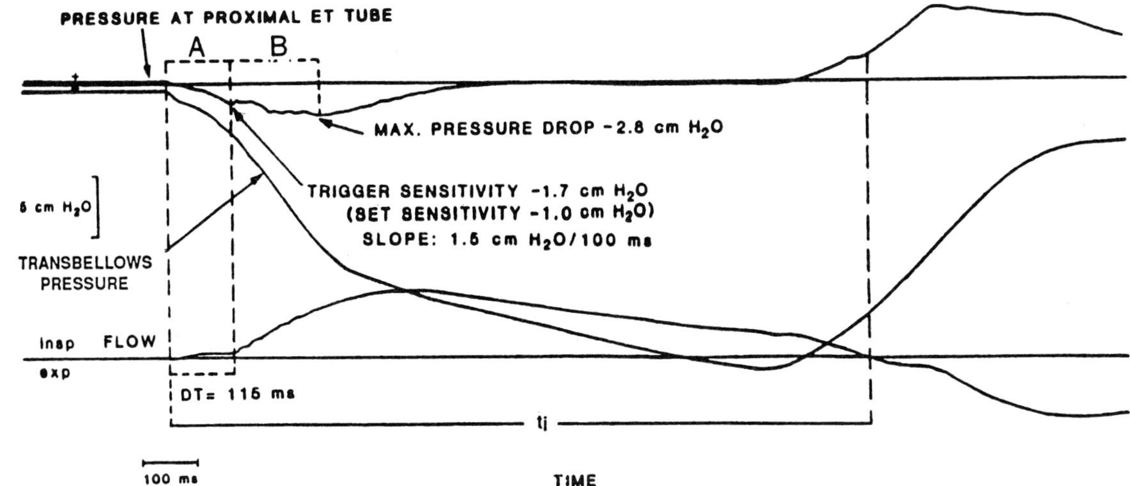

FIGURE **40–14.** Pressure-triggered demand-flow system applied to a mechanical lung model. Pressure is measured at the proximal end of the endotracheal tube (7.5 mm), and transbellows pressure and flow tracings are generated using a one-compartment computer-driven mechanical lung model (tidal volume of 500 ml, a rapid ascending and gradual descending ramp flow waveform at a rate of 45 L/min, and compliance of 25 ml/cm H_2O) ventilated with a demand-flow CPAP system at a CPAP level of 0 cm H_2O without a humidifier (Puritan-Bennett 7200a). *Part A*, Trigger phase is from onset of inspiratory effort to onset of flow delivery. Flow is slightly detectable during *part A* as a result of circuit length and compliance. *Part B*, Posttirgger phase is from measured trigger sensitivity to maximum pressure drop. CPAP, continuous positive airway pressure; DT, time delay from onset of inspiratory effort (negative deflection of transbellows pressure) to onset of flow; t_i, inspiratory time. (From Sassoon CSH: Mechanical ventilator design and function: The trigger variable. Respir Care 37:1056, 1992, with permission.)

−1 cm H_2O) but targets baseline system pressure during CPAP and flow triggering.[75] Although no advantage exists during partial ventilatory support, because of the advantage during CPAP and the difficulty setting pressure triggers approximately (−0.5 to −1.0 cm H_2O) without self-cycling, flow triggering is the ideal trigger to minimize effort and improve synchrony.

Humidification

With the current generation of mechanical ventilators, the use of heated humidifiers or heated wire circuits imposes no additional effort on patients maintained in partial ventilatory support.[81] However, the use of artificial noses can impose a resistive load during partial ventilatory support.[82,83] After 24 hours of use up to 5 cm H_2O pressure gradient is needed to maintain a flow of 60 L/min across these devices.[82] When this load is added in series with that of artificial airways and ventilator triggering, the potential for excessive imposed effort clearly exists in patients on CPAP. Even in those receiving partial ventilatory support, effort to trigger in some patients may be excessive. Despite this, the use of heat and moisture exchangers is reasonable in patients requiring short-term postoperative ventilatory support.[84–86] Use for longer than 48 to 72 hours in patients especially with chronic pulmonary disease who are receiving partial ventilatory support is discouraged because of the imposed ventilatory load and other problems common to heat and moisture exchangers (Table 40–6).[81] However, some clinicians do recommend the use of heat and moisture exchanges on all ventilated patients regardless of the length of ventilatory support.[87–89]

Peak Flow

Inability of the ventilator to meet patient demand results in patient ventilator dyssynchrony and markedly increased patient effort.[31,90,91] This is particularly true during volume ventilation, for as shown in Figure 40–17, if peak flow is less than patient demand, patient effort during volume ventilation may be as high as during unsupported ventilation.[91] To minimize the effect of inadequate peak flow with spontaneously breathing patients, peak flow should be set greater than or equal to 60 L/min and inspiratory time set at 1.0 second or less.[74,81]

Mode of Ventilation

Mode of ventilation can have a dramatic effect on patient ventilator dyssynchrony.[52] As illustrated in Figure 40–18, SIMV has the potential of markedly increasing patient effort as the mandatory rate is decreased.[52] It would appear that there is a level of support in all patients where ventilatory pattern will be dependent upon the mandatory breath delivery pattern, and a level where dependence is on the spontaneous breathing pattern.[74] From the data of Marini et al.,[52] it appears that at less than or equal to 60% support provided by mandatory breaths, effort on all breaths increases markedly as compared to controlled ventilation.

As discussed earlier, there is debate over the effective use of volume- versus pressure-targeted ventilation. Since pressure-targeted ventilation is better able to meet patient ventilatory demand than volume-targeted ventilation,[31,39,41] it is the choice of target during partial ventilatory support. Not only does pressure-targeted ventilation meet patient demand at onset because of its high

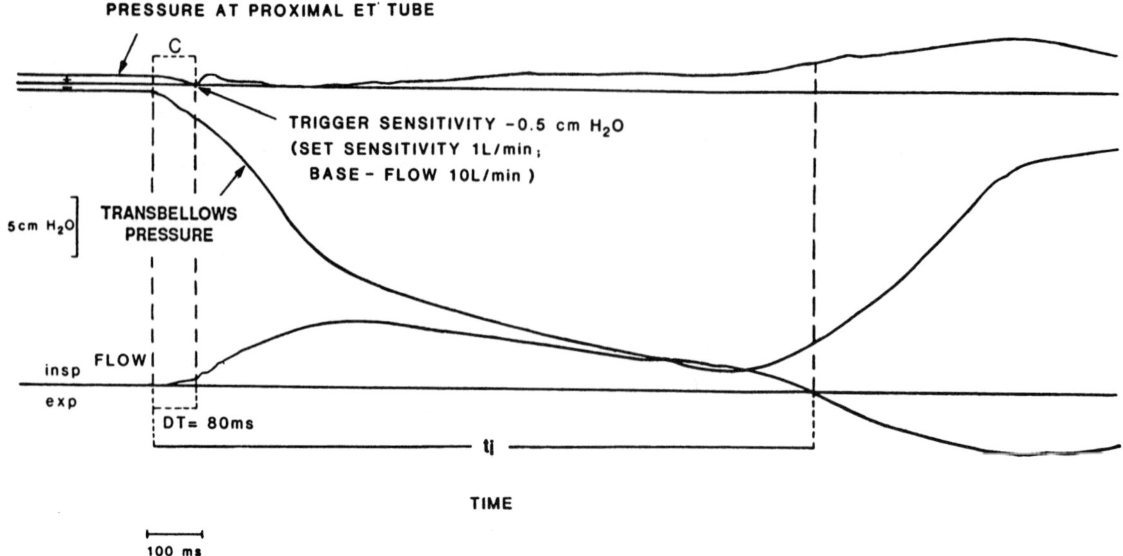

FIGURE **40–15.** Flow-triggered or flow-by system applied to a mechanical lung model at a CPAP level of 0 cm H_2O. Settings of mechanical lung model are the same as in Figure 40–14. *Part C*, From inspiratory effort to opening of the pneumatic system. Flow during *part C* is provided by the base flow. *Note*: Airway pressure remains at or above baseline pressure, acting as a small inspiratory pressure-assist due to the flow-control algorithm. The measured trigger sensitivity of 0.5 cm H_2O is not the actual sensitivity that triggers the pneumatic system to open. See Figure 40–14 for definition of abbreviations. (From Sassoon CSH: Mechanical ventilator design and function: The trigger variable. Respir Care 37:1056, 1992, with permission.)

flow but it is capable of responding to changes in demand over time. This capability is not available with volume ventilation. Whether to use pressure support or pressure control is dependent on the patient's ability to cycle to exhalation without activation of accessory muscles of exhalation.[37] When pressure control is used, care in setting inspiratory time must be exercised. Inspiratory time should be set equal to the patient's spontaneous inspiratory time, usually 1.0 second or less but greater than or equal to 0.6 second.

It must also be emphasized that any mode of ventilation is usually adequate for short-term (12 to 48 hours) ventilation of the average postoperative patient. It is primarily in those patients with long-term ventilatory support that the use of pressure-targeted ventilation becomes critical for patient-ventilator synchrony.

Auto-PEEP

One of the most overlooked causes of patient-ventilator dyssynchrony is auto-PEEP, primarily because it is not observable or measurable during normal ventilation.[92,93] Auto-PEEP is intrinsic PEEP or identified PEEP that develops as a result of incomplete emptying of local lung units and air trapping.[94] Two general settings increase the probability of auto-PEEP developing: (1) acute or chronic pulmonary disease where dynamic airway compression is present, and (2) a rapid respiratory rate with large VT where expiratory time is inadequate.[95] As noted in Figure 40–19, with auto-PEEP central airway pressure and ventilator circuit pressure do not reflect the auto-PEEP level unless an end-expiratory hold is established.[96] Thus, unless auto-PEEP is looked for, its pres-

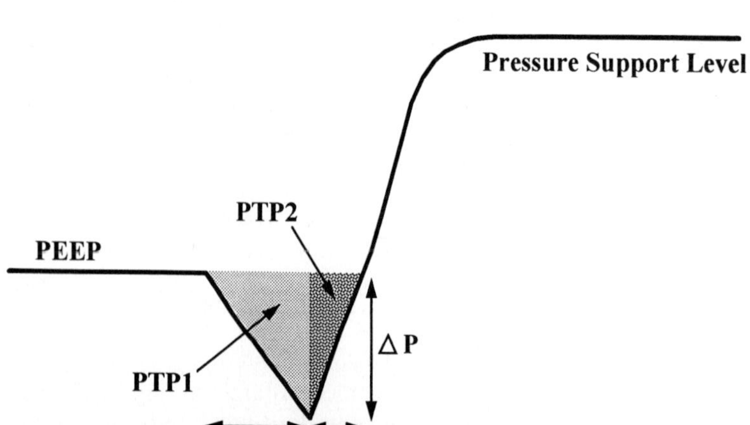

FIGURE **40–16.** Airway pressure-versus-time tracing during triggering of pressure support. ΔP, pressure change to trigger; ΔT1, time from beginning of inspiration to trigger of ventilator; ΔT2, time for return of pressure to baseline (posttrigger period); PTP1, pressure time product of trigger phase; PTP2, pressure time produce of post-trigger period. (From Goulet R, Hess D, Kacmarek RM: Pressure vs. flow triggering during pressure support ventilation. Chest 111:1997 [in press], with permission.)

TABLE 40–6
Concerns Associated with the Use of Heat of Moisture Exchangers

Increased ventilatory load
Increased dead space (up to 100 ml depending on device)
Reduced efficacy at low (<100 ml) or high (>1,000 ml) VT
Occlusion of exchanger with secretion
Obstruction of artificial airway because on inadequate humidification

ence is not identified. Auto-PEEP results in the same localized or global (if extensive) effects seen with applied PEEP,[96] except that it is established in lung units with high or normal compliance and normal or high airway resistance.[94] Auto-PEEP is primarily a problem in patients with intrinsic lung disease—COPD or asthma.

Patient-ventilatory synchrony is affected by auto-PEEP because auto-PEEP markedly increases patient effort to ventilate (Fig. 40–20). Patients must decompress auto-PEEP in order to trigger the ventilator.

Identification of Auto-PEEP

Auto-PEEP can be identified from the airway pressure waveform but only after the application of an end-expiratory hold (Fig. 40–21).[93] Generally patients must be passively ventilated in order to allow accurate evaluation, however, in some patients actively triggering the ventilator, an estimate of auto-PEEP is occasionally possible using this method.[97] The auto-PEEP reflected on

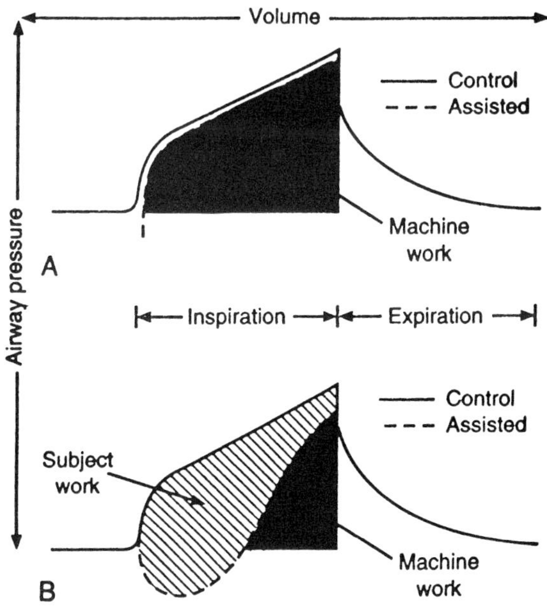

FIGURE **40–17.** Estimation of patient work of breathing during assisted, volume-limited (square waveflow) ventilation. *A*, Actual total work of breathing during controlled ventilation and ideal assisted ventilation. *B*, Controlled ventilation compared to actual assisted ventilation. The *hatched area* represents work performed by a patient during assisted ventilation. (From Marini JJ, Rodriguez M, Lamb V: The inspiratory workload of patient initiated mechanical ventilation. Am Rev Respir Dis 134:902, 1986. © American Lung Association, with permission.)

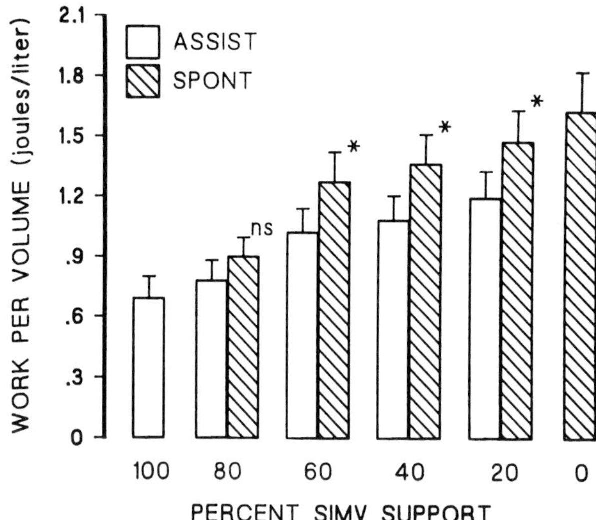

FIGURE **40–18.** Inspiratory work per unit volume (work per liter [W_p/L]) done by the patient during assisted cycles (*open bars*) and spontaneous cycles (*reversed cross-hatched bars*). W_p/L increased monotonically with decreasing SIMV percentage for both types of breath. W_p/L for spontaneous breaths tended to exceed W_p/L for machine-assisted breaths. (*$p < .01$.) (From Marini JJ, Smith TC, Lamb VJ: External work output and force generation during synchronized intermittent mechanical ventilation. Am Rev Respir Dis 138: 1169, 1988. © American Lung Association, with permission.)

the system manometer or pressure waveform is the mean auto-PEEP level, since it reflects the end-expiratory equilibration pressure within the patient/ventilator system; the maximum local auto-PEEP level always exceeds that measured.[95] Auto-PEEP measurement can only occur if no continuous system flow is present. Even systems utilizing low-level flow triggering must be turned off or the auto-PEEP level is overestimated. During assisted or controlled ventilation, auto-PEEP can be identified but not quantified by evaluating end-expiratory flow (Fig. 40–22).[94] If end-expiratory flow has not reached zero prior to the next inspiration, auto-PEEP is present. However, in patients with severe dynamic airway obstruction, the end-expiratory flow may be too low to accurately measure by the crude flow measurement technology on ventilators. In patients with auto-PEEP, expiratory breath sounds continue until they are interrupted by inspiratory sounds, and physical examination and chest x-ray show hyperinflation. In spontaneously breathing patients, the only way to accurately measure auto-PEEP is to evaluate esophageal pressure change (Fig. 40–23) during inspiration at the same time airway opening pressure or flow is evaluated.[95] With auto-PEEP a drop in esophageal pressure occurs before flow is measured at the airway. The magnitude of the drop is equal to the auto-PEEP level. In patients activating abdominal muscles during exhalation, the estimate of auto-PEEP may be inaccurately increased.

As illustrated in Figure 40–24, the volume of gas trapped but not the auto-PEEP level can be estimated by allowing a prolonged uninterrupted expiratory phase (30 to 60 seconds).[98] This maneuver is only possible in patients who are apneic, receiving controlled ventilation. Particularly in patients with asthma whose lungs are

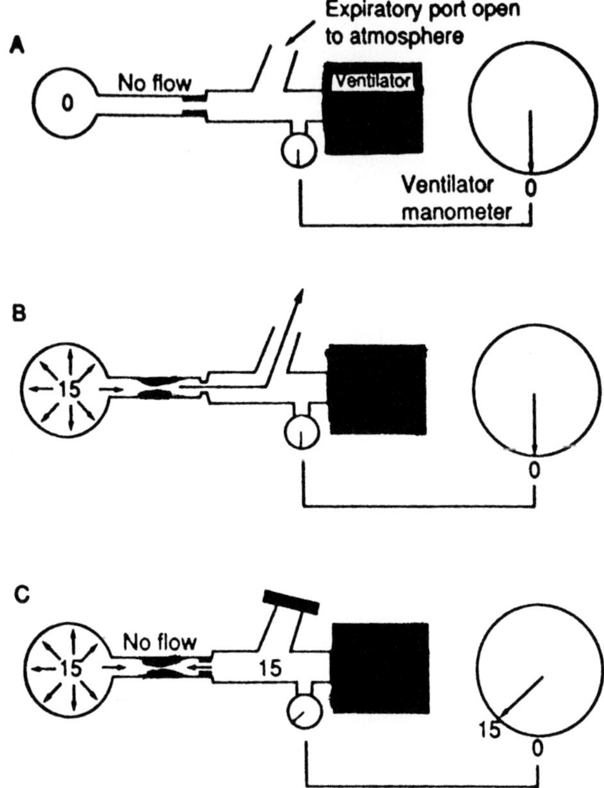

FIGURE **40–19.** Relationship between alveolar, central airway, and ventilator circuit pressure under (*A*) normal conditions and in the presence of severe dynamic airway obstruction, (*B*) with expiratory port open, and (*C*) with expiratory port occluded. Auto-PEEP level is identified by creating an end-expiratory hold, allowing alveolar, central airway, and ventilator circuit pressure to equilibrate. Note that during equilibration auto-PEEP level can be read on the system manometer. (From Pepe PE, Marini JJ: Occult positive end-expiratory pressure in mechanically ventilated patients with airflow obstruction: The auto-PEEP effect. Am Rev Respir Dis 126:166, 1982. © American Lung Association, with permission.)

highly compliant, adjusting the ventilator to reduce trapped volume may be more useful than attempting to measure auto-PEEP by an end-expiratory hold.[99] In some asthmatic patients, airways may completely occlude at end-expiration and precise estimation of auto-PEEP may be impossible.[100]

In addition, because of the large intrathoracic pressure gradient that must be established to cause airflow and triggering of the ventilator in the presence of auto-PEEP, many patients are unable to trigger assisted breaths.[95] Whenever the patient's actual respiratory rate exceeds the ventilator response rate, auto-PEEP is present.

Management of Auto-PEEP

Table 40–7 lists the various techniques used to minimize the level of auto-PEEP. With dynamic airway compression or secretion accumulation, aggressive bronchial hygiene and aerosolized pharmacology should be employed. In addition, respiratory rate and tidal volume should be decreased and inspiratory time shortened in order to maximize expiratory time.[101] In spontaneously breathing patients, PEEP can be applied to balance the auto-PEEP. This allows alveolar, airway, and ventilatory circuit pressure to equilibrate.[95,102] Provided the auto-PEEP is a result of dynamic airway obstruction and applied PEEP does not exceed about 80% of the auto-PEEP, pulmonary mechanics should not be altered when PEEP is applied.[103] If peak and plateau pressures increase with volume-targeted ventilation, or if V_T decreases with pressure-targeted ventilation, the applied PEEP has caused greater overdistention.

Ventilator-Induced Lung Injury

Mechanical ventilation is a nonphysiologic process. Pressure, volume, and F_{IO_2} beyond the levels that the lung normally tolerates are frequently used. As a result, lung injury may be caused or extended by the process of mechanical ventilation. Lung injury generally manifests itself in two forms: gross barotrauma (volutrauma) or parenchymal injury similar to adult respiratory distress syndrome (ARDS).

Barotrauma (Volutrauma)

The term "barotrauma" has been used to describe the gross air leak associated with mechanical ventilation. However, more recently, the term "volutrauma" has been preferred.[104] Since it is now believed that the primary mechanical phenomenon that precipitates injury is localized overdistention of a lung, not pressure per se.[105] Generally, three conditions must be present for volutrauma to develop: disease, high transpulmonary pressure, and overdistention. The precise pressure and volume that increase the likelihood for volutrauma is unknown; however, the maximum transpulmonary pressure developed by healthy individuals is about 30 cm H_2O.[106] Thus, it seems reasonable to expect that the probability of volutrauma will increase if pressure is applied above this level.

Pneumothorax is the most commonly reported acute form of volutrauma. In adult patients, the incidence varies from 0.5 to 44% of ventilated patients.[107–109] The consequences of a pneumothorax may be benign or catastrophic. Small air collections may be asymptomatic. Large collections of air may cause cardiac tamponade. The most dramatic and fatal air leak syndrome occurs with rupture into a bronchial vein producing air embolism.[110] Bronchopleural fistula frequently occurs if air leaks persist for greater than 24 hours.[111]

Precise guidelines for the avoidance of volutrauma are unavailable, although volutrauma is rare when peak inspiratory pressure (PIP) is less than 30 cm H_2O.[112] Cullen and Caldera[113] reported that no patient whose peak airway pressure was less than 60 cm H_2O experienced an air leak, while a 44% incidence was observed when peak airway pressure exceeded 70 cm H_2O. More recently, Hickling et al.[114] reported no air leaks in a series of ARDS patients ventilated at PIP less than 45 cm H_2O. Darioli et al.[115] also reported a zero incidence of pneu-

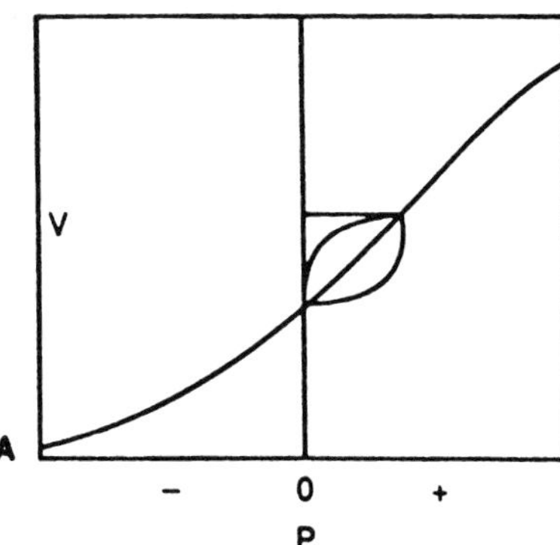

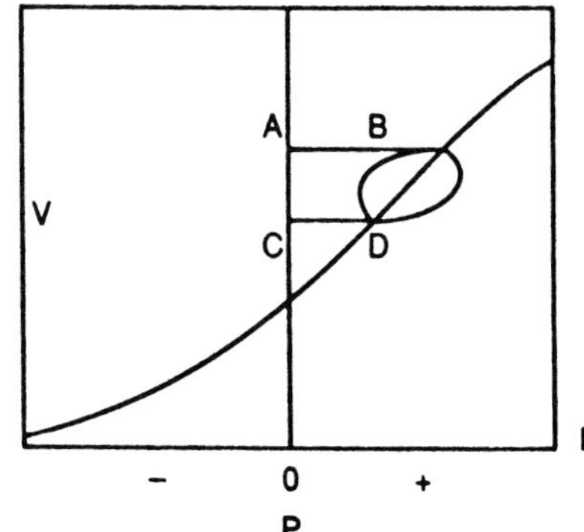

FIGURE **40–20.** *A*, Normal spontaneously breathing esophageal pressure-volume (P-V) loop. *B*, Effect of auto-PEEP on area of P-V loop, reflecting marked increase in work of breathing as a result of the need to decompress the auto-PEEP prior to changing lung volume. Central airway pressure at end-exhalation is depicted by *C*; the pressure change from *C* to *D* must occur before gas movement to the lung periphery is possible. The area of the rectangle CDBA represents the increased workload with auto-PEEP. (From Otis AB: Work of breathing. In Finn WU, Rahn H [eds]: Handbook of Physiology: The Respiratory System, Vol 1. Washington, DC, American Physiological Society 1964, with permission.)

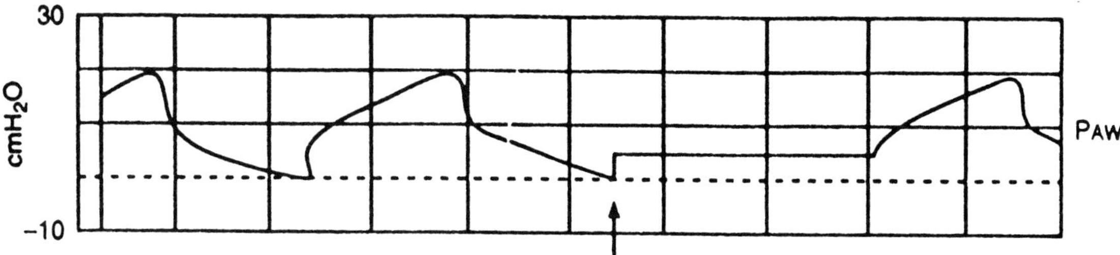

FIGURE **40–21.** Measurement of auto-PEEP (*arrow*) using an end-expiratory hold on the Servo 900C ventilator. Note that peak airway pressure is not affected on the inspiration following measurement, since auto-PEEP is present even though unnoticed on every breath. (From Pierson DJ, Kacmarek RM [eds]: Foundations of Respiratory Care. New York, Churchill Livingstone, 1992, with permission.)

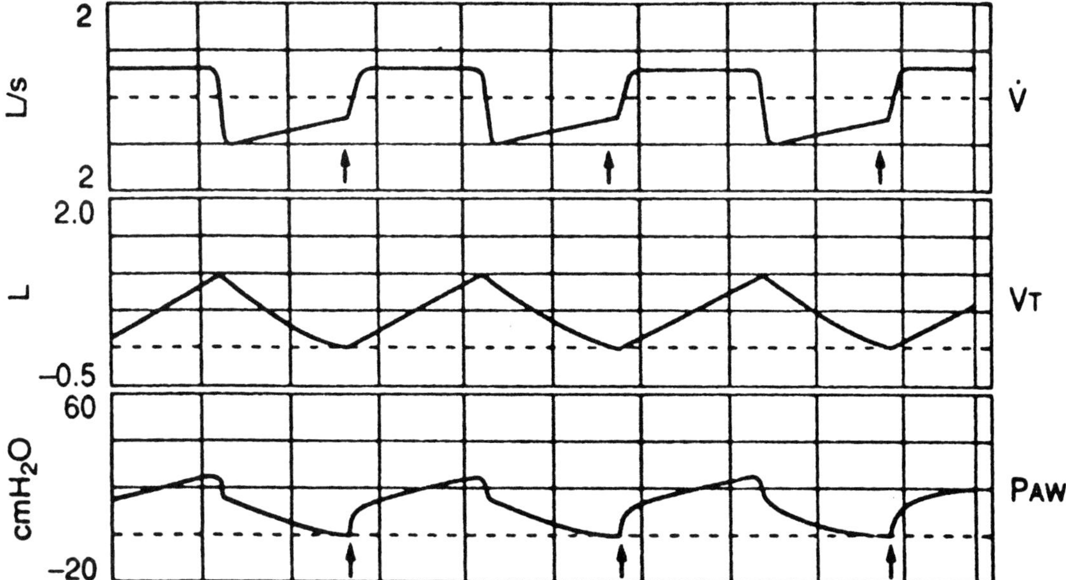

FIGURE **40–22.** Airway pressure (PAW) and flow waveforms during volume-limited controlled ventilation in the presence of auto-PEEP. The initial airway pressure demonstrates a rapid initial increase (*arrow*), approximating the auto-PEEP level and then gradually increasing to peak airway pressure. Expiratory gas flow does not return to zero (*arrow*) in the presence of auto-PEEP. (From Pierson DJ, Kacmarek RM [eds]: Foundations of Respiratory Care. New York, Churchill Livingstone, 1992, with permission.)

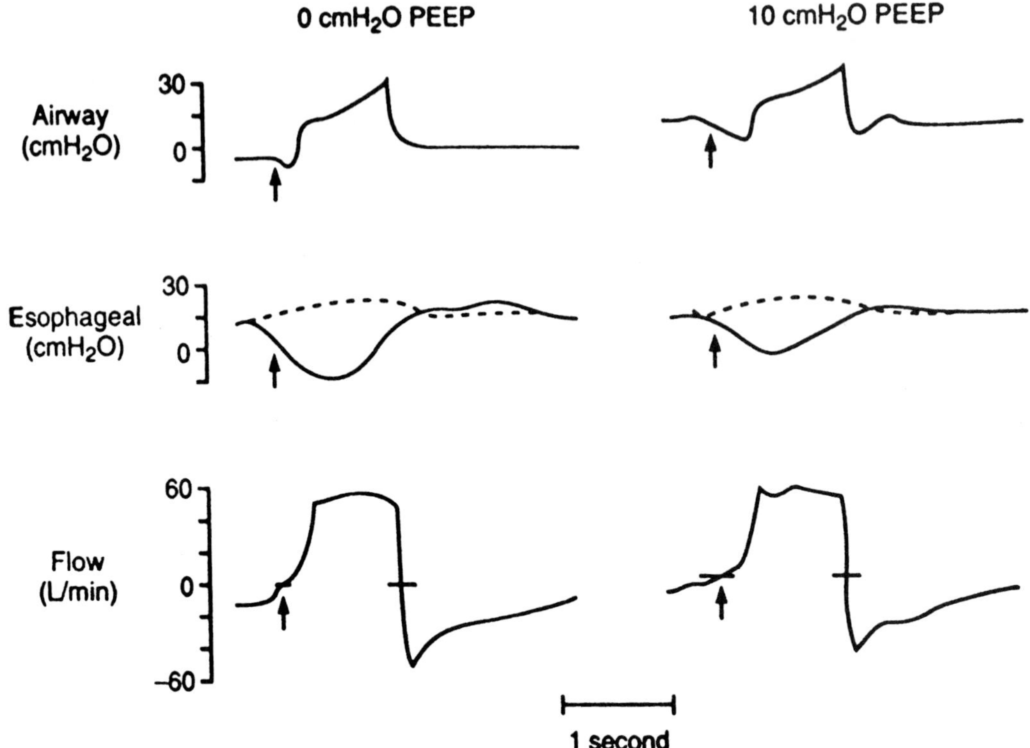

FIGURE **40–23.** Assessment of the level of auto-PEEP in spontaneously breathing patients by evaluation of esophageal pressure change relative to either airway opening pressure or flow at airway opening. *Arrows* indicate pressure and flow change at airway opening. The change in esophageal pressure between baseline and the level that allows change in airway opening pressure or in flow is equal to the auto-PEEP level. Note the effect of 10 cm H_2O applied PEEP on the level of auto-PEEP (left side). (From Smith TC, Marini JJ: Impact of PEEP on lung mechanics and work of breathing in severe airflow obstruction. J Appl Physiol 65:1499, 1988, with permission.)

mothorax in a series of 34 patients with severe asthma ventilated at PIP less than 60 cm H_2O. Both Hickling et al.[114] and Darioli et al.[115] allowed permissive hypercapnia. Analysis of these data makes it difficult to define a precise pressure limit because of the varying approaches used to ventilate patients. Some used volume-targeted ventilation with a square waveform, other employed sign waveforms, and still others used pressure-targeted ventilation. The best overall guidelines to date have been provided by the American College of Chest Physicians, who recommended limiting end-inspiratory plateau pressure to 35 cm H_2O.[116] Recently, a number of authors have recommended measuring and plotting classic pressure-volume curves to determine the upper deflection point or that specific pressure that causes overdistention (Fig. 40–25).[117,118]

Parenchymal Lung Injury

Numerous animal studies (e.g., rats, sheep, dogs, and pigs) have demonstrated parenchymal lung damage (Table 40–8) similar to acute lung injury after relatively short periods of mechanical ventilation when high peak airway pressures were maintained.[119–125] Webb and Tierney[119] noted gross pulmonary edema and hemorrhage in rats after 60 minutes of ventilation with a PIP of 45 cm H_2O (Fig. 40–26). Similar results were reported by Her-

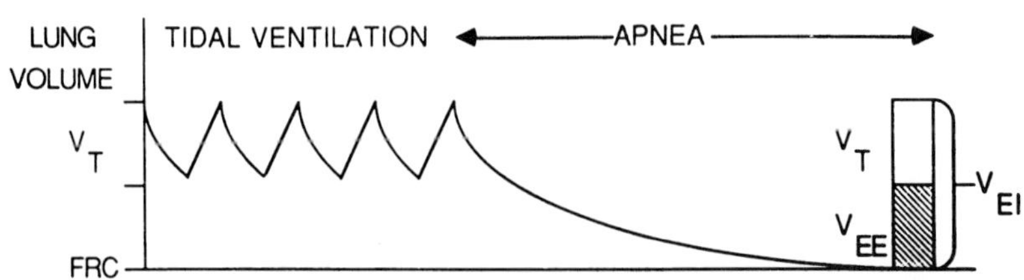

FIGURE **40–24.** Schematic representation of the measurement of end-inspiratory volume (V_{EI}) in a patient with acute asthma. V_{EE} is end-expiratory lung volume above FRC. (From Tuxon DV, Lane S: The effects of ventilatory pattern on hyperinflation, airway pressure, and circulation in mechanical ventilation of patients with severe air-flow obstruction. Am Rev Respir Dis 136:872, 1987. © American Lung Association, with permission.)

TABLE 40–7
Approaches Used to Modify the Level of Auto-PEEP

Decrease dynamic airflow obstruction
  Aggressive bronchodilation
  Chest physical therapy
  Airway suctioning
  Large-size endotracheal tube

Modify ventilatory pattern
  Increase expiratory time
    Decrease rate
    Decrease VT
  Decrease inspiratory time
    Increase peak inspiratory flow
    Use low compressible volume circuit
  Use low rate SIMV

Allow P_{CO_2} to rise >60 mm Hg
  Decrease rate
  Decrease VT

Normalize pH
  Administer $NaHCO_3$ during metabolic acidosis
  Avoid purposeful hyperventilation
Apply PEEP/CPAP to reduce work of breathing

PEEP, positive end-expiratory pressure; VT, tidal volume; SIMV, synchronized intermittent mandatory ventilation; P_{CO_2}, partial pressure of carbon dioxide; $NaHCO_3$, sodium bicarbonate; CPAP, continuous positive airway pressure.

TABLE 40–8
The Spectrum of Lung Injury Induced by Mechanical Ventilation*

Atelectasis
Alveolar hemorrhage
Alveolar neutrophil infiltration
Alveolar macrophage accumulation
Decreased compliance
Detachment of endothelial cells
Denuding of basement membranes
Emphysematous changes
Gross pulmonary edema
Hyaline membrane formation
Interstitial edema
Increased interstitial albumin levels
Interstitial lymphocyte infiltration
Intracapillary bleeding
Pneumothorax
Severe hypoxemia
Subcutaneous emphysema
Systemic gas embolism
Tension cyst formation

*Modified from Kacmarek RM, Hickling KG: Permissive hypercapnia. Respir Care 38:373, 1993, with permission.

nandez et al.[120] in rabbits following ventilation also at PIP of 45 cm H_2O. Kolobow et al.[121] ventilated normal sheep with 40% oxygen at peak airway pressures of 50 cm H_2O. All animals developed severe respiratory failure and at necropsy had pulmonary consolation. Similar injury in rats was shown by Dreyfuss et al.[106,122] (Fig. 40–27), who also demonstrated the same effect with equal levels of negative-pressure ventilation.[105] More recent data by Dreyfuss et al.[123] indicate that high peak airway pressure extends pre-existing lung injury

The key factor that prevents the development of ventilator-associated parenchymal lung injury or the extension of existing injury appears to be the application of PEEP above the low inflection point on the pressure volume curve (Fig. 40–25). The repetitive recruitment and subsequent derecruitment of unstable lung units when PEEP is below the inflection point appears to cause parenchymal lung injury.[119,124,125] The most striking data to support this are that of Webb and Tierney (Fig. 40–26), where at the same peak airway pressure the lung injury was greatly reduced after 60 minutes of ventilatory support when PEEP was applied. Similar data are provided by Corbridge et al.[125] in sheep ventilated at the

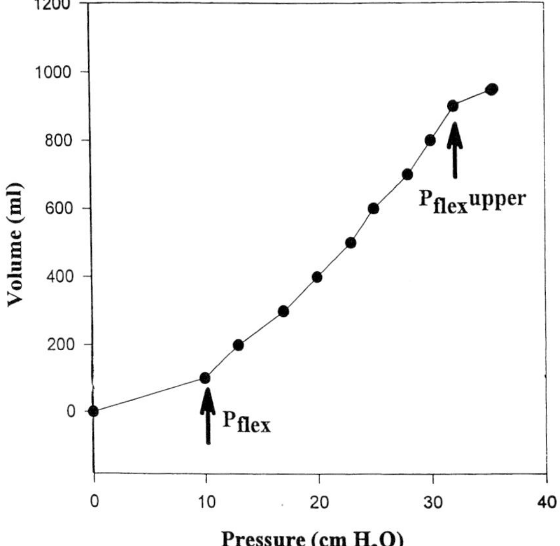

FIGURE 40–25. Classic static pressure-volume curve from a ventilated patient with ARDS. P_{flex}, lower inflection point; P_{flex} upper, upper deflection point.

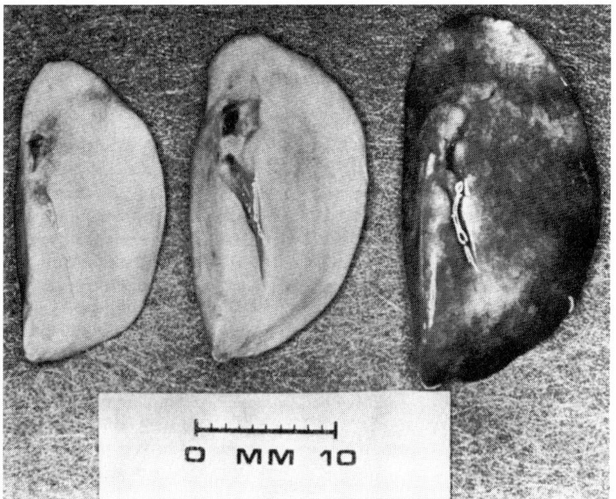

FIGURE 40–26. Comparison of left lungs from rats ventilated, from left to right: peak inspiratory pressure 14 cm H_2O, PEEP 0 cm H_2O; peak inspiratory pressure 45 cm H_2O, PEEP 10 cm H_2O; peak inspiratory pressure 45 cm H_2O, PEEP 0 cm H_2O. The perivascular groove is distended with edema in the lung ventilated at 45/10. Gross hemorrhage edema is present in the lung ventilated with 45/0. (From Webb HH, Tierney DF: Experimental pulmonary edema due to intermittent positive pressure ventilation with high inflation end expiratory pressure. Am Rev Respir Dis 110:556, 1994. © American Lung Association, with permission.)

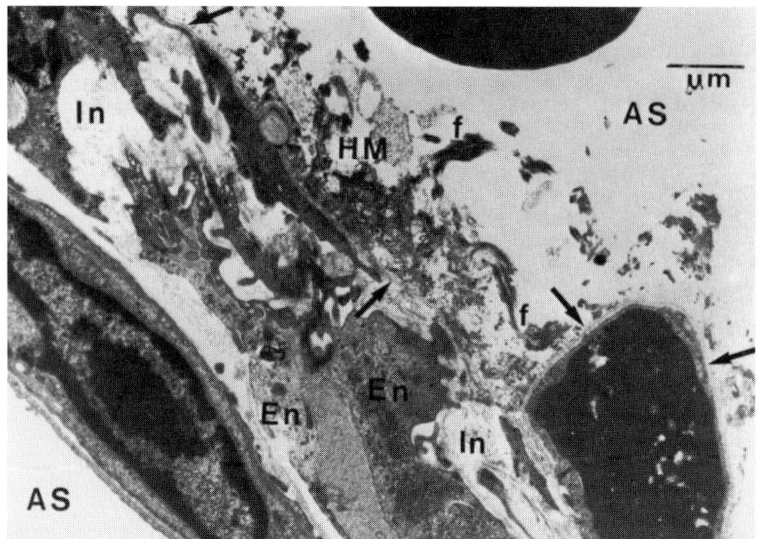

FIGURE **40–27.** Alveolar septum with three capillaries of an adult rat after 20 minutes of ventilation at 45 cm H_2O. At the right side, the epithelial lining is destroyed, denuding the basement membrane (*arrows*). Hyaline membranes (HM) composed of cell debris and fibrin (f) are present. Two endothelial cells (En) of another capillary are visible inside the interstitium (In). At the lower left side, a monocyte fills the lumen of a third capillary with a normal blood-air barrier. (From Dreyfuss D, Basset G, Soler P, Saumon G: Intermittent positive-pressure hyperventilation with high inflation pressure produces pulmonary microvascular injury in rats. Am Rev Respir Dis 132:880, 1985, with permission.)

same peak airway pressure but with different levels of PEEP. PEEP applied at 12.5 cm H_2O with low VT resulted in markedly less injury than low PEEP (2.5 cm H_2O) and a large VT (Fig. 40–28).

Based on these data it appears the best approach in managing patients with acute lung injury is to maintain PEEP above the lower inflection point on the pressure-volume curve of the lung and the peak alveolar pressure (end-inspiratory plateau pressure) below the upper deflection point (Fig. 40–25). However, these pressure targets often result in compromised alveolar ventilation, since ventilatory pressures can be as low as 20 cm H_2O and VT's as small as 5 to 6 ml/kg. When the targeted upper inflection point is reached and gas exchange is still poor, a decision to exceed or not exceed the limit must be made based on the potential detrimental effects of elevated peak alveolar pressure versus permissive hypercapnia.

Gas Exchange Targets

As a result of the potential of ventilatory-induced lung injury, the concept of normal gas exchange during mechanical ventilation is being challenged. Of particular concern are patients presenting with acute lung injury,

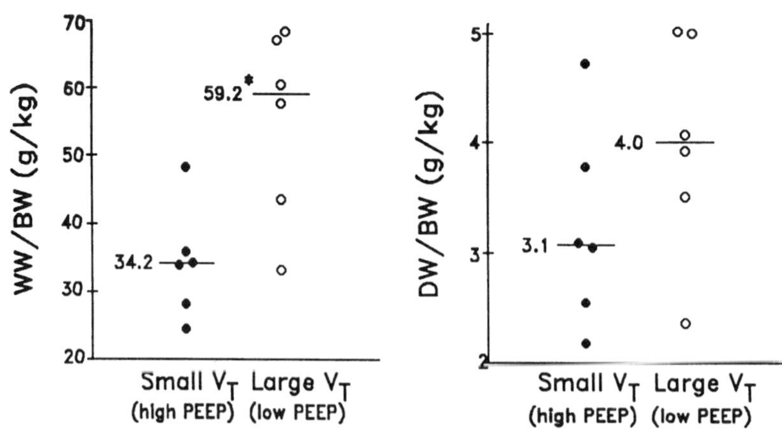

FIGURE **40–28.** Gravimetric estimates of edema. Wet weight to body weight ratios (WW/BW) (gm/kg) and dry weight to body weight ratios (DW/BW) (gm/kg) with median values shown for all animals in both groups. *Median WW/BW was statistically higher in the large VT–low PEEP group by the Mann-Whitney rank sum test (p = .041). Median DW/BW ratios were not significantly different between groups. (From Corbridge TC, Wood DH, Crawford GP, et al: Adverse effects of large tidal volume and low PEEP in canine acid aspiration. Am Rev Respir Dis 142:311, 1990, with permission.)

asthma, or chronic lung disease with high impedance to ventilation.

Permissive Hypercapnia

Permissive hypercapnia is the deliberate limitation of ventilatory support to avoid alveolar overdistention (e.g., adult respiratory distress syndrome [ARDS]) or auto-PEEP (e.g., acute asthma), allowing $Pa{CO_2}$ to rise to levels greater than normal (50 to 100 mm Hg).[126] Allowing the $Pa{CO_2}$ to rise to these levels is considered when the only alternative is a potentially dangerous increase in peak alveolar pressure or auto-PEEP. The potential adverse effects of an elevated $Pa{CO_2}$ are listed in Table 40–9. Most of the clinical problems with permissive hypercapnia occur at $Pa{CO_2}$ levels above 150 mm Hg.[127] However, even small increases in $Pa{CO_2}$ increase cerebral blood flow, and permissive hypercapnia is generally contraindicated when intracranial pressure is increased.[128] Elevated $Pa{CO_2}$ also stimulates ventilation, but patients are usually sedated with some paralyzed in settings where permissive hypercapnia is considered.[129]

Permissive hypercapnia may adversely affect the oxygenation status of some patients. Elevated $Pa{CO_2}$ and low pH shift the oxyhemoglobin dissociation curve to the right.[106] This decreases the affinity of hemoglobin for oxygen, decreasing oxygen loading in the lungs, but facilitating the unloading of oxygen at the tissues.[106] As illustrated by the alveolar gas equation, an increase in the alveolar $P{CO_2}$ results in a decrease in alveolar $P{O_2}$. For each $PA{CO_2}$ rise of 1 mm Hg, the $PA{O_2}$ decreases by about 1 mm Hg.[106]

The effect of carbon dioxide on the cardiovascular system is difficult to predict. As illustrated in Figure 40–29, carbon dioxide elicits competing responses from the cardiovascular system.[130] Carbon dioxide directly stimulates or depresses specific aspects of the cardiovascular system, but opposite effects can occur via stimulation of the autonomic nervous system.[130] It is thus difficult to predict the precise response of the cardiovascular system to permissive hypercapnia in any given patient. However, the most common response is an increase in pulmonary hypertension[131] and potentially the most significant is myocardial depression associated with an increased or decreased cardiac output.[132] Dosages of pharmaceutical agents affecting the cardiovascular and autonomic nervous system may need to be adjusted in the presence of permissive hypercapnia, when a marked acidosis is present.[133]

The primary factor limiting permissive hypercapnia is the pH.[125] Patients without primary cardiovascular disease or renal failure can usually tolerate a pH of 7.20 or higher, and some may tolerate an even lower pH.[114,126,134] The specific minimal pH acceptable needs to be determined for the individual patient. Allowing $P{CO_2}$ to gradually rise from the onset of ventilation allows gradual renal compensation, minimizing marked pH change. Abrupt changes in ventilatory strategies that result in rapid and marked elevation of $Pa{CO_2}$ are usually poorly tolerated.

Whether alkalizing agents should be administered to manage the acidosis induced by permissive hypercapnia is debatable.[114,135] In the setting of cardiac arrest, sodium bicarbonate is contraindicated because of the resulting increased intracellular acidosis.[135] However, intracellular pH does return to 90% of normal within 3 hours of the development of an acute systemic acidosis.[130,136] The use of sodium bicarbonate in permissive hypercapnia, however, has not been extensively studied. One can expect a short-term increase in carbon dioxide load when sodium bicarbonate is administered, which is exhaled over time if the level of ventilation is held constant. Whether the use of alkalizing agents has any effect on an overall tolerance of permissive hypercapnia is not known.

TABLE 40–9
Potential Adverse Physiologic Effects of Permissive Hypercapnia

Shift in the oxyhemoglobin dissociation curve to the right
Decreased $PA{O_2}$
Both stimulation and depression of the cardiovascular system
Central nervous system depression
Simulation of ventilation
Dilation of vascular bed
Increased intracranial pressure
Anesthesia ($Pa{CO_2}$ 200 mm Hg)
Decreased renal blood flow ($Pa{CO_2}$ 150 mm Hg)
Leakage of intracellular potassium ($Pa{CO_2}$ 150 mm Hg)
Alteration of the action of pharmacologic agents (a result of intracellular acidosis)

$PA{O_2}$, partial pressure of oxygen, alveolar; $Pa{CO_2}$, partial pressure of carbon dioxide, arterial.

Oxygenation

Achievement of a normal $Pa{O_2}$ (≥80 mm Hg) is desired in all patients mechanically ventilated. However, the cost of maintaining this level of oxygenation may exceed the benefit in some patients. Provided cardiovascular function is normal and adequate oxygen-carrying capacity is present, a lower $Pa{O_2}$ target becomes acceptable the more acutely ill the patient (Table 40–10).

Management of Oxygenation

Oxygenation status, although dependent on $FI{O_2}$, is also intimately affected by the level of cardiovascular function, PEEP, and mean airway pressure ($\bar{P}aw$). Increasing $FI{O_2}$ is the primary approach used to manage hypoxemia that is a result of $\dot{V}/\dot{Q}$ mismatch and diffusion deficit, while an appropriate level of ventilation corrects hypoxemia resulting from hypoventilation, and PEEP along with $\bar{P}aw$ adjustments are the primary approaches used to manage intrapulmonary shunt.[137] Decreased cardiovascular dysfunction can extend the hypoxemia resulting from any of these causes.[137] When cardiac output is low, tissue O_2 extraction rate is high and mixed venous $P{O_2}$ and O_2 content are usually low. When shunt, $\dot{V}/\dot{Q}$ mismatch, or diffusion deficit is present with low cardiac output, blood with a lower O_2 content from affected

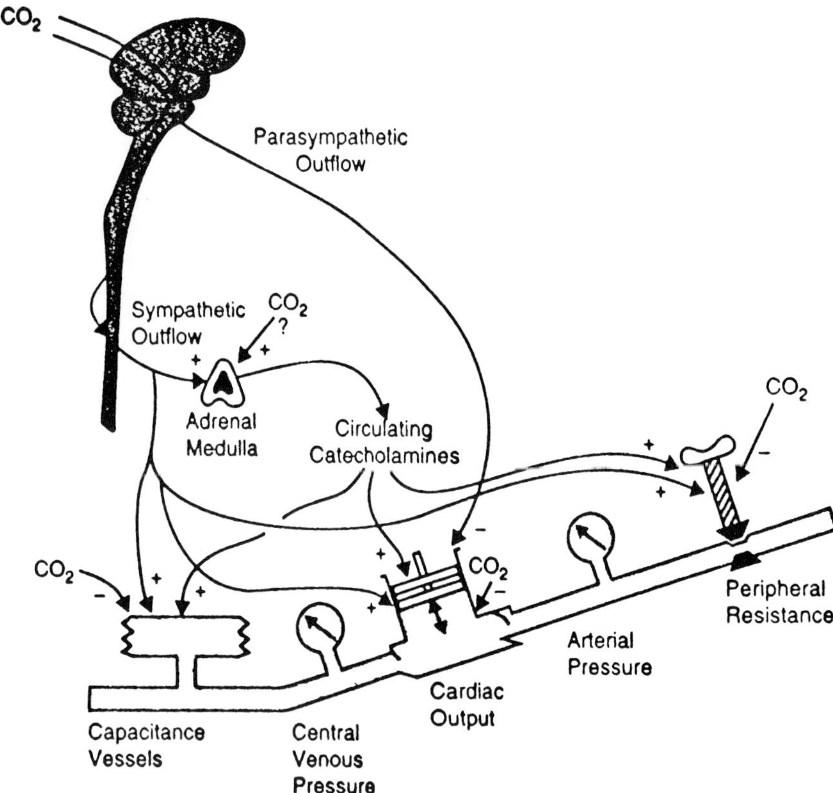

FIGURE **40–29.** This diagram shows the complexity of the mechanisms by which carbon dioxide can influence the circulatory system. See text for details. (From Nunn JF [ed]: Applied Respiratory Physiology, 2nd ed. London, Butterworth Heinemann 1977, with permission.)

areas mixes with blood from unaffected lung units, resulting in a greater degree of hypoxemia than if cardiac output were optimal.[137] Regardless of the cause of hypoxemia or approach used to manage it, for therapy to be most effective cardiovascular function must also be optimized. Throughout the remainder of this section it is assumed cardiovascular function is optimal.

FIO_2

In general, the lowest FIO_2 that results in an acceptable PaO_2 should be set. However, because of concerns regarding oxygen toxicity, FIO_2's above 0.6 for lengthy periods should be avoided when possible.[183–141] In normal, healthy, small mammals inspiration of 100% O_2 for about 24 hours results in structural changes at the alveolar-capillary membrane, pulmonary edema, atelectasis, and a decreased PaO_2.[138,139] In healthy humans, chest pain and tightness develop, but no edema, atelectasis, or decreased PaO_2 has been observed following 24-hour administration of 100% O_2.[140] In the severely diseased lung, antioxidants capable of minimizing the effects of high FIO_2's may be induced, allowing the lung to tolerate high FIO_2 without further damage.[141] Considering the potential damaging effects of high peak alveolar pressure, it is recommended that a higher FIO_2 be applied before the application of high peak alveolar pressure (above upper deflection point).[127,134,142]

In addition to the potential for O_2 toxicity, high FIO_2 may cause absorption atelectasis in poorly ventilated, unstable lung units due to denitrogenation. This does not mean that 100% O_2 should never be used. Whenever oxygenation status is in question or generalized cardiopulmonary instability occurs, 100% O_2 should be administered. FIO_2 should be reduced as rapidly as possible to more appropriate levels when the acute concerns have been resolved. The use of 100% O_2 during patient transport, bronchoscopy, suctioning, chest physical therapy, and any other stressful procedure is also recommended. Unless the required FIO_2 is already established, 100% O_2 should be administered during initial ventilator setup but quickly reduced when appropriate PaO_2 or SpO_2 are established.

TABLE **40–10**
PaO_2 Targets in Acute Lung Injury

>80 mm Hg normal lungs
>70 mm Hg mild lung injury
>60 mm Hg moderate lung injury
>50 mm Hg severe lung injury

PaO_2, partial pressure of oxygen, arterial.

PEEP

Positive end-expiratory pressure increases $\bar{P}aw$ and mean intrathoracic pressure while affecting many other physiologic responses (Table 40–11). When applied to appropriate levels for the clinical setting, PEEP generally improves pulmonary mechanics and gas exchange, but may have varying effects on the cardiovascular system.[143]

TABLE 40–11
Potential Physiologic Effects of Appropriately and Excessively Applied PEEP*

	Appropriate Level	Excessive Level
Intrapulmonary pressure	Increased	Increased
Intrathoracic pressure	Increased	Increased
FRC	Increased	Increased
Lung compliance	Increased	Increased or decreased
Closing volume	Decreased	Decreased
Pa_{O_2}	Increased	Increased or decreased
Pa_{CO_2}	No change or decreased	Increased
$\dot{Q}s/\dot{Q}T$	Decreased	Decreased or increased
$P(A-a)_{O_2}$	Decreased	Decreased or increased
$C(a-\bar{v})_{O_2}$	Decreased	Decreased or increased
$P\bar{v}_{O_2}$	Increased	Increased or decreased
$P(a-ET)_{CO_2}$	Decreased	Increased
VD/VT	Decreased	Increased
Work of breathing	Decreased	Increased
Extravascular lung water	No change or increased	No change or increased
Pulmonary vascular resistance	Increased	Increased
Total pulmonary perfusion	No change or decreased	Decreased
Cardiac output	No change or decreased	Decreased
Pulmonary artery pressure	No change or increased or decreased	Decreased
Pulmonary capillary wedge pressure	No change or increased or decreased	Decreased
Central venous pressure	No change or increased or decreased	Decreased
Arterial pressure	No change or increased or decreased	Decreased
Intracranial pressure	No change or increased	Increased
Urinary output	No change or decreased	Decreased

*From Pierson DJ, Kacmarek RM (eds): Foundations of Respiratory Care. New York, Churchill Livingstone, New York, 1992, with permission.

FRC, functional residual capacity; $\dot{Q}s/\dot{Q}T$, shunt fraction; $P(A-a)_{O_2}$, alveolar–arterial O_2 pressure difference; $C(a-\bar{v})O_2$, arterial–mixed venous O_2 content difference; $P\bar{v}O_2$, mixed venous O_2 pressure; $P(a-ET)_{CO_2}$, arterial–end tidal CO_2 pressure difference, VD/VT, dead space/tidal volume ratio.

Pulmonary Mechanics

PEEP increases FRC regardless of the level applied or the setting used (Fig. 40–30). In acute lung injury where unstable lung units have collapsed, PEEP stabilizes lung units once expanded, preventing their collapse.[144] When recruitment of lung units is stabilized with PEEP, lung compliance improves (Fig. 40–31).[145,146] Along with the improvement in compliance is a reduction in intrapulmonary shunt, an increase in Pa_{O_2}, and a decrease in work of breathing in spontaneously breathing patients.[145] Excessive PEEP further increases FRC, although at a smaller volume/unit pressure change, since excessive PEEP places the lung on the flat portion of the compliance curve.[146] As a result, with pressure-targeted ventilation appropriate adjustment of PEEP can be expected to result in an increase in VT, whereas excessive application causes the VT to decrease.[18] In volume-targeted ventilation, appropriate application of PEEP maintains or may decrease peak alveolar and airway pressure and excessive application increases peak alveolar and airway pressure.[18]

Gas Exchange

In most clinical applications, PEEP is applied to improve arterial P_{O_2}. Appropriate setting of PEEP usually results in increased Pa_{O_2} and decreased intrapulmonary shunt.[145] PEEP may also improve the $P(a\text{-}ET)_{CO_2}$ (end-tidal CO_2) and Pa_{O_2}, by decreasing dead space.[147] However, excessive PEEP can decrease perfusion to well-ventilated areas, causing an increase in $P(a\text{-}ET)_{CO_2}$, Pa_{CO_2} itself, and dead space.[147] Depending on the overall $\dot{V}/\dot{Q}$, excessive PEEP may or may not adversely affect Pa_{O_2} and shunt.

Cardiovascular Function

The effect of PEEP on the cardiovascular system is dependent upon the level of PEEP, the compliance of the lung-thorax system, and cardiovascular status. Because PEEP increases $\bar{P}aw$ and mean intrathoracic pressure, venous return and cardiac output may decrease as PEEP is applied.[148] PEEP has the greatest effect on cardiac output in a setting where lung compliance is high and thoracic compliance and cardiovascular reserve are low.[149] High levels of PEEP increase right ventricular afterload[150] (increased pulmonary vascular resistance), which increases end-diastolic volume,[151] decreases ejection fraction,[152] and shifts the interventricular septa to the left.[153] This, along with a reduction in the pericardial pressure gradient, limits left ventricular distensibility, reducing left ventricular end-diastolic volume and stroke volume.[154] Thus, both intrathoracic and systemic vascular pressures are affected by PEEP. If flow is maintained when PEEP is applied, vascular pressures remain unchanged or increase. However, if pulmonary perfusion is decreased, vascular pressures generally decrease as PEEP is applied. The result is decreased cardiac output, arterial blood pressure, urine output, and tissue oxygenation. Thus, PEEP may increase arterial oxygenation, but decrease tissue oxygenation.

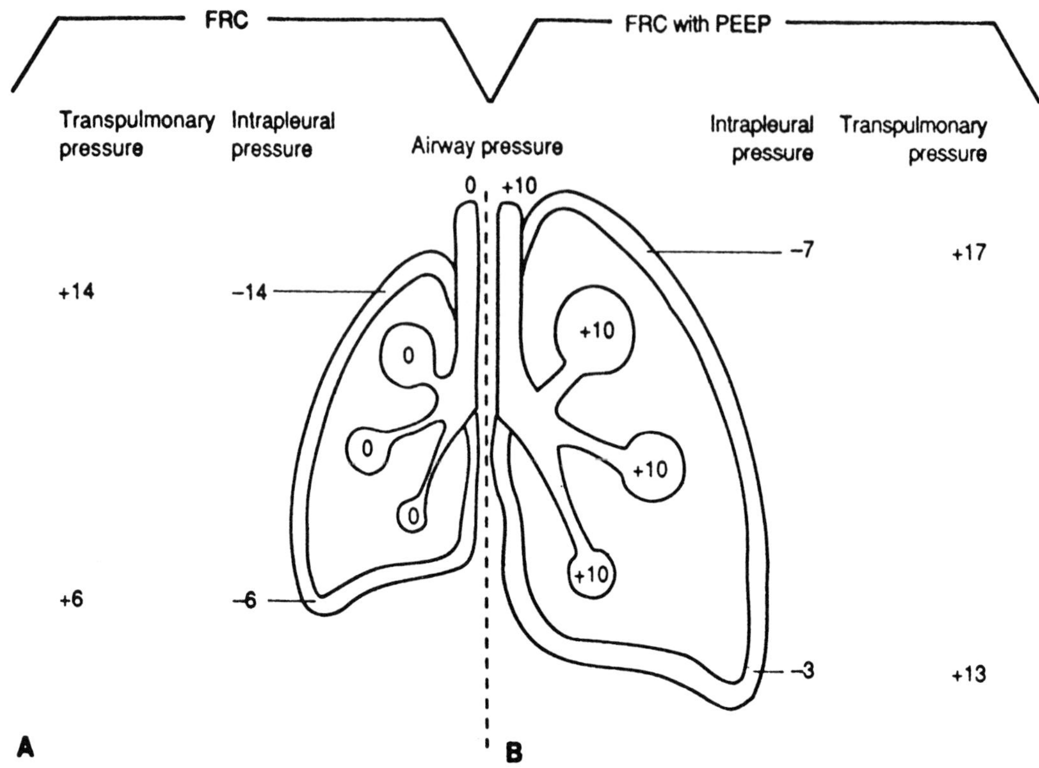

FIGURE **40–30.** *A*, Acute restrictive lung disease without PEEP results in greater than normal negative intrapleural pressures at functional residual capacity (FRC). *B*, With 10 cm H_2O PEEP, more pressure is transmitted to the pleural space at the apex (7 cm H_2O transmitted) because of the normal apex-to-base variation in compliance than at the base (3 cm H_2O transmitted). Thus, transpulmonary pressure is increased by 7 cm H_2O at the base and only 3 cm H_2O at apex. (From Shapiro BA, Kacmarek RM, Cane RD, et al: Clinical Applications of Respiratory Care, 4th ed. Chicago, Mosby-Yearbook Medical Publishers, 1991, with permission.)

Acute Lung Injury

The primary use of PEEP is in the management of acute lung injury, The pressure-volume curve of the lung-thorax system in acute lung injury is illustrated in Figure 40–32.[155] This curve is characterized by a shift to the right, the appearance of an inflection point, and marked hysteresis, when compared to the normal pressure-volume curve. The inflection point on the curve represents a critical level of end-expiratory pressure. PEEP applied at or above this level prevents derecruitment of unstable lung units.[156] In most adults, the inflection point is reached with about 8 to 18 cm H_2O PEEP.[117,118] As noted by Gattinoni et al.[157] on serial computed tomography (CT) scans of the chest with PEEP, the critical closing pressure of lung units is gravity dependent. Generally, as PEEP is slowly titrated, a large improvement in gas exchange (>15 mm Hg increase in Po_2 or >2% increase in Sao_2) is observed and system compliance improved as the inflection point is reached.[156,157] Once PEEP is above the inflection point, a linear relationship generally exists between Pao_2 and mean airway pressure,[158] although the Pao_2 increase per cm H_2O $\bar{P}aw$ increase may be very small. In later stages of acute lung injury, marked consolidation and fibrosis are observed with a loss of the inflection point and grossly decreased lung volume. A PEEP level lower than that applied in early injury is frequently appropriate; however, $\bar{P}aw$ may still need to be elevated.[149]

Mean Airway Pressure

$\bar{P}aw$ is the average pressure applied to the lung over the entire ventilatory cycle. The magnitude of $\bar{P}aw$ is dependent upon numerous factors that affect gas delivery (Table 40–12). In acute lung injury, $\bar{P}aw$ and oxygenation are directly related if PEEP is applied above the inflection point on the pressure-volume curve.[156] Extending inspiratory time is a useful method of increasing $\bar{P}aw$ without elevating peak alveolar pressure and maintaining a constant level of ventilation.[18,159] This is true provided no auto-PEEP is developed. If auto-PEEP develops, either peak alveolar pressure or tidal volume is affected. With volume-targeted ventilation, auto-PEEP increases peak alveolar pressure because VT is constant, while with pressure-targeted ventilation, tidal volume is decreased as auto-PEEP develops. Because peak airway pressure and peak alveolar pressure are kept constant with pressure-targeted ventilation, the pressure gradient establishing VT decreases when auto-PEEP occurs. Auto-PEEP also causes a less uniform distribution of PEEP and FRC than applied PEEP.[160] As a result of the heterogeneous lung disease in adult respiratory distress syndrome (ARDS), pulmonary time constants can vary considerably from one lung unit to another.[161,162] With auto-PEEP, FRC and total PEEP will be largest in the most compliant lung units (longest expiratory time constant) and lowest in the least compliant lung units (short-

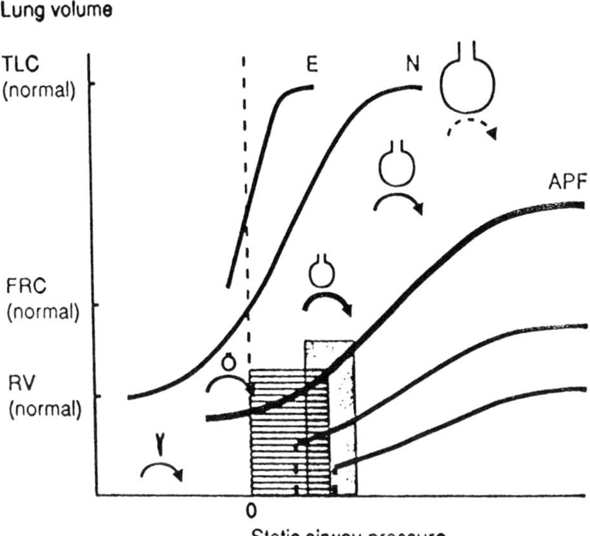

FIGURE **40–31.** Family of regional pressure-volume curves of the respiratory system, in normal lungs (N) and in lungs of patients with emphysema (E) and acute pulmonary failure (APF). The whole lung APF curve is the sum of multiple regional compliance curves, some resembling normal and others very low compliance regions, two of which are shown in the diagram. *Shaded areas* show the pressure-volume relationship during the same tidal ventilation with and without PEEP. *Broken vertical line* denotes regional volume (RV) at which alveoli are unstable and readily "open" or "close." TLC, total lung capacity. (From Suter PM, Fairley HB, Isenberg MD: Optimum end-expiratory airway pressure in patients with acute pulmonary failure. N Engl J Med 292:284, 1975, with permission.)

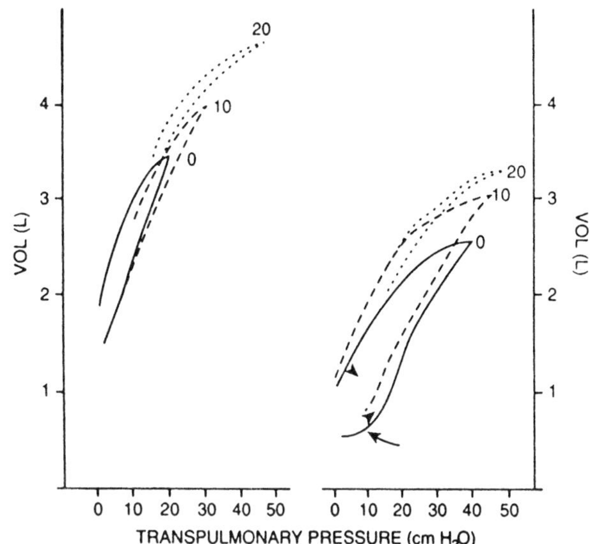

FIGURE **40–32.** Static pressure-volume curves of the respiratory system for two patients at 0, 10, and 20 cm H_2O PEEP. The curves on the left are from a patient with a normal chest radiograph who was intubated for coma. There is little hysteresis, and the FRC is normal. The curves on the right are from a patient early in the course of ARDS. Without PEEP applied, the pressure-volume curve demonstrates marked hysteresis (*arrowheads*) and an inflection point on the inflation limb (*arrow, right*). At the highest level of PEEP (20 cm H_2O), the inflection point is lost and the pressure-volume curve assumes a monotonic profile with a P-V slope (compliance) similar to that of patients with normal lungs. (From Benito S, Lemaine F: Pulmonary pressure-volume relationship in acute respiratory distress syndrome in adults: Role of positive end-expiratory pressure. J Crit Care 5:27, 1990, with permission.)

est expiratory time constant).[159] Inspiratory time should be limited to the maximum level that does not create auto-PEEP. However, as noted earlier no controlled, randomized, prospective study has shown improved physiologic response with inverse ratio ventilation.[23–28] All references illustrating a beneficial physiologic response from inverse ratio ventilation have been case presentation series.[14,21,22]

Optimizing Oxygenation

Assuming appropriate cardiovascular function, increasing FIO_2 is the recommended first step in managing oxygenation. In acute lung injury, once FIO_2 exceeds 0.40, PEEP should be applied above the inflection point. If oxygenation is still compromised, the FIO_2 is slowly increased to 0.60, after which the inspiratory time is increased to further increase $\bar{P}aw$ until auto-PEEP develops. If further therapy is needed once inspiratory time is maximized, either FIO_2 or PEEP should be further increased. It is at this point in the management of oxygenation when decisions regarding which maneuver is considered least detrimental in the specific patient, high FIO_2 or high peak alveolar pressure, must be made.

Weaning

The ultimate goal of mechanical ventilation is discontinuation of support, and in the vast majority of patients this is a simple process. About 75 to 80% of patients mechanically ventilated can simply have the ventilator discontinued when the physiologic reason for ventilatory support is reversed.[68,163,164] Another 15 to 20% of patients may require the use of a specific weaning protocol applied over an 8- to 72-hour period before discontinuation is possible.[68] But it is the remaining small percentage of mechanically ventilated patients that require gradual weaning, sometimes requiring weeks or months before discontinuation, that are most problematic.[165–167] This is the group where the term "weaning" is most properly applied. There is also a very small percentage of these patients who may never be physiologically ready to

TABLE **40–12**
Factors Affecting Mean Airway Pressure

Applied PEEP
Auto-PEEP
Vital volume
Pressure control level
Gas flow waveform*
Rate*
Inspiratory time/I:E ratio*

*Do not increase peak alveolar pressure unless auto-PEEP develops.
PEEP, positive end-expiratory pressure; I:E, inspiratory to expiratory.

"wean" and should be considered chronically ventilator dependent.[168–170]

Readiness to Wean

Before weaning is considered, the specific indication for ventilatory support must be reversed. The patients should be able to maintain a Pa_{O_2} of 60 mm Hg or greater with an F_{IO_2} 0.40 or less and PEEP of 5 cm H_2O or less.[68,165,171] Excess minute ventilation during ventilatory support should not be required to maintain a normal Pa_{CO_2}, and V_D/V_T should be less than 0.6.[68,165] The patient should also have an intact ventilatory drive. Cardiovascular function should be optimized,[172,173] fever should be managed, electrolytes in balance,[174,175] nutritional status normalized,[176,177] and all other major organ systems functioning appropriately. Without this level of readiness, weaning trials frequently fail.

Predictors of Weaning Outcome

Various indices have been used to predict successful weaning outcome (Table 40–13). Unfortunately, few of these have demonstrated clinical efficacy. Maximal inspiratory pressure (MIP) and vital capacity (VC) have been proposed by many as useful predictors of ability to ventilate spontaneously[178]; however, the results of other groups have been conflicting.[179–181] Sahn and Lakshminarayan[178] found an MIP of less than 20 cm H_2O predicted weaning failure and an MIP greater than 30 cm H_2O predicted weaning success. Tahvanainen et al.[179] and others[180,181] identified high percentages of false-positives and false-negatives using Sahn and Lakshminarayan's guidelines. Similar controversy exists over the use of a VC of greater than 10 ml/kg[182] or a minute ventilation of less than or equal to 10 L/min[178,180] as predictors of weaning success. Others have recommended the use of maximal voluntary ventilation,[178] dead space–to–tidal volume ratio,[183] and P_{100}[184] as predictors of weaning capability; however, all have subsequently demonstrated poor sensitivity and specificity.[179,185–187] The single index that has demonstrated both sensitivity and specificity is the rapid/shallow breathing index (f/V_T) proposed by Yang and Tobin (Fig. 40–33).[188] These authors compared the f/V_T to other traditional weaning indexes and found that f/V_T was the best predictor of weaning success, while the maximum inspiratory pressure measurement (<20 cm H_2O) and the f/V_T were the best predictors of weaning failure. The f/V_T is evaluated 1 minute after both ventilation and oxygenation support are removed. An f/V_T of less than 105 is predictive of successful weaning.[188]

TABLE 40–13
Proposed Indexes of Successful Weaning

Measurement	Predictor of Success
Maximum inspiratory pressure	$\geq$30 cm H_2O
Vital capacity	>10 ml/kg
Minute ventilation	$\leq$10 L/min
Dead space to tidal volume	$\leq$60%
Rapid shallow breathing index	$\leq$105
P_{100}	$\leq$5 cm H_2O

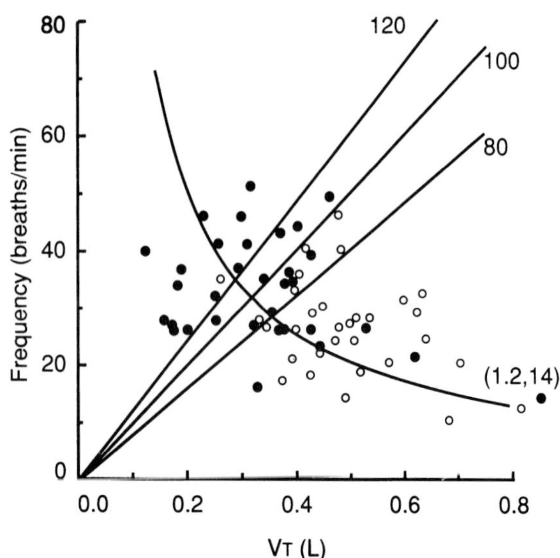

FIGURE **40–33.** Isopleths for the breathing frequency/V_T(f/V_T) ratio representing different degrees of rapid shallow breathing. For the patients indicated by the points to the left of the isopleth, representing 100 breaths/min/L, the likelihood that a weaning trial would fail was 95%, whereas for the patients indicated by the points to the right of this isopleth, the likelihood of a successful weaning outcome was 80%. This hyperbola represents a minute ventilation of 10 L/min. Values for successfully weaned patients (*open circles*) and for patients in whom weaning failed (*solid circles*) are indicated. Values for one patient (V_T 1.2 L and respiratory frequency of 14 breaths/min) lay outside the graph. (From Yang KL, Tobin MJ: A prospective study of indexes predicting the outcome of trials of weaning from mechanical ventilation. N Engl J Med 324:1445, 1991, with permission.)

On a more global perspective most have recommended that a patient's oxygen requirements are low (Pa_{O_2}/F_{IO_2} ratio >200 mm Hg, F_{IO_2} $\leq$0.40, PEEP $\leq$5 cm H_2O), their use of sedatives and narcotics as well as vasopressors are minimized, that they have intact upper airway reflexes, and an intact and responsive ventilatory drive to be considered candidates for weaning trials.[165,171,189–191] Most recently it has been recommended that patients meeting these criteria receive a spontaneous weaning trial of as long as 2 hours (T-piece or CPAP [$\leq$5 cm H_2O] trial) to determine if they can sustain spontaneous ventilation.[189–191] Criteria for failure of the trial include a respiratory rate greater than 35 breaths/min for 5 minutes or longer; a heart rate that exceeds 140 bpm; or sustained changes in the heart rate of 20% in either direction, a systolic blood pressure greater than 180 mm Hg or less than 90 mm Hg, increased anxiety, and diaphoresis.[191]

Weaning Failure

One of the biggest mistakes made when weaning patients is to push patients to the point of exhaustion. When this occurs, it normally delays weaning progress.[192] Whether exhaustion of patients failing weaning is syn-

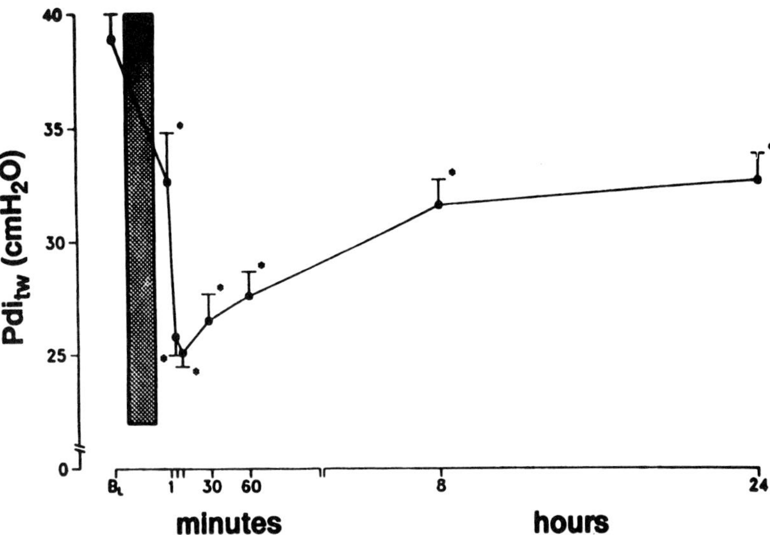

FIGURE **40–34.** Induction of diaphragmatic fatigue (*stippled bar*) produced a significant fall in Pdi_{tw} (twitch transdiaphragmatic pressure). Nadir of Pdi_{tw} was reached 10 minutes after conclusion of fatigue protocol, and Pdi_{tw} values at 8 and 24 hours remain lower than at B_L (baseline). Values are means ± SE. *Significant difference compared with B_L values, $p < .01$. (From Laghi F, D'Alfonso N, Tobin MJ: Pattern of recovery from diaphragmatic fatigue over 24 hours. J Appl Physiol 79:539, 1995, with permission.)

onymous with fatigue is debatable.[193] However, if fatigue does occur it requires greater than 24 hours for recovery.[194] Recent data from Laghi et al.[194] in volunteers indicates that ventilatory muscle fatigue only recovers to about 75% of maximal capacity in healthy young adults after 24 hours (Fig. 40–34). As a result it can be assumed that ventilatory muscle fatigue in acutely ill patients would require at least a similar period for recovery.

Although work of breathing is not a good predictor of weaning success, an excessive workload may be the primary reason why a patient fails a trial of weaning.[181,195] High airway resistance and low compliance contribute to the increased effort necessary to breathe. Aerosolized sympathomimetics, bronchial hygiene therapy, and a normalized fluid balance all assist in normalizing compliance, resistance, and work of breathing. In a large percentage of patients with chronic lung disease who require lengthy weaning periods, auto-PEEP is a primary problem.[196–198] If present, auto-PEEP increases the pressure gradient needed to inspire if patients are assisting or spontaneously breathing. The use of CPAP/PEEP balances alveolar pressure with central airway pressure, decreasing the pressure gradient required to ventilate.[95,102]

Imbalance of serum electrolytes causes muscular weakness. Specifically, decreased potassium, magnesium, phosphate, and calcium levels impair ventilatory muscle function.[199–201] Patients with a negative nitrogen balance rarely are capable of weaning.[202] However, care should be exercised to avoid overfeeding, since excessive carbohydrate ingestion markedly elevates CO_2 production.[202] Failure of any other major organ system can also precipitate weaning failure. Fever and infection are of particular concern, since both O_2 consumption and CO_2 production are increased, resulting in an increased ventilatory requirement (Table 40–14).

Of particular concern in patients with cardiopulmonary disease is poorly managed left heart failure.[203,204] A delicate balance between mean airway pressure and pulmonary hemodynamics may exist that is easily disrupted by the decreasing of mean airway pressure during weaning trials (Fig. 40–35). These patients may rapidly develop pulmonary edema during weaning. Appropriate management of cardiovascular status is necessary before weaning is successful.

Approaches to Weaning

In general, approaches to weaning can be grouped into three categories: (1) pressure-support ventilation (PSV), (2) SIMV, and (3) T-piece/CPAP trials, although combinations of these are also employed.[45] In those patients requiring a lengthy period of weaning (>12 hours), it is important to adjust ventilatory support to ensure ventilatory muscle rest at night and a good night's sleep. Successful weaning approaches appropriately mix work with rest periods and ensure proper nutrition and sleep.

Pressure Support

Many recommend the use of a gradual reduction in the level of PSV, provided the patient can maintain a target respiratory rate and V_T, as the most appropriate approach to weaning.[32,39,41,189] The process is begun by setting the pressure support at a level that achieves a respiratory rate (RR) and tidal volume consistent with the level expected on discontinuation (RR ≤30 breaths/min, V_T ≥5 ml/kg).[189] Generally, the minimum level of pressure support

TABLE **40–14**
Common Reasons for Failure to Wean

Weaning to exhaustion
Auto-PEEP
Excessive work of breathing
Poor nutritional status
Overfeeding
Left heart failure
Decreased magnesium and phosphate levels
Infection/fever
Major organ system failure
Technical limitations

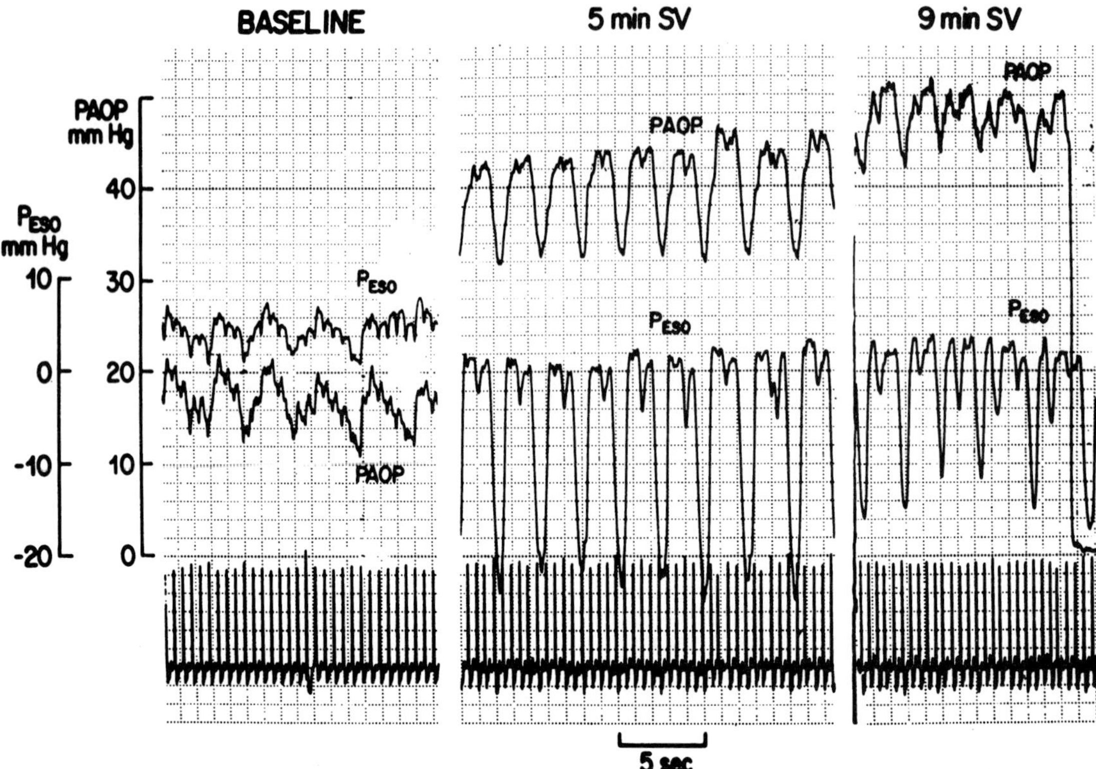

FIGURE **40–35.** Weaning of patient 6 from mechanical ventilation (baseline) to spontaneous ventilation (SV). There is a progressive increase of pulmonary artery occlusion pressure (PAOP) from 14 mm Hg (baseline) to 50 mm Hg (9-minute SV). The esophageal pressure is reduced during SV with marked negative inspiratory excursions. (From Lemaire F, Teboul JL, Cinotti L, et al: Acute left ventricular dysfunction during unsuccessful weaning from mechanical ventilation. Anesthesiology 69:171, 1988, with permission.)

that prevents activation of accessory muscles is appropriate.[40] PSV is then decreased on a regular basis (hours or days) until some minimum level (5 to 8 cm H_2O) is reached that unloads the work of breathing imposed by the ventilator/artificial airway system, but still maintains the desired ventilatory pattern.[190,192] Once the patient is capable of maintaining the target ventilatory pattern and gas exchange at this minimal level, mechanical ventilation is discontinued.

Although this approach works well with most patients requiring short-term weaning (8 to 72 hours), this approach can be problematic in patients who require weeks to wean, since it does not allow the patient to rest. Maintaining the level of ventilatory support continually at the minimal level necessary may not be appropriate in patients requiring lengthy weaning periods.[165]

SIMV

SIMV was introduced as a ventilatory mode to facilitate weaning.[50] Like PSV, a gradual reduction in SIMV rate to a predefined minimal level is commonly the approach used during weaning.[189,190] However, contrary to PSV, with SIMV two very distinct types of breaths are established: a pressure- or volume-targeted mandatory breath and an unassisted spontaneous breath. As a result, some patients may experience dyssynchrony with low SIMV rates.[52] As with PSV, an SIMV wean does not allow for rest periods at a level of support greater than the minimal set level. SIMV is most useful for the rapid weaning of short-term mechanical ventilation (e.g., postoperatively, overdose). When SIMV is used during weaning of patients with longer ventilatory courses, it is essential that the level of ventilatory support be increased during the night to ensure rest and sleep.[10] Generally, an SIMV rate at night that provides near 100% support if recommended. Because of the work of breathing imposed by the ventilator and the endotracheal tube, patients should not be maintained on an SIMV rate of 4 or less without PSV unloading the spontaneous breaths.[10,33]

T-Piece/CPAP Trials

The classic approach to weaning is the T-piece or CPAP trial.[165,205] With this approach, increasing periods of unsupported spontaneous breathing are interspersed between periods of full ventilatory support. In long-term mechanically ventilated patients, the trial period may begin with periods as short as 5 minutes several times per day. The length of the trials is then increased over time as the patient's tolerance improves, always allowing periods of complete rest between trials and during the night. How long a spontaneous breathing trial should extend before ventilatory discontinuation is dependent upon the type of airway. In patients with tracheostomy tubes and long-term ventilatory support, T-piece/CPAP trials may extend for as much as 24 hours before ventilator discontinuation is complete. However, with endotracheal tubes, unsupported spontaneous ventilation for more than 30 to 120 minutes is poorly tolerated.[165] Patients with endotracheal tubes ventilated short term who can tolerate spontaneous breathing without blood-gas or ventilatory pattern changes for 30 minutes should be considered weaned from ventilatory support and candidates for extubation.[165,188]

The Optimal Weaning Approach

Unfortunately, no single optimal approach to weaning has been clearly defined, and it is doubtful that any specific approach facilitates weaning; however, all approaches applied inappropriately may delay weaning. Patients wean from ventilatory support when they are physiologically ready to wean, not because a particular approach had been used in the process. The goal of any weaning protocol is to ensure that patients who are ready for ventilator independence are rapidly identified. Two multicenter studies evaluating different approaches to weaning have been recently published,[190,191] unfortunately with opposite results. One study[190] demonstrated that pressure support was the optimal approach, the other[191] T-piece/CPAP trials, however, both identified SIMV as the approach that most prolonged ventilatory support. Protocol differences reflective of investigators' bias may account for some of the differences, but which approach—pressure support or T-piece/CPAP trial—is best has not been defined.

More recently, Ely et al.[191] compared in a randomized prospective manner a well-defined therapist/nurse-driven protocol for weaning to standard physician ordering practices. Patients in the treatment group were evaluated daily. Those whose $Pa{O_2}/F{IO_2}$ ratio was greater than or equal to 200, PEEP was 5 cm H_2O or less, f/VT was 105 or less, and who were not receiving significant vasopressors or sedatives with intact upper airway reflexes underwent an up to 2-hour T-piece/CPAP trial. If they completed the trial with their RR 35 or fewer breaths/min, SaO_2 90% or greater, heart rate of 140 bpm or less with no sustained changes of greater than 20% in either direction, systolic blood pressure above 90 mm Hg but less than 180 mm Hg and no increased anxiety or diaphoresis, the patient was considered weaned. They found a significant decrease in weaning time, mechanical ventilator days, and complications (frequency of reintubation) in the treatment group. These data along with those of Brochard[190] and Esteban[191] point to the need for establishing well-defined literature-based protocols as the best method of ensuring that weaning is not prolonged by the approach used.

Ventilatory Support

The majority of patients requiring ventilatory support in the postoperative period are apneic because of unreversed anesthetic agents, and most are without significant pulmonary disease. These patients generally require a short (<24 hours) course of ventilatory support without complicating issues. They can be ventilated successfully with any of the current modes of ventilatory support (Table 40–15).[206]

Postoperative patients with a history of chronic lung disease are more challenging. These patients generally fall into two groups: those with chronic obstructive and those with chronic restrictive lung disease. In patients with chronic obstructive lung disease the major concern is air trapping and auto-PEEP. As a result, ventilatory rates are kept low and tidal volume maintained at a moderate level with peak alveolar pressure kept below 30 cm H_2O where possible. Once these patients begin to breathe spontaneously PEEP should be applied at low levels to balance auto-PEEP and reduce effort to trigger the ventilator (Table 40–15).

In patients with chronic restrictive pulmonary disease, rapid rates, small tidal volume, and very short inspiratory time are necessary to ensure peak alveolar pressure is not excessive. Frequently VT's of 4 ml/kg with inspiratory time of less than 1.0 second are necessary to ensure patient/ventilatory synchrony.

The most difficult patient to manage in the postoperative period is the one with single-lung pathology or obstructive pathology in one lung and restrictive pathology in the other lung (e.g., single-lung transplantation; native lung obstructed, transplanted lung stiff). In these situations, the final ventilator settings are generally a compromise between the conflicting ventilatory requirements of each lung. In all patients, appropriate setting of PEEP and limiting of peak airway pressure along with the avoidance of auto-PEEP are the overriding management concerns. Generally, either moderate VT's with slow rates or small VT's with rapid rates result in the best gas exchange. In both settings inspiratory times are kept short (1.0 second) to avoid air trapping in the obstructed lung.

The postoperative patient developing ARDS is generally managed as described with PEEP set above the inflection point on the pressure-volume curve and peak alveolar pressure maintained below the deflection point. This generally means a low VT ($\leq$8 ml/kg) with moderate set respiratory rates ($\leq$20 breaths/min) and permissive hypercapnia. Extending inspiratory time is used by some to elevate mean airway pressure without increasing peak alveolar pressure and high $F{IO_2}$ ($\geq$0.6) may be required in severe ARDS to keep PaO_2 above 50 mm Hg.

Adjuncts to Ventilatory Support

Over the last 5 to 10 years much of the research regarding support of the patient with acute respiratory failure has moved from emphasis on ventilatory methodology to the use of adjuncts to ventilatory support. A number of specific techniques have demonstrated improved physiologic response in ARDS. The use of prone positioning,[207] tracheal gas insufflation,[208] inhaled nitric oxide,[209] and partial liquid ventilation[210] show the greatest promise of affecting patient outcome.

TABLE 40–15
Recommended Initial Ventilator Settings for Postoperative Patients*

Setting	Recommendation
	Postoperative Patients with No Prior Pulmonary Disease
Mode	A/C or SIMV
Rate	8–12/min
Volume/pressure target	Volume or pressure
Tidal volume	12–15 ml/kg and plateau pressure <35 cm H_2O
Inspiratory time	1–1.2 sec
PEEP	≤5 cm H_2O
FI_{O_2}	Sufficient to maintain PaO_2 ≥80 mm Hg
Flow waveform	Decelerating
	Postoperative Patients with Prior Obstructive Lung Disease
Mode	A/C or SIMV
Rate	6–8/min
Volume/pressure target	Pressure
Tidal volume	8–12 ml/kg and plateau pressure <30 cm H_2O
Inspiratory time	0.8–1.25 sec (peak flow ≥60 L/min with volume ventilation)
PEEP	≥5 cm H_2O to offset auto-PEEP
FI_{O_2}	Sufficient to maintain PaO_2 ≥60 mm Hg
Flow waveform	Decelerating
	Postoperative Patients with Prior Restrictive Lung Disease
Mode	A/C or SIMV
Rate	12–20/min
Volume/pressure target	Pressure
Tidal volume	4–8 ml/kg and plateau pressure <35 cm H_2O
Inspiratory time	≤1 sec (peak flow ≥60 L/min with volume ventilation)
PEEP	≤5 cm H_2O
FI_{O_2}	Sufficient to maintain Pa_{O_2} ≥60 mm Hg
Flow waveform	Decelerating

*Modified from Hess DR, Kacmarek RM: Essentials of Mechanical Ventilation. New York, McGraw-Hill, 1996, with permission.
A/C, assist/control; SIMV, synchronized intermittent minute ventilation; PEEP, positive end-expiratory pressure.

Prone Positioning

Adult respiratory distress syndrome has been defined as a homogenous severe lung injury associated with atelectasis, decreased compliance, intrapulmonary shunting, and severe hypoxemia.[68] However, more detailed analysis of ARDS shows a lung that demonstrates a very heterogenous pattern of injury with areas of normal lung, recruitable lung, and consolidated lung.[161,162] This pattern of consolidation frequently presents in a gravity-dependent distribution.[161,162] Since blood flow is primarily distributed to gravity, marked $\dot{V}/\dot{Q}$ mismatch and intrapulmonary shunting is the result. Placing the patient with this pattern of injury in the prone position can result in marked improvement in oxygenation (Fig. 40–34).[207,211–217] Recently, Chatte et al.[207] reported on 32 consecutive patients with severe acute respiratory failure who were placed in the prone position. Seven of the 32 had no response to prone positioning (<20 mm Hg PaO_2 improvement); however, 25 (78%) showed an increase in PaO_2/FIO_2 from 117 ± 24 to 164 ± 44 mm Hg after prone positioning.

The mechanism by which prone positioning improved oxygenation relates directly to its effects on regional pleural pressure gradients.[218] In the supine position a marked pleural pressure gradient exists anterior to posterior as a result of the interrelationships among the structures in the thoracic cavity. The gravitational gradient of pleural pressure is more uniform in the prone position than in the supine position, causing a more uniform distribution of ventilation.[213–219] Since perfusion is still distributed based on gravity, the prone position results in reduced shunt and improved $\dot{V}/\dot{Q}$ relationships.[219]

With time some of the initial benefits of the prone position is lost in all patients. This requires a repetitive repositioning of patients from supine to prone to supine. The precise frequency of this rotation has not been well defined but in most patients seems to be between 4 and 8 hours.

Prone positioning is not without risks; the potential adverse effects must be carefully compared to potential benefits in a given patient before turning. Chattle et al.[207] reported minor skin injury and edema, two instances of apical atelectasis, one catheter removal, one catheter compression, one extubation, and one transient supraventricular tachycardia in 32 patients experiencing 294 periods of prone positioning.

Tracheal Gas Insufflation

Concern regarding ventilator-induced lung injury has resulted in the use of lower peak alveolar pressures and VT's and the frequent maintenance of permissive hypercapnia.[116] Although many patients tolerate permissive hypercapnia, many experience adverse responses from the associated acidosis.[128] Tracheal gas insufflation (TGI) is a method of reducing arterial Pa_{CO_2} without increasing peak alveolar pressure.[220] A secondary flow of gas either continuous or intermittent is injected distal to the tip of the endotracheal tube.[221] The direction of injection may be toward the carina or toward the mouth.[222] TGI improves CO_2 elimination by washing CO_2 from the dead space of the upper airway, endotracheal tube, and ventilator circuit, and creates turbulence about the tip of the catheter enhancing gas mixing.[220] In both animal models[220–225] and patients[208] TGI has been shown to enhance CO_2 elimination. However, many questions regarding its safe application must be addressed before it can be recommended for routine use. With the crude systems currently available, peak alveolar pressure, V_T, and PEEP can be markedly increased during continuous-flow TGI.[226] Intermittent (expiratory phase only) TGI can eliminate these concerns, but expiratory phase TGI requires intimate interaction of the TGI gas delivery system with the mechanical ventilator.[227] This is not currently available commercially.

Inhaled Nitric Oxide

Nitric oxide (NO) is endogenously produced in multiple organ systems by the conversion of L-arginine to L-citruline in the presence of nitric oxide synthesis.[228] Guanylate cyclase conversion of guanosine triphosphate (GTP) to cyclic guanosine monophosphate (cGMP) is accelerated by the pressure of NO.[228] Although cGMP exerts its effect on many systems, it is the effect of cGMP on vascular smooth muscle that is of interest in ARDS.[229] NO via cGMP dilates vascular smooth muscle.[230] Many systemically administered vasodilators release NO for this effect. When NO is inhaled, its effects on pulmonary vascular smooth muscle only occur in areas of the lung where ventilation is present, and since NO rapidly reacts with hemoglobin, its effects when inhaled are localized to the lung.[231] Inhaled NO is thus classified as a selective pulmonary vasodilator that decreases pulmonary artery pressure and improves intrapulmonary shunt and oxygenation.[232]

The beneficial physiologic effects of inhaled NO are well documented.[209,233–236] Patients with severe acute respiratory failure have shown improved Pa_{O_2} and decreased pulmonary artery pressure with inhaled nitric oxide. Whether these effects in adults will have an impact on overall outcome is still debatable. However, preliminary data from phase II trials in adults[237] and phase III data in infants with persistent pulmonary hypertension,[238,239] seem to indicate that low levels of inhaled NO ($\leq$10 ppm) do have a positive effect on outcome. The effect in adults may be related to the anti-inflammatory effect of NO noted in animal[240,241] and preliminary human studies.[242]

Not all patients receiving inhaled NO respond to its administration.[243] The specific populations of patients where inhaled NO is most useful are yet to be defined. However, in patients with sepsis, response rate is markedly reduced.[243]

Unfortunately, no commercially designed NO delivery system is available in the United States. Current administration methodologies are less than optimal.[244,245] However, it is anticipated that appropriate technology will be available in the near future.

Partial Liquid Ventilation

The most recent adjunct to management of severe acute respiratory failure that shows promising preliminary results is partial liquid ventilation (PLV).[210,246–251] During PLV a perfluorocarbon (perfluoroctyl bromide [$C_8F_{17}BR$]) is slowly instilled into the lung (~15 to 30 ml/kg) during ventilatory support.[246,247] Perfluoroctyl bromide is odorless, colorless, insoluble in water, chemically stable, and biologically inert. It has a very low surface tension (18 dyne/cm), high density (1.92 gm/ml), and a high spreading coefficient (2.7 dyne/cm).[210] PLV has been referred to as "liquid PEEP" because of its ability to recruit collapsed lung units.[248] It also causes lavage of distal lung.[249] As a result of its high density, cellular debris and mucus float to the top of the column of perfluoroctyl bromide and can easily be suctioned from the airway.

Animal data indicate a dose-dependent improvement in arterial oxygenation.[248] However, few data evaluating the cardiovascular effects of PLV are available, nor are data defining optimal approaches to ventilation during PLV. Preliminary human data in infants during extracorporeal membrane oxygenation (ECMO)[250] and conventional ventilation[210] demonstrate improved gas exchange and pulmonary compliance. Only limited data in adults are currently available.[251] Use of PLV in neonates, pediatrics, and adults is in various phases of FDA-regulated trials.

References

1. Maier HC, Cournand A: Studies of arterial oxygen saturation in the postoperative period after pulmonary resection. Surgery 13: 199, 1943.
2. Gale GD, Sanders DE: The Bartlett-Edwards incentive spirometer: A preliminary assessment of its use in the prevention of atelectasis after cardiopulmonary bypass. Can Anesth Soc J 24: 408, 1977.
3. Gale GD, Teasdale SJ, Sanders DE, et al: Pulmonary ateletasis and other respiratory complications after cardiopulmonary bypass and investigation of etiological factors. Can Anesth Soc J 26:15, 1979.
4. Brown SR, Birnbaum ML, Chopra PS: Pre- and postoperative pulmonary function abnormalities in coronary artery revascularization in surgery. Chest 23:316, 1978.
5. Rehder K, Sessler Ad, Marsh HM: General anesthesia and the lung. Am Rev Respir Dis 112:541, 1975.
6. Catley DM, Thornton C, Jordan C, et al: Pronounced episodic oxygen desaturation in the postoperative period: Its association with ventilatory pattern and analgesic regimen. Anesthesiology 63:20, 1985.
7. Kacmarek RM, Hess D: Basic principles of ventilatory machinery. In Tobin MJ (ed): Principles and Practice of Mechanical Ventilation. New York, McGraw Hill, 1994, p 65.
8. Marini JJ: Pressure-controlled ventilation. In Tobin MJ (ed): Principles and Practice of Mechanical Ventilation. New York, McGraw-Hill, 1994, p 305.
9. Ravencraft SA, Burke WC, Marini JJ: Volume cycled decelerating flow: An alternate form of mechanical ventilation. Chest 101:1342, 1992.

10. Kacmarek RM: Management of the patient ventilator system. In Pierson DJ, Kacmarek RM (ed). Foundations of Respiratory Care. New York, Churchill Livingstone, 1992, p 973.
11. Truwitt JP, Marini JJ: Evaluation of thoracic mechanics in the ventilated patient. Part II, applied mechanics. J Crit Care 3:199, 1988.
12. Marcy T, Marini J: Inverse ratio ventilation: Rationale and implementation. Chest 100:494, 1991.
13. Marcy T, Burke W, Adams A, et al: Mean alveolar pressure is higher during ventilation with constant pressure than with constant flow or sinusoidal flow wave forms (Abstract). Am Rev Respir Dis 141:A239, 1990.
14. Abraham E, Yoshihara G: Cardiorespiratory effects of pressure controlled ventilation in severe respiratory failure. Chest 98: 1445, 1990.
15. Al-Saady N, Bennett ED: Decelerating flow waveform improves lung mechanics and gas exchange in patients on intermittent positive pressure ventilation. Intensive Care Med 11:68, 1985.
16. Baker AB, Babington PCB, Colliss, Cowie RW: Effects of varying inspiratory flow waveform and time in intermittent positive pressure ventilation. Br J Anaesth 49:1221, 1977.
17. Baker AB, Restall R, Clark BW: Effects of varying inspiratory flow waveform and time in intermittent positive pressure ventilation: Emphysema. Br J Anaesth 54:547, 1982.
18. Kacmarek RM: Inverse ratio ventilation (IRV) in the critically ill. Curr Opin Crit Care 1998 (in press).
19. Rossi A, Ranieri VM: Positive end inspiratory pressure. In Tobin MJ (ed): Principles and Practice of Mechanical Ventilation. New York, McGraw-Hill, 1994, p 259.
20. Marini JJ, Cooke PS, Truwitt JD: Determinants and limits of pressure preset ventilation: A mathematical model of pressure control. J Appl Physiol 67:1081, 1989.
21. Tharratt R, Allen R, Albertson T: Pressure controlled inverse ratio ventilation in severe adult respiratory failure. Chest 94:755, 1988.
22. Gurevitch M, Van Dyke J, Young E, Jackson K: Improved oxygenation and lower peak airway pressure in severe adult respiratory distress syndrome: Treatment with inverse ratio ventilation. Chest 89:211, 1986.
23. Cole A, Weller S, Sykes M: Inverse ratio ventilation compared with PEEP in adult respiratory failure. Intensive Care Med 10: 227, 1984.
24. Mang H, Kacmarek RM, Ritz R, et al: Cardiopulmonary effects of volume and pressure controlled CPPV at various I:E ratios in an acute lung injury model. Am J Respir Crit Care Med 151: 731, 1995.
25. Lessard MRE, Guerot H, Lorino F, et al: Effects of pressure controlled with different I:E ratios versus volume-controlled ventilation on respiratory mechanics, gas exchange, and hemodynamics in patients with adult respiratory distress. Anesthesiology 80:983, 1994.
26. Munoz J, Guerrero JE, Escalante JL, et al: Pressure-controlled ventilation with decelerating inspiratory flow. Crit Care Med 21: 1143, 1993.
27. Mercat A, Graini L, Teboul J-L, et al: Cardiorespiratory effects of pressure controlled ventilation with and without inverse ratio in the adult respiratory distress syndrome. Chest 104:871, 1993.
28. Brandolese R, Broseghini C, Polese G, et al: Effects of intrinsic PEEP on pulmonary gas exchange in mechanically-ventilated patients. Eur Respir J 6:358, 1993.
29. Kacmarek RM, Hess D: Airway pressure, flow and volume waveforms and lung mechanics during mechanical ventilation. In Kacmarek RM, Hess D, Stoller JR (eds): Monitoring in Respiratory Care. Chicago, Mosby-Yearbook Medical Publishers, 1993, p 497.
30. Kacmarek RM: Methods of providing mechanical ventilatory support. In Pierson DJ, Kacmarek RM (eds): Foundations of Respiratory Care. New York, Churchill Livingstone, 1992, p 953.
31. Cinnella G, Conti G, Lofaso, et al: Effects of assisted ventilation on the work of breathing: Volume-controlled versus pressure-controlled ventilation. Am J Respir Crit Care Med 153:1025, 1996.
32. MacIntyre NR: Respiratory function during pressure support ventilation. Chest 89:677, 1986.
33. Kacmarek RM: the role of pressure support ventilation in reducing the work of breathing. Respir Care 33:99, 1988.
34. MacIntyre NR, Ho Li: Effects of initial flow rate and breath termination criteria on pressure support ventilation. Chest 99: 134, 1991.
35. MacIntyre NR, Nishimuron M, Usada Y, et al: The Nagoya Conference on system designs and patient-ventilator interactions during pressure support ventilation. Chest 97:1463, 1990.
36. Bunburaphong T, Imanaka H, Nishimura M, et al: Performance characteristics of Bilevel Pressure Ventilators: A lung model study. Chest 1998 (in press).
37. Jubran A, Van de Graaf WB, Tobin MJ: Variability of patient-ventilator interaction with pressure support ventilation in patients with chronic obstructive pulmonary disease. Am J Respir Crit Care Med 152:129, 1995.
38. Prakash O, Meji S: Cardiopulmonary response to inspiratory pressure support during spontaneous ventilation vs conventional ventilation. Chest 88:403, 1985.
39. Brochard L, Pluskwa F, Lemaire F: Improved efficacy of spontaneous breathing with inspiratory pressure support. Am Rev Respir Dis 136:411, 1987.
40. Murphy DF, Dobb GD: Effect of pressure support of spontaneous breathing during intermittent mandatory ventilation. Crit Care Med 15:612, 1987.
41. Brochard L, Harf A, Lorino H, Lemaire F: Inspiratory pressure support prevents diaphragmatic fatigue during weaning from mechanical ventilation. Am Rev Respir Dis 139:513, 1989.
42. Ershowsky P, Krieger B: Changes in breathing pattern during pressure support ventilation. Respir Care 32:1011, 1987.
43. Tokioka H, Saito S, Kosaka F: Effect of pressure support ventilation on breathing pattern and respiratory work. Intensive Care Med 15:491, 1989.
44. Van de Graaf WB, Gordey K, Dornseif SE, et al: Pressure support: Changes in ventilatory pattern and components of the work of breathing. Chest 100:1082, 1991.
45. Hurst JM, Branson RD, Davis K, Barrette RR: Cardiopulmonary effects of pressure support ventilation. Arch Surg 124:1067, 1989.
46. MacIntyre NR: Pressure support ventilation: Effects on ventilatory reflexes and ventilatory muscle work load. Respir Care 32: 447, 1987.
47. Brochard L, Rua F, Lorino H, et al: Inspiratory pressure support compensates for the additional work of breathing caused by the endotracheal tube. Anesthesiology 75:739, 1991.
48. Kirby RR, Robinson EJ, Shulz J, deLemos R: A new pediatric volume ventilator. Anesth Analg 50:533, 1971.
49. Kirby RR, Robinson EJ, Shulz J, deLemos R: Continuous flow as an alternative to assisted or controlled ventilation in infants. Anesth Analg 18:179, 1972.
50. Downs JB, Klein EF, Desautels RS: Intermittent mandatory ventilation: A new approach to weaning patients from mechanical ventilation. Chest 64:331, 1973.
51. Luce JM, Pierson DJ, Hudson LD: Intermittent mandatory ventilation. Chest 79:678, 1991.
52. Marini JJ, Smith TC, Lamb VJ: External work output and force generation during synchronized intermittent mechanical ventilation: Effect of machine assistance on breathing effort. Am Rev Respir Dis 138:1169, 1988.
53. Quan SF: Mandatory minute ventilation. In Tobin MJ (ed): Principles and Practice of Mechanical Ventilation. New York, McGraw-Hill, 1994, p 333.
54. Hewlett AM, Platt AS, Terry VG: Mandatory minute ventilation. Anesthesiology 32:163, 1977.
55. Chapin C, Fourier F, Chambrin MC, et al: A new method of weaning from mechanical ventilation: CO_2-regulated ventilation. Presse Med 12:495, 1983.
56. Kacmarek RM, Hess D: Equipment required for home mechanical ventilation. In Tobin MJ (ed): Principles and Practices of Mechanical Ventilation. New York, McGraw-Hill, 1994, p 111.
57. Hill NS, Eveloff SE, Carlisle CC, Goff SG: Efficacy of nocturnal mask ventilation in patients with restrictive thoracic disease. Am Rev Respir Dis 145:365, 1992.
58. Downs JB, Stock MC: Airway pressure release ventilation: A new concept in ventilatory support. Crit Care Med 15:459, 1987.

59. Räsänen J, Downs JB, Stock MC: Cardiovascular effects of conventional positive pressure ventilation and airway pressure release ventilation. Chest 93:911, 1988.
60. Valentine DP, Hammond MD, Downs JB, et al: Distribution of ventilation and perfusion with different modes of mechanical ventilation. Am Rev Respir Dis 143:1262, 1991.
61. Cane RD, Peruzzi WT, Shapiro BA: Airway pressure relief ventilation in severe acute respiratory failure. Chest 100:460, 1991.
62. Walham RE: Nocturnal nasal intermittent positive pressure ventilation with bilevel positive airway pressure (BiPAP) in respiratory failure. Chest 101:516, 1992.
63. Elliott MW, Simondo AK, Carroll MP, et al: Domiciliary nocturnal nasal intermittent positive pressure ventilation in hypercapnia respiratory failure due to chronic obstructive lung disease: Effects on sleep and quality of life. Thorax 47:342, 1992.
64. Restrick LJ, Scott AD, Ward EM, et al: Nasal intermittent positive-pressure ventilation. Respir Med 81:199, 1993.
65. Amato MBP, Barbas CSV, Bonassa J, et al: Volume-assured pressure support ventilation (VAPSV). Chest 102:1225, 1992.
66. Hass CF, Bronson RD, Folk LM: Patient-determined inspiratory flow during assisted mechanical ventilation. Respir Care 40:716, 1995.
67. MacIntyre NR, Gropper C, Westfall T: Combining pressure-limiting and volume-cycling features in a patient-interactive mechanical breath. Crit Care Med 22:353, 1994.
68. Shapiro BA, Kacmarek RM, Cane RD, et al: Clinical Application of Respiratory Care, 4th ed. Chicago, Mosby-Yearbook Medical Publishers, 1991.
69. Pierson DJ: Respiratory failure: Introduction and overview. In Pierson DJ, Kacmarek RM (eds): Fundamentals of Respiratory Care. New York, Churchill Livingstone, 1992, p 295.
70. MacIntyre NR, Leatherman NE: Ventilatory muscle load and the frequency-tidal volume pattern during inspiratory pressure-assisted (pressure supported) ventilation. Am Rev Respir Dis 141:327, 1990.
71. Shapiro W, Wilson RK, Casar G, et al: Work of breathing through different sized endotracheal tubes. Crit Care Med 14: 1028, 1986.
72. Wright PE, Marini JJ, Bernard GR: In vitro versus in vivo comparison of endotracheal tube airflow resistance. Am Rev Respir Dis 142:10, 1989.
73. Bolder PM, Healy TEJ, Bolder AR, et al: The extra work of breathing through endotracheal tubes. Anesth Analg 65:853, 1986.
74. Kacmarek RM: Optimizing ventilatory muscle function during mechanical ventilation. In Pierson DJ, Kacmarek RM (eds): Foundations of Respiratory Care. New York, Churchill Livingstone, 1992, p 1037.
75. Sassoon CSH: Mechanical ventilator design and function: The trigger variable. Respir Care 37:1056, 1992.
76. Sassoon CSH, Codia R, Theeman SH, et al: Inspiratory muscle work of breathing during continuous positive airway pressure, pressure ventilation, and T-piece during weaning from mechanical ventilation. Am Rev Respir Dis 143:489, 1991.
77. Sassoon CSH, Giron AE, Ely EA, Light RW: Inspiratory work of breathing on flow-by and demand-flow continuous airway pressure. Crit Care Med 17:1108, 1989.
78. Hirsch C, Kacmarek RM, Stanek K: Work of breathing during CPAP and PSV imposed by the new-generation mechanical ventilators: A lung model study. Respir Care 36:815, 1991.
79. Nishimura M, Hess D, Kacmarek RM: The response of flow-triggered infant ventilators. Am J Respir Crit Care 152:1901, 1995.
80. Goulet R, Hess D, Kacmarek RM: Pressure vs flow-triggering during pressure support ventilation. Chest 111:1998 (in press).
81. Hess D, Kacmarek RM: Technical aspects of the patient-ventilator interphase. In Tobin MJ (ed): Practice and Principles of Mechanical Ventilation. New York, McGraw-Hill, 1994, p 1039.
82. Ploysongsang Y, Branson RD, Rashkin MC, Hurst JM: Effect of flow rate and duration of use on the pressure drop across six artificial noses. Respir Care 34:902, 1989.
83. Ploysongsang Y, Branson RD, Rashkin MC, Hurst JM: Pressure flow characteristics of commonly used heat-moisture exchangers. Am Rev Respir Dis 138:675, 1988.
84. Conti G, DeBlasi RA, Rocco M, et al: Effects of heat and moisture exchangers on dynamic hyperinflation of mechanically ventilated COPD patients. Intensive Care Med 16:441, 1990.
85. Erkerbom B, Lindholm CE: Heat and moisture exchangers at the body temperature: A peri-operative study. Acta Anaesth Scand 34:538, 1990.
86. Branson RD, Davis K, Campbell RS, et al: Humidification in the intensive care unit. Chest 104:1800, 1993.
87. Roustan JP, Kierlan J, Aubas P, et al: Comparison of hydrophobic heat and moisture exchangers and heated humidification during prolonged mechanical ventilation. Intensive Care Med 18: 97, 1992.
88. Dreyfuss D, Djedaini K, Gros I, et al: Mechanical ventilation with heated humidifiers and heat and moisture exchangers: Effects on patient colonization and incidence of nosocomial pneumonia. Am J Respir Crit Care Med 151:986, 1995.
89. Gallagher J, Stangeways JEM, Allt-Graham: Contamination control in long-term ventilation: A clinical study using a heat and moisture exchanging filter. Anesthesia 41:527, 1987.
90. Marini JJ, Capps JS, Culver BH: The inspiratory work of breathing during assisted mechanical ventilation. Chest 87:612, 1985.
91. Marini JJ, Rodrigues RM, Lamb V: The inspiratory work load of patient-initiated mechanical ventilation. Am Rev Respir Dis 134:902, 1986.
92. Kimball WR, Leith DE, Rolins AG: Dynamic hyperinflation and ventilator dependence in chronic obstructive pulmonary disease. Am Rev Respir Dis 126:991, 1982.
93. Kacmarek RM: Positive end expiratory pressure. In Pierson DJ, Kacmarek RM (eds): Foundations of Respiratory Care. New York, Churchill Livingstone, 1992, p 891.
94. Kacmarek RM, Kirmse M, Nishimara M, et al: The effects of applied vs. auto-PEEP on local lung unit pressure and volume in a four-unit lung model. Chest 108:1073, 1995.
95. Smith TC, Marini JJ: Impact of PEEP on lung mechanics and work of breathing in severe airflow obstruction. J Appl Physiol 65:1488, 1988.
96. Pepe PE, Marini JJ: Occult positive end-expiratory pressure in mechanically ventilated patients with airflow obstruction: The auto-PEEP effect. Am Rev Respir Dis 126:166, 1982.
97. Rossi A, Ranieri VM: Positive end-expiratory pressure. In Tobin MJ (ed): Principles and Practice of Mechanical Ventilation. New York, McGraw-Hill, 1994, p 259.
98. Tuxon D, Lane S: The effects of ventilatory pattern on hyperinflation, airway pressure, and circulation in mechanical ventilation of patients with severe airflow obstruction. Am Rev Respir Dis 136:872, 1987.
99. Tuxon D, William T, Scheinkestel C, et al: Limiting dynamic hyperinflation in mechanically ventilated patients with severe asthma reduces complications. Anaesth Intensive Care 21:718, 1993.
100. Leatherman JW, Ravenscraft SA: Low measure auto-positive end expiratory pressure during mechanical ventilation of patients with severe asthma: Hidden auto-positive end-expiratory pressure. Crit Care Med 24:541, 1996.
101. Brown DG, Pierson DJ: Auto-PEEP is common in mechanically ventilated patients: A study of incidence, severity, and detection. Respir Care 31:1069, 1986.
102. Petrof BJ, Legare M, Goldberg P, et al: Continuous positive airway pressure reduces work of breathing and dyspnea during weaning from mechanical ventilation in severe COPD. Am Rev Respir Dis 141:281, 1990.
103. Ranieri VM, Giuliani R, Cinnella G, et al: Physiologic effects of positive end-expiratory pressure in patients with obstructive pulmonary disease during acute ventilatory failure and controlled mechanical ventilation. Am Rev Respir Dis 149:5, 1993.
104. Dreyfuss D, Saumon G: Ventilator induced injury. In Tobin MJ (ed): Principles and Practices of Mechanical Ventilation. New York, McGraw-Hill, 1994, p 793.
105. Dreyfuss D, Soler P, Basset G, Saumon G: High inflation pressure pulmonary edema: Respective effects of high airway pressure, high tidal volume and positive end-expiratory pressure. Am Rev Respir Dis 137:1159, 1988.
106. West JB: Respiratory Physiology: The Essentials, 4th ed. Baltimore, Williams & Wilkins, 1990.
107. Petersen HP, Baier H: Incidence of pulmonary barotrauma in a medical ICU. Crit Care Med 11:67, 1983.

108. Rohlfing BM, Webb WR, Schlobohm RM: Ventilator-related extra-alveolar air in adults. Radiology 121:25, 1976.
109. Pollack MM, Fields AI, Holbrook PR: Pneumothorax and pneumomediastinum during pediatric mechanical ventilation. Crit Care Med 7:536, 1979.
110. Marini JJ, Culver BH: Systemic gas embolism complicating mechanical ventilation in the adult respiratory distress system. Ann Intern Med 110:699, 1989.
111. Tobin MJ, Dantzker DR: Mechanical ventilation and weaning. In Dantzker DR (ed): Cardiopulmonary Critical Care. New York, Grune & Stratton, 1986, p 908.
112. Hillman K: Pulmonary barotrauma. Clin Anesthesiol 3:777, 1985.
113. Cullen DJ, Caldera DL: The incidence of ventilator induced pulmonary barotrauma in critically ill patients. Anesthesiology 50: 185, 1979.
114. Hickling KG, Walsh J, Henderson S, Jackson R: Low mortality rate in adult respiratory distress syndrome using low-volume, pressure-limited ventilation with permissive hypercapnia: A prospective study. Crit Care Med 22:1568, 1994.
115. Darioli A, Perret C: Mechanical controlled hypoventilation in status asthmaticus. Am Rev Respir Dis 129:385, 1984.
116. Slutsky AS: Mechanical ventilation: ACCP Consensus Conference. Chest 104:1833, 1993.
117. Amato MBP, Barbas CS, Medeiros DM, et al: Beneficial effects of the "open lung approach" with low distending pressure in acute respiratory failure. Am J Respir Crit Care Med 152:1835, 1995.
118. Roupie E, Dambrosio M, Servillo G, et al: Titration of tidal volume and induced hypercapnia in acute respiratory distress syndrome. Am J Respir Crit Care 152:121, 1995.
119. Webb HH, Tierney DF: Experimental pulmonary edema due to intermittent positive pressure ventilation with high inflation pressure: Protection by positive end-expiratory pressure. Am Rev Respir Dis 110:556, 1974.
120. Hernandez LA, Peevy KJ, Moise AA, Parker JC: Chest wall restriction limits high airway pressure-induced lung injury in young rabbits. J Appl Physiol 66:2364, 1989.
121. Kolobow T, Moretti MP, Fumagalli R, et al: Severe impairment in lung function induced by high peak airway pressure during mechanical ventilation: An experimental study. Am Rev Respir Dis 135:312, 1987.
122. Dreyfuss D, Basset G, Soler P, Saumon G: Intermittent positive-pressure hyperventilation with high inflation pressure produces pulmonary microvascular injury in rats. Am Rev Respir Dis 132: 880, 1985.
123. Dreyfuss D, Soler D, Saumon G: Mechanical ventilation–induced pulmonary edema: Interaction with previous lung alterations. Am J Respir Crit Care Med 181:1568, 1995.
124. Muscedere JG, Mullen JBM, Gan K, Slutsky AS: Tidal ventilation at low airway pressure can augment lung injury. Am J Respir Crit Care Med 149:1327, 1994.
125. Corbridge TC, Wood LDH, Crawford GP, et al: Adverse effects of large tidal volume and low PEEP in canine acid aspiration. Am Rev Respir Dis 142:311, 1990.
126. Hickling KG, Henderson SJ, Jackson R: Low mortality associated with low volume, pressure limited ventilation with permissive hypercapnia in severe adult respiratory distress syndrome. Intensive Care Med 16:372, 1990.
127. Kacmarek RM, Hickling K: Permissive hypercapnia. Respir Care 38:373, 1993.
128. Tuxen DV: Permissive hypercapnic ventilation. Am J Respir Crit Care Med 150:870, 1994.
129. Hickling KG, Joyce C: Permissive hypercapnia in ARDS and its effect on tissue oxygenation. Acta Anaesthesiol Scand 39:201, 1995.
130. Nunn JF: Carbon dioxide. In Nunn JF (ed): Applied Respiratory Physiology, 2nd ed. London, Butterworth's, 1977, p 334.
131. Carpellier G, Tolh J, Walker P, et al: Hemodynamic effects of permissive hypercapnia. Am Rev Respir Dis 195:A527, 1992.
132. Wolley K, Lewis T, Wood L: Acute respiratory acidosis decreases left ventricular contractibility but increases cardiac output in dogs. Circ Res 100:102, 1990.
133. Achike F, Dai S: Cardiovascular responses to verapamil and nifedipine in hypoventilated and hyperventilated rats. Br J Pharmacol 100:102, 1990.
134. Hickling K: Ventilatory management of ARDS: Can it affect outcome? Intensive Care Med 16:219, 1990.
135. Graf H, Leach W, Arieff AL: Evidence for a detrimental effect of bicarbonate therapy in hypoxic lactic acidosis. Science 227: 754, 1991.
136. Prys-Roberts C: Hypercapnia. In Gray T, Nunn J, Utting J (eds): General Anesthesia, 4th ed. London, Butterworth's, 1980, p 435.
137. Shapiro BA, Cane RD, Harrison A: Positive end-expiratory pressure therapy in adults with special reference to acute lung injury: A review of the literature and suggested clinical correlations. Crit Care Med 12:127, 1984.
138. Bryan CC, Jenkinson SG: Oxygen toxicity. Clin Chest Med 9: 141, 1988.
139. Duane P: Pulmonary insults due to transfusion radiation and hyperoxia. Semin Respir Infect 3:240, 1988.
140. Comroe JH, Dripps RN, Dunke PR, Deming M: The effect of inhalation of high concentrations of oxygen for 24 hours on normal men at sea level and at a simulated altitude of 18,000 ft. JAMA 128:710, 1945.
141. Lodata RF: Oxygen toxicity. In Tobin MJ (ed): Principles and Practice of Mechanical Ventilation. New York, McGraw-Hill, 1994, p 837.
142. Marini J, Kelsen S: Re-targeting ventilatory objectives in adult respiratory distress syndrome. Am Rev Respir Dis 146:2, 1992.
143. Hurford WE, Teboul JL: Cardiovascular function during acute respiratory failure. In Zapol WM, Lemaire F (eds): Acute Respiratory Distress Syndrome. New York, Marcel Dekker, 1991, p 182.
144. Kumar A, Falke KJ, Geffin B, et al: Continuous positive-pressure ventilation in acute respiratory failure. N Engl J Med 273:1430, 1970.
145. Kirby RR, Perry JC, Calderwood HW, et al: Cardiorespiratory effects of positive end-expiratory pressure. Anesthesiology 43: 533, 1975.
146. Suter PM, Fairley HB, Isenberg MD: Optimal end-expiratory airway pressure in patients with acute pulmonary failure. N Engl J Med 292:284, 1995.
147. Murray IP, Modell JH, Gallagher TJ, Banner MJ: Titration of PEEP by the arterial minus end-tidal CO_2 gradient. Chest 85: 100, 1984.
148. Qvist J, Pontoppidan H, Wilson RS, et al: Hemodynamic responses to mechanical ventilation with PEEP. Anesthesiology 42:45, 1975.
149. Marini JJ, Wheeler AP: Critical Care Medicine: The Essentials. Baltimore, Williams & Wilkins, 1989.
150. Hobelmann CF, Smith DE, Virgillo RW, et al: Hemodynamic alterations with positive end-expiratory pressure: The contribution of the pulmonary vasculature. J Trauma 15:951, 1975.
151. Fewell JE, Abendschein DR, Carslon CJ: Mechanism of decreased right and left ventricular end-diastolic volumes during continuous positive-pressure ventilation in dogs. Circ Res 47: 467, 1980.
152. Lenfant C, Howell BJ: Cardiovascular adjustment in dogs during continuous positive-pressure breathing. J Appl Physiol 15:425, 1960.
153. Robotham JL, Lixfield W, Holland L, et al: The effects of positive end-expiratory pressure on right and left ventricular performance. Am Rev Respir Dis 121:677, 1980.
154. Dorinsky PM, Whitcomb ME: The effects of PEEP on cardiac output. Chest 84:210, 1983.
155. Benito S, Lemaire F: Pulmonary pressure-volume relationship in acute respiratory distress syndrome in adults: Role of positive end-expiratory pressure. J Crit Care 5:27, 1990.
156. Pesenti A, Marcolin R, Prato P, et al: Mean airway pressure vs positive end-expiratory pressure during mechanical ventilation. Crit Care Med 13:34, 1985.
157. Gattinoni L, D'Andrea L, Pelosi P, et al: Regional effects and mechanism of positive end-expiratory pressure in early adult respiratory distress syndrome. JAMA 269:2122, 1993.
158. Ciszek T, Modanlou H, Owings D, Nelson P: Mean airway pressure: Significance during mechanical ventilation in neonates. J Pediatr 99:121, 1981.
159. Marcy TW: Inverse ratio ventilation. In Tobin MJ (ed): Principles and Practices of Mechanical Ventilation. New York, McGraw-Hill, 1994, p 319.

160. Kacmarek RM, Kirmse M, Mang H, Kimball W: The effects of applied vs auto-PEEP on local lung unit pressure and volume in a four-unit lung mode. Chest 108:1073, 1995.
161. Maunder RJ, Shuman WP, McHugh JW, et al: Preservation of normal lung regions in the adult respiratory distress syndrome: Analysis by computed tomography. JAMA 255:2463, 1986.
162. Gattinoni L, Pesenti A, Avalli L, et al: Pressure-volume curve of total respiratory system in acute respiratory failure: Computed tomographic scan study. Am Rev Respir Dis 136:730, 1987.
163. Aps C, Huter JA, Williams BT: Anesthetic management and postoperative care of cardiac surgical patients in a general recovery ward. Anaesthesia 41:533, 1986.
164. Klineberg PL, Geer RT, Hirsh RA, Aukburg SJ: Early extubation after coronary artery bypass graft surgery. Crit Care Med 5:272, 1977.
165. Tobin MJ, Alex CG: Discontinuation of mechanical ventilation. In Tobin MJ (ed): Principles and Practices of Mechanical Ventilation. New York, McGraw-Hill, 1994, p 1177.
166. Demling RH, Read T, Lind LJ, Flanagan HL: Incidence and morbidity of extubation failure in surgical intensive care patients. Crit Care Med 16:573, 1988.
167. Schmidt CD, Elliott CG, Carmelli D, et al: Prolonged mechanical ventilation for respiratory failure: A cost-benefit analysis. Crit Care Med 11:407, 1983.
168. Spicher JE, White DP: Outcome and function following prolonged mechanical ventilation. Arch Intern Med 147:41, 1987.
169. Davis HII, Lefrak SS, Miller D, Malt S: Prolonged mechanically assisted ventilation. An analysis of outcome and charges. JAMA 243:43, 1980.
170. Martin TR, Lewis SW, Albert RK: The prognosis of patients with chronic obstructive pulmonary disease after hospitalization for acute respiratory failure. Chest 82:310, 1982.
171. Higgens TL, Stoller JK: Discontinuing ventilatory support. In Pierson DJ, Kacmarek RM (eds): Fundamentals of Respiratory Care. New York, Churchill Livingstone, 1992, p 1019.
172. Lemaire F, Teboul J-L, Cinotti L, et al: Acute left ventricular dysfunction during unsuccessful weaning from mechanical ventilation. Anesthesiology 69:171, 1988.
173. Mathru M, Tadikonda LK, Rao TLK, et al: Hemodynamic response to changes in ventilatory patterns in patients with normal and poor left ventricular reserve. Crit Care Med 10:423, 1982.
174. Wilson DO, Rogers RM: The role of nutrition in weaning from mechanical ventilation. J Intensive Care 4:124, 1989.
175. Larca L, Greenbaum DM: Effectiveness of intensive nutritional regimes in patients who fail to wean from mechanical ventilation. Crit Care Med 10:297, 1982.
176. Aubier M, Viires N, Piquet J, et al: Effects of hypocalcemia on diaphragmatic strength generation. J Appl Physiol 58:2054, 1985.
177. Aubier M, Murciano D, Lecocguic Y, et al: Effects of hypophosphatemia on diaphragmatic contractility in patients with acute respiratory failure. N Engl J Med 313:420, 1985.
178. Sahn SA, Lakshminarayan S: Bedside criteria for discontinuation of mechanical ventilation. Chest 63:1002, 1973.
179. Tahvanainen J, Salenpera M, Nikki P: Extubation criteria after weaning from intermittent mandatory ventilatory and continuous positive airway pressure. Crit Care Med 11:702, 1983.
180. Morganroth ML, Morganroth JL, Nett LM, Petty TL: Criteria for weaning from prolonged mechanical ventilation. Arch Intern Med 144:1012, 1984.
181. Fiastro JF, Habib MP, Shon BY, Campbell SC: Comparison of standard weaning parameters and mechanical work of breathing in mechanically ventilated patients. Chest 94:232, 1988.
182. Milbern SM, Downs JB, Jumper LC, et al: Evaluation of criteria for discontinuing mechanical ventilation support. Arch Surg 113: 1441, 1978.
183. Tores D, Roizen MF, Bushnell LS: Successful weaning from controlled ventilation despite high deadspace-to-tidal volume ratio. Anesthesiology 39:656, 1973.
184. Sassoon CSH, Te TT, Mahutte CK, Light RW: Airway occlusion pressure: An important indicator for successful weaning in patients with chronic obstructive pulmonary disease. Am Rev Respir Dis 135:107, 1987.
185. Lewis WD, Chwals W, Benotti PN, et al: Bedside assessment of the work of breathing. Crit Care Med 16:117, 1988.
186. Montgomery AB, Holle RHO, Neagley SR, et al: Prediction of successful ventilator weaning using airway occlusion pressure and hypercapnic challenge. Chest 91:496, 1987.
187. Pourriat JL, Baud M, Lamberto C, et al: Effects of doxapram on hypercapnic response during weaning from mechanical ventilation in COPD patients. Chest 101:1639, 1992.
188. Yang K, Tobin MJ: A prospective study of indexes predicting outcome of trials of weaning from mechanical ventilation. N Engl J Med 324:1445, 1991.
189. Brochard L, Rauss A, Beneto S, et al: Comparison of three methods of gradual withdrawal from ventilatory support during weaning from mechanical ventilation. Am J Respir Crit Care Med 150:896, 1994.
190. Esteban A, Frutos F, Tobin MJ, et al: A comparison of four methods of weaning patients from mechanical ventilation. N Engl J Med 332:345, 1995.
191. Ely EW, Baker AM, Dunagan DP, et al: Effect on the duration of mechanical ventilation of identifying patients capable of breathing spontaneously. N Engl J Med 335:1864, 1996.
192. Cohen C, Zagelbaum G, Gross D, et al: Clinical manifestations of inspiratory muscle fatigue. Am J Med 73:308, 1982.
193. Tobin MJ, Guenther SM, Perez W, et al: Konno-Meade analysis of ribcage-abdominal motion during successful and unsuccessful trials of weaning from mechanical ventilation. Am Rev Respir Dis 135:1320, 1987.
194. Laghi F, D'Alfonso N, Tobin MJ: Pattern of recovery from diaphragmatic fatigue over 24 hours. J Appl Physiol 79:539, 1995.
195. Jubran A, Tobin MJ: Pathophysiologic basis of acute respiratory distress in patients who fail a trial of weaning from mechanical ventilation. Am J Respir Crit Care Med 155:906, 1997.
196. Tobin MJ: Respiratory muscles in disease. Clin Chest Med 9: 263, 1988.
197. Rochester DF, Braun NMT: Determinants of maximal inspiratory pressure in chronic obstructive pulmonary disease. Am Rev Respir Dis 132:42, 1985.
198. Jubran A, Tobin J: Passive mechanics of lung and chest wall in patients who failed or succeeded in trials of weaning. Am J Respir Crit Care Med 155:916, 1997.
199. Malloy DW, Dhingra S, Solven FS: Hypomagnesemia and respiratory muscle power. Am Rev Respir Dis 129:497, 1984.
200. Planus RF, McBrayer RH, Koen PA: Effect of hypophosphatemia on pulmonary muscle performance. Adv Exp Med Biol 151:283, 1982.
201. Aubier M, Viires N, Piquet J, et al: Effects of hypocalcemia on diaphragmatic strength generation. J Appl Physiol 58:2054, 1985.
202. Pingleton SK: Nutritional support in the mechanically ventilated patient. Clin Chest Med 9:101, 1988.
203. Lemaire F, Teboul JL, Cinotti L, et al: Acute left ventricular dysfunction during unsuccessful weaning from mechanical ventilation. Anesthesiology 69:171, 1988.
204. Hurford WE, Lynch KE, Strauss HW, et al: Myocardial perfusion as assessed by thathuium-201 scintigraphy during the discontinuation of mechanical ventilation in ventilator-dependent patients. Anesthesiology 74:1007, 1991.
205. Nett LM, Morganroth M, Petty TL: Weaning from mechanical ventilation: A perspective and review of techniques. In Bone RC (ed): Critical Care: A Comprehensive Approach. Park Ridge, IL, American College of Chest Physicians, 1984, p 171.
206. Hess DR, Kacmarek RM: Essentials of Mechanical Ventilation. New York, McGraw-Hill, 1996.
207. Chatte G, Sab JM, Dubois JM: Prone position in mechanically ventilated patients with severe acute respiratory failure. Am J Respir Crit Care Med 155:473, 1997.
208. Ravenscraft SA, Burke WC, Nahum A, et al: Tracheal gas insufflation augments CO_2 clearance during mechanical ventilation. Am Rev Respir Dis 148:348, 1993.
209. Rossaint R, Falke KJ, Lopez F, et al: Inhaled nitric oxide for the adult respiratory distress syndrome. N Engl J Med 328:399, 1993.
210. Leach CL, Greenspan JS, Rubenstein SD, et al: Partial liquid ventilation with perflubron in premature infants with severe respiratory distress syndrome. N Engl J Med 335:761, 1996.
211. Gattinoni L, Pelosi G, Vitale A, et al: Body position changes redistribute lung computed tomographic density in patients with acute respiratory failure. Anesthesiology 74:15, 1991.

212. Douglas WWK, Rehder FM, Beyned AD, et al: Improved oxygenation in patients with acute respiratory failure: The prone position. Am Rev Respir Dis 113:559, 1977.
213. Langer M, Muscarine D, Marcollin R, Gattinoni L: The prone position in ARDS patients: Clinical study. Chest 94:103, 1988.
214. Pappert D, Rossaint R, Slama R, et al: Influence of positioning on ventilation-perfusion relationships in severe adult respiratory distress syndrome. Chest 106:1511, 1994.
215. Albert RK, Leasa D, Sanderson M, et al: The prone position improves arterial oxygenation and reduces shunt in oleic-acid-induced acute lung injury. Am Rev Respir Dis 135:628, 1987.
216. Weiner CM, Kirk W, Albert RK: Prone position reverse gravitational distribution of perfusion in dog lungs with oleic acid-induced injury. J Appl Physiol 68:1386, 1990.
217. Amis TC, Jones HA, Hughes JM: Effect of posture on interregional distribution of pulmonary ventilation in man. Respir Physiol 56:145, 1984.
218. Albert RK: For every thing (turn . . . turn . . . turn) (Editorial). Am J Respir Crit Care Med 155:393, 1997.
219. Mutoh T, Guest RJ, Lamm WJE, Albert RK: Prone position alters the effect of volume overload on regional pleural pressures and improves hypoxemia in pigs in-vivo. Am Rev Respir Dis 146:300, 1992.
220. Nahum A, Ravenscraft SA, Nakos G, et al: Tracheal gas insufflation during pressure-control ventilation: Effect of catheter position, diameter, and flow rate. Am Rev Respir Dis 146:1411, 1992.
221. Burke WC, Nahum A, Ravenscraft SA, et al: Modes of tracheal gas insufflation: Comparison of continuous and phase-specific gas injection in normal dogs. Am Rev Respir Dis 148:562, 1993.
222. Nahum A, Ravenscraft SA, Nakos G, et al: Effect of catheter flow direction on CO_2 removal during tracheal gas insufflation in dogs. J Appl Physiol 75:1238, 1993.
223. Nahum A, Chandra A, Niknam A, et al: Effect of tracheal gas insufflation on gas exchange in canine oleic acid-induced lung injury. Crit Care Med 23:348, 1995.
224. Nahum A, Burke WC, Ravenscraft SA, et al: Lung mechanics and gas exchange during pressure-control ventilation in dogs: Augmentation of CO_2 elimination by an intratracheal catheter. Am Rev Respir Dis 46:965, 1992.
225. Nahum A, Shapiro RS, Ravenscraft SA, et al: Efficacy of expiratory tracheal gas insufflation in a canine model of lung injury. Am J Respir Crit Care Med 152:489, 1995.
226. Imanaka H, Kacmarek RM, Ritz R, Hess D: Tracheal gas insufflation—pressure control vs. volume control ventilation: A lung model study. Am J Respir Crit Care Med 153:1019, 1996.
227. Kirmse M, Imanaka H, Mang H, et al: Tracheal gas insufflation: Effects of the direction of gas flow during pressure control ventilation (Abstract). Am J Respir Crit Care Med 153:A368, 1996.
228. Palmer R, Rees D, Ashton D, Moncada S: L-arginine is the physiological precursor for the formation of nitric oxide in endothelium dependent relaxation. Biochem Biophys Res Commun 153:1251, 1988.
229. Moncada S, Higgs A: Mechanisms of disease: The L-arginine-nitric oxide pathway. N Engl J Med 329:2002, 1993.
230. Moncada S, Higgs EA: Molecular mechanisms and therapeutic strategies related to nitric oxide. FASEB J 9:1319, 1995.
231. Rimar S, Gillis CN: Selected pulmonary vasodilation by inhaled nitric oxide is due to hemoglobin inactivation. Circulation 88: 2884, 1993.
232. Zapol W, Hurford W: Inhaled nitric oxide in the adult respiratory distress syndrome and other lung diseases. New Horizons 1:638, 1993.
233. Pison U, Lopez F, Heidelmeyer C, et al: Inhaled nitric oxide reverses hypoxic pulmonary vasoconstriction without impairing gas exchange. J Appl Physiol 74:1287, 1993.
234. Frostell C, Blomqvist H, Hedebstierna G, et al: Inhaled nitric oxide selectively reverses human hypoxic pulmonary vasoconstriction without causing systemic vasodilation. Anesthesiology 78:427, 1993.
235. Bigatello L, Hurford W, Kacmarek RM, et al: Prolonged inhalation of low concentrations of nitric oxide in patients with severe adult respiratory distress syndrome: Effects on pulmonary hemodynamics and oxygenation. Anesthesiology 80:761, 1994.
236. Rossaint R, Gerlach H, Schmidt-Ruhnke H, et al: Efficacy of inhaled nitric oxide in patients with severe ARDS. Chest 107: 1107, 1995.
237. Dellinger RP, Zimmerman JL, Hyers TM, et al: Inhaled nitric oxide in ARDS: Preliminary results of a multicenter trial. Crit Care Med 24:A29, 1996.
238. The neonatal inhaled nitric oxide group: Inhaled nitric oxide in full-term and nearly full-term infants with hypoxic respiratory failure. N Engl J Med 336:597, 1997.
239. Roberts JD, Fineman JR, Morin FC, et al: Inhaled nitric oxide and persistent pulmonary hypertension of the newborn. N Engl J Med 336:605, 1997.
240. Claney J, Leszcznska-Piziak J, Abramson SB: Nitric oxide and endothelial cell relaxation factor, inhibits neutrophil superoxide alveolar production via a direct action on NADPH oxidase. J Clin Invest 90:1116, 1992.
241. Kavanagh BP, Mouchawan A, Goldsmith J, Pearl RG: Effects of inhaled NO and inhibition of endogenous NO synthesis in oxidant-induced acute lung injury. J Appl Physiol 76:1324, 1994.
242. Chollet-Martin S, Gatecel C, Kermarrec N, et al: Alveolar neutrophil functions and cytokine levels in patients with the adult respiratory distress syndrome during nitric oxide inhalation. Am J Respir Crit Care Med 153:985, 1996.
243. Krafft P, Fridrich P, Fitzgerald RD, et al: Effectiveness of nitric oxide inhalation in septic ARDS. Chest 109:486, 1996.
244. Nishimura, Hess D, Kacmarek RM, et al: Nitrogen dioxide production during mechanical ventilation with nitric oxide in adults. Effects of ventilator internal circuitry. Crit Care Med 152:318, 1995.
245. Imanaka H, Hess D, Kirmse M, et al: Inaccuracies of nitric oxide delivery systems during adult mechanical ventilation. Anesthesiology 86:676, 1997.
246. Hirschl RB, Tooley R, Parent A, et al: Evaluation of gas exchange, pulmonary compliance, and lung injury during total and partial liquid ventilation in the acute respiratory distress syndrome. Crit Care Med 24:1001, 1996.
247. Papo MC, Paczan PR, Fuhrman BP, et al: Perfluorocarbon-associated gas exchange improves oxygenation, lung mechanics, and survival in a model of adult respiratory distress syndrome. Crit Care Med 24:466, 1996.
248. Hernan LJ, Fuhrman BP, Kaiser RE, et al: Perfluorocarbon-associated gas exchange in normal and acid-injured large sheep. Crit Care Med 24:475, 1996.
249. Overbeck MC, Pranikoff T, Yadao CM, et al: Efficacy of perfluorocarbon partial liquid ventilation in a large animal model of acute respiratory failure. Crit Care Med 24:1208, 1996.
250. Hirschl RB, Pranikoff T, Gauger P, et al: Liquid ventilation in adults, children, and full term neonates. Lancet 346:1201, 1995.
251. Kazerooni EA, Pranikoff T, Cascade PN, et al: Partial liquid ventilation with perflubron during extracorporeal life support in adults: Radiographic appearance. Radiology 198:137, 1996.

Index

Note: Page numbers in *italics* indicate figures; page numbers followed by t indicate tables.

ISBN 0-443-08920-5